Schiff's
Diseases of
the Liver

Companion website

Purchasing this book entitles you to access to the companion website:

www.schiffsdiseasesoftheliver.com

The website includes:

- Eighty multiple choice questions of the standard used in ABIM board exams in gastroenterology, to allow the user to self-assess their clinical knowledge
- All 450+ figures from the book in a high-quality, fully transportable and downloadable electronic format
- High-quality video clips of a variety of surgical procedures
- 35 case studies featuring real-life clinical scenarios.

How to access the website:

1. Carefully scratch away the top coating on the label on the inside front cover of the book to reveal PIN code.
2. Go to www.schiffsdiseasesoftheliver.com to register your PIN and access the site.

We dedicate this eleventh edition of *Diseases of the Liver* to Dr Harvey Alter, who has been an outstanding leader in the development of knowledge regarding viral hepatitis. Dr Alter is a gifted scientist, physician, teacher, and mentor. His abilities to create and transmit information with clarity and enthusiasm have inspired and enriched us all.

In addition, we wish to recognize the tremendous contributions to the field of hepatology by the late Dr Baruch Blumberg.

We further dedicate this edition to our wives Dana, Shirley, and Ann for their continuing support of our endeavors.

It has been an honor and a privilege for us to participate in the creation and editing of *Diseases of the Liver*.

E.R.S.
W.C.M.
M.F.S.

Schiff's Diseases of the Liver

EDITED BY

Eugene R. Schiff

MD MACP FRCP
Leonard Miller Professor of Medicine
Nasser Ibrahim Al-Rashid Chair Hepatology
Director, Center for Liver Diseases and Schiff Liver Institute
University of Miami Miller School of Medicine
Miami, FL, USA

Willis C. Maddrey

MD MACP FRCP
Adelyn and Edmund M. Hoffman Distinguished Chair in Medical Science
Professor, Department of Internal Medicine
University of Texas Southwestern Medical Center
Dallas, TX, USA

Michael F. Sorrell

MD FACP
Robert L. Grissom Professor of Medicine
University of Nebraska College of Medicine
Omaha, NE, USA

ELEVENTH EDITION

WILEY-BLACKWELL

A John Wiley & Sons, Ltd., Publication

Library of Congress Cataloging-in-Publication Data

Schiff's diseases of the liver. – 11th ed. / edited by Eugene R. Schiff, Willis C. Maddrey,
Michael F. Sorrell.
p. ; cm.
Diseases of the liver
Includes bibliographical references and index.
ISBN-13: 978-0-470-65468-2 (hardcover : alk. paper)
ISBN-10: 0-470-65468-6 (hardcover : alk. paper)   1. Liver–Diseases.   I. Schiff, Eugene R.
II. Maddrey, Willis C.   III. Sorrell, Michael F.   IV. Schiff, Leon, 1901–1994.   V. Title: Diseases
of the liver.
[DNLM: 1. Liver Diseases. WI 700]
RC845.D53 2011
616.3'62–dc23   2011014998

A catalogue record for this book is available from the British Library.

This book is published in the following electronic formats: ePDF 9781119950479;
Wiley Online Library 9781119950509; ePub 9781119950486; mobi 9781119950493

Set in 9.5/12pt Palatino by Aptara® Inc., New Delhi, India
Printed and bound in Singapore by Markono Print Media Pte Ltd

2   2013

Contents

List of Contributors

Peter L. Abt
MD
Department of Surgery
Division of Transplant Surgery
The Hospital of the University of
Pennsylvania
Philadelphia, PA, USA

Abdullah M. S. Al-Osaimi
MBBS, FACP, FACG
Associate Professor of Medicine and Surgery
Associate Medical Director of Liver
Transplantation
Division of Gastroenterology and Hepatology
Department of Medicine
University of Virginia Health System
Charlottesville, VA, USA

Curtis K. Argo
MD, MS
Assistant Professor
Medical Director, Inpatient Digestive Health
Center
Associate Director, Transplant Hepatology
Fellowship
Division of Gastroenterology and Hepatology
Department of Internal Medicine
University of Virginia Health System
Charlottesville, VA, USA

Carmen Ayuso
MD
Professor of Radiology
Barcelona Clinic Liver Cancer Group
Hospital Clinic
University of Barcelona
Barcelona, Spain

Bruce R. Bacon
MD
Professor of Internal Medicine
Co-Director, Liver Center
Division of Gastroenterology and Hepatology
Saint Louis University School of Medicine
St. Louis, MO, USA

Yannick Bacq
MD
Department of Hepatogastroenterology
Centre Hospitalier de Tours
Hôpital Trousseau
Tours, France

Ranjeeta Bahirwani
Division of Gastroenterology
Department of Internal Medicine
The University of Pennsylvania School of
Medicine
Philadelphia, PA, USA

Alex S. Befeler
MD
Associate Professor of Internal Medicine and
Medical Director of Liver Transplantation
Division of Gastroenterology and Hepatology
Saint Louis University School of Medicine
St. Louis, MO, USA

Paul D. Berk
MD
Professor of Medicine
Division of Digestive and Liver Diseases
Columbia University College of Physicians
and Surgeons
New York, NY, USA

Jean F. Botha
MD
Department of Surgery
University of Nebraska Medical Center
Omaha, NE, USA

Robert S. Britton
PhD
Division of Gastroenterology and Hepatology
Saint Louis University School of Medicine
St. Louis, MO, USA

Jordi Bruix
MD
Senior Consultant
Professor of Medicine
Barcelona Clinic Liver Cancer Group
Hospital Clinic
CIBERehd, Institut d'Investigacions
Biomediques Agusto Pi i Sunyer (IDIBAPS)
University of Barcelona
Barcelona, Spain

Stephen H. Caldwell
MD
Professor and Director of Hepatology
Division of Gastroenterology and Hepatology
Department of Internal Medicine
University of Virginia Health System
Charlottesville, VA, USA

B. Daniel Campos
MD
Division of Transplantation
Department of Surgery
University of Nebraska Medical Center
Omaha, NE, USA

Shivakumar Chitturi
MD
Department of Hepatic Medicine
Australian National University Medical
School
Gastroenterology and Hepatology Unit
Canberra Hospital
Garran, Australia

Jama M. Darling
MD
UNC Liver Center
University of North Carolina School of
Medicine
Chapel Hill, NC, USA

Srinivasan Dasarathy
MD
Department of Pathobiology
Lerner Research Institute
Cleveland Clinic Foundation
Cleveland, OH, USA

Adrian M. Di Bisceglie
MD, FACP
Professor and Chairman
Bander Chair in Internal Medicine
Saint Louis University School of Medicine
St. Louis, MO, USA

Douglas T. Dieterich
MD
Professor of Medicine
Liver Diseases
Mount Sinai School of Medicine
Division of Liver Diseases
New York, NY, USA

Michael A. Dunn
MD
Professor of Medicine and Biomedical
Informatics
University of Pittsburgh
Pittsburgh, PA, USA

Bijan Eghtesad
MD
Cleveland Clinic Foundation
Cleveland, OH, USA

Michael B. Fallon
MD
Professor of Medicine
Division of Gastroenterology, Hepatology and
Nutrition
The University of Texas Health Science Center
at Houston
Houston, TX, USA

Geoffrey C. Farrell
MD, FRACP
Professor of Hepatic Medicine
Australian National University Medical
School
Gastroenterology & Hepatology Unit
The Canberra Hospital
Garran, Australia

Thomas W. Faust
MD, MBE
University of Pennsylvania Health System
Philadelphia, PA, USA

Jonathan M. Fenkel
MD
Division of Gastroenterology and Hepatology
Thomas Jefferson University
Philadelphia, PA, USA

Alejandro Forner
MD
Barcelona Clinic Liver Cancer Group
Hospital Clinic, CIBERehd
Institut d'Investigacions Biomediques Agusto
Pi i Sunyer (IDIBAPS)
University of Barcelona
Barcelona, Spain

Alyson N. Fox
MD, MSCE
Division of Gastroenterology
University of California
San Francisco, CA, USA

Richard B. Freeman, Jr.
MD
William N. and Bessie Alyn Professor and
Chair
Department of Surgery
Dartmouth-Hitchcock Medical Center
Lebanon, NH, USA

Michael W. Fried
MD
Professor of Medicine
Director, UNC Liver Center
University of North Carolina at Chapel Hill
Chapel Hill, NC, USA

Scott Friedman
MD
Chief of Liver Diseases and Professor of
Medicine
Mount Sinai School of Medicine
New York, NY, USA

Lawrence S. Friedman
MD
Chair, Department of Medicine
Newton-Wellesley Hospital
Newton, MA, USA
Assistant Chief of Medicine
Massachusetts General Hospital
Professor of Medicine, Harvard Medical
School
Professor of Medicine, Tufts University School
of Medicine
Boston, MA, USA

John J. Fung
MD, PhD
Cleveland Clinic Foundation
Cleveland, OH, USA

Zachary D. Goodman
MD, PhD
Center for Liver Diseases
Inova Fairfax Hospital
Falls Church, VA, USA

Stuart C. Gordon
MD
Director, Division of Hepatology
Henry Ford Health Systems
Professor of Medicine
Wayne State University School of Medicine
Detroit, MI, USA

Gregory J. Gores
MD
Division of Gastroenterology and Hepatology
Mayo Clinic, College of Medicine
Rochester, MN, USA

Norton J. Greenberger
MD
Clinical Professor of Medicine
Harvard Medical School
Division of Gastroenterology, Hepatology and
Endoscopy
Brigham and Women's Hospital
Boston, MA, USA

H. Franklin Herlong
MD
Associate Professor of Medicine
Department of Gastroenterology
Johns Hopkins Bayview Medical School
Baltimore, MD, USA

Ira Jacobson
MD
Professor of Medicine
New York Presbyterian Hospital
Division of Gastroenterology and Hepatology
Weill Cornell Medical Center
New York, NY, USA

Kunal Jajoo
MD
Associate Physician
Division of Gastroenterology, Hepatology and
Endoscopy
Brigham and Women's Hospital
Harvard Medical School
Boston, MA, USA

Stephen P. James
MD
Division of Digestive Diseases and Nutrition
National Institute of Diabetes & Digestive &
Kidney Diseases
National Institutes of Health
Bethesda, MD, USA

Lennox J. Jeffers
MD
Center for Liver Diseases
Miami, FL, USA

David Kershenobich
MD, PhD
Professor of Medicine
Faculty of Medicine
Experimental Research Unit
Universidad Nacional Autónoma de México
Hospital General de México
Mexico City, Mexico

Rajan Kochar
MD MPH
Assistant Professor of Medicine
Division of Gastroenterology, Hepatology and
Nutrition
The University of Texas Health Science Center
at Houston
Houston, TX, USA

Kiley Kolb
DO
Department of Medicine
Temple University Hospital and School of
Medicine
Philadelphia, PA, USA

Edward L. Krawitt
MD
Professor of Medicine
University of Vermont College of Medicine
Burlington, VT, USA

Anne M. Larson
MD, FACP
Associate Professor of Medicine
Medical Director of Liver Transplant
Director of Clinical Hepatology
University of Texas Southwestern Medical
Center
Dallas, TX, USA

Nicholas F. LaRusso
MD
Chairman, Department of Internal Medicine
Mayo Clinic College of Medicine
Rochester, MN, USA

Marie A. Laryea
MD
Hepatology/Multi-Organ Transplant Program
Assistant Professor of Medicine
Dalhousie University
Halifax, Nova Scotia
Canada

Konstantinos N. Lazaridis
MD
Center for Basic Research in Digestive
Diseases
Division of Gastroenterology and Hepatology
Mayo Clinic College of Medicine
Rochester, MN, USA

Stanley M. Lemon
MD
UNC Liver Center
University of North Carolina School of
Medicine
Chapel Hill, NC, USA

Josh Levitsky
MD, MS
Associate Professor of Medicine & Surgery
Division of Hepatology & Comprehensive
Transplant Center
Northwestern University Feinberg School of
Medicine
Northwestern Memorial Hospital
Chicago, IL, USA

James H. Lewis
MD
Professor of Medicine
Georgetown University School of Medicine
Washington, DC, USA

Anna S.F. Lok
MD
Alice Lohrman Andrews Research Professor
in Hepatology
Division of Gastroenterology
University of Michigan Medical Center
Ann Arbor, MI, USA

Harmeet Malhi
MD
Division of Gastroenterology and Hepatology
Mayo Clinic, College of Medicine
Rochester, MN, USA

Hitoshi Maruyama
MD, PhD
Department of Medicine and Clinical
Oncology
Chiba University Graduate School of
Medicine
Chiba, Japan

Timothy M. McCashland
MD
University of Nebraska Medical Center
Nebraska Medical Center
Omaha, NE, USA

Arthur J. McCullough
MD
Department of Pathobiology
Lerner Research Institute
Cleveland Clinic Foundation
Cleveland, OH, USA

Manuel Mendizabal
MD
Staff Hepatologist
Unidad de Hígado y Trasplante Hepático
Hospital Universitario Austral
Pilar, Argentina

Kevin W. Mennitt
MD
Assistant Professor of Radiology
Weill Cornell Medical College
New York, NY, USA

Mack C. Mitchell, Jr
MD
Medical Director of Ambulatory Services
Johns Hopkins Bayview Medical Center
Baltimore, MD, USA

Kevin D. Mullen
MD
Division of Gastroenterology
MetroHealth Medical Center
Cleveland, OH, USA

Santiago J. Munoz
MD, FACP, FACG
Professor of Medicine
Director, Clinical Hepatology
Temple University School of Medicine
Philadelphia, PA, USA

Francesco Negro
MD
Professor of Medicine
University of Geneva Medical Centre
Switzerland

Douglas L. Nguyen
MD
Center for Basic Research in Digestive
Diseases, Division of Gastroenterology and
Hepatology
Mayo Clinic College of Medicine
Rochester, MN, USA

Marco A. Olivera-Martinez
MD
Assistant Professor of Medicine
Department of Internal Medicine
Section of Gastroenterology and Hepatology
University of Nebraska Medical Center
Omaha, NE, USA

Kim M. Olthoff
MD
Donald Guthrie Professor of Surgery
The Hospital of the University of
Pennsylvania
Philadelphia, PA, USA

Hemal K. Patel
MD
Division of Gastroenterology and Hepatology
Henry Ford Health Systems
Detroit, MI, USA

David H. Perlmutter
MD
Vira I. Heinz Professor and Chair, Department
of Pediatrics
Professor of Cell Biology & Physiology
University of Pittsburgh School of Medicine
Physician-in-Chief and Scientific Director
Children's Hospital of Pittsburgh of UPMC
Pittsburgh, PA, USA

Ponni Perumalswami
MD
Mount Sinai School of Medicine
New York, NY, USA

Ravi K. Prakash
MD MRCP (UK)
Division of Gastroenterology
MetroHealth Medical Center
Case Western Reserve University
Cleveland, OH, USA

K. Rajender Reddy
MD, FACP, FACG, FRCP
Professor of Medicine in Surgery
Director of Hepatology
Medical Director of Liver Transplantation
University of Pennsylvania
Philadelphia, PA, USA

Mark A. Rosen
Division of Gastroenterology
Department of Internal Medicine
The University of Pennsylvania School of
Medicine
Philadelphia, PA, USA

Bruce A. Runyon
MD
Professor of Medicine
Chief of Liver Service
Division of Gastroenterology/Hepatology
Loma Linda University Medical Center
Loma Linda, CA, USA

Arun J. Sanyal
MD
Division of Gastroenterology and Hepatology
Virginia Commonwealth University
Richmond, VA, USA

Michael Schilsky
MD
Yale New Haven Transplant Center
Yale University Medical Center
New Haven, CT, USA

Maria H. Sjogren
MD, MPH
Gastroenterology Service
Department of Medicine
Walter Reed Army Medical Center
Washington, DC, USA

Anthony S. Tavill
MD, FACP, FRCP
Professor Emeritus of Medicine
Case Western Reserve University
Consultant Hepatologist
Cleveland Clinic
Cleveland, OH, USA

James F. Trotter
MD
Medical Director of Liver Transplantation
Baylor University Medical Center
Dallas, TX, USA

Marie-Louise Vachon
MD
Mount Sinai School of Medicine
New York, NY, USA

Natasha Walzer
MD
Assistant Professor of Medicine
Division of Hepatology
University of Illinois at Chicago
Chicago, IL, USA

Ian R. Wanless
MD, CM, FRCPC
Department of Pathology
Dalhousie University
Halifax, Nova Scotia, Canada

Paul B. Watkins
MD
Verne S. Caviness Distinguished Professor of
Medicine
University of North Carolina at Chapel Hill
Chapel Hill, NC, USA

Joshua Watson
MD
Gastroenterology Service
Department of Medicine
Walter Reed Army Medical Center
Washington, DC, USA

Kymberly D.S. Watt
MD
Hepatology & Liver Transplantation
Mayo Clinic Rochester
MN, USA

Russell H. Wiesner
MD
Transplant Center
Mayo Clinic Rochester, MN, USA

Allan W. Wolkoff
MD
Professor of Medicine and Anatomy &
Structural Biology
Marion Bessin Liver Research Center
Division of Gastroenterology and Liver
Diseases
Albert Einstein College of Medicine
Bronx, NY, USA

Florence Wong
MD, FRCPC
Associate Professor, University of Toronto
Staff Hepatologist, Toronto General Hospital
Toronto, ON, Canada

Foreword

At the start of my clinical training three decades ago, the study of hepatology was dominated by two academic phenotypes, including investigators devoted to metabolic biochemistry and bilirubin, and astute diagnosticians capable of artful and accurate prognostication but who possessed few tools to alter clinical outcomes. Fear of bile acid metabolism almost kept many of us out of the laboratory, but the promise of better tools to come was alluring. The progress has been remarkable on both fronts. Transplantation, molecular diagnostics, effective antiviral therapies, and sophisticated supportive treatments have altered the landscape dramatically. Further, advances in understanding the human genetic factors responsible for the substantial person-to-person differences in pharmacokinetics, response to interferon, and susceptibility to liver diseases foreshadows the coming era of personalized hepatology based on a prospective assessment of risk.

Against the scope and pace of these changes, it has been argued that the traditional role of the textbook is challenged by electronic media. An authoritative textbook, however, has a different function. Under the best of circumstances, a textbook provides history, context, and the leavening ability to integrate advances and put them in their proper perspective. This perspective is essential to understanding the implications of science for both physiology and clinical care. It also allows for appropriate humility, since the scientific news of the day fails to withstand scrutiny more often than we would like to admit.

Given these considerations, the timeliness and authority of this new edition of *Schiff's Diseases of the Liver* is remarkable. This is a classic text based solidly in the biochemical origins of our discipline. It also succeeds masterfully in providing the depth and perspective that is essential to students at any stage of their careers. This results in large part from the careful selection of chapters with broad thematic relevance, and to the equally critical selection of authors who are the best in the field. The result is an authoritative statement of where we are today. Beyond the appeal to trainees, this text is one that targets important issues in clinical care. Accordingly, clinicians can use this textbook with confidence to inform and support decisions in patient care. Beyond that, the scientific basis for the presentations assures that investigators also can rely on *Schiff's* for keeping pace with the broader advances in hepatology based on appropriate cell and molecular biology.

The chapters are organized and comprehensive. Opening sections on Clinical Fundamentals, General Considerations, and Consequences of Liver Disease provide a foundation for clinical assessment, pathologic diagnosis, and imaging. The chapter on mechanisms of liver injury has broad implications for the authoritative chapters on the major complications of liver injury that follow, including portal hypertension, hepatorenal syndrome, peritonitis, and encephalopathy. In each case the emphasis on the physiologic basis for management is emphasized. The subsequent sections are organized around more specific groups of disorders, including Cholestasic Disorders, Viral Hepatitis, and Alcohol and Drug-induced Liver Disease. The section on Genetic and Metabolic Disease has benefited from considerable changes as required by the scientific and clinical advances in that area. Finally, emphasis is placed on the emerging challenges in the care of patients with liver tumors and liver transplantation. Collectively, the authors include both future and established leaders of hepatology, and they are to be congratulated for a comprehensive yet disciplined assessment of the state of our field.

The challenges in hepatology are still substantial. Clinical manifestations range from isolated and clinically silent laboratory abnormalities to dramatic and life-threatening complications of liver failure. The incidence of cirrhosis is increasing, but the best estimates suggest that up to 40% of those so affected are without symptoms, resulting in long delays in diagnosis and treatment. The result is unusually high human and economic costs. This new edition of *Schiff's Diseases of the Liver* is solidly grounded in the tradition of the investigators and diagnosticians who have advanced our discipline so far, and provides a timely and comprehensive statement of the current art to prepare a new generation to make advances in the future.

J. Gregory Fitz, MD
Provost and Dean
UT Southwestern Medical School, Dallas, TX

Preface

This eleventh edition of *Schiff's Diseases of the Liver* and a retrospective review of the previous editions attests to the remarkable advances in our understanding of the pathogenesis and treatment of liver diseases. New treatments, particularly of chronic viral hepatitis, are interrupting the progression towards cirrhosis and reducing the risk for hepatocellular carcinoma. An accurate history, physical examination, and standard laboratory chemistries will still make the diagnosis in the majority of patients with hepatobiliary disorders. Worldwide, liver biopsy is gradually being replaced by noninvasive diagnostic modalities. However, histopathologic examination is paramount in establishing the type and degree of liver injury. Antifibrotic therapies are evolving and clinical trials have been initiated. Improvement in the management of acute liver failure and complications of cirrhosis have allowed for more patients to be salvaged with liver transplantation.

There remain a significant number of patients with idiopathic acute and chronic liver disease where the etiology has not yet been established. Autoimmune hepatitis commonly overlaps with both intrahepatic and extrahepatic biliary disease. Successful treatment of primary sclerosing cholangitis is a challenge for the future. The development and implementation of vaccinations for hepatitis A, B, and more recently E, will continue to reduce the incidence of acute viral hepatitis. Yet the spectrum of molecular variants within the sphere of hepatitis C has frustrated the successful development of a hepatitis C vaccine.

Proteonomics and genomics are becoming germane to understanding the pathogenesis of liver disease, particularly drug-induced liver disease. Comorbidities of steatohepatitis, both alcoholic and non-alcoholic, together with genetic predispositions including heterozygous states for alpha-1 antitrypsin deficiency and iron overload are often involved in the pathogenesis of liver disease. With increased life expectancy and an older aged population, cardiac disease and ischemic hepatitis are becoming more prevalent. Earlier detection of hepatocellular carcinoma coupled with more accurate radiologic examination and newer therapeutic options have salvaged many of these patients. As advances in the prevention and treatment of liver disease evolve, the last resort for those with decompensated liver disease remains liver transplantation. Improvement of tolerance for the transplanted liver is a major focus of research.

This eleventh edition of *Diseases of the Liver* is a readily accessible and valuable resource reflecting the talent and expertise of outstanding authors.

Eugene R. Schiff
Willis C. Maddrey
Michael F. Sorrell

PART I

Overview: Clinical Fundamentals of Hepatology

CHAPTER 1

History Taking and Physical Examination for the Patient with Liver Disease

Norton J. Greenberger

Division of Gastroenterology, Hepatology and Endoscopy, Brigham and Women's Hospital, Boston, MA, USA

Key concepts

- In the care of patients with jaundice, a careful history, physical examination, and review of standard laboratory tests should allow a physician to make an accurate diagnosis in 85% of the cases.
- The triad of findings of splenomegaly, ascites, and an increased number of venous collateral vessels on the anterior abdominal wall indicates a diagnosis of portal hypertension.
- The presence of two physical findings (ascites and evidence of portasystemic encephalopathy (asterixis)) and two laboratory findings (hypoalbuminemia (<2.8 g/dL) and a prolonged prothrombin time (international normalized ratio >1.6)) indicates a diagnosis of cirrhosis of the liver.

- Three physical findings (parotid enlargement, gynecomastia, and Dupuytren contracture) indicate that a patient is almost certainly consuming excessive amounts of alcohol.
- In adult patients with a new onset of jaundice, ten disorders account for 98% of the ultimately established diagnoses. They include decompensated chronic liver disease, alcoholic hepatitis, gallstones, malignancy, sepsis/abnormal hemodynamics, drug-induced liver disease, hemolysis (sickle cell anemia), postoperative jaundice, viral hepatitis, and primary biliary cirrhosis and primary sclerosing cholangitis. By the time patients with metastatic liver disease have jaundice, the diagnosis should be obvious because the liver has been extensively replaced by tumor.

Jaundice is a common presentation among patients with liver and biliary tract disease. The terms *jaundice* and *icterus* are used to designate skin and eyes appearing yellow resulting from the retention and deposition of biliary pigments (biliary monoglucuronides and diglucuronides). Although bilirubin stains all tissue, jaundice is most evident in the sclerae, face, and trunk. Jaundice is most commonly caused by parenchymal liver diseases such as viral hepatitis or cirrhosis, obstruction of the extrahepatic biliary tree as in choledocholithiasis and carcinoma of the pancreas, and less commonly, disorders associated with brisk hemolysis such as sickle cell anemia. The late Franz Ingelfinger stated in 1958 that the cause of jaundice can be identified in approximately 85% of patients after a careful study of the history and the performance of a physical examination and review of standard laboratory data. The same applies today. Box 1.1 lists specific questions to ask in relation to the different causes of liver and biliary tract disease.

History taking for patients with jaundice or abnormal liver test results

Anorexia is a cardinal symptom of viral hepatitis and of neoplasms involving the liver, colon, biliary tree, or pancreas. Weight loss of more than 10 pounds (4.5 kg) should always raise the question of a neoplastic disorder.

Chills and fever along with headache and myalgia should raise the question of viral hepatitis. Chills and fever along with right upper quadrant abdominal pain suggest a diagnosis of biliary tract disease, especially choledocholithiasis and ascending cholangitis.

Arthritis can be the harbinger of viral hepatitis, autoimmune chronic hepatitis, inflammatory bowel disease with underlying liver disease, primary sclerosing cholangitis, or granulomatous disorders such as sarcoidosis.

Fleeting skin lesions are often present in patients with viral hepatitis type B. Excoriations, indicating pruritus, should raise the question of either intrahepatic or

---

Schiff's Diseases of the Liver, Eleventh Edition. Edited by Eugene R. Schiff, Willis C. Maddrey and Michael F. Sorrell.
© 2012 John Wiley & Sons, Ltd. Published 2012 by John Wiley & Sons, Ltd.

Box 1.1 Specific questions to ask patients with jaundice or liver disease.

Questions related to viral hepatitis
- Blood transfusions (especially if before 1990)
- Intravenous drug use
- Sexual practices:
    Anal-receptive intercourse
    Sex with a prostitute
    History of sexually transmitted disease
    Multiple sexual partners (>5/year)
    Intercourse with individuals with hepatitis B or C
- Contact with individuals with jaundice
- Changes in taste and smell
- Needlestick exposure
- Work in renal dialysis units
- Surgeons in trauma units or operating rooms exposed to users of intravenous drugs
- Shared razors or toothbrushes
- Body piercing (ears, nose)
- Tattoos
- Intranasal cocaine use

Special risk factors for hepatitis A (if not previously immunized)
- Travel to endemic areas
- Ingestion of raw shellfish (harvested from contaminated waters)
- Exposure to patients in places where clusters of hepatitis may occur (e.g., institutions, prisons, preschool nurseries)

Medication-related questions
- Review all prescription medications
- Ask specifically about all over-the-counter drugs
- Ask specifically about vitamins (especially vitamin A)
- Ask specifically about any foods, herbal preparations, and home remedies purchased in a health food store

Alcohol use questions
- Obtain detailed *quantitative* history of both recent and previous alcohol use from the patient *and* family members
- Question whether patient has experienced withdrawal symptoms or driving-under-the-influence convictions
- CAGE (cut down, annoyed, guilty, eye opener) criteria (see text)
- Check for evidence of alcohol-associated illnesses (pancreatitis, peripheral neuropathy)

Miscellaneous questions
- Pruritus (suggests cholestasis, either intrahepatic or extrahepatic)
- Evolution of jaundice (dark urine, light stools)
- Recent changes in menstrual cycle (amenorrhea suggests chronic liver disease, often cirrhosis)
- History of anemia, sickle cell disease, known hemoglobinopathy, or artificial heart valves
- Symptoms suggestive of biliary colic or chronic cholecystitis
- Family history of liver or gallbladder disease
- History of inflammatory bowel disease (should raise the question of primary sclerosing cholangitis and receipt, if any, of blood transfusions)
- Occupational history and, specifically, exposure to hepatotoxins

extrahepatic cholestasis, particularly primary biliary cirrhosis or primary sclerosing cholangitis. With regard to abdominal pain, the standard questions to ask concern the location, character, radiation, factors precipitating or relieving pain, and whether there are other systemic symptoms that accompany the pain. Patients should be asked to compare current abdominal discomfort with other causes of abdominal pain that they have experienced in the past (e.g., gastroesophageal reflux symptoms, non-ulcer-type dyspepsia).

Questions to be asked in relation to viral hepatitis include specific questions about blood transfusions, especially whether they were received before 1990. The date is important because before that time no serologic tests were available for the detection of infection with hepatitis C virus. Intravenous drug use is currently the most common cause of hepatitis C. It is important to ask specifically about sexual practices, especially high-risk sexual behavior. In this regard, anal-receptive intercourse is known to be a significant risk factor for hepatitis B. Sexual practices associated with an increased risk of hepatitis C include a history of sexual relations with a prostitute, history of a sexually transmitted disease, and multiple sexual partners per year. In addition, intercourse with patients known to be positive for hepatitis B and C (e.g., spouses) is known to be a risk factor for contracting these forms of hepatitis. Contact with jaundiced individuals may be a risk factor for hepatitis A and B. Changes in taste and smell occur fairly frequently in patients with viral hepatitis. They contribute, in a large part, to the anorexia experienced by such patients. This is in part due to a decreased sense of smell (hyposmia), perception of unpleasant smells from foods that are not ordinarily perceived as unpleasant (dysosmia), a decreased sense of taste (hypogeusia), and perception of unpleasant tastes (dysgeusia). Hypogeusia is often reflected in the fact that patients may spontaneously state that they have lost their taste for cigarettes.

Health care professionals are at risk of contracting hepatitis C. This can occur through needlestick exposure, by working in renal dialysis units, and by working in trauma units, emergency departments, or operating rooms through surgical procedures on patients harboring the hepatitis C virus in whom that diagnosis is not immediately apparent. All users of intravenous drugs should be suspected of harboring the hepatitis C virus. Special risk factors for hepatitis C include tattoos, body piercing (e.g., of the ears and nose), a history of snorting cocaine, and the use of shared razors or toothbrushes.

The incidence of hepatitis A and hepatitis B has decreased markedly due to immunization, however, there are special risk factors for hepatitis A that include travel to endemic areas such as Mexico and Latin America and the African subcontinent, ingestion of raw shellfish that may have been harvested from contaminated waters, and exposure to patients in places where clusters of hepatitis may occur. The latter has been well documented in mental institutions, prisons, preschool nurseries, and close living quarters. Hepatitis A can be transmitted parenterally because there is brief viremia.

Medication use, including all prescription drugs and all over-the-counter drugs, should be carefully reviewed. The constellation of clinical features that include fever, arthritis or arthralgia, rash, and eosinophilia in a patient with jaundice or abnormal results of liver tests should always raise the question of medication-induced liver disease. This can be recalled by the mnemonic FARE, which stands for *f*ever, *a*rthritis, *r*ash, and *e*osinophilia. The patient should be asked specifically about intake of vitamins, especially vitamin A, and about any foods, herbal preparations, or home remedies purchased in health food stores. Several herbal preparations have been found to be hepatotoxic.

Detailed quantitative information should be obtained from both the patient and family members about recent and previous alcohol use. For reference purposes, 30 mL (1 ounce) of bourbon whiskey contains 10–11 g of alcohol, as does one 360 mL (12-ounce) container of beer or 120 mL (4 ounces) of red table wine. Each one of these can be considered as 1 unit. Ingestion of more than 3 units/day every day or more than 21 units/week is excessive, especially for women. The threshold for alcohol-induced hepatic injury appears to be 30 g/day for women and 60 g/day for men if ingested over 5–10 years. These numbers may have to be modified if additional risk factors for liver disease are present (e.g., hepatitis C). One also needs to determine whether the patient has experienced withdrawal symptoms. The CAGE criteria are reliable indicators of excessive alcohol use. The CAGE criteria relate to the following four questions:

1 Has the patient tried to *c*ut back on alcohol use?
2 Does the patient become *a*ngry when asked about his or her alcohol intake?
3 Does the patient feel *g*uilty about his or her alcohol use?
4 Does the patient need an *e*ye opener in the morning?

In this regard, many patients with chronic alcoholism experience morning nausea and dry heaves. The examiner should check for evidence of alcohol-associated illnesses (e.g., pancreatitis and peripheral neuropathy).

A history of pruritus suggests cholestasis, either intrahepatic or extrahepatic. Box 1.2 shows the differential diagnosis of jaundice [1]. The patient should be specifically asked about the evolution of jaundice (i.e., the onset of dark urine and light stools), which may provide clues to the duration of illness. Recent changes in the menstrual cycle, particularly amenorrhea, if present, suggest chronic liver disease and often cirrhosis. A history of anemia, sickle cell disease, and hemoglobinopathy

---

Box 1.2 Differential diagnosis of jaundice.

Most common causes
- Decompensation of chronic liver disease
- Alcoholic hepatitis
- Gallbladder disease (cholecystitis, choledocholithiasis)
- Sepsis/abnormal hemodynamics
- Malignancy (pancreatic cancer, liver metastases)

Common causes
- Viral hepatitis
- Drug- or toxin-induced liver disease (especially acetaminophen)
- Hemolysis (especially sickle cell anemia)
- Postoperative (multiple factors)
- Primary biliary cirrhosis
- Primary sclerosing cholangitis

Less common causes
- Hodgkin disease and non-Hodgkin lymphoma
- Total parenteral nutrition
- Gilbert syndrome; while unconjugated hyperbilirubinemia ≥1.2 mg/dL occurs in 2–5% of the population, serum bilirubin levels infrequently exceed 3.0 mg/dL and detectable jaundice is unusual

Causes and presumed sites of intrahepatic cholestasis
- Liver cell (hepatocellular):
  Viral hepatitis
  Alcoholic liver disease
  Chronic active liver disease
  α_1-Antitrypsin deficiency
- Hepatocanalicular:
  Drugs (androgens, phenothiazines)
  Sepsis
  Postoperative state
  Total parenteral nutrition
  Hodgkin and non-Hodgkin lymphoma
  Amyloidosis
  Sickle cell anemia
  Toxic shock syndrome
- Ductular:
  Sarcoidosis
  Primary biliary cirrhosis
- Bile ducts:
  Intrahepatic biliary atresia
  Caroli disease
  Cholangiocarcinoma
  Primary sclerosing cholangitis
- Recurrent cholestasis:
  Benign recurrent intrahepatic cholestasis
  Recurrent jaundice of pregnancy
  Dubin–Johnson syndrome

---

should also be ascertained for African-American patients. Right upper quadrant abdominal pain should prompt detailed questions about whether such pain is consistent with biliary colic or chronic cholecystitis. A history of inflammatory bowel disease should raise the question of primary sclerosing cholangitis or, if the patient has received blood transfusions in the past, hepatitis C. An occupational history should be obtained and questions about specific exposure to a known or suspected hepatotoxin should be asked of industrial workers with jaundice or liver disease.

Physical examination of the patient with jaundice or abnormal results of liver tests

The key elements in the physical examination of a patient with jaundice or abnormal results of liver tests are summarized in Box 1.3. Several important clues are evident on general inspection of the patient. It should be determined whether scleral icterus is present, and this should be done in natural daylight. Scleral icterus can usually be detected if the serum bilirubin level is elevated to values greater than 3.0 mg/dL. The presence of pallor suggests anemia. Wasting suggests advanced chronic liver disease or a neoplastic disorder. Needle tracks or evidence of skin popping suggest intravenous drug abuse. The presence of skin excoriation confirms that the patient has been experiencing pruritus, which can be particularly severe among patients with primary biliary cirrhosis and primary sclerosing cholangitis. The one area where such patients cannot scratch is the interscapular area, and this is usually free of evidence of excoriation. The presence of ecchymosis or petechiae raises the question of clotting problems, especially thrombocytopenia. Muscle tenderness and weakness are not uncommon among patients with chronic alcoholism and alcoholic myopathy. These findings are often overlooked. When associated with severe acute pancreatitis, discoloration of the abdomen is termed the *Grey Turner sign.* This finding implies increased likelihood of death. Other less common causes of ecchymosis include rhabdomyolysis, muscle infarction, mesentery thrombosis, strangulated bowel with extensive intestinal infarction, and massive intraperitoneal bleeding.

The presence of lymphadenopathy, if generalized, suggests a lymphoproliferative disorder such as Hodgkin disease or non-Hodgkin lymphoma. Supraclavicular lymphadenopathy should raise the question of underlying malignant disease of the stomach or bronchopulmonary tract. Patients with pneumonia have jaundice in approximately 3% of cases; this is more likely to be the case among patients with pneumococcal pneumonia. Accordingly, a careful examination of the lungs is in order in the evaluation of patients with jaundice. Patients with congestive heart failure quite frequently have chronic passive congestion of the liver, which can result not only in jaundice but also in signs of portasystemic encephalopathy.

Box 1.3 Physical examination of the patient with jaundice.

General inspection
- Scleral icterus
- Pallor
- Wasting
- Needle tracks
- Evidence of skin excoriations
- Ecchymosis or petechiae
- Muscle tenderness and weakness
- Lymphadenopathy
- Evidence of pneumonia
- Evidence of congestive heart failure

Peripheral stigmata of liver disease
- Spider angiomata
- Palmar erythema
- Gynecomastia[a]
- Dupuytren contracture[a]
- Parotid enlargement[a]
- Testicular atrophy
- Paucity of axillary and pubic hair
- Eye signs mimicking hyperthyroidism

Abdominal examination
- Hepatomegaly
- Splenomegaly
- Ascites
- Prominent abdominal collateral veins
- Bruits and rubs
- Abdominal masses
- Palpable gallbladder

Signs of "decompensated" hepatocellular disease
- Jaundice
- Ascites
- Oliguric hepatic failure
- Hepatic encephalopathy:
    Fetor hepaticus
    Asterixis
    Behavioral alterations (confusion, disorientation, failure to complete simple mental tasks)

[a]This triad suggests chronic alcoholism.

There are several peripheral stigmata of chronic parenchymal liver disease. Spider angiomata are usually found in the distribution of the superior vena cava and most commonly on the upper anterior chest, neck, face, and upper thorax. The presence of more than a dozen spider angiomata should raise the question of portal hypertension. The triad of gynecomastia, Dupuytren contracture, and parotid enlargement should always raise the question of chronic alcoholism. Paucity of axillary and pubic hair and eye signs mimicking those of hyperthyroidism are often found among patients with advanced liver disease. Testicular atrophy, defined by a testicular diameter of less than 3 cm, is also common.

The abdominal examination is important in determining the liver size as well as the presence of an enlarged spleen. Percussion of the abdomen is important for several reasons. First, the size of solid organs such as the liver and spleen can be evaluated with percussion. One can often determine whether an increased amount of intraperitoneal fluid (ascites) is present. The upper and lower borders of liver dullness can be assessed by means of percussion along the right midclavicular line from the midchest to the midabdomen (Fig. 1.1). Liver size can be further assessed by having the patient inspire and observing the descent of the liver (Fig. 1.2). The lower border of liver dullness alerts the examiner to the site where the liver edge should be palpable. The liver span as judged by liver dullness measures 10–12 cm in men and 8–11 cm in women. A sudden decrease in liver dullness can occur in several conditions, such as viral hepatitis with the development of submassive or massive liver cell necrosis, localized dilatation of the transverse colon (as in toxic megacolon), fulminant colitis, and ileus associated with peritonitis or a perforated viscus (e.g., duodenal ulcer or diverticulitis). The spleen is normally not palpable. Percussion over the spleen reveals an area of dullness extending from the 10th rib in the posterior midaxillary aspect to the anterior aspect of the chest (Figs 1.2 and 1.3). When the patient inspires, the area of splenic dullness moves inferiorly and to the right.

The detection of splenic dullness is important for the following three reasons:

1 It may indicate splenic enlargement before the spleen can be palpated.
2 It alerts the examiner to the site where the spleen may be palpated.
3 Increasing dullness of the left flank may be a valuable clue to the diagnosis of traumatic rupture of the spleen or subcapsular hematoma.

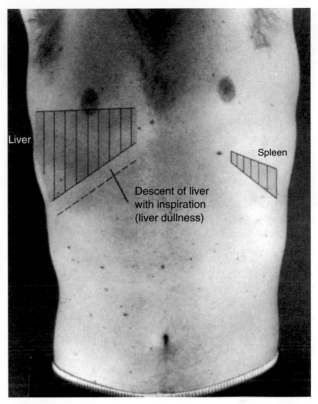

Figure 1.2 Abdomen and chest showing the location of the liver and the spleen as outlined by means of percussion. The liver descends 1–3 cm with inspiration, which is reflected by a change in liver dullness.

All quadrants of the abdomen must be palpated in an orderly manner. When palpating the abdomen, the hand should be warm and the palm and extended fingers of the right hand placed flat in a plane parallel to the surface of the abdomen (Fig. 1.4). The pads of the fingers are used together to perform light general palpation. Light palpation is used on the abdomen first, and as tense

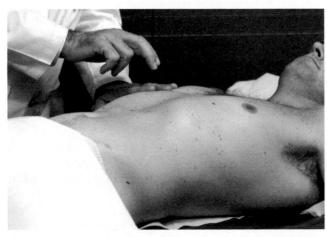

Figure 1.1 Determination of liver size by means of percussion over the lower right anterior chest and the right upper quadrant of the abdomen.

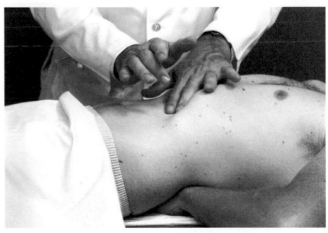

Figure 1.3 Technique for percussion of the spleen. If splenomegaly is present, the percussion note is dull, and with inspiration the spleen moves downward and medially and the percussion note changes accordingly.

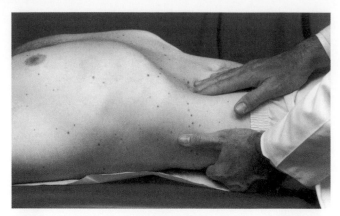

Figure 1.4 Technique for palpation of the liver.

muscles relax, deeper palpation should be tried. Quick jabbing movements should be avoided. Any area of tenderness or any increased muscular resistance should be recognized and examined in detail.

Percussion should alert the examiner to the approximate size and lower edge of the liver. Beginning at the right iliac fossa, the right hand is moved gradually upward until the edge of the liver is appreciated (Fig. 1.4). The patient can be asked to slowly take a deep breath. The descent of the diaphragm carries the liver down, which facilitates palpation of the liver edge. The edge of the liver can be felt in most healthy individuals if the patient's abdominal wall muscles are relaxed and the patient takes a slow, deep breath. In some healthy individuals, a very low lying thin segment of the liver can be palpated in the right lower quadrant. This is termed the *Riedel lobe of the liver.* An alternative approach to feeling the edge is to gently curl the fingers of the right hand below the costal margin and ask the patient to inspire slowly (Fig. 1.5). This is termed the *Middleton method.* In this manner,

the liver descent is appreciated by eight fingertips. This method is important in determining minimal enlargement of the liver or a liver palpable only in the epigastrium, as can occur in advanced cirrhosis.

The examiner should determine whether the liver is soft, firm, hard, or irregular; whether the edge is rounded or sharp; whether discrete masses are present; and whether the left lobe is palpable across the midline. The presence of a palpable left lobe always denotes an abnormality, usually chronic liver disease. The size of the liver should be assessed as judged by the location of the edge below the right midclavicular line and the xiphoid. A normal liver edge is sharp, smooth, and not hard, and the left lobe is not palpable. A rounded edge suggests liver disease; a palpable left lobe suggests either chronic infiltrative or neoplastic liver disease. Modest enlargement of the liver occurs in several disorders, most notably viral hepatitis, chronic liver disease (all causes), chronic hepatitis, cirrhosis, choledocholithiasis, and extrahepatic biliary tract obstruction. Marked enlargement of the liver (edge >10 cm below the costal margin) occurs in relatively few disorders, which include: (i) primary and metastatic tumors of the liver, including lymphoma; (ii) alcoholic liver disease (fatty liver, alcoholic hepatitis, cirrhosis); (iii) severe congestive heart failure; (iv) infiltrative diseases of the liver, such as amyloidosis and myelofibrosis; and (v) chronic myelogenous leukemia. Finally, a pulsatile liver should raise the question of tricuspid regurgitation, which can occur with advanced mitral stenosis, endocarditis of the tricuspid valve, and severe pulmonary hypertension.

Percussion of the left upper quadrant may have alerted the examiner to the presence of an enlarged spleen. Palpation of the spleen should begin in the left iliac fossa and move up to the left costal margin (Fig. 1.6). If the spleen is not felt while the patient is supine, the patient should roll onto his or her right side so the examiner can again examine the left upper quadrant (Fig. 1.7). This method

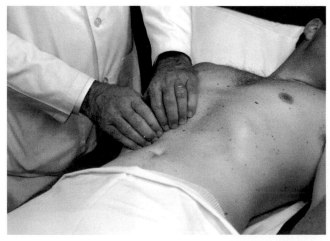

Figure 1.5 Alternative technique for palpation of the liver. The best results are obtained with gentle pressure of the curled fingers on the anterior abdominal wall.

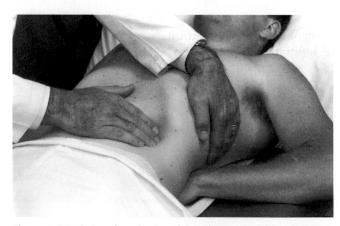

Figure 1.6 Technique for palpation of the spleen.

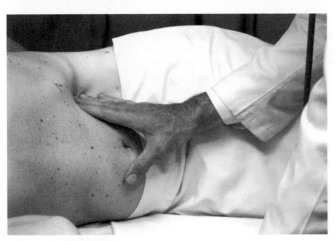

Figure 1.7 Palpation with the patient in the right lateral decubitus position. This should be performed on all patients with suspected splenomegaly if the spleen is not felt with the patient in the supine position.

takes advantage of the fact that when the spleen enlarges, it becomes more easily palpable inferiorly and medially. This enlargement is better appreciated when the patient is in the right lateral decubitus position. An alternative is for the examiner to stand at the patient's right side with the patient's left hand placed under the 11th rib to elevate the thorax. The examiner then curls the fingers of either one or both hands below the costal margin and asks the patient to inspire. The splenic margin may then be felt by the fingertips.

A common problem in evaluating left upper quadrant masses is differentiating the spleen and the left kidney. Palpation of a notch on the medial surface suggests that the organ being palpated is the spleen. Differentiation of the left lobe of the liver from the spleen can be difficult if massive hepatomegaly is present. One can usually discern a space or open area between the two organs. Common causes of splenomegaly include the following:

1 Portal hypertension caused by cirrhosis of the liver.
2 Infections (viral, bacterial, fungal).
3 Leukemia, lymphoma, and Hodgkin disease.
4 Connective tissue diseases (systemic lupus erythematosus and rheumatoid arthritis).
5 Infiltrative disorders (amyloidosis and sarcoidosis).
6 Hemolytic disorders.
7 Myelofibrosis.

Gallbladder

The gallbladder, when enlarged, can often be palpated in the right upper quadrant at the angle formed by the lateral border of the rectus abdominis muscle and the right costal margin. The gallbladder is palpable in approximately 25% of cases of carcinoma of the head of the pancreas (Courvoisier's law) because of painless distention of the gallbladder. The gallbladder is also palpable in approximately 30% of patients with acute cholecystitis, often because stones are impacted in the neck of the gallbladder. Often in acute cholecystitis, rather marked right upper quadrant tenderness is present, and palpation can be difficult because of intense involuntary spasms of the abdominal muscles. Percussion over the right lower anterior chest and right upper quadrant often elicits pain.

Another sign pointing to acute cholecystitis is right upper quadrant abdominal pain aggravated by inspiration (Murphy's sign). The patient is asked to inspire after the examining fingers are placed high in the right upper quadrant; inspiration causes the gallbladder to descend and come in contact with the extended fingers, causing pain and inspiratory arrest.

Bruits

Bruits are systolic sounds usually produced by the turbulence of blood flowing through diseased or compressed blood vessels. The many causes of abdominal bruits are listed in Table 1.1. The most common causes of such bruits include calcification of the aorta, celiac axis compression, and alcoholic hepatitis. An epigastric bruit can be appreciated in 20% of healthy thin young adults, especially if auscultation is performed after a meal. Such bruits are usually caused by the compression of the celiac axis artery by muscle fibers of the crus of the diaphragm. Abdominal bruits are often important clues leading to the diagnosis of hepatocellular carcinoma, renal artery stenosis, fibromuscular hyperplasia of the renal arteries, intestinal angina, aortic aneurysm, and pancreatic cancer.

Peritoneal friction rub

A friction rub heard over the liver suggests the diagnosis of liver metastasis or primary hepatocellular carcinoma. Other causes of hepatic friction rub include infarction of the liver (as in sickle cell anemia and polyarteritis nodosa) and liver abscess. A transient friction rub caused by a hematoma around the puncture site is common after liver biopsy but is usually not audible 4–6 hours after biopsy.

Ascites

Assessment of shifting dullness is often used to determine whether ascites is present. When free fluid is present in the abdomen, such fluid gravitates to the flanks, and the intestines float upward when the patient lies on his or her back. Percussion with the patient in this position discloses tympany over the anterior abdomen and dullness over the flanks. If the patient is turned to one side, the dullness shifts, and the percussion on the side that is uppermost becomes tympanic, because that area becomes occupied by gas-filled intestine.

Another physical finding pointing to the diagnosis of ascites is the fluid wave. A fluid wave is demonstrated

Table 1.1 Causes of abdominal bruit [3].

Location of bruit	Diagnostic considerations	Comment
Liver	Alcoholic hepatitis Hepatocellular carcinoma	Bruits may change day to day Suspect hepatocellular carcinoma in decompensated cirrhosis with a disproportionately increased serum level of alkaline phosphatase
	Effect of surgery Portosystemic shunt Hepatic artery aneurysm Hepatic arteriovenous fistula (trauma)	
Spleen	Splenic artery aneurysm	May see calcification in left upper quadrant on plain radiographs of the abdomen
	Splenorenal shunt Splenic arteriovenous fistula Calcified aorta	
Aorta	Aortic aneurysm Celiac axis compression Celiac or superior mesenteric artery disease (atheroma, thrombi)	Bruits common in thin individuals, especially after meals Intestinal angina characterized by the triad of: (i) bruit, (ii) weight loss, and (iii) postprandial abdominal pain
Left upper quadrant	Pancreatic cancer (body or tail)	Bruit caused by encasement of splenic artery or vein by tumor; present in 25% of cases
Umbilicus	Cruveilhier–Baumgarten syndrome	Bruit caused by increased flow through umbilical veins secondary to portal hypertensions
	Renal artery stenosis (atheroma, emboli) Renal artery fibromuscular hyperplasia Renal artery aneurysm	Bruit may be unilateral or bilateral

by tapping the left flank sharply with the right hand while the left hand is placed against the opposite flank (Fig. 1.8). Either the patient or a second examiner must place the ulnar surface of his or her hand along the midline of the abdomen. A positive test result is one in which an impulse on the opposite flank is percussed after the right flank is tapped. Neither the test for shifting dullness nor the test for a fluid wave uniformly reveal modest amounts of ascitic fluid (<1,000 mL). Indeed, both tests have a sensitivity of only approximately 60% compared with ultrasound examination [2]. Furthermore, the test results can be spuriously positive in examinations of obese patients.

A third sign, bulging flanks, although often present in ascites, is frequently present in obese patients as well. A fourth test of ascites is elicitation of the puddle sign. In this test, the patient lies prone for a few minutes and then moves to hands and knees. The diaphragm of the stethoscope is placed over the most dependent part of the abdomen, where puddling would be expected to occur. The examiner then repeatedly flicks the near flank of the abdomen while moving the stethoscope toward the opposite flank. A positive test result consists of a definite

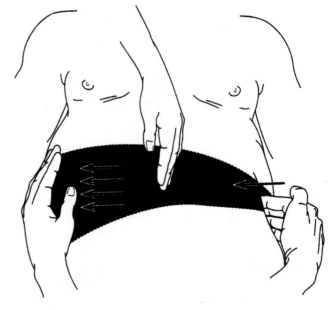

Figure 1.8 Technique for eliciting a fluid wave. The examiner's left hand is placed on the right lateral abdomen, and the right hand taps the left flank or loin while a second examiner or the patient's hand compresses the abdomen in the midline.

change in the intensity and character of the percussion note as the stethoscope is moved.

The presence or absence of ascites can be confirmed most reliably with imaging procedures such as ultrasonography and computed tomography (CT). The urinary bladder is often percussed in the hypogastrium, especially if urinary retention is present.

Abdominal masses

All nine areas of the abdomen should be palpated carefully for the presence of abdominal masses. In addition, the examiner should palpate the periumbilical area for the presence of lymph nodes. Such lymph nodes, termed Sister Mary Joseph nodes, reflect intraperitoneal tumor and are the harbinger of peritoneal carcinomatosis.

Signs and symptoms of decompensated liver disease

Signs of decompensated liver disease in patients with cirrhosis include jaundice, ascites, portal hypertension with bleeding esophageal or gastric varices, oliguric hepatic failure, and hepatic encephalopathy. These are discussed in detail in Chapters 11, 13, and 18. A bedside diagnosis of cirrhosis of the liver can be made on the basis of two physical findings and two laboratory findings. The physical findings are ascites and asterixis, and the laboratory findings are a serum albumin level of less than 2.8 g/dL and a prolongation of the prothrombin time of more than 16 seconds.

The topic of hepatic encephalopathy is discussed in detail in Chapter 18. However, this diagnosis can be made readily at physical examination when the following findings are present, especially in a jaundiced patient:

1 Hypothermia, with a temperature of less than 36°C.
2 Fetor hepaticus, which is a pungent odor in the breath caused by the excretion of sulfur-containing amino acid by-products such as dimethyl sulfide, methanethiol, and ethanethiol.
3 Asterixis, which can be elicited by two techniques (Fig. 1.9), and abnormal cognitive functioning as evidenced by an abnormal result of a Reitan trial test or A-deletion test. The latter is performed by asking the patient to delete all the As in one or two paragraphs of newsprint; the examiner tabulates how many As were not deleted.

Asterixis, although characteristic of hepatic encephalopathy, is not pathognomonic of this disorder. Asterixis is also found in patients with renal failure, pulmonary insufficiency, and congestive heart failure. Patients with hepatic encephalopathy may have difficulty with seemingly simple tasks such as drawing a square, spiral, or five-cornered star or signing their name.

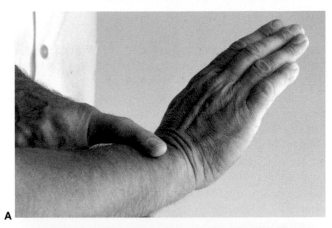

A

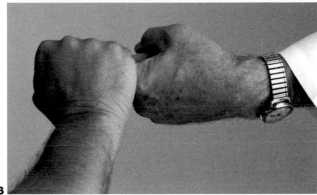

B

Figure 1.9 Techniques for eliciting asterixis. (A) The examiner applies his index finger over the dorsum of the patient's wrist while asking the patient to dorsiflex the wrist. Asterixis is the downward drift and abnormal recovery motion of the hand with the fingers either together or outstretched. (B) Alternative method for eliciting asterixis in patients who may not have the requisite extensor tonus. The examiner asks the patient to clench his fingers around the examiner's fingers. Asterixis is elicited with subtle movements of the examiner's wrist. In this manner, one can both feel and see the asterixis movement.

The diagnosis of chronic portosystemic encephalopathy is usually established on the basis of the following criteria:

1 Documented chronic parenchymal liver disease.
2 Evidence of portosystemic shunting, occurring either naturally (varices) or following the insertion of a transjugular intrahepatic portosystemic shunt (TIPS).
3 Behavioral alterations that can range from subtle abnormalities in cognitive functioning to frank unresponsive coma.
4 Improvement in mental status after measures directed at altering gastrointestinal ammonia metabolism, such as with dietary protein restriction or lactulose therapy.
5 An abnormal result of an electroencephalogram showing a decrease in mean cycle frequency. This is not routinely done.

Role of noninvasive imaging

Noninvasive imaging of the liver and biliary tree in the evaluation of the patient with jaundice and/or liver disease

As noted earlier, in patients with jaundice, a careful history, physical examination, and review of standard laboratory tests should allow a physician to make an accurate clinical diagnosis in 85% of cases. All too often, however, an imaging procedure is done before these basic steps have been completed and such omissions may actually delay establishing the correct diagnosis. The following are offered as guidelines to be considered for ordering imaging procedures:

1 Liver imaging procedures are not indicated in a patient with acute viral hepatitis.
2 Liver imaging procedures are not necessary in a patient with a firm clinical diagnosis of nonalcoholic fatty liver disease.
3 In a patient with jaundice and obstructive-type liver test abnormalities, that is, a disproportionately elevated serum alkaline phosphatase level and serum aminotransferases of less than 300 units, ultrasonography is the usual initial imaging procedure. Ultrasonography is reliable for differentiating medical jaundice, that is, intrahepatic cholestasis, from extrahepatic obstructive jaundice. In a patient with a serum bilirubin greater than 10 mg/dL that has been present for more than 2 weeks, ultrasound has a sensitivity of 95% and a specificity of 95% in differentiating intrahepatic versus extrahepatic causes of jaundice. Box 1.2 lists several causes of intrahepatic cholestasis. In some cases, the level and cause of bile duct obstruction can be identified.
4 If an ultrasound examination in a patient with jaundice reveals evidence of dilated intrahepatic ducts, additional imaging procedures such as CT scanning, magnetic resonance cholangiopancreatography (MRCP), endoscopic retrograde cholangiopancreatography (ERCP), and endoscopic ultrasonography (EUS) with biopsies are often necessary to establish the cause of obstruction. If no dilated ducts are found and the cause of jaundice is deemed to be "medical," a liver biopsy is frequently in order.
5 In patients with suspected cholelithiasis, ultrasonography is the primary diagnostic imaging procedure. In patients with suspected choledocholithiasis MRCP is often the next step. However, if there is a question of ascending cholangitis, ERCP is the preferred diagnostic procedure as papillotomy may be indicated.
6 In a patient with new onset of ascites, Doppler ultrasonography is indicated to determine the patency of the portal and hepatic venous systems.

7 In patients with obstructive jaundice due to suspected pancreatic carcinoma, EUS is superior to CT scanning with regard to detecting a pancreatic mass but comparable with regard to tumor staging and predicting either resectability or nonresectability.
8 In patients with unexplained hepatomegaly, either ultrasound or CT scanning are appropriate initial imaging procedures.

Case vignettes: practical considerations

The following are vignettes in which the salient features of a patient's illness alert the clinician to the most likely diagnosis.

1 A 35-year-old woman is referred with the diagnosis of acute viral hepatitis. Liver tests reveal a total serum bilirubin level of 3.0 mg/dL; serum aspartate aminotransferase (AST), 900 U/L; serum alanine aminotransferase (ALT), 880 U/L; serum alkaline phosphatase, 180 U/L; serum albumin, 3.6 g/dL; serum globulins, 5.8 g/dL; and prothrombin time, 15 seconds (international normalized ratio (INR), 1.9).
Key: The presence of marked hypergammaglobulinemia along with prolongation of the prothrombin time suggests that this patient has *chronic* rather than acute hepatitis. The most likely diagnosis for this 35-year-old woman would be autoimmune chronic hepatitis.
2 A 30-year-old man is referred for evaluation of elevated serum aminotransaminase levels. The patient weighed 230 pounds (103.5 kg) as a high school football player, 250 pounds (112.5 kg) after graduating from college, and 300 pounds (135 kg) 5 years later. Results of all liver tests are normal except for a serum AST level of 65 U/L and a serum ALT level of 80 U/L.
Key: If a patient has no symptoms except that the transaminase values are elevated approximately twice the normal value, six considerations should come to mind. They include: (i) excessive alcohol use; (ii) obesity with a body mass index (BMI) greater than 30; (iii) hepatitis C; (iv) excessive doses of acetaminophen (>4.0 g/day); (v) use of statin-type cholesterol-lowering agents; and (vi) celiac sprue. In this patient, the most likely explanation is obesity, and he may well have nonalcoholic steatohepatitis.
3 A 30-year-old man has severe flu symptoms for 5 days. Cough, myalgia, headache, and anorexia have resulted in markedly diminished intake of food and liquid. He has been ingesting generic acetaminophen 4.0 g/day and acetaminophen plus diphenhydramine (Tylenol PM™) to facilitate sleep. He was found to have a serum AST level of 5,000 U/L and an ALT level of 5,500 U/L.

Key: Ingestion of seemingly therapeutic doses of acetaminophen by a patient who has in essence fasted for 4 or 5 days can result in drug-induced hepatotoxicity. Results of early studies indicated that concurrent ingestion of alcohol and acetaminophen was the most common cause of this presentation. However, the scenario in this case is the more common presentation now. In patients who come to medical attention with serum aminotransaminase values of approximately 5,000 U/L, the differential diagnosis is limited to viral hepatitis, effects of drugs and toxins, and ischemia with shock liver. In the United States, approximately one half of cases of fulminant hepatic failure are related to acetaminophen ingestion.

4 A 63-year-old woman with non-insulin-requiring diabetes mellitus and hypercholesterolemia has been found to have abnormal results of liver tests. Results of liver biopsy establish the diagnosis of cirrhosis, but there is no obvious cause, and the patient is considered to have cryptogenic cirrhosis.

Key: A detailed history reveals that the patient was obese through much of her adult life, weighing in excess of 300 pounds (135 kg; BMI >35). Although she weighed only 200 pounds (90 kg) when she sought medical attention, many years of obesity coupled with diabetes and hypercholesterolemia most likely caused nonalcoholic steatohepatitis, which progressed to cirrhosis. The most common cause of cryptogenic cirrhosis is antecedent nonalcoholic steatohepatitis.

5 A 28-year-old man who has had ulcerative colitis for 10 years is found through routine screening to have a serum alkaline phosphatase level of 500 U/L. Results of all other liver tests are normal.

Key: Persistent elevation of serum alkaline phosphatase level to values greater than twice the normal value in patients with inflammatory bowel disease, especially those with ulcerative colitis, should raise the question of occult primary sclerosing cholangitis. This patient needs an MRCP as the initial screening procedure.

6 A 40-year-old woman is admitted to hospital for therapy for alcohol withdrawal and impending delirium tremens. Laboratory studies reveal serum bilirubin, 2.0 mg/dL; AST, 225 U/L; serum ALT, 45 U/L; prothrombin time, 14 seconds (INR, 1.3); serum iron level, 170 μg/dL; total iron-binding capacity, 200 μg/dL; iron saturation, 85%; and serum ferritin, 700 μg/dL.

Key: The increased percentage of iron saturation and elevated serum ferritin level in this case are not indicative of a diagnosis of hemochromatosis. Serum iron levels and serum ferritin levels are frequently elevated in patients with acute liver disease and marked liver cell necrosis.

7 A 17-year-old boy is referred for evaluation of hepatosplenomegaly and thrombocytopenia. On examination, he is found to have a peculiar "wing-beating" tremor. When the patient abducts his arms and flexes his forearms, a sustained tremor develops. The patient does not have Kayser–Fleischer rings. The serum ceruloplasmin level is 30 mg/dL.

Key: The presence of a wing-beating tremor in a young man with apparent chronic liver disease is almost pathognomonic of Wilson disease. Examination of a 24-hour urine collection for copper revealed excretion of 1,100 μg of copper. Of the three standard screening tests for Wilson disease – that is, Kayser–Fleischer rings, low serum ceruloplasmin level, and increased urinary excretion of copper – results of all three are abnormal in only one third of patients. In the remaining two thirds of patients, only one test may have a positive result. The clue in this case was the unusual tremor.

8 A 25-year-old Guatemalan man who does not speak English is visiting relatives in the United States. After a large meal, he develops retching and hematemesis. Esophagogastroduodenoscopy reveals esophageal varices. The patient is admitted to hospital and found to have hepatosplenomegaly, thrombocytopenia, a normal serum albumin level, and minimal hyperbilirubinemia (serum bilirubin, 2.0 mg/dL). Through interpreters, it is learned that the patient had his first episode of hematemesis at 10 years of age. He had several subsequent episodes managed by means of banding of varices.

Key: The onset of variceal bleeding at 10 years of age with stigmata of chronic liver disease but with well-preserved liver function indicates that the most likely diagnosis is congenital hepatic fibrosis.

9 A 55-year-old man is referred for evaluation of asymptomatic hepatosplenomegaly. The patient's liver span is over 20 cm with a smooth, rounded edge felt 14 cm below the costal margin with a prominent left lobe. The spleen is palpable 4 cm below the left costal margin. Serum bilirubin, alkaline phosphatase, AST, and ALT levels are normal. The serum albumin level is 3.5 g/dL and serum globulin levels are 3.0 g/dL. The prothrombin time and partial thromboplastin time are normal. The results of a complete blood cell count and routine chemical analyses are normal. Urinalysis is unremarkable except for 2+ proteinuria. Blood glucose levels are normal, and the patient is not overweight.

Key: The finding of marked hepatomegaly with normal liver test results in the evaluation of a patient without symptoms should raise the question of infiltrative liver disease, such as amyloidosis. In addition to amyloidosis, relatively few disorders give rise to marked hepatomegaly. These include primary and metastatic tumors of the liver, alcoholic liver disease, severe congestive heart failure, and advanced chronic myelogenous leukemia.

10 A 49-year-old man has documented end-stage chronic liver disease due to hepatitis C and alcohol ingestion. He has had previous hospital admissions for bleeding esophageal varices and ascites. Because of lack of compliance with a salt- and fluid-restricted diet, the patient has recurrent ascites despite treatment with diuretics. He is known to have diverticular disease, having had one previous episode of diverticulitis. He is admitted to the hospital with a 2-day history of severe abdominal pain, chills, fever, and anorexia. Diagnostic paracentesis reveals the following: white blood cell count, $10,000/\mu L$ with 90% polymorphonuclear leukocytes; ascitic fluid protein, $4.0\,g/dL$; ascitic fluid glucose, $35\,mg/dL$ with a simultaneous serum glucose level of $120\,mg/dL$ and peritoneal fluid of pH 7.1.

Key: This patient does not have spontaneous bacterial peritonitis. Rather, he has *primary* bacterial peritonitis. The triad of findings of a white blood cell count of $10,000/\mu L$ with a left shift, increased serum protein level, and low glucose level points to primary bacterial contamination of the peritoneal cavity, rather than spontaneous bacterial peritonitis, most likely from a perforated viscus. If a flat abdominal radiograph does not reveal evidence of free air, a CT scan should be obtained. If perforation is confirmed, the patient, despite the advanced liver disease, needs surgical exploration.

11 A 47-year-old man is referred for evaluation of ascites believed to be caused by chronic liver disease. There is no history of excessive alcohol use, risk factors for hepatitis B and C, or other gastrointestinal symptoms. There is a remote history of tuberculosis 20 years earlier managed appropriately. Previous physical examinations are said to be unremarkable except for ascites. Repeated physical examination reveals normal vital signs except for pulsus paradoxus of $20\,mmHg$. Inspiratory distention of the cervical neck veins is noticed. A third heart sound is heard to the left of the sternal border. The lungs are clear to auscultation. Abdominal examination reveals obvious ascites with a fluid wave. There is no peripheral edema. Ultrasound examination confirms the presence of ascites, reveals a liver that spans $15\,cm$, and a normal-sized spleen. The portal and hepatic veins are patent.

Key: The presence of pulsus paradoxus and a Kussmaul sign (inspiratory distention of the cervical neck veins) point to a diagnosis of constrictive pericarditis manifesting as ascites and masquerading as chronic

liver disease. Results of an echocardiogram confirmed the diagnosis.

12 A 47-year-old woman is referred for evaluation of hepatosplenomegaly. The patient has no risk factors for chronic liver disease. These include absence of alcohol intake, no risk factors for hepatitis B and C, and no excessive use of vitamins or herbal teas. Urinalysis, however, reveals the presence of hematuria; a CT scan shows a lesion in the right kidney consistent with renal cell carcinoma. What is the cause of the patient's hepatosplenomegaly?

Key: Although one would be tempted to consider metastatic liver disease to be the most likely explanation for the hepatosplenomegaly, a rare syndrome termed *Stauffer syndrome* is a form of nephrogenic hepatosplenomegaly. Hypernephroma, in some ill-defined way, may elaborate hepatotropic growth factors that cause enlargement of the liver and spleen. Such patients do not usually have evidence of metastatic liver disease, and with nephrectomy the liver may actually regress in size.

13 A 57-year-old woman is referred for evaluation of ascites. She initially visited her gynecologist, who suspected that she might have ovarian carcinoma. However, a pelvic examination and pelvic and abdominal CT scans did not reveal any evidence of tumor. There is no history to explain the development of ascites except that the patient has been drinking enormous quantities of herbal tea, ingesting 18–24 cups/day for the last 2 years.

Key: An ultrasound examination with determination of portal and hepatic venous flow velocity revealed findings consistent with hepatic venous occlusion. Tumors (hepatocellular carcinoma, pancreatic carcinoma, hypernephroma, and gastric carcinoma) are infrequent causes of Budd–Chiari syndrome. The most common cause is an obvious or incipient myeloproliferative syndrome. Herbal teas may contain alkaloids that can cause both intrahepatic and extrahepatic venoocclusive disease.

14 A 62-year-old woman has been to the hospital because of pruritus and is found to have jaundice. Except for scleral icterus, the findings of the physical examination are unremarkable. The liver span measures $12\,cm$ at percussion. Liver tests reveal the serum bilirubin level to be $8.0\,mg/dL$; AST, $400\,U/L$; ALT, $420\,U/L$; serum alkaline phosphatase, $500\,U/L$; normal serum prothrombin time; and normal serum albumin and globulin levels. Results of serum albumin, globulin, and antinuclear antibody tests are all either negative or within normal limits. An ultrasound examination shows a normal liver, gallbladder, and pancreas.

Key: A detailed history interview reveals that this woman took amoxicillin–clavulanic acid at a dosage of 2.0 g/day for 2 weeks, but this medication was discontinued 3 weeks earlier. Amoxicillin–clavulanic acid has been frequently reported to cause a cholestatic hepatitis. Jaundice and abnormal results of liver tests can develop 1–4 weeks after discontinuation of treatment. Histologic examination of the liver usually shows evidence of centrilobular (zone 3) or panlobular cholestasis, which, on rare occasions, is associated with a granulomatous hepatitis. The prognosis is excellent.

15 A 43-year-old man with a history of excessive alcohol ingestion (6 to 12 bottles of beer per day for many years) is admitted to the hospital with right upper quadrant pain, chills, fever, dark urine, and pruritus. Physical examination reveals right upper quadrant tenderness, the liver measuring 14 cm with a round, smooth, tender edge palpable 3 cm below the right costal margin. Liver tests reveal serum bilirubin, 8.0 mg/dL; AST, 220 U/L; ALT, 400 U/L; serum albumin, 3.8 g/dL; serum globulins, 3.2 g/dL; serum alkaline phosphatase, 400 U/L; mean corpuscular volume, 94 μm^3; white blood cell count, 14,000/μL with a left shift; and prothrombin time, 13 seconds (INR, 1.2).

Key: In patients with alcoholic hepatitis, the AST:ALT ratio is almost invariably 2:1 or greater. In this case, although the patient has consumed excessive amounts of alcohol, the disproportionately higher ALT:AST ratio suggests a cause of jaundice other than alco-

holic hepatitis. An ultrasound examination showed cholelithiasis and a dilated common bile duct. This patient, although with a history of alcoholism, had biliary tract disease. A clue to the correct diagnosis was the unanticipated reversal of the AST:ALT ratio.

Further reading

Cattau EL Jr, Benjamin SB, Knuff TE, et al. The accuracy of the physical examination in the diagnosis of suspected ascites. *JAMA* 1982;247:1146. *Report of a study that shows that the bedside diagnosis of ascites is inaccurate in approximately one third of cases and that ultrasound examination is helpful in detecting moderate amounts of ascitic fluid.*

Greenberger NJ, Hinthorn DH. *History Taking and Physical Examination: essentials and clinical correlates.* St Louis: Mosby-Year Book, 1992:220–61. *A detailed presentation of history taking and physical examination of the abdomen and description of acute and chronic abdominal pain syndromes. Much of the information is directly applicable to patients with diseases of the liver, biliary tree, or pancreas.*

Vuppalanchi R, Liangpunsakul S, Chalsani N. Etiology of new-onset jaundice: how often is it caused by idiosyncratic drug-induced liver injury in the United States? *Am J Gastroenterol* 2007;102:558–62. *A detailed analysis of the causes of jaundice in 732 cases with a serum bilirubin ≥ 3.0 mg/dL.*

References

1. Vuppalanchi R, Liangpunsakul S, Chalsani N. Etiology of new-onset jaundice: how often is it caused by idiosyncratic drug-induced liver injury in the United States? *Am J Gastroenterol* 2007; 102: 558–62.
2. Cattau EL Jr, Benjamin SB, Knuff TE, et al. The accuracy of the physical examination in the diagnosis of suspected ascites. *JAMA* 1982; 247: 1146.
3. Greenberger NJ, Hinthorn DH. *History Taking and Physical Examination: essentials and clinical correlates.* St Louis: Mosby-Year Book, 1992: 220–61.

Multiple choice questions

1.1 Each unit of packed red blood cells transfused to a patient contains bilirubin. Which of the following best approximates the amount infused in one unit?

    a 25 mg.
    b 50 mg.
    c 100 mg.
    d 150 mg.
    e 200 mg.

1.2 A 20-year-old woman is transferred to your hospital because of the onset of jaundice and acute liver failure over a period of 7 days. There is no history of antecedent medication use except for acetaminophen 1.8 g/day for 2 days, no exposure to jaundiced patients, and no recreational drug use. Physical examination revealed marked jaundice, hepatomegaly, and asterixis. Laboratory studies revealed: hemoglobin 8 g/dL, hematocrit 24%, serum bilirubin 15.1 mg/dL, AST 120 U/L, ALT 150 U/L, serum albumin 1.9 g/dL, and hemoglobinuria. What is the most likely etiology of her liver failure?

    a Autoimmune hepatitis.
    b Wilson disease.
    c Leptospirosis.
    d Acetaminophen hepatoxicity.
    e Herpes simples virus.

Answers to the multiple choice questions can be found in the Appendix at the end of the book.

These multiple choice questions are also available for you to complete online.
Visit http://www.schiffsdiseasesoftheliver.com/

CHAPTER 2

Laboratory Tests

H. Franklin Herlong & Mack C. Mitchell Jr

Department of Gastroenterology, Johns Hopkins Bayview Medical School, Baltimore, MD, USA

Key concepts

- Biochemical tests can be used to detect acute injury to the liver and chronic diseases of the liver before development of symptoms.
- Elevations in serum levels of aminotransferases (aspartate aminotransferase and alanine aminotransferase) reflect hepatocellular injury and/or permeability of the liver cell membrane, but do not correlate with the extent of fibrosis or measures of metabolic functions of the liver.
- An elevation of serum alkaline phosphatase occurs in response to intrahepatic cholestasis, extrahepatic obstruction of bile ducts, or infiltration of the liver with granulomatous inflammation, amyloidosis, or venous congestion.
- The rate-limiting step in metabolism and disposition of bilirubin is the transport of conjugated bilirubin from the hepatocyte into the bile.

- An elevation in the conjugated (direct-reacting) fraction of bilirubin is evidence of intrahepatic cholestasis or extrahepatic obstruction of the bile ducts.
- Serum levels of albumin may be low in patients with acute or chronic liver disease, but very often drop in response to the "acute phase response," making it difficult to evaluate hepatic metabolic function in clinical situations such as infection.
- Although single laboratory tests are generally not useful in evaluating the severity of acute or chronic liver diseases, the use of mathematical equations combining tests may be effective as surrogate markers for the extent of fibrosis, steatosis, and inflammation as well as to predict the short-term prognosis in patients with liver disease.

The use of laboratory tests is an important component of the assessment of patients with liver disease. With increasing frequency, elevations in the hepatic enzymes detected on routine screening tests provide the first evidence of liver disease in otherwise asymptomatic patients. In those patients with previously recognized hepatic dysfunction, laboratory tests can help establish the etiology of liver disease and provide valuable prognostic information. Rarely does a single test provide sufficient information to establish a diagnosis or assess severity of liver disease. A combination of tests such as serum bilirubin, albumin, aminotransferases, and alkaline phosphatase is sometimes referred to "liver function tests" or a "liver panel." These tests, in combination with the prothrombin time can provide an initial characterization of the etiology and severity of liver disease. However, one should recognize that the aminotransferases and alkaline phosphatase are tests that reflect hepatic injury not function. Traditionally liver diseases have been characterized as primarily hepatocellular or cholestatic based on the predominance of elevated aminotransferases or alkaline phosphatase. While an individual laboratory test may not provide a specific diagnosis, the pattern of abnormalities can suggest a general category of hepatic dysfunction. Although this distinction helps direct the initial evaluation there is often considerable overlap so that aggregating the diseases is less useful, as in the case of hepatotoxic drug reactions. With regard to drug-induced liver injury (DILI), those instances where the alanine aminotransferase (ALT) is greater than two times the upper limits of normal (ULN) and the ALT:alkaline phosphatase ratio is greater than 5 are considered primarily hepatocellular injuries. Those where the alkaline phosphatase is greater than two times the ULN and the ALT:alkaline phosphatase ratio is less than 2 are considered primarily cholestatic injuries. If the ALT and alkaline phosphatase are more than two times the ULN and the ratio is >2 or <5, the disorder is considered mixed hepatocellular/cholestatic. On occasion, minor elevations in the hepatic enzymes result from metabolic adaptation to drug metabolism and do not represent hepatic injury.

Laboratory tests can sometimes be helpful in assessing the severity of a liver disease, as is the case for using the prothrombin time to identify acute liver

Schiff's Diseases of the Liver, Eleventh Edition. Edited by Eugene R. Schiff, Willis C. Maddrey and Michael F. Sorrell.
© 2012 John Wiley & Sons, Ltd. Published 2012 by John Wiley & Sons, Ltd.

failure in a patient with acute liver disease or injury. However, for chronic conditions such as alcoholic liver disease, commonly measured tests of "liver function" such as the serum albumin can be affected significantly by factors other than extent of liver disease such as malnutrition, malabsorption, or chronic inflammation. The commonly used laboratory tests also lack specificity, which may limit their effectiveness in establishing a diagnosis. For example, an elevation in the alkaline phosphatase can reflect disorders of bone or liver, while elevated aminotransferases can be seen in cardiac disease or disorders of skeletal muscle as well as liver diseases. Unfortunately the commonly measured liver enzymes do not correlate with the extent of fibrosis or measures of metabolic functions of the liver. Consequently, patients with cirrhosis may have no abnormalities in laboratory tests.

Finally laboratory tests provide an important tool to assess the effectiveness of therapy in diseases like viral or autoimmune hepatitis or when injury has resolved after discontinuing a hepatotoxic drug. Serial determinations of liver enzymes are useful in identifying particular causes of liver injury. For example, ischemic necrosis will cause a marked elevation in the aminotransferases that returns to normal within a matter of days, whereas acute viral hepatitis will cause sustained elevations for several weeks. In the evaluation of patients for liver disorders, it is helpful to group these tests into general categories. We have found the following classification most useful:

- *Tests to detect injury to hepatocytes*: these include all the enzyme tests, of which the aminotransferases and alkaline phosphatase are the most useful.
- *Tests of the biosynthetic capacity of the liver*: included in this group are coagulation factors (prothrombin time/international normalized ratio (INR)) serum albumin, ceruloplasmin, ferritin, α_1-antitrypsin, and lipoproteins. These substances are synthesized in the liver and transported into the circulation.
- *Tests of the capacity of the liver to transport organic anions and metabolize drugs*: within this category, the serum bilirubin is the most useful. Other tests that assess clearance of organic compounds from the circulation by the liver include indocyanine green (ICG), bile acids, caffeine, lidocaine, and breath tests. These tests are rarely used in clinical medicine, but may have a limited role in some research studies.
- *Tests to detect fibrosis in the liver*: these include proprietary tests such as Fibrosure®, FibroTest®, and the Enhanced Liver Fibrosis® (ELF) test. These tests rely on the use of several biochemical markers that are mathematically combined to estimate the degree of fibrosis assessed by histopathology of the liver (see Chapter 12).
- *Tests that reflect chronic inflammation or altered immunoregulation*: these include specific autoantibodies and immunoglobulins, proteins that are made by B lym-

phocytes, not hepatocytes. Some of these tests may be helpful in diagnosing autoimmune liver diseases such as autoimmune hepatitis and primary biliary cirrhosis.

Tests for detection of injury to hepatocytes (serum enzyme tests)

The liver contains thousands of enzymes, some of which are also present in serum in very low concentrations. Most of these enzymes have no known function in the serum. They are distributed in the plasma and interstitial fluid and have characteristic half-lives of disappearance, usually measured in days. Little is known about their catabolism or clearance. The elevation of activity for a given enzyme in serum is thought to primarily reflect its increased rate of entry into serum from injured liver cells. Serum enzyme tests can be grouped into two categories: (i) enzymes whose elevation in serum reflects generalized damage to hepatocytes; and (ii) enzymes whose elevation in serum primarily reflects cholestasis.

Enzymes that indicate the presence of hepatocellular necrosis

Aminotransferases

The serum aminotransferases (formerly called transaminases) are sensitive indicators of liver cell injury and are most helpful in recognizing acute hepatocellular diseases like hepatitis. The activities of ALT, formerly serum glutamic-pyruvic transaminase, and aspartate aminotransferase (AST), formerly serum glutamic-oxaloacetic transaminase, in serum are the most frequently measured indicators of liver disease. These enzymes catalyze the transfer of the α-amino groups of alanine and aspartic acid, respectively, to the α-keto group of ketoglutaric acid. This reaction results in the formation of pyruvic acid and oxaloacetic acid (Fig. 2.1). Of the numerous methods developed for measuring ALT and AST activity in serum, the most specific method couples the formation of pyruvate and oxaloacetate – the products of the aminotransferase reactions – to their enzymatic reduction to lactate and malate. The reduced form of nicotinamide adenine dinucleotide (NADH), the cofactor in this reduction, is oxidized to nicotinamide adenine dinucleotide (NAD). Because NADH (but not NAD) absorbs light at 340 nm, the event can be followed spectrophotometrically by means of the loss of absorptivity at 340 nm.

Both aminotransferases are normally present in serum in low concentration. The precise source of these enzymes in serum has never been firmly identified, although presumably they originate in tissues rich in ALT and AST. AST is present in liver, cardiac muscle, skeletal

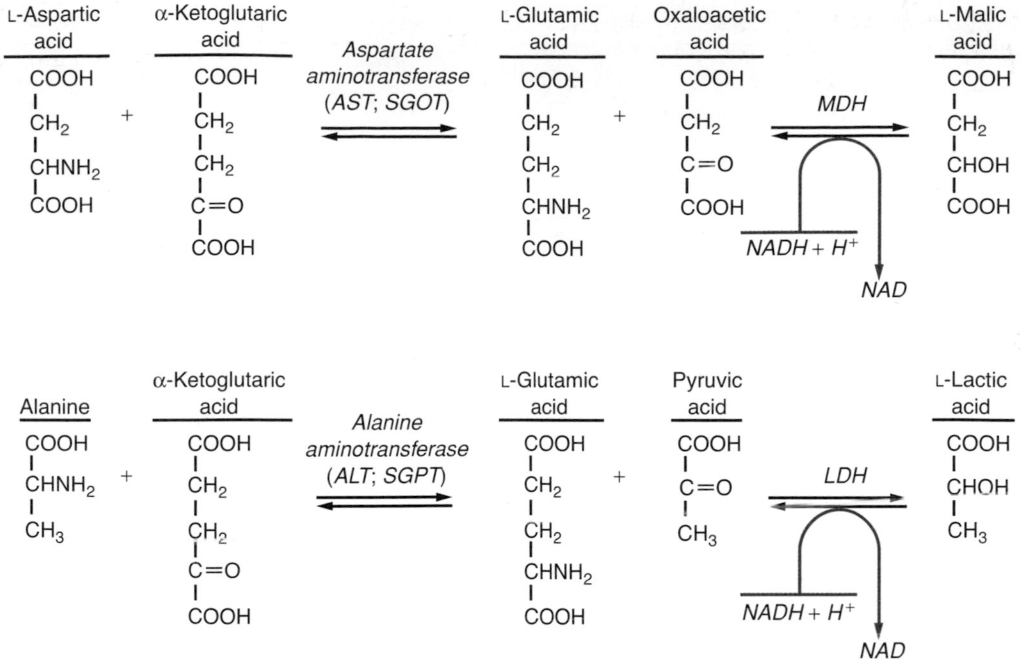

L-Aspartic acid   α-Ketoglutaric acid   Aspartate aminotransferase (AST; SGOT)   L-Glutamic acid   Oxaloacetic acid   MDH   L-Malic acid

L-Aspartic acid:
COOH
|
CH_2
|
$CHNH_2$
|
COOH

+

α-Ketoglutaric acid:
COOH
|
CH_2
|
CH_2
|
C=O
|
COOH

→ Aspartate aminotransferase (AST; SGOT) ⇌

L-Glutamic acid:
COOH
|
CH_2
|
CH_2
|
$CHNH_2$
|
COOH

+

Oxaloacetic acid:
COOH
|
CH_2
|
C=O
|
COOH

— MDH →

L-Malic acid:
COOH
|
CH_2
|
CHOH
|
COOH

$NADH + H^+$ → NAD

Alanine   α-Ketoglutaric acid   Alanine aminotransferase (ALT; SGPT)   L-Glutamic acid   Pyruvic acid   LDH   L-Lactic acid

Alanine:
COOH
|
$CHNH_2$
|
CH_3

+

α-Ketoglutaric acid:
COOH
|
CH_2
|
CH_2
|
C=O
|
COOH

→ Alanine aminotransferase (ALT; SGPT) ⇌

L-Glutamic acid:
COOH
|
CH_2
|
CH_2
|
$CHNH_2$
|
COOH

+

Pyruvic acid:
COOH
|
C=O
|
CH_3

— LDH →

L-Lactic acid:
COOH
|
CHOH
|
CH_3

$NADH + H^+$ → NAD

Figure 2.1 Enzymatic assay of aspartate aminotransferase (AST) and alanine aminotransferase (ALT). LDH, lactate dehydrogenase; MDH, malic dehydrogenase; NAD, nicotinamide adenine dinucleotide; NADH, reduced nicotinamide adenine dinucleotide; SGOT, serum glutamic-oxaloacetic transaminase; SGPT, serum glutamic-pyruvic transaminase.

muscle, kidneys, brain, pancreas, lung, leukocytes, and erythrocytes, in decreasing order of concentration. ALT is present in highest concentration in the liver. ALT and AST both require pyridoxal 5'-phosphate as a cofactor, and both may be present in serum in apoenzyme as well as holoenzyme form [1]. In tissues, ALT is present in the cytosol; whereas AST occurs in two locations, the cytosol and mitochondria. The cytosolic and mitochondrial forms of AST are true isoenzymes and are immunologically distinct. Approximately 80% of AST activity in human liver is contributed by the mitochondrial isoenzyme, whereas most of the circulating AST activity in healthy individuals is derived from the cytosolic isoenzyme. Neither ALT nor AST has isoenzymes that are tissue-specific. Hence, isoenzyme analysis of serum ALT or AST seldom is useful. Patients with acute myocardial infarction and chronic alcoholic liver disease may be exceptions. Large increases in mitochondrial AST occur in serum after extensive tissue necrosis. Because of this, assay of mitochondrial AST has been advocated as an accurate test for the detection of myocardial infarction, but is not widely used. The level of mitochondrial AST is also increased in chronic, but not acute, alcoholic liver disease. AST and ALT levels are equally elevated in most hepatobiliary disorders, with the ALT level usually being somewhat higher than the AST level. ALT appears to be a more sensitive and specific test of liver injury than AST and is commonly used in epidemiologic studies to document the incidence of viral hepatitis.

Aminotransferase levels are typically elevated in all liver disorders (Tables 2.1 and 2.2). These include all types of acute and chronic hepatitis, cirrhosis, acute and chronic heart failure, various infections, metastatic carcinoma, and granulomatous and alcoholic liver diseases. The highest elevations occur in disorders associated with extensive hepatocellular injury, such as drug and viral hepatitis, acute ischemia, and exposure to hepatotoxins such as acetaminophen. Values are commonly in the range of several hundred to the low thousands, although values in the range of 10,000 to 15,000 IU/L (167–250 µkat/L[1] – see subsequent text) can occur in rare patients with viral hepatitis who make uneventful recoveries. Levels of aminotransferases are seldom elevated above 500 IU/L (8.34 µkat/L) in obstructive jaundice, in viral hepatitis in patients with acquired immune deficiency syndrome (AIDS), and in cirrhosis (Tables 2.1 and 2.2) [2].

The increase in the serum values of ALT and AST is related to injury to cells rich in the aminotransferases or

[1]SI units (Le Système International d'Unites) are gradually replacing other units to have one common, worldwide system for reporting scientific data. The SI unit for enzymatic reactions is the katal, abbreviated kat. It replaces the international unit (IU/L) and denotes moles of substrate converted per second. For example, to convert alkaline phosphatase in IU/L to SI units (µkat/L), multiply the IU/L value by 0.01667. The SI reference range for alkaline phosphatase is 0.5–2 µkat/L. This value may vary somewhat among laboratories.

Table 2.1 Evaluation of acute elevations in aminotransferases.

Diagnosis	Range of ALT (IU/L)	AST : ALT ratio	Additional tests
Viral hepatitis	N l–3,000	<1	Hepatitis serologies: HBsAg, anti-HCV, anti-HDV, HCV RNA, HBV DNA
Drug-induced liver injury	N l–15,000	>1	Acetaminophen level, acetaminophen adducts, serial determinations of aminotranserases
Ischemic necrosis	N l–10,000	>1	–
Rhabdomyolysis	N l–5,000	>1	CPK
Myocardial infarction	N l–400	>1	CPK, troponin
Sepsis	N l–400	<1	Blood, urine cultures
Acute biliary obstruction	N l–2,000	<1	Imaging
Aminita phalloides poisoning	N l–5,000	<1	–

ALT alanine aminotransferase; AST, aspartate aminotransferase; CPK, creatine phosphokinase; HBsAg, hepatitis B surface antigen; HBV, hepatitis B virus; HCV, hepatitis C virus; HDV, hepatitis D virus; N, normal.

to changes in cell membrane permeability. The activity of any of the liver enzymes in serum reflects the rate of release of the enzyme from the liver into the circulation and the clearance of the enzyme from the circulation. The activity of AST and ALT in liver cells is more than 1,000 times greater than the activity in serum, so that, as liver cells die, the activity of aminotransferases increases in plasma. Under most circumstances the rate of clearance from the circulation remains relatively constant. An acute hepatocellular injury that takes place within a short period of time, such as necrosis due to acetaminophen poisoning, will result in a rapid rise in the serum levels of the enzymes as the enzyme activity from the dying cells enters the circulation. In patients with acetaminophen poisoning or ischemic injury, the peak level of AST exceeds that of ALT in the first 24 hours. Once there is no further injury to cells, the serum activity of both AST and ALT will return to the normal range. The rate of decline in the level of the enzymes depends on the clearance from the circulation, in much the same fashion as drugs are

Table 2.2 Evaluation of chronically elevated aminotransferases.

Diagnosis	Range of ALT (IU/L)	AST : ALT ratio	Additional tests
Viral hepatitis	N l–500	<1	Hepatitis serologies: HBsAg, anti-HCV, anti-HDV, HCV RNA, HBV DNA
Cirrhosis	N l–500	>1	Tests for advanced fibrosis, imaging
NAFLD	N l–300	<1	Imaging, elevated triglycerides, tests for insulin resistance
Cirrhosis	N l–300	>1	Tests for advanced fibrosis, imaging
Alcoholic liver disease	N l–400	>2	GGT, CAGE, or AUDIT questions, carbohydrate-deficient transferrin
Hemochromatosis	N l–200	>1	Ferritin, iron saturation, genetic testing
Autoimmune hepatitis	N l–2,000	<1	Antismooth muscle antibody, ANA, elevated IgG
Wilson disease	N l–2,000	<1	Ceruloplasmin, elevated serum copper, elevated urinary copper
Celiac disease	N l–100	<1	Tissue transglutaminase antibody, antiendomysial antibody
α_1-Antitrypsin deficiency	N l–100	<1	α_1-Antitrypsin phenotype
Hyperthyroidism	N l–200	<1	Elevated free T4, low TSH
Granulomatous liver disease	N l–500	<1	Various
Drug-induced liver injury	N l–2,000	<1	–
Myositis	N l–5,000	Usually >1	Elevated CPK, elevated aldolase
TPN	N l–300	<1	–

ALT alanine aminotransferase; ANA, antinuclear antibodies; AST, aspartate aminotransferase; CPK, creatine phosphokinase; GGT, γ-glutamyltransferase; HBsAg, hepatitis B surface antigen; HBV, hepatitis B virus; HCV, hepatitis C virus; HDV, hepatitis D virus; IgG, immunoglobulin G; N, normal; NAFLD, nonalcoholic fatty liver disease; TSH, thyroid-stimulating hormone.

eliminated. ALT and AST are both catabolized by the liver with a resulting plasma half-life of 47 ± 10 hours for ALT and 17 ± 5 hours for AST [3]. The enzymes are presumably catabolized by cells in the reticuloendothelial system. Hepatic sinusoidal cells appear to be the main site for AST clearance. Almost no aminotransferases are present in urine and only a very small amount is present in bile. It is therefore unlikely that biliary or urinary excretion plays a role in the clearance of ALT or AST.

Chronic injury to the liver results in significant variability in the rate of release of enzymes into the circulation. Many studies have shown a poor correlation between the severity of necrosis or inflammation and the serum level of ALT. Since the plasma level of ALT is affected by both the rate of release of the enzyme into the plasma and the rate of clearance of ALT from the plasma, both parameters could potentially affect the plasma level of ALT. Unfortunately, there is little information regarding the effect of chronic liver disease on the plasma clearance of aminotransferases. The level of ALT in serum varies considerably over time in patients with chronic viral hepatitis [4], presumably as a result of variable degrees of inflammation and/or necrosis in the liver. Only rarely does the level of ALT in chronic viral hepatitis exceed 500 IU/L. Although the level of ALT is variable in patients with chronic hepatitis, there is not a consistent and predictable decline in the serum level as observed after acetaminophen poisoning or ischemia. These random fluctuations can easily be distinguished from the first-order decay in the level of AST and ALT seen after massive necrosis from drug-induced or ischemic injury helping to distinguish a short-term acute injury from a more chronic one.

For any laboratory test, the mean value ± 2 standard deviations (SD) in a presumably healthy population constitutes the normal range for those tests with a normal, Gaussian distribution. In the 1950s the standard range was established using 88 healthy individuals [5]. Testing on a larger population of over 12,000 volunteers defined the "reference range" for AST to be 13–31 IU/mL and for ALT to be 13–40 IU/mL [6]. The distribution of serum AST and ALT activity in healthy volunteers is asymmetric and does not follow a normal, Gaussian distribution. For serum ALT activity, the distribution is linear after a log transformation. Therefore, the normal range is more often defined by excluding the top 2.5% of the values from presumably healthy volunteers, rather than using the mean ± 2 SD [7]. Local clinical laboratories have also independently defined the range of "normal" ALT based on measurements in specific populations [7]. However, this approach may not accurately reflect the "true normal" values since there are many factors that can influence serum ALT activity, including gender, obesity, and the presence of undiagnosed liver diseases in asymptomatic individuals. Men have higher serum activity of ALT than women [6–9]. In recent years, considerable attention has been focused on the role of obesity as a factor contributing to a higher upper limit of the "normal" range for ALT. Nonalcoholic fatty liver disease (NAFLD) is widely recognized as the most common reason for abnormal liver enzymes in the population. Individuals with NAFLD may have only slight elevations in ALT. Failure to exclude them from a population used to define the "normal" range could lead a higher than expected upper limit. Since many diseases of the liver are asymptomatic in early stages, careful definition of the true normal range of ALT and AST is important in screening patients for the presence of liver disease.

In a cohort of 1,033 blood donors, the upper limit of the normal range of ALT was found to depend on body mass index (BMI) and gender; the authors therefore recommended adjusting the ULN for these factors to reduce the artificial heterogeneity in selecting blood donors [8]. Interestingly, an effect of alcohol consumption on ALT was not observed. Based on these findings, a value was recommended of 31 IU/L for the ULN in females with a BMI $<23 \, kg/m^2$ and of 42 IU/L for males with a BMI $<23 \, kg/m^2$, and of 44 IU/L for females with a BMI $>23 \, kg/m^2$ and of 66 IU/L for males with a BMI $>23 \, kg/m^2$. A similar study of 6,835 volunteer blood donors in Italy also identified gender and BMI as the primary factors that were associated with a higher ALT [9]. In addition, laboratory parameters indicating abnormal lipid or glucose metabolism were associated with a higher ALT, consistent with what is known about the risk factors for NAFLD. The authors recommended a ULN of 30 IU/L for men and 19 IU/L for women, based on the 95 percentile of subjects (top 5% were excluded). The sensitivity for identifying individuals with hepatitis C virus (HCV) viremia improved from 55% to 76.3% using these limits, compared with 40 and 30 IU/mL for men and women, respectively. Data from a Korean population of healthy, voluntary liver donors found a similar ULN threshold (29 IU/L in men and 22 IU/L in women for the 95 percentile) to those of other recent studies [10]. Using the 97.5 percentile would produce a ULN of 33 IU/L for men and 25 IU/L for women. The voluntary donors all had liver biopsies documenting normal histology (Table 2.3).

Beyond defining the normal range for a population, knowing the "true normal value" for serum ALT is important in making treatment decisions for diseases such as chronic viral hepatitis, particularly hepatitis B. Guidelines published by the American Association for the Study of Liver Diseases (AASLD), the European Association for the Study of the Liver (EASL), and the Asia–Pacific Association for the Study of the Liver (APASL) all use elevation in ALT above the ULN as a factor to

Table 2.3 Population studies of normal alanine aminotransferase (ALT).

Number of subjects	95% ULN	97.5% ULN	Variables affecting ALT	Reference
12,682 Presumably healthy individuals	61 IU/L (men)	38 IU/L (men)	Age, gender, weight	Siest et al. [6]
	38 IU/L (women)	51 IU/L (women)	–	
Voluntary HCV-negative blood donors 3,856 men	36 IU/L (men)	–	BMI, triglycerides, by multiviariate analysis	Prati et al. [9]
2,970 women	21 IU//L (women)	–	–	
1,085	42 (men with BMI <23 kg/m^2)	–	BMI, GGT	Piton et al. [8]
–	31 (women with BMI <23 kg/m^2)	–	–	
Voluntary liver donors with normal histology, 643 men	31 IU/L (men)	35 IU/L (men)	BMI, age	Lee et al. [10]
462 women	24 IU/L (women)	26 IU/L (women)	–	

ALT alanine aminotransferase; BMI, body mass index; GGT, γ-glutamyltransferase; HCV, hepatitis C virus; ULN, upper limit of normal.

determine appropriateness for treatment of chronic hepatitis B [11–13]. In several of the guidelines, the panels recommend treatment based on values that exceed twice the ULN for ALT. The absolute value could be considerably higher if the ULN was 30 versus 19 or 40 versus 30 IU/L. The importance of defining the true normal ALT in considering treatment for chronic hepatitis B was addressed by a group of experts who recommended using 19 IU/L for women and 30 IU/L for men [14]. A population-based study in Korea, where there is a high prevalence of chronic hepatitis B infection, showed an increase in the relative risk of liver-related mortality in both men and women with an AST or ALT of greater than 20 IU/L [15]. The mean ALT activity in Japanese patients who achieved a sustained remission following treatment for chronic hepatitis C was 14.4 ± 3.2 IU/L for men and 9.9 ± 3.5 IU/L for women. These values were slightly lower than those of the healthy population although the reasons for this were unclear [16]. Of interest, serum ALT activity that is within the normal range may drop lower in response to oral nucleos(t)ide analog treatment of patients with chronic hepatitis B infection. These observations suggest that the true normal value in those individuals may be even lower than previously thought. The issue of what level of serum ALT activity should be considered normal in a population with chronic hepatitis has not been fully resolved.

There is a poor correlation between the extent of liver cell necrosis and the elevation of serum aminotransferases levels in chronic liver diseases. Similarly, absolute elevation of aminotransferase levels is of little value in predicting the outcome of acute hepatocellular disorders. Rapid decreases in serum aminotransferase levels are usually a sign of recovery from disease, but may be a poor prognostic sign in acute liver failure.

Elevated aminotransferase activity is among the first laboratory abnormalities to be detected in the early phases of viral hepatitis. In patients with jaundice due to hepatitis, the elevation of serum bilirubin level usually lags behind the increase in aminotransferase levels by approximately 1 week. Therefore, aminotransferase levels are frequently declining as the bilirubin level is increasing. Aminotransferase levels typically decline steadily during recovery from viral hepatitis. Secondary increases in aminotransferase levels or persistent elevation may indicate recrudescence of acute hepatitis or the development of chronic active hepatitis.

Hepatitis C is commonly associated with fluctuations in ALT and AST levels [4]. Some chronic hepatitis C patients with persistently normal ALT and AST levels have histologic evidence of chronic hepatitis on liver biopsy. The measurement of aminotransferases is one of the important means of evaluating the response to therapy for chronic hepatitis.

The AST : ALT ratio may be helpful in the recognition of alcoholic liver disease. If the AST is less than 400 IU/L (5.1 μkat/L), an AST : ALT ratio of more than 2 suggests alcoholic liver disease; a ratio greater than 3 is highly suggestive of alcoholic liver disease (Fig. 2.2) [17]. The increased ratio primarily reflects the low serum activity of ALT in patients with alcoholic liver disease [2]. This is secondary to a deficiency of pyridoxal 5'-phosphate in

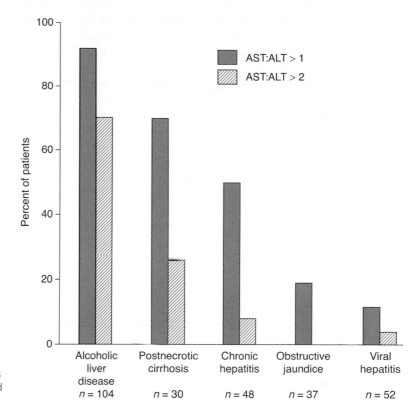

Figure 2.2 Percentage of patients with aspartate aminotransferase (AST): alanine aminotransferase (ALT) ratios greater than 1 and greater than 2. (Adapted from Cohen and Kaplan [17] with permission from Plenum.)

patients with alcoholic liver disease [1]. ALT synthesis in the liver requires pyridoxal phosphate more than AST synthesis does [1]. The altered AST:ALT ratio in the serum appears to reflect the altered ratios in the liver [2]. The less than expected increase in serum ALT and AST values in alcoholic liver disease – usually less than 200 IU/L (3.3 μkat/L) and 300 IU/L (5.1 μkat/L), respectively – cannot be explained simply by the decreased hepatic concentrations. This becomes evident whenever a patient with alcoholic liver disease has concomitant heart failure, viral hepatitis, or drug hepatotoxicity, particularly with acetaminophen; when this occurs, serum AST and ALT levels may soar to the thousands (>20 μkat/L). Despite striking elevations, the AST:ALT ratio remains increased and typical of alcoholic liver disease.

The AST:ALT ratio has been studied as a noninvasive indicator of cirrhosis in patients with chronic hepatitis C infection [18–21]. These studies have shown that an AST:ALT ratio greater than 1 indicates the presence of cirrhosis with a very high specificity (94–100%) but with a relatively low sensitivity (44–75%). Researchers identified a possible contributing factor to the AST:ALT ratio seen in both alcoholics and cirrhotics [22]. AST–immunoglobulin (Ig) complexes were studied in 128 patients with liver disease. AST was found to bind to Ig of the IgA class, but not to either IgG or IgM. This complex was seen in 41.8% of patients with chronic hepatitis, 62.2%

of patients with cirrhosis, and 66.7% of patients with alcohol-related liver disease. The high level seen in the final group likely reflected the high levels of IgA seen in patients with alcoholic liver disease. The AST:ALT ratio was significantly higher in the patients with the AST–Ig complex, rather than those without, and this observation probably contributes to the higher AST:ALT ratio seen in patients with cirrhosis and alcoholic liver disease.

Elevated serum aminotransferase values are not specific for hepatobiliary disorders. They are also found in patients with severe cardiac and skeletal muscle damage. AST level is more often increased in patients with myocardial infarction than ALT, and is undoubtedly of cardiac origin. Marked increases in AST and ALT (>5000 IU/L) in patients with severe cardiac disease likely represent hepatic ischemia with centrilobular (zone 3) necrosis. AST and ALT values in muscle disease are typically less than 300 U/L (5.1 μkat/L) but have been reported to be much higher [23]. Except in instances of acute rhabdomyolysis, values rarely reach the range observed in patients with acute hepatocellular disorders. Serum AST and, occasionally, ALT activity can increase after vigorous exercise, with an AST level of greater than 1,000 U/L reported. In such cases the AST:ALT ratio is initially greater than 3:1, but the ratio rapidly approaches 1:1 given the shorter half-life of AST [23]. The ratio is typically close to 1:1 in patients with chronic muscle diseases or injury. This may account for the slight, usually unexplained, increases in aminotransferase values observed among some runners.

Levels of the aminotransferases can be falsely elevated or diminished under certain circumstances. Drugs such as erythromycin and para-aminosalicylic acid can yield falsely elevated aminotransferase values if older colorimetric tests are used. Conversely, low AST values can occur in patients with uremia. These low values increase after dialysis; this finding suggests that a dialyzable inhibitor of the aminotransferase reaction is present in the serum of patients with uremia.

The cost-effectiveness of evaluating minimal elevations in ALT has been a subject of controversy. Many experts have argued that the lack of specificity of ALT and the number of conditions that do not require treatment, such as uncomplicated NAFLD, support a conservative approach to the evaluation and follow-up of these individuals [24–26]. However, several large epidemiologic studies have shown that an elevation in serum ALT activity is associated with an increase in the relative risk of death from chronic liver disease [15,27,28]. Some studies have also suggested that an elevation in serum ALT may predict an increased risk of overall mortality [15,27,29,30], whereas other studies have not found an association with increased risk of mortality from diseases other than liver ones [28]. Interestingly, a lower than normal ALT was also found to be associated with increased mortality and frailty in a geriatric population [31]. The increased mortality rate in this population appeared to be due to the association with frailty, a known risk factor for increased mortality in older individuals. Unfortunately, the disparities of opinion regarding the significance of minimal elevations of ALT are not likely to be resolved soon.

Other enzyme tests of hepatocellular necrosis

A number of other serum enzyme tests have been promulgated as being either more specific or more sensitive in the detection of hepatocellular necrosis than is the measurement of aminotransferases. Some of these enzymes are found only in liver tissues and, theoretically, the tests could be more specific for liver disease than are the aminotransferase tests. None of these enzymes have proved more useful in practice than the aminotransferase tests, and none are more widely used. Furthermore, some of these tests are not commercially available. A brief description of some of these enzyme tests follows.

Glutamate dehydrogenase

Glutamate dehydrogenase, a mitochondrial enzyme, is present primarily in the liver, heart, muscle, and kidneys. In the liver, it is present in its highest concentration in the centrilobular (zone 3) hepatocytes. Because of this location and the fact that the level is particularly elevated after acute right-sided heart failure, serum glutamate dehy-

drogenase was investigated as a specific marker for liver disorders that primarily affect centrilobular hepatocytes, such as alcoholic hepatitis. An initial report suggested that glutamate dehydrogenase may be a sensitive and relatively specific marker for alcoholic hepatitis, but this has not been confirmed [32].

Isocitrate dehydrogenase

Isocitrate dehydrogenase (ICDH), a cytoplasmic enzyme, is present in the liver, heart, kidneys, and skeletal muscle. Its activity in serum parallels that of the aminotransferases in acute and chronic hepatitis, but it is less sensitive. Although elevations in serum ICDH are relatively specific for liver disorders, increased levels have also been reported in disseminated malignant disease without detectable hepatic involvement. Like glutamate dehydrogenase, ICDH is predominantly found in hepatocytes in the centrilobular zone [33]. The measurement of ICDH does not yet offer any diagnostic advantage over the measurement of aminotransferases.

Lactate dehydrogenase

Lactate dehydrogenase (LDH) is a cytoplasmic enzyme present in tissues throughout the body. Five isoenzymes of LDH are present in serum, and are readily separated by various electrophoretic techniques. The slowest migrating band predominates in the liver. This test is not as sensitive as aminotransferase tests in the detection of liver disease and has poor diagnostic specificity, even when isoenzyme analysis is used. The LDH test is more useful as a marker of myocardial infarction and hemolysis. Marked elevations in serum LDH are sometimes seen in patients with acute liver failure due to ischemia or to infiltration of the liver with tumors such as melanoma or small cell carcinoma of the lung.

Sorbitol dehydrogenase

Sorbitol dehydrogenase is a cytoplasmic enzyme predominantly present in the liver; only relatively low concentrations are found in the prostate gland and kidneys. The activity of sorbitol dehydrogenase in serum parallels that of the aminotransferases in hepatobiliary disorders [34]. The measurement of sorbitol dehydrogenase appears to be less sensitive, however, and values may be normal in cirrhosis and other chronic liver disorders. The instability of this enzyme in serum further limits its diagnostic usefulness.

Enzymes for the detection of cholestasis

Alkaline phosphatase

Alkaline phosphatase is the name given to a group of zinc metalloenzymes that catalyze the hydrolysis of a large number of organic phosphate esters, optimally at an alkaline pH. The alkaline phosphatases of different tissues are true isoenzymes because they catalyze the same reaction, but differ in certain physicochemical properties [35]. Most of the alkaline phosphatase isoenzymes of clinical interest are coded by one gene: the liver/bone/kidney enzyme, also known as *tissue-unspecific alkaline phosphatase*. They have the same immunologic properties and amino acid sequence. Their unique physicochemical properties are conferred by the different carbohydrate and lipid side chains added by post-translational modification. A second gene codes for intestinal alkaline phosphatase; a third gene codes for placental alkaline phosphatase and an isoenzyme made in certain cancers, the Reagan isoenzyme; and a fourth gene encodes a placental like isoenzyme [36].

The precise function of alkaline phosphatase remains unknown. Alkaline phosphatases are found in the membrane of bone osteoblasts, the canalicular membranes of hepatocytes, the brush border of mucosal cells of the small intestine, the proximal convoluted tubules of the kidney, the placenta, and white blood cells [37]. In rat liver, alkaline phosphatase appears to have an active role in downregulating the secretory activities of the intrahepatic biliary epithelium [38]. In bones, the enzyme appears to be concerned with calcification, although its precise function is unknown. At other sites, it may participate in transport processes, but its actual physiologic purpose is largely unknown. There is good evidence that serum alkaline phosphatase in the normal adult is primarily derived from three sources: the liver, bone, and intestinal tract. The liver and bone are the major sources [39]. Contribution from the intestine (approximately 10–20%) is of importance, primarily in individuals with blood groups O and B, and the blood level of alkaline phosphatase is enhanced after the consumption of a fatty meal [40]. Studies with infused placental alkaline phosphatase have shown that the circulating enzyme appears to behave as other serum proteins do. The half-life is 7 days, and clearance from the serum is independent of the functional capacity of the liver or the patency of the bile ducts. The sites of degradation are unknown.

In the 15–50-year-old group, mean serum alkaline phosphatase activity is somewhat higher in men than in women (Fig. 2.3). In contrast, among individuals older than 60 years, the enzyme activity of women equals or exceeds that of men, and both sexes have somewhat higher values than younger adults [41]. The reasons for these differences are not known. In children, serum alkaline phosphatase activity is considerably elevated in both sexes, correlates well with the rate of bone growth, and appears to be accounted for by the influx of enzyme from osteoid tissue. Serum alkaline phosphatase in healthy adolescent males may reach mean levels three times greater than in healthy adults, without implying the pres-

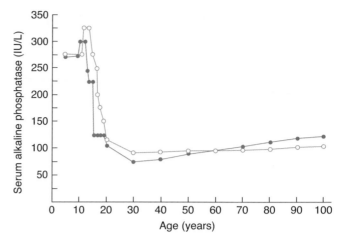

Figure 2.3 Normal serum alkaline phosphatase values at various ages for men (open circles) and women (closed circles). (Multiply by 0.01667 to convert to SI units, μkat/L.) (Data from Clarke and Beck [104] and Wolf [105].)

ence of hepatobiliary disease. Enzyme activity in serum may double late in normal pregnancy, primarily because of the influx of placental phosphatase. Although elevation of serum alkaline phosphatase activity is observed in various hepatobiliary diseases, similar elevations are seen in disorders of bone characterized by increased osteoblastic activity, and normally occur during growth and pregnancy. The intestinal tract may occasionally and the kidneys may rarely be the sources of an elevated serum enzyme level [42].

Identification of the specific isoenzymes of alkaline phosphatase could be helpful if an elevated serum alkaline phosphatase level is the only abnormal finding in an asymptomatic individual, or if the degree of elevation is higher than expected in the clinical setting. Although alkaline phosphatases derived from the liver, bone, intestine, and placenta have different electrophoretic mobilities [43], unfortunately electrophoresis and other methods of testing such as stability after heating are not sufficiently accurate to provide reliable differentiation of the isoenzymes. Therefore, the best substantiated approach to identifying the source of an isolated elevation in alkaline phosphatase is to measure the activity of enzymes that are released in parallel to liver alkaline phosphatase – such as serum leucine aminopeptidase, 5'-nucleotidase, and γ-glutamyltransferase (GGT) (Fig. 2.4). The levels of these enzymes, discussed later, are not elevated in bone disorders but only in those patients with liver dysfunction or, in the case of leucine aminopeptidase and 5'-nucleotidase, possibly in pregnancy. An increase of these enzymes in the serum of nonpregnant patients indicates that an elevated serum alkaline phosphatase is caused at least in part by hepatobiliary disease. In contrast, the lack of an increased level of 5'-nucleotidase in serum in the presence

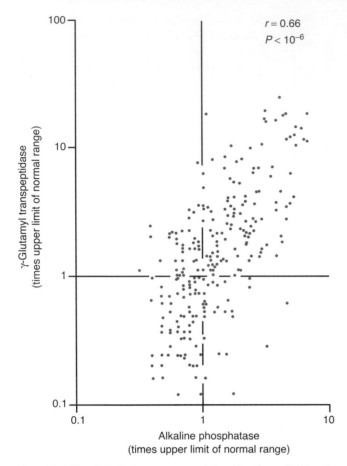

Figure 2.4 Correlation between serum γ-glutamyltransferase (GGT) and serum alkaline phosphatase levels in 245 healthy subjects and patients with hepatobiliary diseases. The units on the abscissa and ordinate are the logarithms of the multiples of the upper limits of normal for each test. Each point represents one patient. Although the correlation between the logarithmic values of the population is good ($r = 0.66$), a considerable variation exists between the percentage of GGT and alkaline phosphatase elevations in individual patients. (Reproduced from Whitefield et al. [106] with permission from British Medical Journal.)

bound to such membranes [45]. The precise manner in which the phosphatase reaches the circulation is unclear. In some patients with cholestasis, small vesicles that contain many basolateral (sinusoidal) membrane enzymes – including alkaline phosphatase – still bound to these membranes have been found in serum [46]. These observations may explain the delayed elevation of serum alkaline phosphatase after acute obstruction of the biliary tract.

The principal value of serum alkaline phosphatase in the diagnosis of liver disorders is in the recognition of cholestatic disorders. Approximately 75% of patients with prolonged cholestasis have alkaline phosphatase values increased four-fold or greater. Such elevations occur in both extrahepatic and intrahepatic obstruction, and the extent of the elevation does not differentiate the two. There is essentially no difference among the values found in obstructive jaundice due to cancer, common duct stone, sclerosing cholangitis, or bile duct stricture. Values are similarly increased in patients with intrahepatic cholestasis due to drug-induced hepatitis, primary biliary cirrhosis, rejection of transplanted liver, and, rarely, alcohol-induced steatonecrosis. Values are also greatly elevated in hepatobiliary disorders in patients with AIDS (e.g., primary sclerosing cholangitis due to cytomegalovirus infection and tuberculosis with hepatic involvement) [47].

Lesser increases in alkaline phosphates activity – up to three times the upper limit of normal – are nonspecific and may occur in all types of liver disorders (including viral hepatitis, chronic hepatitis, cirrhosis, and infiltrative diseases of the liver) and congestive heart failure.

Isolated elevations of hepatic alkaline phosphatase or a disproportionate elevation compared with the results of other tests, such as the measurement of aminotransferases and serum bilirubin, may occur in partial bile duct obstruction due to gallstones or tumor, as well as in infiltrative disease (such as sarcoidosis, hepatic abscesses, tuberculosis, and metastatic carcinoma) [39]. The mechanism is unknown, but probably represents local areas of bile duct obstruction with induction and leakage of hepatic alkaline phosphatase into serum, from these obstructed areas. An elevated serum alkaline phosphatase level in patients with primary extrahepatic cancer does not necessarily imply metastasis to the liver or bone. Some cancers secrete their own alkaline phosphatase into serum or cause leakage of hepatic alkaline phosphatase into serum by an unknown mechanism [48].

Moderate elevations in the level of alkaline phosphatase of hepatic origin can occur in disorders that do not directly involve the liver, such as stage I or II Hodgkin disease, myeloid metaplasia, congestive heart failure, intra-abdominal infections, and osteomyelitis [48]. Certain families may also have increased levels of serum alkaline phosphatase that are genetic in origin [42].

of an elevated level of alkaline phosphatase does not rule out liver disease, because these enzymes do not necessarily increase in parallel in early or modest hepatic injury.

Hepatobiliary disease leads to an increased serum activity of alkaline phosphatase that is paralleled by a striking increase in hepatic enzyme activity. The increased hepatic activity cannot be accounted for by the biliary retention of alkaline phosphatase [44]. Most evidence suggests that this elevation primarily occurs because of enhanced translation of mRNA rather than increased synthesis of mRNA in the liver, with subsequent release of the phosphatase into the circulation (44,45). This process appears to be mediated by the action of bile acids, which induce the synthesis of the enzyme and may cause it to leak into the circulation, perhaps by the disruption of hepatic organelles and the solubilization of phosphatase

Finally, extremely low levels of alkaline phosphatase can be present in patients with fulminant Wilson disease complicated by hemolysis [49,50].

5'-Nucleotidase

5'-Nucleotidase specifically catalyzes the hydrolysis of nucleotides such as adenosine 5'-phosphate and inosine 5'-phosphate, in which the phosphate is attached to the 5-position of the pentose moiety. 5'-Nucleotidase is found in the liver, intestines, brain, heart, blood vessels, and endocrine pancreas. In the liver, the enzyme is primarily associated with canalicular and sinusoidal plasma membranes. The physiologic purpose is unknown. In most laboratories, 5'-nucleotidase activity is assayed by the use of adenosine 5'-phosphate as a substrate, and the measurement of either the released inorganic phosphate or the free adenosine. The presence of alkaline phosphatase in serum complicates the assay because it also hydrolyzes the 5'-nucleotide substrates. Corrections for alkaline phosphatase activity can be made in two ways: (i) preliminary incubation of serum with appropriate concentrations of ethylenediaminetetra-acetic acid, which selectively inactivates only alkaline phosphatase; or (b) assay in the presence and absence of nickel (Ni^{2+}), a heavy metal that specifically inhibits 5'-nucleotidase. In most clinical laboratories, free inorganic phosphate is measured. A unit of 5'-nucleotidase activity is designated as an equivalent to the amount of enzyme that liberates 1 mg of phosphate per 100 mL of serum per hour. These units are analogous to the old Bodansky units of alkaline phosphatase activity and are expressed as such. In most series of healthy adults, the serum 5'-nucleotidase level ranges from 0.3 to 3.2 Bodansky units, and is not clearly influenced by sex or race. Values are substantially lower in children than in adults, increase gradually with adolescence, and reach a plateau after 50 years of age.

Serum values of 5'-nucleotidase are primarily elevated in hepatobiliary disease with a spectrum of abnormal values similar to that for alkaline phosphatase. The parallel behavior of these two enzymes in hepatobiliary disease probably reflects their similar subcellular location in hepatocytes [51]. Both enzymes are bound to bile canalicular and sinusoidal membranes, and must be solubilized to gain access to the circulation. Bile acids may act as detergents and solubilize them. In experimental bile duct obstruction in rats, bile acid concentrations rapidly reach levels sufficient to disrupt plasma membranes and solubilize both these enzymes. The same may occur in hepatobiliary disorders in which any degree of cholestasis develops [51].

The results of most studies indicate that alkaline phosphatase and 5'-nucleotidase are equally valuable in demonstrating biliary obstruction or hepatic infiltrative and space-occupying lesions. In selected patients, however, the level of one enzyme may be elevated and that of the other normal. Although the coefficient of correlation between the two enzymes is high, the values may not increase proportionately in individual patients [52].

Most data suggest that the 5'-nucleotidase and serum alkaline phosphatase are of equal value in differentiating obstructive from parenchymal liver disease. All investigators have shown some overlap in 5'-nucleotidase values in obstructive and hepatocellular jaundice. Some investigators have found this overlap to be small, and have concluded that this assay is equal to or better than the measurement of serum alkaline phosphatase for differentiating these two types of jaundice. Others have reported that the measurement of alkaline phosphatase has greater selective value [52].

Conflicting data have been reported for values of 5'-nucleotidase activity in serum during normal pregnancy. Some investigators have found an increase in enzyme activity in the third trimester, and others have reported no change during pregnancy. It is not clear whether these experiences are accounted for by differences in the methods used to measure 5'-nucleotidase activity. The major advantage of 5'-nucleotidase over the nonspecific alkaline phosphatase measurement in serum is enhanced specificity. Most studies show that the serum level of 5'-nucleotidase does not increase in bone disease; in the few instances in which an increase was observed, it was of low magnitude [52]. This is in striking contrast to results with alkaline phosphatase [52].

The greatest value of the 5'-nucleotidase assay is its specificity for hepatobiliary disease. An increased serum 5'-nucleotidase level in a nonpregnant individual suggests that a concomitantly increased serum alkaline phosphatase level is of hepatic origin. A normal nucleotidase level in the presence of an elevated serum alkaline phosphatase level does not rule out the liver as the source of the elevated phosphatase level. The level of one enzyme may occasionally be normal and the other elevated in liver disease.

Gamma-glutamyltransferase

γ-Glutamyltransferase catalyzes transfer of the γ-glutamyl group from γ-glutamyl peptides such as glutathione (GSH) to other peptides and to L-amino acids. GGT is present in many tissues in cell membranes, including the ductular side in the proximal tubule of the kidneys, intestine, and epididymis. A lower activity of GGT is found in the pancreas, liver, spleen, heart, brain, and seminal vesicles. GGT plays an important role in the hydrolysis of GSH and may also play a role in amino acid transport across membranes as part of the γ-glutamyl cycle. Within the liver, GGT is localized predominantly on biliary epithelial cells and on the apical membrane of hepatocytes. Although the activity of GGT in liver is relatively low in comparison to kidney and other tissues, the liver is the predominant source of the enzyme in the serum. Serum enzyme values are usually comparable for men and women, although some investigators have found higher values in men [53]. Children more than 4 years old have serum values of healthy adults. Serum enzyme activity does not increase during the course of normal pregnancy. The normal range is 0–30 IU/L (0–0.5 μkat/L).

Elevated serum GGT enzyme activity is found predominantly in diseases of the liver, biliary tract, and pancreas [53]. Abnormal values appear in approximately the same spectrum of hepatobiliary diseases as for alkaline phosphatase, leucine aminopeptidase, and 5′-nucleotidase. Some investigators find the GGT test more sensitive than alkaline phosphatase and leucine aminopeptidase tests in the detection of liver disease [53]. Others find little difference in sensitivity between GGT and alkaline phosphatase tests. A reasonably good, albeit far from perfect, correlation exists between GGT levels and those of 5′-nucleotidase and alkaline phosphatase in liver disease (Figs 2.4 and 2.5). The mechanism underlying the elevation of GGT in hepatobiliary diseases remains uncertain, but solubilization and release of membrane-bound GGT is one possible mechanism. Alternatively, death of biliary epithelial cells is another possibility [54].

High values of serum GGT are also found in patients who take medications such as barbiturates or phenytoin, or in those who ingest large quantities of alcohol [55,56], even when other serum enzyme and bilirubin values are normal. An isolated elevation in GGT level, or an elevation in GGT level out of proportion with that of other enzymes such as alkaline phosphatase or ALT, particularly in an asymptomatic patient, may be an indicator of heavy alcohol consumption. The induction of hepatic microsomal GGT by alcohol and other drugs may account for some of these observations. This is not the only explanation, however, because neither elevated serum GGT levels, nor a history of recent alcohol ingestion, correlates with hepatic GGT activity in patients with biopsy-proven alcoholic liver disease [57]. In addition, the alkaline phosphatase and hepatic GGT activities are similarly increased in patients with alcoholic hepatitis, yet serum GGT levels were 1,300% of normal while alkaline phosphatase serum levels were only slightly above normal [57]. Aside from its value in conferring liver specificity to an elevated alkaline phosphatase level and its possible use in identifying that a patient abuses alcohol, the measurement of serum GGT offers little advantage over aminotransferase and alkaline phosphatase testing in the evaluation of patients with suspected liver disease. In a prospective study with 1,040 nonselected inpatients, 139 patients (13.4%) had elevated serum GGT activity. Only 32% of these patients had hepatobiliary disease; the other 68% had other diseases that

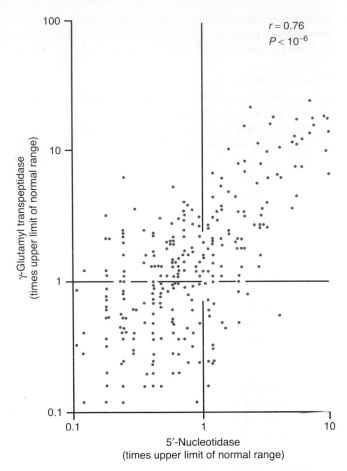

Figure 2.5 Correlation between serum γ-glutamyltransferase (GGT) and serum 5′-nucleotidase values in 245 healthy subjects and patients with hepatobiliary diseases. The units on the abscissa and ordinate are the logarithms of the multiples of the upper limits of normal for each test. Although the correlation between the logarithmic values of the population is good ($r = 0.76$), there is considerable variation between the percentage of GGT and 5′-nucleotidase elevations in individual patients. (Reproduced from Whitefield et al. [106] with permission from British Medical Journal.)

did not involve the liver [58]. The clinical value of GGT lies in its use in conferring organ specificity to an elevated value of alkaline phosphatase, because GGT activity is not elevated in patients with bone disease.

Leucine aminopeptidase

Leucine aminopeptidase, a proteolytic enzyme, hydrolyzes tissue amino acids from the N-terminal of proteins and polypeptides. It is most active when leucine is the N-terminal residue – hence, its name. Leucine aminopeptidase is found in all human tissues assayed; it has high activity in the liver, where it is primarily localized in the biliary epithelium. The function of this enzyme is not known, although it possibly involves hydrolysis of a peptide bond near an L-leucine residue, or the transfer of L-leucine from one peptide to another. The leucine aminopeptidase of normal serum, as a rule, is electrophoretically homogenous and probably originates in the liver. In hepatobiliary disease, several peaks of activity are detected, and they probably represent isoenzymes.

The prevalent method for measuring serum leucine aminopeptidase involves α-leucyl-β-naphthylamine hydrochloride as a substrate; the liberated β-naphthylamine is assayed colorimetrically. Some evidence exists that the peptidase responsible for this reaction differs from the peptidases that hydrolyze other leucine compounds. Accordingly, in extrapolating data from one study to another, one should carefully consider the substrate used. Normal values when α-leucyl-β-naphthylamine is used usually range from 50 to 220 IU/L without a significant difference due to sex, age (18–75 years), or fed state.

Elevation in the leucine aminopeptidase level, like that of 5′-nucleotidase and to a lesser degree GGT, appears to be specific for liver disorders. The level of leucine aminopeptidase is not elevated in patients with bone disease [59], and enzyme values in children, although based on a small number of determinations, are comparable with those of adults. The only condition other than hepatobiliary disease known to result in an increase in this enzyme is pregnancy [59]. The level of serum leucine aminopeptidase progressively increases during gestation and reaches a peak at term. After delivery, the enzyme level falls, decreasing approximately 35% in 4 days. Electrophoresis of serum leucine aminopeptidase from pregnant women and from individuals with liver disease shows much overlap among the isoenzymes. This procedure is probably of no practical value in differentiating these two sources of the enzyme.

Serum leucine aminopeptidase testing is as sensitive as the measurement of alkaline phosphatase and 5′-nucleotidase in the detection of obstructive, infiltrative, or space-occupying lesions of the liver. Some investigators consider leucine aminopeptidase to be a more sensitive indicator of infiltrative diseases, rather than alkaline phosphatase, in nonjaundiced patients [59]. Contrary to the findings described in the original reports, pancreatic cancer without hepatobiliary disease does not cause an elevation in the level of serum leucine aminopeptidase.

Leucine aminopeptidase activity is elevated in most types of liver disease, but values are highest in biliary obstruction. Some investigators have promulgated it as a reliable test for differentiating obstructive and hepatocellular liver disease [56]. Others have observed a considerable overlap in values among patient groups, and found serum alkaline phosphatase to be at least as selective. The controversy regarding the specificity of measurement of leucine aminopeptidase as a test of biliary obstruction has never been resolved. Because of the availability of other equally sensitive, convenient, and specific tests, leucine aminopeptidase is not widely used. Its possible value is

its specificity only for liver disease. In this regard, 5′-nucleotidase and GGT seem to have comparable merit.

Tests of the liver's biosynthetic capacity

Serum contains a complex mixture of proteins that have been extensively studied with various techniques. A schematic representation of the results of some of these methods is shown in Fig. 2.6. The liver is the main source of most of these serum proteins. The parenchymal cells are responsible for the synthesis of albumin, fibrinogen, and other coagulation factors, and most of the α- and β-globulins. γ-Globulins are an important exception, being synthesized by B lymphocytes [60].

In this section, we only discuss proteins used in the diagnosis of liver disease: albumin and coagulation factors, which are synthesized exclusively by hepatocytes. Additional diagnostic proteins include lipoproteins, ceruloplasmin (the blue copper-containing protein), ferritin, and α₁-antitrypsin.

Albumin

Albumin, which is quantitatively the most important plasma protein, is synthesized exclusively by the liver. Normal serum values range from 3.5 to 4.5 g/dL (35–45 g/L). The average adult has approximately 300–500 g of albumin distributed in body fluids, and synthesizes approximately 15 g/day (200 mg/kg/day). The synthesis rate may double in conditions in which rapid albumin loss or a decrease in serum albumin concentration occurs because of dilution, such as during the rapid accumulation of ascitic fluid [61]. Albumin has a long half-life, about 20 days. Approximately 4% is degraded each day, but little is known about the site of degradation. The serum level at any time reflects the rate of synthesis and degradation, and the volume of distribution. Albumin synthesis is regulated by changes in nutritional status, osmotic pressure, systemic inflammation, and hormone levels [61,62]. The precise mechanism is not entirely known, but appears to be related to the formation of albumin mRNA polysomes within the liver [62]. Substances that stimulate albumin synthesis cause individual ribosomes to bind to the albumin mRNA to form polysomes, which synthesize albumin more efficiently [62]. Amino acids such as tryptophan, phenylalanine, glutamine, and lysine function in this way and increase albumin synthesis in vitro [62]. Albumin synthesis is also stimulated by the amino acids that increase urea synthesis, that is, ornithine and arginine [63]. Ornithine serves as a precursor of the polyamine spermine, a compound that promotes polysome formation [63]. Corticosteroids and thyroid hormone stimulate albumin synthesis by increasing the concentration of albumin mRNA and transfer RNA in

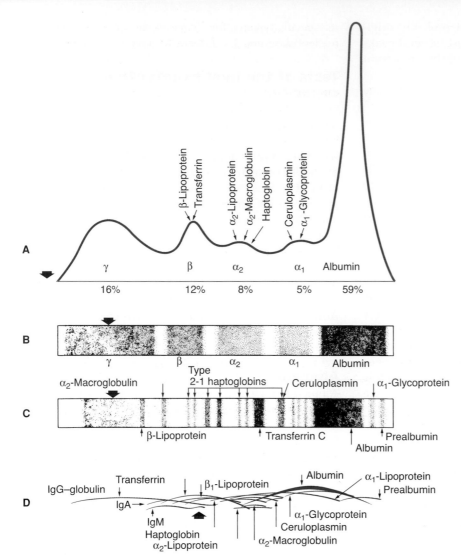

Figure 2.6 Schematic representation of the electrophoretic pattern of normal human serum in pH 8.6 buffer obtained with four methods: (A) tiselius or free boundary electrophoresis; (B) paper electrophoresis; (C) starch-gel electrophoresis; and (D) immunoelectrophoresis. The arrow indicates the starting point with each method. α_2-Macroglobulin remains at the origin in starch-gel electrophoresis, but moves in the γ- to β-range with other methods. Ig, immunoglobulin. (Reproduced from Putnam [107] with permission from Elsevier.)

hepatocytes either by increasing its synthesis or decreasing its degradation [64]. In vitro, alcohol decreases albumin synthesis by inhibiting the formation of polysomes [62], whereas inflammation decreases albumin synthesis [65] through the inhibitory effects of interleukin 1 and tumor necrosis factor [66].

Serum albumin levels tend to be normal in patients with liver disease such as acute viral hepatitis, drug-related hepatoxicity, and obstructive jaundice. Albumin levels of less than 3 g/dL associated with hepatitis should raise the suspicion of chronic hepatitis. Hypoalbuminemia is more common among individuals with chronic liver disorders, such as cirrhosis, and usually reflects severe liver damage and decreased albumin synthesis. One exception is patients with ascites, in whom synthesis may be normal or even increased, but serum levels are low because of the increased volume of distribution [61]. Heavy alcohol ingestion, chronic inflammation, and pro-

tein malnutrition can inhibit albumin synthesis. Hypoalbuminemia is not specific for liver disease and may occur in protein malnutrition of any cause, such as protein-losing enteropathy, chronic infection, or nephrotic syndrome. Serum albumin should not be measured when screening patients with no suspicion of liver disease. A study of patients consecutively examined in a general medical clinic, showed that in 56 of 449 patients in whom no indications for albumin measurement were present, the results were abnormal. However, in only two patients (0.4%) was the finding of any clinical significance [67].

Prothrombin time

Clotting is the end result of a complex series of enzymatic reactions that involve at least 13 factors. The liver is the major site of synthesis of 11 blood coagulation proteins:
- Factor I: fibrinogen [68].
- Factor II: prothrombin [69].

- Factor V: proaccelerin and labile factor [69].
- Factor VII: serum prothrombin conversion accelerator and stable factor [69].
- Factor IX: plasma thromboplastin component and Christmas factor [69].
- Factor X: Stuart–Prower factor [68].
- Factors XII and XIII: prekallikrein and high molecular weight kininogen.

Tissue factor (factor III) is present in subendothelial tissue, platelets, and leukocytes. Factor VIII is made in endothelial cells and the sinusoidal cells within the liver. The liver is involved in clearing some of the clotting factors from serum. The levels of components of the clotting mechanism are frequently abnormal in the course of hepatic disease [70]. These abnormalities can be assessed with tests in which one factor or the interplay of a number of factors is measured. The one-stage prothrombin time of Quick is one of the most useful tests available. It is used to measure the rate at which prothrombin is converted to thrombin. This occurs in the presence of a tissue extract (thromboplastin), calcium ions, and a series of activated coagulation factors (factors I, II, V, VII, and X), and is followed by the polymerization of fibrinogen to fibrin by thrombin (Fig. 2.7). The results may be expressed in seconds or as a ratio of the plasma prothrombin time to a control plasma time. A normal control is usually in the range of 9 to 11 seconds. A prolongation of 2 seconds or more is considered abnormal, and values of more than 4 seconds indicate a patient at risk of uncontrolled bleeding. The prothrombin time is prolonged if any of the involved factors are deficient, either singly, or in combination.

The INR is often used to express the degree of anticoagulation in patients receiving warfarin sodium (Coumadin®). The INR standardizes prothrombin time measurement according to the characteristics of the thromboplastin reagent used in the laboratory. The INR may not be the best expression of coagulation derange-ment in patients with liver failure, unless the same thromboplastin reagent is consistently used for measurement.

Hepatic synthesis of biologically active forms of factors II, VII, IX, and X requires vitamin K for the γ-carboxylation of glutamic acid residues in these proteins. The γ-carboxylation step is a post-translational process that allows these proteins to bind Ca^{2+} avidly, a necessity for them to function as clotting factors [71]. The absence of vitamin K, the ingestion of vitamin K antagonists, or the presence of certain hepatic disorders (hepatocellular carcinoma) inhibits vitamin K-dependent carboxylation and allows the release of des-γ-carboxy (abnormal) prothrombin into serum [71]. This can be detected with a specific radioimmunoassay [72]. Healthy individuals have no des-γ-carboxy prothrombin in serum. Plasma levels of des-γ-carboxy prothrombin do not correlate with α-fetoprotein levels in patients with established hepatocellular carcinoma, but the two tests have a combined sensitivity of 85% [73]. The des-γ-carboxy prothrombin level can return to normal with excision of, or therapy for, hepatocellular carcinoma, and will increase again with a recurrence of the tumor [74]. However, elevated des-γ-carboxy prothrombin levels were detected only in 20% of hepatocellular carcinomas less than 3 cm in diameter; therefore, the measurement of this substance is not a satisfactory screening test [75].

A prolonged prothrombin time is not specific for liver disease and is seen in various congenital deficiencies of coagulation factors and in acquired conditions, including the consumption of clotting factors and ingestion of drugs that affect the prothrombin complex. In these instances, the underlying cause can usually be elucidated. When the aforementioned conditions are excluded, a prolonged prothrombin time may be the consequence of either hypovitaminosis K – as is found in patients with prolonged obstructive jaundice, steatorrhea, dietary deficiency, or an intake of antibiotics that alter the intestinal flora – or poor utilization of vitamin K owing to parenchymal liver disease. These two situations can usually be differentiated by means of parenteral administration of vitamin K_1. If the prothrombin time returns to normal or improves at least 30% within 24 hours of a single parenteral injection of vitamin K_1 (doses of 5–10 mg are usually given), it can be surmised that parenchymal function is good and that hypovitaminosis K was responsible for the original prothrombin time. In contrast, slight (if any) improvement occurs in most patients with parenchymal liver disease. Most patients with extrahepatic obstruction respond promptly to vitamin K. In patients with jaundice, the type of response to vitamin K_1 is therefore of some value in differential diagnosis. Observations of sluggish responses to vitamin K_1 – prolonged values are still recorded 24 hours before normalization at 48–72 hours in some patients with obstructive jaundice – and of good

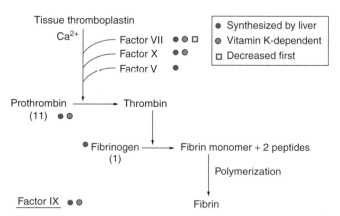

Figure 2.7 Factors involved in the Quick one-stage prothrombin time test.

responses among some patients with hepatocellular disease have been reported and complicate interpretation.

The prothrombin test is not a sensitive index of chronic liver disease because, even in severe cirrhosis, prothrombin levels can be normal or the prothrombin time only slightly prolonged. On the other hand, the test has high prognostic value, particularly for patients with acute hepatocellular disease. Prolongation of the prothrombin time to more than 5–6 seconds above the control value is the single laboratory test that draws attention to the possible development of acute liver failure in the course of acute viral hepatitis. Such a prolonged prothrombin time often precedes by days the manifestations of liver failure. Not all patients with abnormal prothrombin times of this extent have evidence of acute liver failure. Progressive shortening of the prothrombin time to normal usually precedes or accompanies other evidence of clinical improvement in the latter group. The degree of prolongation of the prothrombin time is a prognostic factor for patients with alcoholic steatonecrosis. A prothrombin time greater than 4 seconds above the control value occurred six times as often in a group of patients who died (60%) than in a group who survived (10%). In patients with hepatocellular disease, an abnormal prothrombin time, particularly one prolonged by more than 4–5 seconds that does not respond to parenteral administration of vitamin K_1, indicates extensive parenchymal damage and a poor long-term prognosis. The test is also used as an early predictor of outcome after acetaminophen overdose.

The prothrombin test is particularly important in the treatment of patients with liver disease. It allows assessment of the tendency to bleed before any contemplated surgical or diagnostic procedure, such as closed liver biopsy, splenic puncture, or transhepatic cholangiography. When the prothrombin time is prolonged, vitamin K_1 should be administered routinely in doses of 5–10 mg/day parenterally in up to three doses. It is difficult to identify the prothrombin time at which diagnostic procedures such as a needle biopsy of the liver are contraindicated, because the risk of bleeding has not been well correlated with the values of this test. Furthermore, vascular reactivity and coagulation factors, such as platelets, play an important contributory role. The prothrombin time can often be corrected by infusions of fresh frozen plasma in those situations in which surgery or procedures are required.

Tests of the liver's capacity to transport organic anions and to metabolize organic compounds

Bilirubin

See also Chapter 8.

Bilirubin metabolism

Bilirubin is a tetrapyrrole pigment derived from the breakdown of ferroprotoporphyrin IX (heme), an integral part of heme-containing proteins. Approximately 70–80% of the 250–300 mg of bilirubin produced each day is derived from the breakdown of hemoglobin in senescent red blood cells [76]. The remainder comes from prematurely destroyed erythroid cells in bone marrow and from the turnover of hemoproteins in tissues throughout the body [77]. The liver is the main source of the latter because of its high concentration of hemoproteins with relatively high turnover rates, such as cytochrome P_{450}. The initial steps leading to the formation of bilirubin occur in reticuloendothelial cells, primarily in the spleen and liver. The first reaction, catalyzed by the microsomal enzyme heme oxygenase, oxidatively cleaves the α-bridge of the porphyrin group, opens the heme ring, and produces equimolar amounts of biliverdin and carbon monoxide (Fig. 2.8) [78]. The second reaction, catalyzed by the cytosolic enzyme biliverdin reductase, reduces the central methylene bridge of biliverdin, converting it to bilirubin [79]. Bilirubin formed in the reticuloendothelial cells is lipid-soluble and almost insoluble in water. To be transported in blood, it must be solubilized, which is accomplished by reversible, noncovalent binding to albumin. Bilirubin is then transported to the liver, where it, but not the albumin, is taken up by hepatocytes in a process that involves carrier-mediated membrane transport (Fig. 2.9) [80]. Although several potential transporters have been identified, none has yet been cloned. In the hepatocyte, bilirubin is coupled to glutathione-*S*-transferases

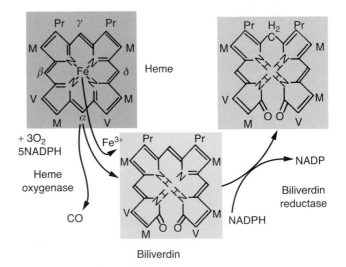

Figure 2.8 Formation of bilirubin from heme by the sequential actions of the enzymes heme oxygenase and biliverdin reductase. CO, carbon monoxide; M, methyl; NADP, nicotine adenine dinucleotide phosphate; NADPH, reduced form of nicotine adenine dinucleotide; Pr, propionic acid side chains; V, vinyl. (Adapted from Ostrow [108] with permission from American Gastroenterological Association.)

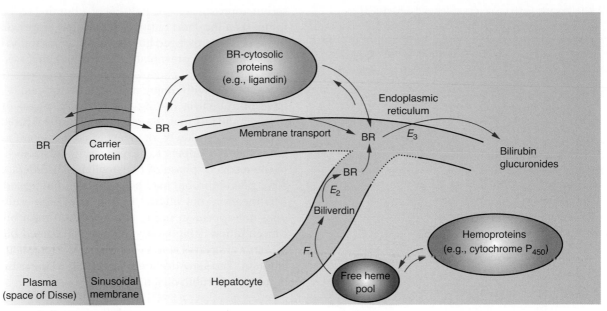

Figure 2.9 Scheme of bilirubin uptake, hepatocellular transport, and metabolism. Exogenous bilirubin is taken up by the hepatocyte at the sinusoidal membrane by an unidentified carrier protein (as depicted) or by transmembrane "flip-flop." The bilirubin is delivered to the endoplasmic reticulum by means of membrane–membrane transfer, with cytosolic-binding proteins serving as a potential means to preclude the diffusion of bilirubin back to the plasma. Heme generated within the liver from endogenous hemoproteins also gives rise to bilirubin. Glucuronidation occurs primarily within the endoplasmic reticulum. BR, bilirubin; E_1, heme oxygenase; E_2, biliverdin reductase; E_3, bilirubin uridine diphosphate glucuronosyltransferase 1. (Reproduced from Crawford et al. [109] with permission from Thieme.)

(formerly called ligandins). Bilirubin is then solubilized by means of conjugation to glucuronic acid; bilirubin monoglucuronide and diglucuronide are formed, both of which are called *direct-acting bilirubins*. The conjugation of glucuronic acid to bilirubin is catalyzed by an enzyme system in the endoplasmic reticulum of the hepatocyte that transfers glucuronic acid from uridine diphosphate–glucuronic acid to the acyl groups of the propionic acid side chains of bilirubin. The bilirubin conjugates are then actively transported from the hepatocyte into canalicular bile by an adenosine triphosphate-dependent transport process that is the rate-limiting step in hepatic bilirubin excretion. This process is mediated by a protein in the bile canalicular membrane called *multidrug resistance-associated protein 2*. The conjugated bilirubins drain from the bile duct into the duodenum and are carried distally through the intestine. In the distal ileum and colon, the conjugated bilirubins are hydrolyzed to unconjugated bilirubin by bacterial β-glucuronidases. The unconjugated bilirubin is reduced by normal intestinal bacteria to form a group of colorless tetrapyrroles called *urobilinogens*. Approximately 80–90% of these products are excreted in feces, either unchanged or oxidized to orange derivatives called *urobilins*. The remaining 10–20% of the urobilinogens are passively absorbed, enter the portal-venous blood, and are reexcreted by the liver. A small fraction, usually less than 3 mg/dL, escapes hepatic uptake, filters across the renal glomerulus, and is excreted in urine. The renal excretion of urobilinogen is complicated, partly because urobilinogen is a weak acid that passively diffuses across the renal tubule when in its undissociated form. The appearance of urobilinogen in urine depends on many factors, including urine pH and the rate of urine flow.

Measurement of serum bilirubin

The terms direct- and indirect-reacting bilirubin are based on the original van den Bergh method of measuring unconjugated bilirubin [81]. This method is still used in some clinical chemistry laboratories to determine the serum bilirubin level. In this assay, bilirubin reacts with diazotized sulfanilic acid and splits into two relatively stable dipyrryl azopigments that absorb light maximally at 540 nm. The direct fraction is that which reacts with diazotized sulfanilic acid in 1 minute in the absence of alcohol [81]. This fraction provides an approximate determination of the amount of conjugated bilirubin in serum. The total serum bilirubin level is the amount that reacts in 30 minutes after the addition of alcohol. The indirect fraction is the difference between the total and the direct bilirubin levels, and provides an estimate of the amount of unconjugated bilirubin in serum. With the van den Bergh method, the normal serum bilirubin concentration is usually less than 1 mg/dL (18 mmol/L). As much as 30% or 0.3 mg/dL (5.1 mmol/L) of the total is direct-reacting bilirubin [81]. Total serum bilirubin

Table 2.4 Differences between unconjugated and conjugated bile pigments.

Property	Unconjugated bilirubin	Conjugated bilirubin
van den Bergh reaction	Indirect (+ alcohol)	Direct
Water-soluble	−	+
Fat-soluble	+	−
Attachment to plasma albumin	+	+
Presence in icteric urine	−	+
Presence in bile	−[a]	+
Affinity for brain tissue	+	−
Association with hemolytic jaundice	++	±
Association with obstructive and hepatocellular jaundice	+	+++

[a]A small quantity of unconjugated bilirubin may be present in the common duct bile. There is a relative increase in unconjugated bilirubin in bile in conditions associated with severe unconjugated hyperbilirubinemia, such as Crigler–Najjar syndrome [7].

+, present or positive; −, absent or negative; ±, present or absent; ++, strong; +++, very strong.

concentrations are between 0.2 and 0.9 mg/dL (2.0–15.4 mmol/L) in 95% of a healthy population, and less than 1 mg/dL (18 mmol/L) in 99% [81]. Some differences in the properties of unconjugated and conjugated bilirubin are listed in Table 2.4.

Newer techniques for measuring serum bilirubin using high-performance liquid chromatography (HPLC) have contributed considerably to our understanding of bilirubin metabolism. First, they show that almost 100% of the serum bilirubin in healthy individuals, or those with Gilbert syndrome, is unconjugated, and less than 3% is monoconjugated bilirubin. Second, in patients with jaundice and hepatobiliary disease, the total serum bilirubin concentration measured with these newer, more accurate methods is lower than the values found with diazo methods [82]. This suggests that diazo-positive compounds distinct from bilirubin exist in the serum of patients with hepatobiliary disease. Third, the results of these studies indicate that in patients with jaundice and hepatobiliary disease, monoglucuronides of bilirubin predominate over the diglucuronides. Fourth, part of the direct-reacting bilirubin fraction includes conjugated bilirubin that is covalently linked to albumin [83]. This albumin-linked bilirubin fraction represents an important fraction of total serum bilirubin in patients with cholestasis and hepatobiliary disorders [83]. Albumin-bound bilirubin is formed in serum when hepatic excretion of bilirubin glucuronides is impaired, and the glucuronides are present in serum in increasing amounts. Because of its tight binding to albumin, the clearance rate of albumin-bound bilirubin from

serum approximates the half-life of albumin (12–14 days) rather than the short half-life of bilirubin (approximately 4 hours). The prolonged half-life of albumin-bound bilirubin explains two previously unexplained enigmas in the care of jaundiced patients with liver disease: (i) that some patients with conjugated hyperbilirubinemia do not have bilirubinuria during the recovery phase of their disease; and (ii) that the elevated serum bilirubin level declines more slowly than expected in some patients who otherwise appear to be recovering satisfactorily. Late in the recovery phase of hepatobiliary disorders, all the conjugated bilirubin may be in the albumin-linked form. It is therefore not filtered by the renal glomerulus and does not appear in urine, although the serum bilirubin concentration is high. The value of conjugated bilirubin in serum decreases slowly because of the long half-life of albumin. The slow decline is unrelated to the actual rate of hepatic bilirubin metabolism.

Diagnostic value of serum bilirubin

The bilirubin normally present in serum represents a balance between the input from production and the hepatic removal of the pigment. Hyperbilirubinemia may therefore result from: (i) overproduction of bilirubin; (ii) impaired uptake, conjugation, or excretion of bilirubin; or (iii) regurgitation of unconjugated or conjugated bilirubin from damaged hepatocytes or bile ducts. One may anticipate that an increase in unconjugated bilirubin in serum results from overproduction or from impairment of uptake or conjugation, whereas an increase in the conjugated moiety is caused by decreased excretion or backward leakage of the pigment.

The total serum bilirubin level is not a sensitive indicator of hepatic dysfunction and may not reflect accurately the degree of liver injury. Hyperbilirubinemia may not be detected in instances of moderate to severe hepatic parenchymal damage or a partially or briefly obstructed common bile duct. This lack of sensitivity is partly explained by observations obtained in healthy persons given infusions of unconjugated bilirubin and in patients with uncomplicated hemolysis. These observations suggest that the capacity of the human liver to remove bilirubin from serum before hyperbilirubinemia occurs is at least two-fold greater than the daily pigment load (250–300 mg or 4,275–5,130 mmol) normally presented to this organ. This capacity may be even higher, according to the maximal rate of excretion of bilirubin into bile – approximately 55.2 mg/kg/day [84] – and the average amount of bilirubin formed from the destruction of senescent red blood cells, 3.9 mg/kg/day. In the steady state, the serum bilirubin concentration usually reflects the intensity of jaundice and the increase in total-body bile pigment. The serum bilirubin concentration may occasionally decrease transiently with the presence in serum of substances such as salicylates, sulfonamides, or free fatty acids, which displace bilirubin from its attachment to plasma albumin and enhance the transfer of the pigment into the tissues [85]. Conversely, an increase in serum albumin concentration may induce a temporary shift of bilirubin from tissue sites into the circulation.

Total serum bilirubin concentration is seldom of value in specifying the cause of jaundice in individual patients because values among the various types of jaundice overlap considerably. On the average, uncomplicated hemolysis seldom causes a serum bilirubin value in excess of 5 mg/dL (85.5 mmol/L), and parenchymal liver disease or incomplete extrahepatic obstruction due to biliary calculi gives lower serum bilirubin values than those that occur with malignant obstruction of the common bile duct.

Few controlled studies have critically assessed the prognostic value of magnitude and duration of hyperbilirubinemia in liver disease. In general, the higher the serum bilirubin concentration in viral hepatitis, the greater the histologic evidence of hepatocellular damage and the longer the course of disease. Nevertheless, patients may die of acute liver failure with only a modest elevation in serum bilirubin level. The presence of concomitant hemolysis with overproduction of bilirubin and diminished glomerular filtration rate causing decreased excretion of the pigment may also confuse the issue by causing higher serum bilirubin values than would be expected for any degree of hepatocellular damage present. In acute alcoholic hepatitis, hyperbilirubinemia in excess of 5 mg/dL (85.5 mmol/L) is one of the findings that suggests a poor prognosis [86].

The major value of fractionating total serum bilirubin into unconjugated and direct-reacting moieties is in the detection of states characterized by unconjugated hyperbilirubinemia (Table 2.5). Such a diagnosis appears warranted when the serum level of indirect-reacting bilirubin is in excess of 1.2 mg/dL (20.5 mmol/L) and the direct-reacting fraction constitutes less than 20% of the total serum bilirubin value. Unfortunately, when the total serum bilirubin concentration is minimally elevated, it may be difficult to differentiate the cause of the bilirubin elevation. This difficulty reflects the inaccuracy of the diazo methods in differentiating conjugated from unconjugated bilirubin at low total serum bilirubin concentrations. This is one of the instances in which the newer, more precise methods of bilirubin determination may provide clinically useful information that is not attainable with the older diazo methods. This is particularly true in the detection of early or mild liver injury. Total bilirubin concentration may be normal in some patients with cirrhosis, hepatitis, hemochromatosis, congestive heart failure, and other disorders. An increase in the direct fraction above 0.3 mg/dL (5.1 mmol/L) should alert one to the

Table 2.5 Causes of unconjugated hyperbilirubinemia.

Cause	Mechanism
Hemolytic disorders	
Inherited: spherocytosis, elliptocytosis, glucose-6-phosphate dehydrogenase deficiency, sickle cell anemia	Overproduction of bilirubin
Acquired: microangiopathic hemolytic anemias, paroxysmal nocturnal hemoglobinuria, immune hemolysis	Overproduction of bilirubin
Ineffective erythropoiesis	
Cobalamin, folate and severe iron deficiencies, thalassemia	Overproduction of bilirubin
Drugs	
Rifampicin, probenecid	Impaired hepatic uptake
Inherited conditions	
Gilbert syndrome	Impaired conjugation
Crigler–Najjar, types I and II	Impaired conjugation
Neonates	
Neonatal (physiologic)	Overproduction of bilirubin, impaired conjugation, increased intestinal absorption
Breast milk	Impaired conjugation and increased intestinal absorption
Other	
Hematoma	Overproduction of bilirubin

possibility of mild liver injury. If the newer, more accurate techniques are used, conjugated bilirubin concentrations greater than 0.1 mg/dL (1.7 mmol/L) should be accurate in the detection of early liver injury, because bilirubin glucuronides are normally undetectable in serum, except in hepatobiliary disorders [82].

The measurement and fractionation of serum bilirubin concentration in patients with jaundice does not differentiate accurately parenchymal (hepatocellular) from cholestatic (obstructive) jaundice. The accurate HPLC methods for measuring serum bilirubin show that the levels of both unconjugated and conjugated bilirubins are increased in hepatobiliary disease. No consistent pattern of elevation of these fractions differentiates hepatocellular from cholestatic liver disease [82]. Levels of both monoglucuronide and diglucuronide are elevated, with the monoglucuronides predominating.

Urinary bilirubin

The presence of bilirubin in the urine indicates the presence of hepatobiliary disease. Unconjugated bilirubin is tightly bound to albumin, is not filtered by the glomerulus, and is not excreted into the urine. Consequently, only conjugated bilirubin is found in urine. This occurs only when conjugated bilirubin is in the serum, that is, when there is hepatobiliary dysfunction. The new, more precise methods for measuring serum bilirubin indicate that 100% of the serum bilirubin in healthy persons and those with Gilbert syndrome is unconjugated bilirubin. Measurable amounts of conjugated bilirubin in serum are found only in hepatobiliary disease. Because the renal threshold for conjugated bilirubin is low and the laboratory methods used can detect bilirubin concentrations as low as 0.05 mg/dL (0.9 mmol/L) of urine, conjugated bilirubin may be found in urine when the total serum bilirubin value is normal and the patient does not have clinical jaundice. This can occur early in the course of viral hepatitis or other hepatobiliary diseases when conjugated bilirubin first appears in the serum. Conversely, the urine can become free of bilirubin long before the level of conjugated serum bilirubin falls to normal in patients recovering from hepatobiliary diseases [83]. When this occurs, all the conjugated bilirubin is in the albumin-bound form and is not filtered by the glomerulus.

Bile acid tests

Although sensitive tests to measure serum bile acid concentration (see Chapter 9) have been available for more than 25 years, the role for these tests in the evaluation of patients with suspected liver disease remains uncertain. Bile acids are synthesized from cholesterol in hepatocytes, conjugated to glycine or taurine, and then secreted into bile. Serum bile acids are sensitive but nonspecific indicators of hepatic dysfunction. They allow some quantification of functional hepatic reserve.

Serum bile acid tests are most elevated in certain cholestatic liver diseases, such as primary biliary cirrhosis and primary sclerosing cholangitis. Serum bile acid levels are elevated in pregnant women, particularly in those with the pruritus of cholestasis. Serum bile acid levels are normal in patients with Gilbert syndrome and Dubin–Johnson syndrome, an observation that reinforces the separate pathways of transport for bilirubin and bile acids.

The attempt to improve the sensitivity and specificity of the serum bile acid tests with intravenous or oral tolerance tests has not proved successful. The ratio of cholic acid to chenodeoxycholic acid has also been considered a means of increasing the sensitivity and specificity of bile salt testing. Unfortunately, a marked overlap exists, both between the healthy control and various hepatic disease states. Serum bile acid tests offer the advantage of being highly specific indicators of liver dysfunction, but they are less sensitive than they were originally hoped to be and they are nonspecific in differentiating the various types of liver disease.

Clearance tests

Because serum bilirubin is an insensitive indicator of hepatic dysfunction and at low serum levels the measurement of total and direct bilirubin lacks biochemical precision, an effort was made to develop other tests of hepatic excretory capacity that were more sensitive and specific. The goal was to develop tests that could be used for more critical and specific evaluations of the excretory or detoxification capacity of the liver. Although these clearance tests are more sensitive than the serum bilirubin test, they have limited value because of their lack of specificity in diagnosing specific hepatobiliary disorders.

Dye clearance tests using sulfobromophthalein sodium (BSP) are not widely used because the test is difficult to perform and the substrate may be toxic and is no longer available. ICG dye is nontoxic and has a higher hepatic extraction ratio than BSP (70–96%). Ninety-seven percent of an administered dose is excreted unchanged in bile and the liver appears to be the only site of ICG clearance in humans. ICG is used primarily to estimate hepatic blood flow because the first-pass extraction of ICG by the liver is high. The elimination of ICG has been shown to correlate with mortality and morbidity after hepatic resections [87] and in intensive care unit patients [88].

Use of drug metabolism to assess liver function

Measurement of the clearance of drugs by the liver has the potential to provide an accurate method of measuring hepatic function. A number of candidate compounds have been studied in various clinical states, including acute and chronic viral hepatitis, cirrhosis from various causes, and before and after liver transplantation. Most of the compounds that have been studied, including aminopyrine, antipyrine, caffeine, and lidocaine, are metabolized by one or more of the isoenzymes of cytochrome P_{450}. Breath tests using ^{13}C- or ^{14}C-labeled aminopyrine as a way to measure the metabolism of aminopyrine are used infrequently although they have been available for more than 25 years in the United States. There are several reasons for this. They are less convenient to perform than are simple blood tests and the use of ^{13}C or ^{14}C isotopes is cumbersome and expensive.

Lidocaine is an example of a drug that is highly extracted by the liver (high first-pass effect) and oxidized by cytochrome P_{450} 3A/4A [89]. After intravenous administration, clearance of lidocaine is therefore a good measure of hepatic blood flow in healthy individuals. However, in patients with advanced liver disease, the compound is not highly extracted, most likely because of portal-venous shunting and changes in the intrinsic activity of the P_{450} drug-metabolizing enzymes in the liver. Measurement of the appearance of metabolites of lidocaine (monoethylglycinxylidide or MEGX) in plasma has been used as a measure of hepatic function in patients with more advanced liver diseases, but the clearance of lidocaine can be altered by drugs that inhibit the specific isoenzymes of P_{450}. The MEGX test has been evaluated in a number of clinical situations: before and after liver transplantation [90], in patients with chronic hepatitis C with or without cirrhosis [91], and after prolonged treatment with pegylated interferon [92]. It has been shown to correlate well with histology but it is unclear whether it offers significant advantages over the model for end-stage liver disease (MELD) test [93]. The test requires HPLC, enzyme-linked immunosorbent assay (ELISA), or other methods of measuring MEGX.

Caffeine clearance and morning salivary caffeine levels

Caffeine clearance tests have been used to quantify functional hepatic capacity by asssessing the activity of cytochrome P_{450} 1A2, N-acetyltransferase, and xanthine oxidase [94]. Several variations in these tests have been described. In all studies, caffeine (200–366 mg) is taken orally. Early studies required that plasma caffeine concentrations be measured at multiple time points over 24 hours. In more recent studies, caffeine and its metabolites have been measured in 24-hour urine collections, in saliva, and in scalp hair. Results with these alternative methods are similar to those of the plasma clearance method. Overnight salivary caffeine clearance has been shown to correlate with ICG and galactose clearance and the aminopyrine breath test [95]. The measurement of a single level of caffeine in saliva in the morning after overnight abstinence was shown to correlate well with salivary caffeine clearance and is considerably easier to obtain [96]. Concomitant tobacco use is a confounding factor in these tests because it increases caffeine clearance [97]. The results of caffeine clearance tests correlate well with the ^{14}C aminopyrine test.

Tests used to detect fibrosis in the liver

Liver biopsy remains the standard for grading (inflammation) and staging (fibrosis) the severity of chronic liver disease. There is considerable interest in identifying biochemical markers that can be used as noninvasive surrogate markers for both liver fibrosis and inflammation to permit longitudinal assessment of disease progression as well as measuring responses to therapy. Thus far, no single biochemical test or marker has been identified as a perfect marker for fibrosis. A number of biochemical markers including hyaluronan, type IV collagen, procol-

lagen III, and laminin have been studied. As discussed in Chapter 12 these tests are surrogates, not true biomarkers of fibrosis and their value is limited since they reflect the rate of matrix turnover rather than the deposition of matrix proteins. Multiparameter tests have also been examined; these include the well-studied FibroTest®, a multiparameter test that includes haptoglobin, bilirubin, GGT, apolipoprotein A-I, and α_2-macroglobulin [98]. Another multiparameter test is the ELF test that utilizes a diagnostic algorithm [99].

Tests used to detect chronic inflammation or fibrosis in the liver or altered immunoregulation

Immunoglobulins

Serum immunoglobulins are produced by stimulated B lymphocytes, and elevated levels in many patients with chronic liver disease are believed to indicate the impaired function of reticuloendothelial cells in hepatic sinusoids or shunting of portal-venous blood around the liver [100]. Antibodies directed against antigens of the normal colonic flora account for much of the increased serum immunoglobulin levels in patients with cirrhosis [100]. Because of portosystemic shunting, these antigens escape degradation by hepatic reticuloendothelial cells and reach lymphoid tissue outside the liver where they elicit an inflammatory response.

In most cases of acute hepatitis, immunoglobulin levels are normal or minimally increased. Mild to moderate hypergammaglobulinemia is present in many patients with chronic viral hepatitis or cirrhosis, while a striking increase in serum IgG suggests autoimmune hepatitis [101]. Diffuse polyclonal increases in IgG and IgM in most types of cirrhosis are nonspecific [101]. Increases in IgM levels suggest primary biliary cirrhosis, whereas increases in IgA may occur in patients with alcoholic cirrhosis or alcoholic hepatitis. Immunoglobulin levels are usually normal in patients with obstructive jaundice. Serial determination of serum IgG levels is useful in monitoring the response to immunosuppressive therapy in patients with autoimmune hepatitis. Hypergammaglobulinemia, with or without hypoalbuminemia, is not specific for liver disease and can be found in malignancy and chronic inflammatory diseases, particularly human immunodeficiency virus (HIV) infection.

Use of liver function tests

We have found it useful to order the tests listed in Table 2.6 during the initial encounter with a patient with jaundice or suspected liver disease. The use of these

Table 2.6 Liver function test patterns in hepatobiliary disorders and jaundice.

Type of disorder	Bilirubin	Aminotransferases	Alkaline phosphatase	Albumin	Globulin	Prothrombin time
Hemolysis	Normal	Normal	Normal	Normal	Normal	Normal
Gilbert syndrome	5 mg/dL; >85% due to indirect fraction No bilirubinuria	Normal	Normal	Normal	Normal	Normal
Acute hepatocellular necrosis (viral and drug hepatitis, hepatotoxins, acute heart failure)	Both fractions may be elevated; peak usually follows aminotransferases Bilirubinuria	Elevated, often >500 IU/L; ALT ≥ AST	Normal to three times normal	Normal	Normal	Usually normal; >5 seconds above control and not corrected with parenteral vitamin K suggests massive necrosis and poor prognosis
Chronic hepatocellular disorders	Both fractions may be elevated	Elevated, but usually <400 IU/L	Normal to three times normal	Often decreased	Increased γ-globulin	Often prolonged; is not corrected with parenteral vitamin K
Alcoholic hepatitis or cirrhosis	Bilirubinuria	AST : ALT >2 suggests alcoholic hepatitis or cirrhosis	—	—	—	—
Intrahepatic cholestasis	Both fractions may be elevated	Normal to moderate elevations; rarely >500 IU/L	Elevated, often over four times normal	Normal, unless chronic	γ-Globulin normal	Normal; if prolonged, is corrected with parenteral vitamin K
Obstructive jaundice	Bilirubinuria	Normal to moderate elevations; rarely >500 IU/L	Elevated, often over four times normal	Normal, unless chronic	β-Globulin may be increased	Normal; if prolonged, is corrected with parenteral vitamin K
Infiltrative diseases (tumor, granuloma)	Usually normal	Normal to slightly elevated	Elevated, often over four times normal	Normal	Usually normal; γ-globulin may be increased in granulomatous disease	Normal
Partial bile duct obstruction	—	—	Fractionate, or confirm liver origin with 5'-nucleotidase or γ-glutamyl transpeptidase	—	—	—

ALT, alanine aminotransferase; AST, aspartate aminotransferase.
From Kaplan [103] with permission from Elsevier.

tests, which include total and direct bilirubin, aminotransferases, alkaline phosphatase, albumin, globulin, and prothrombin time, as a battery improves accuracy in the diagnosis of liver disease and makes it unlikely that any case of clinically important liver disease will not be identified.

It is helpful to divide the causes of jaundice and liver dysfunction into the broad categories shown in Table 2.6, that is, disorders of bilirubin metabolism, acute parenchymal or hepatocellular disease, cholestasis, infiltrative diseases, chronic hepatocellular diseases such as cirrhosis, and others. Because the pattern of abnormalities may be similar in patients with infiltrative diseases and patients with partial bile duct obstruction, these two types of disorders are listed together.

Patients with hemolysis or Gilbert syndrome may have a total serum bilirubin level as high as 5 mg/dL (85.5 mmol/L). Bilirubinuria is absent and more than 85% of the bilirubin is in the indirect fraction using the van den Bergh reaction. Results of the remaining liver chemistry tests, listed in Table 2.6, are normal. An elevated reticulocyte count and/or a low serum haptoglobin level suggests hemolysis. If bilirubinuria is present and more than 20% of the elevation in bilirubin is in the direct-reacting fraction of bilirubin, Dubin–Johnson syndrome and Rotor syndrome should be considered. Serum bile acids levels are normal in Dubin–Johnson syndrome. Both Dubin–Johnson syndrome and Rotor syndrome are benign conditions that require no further investigation.

The serum aminotransferase levels are the most sensitive tests for detecting acute hepatocellular disorders, such as viral or drug-induced hepatitis. Aminotransferase levels greater than 500 IU/L (8.3 μkat/L) make such a diagnosis probable. Depending on the severity of the underlying hepatocellular disorder, the bilirubin level may be normal or elevated. If the bilirubin level is elevated, both the direct and the indirect bilirubin fractions will be elevated and bilirubinuria should be present. Alkaline phosphatase elevations as high as three times the upper limit of normal are common for patients with acute hepatocellular disorders; however, values greater than three times normal are unusual, except in some patients with drug-induced hepatitis. Serum albumin level is usually normal, and globulin levels are normal or minimally elevated. The prothrombin time is typically normal in most patients with viral or drug-induced hepatitis. Prolongation of the prothrombin time to more than 5 seconds above the control value and failure of prothrombin time to correct within 24–48 hours of parenteral administration of vitamin K suggest a poor prognosis. This should alert the clinician to the possibility of impending liver failure. If the liver function tests are typical of acute hepatitis, a careful medication history must be obtained along with serologic tests for viral hepatitis

(see Table 2.1). The possibility of hepatic ischemia should also be considered.

Serial determinations of aminotransferases may prove useful in patients with acute hepatocellular disorders. For example, following acute necrosis due to acetaminophen poisoning, the level of AST will decline more rapidly than ALT assuming the injury does not continue. Based on the relative difference in the plasma half-life of the two enzymes, one would predict that the level of ALT would exceed that of AST within the next 1–2 days. The decline in serum activity follows first-order kinetics (Fig. 2.10). This conceptual explanation can be applied to other acute, short-term injuries to the liver, such as necrosis from other drugs, ischemia, blunt trauma to the liver, and transient injury from passage of common duct stones [102]. Therefore, serial determinations of AST and ALT can provide a clue as to whether an injury to the liver is due to acute necrosis or an ongoing injury, such as inflammation.

Liver enzymes may be highly insensitive in chronic hepatitis or cirrhosis. Patients with advanced postnecrotic or alcoholic cirrhosis may have shrunken livers and striking portal hypertension, yet have liver enzymes that are almost normal. Even those patients with active chronic diseases such as chronic hepatitis B or C, autoimmune hepatitis, alcoholic or NAFLD and hemochromatosis have relatively low levels of AST and ALT (<400 IU/L) (see Table 2.2). An AST : ALT ratio greater than 2 raises the possibility of alcoholic liver disease, and an AST : ALT ratio greater than 3 is highly suggestive of this possibility [17]. Alkaline phosphatase level is seldom helpful in the diagnosis of cirrhosis. While there may be clues – such as thrombocytopenia, an AST : ALT ratio greater than 1, low serum albumin, and prolongation of the prothrombin time – suggesting the presence of cirrhosis, a definitive diagnosis depends on demonstrating significant fibrosis in the liver. Although liver biopsy remains the most reliable test for cirrhosis, FibroTest and ELF may be considered as surrogate indicators in patients in whom there is concern for the presence of cirrhosis.

There is a characteristic pattern of liver function tests in cholestasis, although the routine laboratory tests listed in Table 2.6 do not differentiate intrahepatic and extrahepatic disorders. Alkaline phosphatase level is usually elevated out of proportion to the levels of other enzymes. Values four or more times greater than normal suggest some type of cholestasis. Depending on the severity of the underlying condition, the bilirubin level is either normal or elevated. If elevated, the direct fraction is increased and bilirubinuria is present. Aminotransferase levels are usually elevated, but values greater than 500 IU/L (8.3 μkat/L) are rare. Aminotransferase levels are usually less than 300 IU/L (5 μkat/L), unless the tests are performed within 24 hours of the development of acute bile duct obstruction due, for example, to the

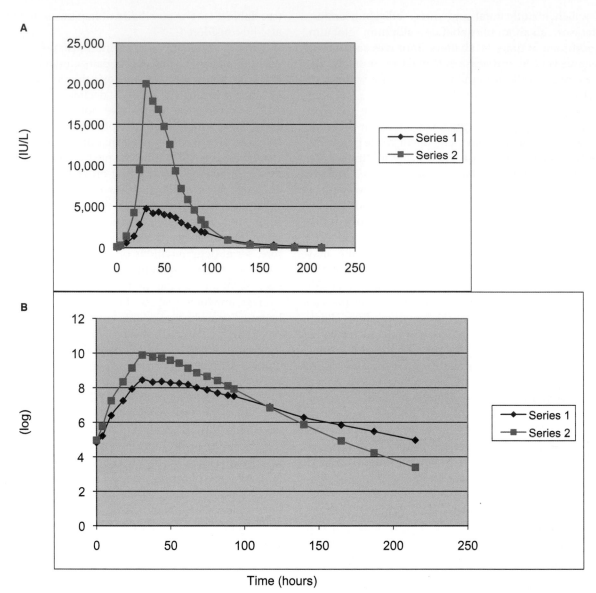

Figure 2.10 Kinetics of aspartate aminotransferase (AST) (pink, series 2) and alanine aminotransferase (ALT) (blue, series 1) following acute hepatic necrosis. AST and ALT are released into serum following acute hepatic necrosis. The level of both AST and ALT will decline over the next few days proportional to the half-life of the enzymes in the serum. The plasma half-life for ALT has been estimated to be 47 ± 10 hours and for AST, 17 ± 5 hours. Initially the AST is greater than the ALT, but 36–72 hours after an episode of acute hepatic necrosis, the ALT will be higher than the AST. (A) AST and ALT levels in IU/mL over time; (B) log AST and log ALT values over time.

passage of a common duct stone [102]. Albumin and globulin levels are usually normal. An increase in serum IgM in a patient with an elevated alkaline phosphatase suggests primary biliary cirrhosis. The antimitochondrial antibody test is helpful in this situation. The result is positive in 90–95% of patients with primary biliary cirrhosis, and is negative in patients with extrahepatic bile duct obstruction or sclerosing cholangitis. The prothrombin time is usually normal. If elevated, it is commonly due to vitamin K deficiency and should correct with parenteral administration of vitamin K.

Infiltrative liver diseases often only produce elevations in the alkaline phosphatase. Minimal elevations in aminotransferases may be observed, but the increase in alkaline phosphatase is much more dramatic. Measurement of 5'-nucleotidase or GGT can be used to confirm the hepatic origin of the alkaline phosphatase. The bilirubin level is almost always normal in infiltrative disease.

In summary, liver enzyme tests are useful in detecting liver disease in asymptomatic individuals and in evaluating patients with jaundice or other clinical evidence of liver disease. The pattern of abnormalities is often helpful in classifying diseases of the liver and suggesting a direction for further evaluation, including serologic testing for hepatitis, genetic markers, ultrasound, computed tomography, magnetic resonance imaging, and percutaneous liver biopsy.

Further reading

Diehl AM, Boitnott J, Van Duyn MA, et al. Relationship between pyridoxal 5′-phosphate deficiency and aminotransferase levels in alcoholic hepatitis. *Gastroenterology* 1984;86:632.

This paper demonstrates that the AST : ALT ratio is greater than 2 : 1 in alcoholic liver disease. The altered ratio is due, in part to a deficiency in pyridoxal phosphate. Addition of pyridoxal 5-phosphate to serum corrected the ratio in vitro.

Kaplan MM, Rhigetti A. Induction of rat liver alkaline phosphatase: the mechanism of the serum elevation in bile duct observation. *J Clin Invest* 1970;49:508.

This paper showed that the mechanism of the elevated serum alkaline phosphatase level in cholestasis is the induction of liver alkaline phosphatase and the leakage of liver alkaline phosphatase in serum. The authors clearly showed that the alternative theory popular at the time – that the liver clears alkaline phosphatase made in other organs from serum and excretes it into bile much as the liver excretes bilirubin – was incorrect. This paper resolved a controversy that had existed in medicine for more than 50 years.

Kim WR, Flamm S, DeBisceglie A, Bodenheimer H Jr. Serum activity of alanine aminotransferase (ALT) as an indicator of health and disease. *Hepatology* 2008;47:1363.

This paper presents the official position of the American Association for the Study of Liver Diseases on the application of serum alanine aminotransferase activity. Issues including the use of ALT as an indicator of liver disease, ALT as an indicator of overall health and mortality, and ALT as a screening test in the population are discussed.

Pratt D, Kaplan M. Evaluation of abnormal liver-enzyme results in asymptomatic patients. *N Engl J Med* 2000;342:1266.

This paper outlines a practical approach to the evaluation of liver enzymes in asymptomatic patients. Information regarding the pattern of liver enzyme abnormalities in various conditions is presented.

Sotil F, Jensen D. Serum enzymes associated with cholestasis. *Clin Liver Dis* 2004;8:41.

This paper discusses the use of alkaline phosphatase, 5′-nucleotidase, and γ-glutamyltranspeptidase in the evaluation of cholestatic liver disorders. The biochemistry of the each enzyme as well as its application in clinical situations is presented.

References

1. Diehl AM, Boitnott J, Van Duyn MA, et al. Relationship between pyridoxal 5′-phosphate deficiency and aminotransferase levels in alcoholic hepatitis. *Gastroenterology* 1984;86:632.
2. Matloff DS, Selinger MJ, Kaplan MM. Hepatic transaminase activity in alcoholic liver disease. *Gastroenterology* 1980;78:1389.
3. Price C, Alberti K. Biochemical assessment of liver function. In: Wright JG, Alberti MM, Karran S, Millward-Sadler GH, eds. *Liver and Biliary Diseases – pathophysiology, diagnosis, management.* London: WB Saunders, 1979:381.
4. Inglesby T, Rai R, Astemborski J, Gruskin L, Nelson K. A prospective, community-based evaluation of liver enzymes in individuals with hepatitis c after drug use. *Hepatology* 1999;29:590.
5. Karmen A, Wroblewksi F, LaDue J. Transaminase activity in human blood. *J Clin Invest* 1955;34:126.
6. Siest G, Schelele F, Marie-Madaleine G, et al. Aspartate aminotransferaser and alanine aminotransferase activities in plasma: statistical distributions, individual variations, and reference values. *Clin Chem* 1975;21:1077.
7. Sherman K. Alanine aminotransferase in clinical practice. *Arch Intern Med* 1991;151:260.
8. Piton A, Poynard T, Imbert-Bismut F, et al. Factors associated with serum alanine transaminase activity in healthy subjects: consequences for the definition of normal values, for selection of blood donors, and for patients with chronic hepatitis C. *Hepatology* 1998;27:1213.
9. Pratti D, Taloli E, Zanella A, et al. Updated definitions of healthy ranges for serum alanine aminotransferase levels. *Ann Int Med* 2002;137:1.
10. Lee JK, Shim JH, Lee HC, et al. Estimation of the healthy upper limites for serum alanine aminotranferase in asin populations with norman liver hepatology. *Hepatology* 2010;51:1577.
11. Lok A, McMahon B. Chronic hepatitis B. *Hepatology* 2007;45:507.
12. Liaw Y-F, Leung N, Kao J-H, et al. Asian-Pacific consensus statement on the management of chronic hepatitis B: a 2008 update. *Hepatol Int* 2008;2:263.
13. Marcellin P, Dusheiko G, Zoulim F, et al. EASL clinical practice guidelines: management of chronic hepatitis B. *J Hepatol* 2009;50:227.
14. Keeffe E, Dieterich D, Han S, et al. A treatment algorithm for the management of chronic hepatitis B virus infection in the United States: 2008 update. *Clin Gastro Hep* 2008;6:1315.
15. Kim HC, Nam CM, Jee SH, et al. Normal serum aminotransferase concentration and risk of mortality from liver disease: prospective cohort study. *Br Med J* 2004;doi:10.1136/bmj.38050.593634.63:1–6.
16. Yagura M, Tanaka A, Kamitsukasa H, et al. Re-evaluation of the serum alanine aminotransferase upper normal limit in chronic hepatitis C patients. *Intern Med* 2010;49:525.
17. Cohen JA, Kaplan MM. The SGOT/SGPT ratio. an indicator of alcoholic liver disease. *Dig Dis Sci* 1979;24:8335.
18. Sheth SG, Flamm SL, Gordon FD, et al. AST/ALT ratio predicts cirrhosis in patients with chronic hepatitis C virus infection. *Am J Gastroenterol* 1998;93:44.
19. Reedy DW, Loo AT, Levine RA. AST/ALT ratio greater than 1 is not diagnostic of cirrhosis in patients with chronic hepatitis C. *Dig Dis Sci* 1998;43:2156.
20. Giannini E, Botta F, Fasoli A, et al. Progressive liver functional impairment is associated with an increase in AST/ALT ratio. *Dig Dis Sci* 1999;44:1249.
21. Park GJ, Lin BP, Ngu MC, et al. Aspartate aminotransferase: alanine aminotransferase ratio in chronic hepatitis C infection: is it a useful predictor of cirrhosis? *J Gastroenterol Hepatol* 2000;15:386.
22. Tameda M, Shirak K, Ooi K, et al. Aspartate aminotransferase–immunoglobulin complexes in patients with chronic liver disease. *World J Gastroenterol* 2005;11:1529.
23. Nathwani RA, Pais S, Reynolds TB, et al. Serum alanine aminotransferase in skeletal muscle diseases. *Hepatology* 2005;41:380.
24. Pratt D, Kaplan M. Evaluation of abnormal liver-enzyme results in asymptomatic patients. *N Engl J Med* 2000;342:1266.
25. Kaplan M. Alanine aminotransferase levels: what's normal. *Ann Int Med* 2002;137:49.
26. Aragon G, Younossi ZM. When and how to evaluate mildly elevated liver enzymes in apparently healthy patients. *Cleveland Clin Med* 2010;77:195.
27. Kim WR, Flamm S, DeBisceglie A, Bodenheimer H Jr. Serum activity of alanine aminotransferase (ALT) as an indicator of health and disease. *Hepatology* 2008;47:1363.
28. Ruhl C, Everhard J. Elevated serum alanine aminotransferase and γ-glutamyltransferase and mortality in the United States population. *Gastroenterology* 2009;136:477.
29. Lee TH, Kim W, Benson J, Therneau T, Melton LJ. Serum aminotransferase activity and mortality risk in a United States community. *Hepatology* 2008;47:880.

30. Ioannao G, Weiss N, Boyko E, Mozaffarian D, Lee SP. Elevated serum alanine aminotransferase activity and calculated risk of coronary heart disease in the United States. *Hepatology* 2006;43:1145.

31. Le Couteur D, Blyth F, Creasey H, et al. The association of alanine transaminase with aging, frailty, and mortality. *J Gerontol A Biol Sci Med Sci* 2010;65:712.

32. Jenkins W, Rosalki S, Foo Y, et al. Serum glutamate dehydrogenase is not a reliable marker of liver cell necrosis in alcoholics. *J Clin Pathol* 1982;35:207.

33. Chung YH, Jung SA, Song BC, et al. Plasma isocitrate dehydrogenase as a marker of centrilobular hepatic necrosis in patients with hyperthyroidism. *J Clin Gastroenterol* 2001;33:118.

34. Khayrollah A, Al-Tamer M, Taka M, et al. Serum alcohol dehydrogenase activity in liver diseases. *Ann Clin Biochem* 1982;19:35.

35. Naryham, S. Serum alkaline phosphatase isoenzymes as markers of liver disease. *Ann Clin Lab Sci* 1991;21:12.

36. Harris H. The human alkaline phosphatases: what we know and what we don't know. *Clin Chim Acta* 1989;186:133.

37. Henny J, Shiele F. Alkaline phosphatase. In: Siest G, Henny J, Shiele F, Young DS, eds. *Interpretation of Clinical Laboratory Tests. Reference values and their biological variation.* Foster City, CA: Biomedical Publications, 1985: 96–118.

38. Alvaro D, Benedetti A, Marucci L, et al. The function of alkaline phosphatase in the liver: regulation of intrahepatic biliary epithelium secretory activities in the rat. *Hepatology* 2000;32:174.

39. Kaplan M. Alkaline phosphatase. *Gastroenterology* 1972;62:452.

40. Bamford KF, Harris H, Luffman J, et al. Serum-alkaline-phosphatase and the ABO blood groups. *Lancet* 1965;1:530.

41. Heino AE, Jokipii SG. Serum alkaline phosphatase levels in the aged. *Am Med Intern Med* 1962;51:105.

42. Siraganian PA, Mulvihill JJ, Mulivor RA, et al. Benign familial hyperphosphatasemia. *JAMA* 1989;261:1310.

43. Kaplan MM, Rogers L. Separation of serum alkaline phosphatase isoenzymes by polyacrylamide gel electrophoresis. *Lancet* 1968;2:102.

44. Kaplan MM, Righetti A. Induction of rat liver alkaline phosphatase: the mechanism of the serum elevation in bile duct obstruction. *J Clin Invest* 1970;49:508.

45. Seetharam S, Sussman NL, Komoda T, Alpers DH. The mechanism of elevated alkaline phosphates activity afterbile duct ligation in the rat. *Hepatology* 1986;6:374.

46. Debroe ME, Roels F, Nouwen EJ, et al. Liver plasma membrane is the source of high-molecular-weight alkaline phosphatase in human serum. *Hepatology* 1985;5:118.

47. Margulis SJ, Honig CL, Soave R, et al. Biliary tract obstruction in the acquired immunodeficiency syndrome. *Ann Intern Med* 1986;105:207.

48. Brensilver HL, Kaplan MM. Significance of elevated liver alkaline phosphatase in serum. *Gastroenterology* 1975;68:1556.

49. Shaver WA, Bhatt H, Combes B. Low serum alkaline phosphatase activity in Wilson's disease. *Hepatology* 1986;6:859.

50. Wilson RA, Clayson KJ, Leon S. Unmeasurable serum alkaline phosphatase activity in Wilson's disease associated with fulminant hepatic failure and hemolysis. *Hepatology* 1987;7:613.

51. Righetti ABB, Kaplan MM. Disparate responses of serum and hepatic alkaline phosphatase and 5'-nucleotidase to bile duct obstruction in the rat. *Gastroenterology* 1972;62:1034.

52. Eshchar J, Ruzki C, Zimmerman HJ, et al. Serum levels of 5'-nucleotidase in disease. *Am J Clin Pathol* 1967;47:598.

53. Rutenberg AM, Goldbarg JA, Pineda GP, et al. Serum γ-glutamyl transpeptidase activity in hepatobiliary pancreatic disease. *Gastroenterology* 1963;45:43.

54. Sotil E, Jensen D. Serum enzymes associated with cholestasis. *Clin Liver Dis* 2004;8:41.

55. Rollason JG, Pincharle G, Robinson D, et al. Serum gamma-glutamyl transpeptidase in relation to alcohol consumption. *Clin Chim Acta* 1972;39:75.

56. Rosalki S, Rau D. Serum gamma-glutamyl transpeptidase activity in alcoholism. *Clin Chim Acta* 1972;39:41.

57. Selinger MJ, Matloff DS, Kaplan MM, et al. γ-Glutamyl transpeptidase activity in liver disease: serum elevation is independent of hepatic GGTP activity. *Clin Chim Acta* 1982;125:283.

58. Burrows S, Feldman W, McBride F, et al. Serum gamma-glutamyl transpeptidase: evaluation in screening of hospitalized patients. *Am J Clin Pathol* 1975;64:311.

59. Rutenberg AM, Banks BM, Pineda EP, et al. A comparison of serum aminopeptidase and alkaline phosphatase in the detection of hematobiliary disease in anicteric patients. *Ann Intern Med* 1964;61:50.

60. Triger DR, Wright R. Hypergammaglobulinemia in liver disease. *Lancet* 1973;1:1494.

61. Rothschild MA, Oratz M, Zimmon D, et al. Albumin synthesis in cirrhotic subjects studied with carbonate 4C. *J Clin Invest* 1969;48:344.

62. Rothschild MA, Oratz M, Schreiber SS. Serum albumin. *Hepatology* 1988;8:385.

63. Oratz M, Rothschild MA, Schreiber SS, et al. The role of the urea cycle and polyamines in albumin synthesis. *Hepatology* 1983;3:567.

64. Jefferson DM, Reid LM, Giambrone MA, et al. Effects of dexamethasone on albumin and collagen gene expression in primary cultures of adult rat hepatocytes. *Hepatology* 1985;5:14.

65. Bernau D, Rogier E, Feldmann G, et al. Decreased albumin and increased fibrinogen secretion by single hepatocytes from rats with acute inflammatory reaction. *Hepatology* 1983;3:29.

66. Dinarello C. Interleukin-1 and the pathogenesis of the acute phase response. *N Engl J Med* 1984;311:1413.

67. van Zanten SJO, Depla ACTM, Dekker PC, et al. The clinical importance of routine measurement of liver enzymes, total protein, and albumin in a general medicine outpatient clinic: a prospective study. *N Engl J Med* 1992;40:53.

68. Olson JP, Miller LL, Troup SB. Synthesis of clotting factors by the isolated perfused rat liver. *J Clin Invest* 1966;45:690.

69. Mattii R, Ambrus JL, Sokal JE, et al. Production of members of the blood coagulation and fibrinolysin systems by the isolated perfused liver. *Proc Soc Exp Biol Med* 1964;116:69.

70. Rapaport SI, Ames SB, Mikkelsen S, et al. Plasma clotting factors in chronic hepatocellular disease. *N Engl J Med* 1960;263:278.

71. Liebman HA, Furie BC, Furie B, et al. Hepatic vitamin K-dependent carboxylation of blood-clotting proteins. *Hepatology* 1982;2:488.

72. Blanchard RA, Furie BC, Jorgensen M, et al. Acquired vitamin K-dependent carboxylation deficiency in liver disease. *N Engl J Med* 1981;305:242.

73. Weitz IC, Liebman HA. Des-γ-carboxy (abnormal) prothrombin and hepatocellular carcinoma: a critical review. *Hepatology* 1993;18:990.

74. Liebman HA, Furie BC, Tong MJ, et al. Des-γ-carboxy (abnormal) prothrombin as a serum marker of primary hepatocellular carcinoma. *N Engl J Med* 1984;310:1427.

75. Suehiro T, Sugimachi K, Matsumata T, et al. Protein induced by vitamin K absence or antagonist II as a prognostic marker in hepatocellular carcinoma: comparison with alpha-fetoprotein. *Cancer* 1994;73:2464.

76. Lester R, Schmid R. Bilirubin metabolism. *N Engl J Med* 1964;270:779.

77. Robinson S, Lester R, Crigler JF Jr, et al. Early-labeled peak of bile pigment in man: studies with glycine-14C and delta aminolevulinic acid-3H. *N Engl J Med* 1967;277:1323.

78. Landow SA, Callahan EW Jr, Schmid R. Catabolism of heme in vivo: comparison of the simultaneous production of bilirubin and carbon monoxide. *J Clin Invest* 1970;49:914.

79. Tenhunen R, Ross ME, Marver HS, et al. Reduced nicotinamide-adenine dinucleotide phosphate-dependent biliverdin reductase:

partial purification and characterization. *Biochemistry* 1970;9: 288.

80. Scharschmidt BF, Waggoner JG, Berk PD. Hepatic organic anion uptake in the rat. *J Clin Invest* 1975;56:1280.

81. Zieve L, Hill E, Hanson M, et al. Normal and abnormal variations and clinical significance of the one-minute and total serum bilirubin determinations. *J Lab Clin Med* 1951;38:446.

82. Blanckaert N, Kabra PM, Farina FA, et al. Measurement of bilirubin and its monoconjugates and diconjugates in human serum by alkaline methanolysis and high-performance liquid chromatography. *J Lab Clin Med* 1980;96:198.

83. Weiss JS, Gautam A, Lauff JJ, et al. The clinical importance of a protein-bound fraction of serum bilirubin in patients with hyperbilirubinemia. *N Engl J Med* 1983;309:147.

84. Raymond GD, Galambos JT. Hepatic storage and excretion of bilirubin in man. *Am J Gastroenterol* 1971;55:135.

85. Schmid R, Diamond I, Hammaker L, et al. Interaction of bilirubin with albumin. *Nature* 1965;206:1041.

86. Hardison WG, Lee FI. Prognosis in acute liver disease of the alcoholic patient. *N Engl J Med* 1966;275:61.

87. Lau H, Man K, Fan SCW, et al. Evaluation of preoperative hepatic function in patients with hepatocellular carcimona undergoing hepatectomy. *Br J Surg* 1997;84:1255.

88. Sakka, S. Assessing liver function. *Curr Opin Crit Care* 2007;13:207.

89. Oellerich M, Armstrong VW. The MEGX test: a tool for the real-time assessment of hepatic function. *Ther Drug Monit* 2001;23:81.

90. Shiffman M, Fisher R, Sanyal A, et al. Hepatic lidocaine metabolism and complications of cirrhosis. *Transplantation* 1993;55:830.

91. Shiffman M, Luketic V, Sanyal A, et al. Hepatic lidocaine metabolism and liver histology in patients with chronic hepatitis and cirrhosis. *Hepatology* 1994;19:933.

92. Everson G, Hiffman M, Morgan T, Sterling R, Wagners D. Quantitative tests of liver function measure hepatic improvement after sustained virological response: results from the HALT-C trial. *Aliment Pharmacol Ther* 2008;29:589.

93. Botta F, Gianni E, Romagnoli P, et al. MELD scoring system is useful for predicting prognosis in patients with liver cirrhosis and is correlated with residual liver function: a European study. *Gut* 2003;52:134.

94. Renner E, Wietholtz H, Huguenin P, et al. Caffeine: a model compound for measuring liver function. *Hepatology* 1984;4:38.

95. Jost G, Wahllander A, von Mandach U, et al. Overnight salivary caffeine clearance: a liver function test suitable for routine use. *Hepatology* 1987;7:338.

96. Tarantion G, Conca P, Capone D, Gentile A. Reliability of total overnight salivary caffeine assessment (TOSCA) for liver function evaluation in compensated cirrhotic patients. *Eur J Clin Pharm* 2006;62:605.

97. Joeres R, Klinker H, Heusler H, et al. Influence of smoking on caffeine elimination in healthy volunteers and in patients with alcoholic liver disease. *Hepatology* 1988;8:575.

98. Castera L, Vergniol J, Foucher J, et al. Prospective comparison of transient elastography, Fibrotest, APRI and liver biopsy for the assessment of fibrosis in chronic hepatitis C. *Gastorenterology* 2005;128:343.

99. Parkes J, Guha IN, Roderick P, et al. Enhanced liver fibrosis (ELF) test accurately identifies liver cirrhosis in patients with chronic hepatitis C. *J Viral Hepat* 2010;18:23.

100. Triger DR, Wright R. Hypergammaglobulinemia in liver disease. *Lancet* 1973;1:1494.

101. Machlachlan MJ, Rodnan CP, Cooper WM, et al. Chronic active (lupoid) hepatitis. *Ann Intern Med* 1965;62:425.

102. Nathwani R, Kumar S, Reynolds T, Kaplowitz N. Marked elevation in serum transaminases: an atypical presentation of choledocholithiasis. *Am J Gastroenterol* 2005;100:295.

103. Kaplan M. Evaluation of hepatobiliary diseases. In: Stein JH, ed. *Internal Medicine*. Boston: Little, Brown, 1998: 443.

104. Clarke LC, Beck EJ. Plasma "alkaline" phosphatase activity, I: normative data for growing children. *J Pediatr* 1950;36:335.

105. Wolf PL. Clinical significance of an increased or decreased serum alkaline phosphatase level. *Arch Pathol Lab Med* 1978;102:497.

106. Whitefield JB, Pounder RE, Neale G, et al. Serum γ-glutamyl transpeptidase activity in liver disease. *Gut* 1972;13:702.

107. Putnam FW. *The Proteins*, 2nd edn, Vol. 1. Orlando: Academic Press, 1975: 18.

108. Ostrow JD, Aria I, Carey M, Forker L. *Unit 1. Hepatic excretory function: undergraduate teaching project*. Baltimore, MD: American Gastroenterological Association, Milner-Fenwick Slides Company.

109. Crawford J, Hauser S, Gollan J. Formation, hepatic metabolism, and transport of bile pigments: a status report. *Semin Liver Dis* 1988;8:105.

CHAPTER 3
Liver Biopsy and Laparoscopy

Alyson N. Fox[1], Lennox J. Jeffers[2], & K. Rajender Reddy[3]

[1]Division of Gastroenterology, University of California, San Francisco, CA, USA
[2]Center for Liver Diseases, University of Miami, Miami, FL, USA
[3]Division of Gastroenterology, University of Pennsylvania, Philadelphia, PA, USA

Key concepts

- Although the standard percutaneous liver biopsy allows for a sample of only 1/50,000 of the liver parenchyma, it continues to serve as the gold standard in the diagnosis and management of liver disease.
- Percutaneous liver biopsy is a safe procedure, with a low mortality rate. Safety of the procedure can possibly be enhanced with the addition of ultrasound guidance or biopsy tract plugging techniques.
- In those with contraindications to percutaneous liver biopsy such as bleeding tendency or ascites, the transjugular approach is an alternative that offers the added benefit of portosystemic pressure gradient measurement.
- Diagnostic laparoscopy affords the clinician the ability to observe the gross appearance of the liver, perform directed biopsies, and obtain peritoneal tissue when indicated.
- While there are a number of noninvasive biomarkers and radiographic techniques in use to assess hepatic fibrosis, liver biopsy continues to have a role, although in a selected manner.

Liver biopsy has been used as a diagnostic tool since the late 1800s, when Paul Ehrlich performed the first percutaneous liver biopsy [1]. The described procedure was lengthy and precarious owing to a long hepatic puncture time. However in 1958, Menghini reported a "one second" technique that defined the procedure as we now know it [2]. Today, liver biopsy continues to serve as an important tool for those who diagnose and treat liver diseases. Biopsy specimens can provide prognostic information for several pathologic processes and the information gleaned can often be used to guide treatment decisions.

While percutaneous liver biopsy remains the most common practice, advances in radiographic and surgical techniques have allowed for the performance of liver biopsy via transvenous and laparoscopic routes, especially in patients with contraindications to a percutaneous approach. Alternatively, noninvasive techniques and serologic markers of liver histology are being validated, and in some cases may obviate the need for invasive procedures. In general, liver biopsies continue to be safe procedures, however infrequently life-threatening events can ensue.

Indications for liver biopsy (Box 3.1)

Abnormal hepatic biochemical tests and acute liver failure

Health care providers are frequently asked to evaluate patients with abnormal hepatic biochemical tests. Typically, the combination of a comprehensive history, physical examination, and laboratory analysis can yield a diagnosis. However, a small proportion of patients will have a negative workup and may require a histologic exam to determine a diagnosis. Histology in the majority of these cases will lead to a diagnosis of nonalcoholic fatty liver disease (NAFLD), however diseases such as primary and secondary biliary cirrhosis, autoimmune hepatitis, primary sclerosing cholangitis, and hemochromatosis have been identified through biopsy, when serologic studies were inconclusive [3]. The clear advantage to pursuing biopsy in this situation is the potential to recognize a disease process for which there is a specific treatment.

Liver biopsy is also indicated to identify the cause of acute liver failure when an obvious precipitant is not clear. The most recent guidelines on the management of acute liver failure (ALF) recommend pursuing biopsy via the transjugular route when the etiology of ALF cannot be determined from history or serology alone [4]. In these cases, biopsy may identify entities such as diffuse malignancy, Wilson disease, autoimmune hepatitis, or viral infection.

Hepatitis C

Currently available treatment for chronic hepatitis C with pegylated interferon and ribavirin is associated with high costs, undesirable side effects, and modest response rates, especially in those with genotype 1 infection. Given these facts, candidates for hepatitis C virus (HCV) therapy need to be carefully selected. A pretreatment liver biopsy was for many years the norm. However, the role of liver biopsy in hepatitis C has been questioned over more recent years, with the advent of noninvasive markers of disease severity becoming more of a reality. Although there are several arguments for performing a liver biopsy in this population, the two main advantages to biopsy are to assess the necessity of antiviral therapy and to predict response to therapy [5].

The role of liver biopsy in prognostication and necessity of treatment is based on the premise that most patients with moderate inflammation from chronic hepatitis C develop cirrhosis within 20 years and nearly all patients with severe inflammation or bridging fibrosis develop cirrhosis within 10 years [6]. Patients with mild inflammation and/or minimal fibrosis have a low risk of progression to cirrhosis. Therefore, the urgency of treating someone with mild inflammation or minimal fibrosis is certainly not as great relative to treating someone with a more advanced histologic stage or grade. With the expectation that better tolerated agents may soon enter the arsenal for HCV therapy, it might make sense to delay treatment in less severe cases until better therapies are available.

Liver biopsy can help to identify a subset of patients with normal alanine aminotransferase (ALT) levels and significant histology that would benefit from therapy. Approximately 30% of patients with chronic hepatitis C have persistently normal ALT levels and only 42% develop peak levels twice the upper limit of normal [7]. Despite the fact that patients with normal ALT

levels have been demonstrated to have significantly lower inflammation and fibrosis scores on liver biopsy examination than patients with elevated ALT levels, almost two thirds have evidence of portal fibrosis and 10% had bridging fibrosis [8]. Therefore, identification of those with clinically silent disease (i.e., those with normal serum aminotransferase levels) but histologic progression is critical for the treatment of a group at high risk of sequelae from HCV infection.

The presence of advanced fibrosis is also negatively associated with the probability of response to hepatitis C therapy. A recent study sought to examine the efficacy of peg interferon alfa and ribavirin therapy in patients with advanced fibrosis [9]. Sustained virological response (SVR) rates decreased according to level of fibrosis, such that in subjects without advanced fibrosis, SVR was 60% in patients with genotype 1 to 4, 51% in those with bridging fibrosis, and 33% in those with cirrhosis ($P = 0.0028$). The same trend held true for subjects with genotype 2/3. Lastly, liver biopsy may also reveal unsuspected cirrhosis, which would prompt initiation of a surveillance strategy for hepatocellular carcinoma and esophageal varices.

Although the information obtained from liver biopsy is useful, it is not mandatory to perform biopsy before treating hepatitis C. Biopsy is certainly more useful in guiding decision making for genotype 1 patients, since the treatment response rates are less than ideal and knowledge of their histologic risk of progression may influence the decision to treat or withhold therapy until better tolerated agents are available. In contrast, patients with genotype 2 or 3 may elect to undergo therapy regardless of findings on liver biopsy because the rates of sustained virological response are much better than seen in their genotype 1 counterparts.

Hepatitis B

The guidelines for initiating treatment of hepatitis B are largely based on the presence of abnormal transaminase levels and levels of viral replication. In many, antiviral therapy can be initiated without a pretreatment biopsy. Knowledge of underlying histology in those infected with hepatitis B can help guide treatment decisions when patients do not meet the guidelines and treatment may be of benefit. Liver biopsy should be considered in patients with modest elevations in transaminases based on the presence of hepatitis E antigen, viral load, and age [10]. Those with evidence of inflammation and/or fibrosis may benefit from initiation of therapy, which may lead to histologic improvement and subsequent clinical outcomes.

Nonalcoholic fatty liver disease

Nonalcoholic fatty liver disease represents a spectrum of liver disease ranging from minimal inflammation to cirrhosis. Most patients afflicted with NAFLD have a silent course, marked by asymptomatic elevations in transaminases; however a subset can develop nonalcoholic steatohepatitis (NASH), a potentially progressive form that can evolve to cirrhosis, end-stage liver disease, and even hepatocellular carcinoma. The role of liver biopsy in NAFLD is primarily to distinguish between steatosis and NASH in order to offer more aggressive risk factor reduction to those with evidence of NASH, as well as to define the presence of cirrhosis, which would prompt initiation of cirrhosis care. Similar to other conditions, there exists a great deal of sampling variability in those with NAFLD, so biopsy likely represents a flawed gold standard for diagnosis [11].

Focal lesions

Focal hepatic lesions identified by radiographic techniques are often easily identifiable by their characteristic appearances. Diagnosis of specific liver masses is routinely made by radiography alone, and techniques and diagnostic experience have advanced to such an extent that biopsy is often unnecessary to make a diagnosis of the nature of the focal lesions. Biopsy becomes useful when there are atypical radiographic features.

Prior to pursuing biopsy for a mass lesion, it is crucial have an appreciation for the context in which the lesion arises. Clearly, a lesion arising in a patient with known cirrhosis makes hepatocellular carcinoma (HCC) a major concern. Biopsy of a suspected HCC is not without risk. HCCs tend to be highly vascular tumors so there is a risk of hemorrhage [12]. The risk of seeding the needle tract with tumor cells and causing spread of disease has been reported in up to 2.7–5% of cases of percutaneous biopsy [13]. Further there is a concern of sampling error when attempting to biopsy a small lesion that may give a false sense of security. Most importantly, the diagnosis of HCC can often be made readily in a patient with cirrhosis based on characteristic radiologic features.

Other lesions not characteristic on imaging such as adenomas, hemangiomas, focal nodular hyperplasia, cysts, abscesses, and lesions that are concerning for metastases, should only be considered for image-guided biopsy after careful review with a radiologist and an alternative imaging technique has failed to give a diagnosis.

Liver transplantation

Liver biopsy is helpful in making a specific diagnosis in both early and late allograft dysfunction. Diagnoses such as allograft rejection, viral infection (such as due to cytomegalovirus), drug-induced liver injury, bile duct injury, or recurrence of the original disease can be made with a liver biopsy. In addition, liver histology is helpful in determining the prognosis and course of recurrent hepatitis C-related fibrosis progression and clinical decompensation [14].

Considerations prior to percutaneous liver biopsy

Contraindications to having a percutaneous liver biopsy are listed in Box 3.2.

Coagulopathy/thrombocytopenia

Many patients undergoing liver biopsy have advanced liver disease complicated by coagulopathy and thrombocytopenia. Although the risk of major hemorrhage after liver biopsy is fairly low, hemorrhage remains the most feared complication of liver biopsy, despite the fact that there is no definitive correlation between risk of bleeding and level of coagulation abnormality. Traditionally, percutaneous biopsy has been avoided in patients with a prothrombin time elevated in excess of 4 seconds over control, an international normalized ratio (INR) greater than 1.5, or a platelet counts less than $60,000/\mu L$. Prothrombin time, partial thromboplastin time, and platelet count should be measured within 4 weeks of biopsy. Patients with any of these derangements or a combination of them are typically sent for transjugular liver biopsy and given preprocedure fresh frozen plasma or platelet transfusions to correct coagulation abnormalities.

Patients taking oral anticoagulants should be counseled on discontinuation of the drugs at least 5 days before the biopsy, and a preprocedure prothrombin time INR is preferred to ensure that the INR is within acceptable limits. The indication for anticoagulation should be reviewed to ensure that discontinuation is appropriate and safe. Oral anticoagulation should not be restarted immediately, but can be resumed 48–72 hours after the biopsy since delayed bleeding has been reported in patients on

---

Box 3.2 Contraindications to percutaneous liver biopsy.

Absolute
- Uncooperative patient
- Bleeding tendency:
    Prothrombin time (PT) $\geq$4 seconds over control or
        international normalized ratio (INR) >1.5
    Platelet count <60,000/mm^3
- Inability to transfuse blood products
- Serious consideration of echinococcal disease
- Presumed hemangioma or other vascular tumors

Relative
- Ascites
- Obesity
- Infection in right pleural cavity and/or below right diaphragm

oral anticoagulants [15,16]. A recent study evaluated the role of aspirin in biopsy-related complications [17]. The authors reported that in over 15,000 image-guided core biopsies of many organs, aspirin did not seem to confer an increased risk of bleeding. Despite this new information, we still advise discontinuation of aspirin and nonsteroidal agents for approximately 7 days prior to the planned procedure, which may be restarted 48–72 hours after the procedure. Data are lacking on the management of newer antiplatelet agents; however, it would seem prudent that these agents be discontinued for a brief period of time before and after biopsy.

Ascites

The presence of ascites precludes percutaneous liver biopsy in many patients. The midaxillary approach is technically hindered as tense ascites causes a separation of the liver from the costal surface. Those with moderate ascites may be able to undergo a therapeutic paracentesis prior to biopsy, but in most cases a transjugular approach is used since many of these patients will have coexisting coagulation impairment.

Other contraindications

Successful percutaneous biopsy requires that the patient is able to cooperate with the procedure. Lack of patient cooperation may increase the risk of complications. Uncooperative patients needing biopsy should get biopsies via the transvenous routes using sedation. Marked obesity should also prompt a transjugular approach, as a percutaneous approach is hindered by adipose tissue. Patients suspected of having either infectious lesions or vascular lesions in the liver should not undergo routine percutaneous biopsy, as puncture of that tissue may cause dissemination of infection or hemorrhage.

Percutaneous liver biopsy

Technique

Percutaneous liver biopsy is the most common technique used to acquire liver tissue. Prior to setting up for the procedure, it is critical to confirm that the patient undergoing the procedure is an appropriate candidate. This entails a complete history and physical examination, a review of medications, and measurement of clotting parameters in order to assess for any contraindications to biopsy. A light meal at least 3 hours before the procedure may facilitate gallbladder emptying and reduce the risk of gallbladder puncture. Alternatively, an overnight fast can reduce the risk of aspiration in case of vomiting.

Prior to initiating the procedure, it is mandatory to clearly explain the procedure and any potential complications that could result from it. Written consent documenting this discussion with the patient and/or a proxy should be obtained. After this is accomplished it is appropriate to prepare the patient for the procedure.

Venous access should be established, preferably in the left arm, so that the patient can lie comfortably in the right lateral decubitus position after the biopsy. Patients are frequently anxious, and intravenous fentanyl and midazolam can alleviate apprehension, facilitate the procedure, provide some postprocedure relief of pain, and achieve some degree of amnesia. Most patients do well with approximately $50\,\mu g$ of fentanyl and $2\,mg$ of midazolam without impairment of their ability to cooperate with the biopsy. Older patients may require less sedation.

The patient should be positioned supine with the right hand placed under the head. The point of maximum liver dullness is percussed over the right hemithorax between the anterior and midaxillary lines and is usually found between the sixth and ninth intercostal spaces. In certain situations, it may be higher (e.g., obesity) or lower (e.g., emphysema). Dullness should be present in both inspiration and expiration as some patients may inadvertently take a deep breath during the procedure and thereby risk a pneumothorax. The routine use of real time ultrasound is helpful in establishing the best location for biopsy, and allows the operator the advantage of visualizing the liver during inspiration and expiration and identifying neighboring organs (i.e., lung, kidney, gut) that may be at risk of inadvertent puncture. The location for biopsy should be marked clearly, and then the area should be prepped and draped in a sterile fashion. A local anesthetic agent, such as 1% lidocaine is injected over the upper border of a rib, avoiding the intercostal nerve and vessels that run along the lower border. A small incision is made with a scalpel in order to accommodate the larger needle used to actually obtain the tissue. The biopsy needle should then be inserted at the incision site and the procedure performed.

Devices

Needles used to perform percutaneous liver biopsy are broadly categorized as aspiration needles (Menghini, Klatskin, and Jamshidi needles) and cutting needles (Vim Silverman and Tru-Cut needles and spring-loaded needles with triggering mechanisms). The aspiration-type devices are attached to a syringe. When the needle is inserted into the liver parenchyma, suction is applied to the syringe and tissue is aspirated into the needle for collection. The cutting-type needles, whether manual or automatic, employ a needle and outer cutting sheath that when propelled beyond the needle cuts and traps tissue within the needle hollow.

Different needles acquire various lengths and diameters of hepatic tissue. Comparisons of Menghini aspiration and Tru-Cut needles have shown increased rates of tissue sample fragmentation with the aspiration needles compared with the cutting-type needles, especially in the presence of cirrhosis [18,19]. Likewise it has been reported that Tru-Cut biopsies were significantly longer (12 mm versus 8 mm; $P <0.001$) and contain a greater number of portal tracts (16 versus 6; $P <0.001$) than aspiration-type needles [18]. Amongst the cutting-type devices, it has been reported that the automated needles acquire slightly longer tissue samples (1.7 mm versus 1.5 mm; $P = 0.05$) [20]. It has also been noted that the nonautomatic cutting needles remain in the liver for a modestly longer time during the biopsy and may pose additional bleeding risk due to this added time [12]. Likewise, larger bore needles may confer a higher risk of bleeding [21].

Imaging

Ultrasonography can be used to guide the operator with respect to location for the percutaneous liver biopsy. Ultrasound can occur either in advance of the procedure, such that the biopsy site is "marked" by an ultrasonographer, or the ultrasound can occur in real time by the operator. The relative ease and availability of real time ultrasound have made its pre-biopsy use routine in some centers [22]. However, use of ultrasonography to guide a percutaneous biopsy is not mandatory. The lack of consensus on the matter is apparent in individual practice. A survey of 112 gastroenterologists associated with a major North American academic center revealed that over half performed liver biopsies without the use of ultrasound guidance [23]. Another survey found that 64% of gastroenterologists used ultrasound prior to biopsy [24].

To examine differences in diagnostic yield and safety, Lindor *et al.* performed a prospective, randomized study of 836 patients, who were randomized to either automatic or traditional cutting needles with or without ultrasound guidance [20]. Those who underwent pre-biopsy ultrasound had lower rates of hospitalization (2 versus 9; $P = 0.04$), lower rates of bleeding or hypotension (9 versus 18; $P = 0.07$), and lower frequency of pain requiring non-narcotic treatment (37% versus 50%; $P = 0.003$). There was no difference in pain requiring narcotic analgesia between those who had and did not have pre-biopsy ultrasonography. In contrast to these findings, a large British survey failed to demonstrate differences in major complications or pain between biopsies performed with and without ultrasonographic guidance [25]. With respect to diagnostic yield, a recent retrospective analysis of 205 patients who underwent liver biopsy found that there were no statistically significant differences between the specimens in terms of tissue fragmentation or number of portal tracts and central veins whether ultrasound guidance was or was not used [26]. Mean specimen length in the ultrasound-guided liver biopsy group was 12.58 mm and in the blind biopsy group was 16.22 mm ($P <0.005$). Neither group experienced major complications.

Another prospective study showed that ultrasonography changed the site of liver biopsy determined by the percussion technique in as many as 15% of patients [27]. If the site had not been moved, what complications may have resulted is not known. A follow-up study showed that ultrasonography may not be of any greater utility in selected patients, such as those with difficult percussion, obesity, or chest wall deformity [28]. Ultrasonography was just as likely to mandate movement of the biopsy site in patients with these features compared with unselected patients.

Cost-effectiveness analysis has suggested that the use of ultrasonography to prevent major complications is cost effective [29]. The use of ultrasonography has resulted in better outcomes, is cost effective, and is already widely utilized. Given the fact that real time ultrasound is widely available, its use is preferred by many over blind percussion technique; however its use is not obligatory [30].

Plugged biopsy

While ultrasound guidance may provide a radiographic technique to enhance the safety of percutaneous biopsy, there is another technique that has been described. Plugged biopsies were first described in the mid 1980s and provide a technique whereby percutaneous biopsy may be considered in a patient with mild coagulopathy and/or ascites [31]. A recent trial studied the safety and efficacy of plugged percutaneous liver biopsies done with ultrasound guidance [32]. In 36 patients undergoing percutaneous biopsy, the needle tract was injected with a foam embolization particle. None of the patents had bleeding complications and specimens were adequate for diagnosis in all cases. Since then, transjugular biopsy has become a common approach for obtaining liver tissue in those with coagulopathy, and this technique has been compared with plugged percutaneous liver biopsy. One study reported bleeding requiring transfusion in two patients undergoing a plugged procedure [33]. The biopsy specimens obtained via the percutaneous route were significantly larger, although both techniques provided specimens adequate for diagnosis. More recently, the two techniques were again compared in a population with coagulopathy and/or ascites and neither group suffered complications of hemorrhage [34]. When available, plugged percutaneous biopsy may provide an alternative in those with mild coagulation abnormalities and ascites, especially given a low reported risk of bleeding and the potential of obtaining larger specimens.

Postprocedural considerations

After the successful completion of the biopsy procedure, the patient should be observed for a period of time with vital signs being taken every 15 minutes for the first hour, then every 30 minutes for the second hour. Conventionally, the patient should remain in the right lateral decubitus position during this time. The duration of observation after biopsy has been arbitrary for several years, with the recognition that postprocedural monitoring is to assess for complications related to bleeding – an event that if it occurs, should occur soon after biopsy. A recent retrospective evaluation of monitoring practices found that the majority of complications occurred within 1 hour postprocedure [35]. As recovery time decreased from 6 hours before 1997 to 1 hour in 2002, the major complication rate was 1.7% regardless of duration of observation. The majority of complications occurred within 1 hour during the observation period or within 24 hours after discharge. Based upon this study, it would be reasonable to conclude that a shorter observation time of 2 hours after ambulatory percutaneous liver biopsy is safe.

Adequacy of sample

A liver biopsy samples approximately 1/50,000th of the liver, and therefore may not be representative of the entire liver, especially given the fact that many diseases cause heterogeneous injury. Standard practice would mandate the presence of at least six portal triads in order to consider the specimen adequate for diagnosis in diffuse liver disease [36]. However, more recent data suggest that these criteria are inadequate for the grading of fibrosis and staging of inflammation in chronic liver disease.

A recent study in patients with chronic hepatitis B and C sought to examine the diagnostic yield of biopsies when the length and width of specimens were varied [37]. Shorter lengths of biopsy specimens yielded more mild estimates of inflammation grade, such that when only 1 cm of length was viewed 86.6% were interpreted as mild whereas when at least 3 cm of biopsy was viewed only 49.7% were graded as such. Similarly, more specimens were reported to show mild fibrosis with shorter length of specimens. As for the width, both grade and stage were significantly underscored in the 1 mm samples, regardless of their length. The study also reported that 11 portal tracts seemed to be the threshold below which disease grade and stage were significantly underestimated. Likewise, a biopsy of 2 cm in length and 1.4 mm in width tended to guarantee this number of portal tracts in 94% of cases. Another more recent study showed that intraobserver agreement was significantly better with longer length (2 cm) specimens than with shorter length (1.5, 10, or 5 mm) [38].

It has been reported that even large biopsy samples may not be reliable for the evaluation of NAFLD. A study

examining two biopsies from patients with NAFLD, using large bore (16 gauge) cutting needles of average length 2 cm, showed surprising variability between the two biopsies, with 41% discordance rate for one or more stages [39]. However, a more recent paper showed that length of the biopsy sample positively correlated with the percentage of patients found to have definite NASH, such that 29% were diagnosed to have NASH in biopsies measuring less than 10 mm and 65% in biopsies measuring ≥25 mm [35].

We can therefore conclude that larger bore biopsies of longer length are desirable to reliably grade and stage chronic liver disease. However, liver biopsy must be regarded to some extent as a flawed gold standard for the evaluation of chronic liver diseases because of significant problems with sampling variability and the heterogeneous nature of liver diseases.

Complications of percutaneous liver biopsy

Complications resulting from liver biopsy range from pain, which is common, to more serious events such as bleeding, perforation of a neighboring organ, infection, or death, all of which are uncommon (Box 3.3). Sixty percent

Box 3.3 Complications of percutaneous liver biopsy.

- Pain (0.056–83%):
    Pleuritic
    Peritoneal
    Diaphragmatic
- Hemorrhage:
    Intraperitoneal (0.03–0.7%)
    Intrahepatic[a] and/or subcapsular (0.59–23%)
    Hemobilia (0.006–0.2%)
- Bile peritonitis (0.03–0.22%)
- Bile pleuritis
- Perforated viscous
- Transient bacteremia (13.5%)
- Sepsis (0.088%) and abscess formation
- Pneumothorax and/or pleural effusion (0.08–0.28%)
- Hemothorax (0.18–0.49%)
- Arteriovenous fistula (5.4%)[b]
- Subcutaneous emphysema (0.014%)
- Reaction to anesthetic (0.029%)
- Breaking of needle (0.02–0.059%)
- Biopsy of other organs:
    Lung (0.001–0.014%)
    Gallbladder (0.034–0.117%)
    Kidney (0.029–0.096%)
    Colon (0.0038–0.044%)
- Mortality (0.0088–0.3%)

[a] Symptomatic and asymptomatic.
[b] Asymptomatic.
Data from references [12,26,47–56,59–64,68–70].

of complications are recognized within 2 hours after the procedure, and 96% within 24 hours [21,40]. Fatal complications typically occur within 6 hours. A hospitalization rate of 1.4–3.2% for the management of complications following a liver biopsy has been reported, with pain or hypotension being the predominant cause [41,42]. Mortality after liver biopsy has been reported to vary from 0.0088% to 0.3% [12,43].

Up to 84% of patients experience pain after percutaneous biopsy, either at the biopsy site, in the right shoulder, or in both locations [44]. The pain is usually mild, dull, and responsive to analgesics. Pain medications are required in approximately one third of patients after biopsy, approximately one half of whom are given narcotics [45]. While pain typically resolves within a few hours of biopsy, one group found that it may persist up to 24 hours after biopsy [44]. Ongoing severe abdominal pain should alert the physician to the possibility of bleeding or peritonitis and warrants radiographic evaluation and/or hospital admission.

The most dreaded complication of liver biopsy is hemorrhage. Hemorrhage after liver biopsy can manifest as a free intraperitoneal bleed, intrahepatic or subcapsular hematoma, or hemobilia. The risk of fatal hemorrhage in patients without malignant disease is 0.04% and the risk of nonfatal hemorrhage is 0.16%. In those with malignancy, the risk of nonfatal hemorrhage is 0.4%, and 0.57% for nonfatal hemorrhage [12]. Risk factors for hemorrhage after liver biopsy include presence of malignancy, performance of multiple passes, advanced age, mycobacterial infection, requirement for pre-biopsy platelet transfusion, acute liver failure, cirrhosis, heparin administration on the day of biopsy, treatment with corticosteroids, use of nonsteroidal anti-inflammatory agents, use of large diameter needles, and when the procedure is performed by a less experienced operator [12,21,46]. Free intraperitoneal hemorrhage may be related to a laceration sustained during deep inspiration or to a penetrating injury of a large vessel. Significant intraperitoneal hemorrhage is manifest by abdominal pain, tachycardia, and hypotension. Typically, these symptoms develop within the first 2–3 hours after the procedure. Patients with these symptoms should ideally undergo radiographic imaging in order to confirm clinical suspicion. If hemorrhage is present, volume resuscitation must be undertaken immediately. If hemodynamic instability persists despite aggressive resuscitation over a couple of hours, then angiography with embolization of the bleeding site is the preferred approach to stop the bleeding. In some cases, surgical exploration is required. The use of prophylactic or rescue strategies such as plasma, fibrinolytic inhibitors, or recombinant factors can be considered, although their effectiveness and use has not been established in the situation of bleeding following a liver biopsy.

Intrahepatic or subcapsular hematomas have been reported in 0.59–23% of cases when ultrasonography is performed after a liver biopsy [47]. These are usually asymptomatic, and the frequency is similar in both laparoscopically guided and "blind" liver biopsies [48]. Large hematomas may cause pain, liver enlargement, tachycardia, hypotension, and a delayed drop in the hematocrit. Conservative treatment generally suffices, and angiography is rarely required.

Hemobilia is a rare complication of percutaneous liver biopsy that presents with the classic triad of right upper quadrant pain, jaundice, and gastrointestinal bleeding. In a series of 68,276 percutaneous biopsies, hemobilia occurred in only four (0.006%) procedures [21]. While some cases of hemobilia may present acutely, most present at least 5 days after the biopsy [49,50], an approximate time period for the erosion of a hematoma or pseudoaneurysm into a bile duct. Bleeding is usually arterial in origin, but can be venous. The severity ranges from life-threatening hemorrhage to occult bleeding with chronic anemia. Endoscopy may reveal blood flowing from the ampulla of Vater. Endoscopic retrograde cholangiopancreatography (ERCP) demonstrates linear, irregular densities in the biliary tree and gallbladder that do not have the configuration of gallstones, and endoscopic sphincterotomy may facilitate the removal of these clots [51]. However, angiography is the preferred modality for diagnosis and embolization therapy.

Transient bacteremia has been reported in up to 13.5% of patients after liver biopsy [52]. This is usually of no clinical significance, although sepsis can sometimes occur in patients with biliary tract disorders. Evaluation of a post-transplant population (a high-risk group on immunosuppressive agents) found that of 1,136 percutaneous liver biopsies, only seven infections resulted [53]. No recommendations are currently available regarding prophylactic antibiotics for those with risk factors for endocarditis. Infection complications in the post-transplant patient are relatively more common in patients with biliary-enteric anastomosis, and antibiotic prophylaxis in such patients prior to the procedure appears prudent.

Other complications of liver biopsy include asymptomatic intrahepatic arteriovenous fistula, bile pleuritis, and bile peritonitis [54–57]. The most common cause of bile peritonitis is puncture of the gallbladder, which becomes apparent immediately and is characterized by severe pain and vasovagal hypotension. Bile peritonitis is also more likely if biliary obstruction is present. Pain may be followed by fever, abdominal pain, leukocytosis, and ileus. Ultrasonography or a computed tomography (CT) scan may identify an intra-abdominal collection of bile, and ERCP or biliary scintigraphy may demonstrate a bile leak. Surgery is indicated when clinical deterioration occurs despite the administration of intravenous antibiotics, fluid, and pain control. Pneumothorax and hemothorax after liver biopsy often spontaneously resolve, and placement of a chest tube is seldom required.

Transjugular liver biopsy

Transjugular liver biopsy (TJLB) was first performed successfully in 1970 [58]. Since that time, it has continued to provide an alternative mechanism of obtaining liver tissue in patients with contraindications to percutaneous biopsy. Despite the fact that TJLB specimens have traditionally been thought of as inferior to those obtained by conventional methods, the transjugular approach offers the added benefit of being able to obtain a hepatic venous pressure gradient, a parameter which is increasingly recognized as an important clinical and prognostic marker.

Indications

Significant ascites and bleeding tendency are the most common indications for transjugular liver biopsy (Box 3.4) [59]. Bleeding is the most feared complication in patients undergoing liver biopsy, especially in those who have altered coagulopathy as a result of impaired synthetic function or thrombocytopenia. Coagulopathy, defined as a prothrombin time greater than 3 seconds over control and/or a platelet count less than 60,000 cm^3, accounts for almost half of all cases [59]. Due to the controlled circumstances of the transjugular approach, the risk of bleeding is minimal and appears to be safe even in those with congenital bleeding disorders when done on an outpatient basis [60,61].

TJLB has been shown to have a diagnostic and prognostic role in those with acute hepatic failure. A report of 17 patients with acute liver failure found that TJLB was technically successful in all patients and that there were no complications due to the procedure [62]. In those found to have submassive or massive necrosis, prognosis was poor. TJLB has also been reported to be safe and helpful in the early postoperative period after liver transplant due to coagulopathy or ascites [63]. Other common indications for TJLB are obesity, failure of percutaneous biopsy, or post liver transplant.

A clear advantage of the transjugular approach is the ability to measure the hepatic venous pressure gradient (HVPG). The measurement of the HVPG has a clear application in the management of portal hypertension. A reduction in the HVPG to a value under 12 or by 20% of baseline has been shown to reduce rates of variceal bleeding and mortality [64]. The measurement of HVPG will likely be used increasingly as its utility in the management of other conditions is demonstrated. For example, there is now evidence that knowledge of the HVPG may be informative in patients with hepatitis C. In a pretransplant setting, improved HVPG measurements have been demonstrated to relate to response to therapy of chronic hepatitis C [65]. In the post-transplant setting, HVPG measurement during TJLB was evaluated as a predictor for severe HCV recurrence after transplant [66]. An HVPG of 6 mmHg or greater was found to accurately identify patients at risk of disease progression after transplant. Additionally, it has been noted that patients with cirrhosis and increased HVPG measurements were at high risk of hepatic decompensation after resection of hepatocellular carcinoma [67].

Technique

Transjugular liver biopsy is performed under fluoroscopic guidance, often by an interventional radiologist, although hepatologists have performed it as well. As with percutaneous biopsy, modest amounts of conscious sedation can be used. The patient is placed in the supine position and is given supplemental oxygen via a nasal cannula. Pulse oximetry and electrocardiographic monitoring is recommended since the passage of the catheter through the heart can trigger cardiac arrhythmias.

A local anesthetic (1% lidocaine) is injected at the puncture site (typically the right internal jugular vein). Once the internal jugular vein is accessed, a sheath introducer is placed into the vein and, under fluoroscopic guidance, a catheter is advanced to the level of the right hepatic vein. Once the hepatic vein has been adequately visualized with venography, a biopsy needle is threaded down the catheter and advanced into the liver parenchyma. Two types of needles can used in TJLB: the Menghini (aspiration) or Tru-Cut (cutting) needle. The total procedure time is usually 30–60 minutes.

Specimens

The necessity of larger biopsy specimens containing a greater number of portal tracts for the evaluation of inflammation and fibrosis has called into question the adequacy of the specimens obtained from TJLB. Traditionally, these specimens have been noted to be suboptimal in size and subject to fragmentation owing to

---

Box 3.4 Indications for transjugular liver biopsy.

- Ascites
- Coagulopathy
- Thrombocytopenia
- Fulminant hepatic failure
- Obesity
- Postoperative liver transplant
- Assessment of hepatic venous pressure gradient (HVPG)
- Refusal or failure of percutaneous biopsy

the method by which they are obtained. However, smaller sample size and fragmentation problems have been overcome since aspiration techniques have given way to Tru-Cut TJLB methods [68]. While grading of inflammation and staging of fibrosis may be impaired in smaller samples, the ability to diagnose using these specimens (i.e., sample length at least 15 mm with at least six portal tracts) does not appear to be impaired.

The adequacy of Tru-Cut-type TJLB specimens was recently evaluated [69]. With three passes; the mean length of specimens obtained was 22 mm, with 65% of samples measuring over 20 mm. Twenty-six percent of specimens obtained had the requisite 11 complete portal tracts, which may limit the utility of TJLB specimens for accurate grading and staging of hepatitis. In a follow-up study, the consequence of doing four passes as opposed to three during TJLB was evaluated [70]. Performing four passes increased the percent of specimens containing at least 11 portal tracts to 40% (as compared to 26%; $P = 0.027$). There were no reported serious complications seen. It was thus concluded that when TJLBs are needed to assess grade and stage, four passes should be used.

Few studies have compared laparoscopic, transjugular, and percutaneous techniques. However, when compared with laparoscopic and percutaneous procedures, transjugular biopsies have been found to have significantly fewer portal tracts (average portal tracts 4.3 versus 11 and 11.7, respectively) [71]. Despite this fact, when these samples were evaluated to assess the grade and stage of chronic liver disease, the investigators did not find decreased levels of grade and stage reported compared with those biopsies obtained via percutaneous or laparoscopic routes.

The consistent observation that TJLB specimens yield decreased numbers of portal tracts may limit its use in the grading and staging of chronic liver disease, however when contrasted with the risk of percutaneous biopsy in those with contraindications, TJLB provides a valuable alternative for assessment of liver histology. Consideration should be given to performing four passes if an assessment of disease severity is the goal.

Complications

Complications due to TJLB are uncommon and range from arteriovenous fistula formation with hemobilia, to hematoma at the jugular access site (Box 3.5). In a recent review of over 7,000 transjugular biopsies, major complications occurred in 0.6% of cases. The majority of complications were intraperitoneal hemorrhage (15), hepatic hematoma (4), ventricular arrhythmia (4), and pneumothorax (4). Minor complications occurred in 6.6% of cases and typically were abdominal pain, fever, or subclinical capsular perforation. Eight deaths (mortality rate, 0.09%)

Box 3.5 Complications of transjugular liver biopsy.

- Hematoma at jugular access site
- Intraperitoneal hemorrhage
- Hepatic hematoma
- Ventricular arrhythmia
- Pneumothorax
- Abdominal pain
- Subclinical capsular perforation

occurred, five were due to hemorrhage and three were due to ventricular arrhythmia [59].

Laparoscopic liver biopsy

Diagnostic laparoscopy can be performed for a variety of indications (Box 3.6). The major advantage of laparoscopy is that it allows for a direct visualization of the liver and affords us an opportunity to take directed biopsies. Diagnostic laparoscopy can be performed safely in patients with liver disease.

Indications

Due to the fact that percutaneous and transvenous biopsy methods are subject to sampling error, a laparoscopic approach can be used to study the gross appearance of the liver. A spectrum of macroscopic changes can occur in the presence of chronic liver disease. Whereas in patients with early disease the surface of the liver tends to appear smooth, in more advanced states the liver surface can appear granular. Cirrhosis is associated with diffuse nodularity and features of portal hypertension. In contrast to laparoscopic evaluation, it has been noted that percutaneously obtained liver biopsy specimens tend to understage the degree of fibrosis. In a study comparing histology with laparoscopic appearance of the liver, laparoscopic appearance was found to be 100% sensitive and 97% specific in identifying cirrhosis, compared with histological evaluation alone, which missed 6% of the cases of cirrhosis [72]. Liver biopsy, while specific for cirrhosis, may be associated with a 32%

Box 3.6 Indications for laparoscopic liver biopsy.

- Evaluation of liver disease after nondiagnostic radiologic examination
- Biopsy in patients with coagulopathy and/or thrombocytopenia
- Biopsy of discrete lesions difficult to access percutaneously
- Staging for primary hepatic tumors
- Evaluation of unexplained hepatomegaly
- Evaluation of unexplained portal hypertension
- When other less invasive modalities fail to provide a diagnosis

sampling error in the diagnosis of cirrhosis compared with laparoscopy [73].

Laparoscopy has been shown to enhance diagnostic yield not only in the case of cirrhosis, but in other disorders as well. Crantock et al. reported on 200 consecutive patients who underwent laparoscopy and biopsy [74]. Twenty-five patients had a malignancy diagnosed by the laparoscopically guided biopsy, eight of which were not seen on ultrasound prior to the laparoscopy. When compared with traditional histology, laparoscopy had >94% sensitivity and specificity at diagnosing fatty change, fibrosis, and inflammatory activity [72]. Laparoscopic appearance of the liver has also been evaluated as a prognostic indicator for treatment of chronic hepatitis C [75]. Worse macroscopic appearance was correlated with a lower sustained virological response.

When routine testing does not reveal a source for ascites, laparoscopy can be an invaluable tool for diagnosis. Laparoscopy can also identify the presence of multiple causes of ascites and is useful in obtaining peritoneal biopsies to confirm the diagnosis of malignancy or infection when suspected [76]. The diagnostic utility of laparoscopy and peritoneal biopsy has been demonstrated in several series and has determined the cause of ascites in up to 86% of cases of ascites of unclear etiology [77]. Special consideration should be given to the role of laparoscopy and peritoneal biopsy in those suspected of having tuberculous peritonitis. In a series of 14 patients with high protein content and elevated lymphocytes measured by paracentesis, all had negative Ziehl–Neelsen stains and culture of ascites after simple paracentesis [78]. Tuberculous peritonitis was only confirmed after laparoscopy demonstrated multiple white tubercles and adhesions. Biopsy specimens demonstrated caseating granulomas.

Laparoscopy can be used in the management of HCC. Diagnostically, a laparoscopic view of the liver surface may demonstrate changes suggestive of malignancy, such as hypervascular nodules and hyperemic, pigmented lesions [79]. Specific laparoscopic features, including the presence of irregular regenerative nodules, a high degree of nodular regeneration, and an atrophic right lobe, have been described to predict the development of HCC in patients with hepatitis C cirrhosis [80]. Therapeutically, laparoscopy can also be used in patients with suspected HCC to assess the extent of the primary lesion and to examine other areas for synchronous tumors [81]. In addition, it may be helpful to perform laparoscopy in patients with an elevated α-fetoprotein and unrevealing imaging studies.

Technique

Previously, patients undergoing diagnostic laparoscopic procedures were required to be admitted for observa-

tion after the procedure. Currently, outpatient diagnostic laparoscopy using conscious sedation has been demonstrated to be safe and effective [82]. Patients should receive oxygen via a nasal cannula and should be monitored during the procedure. Intravenous access is required to give conscious sedation.

With the patient in a supine position, the abdomen is prepped and draped. A Veress needle and trocar are usually placed in the left paramedian area; however, a right paramedian or subumbilical approach can be used in patients with an enlarged left hepatic lobe, splenomegaly, or previous splenectomy. A local anesthetic such as1% lidocaine is injected intradermally 2 cm above and to the left of the umbilicus. Then, a 16 gauge needle is inserted through the center of the wheal to the parietal peritoneum, which usually provokes some pain. Approximately 15–20 mL of 1% lidocaine is applied to the subcutaneous tissue and fascia within a 2 cm radius. It is important that sufficient local anesthesia be applied. A small incision is made in the center of the wheal, and the patient is asked to distend the abdominal wall without arching their back. The Veress needle is then inserted into the abdominal cavity. Aspiration with a 10 mL syringe may avoid air embolism or inadvertent entry into the intestines, both of which are rare complications [83].

Whereas carbon dioxide used for insufflation during therapeutic laparoscopy is a peritoneal irritant and provokes pain, the nitrous oxide commonly used for diagnostic laparoscopy is better tolerated [84]. Insufflation to an abdominal cavity pressure of 20 mmHg is accomplished by delivering 3–6 L of nitrous oxide through the Veress needle. A 20 mL syringe, half filled with saline solution, is then inserted and rotated within the abdominal cavity. Gas bubbles within the syringe indicate an unobstructed area for trocar placement.

The patient is then instructed to distend the abdomen, and the trocar is inserted into the peritoneal cavity. Two distinct "pops" confirm placement. An oblique-view laparoscope is then inserted into the abdominal cavity under direct vision. The area perpendicular to the scope is inspected for insertion-related damage. With the patient in the Trendelenburg position, the bladder and other pelvic structures can be visualized. Placement of the patient in the reverse Trendelenburg position allows thorough inspection of the right and left upper quadrants. A second trocar is inserted into the right midclavicular line to allow, via another laparoscope, inspection of the superior aspect of the right lobe and the delivery of accessory equipment, such as the biopsy needle and palpating probe. Liver specimens are obtained with a biopsy gun or, less commonly, a Tru-Cut needle from left of the falciform ligament, and the medial and lateral aspects of the right lobe to avoid sampling error. To avoid large blood vessels, a tangential approach to the liver left of the falciform ligament is recommended. Pressure is applied with a palpating probe on both the biopsy sites to tamponade the bleeding site and establish hemostasis. Towards the end of the procedure, the initial trocar site (left of the umbilicus) is observed using the laparoscopic camera on the right side to look for any bleeding while the trocar is being removed. If bleeding occurs at the initial trocar site, an Avotin® pellet is inserted into the site to achieve hemostasis.

After the examination is completed, the trocar and biopsy sites can be closed with Steri-strips® or by sutures if a larger incision is made to accommodate larger trocars and laparoscopes. Patients are observed for approximately 18–24 hours postprocedure and discharged to resume regular activity in 3–4 days. Right shoulder pain for 6–8 hours after the procedure is common.

As with percutaneous and transvenous biopsies, patients should avoid nonsteroidal anti-inflammatory drugs and salicylate compounds for 1 week before and after the procedure. Recommendations for patients with clotting factor and platelet count abnormalities are similar to those of percutaneous liver biopsy. Recently, the use of recombinant factor VIIa before laparoscopic liver biopsy has been reported [85]. Moreover, minilaparoscopy appeared safe in a small study of 61 patients with a platelet count less than $50,000/\mu L$ and/or an INR greater than 1.5; however most patients required the application of argon plasma coagulation directly to the liver to stop post-biopsy bleeding [86].

Advances in technology have allowed for the use of mini-laparoscopy, in which a smaller diameter trocar (1.9 mm) is used. This technique has been noted to be extremely safe, less invasive, and well tolerated by patients [87]. When compared with conventional laparoscopy, the mini-laparoscopic technique demonstrated similar success and had the advantage of a shorter procedure time [88]. When compared with a percutaneous approach, mini-laparoscopy has been noted to have the advantage of offering both macroscopic and histologic results that can improve the diagnosis of cirrhosis [89].

Laparoscopic ultrasonography is another technologic advance that has allowed for improved visualization of the liver parenchyma, targeted biopsies, and staging of both primary and metastatic hepatic lesions [90]. Performance of laparoscopic ultrasound can help to identify lesions not seen on conventional preoperative imaging and in this regard has been noted to help in avoiding unnecessary laparotomy [91]. Therapeutically, laparoscopic ultrasound can be used to direct radiofrequency ablation of unresectable lesions [92]. An exciting and recent technical advance involves an extension of the natural orifice transluminal endoscopic surgery (NOTES) procedure to perform a liver biopsy [93].

Box 3.7 Complications of laparoscopic liver biopsy.

- Pain
- Perforated viscous
- Hemobilia
- Splenic laceration
- Bleeding from biopsy site
- Ascitic fluid leak
- Abdominal wall hematoma
- Pneumoperitoneum and/or subcutaneous emphysema

Complications

A large series of 1,794 diagnostic laparoscopies done to evaluate abnormal hepatic biochemical tests, organomegaly, unexplained portal hypertension, and ascites reported that major complications occurred in only eight patients (0.44%) [83]. These major complications included perforation, hemobilia, splenic laceration, and bleeding from the biopsy site (Box 3.7). Minor complications included ascitic fluid leakage, abdominal wall hematoma, and postoperative fever. Subcutaneous emphysema and abdominal pain were observed in 31 patients (1.73%), and one death occurred.

Noninvasive markers of fibrosis

Liver biopsy remains the gold standard for histological assessment of liver disease. As the purpose of liver biopsy has changed from being simply a diagnostic test to a more comprehensive test that is able to provide pivotal information on prognosis and therapeutics, the role of liver biopsy remains central. However, because the procedure is invasive and associated with risk, and because it provides a flawed gold standard and because multiple biopsies may be necessary to chart the course of a disease, there is an obvious need to develop and use noninvasive markers of liver injury. There are currently several biochemical markers and radiographic techniques under evaluation to assess the degree of liver fibrosis in a variety of liver diseases.

Conclusions

Liver biopsy is a time-honored and safe method of evaluating diseases of the liver. Since the late 1800s, liver biopsies have aided practitioners with making accurate diagnoses. The role of biopsy has grown, and we can now glean information on prognosis and therapeutic options in a variety of liver diseases. It is clear that biopsy specimens may be subject to significant variability, and consideration should be given to that prior to performing a biopsy.

Table 3.1 Advantages and disadvantages of the different types of liver biopsy.

	Percutaneous	Transjugular	Laparoscopic
Advantages	Common procedure, widely available	Safe in those with bleeding tendency Safe in acute liver failure	Safe in those with bleeding tendency Macroscopic view Directed biopsy Peritoneal biopsy Can perform radiofrequency ablation
Disadvantages	Limited in specimen adequacy	Limited in specimen adequacy especially with suction-type needles	Infrequently performed by hepatologists in many countries Invasive
Special considerations	Ultrasound guidance	Hepatic venous pressure gradient measurement	Ultrasound guidance and evaluation
	Plugged biopsy		Therapeutic interventions

Percutaneous biopsy continues to be the most common method of obtaining liver tissue. However, when contraindications to percutaneous biopsy exist, transjugular or laparoscopic approaches offer reasonable alternatives (Table 3.1). Complications related to liver biopsy while severe in some cases are fortunately rare and in most cases are able to be managed. While the future promises to include several noninvasive markers of liver injury, it is unlikely that liver biopsy will fall by the wayside.

Further reading

Kalambokis G, Manousou P, Vibhakorn S, et al. Transjugular liver biopsy – indications, adequacy, quality of specimens, and complications: a systematic review. *J Hepatol* 2007;47(2):284–94.
A systemic review on the experience and role of transjugular liver biopsy.

Piccinino F, Sagnelli E, Pasquale G, Giusti G. Complications following percutaneous liver biopsy. A multicentre retrospective study on 68,276 biopsies. *J Hepatol* 1986;2(2):165–73.
A large amount of experience on complications related to percutaneous liver biopsy.

Rockey DC, Caldwell SH, Goodman ZD, Nelson RC, Smith AD. Liver biopsy. *Hepatology* 2009;49(3):1017–44.
Guidelines of the American Association of the Study of Liver Diseases on liver biopsy.

Vargas C, Jeffers LJ, Bernstein D, et al. Diagnostic laparoscopy: a 5-year experience in a hepatology training program. *Am J Gastroenterol* 1995;90(8):1258–62.
A large amount of experience on the safety and utility of diagnostic laparoscopy.

References

1. von Frerichs F. *Uber den Diabetes*. 1884.
2. Menghini G. One-second needle biopsy of the liver. *Gastroenterology* 1958;35(2):190–9.
3. Skelly MM, James PD, Ryder SD. Findings on liver biopsy to investigate abnormal liver function tests in the absence of diagnostic serology. *J Hepatol* 2001;35(2):195–9.
4. Polson J, Lee WM. AASLD position paper: the management of acute liver failure. *Hepatology* 2005;41(5):1179–97.
5. Dienstag JL. The role of liver biopsy in chronic hepatitis C. *Hepatology* 2002;36(5 Suppl 1):S152–60.
6. Yano M, Kumada H, Kage M, et al. The long-term pathological evolution of chronic hepatitis C. *Hepatology* 1996;23(6):1334–40.
7. Conry-Cantilena C, VanRaden M, Gibble J, et al. Routes of infection, viremia, and liver disease in blood donors found to have hepatitis C virus infection. *N Engl J Med* 1996;334(26):1691–6.
8. Shiffman ML, Diago M, Tran A, et al. Chronic hepatitis C in patients with persistently normal alanine transaminase levels. *Clin Gastroenterol Hepatol* 2006;4(5):645–52.
9. Bruno S, Shiffman ML, Roberts SK, et al. Efficacy and safety of peginterferon alfa-2a (40KD) plus ribavirin in hepatitis C patients with advanced fibrosis and cirrhosis. *Hepatology* 2010;51(2):388–97.
10. Lok AS, McMahon BJ. Chronic hepatitis B: update 2009. *Hepatology* 2009;50(3):661–2.
11. Ratziu V, Bugianesi E, Dixon J, et al. Histological progression of non-alcoholic fatty liver disease: a critical reassessment based on liver sampling variability. *Aliment Pharmacol Ther* 2007;26(6):821–30.
12. McGill DB, Rakela J, Zinsmeister AR, Ott BJ. A 21 year experience with major hemorrhage after percutaneous liver biopsy. *Gastroenterology* 1990;99(5):1396–400.
13. Takamori R, Wong LL, Dang C, Wong L. Needle-tract implantation from hepatocellular cancer: is needle biopsy of the liver always necessary? *Liver Transpl* 2000;6(1):67–72.
14. Meriden Z, Forde KA, Pasha TL, et al. Histologic predictors of fibrosis progression in liver allografts in patients with hepatitis C virus infection. *Clin Gastroenterol Hepatol* 2010;8(3).289–96, e1–8.
15. Scott DA, Netchvolodoff CV, Bacon BR. Delayed subcapsular hematoma after percutaneous liver biopsy as a manifestation of warfarin toxicity. *Am J Gastroenterol* 1991;86(4):503–5.
16. Kowdley KV, Aggarwal AM, Sachs PB. Delayed hemorrhage after percutaneous liver biopsy. Role of therapeutic angiography. *J Clin Gastroenterol* 1994;19(1):50–3.
17. Atwell TD, Smith RL, Hesley GK, et al. Incidence of bleeding after 15,181 percutaneous biopsies and the role of aspirin. *AJR Am J Roentgenol* 2010;194(3):784–9.
18. Judmaier G, Prior C, Klimpfinger M, et al. Is percutaneous liver biopsy using the Trucut (Travenol) needle superior to Menghini puncture? *Z Gastroenterol* 1989;27(11):657–61.
19. Colombo M, Del Ninno E, de Franchis R, et al. Ultrasound-assisted percutaneous liver biopsy: superiority of the Tru-Cut over the Menghini needle for diagnosis of cirrhosis. *Gastroenterology* 1988;95(2):487–9.
20. Lindor KD, Bru C, Jorgensen RA, et al. The role of ultrasonography and automatic-needle biopsy in outpatient percutaneous liver biopsy. *Hepatology* 1996;23(5):1079–83.

21. Piccinino F, Sagnelli E, Pasquale G, Giusti G. Complications following percutaneous liver biopsy. A multicentre retrospective study on 68,276 biopsies. *J Hepatol* 1986;2(2):165–73.

22. Padia SA, Baker ME, Schaeffer CJ, et al. Safety and efficacy of sonographic-guided random real-time core needle biopsy of the liver. *J Clin Ultrasound* 2009;37(3):138–43.

23. Muir AJ, Trotter JF. A survey of current liver biopsy practice patterns. *J Clin Gastroenterol* 2002;35(1):86–8.

24. Mayoral W, Lewis JH. Percutaneous liver biopsy: what is the current approach? Results of a questionnaire survey. *Dig Dis Sci* 200;46(1):118–27.

25. Gilmore IT, Burroughs A, Murray-Lyon IM, Williams R, Jenkins D, Hopkins A. Indications, methods, and outcomes of percutaneous liver biopsy in England and Wales: an audit by the British Society of Gastroenterology and the Royal College of Physicians of London. *Gut* 1995;36(3):437–41.

26. Akkan Cetinkaya Z, Sezikli M, Guzelbulut F, et al. Liver biopsy: ultrasonography guidance is not superior to the blind method. *J Gastrointest Liver Dis* 2010;19(1):49–52.

27. Riley TR, 3rd. How often does ultrasound marking change the liver biopsy site? *Am J Gastroenterol* 1999;94(11):3320–2.

28. Ahmad M, Riley TR, 3rd. Can one predict when ultrasound will be useful with percutaneous liver biopsy? *Am J Gastroenterol* 2001;96(2):547–9.

29. Pasha T, Gabriel S, Therneau T, Dickson ER, Lindor KD. Cost-effectiveness of ultrasound-guided liver biopsy. *Hepatology* 1998;27(5):1220–6.

30. Rockey DC, Caldwell SH, Goodman ZD, Nelson RC, Smith AD. Liver biopsy. *Hepatology* 2009;49(3):1017–44.

31. Riley SA, Ellis WR, Irving HC, Lintott DJ, Axon AT, Losowsky MS. Percutaneous liver biopsy with plugging of needle track: a safe method for use in patients with impaired coagulation. *Lancet* 1984;2(8400):436.

32. Kamphuisen PW, Wiersma TG, Mulder CJ, de Vries RA. Plugged-percutaneous liver biopsy in patients with impaired coagulation and ascites. *Pathophysiol Haemost Thromb* 2002;32(4):190–3.

33. Sawyerr AM, McCormick PA, Tennyson GS, et al. A comparison of transjugular and plugged-percutaneous liver biopsy in patients with impaired coagulation. *J Hepatol* 1993;17(1):81–5.

34. Atar E, Ben Ari Z, Bachar GN, et al. A comparison of transjugular and plugged-percutaneous liver biopsy in patients with contraindications to ordinary percutaneous liver biopsy and an "in-house" protocol for selecting the procedure of choice. *Cardiovasc Intervent Radiol* 2010;33(3):560–4.

35. Vuppalanchi R, Unalp A, Van Natta ML, et al. Effects of liver biopsy sample length and number of readings on sampling variability in nonalcoholic fatty liver disease. *Clin Gastroenterol Hepatol* 2009;7(4):481–6.

36. Bravo AA, Sheth SG, Chopra S. Liver biopsy. *N Engl J Med* 2001;344(7):495–500.

37. Colloredo G, Guido M, Sonzogni A, Leandro G. Impact of liver biopsy size on histological evaluation of chronic viral hepatitis: the smaller the sample, the milder the disease. *J Hepatol* 2003;39(2):239–44.

38. Schiano TD, Azeem S, Bodian CA, et al. Importance of specimen size in accurate needle liver biopsy evaluation of patients with chronic hepatitis C. *Clin Gastroenterol Hepatol* 2005;3(9):930–5.

39. Ratziu V, Charlotte F, Heurtier A, et al. Sampling variability of liver biopsy in nonalcoholic fatty liver disease. *Gastroenterology* 2005;128(7):1898–906.

40. van Leeuwen DJ, Wilson L, Crowe DR. Liver biopsy in the mid-1990s: questions and answers. *Semin Liver Dis* 1995;15(4):340–59.

41. Garcia-Tsao G, Boyer JL. Outpatient liver biopsy: how safe is it? *Ann Intern Med* 1993;118(2):150–3.

42. Janes CH, Lindor KD. Outcome of patients hospitalized for complications after outpatient liver biopsy. *Ann Intern Med* 1993;118(2):96–8.

43. Van Thiel DH, Gavaler JS, Wright H, Tzakis A. Liver biopsy. Its safety and complications as seen at a liver transplant center. *Transplantation* 1993;55(5):1087–90.

44. Eisenberg E, Konopniki M, Veitsman E, Kramskay R, Gaitini D, Baruch Y. Prevalence and characteristics of pain induced by percutaneous liver biopsy. *Anesth Analg* 2003;96(5):1392–6.

45. Riley TR, 3rd. Predictors of pain medication use after percutaneous liver biopsy. *Dig Dis Sci* 2002;47(10):2151–3.

46. Terjung B, Lemnitzer I, Dumoulin FL, et al. Bleeding complications after percutaneous liver biopsy. An analysis of risk factors. *Digestion* 2003;67(3):138–45.

47. Minuk GY, Sutherland LR, Wiseman DA, MacDonald FR, Ding DL. Prospective study of the incidence of ultrasound-detected intrahepatic and subcapsular hematomas in patients randomized to 6 or 24 hours of bed rest after percutaneous liver biopsy. *Gastroenterology* 1987;92(2):290–3.

48. Sugano S, Sumino Y, Hatori T, Mizugami H, Kawafune T, Abei T. Incidence of ultrasound-detected intrahepatic hematomas due to Tru-Cut needle liver biopsy. *Dig Dis Sci* 1991;36(9):1229–33.

49. Ormann W, Starck E, Pausch J. [Arterial embolization of an arteriovenous fistula with hemobilia after blind liver puncture]. *Z Gastroenterol* 1991;29(4):153–5.

50. Rossi P, Sileri P, Gentileschi P, et al. Delayed symptomatic hemobilia after ultrasound-guided liver biopsy: a case report. *Hepatogastroenterology* 2002;49(48):1659–62.

51. Worobetz LJ, Passi RB, Sullivan SN. Hemobilia after percutaneous liver biopsy: role of endoscopic retrograde cholangiopancreatography and sphincterotomy. *Am J Gastroenterol* 1983;78(3):182–4.

52. Le Frock JL, Ellis CA, Turchik JB, Zawacki JK, Weinstein L. Transient bacteremia associated with percutaneous liver biopsy. *J Infect Dis* 1975;131(Suppl):S104–7.

53. Larson AM, Chan GC, Wartelle CF, et al. Infection complicating percutaneous liver biopsy in liver transplant recipients. *Hepatology* 1997;26(6):1406–9.

54. Dosik MH. Bile pleuritis: another complication of percutaneous liver biopsy. *Am J Dig Dis* 1975;20(1):91–3.

55. Avner DL, Berenson MM. Asymptomatic bilious ascites following percutaneous liver biopsy. *Arch Intern Med* 1979;139(2):245–6.

56. Ruben RA, Chopra S. Bile peritonitis after liver biopsy: nonsurgical management of a patient with an acute abdomen: a case report with review of the literature. *Am J Gastroenterol* 1987;82(3):265–8.

57. Okuda K, Musha H, Nakajima Y, et al. Frequency of intrahepatic arteriovenous fistula as a sequela to percutaneous needle puncture of the liver. *Gastroenterology* 1978;74(6):1204–7.

58. Weiner M, Hanafee WN. A review of transjugular cholangiography. *Radiol Clin North Am* 1970;8(1):53–68.

59. Kalambokis G, Manousou P, Vibhakorn S, et al. Transjugular liver biopsy – indications, adequacy, quality of specimens, and complications: a systematic review. *J Hepatol* 2007;47(2):284–94.

60. Dawson MA, McCarthy PH, Walsh ME, et al. Transjugular liver biopsy is a safe and effective intervention to guide management for patients with a congenital bleeding disorder infected with hepatitis C. *Intern Med J* 2005;35(9):556–9.

61. Shin JL, Teitel J, Swain MG, et al. A Canadian multicenter retrospective study evaluating transjugular liver biopsy in patients with congenital bleeding disorders and hepatitis C: is it safe and useful? *Am J Hematol* 2005;78(2):85–93.

62. Miraglia R, Luca A, Gruttadauria S, et al. Contribution of transjugular liver biopsy in patients with the clinical presentation of acute liver failure. *Cardiovasc Intervent Radiol* 2006;29(6):1008–10.

63. Azoulay D, Raccuia JS, Roche B, Reynes M, Bismuth H. The value of early transjugular liver biopsy after liver transplantation. *Transplantation* 1996;61(3):406–9.

64. D'Amico G, Garcia-Pagan JC, Luca A, Bosch J. Hepatic vein pressure gradient reduction and prevention of variceal bleeding in cirrhosis: a systematic review. *Gastroenterology* 2006;131(5):1611–24.

65. Roberts S, Gordon A, McLean C, et al. Effect of sustained viral response on hepatic venous pressure gradient in hepatitis C-related cirrhosis. *Clin Gastroenterol Hepatol* 2007;5(8):932–7.

66. Blasco A, Forns X, Carrion JA, et al. Hepatic venous pressure gradient identifies patients at risk of severe hepatitis C recurrence after liver transplantation. *Hepatology* 2006;43(3):492–9.

67. Bruix J, Castells A, Bosch J, et al. Surgical resection of hepatocellular carcinoma in cirrhotic patients: prognostic value of preoperative portal pressure. *Gastroenterology* 1996;111(4):1018–22.

68. Bull HJ, Gilmore IT, Bradley RD, Marigold JH, Thompson RP. Experience with transjugular liver biopsy. *Gut* 1983;24(11):1057–60.

69. Cholongitas E, Quaglia A, Samonakis D, et al. Transjugular liver biopsy: how good is it for accurate histological interpretation? *Gut* 2006;55(12):1789–94.

70. Vibhakorn S, Cholongitas E, Kalambokis G, et al. A comparison of four- versus three-pass transjugular biopsy using a 19-G Tru-Cut needle and a randomized study using a cassette to prevent biopsy fragmentation. *Cardiovasc Intervent Radiol* 2009;32(3):508–13.

71. Beckmann MG, Bahr MJ, Hadem J, et al. Clinical relevance of transjugular liver biopsy in comparison with percutaneous and laparoscopic liver biopsy. *Gastroenterol Res Pract* 2009;2009:947014.

72. Jalan R, Harrison DJ, Dillon JF, Elton RA, Finlayson ND, Hayes PC. Laparoscopy and histology in the diagnosis of chronic liver disease. *Q J Med* 1995;88(8):559–64.

73. Poniachik J, Bernstein DE, Reddy KR, et al. The role of laparoscopy in the diagnosis of cirrhosis. *Gastrointest Endosc* 1996;43(6):568–71.

74. Crantock LR, Dillon JF, Hayes PC. Diagnostic laparoscopy and liver disease: experience of 200 cases. *Aust NZ J Med* 1994;24(3):258–62.

75. Bajaj JS, Molina E, Regev A, Schiff ER, Jeffers LJ. Pretreatment laparoscopic appearance of the liver can predict response to combination therapy with interferon alpha 2B and ribavirin in chronic hepatitis C. *Gastrointest Endosc* 2003;58(3):380–3.

76. Inadomi JM, Kapur S, Kinkhabwala M, Cello JP. The laparoscopic evaluation of ascites. *Gastrointest Endosc Clin N Am* 2001;11(1):79–91.

77. Chu CM, Lin SM, Peng SM, Wu CS, Liaw YF. The role of laparoscopy in the evaluation of ascites of unknown origin. *Gastrointest Endosc* 1994;40(3):285–9.

78. Rodriguez de Lope C SMJG, Pons Romero F. Laparoscopic diagnosis of tuberculous ascites. *Endoscopy* 1982;14(5):178–9.

79. Kameda Y, Shinji Y. Early detection of hepatocellular carcinoma by laparoscopy: yellow nodules as diagnostic indicators. *Gastrointest Endosc* 1992;38(5):554–9.

80. Shiraki K, Shimizu A, Takase K, Suzuki A, Tameda Y, Nakano T. Prospective study of laparoscopic findings with regard to the development of hepatocellular carcinoma in patients with hepatitis C virus-associated cirrhosis. *Gastrointest Endosc* 2001;53(4):449–55.

81. Jeffers L, Spieglman G, Reddy R, et al. Laparoscopically directed fine needle aspiration for the diagnosis of hepatocellular carcinoma: a safe and accurate technique. *Gastrointest Endosc* 1988;34(3):235–7.

82. Unal G, van Buuren HR, de Man RA. Laparoscopy as a day-case procedure in patients with liver disease. *Endoscopy* 1998;30(1):3–7.

83. Vargas C, Jeffers LJ, Bernstein D, et al. Diagnostic laparoscopy: a 5-year experience in a hepatology training program. *Am J Gastroenterol* 1995;90(8):1258–62.

84. Tsereteli Z, Terry ML, Bowers SP, et al. Prospective randomized clinical trial comparing nitrous oxide and carbon dioxide pneumoperitoneum for laparoscopic surgery. *J Am Coll Surg* 2002;195(2):173–9; discussion 9–80.

85. Jeffers L, Chalasani N, Balart L, Pyrsopoulos N, Erhardtsen E. Safety and efficacy of recombinant factor VIIa in patients with liver disease undergoing laparoscopic liver biopsy. *Gastroenterology* 2002;123(1):118–26.

86. Denzer U, Helmreich-Becker I, Galle PR, Lohse AW. Liver assessment and biopsy in patients with marked coagulopathy: value of mini-laparoscopy and control of bleeding. *Am J Gastroenterol* 2003;98(4):893–900.

87. Helmreich-Becker I, Meyer zum Buschenfelde KH, Lohse AW. Safety and feasibility of a new minimally invasive diagnostic laparoscopy technique. *Endoscopy* 1998;30(9):756–62.

88. Schneider AR, Benz C, Adamek HE, Jakobs R, Riemann JF, Arnold JC. Minilaparoscopy versus conventional laparoscopy in the diagnosis of hepatic diseases. *Gastrointest Endosc* 200;53(7):771–5.

89. Denzer U, Arnoldy A, Kanzler S, Galle PR, Dienes HP, Lohse AW. Prospective randomized comparison of minilaparoscopy and percutaneous liver biopsy: diagnosis of cirrhosis and complications. *J Clin Gastroenterol* 2007;41(1):103–10.

90. Berber E, Garland AM, Engle KL, Rogers SJ, Siperstein AE. Laparoscopic ultrasonography and biopsy of hepatic tumors in 310 patients. *Am J Surg* 2004;187(2):213–18.

91. Lo CM, Fan ST, Liu CL, et al. Determining resectability for hepatocellular carcinoma: the role of laparoscopy and laparoscopic ultrasonography. *J Hepatobiliary Pancreat Surg* 2000;7(3):260–4.

92. Santambrogio R, Podda M, Zuin M, et al. Safety and efficacy of laparoscopic radiofrequency ablation of hepatocellular carcinoma in patients with liver cirrhosis. *Surg Endosc* 2003;17(11):1826–32.

93. Tagaya N, Kubota K. NOTES: approach to the liver and spleen. *J Hepatobiliary Pancreat Surg* 2009;16(3):283–7.

CHAPTER 4

Noninvasive and Invasive Imaging of the Liver and Biliary Tract

Kunal Jajoo[1], Kevin Mennitt[2], & Ira Jacobson[3]

[1]Division of Gastroenterology, Hepatology, and Endoscopy, Brigham and Women's Hospital and Harvard Medical School, Boston, MA, USA
[2]Department of Radiology, Weill Medical College of Cornell University, New York, NY, USA
[3]Department of Gastroenterology and Hepatology, Weill Medical College of Cornell University, New York, NY, USA

Key concepts

- Ultrasonography is often the first hepatic imaging performed in patients with liver abnormalities, however it is limited by sensitivity and user dependence.
- Computed tomography (CT) and magnetic resonance imaging (MRI) are similar in sensitivity, however radiation is an issue with CT and MRI has lower spatial resolution.
- The role of positron emission tomography in liver imaging is still being investigated.
- Magnetic resonance imaging is very helpful in qualitatively and quantitatively assessing steatosis but none of the imaging modalities can accurately distinguish between steatosis and steatohepatitis.

- Magnetic resonance angiography and CT angiography have largely replaced diagnostic angiography. However catheter angiography still plays a role in equivocal cases and in conjunction with treatment.
- Endoscopic retrograde cholangiopancreatography has evolved into a primarily therapeutic procedure that allows for removal of common bile duct stones, palliation of obstructive jaundice, and treatment of biliary injury.
- Endoscopic ultrasound provides high resolution imaging of the hepatobiliary system that is complementary to cross-sectional imaging techniques and allows for fine needle aspiration for tissue or fluid acquisition.

Noninvasive imaging

Magnetic resonance imaging (MRI), computed tomography (CT), and ultrasound each have strengths and weaknesses in imaging the liver. Considerations to keep in mind are availability, clinical questions, radiation, contrast allergies, and the patient's overall health. Fortunately, technologic advances have made all of these modalities more widely available and accurate, decreasing the need for more invasive testing.

Ultrasound

Ultrasound is widely available and often the first study performed. However, relative to CT or MRI it has lower sensitivity for the diagnosis of metastatic lesions or detection of hepatocellular carcinoma (HCC). This sensitivity decreases with hepatic parenchymal abnormalities, especially cirrhosis and steatosis.

Ultrasound Doppler imaging is a method of quantifying blood flow, including direction, as well as assessing patency of vessels (Fig. 4.1). It is a fast method for the evaluation of vasculature in the post-transplant patient and monitoring for change. Doppler data can be displayed in a number of different ways including color, spectral, and power. Spectral Doppler is a tracing of the wave from peak systolic velocity, and resistive indices can be calculated. Ultrasound machines with these capabilities are standard and it is important for the clinician to indicate what questions need to be answered so that the appropriate examination is performed.

There are no absolute contraindications to ultrasound; it is very safe and without radiation. While it is recommended that the patient fast for 4–6 hours prior to the examination to decrease bowel gas, the exam can be performed at any time, with the knowledge that the images may be suboptimal in a patient who has just eaten. Morbidly obese patients can be a challenge to evaluate with ultrasound given the increased echogenicity of subcutaneous fat. Additionally, it should always be kept in mind that cirrhosis and steatosis also make the detection of liver lesions more challenging, such that a negative study may

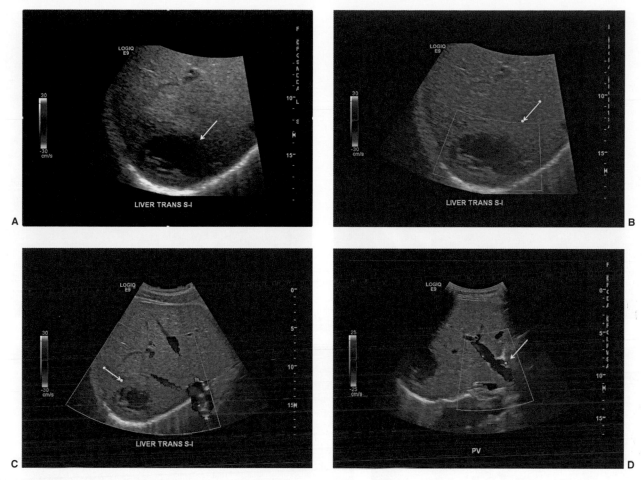

Figure 4.1 Ultrasound of the liver in a patient with hepatic abscess. (A) An irregular margined hypoechoic mass is indicated by the arrow. (B–D) Color Doppler shows no flow within the lesion (B), a patent hepatic vein (arrow) (C), and a patent portal vein (D).

still need to be followed with CT or MRI in a patient with high clinical concern of cancer.

Computed tomography

When CT was first introduced, images were obtained in a painstaking manner of one slice at a time and this is known as "conventional CT." Advances in technology have led to the ability to have the CT tube move in a continuous fashion to generate helical images. This is what is referred to as "multislice" or "helical CT." As a result, CT examinations can be performed rapidly to obtain images in multiple phases of contrast enhancement. Additionally, the acquired images are exceedingly thin (near isometric imaging) and can be manipulated to create sagittal, coronal, and 3D reconstructions (Fig. 4.2). This has become increasing important in evaluating potential living related liver donors, as accurate volumetric calculations can be made and the vasculature mapped.

Perhaps the greatest advance conferred by helical technology has been the ability to obtain post-contrast images in the arterial, portal-venous, and equilibrium (or parenchymal) phases. Hepatocellular carcinoma has an arterial blood supply such that intense enhancement occurs early. However, most metastatic lesions are seen in the later portal-venous or parenchymal phases. This multiphase imaging allows for both increased detection of lesions as well as characterization. The result is what is referred to as "temporal resolution."

It should be noted that while the CT examination only takes a few minutes (approximately 5 minutes with contrast injection), the patient's actual visit to the department will be much longer. Most centers advocate oral contrast to opacify the bowel. Patients are usually asked to ingest approximately 2 L of a barium or iodinated liquid suspension and the contrast is given 90–120 minutes prior to scanning to opacify the bowel. Patients should also be aware that an intravenous cannula will also be placed so that IV contrast can be given.

Relative contraindications include pregnancy, allergy to iodinated contrast, renal failure, or elevated creatinine, and patients with end-stage cirrhosis who are at risk

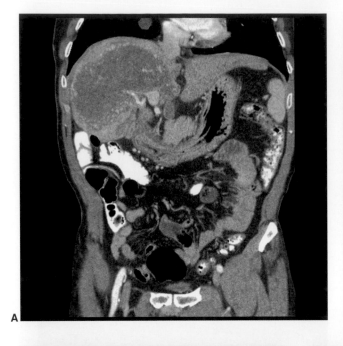
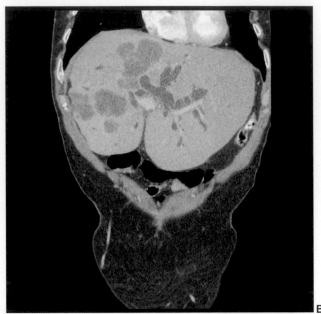
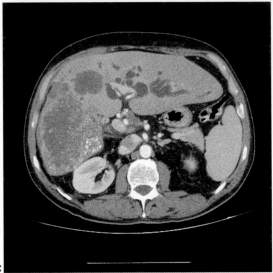
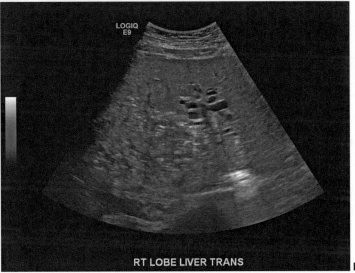

Figure 4.2 (A) Coronal contrast-enhanced CT image (reformatted from original axial images) showing a large partially calcified mass in the liver. Mucinous metastatic disease (from colon cancer) can contain dystrophic calcifications. (B) Coronal CT image from the same patient showing that not all of the metastatic lesions contain calcification, but that these are compressing and obstructing the intrahepatic biliary ducts. (C) Axial CT image showing all three findings: partially calcified mass, hypodense metastastic colonic carcinoma metastatic deposits, and secondary biliary dilatation. (D) Axial ultrasound image obtained as part of an evaluation for percutaneous biopsy and decompression of biliary obstruction.

for hepatorenal syndrome. A recent creatinine should be available prior to the patient receiving contrast.

Radiation and nephrotoxicity

Radiation from medical imaging has rightly become a major concern of patients, fueled in part by media coverage. While children and young women were initially the populations most thought to be potentially affected, with patients receiving multiple exams and living longer, radi-

ation exposure is a concern for all patients and should be kept to the minimum possible [1,2].

The millisievert (mSv) is the unit for assessing the risk of cancer from an exam, known as the effective dose. Table 4.1 lists some common radiology examinations and their associated effective doses. As dose can be altered by the CT scanner used and the settings, it should be noted that the relative dose between imaging modalities is most important. While radiology departments should

Table 4.1 Radiation doses to organs from common radiologic procedures.

Procedure	Approximate order of increasing dose
Dental X-ray (brain)	1×
Chest X-ray (one view) (chest)	10×
Mammography (breasts)	300×
Abdomen CT in adult (stomach/gastrointestinal)	1,000×
Abdomen CT in infant	2,000×

CT, computed tomography.
Adapted from Brenner and Hall [114].

have up-to-date policies ensuring a safe examination in terms of radiation dose, the radiologist is usually not familiar with the patient and may not know how many exams they have already had. Therefore, it is important for the patient's physician to be cognizant of the risk of radiation and weigh the risks and benefits of the procedure.

The newer iodinated contrast agents have osmolarity similar to that of blood. Early contrast agents were hyperosmolar but with the new near-osotonic agents decreased nephrotoxicity has been observed [3]. In patients with borderline renal function or in patients with renal insufficiency where the benefit of the exam outweighs the potential risk of contrast-induced nephropathy, N-acetylcysteine should be considered [4]. While some recent studies have questioned the utility of N-acetylcysteine in reducing contrast-induced nephropathy, it is safe and inexpensive and has not been shown to be of any harm to the patient [5].

Positron emission tomography

Positron emission tomography (PET) uses positron emitters attached to a molecule, such as glucose, to obtain a functional image. There are many positron emitters; however most are of limited clinical use because of their short half-life. Fluorodeoxyglucose (FDG) has a half-life of 110 minutes, which in practice is enough time for the pharmaceutical to be made and delivered. FDG is taken up by tissues with glucose metabolism. This glucose metabolism is generally high in cancers making them "FDG avid." However, other pathologies such as infection or inflammation will also have increased FDG uptake, which can cause diagnostic confusion [6].

While PET alone can be used, it is more usual to use a PET-CT procedure, fusing a CT examination with overlaid PET images (Fig. 4.3). This improves anatomic localization of lesions and therefore accuracy of diagnosis. Additionally, it means that patients can obtain both stud-

ies during the same visit to the radiology department. In actuality the studies are performed separately, but with the patient on the same exam table.

PET-CT is particularly useful in metastatic hepatic lesions. Patients thought to have a solitary hepatic lesion are often found to have multiple lesions on PET [7]. Thus PET often changes the stage and management of patients. Currently in the United States, Medicare pays for PET in the staging of lung, lymphoma, and melanoma; the evaluation of recurrence in melanoma and colorectal cancers; and the initial evaluation of a solitary pulmonary nodule. It is hoped that this list will expand in the future as evidence supports this modality's wider utility.

PET has been an immensely powerful tool in the diagnosis and treatment of certain tumors, such as lung and breast. Based on these experiences, it has been hoped that it would be as helpful in other cancers that are notoriously more difficult to detect and stage. Cholangiocarcinoma is one such neoplasm, which is often diagnosed after the window of opportunity for potential surgical resection. The literature has been scarce, presumably in part due to the relatively small number of cases, but a recent study indicated that PET is no better than CT alone for the detection of the primary cholangiocarcinoma [8]. This is disappointing as it was hoped that PET-CT might serve a surveillance role in patients with primary sclerosing carcinoma. However PET does appear to be clinically useful in the staging of patients with cholangiocarcinoma, as PET can better identify the involvement of regional lymph nodes and distant metastases [9].

PET has a relatively low detection rate for hepatocellular carcinoma, and more recently it has been suggested that it has limited utility in the post-transplant patient for recurrence surveillance [10,11]. Recent experience indicates that PET can be helpful in avoiding a clinically risky biopsy in cirrhotic patients with a known lesion. In this case, multiple lesions may be found and some may be more amenable to biopsy or the number of lesions may preclude treatment.

A PET-CT scan takes longer to perform than MRI, CT, or ultrasound, typically several hours. The patient will first have their blood sugar tested; elevated glucose in the blood competes with FDG and must be monitored. All patients should fast for 6 hours and diabetic patients should not take insulin prior to the exam. Patients should also refrain from exercising the day prior to the examination as the muscles will have greater than normal uptake.

Radiation dose

The increasing number of fused PET-CT scans performed, as opposed to PET alone, as well as the increasing utilization of PET, has raised concerns about its safety. The effective dose of PET-CT exceeds that of other clinically used imaging modalities [12].

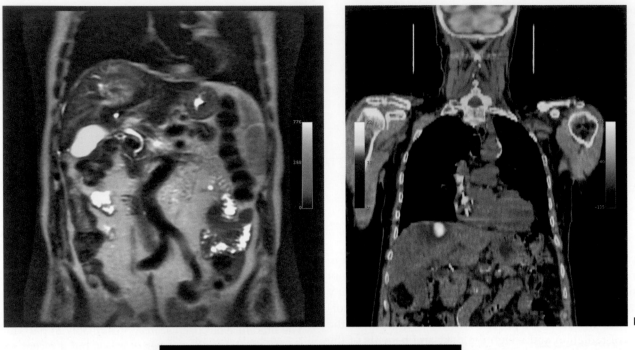

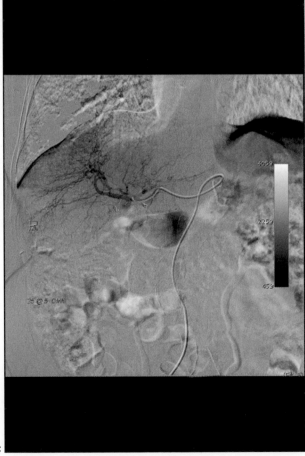

Figure 4.3 (A) MRI of the liver of a patient with known colon cancer; the coronal T2 image shows a mass suspicious for metastatic disease. (B) The patient subsequently had PET-CT to assess for further disease and this fused image shows an area of glucose avidity consistent with metastatic disease in the liver. (C) The patient subsequently underwent catheter angiography for percutaneous embolotherapy.

Magnetic resonance imaging

Magnetic resonance imaging has been increasingly used in screening and follow-up in patients with metastatic hepatic lesions and HCC (Fig. 4.4). It is important to note that while image quality has improved with newer machines, it is essential that the imaging center's knowl-edge of scanning parameters is up to date as well. For instance, changes in time to echo (T_E), time to repetition (T_R), and number of excitations (N_{EX}) must be made if the MRI is 1.5T as opposed to 3.0T (strength of magnet) to maintain image quality and ensure patient safety [13]. The main advantages of MRI over CT and PET are the

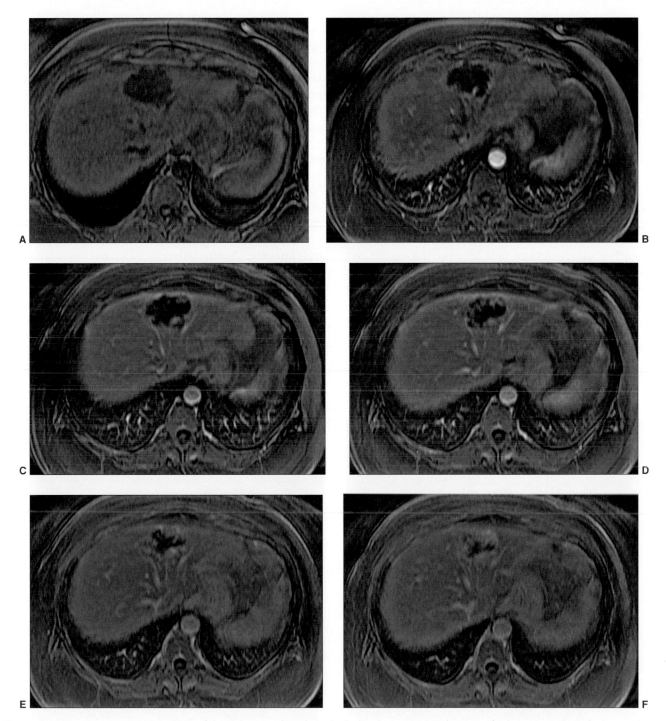

Figure 4.4 Dynamic contrast-enhanced MRI of the abdomen. A large lesion in the liver has a centripetal pattern of enhancement classic for hemangioma. Other lesions including neoplasms such as hepatocellular carcinoma and focal nodular hyperplasia have their own characteristic enhancement patterns. (A) Noncontrast; (B) early arterial phase; (C) late arterial phase; (D) portal-venous phase; (E) 90-second delay; (F) 5-minute delay.

lack of radiation and the use of relatively non-nephrotoxic contrast material (gadolinium). Compared to CT, MRI has higher contrast resolution, making lesions easier to identify, but lower spatial resolution, decreasing the conspicuousness of smaller lesions. Generally, contrast is administered during the MRI examination. The contrast agent is a form of gadolinium chelate that has a desirable safety profile when compared with iodinated contrast agents.

Contrast agents

The gadolinium-based agents can be classified into nonspecific gadolinium chelates, mixed vascular and hepatocellular-specific agents, and blood pool agents. Another group of contrast agents used in liver imaging are the superparamagnetic iron oxide particles, which are taken up by the reticuloendothelial system. For a number of reasons, including a slow infusion rate, they are not routinely used in clinical imaging.

Nonspecific gadolinium chelates are routinely used in all MRI examinations. After injection, the gadolinium distributes into the intravascular component and eventually reaches an equilibrium state between the vessels and extracellular space. As a result, tumor vascularity can be assessed. Lesions with increased vascularity appear "white" on T1-weighted images.

The perfusion/hepatocellular agents approved for use in the United States by the Food and Drug Administration (FDA) include gadobenate dimeglumine (MultiHance®, Bracco Diagnostics, Princeton, NJ) and gadoxetate disodium (Eovist®, Schering, Berlin). After distributing in the vascular interstitial compartment they are taken up by hepatocytes and excreted into the biliary system. Eovist has greater biliary excretion and is a more stable compound, however it is also more expensive, thus limiting its use [14]. In our practice, we routinely administer gadoxetate disodium during MRI examinations performed for the purpose of HCC screening. Since gadoxetate disodium is taken up by normal hepatocytes and excreted into the biliary system, it is useful in the detection of focal nodular hyperplasia (FNH) and its differentiation from hepatocellular adenoma [15]. Hepatocellular adenoma and FNH both enhance during the arterial phase of contrast-enhanced imaging. However, on delayed imaging, usually performed 20 minutes after the administration of gadoxetate disodium intravenously, the FNH will show greater enhancement than the surrounding normal hepatic parenchyma whereas the adenoma will show "wash out" or decreased relative enhancement [16]. This is because hepatic adenomas do not contain normal functional bile canaliculi, while FNH has bile ducts that may have decreased flow.

Gadofosveset trisodium (Ablavar®, Lantheus Medical Imaging, North Billerica, MA) has recently been approved by the FDA for magnetic resonance angiography as a blood pool agent. The role of Ablavar in the imaging of hepatic neoplasm has yet to be determined, so for now more conventional gadolinium preparations should be used. However, it is particularly useful in patients for whom the patency of the portal vein is in doubt after performing other imaging techniques such as ultrasound (Fig. 4.5).

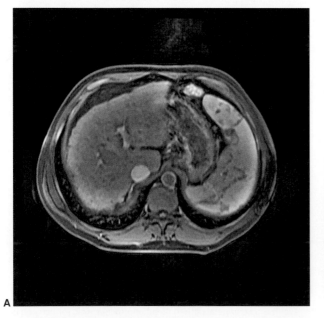 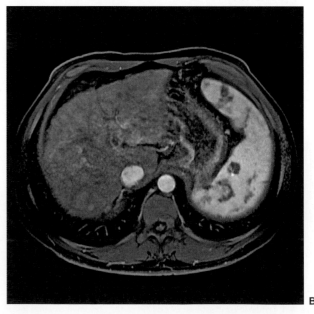

A   B

Figure 4.5 (A) MRI of the liver in a patient with a normal contrast-enhanced left portal vein. (B) Axial MRI with contrast showing tumor thrombus invading the main and right portal vein.

Recently, gadolinium chelates have been linked to nephrogenic sclerosing fibrosis when patients with impaired renal function are given high doses of gadolinium. The exact relationship of gadolinium to the development of nephrogenic sclerosing fibrosis is unclear, but caution should be used in this subset of patients [17,18]. Glomerular filtration rate (GFR) is routinely used to determine which, if any, gadolinium should be administered. For patients with a GFR greater than 60 mg/dL we simply adhere to the dosage allowed by the FDA and printed on the package insert. If the GFR is between 30 and 60 mg/dL we use the gadolinium preparation that has been shown to have the greatest stability, gadobenate dimeglumine [19]. In patients with a GFR of less than 30 mg/dL we do not administer gadolinium unless the benefits outweigh the risks. In all cases, a radiologist reviews the indications for MRI contrast before the examination is performed.

Summary of noninvasive techniques

Computed tomography and MRI are increasingly being used in evaluating patients with suspected or known liver neoplasms over ultrasound. The lack of radiation makes MRI more attractive, particularly in young patients. However, the speed of image acquisition in CT is particularly helpful in older patients or those for whom breath-holding and lying still are difficult or impossible. While CT generally requires approximately 5 minutes lying on a table, MRI takes about 15–20 minutes. The lower nephrotoxicity of gadolinium is also an advantage of an MRI examination over CT. In the selection of MRI scanners, it should be noted that so-called "open" scanners generate lower quality images as compared with the more widespread "closed bore" ones. Many manu-

facturers now offer a compromise with a larger bore magnet, often marketed as large or wide bore. A knowledge of common contraindications to MRI is most important. It is widely appreciated that small internal ferromagnetic objects, such as pacemakers and aneurysm clips, are contraindicated in MRI. If there is any doubt, the wisest approach is to use a reference such as the free online resource mrisafety.com or to reference the manufacturer's web site. Any patient with internal foreign bodies should be brought to the attention of the radiologist prior to scheduling so that the appropriate assessment is done before the patient arrives at the MRI facility.

Noninvasive imaging: selected topics

Nonalcoholic fatty liver disease

Nonalcoholic fatty liver disease (NAFLD) occurs in about 20% of people in the United States and is the most prevalent type of liver disease (Fig. 4.6) [20]. Current evidence supports the concept that NAFLD can progress to progressive hepatic fibrosis with attendant complications, including HCC [21]. Therefore, a distinction has been made between the more commonly occurring steatosis alone, which has a relatively benign prognosis, and nonalcoholic steatohepatitis (NASH), which has greater potential for progressive fibrosis [22]. The challenge then is distinguishing between steatosis and steatohepatitis in the evaluation of patients with NAFLD.

Ultrasound is sensitive for the detection of parenchymal distortion resulting from steatosis and fibrosis. In patients with moderate to severe steatosis, one study showed ultrasound to be 100% sensitive but the positive predictive value was only 62% [23]. However, the

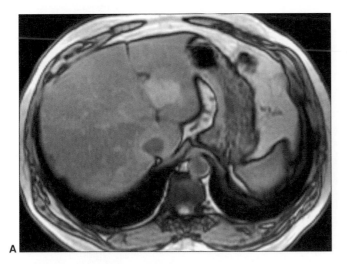
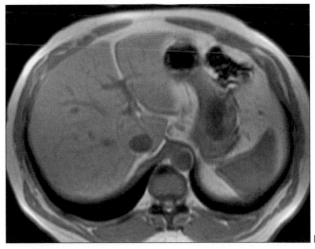

Figure 4.6 A common MRI technique to detect liver steatosis is to use in-phase and opposed-phase T1 gradient echo imaging. (A, B) Axial noncontrast images obtained at different times after the initial pulse. The image in (A) was obtained 2.1 ms earlier than the image in (B), and microscopic fat is demonstrated by loss of signal (darker) on image (A) as compared with (B).

increased echogenicity found in these and other disorders is nonspecific, limiting the accurate diagnosis of steatosis. It is widely accepted that if CT is used for the detection of steatosis, noncontrast images should be used as contrast increases the density measurements of the liver. Furthermore, the spleen is used for an internal reference and is a relatively vascular organ. MRI is the modality of choice given its sensitivity and lack of radiation. Additionally, MRI can quantify fatty deposition, which is particularly helpful in longitudinally evaluating patients during treatment [24,25]. Magnetic resonance spectroscopy is a more elegant technique for serial evaluation of steatosis, but is not as widely available or performed.

Therefore, in the absence of contraindications or expense considerations, MRI should be the initial imaging of a patient with suspected NASH. Unfortunately, distinguishing between NASH and NAFLD is more difficult. A prudent start begins with a history to discover any predisposing patient conditions, such as obesity or alcoholism. If the qualitative or quantitative MRI markers for steatosis do not normalize after change in lifestyle or diet or if there are no known risk factors, a biopsy may be warranted if physical exam and laboratory values do not reveal any clues to the etiology.

In practice, the simplest and most cost-effective imaging study to screen for steatosis is ultrasound. In a patient with steatosis and suspected liver neoplasm, MRI, given its greater lesion sensitivity and lack of radiation, should be considered [26].

Hepatic iron deposition

For many years, liver biopsy was the only way to assess hepatic iron status in patients with primary and secondary hemochromatosis. Routine CT and ultrasound are, in routine practice, ineffective in these patients. Furthermore, superconducting quantum interference device (SQUID) biomagnetic liver susceptometry testing is cumbersome and not widely available [27]. While the technique of quantifying iron using MRI is not new, there has been a recent increase in simple to use software packages and services, including those supplied by the MRI manufacturers themselves. Most importantly, the MRI methods have been validated by comparing them with liver iron concentration obtained by biopsy, the gold standard (Fig. 4.7) [28,29]. One company, Resonance Health, has marketed a product that will do everything but scan the patient and is FDA approved (Ferriscan®, Resonance Health, Claremont, Australia).

An added benefit of using MRI for liver iron concentration measurements is the ability to also quantify myocardial iron during the same MRI examination. In practice, screening for elevated iron deposition, as well as monitoring during chelation therapy, are routinely performed with MRI. Such a study does not require intravenous contrast and can be performed in less than 10 minutes, although a full liver MRI may be indicated to assess for other liver pathology.

Noninvasive hepatic vascular imaging

Ultrasonography is an excellent tool for the evaluation of hepatic vasculature. Routinely, hepatic imaging includes interrogation of the hepatic veins and portal vein, including velocity and direction of flow. This is particularly useful in evaluation for a transjugular intrahepatic portosystemic shunt (TIPS) procedure in cirrhotic patients. Prior to undergoing a TIPS procedure, a patient should undergo ultrasound with Doppler to assess the patency of the portal vein and hepatic artery. This exam is also

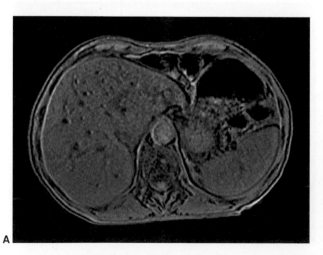 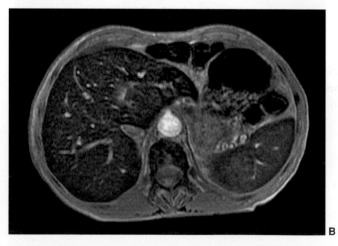

A   B

Figure 4.7 (A, B) Axial noncontrast MRI through the liver. A relatively simple MRI technique for quantifying iron in the liver utilizes the fact that the iron particles cause the signal in the liver to decrease the longer you wait to obtain the image. Image (A) was obtained milliseconds before (B), yet note how the liver signal (brightness) decreases from (A) to (B).

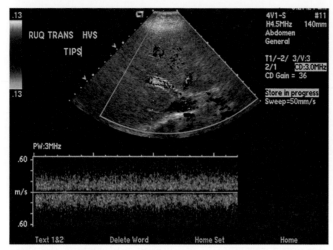

Figure 4.8 Axial ultrasound with spectral/color Doppler showing a patent TIPS.

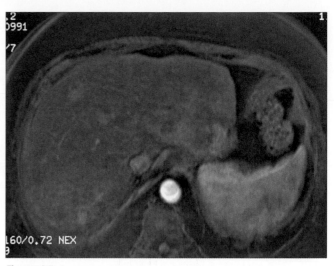

Figure 4.9 Axial post-contrast Image through the liver during a late arterial phase (about 20 seconds after giving contrast) showing a transient hepatic enhancement difference. Patches of enhancement on this axial MRI image are the result of arteriovenous shunting.

useful in examining the hepatic veins and documenting any anatomic variants. Following a TIPS procedure, ultrasound is routinely used to assess the patency and flow within the graft. A Doppler technique can be used to document the velocity as well as direction of flow in the TIPS graft.

The metallic stents commonly used in TIPS cause artifacts on all imaging modalities, but ultrasound's ability to directly evaluate the blood flow is a distinct advantage (Fig. 4.8). A newer, expandable polytetrafluoroethylene-covered stent graft (Viatorr®, Gore, Flagstaff, AZ) has shown decreased artifact and, in a recent trial, good outcomes when evaluated with CT [30].

The increasingly rapid image acquisition of new CT and MRI machines has resulted in an increased number of visualized cases of so-called "transient hepatic enhancement difference". These are almost clinically insignificant areas in the liver where there is arteriovenous shunting and are usually only seen on arterial phase imaging. However, on CT or MRI after contrast, they appear as hypervascular regions in the liver, sometimes wedge-shaped and often peripheral and commonly mistaken for neoplasm (Fig. 4.9) [31]. Arteriovenous shunts can be seen in conjunction with neoplasm; however, in this case an actual mass is identified separate from the flow phenomena. The difficulty arises in patients who have undergone single-phase contrast-enhanced CT and MRI with an area of shunting detected. In those cases a repeat exam with multiphase image acquisition after contrast should clarify the issue. Diffusion-weighted imaging has also been used to distinguish benign or nontumorous shunting from more malignant causes.

In the evaluation of patency of the hepatic veins and portal vein, CT and MRI are superb. However, in rare cases these studies can be inconclusive. In our own

experience, this occurs where there is documented portal vein thrombosis with recanalization in the past and current exams show possible revascularization of the portal vein. In these cases, we have found high resolution MRI after the administration of a blood pool gadolinium agent such as Ablavar to provide the information required. In any case of venous thrombosis, one should carefully inspect the arterial phase to assess for arterial enhancement within the vein that would indicate malignant thrombus (the neoplasm thrombus enhances earlier than a normal portal vein would expect to).

Screening for hepatocellular carcinoma

Screening for HCC commonly employs ultrasound, CT, and/or MRI, depending on the center. In Asia, in particular, there has been more interest and experience with using ultrasound. A recent review article details some of the newest ultrasound techniques, such as elastography, in the evaluation of patients with risk factors for development of HCC [32]. Despite higher financial costs, in the United States more attention has been focused on CT and MRI and faster image acquisition, and the development of novel contrast agents (particularly in MRI) have added to their appeal [33,34]. However, many physicians prefer to screen with ultrasound and then if there are abnormal findings obtain follow-up imaging with either CT or MRI.

A recently published study comparing the sensitivity of contrast-enhanced CT and MRI in detecting HCC lesions <1 cm found the sensitivity of CT to be 56–62% and the sensitivity of MRI to be 62–75% [35]. The sensitivity of ultrasound for the detection of small lesions

(<2 cm) has previously been shown to be lower than CT or MRI but a new study comparing contrast-enhanced ultrasound with MRI and CT found a 59% sensitivity for CT, 69% for contrast-enhanced ultrasound, and 76% for MRI [36]. Targeted ultrasound after positive CT or MRI showed that ultrasound without contrast had a detection rate of 36.4% for HCC lesions ≤1.0 cm, 77.6% for lesions between 1.1 and 2.0 cm, and 93.9% for lesions between 2.1 and 3.0 cm [37]. Overall, the literature suggests that MRI is most sensitive for the detection of small HCCs, with CT having slightly lower sensitivity. Ultrasound is most useful as an initial screening tool, however small lesions will be missed more commonly than if CT or MRI are utilized. Contrast-enhanced ultrasound shows promising initial results, however it is not widely used, particularly in the United States.

Primary sclerosing cholangitis

Primary sclerosing cholangitis (PSC) is a challenging disease to diagnose and follow with imaging (Fig. 4.10) [38,39]. Magnetic resonance cholangiopancreatography (MRCP) techniques continue to improve. In fact, respiratory-gated volumetric techniques have resulted

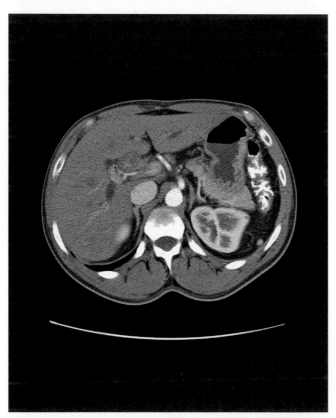

Figure 4.10 Cholangiocarcinoma complicating primary sclerosing cholangitis. Axial CT image through the liver showing dilated intrahepatic biliary ducts and a Klatskin tumor (dark nonenhancing region in the portohepatitis; the cholangiocarcinomas tend to mostly enhance late – minutes as opposed to seconds).

in 3D images of the intrahepatic and extrahepatic biliary system that rival traditional cholangiograms. In practice, endoscopic retrograde cholangiopancreatography (ERCP) and MRCP complement each other, with the former being more dynamic and user dependent and the later allowing for post-processing and reconstructions on a workstation [40].

An advantage of MRCP is the ability to perform a complete dynamic contrast-enhanced liver MRI scan at the same time with little increase in duration of the procedure. Studies utilizing newer hepatocyte-specific gadolinium agents such as gadoxetate disodium are needed as these agents can be used to generate both post-contrast MRCP images as well to potentially improve neoplasm detection rates. Unfortunately, screening for cholangiocarcinoma remains disappointing and lesions detected may not alter ultimate prognosis [41]. ERCP, and its utility in patients with PSC, will be discussed more fully in a separate section.

Choledocholithiasis

For patients with laboratory and clinical findings suggesting choledocholithiasis or cholecystitis, ultrasound is rightfully the first study of choice. Ultrasound can readily detect gallbladder wall thickening and adjacent fluid collections suggesting inflammation from obstructed bilious contents. Calculi in the gallbladder and cystic duct are easily detected, however calculi in the common bile duct are often obscured by adjacent bowel gas. When choledocholithiasis is suspected, either a nuclear medicine biliary scintigraphy scan or MRCP may be helpful, The former provides physiologic information, including possible cholestasis and obstruction. Unfortunately, information such as the number and size of obstructing stones or strictures are not available. MRCP conversely provides direct visualization of calculi along with the number of stones and their position. This information is very helpful to the endoscopist or surgeon.

MRCP uses the same MRI equipment as a routine liver MRI scan. The magnetic resonance sequences are merely tailored to better image the biliary ducts. Gadolinium contrast is not essential but some radiologists prefer to administer it routinely as part of a total abdominal MRI examination (Fig. 4.11).

CT is not a primary imaging tool for the diagnosis of cholecystitis or choledocholithiasis in our practice. However, CT has become the initial study for many patients arriving in the emergency department with abdominal pain and many hospitals do not have 24/7 access to nuclear medicine or MRI equipment. Fortunately, most calculi are visualized on CT and secondary signs and complications (e.g., abscess, gangrenous gallbladder) are readily detected.

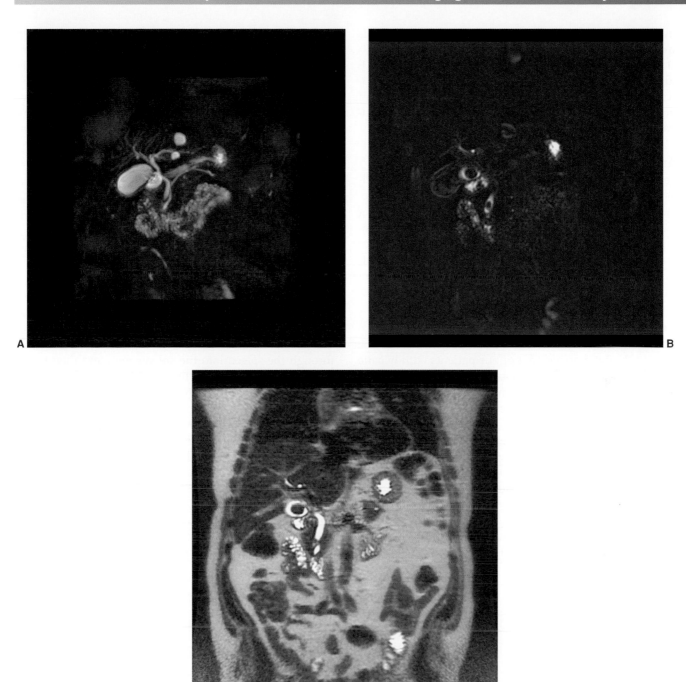

Figure 4.11 Choledocholithiasis. (A) The calculi in the gallbladder neck and common bile duct are difficult to see on this 3D reconstruction. (B) However, when only a portion of the 3D volume set is reviewed, the calculi are easily visualized. (C) A single coronal T2-weighted image also clearly shows the gallbladder neck and distal common bile duct stones.

Invasive imaging of liver and biliary disease

Noninvasive and minimally invasive imaging and procedures have undergone technologic advances in the past few years with noninvasive CT angiography (CTA) and magnetic resonance angiography (MRA) assuming larger roles in diagnosis, and catheter and percutaneous tools pushing the envelope of treatment.

Many percutaneous interventional procedures have been developed to ablate hepatic malignancies, including hepatocellular carcinoma. While selective internal radiation therapy (SIRT) continues to develop, transarterial chemoembolization (TACE) percutaneous ablative tools are more firmly established and are routinely used in radiology departments [42,43]. Recent experience with TACE suggests that it is not only helpful as a bridge until hepatic transplant can be performed but also as a course of treatment for those in whom surgery or transplant is contraindicated [44].

Angiography

Perhaps one of the largest changes in interventional radiology over the past decade has been the continued refinement of MRA, CTA, and Doppler ultrasound allowing high resolution imaging to replace catheter-based angiography. Aside from being noninvasive, these technologies are generally cheaper and also provide information outside the vessels. They can be performed as part of or concurrent with CT or MRI that is already being performed.

Hepatic arteriography

Hepatic arteriography continues to play a role in the state-of-the-art management of our patients with hepatic diseases. Catheter sizes continue to become smaller and more agile allowing the interventionist the ability to selectively inject very small vessels. In turn, this allows the rapid acquisition of images once contrast is administered such that a small area of the liver is evaluated. This is particularly helpful in cases where a MRA or CTA study is inconclusive. Further, if a suspected neoplasm is found it can be treated at the same sitting with catheter-guided embolotherapy (Fig. 4.12).

The contrast administered with catheter studies is the same used for CTA, thus care should be taken to minimize the contrast load if both procedures are done. In the past, patients with renal insufficiency who required catheter-based angiography may have received gadolinium chelate contrast as opposed to iodinated contrast to decrease the risk of contrast-induced nephropathy. However, given the association of nephrogenic systemic fibrosis (NSF) and large doses of gadolinium in the patient with renal insufficiency, this practice has become less common.

Portal and hepatic venography

There are several techniques the interventionist can use to opacify the portal vein (portography) including arteriographic portography, transvenous portography, transabdominal–transhepatic portography, and transabdominal–transplenic portography (Fig. 4.13). The latter two, as the names imply, require localization of the vein or spleen prior to the percutaneous introduction of a catheter. Thus they can be somewhat cumbersome. A catheter placed in the splenic artery via an initial femoral access is simpler – the contrast is injected and travels through the spleen into the splenic vein and then to the portal vein. There is very limited dilution of the contrast and excellent opacification of the portal vein is achieved through this indirect portography approach.

In practice, portography remains important as portal vein pressures can be obtained in the preoperative patient requiring either TIPS or surgical decompression. After TIPS, of course, the stent and portal vein can be easily catheterized via a transjugular approach. Prior to TIPS, portal pressure can be acquired by a transvenous approach. A catheter is introduced retrogradely into small splenic venous branches from an initial jugular approach. Wedge pressures are obtained after injection of carbon

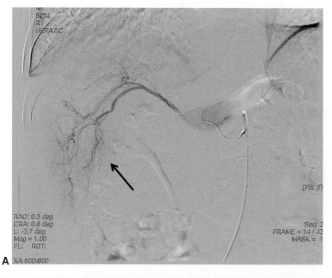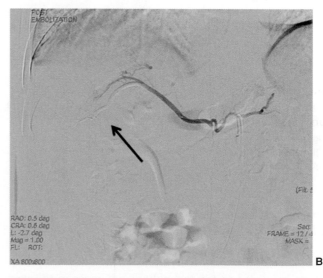

Figure 4.12 Hepatic catheter angiography. (A) Catherization of a branch of the right hepatic artery demonstrating tumor blush in this patient with hepatocellular carcinoma. (B) Postembolization shows no arterial enhancement of the mass.

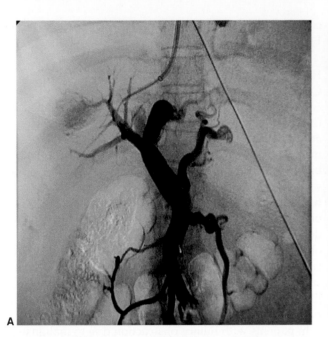
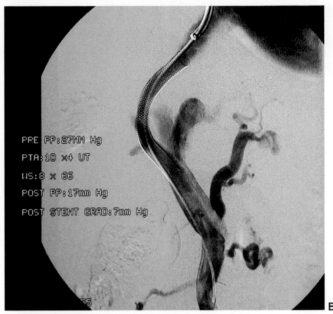

Figure 4.13 (A) Portal venogram with the catheter tip in the superior mesenteric vein demonstrating a prominent collateral vasculature extending from the superior and inferior mesenteric veins as well as a prominent coronary vein. (B) Post-TIPS portal venogram. A stent is identified traversing the right portal and hepatic veins. A repeat venogram demonstrates decreased collateral vasculature within the portal system.

dioxide. Contrast images of the portal vein can also be obtained by retrograde filling of small portal veins via their proximity to capillary veins. Improved techniques and operator experience have decreased complications, but systematic attention to detail and utmost care are essential to ensure patient safety [45].

Percutaneous transhepatic cholangiography

Similar to any percutaneous therapy, percutaneous transhepatic cholangiography (PTHC) is not without risks, including iatrogenic cholangitis, infection, and bleeding. Endoscopic methods of evaluating the bile ducts and, more recently, the continued improvement of MRCP techniques have led to a decrease in the number of PTHC procedures done. Most recently, certain gadolinium chelates such as gadobenate dimeglumine (MultiHance) and gadoxetate disodium (Eovist) have been developed and are partially excreted into the bile ducts. Delayed (20 minutes or later) T1 images produce contrast-enhanced bile ducts. However, this technique has not yet been proven to be superior to T2 MRCP sequences.

A patient who is to undergo PTHC should be properly prepped. This includes a thorough physical examination and history taking. In particular, signs of clotting disorder should be sought as well as uncovering any medications that may prolong the bleeding time. History of allergies should be also elicited and proper preprocedure antibiotic therapy should be administered to cover both Gram-positive and Gram-negative flora. Consultation with infectious disease professionals may be warranted for adequate prophylaxis.

Articles pictorializing the "characteristic" findings of benign versus malignant strictures and filling defects have been widely published. However, the accuracy of distinguishing these entities is far from satisfactory. Therefore, care should be taken to adequately scrutinize any pathology and make certain that air bubbles do not complicate the matter. In the presence of biliary obstruction, most radiologists choose to exchange the diagnostic catheter for a percutaneous drainage tube as there is often high pressure and inflammation as a result of the stasis. More definitive treatment can be attempted several days later, including internalization of the drain (Fig. 4.14).

Endoscopic imaging of the hepatobiliary system

Endoscopic imaging of the liver and biliary tree by ERCP and endoscopic ultrasound (EUS) complements the clinical information obtained by the radiologic modalities described above and allows for further evaluation and treatment of a variety of hepatobiliary abnormalities. Suspected choledocholithiasis can be confirmed or excluded by EUS and treated by ERCP with sphincterotomy. Biliary strictures seen on MRCP can be evaluated and sampled by ERCP with choledochoscopy to differentiate between

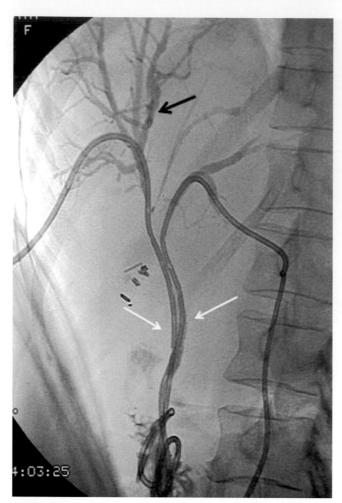

Figure 4.14 Patient with cholangiocarcinoma with intrahepatic biliary ductal dilatation (black arrow) who underwent percutaneous placement of biliary drains (left and right indicated by white arrows). The catheters drain both internally into the duodenum and externally.

benign and malignant processes, or further visualized by EUS and sampled by fine needle aspiration, depending upon the clinical situation. In this way, noninvasive radiologic imaging and minimally invasive endoscopic imaging can be used in conjunction to arrive at the final diagnosis and often provide the definitive therapy.

Endoscopic retrograde cholangiopancreatography

First described in 1968, ERCP provides minimally invasive access to the biliary tree and pancreatic duct to diagnose and treat a wide variety of pancreatobiliary diseases. The introduction of endoscopic sphincterotomy in 1974 allowed for the development of an increasing array of therapeutic modalities [46,47]. Technologic enhancements in MRI, particularly MRCP, have led to the evolution of ERCP from a diagnostic to a primarily therapeutic pro-

cedure. The following section will focus upon the use of ERCP in hepatobiliary disorders.

Hepatobiliary indications

Codified indications for ERCP have been set forth in a consensus statement by the National Institutes of Health (NIH) [48] and a practice guideline by the American Society of Gastrointestinal Endoscopy (ASGE) [49]. The primary indication for ERCP is the treatment of symptomatic biliary obstruction (Box 4.1). In patients who present with jaundice, the delineation between biliary obstruction and other forms of cholestasis is usually made based on clinical history and noninvasive imaging. When choledocholithiasis is found to be the likely cause of biliary obstruction, urgent ERCP for stone extraction is indicated (within 48 hours) when cholangitis or severe acute pancreatitis with persistent ampullary obstruction is present. ERCP is not indicated in mild or moderate acute gallstone pancreatitis without cholangitis [50,51].

In patients with biliary obstruction due to malignancy, ERCP is not required in all cases. Intractable pruritus, cholangitis, and cholestasis preventing the administration of chemotherapy are clear indications for biliary decompression by ERCP. Recent studies have demonstrated that routine ERCP for preoperative biliary decompression of malignant obstruction due to pancreatic cancer is not universally indicated as it is associated with increased morbidity [52,53]. In patients with malignant biliary obstruction who are deemed unresectable, endoscopic biliary decompression is safe and effective and results in less morbidity than palliative surgical by-pass [54]. Self-expanding metal stents are superior to plastic stents for this palliative application [55].

Endoscopic therapy is the preferred treatment modality for postoperative biliary leaks and strictures. The high volume of laparoscopic cholecystectomy and the increasing frequency of liver transplantation have been associated with an increased prevalence of these biliary disorders. Previously, altered surgical anatomy such as Roux-en-Y reconstruction, Whipple resection, and

---

Box 4.1 Indications for endoscopic retrograde cholangiopancreatography (ERCP).

- Obstructive jaundice
- Cholangitis
- Choledocholithiasis
- Severe acute gallstone pancreatitis with persistent ampullary obstruction
- Postoperative or traumatic biliary complications (i.e., leak, stricture)
- Evaluation of the sphincter of Oddi in patients with moderate to high suspicion of sphincter dysfunction

Billroth II anastomosis precluded or greatly hindered the ability to perform ERCP. With the advent of balloon enteroscopy, ERCP can be performed with a greater rate of success in patients with altered enteral anatomy [56].

Recurrent biliary pain or recurrent acute pancreatitis in the absence of gallstones or after cholecystectomy can be caused by sphincter of Oddi dysfunction (SOD). In patients with SOD who demonstrate elevated serum liver tests, a dilated common bile duct, and poor biliary drainage (type I SOD), endoscopic sphincterotomy is effective. In patients with one or two of these clinical findings (type II SOD), sphincter of Oddi manometry should be used to determine if basal sphincter pressures are elevated above 40 mmHg and only then should sphincterotomy be performed. Patients with SOD who do not demonstrate any of these objective findings (type III SOD) should be treated conservatively.

Complications

Endoscopic retrograde cholangiopancreatography carries a higher risk of complications than most other gastrointestinal endoscopic procedures. In 1991, a consensus conference was convened to establish a classification system of ERCP-related complications that would be used for future study (Table 4.2) [57].

In the largest single-center study to date [58], the outcomes of almost 11,500 ERCP procedures were analyzed for rate and predictors of complications. The overall complication rate was 4.0%, with severe complications in 0.36% of cases. Pancreatitis occurred in 2.6% of cases and bleeding in 0.3%. Independent predictors of complications by multivariate analysis included suspected

SOD and biliary sphincterotomy. Independent predictors of post-ERCP pancreatitis included performance of a pancreatogram and suspected SOD. Severe complications were associated with co-morbid illness, obesity, choledocholithiasis, pancreatic manometry, and complex interventions. Placement of a prophylactic small diameter pancreatic stent and the presence of pancreatitis prior to the ERCP were each independent predictors of fewer overall complications. Perforation occurred in only 16 patients, too few to perform multivariate regression analysis.

Pancreatitis is the most common complication of ERCP. Patients present with epigastric pain radiating to the back and are found to have elevated serum pancreatic enzymes greater than three times the normal value. The rate of post-ERCP pancreatitis ranges from 1% to 7% in large studies. Elevation of serum amylase is common after ERCP and in the absence of concurrent abdominal pain is neither predictive nor diagnostic of post-ERCP pancreatitis [59]. In addition to the factors listed above, normal serum bilirubin, difficult or failed cannulation, history of post-ERCP pancreatitis, pre-cut sphincterotomy, pancreatic sphincterotomy, and younger age of patient have each been shown to be risk factors for post-ERCP pancreatitis in multivariate analysis [60].

A multitude of pharmacologic agents have been studied for the prevention of post-ERCP pancreatitis including corticosteroids, nonsteroidal anti-inflammatory drug (NSAID) suppositories, antisecretory agents such as octreotide and somatostatin, protease inhibitors such as gabexate and ulinstatin, and other medications with inconsistent results. Suppository NSAIDs such as diclofenac seem to have the most promise, including

Table 4.2 Grading system for the major complications of ERCP and endoscopic sphincterotomy.

Complication	Mild	Moderate	Severe
Pancreatitis	Amylase at least three times normal at more than 24 hours after the procedure, requiring admission or prolongation of planned admission to 2–3 days	Hospitalization of 4–10 days	Hospitalization of more than 10 days, hemorrhagic pancreatitis, phlegmon or pseudocyst, or intervention required (percutaneous drainage or surgery)
Bleeding	Clinical evidence of bleeding, hemoglobin drop <3 g, and no need for transfusion	Transfusion (4 units or less), no angiographic intervention or surgery	Transfusion (5 units or more), or intervention required (angiographic or surgical)
Cholangitis	>38°C for 24–48 hours	Febrile or septic illness requiring more than 3 days of hospital treatment or endoscopic or percutaneous intervention	Septic shock or surgery
Perforation	Possible, or only very slight leak, treatable by conservative management for 3 days or less	Any definite perforation treated medically for 4–10 days	Medical treatment for more than 10 days, or intervention required (percutaneous or surgical)

Adapted from Cotton et al. [57] with permission from Elsevier.

in meta-analysis [61], but its routine use has not been adopted to date. Placement of a prophylactic pancreatic duct stent during difficult procedures reduces the risk of pancreatitis and also reduces the risk of pancreatitis being severe should this complication occur. The optimal type of stent, and precise indications for use of this prophylactic measure, are yet to be determined [62].

Clinically significant post-sphincterotomy hemorrhage can occur in up to 2% of cases and can be seen as late as 10 days after the procedure. Thrombocytopenia, coagulopathy, and initiation of anticoagulants within 3 days of sphincterotomy are risk factors for post-sphincterotomy hemorrhage [63]. Aspirin and NSAIDs have not been shown to increase the risk of hemorrhage in this setting. There are insufficient published data to determine if antiplatelet agents such as clopidogrel increase this risk [64].

Perforation is rare during ERCP, reported in less than 1% of cases. Perforation can occur due to excess extension of a sphincterotomy, trauma from the endoscope, or migration of stents or guidewires. Bowel wall perforation is much more likely to occur in patients who have a history of biliary diversion surgery such as a Whipple resection [58]. Retroperitoneal perforation from sphincterotomy is the most common type of perforation resulting from ERCP, and can generally be managed conservatively with antibiotics and withholding oral feeding. However, surgery may be necessary for large perforations or for failure to improve after initial conservative management. Other infrequent complications of ERCP include cholecystitis, cholangitis, and papillary stenosis

Technique

Selective cannulation of the biliary tree requires high-volume training in order to opitimize the success rate and minimize the complication rate. ASGE training guidelines state that gastroenterology fellows must complete 180 ERCP procedures, with one half utilizing therapeutic modalities, to achieve competency. This generally requires 12 months dedicated to advanced techniques, either integrated within the traditional 3-year gastroenterology fellowship or, increasingly, in a dedicated additional (fourth) year advanced fellowship [65].

After obtaining informed consent by discussing the risks, benefits, and alternatives to the planned procedure, the patient is placed in the prone position with the head facing the endoscopist ("swimmer's position"). Sedation for ERCP varies broadly across regions ranging from moderate sedation with a benzodiazepine (midazolam) and a narcotic (fentanyl) to deep sedation with propofol to general anesthesia. There is an overall trend toward the more routine use of propofol and general anesthesia. Continuous monitoring of blood pressure, pulse rate, cardiac rhythm, and pulse oximetry is performed as in other endoscopic procedures. Additional respiratory monitoring by capnography has been shown to improve patient safety during ERCP [66].

The biliary tree is cannulated through the major papilla with a cannula or sphincterotome passed through a side-viewing duodenoscope. The duodenoscope allows an en face view of the major papilla, thereby facilitating visualization and cannulation (Fig. 4.15). The majority of patients will have a single ampullary orifice with a short common channel that bifurcates into the common bile duct and the main pancreatic duct. Conventional cannulation involves injection of contrast when the catheter is positioned toward the bile duct. An alternative method involves advancing a hydrophilic tip guidewire and achieving biliary cannulation prior to injecting contrast. We favor the latter approach as this has been shown

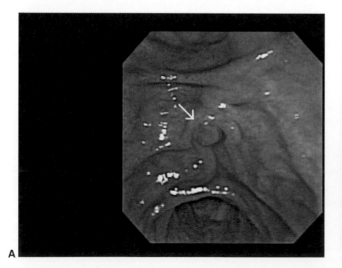
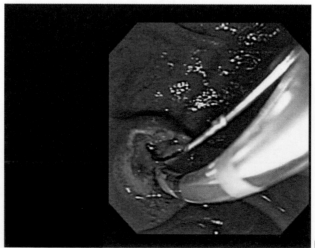

Figure 4.15 (A) Endoscopic view of a normal major papilla (white arrow). (B) Endoscopic view during sphincterotomy.

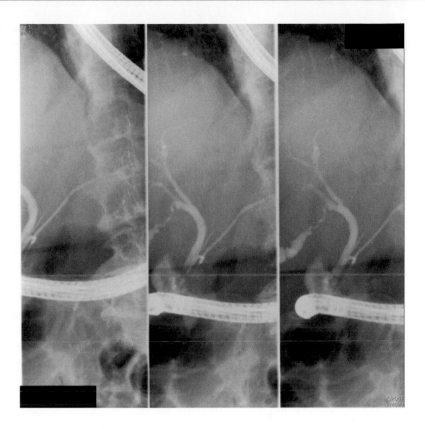

Figure 4.16 Normal ERCP image.

to decrease the risk of post-ERCP pancreatitis, likely by minimizing unintended contrast injection into the pancreatic duct and minimizing trauma to the papilla [67]. Once biliary access is achieved, sphincterotomy and additional therapeutic modalities can be utilized.

Much debate persists regarding the routine use of antibiotics to prevent infection in patients undergoing ERCP. Practice guidelines have been set forth by the ASGE and rely heavily upon expert opinion [68]. These guidelines recommend antibiotic prophylaxis be used when: (i) complete biliary drainage may not be achieved (hilar obstruction, primary sclerosing cholangitis); (ii) incomplete biliary drainage after ERCP; and (iii) drainage of post-transplant biliary strictures is being attempted. These guidelines do not recommend the use of prophylactic antibiotics when complete biliary drainage is expected or biliary obstruction is not suspected.

Cholangiogram

With the evolution of ERCP from a diagnostic to a primarily therapeutic procedure, an entirely normal cholangiogram is seen less frequently than previously. Despite this, it is important to fully understand the normal expected anatomy in order to interpret abnormalities. A scout film is obtained in many centers to demonstrate any tubes, drains, surgical clips, calcifications, or stents. The distal common bile duct fills readily once cannulation is achieved. The normal caliber of the common bile duct after contrast injection ranges from 3 to 9 mm. With the patient in the usual prone position the left main hepatic duct fills preferentially due to gravity. The patient's position may need to be altered or the cannula or a balloon selectively placed in order to achieve filling of the right posterior and right anterior ducts. The cystic duct insertion point can vary significantly from patient to patient (Fig. 4.16).

Choledochoscopy

Very thin endoscopes have been developed to allow direct visualization of the biliary tree (Fig. 4.17). These scopes are advanced through the working channel of the duodenoscope and into the common bile duct for additional evaluation of biliary strictures and treatment of large stones with choledochoscopy. The newest instruments are capable of four-way tip deflection with wheels analogous to those of the duodenoscope and have their own working channels to allow for intraductal biopsy and irrigation

Choledocholithiasis

In the National Health and Nutrition Examination Survey (NHANES III) of 1999, it was estimated that 20 million Americans have gallstone disease [69]. It is estimated that 15–20% of patients with gallstones will have or develop choledocholithiasis. The natural history of choledocholithiasis is not fully understood. While some patients can pass small common bile duct (CBD) stones

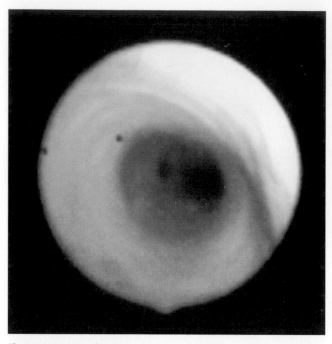

Figure 4.17 Normal endoscopic choledochoscopy.

without symptoms, others can develop life-threatening cholangitis and/or severe acute pancreatitis [70]. Determining which patients are most likely to have CBD stones allows for prompt treatment and avoidance of unnecessary ERCP and its attendant risks.

Several studies have evaluated the clinical predictors that indicate the presence of choledocholithiasis. The strongest predictors in patients with suspected CBD stone(s) include a dilated common bile duct on sonogram (>6 mm), advanced age, and pattern of liver enzyme elevation. In patients with clinically suspected choledocholithiasis whose serum liver enzymes normalized prior to ERCP, the likelihood of recovering a CBD stone at ERCP is less than 13%; whereas in patients with rising serum liver enzymes, the likelihood of a CBD stone is greater than 90% [71]. MRCP is highly sensitive and specific in detecting CBD stones and is particularly useful in those patients who demonstrate intermediate risk of having a CBD stone. A recent meta-analysis demonstrated that MRCP has a pooled sensitivity of 95% for the detection of biliary obstruction and 92% for the detection of a CBD stone. The accuracy of MRCP diminishes with stones that are smaller than 5 mm and in the presence of pneumobilia and surgical clips [72]. Endoscopic ultrasound demonstrates equally high sensitivity and specificity as MRCP, can prevent unnecessary ERCP [73], and is an excellent minimally invasive alternative for those patients who cannot undergo MRI due to the presence of a permanent pacemaker or automated implantable cardioverter-defibrillator.

In patients with choledocholithiasis seen on imaging or a high suspicion of such, as described above, ERCP with endoscopic sphincterotomy and stone extraction should be performed promptly. CBD stones are seen as a filling defect on an endoscopic cholangiogram (Fig. 4.18A). Sphincterotomy is performed by bowing the sphincterotome in order to bring the cutting wire into contact with the roof of the papilla and electrocautery is applied, generally with a blend of high cutting current and low coagulation current, along the direction of the bile duct. The bile duct is outlined by the longitudinal bulge above the ampullary orifice corresponding to the intramural

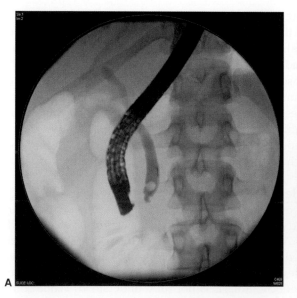

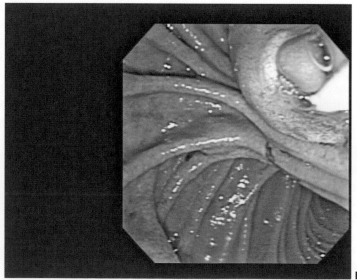

Figure 4.18 (A) ERCP demonstrating a distal common bile duct stone. (B) Endoscopic view of stone extraction.

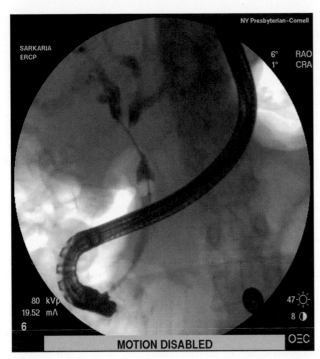

Figure 4.19 ERCP showing obstruction at the hepatic hilum in a patient with cholangiocarcinoma. (Courtesy of Dr Savreet Sarkaria, Weill Cornell Medical College.)

balloon or Dormia basket can be used to remove the stone (Fig. 4.18B). In difficult or multiple stones, mechanical lithotripsy with a crushing basket or electrohydraulic lithotripsy may be necessary. Alternatively, a plastic biliary stent can be placed to allow for slow fragmentation by mechanical erosion, which is removed in approximately 2 months. This has been shown to have a success rate of 90% in patients with multiple or large stones [76]. In patients who are deemed unfit for surgery, these therapeutic modalities significantly reduce the risk of recurrent biliary pancreatitis and cholangitis, but not cholecystitis.

Malignant biliary obstruction

Malignant biliary obstruction is generally detected by cross-sectional imaging performed in patients presenting with jaundice. This obstruction may be caused by cholangiocarcinoma within the bile duct (Fig. 4.19), adjacent pancreatic cancer (Fig. 4.20), or hepatic metastases obstructing the hilum or intrahepatic ducts. ERCP, often in conjunction with EUS, can be used to obtain a tissue diagnosis and treat these obstructing lesions. Once the level of obstruction is identified on cholangiography, a cytology brush can be used to sample the stricture for microscopic analysis. The cytologic yield is fairly low (~35%), but can be increased by using multiple brushes or adding intraductal biopsies. In addition, advanced imaging and molecular techniques have been developed to increase yield. These include choledochoscopy with a miniature scope advanced through the duodenoscope; intraductal ultrasound; digital image analysis (DIA); and fluorescence in situ hybridization (FISH). These

portion of the distal bile duct [74]. In patients who are at increased risk of bleeding due to anticoagulants, antiplatelet agents, or cirrhosis, balloon sphincteroplasty can be utilized instead. This carries a higher risk of pancreatitis than endoscopic sphincterotomy (relative risk, 1.95) [75]. Once the sphincter is ablated, an extraction

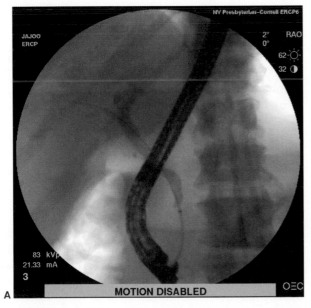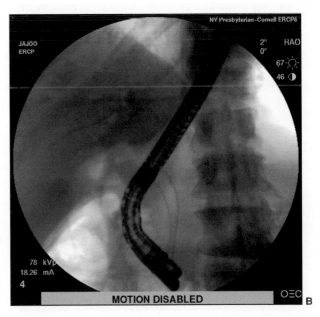

Figure 4.20 ERCP. (A) Obstruction of the distal bile duct by a mass in the head of the pancreas. (B) Immediately after the placement of a self-expanding metal stent (SEMS); note the narrowing of the stent at the level of the mass.

modalities significantly improve the diagnostic yield of indeterminate stricture sampling [77].

Endoscopic therapy of malignant biliary obstruction primarily involves stent placement for decompression. In patients who may be surgical candidates for resection, or for whom the clinical staging is incomplete at time of ERCP, 10 or 11.5 Fr temporary plastic stents are placed across the stricture. These stents generally occlude after about 3–4 months and must be replaced preemptively or removed at the time of surgery. In patients who are not candidates for resection and the diagnosis of malignancy is confirmed, self-expanding metal stents (SEMS) are placed across the obstruction for palliation. Metal stents have higher patency rates extending to 12 months and beyond and are cost-effective, averting the need for repeat ERCP stent change procedures. A multitude of SEMS are commercially available in various sizes. The size of the stent is determined by the endoscopist at the time of ERCP, taking into account the length and location of obstruction. Uncovered metal stents can occlude due to mucosal hyperplasia and tumor ingrowth, prompting the development of covered metal stents. In the studies available to date, there is a trend toward higher patency rates, but increased rates of stent migration and cholecystitis have been seen with covered metal stents [55].

Primary sclerosing cholangitis

Primary sclerosing cholangitis is an idiopathic, progressive cholestatic disease of the biliary tree that is characterized by diffuse structuring, dilatation, and beading of the bile ducts on cholangiography (Fig. 4.21). The vast

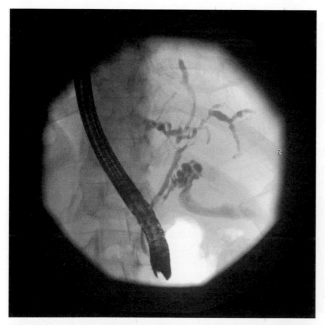

Figure 4.21 ERCP showing intra- and extrahepatic beading and stricturing of PSC. (Courtesy of Dr S. Ian Gan, Virginia Mason Medical Center.)

majority of patients with PSC have concomitant ulcerative colitis. Conversely, approximately 5% of patients with ulcerative colitis will develop PSC. The inflammation and fibrosis of PSC results in cirrhosis and portal hypertension, and predisposes patients to cholangiocarcinoma, with a lifetime risk of 10–15%. This risk may be higher in patients with ulcerative colitis or cirrhosis [78,79]. The natural history of PSC is variable. In recent studies, the median time to death or liver transplantation is approximately 10–18 years from time of diagnosis [80,81]. ERCP was instrumental in the initial understanding of the disease, but MRCP has supplanted ERCP in the initial diagnosis of suspected PSC given the very low risk profile and equivalent diagnostic performance characteristics [82]. The major roles of ERCP in patients with PSC are in the diagnosis of suspected progression to cholangiocarcinoma and to provide biliary drainage in selected patients with dominant strictures (see below) or choledocholithiasis.

A clinical subset of patients with PSC will develop a dominant stricture leading to jaundice, pruritus, and recurrent bouts of acute cholangitis. This is felt to result in further progression of the disease. Endoscopic stricture dilatation and stent placement have been studied as minimally invasive treatment modalities for this type of symptomatic dominant stricture. Balloon dilatation and short- or long-term stent placement have been shown to result in improved liver chemistries, improved pruritus, and improved appearance of the cholangiogram [83,84]. Controlled prospective studies are not available, therefore it remains unclear which treatment modality has greatest efficacy. As discussed above, antibiotic prophylaxis should be given in patients undergoing ERCP for PSC. Unfortunately, this prophylaxis does not eliminate the risk of procedure-related cholangitis [85].

The nonoperative diagnosis of cholangiocarcinoma in patients with PSC can be elusive. Brush cytology during ERCP demonstrates a sensitivity of approximately 50%. Combining serum carbohydrate antigen 19-9 (CA 19-9) results, radiologic imaging, brush cytology, and molecular techniques such as DIA and FISH increases this sensitivity to 86% [86]. Despite these advances, screening for cholangiocarcinoma has not been demonstrated to improve outcomes in patients with PSC and routine screening is not recommended at this time.

Biliary complications of cholecystectomy

Laparoscopic cholecystectomy is one of the most common surgical procedures performed worldwide. Biliary leaks are more common with laparoscopic cholecystectomy than open cholecystectomy, occurring in approximately 1.1% of procedures. Most of these leaks occur from the cystic duct stump (Fig. 4.22), but biliary leaks can also occur from accessory bile ducts that enter the

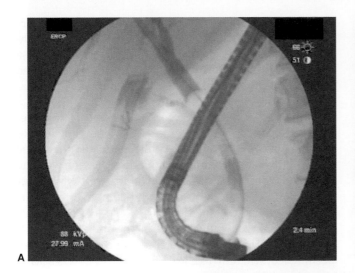
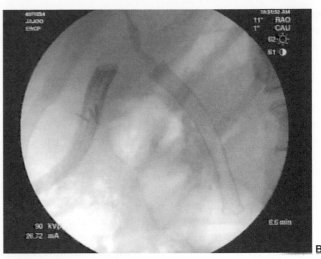
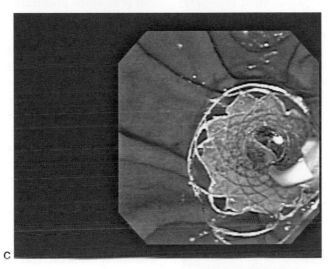

Figure 4.22 ERCP. (A) Bile leak from the cystic duct stump after laparoscopic cholecystectomy. (B) Covered SEMS placement to treat the bile leak. (C) Endoscopic view of covered SEMS deployment.

gallbladder bed (ducts of Luschka) or, less commonly, the common bile duct. Patients present with fever, right upper quadrant abdominal pain, and often an elevation in serum liver chemistries. Although this can be seen in the immediate postoperative period, the average time to presentation is approximately 5 days [87]. Bile leak can be diagnosed by transabdominal ultrasound, CT, or biliary scintigraphy scan. Once a postoperative biliary leak has been diagnosed or it is clinically suspected but imaging is nondiagnostic, ERCP is the primary modality for therapy and is effective in 90% of patients.

ERCP provides confirmation of the bile leak and readily demonstrates the location of the leak. Bile leaks are often associated with retained CBD stone(s), which can be identified and then treated by ERCP with sphincterotomy. The ideal initial endoscopic therapy for post-cholecystectomy bile leak has not been determined. The primary goal of

any therapy for bile leak is to diminish the transpapillary pressure gradient and allow for preferential flow of bile into the duodenum instead of the site of leakage. This can be achieved by sphincterotomy alone, transpapillary stent placement, or both. When a retained stone is found, sphincterotomy is generally necessary for removal. If no stone or other obstruction is present, the less invasive approach of stent placement alone is effective [88]. The interval for stent removal is generally 4–6 weeks, though no controlled studies exist. Endoscopic sphincterotomy combined with nasobiliary drainage has also been shown to be effective in hospitalized patients and provides rapid diversion of bile flow, access for a follow-up cholangiogram, and obviates the need for repeat ERCP for stent removal [89]. Patient discomfort and the need for ongoing hospitalization have limited this approach. In patients who do not respond to these initial treatment modalities, partially covered metal biliary stents have been shown to be very effective [90]. Rarely, surgical repair is required.

Postoperative biliary strictures are also seen as a complication of laparoscopic cholecystectomy as a result of unexpected ischemic injury or a misplaced surgical clip. Patients can present several years after surgery as the injury evolves into a stricture. These strictures are generally focal and can occur anywhere in the extrahepatic biliary tree above the level of the pancreas. Highly effective surgical, percutaneous, and endoscopic treatment options exist for the treatment of post-cholecystectomy strictures. The endoscopic route minimizes procedural morbidity and obviates the need for percutaneous drain placement. Stricture dilatation can be performed with a balloon dilator or graduated catheter dilator over a guidewire. At initial therapy, a plastic stent (8.5–10 Fr) is generally placed to provide drainage and allow for slow, constant dilatation. At times, several stents placed side by side are used to eliminate the stenosis. This may require multiple sessions at 2–3-month intervals over 1 year [91,92]. Recently, covered metal stents have been shown to be highly effective and safe in the management of benign biliary strictures and may be cost-effective by reducing the need for repeated procedures [93,94].

Complications of liver transplant

Biliary complications of orthotopic liver transplantation (OLT) include bile leak, strictures (Fig. 4.23), bil-

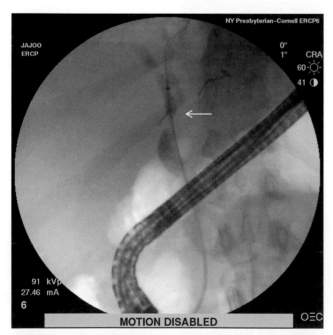

Figure 4.23 ERCP showing a stricture at a choledocho-choledochostomy anastomosis 3 months after orthotopic liver transplantation (white arrow).

iary casts, choledocholithiasis, and sphincter dysfunction due to denervation. Improvements in surgical techniques and organ selection have lead to a decrease in post-transplantation biliary complications; however, the overall rate of biliary stricture remains high at 10–15% and reaches 32% in living donor OLT [95]. Strictures may be more common in Roux-en-Y choledochojejunostomy anastomoses than in end-to-end choledocho-choledochostomy connections. It is postulated that these and additional biliary complications may be seen with the increased use of extended criteria donor grafts, split liver grafts, and other modalities used to compensate for the severe shortage of cadaveric grafts.

Biliary leak generally occurs in the immediate post-transplant period and is treated as discussed above for post-cholecystectomy bile leak. Biliary leak in this setting can arise at the ductal anastomosis or at the insertion site of the T-tube, if one is placed. Endoscopic therapy with stent placement with or without sphincterotomy is effective and safe in the transplant setting.

Biliary strictures after liver transplantation are classified as either anastomotic or nonanastomotic strictures. Anastomotic strictures are related to technical aspects of the ductal reconstruction such as size mismatch between the donor and recipient, tension on the anastomosis due to distance between the cut ends, and bile leak at the anastomosis. Nonanastomotic strictures are often related to ischemia due to hepatic artery occlusion or prolonged ischemia times, immunologic injury due to rejection, and cytotoxic injury from bile salts [95].

Anastomotic strictures are more likely to respond to endoscopic therapy than nonanastomotic ones. Balloon dilatation and stent therapy are often required. Multiple stents may be used over months with a technical success rate approaching 90% [96]. Some authors have argued that balloon dilatation alone is sufficient and stent therapy only adds increased risk due to the possibility of stent occlusion [97]. Emerging data regarding the use of covered metal stents in the post-transplant setting are promising [93,98].

Choledocholithiasis can occur in the post-transplant setting due to stasis from a biliary stricture or related to alterations in bile composition resulting from the transplantation [99]. Biliary cast syndrome, in which sludge and debris from sloughed biliary epithelium results in obstruction, occurs in up to 18% of OLT patients, usually within the first year after surgery. Prolonged warm ischemia time and stricture formation are independent risk factors for cast formation [100,101]. ERCP is the treatment of choice for cast extraction, but success rates are lower than for stone extraction and up to 22% of patients with biliary casts will require repeat transplantation when endoscopic and percutaneous means of treatment fail [100].

Other benign biliary strictures

Chronic pancreatitis is associated with biliary strictures in up to 30% of cases [102]. Surgical biliary diversion was the mainstay of treatment for these strictures, but carries a high morbidity. Stent placement, including multiple side-by-side stents and covered metal stents, has been shown to be effective in biliary strictures due to chronic pancreatitis as in other benign biliary strictures [93].

Benign biliary strictures and leaks can also be seen as a result of blunt abdominal trauma or after nonsurgical interventional procedures such as TIPS. Ischemic strictures have been seen with hepatic artery infusions of antineoplastic agents and sclerosants such as 5-fluorodeoxyuridine and sodium morrhuate or ethanol. Endoscopic therapies as described above have demonstrated efficacy in these rare situations [103].

Endoscopic ultrasound

The close proximity of the biliary tree and liver to the stomach and duodenum allows for high resolution imaging of these structures by EUS. In addition, EUS allows for the visualization of these structures without the acoustic interference of intestinal gas and subcutaneous adipose that is inherent to transabdominal ultrasound. Fine needle aspiration (FNA) can be performed through the EUS scope to further enhance the diagnostic capability of this procedure.

Technique

Specialized endoscopic training is required to proficiently obtain and interpret EUS images. ASGE guidelines have been set forth [104] to serve as a basis for assessing competency and granting procedure privileges. This training should include a stepwise progression of FNA difficulty and adequate FNA experience. As with training for ERCP, EUS training may be best achieved during an additional fellowship year on therapeutic endoscopy.

After obtaining informed consent by discussing the risks, benefits, and alternatives to the planned procedure, the patient is placed in the left lateral decubitus position. Sedation for EUS is generally moderate sedation with a benzodiazepine (midazolam) and a narcotic (fentanyl). Increasingly, intravenous propofol sedation administered by an anesthesiologist or nurse anesthetist is utilized given the generally longer procedure time for EUS compared with general upper endoscopy. Continuous monitoring of blood pressure, pulse rate, cardiac rhythm, and pulse oximetry is performed as in other endoscopic procedures. Additional respiratory monitoring by capnography has been shown to improve patient safety during EUS [66]. Sequential EUS and ERCP can be performed safely on the same day with a risk profile similar to either procedure alone [105].

Two general types of echoendoscopes are available for EUS of the hepatobiliary anatomy: radial array and curvilinear array. Each of these has videoendoscopy capability in addition to an ultrasound transducer at the tip of the endoscope to allow for ultrasound imaging of the gastric and duodenal wall and surrounding structures. Radial array echoendoscopes provide a 360° image plane that is perpendicular to the long axis of the endoscope. This view is analogous to the axial images of a CT scan. The linear array echoendoscope provides a 120–150° image in the same plane as the long axis of the endoscope. This allows for direct sonographic visualization of instruments such as FNA needles as they are advanced through the enteral wall into the lesion being evaluated.

Complications

The complications of general endoscopy can occur with EUS, including sedation-related complications and rarely perforation. FNA carries a risk of bleeding and infection. The risk of bleeding is minimized by utilizing color flow ultrasound prior to advancement of the FNA needle to assess for the presence of blood vessels in the expected needle path. The risk of infection is minimal when solid lesions are sampled.

Indications for hepatobiliary EUS

A primary role for biliary EUS is the evaluation of choledocholithiasis. CBD stones can be difficult to diagnose, particularly in patients who do not demonstrate overt cholangitis or have fluctuating serum liver enzyme values. Transabdominal ultrasound and CT scans are highly specific for the finding of CBD stones, but lack high sensitivity. MRCP is highly sensitive and specific in the diagnosis of choledocholithiasis [77], but is limited for stones smaller than 5 mm. On EUS, CBD stones are seen as hyperechoic objects with shadowing within the anechoic duct (Fig. 4.24). EUS demonstrates similarly high test characteristics as MRCP (sensitivity 93% and 85%; specificity 96% and 93%, respectively) and both can help to avert the risks of unnecessary ERCP [106].

As discussed above, the differentiation between benign and malignant extrahepatic biliary strictures can be quite difficult. EUS with FNA has been shown to be sensitive and specific in the diagnosis of malignant biliary strictures, even when no mass was seen on cross-sectional imaging and ERCP with tissue sampling failed to provide a diagnosis [107,108]. Intraductal ultrasound, using a high-frequency catheter probe passed over a guidewire during ERCP, has also been used to provide additional imaging of indeterminate biliary strictures. EUS can be helpful in determining the cause of benign biliary strictures, such as chronic calcific pancreatitis (Fig. 4.25).

Solid liver lesions are generally approached by percutaneous means given the ready accessibility and safety

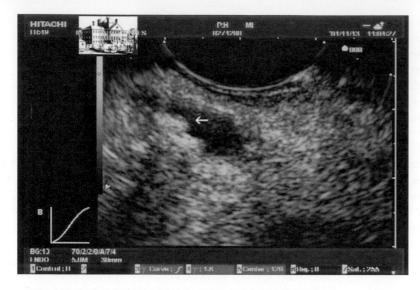

Figure 4.24 EUS demonstrating hyperechoic stones (white arrow) in the common bile duct.

of this approach. EUS with FNA has been shown to be highly sensitive for solid liver lesions and demonstrates the ability to identify and diagnose lesions that may not have been seen on transabdominal ultrasound or CT scan [109]. In cases where metastatic disease is suspected despite negative radiologic imaging or the primary tumor requires EUS evaluation, EUS of the liver with FNA of any solid lesions is advised (Fig. 4.26).

EUS is also useful in the identification and sampling of ascites (Fig. 4.27). EUS can detect ascites that was not seen on other imaging studies such as transabdominal ultrasound and CT scan [110]. Paracentesis of suspected malignant ascites by EUS-FNA is highly sensitive and specific

for malignancy (94% and 100%, respectively) and may significantly affect management decisions [111].

Portal vein thrombosis is generally diagnosed with noninvasive imaging such as transabdominal Doppler ultrasound or triphase CT scan. In cases of suspected portal vein thrombosis not identified by the usual means, EUS can provide the diagnosis with high sensitivity and excellent specificity (81% and 93%, respectively) [112]. Thrombus is generally seen as hyperechoic material within an otherwise hypoechoic or anechoic vessel.

As with the increasingly therapeutic focus of ERCP, the role of EUS has come to include interventional therapeutic indications that can avert surgical or percutaneous

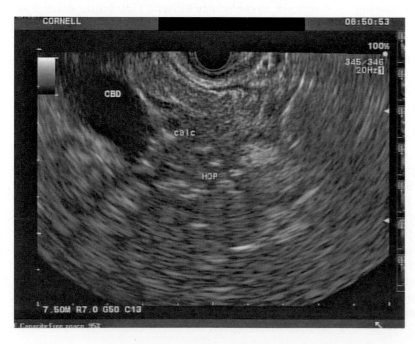

Figure 4.25 EUS showing obstruction of the distal common bile duct (CBD) due to chronic calcific pancreatitis (calc) in the head of the pancreas (HOP).

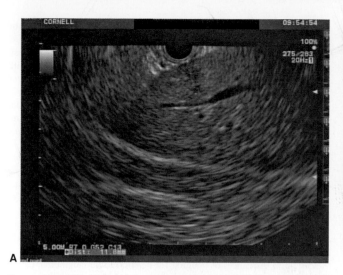 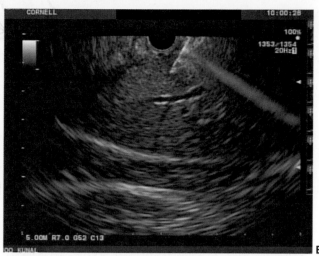

Figure 4.26 EUS. (A) An 11.8 mm hypoechoic liver mass (dashed green line) in a patient with pancreatic cancer. (B) Fine needle aspiration of the lesion to confirm metastasis.

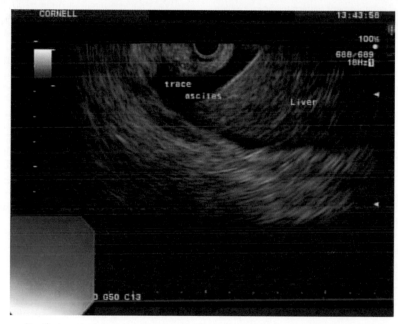

Figure 4.27 EUS showing trace ascites that was not seen on other imaging in a patient with concurrently diagnosed pancreatic cancer.

procedures. In cases where transpapillary access to the biliary tree is not possible due to altered surgical anatomy or enteral obstruction, EUS with FNA access of the biliary tree can allow for antegrade placement of a biliary stent through the gastric or duodenal wall [113]. This has only been described in small series and requires further investigation.

References

1. Fazel R, Krumholz H, Wang Y, et al. Exposure to low-dose ionizing radiation from medical imaging procedures. *N Engl J Med* 2009;361(9):849–57.
2. Brenner D. Medical imaging in the 21st century – getting the best bang for the rad. *N Engl J Med* 2010;362(10):943–5.
3. Aspelin P, Aubry P, Fransson S, et al. Nephrotoxic effects in high-risk patients undergoing angiography. *N Engl J Med* 2003;348(6):491–9.
4. Trivedi H, Daram S, Szabo A, Bartorelli A, Marenzi G. High-dose N-acetylcysteine for the prevention of contrast-induced nephropathy. *Am J Med* 2009;122(9):874.e9–15.
5. Brown J, Block C, Malenka D, O'Connor G, Schoolwerth A, Thompson C. Sodium bicarbonate plus N-acetylcysteine prophylaxis: a meta-analysis. *JACC Cardiovasc Interv* 2009;2(11): 1116–24.
6. Bakheet S, Powe J. Benign causes of 18-FDG uptake on whole body imaging. *Semin Nucl Med* 1998;28(4):352–8.

7. Arulampalam T, Francis D, Visvikis D, Taylor I, Ell P. FDG-PET for the pre-operative evaluation of colorectal liver metastases. *Eur J Surg Oncol* 2004;30(3):286–91.

8. Lee S, Kim H, Park J, et al. Clinical usefulness of 18F-FDG PET-CT for patients with gallbladder cancer and cholangiocarcinoma. *J Gastroenterol* 2010;45(5):560–6.

9. Li J, Kuehl H, Grabellus F, et al. Preoperative assessment of hilar cholangiocarcinoma by dual-modality PET/CT. *J Surg Oncol* 2008;98(6):438–43.

10. Kim Y, Lee K, Cho S, et al. Usefulness 18F-FDG positron emission tomography/computed tomography for detecting recurrence of hepatocellular carcinoma in posttransplant patients. *Liver Transpl* 2010;16(6):767–72.

11. Wolfort R, Papillion P, Turnage R, Lillien D, Ramaswamy M, Zibari G. Role of FDG-PET in the evaluation and staging of hepatocellular carcinoma with comparison of tumor size, AFP level, and histologic grade. *Int Surg* 2010;95(1):67–75.

12. Brix G, Lechel U, Glatting G, et al. Radiation exposure of patients undergoing whole-body dual-modality 18F-FDG PET/CT examinations. *J Nucl Med* 2005;46(4):608–13.

13. Merkle E, Dale B. Abdominal MRI at 3.0 T: the basics revisited. *AJR Am J Roentgenol* 2006;186(6):1524–32.

14. Karam A, Shankar S, Surapaneni P, Kim Y, Hussain S. Focal nodular hyperplasia: central scar enhancement pattern using gadoxetate disodium. *J Magn Reson Imaging* 2010;32(2):341–4.

15. Ringe K, Husarik D, Sirlin C, Merkle E. Gadoxetate disodium-enhanced MRI of the liver: part 1, protocol optimization and lesion appearance in the noncirrhotic liver. *AJR Am J Roentgenol* 2010;195(1):13–28.

16. Grazioli L, Morana G, Kirchin M, Schneider G. Accurate differentiation of focal nodular hyperplasia from hepatic adenoma at gadobenate dimeglumine-enhanced MR imaging: prospective study. *Radiology* 2005;236(1):166–77.

17. Sena B, Stern J, Pandharipande P, et al. Screening patients to assess renal function before administering gadolinium chelates: assessment of the choyke questionnaire. *AJR Am J Roentgenol* 2010;195(2):424–8.

18. Chen A, Zirwas M, Heffernan M. Nephrogenic systemic fibrosis: a review. *J Drugs Dermatol* 2010;9(7):829–34.

19. Laurent S, Elst L, Muller R. Comparative study of the physicochemical properties of six clinical low molecular weight gadolinium contrast agents. *Contrast Media Mol Imaging* 2006;1(3):128–37.

20. Pasumarthy L, Srour J. Nonalcoholic steatohepatitis: a review of the literature and updates in management. *South Med J* 2010;103(6):547–50.

21. Matteoni C, Younossi Z, Gramlich T, Boparai N, Liu Y, McCullough A. Nonalcoholic fatty liver disease: a spectrum of clinical and pathological severity. *Gastroenterology* 1999;116(6):1413–9.

22. Neuschwander-Tetri B, Caldwell S. Nonalcoholic steatohepatitis: summary of an AASLD Single Topic Conference. *Hepatology* 2003;37(5):1202–19.

23. Saadeh S, Younossi Z, Remer E, et al. The utility of radiological imaging in nonalcoholic fatty liver disease. *Gastroenterology* 2002;123(3):745–50.

24. Bohte A, van Werven J, Bipat S, Stoker J. The diagnostic accuracy of US, CT, MRI and (1)H-MRS for the evaluation of hepatic steatosis compared with liver biopsy: a meta-analysis. *Eur Radiol* 2010 (Epub ahead of print, PubMed PMID 20680289).

25. Cesbron-Métivier E, Roullier V, Boursier J, et al. Noninvasive liver steatosis quantification using MRI techniques combined with blood markers. *Eur J Gastroenterol Hepatol* 2010;22(8):973–82.

26. Ma X, Holalkere N, Kambadakone RA, Mino-Kenudson M, Hahn P, Sahani D. Imaging-based quantification of hepatic fat: methods and clinical applications. *Radiographics* 2009;29(5):1253–77.

27. Sheth S. SQUID biosusceptometry in the measurement of hepatic iron. *Pediatr Radiol* 2003;33(6):373–7.

28. Chandarana H, Lim R, Jensen J, et al. Hepatic iron deposition in patients with liver disease: preliminary experience with breath-hold multiecho T2*-weighted sequence. *AJR Am J Roentgenol* 2009;193(5):1261–7.

29. Ramazzotti A, Pepe A, Positano V, et al. Multicenter validation of the magnetic resonance T2* technique for segmental and global quantification of myocardial iron. *J Magn Reson Imaging* 2009;30(1):62–8.

30. Fanelli F, Bezzi M, Bruni A, et al. Multidetector-row computed tomography in the evaluation of transjugular intrahepatic portosystemic shunt performed with expanded-polytetrafluoroethylene-covered stent-graft. *Cardiovasc Intervent Radiol* 2010 (Epub ahead of print, PubMed PMID 20532776).

31. Ahn J, Yu J, Hwang S, Chung J, Kim J, Kim K. Nontumorous arterioportal shunts in the liver: CT and MRI findings considering mechanisms and fate. *Eur Radiol* 2010;20(2):385–94.

32. Choi B. Advances of imaging for hepatocellular carcinoma. *Oncology* 2010;78(Suppl 1):46–52.

33. Kudo M. Will Gd-EOB-MRI change the diagnostic algorithm in hepatocellular carcinoma? *Oncology* 2010;78(Suppl 1):87–93.

34. Colombo M. Screening and diagnosis of hepatocellular carcinoma. *Liver Int* 2009;29(Suppl 1):143–7.

35. Akai H, Kiryu S, Matsuda I, et al. Detection of hepatocellular carcinoma by Gd-EOB-DTPA-enhanced liver MRI: comparison with triple phase 64 detector row helical CT. *Eur J Radiol* 2010 (Epub ahead of print, PubMed PMID 20732773).

36. Mita K, Kim S, Kudo M, et al. Diagnostic sensitivity of imaging modalities for hepatocellular carcinoma smaller than 2 cm. *World J Gastroenterol* 2010;16(33):4187–92.

37. Lee M, Kim Y, Park H, et al. Targeted sonography for small hepatocellular carcinoma discovered by CT or MRI: factors affecting sonographic detection. *AJR Am J Roentgenol* 2010;194(5):W396–400.

38. Dave M, Elmunzer B, Dwamena B, Higgins P. Primary sclerosing cholangitis: meta-analysis of diagnostic performance of MR cholangiopancreatography. *Radiology* 2010;256(2):387–96.

39. Maccioni F, Martinelli M, Al Ansari N, et al. Magnetic resonance cholangiography: past, present and future: a review. *Eur Rev Med Pharmacol Sci* 2010;14(8):721–5.

40. Thomson A. MRCP versus ERCP in the diagnosis of primary sclerosing cholangitis. *Gastrointest Endosc* 2007;65(3):558; author reply.

41. Alvaro D, Cannizzaro R, Labianca R, Valvo F, Farinati F. Cholangiocarcinoma: a position paper by the Italian Society of Gastroenterology (SIGE), the Italian Association of Hospital Gastroenterology (AIGO), the Italian Association of Medical Oncology (AIOM) and the Italian Association of Oncological Radiotherapy (AIRO). *Dig Liver Dis* 2010 (Epub ahead of print, PubMed PMID 20702152).

42. Wang N, Guan Q, Wang K, et al. TACE combined with PEI versus TACE alone in the treatment of HCC: a meta-analysis. *Med Oncol* 2010 (Epub ahead of print, PubMed PMID 20632218).

43. Kudo M. Radiofrequency ablation for hepatocellular carcinoma: updated review in 2010. *Oncology* 2010;78(Suppl 1):113–24.

44. Biolato M, Marrone G, Racco S, et al. Transarterial chemoembolization (TACE) for unresectable HCC: a new life begins? *Eur Rev Med Pharmacol Sci* 2010;14(4):356–62.

45. Yamagami T, Tanaka O, Yoshimatsu R, et al. Hepatic artery guide wire targeting technique during transjugular intrahepatic portosystemic shunt. *Br J Radiol* 2010 (Epub ahead of print, PubMed PMID 20716652).

46. Classen M, Demling L. Endoscopic sphincterotomy of the papilla of vater and extraction of stones from the choledochal duct. *Dtsch Med Wochenschr* 1974;99:496–7.

47. Kawai K, Akasaka Y, Murakami K, et al. Endoscopic sphinctero-tomy of the ampulla of Vater. Gastrointest Endosc 1974;20:148–51.

48. Cohen, S, Bacon, BR, Berlin, JA, et al. National Institutes of Health State-of-the-Science Conference Statement: ERC for diagnosis and therapy, January 14–16, 2002. Gastrointest Endosc 2002;56:803.

49. Adler DG, Baron TH, Davila RE, et al. ASGE guideline: the role of ERC in diseases of the biliary tract and the pancreas. Gastrointest Endosc 2005;62:1.

50. Petrov MS, van Santvort HC, Besselink MG, et al. Early endo-scopic retrograde cholangiopancreatography versus conservative management in acute biliary pancreatitis without cholangitis: a meta-analysis of randomized trials. Ann Surg 2008;247:250–7.

51. Ayub K, Slavin J, Imada R. Endoscopic retrograde cholangiopan-creatography in gallstone-associated acute pancreatitis. Cochrane Database Syst Rev 2004;4:CD003630.

52. van der Gaag NA, Rauws EA, van Eijck CH, et al. Preoperative bil-iary drainage for cancer of the head of the pancreas. N Engl J Med 2010;362:129–37.

53. Povoski SP, Karpeh MS Jr, Conlon KC, et al. Association of preop-erative biliary drainage with postoperative outcome following pan-creaticoduodenectomy. Ann Surg 1999;230:131–42.

54. Moss AC, Morris E, Leyden J, et al. Malignant distal biliary obstruc-tion: a systematic review and meta-analysis of endoscopic and sur-gical bypass results. Cancer Treat Rev 2007;33:213–21.

55. Moss AC, Morris E, MacMathuna P. Palliative biliary stents for obstructing pancreatic carcinoma. Cochrane Database Syst Rev 2006;1:CD004200.

56. Koornstra JJ, Fry L, Mönkemüller K. ERCP with the balloon-assisted enteroscopy technique: a systematic review. Dig Dis 2008;26:324–9.

57. Cotton PB, Lehman G, Vennes J, et al. Endoscopic sphincterotomy complications and their management: an attempt at consensus. Gas-trointest Endosc 1991;37:383–93.

58. Cotton PB, Garrow DA, Gallagher J, et al. Risk factors for complica-tions after ERCP: a multivariate analysis of 11,497 procedures over 12 years. Gastrointest Endosc 2009;70:80–8.

59. Testoni PA, Bagnolo F. Pain at 24 hours associated with amy-lase levels greater than five times the upper normal limit as the most reliable indicator of post-ERCP pancreatitis. Gastrointest Endosc 2001;53:33–9.

60. Freeman ML. Complications of ERCP: prediction, prevention and management. In: Baron TH, Kozarek R, Carr-Locke DL, eds. ERCP. Philadelphia: Saunders Elsevier, 2008;51–9.

61. Elmunzer BJ, Waljee AK, Elta GH, et al. A meta-analysis of rectal NSAIDs in the prevention of post-ERCP pancreatitis. Gut 2008;57:1262–7.

62. Freeman ML. Pancreatic stents for prevention of post-endoscopic retrograde cholangiopancreatography pancreatitis. Clin Gastroen-terol Hepatol 2007;5:1354–65.

63. Freeman ML, Nelson DB, Sherman S, et al. Complications of endo-scopic biliary sphincterotomy. N Engl J Med 1996;335:909–18.

64. Hussain N, Alsulaiman R, Burtin P, et al. The safety of endo-scopic sphincterotomy in patients receiving antiplatelet agents: a case-control study. Aliment Pharmacol Ther 2007;25:579–84.

65. Chutkan RK, Ahmad AS, Cohen J, et al. ERC core curriculum. Gas-trointest Endosc 2006;63:361–76.

66. Qadeer MA, Vargo JJ, Dumot JA, et al. Capnographic monitor-ing of respiratory activity improves safety of sedation for endo-scopic cholangiopancreatography and ultrasonography. Gastroen-terology 2009;136:1568–76.

67. Cheung J, Tsoi KK, Quan WL, et al. Guidewire versus conventional contrast cannulation of the common bile duct for the prevention of post-ERCP pancreatitis: a systematic review and meta-analysis. Gas-trointest Endosc 2009;70:1211–19.

68. ASGE Standards of Practice Committee, Banerjee S, Shen B, Baron TH, et al. Antibiotic prophylaxis for GI endoscopy. Gastrointest Endosc 2008;67:791–8.

69. Everhart JE, Khare M, Hill M, et al. Prevalence and ethnic differ-ences in gallbladder disease in the United States. Gastroenterology 1999;117:632–9.

70. Frossard JL, Hadengue A, Amouyal G, et al. Choledocholithiasis: a prospective study of spontaneous common bile duct stone migra-tion. Gastrointest Endosc 2000;51:175–9.

71. Roston AD, Jacobson IM. Evaluation of the pattern of liver tests and yield of cholangiography in symptomatic choledocholithiasis: a prospective study. Gastrointest Endosc 1997;45:394–9.

72. Romagnuolo J, Bardou M, Rahme E, et al. Magnetic resonance cholangiopancreatography: a meta-analysis of test performance in suspected biliary disease. Ann Intern Med 2003;139:547–57.

73. Petrov MS, Savides TJ. Systematic review of endoscopic ultrasonog-raphy versus endoscopic retrograde cholangiopancreatography for suspected choledocholithiasis. Br J Surg 2009;96:967–74.

74. Neuhaus H. Biliary sphincterotomy In: Baron TH, Kozarek R, Carr-Locke DL, eds. ERCP. Philadelphia: Saunders Elsevier, 2008;109–18.

75. Weinberg BM, Shindy W, Lo S. Endoscopic balloon sphincter dila-tion (sphincteroplasty) versus sphincterotomy for common bile duct stones. Cochrane Database Syst Rev 2006;4:CD004890.

76. Horiuchi A, Nakayma Y, Kajiyama M, et al. Biliary stenting in the management of large or multiple common bile duct stones. Gastroin-test Endosc 2010;71:1200–3.

77. Levy MJ, Baron TH, Clayton AC, et al. Prospective evalua-tion of advanced molecular markers and imaging techniques in patients with indeterminate bile duct strictures. Am J Gastroenterol 2008;103:1263–73.

78. Lee, YM, Kaplan, MM. Primary sclerosing cholangitis. N Engl J Med 1995;332:924–33.

79. Jesudian AB, Jacobson IM. Screening and diagnosis of cholangio-carcinoma in patients with primary sclerosing cholangitis. Rev Gas-troenterol Disord 2009;9:E41–7.

80. Ponsioen CY, Vrouenraets SM, Prawirodirdjo W, et al. Natural history of primary sclerosing cholangitis and prognostic value of cholangiography in a Dutch population. Gut 2002;51:562–6.

81. Tischendorf JJ, Hecker H, Krüger M, et al. Characterization, out-come, and prognosis in 273 patients with primary sclerosing cholan-gitis: a single center study. Am J Gastroenterol 2007;102:107–14.

82. Dave M, Elmunzer BJ, Dwamena BA, et al. Primary sclerosing cholangitis: meta-analysis of diagnostic performance of MR cholan-giopancreatography. Radiology 2010;256:387–96.

83. van Milligen de Wit AW, van Bracht J, Rauws EA, et al. Endoscopic stent therapy for dominant extrahepatic bile duct strictures in pri-mary sclerosing cholangitis. Gastrointest Endosc 1996;44:293–9.

84. Kaya M, Petersen BT, Angulo P, et al. Balloon dilation compared to stenting of dominant strictures in primary sclerosing cholangitis. Am J Gastroenterol 2001;96:1059–66.

85. Bangarulingam SY, Gossard AA, Petersen BT, et al. Complica-tions of endoscopic retrograde cholangiopancreatography in pri-mary sclerosing cholangitis. Am J Gastroenterol 2009;104:855–60.

86. Charatcharoenwitthaya P, Enders FB, Halling KC, et al. Utility of serum tumor markers, imaging, and biliary cytology for detecting cholangiocarcinoma in primary sclerosing cholangitis. Hepatology 2008;48:1106–17.

87. Barkun AN, Rezieg M, Mehta SN, et al. Postcholecystectomy biliary leaks in the laparoscopic era: risk factors, presentation, and man-agement. McGill Gallstone Treatment Group. Gastrointest Endosc 1997;45:277–82.

88. Kaffes AJ, Hourigan L, De Luca N, et al. Impact of endoscopic inter-vention in 100 patients with suspected postcholecystectomy bile leak. Gastrointest Endosc 2005;61:269–75.

89. Elmi F, Silverman WB. Nasobiliary tube management of postcholecystectomy bile leaks. *J Clin Gastroenterol* 2005;39:441–4.

90. Kahaleh M, Sundaram V, Condron SL, et al. Temporary placement of covered self-expandable metallic stents in patients with biliary leak: midterm evaluation of a pilot study. *Gastrointest Endosc* 2007;66:52–9.

91. Bergman JJ, Burgemeister L, Bruno MJ, et al. Long-term follow-up after biliary stent placement for postoperative bile duct stenosis. *Gastrointest Endosc* 2001;54:154–61.

92. Costamagna G, Pandolfi M, Mutignani M, et al. Long-term results of endoscopic management of postoperative bile duct strictures with increasing numbers of stents. *Gastrointest Endosc* 2001;54:162–8.

93. Kahaleh M, Behm B, Clarke BW, et al. Temporary placement of covered self-expandable metal stents in benign biliary strictures: a new paradigm? *Gastrointest Endosc* 2008;67:446–54.

94. van Boeckel PG, Vleggaar FP, Siersema PD. Plastic or metal stents for benign extrahepatic biliary strictures: a systematic review. *BMC Gastroenterol* 2009;9:96.

95. Williams ED, Draganov PV. Endoscopic management of biliary strictures after liver transplantation. *World J Gastroenterol* 2009;15:3725–33.

96. Morelli J, Mulcahy HE, Willner IR, et al. Long-term outcomes for patients with post-liver transplant anastomotic biliary strictures treated by endoscopic stent placement. *Gastrointest Endosc* 2003;58:374–9.

97. Kulaksiz H, Weiss KH, Gotthardt D, et al. Is stenting necessary after balloon dilation of post-transplantation biliary strictures? Results of a prospective comparative study. *Endoscopy* 2008;40:746–51.

98. Traina M, Tarantino I, Barresi L, et al. Efficacy and safety of fully covered self-expandable metallic stents in biliary complications after liver transplantation: a preliminary study. *Liver Transpl* 2009;15:1493–8.

99. Xu HS, Pilcher JA, Jones RS. Physiologic study of bile salt and lipid secretion in rats after liver transplantation. *Ann Surg* 1993;217:404–12.

100. Gor NV, Levy RM, Ahn J, et al. Biliary cast syndrome following liver transplantation: predictive factors and clinical outcomes. *Liver Transpl* 2008;14:1466–72.

101. Shah JN, Haigh WG, Lee SP, et al. Biliary casts after orthotopic liver transplantation: clinical factors, treatment, biochemical analysis. *Am J Gastroenterol* 2003;98:1861–7.

102. Ng C, Huibregtse K. The role of endoscopic therapy in chronic pancreatitis-induced common bile duct strictures. *Gastrointest Endosc Clin N Am* 1998;8:181–93.

103. Huang ZQ, Huang XQ. Changing patterns of traumatic bile duct injuries: a review of forty years experience. *World J Gastroenterol* 2002;8:5–12.

104. Van Dam, J, Brady, PG, Freeman, M, et al. Guidelines for training in endoscopic ultrasound. *Gastrointest Endosc* 1999;49:829–33.

105. Che K, Muckova N, Olafsson S, et al. Safety of same-day endoscopic ultrasound and endoscopic retrograde cholangiopancreatography under conscious sedation. *World J Gastroenterol* 2010;16:3287–91.

106. Verma D, Kapadia A, Eisen GM, at al. EUS vs MRCP for detection of choledocholithiasis. *Gastrointest Endosc* 2006;64:248–54.

107. Eloubeidi MA, Chen VK, Jhala NC, et al. Endoscopic ultrasound-guided fine needle aspiration biopsy of suspected cholangiocarcinoma. *Clin Gastroenterol Hepatol* 2004;2:209–13.

108. DeWitt J, Misra VL, Leblanc JK, et al. EUS-guided FNA of proximal biliary strictures after negative ERCP brush cytology results. *Gastrointest Endosc* 2006;64:325–33.

109. DeWitt J, LeBlanc J, McHenry L, et al. Endoscopic ultrasound-guided needle fine aspiration cytology of solid liver lesions: a large single-center experience. *Am J Gastroenterol* 2003;98:1976–1981.

110. DeWitt J, LeBlanc J, McHenry L, et al. Endoscopic ultrasound-guided fine-needle aspiration of ascites. *Clin Gastroenterol Hepatol* 2007;5:609–15.

111. Kaushik N, Khalid A, Brody D, et al. EUS-guided paracentesis for the diagnosis of malignant ascites. *Gastrointest Endosc* 2006;64:908–13.

112. Lai L, Brugge WR. Endoscopic ultrasound is a sensitive and specific test to diagnose portal venous system thrombosis (PVST). *Am J Gastroenterol* 2004;99:40–4.

113. Nguyen-Tang T, Binmoeller KF, Sanchez-Yague A, et al. Endoscopic ultrasound (EUS)-guided transhepatic anterograde self-expandable metal stent (SEMS) placement across malignant biliary obstruction. *Endoscopy* 2010;42:232–6.

114. Brenner D, Hall E. Computed tomography – an increasing source of radiation exposure. *N Engl J Med* 2007;357:2277–84.

PART II
General Considerations

CHAPTER 5
Physioanatomic Considerations

Ian R. Wanless

Department of Pathology, Dalhousie University, Halifax, Nova Scotia, Canada

Key concepts

- The branching pattern of large vessels and ducts is used for defining the segmental nomenclature used by radiologists and surgeons.
- Anomalies of the vessels and ducts are of importance to surgeons.
- Bile ducts are supplied by arteries. Arterial injury may lead to ischemic strictures of the ducts, especially after transplantation.
- The liver receives most of the splanchnic blood flow. After severe obstruction at any level of the hepatic vasculature, collateral channels become a source of bleeding and are partly responsible for hepatic encephalopathy.
- The microvasculature of the liver consists of small branches of portal and hepatic veins that interdigitate in a regular pattern, allowing the definition of parenchymal subunits called acini or lobules.
- Arterioles communicate with portal veins near the periportal end of the sinusoids. In cirrhosis, these communications dilate and therefore contribute to portal hypertension.
- Hepatocytes are exposed to gradients of nutrients and waste products leading to zonal metabolic specialization and zonal variation in susceptibility to ischemia and drug toxicity.

- The sinusoids are lined by fenestrated endothelial cells that lack basement membranes. This anatomy facilitates rapid exchange between plasma and hepatocytes.
- Hepatic lymph is formed at the sinusoidal level when there is increased sinusoidal pressure, especially with outflow obstruction. This lymph may accumulate as ascites.
- Sinusoidal macrophages (Kupffer cells) are important in host defense.
- Perisinusoidal stellate cells store vitamin A and, when activated, produce collagen that contributes to the pathogenesis of cirrhosis.
- There are two major anatomic forms of chronic liver disease: nodular regenerative hyperplasia and cirrhosis. These forms are determined by microvascular obliteration. In nodular regenerative hyperplasia, obliteration of portal veins is dominant. In cirrhosis, both portal vein and hepatic vein obliteration are prominent.
- Microvascular obliteration in cirrhosis is usually initiated by necroinflammation adjacent to terminal hepatic venules. Secondary congestion occurs in proximal tissue leading to parenchymal extinction and obliteration of portal veins, followed by angiogenesis, exacerbation of in-out imbalance, and a positive feedback loop that causes progression and slows regression of disease.

Anatomic knowledge is required for understanding normal hepatic physiology and the pathogenesis of disease. This chapter presents a summary of normal anatomy, some physiologic correlates, and a description of the major anatomic abnormalities found in human liver disease.

Surface anatomy

The liver is shaped like a wedge with its base against the right abdominal wall and its tip pointing to the spleen. The normal liver extends from the fifth intercostal space in the midclavicular line down to the right costal margin. It measures 12–15 cm coronally and 15–20 cm transversely. The lower margin can usually be felt below the costal margin during inspiration.

Transcutaneous puncture for liver biopsy is commonly located in the midaxillary line in the third interspace below the upper limit of liver dullness during full expiration, commonly in the ninth intercostal space. The median liver weight is 1,800 g in men and 1,400 g in women [1]. The adult liver weight is between 1.8% and 3.1% of body weight in 80% of individuals [2,3]. Liver weights in fetuses and children are relatively greater, being 5.6% at 5 months' gestational age, 4–5% at birth, and 3% at 1 year of age [4,5].

Impressed by the molding against adjacent organs, William Osler quipped that the liver was present only for packing purposes. Thus, the superior, anterior, and lateral surfaces are smooth and convex to fit against the dome of the diaphragm. The muscle bundles of the diaphragm often impress grooves in the superior surface. The costal margin often marks a transverse groove on the

Schiff's Diseases of the Liver, Eleventh Edition. Edited by Eugene R. Schiff, Willis C. Maddrey and Michael F. Sorrell.
© 2012 John Wiley & Sons, Ltd. Published 2012 by John Wiley & Sons, Ltd.

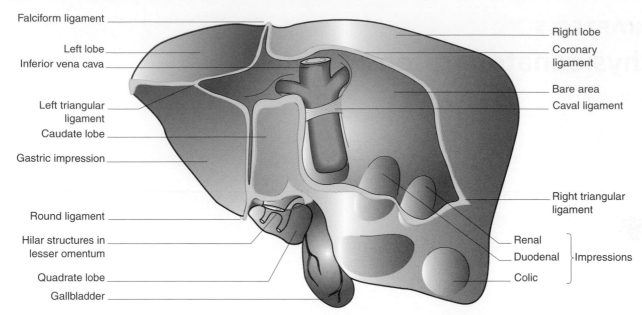

Falciform ligament

Left lobe

Inferior vena cava

Left triangular ligament

Caudate lobe

Gastric impression

Round ligament

Hilar structures in lesser omentum

Quadrate lobe

Gallbladder

Right lobe

Coronary ligament

Bare area

Caval ligament

Right triangular ligament

Renal

Duodenal

Colic

Impressions

Figure 5.1 Posterior view of the liver. The marks impressed on the liver surface by neighboring organs mirror its topographic relations. (Reproduced from Wanless [207] with permission from Elsevier.)

anterior surface (corset deformity). The posterior surface has indentations from the colon, kidney, and duodenum on the right and the stomach on the left (Fig. 5.1). Deeper grooves, called fissures, are formed where extrahepatic vessels or cords press against the developing liver. Three of these structures, the umbilical portion of the left portal vein, the ductus venosus (ligamentum venosum), and the umbilical vein (ligamentum teres), form the umbilical fissure.

The liver is covered by the fibrous capsule of Glisson (or Walaeus). At the porta hepatis, the connective tissue of the capsule is continuous with the fibrous sheath, which invests the portal vessels and ducts and follows them to their smallest ramifications. The capsular peritoneum reflects onto the diaphragm and continues as the parietal peritoneum. The reflections form the coronary ligaments, the right and left triangular ligaments, and the falciform ligament (Fig. 5.1). These ligaments hold the liver firmly in its place and allow passage of the lymphatics, small vessels, and nerves. There is a large bare area where the liver is attached to the diaphragm and retroperitoneum. The vena cava, being retroperitoneal, lies on the bare area and is held to the liver by a ligament or bridge of liver parenchyma between the caudate and right lobes.

The falciform ligament connects the liver to the diaphragm and anterior abdominal wall. The lower free edge of the falciform ligament, called the round ligament, contains the obliterated umbilical vein. The falciform ligament ascends the anterior surface of the liver, joins the reflections of peritoneum left of the vena cava, continues posteriorly as the lesser omentum in the fissure of the

ductus venosus, and finishes at the hilum. Thus, the falciform ligament anteriorly and the lesser omentum and umbilical fissure posteriorly divide the liver into the conventional right and left lobes.

On the posterior surface, the transverse portal fissure contains the hilar vessels and demarcates the conventional right lobe anteriorly from the caudate lobe posteriorly (Fig. 5.1). The quadrate lobe is the portion of the right lobe anterior to the transverse fissure and is delimited on the right by the gallbladder and on the left by the umbilical fissure.

The hepatoduodenal ligament connects the liver to the superior part of the duodenum. It is part of the lesser omentum, which sheathes the hepatic artery (HA), portal vein (PV), nerves, bile duct, and lymph vessels, all present within the porta hepatis. In the ligament the common bile duct lies to the right, the HA to the left, and the PV behind them. However, variations in the topography of the HA are common.

There are several variations in the gross anatomy and topography of the liver [6,7]. The relative size of the right and left conventional lobes is variable, being equal in size in 7% and greater on the left in 4% [7]. The Riedel lobe is a caudal prolongation of the right lobe, which may give a false impression of hepatomegaly (Fig. 5.2). The falciform left lobe is an elongated lobe that extends laterally and posteriorly like a scythe, found in 19% [7]. Extreme atrophy of the left lobe (4%) may be a result of vascular anomalies occurring early in life [8] or extinction of parenchyma occurring after acquired vascular obstruction. The left lobe may be attached to the rest of the liver

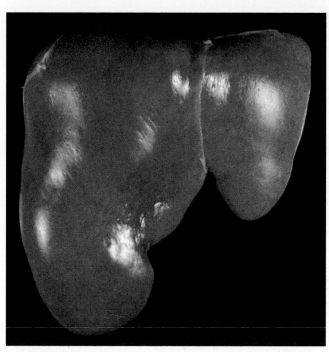

Figure 5.2 Liver with Reidel lobe, a prominent caudal extension of the right lobe.

by a narrow pedicle. Accessory livers may be found in the ligaments or mesentery or on the surface of the gallbladder, spleen, or adrenal glands [6]. Conversely, adrenal rests may be embedded in the right lobe, providing a source for the formation of intrahepatic adrenal cortical adenoma or myelolipoma [9].

Segmental anatomy

Division of the liver at the falciform ligament and umbilical fissure does not correspond to division based on branch points in the vascular supply. Surgical imperative has led to the search for functional divisions within the liver. The anatomic studies of Rex and others [10–13] demonstrated that the liver can be divided on a different plane into right and left livers (or hemilivers), each with its own blood supply and duct drainage. The right hemiliver comprises 50–70% of the liver mass. The liver can be further divided into a total of eight segments based on the vascular or bile duct distribution (Figs. 5.3 and 5.4) [7,13–17]. The segmental nomenclature devised by Couinaud has received the widest acceptance. This classification was based on the divisions of the portal veins. However, the branching of the PVs to the left lobe is irregular because of the entry of the umbilical vein, making it desirable to adopt a nomenclature based on the divisions of the arteries or ducts, as suggested by Strasberg [18]. This can be done without modification of the segments defined by

Couinaud and rationalizes the diverse nomenclature used in different parts of the world. The Strasberg nomenclature is summarized in Figure 5.3 and Table 5.1.

Most hepatic resections can be achieved by division either on the Cantlie line (between the gallbladder and vena cava) or near the falciform ligament. Surgical dissection along the planes between segments is relatively bloodless. Because the segments do not have surface landmarks, small resections are usually performed without attempting to identify the segmental boundaries [17]. The segments vary greatly in size and shape among individuals [19], so that each operation is empirical and may be based on ultrasonography [20,21].

Embryology

The liver arises from the hepatic diverticulum of the foregut during the fourth week of gestation (Fig. 5.5) [7,22]. As the embryo develops, the blood supply to this region evolves in an elaborate fashion to deliver nutrients from three different sources in the sequence: yolk sac, placenta, and gut [7,18].

Hepatocyte precursors, the hepatoblasts, arise from endodermal cells at the advancing front of the diverticulum and invade the mesoderm of the caudal portion of the septum transversum. The vitelline veins traverse the region, bringing blood from the yolk sac and digestive tube to the heart. As hepatoblasts invade the mesenchyme, they disrupt the vitelline veins, tapping their blood supply. This supply is from the vitelline veins, segments of which later become the PVs. The hepatic bud is subdivided into cords by new capillaries called sinusoids. The sinusoidal flow coalesces into three major hepatic veins. At the time the main hepatic veins are developing, the entire liver is composed of only two lobules, and there is no artery and no left or right bile duct. As the hepatic and portal veins begin to branch, the branches interdigitate to remain equidistant from each other, and the parenchyma is subdivided into numerous lobules or acini. It has been suggested that the portal and hepatic vessels invade the most ischemic parenchyma, which is located at the nodal point of Mall, the point most distant from both PVs and hepatic veins [23,24].

The hepatoblast cords develop into anastomosing tubular structures with central bile canaliculi that eventually communicate with the bile ducts. Most hepatoblasts differentiate into hepatocytes, but those adjacent to the portal mesenchyme differentiate into a layer of duct progenitors called the ductal plate [25,26]. The ductal plate becomes bilayered and gradually forms segments with lumina. These segments form ducts that migrate away from the limiting plate to a more central location in the portal tracts near the portal vein. Portions of the ductal

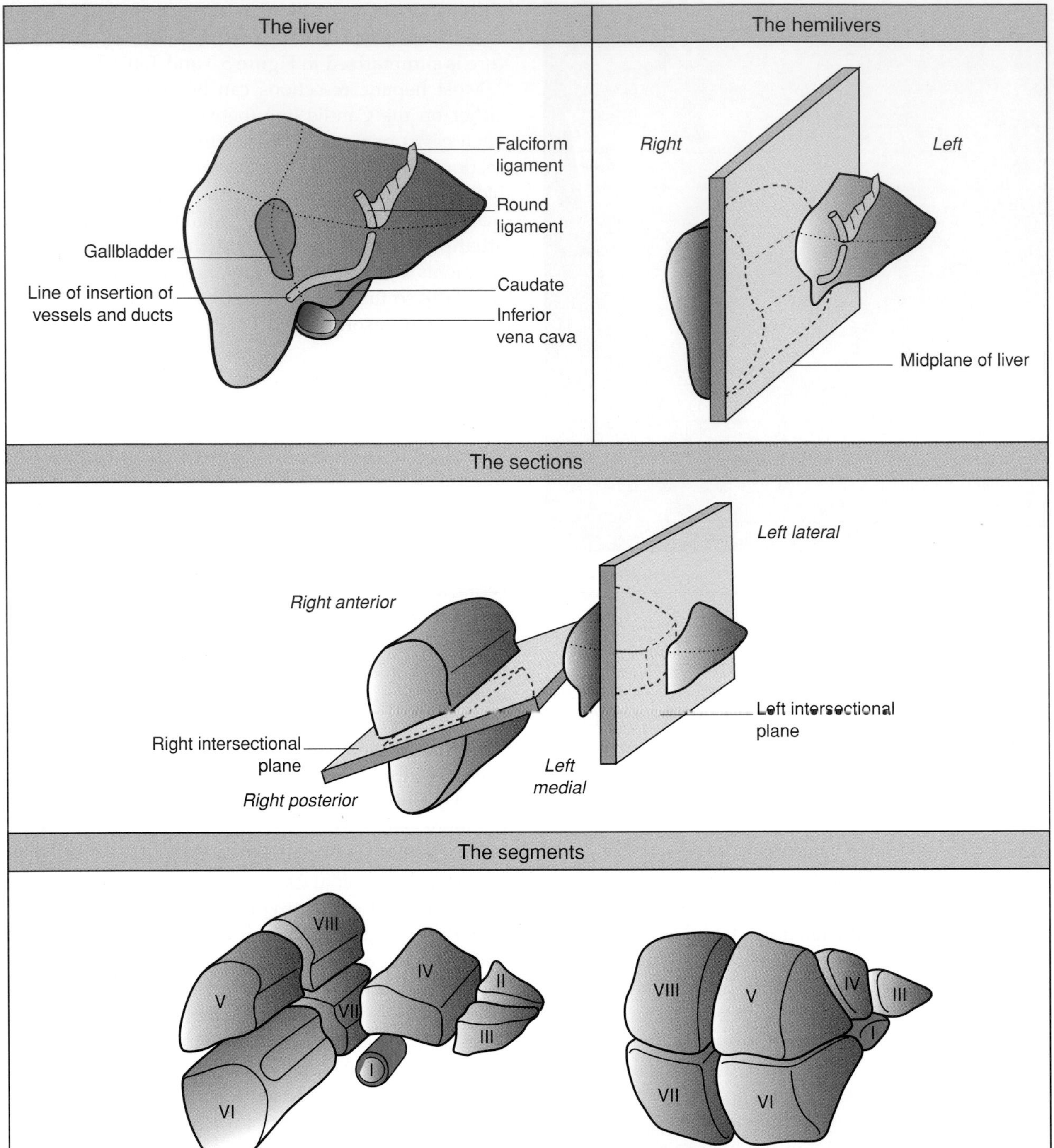

Figure 5.3 Schematic diagram of planes of division in the liver. The liver can be visualized as being divided into two hemilivers by the midplane of the liver. The hemilivers are each subdivided into two sections by right and left intersectional planes. Three of the sections are further subdivided into two segments each by intersegmental planes, based on the divisions of the ducts and arteries. The left medial section does not have a regular duct and artery division and is therefore called one segment (IV). However, for surgical convenience, it is subdivided into the posterior and anterior portions (segments IVa and IVb, respectively, not shown). The caudate lobe is a separate segment (I) that is not part of the four main sections. IVC, inferior vena cava. (Courtesy of Dr Strasberg; reproduced from Strasberg [18] with permission from Elsevier.)

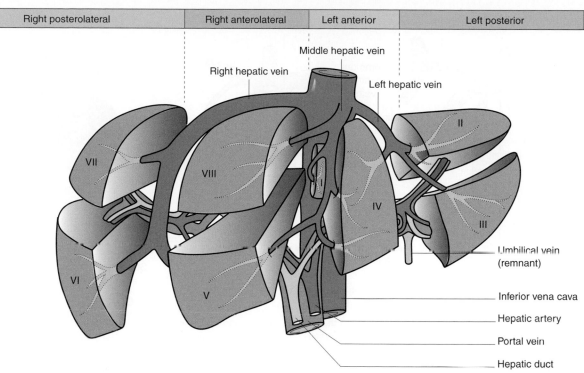

Figure 5.4 Schematic demonstration of the vascular relations of the segments. The segments are numbered using the nomenclature of Couinaud. The remaining elements of nomenclature are those of Strasberg. The midplane extends along the Cantlie line from the vena cava to the gallbladder. The middle hepatic vein runs in this plane. The right and left intersectional planes contain the right and left hepatic veins, respectively. Each section is supplied by one of the four major arteries and bile ducts. The portal pedicles and hepatic veins interdigitate, so they do not lie in the same planes except for the umbilical portion of the left portal vein and the umbilical vein (a medial branch of the left hepatic vein), both of which are found in the umbilical fissure (also known as the left intersectional plane). The *sections* of Strasberg coincide exactly to the *segments* of Healey and Schroy. The two *sections* of the right hemiliver correspond to the two right *sectors* of Couinaud. The tertiary structures of Strasberg and of Couinaud are called *segments*; these coincide to the *areas* of Healey and Schroy, except that segment IV is divided into two *areas* by these authors. (Drawn by M. Thompson; adapted from Wanless [206].)

Table 5.1 Nomenclature for resections of liver.

	Name of operation	
Portion of liver excised	**Strasberg**	**Couinaud, Goldsmith, and Woodburne**
Single segment	Segmentectomy (e.g., segmentectomy III)	–
Two adjacent segments	Bisegmentectomy (e.g., bisegmentectomy V, VIII)	–
Multiple segments	Segmentectomy (e.g., segmentectomy IV, V, VI)	–
One fourth of liver (e.g., left lateral section	Left lateral sectionectomy	Left lobectomy (segments II, III), left lateral segmentectomy
One half of liver, right hemiliver	Right hemihepatectomy (may or may not include segment I; e.g., right hemihepatectomy with segment I[a])	Right hepatectomy (segments V, VI, VII, VIII), right hepatic lobectomy
One half of liver, left hemiliver	Left hemihepatectomy	Left hepatectomy (segments II, III, IV), left hepatic lobectomy
Three fourths of liver, right hemiliver, and left medial section	Right trisectionectomy or right hemihepatectomy with left medial sectionectomy	Right lobectomy (segments IV, V, VI, VII, VIII, ± I), extended right hepatic lobectomy, right trisegmentectomy (Starzl)
Three fourths of liver, left hemiliver, and right anterior section	Left trisectionectomy or left hemihepatectomy with right anterior sectionectomy	Extended left hepatectomy, extended left lobectomy, left trisegmentectomy (Starzl)

[a]This comment also applies to left hemihepatectomy and the trisectionectomies.
Adapted from Strasberg [18].

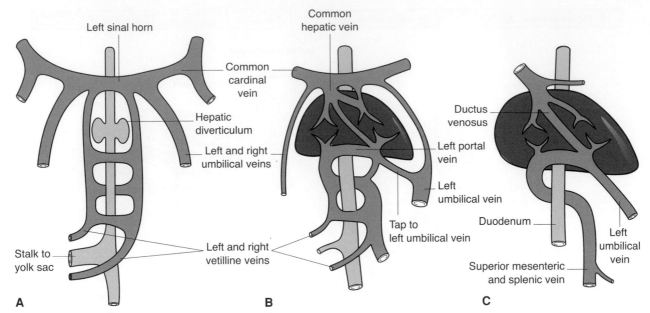

Figure 5.5 Drawing to show three stages in the development of the hepatic vasculature. (A) In the embryo, there are three paired venous beds that drain the placenta (umbilical veins), yolk sac, and intestinal tract (omphalomesenteric or vitelline veins), and the remainder of the body (cardinal veins). These beds converge on the sinal horns before entering the heart. The left and right vitelline veins are joined by three anastomoses to form a ladder-like structure with the intestinal tract intertwined. The extrahepatic portal vein develops from these vessels after selective obliteration of portions of the ladder (B, C). (B) The left vitelline vein receives a tap from the left umbilical vein. The intrahepatic segment of this tap becomes the umbilical portion of the left portal vein. Flow in this segment reverses after birth and supplies segments of the left hemiliver. As the liver develops, the venous drainage of the parenchyma becomes focused into two vessels, the future right and left hepatic veins, and later the middle vein (not shown), which usually drains into the left hepatic vein. The ductus venosus develops as a through-channel from the left portal vein to the common hepatic vein. The remainder of the portal vein blood perfuses sinusoids before reaching the hepatic veins. (C) The vasculature has been simplified with the removal of several segments including the most caudal anastomosis between the vitelline veins, the rostral portions of the left vitelline and left umbilical veins, and the right umbilical vein. The right lobe has grown faster than the left as the left lobe has lost the supply from the left vitelline vein and left umbilical vein blood is shunted through the ductus venosus. The left umbilical vein actually lies in the midline and later shifts to the right of midline.

plate resorb, leaving a complex anastomosing network of ducts that continues to simplify in the weeks after birth [27]. The common bile duct, left and right hepatic ducts, and gallbladder develop in the stalk region of the hepatic diverticulum. These ducts are continuous with the ductal plate in the cranial end of the diverticulum. As bile ducts develop, they become highly vascularized by arterioles and capillaries of the periductal plexus.

The liver occupies most of the abdominal cavity in the third month of gestation, in part because of large masses of sinusoidal hematopoietic cells. Thereafter, the right lobe grows faster than the left lobe but less than the rest of the body. The liver cell cords remain tubular until birth, when they begin to remodel into double-cell plates and finally into single-cell plates by 5 years of age. Hematopoietic cells are still found in the sinusoids at birth and are largely gone from the liver by 4 weeks of age.

The hepatoblast is a bipotential progenitor cell that is positive for cytokeratin CK19 and HepPar1. During organogenesis, these cells differentiate into hepatocytes (CK19-negative and HepPar1-positive) and small bile ducts (CK19-positive and HepPar1-negative) [26,28]. CK7 is expressed later and continues to increase in the weeks after birth. Severe injury to the adult liver causes a return to the pattern of expression seen in hepatoblasts. Thus, regenerating epithelial cells in the liver may have features of both ducts and hepatocytes [29].

Large vessels of the liver

The liver receives blood through the PV and through the HA, a branch of the celiac axis. Because the PV drains the blood of an area supplied by other branches of the celiac axis and by the superior and the inferior mesenteric arteries, the hepatic blood flow depends on the flow in these arteries [30].

Portal veins

The PV is an afferent nutrient vessel of the liver that carries blood from the entire capillary system of the digestive tract, spleen, pancreas, and gallbladder. It is constant in length, but the branches are variable (Fig. 5.6) [31,32]. The PV is formed behind the neck of the pancreas by the

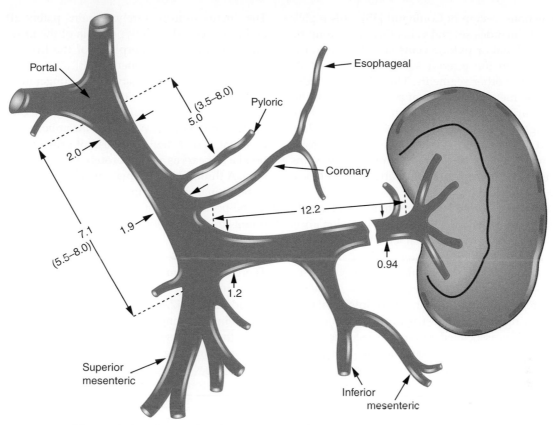

Figure 5.6 Measurements of the portal vein and its main branches, in centimeters. (Reproduced from Gilfillan [31] with permission from American Medical Association.)

confluence of the splenic and superior mesenteric veins. It also receives the superior pancreaticoduodenal vein, the left gastric (coronary) vein, and the cystic vein. Usually the upper 5 cm of the PV is devoid of major branches, allowing easy surgical dissection.

The splenic vein commences with five to six branches that return the blood from the spleen and unite to form a single nontortuous vessel. In its course across the posterior abdominal wall, it grooves the upper part of the pancreas, from which it collects numerous short tributaries. It runs close to the hilum of the left kidney and terminates behind the neck of the pancreas, where it joins at a right angle the superior mesenteric vein. Because of its nearness to the vessels of the left kidney, the splenic vein can be anastomosed to the renal vein. Its tributaries are the short gastric veins, the pancreatic veins, the left gastroepiploic vein, and the inferior mesenteric vein. In the distal splenorenal shunt operation, the short gastric veins are used for collateral drainage of the gastroesophageal varices.

The superior mesenteric vein carries blood from the small intestine, ascending colon, and transverse colon. The inferior mesenteric vein returns blood from the area drained by the superior and the inferior left colic and the superior rectal veins.

An important tributary of the portal trunk is the coronary vein. It runs upward along the lesser curvature of the stomach, where it receives some esophageal veins. In patients with portal hypertension, these enlarge to form varices.

The portal trunk runs in the hepatoduodenal ligament in a plane dorsal to the bile duct and the HA and divides into two lobar veins before entering the portal fissure. The right lobar vein, short and thick, receives the cystic vein. The left lobar vein, longer and smaller, is joined by the umbilical vein and the paraumbilical veins. It connects by the venous ligament with the inferior vena cava. The left lobar vein gives branches to the quadrate lobe and also to the caudate lobe before entering the parenchyma at the left end of the porta hepatis. A separate branch may arise near the bifurcation to supply the caudate lobe. This vein is easily injured during dissection. The paraumbilical veins arise from the umbilical portion of the left PV and travel in the round ligament, where they may become evident as umbilical varices in the presence of portal hypertension. The umbilical vein is easily recanalized in infants, allowing access for blood sampling and angiographic visualization of the portal system.

In addition to the main PV and its branches, the liver receives other veins from the splanchnic circulation, the parabiliary venous system of Couinaud [33]. This highly variable plexus includes several veins that arise from the pancreaticoduodenal or pyloric veins and drain into the PV or directly into the inferior surface of segment IV and less often into other segments. This plexus provides examples of the metabolic effects of proximity to insulin source. Veins arising from the pancreatic region carry blood with high insulin levels and pyloric veins carry low insulin blood. Because insulin determines the propensity of liver to store triglycerides, the anatomy of these veins could explain some examples of focal fatty liver and focal fatty sparing [34].

Anomalies of the portal-venous system are relatively rare. The anterior segment of the right liver occasionally is supplied by a branch of the proximal left PV [35]. Preduodenal PV may be a result of persistence of the most caudad anastomotic channel between the vitelline veins (see Fig. 5.5). It may be associated with duplication of the PV, annular pancreas, duodenal diaphragm, or intestinal malrotation producing duodenal obstruction [36]. Congenital absence of the PV is associated with portosystemic shunting, as the superior mesenteric vein and the splenic vein drain directly to the vena cava or left renal vein, usually separately [37]. This may be associated with hepatoblastoma or nodular hyperplasia of the liver (often simulating a neoplasm), cardiac anomalies, and biliary atresia.

The ductus venosus rarely remains patent after infancy and is associated with hypoplasia of the intrahepatic PV branches, nodular hyperplasia of the liver, atrial septal defect, and hyperammonemia [38].

Atresia of the PV may be a congenital malformation often associated with other vascular anomalies or a response to neonatal injury such as omphalitis or PV thrombosis [39]. When PV thrombosis occurs in the neonatal period the vein does not grow so that in adulthood it appears as a thin fibrous cord (hypoplasia or agenesis). A thrombosed PV may develop numerous irregular intraluminal channels in addition to a leash of collaterals in the porta, giving a radiologic appearance called cavernous transformation of the PV.

Hepatic veins

There are three main hepatic veins. The middle and left veins unite before entering the vena cava in 65–85% of individuals [7,40]. In 18%, there are two right hepatic veins draining into the vena cava [21]. In another 23%, there is a separate middle or inferior right hepatic vein draining segments V or VI, respectively. The veins have variable branching patterns. There are axial veins with four to six orders of dichotomous branching at acute angles, as well as numerous much smaller branches nearly at right angles (Fig. 5.7).

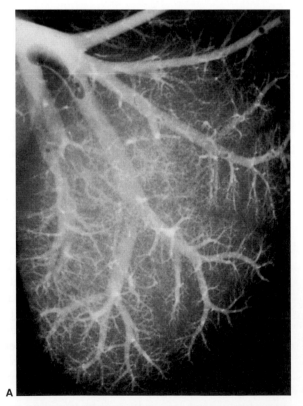
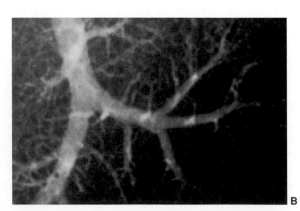

Figure 5.7 Hepatic veins shown on a postmortem angiogram. The major rami branch dichotomously and receive smaller branches nearly at right angles (see magnified portion on right).

The caudate lobe and adjacent parenchyma are usually drained by one or two small veins directly into the vena cava caudal to the main hepatic veins. When thrombosis of the main hepatic veins occurs, the veins of the caudate lobe are often spared, allowing survival and compensatory hyperplasia of this lobe [41]. Anastomoses between branches of the hepatic veins are uncommon in normal liver [42] but may be more frequent in the presence of diseases with portal hypertension [43]. Anastomoses of veins to other lobes become enlarged and may be mistaken for the original hepatic veins on Doppler interrogation. Partial recanalization occurs, often leaving webs in the hepatic veins or vena cava. These webs were formerly thought to be congenital, although now most are considered to be acquired [44,45].

Hepatic arteries

The common HA is the second major branch of the celiac axis [46]. It courses to the right along the upper border of the pancreas in the right gastropancreatic fold, which conducts the artery to the medial border of the hepatoduodenal part of the lesser omentum. It ascends in front of the PV in 91% of humans and to the left of and behind the bile duct in 64% of cases. It gives off the left and the right HAs to supply the corresponding hemilivers, The right and left HAs each divide into two arteries that supply the right anterior and posterior sections and the left medial and lateral sections, respectively. The middle HA arises from the left or right HA and supplies the quadrate lobe.

The cystic artery arises from the right HA in the upper part of Calot's triangle (formed by the cystic duct, common hepatic duct, and inferior surface of liver). The cystic artery divides into a superficial branch that is distributed to the peritoneal surface of the gallbladder and a deep branch that supplies the attached wall of the gallbladder and adjacent liver. In 75% of cases, the artery is single, and in 25%, there are two arteries with separate origins of the deep and superficial branches.

Anomalies of the HA are frequent, occurring in half of individuals [47]. Angiographic studies of the HA have demonstrated that the course of the arterial branches in the hilum deviates markedly from those of the PV, and in some cases the arteries may even cross the segmental fissures [48]. However, the more distal arterial branches follow the PVs closely, "climbing along them like a vine on a tree" [49].

Anomalies of the HA have gained new importance because of the advent of transplantation, aggressive resections, and intra-arterial chemotherapy. The most important anomaly is a right HA arising from the superior mesenteric artery to supply the entire right liver (14%) [50]. As this vessel may appear in Calot's triangle it is at risk during cholecystectomy. The left HA arises from the left gastric artery in 14–25% of people [46,50,51]. This vessel enters the liver at the left end of the hilum and may fail to be ligated during resections, leading to hemorrhage. Each of the aberrant arteries may be the only HA so that their injury can damage the liver severely. The PV and HA to segment IV may cross to the left of the umbilical fissure before turning medial and thus may be injured during left lateral segmentectomy. Ducts or small vessels cross this fissure in 20% [14].

There are extensive communications between the ultimate and penultimate branches of the right, the middle, and the left HAs in the umbilical fossa and in the region around the caudate lobe. The HA is provided with collateral flow through its anastomoses with arteries arising from the celiac axis and superior mesenteric artery. Anastomoses between the left and right HAs may occur. The main collaterals of the common HA are the right and left gastrics, right and left gastroepiploics, gastroduodenal, supraduodenal, retroduodenal, superior and inferior pancreaticoduodenals, aberrant HAs, and inferior phrenic arteries [52].

If ligation of an artery is necessary for the control of hemorrhage, ligation of the left or right artery is safe. Ligation of the HA proximal to potential collaterals such as the right gastric artery or gastroduodenal artery is better than ligation of the proper HA. After ligation of an HA, anastomotic channels enlarge and reestablish flow within a day [53].

Hepatic collateral circulation

Portal hypertension leads to the development of intra- and extrahepatic venous collaterals (Fig. 5.8) [54,55]. Extrahepatic collaterals are important, because when dilated to form varices, they are susceptible to rupture and massive bleeding. Varices in the submucosa of the gastrointestinal tract are most often a problem, especially in the esophagus and stomach but also in the rectum and duodenum and at ostomy sites.

Dilated umbilical or paraumbilical veins are found in 11% of patients with cirrhosis (veins of Sappey) [56]. They may cause a venous hum and caput medusa at the umbilicus (Cruveilhier–Baumgarten syndrome). Their presence implies high pressure in the left PV and therefore intrahepatic vascular obstruction. The direction of flow in lower abdominal wall collaterals is caudad if the inferior vena cava is obstructed, as in some patients with Budd–Chiari syndrome.

Varices may be found at sites where the gastrointestinal tract or pancreas becomes retroperitoneal or adherent to the abdominal wall because of pathologic processes. These "veins of Retzius" establish connections between the portal bed and the ascending lumbar azygos and renal and adrenal veins.

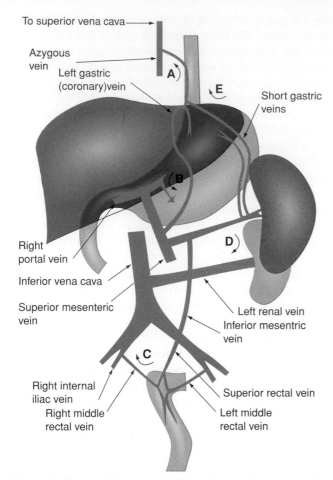

Figure 5.8 Diagram of the portal circulation. The most important sites for the potential development of portosystemic collaterals are shown. (A) Esophageal submucosal veins, supplied by the left gastric vein and draining into the superior vena cava via the azygous vein. (B) Paraumbilical veins, supplied by the umbilical portion of the left portal vein and draining into abdominal wall veins near the umbilicus. These veins may form a *caput medusa* at the umbilicus. (C) Rectal submucosal veins, supplied by the inferior mesenteric vein via the superior rectal vein and draining into the internal iliac veins via the middle rectal veins. (D) Splenorenal shunts, created spontaneously or surgically. (E) Short gastric veins communicate with the esophageal plexus. (Reproduced from Wanless [206] with permission from Elsevier.)

Within cirrhotic parenchyma, shunts are formed by anastomoses between smaller branches of the portal and hepatic veins, as discussed later [57]. These shunts allow blood to by-pass the sinusoidal exchange surface, leading to functional impairment. This effect is made worse by the creation of large shunts. In addition, any procedure that decreases portal flow to the sinusoids increases the likelihood of thrombosis, further increasing intrahepatic resistance. Titration of these benefits and liabilities is an important feature of surgical management. Large spontaneous shunts may be beneficial in lowering portal pressure and should not be disturbed without due consideration.

Portosystemic shunting appears to be responsible for reduced peripheral vascular resistance, possibly through the enhanced release of nitric oxide [58]. Dilated vascular channels in the lungs lead to intrapulmonary shunting with hypoxemia and increased cardiac output.

Lymphatics

Lymphatic channels are divided into deep and superficial networks [42,59,60]. The former run parallel to the branches of the portal vessels and hepatic veins, and the latter are found in the capsule. There are numerous anastomoses between these networks through small branches percolating through the capsule. The superficial lymphatics from the convexity form a dense network that coalesces into 14 groups of lymphatic trunks that drain through the coronary and falciform ligaments, through the diaphragm, and into the esophageal and xiphosternal nodes. From the undersurface of the liver, they drain into hepatic hilar nodes. The deep lymphatics following the portal tracts reach the hepatic nodes at the left side of the porta hepatis, and the lymphatics along the hepatic veins drain to lymph nodes near the vena cava. The portal lymphatic trunks drain 80% of the hepatic lymph.

Lymphatics can be identified by positive endothelial staining with antibodies to podiplanin (D2-40), Prox-1, and LYVE-1 [60]. Basement membranes, pericytes, and smooth muscle cells are scanty or absent [61]. The larger lymphatic vessels and trunks have valves; the walls contain smooth muscle cells.

The formation of lymph is discussed in the microanatomy section.

Nerves

The liver has a rich sympathetic and parasympathetic innervation [62]. Fibers derive from lower thoracic ganglia, the celiac plexus, the vagi, and the right phrenic nerve to form the plexuses about the HA, PV, and bile duct. The majority of fibers are organized into the anterior and posterior trunks, which enter the liver at the hilum. A few fibers enter at the hepatic veins and ligaments. The arteries are innervated mainly by sympathetic fibers. The bile ducts are innervated by both sympathetic and parasympathetic fibers. Unmyelinated sympathetic fibers send branches to individual hepatocytes in zone 1. Nerve discharges are propagated from one hepatocyte to another through gap junctions [63].

Most hepatic nerve fibers are aminergic or peptidergic, with a few cholinergic fibers; while intra-acinar cholinergic fibers have been found to occur in the guinea pig. Immunohistochemical studies have demonstrated many other substances in some hepatic nerve fibers, including vasoactive intestinal peptide, neuropeptide Y, glucagon, somatostatin, neurotensin, and calcitonin gene-related peptide. The effects of nerve stimulation are partially mediated by prostaglandins synthesized in nonparenchymal cells of the liver. There may be local baroreceptors capable of detecting sinusoidal hypertension and leading to reflex renal artery vasoconstriction [64,65]. Afferent nerves may be responsible for pain when the liver is distended.

Stimulation of the nerve bundles around the HA and PV results mainly in a sympathetic discharge that alters metabolism and hemodynamics of the liver [66]. Glucose and lactate output are increased. Ketone and urea production, ammonia uptake, oxygen consumption, arterial and portal blood flow, and bile flow are reduced. Sympathetic nerve stimulation may exacerbate the effect of toxins [67]. Parasympathetic stimulation is thought to increase glycogen synthesis and reduce glucose release. Hepatic parasympathetic activity has an important effect on skeletal muscle insulin resistance [68]. Nerve action is modified by prevailing levels of hormones, especially insulin and glucagon.

Denervation experiments have demonstrated depletion of hepatic norepinephrine, altered blood flow response to stress, a decrease in cholesterol and phospholipid output, a decrease in progenitor cell number and function, altered glycemic control and feeding behavior, and sodium retention [69,70]. The clinical importance of nerve function is uncertain. After transplantation, the denervated state of the liver persists [71], although functional abnormalities appear to be minor [69]. These include increased liver blood flow, decreased postprandial PV flow, a decrease in hepatic progenitor cells, insulin resistance with postprandial hyperglycemia, hyperphagia, and loss of hepatic pain response.

Biliary system

The biliary system includes the bile canaliculi, intrahepatic and extrahepatic bile ducts, peribiliary glands, gallbladder, and ampulla of Vater [28]. The intrahepatic ducts begin at the bifurcation of the common hepatic duct.

Large ducts and gallbladder

The nomenclature of the large intrahepatic ducts will vary with the system used for naming the hepatic subunits (see above). Each hepatic segment has a bile duct that drains into a sectoral duct that drains into the right or left hepatic duct, which drains the right or left hemilivers, respectively. Caudate lobe drainage is variable, with ducts usually entering both the right and left ducts. The junctions of the segmental, hepatic, and common hepatic ducts are also highly variable [72]. The right and left hepatic ducts join to form the common hepatic duct at the right end of the portal fissure. The common hepatic duct is 1–5 cm long (mean, 2 cm), is 0.4–1.3 cm in diameter (mean, 0.66 cm), and is situated to the right of the hepatic artery and in front of the PV [73]. It is joined by the cystic duct at its right side to form the common bile duct (ductus choledochus) that runs another 5–8 cm to the ampulla of Vater. The supraduodenal part of the common bile duct lies in the right border of the lesser omentum. The pancreatic part of the common bile duct passes retroperitoneally behind the first portion of the duodenum. It then runs in a groove on the posterior surface of the head of the pancreas, anterior to the inferior vena cava. At the left side of the duodenum, it is joined in 70–85% of cases by the pancreatic duct (of Wirsung) and forms a common channel of variable length [74]. When a dilatation is present, it is called the ampulla of Vater [75]. The common channel resides within an elevation of the duodenal mucosa called the major papilla (of Vater).

The sphincter of Oddi consists of circular muscle fibers that surround the common bile duct in its course through the duodenal wall [76]. Circular muscle fibers are also present around the end of the pancreatic duct and around the tip of papilla; longitudinal fibers are also present. The sphincter of Oddi is inhibited by cholecystokinin, assisting the expulsion of bile into the duodenum. An elongated common channel has been associated with congenital bile duct dilatation [77]. Bile reflux may occur after papillotomy or surgical anastomoses with the intestine, resulting in recurrent cholangitis.

The gallbladder is a receptacle that receives up to a liter of bile daily, concentrating it by sodium-coupled water transport, and expelling it on stimulation by cholecystokinin. The gallbladder is a pear-shaped sac with a volume of 30–70 mL, measuring 3 cm wide and 7–10 cm long. Its parts are designated as the fundus, body, and neck. It lies on the undersurface of the right liver lobe, with the fundus projecting beyond the inferior border of the liver where the lateral margin of the rectus crosses the costal margin. The body is directed upward and to the left. Posteriorly, the fundus and body are in close relation with the transverse colon and duodenum, respectively. Gallstones can perforate into these viscera. The neck of the gallbladder is curved anteriorly and, when enlarged, forms the so-called Hartmann pouch. The mucosa of the neck forms a spiral valve of Heister that continues into the cystic duct. The spiral valve has the function of regulating bile flow into and out of the gallbladder. The cystic duct measures 4–65 mm in length (mean, 30 mm) and 4 mm in average diameter [78].

The arterial supply of the bile ducts comes mainly from many branches of the common HA, especially the retroduodenal artery and the right HA [46,79]. The gallbladder may be supplied by one, two, or three arteries. The cystic artery usually arises from the right HA. The veins of the gallbladder are variable, draining into the liver at the gallbladder bed or into veins from the common bile duct but eventually draining into branches of either the left and/or right PV [7]. The lymph vessels of the gallbladder, hepatic ducts, and upper parts of the common bile duct empty into lymph nodes of the hilum. Those of the lower common bile duct drain into nodes near the head of the pancreas.

Nerve fibers supplying the extrahepatic ducts and gallbladder derive mainly from the sympathetic hepatic plexus laced around the hepatic artery. These also receive filaments from the right and left vagus nerves. Some nerve fibers deriving from the plexus can be seen running along the common bile duct. Sparse ganglion cells are present in the muscularis and the mucosa of the gallbladder. Nervous connection with the spinal system is brought about by fibers from the right phrenic and musculophrenic nerves. Because these nerves derive from the third or fourth cervical nerve, the anatomic basis for shoulder pain in gallbladder disease is evident. Vagal stimulation causes gallbladder contraction [80].

Histology of the bile ducts and gallbladder has been reviewed by Frierson [81] and Nakanuma et al. [28]. The walls of the extrahepatic ducts are formed by fibrous tissue with elastic fibers; smooth muscle is scanty or absent [82], except at the lower end of the common duct where muscle rings are conspicuous. The gallbladder wall contains abundant smooth muscle and little fibrous tissue. Rokitansky–Aschoff sinuses are outpouchings of the gallbladder mucosa through defects of the muscularis and are found in almost all gallbladders having calculi. The ducts of Luschka are small ducts in the areolar tissues of the hepatic surface of the gallbladder. These ducts communicate with intrahepatic bile ducts, but not usually with the gallbladder cavity, and may leak hepatic bile after cholecystectomy.

The mucosa has numerous papillary folds in the gallbladder, distal pancreatic duct, distal common bile duct, and ampulla. The mucosa of the bile ducts and gallbladder consist of a single layer of columnar epithelium and a lamina propria. A few goblet cells are present, especially in the ampulla. Somatostatin-containing cells may be present in the ampulla, a possible source for the development of somatostatinomas arising at this site.

Mucus-secreting accessory glands (peribiliary glands) are in the lamina propria of the gallbladder neck and extrahepatic bile ducts and adjacent to the large intrahepatic ducts [83].

Intrahepatic ducts

The intrahepatic ducts have been defined as ductules (less than 0.02 mm), interlobular ducts (0.02–0.1 mm), septal

ducts (0.1–0.4 mm), and large ducts (more than 0.4 mm) [28]. These measurements are approximate, as the definition is also dependent on relation to the segmental boundaries and on histologic pattern.

The large and septal bile ducts have a well-demarcated dense fibrous wall and high columnar epithelium with basal nuclei and small mucin droplets. These ducts express blood group antigens. Interlobular ducts are located near the center of portal tracts and have minimal or no fibrous investment, and the epithelium is low columnar or cuboidal and lacks mucin. There is a periodic acid–Schiff (PAS)-positive basement membrane. Ductules are located near the limiting plate and have cuboidal epithelial cells. The presence of a few ductules may be considered normal, but large numbers are a feature of cholestatic or regenerating liver. Throughout the biliary tree, each duct is usually accompanied by an artery of similar diameter, a helpful guide when evaluating the absence of ducts.

The peribiliary glands accompanying large intrahepatic and septal ducts may be located within the walls (intramural) or form clusters outside the fibrous wall (extramural). Intramural glands are mucin rich, and extramural glands may be mucinous or serous, rarely with focal pancreatic acinar differentiation. Peribiliary glands are hypertrophied in patients with clonorchis infestation and may be the origin of some cholangiocarcinomas arising in that disease [84]. These glands may form retention cysts at the hilum in cirrhosis, portal vein obstruction, and polycystic kidney disease [85], rarely causing obstructive jaundice [86].

Intrahepatic bile ducts are the site of injury in many diseases, resulting in duct destruction, secondary cholestasis, and eventually cirrhosis in severe cases. In primary biliary cirrhosis, ducts up to 0.3 mm in diameter are destroyed by an immune process. In primary sclerosing cholangitis, the most severely involved ducts are extrahepatic and large intrahepatic ducts with less severe duct destruction in the smaller branches. Ducts less than 0.1 mm are the focus in chronic allograft rejection, graft-versus-host disease, Alagille syndrome, and reactions to a variety of drugs and toxins. Neonatal biliary atresia, polycystic liver disease, and several other syndromes may be a result of a variety of insults to the developing ducts at the ductal plate stage [87].

The peribiliary vascular plexus is hypertrophied in livers with cirrhosis or with PV obstruction and is especially prominent in congenital hepatic fibrosis, where it may fill on portal venogram and appear to form a duplication of the portal tree [86].

Variations and surgical implications

A portion of the right liver may drain into the left duct system in 6% of cases [7]. In 25%, a branch of the right duct drains into the left duct [88]. The common hepatic duct may receive accessory hepatic ducts. If the common hepatic duct is absent, the right and left hepatic ducts may run separately and join close to the duodenum; the right duct receives the cystic duct. Other variations include a main duct draining into the gallbladder, the cystic duct draining into the right hepatic duct, and the right hepatic duct draining into the cystic duct [7,72,89,90]. The cystic duct usually enters the bile duct at an angle but may run parallel or curve behind the duct in a spiral fashion. The relations of the large ducts and vessels near the hilum are variable, but the peripheral branches of these structures run together within portal tracts.

Because ducts depend on arterial supply, ischemic necrosis, with or without stricture, may occur in the large bile ducts after transplantation, especially if the hepatic artery is compromised. Duct strictures, rupture, and infarction of the gallbladder have also been found after hepatic arterial injection of alcohol or chemotherapeutic agents, possibly because of injury to the peribiliary vascular plexus [28].

Numerous conditions are characterized by congenital or acquired anomalies of the duct system. Aberrant biliary ducts, the vasa aberrantia, form anastomoses between the gallbladder and small ducts in the adjacent liver. These ducts are liable to leak bile after cholecystectomy. Accessory mucus-secreting periductal glands are located all along the duct system. These may develop retention cysts that, rarely, encroach on the duct lumen to produce obstructive jaundice [86]. Congenital dilatation of the intrahepatic and/or extrahepatic ducts, known as choledochal cysts, is a rare cause of cholangitis or obstructive jaundice, usually presenting in childhood (see Chapter 42). Caroli disease is a subset of this condition, with dominant dilatation of the intrahepatic ducts. Congenital fibrocystic disease occurs in a variety of anatomic patterns, often with coexistent renal disease. Von Meyenburg complexes, clusters of dilated ducts within the portal tracts, are markers for adult polycystic kidney disease and polycystic liver disease [91]. Biliary atresia, the absence or obliteration of the extrahepatic bile ducts, is one of the most common causes of cirrhosis in childhood.

Anomalies of the gallbladder have been reviewed [92]. Absent gallbladder and double gallbladder are rare (0.05% and 0.02%, respectively). Duplication may be accompanied by two separate cystic ducts. Agenesis is associated with other congenital defects of the intestines or bones. Bilobed, hourglass-constricted gallbladders and those with a folded fundus (phrygian cap), persistent septum, or diverticulum favor retention and inflammation. The gallbladder can be completely buried in liver substance (intrahepatic gallbladder) or attached loosely to it by a mesentery (floating gallbladder). An ectopic gallbladder may be found attached to the left hepatic duct. Ectopic gastric mucosa within the gallbladder predisposes to perforation or hemorrhage.

Microanatomy

Normal human histology

When viewed histologically, the normal liver displays a uniform arrangement of portal tracts separated by parenchyma composed of hepatocellular plates and sinusoids. Terminal hepatic venules are located equidistant from portal tracts. The portal tracts contain arteries, ducts, nerves, and PVs in a connective tissue stroma (Fig. 5.9). Stroma within the portal tracts normally contains a small number of macrophages, plasma cells, and lymphocytes.

Although often called portal triads, the number of each of these elements varies with the size of the tract. In a study of needle biopsies, the average number of profiles per portal tract was 2.3 ducts, 2.6 arteries, and 0.7 veins [93]. The average minimum diameters were 13 μm for ducts, 12 μm for arteries, and 35 μm for PVs. In normal infants, the number of ducts per portal tract is less than in adults. The average number of portal tracts in adults was 19 per biopsy, with a mean biopsy length of 1.8 cm, although the interpretation of liver biopsies requires an assessment of sampling error. Biopsies obtained by the transjugular route were half this size, and in fibrotic

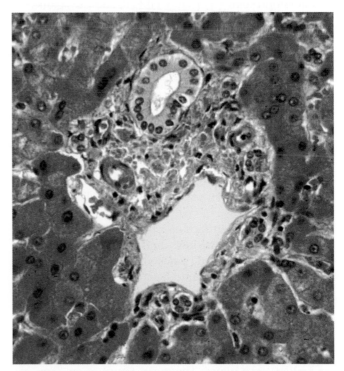

Figure 5.9 Normal portal tract from a human liver, showing several small ducts, two arteries, a portal vein, and occasional lymphocytes. Hematoxylin and eosin (H&E).

conditions the number of portal tracts available was often less than half a dozen.

Hepatocytes

Hepatocytes comprise 65% of the cells in the liver and 80% of hepatic volume. Hepatocytes are polyhedral with a central spherical nucleus. They are arranged in plates one cell in thickness, with blood-filled sinusoids on each side of the plates (Fig. 5.10) [94]. The cytoplasmic membrane has specialized domains providing a canalicular region on the lateral walls and numerous microvilli on the sinusoidal (basolateral) surfaces. The canalicular domains of adjacent hepatocytes are bound together by tight junctions to form bile canaliculi that coalesce and ultimately drain into ducts within portal tracts. Hepatocytes are also attached by gap junctions that have a role in transmission of nerve impulses from zone 1 to zone 3. Normal and abnormal ultrastructure of hepatocytes has been reviewed elsewhere [95,96].

Hepatocytes can be identified by evidence of albumin or α-fetoprotein synthesis using molecular techniques. It is more convenient to use immunohistochemical techniques. HepPar1 (carbamoyl phosphate synthetase), arginase-1, and CK18 stain the cytoplasm of all hepatocytes [97,98]. Glutamine synthetase stains the cytoplasm of hepatocytes near the terminal hepatic venules and regenerating hepatocytes [99,100]. Polyclonal carcinoembryonic antigen (CEA) and CD10 stain bile canaliculi. Alpha-fetoprotein, glypican-3, HSP70, and p28/gankyrin are often expressed in malignant hepatocytes [97,101,102].

Endothelial cells and sinusoids

The length of a human sinusoid varies between 223 and 477 μm. The diameter of the sinusoids can vary from 6 to 30 μm and can increase to 180 μm when necessary. Zone 1 sinusoids are smaller than those in zone 3 [103]. Caliber depends on active contraction of endothelial cells and stellate cells as well as passive distension [104]. Leukocytes are large compared with sinusoidal diameter, so that blood flow compresses the sinusoidal wall, promoting exchange between plasma, subendothelial fluid, and hepatocytes [103].

The sinusoidal surface is covered with a layer of endothelial cells to enclose the extravascular space of Disse (Fig. 5.10). Hepatic sinusoids differ from systemic capillaries in that the endothelial cells are fenestrated, subendothelial basement membrane material is scanty, Weibel–Palade bodies are absent in most species, and intercellular junctions are absent, permitting passage of large macromolecules including lipoproteins but not chylomicrons [94,105]. Fenestrations are grouped into clusters called sieve plates. The mean fenestration diameter in the rat is 150–175 nm, occupying 6–8% of the endothelial surface area [105]. The fenestrations can change in

size in response to various stimuli, including pressure, neural impulses, endotoxins, alcohol, serotonin, and nicotine [106]. They are large in zone 1 and smaller and more numerous in zone 3. Agents that disrupt actin filaments can almost double the number of fenestrations within minutes [106]. The permeability of fenestrations has been studied with marker particles. In the rat, liposomes 400 nm in diameter are readily engulfed by hepatocytes. The ability to traverse fenestrations may depend on deformability or surface charge of the particles [107].

Sinusoidal endothelial cells also differ from continuous endothelial cells in their immunohistochemical phenotypes. Factor VIII-related antigen, *Ulex europaeus* agglutinin I binding, PECAM-1, CD34, and 1F10 are features of continuous endothelial cells but not sinusoidal endothelial cells [108]. Sinusoidal endothelial cells express low affinity Fc γ-receptors (CD32, FcR), lipopolysaccharide-binding protein complex receptors (CD14), thrombospondin receptors (CD36), class II histocompatability receptors (CD4), and ICAM-1, stabilin-1, and stabilin-2 [109–111]. Stabilin-1 and stabilin-2 have roles in endocytosis of proteins by sinusoidal endothelial cells [112].

During embryogenesis, transition from a continuous to fenestrated phenotype occurs between 5 and 20 weeks' gestation [109]. The fenestrated phenotype partially reverts to the continuous endothelial phenotype in chronic hepatitis, cirrhosis, and hepatocellular carcinoma [110], including the expression of CD34, PECAM-1, and laminin receptors α6β1 and α2β1 [108,113]. Stabilin-2 expression is lost when the sinusoidal endothelium acquires CD34 expression [111]. These phenotypic changes may be an indication of arterialization of the sinusoids that occurs during the development of severe cirrhosis. Morphologically, cirrhosis may be accompanied by widening of the space of Disse, subendothelial deposition of collagen and basement membrane material, defenestration, and effacement of hepatocellular microvilli. These changes, often called "capillarization of sinusoids" [114] likely reduce transport across the sinusoidal walls and explain some of the hepatocellular dysfunction seen in cirrhosis.

Nitric oxide produced by hepatocytes, Kupffer cells, and sinusoidal and arterial endothelial cells may cause increased sinusoidal blood flow, thereby protecting the liver during various injuries [115–117]. Increased blood flow may be beneficial by preventing adhesion of leukocytes and platelets that might otherwise injure the endothelium [118]. Nitric oxide production may have a role in the hepatopulmonary syndrome [119] and hepatorenal syndrome [120]. Endothelin-1 is produced by activated stellate cells and causes these cells to contract [121]. Circulating endothelin-1 may have a role in the hepatorenal syndrome [120].

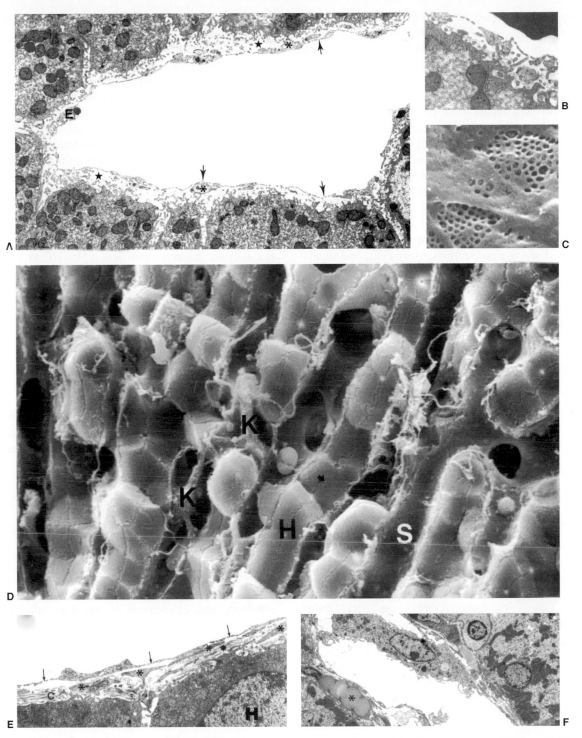

Figure 5.10 Ultrastructure of sinusoids. (A) Sinusoid showing endothelium (E) covering the subendothelial space of Disse (stars). This space contains stellate cell processes (asterisks) and hepatocellular microvilli. Note that the microvilli extend into recesses between hepatocytes. The endothelial cells are fenestrated (arrows). Transmission electron micrograph (TEM), original ×4,840. (B) Closer view showing endothelial fenestrations and microvilli of a hepatocyte. TEM, original ×10,000. (C) Endothelial fenestrations are clustered into sieve plates. Scanning electron micrograph (SEM), original ×29,400. (D) Hepatocellular plates are one cell in width with bile canaliculi (short black arrow) visible on the fractured edges of the plates. Hepatocytes (H), sinusoids (S), and Kupffer cells (K) are seen. Collagen fibers have been pulled from the spaces of Disse. SEM, original ×2,000. (E) The space of Disse (eight-pointed star) contains several stellate cell processes (asterisks) and collagen bundles (C). Endothelial fenestrations are labeled (arrows). H, hepatocyte nucleus. TEM, original ×6,000. (F) Sinusoid with a Kupffer cell in the lumen and a stellate cell containing lipid (asterisk) in the space of Disse. TEM, original ×2,000. (A, B, courtesy of Dr P. Bioulac-Sage. C, from Bioulac-Sage et al. [94] with permission from Springer-Verlag.)

Endothelial cell injury is important in endotoxemia, hypotensive shock, and cold perfusion of donor livers [122,123]. Donor livers may develop rounding-up and detachment of endothelial cells that may be responsible for some instances of primary nonfunction after transplantation [124,125].

It has been suggested that thickening of the space of Disse may contribute to poor transport of materials to the hepatocellular surface [126], as well as possibly contributing to portal hypertension [127]. Amyloid fibril deposition may widen the space of Disse dramatically and cause severe atrophy of subjacent hepatocytes. With severe amyloidosis, hepatomegaly, cholestasis, and noncirrhotic portal hypertension have been reported [128]. Cellular infiltration within the lumina of sinusoids occurs in Gaucher disease, mastocytosis, leukemias, and myeloproliferative disorders, but such infiltration does not correlate with clinical evidence of portal hypertension [129]. Obstruction of small veins is more likely to cause portal hypertension in these diseases, because sinusoids are distensible and able to regenerate [39].

Formation of lymph

Most hepatic lymph derives from the subendothelial space of Disse, and a minority, perhaps 10%, is formed by leakage from capillaries of the peribiliary plexus. The smallest recognizable lymph capillaries are found in the interstitial tissue in terminal portal tracts and adjacent to terminal hepatic venules (Fig. 5.11) [130]. The pathways that join these lymph capillaries to the space of Disse have been demonstrated [60]. It is believed that

lymph percolates through the collagen and proteoglycan matrix located between the periportal hepatocytes and within the portal interstitium. Lymph could also flow in the matrix investing the portal inlet venules and arterioles that penetrate the limiting plate.

Because of the large endothelial fenestrations in sinusoidal (and presumably lymphatic) endothelial cells, there is little or no oncotic pressure gradient between plasma and subendothelial tissue fluid, and the protein content of hepatic lymph is approximately 80% that of plasma. With a very low oncotic pressure gradient, the main stimulus for the formation of lymph is sinusoidal pressure. A 1 mm rise in efferent pressure doubles hepatic lymph flow. The liver normally produces 1–3 L per day but this may increase to 11 L per day in cirrhosis or extrahepatic outflow obstruction [131]. Communications between small bile ducts and lymphatics may allow for the increased formation of lymph seen after biliary tract obstruction [132].

Biliary tree

The biliary tree begins with a network of bile canaliculi that empty into bile ducts via the canal of Hering (Fig. 5.12) [133]. The small bile ducts are supplied by

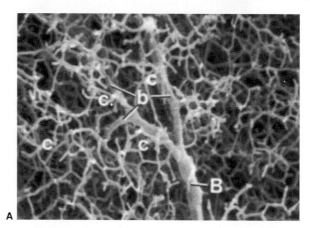

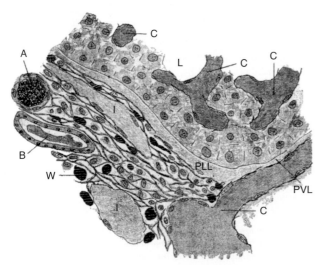

Figure 5.11 Mall's original drawing of portal and periportal tissue showing the space of Disse (perivascular lymph space, PVL), the space of Mall (perilobular lymph space, PLL), and a lymph vessel (l) after injection with gelatin. The space of Disse is continuous with the space of Mall. In life, the space of Mall may be a virtual space where lymph percolates among interstitial matrix fibers. Also shown are lobule (L), sinusoids (C), connective tissue fibers (W), bile duct (B), and artery (A). (Reproduced from Mall [130] with permission from Johns Hopkins University Press.)

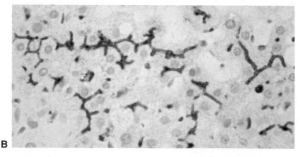

Figure 5.12 Bile canaliculi. (A) Scanning electron micrograph of a methacrylate injection cast of a rat biliary tree (×860). B, terminal twig of the bile duct; b, canal of Hering; c, bile canaliculi emptying into canals of Hering. (B) Photomicrograph of human liver stained for polyclonal carcinoembryonic antigen (CEA). CEA is present in the distribution of the bile canaliculi that could not be seen on H&E. A similar pattern may be seen with CD10 staining. (A, from Murakami et al. [208] with permission from Japanese Society of Histological Documentation.)

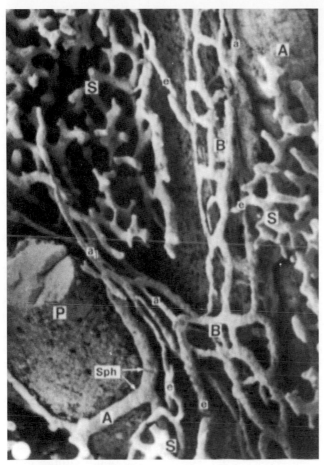

Figure 5.13 Scanning electron micrograph of cast blood vessels in the liver of a rhesus monkey. Peribiliary arterial plexus (B) receives blood from arterial branches (A) by means of afferent arterioles (a). The plexus supplies sinusoids (S) through efferent arterioles (e). Note the grooves indicating arteriolar sphincters (Sph). Arterioles (a₁) bypass the plexus and empty directly into sinusoids. P, portal vein. Methyl methacrylate cast, original ×135. (Courtesy of Dr T. Murakami, Okayama University.)

arteries (Fig. 5.13) [134]. Terminal branches of the hepatic artery supply a general capillary plexus within the portal tract, a peribiliary vascular plexus, and also empty directly into zone 1 sinusoids [135]. The general and peribiliary vascular plexuses eventually drain into sinusoids through capillary connections known as the "internal roots of the portal vein." The peribiliary vascular plexus has been divided into inner, intermediate, and outer layers. The inner layer has fenestrated endothelium, suggesting a role in water exchange. Similar fenestrated endothelium is found in the gallbladder mucosa.

Canaliculi have contractile and secretory properties. Canaliculi in isolated hepatocyte doublets have been shown to undergo rhythmic contraction thought to represent peristaltic activity in the intact liver [136]. These contractile functions are provided by a pericanalicular band of microfilaments composed of actin, myosin II, tropomyosin and α-actinin, and associated proteins,

stabilized by a sheath of noncontractile intermediate filaments [137].

The cholangiocytes lining the small ducts transport water and solutes under hormonal control [138–140]. Peribiliary glands also participate in the concentration of bile. Chloride transport is dependent on the cystic fibrosis transmembrane conductance regulator (CFTR), explaining the decreased water content of bile, hepatolithiasis, and secondary biliary cirrhosis seen in some patients with cystic fibrosis. In polycystic liver disease there is a genetic abnormality in cholangiocytic cilia leading to disruption of fluid transport and cholangiocyte proliferation [141].

Stellate cells

The stellate cells (fat-storing cells or Ito cells) are located within the spaces of Disse. Their cytoplasmic droplets normally contain abundant vitamin A, mostly as retinoyl palmitate [142]. These cells can be identified by the presence of immunoreactivity for smooth muscle actin, transient autofluorescence, and histochemical affinity for gold and silver.

When activated by various cytokines, stellate cells are transformed into myofibroblast-like cells that have reduced vitamin A storage, increased content of myofilaments and α-smooth muscle actin, and increased expression of procollagen gene transcripts [143–145]. Stellate cells, in their activated state, are the principal hepatic fibroblasts. Evidence has been presented that many forms of hepatic injury activate hepatic macrophages and that these cells release cytokines capable of activating stellate cells. Stellate cells can also secrete matrix metalloproteinases that degrade matrix proteins. Activated stellate cells contract under stimulation by sympathetic discharge or endothelin-1 secretion. They also secrete angiogenic factors such as ang1 [146,147]. By these mechanisms, stellate cells could exacerbate portal hypertension.

Kupffer cells

Kupffer cells are the resident macrophages in the liver. They comprise more than 80% of tissue macrophages in the body and 15% of cells in the liver. Although capable of proliferation in situ, they are also recruited from the peripheral blood [148]. Kupffer cells reside in the sinusoids, with pseudopodia anchored to endothelial cells or occasionally hepatocytes. They may form part of the sinusoidal wall. Macrophages in the liver are important in host response to various injuries including that induced by toxins and infectious agents [149].

Liver-associated lymphocytes

A few lymphocytes are normally found in portal tracts and sinusoids, even after washout with saline. Portal lymphocytes are 90% T cells with a CD4 : CD8 ratio of 1.6, whereas sinusoidal lymphocytes are 60% T cells with a CD4 : CD8 ratio of 0.4 and 30% natural killer (NK) cells (CD56+). Sinusoidal lymphocytes reside in the lumen adherent to Kupffer cells and endothelial cells [148]. Many sinusoidal lymphocytes are large, with cytoplasmic granules, and are also called pit cells because of the resemblance of the granules to grape seeds [150]. Pit cells are most numerous in zone 1 sinusoids. These cells are thought to have a role in killing tumor cells and virus-infected cells. The granules of pit cells contain perforin, a protein that injures cell membranes [150]. Traffic of lymphocytes and other leukocytes is largely controlled by chemokines elaborated during inflammatory reactions [151].

Stroma

Connective tissue stroma supports the capsule, the portal tracts from the hilum to periphery, and the sinusoidal walls. The composition of the stroma varies with location. Connective tissue of the capsule and portal tracts is mostly collagen type I and III and elastin. Reticulin fibers, defined by their histochemical affinity for silver, are largely composed of collagen type III and fibronectin [152]. They are located in the spaces of Disse, where they give tensile strength to the parenchyma. Type IV collagen forms a basal lamina around small vessels.

Many noncollagenous glycoproteins are in the matrix, including laminin, fibronectin, tenascin, entactin, vitronectin, undulin, osteonectin, and von Willebrand factor [153]. Laminin links basement membrane collagen to the integrins attached to endothelial cells and epithelial cells. Tenascin function is uncertain, but it is mitogenic for a variety of cell types. Vitronectin stimulates fibroblast migration. Von Willebrand factor is found within endothelial Weibel–Palade bodies and in basement membranes [153]. Proteoglycans bind to cells and matrix proteins and have roles in matrix–cell and cell–cell interaction.

In scarred livers, there is an absolute increase in many matrix proteins. The bulk of the scar tissue is type I collagen. After hepatocellular necrosis, the connective tissue framework is rapidly repopulated with hepatocytes in an orderly fashion. If regeneration is delayed, the deposition of collagen by stellate cells destroys the framework and prevents restitution to normal.

The stromal collagen is important to prevent tears in the blood vessels and sinusoidal walls. Focal rupture of reticulin leads to parenchymal hemorrhage and blood-filled cysts (peliosis hepatis) [154,155]. Mineral oil deposits are present in portal tracts and adjacent to hepatic venules in more than half of human livers and are usually accompanied by a slight mononuclear infiltrate [156].

Three-dimensional organization of the liver

The organization of the hepatic parenchyma has been conceptualized in two contrasting models: the acinus and the lobule [157–159]. Terminal PVs interdigitate with the terminal hepatic venules, with sinusoids bridging the gaps between these vessels. The terminal hepatic venules can be considered as being the center of a lobule or the periphery of several acini. The acinar approach is discussed in detail here.

The simple liver acinus is a small parenchymal mass, irregular in size and shape, arranged around an axis consisting of a terminal hepatic arteriole, portal venule, bile ductule, lymph vessels, and nerves that grow out together from a small portal field (Fig. 5.14). The simple liver acinus lies between two (or more) terminal hepatic venules with which its vascular and biliary axis interdigitate. In a 2D view, it occupies sectors of two adjacent hexagonal or pentagonal fields.

The plates and cords of the simple acini are in continuity with adjacent acini in three dimensions; there is no capsule separating the acini from one another. It can be assumed that the dividing line between the acini is the watershed of biliary drainage, so that each acinus empties its biliary secretion into the axial bile ductule.

A complex acinus is a clump of tissue composed of at least three simple acini whose axial channels branch in three dimensions from the preterminal stalk (Fig. 5.15). Each of its terminal branches forms the axis of a simple acinus. A sleeve of tissue composed of tiny clumps (acinuli) surrounds the preterminal channels. These acinuli are nourished by axial venules and arterioles branching off

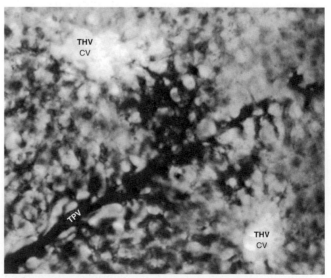

Figure 5.14 Liver acinus in a human. The acinus occupies sectors of only two adjacent hexagonal fields and reaches their central veins (CV). The terminal portal branch (TPV) is injected with India ink and runs perpendicular to the two terminal hepatic venules (THV) with which it interdigitates. Thick cleared section, original ×300.

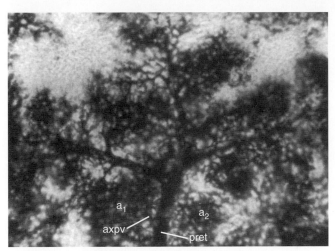

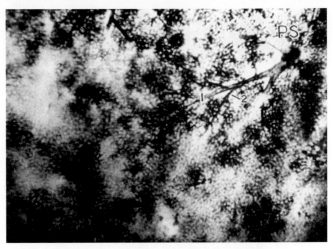

Figure 5.15 Complex acinus in a human. The sinusoids injected with India ink are supplied by three terminal portal branches and their parent preterminal vessel (pret). These portal venules help form the axial channels of a complex acinus cut longitudinally. The sleeve of parenchyma around the preterminal vessel is formed by acinuli (a_1, a_2). axpv, axial portal venule supplying the sinusoids of a_1. The poorly injected white areas (in the upper corners) are parts of zone 3 around the terminal hepatic venules, which are not shown. 150 μm thick cleared section, original ×88.

Figure 5.16 Group of acinar agglomerates in a human liver injected with India ink. Three large portal branches grow out in different directions from a portal space (PS). One of these runs diagonally through the field and represents the axis of an acinar agglomerate. From this portal branch, preterminal (1) and terminal (2) branches grow out and form the axes of complex and simple acini, respectively. 100 μm thick cleared section, original ×18.

the preterminal vessels. Structural and functional unity in a complex acinus can be demonstrated by injection of colored materials [160]. The axial vessels of the simple acini are always the same color as the parent vessels of the complex acinus. Three or four complex acini form larger clumps of tissue, the acinar agglomerates. Acini or acinuli also form a sleeve of parenchyma around the axial stem servicing the agglomerate.

The acinar agglomerate has unity because the main route of vascular supply and the biliary drainage are common to the whole clump as well as to its subdivisions. The hierarchy can be continued because several agglomerates are supplied by a single macroscopic portal tract. The PVs supplying agglomerates in the human liver are approximately 150 μm in diameter (Fig. 5.16) [160]. All branches of the hepatic vein interdigitate with HA and PV branches of similar order; this creates a hexagonal or pentagonal pattern when seen histologically in cross-section (Figs. 5.17 and 5.18).

The acinus is an ideal physiologic unit for the understanding of many vascular and biliary events in human biology (see discussion of cirrhosis below). The conceptual advantage of the acinus is that the blood supply of a portion of parenchyma and the bile duct draining that same parenchyma reside in the same portal triad. "Thus, structural, circulatory, and functional unity is established in this small clump of parenchyma" (Fig. 5.19) [161]. By contrast, the classic hexagonal lobule is supplied by several separate PV branches, arteries, and ducts, each of which also supplies other adjacent lobules [160].

McCuskey [162] notes that all the essential relationships are present within a smaller unit called hepatic microvascular subunits. The smallest useful unit is that in which there is a significant barrier to blood flow between adjacent units.

Recent studies show that PV blood is distributed by numerous small inlet venules, giving a portal supply that is more diffuse and less granular than that pictured by the original description of the acinus [157–159]. These analyses suggest that isobars of oxygen tension are

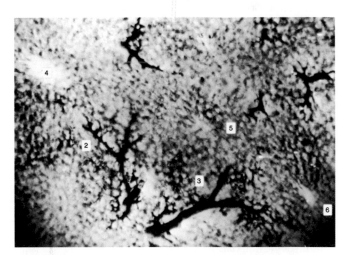

Figure 5.17 Interdigitation of portal and hepatic vein branches in a human liver injected with India ink. Two horizontal terminal portal branches (2, 3), forming the axes of acini, interdigitate with three vertical terminal hepatic venules (4, 5, 6), around which they arch. Thick cleared section, original ×110.

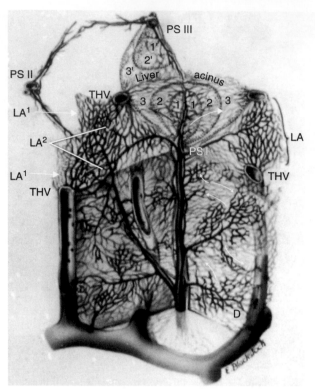

Figure 5.18 Vascular and biliary architecture of an acinar agglomerate and the relation of the acini to the adjacent hexagonal lobule. Note the arcuate courses of the terminal portal branches, the irregularly arranged simple acini, and the short portal vessels that form the axes of tiny acinuli constituting the mantle of parenchyma around the longitudinally cut portal space. Intercommunicating paths of acini and acinuli are shown by white arrows. D, channels of Deysach; LA, LA¹, simple liver acinus; LA², simple acinus penetrating a hexagonal field situated well above the level of origin of the acinus; PS I, PS II, PS III, portal spaces; THV, terminal hepatic venule; 1, 2, 3, circulatory zones of the simple liver acinus.

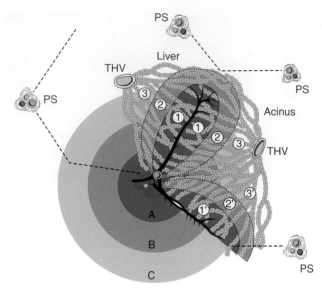

Figure 5.19 Blood supply of the simple liver acinus and the zonal arrangement of cells. The acinus occupies adjacent sectors of neighboring hexagonal fields. Zones 1, 2, and 3, respectively, represent areas supplied with blood of first, second, and third quality with regard to substrate, oxygen, and nutrients. These zones center around the terminal afferent vascular branches, terminal bile ductules, lymph vessels, and nerves and extend into the triangular portal field from which these branches crop out. Zones 1′, 2′, and 3′ designate corresponding areas in a portion of an adjacent acinar unit. In zones 1 and 1′, portal inlet venules empty into sinusoids. Note that zone 3 approaches the preterminal portal tract, nearly reaching the inner circle (A). PS, portal space; THV, terminal hepatic venules (central veins).

sickle-shaped (Fig. 5.20), with the parenchymal subunits being components of a hedge rather than individual grapes on a vine. Although parenchymal subunits are difficult to visualize in the normal human liver, they become evident in pathologic conditions such as nodular regenerative hyperplasia, in which there is a pruning of the portal-venous supply. As with a hedge, when individual portal units are pruned, the remaining units undergo hyperplasia to form an array of spherical units, revealing the underlying acinar structure. The hierarchical arrangement of simple, complex, and agglomerate acini can be appreciated in livers with prominent atrophy or necrosis [161]. In this century-long debate, it is useful to note that parenchymal subunits in the human liver do not exist. The debate concerns the best way to imagine their structure if they did exist.

Hepatocellular heterogeneity

The liver is anatomically situated to receive high concentrations of nutrients and certain hormones from the intestines and pancreas. Gradients of these substances, as well as oxygen and waste products, are found across the functional units of liver. These gradients are not constant but vary with cycles of feeding and exercise.

The position of hepatocytes within the acinus is reflected in the specialized functions of these hepatocytes (Fig. 5.21) [158,163–165]. Zone 1 hepatocytes are adapted to high oxidative activities, having numerous large mitochondria. Dominant processes in zone 1 are gluconeogenesis, β-oxidation of fatty acids, amino acid catabolism and ureagenesis, cholesterol synthesis, and bile acid secretion. Zone 3 is an ideal location for exergonic processes, including glycolysis and lipogenesis. There is a narrow rim of hepatocytes adjacent to terminal hepatic venules that remove ammonia from the blood by synthesizing glutamine. Zone 3 is also the site of general detoxification and biotransformation of drugs.

Metabolic zonation is accompanied by gradients of some anatomic features [161]. Mitochondria are larger and more numerous and lysosomes and Golgi are more abundant in zone 1. Smooth endoplasmic reticulum is more abundant and nuclear volumes are larger in zone 3. Endothelial fenestra are larger and less numerous in zone 1. Kupffer cells, large granular lymphocytes, stellate

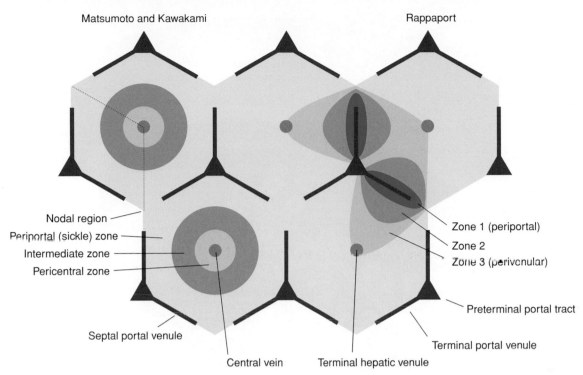

Matsumoto and Kawakami

Rappaport

Nodal region
Periportal (sickle) zone
Intermediate zone
Pericentral zone

Zone 1 (periportal)
Zone 2
Zone 3 (perivenular)

Preterminal portal tract

Septal portal venule

Terminal portal venule

Central vein   Terminal hepatic venule

Figure 5.20 The acinar structure of the hepatic microcirculation, as conceived by Rappaport [160] and modified by Matsumoto and Kawakami [157]. In both models, the margins of the shaded zones represent planes of equal blood pressure (isobars), oxygen content, or other characteristics. The models differ in the shape of the isobars surrounding the terminal portal venules. The acinus is bulb-shaped, and the classic hexagonal lobule is comprised of several wedge-shaped portions (called primary lobules, indicated by dotted lines, upper left), which have cylindrical (sickle-shaped) isobars. The nodal region is the nodal point of Mall [23]. (Reproduced from Wanless [207] with permission from Elsevier.)

cells, and sympathetic nerve endings are all more numerous in zone 1. There are also gradients in the composition of matrix proteins [166]

The control of metabolic zonation has been found to operate at the pretranslational level, with a few exceptions. Thus the gradients of the enzyme protein and the enzyme mRNA tend to parallel each other. Enzyme expression usually varies during the feeding cycle or changes in oxygen tension, and the zonation is said to be dynamic. It is likely that many signals interact to produce dynamic zonation. Glucose and oxygen gradients each have an effect on various enzymes, and these gradients are interdependent [167,168]. Genes in the Wnt/β-catenin pathway appear to mediate metabolic zonation [169,170].

Stable zonation that does not vary with metabolic signals is a result of intercellular or cell–matrix interactions. For example, glutamine synthetase activity may depend on close approximation of hepatocytes with some element of the venules [164,171]. Glutamine synthetase expression becomes undetectable in late cirrhosis [99] possibly because of the destruction of hepatic venules and secondary necrosis of zone 3 hepatocytes during the development of cirrhosis [100].

Clinical importance of hepatocellular heterogeneity

Metabolic heterogeneity is responsible for zonal injuries that are of diagnostic value to the pathologist. The distribution of necrosis and steatosis in response to chemical injury is often zonal. Sharply defined zone 3 necrosis is characteristic of toxicity from acetaminophen, *Amanita phalloides*, pyrrolizidine alkaloids, and various hydrocarbons such as halothane and carbon tetrachloride. Zone 1 necrosis has been found with allyl alcohol, phosphorus, and high-dose iron ingestion. Zone 2 toxicity is rare in humans but has been produced in animals with ngaione, furosemide, and beryllium. Cocaine toxicity in rodents may affect different zones depending on preexisting enzyme induction [172].

Systemic hypoperfusion generally produces zone 3 necrosis. This pattern may be altered by local factors. For example, in disseminated intravascular coagulation, zone 1 sinusoidal fibrin deposition causes maximum ischemia to be located in zone 1 or 2. Zone 2 necrosis has been reported in some patients with hypotensive shock [173]. Viral hepatitis usually produces spotty necrosis in all zones but often with an ill-defined zone 3 predominance. Yellow fever often produces zone 2 necrosis. Herpes virus

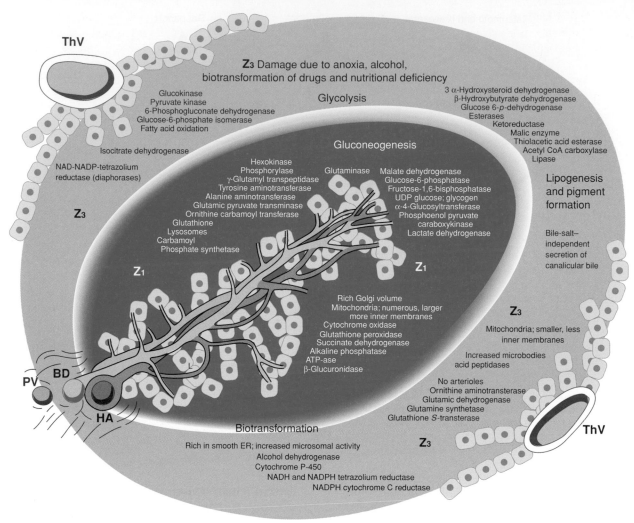

Figure 5.21 Schematic diagram of various metabolic processes that show zonal differences across the acinus. BD, bile duct; hep art, hepatic arteriole; PV, portal vein; ThV, terminal hepatic venule; Z1, periportal area; Z3, periacinar and perivenular area (the latter is derived from portions of zone 3 of several adjacent acini). For description, see text; for references see [161] and [164]. ATP, adenosine triphospate; CoA, coenzyme A; ER, endoplasmic reticulum; NAD, NADH, nicotinamide-adenine dinucleotide (and reduced form); NADP, NADPH, nicotinamide-adenine dinucleotide phosphate (and reduced form). (Adapted from Rappaport and Wanless [161] and Jungermann and Kietzmann [164].)

produces well-demarcated necrosis that does not follow a zonal distribution.

In hemochromatosis, hemosiderin is deposited predominantly in zone 1 hepatocytes. This is useful to distinguish hemosiderin from lipofuscin, the latter occurring predominantly in zone 3 hepatocytes. Proximity to a source of insulin favors the development of steatosis, as seen after instillation of insulin in the peritoneal cavity during dialysis, and decreased steatosis is seen in infarcts of Zahn, where PV supply to the tissue is obstructed.

Control of hepatic microcirculation

The terminal PVs supply sinusoids directly, giving a constant but sluggish blood flow [160,161]. In contrast, arterioles drain into terminal portal venules and zone 1 sinusoids, giving a pulsatile but small volume flow that appears to enhance sinusoidal flow, especially in periods of reactive arterial flow, as in the postprandial state. Groups of sinusoids shift their work asynchronously. The change from storage phase of inactive sinusoids to flow activity demonstrates at the microscopic level the function of the liver as a "venesector and blood giver of the circulatory system" [174].

Arterial flow varies inversely with PV flow. The mechanism of this *hepatic arterial buffer response* is based on washout of locally produced adenosine [175]. When portal-venous flow is reduced, adenosine accumulates and causes dilatation of the arterial resistance vessels; the reverse also occurs. The relative contribution of arterial and portal-venous flow varies between regions of the liver and this varies with gravity and other physiologic variables [176]. The conductance of PVs increases with distention, causing portal pressure to be little altered by large changes in PV flow [177]. In addition to arteriolar tone, local control of the microcirculation may depend on the contraction state of sinusoidal endothelial cells and stellate cells [104].

Regional blood flow is of practical importance when investigating focal lesions such as focal nodular hyperplasia and neoplasms. The venous and arterial circulation can be differentially imaged by using computed tomography (CT) with arterial portography (CTAP) or CT with intravenous contrast injection. Cirrhotic nodules, dysplastic nodules, and small hepatocellular carcinomas may have a portal-venous supply and are usually isodense on contrast CT. Hepatocellular carcinoma, hepatic adenomas, metastases, and focal nodular hyperplasia are mostly supplied by arteries and are therefore hyperdense with contrast CT [178–181].

Physioanatomic aspects of human liver disease

Regeneration of hepatocytes

The normal liver maintains a constant mass that is determined by the needs of the host [182]. If a partial hepatectomy is performed, the organ grows to regain much of the original mass in 10 days in rodents and in a few weeks or months in humans [183]. If a liver is transplanted into a new host, the new liver grows (by mitosis) or shrinks (by apoptosis) to the size of liver expected for that host's body size. Hepatocyte dysfunction, such as chronic cholestasis in primary biliary cirrhosis or primary sclerosing cholangitis, appears to be a signal to initiate cell proliferation, as the liver may be twice the normal weight in the early stages of these diseases.

There is controversy concerning the source of hepatocytes participating in regeneration. The normal resting liver has a very low mitotic rate. After many types of injury, mitoses become readily visible in hepatocytes from all acinar zones. However, some labeling studies have suggested that mitosis is particularly active in the periportal region, giving rise to the hypothesis that hepatocytes are born in zone 1 and migrate in their lifetimes to zone 3 [184]. This "streaming liver" concept implies the presence of stem cells, now considered to be located in the smallest radicles of the biliary tree, the canals of Hering [133,185]. Cells in this location are thought to be able to differentiate into cholangiocytes and hepatocytes [186–188]. The direction of differentiation between these two compartments may be directed by the Wnt and Notch pathways [189]. It appears that the bulk of cell replacement, in acute and subacute injury models, is by panacinar mitosis. The stem cell and streaming liver mechanisms may be important in severe injury states [190]. The stem cell population may be replenished by cells migrating from bone marrow [182,191–193].

In normal human liver, half of hepatocytes are diploid and the remainder are polyploid [194]. One third of hepatocytes are binuclear. The processes of polyploidization and binucleation are irreversible so that polyploidy increases with age. These processes may protect long-lived hepatocytes against mutation. During a regenerative stimulus, binucleation and polyploidy decrease as binucleating growth is suppressed. Thus, after regeneration, freshly divided cells have small and uniform nuclei, in contrast to the polyploid resting cells.

Putative signals for initiation of the cell cycle in hepatocytes include hepatocyte growth factor (HGF), made in all the major types of nonparenchymal liver cells, epithelial growth factor (EGF), made in salivary glands and hepatocytes, transforming growth factor α (TGF-α), made in hepatocytes, and tumor necrosis factor (TNF) [195]. Endotoxin stimulates TNF secretion and TNF stimulates Kupffer cells to secrete interleukin-6, which is an important mediator of hepatocellular regeneration. HGF and TGF-β are bound to extracellular matrix [196]. Insulin and glucagon support hepatocyte growth in culture and in vivo, although they are not complete mitogens for hepatocytes. Although the details of this complex system are not fully understood, it is clear that cytokines and growth factors derived from multiple cells types are involved. Thus, gut-derived endotoxin, pancreatic hormones, activated Kupffer cells, and sinusoidal blood flow will influence hepatocellular regeneration [197].

Pathogenesis of chronic liver disease

Chronic liver disease is usually defined as hepatic injury lasting for at least 6 months. The late stages of chronic liver disease have often been divided in two clinicoanatomic forms: cirrhosis and noncirrhotic portal hypertension, the former associated with portal hypertension and hepatic dysfunction and the latter with portal hypertension and nearly normal function. While these categories are often sufficient for clinical management, the anatomic features allow further subdivision, which is necessary to interpret liver biopsies and understand the pathogenesis of progressing and regressing liver disease (Table 5.2). All types of chronic liver disease are associated with vascular obstruction and the various anatomic patterns in Table 5.2 can be explained by the distribution and severity of the obstructive lesions (Fig. 5.22).

Hemodynamic changes in the parenchyma can be understood in terms of inflow and outflow imbalance. When either inflow is increased (by hyperemia or angiogenesis) or outflow capacity is decreased (by hepatic vein obstruction), the tissue becomes congested and suffers

Table 5.2 Clinical and anatomic features of the major forms of chronic liver disease.

Anatomic diagnosis	Portal hypertension	Hepatocellular dysfunction	Parenchymal extinction and fibrous septa	Description of fibrous septa	Obliteration of small portal veins	Extrahepatic or large intrahepatic portal vein block	Obliteration of small hepatic veins
Cirrhosis, venocentric[a]	++	++	+++	Between hepatic veins, portal tracts not involved	+	− or +[d]	+++
Cirrhosis, micronodular	++	++	+++	Many, broad	+++	− or +[d]	+++
Cirrhosis, macronodular	+	+	++	Many, thin	++	− or +[d]	++
Cirrhosis, incomplete septal	+	+/−	+	Moderate, thin, or incomplete	++	−	+
Chronic obliterative microvascular disease	+	+/−	+/−	Thin or absent	++	−	+
Obliterative portal venopathy[b]	+	+/−	−	−	++	−	− or +
Extrahepatic portal vein obstruction[c]	++	+/−	−	−	++	++	−

Gradings are for typical examples but gradings can vary within each anatomic category.

[a] Also known as reversed-nodularity cirrhosis of Budd–Chiari syndrome.

[b] Often with nodular regenerative hyperplasia.

[c] For example, portal vein thrombosis, portal vein agenesis, or cavernous transformation of the portal vein.

[d] Present with secondary portal vein thrombosis.

injury. This injury involves all components of the tissue, including the portal veins, sinusoidal walls, hepatocytes, and hepatic veins. Congestive injury to the sinusoids leads to atrophy or parenchymal extinction. Congestive injury to the hepatic veins causes obstruction of these veins and a worsening of congestion and a positive feedback loop of parenchymal extinction. Congestive injury to the portal veins causes hepatic inflow to be converted from a predominantly low pressure venous supply to a high pressure arterial supply. Thus, the hemodynamic effects of chronic liver disease can be summarized as *in–out imbalance,* a state that leads to progressive destruction of parenchyma and evolution to cirrhosis [198].

The effects of these flow changes can be recognized histologically. When regions of parenchymal extinction occur, there is collapse of the architecture so that hepatic veins and portal tracts become approximated (Fig. 5.23). If parenchymal extinction lesions are sufficiently large, linear regions lacking hepatocytes are produced that are recognized as "fibrous" septa. Regeneration of hepatocytes adjacent to septa causes curved deformity of the septa. When numerous curved septa are present, the histologic pattern of cirrhosis can be appreciated. If obstruction is greater in portal veins than hepatic veins, tissue injury is not sufficient to cause extensive parenchymal extinction and the result is noncirrhotic portal hypertension, often with nodular regenerative hyperplasia [199].

The histologic appearance of the liver varies with time after injury. If chronic injury abates, as with successful suppression of viral activity or abstinence from alcohol, venous drainage sites improve and in–out imbalance resolves. This allows collagen to be resorbed and hepatocytes to fill-in septal regions [200]. Thus, micronodular cirrhosis can remodel progressively into macronodular cirrhosis, incomplete septal cirrhosis, and eventually a state of regressed cirrhosis (Figs. 5.23 and 5.24). Because portal vein obliteration is difficult to reverse, [201] patients with regressed cirrhosis commonly have noncirrhotic portal hypertension and a histologic appearance described as *chronic obliterative microvascular disease.*

The mechanism of vascular obstruction in chronic liver disease depends on the nature of the primary disease. In most forms of chronic hepatitis, portal and hepatic vein phlebitis occurs as a bystander effect of inflammation in adjacent tissue [202]. In Budd–Chiari syndrome thrombosis is important [203]. In chronic biliary disease, bile salt

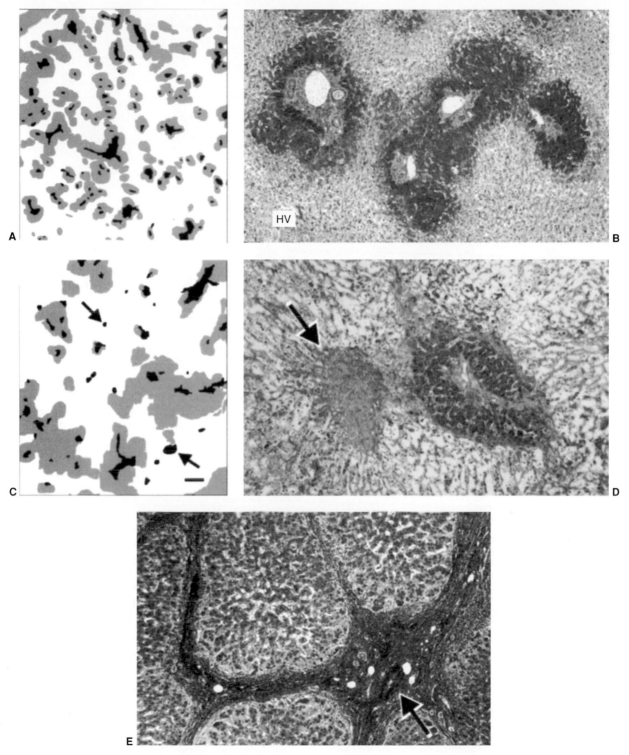

Figure 5.22 The histogenesis of cirrhosis. There are two basic types of cirrhosis, venocentric and venoportal. The type is determined by the distribution of vascular obstruction as illustrated by these examples with Budd–Chiari syndrome. (A, B) Venocentric cirrhosis occurs when parenchyma near obstructed hepatic veins (HV) shows contiguous cell loss (extinction) and fibrosis and cirrhotic nodules (dark tissue) contain portal tracts with patent veins. The periportal tissue survives because of retrograde portal vein drainage. (C, D) When hepatic vein obstruction is followed by portal vein obstruction, retrograde portal vein flow is not possible and the periportal tissue cannot support hepatocytes. This is shown in (C) where portal tracts (black) are usually accompanied by periportal tissue (gray) except in regions affected by portal vein obstruction (arrows) (bar = 1 mm). In (D) the arrow indicates a portal tract with an obstructed portal vein and absent periportal tissue. (E) Venoportal cirrhosis occurs when portal tracts are incorporated into the septa located adjacent to the cirrhotic nodules. Arrow shows obliterated portal vein. (B, D, E) Elastic-trichrome stain. (Adapted from Tanaka and Wanless [203] with permission from Elsevier.)

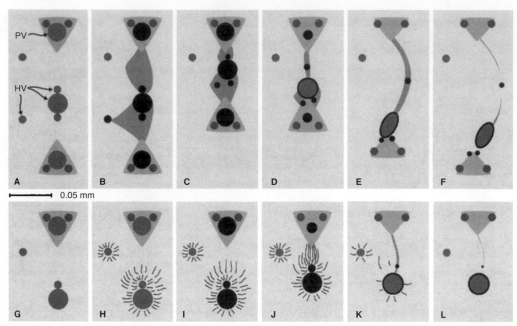

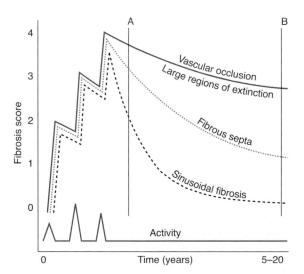

Figure 5.23 Diagram of tissue remodeling in chronic hepatitis (A–F) and in alcoholic liver disease (G–L) during the development and regression of cirrhosis. Normal acini are shown in (A) and (G) with the sequence of events leading to small regions of parenchymal extinction in the following panels. Obstructed veins are shown as black circles. (B) Obliteration of small portal and hepatic veins occurs early in the development of cirrhosis in response to local inflammatory damage. The supplied parenchyma becomes ischemic. (C, D) Ischemic parenchyma shrinks and is replaced by fibrosis (process of parenchymal extinction). The shrinkage is accompanied by close approximation of adjacent vascular structures. (E) Septa are deformed and stretched by expansion of regenerating hepatocytes. (F) As septa are resorbed, they become delicate and perforated before disappearing. Trapped portal structures and hepatic veins are released from the septa and are recognizable as obstructed and ectopic remnants. Note the absence of portal veins. In alcoholic disease (G–L), the sequence of events may differ from other forms of chronic liver disease. (H) Sinusoidal fibrosis is often prominent in advance of parenchymal collapse, leading to a pericellular pattern of fibrosis. (I, J) Inflammation and fibrosis lead to hepatic and portal vein obliteration with secondary condensation of preformed sinusoidal collagen fibers into a septum. (K, L) After prolonged periods of inactivity, sinusoidal fibrosis and septa are resorbed. HV, hepatic vein; PV, portal vein. (Adapted from Wanless et al. [200] with permission from College of American Pathologists.)

Figure 5.24 The time course of the histologic features of cirrhosis in relation to periods of activity. After cessation of activity, various histologic features regress at different rates. The balance of histologic features varies with the duration of low activity disease, for example between time points A and B. At time B cirrhosis cannot be diagnosed histologically, although vascular obstruction (especially of portal veins) and clinical portal hypertension may remain. (Reproduced from Wanless [209] with permission from College of American Pathologists.)

injury is likely responsible for the hepatic vein obliteration and portal inflammation may explain the PV obliteration. In established cirrhosis of any etiology, stasis and reversed flow commonly lead to portal vein thrombosis. Congestive hepatic venopathy may cause parenchymal extinction even if the original disease is inactive [204,205]. In nodular regenerative hyperplasia and some forms of noncirrhotic portal hypertension, portal vein obstruction occurs by local portal inflammation or thrombosis.

The significance of these thrombotic and congestive mechanisms is that they point to possible therapeutic strategies. Antithrombotic therapy is often recommended in patients with obvious thrombotic disease such as Budd–Chiari syndrome and portal thrombosis [206] but may also be beneficial in selected patients with other types of progressive liver disease. Congestive venopathy might be ameliorated by β-blockers or by portacaval or transhepatic shunt procedures.

Further reading

Arias IM, Alter HJ, Boyer JL, et al., eds. *The Liver: Biology and Pathobiology*, 5th edn. New York: Wiley-Blackwell, 2010.
An admirable summary of hepatic physiology with abundant anatomic details.

Nakanuma Y, Hoso M, Sanzen T, Sasaki M. Microstructure and development of the normal and pathologic biliary tract in humans, including blood supply. *Microsc Res Tech* 1997;38:552–70.
A detailed summary of the anatomy of the biliary tree.

Roskams T, Desmet VJ, Verslype C. Development, structure, and function of the liver. In: Burt AD, Portmann BC, Ferrell LD, eds. *MacSween's Pathology of the Liver*, 6th edn. Oxford: Churchill Livingstone, 2012.
A detailed review, strong on embryology, physiology, and ultrastructure.

Wanless IR. Vascular diseases. In: Burt AD, Portmann BC, Ferrell LD, eds. *MacSween's Pathology of the Liver*, 6th edn. Oxford: Churchill Livingstone, 2012.
A detailed review of vascular pathology of the liver.

References

1. Boyd E. Normal variability in weight of the adult human liver and spleen. *Arch Pathol* 1933;16:350.
2. Furbank RA. Conversion data, normal values, nomograms and other standards. In: Simpson K, ed. *Modern Trends in Forensic Medicine*. New York: Appleton-Century-Crofts, 1967:344–64.
3. Ludwig J. *Current Methods of Autopsy Practice*. Philadelphia: WB Saunders, 1972.
4. Sunderman FW, Boerner F. *Normal Values in Clinical Medicine*. Philadelphia: WB Saunders, 1950.
5. Schulz DM, Giordano DA, Schulz DH. Weights of organs of fetuses and infants. *Arch Pathol* 1962;74:244–50.
6. Villemin F, Dufour R, Rigaud A. Variations morphologiques et topographiques du foie. *Arch Mal Appar Dig* 1951;40:63–8.
7. Couinaud C. *Surgical Anatomy of the Liver Revisited*. Paris: Couinaud, 1989.
8. Benz EJ, Baggenstoss AH, Wollaeger EE. Atrophy of the left lobe of the liver. *Arch Pathol* 1952;53:315–30.
9. Woo HS, Lee KH, Park SY, et al. Adrenal cortical adenoma in adrenohepatic fusion tissue: a mimic of malignant hepatic tumor at CT. *AJR Am J Roentgenol* 2007;188:W246–8.
10. Rex H. Beitrage zur Morphologie der Saugereleber. *Morph Jahrb* 1888;14:517–616.
11. Cantlie J. On a new arrangement of the right and left lobes of the liver. *Proc Anat Soc Great Brit Ireland* 1897;32:4–9.
12. McIndoe AH, Counseller VS. The bilaterality of the liver. *Arch Surg* 1927;15:589–612.
13. Hjortsjo CH. The topography of the intrahepatic duct system. *Acta Anat* 1951;11:599–615.
14. Healey JE Jr, Schroy PC. Anatomy of the biliary ducts within the human liver; analysis of the prevailing pattern of branchings and the major variations of the biliary ducts. *Arch Surg* 1953;66:599–616.
15. Couinaud C. Les enveloppes vasculobiliaires du foie ou capsule de Glisson. Leur interet dans la chirurgie vesiculaire, les resections hepatiques et l'abord du hile du foie. *Lyon Chir* 1954;49:589.
16. Goldsmith NA, Woodburne RT. Surgical anatomy pertaining to liver resection. *Surg Gynecol Obstet* 1957;195:310–18.
17. Bismuth H, Chiche L. Surgical anatomy and anatomical surgery of the liver. In: Blumgart LH, ed. *Surgery of the Liver and Biliary Tract*, 2nd edn. Edinburgh: Churchill Livingstone, 1994:3–9.
18. Strasberg SM. Terminology of liver anatomy and liver resections: coming to grips with hepatic Babel. *J Am Coll Surg* 1997;184:413–34.
19. Fasel JHD, Selle D, Everetsz CJG, et al. Segmental anatomy of the liver: poor correlation with CT. *Radiology* 1998;206:151–6.
20. Lafortune M, Madore F, Patriquin H, Breton G. Segmental anatomy of the liver: a sonographic approach to the Couinaud nomenclature. *Radiology* 1991;181:443–8.
21. Cheng YF, Huang TL, Chen CL, et al. Variations of the middle and inferior right hepatic vein: application in hepatectomy. *J Clin Ultrasound* 1997;25:175–82.
22. Severn CB. A morphological study of the development of the human liver. I. Development of the hepatic diverticulum. *Am J Anat* 1971;131:133–58.
23. Mall FP. A study of the structural unit of the liver. *Am J Anat* 1906;5:227.
24. Ekataksin W, Wake K. Liver units in three dimensions: I. Organization of argyrophilic connective tissue skeleton in porcine liver with particular reference to the "compound hepatic lobule." *Am J Anat* 1991;191:113–53.
25. Jorgensen MJ. The ductal plate malformation. *Acta Pathol Microbiol Scand Suppl* 1977;Suppl 257:1–88.
26. Haruna Y, Saito K, Spaulding S, et al. Identification of bipotential progenitor cells in human liver development. *Hepatology* 1996;23:476–81.
27. Van Eyken P, Sciot R, Desmet VJ. Intrahepatic bile duct development in the rat: a cytokeratin-immunohistochemical study. *Lab Invest* 1988;59:52–9.
28. Nakanuma Y, Hoso M, Sanzen T, Sasaki M. Microstructure and development of the normal and pathologic biliary tract in humans, including blood supply. *Microsc Res Tech* 1997;38:552–70.
29. Haque S, Haruna Y, Saito K, et al. Identification of bipotential progenitor cells in human liver regeneration. *Lab Invest* 1996;75:699–705.
30. Elias H, Petty D. Gross anatomy of the blood vessels and ducts within the human liver. *Am J Anat* 1952;90:59–111.
31. Gilfillan RS. Anatomic study of the portal vein and its main branches. *Arch Surg* 1950;61:449–61.
32. Douglas BE, Baggenstoss AH, Hollinshead WH. The anatomy of the portal vein and its tributaries. *Surg Gynecol Obstet* 1950;91:562–76.
33. Couinaud C. The parabiliary venous system. *Surg Radiol Anat* 1988;10:311–16.
34. Battaglia DM, Wanless IR, Brady AP, Mackenzie RL. Intrahepatic sequestered segment of liver presenting as focal fatty change. *Am J Gastroenterol* 1995;90:238–9.
35. Madding GF, Kennedy PA. Trauma of the liver. In: Calne RY, ed. *Liver Surgery with Operative Color Illustrations*. Philadelphia: WB Saunders, 1982:5.
36. Stevens JC, Morton D, McElwee R, Hamit HF. Preduodenal portal vein: two cases with differing presentation. *Arch Surg* 1978;113:311–13.
37. Morgan G, Superina R. Congenital absence of the portal vein: two cases and a proposed classification system for portasystemic vascular anomalies. *J Pediatr Surg* 1994;29:1239–41.
38. Wanless IR, Lentz JS, Roberts EA. Partial nodular transformation of liver in an adult with persistent ductus venosus. *Arch Pathol Lab Med* 1985;109:427–32.
39. Wanless IR. Noncirrhotic portal hypertension: recent concepts. *Prog Liver Dis* 1996;14:265–78.
40. Honda H, Yanaga K, Onitsuka H, et al. Ultrasonographic anatomy of veins draining the left liver: feasibility of live related transplantation. *Acta Radiol* 1991;32:479–84.
41. Tavill AS, Wood EJ, Creel L, et al. The Budd–Chiari syndrome. Correlation between hepatic scintigraphy and the clinical, radiological and pathological findings in 19 cases of hepatic venous outflow obstruction. *Gastroenterology* 1975;68:509–18.
42. Okudaira M. Anatomy of the portal vein system and hepatic vasculature. In: Okuda K, Benhamou J-P, eds. *Portal Hypertension: Clinical and Physiological Aspects*. Tokyo: Springer-Verlag, 1991:3–12.
43. Okuda K, Takayasu K. Angiography in the study of portal hypertension. In: Okuda K, Benhamou J-P, eds. *Portal Hypertension: Clinical and Physiological Aspects*. Tokyo: Springer-Verlag, 1991:219–29.
44. Sen PK, Kinare SG, Kelkar MD, et al. Congenital membranous obliteration of the inferior vena cava. Report of a case and review of the literature. *J Cardiovasc Surg (Torino)* 1967;8:344–52.

45. Kage M, Arakawa M, Kojiro M, Okuda K. Histopathology of membranous obstruction of the inferior vena cava in the Budd–Chiari syndrome. *Gastroenterology* 1992;102:2081–90.

46. Michels NA. Newer anatomy of liver – variant blood supply and collateral circulation. *JAMA* 1960;172:125.

47. Daseler EH, Anson BJ, Hambley WC, Reimann AF. The cystic artery and constituents of the hepatic pedicle: study of 500 specimens. *Surg Gynecol Obstet* 1947;85:47–63.

48. Lunderquist A. Arterial segmental supply of the liver, an angiographic study. *Acta Radiologica* 1967;Suppl 272:1–86.

49. Elias H. A re-examination of the structure of the mammalian liver: II. The hepatic lobule and its relation to the vascular and biliary systems. *Am J Anat* 1949;85:379.

50. Nelson TM, Pollack R, Jonasson O, Abcarian H. Anatomic variants of celiac, superior mesenteric and inferior mesenteric arteries and their clinical relevance. *Clin Anat* 1988;1:75–91.

51. Bengmark S, Rosengren K. Angiographic study of the collateral circulation to the liver after ligation of the hepatic artery in man. *Am J Surg* 1970;119:620.

52. Michels NA. Collateral arterial pathways to liver after ligation of hepatic artery and removal of celiac axis. *Cancer* 1953;6:708.

53. Mays ET. Critical wounds of liver and juxtahepatic veins. *Am Surg* 1977;43:635.

54. McIndoe AH. Vascular lesions of portal cirrhosis. *Arch Pathol Lab Med* 1928;5:23.

55. Okuda K, Matsutani S. Portal-systemic collaterals: anatomy and clinical implications. In: Okuda K, Benhamou J-P, eds. *Portal Hypertension: Clinical and Physiological Aspects*. Tokyo: Springer-Verlag, 1991:51–62.

56. Schabel SI, Rittenberg GM, Javid LH, et al. The "bull's-eye" falciform ligament: a sonographic finding of portal hypertension. *Radiology* 1980;136:157–9.

57. Popper H, Elias H, Petty DE. Vascular pattern of the cirrhotic liver. *Am J Clin Pathol* 1952;22:717.

58. Bernadich C, Bandi JC, Piera C, et al. Circulatory effects of graded diversion of portal blood flow to the systemic circulation in rats: role of nitric oxide. *Hepatology* 1997;26:262–7.

59. Trutmann M, Sasse D. The lymphatics of the liver. *Anat Embryol (Berl)* 1994;190:201–9.

60. Ohtani O, Ohtani Y. Lymph circulation in the liver. *Anat Rec (Hoboken)* 2008;291:643–52.

61. Masuda T, Oikawa H, Sato S, et al. Distinguishing small lymph vessels in the portal tracts of human liver from portal veins by immunohistochemistry for alpha smooth muscle actin. *Int Hepatol Commun* 1996;4:277–82.

62. Timmermans JP, Geerts A. Nerves in liver: superfluous structures? A special issue of The Anatomical Record updating our views on hepatic innervation. *Anat Rec B New Anat* 2005;282:4.

63. Iwai M, Miyashita T, Shimazu T. Inhibition of glucose production during hepatic nerve stimulation in regenerating rat liver perfused in situ. Possible involvement of gap junctions in the action of sympathetic nerves. *Eur J Biochem* 1991;200:69–74.

64. DiBona GF, Sawin LL. Hepatorenal baroreflex in cirrhotic rats. *Am J Physiol* 1995;269:G29–33.

65. Gardemann A, Puschel GP, Jungermann K. Nervous control of liver metabolism and hemodynamics. *Eur J Biochem* 1992;207:399–411.

66. Jungermann K, Stumpel F. Role of hepatic, intrahepatic and hepatoenteral nerves in the regulation of carbohydrate metabolism and hemodynamics of the liver and intestine. *Hepatogastroenterology* 1999;46(Suppl 2):1414–17.

67. Iwai M, Shimazu T. Exaggeration of acute liver damage by hepatic sympathetic nerves and circulating catecholamines in perfused liver of rats treated with D-galactosamine. *Hepatology* 1996;23:524–9.

68. Xie H, Lautt WW. Insulin resistance of skeletal muscle produced by hepatic parasympathetic interruption. *Am J Physiol* 1996;270:E858–63.

69. Colle I, Van Vlierberghe H, Troisi R, De Hemptinne B. Transplanted liver: consequences of denervation for liver functions. *Anat Rec A Discov Mol Cell Evol Biol* 2004;280:924–31.

70. Hamada T, Eguchi S, Yanaga K, et al. The effect of denervation on liver regeneration in partially hepatectomized rats. *J Surg Res* 2007;142:170–4.

71. Kjaer M, Jurlander J, Keiding S, et al. No reinnervation of hepatic sympathetic nerves after liver transplantation in human subjects. *J Hepatol* 1994;20:97–100.

72. Smadja C, Blumgart LH. The biliary tract and the anatomy of biliary exposure. In: Blumgart LH, ed. *Surgery of the Liver and Biliary Tract*, 2 edn. Edinburgh: Churchill Livingstone, 1994:11–24.

73. Dowdy GS Jr, Waldron GW, Brown WG. Surgical anatomy of the pancreatobiliary ductal system. *Arch Surg* 1962;84:229–46.

74. DiMagno EP, Shorter RG, Taylor WF, Go VL. Relationships between pancreaticobiliary ductal anatomy and pancreatic ductal and parenchymal histology. *Cancer* 1982;49:361–8.

75. Anacker H, Weiss HD, Kamann B. *Endoscopic Retrograde Pancreaticocholangiography (ERCP)*. Berlin: Springer, 1977.

76. Boyden EA. The anatomy of the choledochoduodenal junction in man. *Surg Gynecol Obstet* 1957;104:641–52.

77. Suda K, Matsumoto Y, Miyano T. An extended common channel in patients with biliary tract carcinoma and congenital biliary dilatation. *Surg Pathol* 1988;1:65–9.

78. Moosman DA, Coller FA. Prevention of traumatic injury to the bile ducts. A study of the structures of the cystohepatic angle encountered in cholecystectomy and supraduodenal choledochostomy. *Am J Surg* 1951;82:132–43.

79. Northover JMA, Terblanche J. A new look at the arterial blood supply of the bile duct in man and its surgical implications. *Br J Surg* 1979;66:379–84.

80. Magee DF, Naruse S, Pap A. Vagal control of gallbladder contraction. *J Physiol* 1984;355:65–70.

81. Frierson HF. The gross anatomy and histology of the gallbladder, extrahepatic bile ducts, Vaterian system, and minor papilla. *Am J Surg Pathol* 1989;13:146–62.

82. Mahour GH, Wakim KG, Soule EH, Ferris DO. Structure of the common bile duct in man: presence or absence of smooth muscle. *Ann Surg* 1967;166:91–4.

83. Nakanuma Y, Katayanagi K, Terada T, Saito K. Intrahepatic peribiliary glands of humans. I. Anatomy, development and presumed functions. *J Gastroenterol Hepatol* 1994;9:75–9.

84. Terada T, Sasaki M, Nakanuma Y, et al. Hilar cholangiocarcinoma (Klatskin tumor) arising from intrahepatic peribiliary glands [letter]. *J Clin Gastroenterol* 1992;15:79–81.

85. Terayama N, Matsui O, Hoshiba K, et al. Peribiliary cysts in liver cirrhosis: US, CT, and MR findings. *J Comput Assist Tomogr* 1995;19:419–23.

86. Wanless IR, Zahradnik J, Heathcote EJ. Hepatic cysts of periductal gland origin presenting as obstructive jaundice. *Gastroenterology* 1987;93:894–8.

87. Desmet VJ. Congenital diseases of intrahepatic bile ducts: variations on the theme "ductal plate malformation." *Hepatology* 1992;16:1069–83.

88. Healey JE Jr, Schroy PC. The intrahepatic distribution of the hepatic artery in man. *J Int Coll Surg* 1953;20:133.

89. Prinz RA, Howell HS, Pickleman JR. Surgical significance of extrahepatic biliary tree anomalies. *Am J Surg* 1976;131:755.

90. Hayes MA, Goldenberg IS, Bishop CC. The developmental basis for bile duct anomalies. *Surg Gynecol Obstet* 1985;107:447–56.

91. Redston MS, Wanless IR. The hepatic von Meyenburg complex: prevalence and association with hepatic and renal cysts among 2843 autopsies. *Mod Pathol* 1996;9:233–7.

92. Jessurun J, Albores-Saavedra J. Diseases of the gallbladder. In: Burt AD, Portmann BC, Ferrell L, eds. *MacSween's Pathology of the Liver*, 5th edn. Oxford: Churchill Livingstone, 2007:583–612.

93. Crawford AR, Lin XZ, Crawford JM. The normal adult human liver biopsy: a quantitative reference standard. *Hepatology* 1997;26:281A.

94. Bioulac-Sage P, Saric J, Balabaud C. Microscopic anatomy of the intrahepatic circulatory system. In: Okuda K, Benhamou J-P, eds. *Portal Hypertension: Clinical and Physiological Aspects*. Tokyo: Springer-Verlag, 1991:13–26.

95. Phillips MJ, Poucell S, Patterson J, Valencia P. *The Liver. An Atlas and Text of Ultrastructural Pathology*. New York: Raven Press, 1987.

96. MacSween RNM, Scothorne RJ. Developmental anatomy and normal structure. In: MacSween RNM, Anthony PP, Scheuer PJ, Burt AD, Portmann BC, eds. *Pathology of the Liver*, 3rd edn. Edinburgh: Churchill Livingstone, 1994:1–49.

97. Fu X, Tan L, Liu S, et al. A novel diagnostic marker, p28GANK distinguishes hepatocellular carcinoma from potential mimics. *J Cancer Res Clin Oncol* 2004;130:514–20.

98. Yan BC, Gong C, Song J, et al. Arginase-1: a new immunohistochemical marker of hepatocytes and hepatocellular neoplasms. *Am J Surg Pathol* 2010;34:1147–54.

99. Racine-Samson L, Scoazec JY, D'Errico A, et al. The metabolic organization of the adult human liver: a comparative study of normal, fibrotic, and cirrhotic liver tissue. *Hepatology* 1996;24:104–13.

100. Fleming K, Wanless IR. Hepatic glutamine synthetase expression in cirrhosis, veno-occlusive disease, adjacent to mass lesions, and focal nodular hyperplasia (FNH). *Mod Pathol* 2010;23(Suppl):355A.

101. Capurro M, Wanless IR, Sherman M, et al. Glypican-3: a novel serum and histochemical marker for hepatocellular carcinoma. *Gastroenterology* 2003;125:89–97.

102. Sakamoto M. Early HCC: diagnosis and molecular markers. *J Gastroenterol* 2009;44(Suppl 19):108–11.

103. Wisse E, De Zanger RB, Charels K, et al. The liver sieve: considerations concerning the structure and function of endothelial fenestrae, the sinusoidal wall and the space of Disse. *Hepatology* 1985;5:683–92.

104. Rockey D. The cellular pathogenesis of portal hypertension: stellate cell contractility, endothelin, and nitric oxide. *Hepatology* 1997;25:2–5.

105. Wisse E, Braet F, Luo D, et al. Structure and function of sinusoidal lining cells in the liver. *Toxicol Pathol* 1996;24:100–11.

106. Braet F, De Zanger R, Jans D, et al. Microfilament-disrupting agent latrunculin A induces and increased number of fenestrae in rat liver sinusoidal endothelial cells: comparison with cytochalasin B. *Hepatology* 1996;24:627–35.

107. Daemen T, Velinova M, Regts J, et al. Different intrahepatic distribution of phosphatidylglycerol and phosphatidylserine liposomes in the rat. *Hepatology* 1997;26:416–23.

108. Couvelard A, Scoazec JY, Feldmann G. Expression of cell–cell and cell–matrix adhesion proteins by sinusoidal endothelial cells in the normal and cirrhotic human liver. *Am J Pathol* 1993;143:738–52.

109. Couvelard A, Scoazec JY, Dauge MC, et al. Structural and functional differentiation of sinusoidal endothelial cells during liver organogenesis in humans. *Blood* 1996;87:4568–80.

110. Nakamura S, Muro H, Suzuki S, et al. Immunohistochemical studies on endothelial cell phenotype in hepatocellular carcinoma. *Hepatology* 1997;26:407–15.

111. Bioulac-Sage P, Lepreux S, Schledzewski K, et al. Identification of liver sinusoidal endothelial cells in the human liver. *Liver Int* 2010;30:773–6.

112. Hansen B, Longati P, Elvevold K, et al. Stabilin-1 and stabilin-2 are both directed into the early endocytic pathway in hepatic sinusoidal endothelium via interactions with clathrin/AP-2, independent of ligand binding. *Exp Cell Res* 2005;303:160–73.

113. Chaparro M, Sanz-Cameno P, Trapero-Marugan M, et al. Mechanisms of angiogenesis in chronic inflammatory liver disease. *Ann Hepatol* 2007;6:208–13.

114. Schaffner F, Popper H. Capillarization of hepatic sinusoids in man. *Gastroenterology* 1963;44:239–42.

115. Morales-Ruiz M, Jimenez W, Perez-Sala D, et al. Increased nitric oxide synthase expression in arterial vessels of cirrhotic rats with ascites. *Hepatology* 1996;24:1481–6.

116. Shah V, Haddad FG, Garcia-Cardena G, et al. Liver sinusoidal endothelial cells are responsible for nitric oxide modulation of resistance in the hepatic sinusoids. *J Clin Invest* 1997;100:2923–30.

117. Huang TP, Nishida T, Kamiike W, et al. Role of nitric oxide in oxygen transport in rat liver sinusoids during endotoxemia. *Hepatology* 1997;26:336–42.

118. McCuskey RS, Reilly FD. Hepatic microvasculature: dynamic structure and its regulation. *Semin Liver Dis* 1993;13:1–12.

119. Fallon MD, Abrams GA, Luo B, et al. The role of endothelial nitric oxide synthase in the pathogenesis of a rat model of hepatopulmonary syndrome. *Gastroenterology* 1997;113:606–14.

120. Epstein M, Goligorsky MS. Endothelin and nitric oxide in hepatorenal syndrome: a balance reset. *J Nephrol* 1997;10:120–35.

121. Pinzani M, Milani S, De Franco R, et al. Endothelin 1 is overexpressed in human cirrhotic liver and exerts multiple effects on activated hepatic stellate cells. *Gastroenterology* 1996;110:534–48.

122. McCuskey RS, Urbaschek R, Urbaschek B. The microcirculation during endotoxemia. *Cardiovasc Res* 1996;32:752–63.

123. Eakes AT, Howard KM, Miller JE, Olson MS. Endothelin-1 production by hepatic endothelial cells: characterization and augmentation by endotoxin exposure. *Am J Physiol* 1997;272:G605–11.

124. Upadhya AG, Harvey RP, Howard TK, et al. Evidence of a role for matrix metalloproteinases in cold preservation injury of the liver in humans and in the rat. *Hepatology* 1997;26:922–8.

125. Monbaliu D, van Pelt J, De Vos R, et al. Primary graft nonfunction and Kupffer cell activation after liver transplantation from non-heart-beating donors in pigs. *Liver Transpl* 2007;13:239–47.

126. Mastai R, Laganiere S, Wanless IR, et al. Hepatic sinusoidal fibrosis induced by cholesterol and stilbestrol in the rabbit: 2. Hemodynamic and drug disposition studies. *Hepatology* 1996;24:865–70.

127. Tandon BN, Lakshminarayanan R, Bhargava S, et al. Ultrastructure of the liver in non cirrhotic portal fibrosis with portal hypertension. *Gut* 1970;11:905–10.

128. Melkebeke P, Vandepitte J, Hannon R, Fevery J. Huge hepatomegaly, jaundice, and portal hypertension due to amyloidosis of the liver. *Digestion* 1980;20:351–7.

129. Wanless IR, Peterson P, Das A, et al. Hepatic vascular disease and portal hypertension in polycythemia vera and agnogenic myeloid metaplasia: a clinicopathological study of 145 patients examined at autopsy. *Hepatology* 1990;12:1166–74.

130. Mall FP. On the origin of the lymphatics in the liver. *Bull Johns Hopkins Hosp* 1901;12:146.

131. Dumont AE, Mulholland JH. Flow rate and composition of thoracic-duct lymph in patients with cirrhosis. *N Engl J Med* 1960;263:471.

132. Szabo G, Jakab F, Sugar I. The effect of the occlusion of liver lymphatics on hepatic blood flow. *Res Exp Med (Berl)* 1977;169:1.

133. Roskams TA, Theise ND, Balabaud C, et al. Nomenclature of the finer branches of the biliary tree: canals, ductules, and ductular reactions in human livers. *Hepatology* 2004;39:1739–45.

134. Kobayashi S, Nakanuma Y, Matsui O. Intrahepatic peribiliary vascular plexus in various hepatobiliary diseases: a histological survey. *Hum Pathol* 1994;25:940–6.

135. Kardon RH, Kessel RG. Three dimensional organization of the hepatic microcirculation in the rodent as observed by scanning

electron microscopy of corrosion casts. *Gastroenterology* 1980;79: 72–81.

136. Watanabe N, Tsukada N, Smith CR, Phillips MJ. Motility of bile canaliculi in the living animal: implications for bile flow. *J Cell Biol* 1991;113:1069–80.

137. Tsukada N, Ackerley CA, Phillips MJ. The structure and organization of the bile canalicular cytoskeleton with special reference to actin and actin-binding proteins. *Hepatology* 1995;21:1106–13.

138. Xia X, Francis H, Glaser S, et al. Bile acid interactions with cholangiocytes. *World J Gastroenterol* 2006;12:3553–63.

139. Esteller A. Physiology of bile secretion. *World J Gastroenterol* 2008;14:5641–9.

140. Sirica AE, Nathanson MH, Gores GJ, Larusso NF. Pathobiology of biliary epithelia and cholangiocarcinoma: proceedings of the Henry M. and Lillian Stratton Basic Research Single-Topic Conference. *Hepatology* 2008;48:2040–6.

141. Masyuk T, Masyuk A, LaRusso N. Cholangiociliopathies: genetics, molecular mechanisms and potential therapies. *Curr Opin Gastroenterol* 2009;25:265–71.

142. Mathew J, Geerts A, Burt AD. Pathobiology of hepatic stellate cells. *Hepatogastroenterology* 1996;43:72–91.

143. Rockey DC. Stellate cell/HCV interactions in hepatic fibrosis. *Gastroenterology* 2005;129:2117–18.

144. Friedman SL, Rockey DC, Bissell DM. Hepatic fibrosis 2006: report of the Third AASLD Single Topic Conference. *Hepatology* 2007;45:242–9.

145. Henderson NC, Iredale JP. Liver fibrosis: cellular mechanisms of progression and resolution. *Clin Sci (Lond)* 2007;112:265–80.

146. Taura K, De Minicis S, Seki E, et al. Hepatic stellate cells secrete angiopoietin 1 that induces angiogenesis in liver fibrosis. *Gastroenterology* 2008;135:1729–38.

147. Fernandez M, Semela D, Bruix J, et al. Angiogenesis in liver disease. *J Hepatol* 2009;50:604–20.

148. Bioulac-Sage P, Kuiper J, Van Berkel TJ, Balabaud C. Lymphocyte and macrophage populations in the liver. *Hepatogastroenterology* 1996;43:4–14.

149. Roberts RA, Ganey PE, Ju C, et al. Role of the Kupffer cell in mediating hepatic toxicity and carcinogenesis. *Toxicol Sci* 2007;96: 2–15.

150. Wisse E, Luo D, Vermijlen D, et al. On the function of pit cells, the liver-specific natural killer cells. *Semin Liver Dis* 1997;17:265–86.

151. Oo YH, Adams DH. The role of chemokines in the recruitment of lymphocytes to the liver. *J Autoimmun* 2010;34:45–54.

152. Unsworth DJ, Scott DL, Almond TJ, et al. Studies on reticulin. Stereological and immunohistological investigation of the occurrence of collagen type III, fibronectin and the non-collagenous glycoprotein of Pras and Glynn in reticulin. *Br J Exp Pathol* 1982;63:154–66.

153. Johnson SJ. Extracellular matrix proteins and hepatic fibrosis. *Hepatogastroenterology* 1996;43:44–55.

154. Nadell J, Kosek J. Peliosis hepatis. Twelve cases associated with oral androgen therapy. *Arch Pathol Lab Med* 1977;101:405–10.

155. Degott C, Rueff B, Kreis H, et al. Peliosis hepatis in recipients of renal transplants. *Gut* 1978;19:748–53.

156. Wanless IR, Geddie WR. Mineral oil lipogranulomata in liver and spleen. A study of 465 autopsies. *Arch Pathol Lab Med* 1985;109:283–6.

157. Matsumoto T, Kawakami M. The unit-concept of hepatic parenchyma: a reexamination based on angioarchitectural studies. *Acta Pathol Japonica* 1982;32(Suppl 2):285–314.

158. Lamers WH, Hilberts A, Furt E, et al. Hepatic enzymic zonation: a reevaluation of the concept of the liver acinus. *Hepatology* 1989;10:72–6.

159. Bhunchet E, Wake K. The portal lobule in rat liver fibrosis: a reevaluation of the liver unit. *Hepatology* 1998;27:481–7.

160. Rappaport AM. Hepatic blood flow: morphologic aspects and physiologic regulation. *Int Rev Physiol* 1980;21:1–63.

161. Rappaport AM, Wanless IR. Physioanatomic considerations. In: Schiff L, Schiff ER, eds. *Diseases of the Liver*, 7th edn. Philadelphia: JB Lippincott, 1993:1–41.

162. McCuskey RS. The hepatic microvascular system. In: Arias IM, Boyer JL, Fausto N, Jakoby WB, Schacter D, Shafritz DA, eds. *The Liver: Biology and Pathobiology*, 3 edn. New York: Raven Press, 1994:1089–106.

163. Gumucio JJ. Hepatocyte heterogeneity: the coming of age from the description of a biological curiosity to a partial understanding of its physiological meaning and regulation. *Hepatology* 1989;9:154–60.

164. Jungermann K, Kietzmann T. Zonation of parenchymal and non-parenchymal metabolism in liver. *Annu Rev Nutr* 1996;16:179–203.

165. Lamers WH, Geerts WJ, Jonker A, et al. Quantitative graphical description of portocentral gradients in hepatic gene expression by image analysis. *Hepatology* 1997;26:398–406.

166. Reid LM, Fiorino AD, Sigal SH, et al. Extracellular matrix gradients in the space of Disse: relevance to liver biology. *Hepatology* 1992;15:1198–203.

167. Jungermann K, Kietzmann T. Role of oxygen in the zonation of carbohydrate metabolism and gene expression in liver. *Kidney Int* 1997;51:402–12.

168. Stumpel F, Jungermann K. Sensing by intrahepatic muscarinic nerves of a portal-arterial glucose concentration gradient as a signal for insulin-dependent glucose uptake in the perfused rat liver. *FEBS Lett* 1997;406:119–22.

169. Gebhardt R, Baldysiak-Figiel A, Krugel V, et al. Hepatocellular expression of glutamine synthetase: an indicator of morphogen actions as master regulators of zonation in adult liver. *Prog Histochem Cytochem* 2007;41:201–66.

170. Torre C, Perret C, Colnot S. Transcription dynamics in a physiological process: beta-catenin signaling directs liver metabolic zonation. *Int J Biochem Cell Biol* 2011;43:271–8.

171. Lie-Venema H, de Boer PA, Moorman AF, Lamers WH. Role of the 5′ enhancer of the glutamine synthetase gene in its organ-specific expression. *Biochem J* 1997;323:611–19.

172. Roth L, Harbison RD, James RC, et al. Cocaine hepatotoxicity: influence of hepatic enzyme inducing and inhibiting agents on the site of necrosis. *Hepatology* 1992;15:934–40.

173. de la Monte SM, Arcidi JM, Moore GW, Hutchins GM. Midzonal necrosis as a pattern of hepatocellular injury after shock. *Gastroenterology* 1984;86:627–31.

174. Katz LN, Rodbard S. The integration of the vasomotor responses in the liver with those in other systemic vessels. *J Pharmacol Exp Ther* 1939;67:407.

175. Lautt WW. Intrinsic regulation of hepatic blood flow. *Can J Physiol Pharmacol* 1996;74:223–33.

176. Lautt WW, Schafer J, Legare DJ. Hepatic blood flow distribution: consideration of gravity, liver surface, and norepinephrine on regional heterogeneity. *Can J Physiol Pharmacol* 1993;71:128–35.

177. Lautt WW, Legare DJ. Passive autoregulation of portal venous pressure: distensible hepatic resistance. *Am J Physiol* 1992;263:G702–8.

178. Matsui O. Imaging of multistep human hepatocarcinogenesis by CT during intra-arterial contrast injection. *Intervirology* 2004;47:271–6.

179. Kitao A, Zen Y, Matsui O, et al. Hepatocarcinogenesis: multistep changes of drainage vessels at CT during arterial portography and hepatic arteriography – radiologic-pathologic correlation. *Radiology* 2009;252:605–14.

180. Kojiro M, Wanless I, Alves V, et al. Pathologic diagnosis of early hepatocellular carcinoma: a report of The International Consensus Group for Hepatocellular Neoplasia. *Hepatology* 2009;49:658–64.

181. Iavarone M, Sangiovanni A, Forzenigo LV, et al. Diagnosis of hepatocellular carcinoma in cirrhosis by dynamic contrast

imaging: the importance of tumor cell differentiation. *Hepatology* 2010;52:1723–30.

182. Fausto N, Campbell JS, Riehle KJ. Liver regeneration. *Hepatology* 2006;43:S45–53.

183. Nagino M, Ando M, Kamiya J, et al. Liver regeneration after major hepatectomy for biliary cancer. *Br J Surg* 2001;88:1084–91.

184. Sigal SH, Brill S, Fiorino AS, Reid LM. The liver as a stem cell and lineage system. *Am J Physiol* 1992;263:G139–48.

185. Saxena R, Theise N. Canals of Hering: recent insights and current knowledge. *Semin Liver Dis* 2004;24:43–8.

186. Alison MR, Islam S, Lim S. Stem cells in liver regeneration, fibrosis and cancer: the good, the bad and the ugly. *J Pathol* 2009;217:282–98.

187. Cantz T, Manns MP, Ott M. Stem cells in liver regeneration and therapy. *Cell Tissue Res* 2008;331:271–82.

188. Bird TG, Lorenzini S, Forbes SJ. Activation of stem cells in hepatic diseases. *Cell Tissue Res* 2008;331:283–300.

189. Spee B, Carpino G, Schotanus BA, et al. Characterisation of the liver progenitor cell niche in liver diseases: potential involvement of Wnt and Notch signalling. *Gut* 2010;59:247–57.

190. Kubota H, Reid LM. Stem cell-fed maturational lineages and epithelial organogenesis. *Hum Cell* 1997;10:51–62.

191. Thorgeirsson SS, Grisham JW. Hematopoietic cells as hepatocyte stem cells: a critical review of the evidence. *Hepatology* 2006;43:2–8.

192. Theise ND. Gastrointestinal stem cells. III. Emergent themes of liver stem cell biology: niche, quiescence, self-renewal, and plasticity. *Am J Physiol Gastrointest Liver Physiol* 2006;290:G189–93.

193. Grompe M. The origin of hepatocytes. *Gastroenterology* 2005;128:2158–60.

194. Seglen PO. DNA ploidy and autophagic protein degradation as determinants of hepatocellular growth and survival. *Cell Biol Toxicol* 1997;13:301–15.

195. Fausto N. Liver regeneration. *J Hepatol* 2000;32:19–31.

196. Michalopoulos GK, DeFrances MC. Liver regeneration. *Science* 1997;276:60–6.

197. Fausto N. Liver regeneration and repair: hepatocytes, progenitor cells, and stem cells. *Hepatology* 2004;39:1477–87.

198. Wanless I, Crawford J. Cirrhosis. In: Odze R, Goldblum J, eds. *Surgical Pathology of the GI Tract, Liver, Biliary Tree, and Pancreas*, 2nd edn. Philadelphia: WB Saunders, 2009:1115–46.

199. Wanless IR. Micronodular transformation (nodular regenerative hyperplasia) of the liver: a report of 64 cases among 2500 autopsies and a new classification of benign hepatocellular nodules. *Hepatology* 1990;11:787–97.

200. Wanless IR, Nakashima E, Sherman M. Regression of human cirrhosis. Morphologic features and the genesis of incomplete septal cirrhosis. *Arch Pathol Lab Med* 2000;124:1599–607.

201. Ward NL, Haninec AL, Van Slyke P, et al. Angiopoietin-1 causes reversible degradation of the portal microcirculation in mice: implications for treatment of liver disease. *Am J Pathol* 2004;165:889–99.

202. Wanless IR. Thrombosis and phlebitis in the pathogenesis of portal hypertension and cirrhosis: the 2-hit hypothesis for the pathogenesis of chronic liver disease. In: Arroyo V, Bosch J, Bruguera M, Rodes J, eds. *Therapy in Liver Diseases*. Barcelona: Masson, 1997:47–50.

203. Tanaka M, Wanless IR. Pathology of the liver in Budd–Chiari syndrome: portal vein thrombosis and the histogenesis of veno-centric cirrhosis, veno-portal cirrhosis, and large regenerative nodules. *Hepatology* 1998;27:488–96.

204. Wanless IR, Wong F, Blendis LM, et al. Hepatic and portal vein thrombosis in cirrhosis: possible role in development of parenchymal extinction and portal hypertension. *Hepatology* 1995;21:1238–47.

205. O'Shea A-M, Wanless IR. Congestive hepatopathy: possible role in the formation of tumour capsule in the liver. *Mod Pathol* 2006;19(Suppl 3):124.

206. de Franchis R. Evolving consensus in portal hypertension. Report of the Baveno IV consensus workshop on methodology of diagnosis and therapy in portal hypertension. *J Hepatol* 2005;43:167–76.

207. Wanless IR. Anatomy and developmental anomalies of the liver. In: Feldman M, Scharschmidt BF, Sleisenger MH, eds. *Sleisenger and Fordtran's Gastrointestinal and Liver Disease*, 6th edn. Philadelphia: WB Saunders, 1997:1056.

208. Murakami T, Itoshima T, Hitomi K, Ohtsuka A, Jones AL. A monomeric methyl and hydroxypropyl methacrylate injection medium and its utility in casting blood capillaries and liver bile canaliculi for scanning electron microscopy. *Arch Histol Jpn* 1984;47:223.

209. Wanless IR. Regression of human cirrhosis. In Reply *Arch Pathol Lab Med* 2000;124:1592–3.

CHAPTER 6
Bilirubin Metabolism and Jaundice

Allan W. Wolkoff[1] *& Paul D. Berk*[2]

[1] Marion Bessin Liver Center and Division of Gastroenterology and Liver Diseases, Albert Einstein College of Medicine, New York, NY, USA
[2] Department of Medicine, Division of Digestive and Liver Diseases, Columbia University College of Physicians and Surgeons, New York, NY, USA

Key concepts

- Bilirubin is the final degradation product of heme, which is the prosthetic group of numerous important hemoproteins involved in oxygen transport (e.g., hemoglobin) or metabolism (e.g., P450 cytochromes). The conversion of heme to bilirubin involves two enzymatic steps: opening of the heme ring by heme oxygenase to form biliverdin, with the release of both carbon monoxide (CO) and iron, and reduction of biliverdin to bilirubin by biliverdin reductase.

- Normal adults produce a mean of 4 mg of bilirubin per kologram body weight per day. Degradation in the reticuloendothelial system of the hemoglobin of dying erythrocytes generates 80–85% of daily bilirubin production. The remainder has multiple sources, including ineffective erythropoiesis in the bone marrow and the turnover of short-lived, nonhemoglobin hemoproteins including the various P450 cytochromes. Because synthesis and degradation of these cytochromes occurs throughout the body, both heme biosynthesis and the heme oxygenase/biliverdin reductase pathways are widely distributed.

- Bilirubin was long considered simply a biologic waste product. However, biliverdin and bilirubin have antioxidant properties, CO is important in cell signaling, iron plays a key role in the generation of reactive oxygen species, and both heme biosynthesis and heme degradation are tightly regulated. These observations suggest that, hemoglobin degradation aside, heme synthesis and degradation throughout the body may play a role in cellular antioxidant defenses.

- Bilirubin formed in the periphery is kept in solution during transit to the liver by very tight binding to albumin. Once at the liver, it is transported from the plasma to bile by four distinct steps: hepatocellular uptake; binding to specific intracellular proteins; conversion to a water-soluble form by conjugation to glucuronic acid by the uridine diphosphate (UDP) glucuronosyl-transferase isoform (UGT1A1); and the adenosine triphosphate (ATP)-dependent, carrier-mediated transport of the resultant bilirubin monoglucoronides (BMGs) and diglucuronides (BDGs) across the canalicular domain of the plasma membrane into the bile canaliculus.

- Jaundice is the yellow-orange discoloration of skin, conjunctivae, and mucous membranes that results from an elevated concentration of bilirubin in plasma. Hyperbilirubinemias are usually classified into those that are predominantly unconjugated and those that are mainly conjugated. The latter often, in fact, involve elevations of both the conjugated and unconjugated bilirubin fractions. Instances of hyperbilirubinemia in which other common hepatic biochemical tests are normal often reflect familial hyperbilirubinemias; the combination of hyperbilirubinemia with abnormalities of other hepatic biochemical tests suggests an acquired condition.

- The plasma unconjugated bilirubin concentration reflects a balance between bilirubin turnover and hepatic bilirubin clearance (C_{BR}). Unconjugated hyperbilirubinemia can result from increased bilirubin turnover (e.g., hemolysis), decreased bilirubin clearance (e.g., neonatal hepatic immaturity, familial unconjugated hyperbilirubinemias), or situations in which both processes are occurring (neonatal immaturity in infants with glucose-6-phosphate dehydrogenase (G6PD) deficiency).

- Reduced levels of UGT1A1 on either a congenital (Gilbert and Crigler–Najjar syndromes) or acquired (administration of certain human immunodeficiency virus (HIV) protease inhibitors) basis and shunting of blood around the hepatic parenchyma in cirrhosis are the most frequent causes of a reduction in hepatic bilirubin clearance. Hereditary (Dubin–Johnson syndrome) or acquired (hepatocyte injury) deficiencies of the canalicular transport system, or obstruction to the flow of bile down the biliary tract, are the principal causes of conjugated hyperbilirubinemia.

- Application of molecular technology has led to extensive progress in understanding the pathogenesis of the familial hyperbilirubinemias. Thus, Gilbert syndrome and types I and II Crigler–Najjar syndrome were long considered separate diseases, with separate patterns of inheritance. It is now recognized that they all reflect autosomal recessive disorders characterized by mutations of different severity in the gene encoding UGT1A1. Similarly, Dubin–Johnson syndrome is now known to reflect an inherited abnormality in *MRP2*, encoding an ATP-dependent canalicular plasma membrane transporter for bilirubin conjugates and a number of other non-bile-acid organic anions. Of the five familial hyperbilirubinemias, only Rotor syndrome remains unexplained in terms of molecular pathogenesis.

Schiff's Diseases of the Liver, Eleventh Edition. Edited by Eugene R. Schiff, Willis C. Maddrey and Michael F. Sorrell.
© 2012 John Wiley & Sons, Ltd. Published 2012 by John Wiley & Sons, Ltd.

Bilirubin, a reddish-yellow heme degradation product, is produced principally from the breakdown of the hemoglobin of senescent red blood cells and is eliminated from the circulation by the liver. Jaundice, derived from the French *jaune* (yellow), is the yellow-orange discoloration of the skin, conjunctivae, and mucous membranes that is a consequence of an elevated concentration of bilirubin in plasma. Although mild hyperbilirubinemia may be clinically undetectable, jaundice becomes apparent at plasma bilirubin concentrations of 3–4 mg/dL. The threshold for its recognition depends on the patient's normal pigmentation, the lighting conditions under which the observation is made, and the particular fraction of plasma bilirubin that is elevated. Optimal interpretation of an elevated plasma bilirubin concentration is based on an appreciation of its metabolism, and in particular, its sources and disposition. These are the subject of this chapter.

Sources, structure, and plasma transport of bilirubin

Bilirubin production from heme

Bilirubin is the final, common end-product of the metabolism of heme, the moiety found in hemoglobin, myoglobin, and other hemoproteins (Fig. 6.1). The formation of bilirubin is the result of a multistep, enzymatic process in which the porphyrin ring of heme is first opened at the α-bridge carbon in a stereoselective, enzymatic oxidative process carried out by the microsomal enzyme heme oxygenase. This step leads to the release of an iron atom and to the formation of equimolar quantities

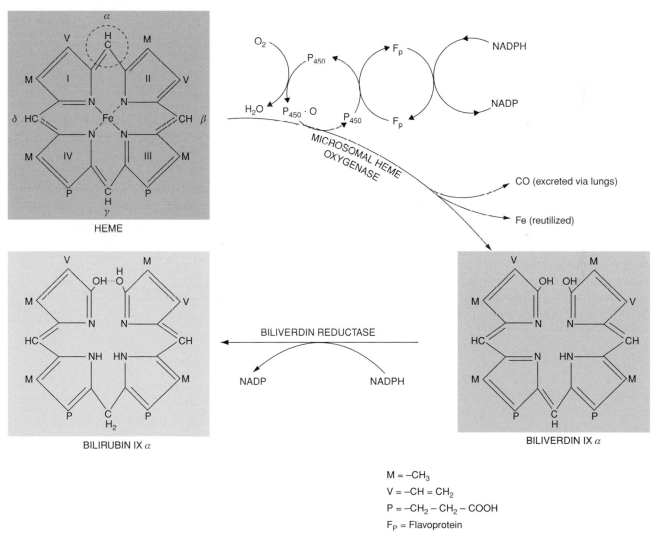

$M = -CH_3$

$V = -CH = CH_2$

$P = -CH_2 - CH_2 - COOH$

$F_P = Flavoprotein$

Figure 6.1 Pathway for the degradation of heme to bilirubin. Stereospecific opening of the heme macrocycle at the α-bridge carbon by the microsomal enzyme heme oxygenase results in the formation of equimolar amount of biliverdin and carbon monoxide. Biliverdin is subsequently reduced to bilirubin by the enzyme biliverdin reductase. NADP, NADPH, nicotinamide adenine dinucleotide phosphate (and reduced form). (Reproduced from Berk et al. [268] with permission from Elsevier.)

of biliverdin, a green tetrapyrrolic pigment, and carbon monoxide [1]. Biliverdin is a water-soluble pigment that is readily excreted unaltered by the liver. It is the principal bile pigment in many amphibia, fish, and birds. However, it does not readily cross the placenta. Accordingly, most mammals rapidly and quantitatively convert biliverdin to the reddish-yellow pigment bilirubin through a reaction that is catalyzed by the enzyme biliverdin reductase [2–4]. Heme oxygenase is present in macrophages throughout the reticuloendothelial system, including Kupffer cells of the liver, and certain epithelial cells including hepatocytes and renal tubular cells [1]. Biliverdin reductase is widely distributed in many cells throughout the body, including macrophages [1,2]. The major sites of bilirubin production are the spleen and other compartments of the reticuloendothelial system, which degrade the hemoglobin of senescent and injured red blood cells. However, the degradation of heme to bilirubin can occur in many sites, including macrophages that migrate into hematomas containing extravasated hemoglobin. Because both heme oxygenase and biliverdin reductase are present in macrophages, the sequential steps in the conversion of heme to bilirubin are readily visualized at the edges of any bruise, where the purplish to green to yellow color changes reflect the conversion of extravasated and deoxygenated hemoglobin first to biliverdin and then to bilirubin.

Possible cytoprotective effects of the heme oxygenase/biliverdin reductase pathway

Heme oxygenase and biliverdin reductase were initially considered to function solely as a heme degradative and waste disposal pathway. However, the widespread distribution of these enzymes in cells outside the reticuloendothelial system, the tight control of heme oxygenase activity achieved through the presence of both an inducible (HO-1) and a constitutive (HO-2) form of the enzyme, and the important biologic effects of the several products of heme degradation led to a growing interest in this pathway [5]. Both biliverdin and bilirubin proved to be potent antioxidants under certain circumstances, and hyperbilirubinemia was reported to have various protective clinical effects (e.g., against ischemic heart disease; reviewed in [1,5]). Carbon monoxide (CO) functions as both a signaling molecule and an important vasoactive regulator; and the iron released during heme degradation contributes to various forms of cellular cytotoxicity by facilitating the formation of reactive oxygen species (ROS). These findings suggested that cells might have evolved fine control over the heme oxygenase/biliverdin reductase pathway specifically to regulate CO production for signaling and heme consumption and the generation of bilirubin and biliverdin for their roles in counteracting *intracellular* oxidative and nitrosative stress [5,6]. The existence of a specific intracellular oxidation/reduction cycle in which lipophilic ROS oxidize bilirubin to biliverdin, which is then re-reduced by biliverdin reductase, was postulated [7] and debated [8]. It was claimed that such a cycle, analogous to the GSH/GSSG (glutathione (reduced form)/glutathione (oxidized form)) cycle for detoxifying soluble oxidants, could potentially permit bilirubin to destroy a 10,000-fold excess of oxidants [7]. However, more recent studies cast serious doubt on the existence and functioning of the proposed intracellular bilirubin/biliverdin redox amplification cycle [2,9]. Although both bilirubin and biliverdin clearly can exhibit antioxidant properties under certain conditions in vitro and extracellularly, it is increasingly doubtful that such conditions occur intracellularly, or that the intracellular oxidation of bilirubin results in its specific, quantitative conversion to biliverdin, which is an essential requirement for the functioning of the proposed cycle.

Quantitative aspects of bilirubin production

In normal human subjects, bilirubin production averages $\sim$4 mg/kg body weight/day (6 μmol/kg body weight/day) [10]. Hemoglobin from senescent or injured erythrocytes is the source of 80–85% of the heme that is eventually catabolized to bilirubin (Fig. 6.2). The remainder

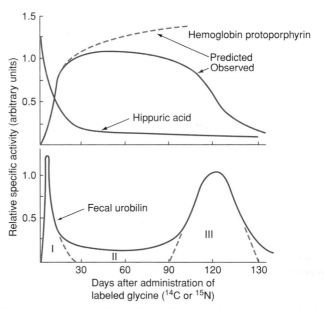

Figure 6.2 Relative specific activities of hemoglobin protoporphyrin, fecal urobilin (stercobilin), and hippuric acid after administration of labeled glycine. The early labeled peak of stercobilin is derived from ineffective erythropoiesis and the turnover of heme enzymes; the late peak reflects the death of senescent erythrocytes. The observed specific activity of hemoglobin protoporphyrin is less than that predicted from the continued availability of labeled glycine for hemoglobin synthesis as determined from the hippuric acid curve. This suggests some random loss of labeled erythrocytes, which may be the source of fraction II of labeled stercobilin. (Reproduced from Berk et al. [268] with permission from Elsevier.)

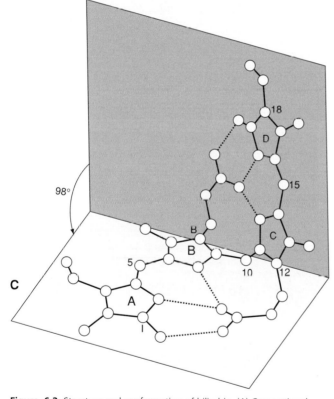

Figure 6.3 Structure and conformation of bilirubin. (A) Conventional "linear tetrapyrrole" structure of the naturally occurring isomer of bilirubin, designated bilirubin IXα. The oxygen functions on the A and D rings are depicted as the lactam tautomers, and the bridge carbons at positions 5 and 15 are shown in the Z configuration. In this configuration they and their attached hydrogens project toward the substituted β-positions on the adjacent pyrrole rings, just as in the protoporphyrin ring from which bilirubin is derived. (B) Planar representation of the 3D conformation of the bilirubin molecule, showing hydrogen bonding (. . .) between each of the –COOH side chains and the –C=O and =NH groups of the end rings (rings A and D) of the opposite half of the molecule. These hydrogen bonds hold the molecule in a rigid 3D conformation.

has multiple sources, including a component of ineffective hemoglobin production in the bone marrow and the turnover of short-lived, nonhemoglobin hemoproteins including the various P450 and b_5 cytochromes, catalase, and peroxidase [11–15]. In normoblastic hemolytic anemias, the bone marrow can increase red blood cell production as much as eight-fold [16], leading to a corresponding increase in the component of bilirubin production derived from erythrocytes [12]. Under these conditions, the amount of bilirubin derived from ineffective erythropoiesis in the marrow may increase in absolute terms, but the proportion of bilirubin production due to ineffective erythropoiesis remains unchanged [12]. By contrast, major increases in the fraction of bilirubin production derived from ineffective erythropoiesis may occur in megaloblastic anemias such as those associated with either folate or vitamin B_{12} deficiency, the thalassemias, and certain dyserythropoietic anemias [12]. Increased bilirubin production also occurs in disorders of heme biosynthesis, including the hereditary erythropoietic porphyrias and lead poisoning [12,13,17]. Finally, administration of phenobarbital and other drugs increases the turnover of heme enzymes, notably hepatic cytochrome P450 isoforms, with a resulting increase in bilirubin production (see below) [14,15,18].

Structure of bilirubin-IXα

Naturally occurring bilirubin is designated bilirubin-4Z,15Z-IXα. This designation indicates that it is derived from protoporphyrin isomer IX, the isomer found in heme and hemoproteins such as hemoglobin, by cleavage of the porphyrin macrocycle at the α-bridge carbon and that the stereochemical arrangement at the 5- and 15-bridge carbons is in the Z configuration (Fig. 6.3) [19,20]. This configuration allows the formation of internal hydrogen bonds between the propionic acid side chain on the B ring and polar groups on the D ring, and between the propionic acid on the C ring and polar groups on the A ring [21]. Although bilirubin is frequently depicted as a linear tetrapyrrole, these hydrogen bonds in fact fix the molecule in a rigid, "ridge tile" configuration [22]. This configuration blocks exposure of the molecule's polar groups to aqueous solvents and of the central bridge carbon to attack by diazo reagents, and is therefore the basis both for bilirubin's hydrophobic behavior and its slow (indirect) diazo reactivity [23,24].

Figure 6.3 (*continued*) (C) Three-dimensional representation of bilirubin-IXα. The molecule takes the form of a ridge tile (i.e., a tile that fits along the top of a roof), with the ridge line defined by the carbons at positions 8, 10, and 12. Rings A and B lie in one plane, and C and D lie in another, with the interplanar angle being approximately 98°. (Reproduced from Berk et al. [268] with permission from Elsevier.)

Other bilirubin isomers

A number of structural (Fig. 6.4A, D) and configurational (Fig. 6.4B, C) (stereo)isomers of bilirubin are of either physiological or clinical interest. Opening of the protoporphyrin-IX ring at bridges other than the α-carbon can occur nonenzymatically, leading to the formation, after reduction, of bilirubin-IXβ, -IXγ, or -1Xδ, respectively (Fig. 6.4A) [25,26]. Stereoisomerization at positions 4 and 15 can lead to formation of -4Z,15E and -4E,15E stereoisomersas illustrated in Fig. 6.4C and D [19,20,27].

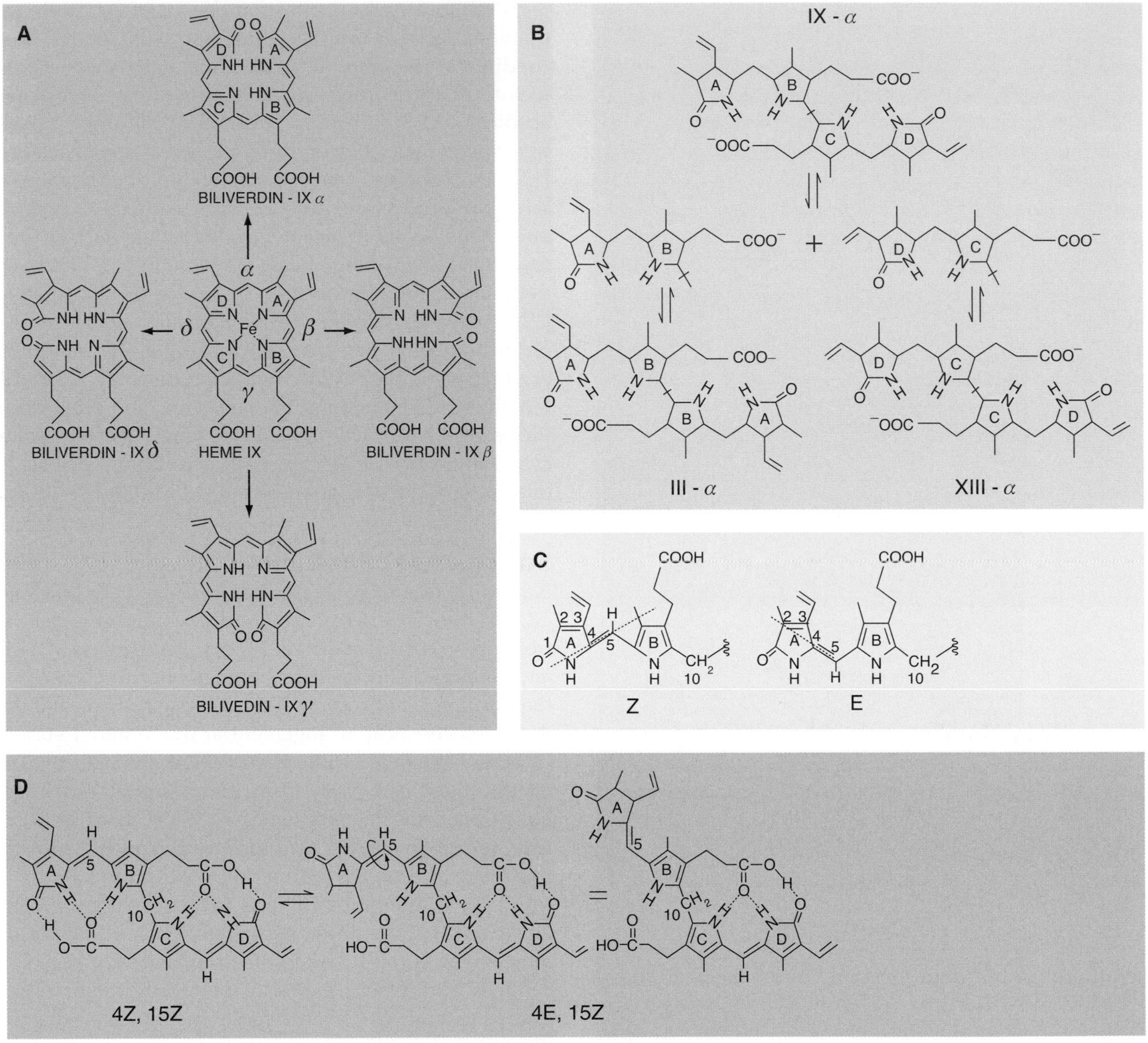

Figure 6.4 Bilirubin isomers. (A) Formation of α-, β-, γ-, and δ-isomers of biliverdin by nonenzymatic cleavage of the protoporphyrin ring of heme at the α-, β-, γ-, and δ-bridge carbons, respectively. (B) Dipyrrolic scrambling. This process involves the nonenzymatic dissociation of the bilirubin tetrapyrrole into dipyrrolic units, which may then reassemble at random into symmetric (bilirubin-IIIα and -XIIIα) and nonsymmetric (bilirubin-IXα) tetrapyrroles. When this process occurs in a mixture of the C8 and C12 isomers of bilirubin-IXα monoglucuronide, final products will include -IIIα, -IXα, and -XIIIα isomers of both unconjugated bilirubin and its mono- and diglucuronides. (C) Nomenclature of the Z and E configurational isomers of bilirubin. If a plane is erected perpendicular to the page along the 4,5 double bond (illustrated by the dashed lines), the B ring may be together (German: *Zuzammen* (Z)) on the same side of the plane or on opposite sides (*Entegegen* (E)) of the plane from the NH group in the A ring. In the Z configuration, the meso hydrogen at position 5 is *trans* to the A-ring lactam hydrogen, while in the E configuration it is *cis*. (D) E,Z isomerization at the 4,5 double bond. In the 4Z,15Z configuration, the molecule is rigidly hydrogen bonded. In the 4E,15Z configuration, the A-ring nitrogen and oxygen groups are not spatially available to form hydrogen bonds with the C12 propionic acid side chain. Because of free rotation about the C5–6 bond, the two 4E,15Z structures are equivalent. Analogous geometric isomerization may occur at the 15,16 double bond. (Reproduced from Berk [269] with permission from Elsevier.)

None of these isomers can form the internal hydrogen bonds characteristic of bilirubin-4Z,15Z-IXα. Accordingly, they behave as more polar molecules, with rapid (direct) diazo reactivity, and can be excreted in bile without conjugation [28–30]. Finally, under certain conditions in vitro, the two nonidentical halves of the bilirubin molecule can dissociate and then reassemble at random [27]. This results in formation of two symmetric isomers, designated bilirubin-IIIα and -XIIIα, in addition to the asymmetric -IXα isomer; the ratio of -IIIα:-IXα:-XIIIα molecules formed is approximately 1:2:1 (Fig. 6.4B). Bilirubin-IIIα and -XIIIα *can* form internal hydrogen bonds. They are, therefore, relatively nonpolar, react slowly with diazo reagents, and require conjugation as a prerequisite to biliary excretion [31–33]. Recognition of the existence and properties of these various bilirubin isomers has increased understanding of the biologic properties of the naturally occurring -4Z,15Z-IXα form, and of the processes involved in its elimination by the liver. However, only the -4Z,15E and -4E,15E photoisomers, which are formed and readily excreted without conjugation during phototherapy of neonatal jaundice [19,20, 29,30], are of clinical significance.

Bilirubin in plasma

Although the bilirubin molecule contains two carboxyls and several other polar groups, internal hydrogen bonding involving these polar moieties constrains the molecule in a rigid, nonpolar and therefore highly insoluble conformation. As an otherwise insoluble molecule, bilirubin formed in the periphery is transported to the liver tightly bound to albumin, at concentrations that far exceed its solubility in protein-free aqueous solutions [34,35]. Adult human albumin has one high-affinity binding site for bilirubin and at least one class of lower affinity sites. Experimental measurements of the affinity of bilirubin for albumin have varied considerably with the methods employed [34], but estimates of a K_d for the high-affinity site have been in the μM range using several different approaches [34,36,37]. The determination of these estimates has been based on the assumption that the affinity of bilirubin for albumin is constant, and is independent of the albumin concentration. Under this assumption, until the bilirubin:albumin molar ratio in the circulation exceeds 1:1, virtually all of the bilirubin present would be bound to the high-affinity site on albumin, and the unbound bilirubin concentration would remain extremely small. This small, unbound bilirubin concentration [38] is, nevertheless, considered to be an important driving force for hepatocellular bilirubin uptake (see below). Under this model, if the 1:1 molar ratio of bilirubin to albumin is exceeded, the unbound bilirubin concentration increases rapidly with further increases in total bilirubin. In the neonatal period,

increased levels of unbound bilirubin can cross the blood–brain barrier, leading to the serious neurologic consequences of kernicterus [39–42]. Similar neurotoxicity may, rarely, occur in adolescents and adults who develop sufficiently high concentrations of unconjugated bilirubin to exceed the critical 1:1 bilirubin:albumin molar ratio [43]. This is, in fact, the only clinically significant potential toxicity of hyperbilirubinemia. Since a normal albumin concentration is ~4 g/dL (600 μM), and a 1 mg/dL bilirubin concentration represents 17.1 μM, the critical 1:1 bilirubin:albumin molar ratio is usually exceeded in otherwise healthy adults only at bilirubin concentrations at or in excess of 35 mg/dL. In catabolic states in which hypoalbuminemia exists, however, the 1:1 ratio may be exceeded at much lower bilirubin concentrations, for example, less than 17 mg/dL in the presence of an albumin concentration of 2 g/dL. Although models of bilirubin binding to albumin that assume a constant affinity independent of the albumin concentration have been the basis for predictions of bilirubin concentrations at which the risk of kernicterus increases, several recent studies have challenged the basic assumptions of the model. Such studies have reported that the affinity of bilirubin for albumin actually varies inversely with the albumin concentration [38,44], making calculation of the critical unbound bilirubin concentration, and hence the risk of kernicterus, even more uncertain than previously. However, the most rapid changes in affinity reportedly occur at quite low albumin concentrations, with only relatively minor further changes occurring as the albumin concentration is increased above 150 μM [44]. Thus, the impact of this new observation on bilirubin to albumin binding within the physiologic range of albumin concentrations, and hence on the risk of kernicterus, has yet to be definitely determined, and may be very small. A variety of xenobiotics may displace or otherwise influence the binding of bilirubin to albumin. The resulting increase in the free bilirubin concentration may increase the risk of kernicterus in susceptible individuals [39,45–47].

Hepatic disposition of bilirubin

Since bilirubin is a potentially toxic waste product, its hepatic disposition is designed to eliminate it from the body via the biliary tract. Transfer of bilirubin from blood to bile involves four distinct but interrelated steps: hepatocellular bilirubin uptake, binding to specific intracellular cytosolic proteins, conjugation with glucuronic acid, and canalicular excretion (Fig. 6.5).

Bilirubin uptake

The fenestrated endothelium that lines the hepatic sinusoids provides the bilirubin–albumin complex with ready

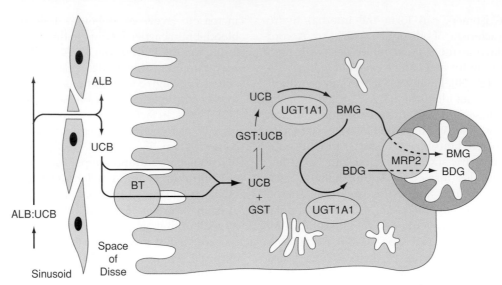

Figure 6.5 Hepatocellular transport of bilirubin. Efficient transfer of bilirubin from blood to bile is dependent on normal sinusoidal architecture, plasma membrane transport processes, and intracellular binding and conjugation. Albumin-bound bilirubin in sinusoidal blood passes through endothelial cell fenestrae to reach the hepatocyte surface, entering the cell by both facilitated and simple diffusional processes. Within the cell it is bound to glutathione-*S*-transferase (GST), and conjugated by bilirubin–uridine diphosphate (UDP) glucuronosyl-transferase (UGT1A1) to mono- and diglucuronides, which are actively transported across the canalicular membrane into the bile. ALB, albumin; BDG, bilirubin diglucuronide; BMG, bilirubin monoglucuronide; BT, proposed bilirubin transporter; MRP2, multidrug resistance-associated protein 2; UCB, unconjugated bilirubin. (Reproduced from Berk and Wolkoff [69] with permission from McGraw-Hill.)

access to the extrasinusoidal space of Disse, where it can come into direct contact with microvilli lining the sinusoidal surface of the hepatocytes [48–50]. In this setting, bilirubin dissociates from albumin and is transported across the hepatocyte plasma membrane into the cell. Numerous in vivo studies of bilirubin uptake kinetics in animals, in isolated, perfused livers, isolated hepatocytes, and plasma membrane vesicles, have all indicated that bilirubin uptake is concentrative, saturable, and competitively inhibited by other organic anions such as sulfobromophthalein (BSP), implying a protein-mediated, facilitated uptake process [51–60]. Subsequent reports, however, showed that BSP and bilirubin uptake could be dissociated under certain conditions, implying the existence of both shared and separate transport processes [55]. Despite an intensive search, the putative bilirubin transporter has not yet been identified, and several candidate transporters [61], including such historical ones as BSP/bilirubin-binding protein (BSP/BR-BP), organic anion-binding protein (OABP), bilirubin translocase (BTL) [56], and the more recently reported human transporter SLC21A6 [57,58] have failed to withstand closer scrutiny. Recent studies have also identified a purely passive, nonsaturable bilirubin uptake process, but its relative magnitude compared with the saturable process remains to be determined [59]. Although transporter mediated unconjugated bilirubin uptake has yet to be definitively identified, it appears that unconjugated bilirubin may be exported from the hepatocyte by the human drug resistance-associated protein MRP1 [60]. MRP2 mediates conjugated bilirubin export.

Intracellular binding
Once within the cell, bilirubin partitions between the cytosol and the lipid bilayer of various intracellular membranes. As with bilirubin binding to albumin in plasma, the cytosolic bilirubin fraction is kept in solution at concentrations that far exceed its aqueous solubility by binding as a nonsubstrate ligand to a number of proteins, of which the most abundant and best characterized are members of the glutathione-*S*-transferase (GST) superfamily [62–65]. This family includes a large number of homodimeric and heterodimeric proteins, previously referred to as ligandins [66], that are principally responsible for bilirubin binding. Kinetic analyses suggest that binding to these proteins is not involved in the initial process of cellular bilirubin uptake, but does increase net bilirubin sequestration by decreasing bilirubin efflux from the cytosol back into the space of Disse [63]. The GSTs have been postulated to play a specific role in presenting bilirubin to the microsomes for conjugation.

Bilirubin glucuronidation
The aqueous insolubility of bilirubin reflects the rigid, highly ordered, molecular structure conferred by internal hydrogen bonding that prevents solvent access to polar components of the molecule. Subsequent conjugation

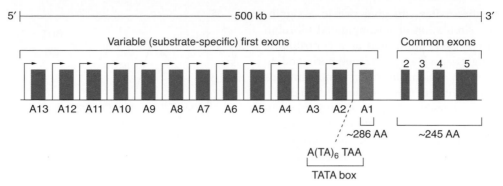

Figure 6.6 Structural organization of the human *UGT1* gene complex. This large complex on chromosome 2 contains at least 13 substrate-specific first exons (A1, A2, etc.), each with its own promoter, that encode the *N*-terminal substrate-specific 286 amino acids of the various *UGT*-encoded isoforms, and common exons 2–5 that encode the 245 carboxyl terminal amino acids common to all of the isoforms. mRNAs for specific isoforms are assembled by splicing a particular first exon such as the bilirubin-specific exon A1 to exons 2–5. The resulting message encodes a complete enzyme, in this particular case bilirubin–uridine diphosphate (UDP) glucuronosyl-transferase (UGT1A1). Mutations in a first exon affect only a single isoform. Those in exons 2–5 affect all enzymes encoded by the UGT1 complex. (Reproduced from Berk and Wolkoff [69] with permission from McGraw-Hill.)

with glucuronic acid residues disrupts this internal hydrogen bonding, rendering the resulting monoglucuronide and diglucuronide conjugates highly soluble in aqueous solutions. The enzyme responsible for bilirubin glucuronidation is the UDP-glucuronosyl-transferase isoform UGT1A1, which is encoded by the *UGT1* gene on chromosome 2 [67,68]. This gene has a complex structure and mutations within it are recognized as the cause of three different disorders characterized by unconjugated hyperbilirubinemia: Gilbert syndrome and types I and II Crigler–Najjar syndrome. The *UGT1* gene (Fig. 6.6) consists of 13 exons (designated A1–A13) each of which encodes a distinct, substrate-specific binding site for one of the multiple protein isoforms produced by this single gene locus [69]. Initiation of RNA transcription at each of these 13 exons is controlled by a separate promoter element immediately upstream of its unique exon. Alternative splicing fuses one of these upstream exons with the four exons (exons 2–5) common to all UGT1 protein isoforms. Exon A1 and the four common exons code for the UGT1A1 protein that is responsible for glucuronidation of bilirubin (Fig. 6.6) [68,70].

Canalicular excretion of bilirubin

Bilirubin glucuronides are transported across the apical plasma membrane into the canaliculus by an ATP-dependent process mediated by a membrane protein initially called canalicular multispecific organic anion transporter (cMOAT), but now designated multidrug resistance-associated protein 2 (MRP2) (see Fig. 6.5) [71–73]. MRP2 is a member of the MRP gene family, other members of which pump drug conjugates, as well as unmodified anticancer drugs, out of cells. In mouse models, effective MRP2 function requires the presence of at least one additional protein, radixin, which localizes to the canalicular membrane and directly binds the carboxy-terminal cytoplasmic domain of MRP2 [74].

Fate of bilirubin in the gastrointestinal tract

Conjugated bilirubin excreted in bile passes through the small intestine without significant absorption and reaches the colon intact [75–77]. There, it is both deconjugated, presumably by bacterial β-glucuronidases [78] and degraded by other bacterial enzymes to a large series of urobilinogens and other products [79,80], the nature and relative proportions of which depend in part on the bacterial flora [79,81,81]. Because of this variability, quantitation of fecal urobilinogen excretion does not provide an accurate measure of heme degradation and bilirubin formation [83] and has largely been abandoned as a clinical test for hemolysis or ineffective erythropoiesis.

Some urobilinogen is reabsorbed from the colon, resulting in small but measurable concentrations of urobilinogen in plasma [84]. Most of this is reexcreted by the liver, but a small fraction is eliminated by the kidney. Increased urinary excretion of urobilinogen is a consequence of an increased plasma level. This in turn may reflect either increased bilirubin production, with a consequent increased formation and enterohepatic circulation of urobilinogen, or decreased hepatic clearance of urobilinogen. Hence, an elevated urine urobilinogen excretion does not distinguish between hemolysis and liver disease [85].

In the neonatal period, the presence of increased levels of intestinal β-glucuronidase [79,86] may result in the presence of appreciable amounts of unconjugated bilirubin within the distal small intestine and upper colon.

Absorption from these sites can give rise to a significant enterohepatic circulation of unconjugated bilirubin [75,76,79], which has been implicated as a contributing factor to physiologic jaundice of the newborn and to the further increase in plasma bilirubin concentrations seen in neonates with intestinal obstruction, delayed passage of meconium, or fasting [78]. In severe unconjugated hyperbilirubinemias such as those occurring in Crigler–Najjar syndrome type I or in the jaundiced Gunn rat (see below), a similar enterohepatic circulation may result from unconjugated bilirubin being excreted both in bile [87,88] and directly across the intestinal lumen into the gut [87]. Efforts to reduce unconjugated hyperbilirubinemia in such situations by interrupting the enterohepatic circulation of unconjugated bilirubin with the use of agents such as oral agar, charcoal, or cholestyramine have had at best limited and inconsistent success [78,79,89]. Recent reports suggest that oral administration of calcium phosphate with or without the lipase inhibitor orlistat may be an efficient means to interrupt bilirubin enterohepatic cycling to reduce serum bilirubin levels [90–92].

Bilirubin in the urine

Because of its very tight binding to albumin, the free fraction of unconjugated bilirubin in plasma is too small to permit efficient ultrafiltration at the glomerulus. Consequently, unconjugated bilirubin never appears in urine no matter what its plasma concentration. By contrast, bilirubin conjugates are appreciably less tightly bound to albumin. In the presence of cholestasis, whether secondary to hepatocellular injury or ductal obstruction, bilirubin conjugates formed in the hepatocyte are diverted back to the circulation, where their weaker albumin binding and larger free fraction permit excretion by the kidney, principally by glomerular filtration [93–97]. A small degree of tubular reabsorption has been demonstrated, but tubular secretion apparently does not occur [97]. The presence of bilirubin in the urine is an absolute indicator of conjugated hyperbilirubinemia.

Clinical physiology of bilirubin

The quantity of unconjugated bilirubin in plasma, and hence the plasma unconjugated bilirubin concentration, reflects a balance between two processes: bilirubin production and hepatic bilirubin clearance (Fig. 6.7) [10,12,48,98]. This balance is indicated by the relationship:

$$BR \cong BRT/C_{BR}, \tag{6.1}$$

where BR represents the plasma unconjugated bilirubin concentration, BRT is plasma bilirubin turnover (which

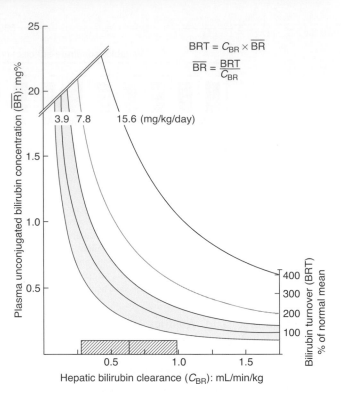

Figure 6.7 Relationship between plasma bilirubin turnover (BRT), hepatic bilirubin clearance (C_{BR}), and plasma concentration of unconjugated bilirubin ($\overline{BR}$). The stippled area represents the normal range for bilirubin turnover; the striped bar on the horizontal axis is the normal range (mean ± 2 standard deviations) for hepatic bilirubin clearance. (Reproduced from Berk et al. [98] with permission from American College of Physicians.)

closely approximates bilirubin production), and C_{BR} is the rate of clearance of unconjugated bilirubin from plasma by the liver. Measurement of C_{BR}, which has units of mL/min/kg, is a quantitative test of hepatic function that is, conceptually, analogous to creatinine clearance, a widely used measure of renal function. Both BRT and C_{BR} can be calculated from the area under the curve of an injected tracer dose of radiolabeled unconjugated bilirubin [10,12,98,99]. Alternatively, the bilirubin production rate can be estimated by isotope dilution from the specific activity of fecal bile pigments following intravenous injection of radiolabeled bilirubin [11,100], or from measurements of the excretion rate of carbon monoxide [101,102]. While estimates of BRT and C_{BR} by any of these methods are not available as routine clinical measurements, an appreciation of the physiologic implications of these two variables is very useful in interpreting data that *are* readily available in clinical settings. Specifically, Eq. (6.1) indicates that BR is directly proportional to the rate of bilirubin turnover and inversely related to hepatic bilirubin clearance in a manner analogous to the relationship between glomerular filtration rate and serum creatinine. Moreover, starting from any given baseline values

Figure 6.8 Relationship between plasma bilirubin turnover and the plasma concentration of unconjugated bilirubin. Normal plasma bilirubin turnover is up to 5 mg/kg body weight/day. Higher values indicate increased bilirubin production, usually from hemolysis. When hepatic bilirubin clearance is within the normal range, the plasma unconjugated bilirubin concentration increases linearly with increases in bilirubin turnover, as indicated by the regression line (stippled area represents ± 2 standard errors of the estimate about the regression line). Extrapolation of the regression line to the maximal rate of steady-state bilirubin production indicates the highest level of unconjugated hyperbilirubinemia that can result from sustained hemolysis in an individual with normal hepatic bilirubin clearance. Since the bone marrow can only increase erythrocyte production by about eight-fold in response to hemolysis, the maximum sustainable rate of bilirubin turnover is ~40 mg/kg/day, and the corresponding value of plasma unconjugated bilirubin is 4 mg/dL. (Reproduced from Berk et al. [90] with permission from American College of Physicians.)

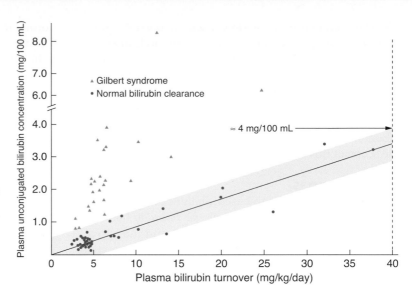

for BRT and C_{BR}, a change in either BRT or C_{BR} will result in a corresponding fractional change in BR. The fractional change in BR will be directly proportional to any fractional change in BRT and inversely proportional to a fractional change in C_{BR} (Figs 6.7 and 6.8) [12,98]. As a result, for any given level of bilirubin production, equal *fractional* changes in hepatic bilirubin clearance can have dramatically different effects on plasma bilirubin concentrations, depending on the initial absolute value of C_{BR}. For example, when bilirubin turnover is normal (~4 mg/kg/day), reducing bilirubin clearance from a normal mean value of ~0.70 mL/min/kg to a lower mean value of ~0.35 mL/min/kg (a reduction of ~50%) will approximately double serum bilirubin, increasing it by ~0.4 mg/dL (from 0.4 to 0.8 mg/dL). This increment may well go unnoticed clinically. By comparison, in a patient whose hepatic clearance is already reduced a corresponding 50% reduction in bilirubin clearance, for example from 0.1 to 0.05 mL/min/kg, will again double the bilirubin concentration. In this instance, however, the interval increase, by ~2.7 mg/dL, will be sufficient to be clinically detectable. Similarly, doubling bilirubin production will double the plasma concentration of unconjugated bilirubin. The absolute magnitude of the increase, in mg/dL, will depend on the value of C_{BR}.

Measurement of plasma bilirubin concentration

Plasma bilirubin is typically measured in clinical laboratories by some modification of the diazo reaction first described by van den Bergh and Müller in 1916 [103] (reviewed in [104]). In this procedure, unconjugated bilirubin in the sample reacts slowly with the diazo reagent (for example, diazotized sulfanilic acid) because the central bridge carbon, which is the site of the attack by the reagent, is rendered sterically inaccessible by the internal hydrogen bonding within the molecule (see Fig. 6.3). In the presence of ethanol, caffeine, or other "accelerators" that disrupt the internal hydrogen bonding, the central bridge carbon becomes more readily accessible to nucleophilic attack and the unconjugated bilirubin molecule reacts more rapidly and completely. Similarly rapid diazo reactivity is displayed by conjugated bilirubin, in which esterification of propionic acid side chains with glucuronic acid prevents hydrogen bond formation and exposes the central bridge carbon. Accordingly, the "prompt" or *direct-reacting bilirubin* in serum or plasma, considered a measure of the amount of conjugated bilirubin present, is determined a short time interval (30–60 seconds) after the addition of the diazo reagent to the sample in the absence of an accelerator. The *total bilirubin* concentration, a measure of both unconjugated and conjugated bilirubin, is typically measured at some more prolonged interval (for example, 30–60 minutes) after the addition of an accelerator substance. The *indirect-reacting bilirubin*, calculated as the total minus the direct-reacting bilirubin, is widely used as a proxy for the amount of unconjugated bilirubin in the sample [104].

Bilirubin can also be estimated in biologic fluids by direct spectrophotometry because of its intense absorption band at approximately 450 nm [33,105]. The method is rapid, requires very small samples, and is therefore often used in neonatal nurseries or in amniotic fluid analyses [106] in which sample availability is limited. The method is nonspecific because turbidity and other yellow-orange materials such as carotenoids interfere. Various devices designed to measure bilirubin levels transcutaneously without blood sampling, by reflectance and/or spectrophotometry, are widely used in neonatal nurseries (e.g., [107]). Accurate alternative methods also exist for quantification of individual bilirubin species [108, 109], including bilirubin conjugates covalently bound to plasma proteins (i.e., δ-bilirubin, see below), not only in plasma but also in bile, urine, and other biologic fluids [110–114]. As they are rarely employed outside research laboratories, a description of these technologies is beyond the scope of this review.

Normal ranges

Using conventional, diazo-based, analytic procedures, the upper limit of normal for *total plasma bilirubin* has been reported to be anywhere between .1.0 and 1.5 mg/dL (17–26 μM), and that for the indirect-reacting fraction from 0.8 to 1.2 mg/dL (14–21 μM) [85,104,115,116]. Differences reported reflect both variations in analytic methods and whether the 95% or 99% confidence limits were used to define the normal range. They also reflect the fact that bilirubin concentrations in the normal population exhibit a log-normal (skewed to the right) rather than a Gaussian (bell-shaped) distribution, which must be accounted for in establishing appropriate normal limits [115].

Many studies have set the upper limit of normal for the *indirect-reacting fraction* at 1.0 mg/dL (17.1 μM), in close agreement with limits predicted on theoretical grounds from a knowledge of the distributions of plasma bilirubin turnover and hepatic bilirubin clearance rates in a normal population [115]. When the total plasma bilirubin concentration is normal, the normal direct-reacting fraction (a proxy for conjugated bilirubin) was traditionally reported to be <0.1 mg/dL, or at most <0.2 mg/dL [104]. Because unconjugated bilirubin does react, albeit slowly, with diazo reagents even in the absence of an accelerator, even this small direct-reacting fraction *overestimates* the miniscule amounts of conjugated bilirubin actually present [117]. Consequently, the calculated indirect-reacting bilirubin *underestimates* the amount of unconjugated bilirubin present. The proportional magnitude of these errors is greatest at total bilirubin concentrations within or near the normal range. Nevertheless, at virtually any total bilirubin level, if the direct-reacting fraction was <15% of the total, the bilirubin in the sample could be considered essentially all unconjugated. Unfortunately, the errors involved appear to be greater with autoanalyzer methods currently in widespread use than they were with the manual methods used in the past. "Normal" values for direct-reacting bilirubin have been creeping upward over the years even as more precise chromatographic methods demonstrate that the actual amounts of conjugated bilirubin in normal serum or plasma are vanishingly small. An informal survey several years ago suggested that few large laboratories in the New York metropolitan area set an upper limit of

normal for direct-reacting bilirubin as low as 0.2 mg/dL. The most commonly reported upper limit was 0.3 mg/dL, with limits of 0.4–0.8 mg/dL being reported not infrequently. Such latitude can lead to considerable error in interpreting the direct- and indirect-reacting fractions as conjugated and unconjugated bilirubin. Because the presence of even modest amounts of true conjugated bilirubin in serum should alert the clinician to the possibility of significant hepatobiliary pathology, this distinction is of more than academic interest [118]. Since conventional bilirubin glucuronide conjugates are water-soluble and bind relatively loosely to albumin, they are readily filtered at the glomerulus and excreted in the urine. Accordingly, uncertainty about the clinical significance of a mildly elevated direct-reacting bilirubin can often be clarified by a simple dipstick test for bilirubin in the urine. Even minimal degrees of conjugated hyperbilirubinemia are associated with bilirubinuria. A negative dipstick test in the presence of a modestly elevated direct-reacting fraction suggests either the presence of δ-bilirubin (see below) or an artifact of the diazotization procedure.

With prolonged conjugated hyperbilirubinemia, some of the conjugated bilirubin in plasma binds *covalently* to albumin and produces what is designated the delta (δ) bilirubin fraction [111–114]. Although δ-bilirubin gives a direct diazo reaction, it is not filterable by the glomerulus and does not appear in the urine; it disappears slowly from the plasma with the 14–21-day half-life of the albumin to which it is bound. δ-Bilirubin accounts for the sometimes slow rate at which conjugated (direct) hyperbilirubinemia resolves as hepatitis improves or biliary obstruction is relieved. Although δ-bilirubin is not easily measured, its presence can be inferred when an elevated direct-reacting bilirubin persists after bilirubinuria resolves.

Hyperbilirubinemia and jaundice

Hyperbilirubinemia is conveniently classified as *unconjugated (indirect-reacting)* or *conjugated (direct-reacting) hyperbilirubinemia.* In practice, pure conjugated hyperbilirubinemia is uncommon; in most cases an elevated plasma conjugated bilirubin is accompanied by an elevation of unconjugated bilirubin resulting in a mixed hyperbilirubinemia. In this setting, because the plasma level of conjugated bilirubin reflects renal as well as hepatic clearance of bilirubin conjugates, the ratio of conjugated to total bilirubin is usually not helpful diagnostically. *Another useful characteristic is whether hyperbilirubinemia is the only abnormality of hepatic function or whether other hepatic biochemical tests such as the activities of serum aminotransferases (aspartate aminotransferase (ALT), alanine aminotransferase (AST)), alkaline phosphatase, or γ-glutamyl-transferase are*

Box 6.1 The familial hyperbilirubinemias.

I. Unconjugated hyperbilirubinemias
  A. *Due to increased bilirubin production*
    1. Hemolytic anemias
      a. Hemoglobinopathies
      b. Thalassemia syndromes
      c. Enzyme defects
      d. Membrane defects, etc.
    2. Shunt hyperbilirubinemias
      a. Congenital dyserythropoietic jaundice syndromes
      b. Miscellaneous
  B. *Due to defective hepatic bilirubin clearance*
    1. Gilbert syndrome
    2. Crigler–Najjar syndrome
      a. Type 1: phenobarbital resistant
      b. Type II: phenobarbital responsive

II. Conjugated hyperbilirubinemias
  A. *Dubin–Johnson syndrome*
  B. *Rotor syndrome*

also abnormal. Absence of abnormalities of other hepatic biochemical tests is one of the features that helps to distinguish the *familial hyperbilirubinemias* from the majority of acquired cases of hyperbilirubinemia. However, certain forms of acquired hyperbilirubinemia such as acquired hemolytic disease and inactive cirrhosis may also occur in the absence of other biochemical abnormalities. The major causes of familial hyperbilirubinemia are listed in Box 6.1.

Causes and consequences of hyperbilirubinemia

Unconjugated hyperbilirubinemia

Unconjugated hyperbilirubinemia is the result of any process that increases bilirubin production, decreases bilirubin clearance, or results in both processes acting in concert [12,98,99]. The reference range for the plasma unconjugated (that is, indirect-reacting) bilirubin concentration is generally reported to be 0.3–1.0 mg/dL, although some laboratories set the upper limit at 1.2 mg/dL and occasionally as high as 1.5 mg/dL. Values above the reference range represent unconjugated hyperbilirubinemia. While scleral icterus may become detectable when the bilirubin concentration exceeds 2.5–3.0 mg/dL, many cases of unconjugated hyperbilirubinemia are subclinical and detectable only by measurement of the plasma bilirubin concentration.

Increased bilirubin production

Hemolysis and increased ineffective erythropoiesis are two of the most common processes responsible for increased bilirubin production. A large number of dis-

tinct hereditary hemolytic disorders have been described, and result from inherited hemoglobinopathies, enzyme deficiencies, or abnormalities in red blood cell membrane structure. There are also many acquired hemolytic conditions, ranging from pure, specific autoimmune hemolytic anemias to the shortened red cell life spans that accompany many chronic diseases. Excessive ineffective erythropoiesis may occur on a congenital basis, as in any subtype of congenital dyserythropoietic anemia [48], or on an acquired basis, in disorders such as erythropoietic porphyria, pernicious anemia, and lead poisoning [13]. Transfusion of old bank blood and massive hematomas or pulmonary infarcts can produce unconjugated hyperbilirubinemia by temporarily increasing bilirubin production. Excessive *hepatic* bilirubin production, while seemingly a potential cause of increased plasma bilirubin turnover, has not been convincingly documented as a cause for clinically evident hyperbilirubinemia. Although hepatic heme turnover has been reported to contribute as much as one quarter of total bilirubin production based on the labeling of plasma bilirubin after administration of radiolabeled heme precursors e (e.g., [119–121]), approximately half of hepatic-derived bilirubin is excreted into the bile without transit through the plasma [10,12,48,100,120,122]. This means that hepatic hemes contribute no more than ~12% of plasma bilirubin turnover. Studies documenting a significant discrepancy between the increase in bilirubin labeling from ^{3}H-or ^{14}C-labeled heme precursors and total bilirubin production suggest that that actual percentage is appreciably lower [123,124]. On this basis, hepatic heme turnover would have to increase many-fold in order to result in a clinically recognizable increase in the plasma unconjugated bilirubin concentration.

Unconjugated hyperbilirubinemia due solely to increased bilirubin production rarely exceeds 4 mg/dL, even in the face of brisk hemolysis (Fig. 6.8), and is generally well tolerated. However, subjects are at an increased risk for the development of pigmented gallstones.

Decreased bilirubin clearance

As noted above, four distinct processes are involved in hepatocellular bilirubin disposition, and each, if defective, can result in a decrease in hepatic bilirubin clearance. Although the precise mechanism(s) by which bilirubin is taken up by hepatocytes remains unclear, several drugs (e.g., rifampin, flavispidic acid, novobiocin, and various cholecystographic contrast agents) are reported to competitively inhibit the bilirubin uptake process (see [48]). The resulting unconjugated hyperbilirubinemia resolves with the cessation of the medication. Reduced hepatic bilirubin uptake (and net clearance) can also result from portosystemic shunting by which blood bypasses the hepatocytes. While this is most commonly thought of as occurring through venous channels such as varices, it may also result from capillarization of the hepatic sinusoids – that is, the loss of sinusoidal endothelial fenestrae and increased perisinusoidal matrix deposition – that occurs in cirrhosis. It is also a consequence of an absolute reduction in hepatic blood flow, or from abnormalities in the net extraction of bilirubin from the circulation by hepatocytes.

Abnormalities in the binding of bilirubin to its cytosolic-binding proteins are at least a hypothetical basis for decreased bilirubin clearance. However, defective glucuronidation is a more common mechanism that results in reduced bilirubin clearance and consequent unconjugated hyperbilirubinemia. Delayed expression of UGT1A1 in neonates is primarily responsible for the physiologic jaundice of otherwise normal newborns. Peak serum bilirubin levels in this setting are typically less than 5–10 mg/dL between days 2 and 5 and decline to normal within 2 weeks. Higher neonatal bilirubin levels that predispose to kernicterus occur in the face of profound prematurity, Gilbert syndrome (see below), hemolysis, or both (e.g., [125]). Three familial disorders of bilirubin conjugation are well recognized: Crigler–Najjar syndrome types I and II and Gilbert syndrome. These are described in greater detail below. Although considered until recently as distinct disorders, these conditions are now all known to result from mutations of different functional severity in the bilirubin-conjugating enzyme UGT1A1. Acquired deficiency of UGT1A1 and consequent unconjugated hyperbilirubinemia also occurs with administration of certain HIV protease inhibitors such as indinavir and atazanavir (reviewed in [126,127]).

Conjugated hyperbilirubinemia

Conjugated hyperbilirubinemias typically reflect abnormalities in hepatocellular excretion of conjugated bilirubin or in biliary tract obstruction. Dubin–Johnson and Rotor syndromes are uncommon, heritable disorders of conjugated bilirubin excretion. In Dubin–Johnson syndrome, mutations in MRP2 result in deficient canalicular transport of bilirubin conjugates [72,128,129]. The molecular defect in Rotor syndrome remains unknown but produces a phenotype similar in many respects to that of Dubin–Johnson syndrome. In both disorders, general hepatocellular function is preserved and liver chemistries other than the bilirubin concentration are typically normal. Bilirubin concentrations in Dubin–Johnson and Rotor syndromes are most often between 2 and 5 mg/dL, although values of <25 mg/dL for prolonged periods have been described. Extensive clinical experience suggests that conjugated hyperbilirubinemia produces no significant adverse consequences, even if prolonged for months at levels of up to 35–40 mg/dL.

Far more common is the defective bilirubin excretion that occurs with a broad spectrum of hepatobiliary diseases. In these conditions, elevations in bilirubin concentration typically occur in association with abnormalities of other hepatic biochemical tests, including elevations in AST, ALT, alkaline phosphatase, and, if severe, reduction in serum albumin and prolongation of clotting times. This broad category of diseases includes hepatocellular and cholestatic liver diseases, benign postoperative jaundice, mechanical intrahepatic or extrahepatic bile duct obstruction, and a rare group of disorders classified under the rubric of familial intrahepatic cholestasis (see below).

Familial hyperbilirubinemias

Familial unconjugated hyperbilirubinemias

The spectrum of familial unconjugated hyperbilirubinemias is indicated in Box 6.1. This review will limit itself to those entities associated with a decrease in hepatic bilirubin clearance: Crigler–Najjar syndrome types I and II and Gilbert syndrome. Important characteristics of these three entities are summarized in Table 6.1. These were once considered distinct genetic and pathophysiologic entities, with Gilbert syndrome reportedly an autosomal dominant and Crigler–Najjar type I an autosomal recessive disorder. However, physiologic observations (see Fig. 6.9) suggested that the three entities might reflect mutations with quantitatively different impact on the functioning of a single gene [130]. Subsequent molecular findings in the specific syndromes and the observation that one *normal* UGT1A1 allele is sufficient to maintain a normal plasma bilirubin concentration [67,70] have established that, in almost all instances, the hereditary unconjugated hyperbilirubinemias are related autosomal recessive disorders.

Crigler–Najjar syndrome type I

Crigler–Najjar syndrome type I is a rare, recessive disorder characterized by profound unconjugated hyperbilirubinemia of 20–45 mg/dL as a result of mutations in UGT1A1 that result in the near total loss of UGT1A1 enzyme activity [67,70,89,131–135]. Mutations most often occur in exons 2–5 of the *UGT1* gene affecting the glucuronidation of a wide spectrum of substrates in addition to bilirubin (type 1a). Less often the mutation occurs in exon 1 and the loss of glucuronidation capacity is largely limited to bilirubin conjugation (type 1b). Crigler–Najjar syndrome type I first appears in the neonatal period and, historically, most patients succumbed from kernicterus in infancy and early childhood. Patients with Crigler–Najjar syndrome type I do not respond to phenobarbital with a reduction in plasma bilirubin concentrations [89,133]. Although survival has been extended with the advent of phototherapy, those who survive beyond early childhood remain at substantial risk for late-onset bilirubin encephalopathy, the onset of which often follows after

Table 6.1 Principal features of the familial unconjugated hyperbilirubinemias.

Feature	Crigler–Najjar syndrome		Gilbert syndrome
	Type I	Type II	
Incidence	Very rare	Uncommon	Up to 12% of population
Total serum bilirubin (mg/dL)	18–45 (usually >20), unconjugated	6–25 (usually ≤20), unconjugated	Typically ≤4 in absence fasting or hemolysis; mostly unconjugated
Defect(s) in bilirubin metabolism	Bilirubin UGT1A1 activity markedly reduced: trace to absent	Bilirubin UGT1A1 activity reduced: ≤10% of normal.	Bilirubin UGT1A1 activity typically reduced to 10–33% of normal; reduced hepatic bilirubin uptake in some cases; mild hemolysis in up to 50% of patients
Routine liver tests	Normal	Normal	Normal
Serum bile acids	Normal	Normal	Normal
Plasma sulfobromophthalein (BSP) removal (% retention of 5 mg/kg dose at 45 minutes)	Normal	Normal	Usually normal (<5%); mildly increased 45-minute retention (<15%) in some patients
Oral cholecystography	Normal	Normal	Normal
Pharmacologic responses/special features	No response to phenobarbital	Phenobarbital reduces bilirubin by ≤75% but not to normal	Phenobarbital reduces bilirubin, often to normal
Major clinical features	Kernicterus in infancy if untreated; may occur later despite therapy	Rare late-onset kernicterus with fasting	None
Hepatic morphology/histology	Normal	Normal	Normal; occasionally increased lipofucin pigment
Bile bilirubin fractions[a]	>90% unconjugated	Largest fraction (mean 57%) monoconjugates	Mainly diconjugates but monoconjugates are increased (mean 23%)
Inheritance (all autosomal)	Recessive	Recessive	Promoter mutation is recessive; missense mutation often dominant
Diagnosis	Clinical and laboratory findings, lack of response to phenobarbital	Clinical and laboratory findings, response to phenobarbital	Clinical and laboratory findings; promoter genotyping may be helpful; liver biopsy rarely necessary
Treatment	Phototherapy or tin protoporphyrin as short-term therapy; liver transplantation definitive	Consider phenobarbital if baseline bilirubin ≥8 mg/dL	None necessary

[a]Bilirubin in normal bile: <5% unconjugated bilirubin, with an average of 7% bilirubin monoconjugates and 90% bilirubin diconjugates.

even mild febrile illnesses (e.g., [89,136]). Although isolated hepatocyte transplantation has been used experimentally in a limited number of cases of Crigler–Najjar syndrome type I [137,138], early liver transplantation remains the best hope to prevent brain injury and death [139–142].

Much of the basis for elucidation of the pathobiology of Crigler–Najjar syndrome type I has arisen from studies that have been performed in the Gunn rat. This mutant Wistar strain of rats was initially described by Gunn in 1938 as having chronic nonhemolytic unconjugated hyperbilirubinemia [143]. As in patients with

Crigler–Najjar syndrome type I, jaundice in these animals is inherited as an autosomal recessive trait. Heterozygotes are anicteric, and liver histology in affected rats is normal. Bilirubin glucuronyl transferase activity is undetectable in livers of affected rats [144].

Crigler–Najjar syndrome type II

In contrast, in Crigler–Najjar type II, UGT1A1 activity is maintained, albeit at a minimal level (<10% of normal), and serum bilirubin concentrations typically vary between 6 and 25 mg/dL [133,145,146]. Induction of UGT1A1 levels with exposure to phenobarbital can

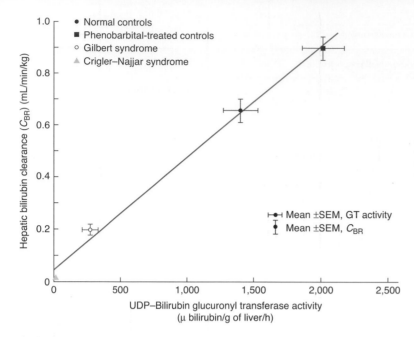

Figure 6.9 Relationship between the mean values for hepatic bilirubin clearance (C_{BR}) and bilirubin–uridine diphosphate (UDP) glucuronsyl-transferase (UDPGT) activity in patients with Crigler–Najjar syndrome type I, Gilbert syndrome, and normal controls. For the control group, data are presented for both untreated and phenobarbital-treated subjects. The line represents a least squares fit to the mean values for the four groups represented. Subsequent data in Crigler–Najjar type II fell on the regression line. Data such as these suggested that Gilbert syndrome and the two Crigler–Najjar syndromes might all reflect mutations with quantitatively differing effects on a single gene, designated at the time bilirubin-UDPGT. (Adapted from Blaschke et al. [130].)

further reduce bilirubin levels by >25% [133,147–150]. Depending on the severity of the molecular defect, either basal or phenobarbital-stimulated enzyme activity is sufficient in most cases to prevent the development of kernicterus. Clinically relevant neurologic sequelae can, however, be precipitated in the setting of intercurrent illnesses, fasting, or any other factor that temporarily raises the serum bilirubin concentration significantly above baseline (e.g., [43]), especially if the resulting bilirubin : albumin molar ratio exceeds 1. Overall, available data in the majority of type II patients indicates that in adolescents and adults with normal serum albumin levels, prolonged exposure to unconjugated bilirubin <16 mg/dL does not result in neurologic injury. Indeed, the majority of patients in the original reports describing the syndrome were healthy adults, many with college-level education [133,145]. To date, a total of 77 different mutations in the *UGT1* gene have been identified in association with either type I or type II Crigler–Najjar syndrome [151]. Chain-terminating mutations have been more commonly associated with a Crigler–Najjar type I phenotype whereas missense mutations have been more frequently observed among less severely affected patients with Crigler–Najjar syndrome type II [151].

Gilbert syndrome

Gilbert syndrome resides at the other end of the spectrum of disorders of bilirubin conjugation. Originally described in 1901 (152), this condition occurs with a phenotypic prevalence of approximately 8% in the general population. It is characterized by a mild, unconjugated hyperbilirubinemia to levels that rarely exceed 4 mg/dL, oth-

erwise normal liver function, and hepatic histology that is also normal other than a modest increase in lipofuscin pigment in some cases. Other than mild icterus in some patients, physical examination is also unremarkable. Bilirubin clearance is reduced to approximately one third of normal (Fig. 6.10) [153], and some patients also exhibit abnormalities in the plasma clearance patterns of other organic anions such as sulfobromophthalein or indocyanine green [53,154], for which the mechanism remains uncertain. By contrast, fasting serum bile acid levels are normal [155]. The most common recognized molecular defect is the addition of an extra dinucleotide sequence, TA, to the transcription initiation sequence (TATAA box) of the promoter for the A1 exon [156]. Thus, compared with the normal A(TA)₆TAA sequence, an A(TA)₇TAA mutation is commonly found in patients with Gilbert syndrome. Much less common A(TA)₅TAA or A(TA)₈TAA mutations are also associated with Gilbert syndrome [157]. In individuals homozygous for one of these variants, enzyme activity is decreased to 10–35% of normal, due to decreased synthesis of a functionally normal enzyme. Homozygosity for the promoter mutation appears to be necessary, but apparently not always sufficient for clinical expression of Gilbert syndrome, as population studies suggest that only about half of A(TA)₇TAA homozygotes have hyperbilirubinemia [158]. It has been suggested that additional variables, such as mild hemolysis (reported in up to 50% of Gilbert patients) or a separate defect in bilirubin uptake [153,156,157,159], might be among the factors enhancing phenotypic expression.

Additional molecular mechanisms result in a phenotype identical to that associated with homozygosity for

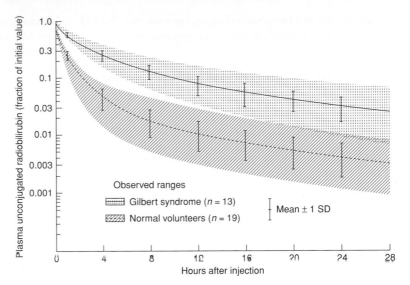

Figure 6.10 Observed ranges of plasma radiobilirubin disappearance curves in patients with Gilbert syndrome and in healthy young adult volunteers. The average curve for each group was calculated by computer from the mean values, for the group, of the intercompartmental rate constants of a compartmental model of bilirubin metabolism. The groups do not overlap for the first 16 hours after injection. Estimates of bilirubin clearance (C_{BR}), calculated from the areas under the curves, were reduced to one third of normal in the Gilbert syndrome patients. (Reproduced from Berk et al. [98] with permission from American College of Physicians.)

the A(TA)$_7$TAA promoter variant (Box 6.2) [156,157]. Consistent with the previously noted observation that one *normal* UGT1A1 allele is sufficient to maintain a normal plasma bilirubin concentration, individuals who are heterozygous for one UGT1A1 allele encoding an enzyme with reduced to absent bilirubin conjugating activity will nevertheless have normal bilirubin concentrations if the second UGT1A1 allele is normal. However, if that second allele has the A(TA)$_7$TAA promoter variant, the patient will have mild unconjugated hyperbilirubinemia with a Gilbert syndrome phenotype. Additionally, a number of instances have been documented in which mutations in the coding regions of the UGT1A1 gene encode proteins with only mildly reduced enzymatic activity. Such missense mutations, which result in a Gilbert syndrome phenotype, have thus far been reported only from Japan [160]. Inheritance has been either recessive or as a dominant negative [156,157]. If a phenotypic reduction in bilirubin clearance is taken as the operational definition of Gilbert syndrome, recognition of these alternative genotypes is important for the appropriate interpretation of mild, nonhemolytic, unconjugated hyperbilirubinemia. While homozygosity for the A(TA)$_7$TAA promoter variant supports a diagnosis of Gilbert syndrome, absence of homozygosity for this variant does not exclude Gilbert syndrome in this setting.

Box 6.2 Alternative molecular bases for the Gilbert syndrome phenotype.

- A(TA)$_7$TAA homozygote
- A(TA)$_7$TAA/structural mutation compound heterozygote
- Structural mutation, for example G71R (homozygous recessive or dominant negative)

The diagnosis of Gilbert syndrome is most often made clinically on the basis of a mild, unconjugated hyperbilirubinemia in the absence of other causes. While a definitive diagnosis can be established by assays of UGT1A1 enzymatic activity or identification of the homozygous A(TA)$_7$TAA promoter mutation, such elaborate studies, like liver biopsies, are rarely necessary [161]. Provocation tests such as a 48-hour fast or the intravenous administration of nicotinic acid augment the bilirubinemia of Gilbert syndrome patients and normal controls by a similar proportion, and are of limited value in establishing a diagnosis of Gilbert syndrome (reviewed in [48]). Bilirubin levels in simple Gilbert syndrome in adults are never sufficiently elevated to pose a risk of neurologic damage. However, neonates with *both* Gilbert syndrome *and* some form of hemolysis are at increased risk of transiently developing dangerous degrees of hyperbilirubinemia [162–165].

Some patients with Gilbert syndrome exhibit abnormalities in the hepatic handling of a variety of xenobiotics metabolized by glucuronidation, including menthol, estradiol benzoate, lamotrigine, tolbutamide, rifamycin SV, acetaminophen [48,166], and HIV protease inhibitors [126]. The HIV protease inhibitors indinavir and atazanavir produce hyperbilirubinemia by specifically inhibiting UGT1A1 [127]. The degree of hyperbilirubinemia is greater with preexisting Gilbert syndrome. Abnormalities in the glucuronidation of other substrates may be attributable to polymorphisms of other UGT isoforms [166]. No significant toxicity has been ascribed to any of these pharmacokinetic abnormalities. Virtually the sole risk from Gilbert syndrome in adults is associated with exposure to the antitumor agent irinotecan (CPT-11), the active metabolite of which is glucuronidated by UGT1A1. Administration of CPT-11 to patients with

Gilbert syndrome has resulted in severe toxicities, including intractable diarrhea and myelosuppression.

Familial conjugated hyperbilirubinemias

Two inherited disorders characterized by conjugated hyperbilirubinemia without cholestasis, the Dubin–Johnson [167] and Rotor [168] syndromes, have been described. Although a third disorder that had been termed hepatic storage disease [169] was also included in this group, more recent evidence indicates that these patients have Rotor syndrome. These disorders are relatively rare. They are clinically benign, but establishment of a precise diagnosis is important to differentiate them from other more serious disorders and to save patients from unnecessary anxiety or surgical intervention. There are several additional familial disorders characterized by conjugated hyperbilirubinemia in association with cholestasis. These include benign recurrent intrahepatic cholestasis, and the progressive familial intrahepatic cholestases, described below.

Dubin–Johnson syndrome

Clinical features

This disorder, independently described in 1954 by Dubin and Johnson [167] and by Sprinz and Nelson [170] is characterized by mild, predominantly conjugated hyperbilirubinemia (Table 6.2). Aside from jaundice, physical examination is normal in most cases, but an occasional patient may be found to have unexplained hepatosplenomegaly [171,172]. Mild constitutional symptoms similar to those observed in Gilbert syndrome (vague abdominal pain, fatigue, weakness) are common [171,172]. However, as in Gilbert syndrome, these symptoms may be related to the anxiety associated with prolonged diagnostic testing. For the most part, newly detected cases are asymptomatic. Hyperbilirubinemia and clinical icterus are typically increased by intercurrent illness, by the administration of drugs that decrease hepatic excretion of organic anions (notably oral contraceptives), and by pregnancy [173]. The condition is rarely observed before the onset of puberty, although occasional cases have been reported in infants [174–176]. Subclinical cases often become manifest during pregnancy or in association with the initiation of oral contraceptive therapy [173]. In contrast to syndromes associated with true cholestasis, pruritus is not seen in Dubin–Johnson syndrome, and serum bile acid levels are characteristically normal [173] as are other routine tests of liver function (e.g., serum alkaline phosphatase) [167,172]. Useful animal models of the Dubin–Johnson syndrome have been described in mutant Corriedale sheep [177–180], golden lion tamarin monkeys [181], and in Tr$^-$/GY [72,182–186], and EHBR [187–189] mutant rat strains. Because of the insights they have provided into the probable pathophysiology of the Dubin–Johnson syndrome, the rat mutants are discussed in detail below.

Frequency

Dubin–Johnson syndrome has been described worldwide in all races, nationalities, and ethnic backgrounds and in both sexes [171,172,190–194]. Uncommon on a worldwide basis, the disorder is highly prevalent (1 : 1300) among Iranian Jews [172]. Its frequent association in this population with a deficiency of clotting factor VII [195,196] appears to represent the coincidental inheritance of two conditions, as factor VII deficiency is not observed as part of the syndrome in other populations, and is caused by a different genetic mutation [197,198].

Table 6.2 Phenotypic features of Dubin–Johnson and Rotor syndromes.

Feature	Dubin–Johnson syndrome	Rotor syndrome
First described	1954	1948
Serum bilirubin	Usually 2–5 mg/dL, predominantly (~60%) direct reacting. Less often ≤25 mg/dL total	Usually 2–5 mg/dL, predominantly (~60%) direct reacting. Less often ≤25 mg/dL total
Other liver function tests	Normal	Normal
Serum bile acids	Normal	Normal
Appearance of liver	Grossly black; coarse, dark centrilobular pigment	Normal
Physical findings	Jaundice ± hepatomegaly	Jaundice
Urine coproporphyrins	Normal total; >80% isomer I	Markedly increased total; isomer I increased, but always <80%
Inheritance	Autosomal recessive	Autosomal recessive

Laboratory findings

Serum bilirubin concentration is typically between 2 and 5 mg/dL, but values as high as 20 or even 25 mg/dL have been reported [171,172]. Fifty percent or more of total serum bilirubin is direct reacting, and, accordingly, bilirubinuria and an increase in the covalently bound δ-bilirubin fraction in plasma are frequently present. The serum bilirubin concentration often fluctuates and occasional bilirubin determinations may be within normal limits. Other routine tests of liver function are normal, including aminotransferases, alkaline phosphatase, and γ-glutamyl transferase activities; serum albumin concentration; cholesterol level; and (except in the Iranian population) prothrombin time. Hematological studies, including complete blood count, reticulocyte count, and red cell survival studies, are also normal [199], indicating no evidence of hemolysis. Fasting and postprandial levels of the common serum bile acids are normal in the majority of patients with Dubin–Johnson syndrome [173,200] although mild elevations have been described in occasional patients [201].

Imaging studies

Cholecystography, even when carried out with supplemental doses of contrast media, does not visualize the gallbladder in Dubin–Johnson syndrome [171,172] but intravenous administration of iodipamide may permit visualization of the gallbladder at 4–6 hours [202,203]. Biliary scintigraphy with agents such as ^{99m}Tc-lidofenin or ^{99m}TC-disofenin may be helpful in the evaluation of patients with Dubin–Johnson and Rotor syndromes [204–206]. In six patients with Dubin–Johnson syndrome, administration of ^{99m}Tc-lidofenin was followed by rapid, intense, homogeneous accumulation of isotope within the liver without visualization of the intrahepatic biliary tree [204]. In the majority of patients with intact gallbladders, this organ was visualized approximately 90 minutes after injection; in all cases, isotopic activity had reached the intestine within 1 hour of injection. However, in a patient with Rotor syndrome, as well as in jaundiced patients with hepatocellular disease, administration of ^{99m}T-lidofenin resulted in no visualization of the liver, gallbladder, or biliary tract and no accumulation of radioactivity in the intestine over 24 hours of observation. The kidneys visualized intensely in these latter conditions, indicating selective excretion of the radionuclide by this route [204].

Histopathology

Gross examination of the liver from typical patients with Dubin–Johnson syndrome shows it to be intensely pigmented to the point of appearing black in color [170, 171]. Light microscopy reveals no scarring, hepatocellular necrosis, or distortion of zonal architecture. Instead,

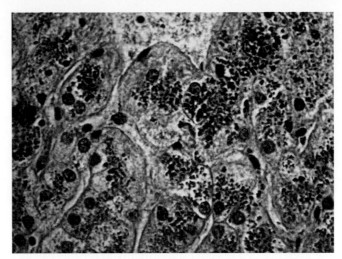

Figure 6.11 Liver biopsy in Dubin–Johnson syndrome showing coarsely granular pigment most pronounced in the centrilobular region. Hematoxylin and eosin, original ×240. (Courtesy of Dr Kamal G. Ishak, Armed Forces Institute of Pathology.)

the characteristic feature is the accumulation of a coarsely granular pigment, most pronounced in the centrilobular zones (Fig. 6.11), with a characteristic appearance of lysosomal distribution [207]. Its nature has been the subject of some debate, with some authors considering it a lipofuscin and others a melanin derivative. The histologically similar pigment observed in mutant Corriedale sheep resembles melanin histochemically and incorporates tritium following infusion of ^{3}H-epinephrine, a finding consistent with a melanin-like origin of the pigment granules [208]. A study of Dubin–Johnson syndrome employing electron spin resonance spectroscopy demonstrated differences in the physicochemical characteristics of the Dubin–Johnson pigment when compared with authentic melanin [209]. Although the nature of the pigment was not clearly defined, the data were consistent with its being composed of polymers of epinephrine metabolites. The degree of hepatic pigmentation may be variable, both within families and in a single individual with the Dubin–Johnson syndrome. Some of the variability may be genetic, but some may be due to the fact that coincidental diseases, such as viral hepatitis, are associated with the complete disappearance of pigment from the liver [210]. Pigment reaccumulates slowly after recovery from the hepatitic episode [211].

Metabolism of organic anions

Following intravenous injection, initial plasma disappearance of organic anions such as bilirubin, sulfobromophthalein (BSP), dibromosulphthalein (DBSP), and indocyanine green (ICG) is normal [212,213]. It should be noted that, with the exception of ICG, these compounds are no longer commercially available for clinical use.

A characteristic feature of Dubin–Johnson syndrome is that the plasma concentration of BSP is higher at 90 minutes as compared with 45 minutes after injection, due to reflux of conjugated BSP back into the circulation from the hepatocyte, where it was conjugated with glutathione (GSH) [172,173,202]. This secondary rise is not seen following the intravenous administration of DBSP or ICG, compounds that are excreted into bile by the hepatocyte without further metabolism [212,213]. A secondary rise, representing reflux of conjugated bilirubin, has been noted following the intravenous administration of unconjugated bilirubin-IXa to patients with this syndrome [209,212]. The defect in the excretion of conjugated BSP has been confirmed by direct studies of the plasma clearance of this metabolite [214], consistent with the presence of a selective abnormality in the bile canalicular excretion of conjugated organic anions with normal excretion of bile salts. Studies of BSP metabolism involving continuous infusion of dye support these findings as they show a marked reduction in the calculated secretory transport maximum with a normal relative storage capacity [172,173]. Even though the secondary rise of BSP levels observed following intravenous administration of a single 5 mg/kg dose is highly suggestive of the syndrome, it is not diagnostic and has occasionally been observed in other hepatobiliary disorders [215].

Urinary coproporphyrin excretion

Patients with Dubin–Johnson syndrome also have a diagnostic abnormality in urinary coproporphyrin excretion [190,216–218]. There are two naturally occurring coproporphyrin isomers, I and III. Normally, approximately 75% of the coproporphyrin in urine is isomer III. In urine from Dubin–Johnson syndrome patients, total coproporphyrin content is normal, but more than 80% is isomer I. Heterozygotes for the syndrome show an intermediate pattern [190,219]. The molecular basis for this phenomenon is not yet known.

Animal models of Dubin–Johnson syndrome

The mutant Corriedale sheep was the first recognized animal model of Dubin–Johnson syndrome [177–180]. These animals have grossly black livers and defects in organic anion and coproporphyrin excretion that are identical to patients with the syndrome. Subsequently two mutant rat models of Dubin–Johnson syndrome were described. These are the TR⁻, also known as GY (Groningen yellow), and EHBR rat strains [72,182–189]. These mutant rat strains exhibit many of the characteristic phenotypic features of the Dubin–Johnson syndrome, including: (i) autosomal recessively inherited conjugated hyperbilirubinemia and bilirubinuria; (ii) defective biliary excretion of conjugated organic anions with normal bile acid excretion; and (iii) normal total urinary coproporphyrin excre-

tion with increased percentage of isomer I. Although these animals do not typically have increased hepatic pigmentation, studies in TR⁻ animals demonstrate accumulation of lysosomal pigment following infusion of epinephrine metabolites, or feeding a diet high in aromatic amino acids [220]. A mutant strain of golden lion tamarins with a Dubin–Johnson phenotype have also been described [181].

Inheritance

The initial descriptions of the Dubin–Johnson syndrome indicated that it was an inheritable disorder [171] and its familial nature has been verified in many subsequent studies [145,191,194,196,202,221,222]. Although it was thought to be inherited as an autosomal recessive trait, there was initially no means to detect heterozygous carriers [223]. This subsequently became available from determination of urinary coproporphyrin excretion [190,219]. As noted above, there is a characteristic abnormality in the pattern of urinary coproporphyrin excretion in patients with Dubin–Johnson syndrome [190,216,217]. Subsequent studies found that in obligate heterozygotes (e.g., phenotypically normal parents and children of Dubin–Johnson syndrome patients), this pattern was intermediate between normal and affected individuals, consistent with autosomal recessive inheritance [190,219]. The pathogenesis of abnormal urinary coproporphyrin excretion in Dubin–Johnson syndrome is not known [224,225].

Genetic defect

The gene responsible for causing Dubin–Johnson syndrome has been identified as *MRP2*, encoding an ATP-dependent canalicular plasma membrane transporter for bilirubin conjugates and a number of other nonbile acid organic anions [226]. Mutations in this gene can result in a Dubin–Johnson syndrome phenotype in rats and humans [194,226–229]. Although it is clear that MRP2 plays a major role in the biliary excretion of conjugated bilirubin, even in its absence bilirubin conjugates are found in bile, implying the existence of other, not yet identified, alternative transport proteins. At least 15 mutations in the *MRP2* gene have been described in patients with the Dubin–Johnson syndrome [228]. These include four splice site mutations, six missense mutations, three nonsense mutations, and one deletion mutation. As noted above, as many as 60% of patients with Dubin–Johnson syndrome in an Israeli series had coexistence of clotting factor VII deficiency. It is now known that the gene for factor VII is located on chromosome 13, in contrast to the localization of *MRP2* to chromosome 10, which has effectively excluded a primary genetic linkage between these two phenotypes.

Treatment

No specific therapy is indicated for Dubin–Johnson syndrome. It is generally considered to be a benign disorder requiring only reassurance of the patient and avoidance of invasive diagnostic procedures. Although phenobarbital has been used in an attempt to reduce the serum bilirubin concentration, the results have been highly variable [230,231]. Although some patients with nonspecific abdominal complaints report amelioration of their vague symptoms during phenobarbital therapy, irrespective of any lowering of the serum bilirubin concentration, chronic phenobarbital administration is not recommended.

Rotor syndrome

This syndrome is characterized by chronic, predominantly conjugated hyperbilirubinemia, phenotypically resembling the Dubin–Johnson syndrome (see Table 6.2), and was initially described in two Philippine families by Rotor et al. in 1948 [168]. Although the incidence of Rotor syndrome remains much less than that of the Dubin–Johnson syndrome, it has a widespread geographic distribution [232–235].

Clinical and laboratory findings

Patients with Rotor syndrome are generally asymptomatic, and their conjugated hyperbilirubinemia is most often discovered incidentally. Some individuals describe mild symptoms such as weakness and vague abdominal pain, but pruritus is not a feature. In contrast to the Dubin–Johnson syndrome, hepatosplenomegaly has not been reported. The serum bilirubin concentration is typically elevated to between 2 and 5 mg/dL but may be as high as 20 mg/dL. More than half of the serum bilirubin is direct-reacting, and bilirubinuria is typically present. Bilirubin levels often fluctuate in a given individual and may be increased by intercurrent illness. Conventional hepatic biochemical tests other than serum bilirubin, such as alkaline phosphatase and aminotransferase activities, serum albumin concentration, and prothrombin time, are typically normal [168,234]. The gallbladder usually visualizes on oral cholecystography, in contrast to findings in the Dubin–Johnson syndrome [232,234]. Liver biopsy also is normal, and there is no increase in hepatic pigmentation.

Organic anion metabolism

Although Rotor syndrome phenotypically resembles the Dubin–Johnson syndrome and both disorders were initially considered to be variants of the same entity, detailed studies of BSP and coproporphyrin metabolism have indicated that they are distinct disorders [232,236]. In addition, while oral cholecystographic agents usually do not visualize the gallbladder in the Dubin–Johnson

syndrome, visualization is usual in Rotor syndrome [234,237]. Following the administration of a 5 mg/kg dose of BSP, a compound that is no longer available for clinical use, the initial plasma disappearance rate in Rotor syndrome is markedly reduced and the 45-minute retention is elevated, often to 30–50% [236]. There is no secondary rise in plasma BSP and conjugated BSP does not accumulate in the plasma [236]. Studies of biliary excretion failed to document a defect in the transport of either free BSP or the BSP glutathione conjugate [214]. In contrast to the Dubin–Johnson syndrome, there is marked retention of ICG and unconjugated bilirubin following intravenous infusion [238]. In addition, during constant infusion, the transport maximum T_m for BSP in Rotor syndrome was only minimally to moderately reduced, while the relative storage capacity (S) was reduced by 75–90% [236,238]. These data are in marked contrast to those in the Dubin–Johnson syndrome in which T_m is virtually 0, while S is normal. These results for BSP T_m and S are identical to those that have been described in a phenotypically disorder that had been termed hepatic storage disease [169,239]. It must be concluded that these two disorders are the same. When plasma BSP disappearance studies were conducted in 11 phenotypically normal obligate heterozygotes for Rotor syndrome, mildly elevated retention at 45 minutes, averaging 11%, was intermediate between results in patients and normal controls [236]. Similarly, during constant BSP infusion studies, T_m and S in obligate heterozygotes were also intermediate between those of Rotor syndrome patients and healthy controls [236]. These findings, suggesting an autosomal recessive mode of inheritance for Rotor syndrome, are in contradistinction to similar studies in Dubin–Johnson syndrome, in which the carrier state is not usually detectable by studies of BSP metabolism.

Urinary coproporphyrin excretion

Rotor syndrome is also differentiated from Dubin–Johnson syndrome with respect to patterns of urinary coproporphyrin excretion [218,232,240]. Total urinary coproporphyrin excretion in patients with Rotor syndrome is increased by 2.5–5-fold compared with healthy controls [232,240]. The proportion of coproporphyrin-I is also increased to an average of 65%. These results are similar to those seen in a variety of acquired hepatobiliary disorders and sharply contrast with those observed in the Dubin–Johnson syndrome [241]. Obligate heterozygotes for Rotor syndrome are phenotypically normal and have a coproporphyrin excretion pattern intermediate between that of Rotor syndrome and healthy controls [232]. On the basis of urinary coproporphyrin excretion studies, Rotor syndrome appears to be inherited as an autosomal recessive characteristic and is clearly distinct from Dubin–Johnson syndrome (Fig. 6.12) [232,240].

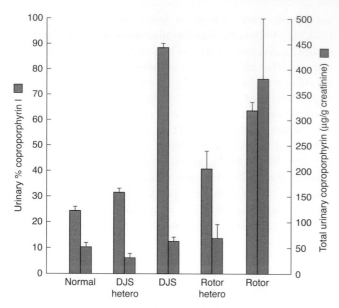

Figure 6.12 Urinary coproporphyrin in Dubin–Johnson and Rotor syndromes. The shaded bars represent the percentage of total urinary coproporphyrin excreted as coproporphyrin I. The open bars represent total urinary coproporphyrin excretion; vertical bars represent ± standard error of the mean. Total urinary coproporphyrin excretion is normal to slightly increased in the Dublin–Johnson syndrome (DJS) with a markedly elevated proportion of coproporphyrin I (approximately 80%). Both variables are markedly elevated in the Rotor syndrome. Thus, with respect to urinary coproporphyrin excretion, the two disorders are distinct. Results in obligate heterozygotes (DJS hetero, Rotor hetero) lie intermediate between results in normal individuals and in individuals manifesting the respective disorder. (Reproduced from Berk et al. [218] with permission from Elsevier.)

Genetic defect

It is clear that Rotor syndrome is an inheritable disorder distinct from the Dubin–Johnson syndrome [232,236,238,240]. However, the genetic defect has not as yet been elucidated.

Treatment

There is no treatment that is required or effective for Rotor syndrome. The majority of patients are, in any case, asymptomatic. In the absence of ill-advised medical or surgical intervention, life expectancy appears to be normal.

Familial cholestasis syndromes

Several rare familial disorders characterized by cholestasis, often in association with conjugated hyperbilirubinemia, have long been recognized, and designated progressive familial intrahepatic cholestasis (PFIC), benign recurrent intrahepatic cholestasis (BRIC), and intrahepatic cholestasis of pregnancy (ICP). In some, notably in PFIC, the cholestasis is associated with the evolution of structural liver damage that may ultimately require liver

transplantation. Over the past two decades advances in molecular cloning and the complete sequencing of the human genome have led to the identification of the major components of the hepatocellular bile secretory apparatus [242]. These advances, applied to genetic studies in individuals and kindreds affected by the various familial forms of cholestasis, established that different mutations in just three proteins – familial intrahepatic cholestasis 1 (FIC1), the bile salt export pump (BSEP), and multidrug resistance protein 3 (MDR3) – located in the canalicular plasma membrane and involved in canalicular bile salt and phospholipid transport, were the basis for the multiple different clinical presentations and manifestations of familial cholestasis observed in neonatal, pediatric, and adult – including obstetric – settings. A small number of patients with a PFIC phenotype do not appear to have a mutation in any of these three genes, suggesting that mutations in additional genes also may produce the phenotype.

Progressive familial intrahepatic cholestasis

This name is applied to three phenotypically related syndromes (Table 6.3). PFIC type 1 presents in early infancy as cholestasis that may be initially episodic [243]. However, in contrast to BRIC (see below), PFIC progresses during childhood to malnutrition, growth retardation, and end-stage liver disease often requiring transplantation. The disorder is a consequence of a mutation in the *ATP8B1* gene encoding the protein designated FIC1 [244]. FIC1 is expressed primarily in the small intestine and weakly in the liver. It is a member of a P-type ATPase family that transports aminophospholipids from the outer to the inner leaflet of a variety of cell membranes, and has little similarity to genes that have been shown to play a role in bile canalicular excretion of compounds such as bilirubin conjugates [244–246]. The precise functional relationship of the FIC1 protein to the pathogenesis of cholestasis is not yet entirely clear. However, under normal circumstances, the distribution of phospholipids in the hepatocyte plasma membrane is asymmetric, with phosphatidyl choline being concentrated in the external leaflet and phosphatidyl serine and phosphatidyl ethanolamine in the cytoplasmic leaflet. The asymmetry, which is important to the physical properties of the canalicular membrane, is actively maintained by inwardly directed phospholipid transporters called flippases and outwardly directed ones called floppases. FIC1 is a phosphatidyl serine flippase. In the presence of deficient FIC1 activity, phosphatidyl serine accumulates in the outer membrane leaflet, increasing membrane flexibility. Subsequent phospholipid rearrangement makes the membrane more sensitive to the extraction of cholesterol and certain ectoenzymes by bile salt micelles. This

Table 6.3 Inheritable disorders characterized by conjugated hyperbilirubinemia.

	Non-cholestatic syndromes		Familial cholestatic syndromes					
	Dubin–Johnson	Rotor	PFIC1	PFIC2	PFIC3	BRIC-1	BRIC-2	ICP-1,2,3
Gene	ABCC2	?	ATP8B1	ABCB11	ABCB4	ATP8B1	ABCB11	ATP8B1 (type 1) ABCB11 (type 2) ABCB4 (type 3)
Protein	MRP2	?	FIC1	BSEP	MDR3	FIC1	BSEP	FIC1 (type 1) BSEP (type 2) MDR3 (type 3)
Cholestasis	No	No	Yes	Yes	Yes	Episodic	Episodic	Yes
Serum γ-glutamyltransferase	Normal	Normal	Normal	Normal	↑↑	Normal	Normal	Normal in types 1 and 2; can be mildly ↑ in type 3
Serum bile acids	Normal	Normal	↑↑	↑↑	↑↑	↑↑ during episodes	↑↑ during episodes	↑↑
Clinical features	Mild conjugated hyperbilirubinemia; otherwise normal liver function; dark pigment in liver; characteristic pattern of urinary coproporphyrins	Mild conjugated hyperbilirubinemia; otherwise normal liver function; liver without abnormal pigmentation	Severe cholestasis beginning in childhood	Severe cholestasis beginning in childhood	Severe cholestasis beginning in childhood. Decreased phospholipids in bile	Recurrent episodes of cholestasis beginning at any age	Recurrent episodes of cholestasis beginning at any age	Symptomatic cholestasis with pruritus but not jaundice starting in third trimester. Resolves after delivery. Increased fetal wastage

leads to impairment of BSEP activity, which is the ultimate cause of cholestasis [247,248]. To date, more than 50 distinct mutations in *ATP8B1* have been reported [249]. Nonsense and frameshift mutations likely to cause severe defects in protein expression or function are typically detected in patients with progressive disease while missense mutations are more common in less clinically severe variants. Homozygosity for the Gly308Val mutation is almost invariably found among old-order Amish in Pennsylvania, where the condition is known as Byler syndrome after the original "founders" of the disease [243]. While other specific mutations are commonly found in several other isolated populations, in the population at large no single mutation is widely detected, so that the entire gene must be sequenced if a diagnosis is to be based on mutational analysis.

Two other types of PFIC (types 2 and 3) have been described. Type 2 is associated with mutations in *ABCB11* [250,251], which encodes BSEP per se. More than 100 mutations have been reported and, as with *ATP8B1* mutations, they produce a clinical spectrum from mild to progressive. The missense mutations Glu297Gly and/or Asp482Gly have been found in more than half of the well-studied European families [249]. PFIC type 3 has been associated with at least 45 different mutations of the *ABCB4* gene encoding MDR3, a protein that is essential for normal hepatocellular excretion of phospholipids across the bile canalicular membrane, where it functions as a phospholipid floppase (i.e., an outwardly directed phospholipid transporter), translocating phosphatidylcholine into the canalicular bile [252–254]. As a result of *ABCB4* mutations, bile phospholipid concentrations in this condition are low. Injury to bile canaliculi and the biliary epithelium in the form of cholangitis is thought to result from their continuous exposure to hydrophobic bile salts, the detergent effects of which are not prevented by the reduced biliary phospholipid levels. Consequently, although all three types of PFIC have similar clinical phenotypes, only type 3 is associated with high serum levels of γ-glutamyltransferase (GGT) activity [249,254]. The activity of this enzyme is normal or only mildly elevated in symptomatic BRIC and PFIC types 1 and 2.

Short of full mutational analysis, distinction among the three forms of PFIC is based on histologic and biochemical differences. All three forms of PFIC exhibit elevated serum bile salt concentrations and abnormalities of standard hepatic biochemical tests. On routine histologic examination, PFIC type 1 tends to show a "bland cholestasis" with little inflammation, whereas PFIC type 2 exhibits features of neonatal hepatitis. Bile ductular proliferation is suggestive of PFIC type 3. Type 3 is distinguishable from types 1 and 2 by having an elevated GGT level. Electron microscopy shows the bile in type 1 to be coarsely granular, while that in type 2 is filamentous.

Overall, most medical therapies are of limited value in PFIC types 1 and 2, especially in patients with progressive disease. Cholestyramine, alone or in combination with rifampicin, may shorten episodes in patients whose cholestasis is intermittent. In contrast, ursodeoxycholic acid (UCDA) therapy may ameliorate symptoms and even normalize hepatic biochemical tests in up to 60% of patients with PFIC type 3 [254,255]. Its mechanism of action in this situation appears to involve the changes it effects in the composition of the bile salt pool with a consequent decrease in hydrophobicity, as well as possible upregulation of the expression of some mutated *MDR3* genes, resulting in some phospholipids being translocated into bile. These two factors may be adequate to protect cell membranes from the toxicity of primary bile salts in some patients [253]. Results with UCDA in PFIC types 1 and 2 are conflicting, varying from no effect to some instances of clear benefit [255].

In many patients with progressive disease who fail medical therapy, partial external biliary diversion may slow disease progression. In those with symptomatically difficult intermittent disease, nasobiliary drainage may bring temporary relief. Ultimately, intolerable pruritus and/or progression to cirrhosis may mandate orthotopic liver transplantation. Although lifelong immunosuppression is often required postoperatively, the procedure usually provides symptomatic relief and correction of the phenotype in type 2 and 3 disease. However, severe recurrence of the phenotype has been reported in type 2 disease due to the formation of autoantibodies against BSEP [256]. In PFIC type 1 disease, diarrhea may appear or worsen after transplantation. Cholestyramine may be of benefit in this situation.

Benign recurrent intrahepatic cholestasis type 1

This rare disorder, also known as Tygstrup or Summerskill and Walshe cholestasis, is characterized by recurrent attacks of pruritus and jaundice. It typically presents with an episode of mild malaise and elevated serum aminotransferases, followed rapidly by rises in alkaline phosphatase and conjugated bilirubin and onset of jaundice, bilirubinuria, and itching [248,257]. Some reports suggest that a fever, even a mild and transient one, is a precipitating event. During the cholestatic episode, hepatic uptake of unconjugated bilirubin has been shown to be normal, but is followed by extensive reflux of conjugated bilirubin to plasma [258]. Initial episodes may be misdiagnosed as acute viral hepatitis. Cholestatic episodes typically begin in childhood or young adulthood, and can last for several weeks to months. In the interval between attacks, lasting from several months to years, there is complete clinical and biochemical resolution. This disorder is familial and has an autosomal recessive pattern of inheritance.

Although BRIC is considered a benign disorder that does not lead to cirrhosis or end-stage liver disease, the prolonged episodes can be highly debilitating, resulting in liver transplantation in some patients. Treatment during the cholestatic episodes is symptomatic and there is no means available to reliably prevent or shorten the occurrence of episodes.

It is now recognized that BRIC type 1 results from mutations in the *ATP8B1* gene encoding FIC1 [244,248,249], the same gene that is mutated in PFIC type 1. There is considerable genetic heterogeneity, and patients with BRIC type 1 may either be heterozygotes for a particular *ATP8B1* gene mutation or homozygotes for a mutation that only partially affects the function of the encoded protein. Interestingly a second phenotypically identical form of BRIC, termed BRIC type 2, has been described resulting from mutations in the bile salt export pump, BSEP [251,259].

Intrahepatic cholestasis of pregnancy

Intrahepatic cholestasis of pregnancy is characterized by the development of pruritus in pregnant women, usually without accompanying clinical jaundice, that most typically presents in the third trimester, becomes more severe as the pregnancy advances, and resolves after delivery [260,261]. Symptoms are typically accompanied by increased serum bile acid, AST, ALT, and alkaline phosphatase concentrations. The syndrome has been associated with heterozygosity for mutations in the genes encoding FIC1 (ICP type 1), BSEP (ICP type 2), and MDR3 (ICP type 3). Serum GGT is typically normal in ICP types 1 and 2, but may be slightly elevated in type 3 [261]. ICP is associated with an increased incidence of fetal distress and prematurity and an unexplained increase in intrauterine deaths, especially after 37 weeks' gestation [24]. Accordingly, the aims of treatment are to reduce maternal symptoms and prevent fetal complications. As the purely obstetric aspects of management are beyond the scope of this chapter, we refer readers to recent reviews of ICP for a detailed overview of management options [24,262].

The most effective medical therapy is UDCA. While not universally approved for use during pregnancy, available data suggest that it is safe and effective in improving both maternal symptoms and biochemical abnormalities [263,264], and may also even diminish fetal complications [265]. A combination of UCDA with S-adenosyl-L-methionine is reported to have synergistic benefits [266]. Since intensive fetal monitoring does not prevent intrauterine death, current literature encourages the induction of labor between 37 and 38 weeks of gestation in women with ICP, with the goal of decreasing the incidence of later intrauterine death [262].

After delivery, the serum biochemical abnormalities normally resolve within 2–8 weeks. Follow-up should be maintained at least long enough to ensure normalization of liver tests, and even longer follow-up should be considered as ICP is associated with the development of hepatobiliary disease later in life, for example gallstones, cholecystitis, and cirrhosis [267]. In addition, recurrence of cholestasis is not uncommon in subsequent pregnancies, and may also occur with the use of oral contraceptives.

Further reading

Kadakol A, Ghosh SS, Sappal BS, Sharma G, Chowdhury JR, Chowdhury NR. Genetic lesions of bilirubin uridine-diphosphoglucuronate glucuronosyltransferase (UGT1A1) causing Crigler–Najjar and Gilbert syndromes: correlation of genotype to phenotype. *Hum Mutat* 2000;16:297–306.

This outstanding review evaluates the available information on the phenotypic consequences of multiple genotypes, including many mutations in both the UGT1A1 coding regions and in the exon 1 promoter, that have been associated with Gilberts syndrome and Crigler–Najjar syndromes I and II. It leads to a much clearer picture of the complex interactions among these three conditions.

Maisels MJ, McDonagh AF. Phototherapy for neonatal jaundice. *N Engl J Med* 2008;358:920–8.

This review details the biochemistry of bilirubin as it relates to treatment of neonatal jaundice. Current treatment guidelines are reviewed, and rational use of this treatment modality for prevention of kernicterus is clearly presented.

McDonagh AF. The biliverdin–bilirubin antioxidant cycle of cellular protection: missing a wheel? *Free Radic Biol Med* 2010;49:814–20.

Earlier observations led to the proposed existence of a specific intracellular oxidation/reduction cycle in which lipophilic reactive oxygen species (ROS) oxidize bilirubin to biliverdin, which is then re-reduced by biliverdin reductase, thus contributing in a regulated fashion to cellular antioxidant defenses. However, existence of such a cycle appears unlikely on the basis of more recent studies summarized in this review.

Nies AT, Keppler D. The apical conjugate efflux pump ABCC2 (MRP2). *Pflugers Arch* 2007;453:643–59.

This is a review of the pathobiology of the bile canalicular efflux pump, MRP2 (ABCC2) and its relationship to normal liver excretory mechanisms. Mutations that result in Dubin–Johnson syndrome are detailed.

Ostrow JD, Pascolo L, Brites D, Tiribelli C. Molecular basis of bilirubin-induced neurotoxicity. *Trends Molec Med* 2004;10:65–70.

The susceptibility of newborns to bilirubin neurotoxicity is highly variable. Furthermore neurologic damage sometimes occurs at plasma unconjugated bilirubin concentrations well below therapeutic guidelines. This paper reviews current information on mechanisms of cellular bilirubin toxicity, and the transport processes determining its access to and accumulation within the central nervous system.

Servedio V, d'Apolito M, Maiorano N, et al. Spectrum of UGT1A1 mutations in Crigler–Najjar (CN) syndrome patients: identification of twelve novel alleles and genotype-phenotype correlation. *Hum Mutat* 2005;25(3):325.

This brief paper is a valuable addition to the Kadakol et al. reference, identifying 12 novel UGT1A1 mutations, reviewing the total spectrum of 77 such mutations identified as of early 2005, and exploring genotype–phenotype correlations.

Strassburg CP, Lankisch TO, Manns MP, Ehmer U. Family 1 uridine-5′-diphosphate glucuronosyltransferases (UGT1A): from Gilbert's syndrome to genetic organization and variability. *Arch Toxicol* 2008;82:415–33.

This is a comprehensive review of the UGT1A gene and its relationship to the pathophysiology of Gilbert syndrome and potential alterations in drug metabolism in these individuals. Genetic variants are detailed as are their clinical sequelae.

Takeuchi K, Kobayashi Y, Tamaki S, et al. Genetic polymorphisms of bilirubin uridine diphosphate-glucuronosyltransferase gene in Japanese patients with Crigler–Najjar syndrome or Gilbert's syndrome as well as in healthy Japanese subjects *J. Gastroenterol Hepatol* 2004;19:1023–8.

This meticulous study analyzed both the UGT1A1 promoter and coding regions of 63 Japanese patients with Gilbert syndrome and 71 normal Japanese controls. The data indicate clearly that the genetic basis for the familial hyperbilirubinemias differs between Japanese and Caucasian populations.

Van der Woerd WL, van Mil SW, Stapelbroek JM, Klomp LW, van de Graaf SF, Houwen RH. Familial cholestasis: progressive familial intrahepatic cholestasis, benign recurrent intrahepatic cholestasis and intrahepatic cholestasis of pregnancy. *Best Pract Res Clin Gastroenterol* 2010;24:541–53.

A combination of advances in molecular technology, sequencing of the human genome, and detailed human genetic studies have established that different mutations in just three proteins, familial intrahepatic cholestasis-1 (FIC1), the bile salt export pump (BSEP), and multidrug resistance protein-3 (MDR3), are the basis for the multiple different clinical presentations and manifestations of familial cholestasis. This review summarizes the clinical features, underlying pathophysiology, molecular genetic bases, and treatment of the major forms of familial cholestasis.

References

1. Abraham NG, Kappas A. Pharmacological and clinical aspects of heme oxygenase. *Pharmacol Rev* 2008;60:79–127.

2. McDonagh AF. The biliverdin–bilirubin antioxidant cycle of cellular protection: missing a wheel? *Free Radic Biol Med* 2010;49:814–20.

3. McDonagh AF. Turning green to gold. *Nat Struct Biol* 2001;8:198–200.

4. Baranano DE, Rao M, Ferris CD, Snyder SH. Biliverdin reductase: a major physiologic cytoprotectant. *Proc Natl Acad Sci USA* 2002;99:16093–8.

5. Kapitulnik J. Bilirubin: an endogenous product of heme degradation with both cytotoxic and cytoprotective properties. *Mol Pharmacol* 2004;66:773–9.

6. Foresti R, Green CJ, Motterlini R. Generation of bile pigments by haem oxygenase: a refined cellular strategy in response to stressful insults. *Biochem Soc Symp* 2004;71:177–92.

7. Sedlak TW, Snyder SH. Bilirubin benefits: cellular protection by a biliverdin reductase antioxidant cycle. *Pediatrics* 2004;113:1776–82.

8. McDonagh A. Bilirubin the beneficent. *Pediatrics* 2004;114:1741–2.

9. Maghzal GJ, Leck MC, Collinson E, Li C, Stocker R. Limited role for the bilirubin–biliverdin redox amplification cycle in the cellular antioxidant protection by biliverdin reductase. *J Biol Chem* 2009;284:29251–9.

10. Berk PD, Howe RB, Bloomer JR, Berlin NI. Studies on bilirubin kinetics in normal adults. *J Clin Invest* 1969;48:2176–90.

11. Berk PD, Blaschke TF, Scharschmidt BF, Waggoner JG, Berlin NI. A new approach to quantitation of the various sources of bilirubin in man. *J Lab Clin Med* 1976;87:767–80.

12. Berlin NI, Berk PD. Quantitative aspects of bilirubin metabolism for hematologists. *Blood* 1981;57:983–99.

13. Berk PD, Tschudy DP, Shepley LA, Waggoner JG, Berlin NI. Hematologic and biochemical studies in a case of lead poisoning. *Am J Med* 1970;48:137–44.

14. Schmid R, Marver HS, Hammaker L. Enhanced formation of rapidly labelled bilirubin by phenobarbital: hepatic microsomal cytochromes as a possible source. *Biochem Biophys Res Commun* 1966;24:319–28.

15. Schmid R. Synthesis and degradation of microsomal hemoproteins. *Drug Metab Dispos* 1973;1:256–8.

16. Crosby WH, Akeroyd JH. The limits of hemoglobin synthesis in hereditary hemolytic anemias. *Am J Med* 1952;13:273–83.

17. Lewis VW, Verwilghen RL. Dyserythropoiesis: definition, diagnosis and assessment. In: Lewis VW, Verwilghen RL, eds. *Dyserythropoiesis.* New York: Academic Press, 1977:3.

18. Bissell DM, Hammaker LE. Cytochrome p-450 heme and the regulation of delta-aminolevulinic acid synthetase in the liver. *Arch Biochem Biophys* 1976;176:103–12.

19. Mreihil K, McDonagh AF, Nakstad B, Hansen TW. Early isomerization of bilirubin in phototherapy of neonatal jaundice. *Pediatr Res* 2010;67:656–9.

20. Maisels MJ, McDonagh AF. Phototherapy for neonatal jaundice. *N Engl J Med* 2008;358:920–8.

21. Fog J, Jellum E. Structure of bilirubin. *Nature* 1963;198:88–9.

22. Bonnett R, Davies JE, Hursthouse MB. Structure of bilirubin. *Nature* 1976;262:327–8.

23. Heirwegh KP, Fevery J, Meuwissen JA, et al. Recent advances in the separation and analysis of diazo-positive bile pigments. *Methods Biochem Anal* 1974;22:205–50.

24. Geenes V, Williamson C. Intrahepatic cholestasis of pregnancy. *World J Gastroenterol* 2009;15:2049–66.

25. Blanckaert N, Heirwegh KP, Compernolle F. Synthesis and separation by thin-layer chromatography of bilirubin-IX isomers. Their identification as tetrapyrroles and dipyrrolic ethyl anthranilate azo derivatives. *Biochem J* 1976;155:405–17.

26. Lim CK, Peters TJ. High-performance liquid chromatographic separation of the bilirubin isomers. *Methods Enzymol* 1986;123: 389–95.

27. McDonagh AF. Thermal and photochemical reactions of bilirubin IX-alpha. *Ann NY Acad Sci* 1975;244:553–69.

28. Blanckaert N, Heirwegh KP, Zaman Z. Comparison of the biliary excretion of the four isomers of bilirubin-IX in Wistar and homozygous Gunn rats. *Biochem J* 1977;164:229–36.

29. Lightner DA, Wooldridge TA, McDonagh AF. Configurational isomerization of bilirubin and the mechanism of jaundice phototherapy. *Biochem Biophys Res Commun* 1979;86:235–43.

30. McDonagh AF, Palma LA, Lightner DA. Blue light and bilirubin excretion. *Science* 1980;208:145–51.

31. Hauser SC, Gollan JL. Bilirubin metabolism and hyperbilirubinaemic disorders. In: Millward-Sadler GH, Wright R, Arthur MJP, eds. *Wright's Liver and Biliary Disease*, 3rd edn. London: WB Saunders, 1992:317–70.

32. Blanckaert N, Fevery J. Physiology and pathophysiology of bilirubin metabolism. In: Zakim D, Boyer TD, eds. *Hepatology: a textbook of liver disease.* Philadelphia: WB Saunders, 1990:254–302.

33. McDonagh AF. Bile pigments: bilatrienes and 5, 15-biladienes. In: Dolphin D, ed. *The Porphyrins.* New York: Academic Press, 1979:293–491.

34. Brodersen R. Binding of bilirubin to albumin. *CRC Crit Rev Clin Lab Sci* 1980;11:305–99.

35. Hahm JS, Ostrow JD, Mukerjee P, Celic L. Ionization and self-association of unconjugated bilirubin, determined by rapid solvent partition from chloroform, with further studies of bilirubin solubility. *J Lipid Res* 1992;33:1123–37.

36. Jacobsen J. Binding of bilirubin to human serum albumin – determination of the dissociation constants. *FEBS Lett* 1969;5:112–14.

37. Athar H, Ahmad N, Tayyab S, Qasim MA. Use of fluorescence enhancement technique to study bilirubin–albumin interaction. *Int J Biol Macromol* 1999;25:353–8.

38. Ahlfors CE. Measurement of plasma unbound unconjugated bilirubin. *Anal Biochem* 2000;279:130–5.

39. Kaplan M, Hammerman C. Understanding severe hyperbilirubinemia and preventing kernicterus: adjuncts in the interpretation of neonatal serum bilirubin. *Clin Chim Acta* 2005;356:9–21.

40. Ahlfors CE, Wennberg RP. Bilirubin–albumin binding and neonatal jaundice. *Semin Perinatol* 2004;28:334–9.

41. Ostrow JD, Pascolo L, Brites D, Tiribelli C. Molecular basis of bilirubin-induced neurotoxicity. *Trends Mol Med* 2004;10:65–70.

42. Cohen RS, Wong RJ, Stevenson DK. Understanding neonatal jaundice: a perspective on causation. *Pediatr Neonatol* 2010;51:143–8.

43. Gordon ER, Shaffer EA, Sass-Kortsak A. Bilirubin secretion and conjugation in the Crigler–Najjar syndrome type II. *Gastroenterology* 1976;70:761–5.

44. Weisiger RA, Ostrow JD, Koehler RK, et al. Affinity of human serum albumin for bilirubin varies with albumin concentration and buffer composition: results of a novel ultrafiltration method. *J Biol Chem* 2001;276:29953–60.

45. Nerli B, Romanini D, Pico G. Structural specificity requirements in the binding of beta lactam antibiotics to human serum albumin. *Chem Biol Interact* 1997;104:179–202.

46. Davies BE. Displacement of bilirubin from cord serum by sulphadimethoxine, amoxycillin, clavulanic acid in combination with either amoxycillin or ticarcillin, temocillin and cloxacillin. *Br J Clin Pharmacol* 1985;20:345–8.

47. Shankaran S, Poland RL. The displacement of bilirubin from albumin by furosemide. *J Pediatr* 1977;90:642–6.

48. Berk PD, Noyer CA. Bilirubin metabolism and the hereditary hyperbilirubinemias. *Semin Liver Dis* 1994;14:321–2.

49. Wisse E. Ultrastructure and function of Kupffer cells and other sinusoidal cells in the liver. *Med Chir Dig* 1977;6:409–18.

50. Grisham JW, Nopanitaya W, Compagno J, Nagel AE. Scanning electron microscopy of normal rat liver: the surface structure of its cells and tissue components. *Am J Anat* 1975;144:295–321.

51. Stremmel W, Tavoloni N, Berk PD. Uptake of bilirubin by the liver. *Semin Liver Dis* 1983;3:1–10.

52. Sorrentino D, Stremmel W, Berk PD. The hepatocellular uptake of bilirubin: current concepts and controversies. *Mol Aspects Med* 1987;9:405–28.

53. Berk PD, Blaschke TF, Waggoner JG. Defective bromosulfophthalein clearance in patients with constitutional hepatic dysfunction (Gilbert's syndrome). *Gastroenterology* 1972;63:472–81.

54. Berk PD, Martin JF, Vierling JM, et al. Heterogeneity of Gilbert's syndrome, as manifested by abnormalities in the hepatic transport of sulfobromophthalein and indocyanine green. In: Preisig R, Bircher G, Paumgartner G, eds. *The Liver: quantitative aspects of structure amd function. Proceedings of the 2nd International Gstaad Symposium.* Aulendorf: Editio Cantor, 1976.

55. Gartner U, Stockert RJ, Levine WG, Wolkoff AW. Effect of nafenopin on the uptake of bilirubin and sulfobromophthalein by isolated perfused rat liver. *Gastroenterology* 1982;83:1163–9.

56. Berk PD, Potter BJ, Stremmel W. Role of plasma membrane ligand-binding proteins in the hepatocellular uptake of albumin-bound organic anions. *Hepatology* 1987;7:165–76.

57. Cui Y, Konig J, Leier I, Buchholz U, Keppler D. Hepatic uptake of bilirubin and its conjugates by the human organic anion transporter SLC21A6. *J Biol Chem* 2001;276:9626–30.

58. Wang P, Kim RB, Chowdhury JR, Wolkoff AW. The human organic anion transport protein SLC21A6 is not sufficient for bilirubin transport. *J Biol Chem* 2003;278:20695–9.

59. Zucker SD, Goessling W, Hoppin AG. Unconjugated bilirubin exhibits spontaneous diffusion through model lipid bilayers and native hepatocyte membranes. *J Biol Chem* 1999;274:10852–62.

60. Rigato I, Pascolo L, Fernetti C, Ostrow JD, Tiribelli C. The human multidrug-resistance-associated protein MRP1 mediates ATP-dependent transport of unconjugated bilirubin. *Biochem J* 2004;383:335–41.

61. Kamisako T, Kobayashi Y, Takeuchi K, et al. Recent advances in bilirubin metabolism research: the molecular mechanism of hepatocyte bilirubin transport and its clinical relevance. *J Gastroenterol* 2000;35:659–64.

62. Levi AJ, Gatmaitan Z, Arias IM. Two hepatic cytoplasmic protein fractions, Y and Z, and their possible role in the hepatic uptake of bilirubin, sulfobromophthalein, and other anions. *J Clin Invest* 1969;48:2156–67.

63. Wolkoff AW, Goresky CA, Sellin J, Gatmaitan Z, Arias IM. Role of ligandin in transfer of bilirubin from plasma into liver. *Am J Physiol* 1979;236:E638–48.

64. Listowsky I, Gatmaitan Z, Arias IM. Ligandin retains and albumin loses bilirubin binding capacity in liver cytosol. *Proc Natl Acad Sci USA* 1978;75:1213–16.

65. Jakoby WB. The glutathione *S*-transferases: a group of multifunctional detoxification proteins. *Adv Enzymol Relat Areas Mol Biol* 1978;46:383–414.

66. Sheehan D, Mantle TJ. Evidence for two forms of ligandin (YaYa dimers of glutathione *S*-transferase) in rat liver and kidney. *Biochem J* 1984;218:893–7.

67. Ritter JK, Chen F, Sheen YY, et al. A novel complex locus UGT1 encodes human bilirubin, phenol, and other UDP-glucuronosyltransferase isozymes with identical carboxyl termini. *J Biol Chem* 1992;267:3257–61.

68. Strassburg CP, Lankisch TO, Manns MP, Ehmer U. Family 1 uridine-5′-diphosphate glucuronosyltransferases (UGT1A): from Gilbert's syndrome to genetic organization and variability. *Arch Toxicol* 2008;82:415–33.

69. Berk PD, Wolkoff AW. Bilirubin metabolism and the hyperbilirubinemias. In: Braunwald E, Fauci AS, Kasper DL, Hauser SL, Longo DL, Jameson JL, eds. *Harrison's Principles of Internal Medicine*, 15th edn. New York: McGraw Hill, 2001:1715–20.

70. Bosma PJ, Seppen J, Goldhoorn B, et al. Bilirubin UDP-glucuronosyltransferase 1 is the only relevant bilirubin glucuronidating isoform in man. *J Biol Chem* 1994;269:17960–4.

71. Gatmaitan ZC, Arias IM. ATP-dependent transport systems in the canalicular membrane of the hepatocyte. *Physiol Rev* 1995;75:261–75.

72. Paulusma CC, Oude Elferink RP. The canalicular multispecific organic anion transporter and conjugated hyperbilirubinemia in rat and man. *J Mol Med* 1997;75:420–8.

73. Nies AT, Keppler D. The apical conjugate efflux pump ABCC2 (MRP2). *Pflugers Arch* 2007;453:643–59.

74. Kikuchi S, Hata M, Fukumoto K, et al. Radixin deficiency causes conjugated hyperbilirubinemia with loss of Mrp2 from bile canalicular membranes. *Nat Genet* 2002;31:320–5.

75. Lester R, Schmid R. Intestinal absorption of bile pigments. I. The enterohepatic circulation of bilirubin in the rat. *J Clin Invest* 1963;42:736–46.

76. Lester R, Schmid R. Intestinal absorption of bile pigments. II. Bilirubin absorption in man. *N Engl J Med* 1963;269:178–82.

77. Gollan J, Hammaker L, Licko V, Schmid R. Bilirubin kinetics in intact rats and isolated perfused liver. Evidence for hepatic deconjugation of bilirubin glucuronides. *J Clin Invest* 1981;67:1003–15.

78. Poland RL, Odell GB. Physiologic jaundice: the enterohepatic circulation of bilirubin. *N Engl J Med* 1971;284:1–6.

79. Billing BH. Intestinal and renal metabolism of bilirubin including enterohepatic circulation. In: Ostrow JD, ed. *Bile Pigments and Jaundice*. New York: Marcel Dekker, 1986:255–69.

80. Elder G, Gray CH, Nicholson DC. Bile pigment fate in gastrointestinal tract. *Semin Hematol* 1972;9:71–89.

81. Moscowitz A, Weimer M, Lightner DA, Petryka ZJ, Davis E, Watson CJ. The in vitro conversion of bile pigments to the urobilinoids by a

rat clostridia species as compared with the human fecal flora. 3. Natural d-urobilin, synthetic i-urobilin, and synthetic i-urobilinogen. *Biochem Med* 1971;4:149–64.

82. Troxler RF, Dawber NH, Lester R. Synthesis of urobilinogen by broken cell preparations of intestinal bacteria. *Gastroenterology* 1968;54:568–74.

83. Bloomer JR, Berk PD, Howe RB, Waggoner JG, Berlin NI. Comparison of fecal urobilinogen excretion with bilirubin production in normal volunteers and patients with increased bilirubin production. *Clin Chim Acta* 1970;29:463–71.

84. Schmidt M, Puttkammer G, Eisenburg J, Stich W. Studies of human urobilinoid metabolism. II. Determination of urobilinoid concentration of human serum and urine at acute viral hepatitis. *Acta Hepatogastroenterol (Stuttg)* 1974;21:134–8.

85. Jones EA, Berk PD. Chemical and immunological tests in the evaluation of liver disease. In: Brown SS, Mitchell FL, Young DS, eds. *Chemical Diagnosis of Disease*. Amsterdam: Elsevier, 1979:525–662.

86. Lee KS, Gartner LM. Fetal bilirubin metabolism and neonatal jaundice. In: Ostrow JD, ed. *Bile Pigments and Jaundice*. New York: Marcel Dekker, 1986:373–94.

87. Schmid R, Hammaker L. Metabolism and disposition of C14-bilirubin in congenital nonhemolytic jaundice. *J Clin Invest* 1963;42:1720–34.

88. Blanckaert N, Fevery J, Heirwegh KP, Compernolle F. Characterization of the major diazo-positive pigments in bile of homozygous Gunn rats. *Biochem J* 1977;164:237–49.

89. Blaschke TF, Berk PD, Scharschmidt BF, Guyther JR, Vergalla JM, Waggoner JG. Crigler–Najjar syndrome: an unusual course with development of neurologic damage at age eighteen. *Pediatr Res* 1974;8:573–90.

90. Hafkamp AM, Havinga R, Sinaasappel M, Verkade HJ. Effective oral treatment of unconjugated hyperbilirubinemia in Gunn rats. *Hepatology* 2005;41:526–34.

91. Van Der Veere CN, Jansen PL, Sinaasappel M, et al. Oral calcium phosphate: a new therapy for Crigler–Najjar disease? *Gastroenterology* 1997;112:455–62.

92. Hafkamp AM, Nelisse-Haak R, Sinaasappel M, Oude Elferink RP, Verkade HJ. Orlistat treatment of unconjugated hyperbilirubinemia in Crigler–Najjar disease: a randomized controlled trial. *Pediatr Res* 2007;62:725–30.

93. Fulop M, Sandson J, Brazeau P. Dialyzability, protein binding, and renal excretion of plasma conjugated bilirubin. *J Clin Invest* 1965;44:666–80.

94. Fevery J, Heirwegh K, De Groote J. Renal bilirubin clearance in liver patients. *Clin Chim Acta* 1967;17:63–71.

95. Monserrate IC, Garcia MDR. Aclaramiento renal de las fracciones glucuronizadas de la bilirubina en las diversas ictericias. *Rev Exp Enferm Aper Dig* 1975;46:1–12.

96. Ali MA, Billing BH. Renal excretion of bilirubin by the rat. *Am J Physiol* 1968;214:1340–5.

97. Gollan JL, Dallinger KJ, Billing BH. Excretion of conjugated bilirubin in the isolated perfused rat kidney. *Clin Sci Mol Med* 1978;54:381–9.

98. Berk PD, Martin JF, Blaschke TF, Scharschmidt BF, Plotz PH. Unconjugated hyperbilirubinemia. Physiologic evaluation and experimental approaches to therapy. *Ann Intern Med* 1975;82:552–70.

99. Berk PD, Bloomer JR, Howe RB, Blaschke TF, Berlin NI. Bilirubin production as a measure of red cell life span. *J Lab Clin Med* 1972;79:364–78.

100. Jones EA, Shrager R, Bloomer JR, Berk PD, Howe RB, Berlin NI. Quantitative studies of the delivery of hepatic-synthesized bilirubin to plasma utilizing aminolevulinic acid-4- 14 C and bilirubin- 3 H in man. *J Clin Invest* 1972;51:2450–8.

101. Berk PD, Rodkey FL, Blaschke TF, Collison HA, Waggoner JG. Comparison of plasma bilirubin turnover and carbon monoxide production in man. *J Lab Clin Med* 1974;83:29–37.

102. Lynch SR, Moede AL. Variation in the rate of endogenous carbon monoxide production in normal human beings. *J Lab Clin Med* 1972;79:85–95.

103. van den Bergh AAH, Muller P. Ueber eine direkte und eine indirekte Diazoreaktion auf Bilirubin. *Biochem Z* 1916;77:90.

104. Dufour DR. Evaluation of liver function and injury. In: Henry JB, ed. *Clinical Diagnosis and Management by Laboratory Methods*, 20th edn. Philadelphia: WB Saunders, 2001:264–80.

105. Hertz H, Dybkaer R, Lauritzen M. Direct spectrometric determination of the concentrations of (unconjugated) bilirubin and conjugated bilirubin in serum. *Scand J Clin Lab Invest* 1974;34:265–73.

106. Lucy A. Liquor amnii analysis in the management of the pregnancy complicated by rhesus sensitization. *Am J Obstet Gynecol* 1961;82:1359–70.

107. Bertini G, Rubaltelli FF. Non-invasive bilirubinometry in neonatal jaundice. *Semin Neonatol* 2002;7:129–33.

108. Blanckaert N, Kabra PM, Farina FA, Stafford BE, Marton LJ, Schmid R. Measurement of bilirubin and its monoconjugates and diconjugates in human serum by alkaline methanolysis and high-performance liquid chromatography. *J Lab Clin Med* 1980;96:198–212.

109. Gordon ER, Goresky CA. A rapid and quantitative high performance liquid chromatographic method for assaying bilirubin and its conjugates in bile. *Can J Biochem* 1982;60:1050–7.

110. Blanckaert N. Analysis of bilirubin and bilirubin mono- and diconjugates. Determination of their relative amounts in biological samples. *Biochem J* 1980;185:115–28.

111. Lauff JJ, Kasper ME, Ambrose RT. Separation of bilirubin species in serum and bile by high-performance reversed-phase liquid chromatography. *J Chromatogr* 1981;226:391–402.

112. Onishi S, Itoh S, Kawade N, Isobe K, Sugiyama S. An accurate and sensitive analysis by high-pressure liquid chromatography of conjugated and unconjugated bilirubin IX-alpha in various biological fluids. *Biochem J* 1980;185:281–4.

113. Sundberg MW, Lauff JJ, Weiss JS, et al. Estimation of unconjugated, conjugated, and "delta" bilirubin fractions in serum by use of two coated thin films. *Clin Chem* 1984;30:1314–17.

114. McKavanagh SM, Billing BH. The use of bond-elut for the estimation of serum bile pigments bonded covalently to albumin. *Biomed Chromatogr* 1987;2:62–5.

115. Bloomer JR, Berk PD, Howe RB, Berlin NI. Interpretation of plasma bilirubin levels based on studies with radioactive bilinibin. *JAMA* 1971;218:216–20.

116. Green RM, Flamm S. AGA technical review on the evaluation of liver chemistry tests. *Gastroenterology* 2002;123:1367–84.

117. Blanckaert NB, Heirwegh KPM. Analysis and preparation of bilirubins and biliverdins. In: Ostrow JD, ed. *Bile Pigments amd Jaundice*. New York: Marcel Dekker, 1986:31–79.

118. Gambino SR, Other A, Burns W. Direct serum bilirubin and the sulfobromophthalein test in occult liver disease. *JAMA* 1967;201:1047–9.

119. Tarao K, Fukushima K, Endo O, Kamiyo A. The effects of acute infectious hepatitis and cirrhosis of the liver on the nonerythropoietic component of early bilirubin. *J Lab Clin Med* 1976;87:240–50.

120. Samson D, Halliday D, Chanarin I. Enhancement of bilirubin clearance and hepatic haem turnover by ethanol [Letter]. *Lancet* 1976;2:256.

121. Robinson SH. Increased bilirubin formation from nonhemoglobin sources in rats with disorders of the liver. *J Lab Clin Med* 1969;73:668–76.

122. Kirshenbaum G, Shames DM, Schmid R. An expanded model of bilirubin kinetics: effect of feeding, fasting, and phenobarbital in Gilbert's syndrome. *J Pharmacokinet Biopharm* 1976;4:115–55.

123. Gisselbrecht C, Berk PD. Failure of phenobarbital to increase bilirubin production in the rat. *Biochem Pharmacol* 1974;23:2895–905.

124. Okuda H, Tavoloni N, Blaschke TF, et al. Phenobarbital does not increase early labeling of bilirubin from 4-[14C]-delta-aminolevulinic acid in man and rat. *Hepatology* 1991;14:1153–60.

125. Bancroft JD, Kreamer B, Gourley GR. Gilbert syndrome accelerates development of neonatal jaundice. *J Pediatr* 1998;132:656–60.

126. Korenblat KM, Berk PD. Hyperbilirubinemia in the setting of antiviral therapy. *Clin Gastroenterol Hepatol* 2005;3:303–10.

127. Rotger M, Taffe P, Bleiber G, et al. Gilbert syndrome and the development of antiretroviral therapy-associated hyperbilirubinemia. *J Infect Dis* 2005;192:1381–6.

128. Kartenbeck J, Leuschner U, Mayer R, Keppler D. Absence of the canalicular isoform of the MRP gene-encoded conjugate export pump from the hepatocytes in Dubin–Johnson syndrome. *Hepatology* 1996;23:1061–6.

129. Paulusma CC, Kool M, Bosma PJ, et al. A mutation in the human canalicular multispecific organic anion transporter gene causes the Dubin–Johnson syndrome. *Hepatology* 1997;25:1539–42.

130. Blaschke TF, Berk PD, Rodkey FL, Scharschmidt BF, Collison HA, Waggoner JG. Drugs and the liver. I. Effects of glutethimide and phenobarbital on hepatic bilirubin clearance, plasma bilirubin turnover and carbon monoxide production in man. *Biochem Pharmacol* 1974;23:2795–806.

131. Crigler JF Jr, Najjar VA. Congenital familial nonhemolytic jaundice with kernicterus. *Pediatrics* 1952;10:169–80.

132. Childs B, Sidbury JB, Migeon CJ. Glucuronic acid conjugation by patients with familial nonhemolytic jaundice and their relatives. *Pediatrics* 1959;23:903–13.

133. Arias IM, Gartner LM, Cohen M, Ezzer JB, Levi AJ. Chronic nonhemolytic unconjugated hyperbilirubinemia with glucuronyl transferase deficiency. Clinical, biochemical, pharmacologic and genetic evidence for heterogeneity. *Am J Med* 1969;47:395–409.

134. Burchell B, Coughtrie MW, Jackson MR, Shepherd SR, Harding D, Hume R. Genetic deficiency of bilirubin glucuronidation in rats and humans. *Mol Aspects Med* 1987;9:429–55.

135. Bosma PJ, Chowdhury NR, Goldhoorn BG, et al. Sequence of exons and the flanking regions of human bilirubin-UDP-glucuronosyltransferase gene complex and identification of a genetic mutation in a patient with Crigler–Najjar syndrome, type I. *Hepatology* 1992;15:941–7.

136. Wolkoff AW, Chowdhury JR, Gartner LA, et al. Crigler–Najjar syndrome (type I) in an adult male. *Gastroenterology* 1979;76:840–8.

137. Fox IJ, Chowdhury JR, Kaufman SS, et al. Treatment of the Crigler–Najjar syndrome type I with hepatocyte transplantation. *N Engl J Med* 1998;338:1422–6.

138. Ambrosino G, Varotto S, Strom SC, et al. Isolated hepatocyte transplantation for Crigler–Najjar syndrome type 1. *Cell Transplant* 2005;14:151–7.

139. Van Der Veere CN, Sinaasappel M, McDonagh AF, et al. Current therapy for Crigler–Najjar syndrome type 1: report of a world registry. *Hepatology* 1996;24:311–15.

140. Schauer R, Stangl M, Lang T, et al. Treatment of Crigler–Najjar type 1 disease: relevance of early liver transplantation. *J Pediatr Surg* 2003;38:1227–31.

141. Morioka D, Kasahara M, Takada Y, et al. Living donor liver transplantation for pediatric patients with inheritable metabolic disorders. *Am J Transplant* 2005;5:2754–63.

142. Shneider BL. Pediatric liver transplantation in metabolic disease: clinical decision making. *Pediatr Transplant* 2002;6:25–9.

143. Gunn CH. Hereditary acholuric jaundice in a new mutant strain of rats. *J Hered* 1938;29:137.

144. Schmid R, Axelrod J, Hammaker L, Swarm RL. Congenital jaundice in rats, due to a defect in glucuronide formation. *J Clin Invest* 1958;37:1123–30.

145. Arias IM. Chronic unconjugated hyperbilirubinemia without overt signs of hemolysis in adolescents and adults. *J Clin Invest* 1962;41:2233–45.

146. Jansen PL. Diagnosis and management of Crigler–Najjar syndrome. *Eur J Pediatr* 1999;158(Suppl 2):S89–94.

147. Yaffe SJ, Levy G, Matsuzawa T, Baliah T. Enhancement of glucuronide-conjugating capacity in a hyperbilirubinemic infant due to apparent enzyme induction by phenobarbital. *N Engl J Med* 1966;275:1461–6.

148. Gollan JL, Huang SN, Billing B, Sherlock S. Prolonged survival in three brothers with severe type 2 Crigler–Najjar syndrome. Ultrastructural and metabolic studies. *Gastroenterology* 1975;68:1543–55.

149. Holstein A, Plaschke A, Lohse P, Egberts EH. Successful photo- and phenobarbital therapy during pregnancy in a woman with Crigler–Najjar syndrome type II. *Scand J Gastroenterol* 2005;40:1124–6.

150. Ito T, Katagiri C, Ikeno S, Takahashi H, Nagata N, Terakawa N. Phenobarbital following phototherapy for Crigler–Najjar syndrome type II with good fetal outcome: a case report. *J Obstet Gynaecol Res* 2001;27:33–5.

151. Servedio V, d'Apolito M, Maiorano N, et al. Spectrum of UGT1A1 mutations in Crigler–Najjar (CN) syndrome patients: identification of twelve novel alleles and genotype–phenotype correlation. *Hum Mutat* 2005;25:325.

152. Gilbert A, Lereboullet P. La cholamae simple familiale. *Semin Med* 1901;21:241.

153. Berk PD, Bloomer JR, Howe RB, Berlin NI. Constitutional hepatic dysfunction (Gilbert's syndrome). A new definition based on kinetic studies with unconjugated radiobilirubin. *Am J Med* 1970;49:296–305.

154. Martin JF, Vierling JM, Wolkoff AW, et al. Abnormal hepatic transport of indocyanine green in Gilbert's syndrome. *Gastroenterology* 1976;70:385–91.

155. Vierling JM, Berk PD, Hofmann AF, Martin JF, Wolkoff AW, Scharschmidt BF. Normal fasting-state levels of serum cholyl-conjugated bile acids in Gilbert's syndrome: an aid to the diagnosis. *Hepatology* 1982;2:340–3.

156. Bosma PJ. Inherited disorders of bilirubin metabolism. *J Hepatol* 2003;38:107–17.

157. Burchell B, Hume R. Molecular genetic basis of Gilbert's syndrome. *J Gastroenterol Hepatol* 1999;14:960–6.

158. Bosma PJ, Chowdhury JR, Bakker C, et al. The genetic basis of the reduced expression of bilirubin UDP-glucuronosyltransferase 1 in Gilbert's syndrome. *N Engl J Med* 1995;333:1171–5.

159. Berk PD, Berman MD, Blitzer BL, et al. Effect of splenectomy of hepatic bilirubin clearance in patients with hereditary spherocytosis. Implications for the diagnosis of Gilbert's syndrome. *J Lab Clin Med* 1981;98:37–45.

160. Takeuchi K, Kobayashi Y, Tamaki S, et al. Genetic polymorphisms of bilirubin uridine diphosphate-glucuronosyltransferase gene in Japanese patients with Crigler–Najjar syndrome or Gilbert's syndrome as well as in healthy Japanese subjects. *J Gastroenterol Hepatol* 2004;19:1023–8.

161. Okolicsanyi L, Fevery J, Billing B, et al. How should mild, isolated unconjugated hyperbilirubinemia be investigated? *Semin Liver Dis* 1983;3:36–41.

162. Kaplan M, Hammerman C. Glucose-6-phosphate dehydrogenase deficiency: a hidden risk for kernicterus. *Semin Perinatol* 2004;28:356–64.

163. Herschel M, Ryan M, Gelbart T, Kaplan M. Hemolysis and hyperbilirubinemia in an African American neonate heterozygous for glucose-6-phosphate dehydrogenase deficiency. *J Perinatol* 2002;22:577–9.

164. Nicolaidou P, Kostaridou S, Mavri A, Galla A, Kitsiou S, Stamoulakatou A. Glucose-6-phosphate dehydrogenase deficiency and Gilbert syndrome: a gene interaction underlies severe jaundice without severe hemolysis. *Pediatr Hematol Oncol* 2005;22:561–6.

165. Kalotychou V, Antonatou K, Tzanetea R, Terpos E, Loukopoulos D, Rombos Y. Analysis of the A(TA)(n)TAA configuration in the promoter region of the UGT1 A1 gene in Greek patients with thalassemia intermedia and sickle cell disease. *Blood Cells Mol Dis* 2003;31:38–42.

166. Miners JO, McKinnon RA, Mackenzie PI. Genetic polymorphisms of UDP-glucuronosyltransferases and their functional significance. *Toxicology* 2002;181/182:453–6.

167. Dubin IN, Johnson FB. Chronic idiopathic jaundice with unidentified pigment in liver cells; a new clinicopathologic entity with a report of 12 cases. *Medicine (Baltimore)* 1954;33:155–97.

168. Rotor AB, Manahan L, Florentin A. Familial nonhemolytic jaundice with direct van den Bergh reaction. *Acta Med Phil* 1948;5:37–49.

169. Dhumeaux D, Berthelot P. Chronic hyperbilirubinemia associated with hepatic uptake and storage impairment. A new syndrome resembling that of the mutant Southdown sheep. *Gastroenterology* 1975;69:988–93.

170. Sprinz H, Nelson RS. Persistent non-hemolytic hyperbilirubinemia associated with lipochrome-like pigment in liver cells: report of four cases. *Ann Intern Med* 1954;41:952–62.

171. Dubin IN. Chronic idiopathic jaundice; a review of fifty cases. *Am J Med* 1958;24:268–92.

172. Shani M, Seligsohn U, Gilon E, Sheba C, Adam A. Dubin–Johnson syndrome in Israel. I. Clinical, laboratory, and genetic aspects of 101 cases. *Q J Med* 1970;39:549–67.

173. Cohen L, Lewis C, Arias IM. Pregnancy, oral contraceptives, and chronic familial jaundice with predominantly conjugated hyperbilirubinemia (Dubin–Johnson syndrome). *Gastroenterology* 1972;62:1182–90.

174. Kondo T, Yagi R, Kuchiba K. Dubin–Johnson syndrome in a neonate {Letter]. *N Engl J Med* 1975;292:1028–9.

175. Nakata F, Oyanagi K, Fujiwara M, et al. Dubin–Johnson syndrome in a neonate. *Eur J Pediatr* 1979;132:299–301.

176. Haimi-Cohen Y, Merlob P, Marcus-Eidlits T, Amir J. Dubin–Johnson syndrome as a cause of neonatal jaundice: the importance of coproporphyrins investigation. *Clin Pediatr (Phila)* 1998;37:511–13.

177. Alpert S, Mosher M, Shanske A, Arias IM. Multiplicity of hepatic excretory mechanisms for organic anions. *J Gen Physiol* 1969;53:238–47.

178. Upson DW, Gronwall RR, Cornelius CE. Maximal hepatic excretion of bilirubin in sheep. *Proc Soc Exp Biol Med* 1970;134:9–12.

179. Mia AS, Gronwall RR, Cornelius CE. Unconjugated bilirubin transport in normal and mutant Corriedale sheep with Dubin–Johnson syndrome. *Proc Soc Exp Biol Med* 1970;135:33–7.

180. Cornelius CE, Arias IM, Osburn BI. Hepatic pigmentation with photosensitivity: a syndrome in Corriedale sheep resembling Dubin–Johnson syndrome in man. *J Am Vet Med Assoc* 1965;146:709–13.

181. Schulman FY, Montali RJ, Bush M, et al. Dubin–Johnson-like syndrome in golden lion tamarins (Leontopithecus rosalia rosalia). *Vet Pathol* 1993;30:491–8.

182. Jansen PL, Peters WH, Lamers WH. Hereditary chronic conjugated hyperbilirubinemia in mutant rats caused by defective hepatic anion transport. *Hepatology* 1985;5:573–9.

183. Elferink RP, Ottenhoff R, Liefting W, de Haan J, Jansen PL. Hepatobiliary transport of glutathione and glutathione conjugate in rats with hereditary hyperbilirubinemia. *J Clin Invest* 1989;84:476–83.

184. Koopen NR, Wolters H, Havinga R, et al. Impaired activity of the bile canalicular organic anion transporter (Mrp2/cmoat) is not the main cause of ethinylestradiol-induced cholestasis in the rat. *Hepatology* 1998;27:537–45.

185. Dijkstra M, Kuipers F, Havinga R, Smit EP, Vonk RJ. Bile secretion of trace elements in rats with a congenital defect in hepatobiliary transport of glutathione. *Pediatr Res* 1990;28:339–43.

186. Paulusma CC, Bosma PJ, Zaman GJ, et al. Congenital jaundice in rats with a mutation in a multidrug resistance-associated protein gene. *Science* 1996;271:1126–8.

187. Naba H, Kuwayama C, Kakinuma C, Ohnishi S, Ogihara T. Eisai hyperbilirubinemic rat (EHBR) as an animal model affording high drug-exposure in toxicity studies on organic anions. *Drug Metab Pharmacokinet* 2004;19:339–51.

188. Fernandez-Checa JC, Takikawa H, Horie T, Ookhtens M, Kaplowitz N. Canalicular transport of reduced glutathione in normal and mutant Eisai hyperbilirubinemic rats. *J Biol Chem* 1992;267:1667–73.

189. Kurisu H, Kamisaka K, Koyo T, et al. Organic anion transport study in mutant rats with autosomal recessive conjugated hyperbilirubinemia. *Life Sci* 1991;49:1003–11.

190. Wolkoff AW, Cohen LE, Arias IM. Inheritance of the Dubin–Johnson syndrome. *N Engl J Med* 1973;288:113–17.

191. Butt HR, Anderson E, Foulk WT, Baggenstoss AH, Schoenfield LJ, Dickson ER. Studies of chronic idiopathic jaundice (Dubin–Johnson syndrome). II. Evaluation of a large family with the trait. *Gastroenterology* 1966;51:619–30.

192. Hashimoto K, Uchiumi T, Konno T, et al. Trafficking and functional defects by mutations of the ATP-binding domains in MRP2 in patients with Dubin–Johnson syndrome. *Hepatology* 2002;36:1236–45.

193. Cebecauerova D, Jirasek T, Budisova L, et al. Dual hereditary jaundice: simultaneous occurrence of mutations causing Gilbert's and Dubin–Johnson syndrome. *Gastroenterology* 2005;129:315–20.

194. Machida I, Wakusawa S, Sanae F, et al. Mutational analysis of the MRP2 gene and long-term follow-up of Dubin–Johnson syndrome in Japan. *J Gastroenterol* 2005;40:366–70.

195. Levanon M, Rimon S, Shani M, Ramot B, Goldberg E. Active and inactive factor VII in Dubin–Johnson syndrome with factor-VII deficiency, hereditary factor-VII deficiency and on coumadin administration. *Br J Haematol* 1972;23:669–77.

196. Seligsohn U, Shani M, Ramot B, Adam A, Sheba C. Dubin–Johnson syndrome in Israel. II. Association with factor-VII deficiency. *Q J Med* 1970;39:569–84.

197. Tamary H, Fromovich Y, Shalmon L, et al. Ala244Val is a common, probably ancient mutation causing factor VII deficiency in Moroccan and Iranian Jews. *Thromb Haemost* 1996;76:283–91.

198. Fromovich-Amit Y, Zivelin A, Rosenberg N, Tamary H, Landau M, Seligsohn U. Characterization of mutations causing factor VII deficiency in 61 unrelated Israeli patients. *J Thromb Haemost* 2004;2:1774–81.

199. Arias IM. Studies of chronic familial non-hemolytic jaundice with conjugated bilirubin in the serum with and without an unidentified pigment in the liver cells. *Am J Med* 1961;31:510–18.

200. Javitt NB, Kondo T, Kuchiba K. Bile acid excretion in Dubin–Johnson syndrome. *Gastroenterology* 1978;75:931–2.

201. Kawasaki H, Yamanishi Y, Kishimoto Y, et al. Abnormality of oral ursodeoxycholic acid tolerance test in the Dubin–Johnson syndrome. *Clin Chim Acta* 1981;112:13–19.

202. Mandema E, de Fraiture WH, Nieweg HO, Arends A. Familial chronic idiopathic jaundice (Dubin–Sprinz disease), with a note on bromsulphalein metabolism in this disease. *Am J Med* 1960;28:42–50.

203. Morita M, Kihara T. Intravenous cholecystography and metabolism of meglumine iodipamide (biligrafin) in Dubin–Johnson syndrome. *Diag Radiol* 1971;99:5760.

204. Bar-Meir S, Baron J, Seligson U, Gottesfeld F, Levy R, Gilat T. 99mTc-HIDA cholescintigraphy in Dubin–Johnson and Rotor syndromes. *Radiology* 1982;142:743–6.

205. Pinos T, Constansa JM, Palacin A, Figueras C. A new diagnostic approach to the Dubin–Johnson syndrome. *Am J Gastroenterol* 1990;85:91–3.

206. Yoo J, Reichert DE, Kim J, Anderson CJ, Welch MJ. A potential Dubin–Johnson syndrome imaging agent: synthesis, biodistribution, and microPET imaging. *Mol Imaging* 2005;4:18–29.

207. Essner E, Novikoff AB. Human hepatocellular pigments and lysosomes. *J Ultrastructure Res* 1960;3:374–91.

208. Arias IM, Bernstein L, Toffler R, Ben-Ezzer J. Black liver disease in Corriedale sheep: Metabolism of tritiated epinephrine and incorporation of isotope into the hepatic pigment in vivo. *J Clin Invest* 1965;44:1026.

209. Swartz HM, Sarna T, Varma RR. On the nature and excretion of the hepatic pigment in the Dubin–Johnson syndrome. *Gastroenterology* 1979;76:958–64.

210. Ware AJ, Eigenbrodt EH, Shorey J, Combes B. Viral hepatitis complicating the Dubin–Johnson syndrome. *Gastroenterology* 1972;63:331–9.

211. Varma RR, Grainger JM, Scheuer PJ. A case of the Dubin–Johnson syndrome complicated by acute hepatitis. *Gut* 1970;11:817–21.

212. Schoenfield LJ, McGill DB, Hunton DB, Foulk WT, Butt HR. Studies of chronic idiopathic jaundice (Dubin–Johnson syndrome). I. Demonstration of hepatic excretory defect. *Gastroenterology* 1963;44:101–11.

213. Erlinger S, Dhumeaux D, Desjeux JF, Benhamou JP. Hepatic handling of unconjugated dyes in the Dubin–Johnson syndrome. *Gastroenterology* 1973;64:106–10.

214. Abe H, Okuda K. Biliary excretion of conjugated sulfobromophthalein (BSP) in constitutional conjugated hyperbilirubinemias. *Digestion* 1975;13:272–83.

215. Rodes J, Zubizarreta A, Bruguera M. Metabolism of the bromsulphalein in Dubin–Johnson syndrome. Diagnostic value of the paradoxical increase in plasma levels at BSP. *Am J Dig Dis* 1972;17:545–52.

216. Koskelo P, Toivonen I, Adlercreutz H. Urinary coproporphyrin isomer distribution in the Dubin–Johnson syndrome. *Clin Chem* 1967;13:1006–9.

217. Ben Ezzer J, Rimington C, Shani M, Seligsohn U, Sheba C, Szeinberg A. Abnormal excretion of the isomers of urinary coproporphyrin by patients with Dubin–Johnson syndrome in Israel. *Clin Sci* 1971;40:17–30.

218. Berk PD, Wolkoff AW, Berlin NI. Inborn errors of bilirubin metabolism. *Med Clin North Am* 1975;59:803–16.

219. Ben Ezzer J, Blonder J, Shani M, et al. Dubin–Johnson Syndrome. Abnormal excretion of the isomers of urinary coproporphyrin by clinically unaffected family members. *Isr J Med Sci* 1973;9: 1431–6.

220. Kitamura T, Alroy J, Gatmaitan Z, et al. Defective biliary excretion of epinephrine metabolites in mutant (TR–) rats: relation to the pathogenesis of black liver in the Dubin–Johnson syndrome and Corriedale sheep with an analogous excretory defect. *Hepatology* 1992;15:1154–9.

221. Wolf RL, Pizette M, Richman A, et al. Chronic idiopathic jaundice. A study of two afflicted families. *Am J Med* 1960;28:32–41.

222. Kondo T, Kuchiba K, Ohtsuka Y, Yanagisawa W, Shiomura T, Taminato T. Clinical and genetic studies on Dubin–Johnson syndrome in a cluster area in Japan. *Jap J Human Genet* 1974;18: 378–92.

223. Shani M, Gilon E, Ben-Ezzer J, Sheba C. Sulfobromophthalein tolerance test in patients with Dubin–Johnson syndrome and their relatives. *Gastroenterology* 1970;59:842–7.

224. Kondo T, Kuchiba K, Shimizu Y. Metabolic fate of exogenous delta-aminolevulinic acid in Dubin–Johnson syndrome. *J Lab Clin Med* 1979;94:421–8.

225. Frank M, Doss M, de Carvalho DG. Diagnostic and pathogenetic implications of urinary coproporphyrin excretion in the Dubin–Johnson syndrome. *Hepatogastroenterology* 1990;37: 147–51.

226. Keppler D, Konig J. Hepatic canalicular membrane 5: expression and localization of the conjugate export pump encoded by the MRP2 (cMRP/cMOAT) gene in liver. *FASEB J* 1997;11:509–16.

227. Toh S, Wada M, Uchiumi T, et al. Genomic structure of the canalicular multispecific organic anion-transporter gene (MRP2/cMOAT) and mutations in the ATP-binding-cassette region in Dubin–Johnson syndrome. *Am J Hum Genet* 1999;64:739–46.

228. Mor-Cohen R, Zivelin A, Rosenberg N, Goldberg I, Seligsohn U. A novel ancestral splicing mutation in the multidrug resistance protein 2 gene causes Dubin–Johnson syndrome in Ashkenazi Jewish patients. *Hepatol Res* 2005;31:104–11.

229. Konig J, Nies AT, Cui Y, Leier I, Keppler D. Conjugate export pumps of the multidrug resistance protein (MRP) family: localization, substrate specificity, and MRP2-mediated drug resistance. *Biochim Biophys Acta* 1999;1461:377–94.

230. Shani M, Seligsohn U, Ben Ezzer J. Effect of phenobarbital on liver functions in patients with Dubin–Johnson syndrome. *Gastroenterology* 1974;67:303–8.

231. Merdler C, Burke M, Shani M, Felner S, Lurie I. The effect of phenobarbital on patients with Dubin–Johnson syndrome. *Digestion* 1976;14:394–9.

232. Wolkoff AW, Wolpert E, Pascasio FN, Arias IM. Rotor's syndrome. A distinct inheritable pathophysiologic entity. *Am J Med* 1976;60:173–9.

233. Schiff L, Billing BH, Oikawa Y. Familial nonhemolytic jaundice with conjugated bilirubin in the serum. A case study. *N Engl J Med* 1959;260:1315–18.

234. Lima JEP, Utz E, Roisenberg I. Hereditary nonhemolytic conjugated hyperbilirubinemia without abnormal liver cell pigmentation. *Am J Med* 1976;40:628–33.

235. Chen YW, Lee IH, Chuang YW, Chang TT, Liu GC. Tc-99m di-isopropyl-iminodiacetic acid cholescintigraphic findings in Rotor's syndrome. *Kaohsiung J Med Sci* 2002;18:529–32.

236. Wolpert E, Fernandez E, Lisker R, Suarez GI, Dehesa M, Robles G. Rotor syndrome, a family study. *Rev Invest Clin (Mex)* 1974;26:363–71.

237. Porush JG, Delman AJ, Feuer MM. Chronic idiopathic jaundice with normal liver histology. *Arch Intern Med* 1962;109:302–9.

238. Kawasaki H, Kimura N, Irisa T, Hirayama C. Dye clearance studies in Rotor's syndrome. *Am J Gastroenterol* 1979;71:380–8.

239. Fedeli G, Rapaccini GL, Anti M, et al. Impaired clearance of cholephilic anions in Rotor syndrome. *Z Gastroenterol* 1983;21: 228–33.

240. Shimizu Y, Naruto H, Ida S, Kohakura M. Urinary coproporphyrin isomers in Rotor's syndrome: a study of eight families. *Hepatology* 1981;1:173–8.

241. Aziz MA, Schwartz S, Watson CJ. Studies of coproporphyrin. VIII. Reinvestigation of the isomer distribution in jaundice and liver diseases. *J Lab Clin Med* 1964;63:596–604.

242. Hofmann AF. Biliary secretion and excretion in health and disease: current concepts. *Ann Hepatol* 2007;6:15–27.

243. Clayton RJ, Iber FL, Ruebner BH, McKusick VA. Byler disease. Fatal familial intrahepatic cholestasis in an Amish kindred. *Am J Dis Child* 1969;117:112–24.

244. Bull LN, van Eijk MJ, Pawlikowska L, et al. A gene encoding a P-type ATPase mutated in two forms of hereditary cholestasis. *Nat Genet* 1998;18:219–24.

245. Eppens EF, van Mil SW, de Vree JM, et al. FIC1, the protein affected in two forms of hereditary cholestasis, is localized in the cholangiocyte and the canalicular membrane of the hepatocyte. *J Hepatol* 2001;35:436–43.

246. Ujhazy P, Ortiz D, Misra S, et al. Familial intrahepatic cholestasis 1: studies of localization and function. *Hepatology* 2001;34:768–75.

247. Folmer DE, Elferink RP, Paulusma CC. P4 ATPases – lipid flippases and their role in disease. *Biochim Biophys Acta* 2009;1791:628–35.

248. Paulusma CC, Elferink RP, Jansen PL. Progressive familial intrahepatic cholestasis type 1. *Semin Liver Dis* 2010;30:117–24.

249. van der Woerd WL, van Mil SW, Stapelbroek JM, Klomp LW, van de Graaf SF, Houwen RH. Familial cholestasis: progressive familial intrahepatic cholestasis, benign recurrent intrahepatic cholestasis and intrahepatic cholestasis of pregnancy. *Best Pract Res Clin Gastroenterol* 2010;24:541–53.

250. Strautnieks SS, Bull LN, Knisely AS, et al. A gene encoding a liver-specific ABC transporter is mutated in progressive familial intrahepatic cholestasis. *Nat Genet* 1998;20:233–8.

251. Lam P, Soroka CJ, Boyer JL. The bile salt export pump: clinical and experimental aspects of genetic and acquired cholestatic liver disease. *Semin Liver Dis* 2010;30:125–33.

252. Deleuze JF, Jacquemin E, Dubuisson C, et al. Defect of multidrug-resistance 3 gene expression in a subtype of progressive familial intrahepatic cholestasis. *Hepatology* 1996;23:904–8.

253. de Vree JM, Jacquemin E, Sturm E, et al. Mutations in the MDR3 gene cause progressive familial intrahepatic cholestasis. *Proc Natl Acad Sci USA* 1998;95:282–7.

254. Davit-Spraul A, Gonzales E, Baussan C, Jacquemin E. The spectrum of liver diseases related to ABCB4 gene mutations: pathophysiology and clinical aspects. *Semin Liver Dis* 2010;30:134–46.

255. Jacquemin E, Hermans D, Myara A, et al. Ursodeoxycholic acid therapy in pediatric patients with progressive familial intrahepatic cholestasis. *Hepatology* 1997;25:519–23.

256. Jara P, Hierro L, Martinez-Fernandez P, et al. Recurrence of bile salt export pump deficiency after liver transplantation. *N Engl J Med* 2009;361:1359–67.

257. Williams R, Cartter MA, Sherlock S, Scheuer PJ, Hill KR. Idiopathic recurrent cholestasis: a study of the functional and pathological lesions in four cases. *Q J Med* 1964;33:387–99.

258. Summerfield JA, Scott J, Berman M, et al. Benign recurrent intrahepatic cholestasis: studies of bilirubin kinetics, bile acids, and cholangiography. *Gut* 1980;21:154–60.

259. van Mil SW, van der Woerd WL, van der Brugge G, et al. Benign recurrent intrahepatic cholestasis type 2 is caused by mutations in ABCB11. *Gastroenterology* 2004;127:379–84.

260. Williamson C, Hems LM, Goulis DG, et al. Clinical outcome in a series of cases of obstetric cholestasis identified via a patient support group. *Br J Obstet Gynaecol* 2004;111:676–81.

261. Bacq Y, Sapey T, Brechot MC, Pierre F, Fignon A, Dubois F. Intrahepatic cholestasis of pregnancy: a French prospective study. *Hepatology* 1997;26:358–64.

262. Mays JK. The active management of intrahepatic cholestasis of pregnancy. *Curr Opin Obstet Gynecol* 2010;22:100–3.

263. Diaferia A, Nicastri PL, Tartagni M, Loizzi P, Iacovizzi C, Di Leo A. Ursodeoxycholic acid therapy in pregnant women with cholestasis. *Int J Gynaecol Obstet* 1996;52:133–40.

264. Palma J, Reyes H, Ribalta J, et al. Ursodeoxycholic acid in the treatment of cholestasis of pregnancy: a randomized, double-blind study controlled with placebo. *J Hepatol* 1997;27:10228.

265. Zapata R, Sandoval L, Palma J, et al. Ursodeoxycholic acid in the treatment of intrahepatic cholestasis of pregnancy. A 12-year experience. *Liver Int* 2005;25:548–54.

266. Nicastri PL, Diaferia A, Tartagni M, Loizzi P, Fanelli M. A randomised placebo-controlled trial of ursodeoxycholic acid and S-adenosylmethionine in the treatment of intrahepatic cholestasis of pregnancy. *Br J Obstet Gynaecol* 1998;105:1205–7.

267. Ropponen A, Sund R, Riikonen S, Ylikorkala O, Aittomaki K. Intrahepatic cholestasis of pregnancy as an indicator of liver and biliary diseases: a population-based study. *Hepatology* 2006;43:723–8.

268. Berk PD, Jones EA, Howe RB, Berlin NI. Disorders of bilirubin metabolism. In: Bondy PK, Rosenberg LE, eds. *Metabolic Control and Disease*, 8th edn. Philadelphia: WB Saunders, 1979:1009–88.

269. Berk PD. Bilirubin metabolism and the hereditary hyperbilirubinemias. In: Berk JE, Haubrich MD, Kalser, Roth JLA, Schaffner F, eds. *Bockus' Gastroenterology*, Vol. 5. Philadelphia: WB Saunders, 1985:2732–97.

Multiple choice questions

6.1 A 36-year-old female nurse presents with a 1-week history of malaise, abdominal discomfort, arthralgias, fatigue, and obvious jaundice. Her past medical history is unremarkable, and she denies any history of a needle-stick. Her family history includes rheumatoid arthritis in her mother and primary biliary cirrhosis in her sister. Her physical examination includes a tachycardia of 120 bpm, icterus, and a spleen that is palpable two finger-breadths below the left costal margin. In the emergency room the hemoglobin (Hgb) is 7.0 g/dL, hematocrit (Hct) 22%, platelets 285,000, and total bilirubin 4.0 mg/dL. During an annual check-up last month her total bilirubin was 0.45 mg/dL and her hemoglobin 12.4 g/dL. The initial differential diagnosis included acute hepatitis, acute biliary obstruction due to gallstones, and chronic liver disease with gastrointestinal bleeding. Which one of the following test results indicates that none of these diagnoses is correct?

   a Stool guaiac: negative.
   b Reticulocytes: 12%.
   c Urine dipstick for bilirubin: negative.
   d Antihepatitis A virus IgM: negative.

6.2 In the same patient as in question 1, new-onset unconjugated hyperbilirubinemia in the presence of new onset of anemia strongly suggests an acute hemolytic process. Given the positive family history for autoimmune disease an autoimmune hemolytic anemia is now suspected. Direct and indirect Coombs tests are ordered and are positive. The patient is begun on prednisone, 40 mg/day, for an autoimmune hemolytic anemia, and returns to the clinic for follow-up after 1 week. At that time, her Hgb is 8.2 g/dL, Hct 25%, reticulocytes 10%, platelets 225,000, and total serum bilirubin 0.4 mg/dL. Her jaundice has disappeared. However, based on her Hgb, Hct, and reticulocyte count, the resident argues that she must still be hemolyzing, and proposes to increase her prednisone to 60 mg/day. By contrast, the attending declares that the hemolysis has essentially ceased, and orders a continuation of the current prednisone dose. He predicts that the results of a similar group of tests at follow-up in a week will allow them to start reducing her prednisone dose. When the patients returns a week later her Hgb is 11.8 mg/dL, Hct 35%, reticulocytes 2%, and total bilirubin 0.5 mg/dL. The strongest indication that hemolysis had appreciably decreased after 1 week of prednisone was which of the following?

   a An increase in hemoglobin from 7.0 to 8.2 g/dL.
   b A fall in reticulocytes from 12% to 10%.
   c A decrease in total bilirubin from 4.0 to 0.4 mg/dL.
   d A fall in platelet count from 285,000 to 240,000.

6.3 The following hereditary syndromes may all exhibit both conjugated hyperbilirubinemia and elevated serum bile acids except which of the following?

   a Progressive familial intrahepatic cholestasis type 1.
   b Progressive familial intrahepatic cholestasis type 3.
   c Benign recurrent intrahepatic cholestasis type 1.
   d Dubin–Johnson syndrome.

Answers to the multiple choice questions can be found in the Appendix at the end of the book.

These multiple choice questions are also available for you to complete online.
Visit http://www.schiffsdiseasesoftheliver.com/

CHAPTER 7

Hepatic Histopathology

Zachary D. Goodman

Center for Liver Diseases, Inova Fairfax Hospital, Falls Church, VA, USA

Key concepts

- Histopathologic examination of a liver biopsy specimen is a source of otherwise unobtainable qualitative information about the structural integrity of the liver tissue, the type and degree of injury, and the host's response to the injury. Histopathologic examination also provides a basis for the diagnosis and classification of tumors.
- Histochemical and immunohistochemical stains are extremely helpful in evaluating the liver biopsy specimen.
- Qualitatively different patterns of injury can be used to distinguish diseases that have similar clinical presentations, such as chronic

hepatitis, alcoholic or nonalcoholic steatohepatitis, and chronic cholestatic syndromes.
- Specific histologic features may allow precise diagnosis or strongly suggest a specific diagnosis. For example, "ground-glass" cells with positive histochemical or immunostaining for hepatitis B surface antigen indicates chronic hepatitis B infection, or florid duct lesions often indicate the early stage of primary biliary cirrhosis.
- Accurate classification of tumors almost always requires histologic examination of tissue obtained by either biopsy or surgical excision.

The liver biopsy is an essential part of the investigation of diseases of the liver. Percutaneous (sometimes laparoscopic or transjugular) needle biopsies provide most of the specimens and the greatest challenge to the pathologist, but open surgical biopsies and resection specimens obtained at laparotomy are also seen from time to time, especially when dealing with tumors, and even total hepatectomies in liver transplantation centers. Despite the many advances in laboratory tests, molecular diagnosis, and radiologic imaging techniques, liver biopsies continue to be performed. This is because histopathologic examination of the biopsy specimen is a source of otherwise unobtainable qualitative information about the structural integrity of the liver tissue, the type and degree of injury, and the host's response to the injury; histopathologic examination also provides a basis for the diagnosis and classification of tumors.

Liver biopsy should only be performed after a thorough noninvasive clinical evaluation. This information, including a history of possible exposure to hepatotoxins and sources of infection, pertinent physical findings, laboratory tests of liver function and integrity, serologic tests to detect infectious agents and autoimmunity, and radiologic studies, when appropriate, should be made available to the pathologist. Many biopsy specimens can be interpreted solely on morphologic grounds, and we

recommend that the pathologist first examine the specimen and make initial observations without being biased by the clinical impression and laboratory data. However, after these initial observations, we strongly recommend that the pathologist review the clinical and laboratory data, preferably with the clinician, and then arrive at the best possible clinical–pathologic correlation as the definitive diagnosis. This will allow the pathologist to avoid embarrassing errors that result from lack of information and will, at the same time, provide the clinician with an interpretation that will allow optimal patient care. In that regard, this chapter emphasizes the morphologic (predominantly light microscopic) aspects of the diseases of the liver, with clinical correlations in some of the major diseases.

Systematic approach to the liver biopsy

A liver biopsy specimen should always be examined using a systematic approach to histopathologic evaluation. All fragments from a given biopsy specimen should be examined because a focal lesion, such as a granuloma, can be easily missed. In an architecturally normal liver it is best to begin by locating the terminal hepatic venules (or "central" veins) and then move in the direction of

Schiff's Diseases of the Liver, Eleventh Edition. Edited by Eugene R. Schiff, Willis C. Maddrey and Michael F. Sorrell.
© 2012 John Wiley & Sons, Ltd. Published 2012 by John Wiley & Sons, Ltd.

the portal areas. In doing so, changes involving the veins themselves and then the liver cells, bile canaliculi, abnormal deposits in spaces of Disse (e.g., collagen, amyloid), hypertrophied stellate cells, the sinusoids and their contents, and the Kupffer cells should be specifically examined. The plates of hepatocytes nearest the portal areas should receive special attention, particularly in chronic necroinflammatory or cholestatic disorders. A proliferation of ductules and fibrosis also occur in this region of the acinus. All structures of the portal areas, namely, the connective tissue, bile ducts, veins, arteries, and lymphatics, as well as the inflammatory response (e.g., granulomas and the various types and relative proportions of inflammatory cells), should be examined. In addition to searching for specific lesions, the absence of various structures in the portal areas such as the destruction and disappearance of bile ducts in primary biliary cirrhosis (PBC) or the obliteration of veins in hepatoportal sclerosis should also be carefully noted.

Special histochemical stains

Although most of the observations that lead to a diagnosis are made using the routine hematoxylin and eosin (H&E) stain, special stains are helpful in evaluating liver biopsy specimens. Staining methods referred to in this chapter can be found in the Armed Forces Institute of Pathology's *Laboratory Methods in Histotechnology* [1].

Fibrosis and connective tissue

Evaluation of the presence, extent, and location of fibrosis is essential in the diagnosis of non-neoplastic liver disease. A Masson trichrome (Fig. 7.1) is useful for demonstrating the degree of fibrosis and cirrhosis in chronic liver disease and is also useful in assessing changes involving arteries and veins, such as the lesions of venoocclusive disease and hepatic vein thrombosis. A Movat

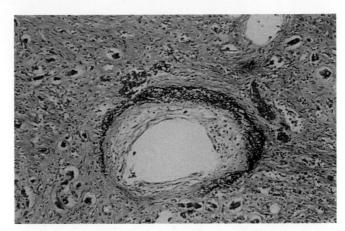

Figure 7.2 The Movat pentachrome stain shows a partially occluded outflow vein in this case of alcoholic cirrhosis. The elastic tissue in the wall of the vein is black, whereas mucopolysaccharides in the hypertrophied intima are pale blue, and collagen in the cirrhotic scars is yellow-green.

pentachrome stain is particularly useful for vascular lesions because it stains elastica and acid mucopolysaccharide, in addition to collagen and smooth muscle (Fig. 7.2). Elastic tissue can also be well demonstrated by orcein or Victoria blue stains that are used to identify ground-glass cells containing hepatitis B surface antigen. A reticulin stain is useful for outlining areas of focal or zonal necrosis (Fig. 7.3), thick liver plates, or nodules of regeneration. It can also be used to demonstrate fibrosis, but in general the Masson stain is preferred because the reticulin stain does not distinguish permanent scarring from stromal collapse.

Complex carbohydrates

Complex carbohydrates are readily demonstrated with the periodic acid–Schiff (PAS) stain, which produces a reddish-violet color. This will demonstrate glycogen in liver cells, both physiologically and in glycogen storage diseases. However, a much more useful procedure is to perform the PAS stain after pretreatment with diastase (DPAS) to remove the glycogen and unmask other complex carbohydrate-containing substances, including metabolic and synthetic products of the liver, and structural components. The DPAS stain strikingly demonstrates the presence of lipofuscin and other cell debris in Kupffer cells and portal macrophages in acute hepatocellular injury (Fig. 7.4). DPAS is also useful for staining bile duct basement membranes to demonstrate ductal injury; fibrin (e.g., in disseminated intravascular coagulation); amyloid; starch; amoebae; and most pathogenic fungi and intracellular carbohydrate-containing material in many inherited and acquired storage diseases, such as α_1-antitrypsin deficiency (Fig. 7.5).

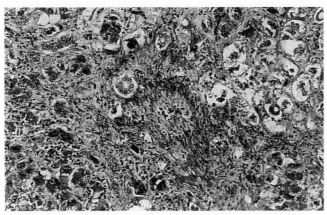

Figure 7.1 The Masson trichrome stains type I collagen blue, revealing zone 3 fibrosis in this case of alcoholic liver disease. An occluded terminal hepatic venule can be seen in the center of the field.

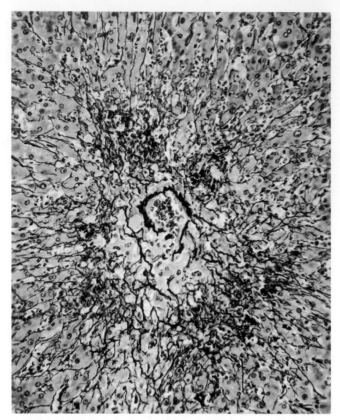

Figure 7.3 The reticulin stain shows the black-staining type III collagen fibers that support the liver cell plates. A terminal hepatic venule in the center of the field is surrounded by collapsed reticulin, indicating zone 3 necrosis.

Iron, copper, and other stains

Iron in the form of hemosiderin granules is readily demonstrated with the Prussian blue stain, which is also useful in bringing out the green color of bile and the golden brown color of lipofuscin, both of which can be

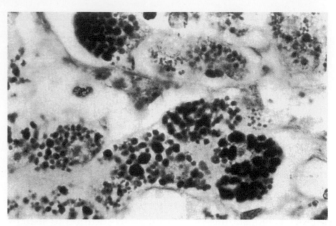

Figure 7.5 Globules of α_1-antitrypsin are strongly PAS-positive and diastase resistant.

masked by overstaining with either eosin or hematoxylin (Fig. 7.6). Copper is best demonstrated using a rhodanine stain (Fig. 7.7), but the orcein and Victoria blue stains, which are technically easier, can also be used because these will stain concentrated deposits of the copper-binding protein, metallothionine. In the past, orcein and Victoria blue were primarily used to demonstrate the ground-glass inclusions of chronic hepatitis B infections (Fig. 7.8), but these have now been largely supplanted by specific immunostains, as discussed later.

Other stains that find occasional use include the Hall stain for bile; the Fontana stain for lipofuscin and Dubin–Johnson pigment; the phosphotungstic acid–hematoxylin stain for fibrin or mitochondria; the Congo red, sirius red, or crystal violet stains for amyloid; an acid-fast stain for mycobacteria, schistosome eggs, or the hooklets in the scolices of echinococcal cysts; and the Warthin–Starry stain for spirochetes, leptospira, or bacilli causing cat scratch disease. A Giemsa stain can be useful

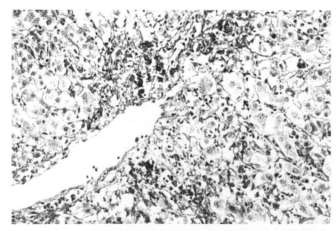

Figure 7.4 The periodic acid–Schiff (PAS) stain after diastase digestion to remove glycogen demonstrates the presence of lipofuscin and other cell debris in Kupffer cells in acute hepatocellular injury.

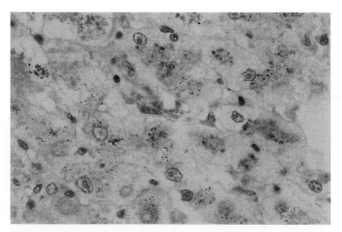

Figure 7.6 The Prussian blue stain for iron demonstrates hemosiderin (blue granules) and also brings out the green color of bile and the golden brown color of lipofuscin.

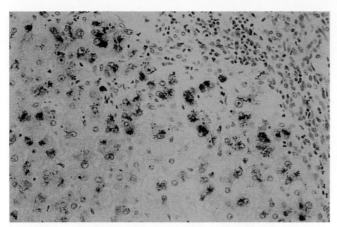

Figure 7.7 The rhodanine stain demonstrates copper as brick-red granules in liver cells in this case of Wilson disease.

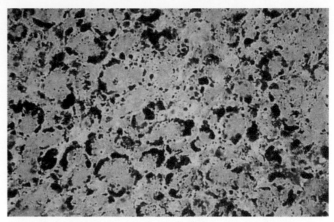

Figure 7.9 The oil red O stain of a frozen section shows microvesicular fat in acute fatty liver of pregnancy.

in studying the morphology of hematopoietic cells or in identifying some microorganisms, such as *Leishmania* or *Cryptosporidia*.

Fat

Fat can be demonstrated histochemically, but this requires unprocessed frozen sections, which must be prepared with a cryostat from fresh or formalin-fixed tissue. Routine processing exposes the tissue to organic solvents, which will extract lipids and render fat stains useless. However, frozen sections prepared and stained with oil red O (Fig. 7.9) can be quite useful for demonstrating neutral lipid in liver cells in a variety of conditions or in cells of benign or malignant tumors. This stain may also be used to demonstrate fat globules of stellate cells, and cholesterol crystals and lipofuscin in liver or Kupffer cells. Cholesterol can be specifically stained in frozen sections by the Schultz modification of the Liebermann–Burchard reaction, a reaction useful for the diagnosis of Wolman

disease or cholesteryl ester storage disease. Metachromatic granules in macrophage cells and bile duct epithelium in metachromatic leukodystrophy are best demonstrated in frozen sections by using stains such as cresyl violet or toluidine blue.

Immunopathology

Immunostains are routinely used in the diagnosis and classification of hepatic neoplasms, but there are fewer practical applications in the study of non-neoplastic diseases of the liver. Nevertheless, these techniques can be used to demonstrate and characterize normal structural components and a number of histopathologic changes; they can also be used to locate viral antigens and other infectious agents.

In the normal liver, bile duct epithelial cells react with monoclonal antibodies to cytokeratins 7, 8, 18, and 19 (Fig. 7.10), whereas the liver cells react only with

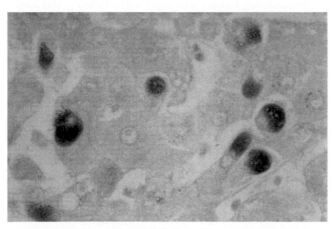

Figure 7.8 The Victoria blue stain shows cells containing large amounts of hepatitis B surface antigen in a chronic carrier.

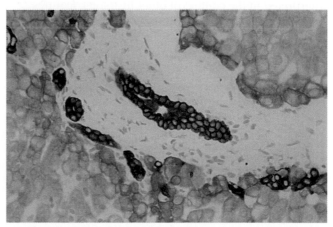

Figure 7.10 Immunostain with a cocktail of monoclonal antibodies that react with cytokeratin types 7, 8, 18, and 19. There is strongly positive staining of the bile duct in the center of the portal area and the ductular cells at the edge, whereas hepatocytes stain only weakly.

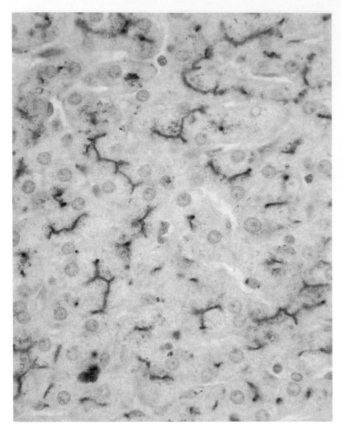

Figure 7.11 Immunostain with polyclonal antibodies to carcinoembryonic antigen demonstrates dark-staining bile canaliculi between hepatocytes.

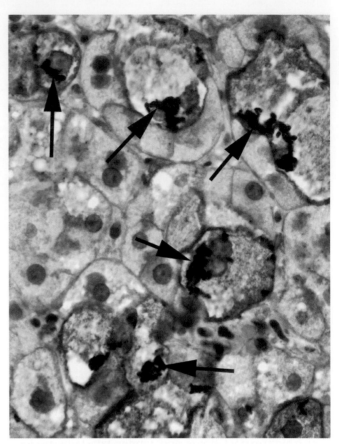

Figure 7.12 Immunostain with antibody to ubiquitin demonstrates dark-staining Mallory–Denk bodies (arrows) in liver cells in alcoholic hepatitis.

monoclonal antibodies to cytokeratins 8 and 18 [2]. Bile canaliculi are demonstrated by polyclonal antibodies to carcinoembryonic antigen (CEA) (Fig. 7.11) because of the presence of a cross-reacting biliary glycoprotein. Tumors derived from hepatocytes and bile ducts often maintain the antigenic characteristics of their normal counterparts, but this is not invariable, hence staining patterns must be interpreted in the context of other histologic features.

A few practical applications for immunohistochemistry have been found in the diagnosis of non-neoplastic diseases. In chronic cholestatic disorders, such as PBC, cytokeratin type 7, which is normally only found in biliary-type cells, appears in periportal hepatocytes [3]. Because cytokeratin proteins are a major component of Mallory–Denk bodies (formerly called Mallory bodies), antibodies to several high and low molecular weight keratins may be used to demonstrate this pathologic feature, but none are as reliable for this purpose as staining with antibodies to the cellular stress proteins ubiquitin [4] or p62 [5] that coat the surface of filamentous tangles such as Mallory–Denk bodies (Fig. 7.12).

Immunostaining for viral antigens in different types of viral hepatitis is extensively used for investigational purposes and, to a lesser extent, for diagnosis. In routine practice, hepatitis B antigens (surface and core: HBsAg

and HBcAg) are readily identified with commercially available antisera (Fig. 7.13). Hepatitis D virus can also be identified in routinely processed tissue, but antibodies are more difficult to obtain. Hepatitis A, C, and E viruses can only be reliably identified in frozen sections, and staining for these is generally limited to research settings. Several viruses, other than those causing viral hepatitis, including herpes simplex virus, cytomegalovirus (CMV), and adenovirus, can be detected in the liver by using commercially available antisera.

Electron microscopy

Transmission electron microscopy has many investigational applications but a limited number of diagnostic ones [6]. Its greatest value is in the interpretation of biopsy specimens from patients with known or suspected metabolic disorders, and it can also be helpful in drug-induced and cholestatic diseases and in some infections. Among the metabolic diseases, distinctive or pathognomonic ultrastructural findings are present in hereditary fructose intolerance, α_1-antitrypsin deficiency, Farber disease, glycogenoses types II and IV, Gaucher disease, metachromatic leukodystrophy, Dubin–Johnson syndrome,

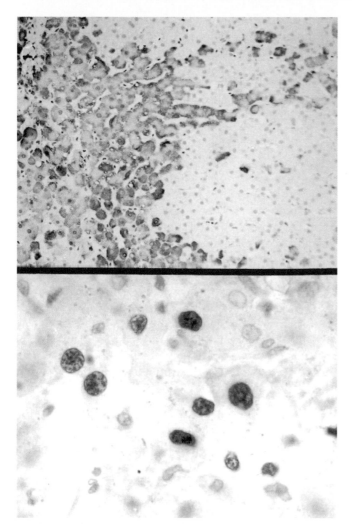

Figure 7.13 Immunostains for hepatitis B antigens. (A) Antibody to hepatitis B surface antigen (HBsAg) shows variable amounts of antigen in the cytoplasm of some hepatocytes. (B) Antibody to hepatitis B core antigen (HBcAg) shows antigen in the nuclei of liver cells with replicative virus.

erythropoietic protoporphyria, Wilson disease, Zellweger syndrome, and many others. Drug-induced injury causes changes in many organelles of the liver depending on the drug, duration of use, and other factors. Many drugs (e.g., phenytoin, phenobarbital) and toxins (e.g., DDT (2,2-bis(*p*-chlorophenyl)-1,1,1,-trichloroethane) and other pesticides) cause proliferation of the smooth endoplasmic reticulum of liver cells ("induced" hepatocytes), which results in a characteristic ground-glass appearance on light microscopy. Megamitochondria, sometimes assuming monstrous forms, are considered typical of drug reactions, while lysosomal phospholipidosis is highly typical of several drugs (e.g., amiodarone). Subtle manifestations of cholestasis due to a variety of causes can be seen ultrastructurally before becoming recognizable by light microscopy. Among infectious agents, viral particles can be visualized directly in herpes simplex, adenovirus, and

CMV infections, and both incomplete and complete particles of hepatitis B can be seen in infected liver cells.

Scanning electron microscopy has also proved more useful for investigation than for diagnosis. The diagnostic applications of this technique are largely limited to particulate material, especially when X-ray spectrophotometry (also called *electron probe analysis*) is combined with scanning electron microscopy [7]. Using this technique, the elements that are present in particulate material, such as talc, Thorotrast, silicone, silica, titanium, gold, and barium sulfate can be positively identified.

Other special techniques

In situ hybridization may be used to detect genomic DNA of the hepatitis B virus (HBV) [8] in chronic hepatitis B, and it has been used to detect early ribonucleic acid of the Epstein–Barr virus (EBV) in both hepatitis and neoplasms related to that virus [9].

Polarizing microscopy is useful in identifying birefringent crystals of talc (Fig. 7.14) in portal macrophages or Kupffer cells in abusers of intravenous drugs [10]. The remnants of previous surgery, such as suture material, talc, or starch from glove powder left on the surface of the liver are also birefringent in polarized light,

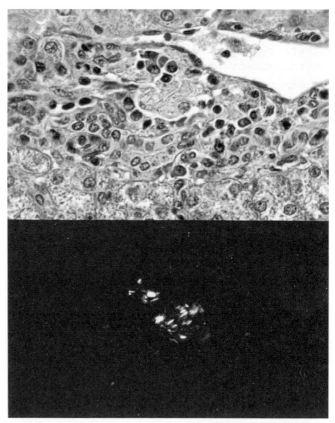

Figure 7.14 Portal macrophages in the center of field (A) contain talc crystals, which are birefringent and easily visualized with polarizing microscopy (B).

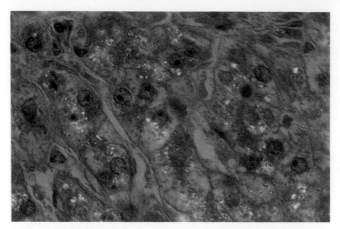

Figure 7.15 Deposits of protoporphyrin are birefringent and appear red in polarized light. Larger deposits show a characteristic Maltese cross.

as is silica in multiorgan silicosis [11]. Type I collagen has a silvery birefringence, and amyloid has a characteristic apple green birefringence when sections stained with Congo red are examined by polarizing microscopy. Formalin pigment (typically in blood vessels) and both malarial and schistosomal pigments (in reticuloendothelial cells) are brown to black deposits of acid hematin and are birefringent under polarized light. Cholesterol crystals (e.g., in the livers of patients with Wolman disease and cholesteryl ester storage disease) in frozen sections, whether stained or unstained, are birefringent, as are cystine crystals in cystinosis. Needle-like uroporphyrin crystals in liver cells can sometimes be visualized by polarizing microscopy of unstained frozen or paraffin sections in porphyria cutanea tarda [12]. Red birefringent Maltese crosses and amorphous materials are characteristic of protoporphyrin accumulation in canaliculi or Kupffer cells in erythropoietic protoporphyria (Fig. 7.15) [13].

Ultraviolet (UV) microscopy is most useful in confirming the diagnosis in the hepatic porphyrias. However, unfixed, air-dried frozen sections are required, so the usefulness of the technique is limited. Nevertheless, frozen sections of the liver in porphyria cutanea tarda and erythropoietic protophorphyria reveal red autofluorescence under UV microscopy because of the presence of porphyrins. Vitamin A stored in stellate cells has a green and rapidly fading autofluorescence in UV light, while a granular yellow autofluorescence is characteristic of lipofuscin.

Morphologic patterns of injury

Acute necroinflammatory disease (acute hepatitis)

Acute necroinflammatory disease is typically seen in cases of acute infection with the hepatitis viruses, but identical injury may occur with hepatitis-like reactions to a number of therapeutic drugs (see Chapter 27). Hepatocellular injury, leading to cell death, is the predominant morphologic feature of acute necroinflammatory diseases, although the term *necroinflammatory* has become something of a misnomer in view of recent advances in pathobiology. The term *necrosis*, previously used for all forms of cell death, is now applied more selectively to certain forms of cell death. Many of the injured and dying cells seen in the various forms of hepatitis are actually in the process of apoptosis, while the "inflammatory" component is at times the effector of apoptosis and at times the response to the hepatocellular injury. Nevertheless, for the purposes of this discussion, the term necroinflammatory will be maintained.

Several basic lesions are seen in various forms of necroinflammatory injury:

1 *Apoptosis* results in shrinkage of the hepatocyte, which often has an angular configuration and is more eosinophilic than its neighbors in the liver plate ("acidophilic degeneration") (Fig. 7.16) [14,15]. The nucleus is often pyknotic and deeply basophilic. The cytoplasm of the liver cell develops protuberances that separate

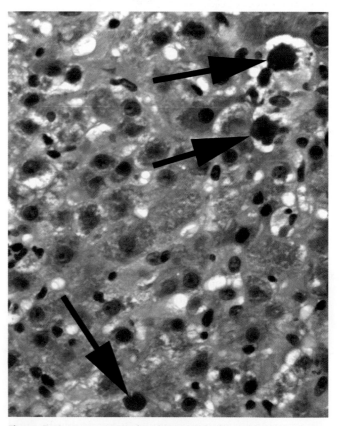

Figure 7.16 Hepatocytes undergoing apoptosis (arrows) become shrunken, angulated and darker than their neighbors, lose their nuclei and begin to fragment, forming acidophilic bodies.

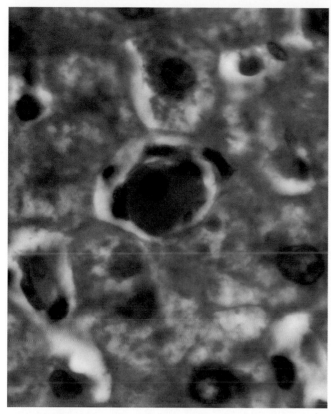

Figure 7.17 High magnification of an acidophilic body that has been extruded from the liver cell plate into a sinusoid. Most of the degenerated nucleus of the dead hepatocyte remains.

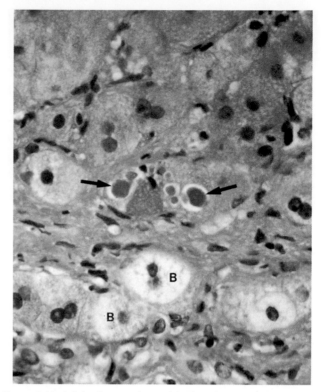

Figure 7.18 Cellular degeneration and death with apoptotic bodies (arrows) and ballooning (B).

and are released into the spaces of Disse and sinusoids. The larger cell fragments, which may contain parts of the nucleus, have been termed *apoptotic, acidophilic,* or *hyaline bodies* (Figs 7.17 and 7.18). The apoptotic bodies are quickly phagocytosed by Kupffer cells or adjoining liver cells, where they undergo degeneration and are reduced to residual bodies.

2 *Ballooning degeneration* refers to the swelling of hepatocytes, often to several times their normal size. Affected cells have an indistinct cell membrane and the cytoplasm is rarefied (Figs 7.18 and 7.19). The ballooned hepatocytes eventually undergo lysis, with disappearance or "dropping out." The remnants of these cells attract lymphocytes and, less often, other types of inflammatory cells ("focal necrosis"), as well as hypertrophied Kupffer cells.

3 *Coagulative necrosis* refers to a form of cell death recognized by deeply eosinophilic, granular cytoplasm with loss of the nucleus and discohesion from the surrounding cells of the tissue (Fig. 7.20). The cell outline may be maintained for some time, but this is eventually lost as the tissue becomes amorphous. This change is typical of anoxic injury, although it may be seen in some forms of necroinflammatory injury.

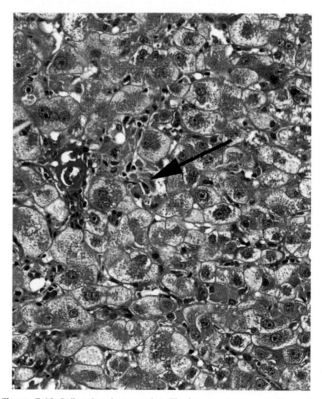

Figure 7.19 Ballooning degeneration. The hepatocytes are swollen and pale. A cluster of inflammatory cells ("focal necrosis") in the center of the field shows the position where a hepatocyte has disappeared from the tissue (arrow).

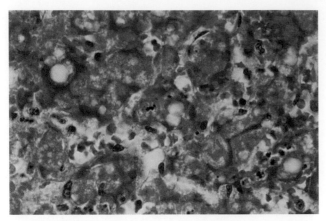

Figure 7.20 Coagulative necrosis in a case of ischemic injury. The cytoplasm of the necrotic cells is eosinophilic and granular, and the nuclei have disappeared.

4 *Regeneration*, recognized by the enlargement of nuclei and nucleoli, mitoses, binucleation, and thickening of the liver cell plates (Fig. 7.21), may be seen shortly after the onset of a necroinflammatory injury such as viral hepatitis. The number of regenerating cells gradually increases as the patient recovers.

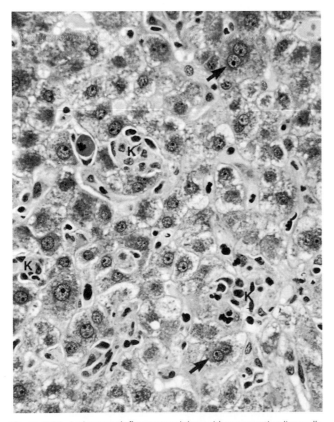

Figure 7.21 Active necroinflammatory injury with regenerating liver cells, recognizable by enlarged nuclei, prominent nucleoli, and binucleate liver cells (arrows). Clusters of hypertrophied Kupffer cells (K) are present at sites of liver cell dropout.

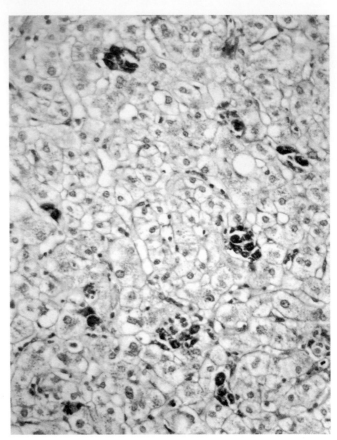

Figure 7.22 The PAS stain after diastase digestion demonstrates clusters of hypertrophied, lipofuscin-filled Kupffer cells (dark staining) at the sites of liver cell dropout.

5 *Kupffer cell hypertrophy* is characteristic of acute necroinflammatory injuries. Sinusoidal macrophages are normally inconspicuous, but in response to liver cell death these enlarge as they perform their phagocytic function. They can be recognized by the presence of cytoplasmic light brown, finely granular lipofuscin presumed to be phagocytosed from necrotic hepatocytes (Figs 7.21 and 7.22).

Acute necroinflammatory patterns

Acute hepatitis

"Classic" acute hepatitis, typical of the common forms of acute viral hepatitis, is characterized by panacinar necroinflammatory disease with spotty necrosis. The appearance of the liver is one of acinar disarray (Fig. 7.23) caused by widespread degeneration and death of individual and small groups of hepatocytes, which display features of both apoptosis and ballooning with focal necrosis. These are seen throughout the acinus in various combinations, and not all hepatocytes in a given acinus are affected. Features of regeneration are invariably present, and there is typically an inflammatory response

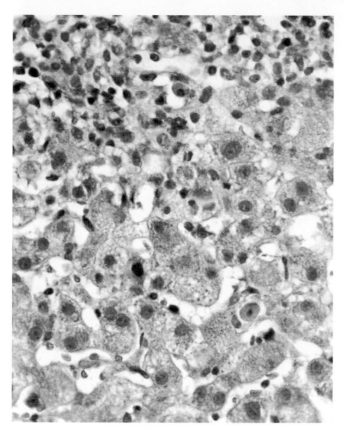

Figure 7.23 Acute viral hepatitis. Note acinar disarray, apoptosis, and focal necrosis, Kupffer cell hypertrophy, and lymphocytic infiltrate.

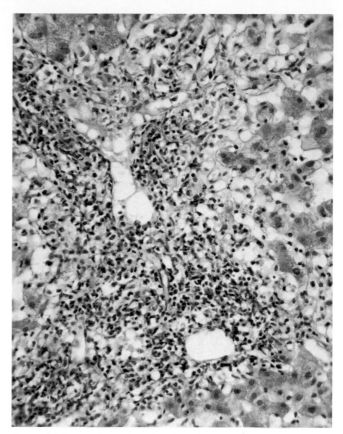

Figure 7.24 Acute hepatitis A, showing marked portal inflammation with extension into the adjacent parenchyma (interface hepatitis), mimicking the appearance of chronic hepatitis.

consisting of hypertrophied Kupffer cells and lymphocytes. The portal areas in typical acute hepatitis are usually infiltrated with inflammatory cells. Lymphocytes predominate, but a small number of plasma cells, as well as eosinophils and neutrophils (especially in drug-induced disease), may be present. Occasionally, plasma cells predominate, especially in hepatitis A [16,17]. The inflammatory response often extends beyond the confines of the portal areas, leading to some blurring of the outline of the limiting plate and creating the appearance of interface hepatitis, as discussed later under chronic hepatitis. This also is especially true in hepatitis A (Fig. 7.24). Cholestasis is not a significant component of the histopathology of "classic" acute viral hepatitis, and when present, it is usually seen as an occasional, haphazardly distributed, canalicular bile plug. Occasional cases may reveal abnormalities of the bile ductal epithelium, including swelling, disruption, and infiltration by lymphocytes, which constitute the hepatitis-associated bile duct lesions that are discussed in the section on chronic hepatitis.

The subsiding phase of viral hepatitis is characterized by a lessening of the injury and inflammation with increased regeneration and repair. The differences between this and the active phase are, however, mainly quantitative. Acinar disarray diminishes and eventually disappears, and the hepatic parenchyma gradually reverts to a normal appearance over a period of several weeks to months, although varying degrees of unrest are still evident. The liver cell plates often appear thickened. Only occasional degenerating cells and small foci of inflammation are evident. A frequent finding is the continuing hypertrophy of Kupffer cells and portal macrophages (see Fig. 7.22). They become relatively more conspicuous because the hepatocytes are less swollen, and they now contain variable amounts of hemosiderin in addition to lipofuscin. The portal area inflammatory response gradually diminishes. Uncomplicated viral hepatitis is not followed by any significant periportal or intra-acinar fibrosis.

Mononucleosis hepatitis

Mononucleosis hepatitis is typical of EBV and CMV infections in immunocompetent patients [9,18–20]. Similar histology can be seen in reactions to some drugs, especially diphenylhydantoin [21], and on occasion in acute hepatitis B or C, so a complete serologic workup is advisable whenever this pattern of injury is seen. In comparison

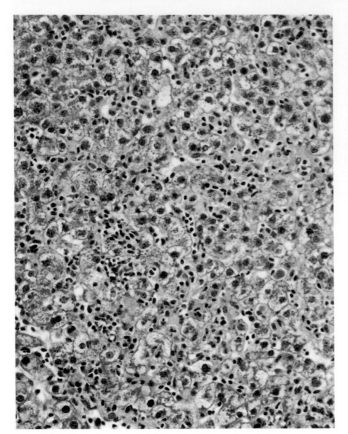

Figure 7.25 Infectious mononucleosis hepatitis. There is a prominent sinusoidal mononuclear cell infiltrate along with the hepatocellular injury of an acute hepatitis.

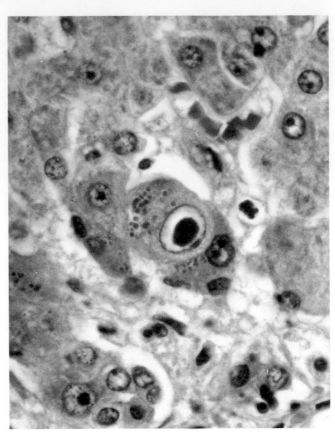

Figure 7.26 Cytomegalovirus infection in an immunodeficient host. The large cell in the center of the field has a characteristic intranuclear inclusion and many small cytoplasmic inclusions.

with "classic" viral hepatitis, the inflammatory response in this variant is more prominent (Fig. 7.25) while the hepatocellular injury is milder. Hepatocellular regeneration is prominent, and mitotic figures are often seen in hepatocytes, Kupffer cells, and portal mononuclear cells. Apoptosis is present but ballooning is absent or minimal. Kupffer cells are often markedly hypertrophied and sometimes form tiny granulomatoid foci or, rarely, true granulomas. The hepatic sinusoids characteristically contain an increased number of lymphocytes, sometimes closely packed together in a "string of beads" pattern (Fig. 7.25). In CMV infection, cytomegaly and viral inclusions are never seen in immunocompetent patients, but in CMV infections of the newborn, and of adults who are immunocompromised, characteristic intranuclear and cytoplasmic inclusions (Fig. 7.26) may be present in the bile duct and liver cells.

Cholestatic hepatitis

Cholestatic hepatitis, or combined hepatocellular and cholestatic injury, is an uncommon complication of most types of acute viral hepatitis, but it is frequent in hepatitis E infection [22]. As a pattern of injury, it is more

frequently seen in reactions to a number of drugs [23]. Synonyms for cholestatic viral hepatitis include "cholangiolitic" or "pericholangitic" viral hepatitis, while drug-induced injury is termed hepatocanalicular or mixed hepatocellular and cholestatic. The clinical and laboratory findings tend to simulate those of obstructive biliary tract disease. The histopathology of cholestatic hepatitis includes hepatocellular and canalicular bile stasis, often with pseudogland formation, and variable degrees of parenchymal injury (Fig. 7.27). There may be periportal ductular proliferation with infiltration by neutrophils (acute cholangiolitis), as well as many neutrophils in the portal inflammatory infiltrate, but the acinar bile ducts are not involved.

Neonatal giant cell hepatitis

Neonatal giant cell hepatitis typically has features of acute hepatitis with transformation of hepatocytes into multinucleate giant cells. Newborns with this disease typically present with jaundice, and the principal differential diagnosis is between this and extrahepatic biliary atresia. The term idiopathic neonatal hepatitis is used for most cases in which no cause is found, but the features seen

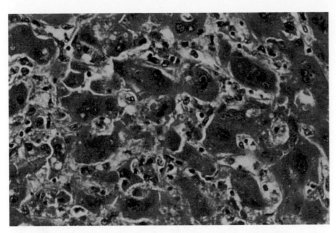

Figure 7.27 Acute cholestatic hepatitis (combined hepatocellular–cholestatic injury). There is prominent cholestasis, as well as hepatocellular injury, acidophilic bodies, liver cell dropout, and inflammation.

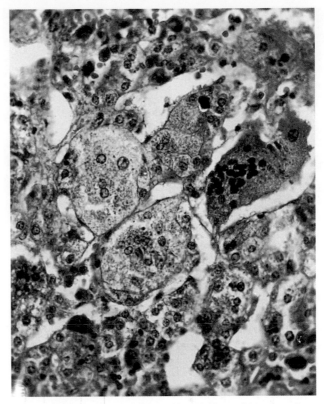

Figure 7.28 Idiopathic neonatal hepatitis with giant cell transformation. Note the enlarged hepatocytes containing numerous nuclei.

in some neonates with α_1-antitrypsin deficiency may be identical to those seen in a number of other metabolic disorders and infections. The "idiopathic" cases are presumably secondary to undiagnosed viruses because most patients recover without sequellae. Histologically, all the features of acute hepatitis are present, along with significant bile stasis, but the most striking feature is giant cell transformation of the hepatocytes (Fig. 7.28). The giant cells appear to result from the fusion of several liver cells to form a syncytium, and there may be up to several dozen nuclei in a single cell. The cholestasis may be quite prominent and there is often extramedullary hematopoiesis. Portal fibrosis and ductular proliferation, typical of biliary atresia, are not seen.

Acute injury with microabscess formation

Acute injury with microabscess formation is typical of a number of bacterial infections complicated by sepsis or hematogenous dissemination. This includes diseases caused by both Gram-positive and Gram-negative organisms, such as listeriosis (Fig. 7.29), melioidosis, and typhoid fever, as well as disseminated mycotic infections such as those caused by *Cryptococcus*, *Candida*, or *Aspergillus* species. Organisms may or may not be demonstrable in the lesions. In the immunocompromised host, CMV infection can also lead to this type of tissue response (with or without viral inclusions) in the liver. In all these diseases, lesions typically consist of varying-sized microabscesses, but they sometimes have a granulomatoid appearance. In CMV infection, the lesions are quite small, often only a single degenerating hepatocyte surrounded by neutrophils (sometimes containing an intranuclear inclusion), whereas bacterial and fungal infections may have grossly visible abscesses. In the later stages, lesions may have a purulent center and an

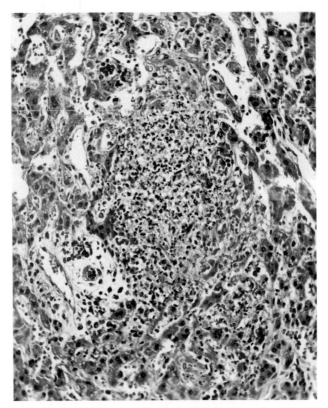

Figure 7.29 Listeriosis. A microabscess is present in the center of the field because of hematogenous dissemination of the infection.

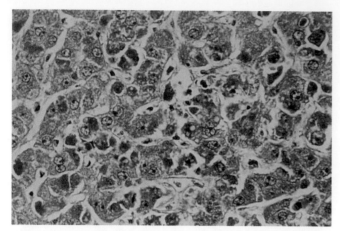

Figure 7.30 Yellow fever. Many individual hepatocytes display coagulative necrosis in a haphazard distribution.

organized granulomatous periphery, with variable fibrosis, especially in diseases such as meliodosis or typhoid. Noninfectious causes of focal necrosis with a neutrophilic response or microabscess formation also include the characteristic reaction to degenerating liver cells harboring Mallory–Denk bodies in steatohepatitis – either alcoholic or nonalcoholic. In addition, perivenular focal necrosis with neutrophilic aggregation is an iatrogenic artifact often observed in open surgical biopsy specimens of the liver.

Acute injury with focal coagulative necrosis

Acute injury with focal coagulative necrosis is seen in some viral infections in children, for example, coxsackie B4 and B9, but more importantly, this type of injury is typical of hepatic involvement in many types of viral hemorrhagic fevers, including yellow fever (Fig. 7.30), dengue, Lassa fever, and others [24]. Haphazardly distributed single liver cells or clusters of liver cells are affected by coagulation necrosis, often with little or no inflammatory response. Viral inclusions are not present in any of these diseases.

Acute injury with patchy or confluent coagulative necrosis

This type of injury is seen in disseminated herpes simplex hepatitis, whether occurring in neonates, children, or adults [25], both immunocompetent and immunocompromised. Similar findings are rarely seen in adenovirus hepatitis in immunocompromised patients [26]. Viral inclusions are most easily identified in the relatively preserved hepatocytes at the margins of the necrotic foci. In herpes simplex, the classic Cowdry type A inclusions are eosinophilic, rounded or irregular, and surrounded by a clear halo with margination of the chromatin (Fig. 7.31). Adenovirus inclusions are more pleo-

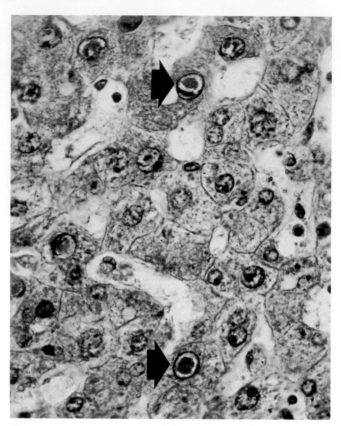

Figure 7.31 Herpes simplex hepatitis. Several of the nuclei have eosinophilic Cowdry type A inclusions surrounded by a clear halo with margination of the chromatin (arrows).

morphic. Some resemble the Cowdry type A inclusions of herpes simplex but many are more basophilic and irregular in contour.

Acute injury with zonal submassive or massive coagulative necrosis

This is typical of toxic injury from a number of direct hepatotoxins, although it may also be produced by ischemic injury. Among toxins, acetaminophen overdose is by far the most frequent cause of this type of injury [27]. The tissue maintains its acinar architecture, but hepatocytes in zone 3 are entirely necrotic (Fig. 7.32), with progressive involvement of zones 2 and 1 with increasing severity of injury. In the most severe cases, only a thin rim of viable hepatocytes surrounds each portal area.

Acute hepatitis with submassive necrosis and stromal collapse

Acute hepatitis with submassive necrosis and stromal collapse can be seen with severe hepatitis of any cause. This pattern of injury is more frequently encountered in biopsy and in surgical material from patients with drug-induced liver disease than with viral hepatitis. This is partly because patients with acute viral hepatitis are rarely

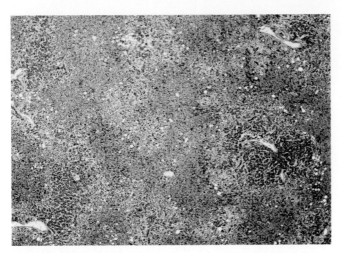

Figure 7.32 Submassive zonal coagulative necrosis in a fatal case of acetaminophen overdose. The necrotic hepatocytes of zones 2 and 3 are present in the section, while some of the zone 1 (periportal) cells survive.

subjected to biopsy and because drug-induced injury tends, on average, to be more severe than viral hepatitis, and also because many drugs are preferentially metabolized by hepatocytes of zone 3, thereby having the greatest toxic effects in this part of the acinus. There are patients who have not been exposed to a drug or chemical but who develop acute liver failure with submassive or massive hepatic necrosis and in whom no evidence for any of the known hepatitis viruses can be found serologically or by polymerase chain reaction (PCR) for viral DNA or RNA [27,28]. These may be caused by some as yet undiscovered viral agent, but for now they remain enigmatic and unclassified. Finally, autoimmune hepatitis, although considered a chronic disease, often has an acute clinical presentation, and biopsies from the patients with this type of hepatitis may also show an appearance of acute hepatitis with submassive necrosis [29].

Submassive necrosis of any cause is due to the simultaneous death of the hepatocytes of an entire zone or more of the hepatic acini, thereby producing confluent necrosis, lysis of the necrotic tissue, and collapse of the supporting stroma. The necrosis usually involves zone 3 and, less often, zone 2 of the hepatic acini (Fig. 7.33), but viral hepatitis A and injury due to some drugs and toxins are characterized by necrosis predominantly involving zone 1 (Fig. 7.34). In various planes of the section, acinar zone 3 necrosis may appear to be entirely around the terminal hepatic venule ("centrilobular"), may appear to extend between the terminal venules of adjacent acini, or may appear to extend from the terminal venule to the edge of the portal area. Consequently, when necrosis affects zone 3, the collapsed reticulin framework may extend between adjacent vascular structures, making them appear linked together ("bridging necrosis"). There

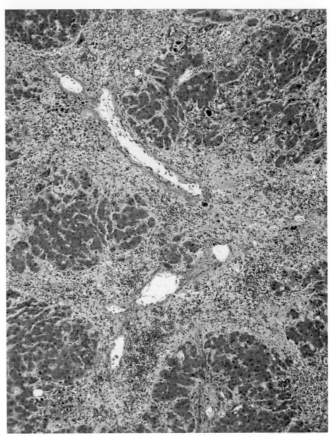

Figure 7.33 Acute submassive necrosis of acinar zones 3 and 2. Surviving liver cells are predominantly periportal in zone 1 of the acini. In contrast to the coagulative necrosis shown in Fig. 7.32, there is a collapse of the stroma where the hepatocytes have been lost

may also be linkage of portal areas with terminal hepatic venules ("portal–central bridging") or of two or more terminal hepatic venules ("central–central bridging"), both due to submassive zone 3 necrosis.

Acute hepatitis with massive necrosis

Acute hepatitis with massive necrosis, the most extreme form of acute hepatocellular injury, may be caused by viral hepatitis or drug-induced liver disease. There is virtually complete loss of hepatocytes (Fig. 7.35), but occasionally the haphazardly distributed cells can survive, as can a cuff of cells around the portal areas. The reticulin framework is usually intact but frequently collapsed because of the loss of liver cells, with resultant approximation of the portal areas. Variable numbers of inflammatory cells are present in the areas of collapse. These include lymphocytes and plasma cells, as well as a lesser number of eosinophils and neutrophils. Central vein endophlebitis may be present. The collapsed parenchyma contains numerous hypertrophied Kupffer cells with cytoplasm packed with lipofuscin. Zone 1 of the

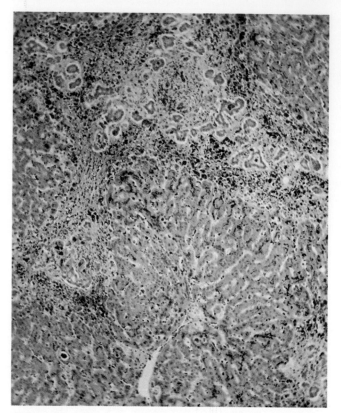

Figure 7.34 Acute submassive necrosis of zone 1. With the Prussian blue stain, hemosiderin-laden macrophages (dark staining) are shown to outline the areas of periportal necrosis and liver cell loss.

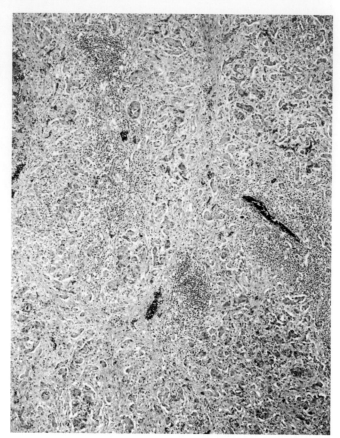

Figure 7.35 Acute hepatitis with massive hepatic necrosis. There is loss of all hepatocytes with proliferation of ductules in the collapsed hepatic stroma.

hepatic acinus typically shows proliferation of the putative hepatic stem cells (Fig. 7.36), forming ductules and ductular hepatocytes [30].

Chronic necroinflammatory injury (chronic hepatitis)

Chronic necroinflammatory disease refers to a morphologic pattern that is seen most often in chronic viral hepatitis and also in autoimmune hepatitis, occasional drug reactions, and, in rare instances, some metabolic diseases. As in acute necroinflammatory disease, there is hepatocellular injury and inflammation, but in the chronic diseases the brunt of the injury tends to be portal and periportal rather than panacinar, and the injury is accompanied by fibrosis that can progress to cirrhosis. Chronic hepatitis, regardless of cause, is characterized by several pathologic changes that are present to a variable extent in each case. These include portal inflammation and sometimes lesions of bile ducts within the portal spaces; periportal injury and inflammation; several forms of degeneration and death by apoptosis of intra-acinar hepatocytes with an associated inflammatory response; and fibrosis that may involve only the portal and periportal areas or that may form septa.

Morphology of chronic hepatitis

In all forms of chronic hepatitis the portal areas are *inflamed* and variably infiltrated by lymphocytes and plasma cells. Lymphoid aggregates or follicles with germinal centers may be present and are now considered typical, although not pathognomonic, of chronic hepatitis C (Fig. 7.37). Immunohistochemical studies have shown that even when germinal centers are not apparent by light microscopy, these are true functional lymphoid follicles [31]. The germinal centers contain activated B cells surrounded by a follicular dendritic cell network and a mantle zone of B cells, which, in turn, is surrounded by a T-cell zone. Patients with autoimmune hepatitis will often have large numbers or plasma cells in the portal inflammatory infiltrate (Fig. 7.38). Biopsy specimens from patients who are affected by chronic hepatitis through intravenous drug abuse may have birefringent talc crystals in portal macrophages (see Fig. 7.14) [10].

Hepatitis-associated bile duct lesions were first described in chronic hepatitis [32], but lesions may also be found in biopsy specimens of acute hepatitis. The lesion is characterized by swelling, vacuolization, nuclear irregularity, and, sometimes, pseudostratification of the biliary

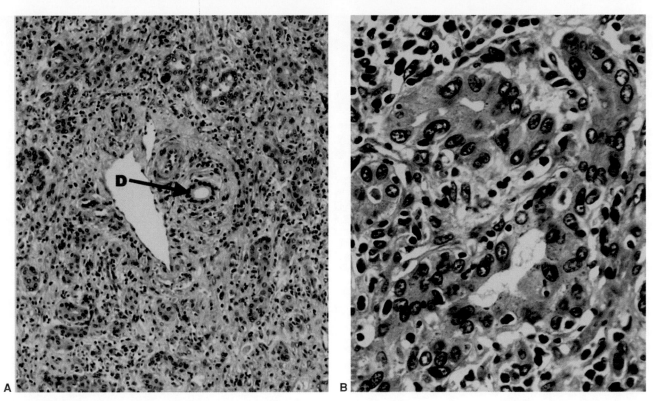

Figure 7.36 Ductular proliferation in massive hepatic necrosis. The putative stem cells of the liver have proliferated, forming ductules and differentiating into hepatocytes in a vain attempt to repopulate the liver. (A) A portal area with an acinar bile duct (D) surrounded by collapsed stroma that contains proliferating ductules and inflammatory cells. (B) The ductules at high magnification. Some of the ductular cells have granular, eosinophilic cytoplasm, indicating differentiation into hepatocytes.

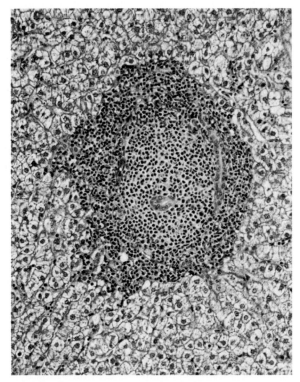

Figure 7.37 Chronic portal inflammation with a lymphoid aggregate that has a germinal center in a patient with chronic hepatitis C.

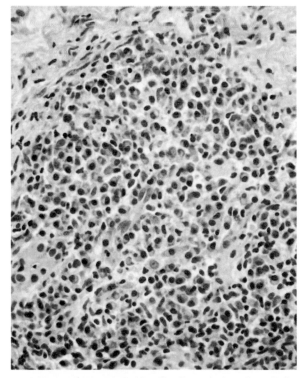

Figure 7.38 Autoimmune hepatitis with a large number of portal plasma cells, recognizable by their eccentric nuclei and clear perinuclear Golgi zone.

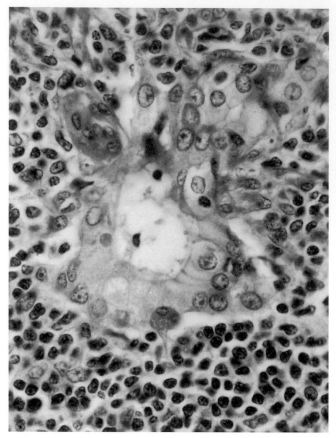

Figure 7.39 Hepatitis-associated bile duct lesion with marked epithelial injury and infiltration by chronic inflammatory cells, similar to the florid duct lesions of primary biliary cirrhosis.

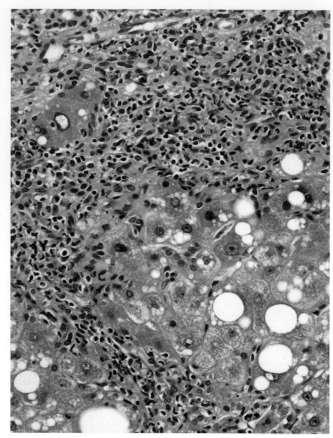

Figure 7.40 Interface hepatitis ("piecemeal necrosis") can be most easily recognized as irregularity of the limiting plate, caused by extension of portal inflammation through the plate into the periportal parenchyma.

epithelial cells (Fig. 7.39). The basement membrane may appear to be ruptured, and lymphocytes, occasional plasma cells, and sometimes neutrophils infiltrate the duct. The lesion is reminiscent of and sometimes indistinguishable from the "florid duct lesions" of PBC. However, in contrast to the lesions of PBC, the ducts are not destroyed, so portal areas without ducts are seldom seen and features of chronic cholestasis do not develop. Serial section reconstruction studies [33] have demonstrated that the most frequently observed lesions are actually blind diverticula arising from injured ducts rather than the ducts themselves. The ductal lesions have been seen in all forms of hepatitis, but most commonly in hepatitis C [34].

Interface hepatitis is now the preferred term for the lesion formerly known as piecemeal necrosis [35]. The original term was defined by an international group as "the destruction of liver cells at an interface between parenchyma and connective tissue, together with a predominantly lymphocytic or plasma cell infiltrate" [36]. It is now apparent that the destruction of liver cells is primarily through apoptosis, and because the dead hepa-

tocytes quickly disappear from the tissue, it is the location of the inflammatory component that permits recognition of the lesion, making interface hepatitis the more accurate term. Interface hepatitis has long been considered to be a key lesion in the progression and pathogenesis of chronic hepatitis, and the degree of periportal injury (mild, moderate, or marked) is still used to grade the degree of activity. Interface hepatitis can be most easily recognized as irregularity of the limiting plate, caused by extension of the portal inflammation through the plate into the periportal parenchyma (Fig. 7.40). The limiting plate becomes irregular and may disappear as the portal area expands. Inflammatory cells surround and invade injured hepatocytes ("emperipolesis"). There may be evidence of hepatocellular degeneration and death, characterized by either acidophilic or ballooning degeneration. As in acute hepatitis, cell death occurs principally by the process of apoptosis, resulting in the formation of apoptotic or acidophilic bodies, which rapidly disappear from the liver plates or sinusoids. As chronic hepatitis progresses, there is continuous erosion of the hepatic parenchyma, with closer and closer approximation of the expanded portal areas, and small groups of hepatocytes ("hepatocytic islets") become trapped in expanded portal zones. The necroinflammatory changes are gradually succeeded by fibrosis, often best appreciated with a Masson or other collagen stain. Delicate collagen fibers laid down in areas of periportal liver cell loss eventually condense into scars. Interface hepatitis may not involve all the portal areas equally in a given biopsy specimen. It may affect either a segment or the entire perimeter of a portal area. Furthermore, even after cirrhosis has developed, interface hepatitis can continue unabated along the fibrous septa, causing further loss of parenchyma and, eventually, clinical decompensation of the cirrhosis.

Parenchymal injury, causing intra-acinar necroinflammatory changes, is present to some degree in most biopsy specimens from patients with any type of chronic hepatitis. This is typically multifocal ("spotty") in distribution and consists mainly of apoptosis, as in acute hepatitis. Scattered apoptotic bodies of varied size are observed, as well as focal aggregates of lymphocytes, plasma cells, and hypertrophied Kupffer cells that have scavenged the apoptotic bodies and other debris, producing lesions traditionally called *focal or spotty necrosis*. More severe intra-acinar injury is generally seen when the biopsy is performed during an acute exacerbation of the chronic hepatitis, even if the patient is asymptomatic. Changes typical of acute hepatitis, superimposed on those of chronic hepatitis, may include an increase in the degree of spotty necrosis; ballooning degeneration, often most severe in zone 3, with dropout of hepatocytes and central–central or central–portal bridging necrosis, especially in autoimmune hepatitis; variable cholestasis, often with associated periportal ductular proliferation and infiltration of the ductules by neutrophils; or (in extreme cases) multiacinar necrosis with stromal collapse. There is simultaneous regeneration of hepatocytes as cells are lost through apoptosis. This is typically seen in the form of two-cell thick plates and an increased number of bi- and trinucleated hepatocytes, but mitotic figures may occasionally be present. There may be some degree of steatosis – generally macrovesicular and of mild to moderate severity – most often in hepatitis C but also in chronic hepatitis of other causes.

Fibrosis is an almost invariable part of chronic hepatitis, although the degree of fibrous tissue deposition is quite variable from patient to patient. Fibrosis is the progressive component of the disease because it is the fibrous scarring that leads to architectural distortion and cirrhosis. It is thought that at least two pathways may lead to the fibrosis of chronic hepatitis. Probably most important in chronic viral hepatitis is the collagen deposition that accompanies the periportal injury of interface hepatitis, causing fibrous expansion of the portal tracts. As the disease progresses, portal–portal fibrous bridges

are formed, filling zone 1 between adjacent acini. There may also be the formation of central–portal and sometimes central–central fibrous bridges, which can develop from superimposed episodes of necrosis involving zone 3. In addition, it is likely that broad areas of fibrosis can result from the healing of bouts of multiacinar necrosis or from ischemic injury due to vascular damage secondary to the inflammation (see Chapter 5). In evaluating needle biopsies, it is important to distinguish tangential cuts through enlarged portal areas, which contain preexisting bile ducts and portal vessels, from true bridging fibrosis, which forms septa through parenchyma that had no preexisting fibrous tissue (Fig. 7.41). The scars of bridging fibrosis contain elastic fibers in addition to collagen. Like scars in any tissue, these tend to contract. Contraction of the fibrous septa in concert with nodular regeneration of the surviving parenchyma produces architectural distortion, and when complete nodules have formed, surrounded by fibrous septa, the result is the development of cirrhosis. Before the architecture is entirely obliterated, parts of the tissue are nodular while adjacent areas maintain an acinar structure, a state that can be regarded as an "incomplete" cirrhosis is present. When necroinflammatory changes continue along the septa and within the nodules, this may be considered to be active cirrhosis, or a term such as chronic hepatitis with cirrhosis may be used.

Morphology of chronic hepatitis due to different causes

There are several known causes of chronic hepatitis, and although the histopathologic features are similar, there are some noteworthy features that are more characteristic of one type than another. Parenterally transmitted forms of viral hepatitis, which account for at least 90% of cases, are discussed in detail in Chapters 24 and 25. Approximately 5–10% of chronic hepatitis is autoimmune (see Chapter 22). Drug-induced liver disease is a rare but well-documented cause of chronic hepatitis [23], and if the other known causes are excluded this should always be considered and evaluated clinically with a complete drug history. Metabolic diseases, such as Wilson disease, α_1-antitrypsin deficiency, and hemochromatosis, are sometimes listed in textbooks and reviews as causes of chronic hepatitis, but because these are usually readily distinguished from chronic hepatitis by liver biopsy and laboratory tests, they are considered separately in this chapter.

Hepatitis B

Hepatitis B can be diagnosed histologically and distinguished from other causes of chronic hepatitis by demonstration of the virus in tissue. HBsAg can be demonstrated by histochemical stains (orcein or Victoria blue, see Fig. 7.8) or the more sensitive immunostains

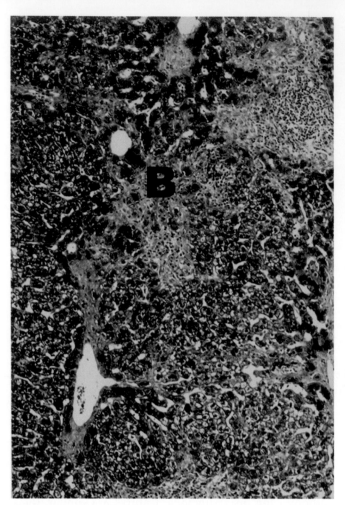 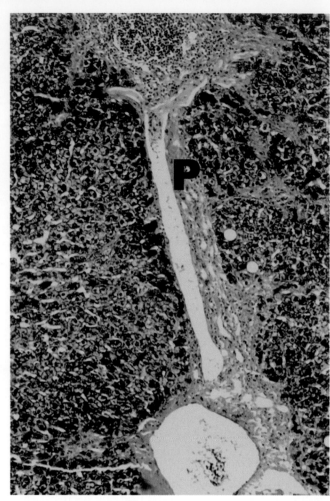

Figure 7.41 Bridging fibrosis (B) is scar tissue that forms across an area of parenchyma that had no preexisting fibrous tissue. It must be distinguished from tangential cuts through fibrotic preexisting portal areas (P), which contain bile ducts and arteries.

(see Fig. 7.13) in 80% or more cases of chronic hepatitis B. Cells containing large quantities of HBsAg have cytoplasm with a uniform, finely granular appearance, the so-called ground-glass cells (Fig. 7.42), which are scattered randomly through the liver, often occurring in clusters. The number of ground-glass cells tends to be inversely related to the activity of the hepatitis. Most cells are found in livers with the least active disease, whereas livers with the most activity tend to have the fewest ground-glass cells. In acute hepatitis B, the immune response eliminates antigen-containing cells and immunostains are entirely negative. Conversely, the presence of stainable surface antigen proves a chronic rather than an acute infection, even when there is severe hepatocellular injury. HBcAg can also usually be immunohistochemically demonstrated in nuclei, and often in cytoplasm when there is chronic disease in HBe-positive patients. The presence of core antigen reflects active viral replication, so the amount of core tends to be proportional to the activity of the hepatitis. Patients with recent acute

exacerbations will have the most core and will often have HBcAg in hepatocyte cytoplasm and in numerous nuclei; while after seroconversion to anti-HBe, no HBcAg is detectable. Strains of virus with precore mutations associated with increased disease severity occasionally have increased cytoplasmic core antigen, but most HBe-negative mutants with active disease have little or no HBcAg [37].

Hepatitis C

Hepatitis C virus (HCV) cannot currently be reliably demonstrated in routinely processed liver biopsies. There are, however, histologic features that are characteristic, although not pathognomonic, of chronic hepatitis C [34], and the finding of these features should prompt a serologic evaluation if not already done. Chronic hepatitis C tends to have more intense chronic portal inflammation than other types of chronic hepatitis, often with lymphoid aggregates and sometimes follicles with germinal centers (see Fig. 7.37). There is also a greater

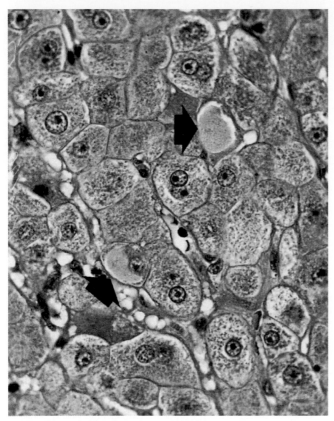

Figure 7.42 Ground-glass cells (arrows) in chronic hepatitis B. The cytoplasm of liver cells containing large quantities of hepatitis B surface antigen has a uniform finely granular appearance.

tendency toward hepatocellular fat accumulation than in other types. Approximately 50% of biopsy specimens have some fat, and in approximately 10% this may be considerable. Patients infected with genotype 3 tend to have even more fat, and it is suggested that this may be due to a cytopathic effect [38]. Hepatitis-associated bile duct lesions (see preceding text) may be found in acute or chronic hepatitis of any cause, but they are most frequent in hepatitis C. Severe degrees of bile duct injury can be seen in approximately 10–15% of biopsy specimens from patients with chronic hepatitis C (see Fig. 7.39). Lesser degrees of duct irregularity and lymphocytic infiltration can be found more often.

Hepatitis D

Hepatitis D can only infect individuals who are also infected with HBV, which serves as an obligatory helper. Simultaneous coinfection with HBV and hepatitis δ virus (HDV) tends to cause more severe disease than HBV alone, with a higher likelihood of fulminant hepatitis. HDV superinfection of a person with previous chronic HBV infection often causes an acute exacerbation of the underlying chronic hepatitis or deterioration in the clin-

ical status of a previously stable patient, or it may cause fulminant liver failure. Morphologically, HDV superimposed on HBV tends to produce more severe disease than hepatitis B alone, but there are no features that specifically implicate hepatitis D [39]. The only way to histologically prove the presence of the virus is to demonstrate δ-antigen in the hepatocyte nuclei by immunohistochemical staining (although commercial antibodies are not widely available) or to detect antibodies to δ-antigen in the blood.

Autoimmune hepatitis

Autoimmune hepatitis tends to be a very severe chronic hepatitis, often with multiacinar collapse and/or cirrhosis at the time of presentation. Numerous plasma cells are often seen in the portal inflammatory infiltrate (see Fig. 7.38). About one third of cases have an acute onset, and, typically, there is severe acute hepatitis-like hepatocellular injury, often with diffuse ballooning of hepatocytes, regeneration with hepatocyte rosette formation, and sometimes confluent zone 3 hepatocellular necrosis [29]. Extensive giant cell transformation [40] is seen in some cases, which have been called postinfantile giant cell hepatitis or syncytial giant cell hepatitis.

Recurrent chronic hepatitis after liver transplantation

Recurrent chronic hepatitis after liver transplantation may resemble the original disease or may have atypical features. Hepatitis B, before antiviral therapy became established as standard post-transplantation therapy, virtually always recurred and in many cases caused a severe, rapidly progressive disease in immunosuppressed patients. The term fibrosing cholestatic hepatitis was proposed for this form of hepatitis B [41]. Liver biopsy specimens show numerous ground-glass hepatocytes with massive amounts of intracellular HBsAg and HBcAg, and it is thought that this represents a cytopathic form of viral infection, in contrast to the usual chronic hepatitis B. As the disease progresses, there is portal and diffuse pericellular fibrosis, hepatocyte dropout, and, in the late stages, nodular regeneration, producing cirrhosis (Fig. 7.43). Cholestasis in the tissue may be severe, but patients typically have elevated serum bilirubin concentrations even when bile pigment is histologically inapparent, hence the "cholestatic" part of the name. Hepatitis C also recurs, but most patients have histologic features of typical chronic hepatitis. Occasionally, however, patients display features of fibrosing cholestatic hepatitis, except for ground-glass cells [42]. It is not clear whether the pathogenesis is the same as that for hepatitis B. Both hepatitis B and C occasionally produce the pattern of fibrosing cholestatic hepatitis in patients who have not undergone liver transplantations but are immunosuppressed or immunodeficient for other reasons [43].

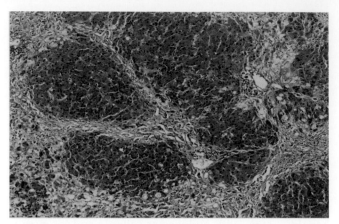

Figure 7.43 Recurrent hepatitis B with fibrosing cholestatic hepatitis progressing to cirrhosis 1 year after liver transplantation. The surviving hepatocytes have abundant cytoplasmic hepatitis B surface antigen, producing a ground-glass appearance, and there is canalicular bile stasis.

Grading and staging of chronic hepatitis

The stage of any disease is a measure of how far it has progressed in its natural history, with the end stage resulting in death of the patient or failure of the organ. The grade of the disease is meant to reflect how quickly the disease is progressing to the end stage. In chronic hepatitis the end stage is cirrhosis with clinical decompensation, whereas earlier stages have lesser degrees of fibrosis or cirrhosis. The grade is considered to be the degree of inflammation and hepatocellular injury, which is thought to lead to fibrosis.

The old terminology classified chronic hepatitis as "chronic persistent hepatitis," implying a benign, nonprogressive disease, or "chronic active hepatitis," implying a disease with a high likelihood of progression to cirrhosis, and was a form of grading. Advances in understanding the causes and elucidating the natural history of the diseases that produce this type of liver injury have rendered this terminology obsolete.

There are several methods, currently in use, of expressing the grade and stage of chronic hepatitis. These can be grouped into: (i) those that are simple verbal descriptions; (ii) those that are relatively simple numeric grades and stages that correspond to the verbal descriptions; and (iii) those that use more complicated numeric scoring of histologic features to generate numbers that correspond to the grade and stage. Each method has advantages and disadvantages, and the system used should be appropriate to its suitability for the task at hand. In general, more complex systems have the capability to provide more information than simple ones but are less reproducible.

For routine diagnosis and patient management a simple system of grading and staging is preferred, and the guidelines proposed by a panel of experts convened by the International Association for the Study of the Liver (IASL) in 1994 [44] are recommended. Grading of chronic hepatitis is accomplished by deciding whether the degree of activity is mild, moderate, or marked. The principal features used to determine grade are the degree of periportal interface hepatitis and spotty parenchymal injury (Table 7.1). Interface hepatitis is mild when one must search to find any in the biopsy specimen; moderate when most portal areas have some interface hepatitis, but it extends around less than 50% of the circumference in the majority; and marked when most portal areas have interface hepatitis extending around more than 50% of the circumference. Parenchymal injury is most easily graded using the 10× (medium power) objective of the microscope with the usual 10× ocular lens. At this magnification it is possible to detect acidophilic bodies, ballooned hepatocytes, and clusters of inflammatory cells at sites of focal necrosis, and it is relatively easy to estimate the amount of injury and form an overall impression of the degree of injury. Parenchymal injury can be considered mild when fewer than five injured cells or clusters of inflammatory cells are seen per 10× field; moderate when there are 5–20 cells; and marked when there are more than 20 cells per 10× field. Portal inflammation can also be considered, but this is more a sign of chronicity than of activity. In grading the overall activity, the chronic hepatitis can be considered as

Table 7.1 Grading activity in chronic hepatitis.

Grade	Interface hepatitis	Parenchymal injury[a]	Activity
Mild	Found only after diligent search	<5 per 10× field	*Both* interface hepatitis and parenchymal injury are *mild* or less
Moderate	Most portal areas have at least some, but most have <50% of circumference	5–20 per 10× field	*Either* interface hepatitis or parenchymal injury is *moderate*
Marked	>50% of circumference of most portal areas	>20 per 10× field	*Either* interface hepatitis or parenchymal injury is *marked*

[a] Apoptotic bodies, ballooned cells, and inflammatory cell aggregates.

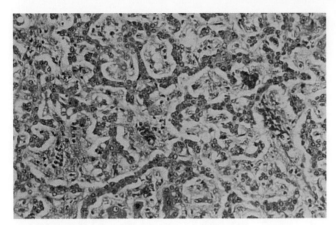

Figure 7.46 Reactive ductules at the margin of an edematous, inflamed portal tract.

in bile ducts [53,54]. Ductules, which are usually more angulated than bile ducts, become prominent and appear to proliferate in response to a variety of injuries [55]. Neutrophils are commonly situated in and around the reactive ductules, but this does not have the same significance as acute cholangitis, which is characterized by neutrophils in or around the acinar bile duct (Fig. 7.47) and

is highly suggestive (but not pathognomonic) of mechanical biliary obstruction. Cholangitis may be present without histologic bile stasis, depending on the degree of obstruction; bile pigment is not usually found without complete obstruction, but acute cholangitis indicates a high likelihood of an obstruction being present. Bile pigment, when present, is seen first in acinar zone 3 and later in zones 2 and 1 as jaundice becomes more profound. Rarely, there is bile in the lumina or epithelium of the acinar bile ducts (see Fig. 7.45), but when present this strongly suggests the presence of obstruction. Other frequent findings include ductular reaction with associated acute inflammation, neutrophilic infiltration of the portal tracts, and bile duct epithelial irregularity or hyperplasia. Severe acute cholangitis is occasionally complicated by rupture, with the development of cholangitic abscesses in the region of the affected bile ducts (Fig. 7.48). Remnants of the disrupted biliary epithelium, bile, and mucin are often located within the abscesses. Xanthomatous cells and foreign body giant cells with phagocytosed bile may also be present. Bile lakes, due to extravasation of bile, and bile infarcts may be seen when there is duct rupture in advanced cases (Fig. 7.49).

Although an acute cholangitis most often denotes extrahepatic biliary tract disease with an ascending

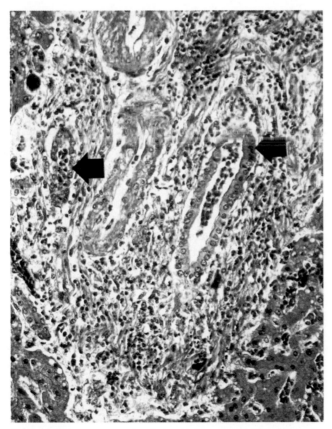

Figure 7.47 Acute suppurative cholangitis in a patient with mechanical biliary obstruction. The portal area is edematous and contains many neutrophils. Neutrophils are present in the lumina of two bile ducts (arrows).

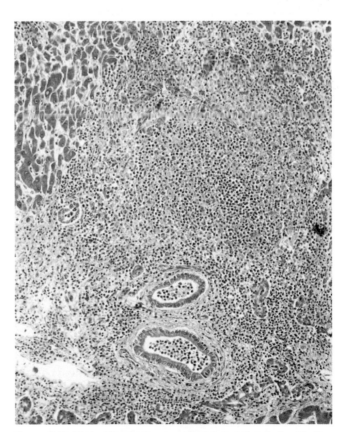

Figure 7.48 Cholangitic abscess, secondary to ascending cholangitis. The two bile ducts at the bottom of the field are filled with neutrophils.

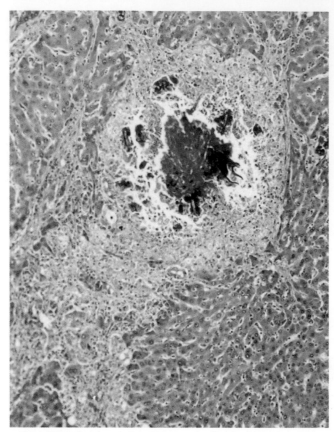

Figure 7.49 Bile lake secondary to rupture of a duct and extravasation of bile in mechanical obstruction.

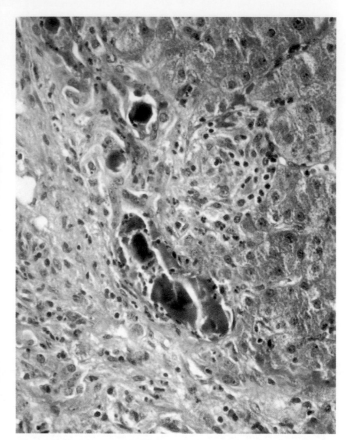

Figure 7.50 "Bile ductular cholestasis." The periportal ductules are markedly dilated and filled with bile in a patient with bacterial sepsis.

infection, there are rare nonobstructive causes, including toxic shock syndrome, several toxins (e.g., paraquat, methylene diamine, and the toxin of toxic oil syndrome), and a number of drugs (e.g., chlorpromazine, allopurinol, and amoxicillin–clavulanate) [56].

Bile ductular cholestasis

Neutrophils may also be associated with inspissated bile in dilated periportal ductules (Fig. 7.50), a lesion called bile ductular cholestasis [57]. This lesion is sometimes seen in severely ill patients with sepsis and/or dehydration [57,58], but like other forms of ductular reaction, it does not necessarily indicate mechanical biliary obstruction.

Chronic cholestasis

Clinical and histologic features of chronic cholestasis appear when there is impaired flow of bile that persists for more than a few weeks. However, most chronic cholestatic disorders are insidious in onset, and chronic cholestasis progresses slowly over the course of years before it becomes clinically apparent. The most reliable histologic sign of chronic cholestasis is the lesion known as cholate stasis [53], which is also called pseudoxan-

thomatous change, xanthomatous change, or feathery degeneration. These terms refer to a foamy transformation of the cytoplasm of hepatocytes, Kupffer cells, and biliary epithelial cells, which is seen when there is any type of prolonged (chronic) cholestasis (Fig. 7.51). The affected cells are foamy and often bile stained, as a result of the accumulation of the bile salt and lipid components of bile. Other changes seen in chronic cholestasis include periportal bile pigment, copper accumulation demonstrated with special stains for copper (rhodanine) or by staining for the copper-binding protein, a metallothionein protein within lysosomes (Victoria blue stain) and, in some cases, periportal Mallory bodies. Although there are a number of causes of chronic cholestasis, the most frequent are PBC (see Chapter 21) and primary sclerosing cholangitis (see Chapter 20). Furthermore, in patients who have undergone liver transplantation, allograft rejection can produce bile duct damage and loss, leading to chronic cholestasis.

Primary biliary cirrhosis

The diagnosis of PBC is usually made on the basis of a constellation of clinical, serologic, and histologic

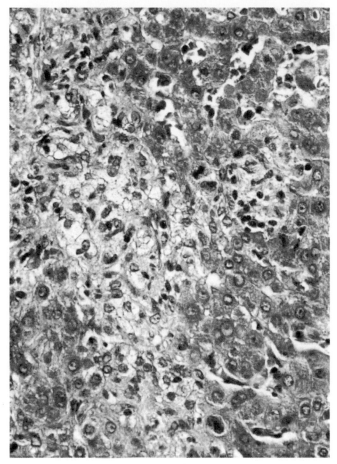

Figure 7.51 Cholate stasis, indicating chronic cholestasis. The affected cells have pale, foamy cytoplasm because of bile lipid retention.

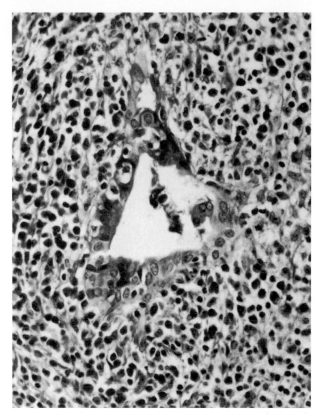

Figure 7.52 Florid duct lesion of early primary biliary cirrhosis. The ductal epithelium is infiltrated with inflammatory cells (predominantly lymphocytes), the epithelial cells are severely injured, and the basement membrane is ruptured.

findings. In a patient known to have a positive antimitochondrial antibody (AMA), liver biopsy is usually performed to confirm the diagnosis and assess the stage of disease. In a patient who has not had a complete workup or in whom the AMA is negative, the biopsy may still be diagnostic of the disease.

In patients with clinical and laboratory features of chronic cholestasis, particular attention paid to the condition of the acinar bile ducts is critical in histologic evaluation. Ducts affected by PBC show variable chronic inflammation and epithelial injury that lead to destruction of the duct, a lesion called chronic nonsuppurative destructive cholangitis [59] or the florid duct lesion [60]. It is this immunologically mediated destruction of ducts that initiates the disease. Lymphocytes and plasma cells penetrate the basement membrane and insinuate themselves between the epithelial cells, causing destruction of epithelial cells (Figs 7.52 and 7.53) and segments of the basement membrane. Eosinophils and even some neutrophils (despite the fact that it is called *nonsuppurative*) may be present, but it is the lymphocytes that appear to be the

primary effectors of the injury. Well-developed lymphoid follicles, sometimes with germinal centers, may be found around or adjacent to the degenerating bile ducts. Epithelioid granulomas (Fig. 7.53), typically less well organized than those of sarcoidosis, are located in the portal areas adjacent to or surrounding the bile ducts, or less often in the parenchyma, in approximately one third of the cases.

Florid duct lesions are generally considered to be pathognomonic of PBC [53,59–61], but they must be distinguished from the hepatitis-associated bile duct lesions (see Fig. 7.39) discussed above under chronic hepatitis. This is most easily accomplished by searching for the features that accompany the destruction of ducts in PBC, namely ductopenia and chronic cholestasis. In chronic hepatitis, the loss of ducts is rare and chronic cholestatic features do not develop. The degree of cholangitis in PBC varies greatly from one portal tract to another. Some ducts can appear completely normal, whereas others exhibit striking inflammation and epithelial injury. Therefore, the active diagnostic lesion can be absent in small biopsy samples, and the pathologist is then compelled to apply other criteria and clinical data to the evaluation.

The number of portal tracts lacking acinar bile ducts should be estimated. With the exception of premature

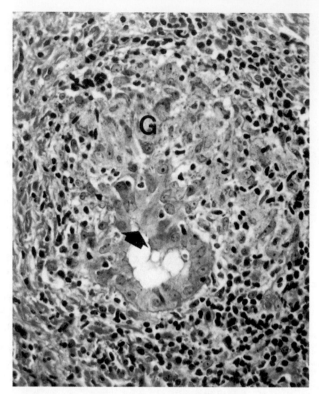

Figure 7.53 Florid duct lesions of early primary biliary cirrhosis. The duct has ruptured (arrow), and there is a poorly formed epithelioid cell granuloma (G) adjacent to the damaged duct.

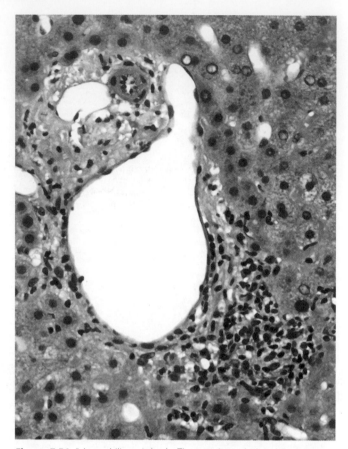

Figure 7.54 Primary biliary cirrhosis. The portal area lacks a bile duct (ductopenia).

infants, a normal liver has a ratio of bile ducts to portal areas of 0.9 or greater [62], usually with the acinar duct running parallel to the hepatic artery branch. In most patients with PBC, more than half of the portal tracts lack bile ducts (i.e., ductopenia) (Fig. 7.54), and it is only in the earliest stages that there are no portal areas with missing ducts. Also helpful is the frequent presence of periportal bile pigment and cholate stasis (see Fig. 7.51). These changes are often subtle and must be sought with care. Small to moderate amounts of copper-binding protein (stainable with Victoria blue) and copper (on rhodanine stain) are frequently detected in hepatocytes in the periportal area (see Fig. 7.7). Periportal (zone 1) Mallory bodies, found in 10–15% of cases, are further evidence of chronic cholestasis. These are identical to the Mallory bodies of alcoholic and nonalcoholic steatohepatitis except for their location – the Mallory bodies of steatohepatitis are in zone 3.

Ductular reaction can be prominent in PBC, particularly in the surrounding portal areas that lack acinar bile ducts. Care must be taken to distinguish the ductules from bile ducts. Hepatocytes are relatively spared, but there is invariably some element of interface hepatitis ("piecemeal necrosis") and hepatitis-like parenchymal injury [61,63]. Some investigators have distinguished what they call "biliary piecemeal necrosis," seen in areas

of cholate stasis, from "lymphocytic piecemeal necrosis" that is typical of chronic hepatitis [64], but in this author's experience, these occur together so often that the distinction is not meaningful. There are cases in which the biopsy specimen shows so much hepatocellular injury and interface hepatitis that an overlap syndrome of PBC and autoimmune hepatitis is considered [65,66]. In such cases, the clinical and laboratory findings may also suggest both disease processes. However, it is the loss of bile ducts and chronic cholestatic injury that is more significant because bile ducts do not regenerate as readily as hepatocytes. Since it is chronic cholestasis that leads to cirrhosis in these patients, the overlap syndrome is best considered to be a hepatitic form of PBC [67].

Primary sclerosing cholangitis

Primary sclerosing cholangitis usually involves the entire biliary tract, but there are occasional cases that affect only extrahepatic or intrahepatic ducts. The extrahepatic ducts are thick and cord-like and have a narrowed lumen. Histologically, a variety of changes may be seen, depending in part on the integrity of the ductal system draining the biopsied area. Changes in the parenchyma are largely due

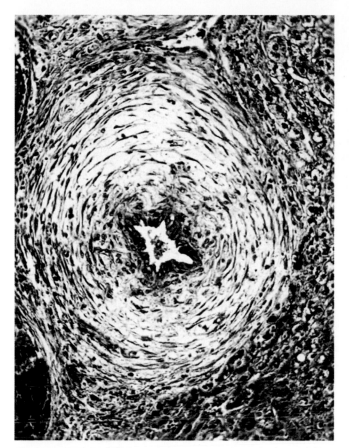

Figure 7.55 Primary sclerosing cholangitis. Note the marked periductal fibrosis with compression and atrophy of the epithelium.

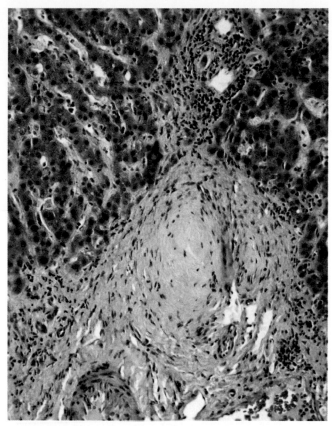

Figure 7.56 Primary sclerosing cholangitis. The acinar bile duct is replaced by a fibrous nodule.

to incomplete chronic mechanical biliary obstruction. Bile pigment is often minimal or absent because obstruction is rarely complete. Clues to the diagnosis can be observed in the portal areas. Some acinar bile ducts may show marked periductal fibrosis with prominent compression and distortion of the epithelium (Fig. 7.55). The epithelium may be almost unidentifiable or even completely atrophic, while a small nodule (cross-section of a cord) of fibrous tissue remains in its place (Fig. 7.56). The basement membrane is intact and often thickened. The bile ducts still may be present, but they are often reduced in number or may be totally absent, depending on the stage of the disease. Ductular proliferation is relatively mild compared with that seen in other types of biliary obstruction. Chronic cholestatic features, with cholate stasis and copper accumulation, become increasingly prominent as the disease progresses and may render its distinction from PBC difficult. Furthermore, granulomas, considered a typical feature of PBC, are occasionally present in primary sclerosing cholangitis [68]. However, periductal fibrosis is not a typical feature of PBC, while florid duct lesions, in particular the destruction of the basement membrane, are not observed in sclerosing cholangitis.

Fibrosis follows the loss of bile ducts in both sclerosing cholangitis and PBC, although the mechanism is not clear. In PBC, at least, both ductular proliferation and interface hepatitis, accompanied by collagen deposition, appear to be important [69], but the possible roles of other factors related to chronic cholestasis have not been studied in detail. The fibrosis extends progressively with portal–portal bridging and septum formation, eventually with nodule formation and development of a micronodular biliary cirrhosis indistinguishable from that caused by chronic mechanical obstruction (Fig. 7.57). Staging of disease, if requested, is best accomplished by estimating the degree of fibrosis because any combination of histologic lesions can be found in an individual biopsy specimen. Ludwig suggested four stages for both PBC [70] and sclerosing cholangitis [71]: stage I (portal), stage II (periportal), stage III (septal), and stage IV (cirrhosis). Early stage, mid stage, and late stage are also acceptable terms, although they sound less scientific.

Allograft rejection

Acute (cellular) rejection is an immunologically mediated attack of the host's defenses against the engrafted liver. The principal targets of the attack are the bile ducts and

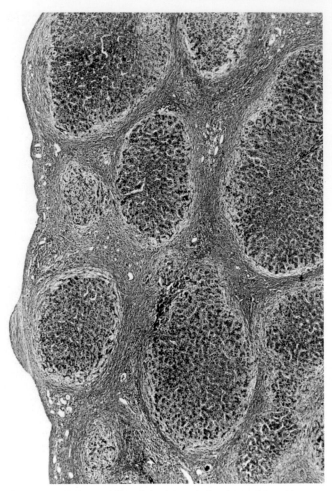

Figure 7.57 End-stage biliary cirrhosis is typically micronodular with chronic cholestatic features in the residual parenchyma and thick bands of collagen between the nodules, imparting a "jigsaw" pattern to the tissue. Bile ducts are absent.

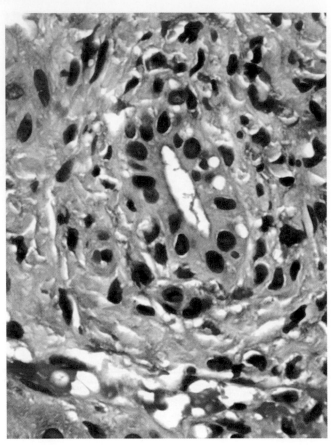

Figure 7.58 Acute cellular allograft rejection. The bile duct is damaged by a lymphoplamacytic inflammatory infiltrate.

the endothelium of veins and arteries but not of sinusoids. Snover's triad, consisting of mixed portal inflammation (involving lymphocytes, plasma cells, neutrophils, and eosinophils), bile duct damage (Fig. 7.58) (e.g., rejection cholangitis), and endothelialitis (usually affecting portal vein branches and sometimes the central veins, in the form of lymphocytes attached to the luminal surface of the endothelial cells or between the cell and its basement membrane), is considered diagnostic of rejection [72]. These features are variable, and diagnostic findings may or may not present on any individual liver biopsy, so the presence of two of the three features is usually considered sufficient for diagnosis. Cholestasis, hepatocyte ballooning, apoptotic or acidophilic bodies, and focal necrosis may also be present.

Chronic (ductopenic) rejection refers to the irreversible damage to the engrafted liver through a combination of immunologically mediated injury and ischemia. It typically follows repeated episodes of acute rejection and so

is usually not diagnosed until at least several months after transplantation. Rapidly progressive cases are sometimes seen (acute vanishing bile duct syndrome) but are uncommon. The changes of chronic rejection are thought to be partly due to the injury associated with repeated acute rejection and partly due to reduced arterial flow caused by foam cell arteriopathy in the large arteries of the graft. Bile ducts require an arterial blood supply, so the loss of the arteries contributes to the loss of ducts. Changes of chronic rejection include bile duct atrophy and pyknosis, loss of bile ducts (ductopenia) with or without loss of hepatic artery branches, and foam cell arteriopathy in larger arteries, particularly those near the hilum [73]. The loss of ducts produces features of chronic cholestasis, and zone 3 fibrosis may also occur because of ischemia.

Other chronic cholestatic syndromes

- *Mechanical obstruction*: any of the microscopic changes observed in acute biliary obstruction may be present in biopsy specimens from patients with longstanding obstruction. Additional changes that point to the chronic nature of the process commonly develop when obstruction persists for more than a few weeks. These include periductal sclerosis, cholate stasis, periportal bile stasis, copper accumulation, and sometimes Mallory body formation. Bile becomes inspissated, appearing dark olive green and laminated in sections. Loss of hepatocytes in zone 1 contributes to periportal fibrosis. Cirrhosis may develop when complete or nearly complete obstruction persists for many months, but most patients will be relieved of the obstruction or will develop complications and death before cirrhosis ensues. Biliary cirrhosis is histologically characterized by fibrous septa, linking portal tracts and outlining irregular islands of parenchyma that resemble the pieces of a jigsaw puzzle (see Fig. 7.57).

- *Extrahepatic biliary atresia* in the neonate is more likely to produce secondary biliary cirrhosis than other causes of mechanical obstruction. In this condition, all the morphologic features of acute and chronic biliary obstruction described in the preceding text can be observed, depending on the stage during which a biopsy specimen is obtained. The same criteria for the diagnosis of biliary obstruction, described in the preceding text, must be used to differentiate biliary atresia from other cholestatic disorders of the neonate and infant. Some degree of portal fibrosis and ductular proliferation are usually present in biliary atresia and help in distinguishing it from neonatal hepatitis. Diagnostic difficulty may be caused by the presence of giant cell transformation, suggesting hepatocellular injury, in some cases of biliary atresia, but giant cell transformation in neonates should be considered a nonspecific pattern of injury, induced by a variety of hepatic and extrahepatic disorders.

- *Sarcoidosis* sometimes causes a syndrome of chronic intrahepatic cholestasis that can mimic PBC or primary sclerosing cholangitis in many clinical, biochemical, and histologic aspects [74]. In such cases, the liver develops confluent granulomas that destroy bile ducts, cause chronic cholestasis, and may lead to biliary cirrhosis. Although depletion of bile ducts is characteristic, florid duct lesions are uncommon. Granulomatous inflammation in the liver can be found in portal, periportal, and parenchymal areas in the active phase of the syndrome, and the granulomas are better formed and a more dominant feature than those in PBC (Fig. 7.59).

- *Secondary sclerosing cholangitis* with features nearly identical to primary sclerosing cholangitis may follow mechanical obstruction from a variety of causes, such as surgical manipulation of the biliary tract or tumors of the extrahepatic ducts. Secondary sclerosing cholangitis may also follow chemical injury, such as intra-arterial injection of floxuridine to treat metastatic colon cancer [75] or the injection of formalin into hydatid cysts. Langerhans cell histiocytosis occasionally affects bile

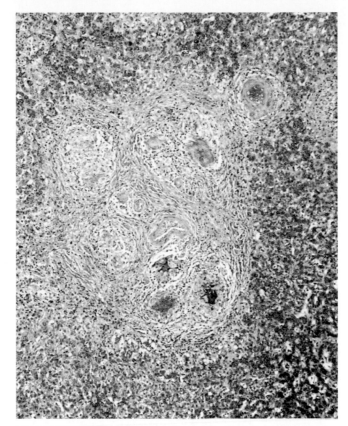

Figure 7.59 Chronic cholestatic syndrome of sarcoidosis. This portal area has several granulomas and considerable fibrosis but lacks a bile duct.

ducts, causing ductal destruction and secondary sclerosing cholangitis [76].

- *Acquired immunodeficiency syndrome (AIDS) cholangiopathy* is a form of secondary sclerosing cholangitis that follows some biliary tract infections such as cryptosporidiosis or CMV in patients with AIDS [77].

- *Drug-induced chronic cholestasis* is an uncommon complication of acute drug injury. A patient with this syndrome develops jaundice, often severe, that does not fully resolve, producing a disorder with some degree of histologic, biochemical, and clinical resemblance to PBC but not with the insidious onset of the idiopathic forms of chronic cholestasis described in the preceding text. In the early stage there is an acute cholangitis, while biopsy specimens in the later stages show ductopenia and chronic cholestatic features [78].

- *Paucity of intrahepatic bile ducts* is a term used for congenital diseases that produce chronic cholestasis associated, as the name implies, with absence of the small acinar ("interlobular") ducts [79]. The best defined of these is arteriohepatic dysplasia or Alagille syndrome. Bile ducts are present at birth but undergo progressive destruction from early infancy to childhood. In later childhood, there is paucity or absence of acinar bile

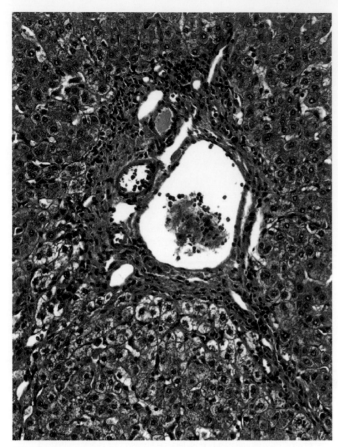

Figure 7.60 Paucity of intrahepatic ducts (Alagille syndrome). This medium-sized, fibrotic portal area lacks a bile duct, but there is very little inflammation or cholestatic features.

ducts (Fig. 7.60), paradoxically with mild cholestatic features [80,81]. Despite the lack of ducts, it is rare to see bile stasis, and progressive fibrosis or cirrhosis is uncommon. By contrast, children who have bile duct paucity without the other anomalies of Alagille syndrome tend to have a much worse disease, often with progression to end-stage liver disease. Such cases are usually idiopathic but are thought to result from various types of in utero injuries that prevent the normal development of acinar ducts, resulting in a diminished number of ducts at birth.

- *Idiopathic adulthood ductopenia* is a term that is suggested for the rare patient who has a chronic cholestatic syndrome with progressive bile duct loss but does not fit into one of the entities listed in the preceding text [82].

Steatosis (fatty liver)

Steatosis can be subclassified into two broad morphologic categories – macrovesicular and microvesicular – on the basis of the size of the fat vacuoles in the liver cells. The distinction is not always sharp, and there are cases where both macrovesicular and microvesicular fat

coexist. In general, steatosis is considered macrovesicular when the hepatocytes contain a single large fat vacuole that displaces the nucleus to the edge of the cell, whereas the steatosis is microvesicular when there are numerous small cytoplasmic fat vacuoles that tend to leave the nuclei centrally placed within the hepatocytes. In routinely processed material, the lipid is dissolved by organic solvents, so frozen sections with special stains (e.g., oil red O) are necessary to confirm its presence in cases where there is doubt.

Macrovesicular steatosis is a reaction to a wide variety of injuries, many of which are subclinical and might be more properly regarded as a physiologic adaptation manifested as an imbalance between the uptake of lipids from the blood and the secretion of lipoproteins by the hepatocyte. Most affected hepatocytes contain a single, medium-sized or large, rounded vacuole that displaces the nucleus and cytoplasm to the periphery of the cell (Fig. 7.61). The vacuoles can be as large as or larger than a normal hepatocyte. Conditions often associated with macrovesicular steatosis include malnutrition, diabetes mellitus, obesity, malabsorption, various debilitating

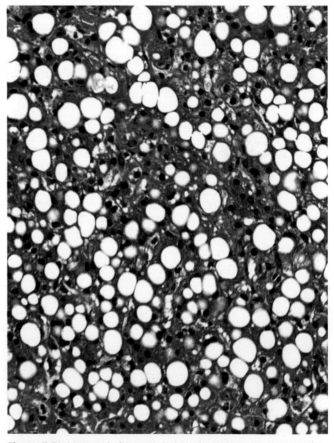

Figure 7.61 Macrovesicular steatosis. Most hepatocytes contain a single, large, rounded vacuole that displaces the nucleus and cytoplasm to the periphery of the cell.

disorders, some metabolic diseases, corticosteroid therapy, and exposure to various other drugs and toxins. Steatosis can be the only change, or it may be associated with other lesions. For example, in chronic hepatitis C, there is often macrovesicular steatosis associated with the other changes described in the preceding text. Steatohepatitis (alcoholic or nonalcoholic), several metabolic diseases (e.g., Wilson disease), and drug-induced injury (e.g., methotrexate) may be associated with fat accumulation, along with other lesions characteristic of the disease. The location of the fat is quite variable; it is usually diffuse but can be predominantly in zone 1 or 3.

Microvesicular steatosis generally connotes a more serious injury than macrovesicular steatosis, although it has been shown that this is a frequent nonspecific finding, especially in autopsy material [83,84]. Consequently, a diagnosis of one of the diseases characterized by microvesicular steatosis cannot be made without compatible clinical and laboratory findings. Hepatocytes with microvesicular steatosis show a central nucleus surrounded by sharply defined small vacuoles (Fig. 7.62). Acute fatty liver of pregnancy [85] and Reye syndrome

[86] are well-recognized causes of microvesicular steatosis. A number of metabolic diseases, including fatty acid oxidation disorders, mitochondrial oxidation chain disorders, and urea cycle disorders, are associated with microvesicular steatosis and can mimic Reye syndrome to varying degrees [87,88]. Toxic injury from drugs such as tetracycline, aspirin, valproic acid, antiretroviral nucleoside analogs, and fialuridine can also produce microvesicular steatosis [50,89–91]. Alcoholic liver injury can also occasionally lead to a toxic microvesicular steatosis, a lesion called alcoholic foamy degeneration [92]. South American epidemics of hepatitis D and B coinfection are found to have marked microvesicular steatosis [93] for unknown reasons. Other forms of viral hepatitis, both acute and chronic, may have some degree of microvesicular steatosis, especially if frozen sections and oil red O stains are used to demonstrate its presence. However, in general, fat stains should be reserved for situations in which there is a high clinical suspicion of one of the diseases in which microvesicular steatosis is a cardinal feature, such as acute fatty liver of pregnancy.

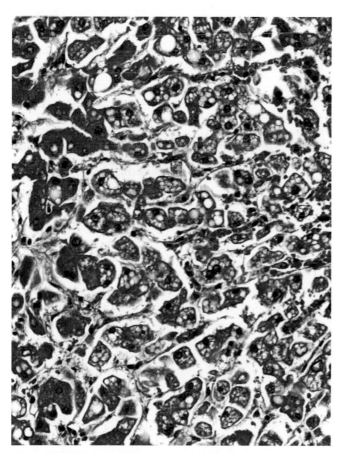

Figure 7.62 Microvesicular steatosis in acute fatty liver of pregnancy. Hepatocytes have a central nucleus surrounded by numerous small fat vacuoles.

Steatohepatitis: alcoholic hepatitis and nonalcoholic (metabolic) steatohepatitis

Steatohepatitis

Steatohepatitis is the term used for the morphologic pattern of injury characteristic of the active phase of alcoholic liver disease. Synonyms include alcoholic steatonecrosis, sclerosing hyaline necrosis, and alcoholic hepatitis, when it is found in persons who consume large quantities of alcohol, and fatty liver hepatitis, metabolic steatohepatitis, and nonalcoholic steatohepatitis, when it occurs in nondrinkers. Because the morphology is so similar, regardless of cause, the term *steatohepatitis* is used here when the lesion is referred to, and alcoholic hepatitis or nonalcoholic steatohepatitis is used for the clinicopathologic entities. Because the pathologist is often unaware of the pertinent clinical information, a diagnosis of steatohepatitis is acceptable until it is known whether the patient consumes alcohol. In patients who are alcoholic, it is presumed that the liver disease represents direct toxicity from ethanol. In those who do not drink, the pathogenesis of the liver disease remains obscure and seems most likely to represent some form of metabolic (probably genetic) disease related to obesity with insulin resistance and/or diabetes (see Chapter 32). It should be emphasized that every liver biopsy specimen with fat and inflammation is not steatohepatitis, despite the name. For example, a patient with preexisting steatosis may have hepatitis-like spotty necrosis and inflammation from an unrecognized drug, undiagnosed virus, or oxidative stress of other unknown cause, but this is not considered steatohepatitis. Only when there are other changes, as described in the subsequent text, is the term steatohepatitis appropriate.

Steatohepatitis, whatever the cause, is a chronic lesion that predominantly affects acinar zone 3 [94]. Microscopically, this is characterized by a constellation of features that vary in degree and extent from patient to patient. In addition to steatosis (usually macrovesicular but sometimes microvesicular or "mixed"), as noted in the preceding text, there is ballooning of liver cells, most prominently in zone 3. Globular cytoplasmic inclusions, representing enlarged, damaged mitochondria, may be present, as well as Mallory–Denk bodies.

Mallory–Denk bodies represent a form of cellular injury that results from a derangement of the intermediate filament component of the cytoskeleton of liver cells [95]. These filaments, which can be seen by electron microscopy (Fig. 7.63), have been shown to be composed of cytokeratin proteins, both those that are normally found in hepatocytes (types 8 and 18) and other types of keratin, mixed with unidentified high molecular weight components and coated with the heat shock protein, ubiquitin, and the regulatory protein, p62. The presence of Mallory–Denk bodies can induce a neutrophilic inflammatory cell response (Fig. 7.64); sometimes a ring of neutrophils surrounds the damaged cell ("satellitosis").

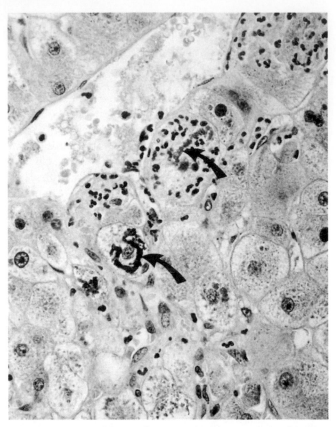

Figure 7.64 Neutrophilic "satellitosis." In this immunostain for ubiquitin, the dark-staining Mallory–Denk bodies (arrows) have incited a neutrophilic inflammatory cell response.

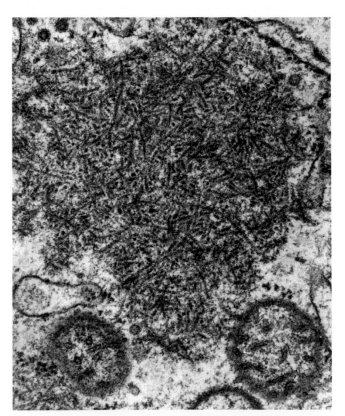

Figure 7.63 Ultrastructural appearance of a Mallory–Denk body. It consists of a tangled mass of intermediate filaments.

Neutrophils migrate into liver cells containing Mallory–Denk bodies, and their degranulation is one of the major factors contributing to the hepatocellular damage. Steatosis resolves within 3–4 weeks of abstinence from alcohol, while Mallory–Denk bodies may take months to disappear. Mallory–Denk bodies are eosinophilic and may be short and irregular or long and rope-like. The cytoplasm around large Mallory–Denk bodies is typically empty or rarified due to hepatocellular ballooning (Fig. 7.65), but sometimes it remains eosinophilic and granular (Fig. 7.66), making the inclusion hard to detect. In mild cases the small Mallory–Denk bodies may be few and particularly hard to see (Fig. 7.67), so immunostains for ubiquitin (see Figs 7.12, 7.64, 7.68) or p62 protein are particularly helpful in this setting. When Mallory–Denk bodies cannot be found despite diligent search, the diagnosis is less certain, but the presence of fat, hepatocellular ballooning, and pericellular fibrosis, described next, strongly suggests steatohepatitis. This is particularly helpful in biopsies from patients with nonalcoholic steatohepatitis, because they tend to have fewer Mallory–Denk bodies and less severe active injury than patients with clinical alcoholic hepatitis [96].

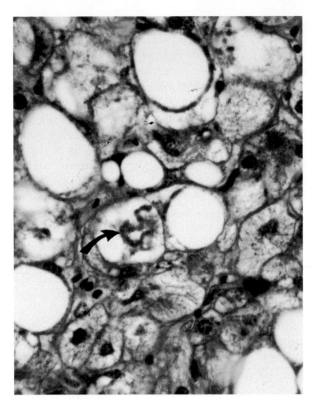

Figure 7.65 A Mallory–Denk body (arrow) in a ballooned hepatocyte is easily detected by routine microscopic examination.

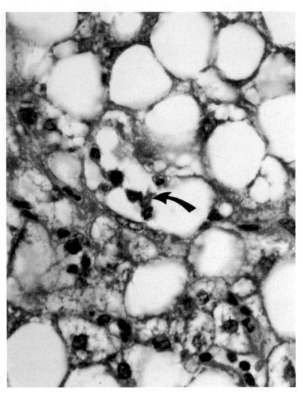

Figure 7.67 Mallory–Denk bodies (arrow) in a case of mild nonalcoholic steatohepatitis. The Mallory–Denk bodies in this case are all small and thin, making them difficult to find. Note the two neutrophils adjacent to the Mallory–Denk body.

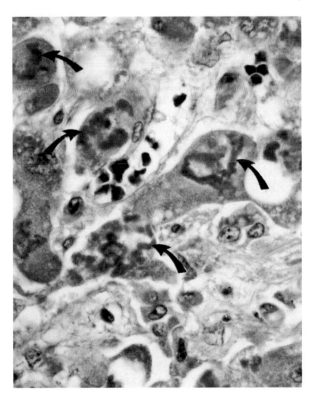

Figure 7.66 Mallory–Denk bodies (arrows) in this case of alcoholic hepatitis are less easily seen because the hepatocytes are not as ballooned, but heavy eosin staining brings them out.

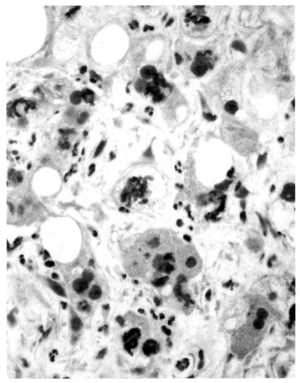

Figure 7.68 Numerous Mallory–Denk bodies in this case of alcoholic hepatitis are easily seen with the immunostain for ubiquitin.

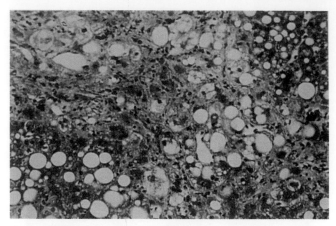

Figure 7.69 Steatohepatitis with early pericellular ("chicken-wire") fibrosis in acinar zone 3, best appreciated with the Masson stain.

Continued activity of steatohepatitis is associated with progressive pericellular fibrosis in acinar zone 3 (Fig. 7.69), with a lattice-like or "chicken-wire" appearance in sections stained with connective tissue stains. Continued scarring also leads to periportal fibrosis and occlusive lesions of terminal hepatic venules [97]. With progression of disease, fibrous septa begin to link the chicken-wire fibrosis in zone 3 to extensions of the periportal fibrosis, eventually leading to complete encirclement of the islets of hepatic parenchyma. The cirrhosis that develops is usually micronodular (Fig. 7.70), but a macronodular pattern can evolve after alcohol withdrawal. In patients with nonalcoholic steatohepatitis, after cirrhosis develops, the underlying steatohepatitis may become quiescent with the disappearance of fat, active injury, and Mallory–Denk bodies, leaving the patient with a histologically cryptogenic cirrhosis [98].

Other diseases with features of steatohepatitis

- *Indian childhood cirrhosis* (which occasionally is diagnosed in other countries) is thought to be due to

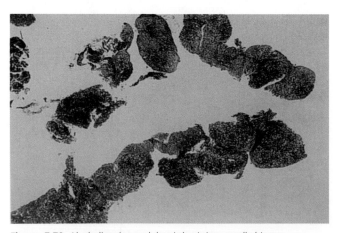

Figure 7.70 Alcoholic micronodular cirrhosis in a needle biopsy.

copper toxicity in susceptible children [99]. Histologically, the liver shows advanced micronodular cirrhosis with marked copper overload. Fat accumulation is generally mild or absent, but there is considerable hepatocellular injury with ballooning, and Mallory–Denk bodies are numerous in many cases.

- *Drug-induced liver disease* from a few drugs may demonstrate Mallory–Denk bodies and other features of steatohepatitis [50]. Amiodarone and perhexiline maleate are the best characterized of these. Mallory–Denk body formation has also been attributed to estrogens, glucocorticoids, calcium channel blockers, and antiretroviral drugs, but the evidence for these is less convincing.

- *After jejunoileal bypass surgery*, some patients developed severe steatohepatitis [100], leading to death from hepatic failure in a few cases. Similarly, steatohepatitis has been reported occasionally in patients with postsurgical short gut syndrome and gastroplasty.

Other diseases with Mallory–Denk bodies include chronic cholestatic syndromes such as PBC and primary sclerosing cholangitis, although in these diseases the Mallory–Denk bodies are in zone 1 rather than zone 3 and other features of steatohepatitis are lacking. Wilson disease may have Mallory–Denk bodies in the cirrhotic stage and can have steatosis as well, making it difficult to distinguish this disease from steatohepatitis. Finally, tumors of hepatocellular origin, including hepatocellular carcinoma, hepatocellular adenoma, and, occasionally, focal nodular hyperplasia may contain Mallory–Denk bodies in the tumor cells.

Granulomatous and suppurative diseases

Space-occupying inflammatory lesions

Abscess is the term used for a collection of neutrophils (i.e., "pus" or purulent inflammation) in a confined space. A microscopic focus of neutrophils may be termed a microabscess. This is the typical lesion of some disseminated infections such as listeriosis and salmonellosis, as discussed in the preceding text under "Acute necroinflammatory disease". Other bacterial infections that gain access to the liver – blood borne, secondary to an intraabdominal infection, or through the biliary tract, secondary to mechanical obstruction and ascending cholangitis – cause a typical pyogenic abscess (see Chapter 38). When the abscess is due to ascending cholangitis and the remnants of a bile duct can be found in the lesion, the term *cholangitic abscess* (see Fig. 7.48) is appropriate. Pylephlebitic abscesses are secondary to an acute ascending pylephlebitis from a focus of abdominal suppuration. As an abscess heals, chronic inflammation and scarring can be seen around the edges, with compression and destruction of the hepatic parenchyma.

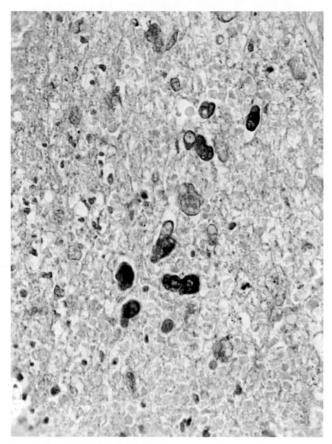

Figure 7.71 Amebic trophozoites (dark staining) are easily seen with the PAS stain. They are present in the amorphous, necrotic tissue at the edge of an amebic abscess.

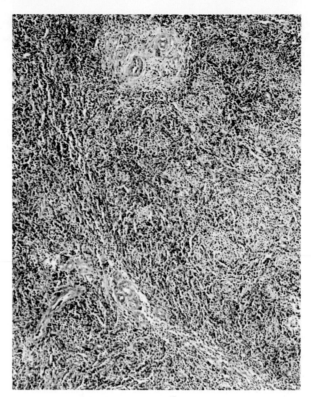

Figure 7.72 An inflammatory pseudotumor is a mass of inflammatory cells, histiocytes, and fibroblasts, presumably the result of a healing inflammatory lesion.

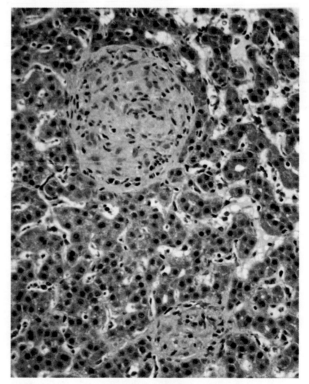

Figure 7.73 Typical noncaseating granulomas in a patient with sarcoidosis. The granulomas are composed predominantly of epithelioid histiocytes. The smaller granuloma in the lower part of the field probably represents a tangential cut through a larger lesion.

Amebic abscess is not a true abscess. It is a mass of amorphous, necrotic tissue infected with amebas. The amebic trophozoites (Fig. 7.71) can be found at the edges of the lesion, but inflammation is minimal unless there is bacterial superinfection.

Inflammatory pseudotumor [101] is a mass of chronic inflammatory cells (in particular plasma cells), xanthomatous histiocytes, myofibroblasts, and fibroblasts (Fig. 7.72). Its pathogenesis is uncertain, but at least some cases result from healing abscesses. Some cases are suspected to be true neoplasms, and the term inflammatory myofibroblastic tumor is used.

A *granuloma* is a compact, organized collection of mature mononuclear phagocytes (Fig. 7.73) that may or may not be accompanied by accessory features, such as other types of inflammatory cells, necrosis, or scarring [102–104]. Granulomatous inflammation is a response to an injury that cannot be contained and eliminated by the usual acute inflammatory response. Granulomas evolve in three stages: (i) an infiltrate of young mononuclear phagocytes; (ii) the maturation and aggregation of these cells into a mature granuloma; and (iii) the potential further maturation of these cells into an epithelioid granuloma [102]. A small focus of granulomatous inflammation, consisting of only a few epithelioid histiocytes, is often called a granulomatoid focus. The term granulomatous hepatitis should be reserved for cases in which there are both granulomas and necroinflammatory hepatocellular injury, as discussed above. The many causes of hepatic granulomas are discussed in Chapter 40. In the broadest sense, granulomas can be classified as infectious or noninfectious.

Infectious granulomas

Infectious granulomas may be due to any class of organism, and these can sometimes be identified in the tissue or there may be other features to provide a clue to the diagnosis.

- *Viruses*: granulomatoid foci or, rarely, true granulomas may be seen in the liver in some viral infections, such as infectious mononucleosis and CMV mononucleosis. Other features of mononucleosis hepatitis are invariably present.
- *Rickettsia*: Q fever (*Coxiella burnetii* infection) typically produces granulomas with a distinctive, although not pathognomonic, appearance (Fig. 7.74) [105,106]. These

lesions have a central fat vacuole surrounded by epithelioid histiocytes and other inflammatory cells. Brightly eosinophilic strands of fibrin form a ring within the granuloma, so these lesions are called *fibrin ring granulomas*. Similar granulomas are described occasionally in patients with a number of other diseases (CMV, EBV, hepatitis A, AIDS, boutonneuse fever, staphylococcal sepsis, toxoplasmosis, visceral leishmaniasis, allopurinol toxicity, giant cell arteritis, Hodgkin disease, and lupus erythematosus) [103,106]. In each case these are unusual manifestations of the diseases, whereas the fibrin ring granulomas are typical of Q fever hepatitis. The organisms cannot be identified in tissue, but finding fibrin ring granulomas should prompt serologic testing for *C. burnetii*.

- *Bacteria*: true granulomas are unusual in most bacterial diseases except in brucellosis and occasionally in syphilis; organisms are almost never demonstrable. Microabscesses or ill-formed granulomas that contain neutrophils suggest a bacterial infection such as catscratch disease, melioidosis, tularemia, or typhoid.
- *Mycobacteria*: caseous necrosis (Fig. 7.75) should suggest miliary tuberculosis, although acid-fast bacilli may be difficult or impossible to find. Absence of caseation,

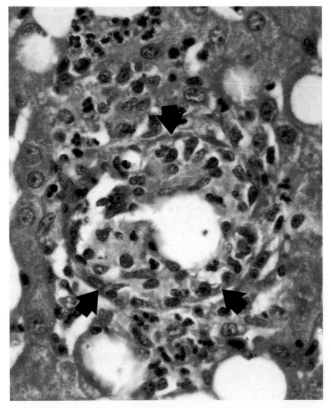

Figure 7.74 Fibrin ring granuloma in Q fever (*Coxiella burnetti* infection) has a central fat globule surrounded by epithelioid cells and a brightly eosinophilic ring of fibrin (arrows).

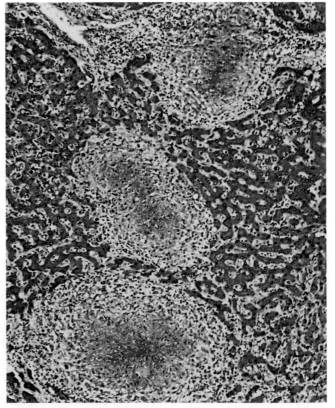

Figure 7.75 Miliary tuberculosis with amorphous, caseous necrosis in the centers of the granulomas.

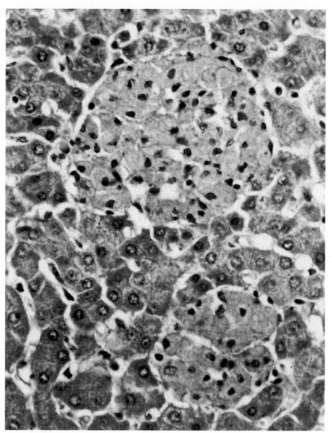

Figure 7.76 Disseminated *Mycobacterium avium intracellulare* in a patient with acquired immunodeficiency syndrome. The liver contains "macrophagic" granulomas composed of hypertrophied, grey–blue macrophages. Acid-fast stains typically show hundreds of acid-fast bacilli.

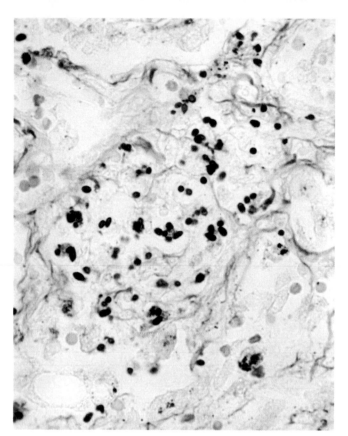

Figure 7.77 Gomori methenamine silver stain is useful for demonstrating fungal organisms in systemic mycoses. Yeast forms can be seen in this case of histoplasmosis.

of course, does not exclude tuberculosis. Lepra bacilli are difficult to find in granulomas in tuberculoid leprosy, but they can be demonstrated in large numbers with special stains in untreated lepromatous leprosy in enlarged reticuloendothelial cells that have a foamy cytoplasm (lepra cells) and are clustered in granuloma-like formations [107]. Similarly, patients with AIDS and disseminated *Mycobacterium avium intracellulare* frequently have hepatic involvement with "macrophagic" granulomas composed of hypertrophied, grey-blue macrophages containing hundreds of acid-fast bacilli (Fig. 7.76) [108]. Giant cells and inflammatory cells are generally absent, as is caseous necrosis.

- *Fungi*: granulomas in the systemic mycoses often contain the fungal spores or hyphae that may be visible with H&E but are best demonstrated with the Gomori methenamine silver stain (Fig. 7.77).
- *Protozoa*: organisms in visceral leishmaniasis are usually found in hypertrophied Kupffer cells, but granulomas may be seen, sometimes with central necrosis and sometimes with fibrin rings [103].

- *Parasites*: several parasitic diseases can involve the liver with a granulomatous response [103]. By far the most important of these is schistosomiasis. The granulomas in this disease usually contain intact eggs (Fig. 7.78) or their chitinous remnants. The granulomas in the same biopsy specimen can be of differing ages, from "active" granulomas with many epithelioid cells and eosinophils to round scars containing fragments of egg chitin. Granular black schistosomal pigment, which is the acid hematin residue from the breakdown of host hemoglobin by the parasite, is usually readily identified in the reticuloendothelial cells in livers harboring active granulomas. Other parasitic diseases in which eggs can be found in association with a granulomatous response include hepatic capillariasis, fascioliasis, paragonimiasis, and ascariasis. Visceral larva migrans, usually attributable to the larvae of *Toxocara* species, produces a characteristic lesion in the liver. The granulomas are associated with a massive outpouring of eosinophils and often reveal areas of central necrosis resulting from degeneration and degranulation of eosinophils (Fig. 7.79); there can be Charcot–Leyden crystals in the necrotic foci, but larvae are only rarely identified [109].

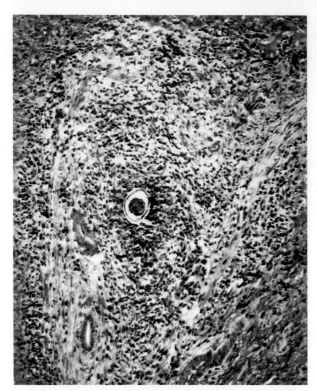

Figure 7.78 Schistosomiasis. This portal granuloma contains an embryonated egg.

Noninfectious granulomas

Sarcoidosis is the prototype of all granulomatous diseases. It is always a diagnosis of exclusion, requiring demonstration of granulomas in two or more tissues with exclusion of all known causes of granulomatous disease. At least 90% of patients with sarcoidosis have hepatic involvement, although in most it is clinically insignificant. Granulomas in sarcoidosis have no specific identifying features, but they do tend to have certain characteristics. The granulomas are scattered throughout the liver tissue, but most tend to be portal or periportal. Granulomas of all ages are typically present. The earliest lesions consist of small, loosely arranged clusters of a few epithelioid cells within the acini. Older lesions are globular or ovoid and sharply defined (see Fig. 7.73), and in cases with severe involvement, the granulomas may be confluent. Young granulomas tend to be composed predominantly of epithelioid cells, often with a few lymphocytes, while giant cells are a sign of aging. The giant cells may contain asteroid bodies (Fig. 7.80), Schaumann bodies, or calcium oxalate crystals. Older granulomas often have many giant cells, and sometimes, when the granulomas have resolved, a few naked giant cells may remain in the tissue. Usually, however, sarcoid granulomas heal by scarring, and often there is a rim of dense collagen around each granuloma (Fig. 7.81). The last remnant is a fibrous

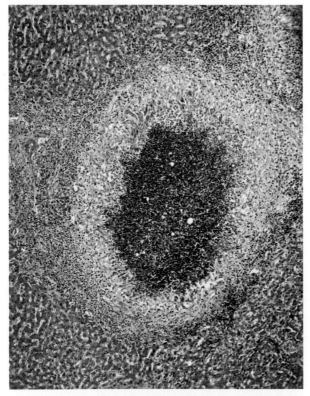

Figure 7.79 Visceral larva migrans. This eosinophilic granuloma consists of a central area of necrotic eosinophils surrounded by a palisade of epithelioid histiocytes and an outer zone that contains many additional eosinophils.

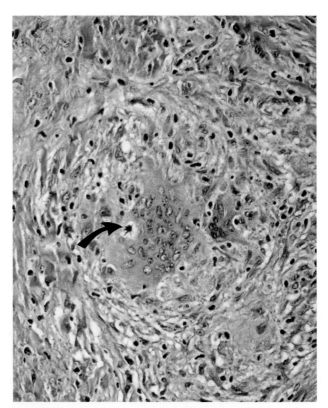

Figure 7.80 Sarcoidosis. An old fibrotic granuloma containing several giant cells, one of which has an asteroid body (arrow).

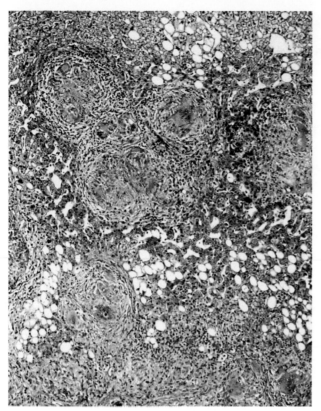

Figure 7.81 Sarcoidosis. Old, partially healed granulomas are surrounded by fibrosis and contain both epithelioid histiocytes and giant cells.

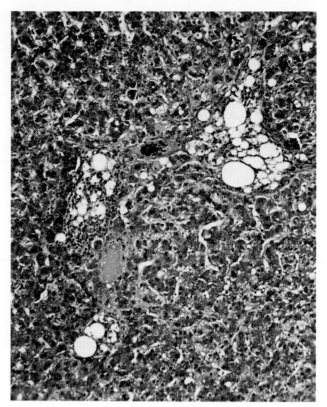

Figure 7.82 Three small lipogranulomas, composed of mineral oil droplets, macrophages, and chronic inflammatory cells.

nodule, sometimes containing one or two giant cells. The granulomas in sarcoidosis are typically noncaseating, but rarely caseous necrosis may be seen in otherwise typical cases [74].

In most patients with sarcoidosis, the hepatic granulomas are clinically silent. An unknown proportion of patients, however, come to clinical attention because of clinical symptoms and signs of cholestatic liver disease, portal hypertension, or abnormal liver test results. Biopsy results in such cases show a spectrum of changes [74]. Some patients have only sarcoid granulomas without other associated changes, but the majority show some degree of associated necroinflammatory injury (e.g., apoptosis, focal necrosis, chronic portal inflammation), features of chronic cholestasis (e.g., cholate stasis, bile duct loss), or some combination of these. Extensive portal fibrosis may cause severe bile duct loss leading to a biliary cirrhosis, or there may be fibrous obliteration of portal vein branches, producing portal hypertension.

In a significant proportion of patients a cause is never found for the sarcoid-like hepatic granulomas, and no extrahepatic granulomas are found to confirm the diagnosis of sarcoidosis. Nevertheless, such cases probably represent the same idiopathic disease, but until the cause of sarcoidosis is discovered these cases will remain undiagnosed.

Sarcoid-like granulomas can be seen in PBC, chronic berylliosis, brucellosis, drug-induced injury, and in many miscellaneous conditions. Some diseases are characterized by lesions other than the granulomas that suggest the diagnosis. For example, the liver in PBC also reveals chronic cholestasis and cholangio destructive lesions in portal areas. Drug-induced granulomas can be accompanied by hepatocellular injury or combined hepatocellular and cholestatic injury, as is typical of the liver injury associated with several drugs [23,50].

Lipogranulomas in the liver are a common finding, the result of the accumulation of ingested mineral oil [110]. They consist of variable numbers of fat vacuoles, histiocytes, mononuclear cells, and sometimes eosinophils or neutrophils, and there can be some associated focal fibrosis (Fig. 7.82). Typically, lipogranulomas are located in portal areas or in the vicinity of terminal hepatic venules.

Metabolic diseases

Identification of storage products

In the broadest sense, the term storage can be used to include various lesions and diseases characterized by the abnormal or excessive accumulation of a metabolite or substance in one of the cellular or extracellular compartments of the liver. This may include storage in

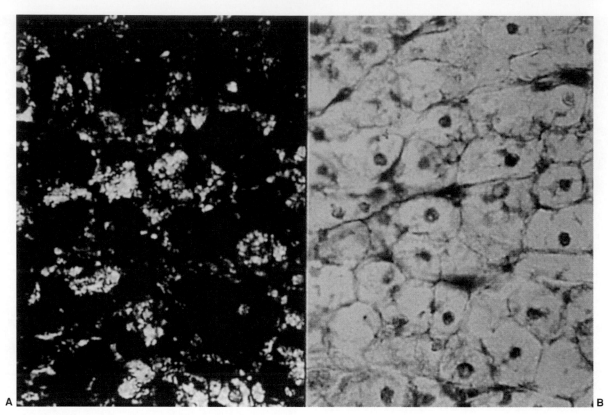

Figure 7.83 Type I glycogen storage disease. PAS stain (A) shows that the enlarged hepatocytes are filled with glycogen, which is removed by diastase digestion (B), showing the liver cells to have a clear, finely vesiculated cytoplasm.

hepatocytes, reticuloendothelial cells (Kupffer cells or other macrophages), stellate cells, and other mesenchymal cells, canaliculi, ductules, bile ducts, space of Disse, and other parts of the vasculature. Storage may indicate an inherited metabolic disease [111], or it may be part of some other process. When an abnormal substance is noted, it can often be identified by its appearance in routine sections and by its reactions with special histochemical stains. Special techniques, such as transmission or scanning electron microscopy, fluorescence or polarizing microscopy, or immunohistochemistry, may help in select cases.

Pigment storage is one of the more common lesions. This can be recognized as brown, green, or black material, which may be stored in hepatocytes, macrophages, or canaliculi. *Bile* pigment varies from brown to green and may be found in canaliculi, ductules, or ducts in cholestatic diseases (see preceding text), which rarely presents an identification problem. Bile pigment in hepatocytes and Kupffer cells can usually be distinguished from other pigments by a characteristic green color in a Hall's stain for bile or by a greenish brown color in a Prussian blue iron stain. Lipofuscin pigment varies from dark brown to golden brown. It is found in hepatocytes ("wear and tear" pigment) as a normal part of aging and in increased amounts in patients with chronic drug inges-

tion and Dubin–Johnson syndrome; it is found in Kupffer cells as the breakdown product of phagocytosed cellular debris when there has been necroinflammatory injury or other forms of tissue necrosis. Lipofuscin stains positively with argentaffin and PAS stains (see Fig. 7.4) and negatively with the iron stain. Hemosiderin is brown and coarsely granular and refractile in routine stains. It accumulates in hepatocytes, Kupffer cells, and mesenchymal cells to varying degrees in hemochromatosis and other iron overload states, and, like lipofuscin, it accumulates in Kupffer cells when there has been necroinflammatory injury. Hemosiderin stains positively with the Prussian blue stain for iron (see Fig. 7.6), so this stain can be easily used in most cases to distinguish the three brown pigments from one another.

Glycogen storage is a physiologic function of hepatocytes. In the fed state, glycogen can be demonstrated in liver cell cytoplasm with the PAS stain, and predigestion with diastase will abolish the staining. If glycogen storage disease is suspected, a portion of the biopsy specimen should be fixed in alcohol, rather than formalin, because this is the most suitable fixative for the histochemical demonstration of glycogen. In glycogen storage diseases, the glycogen often accumulates to such an extent that the hepatocytes appear swollen and plant-like (Fig. 7.83) [111]. Definitive diagnosis, however, depends on

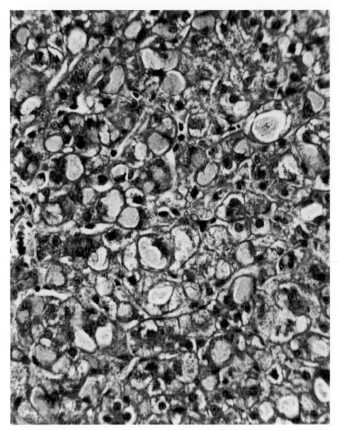

Figure 7.84 Type IV glycogen storage disease. The abnormal glycogen metabolite accumulates in cytoplasmic inclusions.

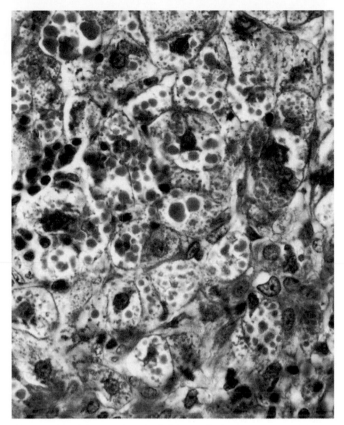

Figure 7.85 Alpha-1 antitrypsin deficiency. The hepatocytes contain eosinophilic globules of α_1-antitrypsin stored in endoplasmic reticulum cisternae.

demonstration of the specific enzymatic defect. Type IV glycogen storage disease differs from the other types and is the only type that can be readily diagnosed on liver biopsy [112]. This type is associated with the accumulation of an abnormal glycogen molecule, an amylopectin-like material, in hepatocytes. This distinctive material is homogeneous and slightly eosinophilic or even colorless. It typically appears as a circumscribed inclusion (Fig. 7.84) displacing the remainder of the cytoplasm and the nucleus to the periphery and stains intensely with PAS, Best's carmine, colloidal iron, and Lugol's iodine. The inclusions resist digestion with diastase or amylase but can be digested with pectinase.

Proteins and glycoproteins are stored in hepatocytes in several conditions. Proteins stain with eosin in routine H&E sections, so they can be recognized as storage material when they form discrete cytoplasmic inclusions. α_1-Antitrypsin (AAT) deficiency (see Chapter 31) is the best-characterized disorder with protein storage. AAT, a major protease inhibitor (Pi) in serum, is a glycoprotein that is synthesized predominantly by the liver to function as a modulator of the inflammatory response by inhibiting proteases. Individuals with one or both AAT alleles of the "Z" phenotype are unable to transport and secrete newly

synthesized AAT molecules normally through the endoplasmic reticulum and Golgi apparatus of the hepatocyte, resulting in low concentrations of AAT in the serum. Faulty secretion of abnormal AAT molecules coupled with defective degradation of these molecules retained in the Golgi apparatus leads to the formation of characteristic eosinophilic globules in hepatocytes (Fig. 7.85) [113]. The globules are PAS-positive and diastase resistant (see Fig. 7.5) due to the carbohydrate moieties of the glycoprotein. These are typically found in patients who are homozygous or heterozygous for PiZ, but they can also occur in other phenotypes, even sometimes in patients with the normal PiM phenotype [114,115]. In the noncirrhotic liver, the characteristic AAT globules are located in periportal hepatocytes. They are round, homogeneous, and eosinophilic, and vary from 1 to 40 μm in diameter. Usually, they are separated from the remainder of the cytoplasm by a halo that is probably artifactual. Immunohistochemical staining can confirm that the globules are composed of AAT but cannot be used to determine the phenotype. PAS-positive globules are usually not detectable in infants younger than 3 months, although some present with neonatal hepatitis or paucity of bile ducts. Liver biopsy specimens from adults with AAT deficiency may reveal only the characteristic globules in periportal regions, or there may be erosion of the limiting plate associated with chronic inflammation and periportal fibrosis, similar to chronic hepatitis of other etiologies, or cirrhosis with globules at the periphery of the nodules.

Other protein storage disorders, both inherited and acquired, may produce cytoplasmic inclusions. α_1-Antichymotrypsin deficiency and antithrombin III deficiency are rare, but both are associated with AAT-like PAS-positive globules [116,117]. Familial fibrinogen storage disease produces globular inclusions that are eosinophilic but only weakly PAS-positive because of a lower carbohydrate content [118]. Plasma protein inclusions [119], consisting of a mixture of circulating proteins imbibed by hepatocytes from the plasma, are seen most often in hepatic congestion. They are variably PAS-positive and may be globular or have a pale eosinophilic appearance that can be confused with the ground-glass inclusions of hepatitis B. PAS-positive, diastase-resistant, ground-glass-appearing inclusions are also seen in patients taking the drug cyanamide [120] (not used in the United States) and in patients with Lafora disease (myoclonus epilepsy) [121].

Lipids, glycolipids, sphingolipids, and other phospholipids accumulate in a number of inherited and acquired conditions. Hepatocytes, Kupffer cells, and stellate cells that contain a lipid storage product generally appear clear, vacuolated, or foamy. Triglyceride is by far the most common storage product, and this is discussed separately in the preceding text under steatosis. All lipids stain positively in unprocessed frozen sections with the oil red O and Sudan black stains. Most, however, do not survive routine processing in organic solvents, so their demonstration requires forethought so that a portion of the specimen can be handled separately. To avoid the artifacts of frozen section, the tissue can be postfixed in osmium tetroxide, which stains the lipid black (Fig. 7.86) [122]. Cholesterol esters are stored along with triglyceride in the two forms of lysosomal acid lipase deficiency, Wolman disease and cholesterol ester storage disease, causing the hepatocytes to appear swollen and pale. Both types of lipid stain with oil red O, but the cholesterol can also be demonstrated in frozen sections with a Schultz stain [1]. Glucosylceramide, a glycolipid, accumulates in Kupffer cells in Gaucher disease (lysosomal glucocerebrosidase deficiency), producing the distinctive striated appearance of Gaucher cells. The PAS stain after diastase digestion provides an excellent demonstration of these cells because enough of the carbohydrate component of the storage product survives processing and stains positively (Fig. 7.87). Sphingomyelin accumulates in Kupffer cells in the many variants of Niemann–Pick disease, producing a foamy appearance (Fig. 7.88). Other phospholipids accumulate in both Kupffer cells and hepatocytes in

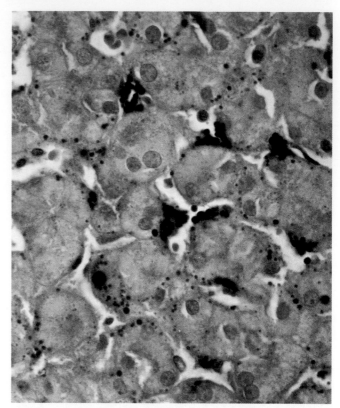

Figure 7.86 Osmium stain for fat. Lipids stain black when the tissue is postfixed in osmium tetroxide. In this patient with hypervitaminosis A, the stellate cells (perisinusoidal lipocytes) are hypertrophied because of vitamin A storage, and there are a few small triglyceride droplets in hepatocytes.

drug-induced phospholipidosis because of chronic ingestion of amphophilic drugs such as amiodarone [50]. The Kupffer cells appear foamy, but the hepatocellular phospholipid storage can generally only be recognized by electron microscopy (Fig. 7.89). Vitamin A is stored in stellate cells, and these become prominent in individuals

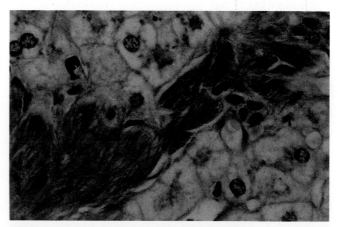

Figure 7.87 Gaucher disease. Striations in the Gaucher cells are nicely demonstrated by the PAS stain after diastase digestion.

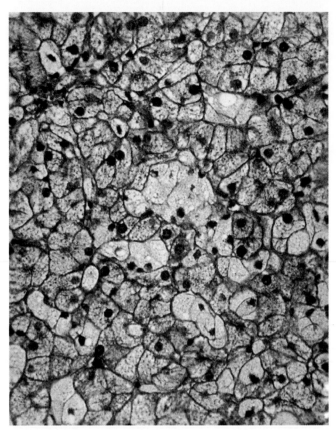

Figure 7.88 Niemann–Pick disease. Sphingomyelin accumulates in Kupffer cells, giving them a foamy appearance. Liver cells appear normal.

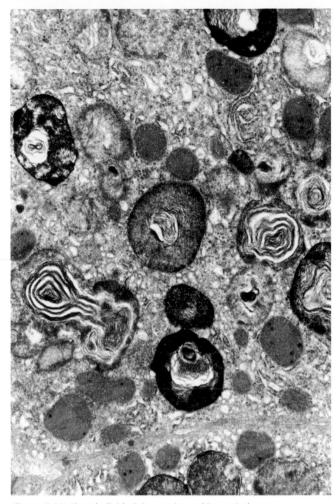

Figure 7.89 Phospholipidosis in a patient taking amiodarone. Ultrastructurally the hepatocyte cytoplasm contains numerous lamellated whorls of phospholipid.

ingesting excess vitamin A (Figs 7.86 and 7.90). Lipid globules containing the vitamin A are apparent with fat stains, and vitamin A is autofluorescent in frozen sections. Mineral oils (paraffins) are common in the western diet, and some are absorbed and stored in portal macrophages or lipogranulomas near terminal hepatic venules (see Fig. 7.82). In frozen sections the mineral oil stains a pale salmon pink with the oil red O stain.

Mucopolysaccharides accumulate in both hepatocytes and Kupffer cells in Hunter disease, Hurler disease (Fig. 7.91), other mucopolysaccharidoses, and mucolipidoses. The affected cells appear swollen and finely vacuolated. Colloidal iron, alcian blue, and other stains for mucopolysaccharides are positive, and the PAS stain after diastase digestion is also positive. Oligosaccharides in diseases such as sialidosis are stored in hepatocyte lysosomes, making the liver cells appear vacuolated.

Porphyrins accumulate in the liver in porphyria cutanea tarda and erythropoietic protoporphyria. Uroporphyrin crystals in hepatocytes are inapparent by routine stains, but can sometimes be demonstrated with a ferric ferricyanide stain [123] in patients with porphyria cutanea tarda. Protoporphyrin deposits in erythropoietic protoporphyria appear as brownish red globular masses in

hepatocytes and bile canaliculi. They are easily mistaken for bile pigment, but with polarized light they are red with characteristic Maltese cross birefringence (see Fig. 7.15) [13].

Copper storage in hepatocytes in chronic cholestatic diseases or in Wilson disease is not visible by light microscopy, but it is often found in association with periportal or periseptal lipofuscin granules. Stains for copper, such as rhodanine (see Fig. 7.7), are needed for demonstrating storage because it can easily be missed.

Crystals of various types may be stored in macrophages under special conditions. Many crystals are birefringent with polarized light, and scanning electron microscopy with X-ray spectrophotometry can specifically identify those that are inorganic. In cystinosis, crystals of cystine can be demonstrated with a polarizer in tissue that has been fixed in alcohol. Birefringent talc crystals (see Fig. 7.14) or black, nonbirefringent titanium dioxide

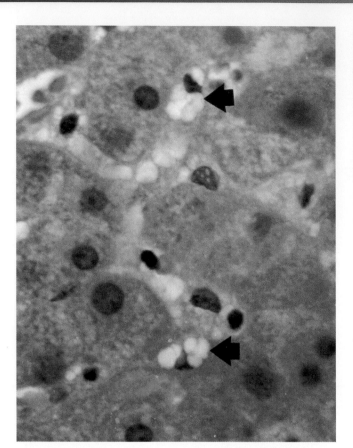

Figure 7.90 Hypervitaminosis A. Stellate cells (arrows) are engorged with stored vitamin A.

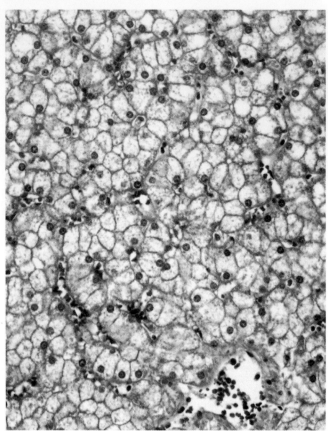

Figure 7.91 Hurler disease. The stored mucopolysaccharide gives the swollen liver cells a finely vacuolated appearance.

pigment granules can sometimes be found in macrophages of some patients who are or have been intravenous drug abusers. Other foreign materials, such as gold (which appears as a black pigment in patients treated with gold for rheumatoid arthritis), thorium dioxide (Thorotrast®, a discontinued radiologic contrast material), polyvinyl pyrrolidone (a discontinued plasma expander), and anthracotic carbon (in coal miners), may be found stored in reticuloendothelial cells.

Genetic hemochromatosis

As the most common hepatic storage disease, biopsy diagnosis of hemochromatosis deserves special mention. Gene analysis and quantification of iron concentration in liver tissue obtained by biopsy are now the preferred method for diagnosis (see Chapter 30), but examination of the biopsy specimen is still useful in distinguishing primary from secondary iron overload and in assessing the degree of fibrosis. Secondary iron overload is the proper term for nongenetic causes of excess tissue iron. This may be due to multiple blood transfusions, chronic hemolysis, or prolonged dietary overload, but it rarely results in tissue damage except in a few extreme instances. Hemosiderosis is the term used for morpholog-

ically identifiable iron accumulation in tissue, whatever the cause. Severe hemosiderosis is usually due to genetic hemochromatosis, but it can be secondary to transfusional or dietary iron or chronic hemolysis. In such cases the hemosiderin accumulation is predominantly in reticuloendothelial cells. Excess iron may accumulate in hepatocytes of patients with damaged livers, especially in alcoholic cirrhosis and also in chronic viral hepatitis. Many of these patients are probably heterozygous for genetic hemochromatosis.

In homozygous genetic hemochromatosis, iron accumulates over the course of the patient's life [124]. In young homozygous patients, this is detected as a progressive increase in hepatocellular hemosiderin pigment (most prominently in periportal regions) with minimal or no other pathologic changes (Fig. 7.92). As the quantity of iron increases, the cells of zones 2 and 3 become affected. Scattered apoptotic bodies and foci of necrosis are found infrequently. Kupffer cells may ingest small quantities of iron. By middle age in men or after menopause in women, enough iron has usually accumulated to cause hepatocellular necrosis, portal inflammation, and portal and bridging fibrosis. Alcohol and intercurrent liver diseases such

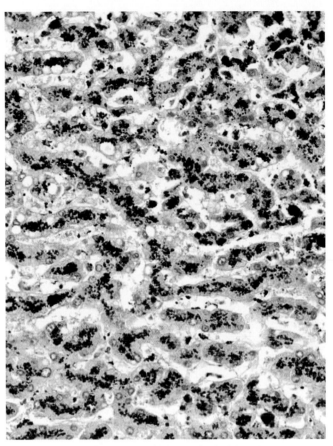

Figure 7.92 Hemochromatosis. This iron stain of a biopsy from a young homozygous patient shows a marked increase in hepatocyte stainable iron (dark granules), most prominently in acinar zone 1. There is no fibrosis as yet.

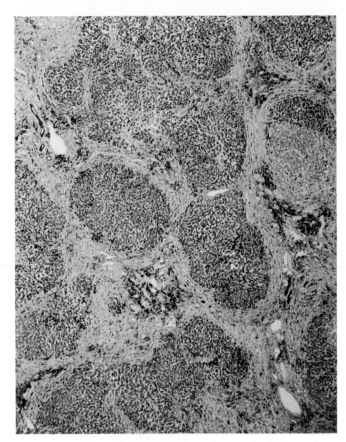

Figure 7.93 Micronodular cirrhosis of hemochromatosis. The iron stain shows marked deposition of hemosiderin (dark granules) in liver cells, bile ducts, and mesenchymal cells of the fibrous septa.

as hepatitis C may accelerate iron accumulation. Fibrous septa eventually creep from the portal areas into the surrounding parenchyma. Evidence of regeneration is not apparent in the precirrhotic stage, but a reticulin stain can demonstrate plates greater than one cell in thickness near the portal tracts. The fibrous septa can show variable ductular proliferation, but inflammation is mild or absent.

Fibrous bands from adjacent portal tracts eventually join and dissect the parenchyma into irregular micronodules (Fig. 7.93). By this stage there is marked hemosiderin deposition with heavy pigment staining of the hepatocytes, bile duct epithelium, ductules, and mesenchymal cells of the fibrous septa and vessels. Relatively less iron is found in Kupffer cells. Regeneration is not usually prominent, but regenerative nodules offer striking contrast to the remaining parenchyma by their lack of stainable iron, so-called iron-free foci [125]. Hepatocellular carcinomas that develop in hemochromatotic livers are also devoid of iron, and there is evidence that the iron-free foci represent preneoplastic lesions.

Wilson disease

Tissue damage in Wilson disease (see Chapter 29) is related to excess copper, and the liver is the earliest site of progressive copper accumulation, after which the copper is released into the blood to accumulate in other organs. The histopathologic changes [126–128] are not specific and must be evaluated in conjunction with clinical and laboratory findings. Hepatic copper concentration can be measured in the tissue obtained by needle biopsy and can provide a definitive diagnosis when other tests are equivocal. Biopsy specimens obtained from young siblings of patients with this disease may show little or no hepatic damage. The earliest microscopic lesions include steatosis, periportal glycogenated nuclei, and rare foci of necrosis or apoptotic bodies. Although the hepatic copper content is elevated, copper is usually not histochemically identifiable at this stage, but ultrastructural changes in hepatic mitochondria, thought to be characteristic if not pathognomonic, are present (Fig. 7.94). These changes include pleomorphism, separation of the inner and outer membranes, enlarged intercristal spaces, and various types of inclusions [6,129]. More advanced cases show lesions that resemble chronic hepatitis of

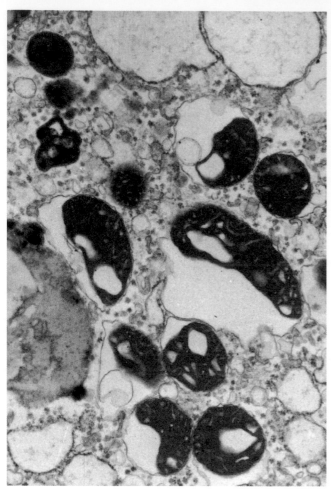

Figure 7.94 Wilson disease. Ultrastructurally, the mitochondria have a dense matrix with separation of the membranes of the cristae.

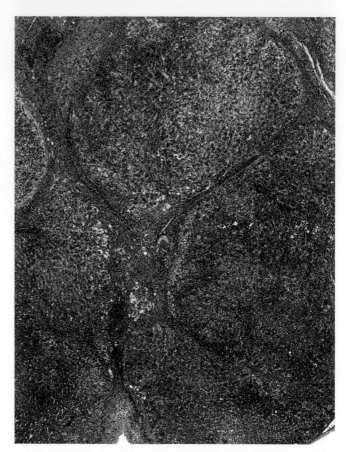

Figure 7.95 End-stage Wilson disease. Macronodular cirrhosis is present with large nodules separated by bands of scar tissue.

other cause. Mallory–Denk bodies, with their characteristic neutrophilic response, may be present in the liver cells in zone 1. Copper may be demonstrable in the periportal areas with appropriate stains. A variety of patterns of cirrhosis can develop in the later stages but a macronodular type is the most common (Fig. 7.95). Regenerative foci lack identifiable copper, so an absence of stainable copper in a cirrhotic biopsy, particularly if the sample is small, does not rule out Wilson disease. On the other hand, a large amount of copper in a cirrhotic liver is strongly suggestive of Wilson disease (see Fig. 7.7).

Vascular disorders

Vascular patterns of injury

Certain patterns of injury in the liver are typical, if not pathognomonic, of a vascular disease. Congestion, atrophy, and coagulative necrosis are all findings that suggest a vascular component to the underlying disorder. A variety of substances, both endogenous and foreign, can be deposited in the vasculature as well.

Acute *ischemic injury* typically produces zone 3 ("centrilobular") coagulative necrosis, similar to that seen in severe injury from certain toxins, such as acetaminophen overdose or mushroom poisoning. Ischemic injury may follow shock, left-sided heart failure, or right-sided failure associated with hypotension [130,131]. Clinically, the presentation may mimic viral hepatitis (ischemic hepatitis) [132]. Liver cells that have undergone coagulative degeneration are shrunken, have an intensely eosinophilic cytoplasm, and show nuclear pyknosis or lysis (see Fig. 7.20). When an inflammatory response is present, it is invariably neutrophilic. Kupffer cells are hypertrophied and usually full of lipofuscin. Clearing of the dead hepatocytes leads to condensation of reticulin fibers and fibrosis in some cases.

Chronic ischemic injury produces *atrophy* of acini or liver cell plates. Mild forms of chronic ischemia are a fairly common consequence of aging. Mild portal fibrosis with some periductal fibrosis and reduction in portal vein diameter is a frequent finding in elderly individuals. Often there will be areas in the liver in which vascular

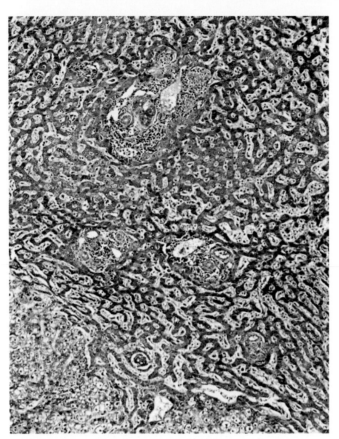

Figure 7.96 Atrophy, secondary to chronic ischemia. Portal areas are fibrotic and close together, indicating atrophy of the acini.

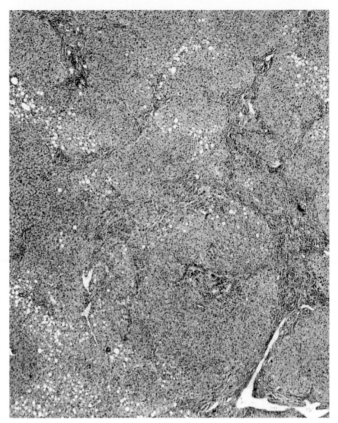

Figure 7.97 Nodular regenerative hyperplasia. The entire hepatic parenchyma is replaced by hyperplastic nodules separated by atrophic liver cell plates.

structures appear close together, indicating that the acini have atrophied (Fig. 7.96). Extreme forms of this phenomenon can result in hepatoportal sclerosis (also called idiopathic portal hypertension, noncirrhotic portal hypertension, or noncirrhotic portal fibrosis) [133] or nodular regenerative hyperplasia [134] when there is heterogeneous blood flow through portal vein branches and hepatic arterioles with atrophy of the affected acini and compensatory hyperplasia of other acini (Fig. 7.97). Both conditions may cause portal hypertension in the absence of cirrhosis. Atrophy of the left lobe and segmental atrophy (Fig. 7.98) [135] are usually due to severe compromise of the vasculature (inflow or outflow) to a portion of the liver, but this may also be due to bile duct occlusion.

Venous outflow obstruction

The terminal hepatic venules ("central veins"), intercalated ("sublobular") veins, hepatic veins, and inferior vena cava form the venous outflow tract, but only the terminal hepatic venules and intercalated veins are commonly sampled by liver biopsy. Obstruction of any portion of the outflow tract can be followed by changes in other vessels, such as sinusoidal dilatation and, rarely, thrombosis of the portal venules. Chronic congestive

heart failure or constrictive pericarditis can mimic outflow tract obstruction when severe.

Hepatic vein thrombosis (Budd–Chiari syndrome) produces histologic findings that are commonly confused with congestive heart failure or drug-induced injury and must be interpreted with care. Many of the changes resemble those of congestive heart failure, but differ by showing variability of involvement among acini, particularly well visualized with open (wedge) biopsy specimens. Those acini with acute changes show severe sinusoidal dilatation and congestion, most pronounced in zone 3 (Fig. 7.99), but sometimes extending to the portal tracts. Coagulative degeneration or necrosis is frequently present. Erythrocytes in the congested areas are packed into the spaces of Disse and crowd the degenerating hepatocytes. The terminal hepatic venules and intercalated veins can show thrombosis, recanalized thrombi (Fig. 7.99), and/or fibrous mural thickening, but in a small biopsy specimen the veins that are sampled may be normal. Some acini are injured in a more gradual manner. Progressive sinusoidal dilatation is accompanied by atrophy of hepatocytes. Zone 3 fibrosis can follow either type of injury and can link adjacent terminal hepatic

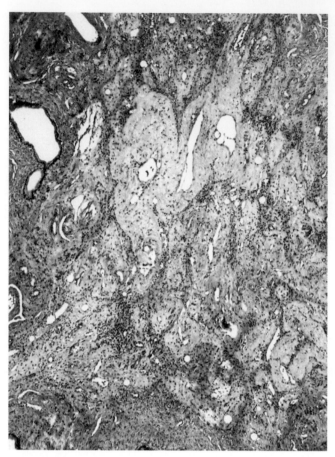

Figure 7.98 Segmental atrophy. The tissue is fibrotic, and there are portal areas and ductules, but hepatocytes are missing, presumably because of chronic ischemia.

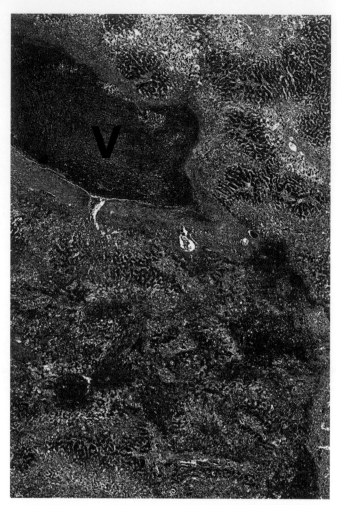

Figure 7.99 Budd–Chiari syndrome. An organizing thrombus in a large intercalated vein (V) is associated with severe sinusoidal dilatation and congestion and necrosis of zone 3 of the surrounding acini.

venules. Small portal veins may also become occluded, further augmenting the injury to parts of the liver [136]. Other acini are entirely spared. The caudate lobe is often uninvolved because of its separate venous drainage and can undergo compensatory hypertrophy.

Venoocclusive disease resulting from toxic injury (e.g., from pyrrolizidine alkaloids) or radiation damage to the endothelium of the small outflow produces parenchymal changes that resemble those of Budd–Chiari syndrome, but in the early stages lesions of the terminal hepatic venules and intercalated veins are distinctive. Intimal edema is followed by the subendothelial deposition of reticulin and collagen fibers and progressive narrowing of the lumen (Fig. 7.100). Extravasated erythrocytes are frequently situated between the fibers. Inflammation is sparse or absent, and superimposed thrombi are not seen. Cases with severe acute injury may show necrosis of the venous walls. With progressive fibrosis of the walls, the veins become difficult to identify, appearing as small hyalinized cylinders. Involvement of hepatic veins or the vena cava does not occur in most cases.

Sinusoidal lesions

Dilatation of sinusoids is a frequent finding in liver biopsy specimens and is often a nonspecific reaction to systemic disease. Chronic congestive heart failure leads to the gradual development of dilatation and congestion of sinusoids and finally to atrophy of hepatocytes, predominantly in zone 3, with secondary fibrosis [130,131]. A characteristic type of periportal (zone 1) sinusoidal dilatation sometimes follows the use of oral contraceptives [137]. Liver plates show variable degrees of atrophy (Fig. 7.101). The change affects all acini, unlike the focal sinusoidal dilatation seen sometimes near hepatic masses. Panacinar sinusoidal dilatation can be found in sickle cell disease; the dilated sinusoids are packed with masses of sickled erythrocytes. Variable dilatation, lacking any particular zonal localization, can be associated with other disorders, notably neoplasms and granulomatous diseases. Sinusoidal dilatation of the liver may be a systemic

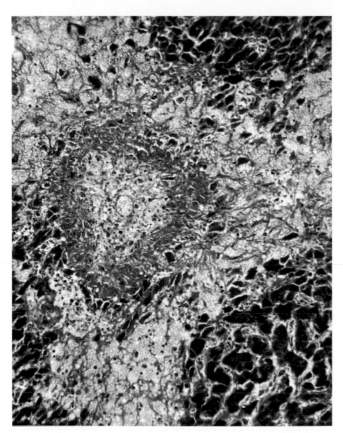

Figure 7.100 Venoocclusive disease associated with *Senecio* alkaloid toxicity. The efferent vein has a markedly narrowed lumen because of intimal thickening with extravasation of erythrocytes. There is zone 3 necrosis and marked congestion.

manifestation of a number of neoplasms. A characteristic triad of histologic changes, consisting of focal sinusoidal dilatation, proliferation of ductules, and infiltration of edematous portal areas by neutrophils, has been observed in the vicinity of space-occupying lesions [138].

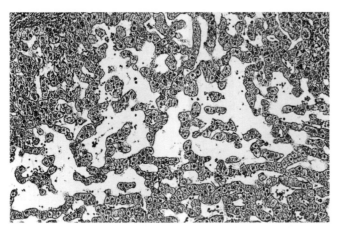

Figure 7.101 Marked periportal sinusoidal dilatation associated with long-term oral contraceptive steroid use. The liver cell plates are atrophic.

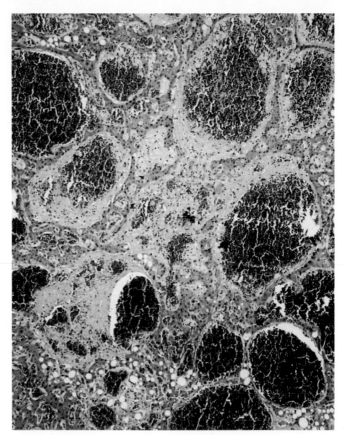

Figure 7.102 Peliosis hepatis associated with anabolic steroid therapy. Variable-sized lakes of blood are scattered throughout the parenchyma.

Peliosis hepatis is characterized by scattered lakes of blood of varying sizes, which appear to represent an extreme degree of localized sinusoidal dilatation (Fig. 7.102). The pathogenesis of the process is now considered to be due to endothelial injury that allows blood to accumulate in the spaces of Disse with a resultant formation of cavities. In the past, peliosis was recognized as a complication of debilitating disorders, such as tuberculosis and malignancies, and was discovered at autopsy as an incidental finding. Currently, the most frequent cause is therapy with androgenic/anabolic steroids [139]. Histologically, the peliotic lakes may have an attenuated endothelial lining. Varying degrees of sinusoidal dilatation can be present near some of the lesions, but the term peliosis hepatis should not be used for simple sinusoidal dilatation. Bacillary angiomatosis due to *Bartonella henselae* in patients with AIDS [140] can mimic peliosis, but stains for bacteria typically demonstrate numerous organisms.

Thrombosis of sinusoids with deposition of fibrin thrombi is unusual, but it happens in some diseases. Patients with toxemia of pregnancy usually have no evidence of liver disease; those who do frequently have deposits of fibrin in periportal sinusoids [141].

Occasionally, the deposits are associated with coagulative-type hepatocellular necrosis. Disseminated intravascular coagulation can be associated with a similar pattern of injury, but the sinusoidal fibrin deposition need not be restricted to the periportal areas.

Fibrosis of sinusoids occurs in many chronic diseases. Collagen is deposited in the space of Disse along with laminin, forming basement membranes and leading to capillarization of the sinusoids. The collagen is well demonstrated with a Masson stain, and many components of basement membranes and extracellular matrix can be demonstrated with specific immunostains. Sinusoidal fibrosis is prominent in zone 3 of the acinus in the early stages of alcoholic hepatitis (see Fig. 7.69), nonalcoholic steatohepatitis, diabetes mellitus, chronic congestive heart failure, and vitamin A hepatotoxicity.

Amyloidosis

Patients with amyloidosis frequently have hepatic involvement, and liver biopsy has been advocated as a means of establishing the diagnosis. Amyloid can be limited to the arteries but can also be found in the parenchyma (Fig. 7.103). In both primary amyloidosis

(type AL) and secondary amyloidosis (type AA), the eosinophilic material gradually accumulates in the space of Disse [142], eventually leading to atrophy of the hepatic plates. The presence of amyloid can be confirmed by an appropriate stain, either histochemical (e.g., Congo red with apple green dichroism under polarized light) or immunohistochemical, with a specific antibody to the amyloid.

Cirrhosis

Cirrhosis is defined as a diffuse process characterized by fibrosis and conversion of the normal liver architecture into structurally abnormal nodules [143]. Three basic morphologic categories are recognized on the basis of the size of the cirrhotic nodules. The micronodular type includes those cases in which almost all nodules are less than 3 mm in diameter. In the macronodular type, most nodules are greater than 3 mm in diameter and usually show striking variation in size. The mixed pattern is characterized by approximately equal numbers of micro- and macronodules. Regenerative nodules are not essential for the diagnosis of cirrhosis; in both biliary cirrhosis and hemochromatosis, for example, regeneration may be minimal or absent.

The diagnosis of cirrhosis may be difficult to establish by percutaneous needle biopsy, particularly if the pattern is macronodular. Cutting needles (e.g., Tru-Cut) are preferred because these obtain specimens that include the fibrous septa and the parenchymal nodules (Fig. 7.104). Suction techniques (e.g., Menghini needles) are limited by preferential sampling of parenchyma as the biopsy needle rebounds from the fibrous septa. There are, however, a number of microscopic clues to the diagnosis, even in this type of specimen. Suction biopsies from cirrhotic livers are commonly fragmented, and the fragments have rounded edges. Fibrous septa can course through the

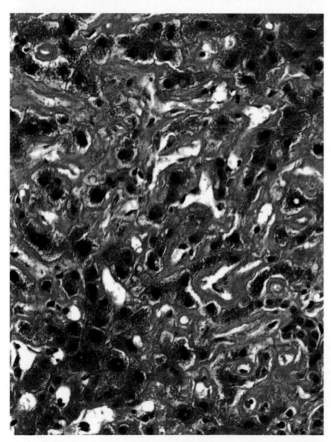

Figure 7.103 Extensive intra-acinar amyloid deposition filling the space of Disse between the hepatocytes and endothelial cells, producing atrophy of the liver cell plates.

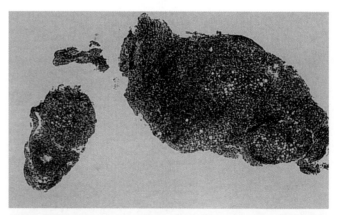

Figure 7.104 Fragmented needle biopsy specimen from a cirrhotic liver. The Masson stain shows collagen of the fibrous septa enveloping and traversing the fragments.

fragments, but these are sometimes represented by thin strips hugging the margins of the fragments. Stains for collagen (Fig. 7.104) are frequently necessary to detect them. Such stains are also valuable for distinguishing collapsed reticulin that follows extensive necrosis from fibrosis and for demonstrating thick liver plates in regenerative nodules of the cirrhotic liver. Reticulin stains usually demonstrate a very irregular pattern because of alterations in the growth of hepatocytes. Many cell plates are more than one cell in thickness, and the compressed sinusoidal spaces may be nearly invisible. Hepatocytes are pleomorphic, unless the process is entirely inactive. An alteration of the spatial relationship between the portal vessels and central veins is typical. Micronodular cirrhosis is less difficult to establish by needle biopsy than is macronodular cirrhosis because the diameter of the biopsy needle usually exceeds that of the small cirrhotic nodules. The capsule of the liver in many noncirrhotic patients is thickened by an increase in fibrous tissue, vessels, and ductules. A small biopsy specimen from such an area (particularly a superficial wedge biopsy) should be interpreted with caution and not diagnosed as cirrhosis.

The morphologic approach in cirrhosis should include an assessment of whether the cirrhosis is fully developed or incomplete, the basic morphologic type (i.e., micronodular, macronodular, or mixed), the degree of activity, and the presumptive cause, if possible. Biopsy specimens showing occasional nodules or extensive fibrosis may be judged to represent early or incomplete cirrhosis, but the designation cirrhosis should be reserved for those with complete loss of acinar architecture. An assessment of the activity should take into account the degree of hepatocellular degeneration and necrosis and the amount of inflammation in the parenchyma of the nodules.

Every effort to establish the underlying cause should be made, although this is not always possible. An etiologic diagnosis can sometimes be established by changes observed in H&E-stained sections alone (e.g., absence of bile ducts and chronic cholestasis indicating biliary cirrhosis, including cirrhosis secondary to PBC or primary sclerosing cholangitis). Special stains, however, are an important auxiliary technique. Particularly useful are copper stains for Wilson disease and PBC, the PAS stain and immunostains for α_1-antitrypsin deficiency, immunostains of the antigens of hepatitis B, and an iron stain for hemochromatosis.

Putative preneoplastic lesions may be found in cirrhotic livers. Large cell change (liver cell dysplasia) is characterized by nuclear and cytoplasmic enlargement, nuclear hyperchromasia, prominent nucleoli, and, occasionally, multinucleation (Fig. 7.105) [144]. Dysplastic nodule is the term used for grossly or radiologically distinctive nodules that are usually larger than the surrounding cirrhotic nodules and that may differ in color

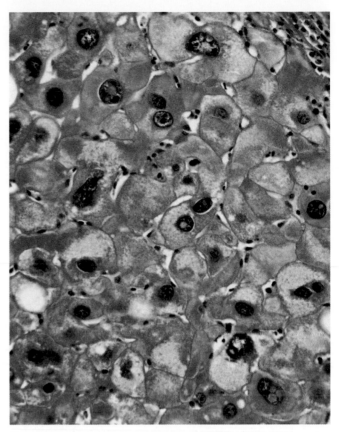

Figure 7.105 Large cell change (liver cell dysplasia) in cirrhosis. The dysplastic cells are large and contain large, dark-stained and sometimes irregular nuclei.

or texture [145]. These are classified microscopically as low-grade dysplastic nodules when there are minimal atypical histologic features. They are classified as high-grade dysplastic nodules when there are atypical features in the hepatocytes of the nodule, such as cytoplasmic basophilia, high nuclear : cytoplasmic ratios, nuclear irregularity, and hyperchromasia. High-grade dysplastic nodules often have ill-defined nodules within the large nodule ("nodule-in-nodule" formation), best recognized by compression of the surrounding reticulin fibers and different orientation of the liver plates. These are often composed of smaller than normal hepatocytes with high nuclear : cytoplasmic ratios, a feature termed small cell change (or small cell dysplasia) (Fig. 7.106). Evidence suggests that this lesion, rather than large cell change, is more likely the precursor of hepatocellular carcinoma in the cirrhotic liver.

Fibropolycystic diseases

Lesions and types of cysts

- *Von Meyenburg complexes* or biliary microhamartomas are a common developmental anomaly in the liver [146,147]. They are typically found adjacent to normal

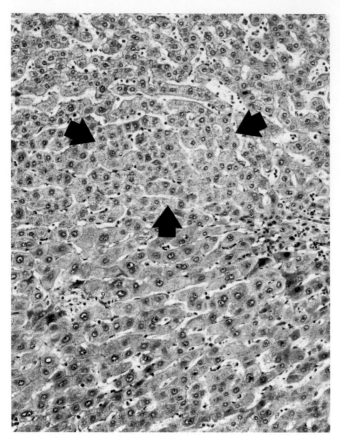

Figure 7.106 Small cell dysplasia in a high-grade dysplastic nodule. There is a nodular growth of small liver cells with high nuclear : cytoplasmic ratios (arrows) within a large cirrhotic nodule.

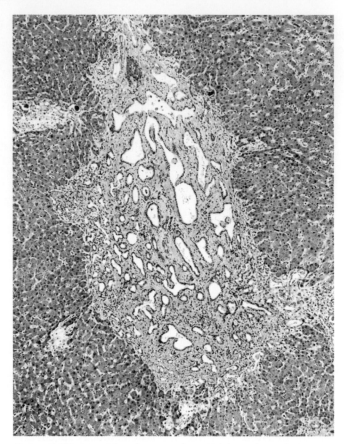

Figure 7.107 A von Meyenburg complex, which has a dense stroma containing irregular small duct-like structures, a few of which are slightly dilated.

portal areas and consist of a fibrous stroma that contains several irregular, duct-like structures lined by biliary epithelium (Fig. 7.107). These are often somewhat dilated and some may be large enough to be considered cysts. They often contain eosinophilic or bile-stained secretions.

- *Bile duct cysts*: these are usually solitary and lined by a cuboidal biliary-type epithelium. These are considered to be of developmental origin, and at least some arise from cystic dilatation of a von Meyenburg complex, although in most cases there are no clues to the exact pathogenesis of the lesion. The cysts typically contain clear fluid, but become infected and contain pus, or when large, there may be hemorrhage and inflammation secondary to minor trauma.
- *Ciliated foregut cyst*: this is an unusual type of developmental cyst that is lined by ciliated columnar epithelium [148]. These cysts are analogous to bronchogenic cysts of the mediastinum. They are extremely rare in the liver.
- *Ductal plate malformation* refers to the persistence of the embryonic ductal plate in the postnatal liver [147]. In embryonic life, before the appearance of the acinar bile

ducts, the portal tracts are surrounded by a layer of biliary-type cells, termed the ductal plate. This structure normally disappears as the true bile duct develops in the center of the portal area. Persistence of parts of the ductal plate may give rise to von Meyenburg complexes, duct-like structures seen in congenital hepatic fibrosis, and cysts of infantile polycystic disease (Fig. 7.108).

Infantile polycystic disease

Infantile polycystic disease, which is an autosomal recessive disease, is part of a spectrum of lesions that includes infantile polycystic kidney disease, congenital hepatic fibrosis, and Caroli disease [149]. Expression varies from individual to individual. The liver in childhood polycystic disease is enlarged and firm, but cysts are not usually visible grossly. Microscopic sections show numerous, irregular, duct-like structures in the portal areas. These have apparent branching and irregular angulated extensions into the acini (Fig. 7.108), and there is often a circular arrangement of the ducts, complete or interrupted, characteristic of the ductal plate malformation. In contrast to congenital hepatic fibrosis, relatively little fibrous tissue is

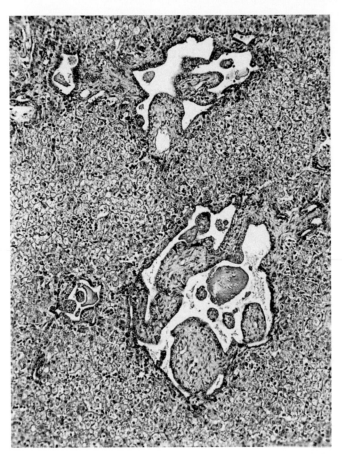

Figure 7.108 Infantile polycystic disease. The ducts are lined by cuboidal epithelium, show polypoid intraluminal projections, and are for the most part empty. They arise from remnants of the embryonic ductal plate.

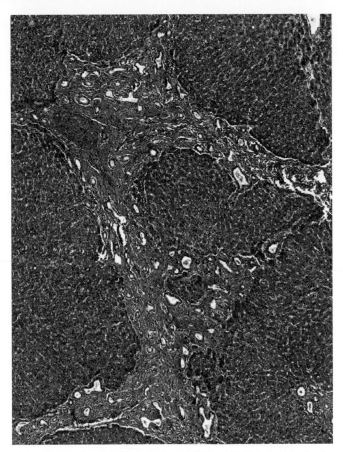

Figure 7.109 Congenital hepatic fibrosis. Masson stain shows islands of parenchyma separated by irregular bands of fibrous tissue that contain numerous small ductal plate remnants.

present. The ducts are slightly dilated, but true cysts are rare. They are lined by a simple, low columnar to cuboidal epithelium.

Congenital hepatic fibrosis

In congenital hepatic fibrosis, thick collagenous bands form an extensive network, usually continuous, that links adjacent portal tracts (Fig. 7.109). Numerous bile duct-like structures, some slightly irregular and dilated, are situated in the fibrous septa and sometimes contain mucin or bile. Although they resemble bile ducts, they actually represent ductal plate remnants. Portal vein branches often appear reduced in size and number, and the sparsity of venous channels might account in part for the portal hypertension. The irregular intervening parenchyma frequently has a "jigsaw" pattern reminiscent of that seen in biliary cirrhosis. However, unlike cirrhosis, congenital hepatic fibrosis does not show evidence of parenchymal destruction or regeneration. The hepatocytic plates are regular and one cell in thickness, and there is an abrupt transition between the normal-appearing hepatocytes and the collagenous septa.

Adult polycystic disease

Adult polycystic disease is frequently associated with adult polycystic kidney disease. Numerous cysts, varying from less than 1 mm to more than 12 cm in diameter, are present, containing clear, colorless or straw-colored fluid, unless infected. Microscopically, the cysts appear to originate in the portal areas. They are lined by low columnar to cuboidal epithelium (Fig. 7.110) and have a collagenous supporting stroma that can be infiltrated by a few inflammatory cells. Von Meyenburg complexes (biliary microhamartomas) are frequently present, and components of the complexes sometimes lie adjacent to the cysts, suggesting that the cysts evolve from progressive dilatation of the biliary channels in the complexes. Occasional cases show many von Meyenburg complexes and no cysts.

Tumors

Hepatocellular tumors

Hepatocellular adenoma

Hepatocellular adenoma is composed of benign hepatocytes arranged in sheets and cords without an

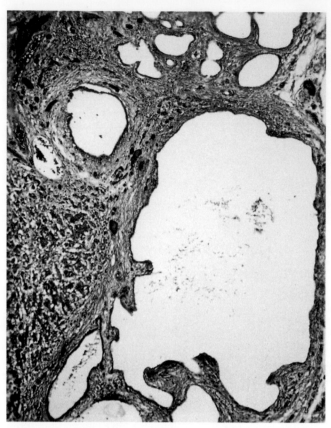

Figure 7.110 Adult polycystic disease. Multiple cysts of varying size are lined by cuboidal to flattened epithelium.

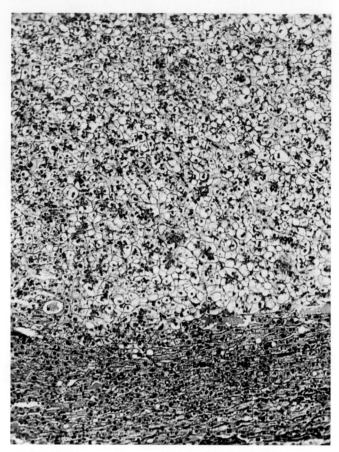

Figure 7.111 Hepatocellular adenoma, composed of a sheet-like growth of large, pale hepatocytes without acinar architecture. Compressed normal liver tissue is present in the lower part of the picture.

acinar architecture (Fig. 7.111) [150]. It is easily mistaken for normal liver if the absence of portal areas is not noticed. The tumor cells are the same size or slightly larger than non-neoplastic hepatocytes and often have a pale cytoplasm because of an increased glycogen and/or fat content. The nuclei are uniform and regular, and the nuclear:cytoplasmic ratio is normal; mitoses are almost never seen. Thin-walled vascular channels are scattered throughout the tumors, but large arteries are only seen around the periphery. The sinusoids are usually compressed with flattened lining cells, contributing to the sheet-like appearance. Sometimes the sinusoids are dilated, a finding that has mistakenly been called peliosis. Kupffer cells are present but are usually inconspicuous, and hematopoietic cells may also be found in sinusoids.

Focal nodular hyperplasia

This is usually a solitary nodule with a typical gross appearance that is extremely useful in making the diagnosis [150]. The lesions are well circumscribed but unencapsulated. When on the surface of the liver, they may appear umbilicated. They are usually of a lighter color than the surrounding liver, ranging from yellow to tan or light brown. The cut surface typically contains a central

"stellate" scar with radiating fibrous septa dividing the lesion into nodules.

The microscopic features correspond to the gross pathology. A section through the center of the lesion nearly always shows the central "stellate" scar that usually contains one or more large arteries, often with abnormal intimal or medial fibromuscular proliferation (Fig. 7.112). Proliferating ductules are usually present but true bile ducts are lacking. Fibrous septa of variable size radiate from the central scar. Between the septa are hyperplastic nodules of normal hepatocytes with cholestatic features, such as cholate stasis, and copper storage, and even bile pigments are usually present to some degree and are occasionally prominent, making the lesion resemble a focal area of biliary cirrhosis. A needle biopsy is easily misinterpreted as cirrhosis unless one is aware that it is from a solitary lesion, but the large artery in an area of scarring provides a valuable clue to the diagnosis.

Hepatocellular carcinoma

The cells of hepatocellular carcinoma resemble normal liver cells to a variable extent [151]. In some tumors,

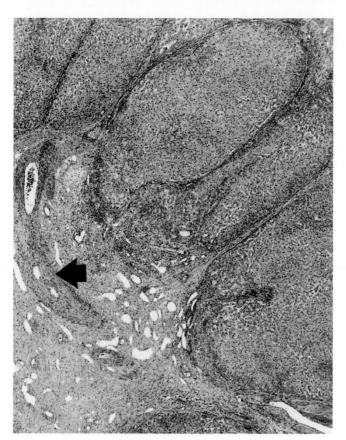

Figure 7.112 Focal nodular hyperplasia. A section through the central scar shows an abnormally thickened large artery (arrow). Cirrhosis-like nodules surround the central scar.

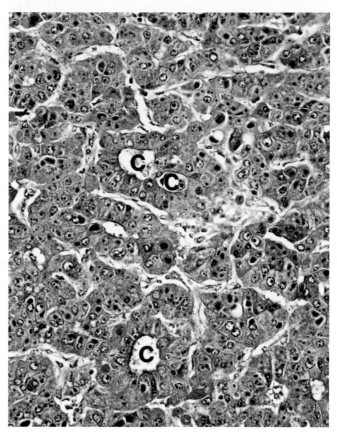

Figure 7.113 Moderately differentiated hepatocellular carcinoma with several dilated canaliculi (C) easily visible between the tumor cells.

the cells are so well differentiated that they are difficult to distinguish from normal hepatocytes or from the cells of hepatocellular adenoma. At the other extreme are tumors with cells that are anaplastic and poorly differentiated, showing only minimal evidence of liver cell origin. Most tumors, however, show definite evidence of hepatocellular differentiation. The tumor cells have distinct cell membranes and an eosinophilic, finely granular cytoplasm. Bile canaliculi are usually present between cells (Fig. 7.113) and, although sometimes hard to find, can usually be seen by light microscopy. Immunostains for CEA are useful for demonstrating canaliculi because of a CEA cross-reacting substance called biliary glycoprotein 1 (BGP-1) located in the canalicular membrane. Bile pigment may be present in tumor cells or in dilated canaliculi and is the most helpful microscopic feature in establishing the diagnosis. The tumor cell nuclei are usually large, producing a high nuclear:cytoplasmic ratio. They show variable degrees of anaplasia and usually have prominent nucleoli.

Several histologic growth patterns may be found in hepatocellular carcinoma, and because the cytologic features can be so variable, recognition of one of these patterns can be helpful in arriving at a diagnosis. Most frequent is the trabecular pattern (Fig. 7.114) in which the tumor cells grow in thick cords that attempt to recapitulate the cell plate pattern of the normal liver. The trabeculae are separated by vascular spaces (sinusoid-like) with very little or no supporting connective tissue. Sometimes the centers of the trabeculae contain dilated canaliculi, producing a pseudoglandular pattern, while solid patterns are produced when the trabeculae grow together, forming sheets of tumor cells.

Fibrolamellar hepatocellular carcinoma

This is usually considered to be a histologic variant of hepatocellular carcinoma, but there is considerable evidence that it is actually a completely different biologic entity, occurring in a different population with a better prognosis than the other types of hepatocellular carcinoma. The pathologic features of fibrolamellar carcinoma are quite distinctive [152]. Microscopically, these tumors appear to be well-differentiated hepatocellular carcinomas but instead of trabeculae separated by sinusoids, they are composed of sheets of large polygonal tumor cells separated by abundant collagen bundles arranged in parallel lamellae (Fig. 7.115), hence the name *fibrolamellar*.

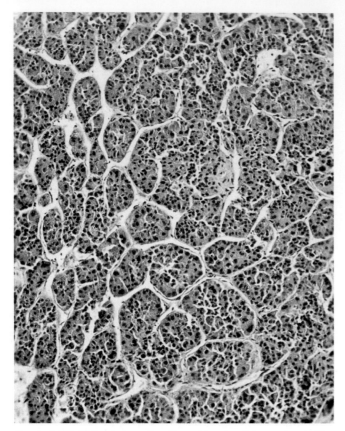

Figure 7.114 Trabecular growth pattern of hepatocellular carcinoma. The tumor cells form thick cords (resembling islands of cells in cross-section), separated by vascular spaces mimicking hepatic sinusoids.

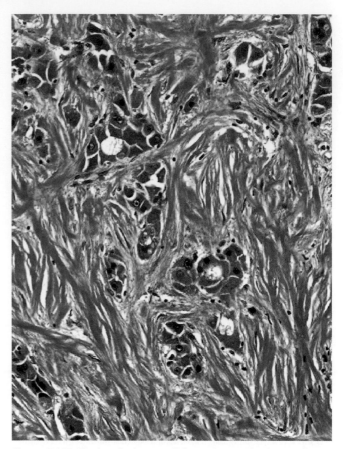

Figure 7.115 Fibrolamellar hepatocellular carcinoma. The tumor cells are large and polygonal and (in contrast to the trabecular hepatocellular carcinoma) are embedded in a fibrous stroma arranged in parallel lamellae.

The tumor cells have a characteristic cytologic appearance with cytoplasm that is deeply eosinophilic and granular due to the presence of numerous mitochondria. Approximately 50% of these tumors have cytoplasmic "pale bodies" that represent intracellular fibrinogen storage.

Hepatoblastoma

Epithelial hepatoblastoma is composed of fetal- or embryonal-type liver cells, or both [153]. Tumors with predominantly fetal cells mimic fetal liver with a distinctive light-and-dark cell pattern and foci of hematopoiesis (Fig. 7.116). Embryonal cells are smaller and more basophilic with a high nuclear:cytoplasmic ratio. They tend to form acini, tubules, or papillary structures. Mixed epithelial–mesenchymal hepatoblastoma has an epithelial component of either fetal or embryonal cells and also a mesenchymal-like element that may consist of primitive mesenchyme, osteoid (with or without calcification), and rarely cartilage or rhabdomyoblasts. An anaplastic type (small cell undifferentiated) and a macrotrabecular type (hepatocellular carcinoma-like) of hepatoblastoma have also been recognized.

Biliary tumors

Bile duct adenoma (peribiliary gland hamartoma)

Bile duct adenoma is usually a solitary subcapsular nodule, although occasional livers have more than one nodule. The lesions may be up to 4 cm in diameter, but 90% are 1 cm or less. They are composed of a proliferation of small, round, normal-appearing ducts with cuboidal, slightly basophilic cells that have very regular nuclei and lack any evidence of dysplasia or mitotic figures (Fig. 7.117). There is always a fibrous supporting stroma that may be dense and hyalinized. Preexisting normal or inflamed portal areas may be present within the tumor. The precise histogenesis of these tumors remains uncertain. Immunophenotypic studies have shown similarities to normal peribiliary glands and to other foregut-derived cell types. The current favored theory is that these lesion represent a biliary proliferative response to localized injury in the liver [154].

Cholangiocarcinoma

Microscopically, these resemble adenocarcinomas arising in other parts of the body [155]. They are glandular

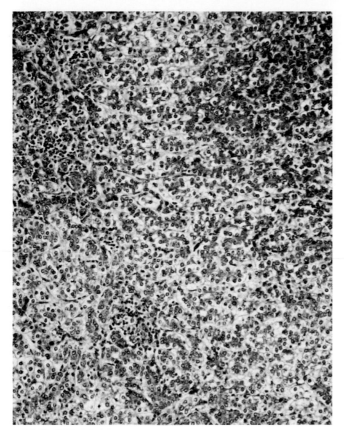

Figure 7.116 Fetal hepatoblastoma mimics fetal liver with a distinctive "light-and-dark" cell pattern and small clusters of hematopoietic cells.

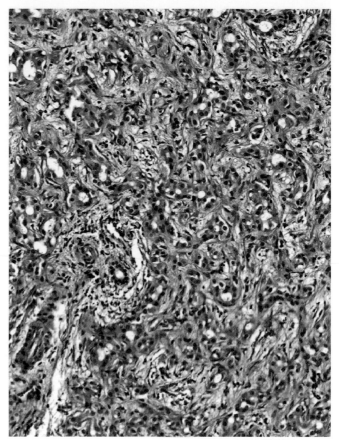

Figure 7.117 Bile duct adenoma (peribiliary gland hamartoma). The tumor is a localized proliferation of small benign glands in a fibrous stroma.

carcinomas (Fig. 7.118) composed of cells resembling biliary epithelium. The cells are low columnar or cuboidal with slightly basophilic cytoplasm and nuclei that are smaller than those of hepatocellular carcinoma; nucleoli are inconspicuous. Mucin can often be demonstrated by special stains but is seldom abundant. There is typically a dense fibrous stroma, which can be helpful in their distinction from hepatocellular carcinoma but not from metastases. Calcifications can sometimes be seen in the fibrous tissue. The tumors are usually well-differentiated gland-forming neoplasms, but they may be poorly differentiated, papillary, or solid, displaying the full range of appearances that can be seen in adenocarcinomas. Occasional tumors show focal squamous differentiation (adenosquamous or mucoepidermoid carcinoma). There are no reliable histologic features distinguishing intrahepatic cholangiocarcinoma from metastatic adenocarcinoma. The diagnosis depends on the reasonable exclusion of an extrahepatic primary.

Biliary cystadenoma and cystadenocarcinoma

These are multilocular cystic neoplasms that arise from intra- and extrahepatic bile ducts [155]. Developmental cysts are never truly multilocular (although secondary

changes occasionally make them seem so). Cystadenomas and cystadenocarcinomas may occur anywhere in the intra- or extrahepatic bile ducts, but nearly all are partly or totally within the liver. Most are over 10 cm in diameter. Microscopically, biliary cystadenoma has a mucin-secreting columnar epithelium lining the cysts (Fig. 7.119). The lining cells have a pale eosinophilic cytoplasm and basally oriented nuclei, typical of biliary-type epithelium. The epithelium is supported by what has been called a *mesenchymal stroma*. This is compact and cellular, and resembles the stroma of the ovary. Biliary cystadenoma is regarded as a premalignant tumor, and when malignancy develops, it is called cystadenocarcinoma. There may only be in situ carcinoma with papillary growth into the cysts, or there may be frank invasive adenocarcinoma.

Biliary papillomatosis

This is an extremely rare disease in which multiple benign papillary adenomas, similar to adenomas of the intestinal tract, arise in the bile ducts [154]. As with intestinal adenomas, invasive carcinoma may develop.

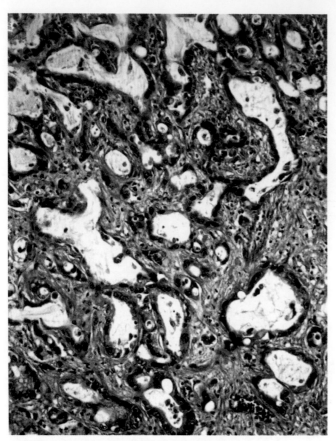

Figure 7.118 Cholangiocarcinoma can resemble an adenocarcinoma arising anywhere in the body. There is typically a dense fibrous stroma infiltrated by irregular glands composed of pleomorphic tumor cells.

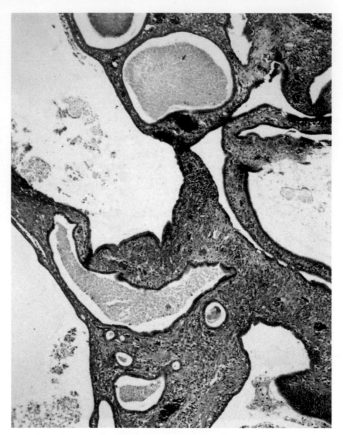

Figure 7.119 Cystadenoma is a multilocular cystic neoplasm with mucinous epithelium overlying a compact mesenchymal stroma.

Hemangiomas and other vascular tumors

Hemangiomas are the only common vascular tumors of the liver. Most are less than 4 cm in diameter, but occasional tumors may be as large as 30 cm. Microscopically these are cavernous hemangiomas with varying-sized vascular channels lined by flattened endothelial cells (Fig. 7.120) [156]. They are usually discrete and well demarcated from the surrounding liver, although an occasional hemangioma may contain trapped bile ducts or foci of parenchyma. Variable amounts of fibrous tissue separate the vascular channels. Many consist of thin, delicate strands, while others have large areas of scarring. Fresh and organizing thrombi may be found in the vascular channels. The dynamics of these thrombi are not known, but they are commonly observed in surgically resected hemangiomas. Because of the sluggish blood flow through these tumors, small thrombi are probably constantly forming and lysing, contributing to the typically heterogeneous appearance on magnetic resonance imaging. Fibroblasts can be found growing into a few thrombi and are probably the source of the scarring that results in the "sclerosing hemangioma." In end-stage

sclerosed and/or calcified hemangiomas, an underlying vascular pattern can usually still be discerned, providing the clue to the diagnosis.

Other vascular tumors are exceedingly rare. *Infantile hemangioendothelioma* is a rare tumor that can occur in the liver in infants [156]. They consist of small proliferating capillary-like vascular channels, similar to the capillary hemangiomas that are common in the skin and mucous membranes of infants. Although histologically benign, they may become large enough to cause hepatic failure or high-output congestive heart failure due to shunting through the tumor. *Angiosarcoma* is a rare, highly malignant tumor in which atypical endothelial cells proliferate in hepatic sinusoids (Fig. 7.121), causing hepatocyte atrophy and the formation of vascular channels and sometimes solid masses of tumor [157]. *Epithelioid hemangioendothelioma* is an equally rare malignant tumor (although not so aggressive as angiosarcoma), in which plump, epithelioid-appearing endothelial cells proliferate in the hepatic vasculature, producing a dense fibrous stroma (Fig. 7.122), similar to that seen in cholangiocarcinoma and metastatic adenocarcinoma [157]. Many of these are misdiagnosed as adenocarcinoma or, if the tumor cells are few, as a benign lesion.

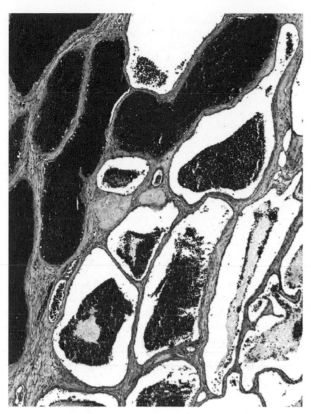

Figure 7.120 Hemangioma consists of a fibrous stroma containing "cavernous" blood-filled spaces lined by flattened endothelial cells.

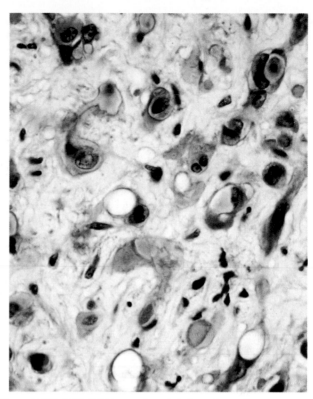

Figure 7.122 Epithelioid hemangioendothelioma is a malignant tumor that forms intracellular capillary lumina and typically produces a dense fibrous stroma as it fills the vascular spaces.

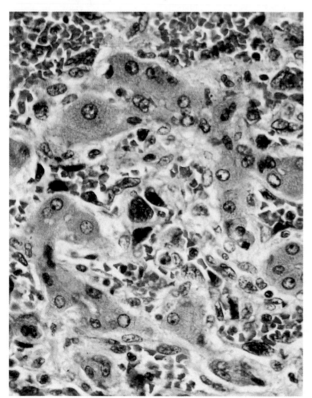

Figure 7.121 Angiosarcoma is a proliferation of malignant endothelial cells that fills the hepatic sinusoids, causing the hepatocytes to atrophy.

Metastases

Metastases far outnumber primary liver tumors, so that any liver mass is more likely to be metastatic than primary. Only if a tumor is benign or shows clear evidence of hepatocellular differentiation, indicating hepatocellular carcinoma, can it be confirmed that it is primary in the liver. Any other malignancy, particularly an adenocarcinoma, should be presumed to be metastatic. Microscopically, metastases usually resemble the primary tumor. If the primary lesion is known and has been biopsied or excised, comparison of the microscopic appearance of the tumor in the liver with that of the primary will confirm whether the hepatic tumor is a metastasis.

Further reading

Burt AD, Portmann BC, Ferrell LD, eds. *MacSween's Pathology of the Liver*, 5th edn. Philadelphia, PA: Churchill Livingstone Elsevier, 2007.
Overall, the best reference book on liver pathology.

Desmet VJ, Gerber M, Hoofnagel JH, et al. Classification of chronic hepatitis: diagnosis, grading and staging. *Hepatology* 1994;19:1513–20.
The preferred classification of chronic hepatitis.

Ishak KG, Goodman ZD, Stocker JT. *Tumors of the Liver and Intrahepatic Bile Ducts. Atlas of tumor pathology*, Third Series, Fascicle 31. Washington, DC: Armed Forces Institute of Pathology, 2001.
The authoritative book on the pathology of liver tumors.

Prophet EB, Mills B, Arrington JB, et al., eds. *Laboratory Methods in Histotechnology*. Washington, DC: Armed Forces Institute of Pathology, 1992.
A book on how to do the special stains.

Scheuer PJ, Lefkowitch JH. *Liver Biopsy Interpretation*, 7th edn. London: WB Saunders, 2006. *A very readable text book.*

References

1. Prophet EB, Mills B, Arrington JB, et al., eds. *Laboratory Methods in Histotechnology*. Washington, DC: Armed Forces Institute of Pathology, 1992.
2. Van Eyken P, Desmet VJ. Cytokeratins and the liver. *Liver* 1993;13:113–22.
3. Goldstein NS, Soman A, Gordon SC. Portal tract eosinophils and hepatocyte cytokeratin 7 immunoreactivity helps distinguish early-stage, mildly active primary biliary cirrhosis and autoimmune hepatitis. *Am J Clin Pathol* 2001;116:846–53.
4. Vyberg M, Leth P. Ubiquitin: an immunohistochemical marker of Mallory bodies and alcoholic liver disease. *APMIS Suppl* 1991;23:46–52.
5. Zatloukal K, French SW, Stumptner C, et al. From Mallory to Mallory–Denk bodies: what, how and why? *Exp Cell Res* 2007;313:2033–49.
6. Phillips MJ, Poucell S, Patterson J, et al. *The Liver. An atlas and text of ultrastructural pathology*. New York: Raven Press, 1987.
7. Ishak KG. Applications of scanning electron microscopy to the study of liver disease. *Prog Liver Dis* 1986;8:1–32.
8. Wu PC, Fang JWS, Lai CL, et al. Hepatic expression of hepatitis B virus genome in chronic hepatitis B virus infection. *Am J Clin Pathol* 1996;105:87–95.
9. Suh N, Liapis H, Misdraji J, Brunt EM, Wang HL. Epstein–Barr virus hepatitis: diagnostic value of in situ hybridization, polymerase chain reaction, and immunohistochemistry on liver biopsy from immunocompetent patients. *Am J Surg Pathol* 2007;31:1403–9.
10. Sherman KE, Lewey SM, Goodman ZD. Talc in the liver of patients with chronic hepatitis C infection. *Am J Gastroenterol* 1995;90:2164–6.
11. Carmichael GP, Targoff C, Pintar K, et al. Hepatic silicosis. *Am J Clin Pathol* 1980;73:720–2.
12. Cortes JM, Oliva H, Paradinas FJ, et al. The pathology of the liver in porphyria cutanea tarda. *Histopathology* 1980;4:471–85.
13. Klatskin G, Bloomer JR. Birefringence of hepatic pigment deposits in erythropoietic protoporphyria. *Gastroenterology* 1974;67:294–302.
14. Benedetti A, Marucci L. The significance of apoptosis in the liver. *Liver* 1999;19:453–63.
15. Jaeschke H, Gujral JS, Bajt ML. Apoptosis and necrosis in liver disease. *Liver Int* 2004;24:85–89.
16. Teixeira MR, Weller IVD, Murray A, et al. The pathology of hepatitis A in man. *Liver* 1982;2:53–60.
17. Abe H, Beninger PR, Ikejiri N, et al. Light microscopic findings of liver biopsy specimens from patients with hepatitis type A and comparison with type B. *Gastroenterology* 1982;82:938–47.
18. Markin RS. Manifestations of Epstein–Barr virus-associated disorders in the liver. *Liver* 1994;14:1–13.
19. Snover DC, Horwitz CA. Liver disease in cytomegalovirus mononucleosis: a light microscopical and immunoperoxidase study of six cases. *Hepatology* 1984;4:408–12.
20. Ten Napel CHH, Houthoff HJ, Teh TH. Cytomegalovirus hepatitis in normal and immune compromised hosts. *Liver* 1984;4:184–94.
21. Mullick FG, Ishak KG. Hepatic injury associated with diphenylhydantoin therapy: a clinicopathologic study of 20 cases. *Am J Clin Pathol* 1980;74:442–52.
22. Peron JM, Danjoux M, Kamar N, et al. Liver histology in patients with sporadic acute hepatitis E: a study of 11 patients from southwest France. *Virchows Arch* 2007;450:405–10.
23. Zimmerman HJ. *Hepatotoxicity: the adverse effects of drugs and other chemicals on the liver*, 2nd edn. Philadelphia, PA: Lippincott Williams and Wilkins, 1999.
24. Ishak KG, Walker DH, Coetzer JAW, et al. Viral hemorrhagic fevers with hepatic involvement: pathologic aspects with clinical correlations. *Prog Liver Dis* 1982;7:495–515.
25. Goodman ZD, Ishak KG, Sesterhenn IA. Herpes simplex in apparently immunocompetent adults. *Am J Clin Pathol* 1986;85:694–9.
26. Varki NM, Bhuta S, Drake T, et al. Adenovirus hepatitis in two successive liver transplants in a child. *Arch Pathol Lab Med* 1990;114:106–9.
27. Schiodt FV, Atillasoy E, Shakil AO, et al. Etiology and outcome for 295 patients with acute liver failure in the United States. *Liver Transpl Surg* 1999;5:29–34.
28. Wright TL. Etiology of fulminant hepatic failure: is another virus involved? *Gastroenterology* 1993;104:640–53.
29. Kessler WR, Cummings OW, Eckert G, et al. Fulminant hepatic failure as the initial presentation of acute autoimmune hepatitis. *Clin Gastroenterol Hepatol* 2004;2:625–31.
30. Demetris AJ, Seaberg EC, Wennerberg A, et al. Ductular reaction after submassive necrosis in humans: special emphasis on analysis of ductular hepatocytes. *Am J Pathol* 1996;149:439–48.
31. Mosnier J-F, Degott C, Marcellin P, et al. The intraportal lymphoid nodule and its environment in chronic active hepatitis C: an immunohistochemical study. *Hepatology* 1993;17:366–71.
32. Poulsen H, Christoffersen P. Abnormal bile duct epithelium in liver biopsies with histological signs of viral hepatitis. *Acta Pathol Microbiol Scand* 1969;76:383–90.
33. Vyberg M. The hepatitis-associated bile duct lesion. *Liver* 1993;13:289–301.
34. Goodman ZD, Ishak KG. Histopathology of hepatitis C virus infection. *Semin Liver Dis* 1995;15:70–81.
35. Ishak KG, Baptista A, Bianchi L, et al. Histological grading and staging of chronic hepatitis. *J Hepatol* 1995;22:696–9.
36. Bianchi L, De Groote J, Desmet VJ, et al. Acute and chronic hepatitis revisited. Review by an international group. *Lancet* 1977;2:914–19.
37. Goodman Z. Histopathology of infection. In: Lai CL, Locarnini S, eds. *Hepatitis B Virus*, 2nd edn. London: International Medical Press, 2008:10.1–10.14.
38. Rubbia-Brandt L, Quadri R, Abid K, et al. Hepatocyte steatosis is a cytopathic effect of hepatitis C virus genotype 3. *J Hepatol* 2000;33:106–15.
39. Verme G, Amoroso P, Lettieri G, et al. A histological study of hepatitis delta virus liver disease. *Hepatology* 1986;6:1303–7.
40. Devaney K, Goodman ZD, Ishak KG. Post-infantile giant cell transformation in hepatitis. *Hepatology* 1992;16:327–33.
41. Davies SE, Portmann BC, O'Grady JG, et al. Hepatic histological findings after transplantation for chronic hepatitis B virus infection, including a unique pattern of fibrosing cholestatic hepatitis. *Hepatology* 1991;13:150–7.
42. Cotler SJ, Taylor SL, Gretch DR, et al. Hyperbilirubinemia and cholestatic liver injury in hepatitis C-infected liver transplant recipients. *Am J Gastroenterol* 2000;95:753–9.
43. Delladetsima JK, Boletis JN, Makris F, et al. Fibrosing cholestatic hepatitis in renal transplant recipients with hepatitis C virus infection. *Liver Transpl Surg* 1999;5:294–300.
44. Desmet VJ, Gerber M, Hoofnagel JH, et al. Classification of chronic hepatitis: diagnosis, grading and staging. *Hepatology* 1994;19:1513–20.
45. Batts KP, Ludwig J. Chronic hepatitis: an update on terminology and reporting. *Am J Surg Pathol* 1995;19:1409–17.
46. Bedossa P, Poynard T. The French METAVIR Cooperative Study Group. An algorithm for grading activity in chronic hepatitis C. *Hepatology* 1996;24:289–93.

47. Knodell RG, Ishak KG, Black WC, et al. Formulation and application of a numerical scoring system for assessing histological activity in asymptomatic chronic active hepatitis. *Hepatology* 1981;1:431–5.

48. The French METAVIR Cooperative Study Group. Intraobserver and interobserver variations in liver biopsy interpretation in patients with chronic hepatitis C. *Hepatology* 994;20:15–20.

49. Westin J, Lagging LM, Wejstal R, et al. Interobserver study of liver histopathology using the Ishak score in patients with chronic hepatitis C virus infection. *Liver* 1999;19:183–7.

50. Lewis JH, Kleiner DE. Hepatic injury due to drugs, chemicals and toxins. In: Burt AD, Portmann BC, Ferrell LD, eds. *MacSween's Pathology of the Liver*, 5th edn. Philadelphia, PA: Churchill Livingstone Elsevier, 2007:649–760.

51. Jansen PLM, Muller M. The molecular genetics of familial intrahepatic cholestasis. *Gut* 2000;47:1–5.

52. Rolfes DB, Ishak KG. Liver disease in pregnancy. *Histopathology* 1986;10:555–70.

53. Review by an International Group. Histopathology of the intrahepatic biliary tree. *Liver* 1983;3:161–75.

54. Roskams TA, Theise ND, Balabaud C, et al. Nomenclature of the finer branches of the biliary tree: canals, ductules, and ductular reactions in human livers. *Hepatology* 2004;39:1739–45.

55. Roskams T, Desmet V. Ductular reaction and its diagnostic significance. *Semin Diagnostic Pathol* 1998;15:259–69.

56. Erlinger S. Drug-induced cholestasis. *J Hepatol* 1997;26(Suppl 1):1–4.

57. Lefkowitch JH. Bile ductular cholestasis: an ominous histopathologic sign related to sepsis and "cholangitis lenta." *Hum Pathol* 1982;13:19–24.

58. Banks JG, Foulis AK, Ledingham IM, et al. Liver function in septic shock. *J Clin Pathol* 1982;35:1249–52.

59. Rubin E, Schaffner F, Popper H. Primary biliary cirrhosis. Chronic non-suppurative destructive cholangitis. *Am J Pathol* 1965;46:387–407.

60. Sherlock C, Scheuer PJ. The presentation and diagnosis of 100 patients with primary biliary cirrhosis. *N Engl J Med* 1983;289:674–8.

61. Goodman ZD, McNally PR, Davis DR, et al. Autoimmune cholangitis: a variant of primary biliary cirrhosis. *Dig Dis Sci* 1995;40: 1232–42.

62. Kahn E, Markowitz J, Aiges H, et al. Human ontogeny of the bile duct to portal space ratio. *Hepatology* 1989;10:21–3.

63. Nakanuma Y. Necroinflammatory changes in hepatic lobules in primary biliary cirrhosis with less well-defined cholestatic changes. *Hum Pathol* 1993;24:378–83.

64. Portmann B, Popper H, Neuberger J, et al. Sequential and diagnostic features in primary biliary cirrhosis based on serial histologic study in 209 patients. *Gastroenterology* 1985;88:1777–90.

65. Terracciano LM, Patzina RA, Lehmann FS, et al. A spectrum of histopathologic findings in autoimmune liver disease. *Am J Clin Pathol* 2000;114:705–11.

66. Woodward J, Neuberger J. Autoimmune overlap syndromes. *Hepatology* 2001;33:994–1002.

67. Lohse AW, Meyer zum Büschenfelde KH, Franz B, et al. Characterization of the overlap syndrome of primary biliary cirrhosis (PBC) and autoimmune hepatitis; evidence for it being a hepatitic form of PBC in genetically susceptible individuals. *Hepatology* 1999;29:1078–84.

68. Ludwig J, Colina F, Poterucha JJ. Granulomas in primary sclerosing cholangitis. *Liver* 1995;15:307–12.

69. Nakanuma Y. Pathology of septum formation in primary biliary cirrhosis: a histological study in the non-cirrhotic stage. *Virchows Archiv A* 1991;419:381–7.

70. Ludwig J, Dickson ER, McDonald GSA. Staging of chronic nonsuppurative destructive cholangitis (syndrome of primary biliary cirrhosis). *Virchows Arch A* 1978;379:103–12.

71. Ludwig J, LaRusso NF, Wiesner RH. The syndrome of primary sclerosing cholangitis. In: Popper H, Schaffner F, eds. *Progress in Liver Disease*, Vol. 9. Philadelphia, PA: WB Saunders, 1990:555–66.

72. International Panel. Banff schema for grading liver allograft rejection: an international consensus document. *Hepatology* 1997;25:658–63.

73. International Panel. Update of the international Banff schema for liver allograft rejection: working recommendations for the histologic staging and reporting of chronic rejection. *Hepatology* 2000;31:792–9.

74. Devaney K, Goodman ZD, Epstein MS, et al. The histologic spectrum of hepatic sarcoidosis – a study of 100 cases. *Am J Surg Pathol* 1993;17:1272–80.

75. Ludwig J, Kim CH, Wiesner RH, et al. Floxuridine-induced sclerosing cholangitis: an ischemic cholangiopathy? *Hepatology* 1995;9:215–18.

76. Kaplan KJ, Goodman ZD, Ishak KG. Liver involvement in Langerhans' cell histiocytosis: a study of nine cases. *Mod Pathol* 1999;12:370–8.

77. Cello JP. Human immunodeficiency virus-associated biliary tract disease. *Semin Liver Dis* 1992;12:213–18.

78. Desmet VJ. Vanishing bile duct syndrome in drug-induced liver disease. *J Hepatol* 1997;26(Suppl 1):31–5.

79. Hadchouel M. Paucity of interlobular bile ducts. *Semin Diagn Pathol* 1992;9:24–30.

80. Dahms BB, Petrelli M, Wyllie R, et al. Arteriohepatic dysplasia in infancy and childhood. A longitudinal study of six patients. *Hepatology* 1982;2:350–8.

81. Kahn EI, Daum F, Markowitz J, et al. Arteriohepatic dysplasia. II. Hepatobiliary pathology. *Hepatology* 1983;3:77–84.

82. Ludwig J. Idiopathic adulthood ductopenia: an update. *Mayo Clin Proc* 1998;73:285–91.

83. Bonnell HJ, Beckwith JB. Fatty liver in sudden childhood death: implications for Reye's syndrome. *Am J Dis Child* 1986;140:30–3.

84. Fraser JL, Antonioli DA, Chopra S, et al. Prevalence and nonspecificity of microvesicular fatty change in the liver. *Mod Pathol* 1995,8:65–70.

85. Rolfes DB, Ishak KG. Acute fatty liver in pregnancy. A clinicopathologic study of 35 cases. *Hepatology* 1985;5:1149–58.

86. Heubi JE, Partin JC, Partin JS, et al. Reye's syndrome: current concepts. *Hepatology* 1987;7:155–64.

87. Treem WR. Inborn defects in mitochondrial fatty acid oxidation. In: Suchy FJ, Sokol RJ, Balistreri WF, et al., eds. *Liver Disease in Children*, 2nd edn. Philadelphia, PA: Lippincott Williams and Wilkins, 2001:735–85.

88. Sokol RJ, Treem WR. Mitochondrial hepatopathies. In: Suchy FJ, Sokol RJ, Balistreri WF, et al., eds. *Liver Disease in Children*, 2nd edn. Philadelphia, PA: Lippincott Williams and Wilkins, 2001:785–809.

89. Starko KM, Mullick FG. Hepatic and cerebral pathology findings in children with fatal salicylate intoxication: further evidence of a causal relationship between salicylate and Reye's syndrome. *Lancet* 1983;1:326–9.

90. Zimmerman HJ, Ishak KG. Valproate-induced hepatic injury. Analyses of 23 fatal cases. *Hepatology* 1982;2:591–7.

91. Kleiner DE, Gaffey MJ, Sallie R, et al. Histopathologic changes associated with fialuridine hepatotoxicity. *Mod Pathol* 1997;10:192–9.

92. Uchida T, Kao H, Quispe-Sjogren M, et al. Alcoholic foamy degeneration. A pattern of acute alcoholic injury of the liver. *Gastroenterology* 1983;84:683–92.

93. Popper H, Thung SN, Gerber MA, et al. Histologic studies of severe delta agent infection in Venezuelan Indians. *Hepatology* 1983;3:906–12.

94. Review by an International Group. Alcoholic liver disease: morphologic manifestations. *Lancet* 1981;3:707–11.

95. Stumptner C, Fuchsbichler A, Heid H, et al. Mallory body – a disease-associated type of sequestrosome. *Hepatology* 2002;35:1053–62.

96. Diehl AM, Goodman ZD, Ishak KG. Alcohol like liver disease in nonalcoholics. A clinical and histological comparison with alcohol induced liver injury. *Gastroenterology* 1988;95:1056–62.

97. Goodman ZD, Ishak KG. Occlusive venous lesions in alcoholic liver disease. A study of 200 cases. *Gastroenterology* 1982;83:786–96.

98. Caldwell SH, Crespo DM. The spectrum expanded: cryptogenic cirrhosis and the natural history of non-alcoholic fatty liver disease. *J Hepatol* 2004;40:578–84.

99. Ludwig J, Farr GH, Freese DK, et al. Chronic hepatitis and hepatic failure in a 14-year-old girl. *Hepatology* 1995;22:1874–9.

100. Peters RL, Thomas G, Reynolds TB. Post-jejunoileal-bypass hepatic disease. Its similarity to alcoholic hepatic disease. *Am J Clin Pathol* 1975;63:318–31.

101. Ishak KG, Goodman ZD, Stocker JT. *Tumors of the Liver and Intrahepatic Bile Ducts. Atlas of tumor pathology*, Third Series, Fascicle 31. Washington, DC: Armed Forces Institute of Pathology, 2001:127–33.

102. Adams DO. The granulomatous inflammatory response: a review. *Am J Pathol* 1976;84:164–91.

103. Ishak KG. Granulomas of the liver. *Adv Pathol Lab Med* 1995;8:247–361.

104. Lamps LW. Hepatic granulomas, with a emphasis on infectious causes. *Adv Anat Pathol* 2008;15:309–18.

105. Qizilbash AH. The pathology of Q fever. *Arch Pathol Lab Med* 1983;107:364–7.

106. Marazuela M, Moreno A, Yebra M, et al. Hepatic fibrin ring granulomas: a clinicopathologic study of 23 patients. *Hum Pathol* 1991;22:607–13.

107. Karat ABA, Job CK, Pao PSS. Liver in leprosy: histological and biochemical findings. *Br Med J* 1971;1:307–10.

108. Klatt EC, Jensen DF, Meyer PR. Pathology of *Mycobacterium avium intercellulare* infection in acquired immunodeficiency syndrome. *Hum Pathol* 1987;18:709–14.

109. Kaplan KJ, Goodman ZD, Ishak KG. Eosinophilic granuloma of the liver: a characteristic lesion with relationship to visceral larva migrans. *Am J Surg Pathol* 2001;25:1316–21.

110. Cruickshank B, Thomas MJ. Mineral oil (follicular) lipidosis. II. Histologic studies of spleen, liver, lymph nodes and bone marrow. *Hum Pathol* 1984;15:731–7.

111. Portmann BC, Roberts EA. Genetic and metabolic liver disease. In: Burt AD, Portmann BC, Ferrell LD, eds. *MacSween's Pathology of the Liver*, 5th edn. Philadelphia, PA: Churchill Livingstone Elsevier, 2007:199–326.

112. Reed GB, Dixon JF, Neustein HB, et al. Type IV glycogenosis. *Lab Invest* 1968;19:546–57.

113. Sharp HL. Alpha-1-antitrypsin deficiency. *Hosp Pract* 1971;6:83–96.

114. Crowley JJ, Sharp HL, Frier E, et al. Fatal liver disease associated with alpha-1-antitrypsin deficiency PiM PiM$_1$/PiMduarte. *Gastroenterology* 1987;93:242–4.

115. Pariente EA, Degott C, Martin JP, et al. Hepatocytic PAS-positive diastase-resistant inclusions in the absence of alpha-1-antitrypsin deficiency – high prevalence in alcoholic cirrhosis. *Am J Clin Pathol* 1981;76:299–302.

116. Callea F, Brisigotti M, Fabbretti G, et al. Hepatic endoplasmic reticulum storage diseases. *Liver* 1992;12:357–362.

117. Mendelsohn G, Gomperts ED, Gurwitz D. Severe antithrombin III deficiency in an infant associated with multiple arterial and venous thrombosis. *Thromb Haemost* 1976;34:495–502.

118. Pfeifer U, Ormanns W, Klinge O. Hepatocellular fibrinogen storage in familial hypofibrinogenemia. *Virchows Arch B Cell Pathol* 1981;36:247–55.

119. Klatt EC, Koss MN, Young TS, et al. Hepatic hyaline globules associated with passive congestion. *Arch Pathol Lab Med* 1988;112:510–13.

120. Bruguera M, Lamar C, Bernet M, et al. Hepatic disease associated with ground-glass inclusions in hepatocytes after cyanamide therapy. *Arch Pathol Lab Med* 1986;110:906–10.

121. Nishimura RN, Ishak KG, Reddick R, et al. Lafora disease: diagnosis by liver biopsy. *Ann Neurol* 1980;8:409–15.

122. Hall P, Gormley BM, Jarvis LR, et al. A staining method for the detection and measurement of fat droplets in hepatic tissue. *Pathology* 1980;12:605–8.

123. Fakan F, Chlumska A. Demonstration of needle-shaped hepatic inclusions in porphyria cutanea tarda using the ferric ferricyanide reduction test. *Virchows Arch A* 1987;411:365–8.

124. Deugnier YM, Loreal O, Turlin B, et al. Liver pathology in genetic hemochromatosis: a review of 135 homozygous cases and their bioclinical correlations. *Gastroenterology* 1992;102:2050–9.

125. Deugnier YM, Charalambous P, Le Quilleuc D, et al. Preneoplastic significance of hepatic iron-free-foci in genetic hemochromatosis: a study of 195 patients. *Hepatology* 1993;18:1363–9.

126. Ludwig J, Moyer TP, Rakela J. The liver biopsy diagnosis of Wilson's disease. *Am J Clin Pathol* 1994;102:443–6.

127. Stromeyer FW, Ishak KG. The histopathology of the liver in Wilson's disease: a study of 34 cases. *Am J Clin Pathol* 1980;73:12–24.

128. Davies SE, Williams R, Portmann B. Hepatic morphology and histochemistry of Wilson's disease presenting as fulminant hepatic failure: a study of 11 cases. *Histopathology* 1989;15:385–94.

129. Sternlieb I. Fraternal concordance of types of abnormal hepatocellular mitochondria in Wilson's disease. *Hepatology* 1992;16:728–32.

130. Lefkowitch JH, Mendez L. Morphologic features of hepatic injury in cardiac disease and shock. *J Hepatol* 1986;2:313–27.

131. Myers RP, Cerini R, Sayegh R, et al. Cardiac hepatopathy: clinical, hemodynamic, and histologic characteristics and correlations. *Hepatology* 2003;37:393–400.

132. Gitlin N, Serio KM. Ischemic hepatitis: widening horizons. *Am J Gastroenterol* 1992;87:831–6.

133. Okudaira M, Ohbu M, Okuda K. Idiopathic portal hypertension and its pathology. *Semin Liver Dis* 2002;22:59–71.

134. Wanless IR. Micronodular transformation (nodular regenerative hyperplasia) of the liver: a report of 64 cases among 2500 autopsies and a new classification of benign hepatocellular nodules. *Hepatology* 1990;11:787–97.

135. Ham JM. Lobar and segmental atrophy of the liver. *World J Surg* 1990;14:457–62.

136. Tanaka M, Wanless IR. Pathology of the liver in Budd–Chiari syndrome, portal vein thrombosis and the histogenesis of veno-centric cirrhosis, veno-portal cirrhosis, and large regenerative nodules. *Hepatology* 1998;27:488–96.

137. Winkler K, Christoffersen P. A reappraisal of Poulsen's disease (hepatic zone 1 sinusoidal dilatation). *APMIS Suppl* 1991;23:86–90.

138. Gerber MA, Thung SN, Bodenheimer HC Jr, et al. Characteristic histologic triad in liver adjacent to metastatic neoplasm. *Liver* 1986;6:85–8.

139. Ishak KG. Hepatic lesions caused by anabolic and contraceptive steroids. *Semin Liver Dis* 1981;1:116–28.

140. LeBoit PE. Bacillary angiomatosis. *Mod Pathol* 1995;8:218–22.

141. Rolfes DB, Ishak KG. Liver disease in toxemia of pregnancy. *Am J Gastroenterol* 1986;81:1138–44.

142. Buck FS, Koss MN. Hepatic amyloidosis: morphologic differences between systemic AA and AL types. *Hum Pathol* 1991;22:904–7.

143. Anthony PP, Ishak KG, Nayak NG, et al. The morphology of cirrhosis. *J Clin Pathol* 1978;31:395–414.

144. Anthony PP, Vogel CL, Barker LF. Liver cell dysplasia: a premalignant condition. *J Clin Pathol* 1973;26:217–23.

145. International Working Party. Terminology of nodular hepatocellular lesions. *Hepatology* 1995;22:983–93.

146. Summerfield JA, Nagaguchi Y, Sherlock S, et al. Hepatic fibropolycystic diseases. A clinical and histological review of 51 patients. *J Hepatol* 1986;2:141–56.

147. Desmet VJ. Congenital diseases of the intrahepatic bile ducts: variations on the theme "ductal plate malformation." *Hepatology* 1992;16:1069–83.

148. Vick DJ, Goodman ZD, Deavers MT, et al. Ciliated hepatic foregut cyst. A study of six cases and review of the literature. *Am J Surg Pathol* 1999;23:671–7.

149. Portmann BC, Roberts EA. Developmental abnormalities and liver disease in childhood. In: Burt AD, Portmann BC, Ferrell LD, eds. *MacSween's Pathology of the Liver*, 5th edn. Philadelphia, PA: Churchill Livingstone Elsevier, 2007:147–98.

150. Ishak KG, Goodman, ZD, Stocker JT. *Tumors of the Liver and Intrahepatic Bile Ducts. Atlas of tumor pathology*, Third Series, Fascicle 31. Washington, DC: Armed Forces Institute of Pathology, 2001; 9–48.

151. Ishak KG, Goodman ZD, Stocker JT. *Tumors of the Liver and Intrahepatic Bile Ducts. Atlas of tumor pathology*, Third Series, Fascicle 31. Washington, DC: Armed Forces Institute of Pathology, 2001;199–230.

152. Ishak KG, Goodman ZD, Stocker JT. *Tumors of the Liver and Intrahepatic Bile Ducts. Atlas of tumor pathology*, Third Series, Fascicle 31. Washington, DC: Armed Forces Institute of Pathology, 2001;231–44.

153. Ishak KG, Goodman ZD, Stocker JT. *Tumors of the Liver and Intrahepatic Bile Ducts. Atlas of tumor pathology*, Third Series, Fascicle 31. Washington, DC: Armed Forces Institute of Pathology, 2001;159–84.

154. Hughes NR, Goodman ZD, Bhathal PS. An immunohistochemical profile of the so-called bile duct adenoma: clues to pathogenesis. *Am J Surg Pathol* 2010;34:1312–18.

155. Ishak KG, Goodman ZD, Stocker JT. *Tumors of the Liver and Intrahepatic Bile Ducts. Atlas of tumor pathology*, Third Series, Fascicle 31. Washington, DC: Armed Forces Institute of Pathology, 2001;245–71.

156. Ishak KG, Goodman ZD, Stocker JT. *Tumors of the Liver and Intrahepatic Bile Ducts. Atlas of tumor pathology*, Third Series, Fascicle 31. Washington, DC: Armed Forces Institute of Pathology, 2001;71–146.

157. Ishak KG, Goodman ZD, Stocker JT. *Tumors of the Liver and Intrahepatic Bile Ducts. Atlas of tumor pathology*, Third Series, Fascicle 31. Washington, DC: Armed Forces Institute of Pathology, 2001;281–323.

CHAPTER 8

Mechanisms of Liver Injury

Harmeet Malhi & Gregory J. Gores

Division of Gastroenterology and Hepatology, Mayo Clinic, College of Medicine, Rochester, MN, USA

Key concepts

- Apoptosis is a prominent feature of acute and chronic liver diseases.
- Injurious stimuli can induce apoptosis in different cellular compartments in the liver.
- Hepatocyte apoptosis is mitochondria dependent.

- Mitochondrial dysfunction in hepatocytes can be secondary to death receptor-mediated extrinsic signals or intrinsic perturbations.
- Apoptosis leads to inflammation and injury in acute liver diseases, and in chronic liver diseases sustained apoptosis begets fibrosis.
- Manipulation of apoptotic pathways has wide therapeutic potential.

The liver is in constant cellular flux with careful removal of senescent or damaged cells and controlled repopulation through a progenitor cell compartment. The unique juxtaposition to the intestine, large resting blood flow, and unfiltered contact with portal blood also provides the liver with a unique sensitivity to various gut-derived, diet-derived, or blood-borne insults. Under basal conditions, removal of hepatocytes occurs mainly through apoptosis without reactive inflammation. Liver injury, on the other hand, is associated with cell death, inflammation, and regeneration.

Cell death in the liver can be apoptotic or necrotic or a combination of the two. Historically, apoptosis, or programmed cell death, has been viewed as a carefully choreographed cascade resulting in protease and endonuclease activation. It has been defined morphologically on the basis of characteristic nuclear appearance, the generation of membrane-bound apoptotic bodies (Councilman bodies), and the absence of an inflammatory reaction. Necrotic cell death has been considered the antithesis of apoptotic cell death. It has been defined on the basis of cellular energy depletion, characteristic morphology of cytoplasmic vacuolation, cell swelling, and the presence of an inflammatory reaction. Cell swelling, a cardinal feature of necrosis, results from an inability to maintain ion gradients, such that the process is in fact called oncotic necrosis. Over the last few years, with better understanding of both pathways of cell death, these arbitrary morphologic definitions have become less important. It is recognized that both apoptosis and necrosis can be triggered by the same stimulus and occur in the same disease process. Furthermore, necroptosis, a form of cell death with necrotic morphology is triggered by apoptotic stimuli in cells deficient in apoptotic signaling, and is a regulated form of cell death. Apoptosis has been shown to be a prominent feature of several liver diseases (Fig. 8.1). The dogma has shifted from apoptosis being a physiologic, bland, noninflammatory process to one that is pathologic, occurs in disease processes, and causes liver inflammation, injury, and fibrosis (Fig. 8.2). This chapter is divided into two sections. The first section provides a general overview of mechanisms of cell death in the liver and the role of the innate immune system in this context. Apoptosis and necrosis are both discussed with emphasis on death receptors and the role of mitochondria in cell fate. The second section focuses on mechanisms of liver injury in some common disorders.

Basic mechanisms

Apoptosis

Apoptosis is a prominent feature of liver injury including drug-induced liver diseases, viral hepatitis, alcoholic liver disease, nonalcoholic fatty liver disease, cholestasis, and vascular liver diseases. Apoptosis of hepatocytes, Kupffer cells, sinusoidal endothelial cells (SECs), hepatic stellate cells (HSCs), and cholangiocytes has been observed in different liver diseases [1]. The initiation of apoptosis occurs via two fundamental pathways: (i) the death receptor or extrinsic pathway; and (ii) the mitochondrial or intrinsic pathway [2]. The extrinsic pathway is triggered by ligation or oligomerization of death receptors. The

Schiff's Diseases of the Liver, Eleventh Edition. Edited by Eugene R. Schiff, Willis C. Maddrey and Michael F. Sorrell.
© 2012 John Wiley & Sons, Ltd. Published 2012 by John Wiley & Sons, Ltd.

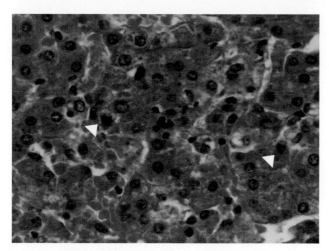

Figure 8.1 Hepatocyte apoptosis in human liver. Hematoxylin and eosin-stained section from the liver of a patient with primary sclerosing cholangitis showing several apoptotic hepatocytes (white arrowheads). Condensed nuclei (pyknosis) surrounded by an eosinophilic cytoplasm can be seen.

mitochondrial pathway is activated by several intracellular perturbations, including DNA damage, lysosomal permeabilization, endoplasmic reticulum stress, chemotherapeutic agents, oxidative stress, toxins, and sustained increases in Ca^{2+} [3]. Cells that die via the extrinsic pathway are classified as type I or type II cells. In type I

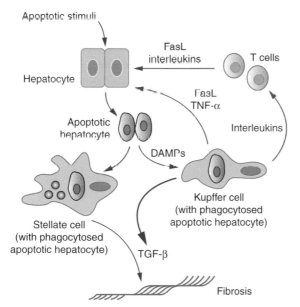

Figure 8.2 Hepatocyte apoptosis is the proximal event in hepatic fibrosis. Apoptotic hepatocytes are engulfed by stellate cells, leading to their activation, and by Kupffer cells, leading to the secretion of several proinflammatory and proapoptotic cytokines. Molecules known as damage-associated molecular patterns (DAMPs) are also released from dead cells and activate cells of the innate immune system, including Kupffer cells. Kupffer cell-derived cytokines promote stellate cell activation and further promote apoptosis. Activated stellate cells play a key role in fibrosis. FasL, Fas ligand; TNF-α, tumor necrosis factor α; TGF-β, transforming growth factor β.

cells amplification and conduction of death signals occurs exclusive of mitochondrial involvement. In type II cells, death receptor activation is not sufficient to propagate into a lethal signal without mitochondrial involvement. Hepatocytes are type II cells and have an obligate need for mitochondria in cell death [4].

In a homeostatic setting, apoptosis is accompanied by activation of phagocytosis leading to efficient removal of cellular corpses without damage to healthy cells [5]. However, apoptosis, if massive or simultaneous, results in liver injury. For example, in the setting of massive apoptosis, such as fulminant hepatic failure, successful hepatocyte repopulation leads to recovery [6]. In such an environment, if hepatocyte repopulation is protracted or delayed liver injury results. Apoptosis is harmful not just in a passive sense of inadequate repopulation, but also as an active inducer of inflammatory processes. In fact, recent data have established a mechanistic link between liver apoptosis, injury, inflammation, and fibrosis in chronic liver disease [7]. Apoptotic body engulfment by phagocytic cells leads to their activation. This results in chemokine secretion, recruitment of leukocytes and inflammatory cells to the liver, and amplification of liver injury. Hepatic stellate cells are activated by phagocytosis of apoptotic bodies as well, leading to fibrosis (see Fig. 8.2) [8].

Death receptors and the liver

Death receptors, transmembrane proteins that belong to the tumor necrosis factor (TNF)/nerve growth factor superfamily, are essential for death ligand mediated cell death. There are several known death receptors (DRs). Fas (CD95/Apo-1), TNF receptor 1 (TNF R1), TNF receptor 2 (TNF-R2), TNF-related apoptosis-inducing ligand (TRAIL) receptor 1 (TRAIL-R1/DR4), TRAIL receptor 2 (TRAIL-R2/DR5/Killer/TRICK2), death receptor 3 (DR3/Apo-3/TRAMP/WSL-1/LARD), and death receptor 6 (DR6). Of these receptors, Fas, TNF-R1, and the TRAIL receptors are thought to be of significance in liver injury [4]. Death receptors are activated by engagement with their cognate ligands, Fas ligand (FasL), TNF-α, and TRAIL. Interaction of these ligands with their cognate receptors triggers intracellular signaling pathways. Receptor ligation brings together the intracellular death domains (DDs) that via adaptor proteins (discussed below) lead to the activation of caspase 8 (an initiator caspase). Once activated, caspase 8 cleaves Bid, a cytoplasmic protein. The cleaved protein, tBid, translocates to mitochondria, leading to release of mitochondrial effectors of apoptosis, ultimately activating caspases 3 and 7 (effector caspases).

Fas is expressed by every cell type in the liver, including hepatocytes, cholangiocytes, sinusoidal endothelial cells, stellate cells, and Kupffer cells [1]. Activation of Fas, in

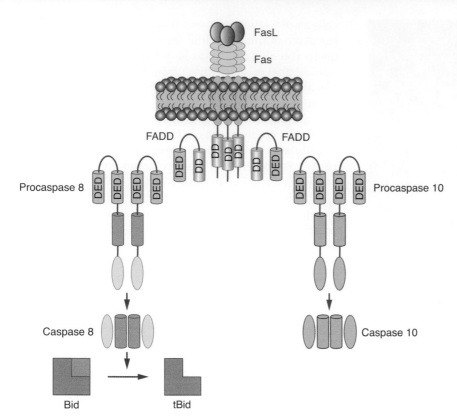

Figure 8.3 Fas receptor and associated signaling. The Fas receptor is activated on ligation with Fas ligand (FasL). The ligated receptor forms homotypic trimers, leading to intracellular signaling initiated by their intracellular death domains (DDs). The DDs of trimerized Fas associate with the protein Fas-associated death domain (FADD) through its DD. FADD in turn possesses death effector domains (DEDs) that bind and activate procaspase 8 by proteolytic cleavage. Caspase 8 leads to the cleavage of Bid to tBid, a form that translocates to the mitochondria and causes mitochondrial dysfunction. Caspase 10 is also activated by FADD, but its intracellular targets remain undefined. This conglomeration of proteins is known as the death-inducing signaling complex (DISC).

most instances, requires binding with membrane-bound FasL-expressing cells or soluble FasL (Fig. 8.3). FasL is expressed in cytotoxic T lymphocytes (CTL) and natural killer (NK) cells. This provides an efficient means of removal of unwanted hepatocytes, such as virus-infected hepatocytes and cancer cells, by T lymphocytes [9]. Mice genetically deficient in Fas exhibit hepatic hyperplasia, proving a role for Fas in hepatic homeostasis in health [10]. Hepatocyte sensitivity to Fas-induced apoptosis is underscored by the fact that the exogenous administration of Fas induces fulminant hepatic failure in mice [11]. Hepatocyte sensitivity to Fas-induced apoptosis is regulated by low cell surface expression levels as well as sequestration by binding with the hepatocyte growth factor (HGF) receptor Met [12]. This inhibitory binding can be overcome by high concentrations of FasL, as well as HGF. Indeed, in diseases such as fatty liver, Fas is dissociated from Met, providing a mechanistic basis for the observed increase in hepatocyte apoptosis [13]. The multifaceted role of Fas in hepatic homeostasis and injury has been introduced in this section, and will be discussed in greater detail in the following sections.

While the significance of Fas in liver disease is undisputed, TNF-α also plays a significant, if somewhat complementary, role. There is clear overlap in the spectrum of liver injury associated with TNF-α and Fas with some features unique to TNF-α receptor-mediated signaling. TNF-R1 and TNF-R2 are both expressed on hepatocytes,

although only TNF-R1 expresses a death domain and executes the apoptotic program. TNF-R1 activation leads to both survival and death signals (Fig. 8.4). Immediate recruitment of TNF receptor-associated protein (TRAF2) and receptor interacting protein 1 (RIP1) to ligated TNF-R1 leads to activation of nuclear factor κB (NF-κB) [14]. This transcription factor activates a variety of survival genes (e.g., Bcl-x_L, A1, XIAP, and cFLIP). Apoptosis is initiated subsequently via adaptor protein TRADD (TNF-R-associated protein with death domain)-mediated FADD (Fas-associated protein with death domain) and caspase 8 activation in a receptor initiated, albeit receptor independent, complex [15]. Thus, TNF-R1 signaling is complex and it usually first activates survival signals and an inflammatory response, but in pathophysiologic states can induce apoptosis.

TRAIL and its receptors add further complexity to death receptors and their role in the liver. TRAIL receptors 1 and 2 induce apoptosis via caspase activation, similar to Fas [4,16], where as TRAIL receptors 3 and 4 are thought to function as decoy receptors, interfering with TRAIL-induced death signaling. Traditionally, TRAIL has been thought of as being harmless to normal hepatocytes but efficiently apoptotic in solid tumors [17,18]. However, recent studies have demonstrated a role for TRAIL in murine hepatocyte apoptosis in several models of hepatitis [19,20]. Circulating TRAIL levels are elevated in chronic viral hepatitis, and in ex vivo experiments

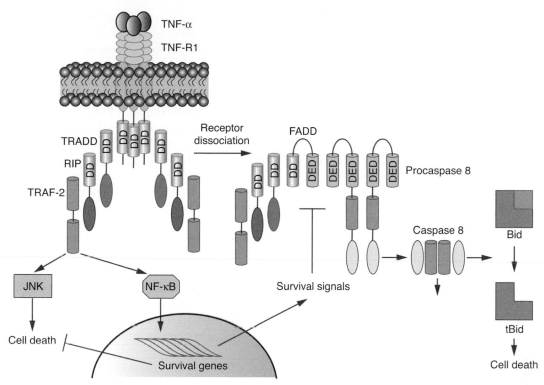

Figure 8.4 Tumor necrosis factor receptor 1 (TNF-R1) and associated signaling. Ligation of tumor necrosis factor α (TNF-α) to its receptor TNF-R1 initiates two distinct set of signals. The initial signaling pathway involves the proteins TRADD (TNF-R-associated protein with death domain), receptor-interacting protein (RIP), and TRAF2 (TNF-associated factor 2), leading to the activation of nuclear factor κB (NF-κB) and c-jun N-terminal kinase (JNK). Following this the receptor undergoes a conformational change, internalization, interaction with FADD, and activation of caspases 8 and 10 with Bid cleavage.

hepatocytes demonstrate enhanced sensitivity to TRAIL-induced apoptosis [21,22]. Steatosis is also associated with enhanced TRAIL receptor expression and ex vivo sensitization to TRAIL-induced apoptosis [22,23]. Thus diseased hepatocytes may be selectively sensitized to TRAIL-induced apoptosis in vivo, and caution should be exercised in using TRAIL-based therapies in patients with underlying liver disease.

Lysosomes

Lysosomes are enzyme-filled, membrane-lined organelles that along with peroxisomes form the acid vesicle system. The intraorganelle pH of lysosomes is acidic, and lysosomal enzymes optimally function at this acidic pH. Abnormal lysosomal morphology is found in acute and chronic liver diseases. The accumulation of phospholipids in lysosomes (phospholipidosis) is associated with drug-induced liver injury by amiodarone, trimethoprin-sulfamethoxazole, alcohol, and ketoconazole. Lipid accumulation in lysosomes is also a feature of hepatocyte steatosis. Iron, copper, and lanthane are also lysomotropic and toxic to lysosomes.

The extent of release of lysosomal contents (permeabilization) leads to either necrotic cell death, if exuberant, or apoptotic cell death, if the release is controlled. Lysosomal permeabilization may simply involve accumula-tion of lysomotropic agents with subsequent disruption and release of their content into the cytoplasm. Additionally, reactive oxygen species, toxic bile salts, sphingosine, free fatty acids, ceramide, and TNF-α lead to selective lysosomal permeabilization with subsequent apoptotic cell death. Lysosomal permeabilization leads to release of lysosomal enzymes into the cytosol, which triggers the mitochondrial pathway of cell death [24,25].

Endoplasmic reticulum

The endoplasmic reticulum (ER) is a network of intracellular membranes, is the largest membranous organelle in a cell, and is abundant in secretory cells such as hepatocytes. Perturbations that interfere with ER function have been collectively called ER stressors. The ER stress pathway is activated by accumulation of misfolded proteins, glycosylation inhibitors, glucose deprivation, ultraviolet irradiation, oxidative stress, and alterations in intracellular calcium. These stimuli lead to the accumulation of misfolded proteins in the ER lumen, and activate the unfolded protein response, which is a hallmark of ER stress [26]. The three sensors of the unfolded protein response are inositol-requiring enzyme 1α (IRE1α), PKR-like ER-localized eIF2α kinase (PERK), and activating transcription factor 6α (ATF6α). Collectively, they mediate adaptive responses aimed at restoring ER homeostasis. However, when sustained, ER stress leads to cell death via at least two known mediators. IRE1α can activate c-jun N-terminal kinase (JNK), which in turn can activate many proapoptotic pathways [27]. Another pathway involves the transcription factor CHOP (C/EBP homologous protein). The downstream effectors of CHOP are not well defined, but it regulates apoptosis transcriptionally and nontranscriptionally via protein–protein interactions [28]. ER stress is described in several liver diseases including chronic viral hepatitis C and nonalcoholic fatty liver disease. The exact role of ER stress in liver disease is not well defined, and is an area of active research.

Oxidative stress

Oxygen and oxidative reactions are an essential part of aerobic oxidative phosphorylation, the process that converts nutrient energy into adenosine triphosphate (ATP), the currency of cellular energy. Oxidative stress is a consequence of this aerobic metabolism. The generation of reactive oxygen species (ROS) (O_2^-, H_2O_2, OH) and subsequent formation of the oxidative products of amino acids, proteins, carbohydrates, lipids, and DNA constitutes oxidative stress. The ROS superoxide (O_2^-) also interacts with nitric oxide to form the reactive nitrogen species, peroxynitrite ($ONOO^-$). Peroxynitrite is a potent oxidizing and nitrating agent. It can nitrate tyrosine residues in several cellular proteins and iron residues in metalloproteins. Given the dependence on aerobic metabolism for energy, cells harbor several antioxidant defense systems to protect from oxidative and nitrative stress. When antioxidant defense systems are overwhelmed, oxidative and nitrative damage ensues. In acute injury models, ROS are associated with the mitochondrial permeability transition in both apoptotic and necrotic cell death. Lipid peroxidation, oxidized DNA, and nitrated proteins are seen in several models of chronic oxidative stress-induced liver injury [29–31]. Iron overload, copper overload, chronic ethanol consumption, nonalcoholic steatohepatitis (NASH), and viral hepatitis are all associated with oxidative cellular constituent damage. The importance of oxidative stress is further underscored by the well-established use of the antioxidant *N*-acetylcyteine in acute acetaminophen-induced liver failure.

Mitochondria

Mitochondria are bound by two membranes, the outer and inner mitochondrial membranes. These two membranes enclose the intermembrane space; the inner membrane is folded into cristae and encloses the mitochondrial matrix. Proapoptotic proteins such as cytochrome *c*, SMAC/DIABLO (second mitochondrial activator of caspase/direct IAP-binding protein with low pI), HtrA2/Omi, AIF (apoptosis-inducing factor), and endonuclease G are located within the intermembrane space. The outer mitochondrial membrane is normally impermeable to these proteins, permitting the cell to survive and function. Mitochondrial permeabilization results in release of these proteins into the cytosol with activation of downstream proteases, which in turn culminate in apoptosis (Fig. 8.5) [32].

Mitochondria are essential for apoptosis in hepatocytes. Apoptosis can be divided arbitrarily into three phases: (i) pre-mitochondrial, (ii) mitochondrial, and (iii) post-mitochondrial. The pre-mitochondrial phase has been discussed in detail in the section on death receptors and other perturbations that culminate on mitochondria. The end result of the mitochondrial phase is selective mitochondrial permeabilization. This process is regulated by the pro- and anti-apoptotic proteins of the Bcl-2 family. Of the anti-apoptotic proteins, Bcl-x_L and Mcl-1 are important in the liver. The proapoptotic proteins are further divided into multidomain (Bak and Bax) and BH-3 domain only (Bid, Noxa, Puma, Bim, and Bad). Bax is located in health in the cytosol but undergoes conformational change and insertion into the mitochondrial membrane upon activation. Bak is an integral mitochondrial membrane protein also activated by conformational change. Bak and Bax then form pores in the outer mitochondrial membrane leading to permeabilization. The BH-3-only protein Bid is cytosolic and involved in the pre-mitochondrial phase of apoptosis. Its activation is mediated by death-receptor-activated caspase 8, and thus it serves as a link from the extrinsic to the intrinsic pathway of apoptosis. Bim is activated by release from the cytoskeletal dynein motor complex, and Bad is activated by dephosphorylation. The goal of the proapoptotic members is mitochondrial permeabilization, and the goal of the anti-apoptotic members is to prevent just that. The manner in which this occurs is complex and not fully known, though not just the sum total of the pro- and anti-apoptotic signals

Mitochondrial abnormalities, both structural and functional, are associated with liver disorders. Drugs and xenobiotics can inhibit the electron transport chain, uncouple oxidative phosphorylation, impair fatty acid oxidation, damage mitochondrial DNA, and impair mitochondrial DNA repair. Mitochondrial abnormalities in alcohol-induced liver disease are well described [30]. Ethanol-driven generation of ROS is associated with oxidative damage to lipids, proteins, and DNA. Moreover, high levels of TNF-α expression, driven by ethanol, also leads to an increase in ROS. Ethanol toxicity thus leads to mitochondrial permeability transition (MPT), which may occur either via death-receptor-mediated pathways or via intrinsic cellular stress. Bile acids, characteristically elevated in cholestatic liver diseases, can also trigger mitochondrial dysfunction [33]. Similarly

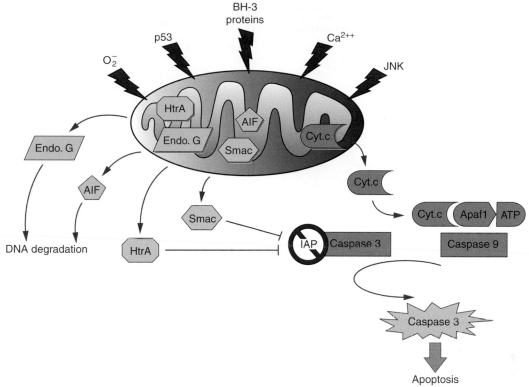

Figure 8.5 The role of mitochondria in cell death. Mitochondrial dysfunction is an obligate event in hepatocellular apoptosis. Intrinsic apoptotic stimuli such as p53, calcium, oxidative stress, and c-jun N-terminal kinase (JNK), as well as extrinsic apoptotic stimuli (BH-3 proteins), converge on mitochondria. Mitochondrial dysfunction leads to the release of several proapoptotic factors. Endonuclease G (Endo. G) and apoptosis-inducing factor (AIF) lead to deoxyribonucleic acid (DNA) degradation. Second mitochondrial activator of apoptosis (Smac) and high temperature requirement A (HtrA) inhibit a set of proteins known as inhibitors of apoptosis (IAP) leading to the release of caspases 3 and 9. Cytochrome c (Cyt. c) complexes with Apaf1 and adenosine-5ʹ-triphosphate (ATP) to form the apoptosome that leads to the activation of caspases 3 and 9 that are released from IAP inhibition.

mitochondrial dysfunction is associated with NASH, though the molecular mediators need to be defined [34].

Necrosis

Necrosis has been defined as an energy-independent process, in which cells swell and lyse, releasing their contents. It has been considered "unprogrammed" compared with apoptosis or programmed cell death. The death signaling in necrosis has been considered absent or disordered, and the cell death equated to a supernova of cellular death phenomenon. Inflammation has been viewed as a consequence of phagocytosis of cellular debris and thought to occur more in necrosis because of the exuberant release of cellular contents. Cellular ATP depletion activates necrotic cell death. During ischemia a lack of oxygen and nutrients leads to a dramatic and absolute inability to generate ATP. This activates processes leading to cellular destruction and necrosis. Exposure to massive ischemia, nitrative/oxidative stress, and xenobiotics can all result in hepatic necrosis [35]. In some instances the magnitude of the noxious stimulus controls the subse-

quent mode of cell death, apoptosis resulting from a lesser stimulus and necrosis occurring with a greater magnitude of hepatic insult (Fig. 8.6). Although historically viewed as distinct, in the past few years similarities between the two processes have surfaced. Morphologically, hepatocytes with dual characteristics have been observed in vivo in injury models such as ischemia–reperfusion. Regulated, albeit caspase independent and death-receptor-independent, cell death has broadened the definition of necrosis and blurred the erstwhile clear-cut distinction from apoptosis.

The cellular protein kinases of the receptor-interacting protein (RIP) family, specifically RIP1and RIP3, are implicated in necrotic signaling [36]. RIP1 has C-terminal death domains and caspase recruitment domains that allow interaction with adaptor proteins such as TRADD and FADD downstream of death receptors. RIP3 interacts with RIP1 via the RIP homotypic interaction motif. Upon activation, the TNF-R1 signaling complex (or other death receptors) recruits RIP1, which can then promote survival and inflammation when polyubiquitinated or

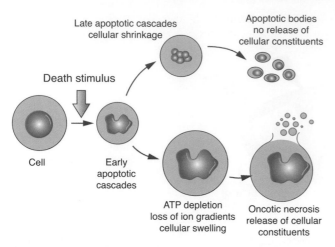

Figure 8.6 Apoptosis and necrosis are divergent end-points of common initiating signals. Death-initiating signals lead to activation of early apoptotic signals. In the milieu of adenosine triphosphate (ATP) depletion, loss of ion gradients, and cellular swelling ensues. This results in mitochondrial and cellular rupture with release of intracellular content. In a controlled and energy-replete environment, the apoptotic cascade proceeds, leading to nuclear condensation and fragmentation of cells into apoptotic bodies. Physiologically, these apoptotic bodies are engulfed and efficiently removed by Kupffer cells.

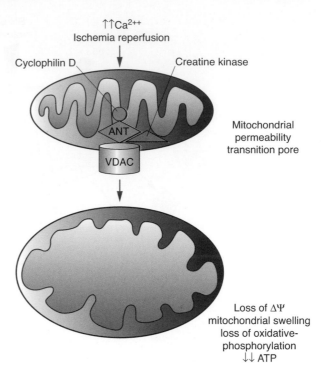

Figure 8.7 The mitochondrial permeability transition pore. Mitochondria mediate necrotic cell death in the liver. The mitochondrial permeability transition pore (PTP) is formed by voltage-dependent anion channel (VDAC) on the outer membrane and adenine nucleotide transporter (ANT) on the inner membrane along with cyclophilin D. Opening of the PTP leads to mitochondrial swelling, rupture, and release of intermembrane proteins. $\Delta\psi$, mitochrondrial membrane potential; ATP, adenosine triphosphate.

programmed necrosis in a deubiquitinated state. Thus, these dichotomous outcomes are determined by the ubiquitination state of RIP1. When apoptosis is inhibited (e.g., by the caspase inhibitor Z-VAD-fmk), RIP1 mediates programmed necrosis or necroptosis downstream of TNF-α. Furthermore, only certain cell lines are susceptible to TNF-α-induced necroptosis; this may be partially explained by RIP3 expression, as it is a downstream mediator of RIP1-induced necropotosis [37]. RIP1 and RIP3 are linked to cellular accumulation of ROS, which correlates with cell death, and reduction of ROS abrogates TNF-α-induced necroptosis. What the role of RIP kinases in hepatocyte cell death and liver injury are, if any, remains to be elucidated, especially given that in a mouse model, TNF-α-induced hepatocyte cell death was caspase 8 dependent [38].

Mitochondria in necrosis
Mitochondria mediate necrotic cell death (Fig. 8.7), in addition to their role in apoptosis. Mitochondrial permeability transition, an abrupt increase in the permeability of the inner and outer mitochondrial membranes, occurs in necrosis. This is mediated by the mitochondrial permeability transition pore (PTP). The PTP is formed by a voltage-dependent anion channel (VDAC) on the outer membrane and adenine nucleotide transporter (ANT) on the inner membrane along with cyclophilin D. The permeability transition leads to dissipation of the electrochemical gradient across the inner mitochondrial membrane, uncoupling of oxidative phosphorylation, and an

inability to synthesize new ATP. Calcium and mitochondrial proteins are released as well. Mitochondrial swelling occurs secondary to an increase in membrane permeability leading to mitochondrial rupture and necrotic cell death [39].

Innate immune system in liver injury
The innate immune system in the liver is characterized by tolerance under physiologic conditions, such as gut-derived low-level lipopolysaccharide, and activation in both acute and chronic liver diseases. This activation is manifest as inflammation, which is a vital component of acetaminophen-induced acute liver injury, acute viral hepatitis, chronic viral hepatitis, alcoholic steatohepatitis, and NASH. Immunologic properties have been ascribed to most of the cell types that comprise the liver, including Kupffer cells, NK cells, natural killer T (NKT) cells, dendritic cells, hepatocytes, cholangiocytes, hepatic stellate cells (HSCs), and liver sinusoidal endothelial cells (LSECs) [40]. The liver is enriched in macrophages, known as Kupffer cells, which are liver resident, and can self-renew or be monocyte-derived. They can phagocytose apoptotic hepatocytes, parasites, and bacteria, secrete

pro- and anti-inflammatory cytokines such as TNF-α and interleukin 6 (IL6), and function as antigen-presenting cells. The liver is also enriched in NK cells and NKT cells. These cells produce death ligands such as Fas and TRAIL, and provide antiviral immunity and tumor surveillance. Dendritic cells function as antigen-presenting cells. Hepatocytes mediate acute phase and inflammatory responses; acute phase proteins are synthesized and secreted by hepatocytes, as are several cytokines. LSECs perform a scavenger function and can present antigens to adaptive immune cells. HSCs too can function as antigen-presenting cells. Given the breadth of innate immune functions, there may be redundancies and possibly proinflammatory and anti-inflammatory roles for different cell types, and the exact contribution of each in a given disease process is not well defined.

Activation and signal transduction in cells of the innate immune system is based on molecular pattern recognition. By being responsive to molecular patterns, and not to specific antigens, the innate immune cells can be activated by stimuli that possess these conserved patterns. Receptors that recognize these molecular patterns are termed pattern recognition receptors (PRRs). Microbial pathogen-associated molecular patterns (PAMPs) and damage-associated molecular patterns (DAMPs) can activate PRRs. PRRs can be found within cell cytoplasm or on the cell surface. Toll-like receptors (TLRs), nucleotide-binding oligomerization domain (NOD)-like receptors (NLRs), and cytoplasmic retinoic acid-inducible gene 1 (RIG-1)-like helicases (RLHs) are examples of PRRs [41]. They can recognize a wide array of molecular patterns derived from microbes or damaged cells such as bacterial lipopolysaccharides, lipoproteins, and peptidoglycans; viral nucleic acids; and uric acid, high mobility group box 1, heat shock protein 70, hyaluronan, cardiolipin, and genomic DNA released from damaged cells [42–44]. The release of DAMPs from apoptotic and necrotic hepatocytes and other target cell death is likely how the innate immune system is activated, and amplifies the subsequent inflammatory response and liver injury. This is exemplified by recent studies using acetaminophen-induced acute liver injury in mice. DAMPs released from dead hepatocytes activate TLR9 with subsequent transcriptional activation of the inflammatory mediators interleukin 1β and interleukin 18 in liver sinusoidal endothelial cells, which are then cleaved to their active forms by the inflammasome [42]. DAMPs from acetaminophen-damaged hepatocytes also activate Kupffer cells [43]. Furthermore, innate immune cells in the liver can distinguish DAMPs released from damaged cells from microbial lipopolysaccharide. Dendritic cells can selectively suppress the inflammatory response to DAMPs released from acetaminophen-damaged hepatocytes while retaining sensitivity to lipopolysaccharide

[44]. Thus, existing evidence points to the complex nature of and multilevel interactions between injurious stimuli in the liver and the resultant activation of innate immune cells.

Disease mechanisms

Alcohol-related liver disease

Alcoholic steatohepatitis is characterized by steatosis, hepatocyte apoptosis, and acute inflammation. The cellular mechanisms and cytokine milieu leading to alcohol-induced liver injury are well defined. The factors that impart each individual's susceptibility to liver damage are less well understood. In experimental models ethanol induces changes in mitochondrial and microsomal function with subsequent apoptosis as well as necrosis [45]. Oxidative stress occurs with acute and chronic ethanol ingestion. Mitochondrial permeability transition occurs as a result of oxidative stress, leading to the release of cytochrome c and other mitochondrial enzymes, activation of effector caspases, and apoptosis [46]. Neutralization of ROS with antioxidants, inhibition of MPT, or inhibition of caspases prevents acute ethanol-induced apoptosis. Oxidative stress also leads to translocation of Bax from cytosol to mitochondria resulting in mitochondrial dysfunction [47]. Induction of cytochrome P450 2E1 (CYP2E1), a well-known effect of ethanol ingestion, also promotes the generation of ROS and may explain how ethanol induces its own toxicity in a feedback loop [48]. Kupffer cells demonstrate increased expression of CYP2E1, oxidative stress, and, more importantly, they become activated in acute alcohol-mediated liver injury. Once activated, they secrete a number of cytokines, including TNF-α, IL6, and transforming growth factor β1 (TGF-β1) [49,50]. The role of these inflammatory cytokines is underscored by studies using endotoxinemia to promote TNF-α expression and liver injury, and on the other hand, selective gut decontamination (with antibiotics to reduce portal vein endotoxin levels) with attenuation of both TNF-α signaling and liver injury [51]. Furthermore, genetic studies in mice demonstrated that TNF-R1 is essential for alcohol-induced liver injury [52].

Apoptosis occurs in patients with alcoholic steatohepatitis, and correlates with bilirubin, aspartate transaminase (AST), and grade 4 steatohepatitis [53,54]. Hepatic Fas receptor expression is enhanced in alcoholic steatohepatitis, compared with normal livers [53]. Studies on sera of patient with alcoholic steatohepatitis demonstrate increased circulating levels of Fas, FasL, and TNF-α. TNF-α levels correlate with mortality in these patients [55,56]. Hepatocyte apoptosis also correlates with the Maddrey score, a prognostic indicator in acute alcoholic hepatitis. The characteristic inflammatory response occurs secondary to hepatocyte apoptosis, and also due to the direct effects of ethanol on Kupffer cells leading to cytokine production [49]. In summary, alcohol-induced liver injury occurs in the setting of oxidative stress and a proinflammatory cytokine environment that together induce hepatocyte apoptosis and consequent inflammation. Apoptosis correlates with the severity of liver injury. Inhibition of the apoptotic signaling pathway holds the potential for future therapies of alcoholic liver disease.

Nonalcoholic steatohepatitis

Nonalcoholic fatty liver disease (NAFLD), the hepatic component of the metabolic syndrome, has become the most common liver disorder in the United States. Hepatocyte apoptosis is a prominent feature of NASH and correlates with disease severity, disease progression, and fibrosis [57]. This association underscores the importance of hepatocyte apoptosis and begs the question why only certain steatotic cells die. Recent mechanistic understanding of hepatocyte apoptosis in NASH has elucidated the role of death receptor ligands, circulating and intrahepatic free fatty acids, inflammatory cytokines, mitochondrial abnormalities, and the genes of fat metabolism [34,57,58].

Early pathogenetic studies have described increased Fas and TNF-R1 expression in the livers of patients with NASH [59]. Furthermore, circulating TNF-α levels are also elevated in patients with NASH. This is confirmed by studies in animal models of steatosis, where apoptosis and inflammation are enhanced following administration of death receptor ligands, Fas and TNF-α [60]. These data demonstrate the sensitivity of the steatotic hepatocyte to a secondary insult. Insulin resistance, a feature of obesity and the metabolic syndrome, leads to elevated plasma free fatty acid (FFA) levels. Recent advances have been made in understanding the cellular mechanisms by which apoptosis occurs by FFAs in steatotic hepatocytes, a process termed lipoapoptosis. Lysosomal permeabilization by FFAs in an in vitro model using HepG2 cells has partially elucidated the role of the intrinsic apoptotic pathway. Indeed this has been confirmed in patients with NASH that show evidence of lysosomal permeabilization and release of cathepsin B [61]. Furthermore, TNF-α expression occurs downstream of, and is partially dependent on, lysosomal permeabilization in this model. In a separate in vitro study, sensitivity of steatotic HepG2 cells to FasL, presumably via upregulation of the Fas receptor, provides another piece of the puzzle that integrates the well-characterized death ligand sensitivity of steatotic livers with the primary metabolic abnormality observed in this syndrome [60]. Mitochondria are central to cell death, and FFA-mediated mitochondrial dysfunction in HepG2 cells as well as primary mouse hepatocytes has been described. One way in which mito-

chondrial dysfunction can be activated is by a family of signaling enzymes, the mitogen-activated protein kinases (MAPKs). FFA-induced activation of JNK, a proapoptotic MAPK, with subsequent JNK-dependent apoptosis in hepatocytes is also an important pathway of FFA-induced lipoapoptosis. Mitochondrial dysfunction in this model results from the upregulation of proapoptotic Bcl-2 family proteins, Bim and Puma, and Bax activation [58,62].

Abnormal mitochondrial structure and function also occur in patients with NASH [34]. Mega-mitochondria with crystalline inclusions, decreased hepatic mitochondrial DNA content, and decreased respiratory chain function occur. CYP2E1 is increased in patients with NASH and there is some evidence for increased oxidative stress, which may be driven by enhanced FFA-driven mitochondrial β-oxidation. Thus, the role of mitochondrial abnormalities and oxidative stress as activators of the intrinsic pathway of apoptosis need to be studied further.

Viral hepatitis

Hepatitis B virus (HBV) and hepatitis C virus (HCV) cause both acute and chronic hepatocellular infection. In acute viral infection, immune-mediated apoptosis leads to elimination of infected cells, and in order for chronic infection to be successful virally infected hepatocytes must evade apoptosis [63]. The cell injury in acute infection occurs in two phases. The first phase in acute HBV and HCV infection involves cytotoxic T lymphocyte (CTL)-induced Fas-mediated hepatocyte apoptosis [64, 65]. The second wave of injury is triggered by apoptosis and occurs as a nonspecific necroinflammatory response that also damages bystander cells that do not express viral antigens [66,67]. Also, the virus has a small direct cytopathic effect.

In chronic infection there is ongoing, low-grade, Fas-mediated apoptosis. Apoptosis correlates with histologic severity of chronic hepatitis [68]. In sera from patients with chronic HBV and HCV infection, soluable Fas levels are increased and correlate with alanine aminotransferase (ALT), histology, and response to therapy [69,70]. Furthermore, at the onset of treatment with interferon, sFas levels increase in parallel with ALT values, suggesting enhanced Fas-mediated immune clearance of infected cells [71]. Active alcohol consumption in hepatitis C leads to a significant increase in hepatocyte apoptosis that correlates with increased Fas levels, pointing towards a convergence of two distinct apoptotic stimuli on the Fas signaling pathway [72]. Not only is there evidence of apoptosis, but also soluble markers of apoptosis hold the promise of surrogacy, decreasing the need for repeated liver biopsies [73]. It is also clear from several experimental models that HCV proteins regulate apoptosis [74]. HCV core protein confers sensitivity to TRAIL-mediated apoptosis in cells previously resistant to its effect [75]. Other HCV proteins such as NS3 can activate caspase 8-mediated apoptosis, independent of Fas [76]. The inhibition of apoptosis of virally infected hepatocytes possibly provides a mechanism for both viral persistence and the development of hepatocellular carcinoma. Indeed, in a mouse model of hepatic carcinogenesis, the introduction of core, E1, and E2 proteins led to the formation of larger tumors [77]. In complementary in vitro experiments, HCV core protein inhibited Fas and TNF-α-mediated apoptosis in HepG2 cells [78].

Similarly in chronic HBV infection both Fas receptor and TNF-R1 expression are increased in hepatocytes [79]. Levels of circulating Fas and TNF-α are increased as well and correlate with severity of infection [70,80]. HBV X protein has complex biologic functions in the host that remain controversial and has been reported to attenuate and promote cell death [81–83]. Thus, both HCV and HBV infection, though cleared by immune-mediated hepatocyte apoptosis, regulate the apoptotic machinery to establish chronic infections predisposing to hepatocarcinogenesis.

Ischemia–reperfusion injury

Ischemia–reperfusion (IR) injury occurs during liver transplantation, liver surgery, and hypotensive states. Hemodynamic changes are an integral part of liver transplantation surgery, therefore understanding the mechanisms of cold ischemia/warm reperfusion (CI/WR) injury should promote therapeutic strategies to minimize injury and improve allograft function. Warm IR occurs in other forms of liver surgery and hypotensive states. Sinusoidal endothelial cells (SECs) are the immediate target of CI/WR injury with hepatocyte injury occurring after prolonged periods of ischemia. In contrast, hepatocytes are the primary target in warm IR injury. Cold storage alone leads to apoptosis of SECs. Use of caspase inhibitors significantly decreases SEC apoptosis and improves survival after orthotopic liver transplantation [84]. Kupffer cells are activated and secrete numerous cytokines that in turn activate apoptosis and attract inflammatory cells. Depletion of Kupffer cells using gadolinium chloride, decreases SEC apoptosis and liver injury in CI/WR [85].

IR injury involves hepatocyte apoptosis, which also correlates with the duration of ischemia and the presence of preexisting liver damage [86]. Activation of NF-κB, TNF-α, and Fas modulate IR-induced hepatocyte apoptosis [87]. NF-κB has a biphasic activation following IR, the initial phase promotes expression of TNF-α leading to apoptosis and inflammation, and the later phase is protective, such that selective inhibition of activation of the later phase enhanced liver injury and nonspecific inhibition attenuated injury [88]. Historically, necrosis and apoptosis both have been thought to mediate IR injury; recent evidence, however, points towards apop-

tosis as the principal mode of hepatocyte cell death in IR [35,89]. In experimental models TNF-α-dependent apoptosis, caspase-dependent hepatocyte apoptosis, and an increase in levels of FasL expression were observed [87]. Stress-activated protein kinases, such as JNK, are also activated soon after orthotopic liver transplantation. Use of JNK inhibitors preserves hepatic architecture and attenuates injury [90]. Expression of Bcl-2, an antiapoptotic protein, by several different modalities, protects hepatocytes against ischemic apoptosis and liver injury [91]. The use of small interfering RNA (siRNA) to decrease the expression of caspase 8 and caspase 3 also reduces IR injury. In summary, ischemia reperfusion injury is mediated by apoptosis of both parenchymal and non-parenchymal liver cells. Inhibition of apoptosis in experimental studies has improved the outcomes of orthotopic liver transplantation; this offers promising interventions to maximize allograft function.

Cholestatic injury

Cholestasis, an impairment in bile flow and/or secretion, is characterized by an increase in hepatocellular bile acid concentrations. At a cellular level, the effects of hydrophobic bile acids are well understood. Glycine conjugated chenodeoxycholic acid (GCDC) is more toxic than taurine-conjugated chenodeoxycholic acid (TCDC) [92]. Toxic bile acids induce hepatocyte apoptosis in vitro and also in animal models of extrahepatic cholestasis (bile duct ligated animal). There is evidence for involvement of the death ligands, Fas, and TRAIL in bile acid-mediated apoptosis [93,94]. The importance of the Fas receptor in this pathway is proved further by studies in mice deficient in Fas receptor (lpr). Following bile duct ligation in these lpr mice, hepatocyte apoptosis was attenuated [95]. Furthermore, in long-term follow-up in these animals, fibrosis was attenuated as well. This study underscores the importance of the paradigm of hepatocyte apoptosis acting as a fibrogenic stimulus resulting ultimately in liver cirrhosis.

Fas-induced apoptosis is not the only mechanism of hydrophobic bile acid toxicity. In cholestatic lpr mice, hepatocyte apoptosis occurs eventually, though delayed and attenuated when compared to wild-type mice. Bax levels and translocation to mitochondria are increased in cholestatic lpr mice and explain the onset of apoptosis [96]. Inhibition of apoptosis by inhibiting Bid prevents both Fas-dependent and Fas-independent bile acid-induced hepatocyte apoptosis [97]. Furthermore, in Fas-deficient cells, the role of TRAIL-R2 has been unmasked in bile acid-induced hepatocyte apoptosis. TRAIL activation by GCDC leads to recruitment of the classic TRAIL death-inducing signaling complex with activation of caspase 8 and caspase 10, involvement of mitochondria, release of cytochrome c, and apoptosis [98].

Primary biliary cirrhosis (PBC) and primary sclerosing cholangitis (PSC) are the two commonest etiologies of adult intrahepatic cholestasis. Immune-mediated apoptosis of biliary epithelial cells (BECs) is well defined in PBC [99]. Pyruvate dehydrogenase complex (PDC), a mitochondrial protein, is expressed on the cell surface membrane of BECs in PBC. Autoantibodies and autoreactive T cells exist against this antigen perpetuating immune-mediated BEC apoptosis. PDC is normally sequestered in the inner mitochondrial membrane. While the perpetuation of autoimmune injury in response to PDC is understood, the initial apoptotic stimulus that leads to mitochondrial dysfunction and expression of PDC on BEC surfaces is unknown. In experimental models it was found that immunoreactive PDC migrated from mitochondria to the plasma membrane of cells after the induction of apoptosis [100]. Thus apoptosis plays a role in bile duct injury, and in the ensuing hepatocellular injury seen in cholestasis.

Wilson disease and hemochromatosis

Wilson disease is characterized by a hepatocellular defect resulting from mutations in a copper transporting P-type ATPase (ATP7B) with an inability to excrete copper in bile. This leads to copper accumulation in hepatocytes, which is cytotoxic [101]. The long evans cinnamon (LEC) rat is a spontaneous mutant that mimics human Wilson disease [102]. These animals show evidence of chronic oxidative damage, such as lipid peroxidation and DNA strand breaks [103,104]. This suggests a role for oxidative stress as copper has redox activity, such as the Fenton and Haber–Weiss reactions, leading to generation of free radicals and oxidative damage to lipids, proteins, and DNA. In vitro data show that copper overload also leads to p53-dependent cell death [105].

The course of Wilson disease in humans runs the gamut from fulminant hepatic failure (FHF) to mild chronic hepatitis. In Wilson disease patients with FHF, high levels of apoptosis, Fas receptor levels, and Fas mRNA levels were detected [106]. Oxidatively damaged DNA and bulky DNA, indicative of damaged DNA with adduct formation, were detected in patients with Wilson disease [29,107]. Thus copper overload causes apoptotic hepatocellular death in patients with Wilson disease.

Oxidative stress is a direct consequence of iron overload, due to the redox activity of iron and the generation of oxygen free radicals. As with copper excess, the generation of ROS occurs via the Fenton and Haber–Weiss reactions. Oxidative damage to all cellular constituents ensues, indeed oxidative DNA adducts are found in patients with hereditary hemochromatosis [108]. Though iron is not a direct carcinogen, iron overload is associated with increased risk for the development of hepatocellular carcinoma [109].

Alpha-1 antitrypsin deficiency

Alpha-1 antitrypsin (A1AT) is normally predominantly secreted by hepatocytes. Patients with A1AT deficiency produce an abnormal variant of the protein, which is aggregation prone, resulting in a failure of hepatocytes to secrete it into serum. This leads to accumulation of the abnormal protein within hepatocytes. This accumulation occurs within the lumen of the ER. The accumulated mutant protein forms aggregates, and a major homeostatic response is to enhance the degradation of the mutant protein via proteasomal degradation and autophagy. Activation of NF-κB occurs secondary to ER accumulation of mutant protein aggregates, and mediates tissue inflammation. Furthermore, mitochondrial dysfunction and caspase 3 activation are associated with ER dysfunction [110]. The exact molecular pathways that mediate A1AT-induced mitochondrial dysfunction and caspase activation are not well defined and are an area for future research.

Fulminant hepatic failure

Several lines of experimental data and human observations point to the importance of death receptor-mediated apoptosis in FHF. In a seminal paper, Lacronique et al. [111] induced massive hepatocyte apoptosis and FHF in mice using an anti-Fas antibody that activates the death signaling cascade, and rescued livers from apoptosis and animals from death by increasing the expression of anti-apoptotic Bcl-2 [11,111]. In patients with FHF, levels of both Fas receptor and FasL expression in hepatocytes are high. FasL levels are elevated in infiltrating lymphocytes, circulating lymphocytes, and sera of patients as well. Hepatocyte apoptosis in addition to enhanced Fas expression has been observed in FHF of different etiologies [112]. In addition to Fas, circulating levels of TNF-α and TNF-α receptors are increased in patients with FHF and correlate with the recovery of native liver function [113]. Besides activation of NF-κB to aid in recovery, the dichotomous role of TNF-α is further developed in FHF, where it increases the expression of FADD protein, perhaps augmenting Fas sensitivity.

In summary, FHF is accompanied by several cytokine changes, of which Fas clearly mediates apoptosis. TNF-α and other cytokines serve dichotomous roles, promoting apoptosis, inflammation, and recovery. Enhancing the milieu in favor of recovery by inhibiting Fas-mediated apoptosis appears to be a promising therapeutic strategy, one that should be developed further with human clinical trials, given the shortage of donor organs.

Therapeutic implications

Understanding apoptotic cascades in liver diseases has unraveled novel therapeutic opportunities (Fig. 8.8). RNA

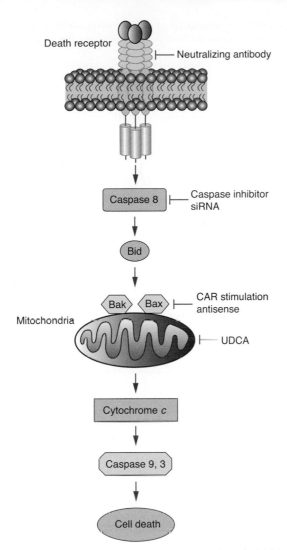

Figure 8.8 Therapeutic targets in apoptosis. Apoptosis can be inhibited at several levels. Death receptor and ligand interaction can be prevented by neutralizing antibodies. Pharmacologic inhibitors, small interfering ribonucleic acid (siRNA), antisense molecules, and modulation of Bcl-2 family pro- and antiapoptotic proteins with nuclear receptor agonists, for example, constitutive androstane receptor (CAR), are all potential therapeutic strategies. Ursodeoxycholic acid (UDCA) has been in clinical use for cholestatic liver disease.

interference (RNAi) therapy selectively manipulates a cell's genetic machinery to reduce expression of the protein of interest. Disruption of Fas and caspase 8 gene expression, using RNAi, ameliorated injury and improved survival in experimental FHF and immune-mediated hepatitis [114,115]. Increased expression of anti-apoptotic Bcl-2 and caspase inhibition protected against FHF [111,116]. Similarly, targeted hepatic delivery of NCX-1,000, a nitric oxide conjugate of urosdeoxycholic acid, which selectively releases nitric oxide in the liver, even after the onset of apoptosis, protects from acetaminophen-induced FHF [117]. In a model of

ischemia–reperfusion injury, silencing initiator and effector caspases had a salutary effect on the liver [89]. Urosdeoxycholic acid has a dual effect, not only preventing mitochondrial permeabilization and apoptosis induced by bile acid, ethanol, Fas, and TGF-β1 [118], but also promoting the activation of survival signals in cells. Furthermore, in animal studies an anti-apoptotic molecule, IDN-6556 (a pan-caspase inhibitor), reduced cholestatic hepatocyte apoptosis, stellate cell activation, liver injury, and resultant fibrosis [119]. At a mitochondrial level, the disruption of proapoptotic Bcl-2 family proteins also prevents bile acid-induced apoptosis [97].

The fact that apoptosis can be modulated temporally after cells have been exposed to apoptotic stimuli is appealing in its applicability to the clinical scenario. Indeed, several studies in experimental models of acute and chronic liver diseases have demonstrated amelioration of liver apoptosis and injury and improved survival with inhibition of apoptosis even after exposure to the apoptogenic stimulus. In patients with chronic hepatitis C, short-term administration of IDN-6556 for 14 days was associated with a reduction in transaminases, suggestive of reduced hepatocyte apoptosis [120]. Future studies should be directed toward the development of rational anti-apoptotic therapies, targeted to the liver.

Acknowledgments

This work was supported by NIH grant DK 41876 and the Mayo and Palumbo Foundations. The authors acknowledge the superb secretarial assistance of Erin Nystuen-Bungum.

Further reading

Canbay A, Higuchi H, Bronk SF, et al. Fas enhances fibrogenesis in the bile duct ligated mouse: a link between apoptosis and fibrosis. *Gastroenterologia* 2002;123:1323–30.
This article is important because it highlights the principle that sustained hepatic injury leads to sustained hepatocyte apoptosis and attendant fibrosis. Interruption of this process prevents apoptosis and mechanistically links two important observations, that is, apoptosis and fibrosis.

Edinger AL, Thompson CB. Death by design: apoptosis, necrosis and autophagy. *Curr Opin Cell Biol* 2004;16:663–9.
Apoptosis and necrosis have classically been viewed as different modes of cell death, with opposite physiologic and pathologic effects. This article explores the gray areas in this erstwhile black or white delineation.

Guicciardi ME, Gores GJ. The death receptor pathway. In: Yin X-M, Dong Z, eds. *Essentials of Apoptosis: a guide for basic and clinical research*, 2nd edn. New York: Humana Press, 2009:119–50.
This is a comprehensive review of death receptors and their signaling pathways. It is essential reading for anyone wishing to understand death receptor-mediated signals.

Parsons MJ, Green DR. Mitochondria in cell death. *Essays Biochem* 2010;47:99–114.
Mitochondria are essential to cell death. Mitochondrial contents need to be released into the cytoplasm for cell death to proceed. This essay describes essential concepts in mitochondrial permeabilization.

Ribeiro PS, Cortez-Pinto H, Sola S, et al. Hepatocyte apoptosis, expression of DRs, and activation of NF-kappaB in the liver of non-alcoholic and alcoholic steatohepatitis patients. *Am J Gastroenterol* 2004;99:1708–17.

The importance of apoptosis, death receptor signaling, and activation of inflammatory pathways in two common and relevant liver diseases are described.

References

1. Malhi H, Gores GJ. Cellular and molecular mechanisms of liver injury. *Gastroenterology* 2008;134(6):1641–54.
2. Scaffidi C, Fulda S, Srinivasan A, et al. Two CD95 (APO-1/Fas) signaling pathways. *Embo J* 1998;17(6):1675–87.
3. Danial NN, Korsmeyer SJ. Cell death: critical control points. *Cell* 2004;116(2):205–19.
4. Guicciardi ME, Gores GJ. The death receptor pathway. In: Yin X-M, Dong Z, eds. *Essentials of Apoptosis: a guide for basic and clinical research*, 2nd edn. New York: Humana Press, 2009: 119–50.
5. Jacobson MD, Weil M, Raff MC. Programmed cell death in animal development. *Cell* 1997;88(3):347–54.
6. Fujino M, Li XK, Kitazawa Y, et al. Selective repopulation of mice liver after Fas-resistant hepatocyte transplantation. *Cell Transplant* 2001;10(4–5):353–61.
7. Faouzi S, Burckhardt BE, Hanson JC, et al. Anti-Fas induces hepatic chemokines and promotes inflammation by an NF-kappa B-independent, caspase-3-dependent pathway. *J Biol Chem* 2001; 276(52):49077–82.
8. Canbay A, Taimr P, Torok N, Higuchi H, Friedman S, Gores GJ. Apoptotic body engulfment by a human stellate cell line is profibrogenic. *Lab Invest* 2003;83(5):655–63.
9. Berke G. The CTL's kiss of death. *Cell* 1995;81(1):9–12.
10. Adachi M, Suematsu S, Suda T, et al. Enhanced and accelerated lymphoproliferation in Fas-null mice. *Proc Natl Acad Sci USA* 1996;93(5):2131–6.
11. Ogasawara J, Watanabe-Fukunaga R, Adachi M, et al. Lethal effect of the anti-Fas antibody in mice. *Nature* 1993;364(6440):806–9.
12. Wang X, DeFrances MC, Dai Y, et al. A mechanism of cell survival: sequestration of Fas by the HGF receptor Met. *Mol Cell* 2002;9(2): 411–21.
13. Zou C, Ma J, Wang X, et al. Lack of Fas antagonism by Met in human fatty liver disease. *Nat Med* 2007;13(9):1078–85.
14. Yamada Y, Webber EM, Kirillova I, Peschon JJ, Fausto N. Analysis of liver regeneration in mice lacking type 1 or type 2 tumor necrosis factor receptor: requirement for type 1 but not type 2 receptor. *Hepatology* 1998;28(4):959–70.
15. Hsu H, Xiong J, Goeddel DV. The TNF receptor 1-associated protein TRADD signals cell death and NF-kappa B activation. *Cell* 1995;81(4):495–504.
16. Schneider P, Thome M, Burns K, et al. TRAIL receptors 1 (DR4) and 2 (DR5) signal FADD-dependent apoptosis and activate NF-kappaB. *Immunity* 1997;7(6):831–6.
17. Hao C, Song JH, Hsi B, et al. TRAIL inhibits tumor growth but is nontoxic to human hepatocytes in chimeric mice. *Cancer Res* 2004;64(23):8502–6.
18. Ganten TM, Koschny R, Haas TL, et al. Proteasome inhibition sensitizes hepatocellular carcinoma cells, but not human hepatocytes, to TRAIL. *Hepatology* 2005;42(3):588–97.
19. Zheng SJ, Wang P, Tsabary G, Chen YH. Critical roles of TRAIL in hepatic cell death and hepatic inflammation. *J Clin Invest* 2004;113(1):58–64.
20. Higuchi H, Bronk SF, Taniai M, Canbay A, Gores GJ. Cholestasis increases tumor necrosis factor-related apoptotis-inducing ligand (TRAIL)-R2/DR5 expression and sensitizes the liver to TRAIL-mediated cytotoxicity. *J Pharmacol Exp Ther* 2002;303(2):461–7.
21. Han LH, Sun WS, Ma CH, et al. Detection of soluble TRAIL in HBV infected patients and its clinical implications. *World J Gastroenterol* 2002;8(6):1077–80.
22. Volkmann X, Fischer U, Bahr MJ, et al. Increased hepatotoxicity of tumor necrosis factor-related apoptosis-inducing ligand in diseased human liver. *Hepatology* 2007;46(5):1498–508.
23. Malhi H, Barreyro FJ, Isomoto H, Bronk SF, Gores GJ. Free fatty acids sensitise hepatocytes to TRAIL mediated cytotoxicity. *Gut* 2007;56(8):1124–31.
24. Canbay A, Guicciardi ME, Higuchi H, et al. Cathepsin B inactivation attenuates hepatic injury and fibrosis during cholestasis. *J Clin Invest* 2003;112(2):152–9.
25. Guicciardi ME, Deussing J, Miyoshi H, et al. Cathepsin B contributes to TNF-alpha-mediated hepatocyte apoptosis by promoting mitochondrial release of cytochrome c. *J Clin Invest* 2000;106(9): 1127–37.
26. Kaufman RJ. Orchestrating the unfolded protein response in health and disease. *J Clin Invest* 2002;110(10):1389–98.
27. Urano F, Wang X, Bertolotti A, et al. Coupling of stress in the ER to activation of JNK protein kinases by transmembrane protein kinase IRE1. *Science* 2000;287(5453):664–6.
28. Oyadomari S, Mori M. Roles of CHOP/GADD153 in endoplasmic reticulum stress. *Cell Death Differ* 2004;11(4):381–9.
29. Bartsch H, Nair J. Oxidative stress and lipid peroxidation-derived DNA-lesions in inflammation driven carcinogenesis. *Cancer Detect Prev* 2004;28(6):385–91.
30. Cahill A, Cunningham CC, Adachi M, et al. Effects of alcohol and oxidative stress on liver pathology: the role of the mitochondrion. *Alcohol Clin Exp Res* 2002;26(6):907–15.
31. James LP, Mayeux PR, Hinson JA. Acetaminophen-induced hepatotoxicity. *Drug Metab Dispos* 2003;31(12):1499–506.
32. Parsons MJ, Green DR. Mitochondria in cell death. *Essays Biochem* 2010;47:99–114.
33. Gores GJ, Miyoshi H, Botla R, Aguilar HI, Bronk SF. Induction of the mitochondrial permeability transition as a mechanism of liver injury during cholestasis: a potential role for mitochondrial proteases. *Biochim Biophys Acta* 1998;1366(1–2):167–75.
34. Pessayre D, Fromenty B. NASH: a mitochondrial disease. *J Hepatol* 2005;42(6):928–40.
35. Jaeschke H, Lemasters JJ. Apoptosis versus oncotic necrosis in hepatic ischemia/reperfusion injury. *Gastroenterology* 2003;125(4): 1246–57.
36. Declercq W, Vanden Berghe T, Vandenabeele P. RIP kinases at the crossroads of cell death and survival. *Cell* 2009;138(2):229–32.
37. He S, Wang L, Miao L, et al. Receptor interacting protein kinase-3 determines cellular necrotic response to TNF-alpha. *Cell* 2009; 137(6):1100–11.
38. Kaufmann T, Jost PJ, Pellegrini M, et al. Fatal hepatitis mediated by tumor necrosis factor TNFalpha requires caspase-8 and involves the BH3-only proteins Bid and Bim. *Immunity* 2009;30(1):56–66.
39. Lemasters JJ, Nieminen AL, Qian T, et al. The mitochondrial permeability transition in cell death: a common mechanism in necrosis, apoptosis and autophagy. *Biochim Biophys Acta* 1998; 1366(1–2):177–96.
40. Crispe IN. The liver as a lymphoid organ. *Annu Rev Immunol* 2009;27:147–63.
41. Beutler B. Microbe sensing, positive feedback loops, and the pathogenesis of inflammatory diseases. *Immunol Rev* 2009;227(1): 248–63.
42. Imaeda AB, Watanabe A, Sohail MA, et al. Acetaminophen-induced hepatotoxicity in mice is dependent on Tlr9 and the Nalp3 inflammasome. *J Clin Invest* 2009;119(2):305–14.
43. Martin-Murphy BV, Holt MP, Ju C. The role of damage associated molecular pattern molecules in acetaminophen-induced liver injury in mice. *Toxicol Lett* 2010;192(3):387–94.

44. Chen GY, Tang J, Zheng P, Liu Y. CD24 and Siglec-10 selectively repress tissue damage-induced immune responses. *Science* 2009;323(5922):1722–5.

45. Lieber CS. The discovery of the microsomal ethanol oxidizing system and its physiologic and pathologic role. *Drug Metab Rev* 2004;36(3–4):511–29.

46. Higuchi H, Adachi M, Miura S, Gores GJ, Ishii H. The mitochondrial permeability transition contributes to acute ethanol-induced apoptosis in rat hepatocytes. *Hepatology* 2001;34(2):320–8.

47. Adachi M, Higuchi H, Miura S, et al. Bax interacts with the voltage-dependent anion channel and mediates ethanol-induced apoptosis in rat hepatocytes. *Am J Physiol Gastrointest Liver Physiol* 2004;287(3):G695–705.

48. Kessova I, Cederbaum AI. CYP2E1: biochemistry, toxicology, regulation and function in ethanol-induced liver injury. *Curr Mol Med* 2003;3(6):509–18.

49. Lin HZ, Yang SQ, Zeldin G, Diehl AM. Chronic ethanol consumption induces the production of tumor necrosis factor-alpha and related cytokines in liver and adipose tissue. *Alcohol Clin Exp Res* 1998;22(Suppl 5):S231–7.

50. Casey CA, Nanji A, Cederbaum AI, Adachi M, Takahashi T. Alcoholic liver disease and apoptosis. *Alcohol Clin Exp Res* 2001;25(Suppl 5 ISBRA):S49–53.

51. Enomoto N, Yamashina S, Kono H, et al. Development of a new, simple rat model of early alcohol-induced liver injury based on sensitization of Kupffer cells. *Hepatology* 1999;29(6):1680–9.

52. Yin M, Wheeler MD, Kono H, et al. Essential role of tumor necrosis factor alpha in alcohol-induced liver injury in mice. *Gastroenterology* 1999;117(4):942–52.

53. Natori S, Rust C, Stadheim LM, Srinivasan A, Burgart LJ, Gores GJ. Hepatocyte apoptosis is a pathologic feature of human alcoholic hepatitis. *J Hepatol* 2001;34(2):248–53.

54. Tagami A, Ohnishi H, Moriwaki H, Phillips M, Hughes RD. Fas-mediated apoptosis in acute alcoholic hepatitis. *Hepatogastroenterology* 2003;50(50):443–8.

55. Bird GL, Sheron N, Goka AK, Alexander GJ, Williams RS. Increased plasma tumor necrosis factor in severe alcoholic hepatitis. *Ann Intern Med* 1990;112(12):917–20.

56. Spahr L, Giostra E, Frossard JL, Bresson-Hadni S, Rubbia-Brandt L, Hadengue A. Soluble TNF-R1, but not tumor necrosis factor alpha, predicts the 3-month mortality in patients with alcoholic hepatitis. *J Hepatol* 2004;41(2):229–34.

57. Feldstein AE, Canbay A, Angulo P, et al. Hepatocyte apoptosis and fas expression are prominent features of human nonalcoholic steatohepatitis. *Gastroenterology* 2003;125(2):437–43.

58. Malhi H, Bronk SF, Werneburg NW, Gores GJ. Free fatty acids induce JNK-dependent hepatocyte lipoapoptosis. *J Biol Chem* 2006;281(17):12093–101.

59. Ribeiro PS, Cortez-Pinto H, Sola S, et al. Hepatocyte apoptosis, expression of death receptors, and activation of NF-kappaB in the liver of nonalcoholic and alcoholic steatohepatitis patients. *Am J Gastroenterol* 2004;99(9):1708–17.

60. Feldstein AE, Canbay A, Guicciardi ME, Higuchi H, Bronk SF, Gores GJ. Diet associated hepatic steatosis sensitizes to Fas mediated liver injury in mice. *J Hepatol* 2003;39(6):978–83.

61. Feldstein AE, Werneburg NW, Canbay A, et al. Free fatty acids promote hepatic lipotoxicity by stimulating TNF-alpha expression via a lysosomal pathway. *Hepatology* 2004;40(1):185–94.

62. Cazanave SC, Elmi NA, Akazawa Y, Bronk SF, Mott JL, Gores GJ. CHOP and AP-1 cooperatively mediate PUMA expression during lipoapoptosis. *Am J Physiol Gastrointest Liver Physiol* 2010;299(1):G236–43.

63. Caronia S, McGarvey MJ, Goldin RD, Foster GR. Negative correlation between intrahepatic expression of hepatitis C antigens and apoptosis despite high-level expression of Fas and HLA antigens. *J Viral Hepat* 2004;11(6):511–18.

64. Takaku S, Nakagawa Y, Shimizu M, et al. Induction of hepatic injury by hepatitis C virus-specific CD8+murine cytotoxic T lymphocytes in transgenic mice expressing the viral structural genes. *Biochem Biophys Res Commun* 2003;301(2):330–7.

65. Kondo T, Suda T, Fukuyama H, Adachi M, Nagata S. Essential roles of the Fas ligand in the development of hepatitis. *Nat Med* 1997;3(4):409–13.

66. Hiramatsu N, Hayashi N, Katayama K, et al. Immunohistochemical detection of Fas antigen in liver tissue of patients with chronic hepatitis C. *Hepatology* 1994;19(6):1354–9.

67. Papakyriakou P, Tzardi M, Valatas V, et al. Apoptosis and apoptosis related proteins in chronic viral liver disease. *Apoptosis* 2002;7(2):133–41.

68. McPartland JL, Guzail MA, Kendall CH, Pringle JH. Apoptosis in chronic viral hepatitis parallels histological activity: an immunohistochemical investigation using anti-activated caspase-3 and M30 cytodeath antibody. *Int J Exp Pathol* 2005;86(1):19–24.

69. Lapinski TW, Kowalczuk O, Prokopowicz D, Chyczewski L. Serum concentration of sFas and sFasL in healthy HBsAg carriers, chronic viral hepatitis B and C patients. *World J Gastroenterol* 2004;10(24):3650–3.

70. Song le H, Binh VQ, Duy DN, et al. Variations in the serum concentrations of soluble Fas and soluble Fas ligand in Vietnamese patients infected with hepatitis B virus. *J Med Virol* 2004;73(2):244–9.

71. Yoneyama K, Goto T, Miura K, et al. The expression of Fas and Fas ligand, and the effects of interferon in chronic liver diseases with hepatitis C virus. *Hepatol Res* 2002;24(4):327–37.

72. Pianko S, Patella S, Ostapowicz G, Desmond P, Sievert W. Fas-mediated hepatocyte apoptosis is increased by hepatitis C virus infection and alcohol consumption, and may be associated with hepatic fibrosis: mechanisms of liver cell injury in chronic hepatitis C virus infection. *J Viral Hepat* 2001;8(6):406–13.

73. Bantel H, Lugering A, Heidemann J, et al. Detection of apoptotic caspase activation in sera from patients with chronic HCV infection is associated with fibrotic liver injury. *Hepatology* 2004;40(5):1078–87.

74. Tan W, Lang Z, Cong Y, Chen G, Miao J, Zhan M. [Core protein of hepatitis C virus expressed in transgenic mice is associated with the expression of Fas molecule.] *Zhonghua Shi Yan He Lin Chuang Bing Du Xue Za Zhi* 1997;11(3):205–7.

75. Chou AH, Tsai HF, Wu YY, et al. Hepatitis C virus core protein modulates TRAIL-mediated apoptosis by enhancing Bid cleavage and activation of mitochondria apoptosis signaling pathway. *J Immunol* 2005;174(4):2160–6.

76. Prikhod'ko EA, Prikhod'ko GG, Siegel RM, Thompson P, Major ME, Cohen JI. The NS3 protein of hepatitis C virus induces caspase-8-mediated apoptosis independent of its protease or helicase activities. *Virology* 2004;329(1):53–67.

77. Kamegaya Y, Hiasa Y, Zukerberg L, et al. Hepatitis C virus acts as a tumor accelerator by blocking apoptosis in a mouse model of hepatocarcinogenesis. *Hepatology* 2005;41(3):660–7.

78. Marusawa H, Hijikata M, Chiba T, Shimotohno K. Hepatitis C virus core protein inhibits Fas- and tumor necrosis factor alpha-mediated apoptosis via NF-kappaB activation. *J Virol* 1999;73(6):4713–20.

79. Mochizuki K, Hayashi N, Hiramatsu N, et al. Fas antigen expression in liver tissues of patients with chronic hepatitis B. *J Hepatol* 1996;24(1):1–7.

80. Akpolat N, Yahsi S, Godekmerdan A, Demirbag K, Yalniz M. Relationship between serum cytokine levels and histopathological changes of liver in patients with hepatitis B. *World J Gastroenterol* 2005;11(21):3260–3.

81. Yun C, Um HR, Jin YH, et al. NF-kappaB activation by hepatitis B virus X (HBx) protein shifts the cellular fate toward survival. *Cancer Lett* 2002;184(1):97–104.

82. Lin N, Chen HY, Li D, Zhang SJ, Cheng ZX, Wang XZ. Apoptosis and its pathway in X gene-transfected HepG(2) cells. *World J Gastroenterol* 2005;11(28):4326–31.

83. Janssen HL, Higuchi H, Abdulkarim A, Gores GJ. Hepatitis B virus enhances tumor necrosis factor-related apoptosis-inducing ligand (TRAIL) cytotoxicity by increasing TRAIL-R1/death receptor 4 expression. *J Hepatol* 2003;39(3):414–20.

84. Natori S, Higuchi H, Contreras P, Gores GJ. The caspase inhibitor IDN-6556 prevents caspase activation and apoptosis in sinusoidal endothelial cells during liver preservation injury. *Liver Transpl* 2003;9(3):278–84.

85. Giakoustidis DE, Iliadis S, Tsantilas D, et al. Blockade of Kupffer cells by gadolinium chloride reduces lipid peroxidation and protects liver from ischemia/reperfusion injury. *Hepatogastroenterology* 2003;50(53):1587–92.

86. Kohli V, Selzner M, Madden JF, Bentley RC, Clavien PA. Endothelial cell and hepatocyte deaths occur by apoptosis after ischemia-reperfusion injury in the rat liver. *Transplantation* 1999;67(8):1099–105.

87. Rudiger HA, Clavien PA. Tumor necrosis factor alpha, but not Fas, mediates hepatocellular apoptosis in the murine ischemic liver. *Gastroenterology* 2002;122(1):202–10.

88. Takahashi Y, Ganster RW, Gambotto A, et al. Role of NF-kappaB on liver cold ischemia–reperfusion injury. *Am J Physiol Gastrointest Liver Physiol* 2002;283(5):G1175–84.

89. Contreras JL, Vilatoba M, Eckstein C, Bilbao G, Anthony Thompson J, Eckhoff DE. Caspase-8 and caspase-3 small interfering RNA decreases ischemia/reperfusion injury to the liver in mice. *Surgery* 2004;136(2):390–400.

90. Uehara T, Xi Peng X, Bennett B, et al. c-Jun N-terminal kinase mediates hepatic injury after rat liver transplantation. *Transplantation* 2004;78(3):324–32.

91. Bilbao G, Contreras JL, Eckhoff DE, et al. Reduction of ischemia–reperfusion injury of the liver by in vivo adenovirus-mediated gene transfer of the antiapoptotic Bcl-2 gene. *Ann Surg* 1999;230(2):185–93.

92. Rust C, Karnitz LM, Paya CV, Moscat J, Simari RD, Gores GJ. The bile acid taurochenodeoxycholate activates a phosphatidylinositol 3-kinase-dependent survival signaling cascade. *J Biol Chem* 2000;275(26):20210–16.

93. Faubion WA, Guicciardi ME, Miyoshi H, et al. Toxic bile salts induce rodent hepatocyte apoptosis via direct activation of Fas. *J Clin Invest* 1999;103(1):137–45.

94. Higuchi H, Yoon JH, Grambihler A, Werneburg N, Bronk SF, Gores GJ. Bile acids stimulate cFLIP phosphorylation enhancing TRAIL-mediated apoptosis. *J Biol Chem* 2003;278(1):454–61.

95. Canbay A, Higuchi H, Bronk SF, Taniai M, Sebo TJ, Gores GJ. Fas enhances fibrogenesis in the bile duct ligated mouse: a link between apoptosis and fibrosis. *Gastroenterology* 2002;123(4):1323–30.

96. Miyoshi H, Rust C, Roberts PJ, Burgart LJ, Gores GJ. Hepatocyte apoptosis after bile duct ligation in the mouse involves Fas. *Gastroenterology* 1999;117(3):669–77.

97. Higuchi H, Miyoshi H, Bronk SF, Zhang H, Dean N, Gores GJ. Bid antisense attenuates bile acid-induced apoptosis and cholestatic liver injury. *J Pharmacol Exp Ther* 2001;299(3):866–73.

98. Higuchi H, Bronk SF, Takikawa Y, et al. The bile acid glycochenodeoxycholate induces trail-receptor 2/DR5 expression and apoptosis. *J Biol Chem* 2001;276(42):38610–18.

99. Tinmouth J, Lee M, Wanless IR, Tsui FW, Inman R, Heathcote EJ. Apoptosis of biliary epithelial cells in primary biliary cirrhosis and primary sclerosing cholangitis. *Liver* 2002;22(3):228–34.

100. Macdonald P, Palmer J, Kirby JA, Jones DE. Apoptosis as a mechanism for cell surface expression of the autoantigen pyruvate dehydrogenase complex. *Clin Exp Immunol* 2004;136(3):559–67.

101. Cuthbert JA. Wilson's disease. Update of a systemic disorder with protean manifestations. *Gastroenterol Clin North Am* 1998;27(3):655–81, vi–vii.

102. Yamaguchi Y, Heiny ME, Shimizu N, Aoki T, Gitlin JD. Expression of the Wilson disease gene is deficient in the Long-Evans cinnamon rat. *Biochem J* 1994;301(1):1–4.

103. Yamamoto H, Hirose K, Hayasaki Y, Masuda M, Kazusaka A, Fujita S. Mechanism of enhanced lipid peroxidation in the liver of Long-Evans cinnamon (LEC) rats. *Arch Toxicol* 1999;73(8–9):457–64.

104. Hayashi M, Kuge T, Endoh D, et al. Hepatic copper accumulation induces DNA strand breaks in the liver cells of Long-Evans cinnamon strain rats. *Biochem Biophys Res Commun* 2000;276(1):174–8.

105. Narayanan VS, Fitch CA, Levenson CW. Tumor suppressor protein p53 mRNA and subcellular localization are altered by changes in cellular copper in human Hep G2 cells. *J Nutr* 2001;131(5):1427–32.

106. Strand S, Hofmann WJ, Grambihler A, et al. Hepatic failure and liver cell damage in acute Wilson's disease involve CD95 (APO-1/Fas) mediated apoptosis. *Nat Med* 1998;4(5):588–93.

107. Carmichael PL, Hewer A, Osborne MR, Strain AJ, Phillips DH. Detection of bulky DNA lesions in the liver of patients with Wilson's disease and primary haemochromatosis. *Mutat Res* 1995;326(2):235–43.

108. Britton RS, Leicester KL, Bacon BR. Iron toxicity and chelation therapy. *Int J Hematol* 2002;76(3):219–28.

109. Harrison SA, Bacon BR. Relation of hemochromatosis with hepatocellular carcinoma: epidemiology, natural history, pathophysiology, screening, treatment, and prevention. *Med Clin North Am* 2005;89(2):391–409.

110. Rudnick DA, Perlmutter DH. Alpha-1-antitrypsin deficiency: a new paradigm for hepatocellular carcinoma in genetic liver disease. *Hepatology* 2005;42(3):514–21.

111. Lacronique V, Mignon A, Fabre M, et al. Bcl-2 protects from lethal hepatic apoptosis induced by an anti-Fas antibody in mice. *Nat Med* 1996;2(1):80–6.

112. Ryo K, Kamogawa Y, Ikeda I, et al. Significance of Fas antigen-mediated apoptosis in human fulminant hepatic failure. *Am J Gastroenterol* 2000;95(8):2047–55.

113. Streetz K, Leifeld L, Grundmann D, et al. Tumor necrosis factor alpha in the pathogenesis of human and murine fulminant hepatic failure. *Gastroenterology* 2000;119(2):446–60.

114. Song E, Lee SK, Wang J, et al. RNA interference targeting Fas protects mice from fulminant hepatitis. *Nat Med* 2003;9(3):347–51.

115. Zender L, Hutker S, Liedtke C, et al. Caspase 8 small interfering RNA prevents acute liver failure in mice. *Proc Natl Acad Sci USA* 2003;100(13):7797–802.

116. Kim KM, Kim YM, Park M, et al. A broad-spectrum caspase inhibitor blocks concanavalin A-induced hepatitis in mice. *Clin Immunol* 2000;97(3):221–33.

117. Fiorucci S, Antonelli E, Distrutti E, et al. Liver delivery of NO by NCX-1000 protects against acute liver failure and mitochondrial dysfunction induced by APAP in mice. *Br J Pharmacol* 2004;143(1):33–42.

118. Rodrigues CM, Fan G, Ma X, Kren BT, Steer CJ. A novel role for ursodeoxycholic acid in inhibiting apoptosis by modulating mitochondrial membrane perturbation. *J Clin Invest* 1998;101(12):2790–9.

119. Canbay A, Feldstein A, Baskin-Bey E, Bronk SF, Gores GJ. The caspase inhibitor IDN-6556 attenuates hepatic injury and fibrosis in the bile duct ligated mouse. *J Pharmacol Exp Ther* 2004;308(3):1191–6.

120. Pockros PJ, Schiff ER, Shiffman ML, et al. Oral IDN-6556, an anti-apoptotic caspase inhibitor, may lower aminotransferase activity in patients with chronic hepatitis C. *Hepatology* 2007;46(2):324–9.

Multiple choice questions

8.1 Fulminant hepatic failure is observed in a mouse upon intravenous administration of a substance. Alanine aminotransferase values are elevated several hundred-fold above normal. Liver tissue is obtained at necropsy and massive hepatocyte apoptosis is observed. Which of the following signaling pathways was activated by the intravenous administration of this substance?

a   TNF-R1 and TNF-α.
b   NF-κB.
c   FasL and Fas.
d   TRAIL-R2 and TRAIL.

8.2 Which of the following statements is true?

a   Necroptosis is the predominant mode of cell death in hepatocytes.
b   Caspase inhibition is associated with increased aminotransferases in patients with hepatitis C.
c   The innate immune system is a critical component of pathways that perpetuate liver injury and inflammation.
d   Hepatocyte apoptosis can only be initiated by agents that directly damage mitochondria.

Answers to the multiple choice questions can be found in the Appendix at the end of the book.

These multiple choice questions are also available for you to complete online.
Visit http://www.schiffsdiseasesoftheliver.com/

CHAPTER 9
Hepatic Manifestations of Systemic Disorders

Stuart C. Gordon & Hemal K. Patel

Division of Hepatology, Henry Ford Hospital, Detroit, MI, USA

Key concepts

- Endotoxin-mediated cytokine release is the likely cause of sepsis-related jaundice, and can occur in the absence of positive blood cultures. High serum bilirubin levels secondary to sepsis is often an unrecognized clinical entity.
- Any infectious organism may involve the liver, and the clinical presentation often mimics other conditions. A disproportionately raised serum alkaline phosphatase level in the presence of fever should raise the possibility of nonviral hepatitis. Sensitive polymerase chain reaction (PCR)-based assays can facilitate a rapid and appropriate diagnosis.

- The porphyria disorders cause liver damage in association with photocutaneous lesions and neurologic dysfunction. Specific causative genetic mutations allow for confident diagnosis.
- Involvement of the liver with lymphoma strongly mimics the various nonviral infectious disorders of the liver, and may cause acute liver failure. A high degree of clinical suspicion is required in order to facilitate the correct histologic diagnosis.
- Diabetes mellitus and celiac disease may independently cause liver disease, or may act to hasten the development of cirrhosis in predisposed individuals. The mechanisms for these recently identified associations remain to be elucidated.

Infectious diseases

Involvement of the liver with various pathogens may be the result of primary infections or represent a component of multisystemic disorders. These conditions, discussed below, often mimic other entities; they therefore mandate a high degree of clinical suspicion in order to establish a potentially life-saving diagnosis.

Independent of infections of the liver itself, jaundice associated with systemic infections is often overlooked among hospitalized patients, and occurs in both pediatric and adult populations [1,2]. A disproportionate increase in serum bilirubin in comparison to aminotransferases and alkaline phosphatase should raise the suspicion of bacteremia, even in the absence of sign/symptoms of infection such as fever, hypotension, tachycardia, or leukocytosis [3].

The mechanism of jaundice in systemic infection remains unclear although endotoxin (i.e., lipopolysaccharide in the outer membrane of Gram-negative bacteria) mediated cytokines, such as tumor necrosis factor α (TNF-α) and interleukin 1 (IL1)-related hyperbilirubinemia have been proposed [3]. Elevated levels of TNF-α and other cytokines are seen in alcoholic hepatitis and total parenteral nutrition (TPN)-associated jaundice [4].

Endotoxemia impairs transport of anions in both sinusoidal and canalicular membranes, resulting in impaired bile flow [5].

Bacterial infections

Salmonella hepatitis (typhoid fever)

According to a 2004 World Health Organization report [6], approximately 26 million new cases and 200,000 deaths from typhoid fever occurred in the year 2000. Both *Salmonella typhi* and *S. paratyphi* can cause typhoid fever. Although clinical hepatitis is unusual (<25%), liver involvement is almost always present in clinical typhoid fever [7]. The term salmonella hepatitis refers to liver injury caused by infection with either *S. typhi* or *S. paratyphi*, and the disease has been documented in both endemic and nonendemic areas. The disease affects people of all ages, and those with immune deficiency are particularly at risk [8].

The clinical presentation of salmonella hepatitis resembles that of viral hepatitis, but certain features help differentiate the two diseases. In particular, high fever (often >40°C) and bradycardia (inappropriate response of heart rate to degree of fever) is more common among patients with salmonella hepatitis. In addition, the biochemical profile in salmonella hepatitis usually suggests the presence of an infiltrative process rather than hepatitis. In a comparison of 27 cases of salmonella hepatitis with acute viral hepatitis, El-Newihi et al. [9] found that patients with salmonella hepatitis were more likely to have a disproportionately increased serum alkaline phosphatase level, and that serum aminotransferase values were far lower than with acute viral hepatitis. Jaundice is unusual, and many cases of salmonella hepatitis are anicteric. In untreated patients, jaundice may be delayed – appearing in the second to the fourth week of the illness. A spectrum of other hepatobiliary disorders secondary to salmonella hepatitis (i.e., acute liver failure, acalculous cholecystitis, spontaneous bacterial peritonitis, liver abscess, etc.) has been reported [10–13].

Establishing a diagnosis of salmonella hepatitis may be difficult because the manifestations are similar to those of other forms of acute hepatitis, including viral hepatitis. One reported series suggested that the alanine aminotransferase (ALT) to lactate dehydrogenase (LDH) ratio is <4 in salmonella hepatitis, >5 in acute viral hepatitis, and <1.5 in central zonal injury, such as hepatic ischemia or acetaminophen injury [9]. Although the diagnosis of typhoid fever is usually established clinically in developing counties, serological tests such as dot enzyme immunoassay (Typhidot-M®) and polymerase chain reaction (PCR)-based tests are widely used; positive blood culture remains the diagnostic standard [14].

The liver histology of salmonella hepatitis is nonspecific. Ballooning degeneration with vacuolation has been reported, as has biliary canalicular injury. Occasionally, S. typhi organisms are found in the liver cells, as are lobular aggregates of Kupffer cells, lesions known as typhoid nodules [15].

Prompt diagnosis and early intervention with appropriate antibiotics generally assure a good prognosis. Because of potential resistant strains of *Salmonella*, antibiotic sensitivity testing is advised. A fluoroquinolone is the therapy of choice for fully sensitive or multidrug-resistant strains of *Salmonella*, while azithromycin or ceftriaxone/cefotaxime should be used in quinolone-resistant strains [14].

Tuberculosis

Hepatic tuberculosis (infection with *Mycobacterium tuberculosis*) as a part of miliary disease may occur in up to 80% of all patients dying of pulmonary tuberculosis. The original description of hepatic tuberculosis classified the disease as either: (i) miliary, a part of generalized disease; or (ii) local, with focal involvement of the liver. The portal of entry of *M. tuberculosis* organisms into the biliary tract and the liver is the hematogenous route or, less commonly, the portal vein or lymphatic vessels. The manifestations of tuberculous liver involvement are protean, and terms in the literature used to describe hepatobiliary system involvement with tuberculosis include tuberculous pseudotumor, tuberculous cholangitis, and tuberculous liver abscess [16]. The term hepatobiliary tuberculosis refers to either isolated hepatic, biliary, or hepatobiliary involvement with other organ system involvement [17].

The clinical manifestations of hepatobiliary tuberculosis are those of the extrahepatic disease; hepatic involvement is usually asymptomatic [18]. Nevertheless, cases of acute liver failure, among both immunosuppressed and immunocompetent persons, are reported [19,20]. Right upper quadrant or nonspecific abdominal pain, fever of unknown origin, and weight loss, are common symptoms. The most common physical finding is hepatomegaly, which is present in most cases. A disproportionately increased serum alkaline phosphatase level is a consistent finding suggestive of an infiltrative hepatic process. The presence of jaundice suggests biliary involvement, and the biochemical profile may simulate extrahepatic biliary obstruction [21].

One variant form of hepatic tuberculosis without active pulmonary or miliary disease is the nodular form, which presents as an isolated liver tumor or abscess [22,23]. In most cases, the clinical presentation is that of neoplasm, with solitary liver lesions of variable size and imaging features, raised alkaline phosphatase values and weight loss in the absence of known previous tuberculosis. Classic histologic findings (see below) and/or PCR assay of the liver tissue help in establishing the diagnosis. Prompt treatment with antituberculous agents leads to complete resolution of symptoms, signs, and radiologic findings.

An unusual manifestation of tuberculosis involves the development of portal hypertension caused by the compression of the portal vein by tuberculous lymph nodes, with resultant variceal hemorrhage [24]. Additionally, isolated pancreatic tuberculosis may manifest in a manner very similar to that of a pancreatic neoplasm, including a mass lesion of the pancreatic head [25]. Similarly, gallbladder tuberculosis is reportedly increasing in incidence and may manifest as biliary colic or acute cholecystitis [26].

Yet another unusual but increasingly reported variant of hepatobiliary tuberculosis is obstructive jaundice caused by involvement of the bile duct, pancreas, or gallbladder. Compression of the biliary tree by involved lymph nodes or possibly by direct involvement of the biliary epithelium, or by rupture of a caseating granuloma into the lumen of the bile duct, may cause jaundice and biochemical cholestasis. Intrahepatic bile duct obstruction may result from granulomatous involvement, often as part of miliary tuberculosis. The entity of bile duct tuberculosis [27] may manifest as bile duct dilation with common hepatic duct strictures (Fig. 9.1). Biliary

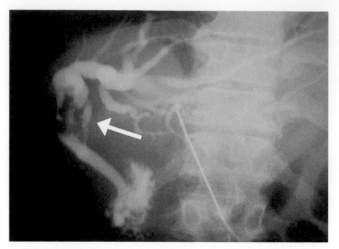

Figure 9.1 A 66-year-old man with abdominal pain and jaundice. Percutaneous transhepatic cholangiogram showing a hilar stricture (arrow) and dilated intrahepatic duct. The diagnosis of tuberculosis was confirmed by fine needle aspiration. (Reproduced from Chong [17] with permission from Wolters Kluwer Health.)

cytologic findings from endoscopic cholangiography may yield the diagnosis. Such patients have painless jaundice and weight loss that mimics pancreatic or cholangiocarcinoma, and dilated bile ducts are found at imaging studies. Experience with therapeutic biliary stenting has been variable, and in unsuccessful cases percutaneous biliary drainage decompresses the obstruction [17,28].

Ultrasonography and computed tomography (CT) may show complex masses, either solitary or multiple. Although the finding of caseating granuloma from a percutaneous biopsy specimen is highly suggestive of tuberculosis (Fig. 9.2), similar pathologic findings occur in brucellosis, coccidioidomycosis, and Hodgkin disease. Giant epitheloid cells and Langhans giant cells are other characteristic histologic findings. The finding of acid-fast bacilli

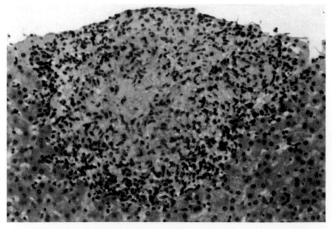

Figure 9.2 Tuberculosis: caseating hepatic granuloma in a patient with fever of unknown origin.

at biopsy occurs infrequently, in <35% of cases. A PCR-based assay on liver tissue has a high sensitivity (overall assay positivity of 88% in one series) with low false negativity among controls [29,30].

The management of hepatic tuberculosis involves the use of at least four antituberculous drugs, usually including isoniazid, rifampicin, pyrazinamide, and ethambutol. Although therapy traditionally lasts at least 6 months, multidrug-resistant organisms and hepatotoxicity of the agents require alternative regimens. Drug-induced liver injury secondary to antituberculous drugs, especially isoniazid, is idiosyncratic and potentially lethal. The American Thoracic Society recommended more vigilant serum ALT monitoring in patients who consume alcohol, take concomitant hepatotoxic drugs, have viral hepatitis or preexisting liver disease or an abnormal baseline ALT, have human immunodeficiency virus (HIV), have a prior history of isoniazid hepatitis, are pregnant, or are within 3 months postpartum [31]. Careful monitoring for drug-induced hepatitis may obviate fatality, especially in the elderly, and once serum bilirubin rises, the prognosis is guarded.

Legionnaires' disease

Hepatic derangements are observed more frequently in *Legionella pneumophila* pneumonia than in other causes of pneumonia. Elevated aminotransferase levels (up to 15 times the upper limit of normal), alkaline phosphatase levels (up to nine times the upper limit of normal), and hyperbilirubinemia (in up to 15% of patients) have been reported. Therefore, the finding of markedly abnormal liver biochemical values in the presence of obvious pneumonia may be a clue to the appropriate diagnosis. Other hepatic manifestations of *L. pneumophila* include acute liver failure as well as liver abscesses [32]. Antigen detection in the urine may serve as a rapid confirmatory test whenever suspicion for *Legionella* infection is high based upon clinical presentation. Antigen detection in respiratory secretions, as well as serologic testing and PCR-based tests may also facilitate diagnosis. The organism can be found with direct immunofluorescence in liver biopsy. Histologic exam of the liver may show necrotic hepatitis with features similar to other forms of viral hepatitis. Antibiotics of choice include flouroquinolones or the newer macrolides.

Brucellosis

Three species of *Brucella* affect humans: *B. melitensis*, *B. abortus*, and *B. suis*. Brucellosis is an occupational disease that affects food handlers, and organisms enter the body through the skin or oropharynx and spread to regional lymph nodes. The disease can also be airborne and transmitted to personnel in microbiology laboratories.

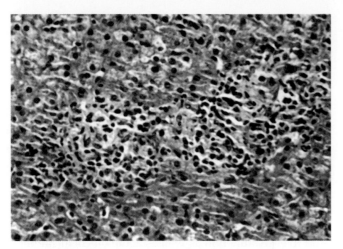

Figure 9.3 *Brucella melitensis*: nonspecific lymphoplasmacytic inflammatory infiltrate in a patient with brucellosis. Hematoxylin and eosin (H&E), original ×510.

The most common clinical manifestation of hepatic involvement by *Brucella* is tender hepatomegaly (20–40%), a modest elevation of aminotransferases (5–40%), and an increase in serum alkaline phosphatase suggesting the presence of an infiltrative process [33]. Spontaneous bacterial peritonitis, acute hepatitis with jaundice, and hepatic abscess have been described [34–36].

Carazo et al. [37] described the imaging features in cases of hepatosplenic brucelloma, and noted that on ultrasound the lesion appears iso- or hypoechogenic with the liver, with focal calcifications. Contrast-enhanced CT scans showed predominantly solid masses with irregular borders, rarely with transdiaphragmatic lung invasion. Histologic examination usually shows granuloma formation with a varying degree of portal and lobular inflammation (Fig. 9.3) [33]. The organism can be isolated from the blood in acute states, but cultures may take 3 weeks to turn positive. Bone marrow aspirate culture is the standard for diagnosis given the very high concentration of the organism in the reticuloendothelial system. Serologic tests are helpful and reliable, and either a titer of 1:320 or demonstration of increasing titers establishes the diagnosis. PCR-based tests are reported to be highly sensitive and specific and offer rapid diagnosis [38].

Combination antibiotic therapy rather than use of a single agent is recommended for *Brucella* infection. Doxycycline combined with streptomycin, rifampin, trimethoprim-sulfamethoxazole, gentamicin, or ciprofloxacilin are various options [38]. In cases of hepatic abscess, percutaneous or surgical drainage may be needed [36].

Tularemia

Infection with *Francisella tularensis*, the causative agent of tularemia, occurs after exposure to jackrabbits and

hares, the main animal reservoir in North America and Europe. Hunters are at risk and may acquire the disease from tick or deer fly bites in the summer months. In Sweden, the lemming is responsible for this disease ("lemming fever"), whereas in Russia the water rat and muskrat may spread tularemia. The disorder usually affects the lungs, and the usual manifestation is a flu-like syndrome occurring between 1 and 10 days after exposure. Liver involvement occurs in up to 75% of patients, in the form of mild to moderate aminotransferase elevation [39]. Jaundice, marked cholestasis, granulomatous hepatitis, ascites, cholangitis, and liver abscesses have been reported.

Histologic examination of the liver in cases of tularemia shows multiple focal areas of coagulative necrosis with a surrounding chronic inflammatory infiltrate. The diagnosis can be established serologically with demonstration of agglutinating antibodies. Enzyme-linked immunosorbent assay (ELISA) tests are available, but a PCR test for *F. tularensis* should enable rapid confirmation of the clinical diagnosis of tularemia. Treatment consists of streptomycin or gentamicin.

Listeriosis

Listeria monocytogenes, a Gram-positive intracellular bacillus, is widely distributed in nature, including soil and plant material, and was thought to be the only causative organism for human listeriosis until recently when *L. ivanovii*-related gastroenteritis and bacteremia was reported in humans [40]. Human *Listeria* infection usually manifests as meningoencephalitis or pneumonitis, although hepatic involvement is reported. A review of 34 cases of *Listeria* related liver disease by Scholing et al. [41] showed that the clinical presentation can be of three different types: a solitary liver abscess, multiple abscesses, or diffuse involvement (hepatitis) with or without granulomas. Patients are often immunosuppressed or at extremes of age. The presence of high fever and leukocytosis tends to differentiate this condition from viral hepatitis, and the diagnosis is confirmed by the isolation of the organism from blood. Radiologic imaging and fine needle aspiration, when applicable, helps in establishing the diagnosis. Treatment consists of drainage of the abscess whenever possible along with systemic administration of antibiotics, usually penicillin in combination with aminoglycosides for 3–4 weeks [41].

Melioidosis

Melioidosis, endemic in northern Australia and Southeast Asia, is a potentially fatal infection caused by the bacterium *Burkholderia pseudomallei*. The mortality may be high, averaging 45%, and in cases of acute septicemia, death occurs within the first 3 days after hospital admission. The liver involvement in melioidosis is common and may manifest as biochemical abnormalities or localized abscesses. Granulomas can be seen on histology. Radiologically, the "honeycomb" appearance has been described as characteristic for large liver abscesses [42]. Immunohistochemistry may play a useful diagnostic role whenever tissue sample is available. Direct immunofluorescence microscopy of the infected material is less sensitive (70%), but highly specific (98%), and confirms diagnosis in 30 minutes [43]. Isolation of the organism from blood remains the most reliable test. Parenteral antibiotics (ceftazidime or amoxicillin-clavulanate) followed by long-term oral antibiotics with a four drug regimen (chloramphanicol, doxycycline, trimethoprim, and sulfamethoxazole) up to 20 weeks may be needed to eradicate the organism [43].

Neisseria and Chlamydia

Nonspecific aminotransferase abnormalities may occur in disseminated gonococcal infection. Cervical and pelvic gonorrhea may be associated with violin-string adhesions between the liver capsule and the peritoneal wall, known as Fitz-Hugh–Curtis syndrome (FHCS). However, such adhesions are not pathognomonic for *Neisseria* infection, and may occur after other infections, including hepatic candidiasis (Fig. 9.4) [44]. Liver abscess from *Neisseria sicca* after repeated radiofrequency ablation of hepatocellular cancer was recently reported [45].

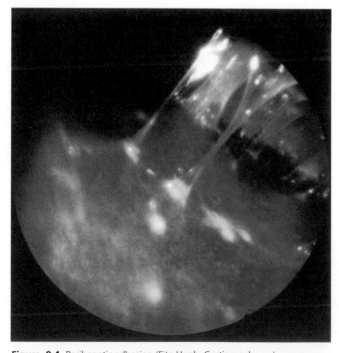

Figure 9.4 Perihepatic adhesion (Fitz-Hugh–Curtis syndrome) may occur in conditions other than gonorrhea. After therapy for hepatic candidiasis, a follow-up laparoscopy showed violin-string adhesions from the focal lesions to the peritoneal wall. Such adhesions may result in marked right upper quadrant pain.

A similar syndrome of perihepatitis occurs with *Chlamydia trachomatis*-related pelvic inflammatory disease (PID) [46]. Various studies have reported the incidence of FHCS to be 4–12% in patients with mild to moderate PID and 20–28% in patients with severe PID [47]. Case reports of Chilaiditi syndrome (colonic or small intestinal interposition between the liver and diaphragm, temporarily or permanently) and right pleural effusion associated with FHCS and *Chlamydia* infection has been reported [48,49]. *Chlamydia pneumoniae* has been purported as a causative agent for primary biliary cirrhosis; however, data on this association are mixed [50].

Campylobacter

Mild liver dysfunction as well as acute biochemical hepatitis may occur after infection with *Campylobacter* organisms. A case of pyogenic liver abscess associated with *Campylobacter curvus* bacteremia was recently reported from Canada [51]. The organism has been isolated from bile during episodes of gallstone-related cholecystitis [52]. Macrolides are the treatment of choice.

Catscratch disease

Hepatosplenic catscratch disease often manifests as fever of unknown origin in children who have had contact with an immature cat. The disease occurs when *Bartonella henselae* causes necrotizing granuloma in the liver or spleen or both. Fleas have also been suggested as vectors for this organism because cat scratches may be absent in some cases. Abdominal pain is common and occasionally is severe. Abdominal ultrasonography shows microabscesses in the liver or spleen. Among HIV-infected patients, a syndrome of peliosis hepatis (bacillary angiomatosis) is caused by *B. henselae* infection. Serologic assays, indirect immunofluorescence, and PCR assays may assist in the diagnosis [53]. Prolonged antibiotic regimens with erythromycin, doxycycline, or macrolides have proved effective in various series [54,55]. In a case report from the United States, *B. henselae*-related liver abscesses developed in a 52-year-old female 3 years following orthotopic liver transplantation [56].

Spirochetal infections

Leptospirosis

Also known as Weil disease, the classic description of leptospirosis – an infection transmitted via exposure to rodent urine – is of febrile headache, jaundice with renal failure, and severe muscle pain. Only a small percentage of patients have these most severe manifestations and most descriptions of liver pathology come from historical autopsy series. Early recognition, with administration of appropriate antibiotics, has resulted in a very low incidence of hepatic manifestations.

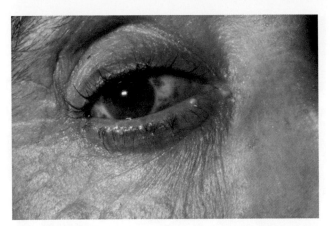

Figure 9.5 Icteric sclera and subconjunctival suffusion in a patient with leptospirosis and liver involvement.

To establish the diagnosis during the first phase, leptospira can be isolated from the cerebrospinal fluid and blood; in the second phase, they are isolated from the urine. Dark-ground microscopic examination of plasma has been found to be a simple and rapid form of early diagnosis of leptospirosis with hepatorenal involvement. PCR based on the *flaB* gene of leptospira has been found to be an efficient tool for rapid detection and identification from clinical specimens. Doxycycline is the treatment of choice. A recent review suggested that the data do not support the practice of doxycycline prophylaxis for all residents of an endemic area, although short-term travelers with a potential for high-risk exposure may be helped [61].

Although often considered a disease of developing nations, cases occur in the United States and may cause a diagnostic dilemma [57]. The initial manifestations are rather nonspecific, i.e., fever, meningism, flu-like illness, abdominal pain, vomiting, and conjunctivitis ("conjunctival suffusion") (Fig. 9.5). The abdominal pain of the acute phase may simulate surgical abdomen and may manifest as biliary colic. During the second phase of illness (usually the second week), severe muscle pain with jaundice and renal failure are common. The serum creatine kinase level may be elevated. The third, or convalescent, stage (third week) shows improvement in mental status and renal function and resolution of jaundice.

When presenting in the late stage of pregnancy, leptospirosis may mimic HELLP syndrome (hemolysis, elevated liver enzymes and low platelets), AFLP (acute fatty liver of pregnancy), or metastatic liver cancer [58–60]. Early intensive care and parenteral antibiotics (penicillin or doxycycline) may be helpful, and therefore early diagnosis is important.

Syphilis

Syphilis is a multisystemic disease caused by the spirochete *Treponema pallidum*. Liver involvement during early syphilis (primary or secondary) presents as biochemical cholestasis with a disproportionate elevation of alkaline phosphatase. An acute cholestatic hepatitis secondary to syphilis occurs among HIV-infected patients – in up to 38% in one series [62].

The gummas of the liver may resemble metastatic disease at autopsy or may resemble cirrhosis because of the nodular configuration of the liver in the later stages. Focal liver lesions with filling defects on CT scans may mimic metastatic disease in a patient with weight loss. Chen et al. [63] reported a case of peliosis hepatis and gummatous syphilis wherein the diagnosis was established by liver biopsy. The pathologic findings generally include lymphocytic and neutrophilic infiltrates in the portal tracts, while pericholangiolar inflammation has also been described (Fig. 9.6). Identification of treponemes in the liver is very uncommon. Additional laboratory studies of the syphilitic hepatitis of secondary stage

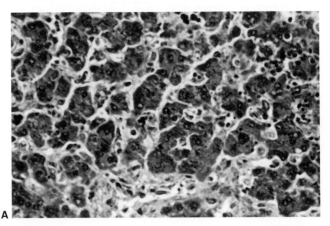
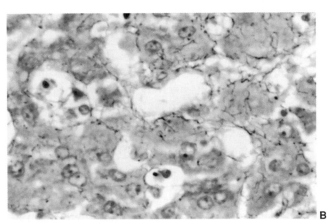

Figure 9.6 Hepar lobatum. (A) Diffuse pericellular sinusoidal fibrosis in congenital syphilis of liver. H&E, original ×485. (B) Numerous spirochetes layered in periphery of sinusoids adjacent to hepatocyte cords. Dieterle stain, original ×1,200. (Courtesy of Dr John Watts.)

disease include a hemagglutination test for *T. pallidum* and a fluorescent treponemal antibody (FTA) absorption (FTA-ABS) test. Treatment with penicillin usually results in symptomatic as well as well biochemical resolution of syphilitic hepatitis.

Lyme disease

Endemic to northeast United States but more recently spreading widely throughout the United States, Lyme disease is caused by the spirochete *Borrelia burgdorferi* and is transmitted to humans by the bite of infected ticks (*Ixodes*). Involvement of the liver is common in the early stage of Lyme disease with a reported incidence of 10–27% [39,64]. The mechanism by which liver injury occurs is not known, but direct toxicity, systemic cytokine release, and immune-mediated damage are proposed theories [65]. Cases of granulomatous hepatitis from Lyme disease have been reported [66].

Histologic examination shows portal inflammation, ballooning of hepatocytes, and sinusoidal mononuclear and neutrophil cell infiltration [65]. Diagnosis is based upon direct tests (microscopy, PCR, and culture) or serological testing. A two-step approach (sensitive enzyme immunoassay or indirect fluorescent antibody assay as the first step, followed by western immunoblots as a confirmatory step) is recommended as *B. burgorferi* shares some antigens with other bacteria and serologic tests can detect nonspecific antibodies. Doxycycline is the treatment drug of choice.

Rickettsial infection

Q fever

The causative rickettsia of Q fever is *Coxiella burnetii*. The organism has been identified in ticks, and the disease has a worldwide distribution. Liver involvement is common. Presentation may vary geographically, as pneumonia is reportedly more common in eastern Canada while hepatitis is more common in southern Spain [67]. A case series of 109 patients reported the prevalence of acute biochemical hepatitis to be as high as 85% [68]. Three main hepatic manifestations of Q fever have been proposed: (i) a clinically acute hepatitis-like illness without respiratory involvement (the most common form of hepatic involvement); (ii) an incidental finding of increased liver biochemical values in a patient with known acute Q fever; or (iii) fever of unknown origin with characteristic hepatic granulomas [69].

The classic "doughnut-like" granuloma of Q fever – a central clear space in the center of the granuloma – is not pathognomonic for the disease and may be seen in Hodgkin disease and infectious mononucleosis (Fig. 9.7). The granuloma is a dense fibrin ring surrounded by a cen-

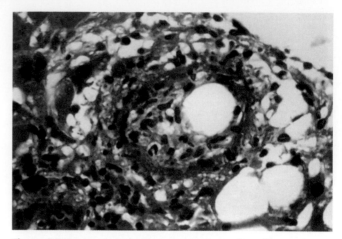

Figure 9.7 Section showing classic doughnut granuloma. The characteristic lesion of Q fever is a doughnut granuloma similar to that shown here. H&E, original ×780. (Courtesy of Dr John Watts.)

tral lipid vacuole and is composed of neutrophils, monocytes, eosinophils, and occasional multinucleated giant cells. Kupffer cells are hypertrophied and there may be a lymphocytic portal inflammation with erosion of the limiting plate.

The diagnosis is established by a serological test (a microimmunofluorescent antibody titer to *C. burnetii*) to phase I and II antigens [67]. PCR can be used to amplify *C. burnetii* DNA from tissue [70]. Doxycycline is considered the treatment of choice, and a fluoroquinolone such as ofloxacin has been used with success [67]. Although controversial, erythromycin may be an appropriate alternative in the treatment of children. Vaccination can be a safe and efficacious tool in decreasing the incidence and hospitalizations associated with Q fever in endemic areas [71].

Ehrlichiosis

Human infection with *Ehrlichia canis*, a tick-borne infection common among dogs, was first reported in 1987. However, human monocytic ehrlichiosis is mostly caused by *E. chaffeensis*, which is transmitted by the lone star tick, *Amblyomma americanum*.

Involvement of the liver in human ehrlichiosis is common and ranges from mildly elevated aminotransferases to fatal hepatitis [72]. Although rare, marked cholestasis and liver failure has been reported, which responds completely to doxycycline therapy [73]. Liver histology may show lobular lymphohistiocytic foci, diffuse lymphohistiocytic infiltration, various degrees of liver cell injury, and cholestasis with bile duct epithelial injury [74]. The organism may be present within the Kupffer cells. The diagnosis is confirmed by indirect immunofluorescence and PCR [75]. Treatment consists of doxycycline or tetracycline [75].

Rocky mountain spotted fever

Rocky mountain spotted fever, a multisystemic disease caused by *Rickettsia rickettsii*, manifests hepatic involvement by mild to moderate derangements in liver biochemistries. Jaundice is rare but when present could predict a poor prognosis. Rickettsiae mostly infect the endothelial lining of liver sinusoids and portal vasculature while sparing hepatocytes; focal hepatitis and periportal inflammation can be seen on liver biopsy [39]. Vasculitis and significant central nervous system (CNS) and pulmonary manifestations are also the result of rickettsial invasion of the endothelial lining. Leukopenia, thrombocytopenia, mild hyponatremia, and elevated liver enzymes are clues to the diagnosis in patients presenting with rash and CNS manifestations. Serology and PCR-based assays are widely available for aid in diagnosis; doxycycline is the treatment of choice.

Fungal infections

Histoplasmosis

Histoplasmosis has a worldwide distribution, and is the most common cause of fungal infection in the Ohio and Mississippi river valleys of the United States. It is usually transmitted after inhalation of the organism *Histoplasma capsulatum*, which is particularly associated with bird droppings, especially those of chickens.

Among 111 patients with systemic histoplasmosis, fever, respiratory symptoms, weight loss, and bone marrow suppression were the predominant presenting symptoms [76]. Liver involvement mainly included raised serum alkaline phosphatase. Bone marrow suppression and elevated liver enzymes are more common in immunocompromised patients with systemic histoplasmosis than in immunocompetent patients. Liver biopsy

may be needed in some cases and hepatic lesions may include widely diffuse granulomas throughout the liver or parenchymal infiltration with macrophages filled with the organism, best seen with fungal staining.

Although liver involvement is common in cases of disseminated histoplasmosis, the disease may also present as an isolated liver mass or as an infiltrative liver disorder. Cases of isolated hepatic histoplasmosis without pulmonary involvement and a solitary right-sided liver lesion invading the diaphragm have been reported [77,78]. A review of the pathologic spectrum of cases of gastrointestinal histoplasmosis showed that 10% of 52 patients had histologic evidence of liver disease, most commonly portal lymphohistiocytic inflammation (Fig. 9.8). Discrete hepatic granulomas were found in fewer than 20% of livers that were involved [79].

Early diagnosis may be life-saving. Fungal culture, histopathology, antibody assays, and histoplasma antigen detection in urine, serum, and other body fluids are the usual modalities to establish the diagnosis. Intravenous itraconazole is recommended for mild to moderate disease, while an amphotericin B formulation is reserved for severe infection [80].

Candidiasis

Caused by infection with fungi of the genus *Candida*, the clinical spectrum of candidal liver disease is varied. The most common species causing human infection is *Candida albicans*, although other species also cause disease. The entity of focal hepatic candidiasis may be part of hepatosplenic candidiasis or chronic disseminated candidiasis [81]. Regular use of antifungal prophylaxis in patients undergoing hematopoietic stem cell transplantation and in neutropenic patients with leukemia undergoing chemotherapy has decreased all-cause mortality from systemic candidiasis [82].

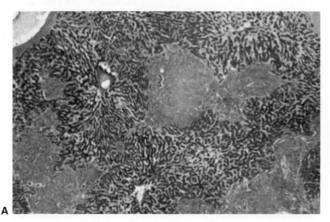
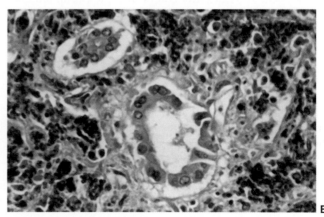

Figure 9.8 An elderly diabetic man living in an area endemic for histoplasmosis with fever and hepatomegaly. (A) Confluent portal granulomas in a patient with hepatic histoplasmosis. H&E. (B) Special stain showing uniform, oval, yeast-like cells morphologically typical of *Histoplasma capsulatum*. H&E, methenamine silver. (Courtesy of Dr Laura Lamps.)

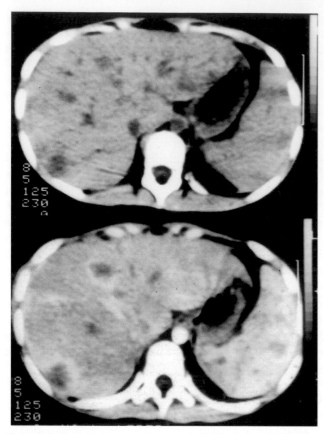

Figure 9.9 Computed tomography scan of a febrile 8-year-old girl with leukemia undergoing chemotherapy. Images before (A) and after (B) administration of contrast material revealing numerous areas of low attenuation throughout the liver and spleen. Rim enhancement of the lesions after injection of contrast material is caused by inflammation. An open biopsy of the hepatic lesion proved the diagnosis of hepatic candidiasis. (Courtesy of Dr Ali Shirkhoda.)

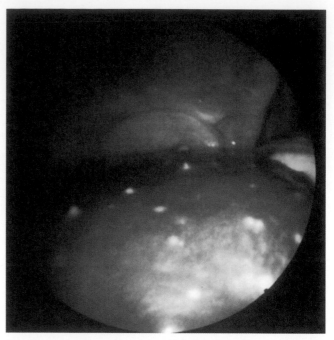

Figure 9.10 A 60-year-old woman with leukemia with fever and jaundice after induction chemotherapy. The computed tomography scan showed no significant pathologic process. At laparoscopy, however, the liver was diffusely infiltrated with small discrete lesions of focal candidiasis.

Jaundice and elevated alkaline phosphatase in leukemic patients after chemotherapy is the usual presentation. The pathogen locally invades the colonic mucosa and subsequently enters into the portal circulation [83]. Results from CT and ultrasonography are often normal in the early stage of neutropenic fever, whereas as the neutrophil count returns to normal, imaging studies may show focal liver lesions with a bull's-eye appearance (Fig. 9.9) [83,84]. However, these lesions may be absent on images in some cases even with jaundice. In such cases, diagnostic laparoscopy may show discrete focal yellowish-white punctate lesions scattered throughout the liver surface with direct-guided liver biopsy revealing granuloma with central necrosis (Figs 9.10 and 9.11) [44]. Cholangitis with common bile duct stenosis secondary to *Candida* colonization of the biliary tract was described in a patient on long-time mechanical ventilation [85].

The diagnosis of hepatic candidiasis can be confirmed by culture, immunofluorescence, or PCR-based testing from histologic specimens. Kirby et al. [86] described a typical case of hepatosplenic candidiasis in which PCR was positive for *Candida* DNA in both the sera and liver biopsy.

Optimal therapy for hepatic candidiasis has not been established, in part because of the rarity of the condition, the paucity of controlled trials, and the absence of established end-points of treatment. A relapse of the infection may be related to either premature discontinuation of therapy or inadequate antifungal treatment of patients

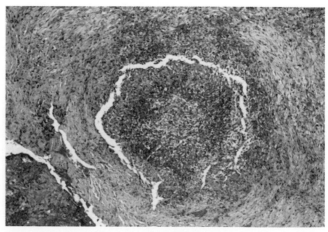

Figure 9.11 Focal hepatic candidiasis (same patient as in Figs 9.4 and 9.10): a centrally necrotic granuloma is surrounded by a thick fibrous capsule. H&E, original ×80. (Courtesy of Dr John Watts.)

with chemotherapy-induced neutropenia [81]. In a review of the treatment of candidiasis [87], it was observed that prior exposure to azoles and the identification of non-*C. albicans* strains can be valuable information, as azole resistance is higher in critically ill patients. Echinocandins are favored for empiric treatment of invasive candidiasis and candidemia [88]. Both fluconazole and caspofungin are as effective as and less toxic than amphotericin B, and can be given orally.

Actinomycosis

Actinomycosis is a chronic, progressive, suppurative disease caused by actinomycetes of the genus *Actinomyces*. The disease occurs worldwide with higher prevalence in areas with low socioeconomic indices and poor dental hygiene. Improved oral hygiene resulted in a decreased incidence of this infection [89]. Involvement of the liver is rare, but primary hepatic actinomycosis may present as hepatocellular carcinoma in endemic areas.

In a recent review of 67 cases of hepatic actinomycosis, the mean age of patients was 44 years (range, 4–85 years) with a male predominance. In 75% of patients, the infection was cryptogenic and 45% of the patients had radiologic findings mimicking liver tumor. Two thirds of the patients had a solitary liver lesion with more than half having right lobe involvement. Elevated serum alkaline phosphatase levels were common. The diagnosis was usually established by microscopic examination of surgical or percutaneous specimens. Antibiotics alone were used in half of the cases, while antibiotics along with surgical/percutaneous drainage were used in the other half. Only two patients required resection as a part of the treatment. The mortality rate was 7.6% in this series [90].

Histologic examination of tissue samples is needed to establish the appropriate diagnosis (Fig. 9.12). The anaerobic *Actinomyces* are difficult to grow in blood culture. Direct fluorescent antibody and immunofluorescence testing can be used but are not readily available in all clinical laboratories [89]. As noted above, most patients respond to prolonged therapy with penicillin (intravenously for 2–6 weeks followed by 6–12 months of oral therapy). Other first-line antibiotics include amoxicillin, tetracycline, erythromycin, and clindamycin. Percutaneous or surgical drainage may be required if an abscess is present [89].

Coccidioidomycosis

The disease known as San Joaquin valley fever is caused by the dimorphic fungus *Coccidioides immitis*. It is endemic in the southwest region of the United States, Central America, and Mexico. The route of infection follows inhalation of the fungus, and the disease may then spread from the primary lung focus to involve the liver. Extrapulmonary disease is rare, but case reports clearly show that both liver and biliary involvement are manifestations of coccidioidomycosis.

The usual clinical features are those of nonspecific anicteric hepatitis, often with biochemical cholestasis, in a person who has recently traveled to Mexico or the American southwest. It commonly presents as a hepatopulmonary syndrome with eosinophilia but may also present as solitary liver mass. Biopsy of the liver shows granulomatous hepatitis. In rare instances, obstructive jaundice may relate to granulomatous involvement of the bile duct epithelium [91].

Among 37 immunosuppressed patients who received liver transplants and later moved to Arizona, the incidence of new coccidioidal infection was 2.7%, suggesting that coccidioidomycosis was not frequent in this population [92]. Nevertheless, among patients with end-stage liver disease listed for transplantation in this same region of Arizona, the incidence of new coccidioidal infection

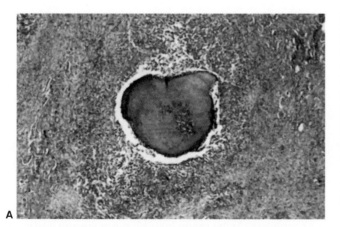
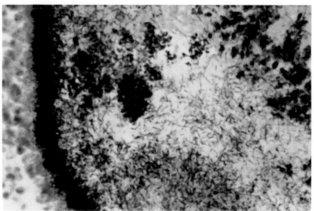

Figure 9.12 (A) A microcolony of *Actinomyces* organisms (sulfur granule) surrounded by acute suppurative inflammation. H&E, original ×80. (B) A high-power Brown–Brenn-stained section of a sulfur granule, composed of Gram-positive filamentous bacteria. The diagnosis of actinomycosis was confirmed with direct immunofluorescence (not shown). Original ×780. (Courtesy of Dr John Watts.)

Table 9.1 Porphyrias: classification and biochemical parameters.

Type of porphyria	Enzyme defect	Site of heme overproduction	Main clinical symptoms	Principal biochemical features
ALA dehydrase deficiency	ALA dehydrase	Liver	Acute attacks and chronic neuropathy	ALA in urine
Acute intermittent porphyria	PBG deaminase	Liver	Acute attacks	ALA and PBG in urine
Congenital erythropoietic porphyria	Uroporphyrinogen III synthase	Erythroid cells	Severe photosensitivity and hemolysis	Uroporphyrin in red cells and urine; coproporphyrin in feces
Porphyria cutanea tarda	Uroporphyrinogen decarboxylase	Liver	Skin fragility and chronic liver disease	Uroporphyrin in urine; isocoproporphyrin in feces
Hepatoerythropoietic porphyria	Uroporphyrinogen decarboxylase	Liver and erythroid cells	Skin fragility and chronic liver disease	Zinc protoporphyrin in red cells; uroporphyrin in urine; isocoproporphyrin in feces
Hereditary coproporphyria	Coproporphyrinogen oxidase	Liver	Acute attacks and skin fragility	ALA, PBG, and coproporphyrin in urine; coproporphyrin in feces
Variegate porphyria	Protoporphyrinogen oxidase	Liver	Acute attacks and skin fragility	ALA, PBG, and coproporphyrin in urine; protoporphyrin in feces
Erythropoietic protoporphyria	Ferrochelatase	Erythroid cells	Photosensitivity and liver damage	Protoporphyrin in red cells and feces

ALA, δ-aminolevulinic acid; PBG, porphobilinogen.

was 4.2%, compared with 0.04% in the same county in the general population [93]. The authors suggested that treatment might alleviate some of the symptoms of coccidioidomycosis originally attributed to disease of the underlying liver disease [93]. Routine surveillance for prior coccidioidal infection and azole prophylaxis (if prior infection is suspected) is advised for patients undergoing solid organ transplantation in endemic areas [94].

Hematology

Porphyrias
Porphyrias represent a group of complex metabolic disorders that result from enzymatic defects in heme biosynthesis. The identification of specific enzyme defects clarified the various subtypes of porphyrias. Subsequently, the identification of specific gene mutations facilitated the screening of relatives and thus early diagnosis and decreased morbidity and mortality. Porphyrias are mostly inherited as autosomal dominants but other patterns (autosomal recessive and complex) are possible. The penetrance of these genes varies and many individuals with genetic defects do not have clinical disease [95].

Heme is synthesized in all human cells, whereas bone marrow (erythroid cells) and liver are the major sites of heme synthesis and therefore porphyrias can be classified as erythropoietic or hepatic, respectively, based

on the principal sites of biochemical abnormalities. Porphyrins are excreted mainly through the liver; however, in patients with advanced liver disease from other etiologies, porphyrins appear in the urine because of the liver's inability to exclusively excrete them. This forms the basis of secondary porphyrias. Clinical manifestations of porphyrias can vary, but the principal manifestations are neurovisceral dysfunction, photosensitivity, and structural liver damage. The biochemical and clinical features are described in Table 9.1 [95,96].

Acute porphyrias
Acute intermittent porphyria, hereditary coproporphyria, and variegate porphyria classically present as acute attacks. Acute attacks may also occur in aminolevulinic acid (ALA) dehydrase-deficiency porphyria. Symptoms usually start after puberty and range from mild behavioral changes to autonomic and sensorimotor neuropathies to CNS involvement [95]. The diagnosis is often delayed in patients presenting with acute attacks without a previously established diagnosis of porphyria. Measurement of the urinary excretion of ALA and porphobilinogen (PBG) leads to prompt diagnosis in acutely ill patients, while the diagnosis of a specific type of porphyria can be made later by more specific testing.

Certain medications, alcohol, infection, and fasting can precipitate an acute attack [97]. Specific treatment with intravenous hematin (3–4 mg/kg daily for 3–4 consecutive days), nutritional support with a high carbohydrate diet or total parenteral nutrition, and symptomatic management are key components of patient care during the acute attack [98]. Liver transplantation can restore normal heme metabolism and has been reported to be curative for acute intermittent porphyria [99,100]. Liver transplantation successfully treated a case of variegate porphyria but cannot be currently recommended for ALA dehydrase-deficiency porphyria [101].

Hepatocellular carcinoma (HCC) has been associated with acute porphyrias and the risk of liver cancer is substantially higher in patients with acute porphyrias compared with the general population [102]. Amongst acute porphyrias, acute intermittent porphyria and porphyria cutanea tarda (PCT) are more commonly associated with HCC. Approximately 5% of patients with porphyria cutanea tarda die of primary liver cancer [102]. The exact pathophysiology remains unexplained, although porphyria-related hepatitis, iron overload, and hepatotoxins are proposed mechanisms [102].

Porphyria cutanea tarda

The most common porphyria worldwide [103], PCT usually manifests after the fourth decade of life although a familial form of PCT may occur early in childhood. PCT is associated with many conditions, including hereditary hemochromatosis, hepatitis C, HIV infection, alcohol consumption, chronic hemodialysis, and estrogen exposure in women.

Patients with symptomatic PCT usually have liver involvement that ranges from mild elevation of aminotransferases to cirrhosis and HCC [104]. If exposed to ultraviolet light, liver biopsy specimens may exhibit red fluorescence. Needle-like cytoplasmic inclusions are found in specimens from untreated patients, which appear to be uroporphyrin crystals. Hemosiderosis is usually demonstrated with iron stains; fatty infiltration is common [105].

The diagnosis is usually made based on clinical presentation and increased urine excretion of uroporphyrin and fecal excretion of isocoproporphyrins. Avoidance of sunlight and fluorescent light, alcohol, contraceptive steroids, and iron supplements should be advised. The mainstay of management are phlebotomies [106]. Urinary excretion of porphyrins usually returns to normal within a year after such therapy, however periodic checks for relapse are required. Patients who continue to have symptoms after phlebotomy, or those who do not tolerate phlebotomies, can be placed on low-dose twice-weekly chloroquine compounds, which enhance porphyrin excretion. Patients with cirrhosis secondary to PCT are at risk for HCC and require screening.

Erythropoietic protoporphyria

Erythropoietic protoporphyria (EPP) is an autosomal dominant condition that usually manifests as acute photosensitivity [103]. Skin symptoms include a burning sensation, edema, and erythema immediately after sun exposure that resolves within a few days. Liver disease is present in 20–30% of symptomatic EPP patients, again ranging from mild disease to cirrhosis [107]. A black pigmentation of the liver results from protoporphyrin deposition in hepatocytes, Kupffer cells, and the biliary system. Birefringence is observed on polarized microscopy as protoporphyrin deposits in the form of crystals [108]. Bile duct destruction (early in the disease), protoporphyrin deposition, portal inflammation, and fibrosis are common findings on liver biopsy. Gallstones are common, again from excessive protoporphyrin accumulation and the resultant excretion that ultimately aggregates – as it is a poorly water-soluble compound – and forms crystalloid deposition.

The biochemical hallmark is an increased level of protoporphyrin in erythroid cells and feces. Excretion of urinary porphyrins is usually normal. No specific therapy is available for patients with liver involvement. Cholestyramine, chenodeoxycholic acid, cysteine, hematin, and blood transfusions have been tried and none has been established as the treatment of choice [107]. A trial of cholestyramine in patients with early liver disease is advised, while monitoring liver chemistries and red cell protoporphyrin levels. Medical treatment followed by bone marrow transplantation was curative in a case of severe cholestatic liver disease [109].

Liver transplantation is well established as a treatment modality for patients with advanced liver disease secondary to EPP [101,110]. Unique complications such as abdominal skin damage from operating room fluorescent lights can be avoided by the use of filters. Perioperative paresis from severe polyneuropathy (a neurotoxic effect of protoporphyrin) can also occur during transplantation. As the ferrochelatase defect in the erythroid cells is not corrected by liver transplantation and because erythroid cells/bone marrow is the major site of biochemical abnormality, protoporphyrin levels remain high after the transplant and can damage the transplanted liver – in up to 65% in a recent series [110]. Bone marrow transplantation after liver transplantation can stabilize recurrent EPP by correcting the biochemical defect [111].

Lymphoma

The neoplastic process of lymphoid tissue commonly involves the liver, as this organ is a part of the reticuloendothelial system. Rarely, however, does lymphoma cause life-threatening hepatic complications. Lymphoma is classified in two broad categories, Hodgkin lymphoma (HL) and non-Hodgkin lymphoma (NHL), with the latter further subdivided as indolent (35–40%), aggressive (~50%), and highly aggressive (~5%) lymphoma.

Hodgkin lymphoma

Hodgkin disease may actually present as acute liver failure [112] or with hepatomegaly (~9% of patients with stage I–II disease compared to 45% with stage III–IV disease). Jaundice may be multifactorial, more commonly from lymphomatous infiltration causing intrahepatic biliary obstruction, however other etiologies, such as paraneoplastic phenomenon and hepatic microsomal function defect, are possible [113]. Vanishing bile duct syndrome with unexplained jaundice may precede the diagnosis of HL [114].

A liver biopsy is recommended for patients with suspected stage IIIE (extralymphatic) or IV disease as this has implications for prognosis and therapy. Histologic abnormalities in patients with HL are nonspecific. In a series of 308 patients with Hodgkin disease who underwent 459 liver biopsies, 35% had normal histology, only 2.4% had classic Reed–Sternberg cells, and the rest had nonspecific findings [115]. A 25-year-old male presented with hepatomegaly and elevated liver enzymes; a diagnostic laparoscopy and biopsy showed peliosis hepatis, followed by a diagnosis of HL from a biopsy of the mediastinal mass [116]. Successful treatment of HL results in the regression of jaundice in a few patients; persistent jaundice despite remission of HL may signify permanent liver damage [117].

Non-Hodgkin lymphoma

Liver involvement is more common in NHL than in HL – in 15–27% of cases and in more than 50% in autopsy studies [118]. The most characteristic findings include hepatomegaly with raised serum alkaline phosphatase levels. Overt jaundice is rare in patients with NHL, but it may occur secondary to extrahepatic biliary obstruction, most commonly at the porta hepatis.

Primary hepatic NHL is rare and may represent around 1% of extranodal NHL [119]; it can be further subdivided into nodular or diffuse types. Initial presentation may be nonspecific and is usually with "B" symptoms (fever, weight loss, and night sweats). In most cases, liver biochemistries are abnormal. A liver biopsy with immunohistochemistry studies is required for the diagnosis of primary hepatic NHL [118]. Median survival has been estimated to be around 15 months [119]. Management options are not standardized and could include surgery, chemotherapy, radiotherapy, or a combined modality [119]. A small subset of patients with primary hepatic NHL may present with acute liver failure, often with high mortality. Prompt diagnosis with liver biopsy followed by aggressive chemotherapy could be a life-saving mea-

sure [120]. Even though generally contraindicated, three patients were treated with orthotopic liver transplantation, with only one out of the three surviving longer than 240 days [119].

Acute liver failure and lymphoma

As noted above, lymphomatous infiltration of the liver may rarely present as acute liver failure. Rowbotham et al. [121] reviewed 4,020 patients with acute liver failure and found only 12 (0.3%) patients (three cases of HL and nine cases of NHL) with lymphoma leading to acute liver failure. NHL appears to be more commonly associated with such presentation than HL. Although a fulminant presentation with acute liver failure (as evidenced by encephalopathy, coagulopathy, and severe lactic acidosis) leading to multisystem organ failure and death is most common, a benign presentation with nonspecific flu-like symptoms and hepatomegaly can also be seen. Replacement of hepatic parenchyma with lymphoid cells, with resultant sinusoidal congestion leading to ischemia and massive hepatocyte necrosis, is the pathophysiology behind such presentation [122]. An antemortem diagnosis is made in less than 50% of cases, attesting to the severity of the presentation [123]. Despite this difficulty, an accurate diagnosis can be established by liver biopsy (transjugular if coagulopathic) and immunohistochemistry and these should therefore be considered in the diagnostic workup of any patient with acute liver failure with negative common etiological evaluation [122]. Histology may show the replacement of hepatic parenchyma with lymphoid cells, sinusoidal congestion, and massive hepatocyte necrosis. In cases with a negative liver biopsy and a high clinical suspicion for lymphoma, a bone marrow biopsy should be pursued [112].

Hepatic lymphoma presenting as acute liver failure carries a grave prognosis, with 83–100% mortality in one series [123]. Systemic lymphoma is a contraindication to liver transplantation as lymphoma frequently recurs [112]. Prompt diagnosis followed by administration of chemotherapy is the only hope for survival in such patients [122].

Sickle cell disease

Sickle cell hepatopathy – liver disorders resulting from the chronic sequelae of sickle cell disease – includes a wide range of clinical syndromes. It is more common in homozygous sickle cell anemia (i.e., sickle cell disease patients) compared with sickle cell trait or hemoglobin sickle cell disease. Hepatic involvement in sickle cell disease can be from the sickling process, which results in acute clinical syndromes (acute sickle hepatic crisis, sickle cell intrahepatic cholestasis, hepatic sequestration crisis, etc.), from multiple transfusions (resulting in iron overload or viral hepatitis), or from chronic hemolysis (resulting in pigment stone production with consequent cholecystitis, choledocholithiasis, and gallstone pancreatitis) [124].

Abnormal liver tests are common in patients with sickle cell disease, especially unconjugated hyperbilirubinemia from hemolysis, as well as raised LDH levels [124]. Alkaline phosphatase levels can also be elevated; however, the source is mostly osseous rather than liver [125,126].

Acute clinical syndromes often manifest as right upper quadrant pain, fever, and jaundice. Acute sickle hepatic crisis usually presents as elevated aspartate aminotransferase (AST) and ALT (less than 300 U/L), and raised serum bilirubin levels (usually less than 15 mg/dL) [125]. Liver biopsy may show sinusoidal obstruction by sickle cell thrombi, Kupffer cell hypertrophy, and engorgement with sickle-shaped red blood cells, mild centrilobular necrosis, and bile stasis [125]. The syndrome is self-limited and usually resolves within 3–14 days with intravenous hydration and analgesics.

Sickle cell intrahepatic cholestasis is a severe variant of acute sickle hepatic crisis and is the result of widespread sickling within sinusoids resulting in massive hepatic ischemia. Patients initially may present with right upper quadrant pain, jaundice, fever, and leucocytosis, but as widespread sickling continues, renal failure, coagulopathy, and encephalopathy ensue. Serum AST and ALT levels are usually greater than 1,000 U/L, and remarkably high serum bilirubin levels may occur because of a combination of hemolysis, renal failure, and severe intrahepatic cholestasis [127]. Liver biopsy may show sickled red blood cells in hepatic sinusoids and dilated canaliculi with bile stasis [125]. Treatment is mostly supportive with the use of exchange transfusion, although successful liver transplantation has been reported [128]. Sequestration of red blood cells in the liver leads to hepatic sequestration crisis and patients usually present with right upper quadrant pain, hepatomegaly, and a falling hematocrit [129]. Death may occur, so rapid initiation of exchange transfusion may be a life-saving measure and is a recommended management strategy [125]. Budd–Chairi syndrome may develop from sickling within the hepatic vein with resultant thrombosis [130].

Cholelithiasis is common in patients with sickle cell disease and gallstones may be present in up to 58% of patients [131]. Approximately 18% of patients are found to have choledocholithiasis at the time of cholecystectomy. Distinguishing acute cholecystitis from acute sickle hepatic crisis may be difficult because of similar presentations. Biliary scintigraphy is more useful than ultrasound in such cases to confirm the diagnosis of acute cholecystitis [132]. Therefore, elective cholecystectomy is recommended in patients with sickle cell disease and gallstones, although such elective surgery carries the risk of development of acute chest syndrome (up to 10%) [133]. This syn-

drome is characterized by the presence of new pulmonary infiltrates in a patient with sickle cell disease presenting with chest pain, fever, tachypnea, wheezing, and cough.

Chronic liver disease associated with sickle cell disease is also common. An autopsy series reveal cirrhosis in 16–29% of patients [125]. Chronic liver disease is mostly due to chronic blood transfusion-related iron overload and hepatitis C exposure before 1990 [124]. Reports of sickle cell disease in association with autoimmune liver disease are described in the pediatric literature [134]. Serum ferritin levels are often raised, usually with poor correlation to the degree of hepatic iron overload; Karam et al. [135] recommended liver biopsy in sickle cell patients with high serum ferritin and abnormal liver enzymes to evaluate for fibrosis and other histologic changes.

Endocrinology

Thyroid diseases

The liver is the major site of thyroid hormone metabolism. The conversion of thyroxine (T_4) to tri-iodothyronine (T_3) and reverse T_3 occurs primarily in the liver (85%). In addition, the liver also produces thyroxine-binding globulin, prealbumin, and albumin, the plasma-binding proteins of the thyroid gland. Both hyper- and hypothyroidism can affect the liver in various manners [136].

Hyperthyroidism

It is estimated that most patients with hyperthyroidism will present with one or more abnormalities in liver function tests, including hypoalbuminemia, elevated aspartate/alanine aminotransferases, elevated alkaline phosphatase, or hyperbilirubinemia [136]. Deep jaundice is relatively rare, however it has been reported in patients with thyroid storm [137,138]. Secondary complications such as sepsis, cardiac failure, or intrinsic liver disease must be ruled out in patients with marked jaundice [139].

Even though cardiac output increases in hyperthyroidism, hepatic blood flow remains the same. Hepatic oxygen consumption, however, is increased in patients with hyperthyroidism, resulting in a diminished oxygen supply mainly to the centrizonal area, and rarely leading to necrosis and shock liver [137,139]. Liver histology findings are nonspecific and may be related to heart failure or weight loss associated with hyperthyroidism. Biopsy may show fatty changes, vacuolization of hepatocytes, bile duct proliferation, focal, diffuse, or centrilobular necrosis, and even fibrosis [136].

Antithyroid medications used to treat hyperthyroidism can also cause liver function abnormalities. Methimazole and carbimazole are rare causes of reversible cholestasis [136]. Propylthiouracil is more commonly associated with mild aminotransferase elevations, which typically normalize with dose adjustment. Clinically significant acute liver failure, resulting in death or transplantation, occurs rarely and is usually seen within the first few months of therapy, often in young women [140,141].

Hypothyroidism

Hypothyroidism can also affect liver function, with a reported decreased hepatic oxygen consumption and decreased bile acid production, flow, and excretion [136]. As a result, elevated bilirubin is common in advanced hypothyroidism. As hypothyroidism also affects lipoprotein synthesis, elevated cholesterol and triglycerides are also common. Hypercholesterolemia along with decreased bile flow may result in an increased risk for gallstone formation. Liver biopsy from patients with longstanding hypothyroidism-related hepatic dysfunction reveals central congestive fibrosis and scarring, likely related to right-sided heart failure [139].

Many of the signs and symptoms of hypothyroidism mimic liver disease, including myalgias, fatigue, elevated liver chemistries, encephalopathy from myxedema coma, and myxedema ascites. Two theories for ascites in myxedema have been proposed: (i) it is secondary to right sided heart failure resulting in central venular scarring; or (ii) it is due to increased permeability of the peritoneal membrane to proteins and mucopolysaccharides along with decreased lymphatic drainage, thus yielding a low serum to ascites albumin gradient. Hypothyroidism mimicking acute liver failure in a patient with known cirrhosis has been described [142]. Differentiating clinical hypothyroidism from the encephalopathy of advanced liver disease is crucial because this form of encephalopathy usually resolves with thyroid replacement therapy.

Diabetes mellitus

The notion that diabetes mellitus is an independent risk factor for the development of liver disease, distinguishable from the recognized risk for nonalcoholic fatty liver disease (NAFLD) associated with obesity or metabolic syndrome, is a relatively new concept. Since 2000 there have been a few small studies [143–146] exploring the association between diabetes and liver disease in US populations that suggest a higher prevalence of type 2 diabetes mellitus in patients with cirrhosis. Such epidemiologic studies were, however, potentially biased because patients with cirrhosis have impaired glucose metabolism.

In 2004, El-Serag et al. [147] from the US Department of Veterans Affairs showed that diabetes doubles the risk not only of liver disease, but also of hepatocellular carcinoma. By excluding patients with any prior history of liver disease and by excluding all patients with chronic viral hepatitis and alcoholism, the authors only examined cases wherein the diagnosis of diabetes mellitus clearly preceded the development of liver disease or liver cancer. The report provided strong evidence that diabetes acts independently as a liver disease risk factor, but did not shed light on the underlying mechanisms. In a recent study from Canada that complements the El-Serag report, Porepa et al. [148] examined administrative health databases over the last decade in the province of Ontario and performed a population-based matched cohort study. Similar to previous reports, these investigators found that adults with newly diagnosed diabetes had a significantly greater risk (adjusted hazard ratio, 1.77; 95% CI, 1.68–1.86) of "serious liver disease," as defined by cirrhosis, liver failure, or need for liver transplantation. This so-called "diabetic hepatopathy" suggests causality, but it remains uncertain whether the liver disease associated with diabetes is distinct from that associated with the other manifestations of the metabolic syndrome, which exists in the majority of diabetic patients [149].

Insofar as diabetes as an independent risk for the development of liver neoplasm, Chen et al. [150] from Taiwan confirmed in a population-based study the association of diabetes and liver neoplasm, adding that diabetic patients with clinical risk factors (especially those with viral hepatitis and cirrhosis) are at especially high risk for hepatocellular carcinoma, and should be screened appropriately. Longer duration of diabetes may likewise increase liver cancer risk [151].

Gastroenterology

Celiac disease

Celiac disease (celiac sprue or gluten-sensitive enteropathy), once thought to be a primary gastrointestinal malabsorption syndrome, is now recognized as a multisystem disorder involving skin, bones, heart, nervous system, and liver [152]. The liver involvement in celiac disease has a wide spectrum that ranges from mild aminotransferase elevations (less than five times the upper limit of normal) to severe liver injury [152]. Conversely, celiac disease was reported to be present in 9% of patients with unexplained chronic liver chemistry abnormalities [153]. The mechanism of liver injury is poorly understood, however an increased permeability of the small intestinal mucosa secondary to inflammation and the resultant accumulation of toxins, antigens, and inflammatory substances in the portal circulation may play a role [153]. Liver biopsy typically reveals nonspecific findings such as periportal inflammation, increased Kupffer cells and mononuclear infiltrates in portal triads, steatosis, fibrosis, and/or cirrhosis [152]. Such patients may be misdiagnosed with NAFLD, thus mandating a heightened clinical suspicion for underlying celiac disease. A gluten-free diet resulted in the normalization of so-called "celiac hepatitis" in 75–95% patients, often with a reversal of histologic changes [152].

In addition to liver dysfunction directly attributable to celiac disease, the condition has also been associated with many other liver disorders, such as primary biliary cirrhosis (PBC), autoimmune hepatitis, primary sclerosing cholangitis (PSC), hemochromatosis, NAFLD, cryptogenic cirrhosis, nodular regenerative hyperplasia, and hepatocellular carcinoma [153]. Celiac disease is not common in patients with inflammatory bowel disease (IBD) compared with the general population, but IBD is in fact more prevalent in patients with celiac disease [154,155]. In contrast to the nonspecific hepatitis associated with celiac disease, the disease courses of PBC, PSC, and autoimmune hepatitis are not changed by the initiation of a gluten-free diet [153].

Inflammatory bowel disease

Hepatobiliary involvement is one of the common extraintestinal manifestations of IBD. Navaneethan and Shen [156] categorized such manifestations into three subtypes: (i) diseases from similar pathogenesis (i.e., PSC, small duct PSC, autoimmune hepatitis, and idiopathic acute or chronic pancreatitis); (ii) diseases from IBD-related damages, (i.e., cholelithiasis and portal vein thrombosis); and (iii) diseases resulting from the medications used to treat IBD, such as drug-induced hepatitis, pancreatitis, cirrhosis, reactivation of hepatitis B, and biologic agent associated hepatosplenic lymphoma. Other less common associated disorders are immunoglobulin G4 (IgG4)-associated cholangitis, PBC, fatty liver, granulomatous hepatitis, and amyloidosis [156]. PSC is the most common

hepatobiliary manifestation associated with IBD, and is discussed in detail elsewhere in this text (Chapter 20).

The prevalence of abnormal liver biochemistries varies from 3% to 50% in patients with IBD [157]. Such abnormalities persist even after colectomy and ileal pouch–anal anastomosis, albeit to a lesser degree, and could be related to coexisting liver disease [157]. Gisbert et al. [158] reported the prevalence of abnormal liver function tests at 20% in their 786 IBD patients, wherein use of azathioprine/6-mercaptopurine and fatty liver were the most common explanations (42.3% and 40.8%, respectively). At least seven cases of hepatocellular carcinoma arising in patients with Crohn disease – without associated viral hepatitis and/or cirrhosis – have been described to date, predominantly among those with early-onset IBD [159].

Rheumatology

Most rheumatologic diseases affect the liver, and various medications used to treat such diseases are potentially hepatotoxic. Distinguishing drug-induced liver disease from liver disease associated with the underlying systemic rheumatic disease may be difficult.

Systemic lupus erythematosus

Liver involvement in patients with systemic lupus erythematosus (SLE) is common, with a spectrum of clinical and biochemical derangements, such as hepatomegaly, splenomegaly, and jaundice [160,161]. Kaw et al. [162] differentiated SLE-associated hepatitis from autoimmune hepatitis (Table 9.2) [162]. Such differentiation is

Table 9.2 Systemic lupus erythematosus hepatitis versus autoimmune hepatitis (AIH).

	Systemic lupus erythematosus hepatitis	Autoimmune hepatitis
Histology	Lobular, rarely periportal	Periportal, piecemeal necrosis
ACR criteria	100%	20%
Hypergammaglobulinemia	Common	Common, IgG elevated
ANA positivity	>99%	80% in type 1 AIH
SMA	30%	60–80%
Serology		
Anti-dsDNA ELISA	Positive	34–64%
Anti-LSP antibody	Negative	Often present
Anti-LKM-1	Negative	Present in type 2 AIH
Response to steroids	Favorable	Favorable

ACR, American College of Rheumatology; ANA, antinuclear antibody; dsDNA, double-stranded deoxyribonucleic antibody lipoprotein; ELISA, enzyme-linked immunoadsorbent assay; LKM, liver kidney microsome; LSP, liver-specific lipoprotein; SMA, smooth muscle antibody.
Reproduced from Kaw et al. [162] with permission from Springer.

important, as autoimmune hepatitis has a more aggressive histologic pattern, low survival without treatment, and increased progression to advanced liver disease as compared with SLE-associated hepatitis. This finding is further corroborated by a recent retrospective review showing favorable liver disease-free survival at 5 years in patients with lupus-associated hepatitis [163].

Nodular regenerative hyperplasia, granulomatous hepatitis, idiopathic portal hypertension, features of PBC, Budd–Chiari syndrome, and hepatic infarction have all been reported in association with SLE [164]. Hemophagocytic syndrome (systemic proliferation of hemophagocytic cells), clinically manifested as fever, cytopenias, lymphadenopathy, and liver dysfunction, may occur in up to 10% of patients with SLE [165].

Treatment of the underlying SLE or cessation of offending medications usually leads to improvement in the biochemical and histologic liver markers [166]. Corticosteroid treatment also improves biochemical abnormalities [161]. Aspirin use may contribute to the abnormal biochemical parameters and is a well-described reversible cause of liver involvement in patients with SLE [166].

Rheumatoid arthritis and Felty syndrome

Abnormal liver biochemistries may occur in anywhere between 6% and 50% of patients with rheumatoid arthritis [164,166,167], but a raised alkaline phosphatase level of bone origin may often be the explanation. Liver biopsy findings are nonspecific [167]. Nodular regenerative hyperplasia may accompany rheumatoid arthritis or Felty syndrome [167]. Felty syndrome is characterized by rheumatoid arthritis in the setting of leukopenia and splenomegaly, often with abnormal liver function tests. This form of noncirrhotic portal hypertension is discussed elsewhere (Chapter 14).

Medications used in the treatment of rheumatoid arthritis, such as methotrexate, gold salts, diclofenac sodium, and immune-modulating agents, have potential drug hepatotoxicity. A case of primary hepatic lymphoma was reported in a 70-year-old male with difficult to control rheumatoid arthritis presenting with elevated liver tests and multiple hypoechoic lesions on liver ultrasound [168].

Sjögren syndrome

The most common liver disease associated with primary Sjögren syndrome (keratoconjunctivitis sicca) is primary biliary cirrhosis in the setting of positive antimitochondrial antibody (AMA) (6.6% of 300 patients with Sjögren syndrome [169]). Patients with primary Sjögren syndrome and abnormal liver tests should undergo AMA testing [164,167]. An association between hepatitis C virus (HCV) infection and Sjögren syndrome is thought to be related to sialotropic properties of HCV and is associated with lymphocytic sialadenitis [164]. In one recent series from Israel, Sjögren syndrome was proved to be the cause of a previously deemed idiopathic granulomatous hepatitis [170].

Scleroderma

Scleroderma is a chronic systemic disease characterized by tissue fibrosis and small vessel vasculopathy. The disease can present as part of the CREST (calcinosis, Raynaud phenomenon, esophageal dysfunction, and sclerodactyly, telangiectasia) syndrome or in a diffuse (systemic scleroderma) form. Although rare, liver involvement has long been described in scleroderma patients, usually in the form of PBC [164]. A positive AMA may be present in >25% of patients with scleroderma; similarly, the anticentromere antibody (a specific antibody of the CREST syndrome) may be positive in approximately 25% of patients with PBC [164]. Powell et al. [171] coined the acronym PACK to describe the association between PBC, anticentromere antibody positivity, CREST syndrome, and keratoconjunctivitis sicca. AMA testing is a sensitive marker for the detection of PBC in patients with scleroderma [172].

Adult Still disease

Adult Still disease (fever, rash, seronegative polyarthritis, lymphadenopathy, and splenomegaly) may involve the liver (hepatomegaly or raised liver enzymes) in up to half of affected individuals [162]. Elevated serum aminotransferase levels occur in up to 92% of patients, and increased serum alkaline phosphatase and bilirubin levels have been described in up to 65% of patients. All biochemical abnormalities resolve either spontaneously or with the treatment of the underlying Still disease. Rare cases of acute liver failure, with death or requiring liver transplantation, have been described [173,174].

Polyarteritis nodosa

Polyarteritis nodosa (PAN) is a focal, segmental, necrotizing vasculitis primarily involving medium-sized arteries. It has been classically associated in hepatitis B virus (HBV) infection, with hepatitis B surface antigen (HBsAg) positivity in about 7% of cases [175]. Anecdotal reports associating chronic HCV infection with PAN are noted, but HCV is primarily associated with mixed cryoglobulinemia [176]. Mild biochemical abnormalities may be noted in 16–55% of patients with PAN, but advanced liver disease is rare [175]. PAN manifesting as acute gastrointestinal hemorrhage in a post-transplant patient has been reported [177]. Liver biopsy in patients with PAN rarely reveals the characteristic lymphocytic infiltration of the intima and media of the hepatic arteries [175] – a finding that can be observed on autopsy specimens (Fig. 9.13). Treatment of HBV-associated PAN

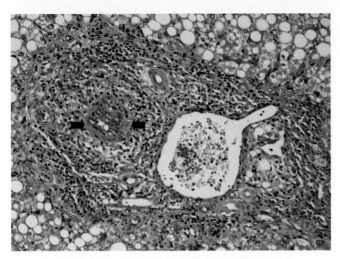

Figure 9.13 Liver biopsy specimen from a patient with hepatic involvement in polyarteritis nodosa revealing a lymphocytic infiltrate in the intima and media of the hepatic artery (arrows). H&E. (Courtesy of Dr John Hart.)

consists of a short course of corticosteroids to decrease the inflammation, along with an oral antiviral agent for HBV treatment [176].

Further reading

Abraham S, Begum S, Isenberg D. Hepatic manifestations of autoimmune rheumatic diseases. *Ann Rheum Dis* 2004;63:123–9.
A comprehensive review of the liver involvement in lupus, rheumatoid arthritis, Sjögren, scleroderma, Felty, and other autoimmune diseases.

Akritidis N, Tzivras M, Delladetsima I, Stefanaki S, Moutsopoulos HM, Pappas G. The liver in brucellosis. *Clin Gastroenterol Hepatol* 2007;5:1109–12.
A topical summary from Greece of the clinical and histopathologic findings in the liver in 14 cases of human brucellosis, with a review of the world literature. The report confirms the universal finding of hepatic granuloma formation in this entity.

Alvarez SZ. Hepatobiliary tuberculosis. *J Gastroenterol Hepatol* 1998;13: 833–9.
Succinct review of the current approach to the classification, clinical spectrum, modern diagnostic techniques, and options in the management of hepatobiliary tuberculosis.

Bhat YM, Krasinskas A, Craig FE, Shaw-Stiffel TA. Acute liver failure as an initial manifestation of an infiltrative hematolymphoid malignancy. *Dig Dis Sci* 2006;51:63–7.
An up-to-date review of lymphoma presenting as acute hepatic failure.

Ebert EC, Nagar M, Hagspiel KD. Gastrointestinal and hepatic complications of sickle cell disease. *Clin Gastroenterol Hepatol* 2010;8(6): 483–9.
Comprehensive discussion outlining the various gastrointestinal and hepatobiliary manifestations of sickle cell disease.

El-Newihi HM, Alamy ME, Reynolds TB. Salmonella hepatitis: analysis of 27 cases and comparison with acute viral hepatitis. *Hepatology* 1996;24:516–19.
This landmark paper from a US medical center summarizes the clinical manifestations and relevance of salmonella (typhoid) hepatitis.

Kauppinen R. Porphyrias. *Lancet* 2005;365:241–52.
Scholarly review of the pathophysiology, clinical manifestations, diagnosis, management, and screening recommendations of the various porphyrias.

Moseley RH. Sepsis and cholestasis. *Clin Liver Dis* 2004;8:83–94.
Comprehensive overview of the pathophysiology of intrahepatic cholestasis in sepsis.

Navaneethan U, Shen B. Hepatopancreatobiliary manifestations and complications associated with inflammatory bowel disease. *Inflamm Bowel Dis* 2010;16:1598–619.
A recent review of the pathogenesis and management recommendations for liver, biliary, and pancreatic disease associated with inflammatory bowel disease.

Robenshtok E, Gafter-Gvili A, Goldberg E, et al. Antifungal prophylaxis in cancer patients after chemotherapy or hematopoietic stem-cell transplantation: systematic review and meta-analysis. *J Clin Oncol* 2007;25:5471–89.
This meta-analysis confirms the reduction in mortality resulting from the antifungal prophylaxis of patients undergoing chemotherapy or bone marrow transplantation.

Rubio-Tapia A, Murray JA. The liver in celiac disease. *Hepatology* 2007; 46:1650–8.
A discussion of the pathogenesis and spectrum of liver involvement in patients with celiac disease and management guidelines for patients with advanced liver disease and celiac disease.

Youssef WI, Mullen KD. The liver in other (nondiabetic) endocrine disorders. *Clin Liver Dis* 2002;6:879–89.
Thorough review of the hepatic manifestations of thyroid and other nondiabetic endocrine disorders.

Zaidi SA, Singer C. Gastrointestinal and hepatic manifestations of tickborne diseases in the United States. *Clin Infect Dis* 2002;34: 1206–12.
A practical review of the hepatic manifestations of tick-borne disorders including Lyme disease.

References

1. Bernstein J, Brown AK. Sepsis and jaundice in early infancy. *Pediatrics* 1962;29:873.
2. Zimmerman HJ, Fang M, Utili R, Seeff LB, Hoofnagle J. Jaundice due to bacterial infection. *Gastroenterology* 1979;77:362–74.
3. Moseley RH. Sepsis and cholestasis. *Clin Liver Dis* 2004;8:83–94.
4. Latham PS, Menkes E, Phillips MJ, Jeejeebhoy KN. Hyperalimentation-associated jaundice: an example of a serum factor inducing cholestasis in rats. *Am J Clin Nutr* 1985;41:61–5.
5. Bolder U, Ton-Nu HT, Schteingart CD, Frick E, Hofmann AF. Hepatocyte transport of bile acids and organic anions in endotoxemic rats: impaired uptake and secretion. *Gastroenterology* 1997;112:214–25.
6. Crump JA, Luby SP, Mintz ED. The global burden of typhoid fever. *Bull World Health Organ* 2004;82:346–53.
7. Morgenstern R, Hayes PC. The liver in typhoid fever: always affected, not just a complication. *Am J Gastroenterol* 1991;86:1235–9.
8. Pramoolsinsap C, Viranuvatti V. Salmonella hepatitis. *J Gastroenterol Hepatol* 1998;13:745–50.
9. El-Newihi HM, Alamy ME, Reynolds TB. Salmonella hepatitis: analysis of 27 cases and comparison with acute viral hepatitis. *Hepatology* 1996;24:516–19.
10. Chou YP, Changchien CS, Chiu KW, Kuo CM, Kuo FY, Kuo CH. Salmonellosis with liver abscess mimicking hepatocellular carcinoma in a diabetic and cirrhotic patient: a case report and review of the literature. *Liver Int* 2006;26:498–501.
11. Khan FY, Elouzi EB, Asif M. Acute acalculous cholecystitis complicating typhoid fever in an adult patient: a case report and review of the literature. *Travel Med Infect Dis* 2009;7:203–6.
12. Khan FY, Kamha AA, Alomary IY. Fulminant hepatic failure caused by *Salmonella paratyphi* A infection. *World J Gastroenterol* 2006;12:5253–5.

13. Lopez-Arce G, Torre-Delgadillo A, Tellez-Avila FI. *Salmonella* sp group A: a rare cause of bacterascites. A case report. *Ann Hepatol* 2008;7:260–1.

14. Bhutta ZA. Current concepts in the diagnosis and treatment of typhoid fever. *Br Med J* 2006;333:78–82.

15. Khosla SN, Singh R, Singh GP, Trehan VK. The spectrum of hepatic injury in enteric fever. *Am J Gastroenterol* 1988;83:413–16.

16. Alvarez SZ. Hepatobiliary tuberculosis. *J Gastroenterol Hepatol* 1998;13:833–9.

17. Chong VH. Hepatobiliary tuberculosis: a review of presentations and outcomes. *South Med J* 2008;101:356–61.

18. Alvarez SZ, Carpio R. Hepatobiliary tuberculosis. *Dig Dis Sci* 1983;28:193–200.

19. Evans RH, Evans M, Harrison NK, Price DE, Freedman AR. Massive hepatosplenomegaly, jaundice and pancytopenia in miliary tuberculosis. *J Infect* 1998;36:236–9.

20. Kushihata S, Yorioka N, Nishida Y, et al. Fatal hepatic failure caused by miliary tuberculosis in a hemodialysis patient: case report. *Int J Artif Organs* 1998;21:23–5.

21. Abascal J, Martin F, Abreu L, et al. Atypical hepatic tuberculosis presenting as obstructive jaundice. *Am J Gastroenterol* 1988;83:1183–6.

22. Huang WT, Wang CC, Chen WJ, Cheng YF, Eng HL. The nodular form of hepatic tuberculosis: a review with five additional new cases. *J Clin Pathol* 2003;56:835–9.

23. Koksal D, Koksal AS, Koklu S, Cicek B, Altiparmak E, Sahin B. Primary tuberculous liver abscess: a case report and review of the literature. *South Med J* 2006;99:393–5.

24. Jazet IM, Perk L, De Roos A, Bolk JH, Arend SM. Obstructive jaundice and hematemesis: two cases with unusual presentations of intra-abdominal tuberculosis. *Eur J Intern Med* 2004;15:259–61.

25. Chen CH, Yang CC, Yeh YH, Yang JC, Chou DA. Pancreatic tuberculosis with obstructive jaundice – a case report. *Am J Gastroenterol* 1999;94:2534–6.

26. Abu-Zidan FM, Zayat I. Gallbladder tuberculosis (case report and review of the literature). *Hepatogastroenterology* 1999;46:2804–6.

27. Kok KY, Yapp SK. Tuberculosis of the bile duct: a rare cause of obstructive jaundice. *J Clin Gastroenterol* 1999;29:161–4.

28. Inal M, Aksungur E, Akgul E, Demirbas O, Oguz M, Erkocak E. Biliary tuberculosis mimicking cholangiocarcinoma: treatment with metallic biliary endoprothesis. *Am J Gastroenterol* 2000;95:1069–71.

29. Akcan Y, Tuncer S, Hayran M, Sungur A, Unal S. PCR on disseminated tuberculosis in bone marrow and liver biopsy specimens: correlation to histopathological and clinical diagnosis. *Scand J Infect Dis* 1997;29:271–4.

30. Alcantara-Payawal DE, Matsumura M, Shiratori Y, et al. Direct detection of *Mycobacterium* tuberculosis using polymerase chain reaction assay among patients with hepatic granuloma. *J Hepatol* 1997;27:620–7.

31. Saukkonen JJ, Cohn DL, Jasmer RM, et al. An official ATS statement: hepatotoxicity of antituberculosis therapy. *Am J Respir Crit Care Med* 2006;174:935–52.

32. Mofredj A, Bahloul H, Mrabet A, Gineyt G, Rousselier P. Fulminant hepatitis during *Legionella* pneumophila infection. *Infect Dis Clin Prac* 2009;17:333.

33. Akritidis N, Tzivras M, Delladetsima I, Stefanaki S, Moutsopoulos HM, Pappas G. The liver in brucellosis. *Clin Gastroenterol Hepatol* 2007;5:1109–12.

34. Erdem I, Cicekler N, Mert D, Yucesoy-Dede B, Ozyurek S, Goktas P. A case report of acute hepatitis due to brucellosis. *Int J Infect Dis* 2005;9:349–50.

35. Gursoy S, Baskol M, Ozbakir O, Guven K, Patiroglu T, Yucesoy M. Spontaneous bacterial peritonitis due to *Brucella* infection. *Turk J Gastroenterol* 2003;14:145–7.

36. Pramateftakis MG, Kanellos D, Kanellos I. Percutaneous drainage of hepatic brucelloma. *Am Surg* 2009;75:1143–4.

37. Carazo ER, Parra FM, Villares MPJ, del García MMC, Calvente SLM, Benitez AM. Hepatosplenic brucelloma: clinical presentation and imaging features in six cases. *Abdom Imaging* 2005;30:291–6.

38. Pappas G, Akritidis N, Bosilkovski M, Tsianos E. Brucellosis. *N Engl J Med* 2005;352:2325–36.

39. Zaidi SA, Singer C. Gastrointestinal and hepatic manifestations of tickborne diseases in the United States. *Clin Infect Dis* 2002;34:1206–12.

40. Guillet C, Join-Lambert O, Le Monnier A, et al. Human listeriosis caused by *Listeria ivanovii*. *Emerg Infect Dis* 2010;16:136–8.

41. Scholing M, Schneeberger PM, van den Dries P, Drenth JP. Clinical features of liver involvement in adult patients with listeriosis. Review of the literature. *Infection* 2007;35:212–18.

42. Lim KS, Chong VH. Radiological manifestations of melioidosis. *Clin Radiol* 2010;65:66–72.

43. White NJ. Melioidosis. *Lancet* 2003;361:1715–22.

44. Gordon SC, Watts JC, Veneri RJ, Chandler FW. Focal hepatic candidiasis with perihepatic adhesions: laparoscopic and immunohistologic diagnosis. *Gastroenterology* 1990;98:214–17.

45. Chung HC, Teng LJ, Hsueh PR. Liver abscess due to *Neisseria sicca* after repeated transcatheter arterial embolization. *J Med Microbiol* 2007;56:1561–2.

46. Peter NG, Clark LR, Jaeger JR. Fitz-Hugh–Curtis syndrome: a diagnosis to consider in women with right upper quadrant pain. *Cleve Clin J Med* 2004;71:233–9.

47. Risser WL, Risser JM, Benjamins LJ, Feldmann JM. Incidence of Fitz-Hugh–Curtis syndrome in adolescents who have pelvic inflammatory disease. *J Pediatr Adolesc Gynecol* 2007;20:179–80.

48. Oh SN, Rha SE, Byun JY, Kim JY, Song KY, Park CH. Chilaiditi syndrome caused by Fitz-Hugh–Curtis syndrome: multidetector CT findings. *Abdom Imaging* 2006;31:45–7.

49. Tajiri T, Tate G, Iwaku T, et al. Right pleural effusion in Fitz-Hugh–Curtis syndrome. *Acta Med Okayama* 2006;60:289–94.

50. Abdulkarim AS, Petrovic LM, Kim WR, Angulo P, Lloyd RV, Lindor KD. Primary biliary cirrhosis: an infectious disease caused by *Chlamydia pneumoniae*? *J Hepatol* 2004;40:380–4.

51. Wetsch NM, Somani K, Tyrrell GJ, Gebhart C, Bailey RJ, Taylor DE. *Campylobacter curvus*-associated hepatic abscesses: a case report. *J Clin Microbiol* 2006;44:1909–11.

52. Verbruggen P, Creve U, Hubens A, Hubens A, Verhaegen J. *Campylobacter fetus* as a cause of acute cholecystitis. *Br J Surg* 1986;73:46.

53. Agan BK, Dolan MJ. Laboratory diagnosis of *Bartonella* infections. *Clin Lab Med* 2002;22:937–62.

54. Bass JW, Freitas BC, Freitas AD, et al. Prospective randomized double blind placebo-controlled evaluation of azithromycin for treatment of cat-scratch disease. *Pediatr Infect Dis J* 1998;17:447–52.

55. Liston TE, Koehler JE. Granulomatous hepatitis and necrotizing splenitis due to *Bartonella henselae* in a patient with cancer: case report and review of hepatosplenic manifestations of bartonella infection. *Clin Infect Dis* 1996;22:951–7.

56. Thudi KR, Kreikemeier JT, Phillips NJ, Salvalaggio PR, Kennedy DJ, Hayashi PH. Cat scratch disease causing hepatic masses after liver transplant. *Liver Int* 2007;27:145–8.

57. Gerasymchuk L, Swami A, Carpenter CF, et al. Case of fulminant leptospirosis in a renal transplant patient. *Transpl Infect Dis* 2009;11:454–7.

58. Covic A, Maftei ID, Gusbeth-Tatomir P. Acute liver failure due to leptospirosis successfully treated with MARS (molecular adsorbent recirculating system) dialysis. *Int Urol Nephrol* 2007;39:313–16.

59. Gaspari R, Annetta MG, Cavaliere F, et al. Unusual presentation of leptospirosis in the late stage of pregnancy. *Minerva Anestesiol* 2007;73:429–32.

60. Granito A, Ballardini G, Fusconi M, et al. A case of leptospirosis simulating colon cancer with liver metastases. *World J Gastroenterol* 2004;10:2455–6.

61. Brett-Major DM, Lipnick RJ. Antibiotic prophylaxis for leptospirosis. *Cochrane Database Syst Rev* 2009;3:CD007342.

62. Crum-Cianflone N, Weekes J, Bavaro M. Syphilitic hepatitis among HIV-infected patients. *Int J STD AIDS* 2009;20:278.

63. Chen JF, Chen WX, Zhang HY, Zhang WY. Peliosis and gummatous syphilis of the liver: a case report. *World J Gastroenterol* 2008;14:1961–3.

64. Horowitz HW, Dworkin B, Forseter G, et al. Liver function in early Lyme disease. *Hepatology* 1996;23:1412–17.

65. Goellner MH, Agger WA, Burgess JH, Duray PH. Hepatitis due to recurrent Lyme disease. *Ann Intern Med* 1988;108:707–8.

66. Zanchi AC, Gingold AR, Theise ND, Min AD. Necrotizing granulomatous hepatitis as an unusual manifestation of Lyme disease. *Dig Dis Sci* 2007;52:2629–32.

67. Tissot-Dupont H, Raoult D. Q fever. *Infect Dis Clin North Am* 2008;22:505–14, ix.

68. Chang K, Lee NY, Chen YH, et al. Acute Q fever in southern Taiwan: atypical manifestations of hyperbilirubinemia and prolonged fever. *Diagn Microbiol Infect Dis* 2008;60:211–16.

69. Marrie TJ, Raoult D. Q fever – a review and issues for the next century. *Int J Antimicrob Agents* 1997;8:145–61.

70. Fournier PE, Raoult D. Comparison of PCR and serology assays for early diagnosis of acute Q fever. *J Clin Microbiol* 2003;41:5094–8.

71. Gidding HF, Wallace C, Lawrence GL, McIntyre PB. Australia's national Q fever vaccination program. *Vaccine* 2009;27:2037–41.

72. Fishbein DB, Dawson JE, Robinson LE. Human ehrlichiosis in the United States, 1985 to 1990. *Ann Intern Med* 1994;120:736–43.

73. Nutt AK, Kauffman J. Gastrointestinal and hepatic manifestations of human ehrlichiosis: 8 cases and a review of the literature. *Dig Dis* 1999;17:37–43.

74. Sehdev AE, Dumler JS. Hepatic pathology in human monocytic ehrlichiosis. *Ehrlichia chaffeensis* infection. *Am J Clin Pathol* 2003;119:859.

75. Olano JP, Walker DH. Human ehrlichioses. *Med Clin North Am* 2002;86:375–92.

76. Assi MA, Sandid MS, Baddour LM, Roberts GD, Walker RC. Systemic histoplasmosis: a 15 year retrospective institutional review of 111 patients. *Medicine (Baltimore)* 2007;86:162–9.

77. Martin RC 2nd, Edwards MJ, McMasters KM. Histoplasmosis as an isolated liver lesion: review and surgical therapy. *Am Surg* 2001;67:430–1.

78. Mazhari NJ, Sakhuja P, Malhotra V, Gondal R, Puri J. Histoplasmosis of the liver: a rare case. *Trop Gastroenterol* 2002;23:90–1.

79. Lamps LW, Molina CP, West AB, Haggitt RC, Scott MA. The pathologic spectrum of gastrointestinal and hepatic histoplasmosis. *Am J Clin Pathol* 2000;113:64–72.

80. Kauffman CA. Histoplasmosis. *Clin Chest Med* 2009;30:217–25, v.

81. Kontoyiannis DP, Luna MA, Samuels BI, Bodey GP. Hepatosplenic candidiasis. A manifestation of chronic disseminated candidiasis. *Infect Dis Clin North Am* 2000;14:721–39.

82. Robenshtok E, Gafter-Gvili A, Goldberg E, et al. Antifungal prophylaxis in cancer patients after chemotherapy or hematopoietic stem-cell transplantation: systematic review and meta-analysis. *J Clin Oncol* 2007;25:5471–89.

83. Cole GT, Halawa AA, Anaissie EJ. The role of the gastrointestinal tract in hematogenous candidiasis: from the laboratory to the bedside. *Clin Infect Dis* 1996;22(Suppl 2):S73–88.

84. Pastakia B, Shawker TH, Thaler M, O'Leary T, Pizzo PA. Hepatosplenic candidiasis: wheels within wheels. *Radiology* 1988;166:417–21.

85. Domagk D, Bisping G, Poremba C, Fegeler W, Domschke W, Menzel J. Common bile duct obstruction due to candidiasis. *Scand J Gastroenterol* 2001;36:444–6.

86. Kirby A, Chapman C, Hassan C, Burnie J. The diagnosis of hepatosplenic candidiasis by DNA analysis of tissue biopsy and serum. *J Clin Pathol* 2004;57:764–5.

87. Pappas PG, Rex JH, Sobel JD, et al. Guidelines for treatment of candidiasis. *Clin Infect Dis* 2004;38:161–89.

88. De Rosa FG, Garazzino S, Pasero D, Di Perri G, Ranieri VM. Invasive candidiasis and candidemia: new guidelines. *Minerva Anestesiol* 2009;75:453–8.

89. Brook I. Actinomycosis: diagnosis and management. *South Med J* 2008;101:1019–23.

90. Kanellopoulou T, Alexopoulou A, Tanouli MI, et al. Primary hepatic actinomycosis. *Am J Med Sci* 2010;339:362–5.

91. Ramirez FC, Walker GJ, Sanowski RA, Manne RK, Stone HH. Obstructive jaundice due to *Coccidioides immitis*. *Gastrointest Endosc* 1996;43:505–7.

92. Blair JE, Douglas DD. Coccidioidomycosis in liver transplant recipients relocating to an endemic area. *Dig Dis Sci* 2004;49:1981–5.

93. Blair JE, Balan V, Douglas DD, Hentz JG. Incidence and prevalence of coccidioidomycosis in patients with end-stage liver disease. *Liver Transpl* 2003;9:843–50.

94. Blair JE, Kusne S, Carey EJ, Heilman RL. The prevention of recrudescent coccidioidomycosis after solid organ transplantation. *Transplantation* 2007;83:1182–7.

95. Kauppinen R. Porphyrias. *Lancet* 2005;365:241–52.

96. Chemmanur AT, Bonkovsky HL. Hepatic porphyrias: diagnosis and management. *Clin Liver Dis* 2004;8:807–38, viii.

97. Kauppinen R, Mustajoki P. Prognosis of acute porphyria: occurrence of acute attacks, precipitating factors, and associated diseases. *Medicine (Baltimore)* 1992;71:1–13.

98. Mustajoki P, Nordmann Y. Early administration of heme arginate for acute porphyric attacks. *Arch Intern Med* 1993;153.2004–8.

99. Dar FS, Asai K, Haque AR, Cherian T, Rela M, Heaton N. Liver transplantation for acute intermittent porphyria: a viable treatment? *Hepatobiliary Pancreat Dis Int* 2010;9.93–6.

100. Soonawalla ZF, Orug T, Badminton MN, et al. Liver transplantation as a cure for acute intermittent porphyria. *Lancet* 2004;363:705–6.

101. Seth AK, Badminton MN, Mirza D, Russell S, Elias E. Liver transplantation for porphyria: who, when, and how? *Liver Transpl* 2007;13:1219–27.

102. Palmieri C, Vigushin DM, Peters TJ. Managing malignant disease in patients with porphyria. *Q J Med* 2004;97:115–26.

103. Murphy GM. The cutaneous porphyrias: a review. The British Photodermatology Group. *Br J Dermatol* 1999;140:573–81.

104. Gisbert JP, Garcia-Buey L, Alonso A, et al. Hepatocellular carcinoma risk in patients with porphyria cutanea tarda. *Eur J Gastroenterol Hepatol* 2004;16:689–92.

105. Lefkowitch JH, Grossman ME. Hepatic pathology in porphyria cutanea tarda. *Liver* 1983;3:19–29.

106. Sarkany RP. The management of porphyria cutanea tarda. *Clin Exp Dermatol* 2001;26:225–32.

107. Murphy GM. Diagnosis and management of the erythropoietic porphyrias. *Dermatol Ther* 2003;16:57–64.

108. Bloomer JR, Phillips MJ, Davidson DL, Klatskin G, Bloomer. Hepatic disease in erythropoietic protoporphyria. *Am J Med* 1975;58:869–82.

109. Wahlin S, Aschan J, Bjornstedt M, Broome U, Harper P. Curative bone marrow transplantation in erythropoietic protoporphyria after reversal of severe cholestasis. *J Hepatol* 2007;46:174–9.

110. McGuire BM, Bonkovsky HL, Carithers RL Jr, et al. Liver transplantation for erythropoietic protoporphyria liver disease. *Liver Transpl* 2005;11:1590–6.

111. Rand EB, Bunin N, Cochran W, Ruchelli E, Olthoff KM, Bloomer JR. Sequential liver and bone marrow transplantation for treatment of erythropoietic protoporphyria. *Pediatrics* 2006;118:e1896–9.

112. Thompson DR, Faust TW, Stone MJ, Polter DE. Hepatic failure as the presenting manifestation of malignant lymphoma. *Clin Lymphoma* 2001;2:123–8.

113. Birrer MJ, Young RC. Differential diagnosis of jaundice in lymphoma patients. *Semin Liver Dis* 1987;7:269–77.

114. Pass AK, McLin VA, Rushton JR, Kearney DL, Hastings CA, Margolin JF. Vanishing bile duct syndrome and Hodgkin disease: a case series and review of the literature. *J Pediatr Hematol Oncol* 2008;30:976–80.

115. Brinckmeyer LM, Skovsgaard T, Thiede T, Vesterager L, Nissen NI. The liver in Hodgkin's disease – I. Clinico-pathological relations. *Eur J Cancer Clin Oncol* 1982;18:421–8.

116. Kleger A, Bommer M, Kunze M, et al. First reported case of disease: peliosis hepatis as cardinal symptom of Hodgkin's lymphoma. *Oncologist* 2009;14:1088–94.

117. Cervantes F, Briones J, Bruguera M, et al. Hodgkin's disease presenting as a cholestatic febrile illness: incidence and main characteristics in a series of 421 patients. *Ann Hematol* 1996;72:357–60.

118. Santos ES, Raez LE, Salvatierra J, Morgenszten D, Shanmugan N, Neff GW. Primary hepatic non-Hodgkin's lymphomas: case report and review of the literature. *Am J Gastroenterol* 2003;98:2789–93.

119. Cameron AM, Truty J, Truell J, et al. Fulminant hepatic failure from primary hepatic lymphoma: successful treatment with orthotopic liver transplantation and chemotherapy. *Transplantation* 2005;80:993–6.

120. Mattar WE, Alex BK, Sherker AH. Primary hepatic Burkitt lymphoma presenting with acute liver failure. *J Gastrointest Cancer* 2010;41:261–3.

121. Rowbotham D, Wendon J, Williams R. Acute liver failure secondary to hepatic infiltration: a single centre experience of 18 cases. *Gut* 1998;42:576–80.

122. Bhat YM, Krasinskas A, Craig FE, Shaw-Stiffel TA. Acute liver failure as an initial manifestation of an infiltrative hematolymphoid malignancy. *Dig Dis Sci* 2006;51:63–7.

123. Lettieri CJ, Berg BW. Clinical features of non-Hodgkins lymphoma presenting with acute liver failure: a report of five cases and review of published experience. *Am J Gastroenterol* 2003;98:1641–6.

124. Ebert EC, Nagar M, Hagspiel KD. Gastrointestinal and hepatic complications of sickle cell disease. *Clin Gastroenterol Hepatol* 2010;8(6):483–9.

125. Banerjee S, Owen C, Chopra S. Sickle cell hepatopathy. *Hepatology* 2001;33:1021–8.

126. Kotila T, Adedapo K, Adedapo A, Oluwasola O, Fakunle E, Brown B. Liver dysfunction in steady state sickle cell disease. *Ann Hepatol* 2005;4:261–3.

127. Stephan JL, Merpit-Gonon E, Richard O, Raynaud-Ravni C, Freycon F. Fulminant liver failure in a 12-year-old girl with sickle cell anaemia: favourable outcome after exchange transfusions. *Eur J Pediatr* 1995;154:469–71.

128. Mekeel KL, Langham MR Jr, Gonzalez-Peralta R, Fujita S, Hemming AW. Liver transplantation in children with sickle-cell disease. *Liver Transpl* 2007;13:505–8.

129. Hatton CS, Bunch C, Weatherall DJ. Hepatic sequestration in sickle cell anaemia. *Br Med J (Clin Res Ed)* 1985;290:744–5.

130. Sty JR. Ultrasonography: hepatic vein thrombosis in sickle cell anemia. *Am J Pediatr Hematol Oncol* 1982;4:213–15.

131. Bond LR, Hatty SR, Horn ME, Dick M, Meire HB, Bellingham AJ. Gall stones in sickle cell disease in the United Kingdom. *Br Med J (Clin Res Ed)* 1987;295:234–6.

132. D'Alonzo WA Jr, Heyman S. Biliary scintigraphy in children with sickle cell anemia and acute abdominal pain. *Pediatr Radiol* 1985;15:395–8.

133. Vichinsky EP, Haberkern CM, Neumayr L, et al. A comparison of conservative and aggressive transfusion regimens in the perioperative management of sickle cell disease. The Preoperative Transfusion in Sickle Cell Disease Study Group. *N Engl J Med* 1995;333:206–13.

134. Lykavieris P, Benichou JJ, Benkerrou M, Feriot JP, Bernard O, Debray D. Autoimmune liver disease in three children with sickle cell disease. *J Pediatr Gastroenterol Nutr* 2006;42:104–8.

135. Karam LB, Disco D, Jackson SM, et al. Liver biopsy results in patients with sickle cell disease on chronic transfusions: poor correlation with ferritin levels. *Pediatr Blood Cancer* 2008;50:62–5.

136. Youssef WI, Mullen KD. The liver in other (nondiabetic) endocrine disorders. *Clin Liver Dis* 2002;6:879–89, vii.

137. Choudhary AM, Roberts I. Thyroid storm presenting with liver failure. *J Clin Gastroenterol* 1999;29:318–21.

138. Soysal D, Tatar E, Solmaz S, et al. A case of severe cholestatic jaundice associated with Graves disease. *Turk J Gastroenterol* 2008;19:77–9.

139. Malik R, Hodgson H. The relationship between the thyroid gland and the liver. *Q J Med* 2002;95:559–69.

140. Primeggia J, Lewis JH. Gone (from the Physicians' desk reference) but not forgotten: propylthiouracil-associated hepatic failure: a call for liver test monitoring. *J Natl Med Assoc* 2010;102:531–4.

141. Testa G, Trevino J, Bogetti D, et al. Liver transplantation for propylthiouracil-induced acute hepatic failure. *Dig Dis Sci* 2003;48:190–1.

142. Khairy RN, Mullen KD. Hypothyroidism as a mimic of liver failure in a patient with cirrhosis. *Ann Intern Med* 2007;146:315–16.

143. Amarapurkar D, Das HS. Chronic liver disease in diabetes mellitus. *Trop Gastroenterol* 2002;23:3–5.

144. El-Serag HB, Richardson PA, Everhart JE. The role of diabetes in hepatocellular carcinoma: a case–control study among United States Veterans. *Am J Gastroenterol* 2001;96:2462–7.

145. Hassan MM, Hwang LY, Hatten CJ, et al. Risk factors for hepatocellular carcinoma: synergism of alcohol with viral hepatitis and diabetes mellitus. *Hepatology* 2002;36:1206–13.

146. Poonawala A, Nair SP, Thuluvath PJ. Prevalence of obesity and diabetes in patients with cryptogenic cirrhosis: a case–control study. *Hepatology* 2000;32:689–92.

147. El-Serag HB, Tran T, Everhart JE. Diabetes increases the risk of chronic liver disease and hepatocellular carcinoma. *Gastroenterology* 2004;126:460–8.

148. Porepa L, Ray JG, Sanchez-Romeu P, Booth GL. Newly diagnosed diabetes mellitus as a risk factor for serious liver disease. *Can Med Assoc J* 2010;11:182–7.

149. Cull CA, Jensen CC, Retnakaran R, Holman RR. Impact of the metabolic syndrome on macrovascular and microvascular outcomes in type 2 diabetes mellitus: United Kingdom Prospective Diabetes Study 78. *Circulation* 2007;116:2119–26.

150. Chen HF, Chen P, Li CY. Risk of malignant neoplasms of liver and biliary tract in diabetic patients with different age and sex stratifications. *Hepatology* 2010;52:155–63.

151. Hassan MM, Curley SA, Li D, et al. Association of diabetes duration and diabetes treatment with the risk of hepatocellular carcinoma. *Cancer* 2010;116(8):1938–46.

152. Rubio-Tapia A, Murray JA. The liver in celiac disease. *Hepatology* 2007;46:1650–8.

153. Abdo A, Meddings J, Swain M. Liver abnormalities in celiac disease. *Clin Gastroenterol Hepatol* 2004;2:107–12.

154. Casella G, D'Inca R, Oliva L, et al. Prevalence of celiac disease in inflammatory bowel diseases: an IG-IBD multicentre study. *Dig Liver Dis* 2010;42:175–8.

155. Leeds JS, Horoldt BS, Sidhu R, et al. Is there an association between coeliac disease and inflammatory bowel diseases? A study of relative prevalence in comparison with population controls. *Scand J Gastroenterol* 2007;42:1214–20.

156. Navaneethan U, Shen B. Hepatopancreatobiliary manifestations and complications associated with inflammatory bowel disease. *Inflamm Bowel Dis* 2010;16:1598–619.

157. Navaneethan U, Remzi FH, Nutter B, Fazio VW, Shen B. Risk factors for abnormal liver function tests in patients with ileal pouch–anal anastomosis for underlying inflammatory bowel disease. *Am J Gastroenterol* 2009;104:2467–75.

158. Gisbert JP, Luna M, Gonzalez-Lama Y, et al. Liver injury in inflammatory bowel disease: long-term follow-up study of 786 patients. *Inflamm Bowel Dis.* 2007;13:1106–14.

159. Murakami A, Tanaka Y, Ueda M, et al. Hepatocellular carcinoma occurring in a young Crohn's disease patient. *Pathol Int* 2009;59:492–6.

160. Runyon BA, LaBrecque DR, Anuras S. The spectrum of liver disease in systemic lupus erythematosus. Report of 33 histologically-proved cases and review of the literature. *Am J Med* 1980;69:187–94.

161. Piga M, Vacca A, Porru G, Cauli A, Mathieu A. Liver involvement in systemic lupus erythematosus: incidence, clinical course and outcome of lupus hepatitis. *Clin Exp Rheumatol.* 2010;28(4):504–10.

162. Kaw R, Gota C, Bennett A, Barnes D, Calabrese L. Lupus-related hepatitis: complication of lupus or autoimmune association? Case report and review of the literature. *Dig Dis Sci* 2006;51:813–18.

163. Chowdhary VR, Crowson CS, Poterucha JJ, Moder KG. Liver involvement in systemic lupus erythematosus: case review of 40 patients. *J Rheumatol* 2008;35.2159–64.

164. Malnick S, Melzer E, Sokolowski N, Basevitz A. The involvement of the liver in systemic diseases. *J Clin Gastroenterol* 2008;42:69–80.

165. Tsuji T, Ohno S, Ishigatsubo Y. Liver manifestations in systemic lupus erythematosus: high incidence of hemophagocytic syndrome. *J Rheumatol* 2002;29:1576–7.

166. Abraham S, Begum S, Isenberg D. Hepatic manifestations of autoimmune rheumatic diseases. *Ann Rheum Dis* 2004;63:123–9.

167. Walker NJ, Zurier RB. Liver abnormalities in rheumatic diseases. *Clin Liver Dis* 2002;6:933–46.

168. Boulton JG, Bax DE. An unusual cause of abnormal liver function in a patient with rheumatoid arthritis. *Rheumatology (Oxford)* 2008;47:226–7.

169. Skopouli FN, Barbatis C, Moutsopoulos HM. Liver involvement in primary Sjogren's syndrome. *Br J Rheumatol* 1994;33:745–8.

170. Miller EB, Shichmanter R, Friedman JA, Sokolowski N. Granulomatous hepatitis and Sjogren's syndrome: an association. *Semin Arthritis Rheum* 2006;36:153–8.

171. Powell FC, Schroeter AL, Dickson ER. Primary biliary cirrhosis and the CREST syndrome: a report of 22 cases. *Q J Med* 1987;62:75–82.

172. Assassi S, Fritzler MJ, Arnett FC, et al. Primary biliary cirrhosis (PBC), PBC autoantibodies, and hepatic parameter abnormalities in a large population of systemic sclerosis patients. *J Rheumatol* 2009;36:2250–6.

173. Taccone FS, Lucidi V, Donckier V, Bourgeois N, Decaux G, Vandergheynst F. Fulminant hepatitis requiring MARS and liver transplantation in a patient with Still's disease. *Eur J Intern Med* 2008;19:e26–8.

174. Thabah MM, Singh KK, Madhavan SM, Gupta R. Adult onset Still's disease as a cause of acute liver failure. *Trop Gastroenterol* 2008;29:35–6.

175. Han SH. Extrahepatic manifestations of chronic hepatitis B. *Clin Liver Dis* 2004;8:403–18.

176. Sharlala H, Adebajo A. Virus-induced vasculitis. *Curr Rheumatol Rep* 2008;10:449–52.

177. Cooper SC, Olliff SP, McCafferty I, Wigmore SJ, Mirza DF. Polyarteritis nodosa, presenting as life-threatening gastrointestinal hemorrhage in a liver transplant recipient. *Liver Transpl* 2008;14:151–4.

Multiple choice questions

9.1 Which of the following clinical presentations represent hepatic manifestations of tuberculosis?

   a Acute liver failure.
   b Isolated hepatic lesion.
   c Signs and symptoms of portal hypertension.
   d Biliary dilatation with strictures.
   e All of the above.
   f None of the above.

9.2 All of the following are true regarding leptospirosis except which one?

   a Presentation as acute abdominal pain simulating a surgical abdomen.
   b Current guidelines advise antibiotic prophylaxis for exposed individuals in endemic regions.
   c The treatment of choice is doxycycline.
   d Headache, myalgia, jaundice, and renal failure are typical findings.

9.3 Which of the following statements is true regarding erythropoietic protoporphyria?

   a Hepatic involvement is present in more than 75% of cases.
   b Liver transplantation results in a cure of the underlying ferrochelatase defect.
   c Increased levels of protoporphyrin in erythroid cells and feces helps establish the diagnosis.
   d The mainstay of management is periodic phlebotomies.
   e Alcoholic beverages may precipitate acute disease flares.

9.4 All of the following are true regarding liver involvement in celiac disease except which one?

   a Celiac disease includes a spectrum of liver disease that may evolve into cirrhosis.
   b A gluten-free diet improves liver histopathologic changes.
   c A gluten-free diet may improve the disease course of primary biliary cirrhosis when underlying celiac disease is present.
   d Celiac disease should be considered in cases of unexplained liver enzyme elevation.

Answers to the multiple choice questions can be found in the Appendix at the end of the book.

These multiple choice questions are also available for you to complete online.
Visit http://www.schiffsdiseasesoftheliver.com/

CHAPTER 10

Hepatobiliary Complications of Hematopoietic Cell Transplantation

Josh Levitsky[1] & Natasha Walzer[2]

[1]Division of Hepatology and Comprehensive Transplant Center, Northwestern University Feinberg School of Medicine, Chicago, IL, USA
[2]Division of Hepatology, University of Illinois at Chicago, Chicago, IL, USA

Key concepts

- An early rise in bilirubin after hematopoietic cell transplantation (HCT) is a negative prognostic indicator for liver-related morbidity and mortality.
- Liver test abnormalities soon after HCT are most commonly caused by acute graft-versus-host disease (GVHD), drug toxicity, and infection.
- Distinguishing sinusoidal obstruction syndrome (SOS) and GVHD may be difficult and require liver biopsy with hepatic venous pressure gradient measurement.

- Liver disease late after HCT is most commonly due to chronic GVHD, hepatitis B virus (HBV), hepatitis C virus (HCV), and iron overload.
- Anti-HBV prophylaxis should be administered before HCT to all HBV surface antigen positive and possibly core positive patients. Donors should be screened for HBV and other transmissible pathogens.
- Life-threatening opportunistic infections (fungus, herpesvirus) typically occur within weeks after HCT and require urgent diagnosis and treatment.

Hematopoietic cell transplantation (HCT) is now a standard procedure to treat patients with malignant and nonmalignant hematologic disorders. Most patients who remain free of their original disease 2 years after HCT are expected to be long-term survivors [1]. Advances in preparative regimens as well as graft-versus-host disease (GVHD) and anti-infective prophylaxis and treatment have brought significant advances in long-term disease-free survival. However, hepatic complications remain a considerable challenge after HCT and are responsible for significant morbidity and mortality after transplantation. Fortunately, they have become far less frequent and detrimental over time with improvements in diagnosis and treatment algorithms. Pretransplant evaluation of donors and recipients and close monitoring of recipients after HCT appears to reduce the incidence of hepatic complications. This chapter will focus on the causes of liver dysfunction following HCT, and the related morbidity, diagnosis and treatment of these conditions.

Prevalence and prognosis

Chronic liver disease in patients being evaluated for HCT is primarily due to viral hepatitis and iron overload. The presence of hepatic fibrosis and cirrhosis can significantly increase the risk of severe liver injury soon after HCT, regardless of the etiology. Long-term survivors of HCT with chronic liver disease may progress to cirrhosis given the interplay of cancer therapy, immunosuppression, and liver disease etiologies [2]. The cumulative incidence of cirrhosis 10 and 20 years after HCT is approximately 0.6% and 3.8%, respectively. Cirrhosis related to chronic hepatitis C virus (HCV) infection is rising in frequency among patients who were transplanted more than 20 years ago [3]. Serum transaminase elevations in the range of 2–10 times normal are fairly common during the first year after HCT [2]. Sinusoidal obstruction syndrome (SOS), GVHD, cholestasis of sepsis, viral hepatitis, drug- and parenteral nutrition-induced liver injury, and biliary complications are the most common causes of early liver dysfunction after HCT (Fig. 10.1). In autologous transplants, hematologic disease recurrence rather than GVHD and sepsis are the main culprits. Liver disease may be responsible for up to 30% of deaths in HCT recipients, and this risk is increased when the donor or recipient have abnormal liver function or are older or unrelated [4]. A bilirubin rise of >3 mg/dL within the first 6 months is associated with a greater than six-fold increase in mortality [5].

Schiff's Diseases of the Liver, Eleventh Edition. Edited by Eugene R. Schiff, Willis C. Maddrey and Michael F. Sorrell.
© 2012 John Wiley & Sons, Ltd. Published 2012 by John Wiley & Sons, Ltd.

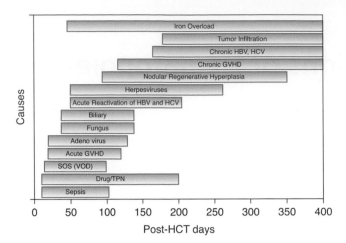

Figure 10.1 Timing of liver disease after hematopoietic cell transplantation. GVHD, graft-versus-host disease; HBV, hepatitis B virus; HCV, hepatitis C virus; SOS, sinusoidal obstruction syndrome; TPN, total parenteral nutrition; VOD, venoocclusive disease.

Donor evaluation

Prospective donors should undergo liver function testing and serologic testing for infections that are potentially transmissible (Table 10.1). Assessment of previous exposure to hepatitis B virus (HBV), HCV, and cytomegalovirus (CMV) provides an important estimate of the risk of transmission and the need for closer monitoring or prophylaxis. Ideally, a donor that

Table 10.1 Donor and recipient assessment prior to hematopoietic cell transplantation.

Donor	Recipient
Liver function tests	Liver function tests
Hepatitis B virus	Hepatitis B virus
Surface antibody and antigen	Surface antibody and antigen
Core IgG	Core IgG
DNA	DNA
Hepatitis C antibody	Hepatitis C antibody
Cytomegalovirus IgG	Cytomegalovirus IgG
Epstein–Barr virus IgG	Epstein–Barr virus IgG
	Varicella zoster virus IgG
	Iron studies
	Iron, TIBC, ferritin
	Hepatobiliary ultrasonography
	with Doppler

DNA, deoxyribonucleic acid; IgG, immunoglobulin G; TIBC, total iron-binding capacity.

has not been infected by a hepatitis virus should be selected.

Recipient diagnosis and evaluation

Before HCT, recipients should also be evaluated with liver function tests, viral hepatitis serologies, and for CMV and Epstein–Barr (EBV) antibodies. Consumption of alcohol and potentially hepatotoxic medications should be avoided. The patient should be monitored clinically for any signs of liver dysfunction (right upper quadrant pain, jaundice, ascites, and weight gain). Any suggestion of liver disease should prompt an immediate diagnostic evaluation that is focused on the specific time period after HCT (Fig. 10.1). Early diagnosis and treatment results in improved prognosis for most etiologies of liver disease post HCT. Infectious causes, including viral hepatitis, should be initially ruled out, preferably with nucleic acid testing, due to the immunosuppressed state. In addition, a thorough medication review should be performed. Imaging tests are primarily useful when there is concern that there may be SOS, complications from gallstones, or the development of portal hypertension. Liver biopsy as a diagnostic tool for abnormal liver function tests in HCT recipients is controversial, although decision making is often altered as a result of liver biopsy findings [6]. Transvenous biopsy is typically required to reduce bleeding complications in patients with coagulopathy or thrombocytopenia [7]. Furthermore, this approach allows an assessment of the hepatic venous pressure gradient (HVPG), which may provide additional support for the diagnosis of SOS or other etiologies [6].

Common complications

Acute graft-versus-host disease

Acute GVHD occurs in up to 70% of allograft recipients, depending on the degree of donor/recipient human leucocyte antigen (HLA) mismatch and the intensity of GVHD prophylaxis [8–10]. Risk factors for the development of acute GVHD include age of over 40 years, degree of HLA disparity, donor/recipient gender disparity, and high-intensity transplant conditioning regimen [11]. Organ involvement is typically less than that of chronic GVHD and is mainly limited to the skin, gastrointestinal tract, and liver. The liver is usually the last organ affected and is characterized by a cholestatic pattern (raised alkaline phosphatase and γ-glutamyltransferase) of liver function tests.

Liver biopsy confirmation of GVHD is almost always justifiable, even in HCT recipients with skin or gastrointestinal GVHD who develop cholestatic parameters.

One study reported that when GVHD was suspected clinically, only 43% of biopsies were confirmatory [12]. In addition, acute GVHD was established on biopsy in 17% of unsuspected cases. Histologic findings of acute GVHD include lymphocytic involvement of intralobular bile ducts, bile duct epithelial cell dropout, and minimal inflammation due to post HCT immunosuppression [13]. A recent review of 48 biopsy specimens demonstrated that bile duct injury was the most common finding [14]. Treatment of acute GVHD can be difficult, and the mortality of steroid-refractory GVHD can exceed 70%. As a result, the development and use of effective prophylaxis is extremely important. Significant risk factors for mortality are a non-HLA-matched sibling donor, absence of methotrexate (MTX) in GVHD prophylaxis, initial liver involvement (versus other organ first), and steroid-refractory GVHD [15].

Prophylactic agents have had varied success in preventing acute GVHD after HCT. Immunosuppression with tacrolimus ± MTX has been found to be superior to cyclosporine + MTX in both sibling and unrelated transplants [16]. Although this regimen has become the standard of care in most transplant centers, it is ineffective in a significant percentage of patients. In addition, MTX is associated with a number of adverse events, including renal, hepatic, and gastrointestinal toxicity [17–19]. One reasonable alternative is to use lower doses of MTX to reduce toxicity, although this may compromise efficacy in preventing acute GVHD. An alternative regimen, using tacrolimus and mycophenolate mofetil (MMF) may have less early toxicity but does not appear to be as effective in preventing severe acute GVHD [20]. Ursodeoxycholic acid (12 mg/kg/day) given up to 90 days post HCT lowers the incidence of severe acute GVHD and is associated with an improved 1-year survival compared with placebo [21].

Prophylaxis for acute GVHD often leads to reduced rates of chronic GVHD. In addition, early-onset (<30 days) acute GVHD portends a worse prognosis in terms of the development and severity of chronic GVHD [22]. Tacrolimus and cyclosporine prophylaxis may reduce the incidence of chronic GVHD to 25–50% [19,23]. While most studies have not shown a survival benefit with prophylaxis, tacrolimus plus MTX has been associated with a 2-year disease-free survival of 50% in one study [24]. A recent study compared tacrolimus plus MTX with tacrolimus plus MMF, and found there were no significant differences between the arms in terms of mortality or overall survival in both acute and chronic GVHD. Ursodeoxycholic acid does not reduce the incidence of chronic GVHD, but 1-year survival is improved mainly due to a reduction in acute GVHD [21].

Corticosteroids are the initial treatment of choice for acute GVHD. Response rates in the range of 24–55% are seen with grade II or greater acute GVHD, with the remaining patients being unresponsive or steroid resistant [25]. Corticosteroids are more effective in treating dermatologic and gastrointestinal manifestations of GVHD than liver involvement [26]. For steroid-refractory acute GVHD, options including MMF, tacrolimus, cyclosporine, interleukin 2 receptor inhibitors (daclizumab), anti-CD54 antibodies (alemtuzumab), and rapamycin [27,28]. In severe, refractory cases, orthotopic liver transplantation (OLT) may be an acceptable treatment option, although recent malignancy may be an absolute contraindication unless the risk of relapse is low. Data from a national database demonstrated reasonable post-OLT 1- and 5-year actuarial survival rates (72.4% and 62.9%, respectively) [29].

Chronic graft-versus-host disease

Chronic GVHD develops in ~50% of long-term survivors of allogeneic HCT. Risk factors include older donor/recipient age, busulfan conditioning, previous acute GVHD, CMV seropositivity, granulocyte colony-stimulating factor use, and receiving an unrelated donor HCT [30–32]. Clinical characteristics differentiating chronic from acute GVHD are as follows: timing (chronic >100 days after HCT), more extensive organ injury, and involvement of other systems (exocrine glands, genitourinary tract, lungs). Portal involvement with lymphocytes and bile duct dropout, periportal fibrosis, piecemeal necrosis, and cholestasis are the predominant histologic features of chronic GVHD (Fig. 10.2). The inflammatory mononuclear cells reacting to mismatched histocompatibility antigens on host biliary epithelial cells lead

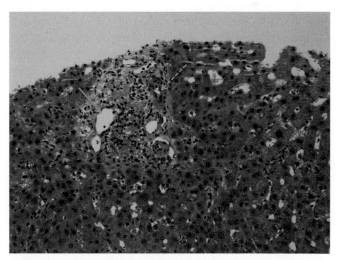

Figure 10.2 Chronic graft-versus-host disease. The portal triad shows the presence of a branch of the hepatic artery (dashed arrow) and portal vein (solid arrow) but no accompanying bile duct. Original ×200. (Courtesy of Simbasiva Rao, Northwestern University Department of Pathology.)

to subsequent obliteration and loss of intrahepatic bile ducts [33].

The liver function tests are predominantly cholestatic, with elevations in the serum alkaline phosphatase, bilirubin, and γ-glutamyltransferase. Rarely, chronic GVHD (>100 days) can present with liver transaminases more than 10 times normal, similar to that of acute viral or drug-induced hepatitis. This classically occurs with recent reduction or cessation of anti-graft-versus-host immunosuppressant therapy. On liver biopsy, lobular hepatitis with hepatocyte necrosis and acidophil bodies are seen in comparison to the characteristic biliary injury features of chronic GVHD [34]. Rapid reinstitution of immunosuppressive therapy and ursodeoxycholic acid generally results in resolution [35]. Interestingly, patients with chronic GVHD may have a clinical and histologic presentation similar to patients with primary biliary cirrhosis (PBC) [36,37]. There is a high frequency of antimitochondrial antibodies in chronic GVHD, although they are often falsely positive. In addition, a bile duct lesion of GVHD can resemble that seen in PBC, without the granulomas [35,38]. Therapy for chronic GVHD is not always indicated, especially when there is stable, mild elevation of liver function tests. Patients with a more severe, cholestatic presentation, are initially treated with corticosteroids ± a calcineurin inhibitor and ursodeoxycholic acid [38]. Most patients require systemic treatment for at least 2 years, but only 50% are able to discontinue therapy after 5 years and 30% are refractory [39]. Salvage treatments result in response rates varying between 19% and 77% [40,41]. MMF has the highest efficacy in refractory cases but may be associated with gastrointestinal side effects and opportunistic infections. Tacrolimus improves and normalizes liver tests in 60% and 33%, respectively [42]. Ursodeoxycholic acid is the only liver specific therapy, and it improves liver tests and long-term hepatic complications [43]. Liver transplantation, including living donor transplantation, for either acute or chronic GVHD appears to be a feasible option in severe, refractory cases [44]. The 5-year survival after OLT for refractory chronic GVHD is reasonable (62.9%) and the rate of retransplantation and recurrent GVHD is fortunately low [29].

Sinusoidal obstruction syndrome

Sinusoidal obstruction syndrome, previously referred to as venocclusive disease, typically occurs within 30 days of HCT and carries a mortality rate of up to 50% in severe cases [45]. The incidence varies widely with the intensity of the conditioning regimen, from <10% with the majority of regimens to as high as 50% after cyclophosphamide 120 mg/kg plus total body irradiation (TBI) >14 Gy [46]. Most series report an incidence of around 20% in HCT

recipients [47,48]. The incidence may also be affected by the use of drugs that alter the metabolism of the myeloablative drugs or cause concomitant liver injury. Recently, the frequency and severity of SOS have fallen significantly for a variety of reasons. The doses of TBI >14 Gy are rarely used anymore, cyclophosphamide has been largely replaced by fludarabine, and the use and efficacy of prophylactic medications have increased. The prognosis depends on the extent of hepatic injury, underlying liver dysfunction, and the presence of multiorgan failure [49]. Multiorgan failure, including fulminant hepatic failure, occurs in about 20–25% of patients and is associated with a near 100% fatality rate [50,51]. Patients typically present with tender hepatomegaly, elevated serum bilirubin (>2 mg/dL), and weight gain (>5%) due to fluid retention and ascites. A continuous increase in bilirubin within 3 weeks after HCT is significantly associated with developing SOS [52]. The diagnosis is secure in patients who meet these clinical criteria, although those with two or less criteria are less likely to have SOS and may need liver biopsy and HVPG measurement for confirmation [53].

Risk factors for SOS are listed in Table 10.2. Busulfan induces oxidative stress by reducing glutathione levels in hepatocytes and sinusoidal endothelial cells [54]. Additional risk factors are female gender, elevated serum ferritin, advanced disease status and high Karnofsky score, total body irradiation, treatment with gemtuzumab ozogamicin, and allogeneic transplantation [55]. Preexisting liver disease significantly increases the risk of developing SOS [56,57]. Patients with chronic hepatitis C can have abnormal sinusoidal endothelium, which could make them more susceptible to the cytoreductive regimen injury.

Table 10.2 Risk factors for sinusoidal obstruction syndrome.

Definite	Suspected
High-dose conditioning	Glutathione-S-transferase M1 polymorphism
Busulfan	
Cyclophosphamide	Intravenous immunoglobulin
Hepatitis C virus	Unrelated or allogeneic transplant
Advanced disease status and Karnofsky score	
Abnormal liver aminotransferases (any cause)	Norethisterone
	Previous abdominal irradiation
Gemtuzumab-ozogamicin	
T-cell depletion	
Low protein C activity	

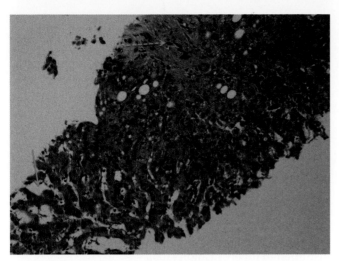

Figure 10.3 Sinusoidal obstruction syndrome showing central vein sclerosis (dashed arrow) and sinusoidal dilatation (solid arrow). Original ×200. (Courtesy of Simbasiva Rao, Northwestern University Department of Pathology.)

Local activation of the coagulation cascade and collagen deposition in the perivenular and subendothelial region results in a reduction in blood flow from the sinusoids to the central veins [58]. Histologically, findings include central vein subendothelial thickening, sinusoidal dilatation, red blood cell extravasation outside the sinusoids, and pericentral hepatocyte necrosis. Activated stellate cells, identified by immunohistochemical staining for alpha smooth muscle actin antibodies, play an important role in the development of luminal narrowing and sinusoidal fibrosis [59]. With ongoing obstruction and necrosis, the fibrosis can extend from these obliterated central veins. Later histologic findings include sclerosis of venular walls (Fig. 10.3) and occlusion of terminal hepatic venules. As such, the term venous occlusive disease has been replaced by sinusoidal obstruction syndrome as not all cases have terminal hepatic venule occlusion. The number and degree of perivenular changes is associated with the clinical severity of SOS and not solely with the presence of occlusion of terminal hepatic venules [60,61].

Rapid diagnosis and intervention are important in the management of SOS. Ultrasonographic findings, such as hepatomegaly, splenomegaly, ascites, an abnormal portal vein waveform, attenuated hepatic venous flow, and an elevated hepatic artery resistive index correlate with the clinical and histologic diagnosis of SOS [62,63]. An HVPG of >10 correlates highly with the histologic diagnosis of SOS and may be useful when the biopsy or clinical features are inconclusive [6].

Because of the absence of specific, effective therapy, prevention of the initial damage to the hepatic sinusoidal endothelial cells is critical. This can be ameliorated via prophylactic strategies or an alteration to the myeloabla-

tive conditioning regimen. The latter strategy, however, may result in either a decrease in the rates of engraftment or an increase in malignancy relapse rates. Once an assessment of the risk of a particular patient has been performed (see Table 10.2), a prophylactic agent should be used in those patients deemed to be at increased risk for the development of SOS. The most promising agents are ursodeoxycholic acid, heparin, and defibrotide [64]. Two of three randomized trials have shown a significant reduction in the incidence of SOS with the use of ursodeoxycholic acid compared with placebo [21,65,66]. Heparin, either unfractionated or low molecular weight or in combination with defibrotide, is also effective in preventing SOS compared with placebo, with a low rate of bleeding complications [67–70]. Based on findings that antithrombin III (ATIII) confers a protective effect on vascular endothelium and ATIII levels are decreased in patients with SOS, a number of trials have tested whether ATIII has activity in SOS. A recent large pediatric trial in which 91 children received preemptive ATIII replacement demonstrated that ATIII administration did not reduce the incidence of SOS compared with the control group who received no SOS prophylaxis [71].

Response rates depend on early diagnosis and severity of the disease. Early intervention has been associated with a complete response in 76% and 50% of all and severe cases of SOS, respectively [63,72]. Those who are deemed to have a mild disease and are likely to recover (>70% of patients) can be treated conservatively with management of fluid balance with sodium restriction, diuretics, and paracentesis as needed for ascites. Those with a poor prognosis can be recognized by rapid rises in serum bilirubin levels, significant weight gain, portal pressures >20 mmHg, and serum alanine aminotransferase (ALT) values >750 U/L [73,74]. Defibrotide is a mixture of porcine oligodeoxyribonucleotides that has local antithrombotic, anti-ischemic, and anti-inflammatory activity. It is able to protect the hepatic sinusoidal endothelium without compromising the antitumor effects of cytotoxic therapy [75]. Previous studies have demonstrated an overall response rate of 55–76% with a severe disease response rate of 36–50% [72,76]. Although not available in the United States, defibrotide is preferred over other thrombolytic agents, such as recombinant tissue plasminogen activator (TPA), that have a significantly higher rate of bleeding complications [77,78]. For refractory cases, transjugular intrahepatic portosystemic shunt (TIPS) improves abdominal pain and ascites but does not result in improved survival [79,80]. In selected cases with a low risk of disease recurrence, liver transplantation may be performed with a potential for long-term survival. A recent review of the literature identified 15 patients with severe SOS who underwent OLT as a life-saving measure [81]. Only 33% of the patients survived more than 2 years, with the remaining dying of overwhelming infections. In the same paper, however, a review of the United Network for Organ Sharing (UNOS) database revealed an additional five cases of SOS where the patients had undergone transplantation with only one death [81].

Hepatitis B virus (de novo and reactivation)

Hepatitis B virus reactivation after HCT is a well-recognized complication in patients who either retain hepatitis B surface antigen (HBsAg) or have resolved infection (hepatitis B core (HBc) antibody) [82]. In addition, HBV can be transmitted from donor to recipient and cause acute hepatitis soon after HCT. For HBV-negative recipients, donors not previously exposed to HBV infection are preferred [83]. The pathophysiology of reactivation is related to impaired cellular immunity because of the underlying hematologic disease and treatment, allowing for viral replication. In addition, subsequent to the withdrawal of the immunosuppressive agents, there is a restoration of immune function that results in the T-cell immune-mediated destruction of the infected hepatocytes.

Donor evaluation

There is a high incidence of HBV-related hepatitis after HCT when HBsAg-positive donors are used, with a mortality rate of up to 17% [84]. Overall, de novo HBV has been reported to occur in 3.2% of recipients [85]. The presence of donor HBsAg and a high viral load predisposes recipients to developing HBV-related hepatitis [86]. HBV carriers (HBsAg without detectable HBV DNA) rarely transmit HBV to the recipient and can be donors if their serum and peripheral stem cells are HBV DNA negative [85,87]. In addition, recipient surface antibody positivity seems to confer protection against HBV [88]. HBsAg-positive donors have been used safely in an HBV endemic area when the donor and recipient are treated with lamivudine, in addition to the recipient being given HBV vaccination before transplantation [89]. Interestingly, adoptive transfer of surface antibody from donor to recipient may result in recipient loss of surface antigen and acquisition of surface antibody [90,91].

Risk of reactivation and acute flare

The degree of immunosuppression and donor/recipient viremia immediately prior to HCT are the most significant risk factors for severe HBV infection or reactivation. Recipients with surface antigen and undetectable HBV DNA have a significantly lower risk of reactivation than those with detectable DNA [92]. Patients with a precore mutant are prone to more severe reactivation episodes and decompensation after HCT [87]. The presence of recipient core antibody also poses a risk, particu-

larly in the setting of detectable DNA and chronic GVHD [93,94]. Reverse seroconversion, that is HBV reactivation in patients with antibodies to HBsAg and/or hepatitis B core antigen, has been reported to occur [86,95,96]. One study demonstrated a 35% risk of HBV reactivation in patients with isolated anti-HBc antibodies [97]. The availability of potent immunosuppressive drugs, like anti-CD20 and anti-CD52 monoclonal antibodies, has further increased the risk of HBV reactivation. It has been reported that patients with surface antibody who have presumed immunity from prior infection can develop acute hepatitis after HCT, potentially related to low surface antibody titers and the presence of viral DNA either in blood or tissues [98,99]. Fulminant hepatic failure can occur if the diagnosis is detected late and therapy is not instituted in timely fashion [100].

Treatment

Acute reactivations of HBV in the setting of immunosuppression tapering or withdrawal are becoming less common with advances in the treatment and prophylaxis of HBV before and after HCT. Lamivudine is typically the first agent selected for HBV flares after HCT, unless the patient has a known lamivudine-resistant strain. Adefovir used in addition to lamivudine or alone is also effective in this situation [101]. In addition, there are multiple new antiviral agents (tenofovir, entecavir) with lower rates of resistance that may be utilized particularly if the patient has cirrhosis or is likely to be on long-term therapy. The length of treatment in all cases is also unknown. Those with reactivation during immunosuppression withdrawal should be treated until immunosuppressive agents are tapered or discontinued and for a time period (~6–12 months) thereafter.

Prevention

Antiviral therapy can prevent most cases of acute hepatitis B after transplant if initiated prior to the start of conditioning therapy in those who are viremic. Patients with known chronic HBV should be treated with antiviral therapy prior to HCT with the goal of undetectable virus at the time of HCT, time permitting. Therapy should continue until long after engraftment and immunosuppression withdrawal. Patients who cannot wait for viral clearance should be given antiviral prophylaxis as soon as possible prior to conditioning. HBsAg-positive recipients who are given lamivudine prophylaxis have a significantly higher 1-year survival (94% versus 54%) and lower incidence of hepatitis flares (5% versus 45%) and acute liver failure (0% versus 15%) compared with those given no prophylaxis [102]. Despite the previously described risk of reactivation, controversy still exists about antiviral prophylaxis in recipients who are anti-HBc positive. In one series, among 25 patients with anti-HBc antibodies, reverse seroconversion and acute hepatitis were not observed in those treated with lamivudine, whereas HBV reactivation developed in three of the untreated patients [103]. The impact of lamivudine resistance in this setting does not appear to be of great concern, as only short-term therapy is needed. Newer antiviral therapies can be used but are probably only required in those requiring long-term therapy.

Hepatitis C virus

Although the risk of acquiring HCV from HCT is relatively low, many patients come to HCT already chronically infected. A large prospective study demonstrated a prevalence of about 6%, although this percentage varies widely in the literature [85]. Prior to the institution of blood product screening, one study demonstrated that a third of patients who had undergone HCT from 1987 to 1988 acquired HCV [104]. Transmission of HCV is currently low due to adequate blood product screening, newer generation HCV antibody testing, and treatment of donors and recipients [105]. Despite this, HCV is the main etiology of chronic liver disease long after HCT [106]. Moreover, a more rapid rate of liver fibrosis has been observed in patients with HCV who received HCT [3].

Risk of acute flare

Although a significant contributor to long-term morbidity, unlike HBV, HCV does not cause severe acute hepatitis or flare upon the withdrawal of immunosuppression after HCT. Mild elevation in liver aminotransferases, limited to a 5–10-fold increase, are not uncommon. The presence of HCV alone is not an independent predictor of liver failure in HCT recipients [107], although the risk of SOS itself is increased with underlying HCV unless the conditioning regimen has little or no liver toxicity. There is no prophylactic agent or antibody for HCV prior to the institution of chemotherapy or HCT to prevent complications.

Long-term prognosis

The influence of chronic HCV on the outcomes for HCT recipients is not fully clear. Some patients can develop progressive fibrosis and clinical decompensation, while other HCV infections lie dormant for years. Studies with long follow-up confirm that HCV leads to a cumulative incidence of cirrhosis of 24% at 20 years, ranking HCV third behind infection and GVHD as a cause of late death after HCT [108]. In addition, iron deposition is thought to be a major cofactor in fibrosis progression. Other potential risk factors for progression are HCV genotype (1a and 1b), hepatic steatosis, insulin resistance, obesity, and the presence of extrahepatic manifestations of HCV.

Treatment

Data regarding HCV treatment after HCT are sparse. One study involved 11 patients 24–65 months post HCT who were treated with interferon for 6–12 months [109]. Ten completed the protocol, 40% had a sustained virological response and 50% had improved liver histology. A more recent evaluation of 22 HCV-infected HCT recipients demonstrated that combined therapy (pegylated or standard interferon with ribavirin) led to a sustained virological response in 4/18 (20%) patients compared with 2/20 (10%) in patients who received interferon alone [110]. Combination therapy led to an increased risk in hematologic toxicity, but only led to drug discontinuation or dose modification in a small percentage.

Iron overload

Iron overload is associated with organ toxicity and can be a cause of significant morbidity in patients with hematologic malignancies [111]. Patients undergoing HCT have ineffective erythropoiesis, increased iron absorption, and often have a need for multiple red blood cell transfusions [112]. Progressive fibrosis due to hepatic iron deposition in HCT recipients is most commonly seen in patients with a pre-HCT history of iron overload from multiple blood transfusions. Pretransplant red blood cell transfusion dependence and/or elevated serum ferritin levels are associated with diminished post-transplant survival among patients with myelodysplastic syndrome and acute leukemia [113]. The presence of severe iron overload significantly impacts survival and transplant-related mortality. As such, those who have hepatomegaly and fibrosis prior to HCT will typically develop progressive iron overload and fibrosis years after HCT [114].

The diagnosis of iron overload is suspected in patients with elevated ferritin and transferrin saturation in association with abnormal liver aminotransferases. A liver biopsy may not be necessary, although other causes of abnormal liver enzymes should be excluded. In addition, biopsy may be of prognostic value, as hepatic iron stores often reflect total body iron stores accurately and may give prognostic information. Iron overload suggested on magnetic resonance imaging is common after HCT and may correlate with the number of previous blood transfusions [115]. Early iron reduction with phlebotomy or iron chelation therapy is safe and may be effective in reducing ferritin levels immediately after HCT, although this is better tolerated when adequate return of red cell production by the bone marrow occurs later after HCT. Studies have shown significant improvements in ferritin, transferrin saturation, liver enzymes, hepatic iron concentration, and fibrosis scores in patients undergoing phelobotomy years following HCT [116].

Causes of cholestasis

Sepsis

Sepsis of any cause, particularly in the setting of neutropenia or high levels of immunosuppression, may lead to biochemical liver abnormalities and cholestasis. The pathophysiologic features of cholestasis due to sepsis are similar in general and transplant populations. Canalicular cholestasis is the most common histologic finding, typically with dilated periportal ductules and occasionally inspissated bile in cholangioles. Other nonspecific findings include steatosis and pericentral ischemic necrosis, the latter related to poor perfusion from sepsis. The serum bilirubin can become quite elevated in severe septic shock. It is thought that the cytokine release that occurs during sepsis downregulates bile acid transport and bile secretion [117]. Ultrasonography can help differentiate cholestasis of sepsis from ductal obstruction. Resolution of sepsis invariably results in slow normalization of bilirubin and cholestasis.

Total parenteral nutrition

Total parenteral nutrition (TPN) as a primary cause of cholestasis after HCT can be a challenging diagnosis to make in the setting of other concurrent factors, including medications, infection, and GVHD. Increases in serum transaminases, alkaline phosphatase, and γ-glutamyltransferase are often seen within 3 weeks of TPN initiation and return to normal in over 75% of patients after withdrawal. The most common histologic abnormalities include intrahepatic cholestasis, portal/periportal fibrosis, and periportal macrovesicular steatosis [118]. Progression to cirrhosis and the development of clinically significant liver disease is uncommon in adults. Reduction of dextrose in the TPN solution with conversion to more lipid-based calories can improve cholestasis. Additionally, cycling infusions to allow "TPN-free" periods can improve biliary flow. TPN should be discontinued, if possible, if cholestasis progresses despite these measures.

Drug hepatotoxicity

Drug-induced liver injury is a cause of liver dysfunction in many patients post HCT, although isolating the culprit drug can often be difficult. Numerous medications can lead to intrahepatic cholestasis and liver test abnormalities. Many chemotherapeutic agents and corticosteroids cause steatosis, SOS, cholestasis, and/or hepatocellular injury. Prophylactic and therapeutic anti-infective agents such as the sulfonamides, macrolides, cephalosporins, penicillins, and azole antifungals can lead to cholestasis, vanishing bile duct syndrome, or phospholipidosis. A recent retrospective review demonstrated a 34% rate of hepatotoxicity with voriconazole therapy, although this is rarely severe [119]. Agents used for GVHD (e.g.,

cyclosporine and less commonly tacrolimus) can cause cholestasis in the setting of high serum and tissue levels. Cyclosporine inhibits bile transport and can often raise the serum bilirubin without affecting the serum ALT or alkaline phosphatase. Histologic changes consist of bile duct epithelial hypertrophy with cytoplasmic vacuoles and foamy deposition within the hepatic sinusoids.

Uncommon complications

Herpesvirus infections

Herpes simplex virus 1 and 2

With the routine prophylactic use of aciclovir or valaciclovir, acute hepatitis due to herpesvirus infections is uncommon [120]. Fulminant hepatitis due to herpes simplex virus (HSV) early after HCT has been reported, although incidence data in this population are not available [121]. Risk factors for reactivation include pretransplant conditioning, HSV seropositivity, and a history of leukemia. Antiviral drug prophylaxis should be given primarily to HSV-seropositive patients. Herpes hepatitis typically causes massive coagulative necrosis with purple nuclear inclusions surrounding the regions of necrosis. HSV DNA detected in peripheral leukocytes is more specific for disseminated infection (esophagitis, hepatitis) and may have predictive value when rapidly rising [122]. When herpesvirus hepatitis is suspected, immediate treatment with intravenous aciclovir is warranted [123]. Prophylactic strategies after HCT, including use of aciclovir and its derivatives, have been shown to lower the incidence of HSV infections in general. Aciclovir- and foscarnet-resistant HSV strains have been reported, but are uncommon in HCT recipients [124].

Varicella-zoster virus

The incidence of varicella-zoster virus (VZV) infections has also been declining, likely due to antiviral prophylaxis and less intensive immunosuppression regimens [125]. Up to one third of patients can have reactivation of VZV after transplantation. Fortunately, the majority of cases are confined to the skin. Visceral presentation has been reported to occur in 1–7% of HCT recipients [126]. Infections typically occur within the first year after transplantation and usually in the setting of GVHD, pretransplant VZV seropositivity, and tapering of antiviral prophylaxis [127]. Immunosuppressed patients may fail to develop a skin rash, especially in the early phase of the infection [128]. Clinically, patients with VZV hepatitis classically present with severe abdominal pain and significant liver aminotransferase elevation. Fulminant hepatic failure from varicella hepatitis has been reported after HCT [129]. Hepatic lesions appear similar to those of HSV with necrosis and minimal inflammation. Electron microscopy, immunocytochemistry, and polymerase chain reaction analysis may help differentiate VZV from other herpesviruses. Prompt antiviral treatment with aciclovir can significantly decrease the high morbidity and mortality associated with the illness. For prophylaxis, aciclovir reduces VZV reactivation significantly, although VZV can occur soon after prophylaxis is discontinued. Longer term prophylaxis may be considered in patients at high risk for VZV (previous zoster infection, GVHD). Varicella vaccination given before HCT has been shown to significantly reduce the incidence of zoster and the potential for viral dissemination [130].

Epstein–Barr virus

Proliferation of EBV occurs in the setting of high immunosuppression, antilymphocyte therapy, and T-cell depletion. Subsequently, this may lead to B-cell proliferation and the potential for post-transplant lymphoproliferative disorder (PTLD). Clinical signs, such as fever, lymphadenopathy, splenomegaly, weight loss, abnormal liver aminotransferases, and bone marrow suppression are common. Histopathology shows a diffuse lymphocytic infiltrate in the sinusoids and focal apoptotic cells [131]. Routine antiviral prophylaxis for EBV has little impact on the development of EBV PTLD. As a serum EBV DNA level of $>10^4$ associated with the development of PTLD after HCT, prospective monitoring of EBV viremia may be recommended in high-risk or pediatric patients [132,133]. In addition, rapid reduction in viremia predicts a successful response [134]. Studies have shown that early intervention with anti-CD20 antibody (rituximab) when EBV DNA is $>10^3$ or CD8+ responses to EBV are detected may prevent the subsequent development of PTLD [135]. Polyclonal EBV infections typically respond to a reduction in immunosuppression. However, rituximab appears to be safe and efficacious for monoclonal or more aggressive EBV PTLD [136].

Cytomegalovirus

There are few reports on the incidence of CMV hepatitis following stem cell transplantation. It is known that recipients of CD34+ peripheral blood stem cell transplants, alemtuzumab infusions, and transfusions without leukocyte depletion or CMV screening have a higher rate of CMV infection [137]. Presenting signs and symptoms include fever, cytopenia, colitis, pneumonitis, and abnormal aminotransferases. The pathognomonic finding is a hepatocyte, bile duct epithelium, or endothelial cell containing cytoplasmic basophilic granules and an intranuclear inclusion surrounded by a clear halo (Fig. 10.4). This is typically positive on CMV immuno-

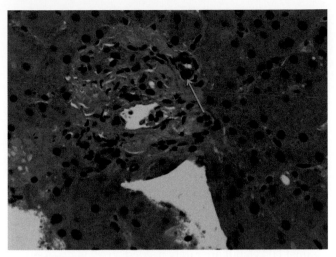

Figure 10.4 Cytomegalovirus hepatitis showing a viral inclusion present in a bile duct epithelial cell (arrow). Original ×600. (Courtesy of Simbasiva Rao, Northwestern University Department of Pathology.)

histochemical staining (Fig. 10.5). Blood CMV DNA testing is more sensitive than culture or antigen testing and may predict the development of CMV end organ disease. Antiviral prophylaxis after HCT, including aciclovir, valaciclovir, ganciclovir, and valganciclovir, are all successful in reducing the incidence of CMV infection. However, prevention of late infections continues to be a challenge in high-risk (donor-positive, recipient-negative) populations [138]. Intravenous ganciclovir is the treatment of choice for confirmed disease, with foscarnet reserved for ganciclovir-resistant strains (<10%). Another preemptive approach is to closely monitor for CMV infection using pp65 antigen or DNA and only treat once CMV is detected before the onset of symptoms

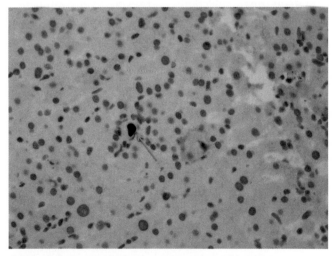

Figure 10.5 Cytomegalovirus hepatitis. Immunostaining for a cytomegalovirus-positive cell (arrow). Original ×600. (Courtesy of Simbasiva Rao, Northwestern University Department of Pathology.)

[139]. Isolation and donor transfer of T cells with specific activity against CMV antigens may reconstitute cellular immunity against CMV and might represent a novel approach [140].

Human herpesvirus 6

Infection with human herpesvirus 6 (HHV6) in transplant recipients, often transmitted from donor to recipient, may result in a lobular, nonspecific hepatitis, marrow suppression, and gastrointestinal symptoms [141]. The detection of HHV6 early after HCT may also be associated with delayed engraftment [142]. A high percentage of HCT recipients have HHV6 viremia, but symptoms and disease specifically related to HHV6 are uncommon. Cidofovir and foscarnet have the highest antiviral activity against HHV6 but are rarely needed.

Adenovirus

Adenovirus infection causing acute hepatitis after HCT is rare and is typically only seen in the setting of induction chemotherapy, high levels of immunosuppression, and GVHD [143]. The clinical presentation is similar to CMV, with pneumonia, gastroenteritis, hepatitis, and occasionally encephalitis and hemorrhagic cystitis. Fulminant hepatic necrosis with intranuclear inclusions appears similar to HSV and VZV. Thus, electron microscopy, immunohistochemical staining, or polymerase chain reaction are often needed to distinguish these etiologies. Treatment with antiviral agents, such as cidofovir and ribavirin, have had limited success.

Fungal infections

In the early days of HCT, fungal organisms were found in up to 10% of liver autopsy specimens. Risk factors after HCT include pre-HCT fungal infection, superficial and deep fungal infections, and severe liver dysfunction either from SOS or GVHD. The most common fungal infections involving the liver are candidiasis, aspergillosis, and zygomycosis, but other mycoses, such as cryptococcosis, histoplasmosis, blastomycocis, and coccidiomycosis can be seen with regional or travel exposures. Hepatosplenic candidiasis can present with multiple portal and periportal abscesses and granulomas, as well as sinusoidal hyphae. Prior to HCT, patients can be treated aggressively with amphotericin to eradicate candidiasis and can still successfully undergo HCT. Aspergilli (*Aspergillus fumigates* and *A. flavus*) and zygomycosis (*Rhizopus*, *Mucor*, and *Absidia*) can cause hemorrhagic hepatic necrosis and local infarction due to blood vessel invasion. Assessing the size, morphology, and special staining on histology typically confirms the specific diagnosis. Specific culture of liver tissue may be necessary. Imaging tests such as ultrasonography and computed tomography scan, particularly for hepatosplenic

candidiasis, may provide additional evidence for fungus, although the sensitivity is low as resolution of neutropenia is required to visualize lesions. The treatment of invasive hepatic infections is usually with amphotericin B or azole agents. Post-HCT prophylaxis with itraconazole, fluconazole, or low-dose amphotericin can significantly reduce the incidence, morbidity, and mortality associated with invasive fungal infections [144,145].

Biliary complications

While gallbladder sludge and stones are typical in HCT recipients, complications such as cholecystitis and cholangitis are uncommon. Gallbladder sludge containing nonspecific residue, calcium-binding protein, and calcium bilirubinate crystals forms early after HCT and often progress to true stone formation [146]. Cholecystitis is treated with either cholecystectomy or nonsurgical measures (antibiotics, percutaneous drainage) in poor surgical candidates. Acalculous cholecystitis is less common and is associated with prolonged fasting, SOS, transfusions, and the use of TPN. This entity usually requires cholecystectomy, as gallbladder wall necrosis and perforation are often present. The incidence of biliary obstruction after HCT was reported to be 0.1% in one large study [147]. The causes were mainly biliary sludge/stones and strictures from recurrent malignancy, EBV PTLD, and GVHD. Endoscopic or percutaneous treatment is usually sufficient to treat and relieve obstruction.

Tumor infiltration

New secondary malignancies can occur in up to 20% of recipients within 10–15 years after HCT. Leukemia and lymphoma can infiltrate the liver, leading to hepatomegaly and high levels of alkaline phosphatase. Secondary solid cancers occur almost twice as frequently in HCT recipients as in the healthy population [1]. In addition, due to exposure to hepatitis B and C before the 1990s, recipients can develop chronic liver disease and hepatocellular carcinoma. Biopsy is the gold standard to differentiate malignancy from infection and other causes of liver dysfunction.

Nodular regenerative hyperplasia

In rare cases, HCT recipients can develop idiopathic non-neoplastic hepatic nodules (nodular regenerative hyperplasia) without fibrosis or liver dysfunction. The etiology is unknown but does not appear to be related to age, underlying disease, or cytoreductive regimen [148]. Even though nodules are less than 1.0 cm in size, they can significantly distort the hepatic architecture enough to cause sinusoidal and presinusoidal portal hypertension (ascites, variceal hemorrhage). The diagnosis can be difficult to determine and is not always apparent on standard liver biopsy, unless a laparoscopic wedge biopsy is taken

[149]. The HVPG may or may not be elevated depending on the region (sinusoidal or presinusoidal) of portal hypertension. Nodular regenerative hyperplasia may resolve spontaneously months after HCT and does not appear to contribute significantly to mortality. Management includes standard therapies for managing portal hypertension (salt restriction, diuretics, primary or secondary prophylaxis of gastrointestinal varices).

Further reading

Angelucci E, Muretto P, Nicolucci A, et al. Effects of iron overload and hepatitis C virus positivity in determining progression of liver fibrosis in thalassemia following bone marrow transplantation. *Blood* 2002;100(1):17–21.
A study on rapid liver fibrosis progression following HCT in patients with HCV and iron overload.

Barshes NR, Myers GD, Lee D, et al. Liver transplantation for severe hepatic graft-versus-host disease: an analysis of aggregate survival data. *Liver Transpl* 2005;11(5):525–31.
A report on excellent outcomes of liver transplantation for refractory cases of GVHD.

Gooley TA, Rajvanshi P, Schoch HG, McDonald GB. Serum bilirubin levels and mortality after myeloablative allogeneic hematopoietic cell transplantation. *Hepatology* 2005;41(2):345–52.
A report showing that an acute rise in bilirubin early after HCT is associated with a significant predictor of mortality.

Hui CK, Lie A, Au WY, et al. Effectiveness of prophylactic anti-HBV therapy in allogeneic hematopoietic stem cell transplantation with HBsAg positive donors. *Am J Transplant* 2005;5(6):1437–45.
Prophylactic antiviral therapy for HCT recipients prevents HBV hepatitis from an HBsAg-positive donor.

Lau GK, Leung YH, Fong DY, et al. High hepatitis B virus (HBV) DNA viral load as the most important risk factor for HBV reactivation in patients positive for HBV surface antigen undergoing autologous hematopoietic cell transplantation. *Blood* 2002;99(7):2324–30.
Study showing that HBV DNA viremia correlates with the risk of HBV reactivation following HCT.

Strasser SI, Myerson D, Spurgeon CL, et al. Hepatitis C virus infection and bone marrow transplantation: a cohort study with 10-year follow-up. *Hepatology* 1999;29(6):1893–9.
Investigation into the association of hepatitis C virus with the development of sinusoidal obstruction syndrome.

Strasser SI, Sullivan KM, Myerson D, et al. Cirrhosis of the liver in long-term marrow transplant survivors. *Blood* 1999;93(10):3259–66.
Largest study on the incidence, etiologies, and outcomes of liver disease following HCT.

References

1. Socie G, Stone JV, Wingard JR, et al. Long-term survival and late deaths after allogeneic bone marrow transplantation. Late Effects Working Committee of the International Bone Marrow Transplant Registry. *N Engl J Med* 1999;341(1):14–21.

2. Strasser SI, McDonald GB. Hepatitis viruses and hematopoietic cell transplantation: a guide to patient and donor management. *Blood* 1999;93(4):1127–36.

3. Peffault de Latour R, Levy V, Asselah T, et al. Long-term outcome of hepatitis C infection after bone marrow transplantation. *Blood* 2004;103(5):1618–24.

4. Locasciulli A, Bacigalupo A, Alberti A, et al. Predictability before transplant of hepatic complications following allogeneic bone marrow transplantation. *Transplantation* 1989;48(1):68–72.

5. Gooley TA, Rajvanshi P, Schoch HG, McDonald GB. Serum bilirubin levels and mortality after myeloablative allogeneic hematopoietic cell transplantation. *Hepatology* 2005;41(2):345–52.

6. Shulman HM, Gooley T, Dudley MD, et al. Utility of transvenous liver biopsies and wedged hepatic venous pressure measurements in sixty marrow transplant recipients. *Transplantation* 1995;59(7):1015–22.

7. Picardi M, Muretto P, De Rosa G, et al. Color ultrasound-guided fine needle cutting biopsy for the characterization of diffuse liver damage in critical bone marrow transplanted patients. *Haematologica* 2002;87(6):652–7.

8. Ratanatharathorn V, Nash RA, Przepiorka D, et al. Phase III study comparing methotrexate and tacrolimus (prograf, FK506) with methotrexate and cyclosporine for graft-versus-host disease prophylaxis after HLA-identical sibling bone marrow transplantation. *Blood* 1998;92(7):2303–14.

9. Mielcarek M, Martin PJ, Leisenring W, et al. Graft-versus-host disease after nonmyeloablative versus conventional hematopoietic stem cell transplantation. *Blood* 2003;102(2):756–62.

10. Chao NJ, Schmidt GM, Niland JC, et al. Cyclosporine, methotrexate, and prednisone compared with cyclosporine and prednisone for prophylaxis of acute graft-versus-host disease. *N Engl J Med* 1993;329(17):1225–30.

11. Hahn T, McCarthy PL Jr, Zhang MJ, et al. Risk factors for acute graft-versus-host disease after human leukocyte antigen-identical sibling transplants for adults with leukemia. *J Clin Oncol* 2008;26(35):5728–34.

12. Carreras E, Granena A, Navasa M, et al. Transjugular liver biopsy in BMT. *Bone Marrow Transplant* 1993;11(1):21–6.

13. Shulman HM, Sharma P, Amos D, Fenster LF, McDonald GB. A coded histologic study of hepatic graft-versus-host disease after human bone marrow transplantation. *Hepatology* 1988;8(3):463–70.

14. Quaglia A, Duarte R, Patch D, Ngianga-Bakwin K, Dhillon AP. Histopathology of graft versus host disease of the liver. *Histopathology* 2007;50(6):727–38.

15. Robin M, Porcher R, de Castro R, et al. Initial liver involvement in acute GVHD is predictive for nonrelapse mortality. *Transplantation* 2009;88(9):1131–6.

16. Nash RA, Antin JH, Karanes C, et al. Phase 3 study comparing methotrexate and tacrolimus with methotrexate and cyclosporine for prophylaxis of acute graft-versus-host disease after marrow transplantation from unrelated donors. *Blood* 2000;96(6):2062–8.

17. Martin PJ, Schoch G, Fisher L, et al. A retrospective analysis of therapy for acute graft-versus-host disease: initial treatment. *Blood* 1990;76(8):1464–72.

18. Yanik G, Levine JE, Ratanatharathorn V, Dunn R, Ferrara J, Hutchinson RJ. Tacrolimus (FK506) and methotrexate as prophylaxis for acute graft-versus-host disease in pediatric allogeneic stem cell transplantation. *Bone Marrow Transplant* 2000;26(2):161–7.

19. Fay JW, Wingard JR, Antin JH, et al. FK506 (tacrolimus) monotherapy for prevention of graft-versus-host disease after histocompatible sibling allogenic bone marrow transplantation. *Blood* 1996;87(8):3514–19.

20. Perkins J, Field T, Kim J, et al. A randomized phase II trial comparing tacrolimus and mycophenolate mofetil to tacrolimus and methotrexate for acute graft-versus-host disease prophylaxis. *Biol Blood Marrow Transplant* 2010;16(7):937–47.

21. Ruutu T, Eriksson B, Remes K, et al. Ursodeoxycholic acid for the prevention of hepatic complications in allogeneic stem cell transplantation. *Blood* 2002;100(6):1977–83.

22. Moon JH, Kim SN, Kang BW, et al. Early onset of acute GVHD indicates worse outcome in terms of severity of chronic GVHD compared with late onset. *Bone Marrow Transplant* 2010;45(10):1540–5.

23. Deeg HJ, Storb R, Thomas ED, et al. Cyclosporine as prophylaxis for graft-versus-host disease: a randomized study in patients undergoing marrow transplantation for acute nonlymphoblastic leukemia. *Blood* 1985;65(6):1325–34.

24. Devine SM, Geller RB, Lin LB, et al. The outcome of unrelated donor bone marrow transplantation in patients with hematologic malignancies using tacrolimus (FK506) and low dose methotrexate for graft-versus-host disease prophylaxis. *Biol Blood Marrow Transplant* 1997;3(1):25–33.

25. MacMillan ML, Weisdorf DJ, Wagner JE, et al. Response of 443 patients to steroids as primary therapy for acute graft-versus-host disease: comparison of grading systems. *Biol Blood Marrow Transplant* 2002;8(7):387–94.

26. Kanojia MD, Anagnostou AA, Zander AR, et al. High-dose methylprednisolone treatment for acute graft-versus-host disease after bone marrow transplantation in adults. *Transplantation* 1984;37(3):246–9.

27. Wandroo F, Auguston B, Cook M, Craddock C, Mahendra P. Successful use of Campath-1H in the treatment of steroid refractory liver GvHD. *Bone Marrow Transplant* 2004;34(3):285–7.

28. Benito AI, Furlong T, Martin PJ, et al. Sirolimus (rapamycin) for the treatment of steroid-refractory acute graft-versus-host disease. *Transplantation* 2001;72(12):1924–9.

29. Barshes NR, Myers GD, Lee D, et al. Liver transplantation for severe hepatic graft-versus-host disease: an analysis of aggregate survival data. *Liver Transpl* 2005;11(5):525–31.

30. Ringden O, Ruutu T, Remberger M, et al. A randomized trial comparing busulfan with total body irradiation as conditioning in allogeneic marrow transplant recipients with leukemia: a report from the Nordic Bone Marrow Transplantation Group. *Blood* 1994;83(9):2723–30.

31. Higman MA, Vogelsang GB. Chronic graft versus host disease. *Br J Haematol* 2004;125(4):435–54.

32. MacDonald KP, Rowe V, Filippich C, et al. Chronic graft-versus-host disease after granulocyte colony-stimulating factor-mobilized allogeneic stem cell transplantation: the role of donor T-cell dose and differentiation. *Biol Blood Marrow Transplant* 2004;10(6):373–85.

33. Miglio F, Pignatelli M, Mazzeo V, et al. Expression of major histocompatibility complex class II antigens on bile duct epithelium in patients with hepatic graft-versus-host disease after bone marrow transplantation. *J Hepatol* 1987;5(2):182–9.

34. Ma SY, Au WY, Ng IO, et al. Hepatitic graft-versus-host disease after hematopoietic stem cell transplantation: clinicopathologic features and prognostic implication. *Transplantation* 2004;77(8):1252–9.

35. Chiba T, Yokosuka O, Kanda T, et al. Hepatic graft-versus-host disease resembling acute hepatitis: additional treatment with ursodeoxycholic acid. *Liver* 2002;22(6):514–17.

36. Wakae T, Takatsuka H, Seto Y, et al. Similarity between hepatic graft-versus-host disease and primary biliary cirrhosis. *Hematology* 2002;7(5):305–10.

37. Siegert W, Stemerowicz R, Hopf U. Antimitochondrial antibodies in patients with chronic graft-versus-host disease. *Bone Marrow Transplant* 1992;10(3):221–7.

38. Strasser SI, Shulman HM, Flowers ME, et al. Chronic graft-versus-host disease of the liver: presentation as an acute hepatitis. *Hepatology* 2000;32(6):1265–71.

39. Stewart BL, Storer B, Storek J, et al. Duration of immunosuppressive treatment for chronic graft-versus-host disease. *Blood* 2004;104(12):3501–6.

40. Kim JG, Sohn SK, Kim DH, et al. Different efficacy of mycophenolate mofetil as salvage treatment for acute and chronic GVHD after allogeneic stem cell transplant. *Eur J Haematol* 2004;73(1):56–61.

41. Busca A, Saroglia EM, Lanino E, et al. Mycophenolate mofetil (MMF) as therapy for refractory chronic GVHD (cGVHD) in chil-

42. Nagler A, Menachem Y, Ilan Y. Amelioration of steroid-resistant chronic graft-versus-host-mediated liver disease via tacrolimus treatment. *J Hematother Stem Cell Res* 2001;10(3):411–17.

43. Vogelsang GB. How I treat chronic graft-versus-host disease. *Blood* 2001;97(5):1196–201.

44. Shimizu T, Kasahara M, Tanaka K. Living-donor liver transplantation for chronic hepatic graft-versus-host disease. *N Engl J Med* 2006;354(14):1536–7.

45. Kumar S, DeLeve LD, Kamath PS, Tefferi A. Hepatic veno-occlusive disease (sinusoidal obstruction syndrome) after hematopoietic stem cell transplantation. *Mayo Clin Proc* 2003;78(5):589–98.

46. Hogan WJ, Maris M, Storer B, et al. Hepatic injury after nonmyeloablative conditioning followed by allogeneic hematopoietic cell transplantation: a study of 193 patients. *Blood* 2004;103(1):78–84.

47. McDonald GB, Sharma P, Matthews DE, Shulman HM, Thomas ED. Venocclusive disease of the liver after bone marrow transplantation: diagnosis, incidence, and predisposing factors. *Hepatology* 1984;4(1):116–22.

48. Jones RJ, Lee KS, Beschorner WE, et al. Venoocclusive disease of the liver following bone marrow transplantation. *Transplantation* 1987;44(6):778–83.

49. McDonald GB, Hinds MS, Fisher LD, et al. Veno-occlusive disease of the liver and multiorgan failure after bone marrow transplantation: a cohort study of 355 patients. *Ann Intern Med* 1993;118(4):255–67.

50. MacQuillan GC, Mutimer D. Fulminant liver failure due to severe veno-occlusive disease after haematopoietic cell transplantation: a depressing experience. *Q J Med* 2004;97(9):581–9.

51. Pihusch R, Salat C, Schmidt E, et al. Hemostatic complications in bone marrow transplantation: a retrospective analysis of 447 patients. *Transplantation* 2002;74(9):1303–9.

52. Litzow MR, Repoussis PD, Schroeder G, et al. Veno-occlusive disease of the liver after blood and marrow transplantation: analysis of pre- and post-transplant risk factors associated with severity and results of therapy with tissue plasminogen activator. *Leuk Lymphoma* 2002;43(11):2099–107.

53. Carreras E, Granena A, Navasa M, et al. On the reliability of clinical criteria for the diagnosis of hepatic veno-occlusive disease. *Ann Hematol* 1993;66(2):77–80.

54. DeLeve LD, Wang X. Role of oxidative stress and glutathione in busulfan toxicity in cultured murine hepatocytes. *Pharmacology* 2000;60(3):143–54.

55. Maradei SC, Maiolino A, de Azevedo AM, Colares M, Bouzas LF, Nucci M. Serum ferritin as risk factor for sinusoidal obstruction syndrome of the liver in patients undergoing hematopoietic stem cell transplantation. *Blood* 2009;114(6):1270–5.

56. El-Sayed MH, El-Haddad A, Fahmy OA, Salama, II, Mahmoud HK. Liver disease is a major cause of mortality following allogeneic bone-marrow transplantation. *Eur J Gastroenterol Hepatol* 2004;16(12):1347–54.

57. Dulley FL, Kanfer EJ, Appelbaum FR, et al. Venocclusive disease of the liver after chemoradiotherapy and autologous bone marrow transplantation. *Transplantation* 1987;43(6):870–3.

58. Shulman HM, Gown AM, Nugent DJ. Hepatic veno-occlusive disease after bone marrow transplantation. Immunohistochemical identification of the material within occluded central venules. *Am J Pathol* 1987;127(3):549–58.

59. Sato Y, Asada Y, Hara S, et al. Hepatic stellate cells (Ito cells) in veno-occlusive disease of the liver after allogeneic bone marrow transplantation. *Histopathology* 1999;34(1):66–70.

60. Shulman HM, Fisher LB, Schoch HG, Henne KW, McDonald GB. Veno-occlusive disease of the liver after marrow transplantation:

histological correlates of clinical signs and symptoms. *Hepatology* 1994;19(5):1171–81.

61. Shulman HM, McDonald GB, Matthews D, et al. An analysis of hepatic venocclusive disease and centrilobular hepatic degeneration following bone marrow transplantation. *Gastroenterology* 1980;79(6):1178–91.

62. Lassau N, Auperin A, Leclere J, Bennaceur A, Valteau-Couanet D, Hartmann O. Prognostic value of doppler-ultrasonography in hepatic veno-occlusive disease. *Transplantation* 2002;74(1):60–6.

63. Sharafuddin MJ, Foshager MC, Steinbuch M, Weisdorf DJ, Hunter DW. Sonographic findings in bone marrow transplant patients with symptomatic hepatic venoocclusive disease. *J Ultrasound Med* 1997;16(9):575–86.

64. Pegram AA, Kennedy LD. Prevention and treatment of veno-occlusive disease. *Ann Pharmacother* 2001;35(7–8):935–42.

65. Ohashi K, Tanabe J, Watanabe R, et al. The Japanese multicenter open randomized trial of ursodeoxycholic acid prophylaxis for hepatic veno-occlusive disease after stem cell transplantation. *Am J Hematol* 2000;64(1):32–8.

66. Essell JH, Schroeder MT, Harman GS, et al. Ursodiol prophylaxis against hepatic complications of allogeneic bone marrow transplantation. A randomized, double-blind, placebo-controlled trial. *Ann Intern Med* 1998;128(12):975–81.

67. Simon M, Hahn T, Ford LA, et al. Retrospective multivariate analysis of hepatic veno-occlusive disease after blood or marrow transplantation: possible beneficial use of low molecular weight heparin. *Bone Marrow Transplant* 2001;27(6):627–33.

68. Attal M, Huguet F, Rubie H, et al. Prevention of hepatic veno-occlusive disease after bone marrow transplantation by continuous infusion of low-dose heparin: a prospective, randomized trial. *Blood* 1992;79(11):2834–40.

69. Forrest DL, Thompson K, Dorcas VG, Couban SH, Pierce R. Low molecular weight heparin for the prevention of hepatic veno-occlusive disease (VOD) after hematopoietic stem cell transplantation: a prospective phase II study. *Bone Marrow Transplant* 2003;31(12):1143–9.

70. Chalandon Y, Roosnek E, Mermillod B, et al. Prevention of veno-occlusive disease with defibrotide after allogeneic stem cell transplantation. *Biol Blood Marrow Transplant* 2004;10(5):347–54.

71. Haussmann U, Fischer J, Eber S, Scherer F, Seger R, Gungor T. Hepatic veno-occlusive disease in pediatric stem cell transplantation: impact of pre-emptive antithrombin III replacement and combined antithrombin III/defibrotide therapy. *Haematologica* 2006;91(6):795–800.

72. Corbacioglu S, Greil J, Peters C, et al. Defibrotide in the treatment of children with veno-occlusive disease (VOD): a retrospective multicentre study demonstrates therapeutic efficacy upon early intervention. *Bone Marrow Transplant* 2004;33(2):189–95.

73. Sakai M, Strasser SI, Shulman HM, McDonald SJ, Schoch HG, McDonald GB. Severe hepatocellular injury after hematopoietic cell transplant: incidence, etiology and outcome. *Bone Marrow Transplant* 2009;44(7):441–7.

74. Coppell JA, Richardson PG, Soiffer R, et al. Hepatic veno-occlusive disease following stem cell transplantation: incidence, clinical course, and outcome. *Biol Blood Marrow Transplant* 2010;16(2):157–68.

75. Eissner G, Multhoff G, Gerbitz A, et al. Fludarabine induces apoptosis, activation, and allogenicity in human endothelial and epithelial cells: protective effect of defibrotide. *Blood* 2002;100(1):334–40.

76. Richardson PG, Murakami C, Jin Z, et al. Multi-institutional use of defibrotide in 88 patients after stem cell transplantation with severe veno-occlusive disease and multisystem organ failure: response without significant toxicity in a high-risk population and factors predictive of outcome. *Blood* 2002;100(13):4337–43.

77. Bajwa RP, Cant AJ, Abinun M, et al. Recombinant tissue plasminogen activator for treatment of hepatic veno-occlusive disease following bone marrow transplantation in children: effectiveness and a scoring system for initiating treatment. *Bone Marrow Transplant* 2003;31(7):591–7.

78. Kulkarni S, Rodriguez M, Lafuente A, et al. Recombinant tissue plasminogen activator (rtPA) for the treatment of hepatic veno-occlusive disease (VOD). *Bone Marrow Transplant* 1999;23(8):803–7.

79. Zenz T, Rossle M, Bertz H, Siegerstetter V, Ochs A, Finke J. Severe veno-occlusive disease after allogeneic bone marrow or peripheral stem cell transplantation – role of transjugular intrahepatic portosystemic shunt (TIPS). *Liver* 2001;21(1):31–6.

80. Azoulay D, Castaing D, Lemoine A, Hargreaves GM, Bismuth H. Transjugular intrahepatic portosystemic shunt (TIPS) for severe veno-occlusive disease of the liver following bone marrow transplantation. *Bone Marrow Transplant* 2000;25(9):987–92.

81. Membreno FE, Ortiz J, Foster PF, et al. Liver transplantation for sinusoidal obstructive syndrome (veno-occlusive disease): case report with review of the literature and the UNOS database. *Clin Transplant* 2008;22(4):397–404.

82. Knoll A, Boehm S, Hahn J, Holler E, Jilg W. Reactivation of resolved hepatitis B virus infection after allogeneic haematopoietic stem cell transplantation. *Bone Marrow Transplant* 2004;33(9):925–9.

83. Locasciulli A, Alberti A, Bandini G, et al. Allogeneic bone marrow transplantation from HBsAg+ donors: a multicenter study from the Gruppo Italiano Trapianto di Midollo Osseo (GITMO). *Blood* 1995;86(8):3236–40.

84. Lau GK, Lie AK, Kwong YL, et al. A case-controlled study on the use of HBsAg-positive donors for allogeneic hematopoietic cell transplantation. *Blood* 2000;96(2):452–8.

85. Locasciulli A, Testa M, Valsecchi MG, et al. The role of hepatitis C and B virus infections as risk factors for severe liver complications following allogeneic BMT: a prospective study by the Infectious Disease Working Party of the European Blood and Marrow Transplantation Group. *Transplantation* 1999;68(10):1486–91.

86. Goyama S, Kanda Y, Nannya Y, et al. Reverse seroconversion of hepatitis B virus after hematopoietic stem cell transplantation. *Leuk Lymphoma* 2002;43(11):2159–63.

87. Chen PM, Yao NS, Wu CM, et al. Detection of reactivation and genetic mutations of the hepatitis B virus in patients with chronic hepatitis B infections receiving hematopoietic stem cell transplantation. *Transplantation* 2002;74(2):182–8.

88. Lau HY, Obata T, Nagakura T, Chow SM. Some characteristics of mast cells cultured from human umbilical cord blood. *Inflamm Res* 2000;49(Suppl 1):S11–12.

89. Hui CK, Lie A, Au WY, et al. Effectiveness of prophylactic Anti-HBV therapy in allogeneic hematopoietic stem cell transplantation with HBsAg positive donors. *Am J Transplant* 2005;5(6):1437–45.

90. Lindemann M, Barsegian V, Runde V, et al. Transfer of humoral and cellular hepatitis B immunity by allogeneic hematopoietic cell transplantation. *Transplantation* 2003;75(6):833–8.

91. Ilan Y, Nagler A, Adler R, et al. Adoptive transfer of immunity to hepatitis B virus after T cell-depleted allogeneic bone marrow transplantation. *Hepatology* 1993;18(2):246–52.

92. Lau GK, Leung YH, Fong DY, et al. High hepatitis B virus (HBV) DNA viral load as the most important risk factor for HBV reactivation in patients positive for HBV surface antigen undergoing autologous hematopoietic cell transplantation. *Blood* 2002;99(7):2324–30.

93. Matsue K, Aoki T, Odawara J, et al. High risk of hepatitis B-virus reactivation after hematopoietic cell transplantation in hepatitis B core antibody-positive patients. *Eur J Haematol* 2009;83(4):357–64.

94. Seth P, Alrajhi AA, Kagevi I, et al. Hepatitis B virus reactivation with clinical flare in allogeneic stem cell transplants with chronic graft-versus-host disease. *Bone Marrow Transplant* 2002;30(3):189–94.

95. Kupeli S, Ozen H, Uckan D, et al. Changes in hepatitis B virus serology in bone marrow transplanted children. *Pediatr Transplant* 2002;6(5):406–10.

96. Onozawa M, Hashino S, Izumiyama K, et al. Progressive disappearance of anti-hepatitis B surface antigen antibody and reverse seroconversion after allogeneic hematopoietic stem cell transplantation in patients with previous hepatitis B virus infection. *Transplantation* 2005;79(5):616–19.

97. Picardi M, De Rosa G, Selleri C, Pane F, Rotoli B, Muretto P. Clinical relevance of intrahepatic hepatitis B virus DNA in HBsAg-negative HBcAb-positive patients undergoing hematopoietic stem cell transplantation for hematological malignancies. *Transplantation* 2006;82(1):141–2.

98. Palmore TN, Shah NL, Loomba R, et al. Reactivation of hepatitis B with reappearance of hepatitis B surface antigen after chemotherapy and immunosuppression. *Clin Gastroenterol Hepatol* 2009;7(10):1130–7.

99. Iwai K, Tashima M, Itoh M, et al. Fulminant hepatitis B following bone marrow transplantation in an HBsAg-negative, HBsAb-positive recipient; reactivation of dormant virus during the immunosuppressive period. *Bone Marrow Transplant* 2000;25(1):105–8.

100. Au WY, Lau GK, Lie AK, et al. Emergency living related liver transplantation for fulminant reactivation of hepatitis B virus after unrelated marrow transplantation. *Clin Transplant* 2003;17(2):121–5.

101. Francisci D, Falcinelli F, Schiaroli E, et al. Management of hepatitis B virus reactivation in patients with hematological malignancies treated with chemotherapy. *Infection* 2010;38(1):58–61.

102. Lau GK, He ML, Fong DY, et al. Preemptive use of lamivudine reduces hepatitis B exacerbation after allogeneic hematopoietic cell transplantation. *Hepatology* 2002;36(3):702–9.

103. Giaccone L, Festuccia M, Marengo A, et al. Hepatitis B virus reactivation and efficacy of prophylaxis with lamivudine in patients undergoing allogeneic stem cell transplantation. *Biol Blood Marrow Transplant* 2010;16(6):809–17.

104. Strasser SI, Myerson D, Spurgeon CL, et al. Hepatitis C virus infection and bone marrow transplantation: a cohort study with 10-year follow-up. *Hepatology* 1999;29(6):1893–9.

105. Akiyama H, Nakamura N, Tanikawa S, et al. Incidence and influence of GB virus C and hepatitis C virus infection in patients undergoing bone marrow transplantation. *Bone Marrow Transplant* 1998;21(11):1131–5.

106. Tomas JF, Pinilla I, Garcia-Buey ML, et al. Long-term liver dysfunction after allogeneic bone marrow transplantation: clinical features and course in 61 patients. *Bone Marrow Transplant* 2000;26(6):649–55.

107. Locasciulli A, Bacigalupo A, Vanlint MT, et al. Hepatitis C virus infection in patients undergoing allogeneic bone marrow transplantation. *Transplantation* 1991;52(2):315–18.

108. Peffault de Latour R, Ribaud P, Robin M, et al. Allogeneic hematopoietic cell transplant in HCV-infected patients. *J Hepatol* 2008;48(6):1008–17.

109. Giardini C, Galimberti M, Lucarelli G, et al. Alpha-interferon treatment of chronic hepatitis C after bone marrow transplantation for homozygous beta-thalassemia. *Bone Marrow Transplant* 1997;20(9):767–72.

110. Peffault de Latour R, Asselah T, Levy V, et al. Treatment of chronic hepatitis C virus in allogeneic bone marrow transplant recipients. *Bone Marrow Transplant* 2005;36(8):709–13.

111. Altes A, Remacha AF, Sureda A, et al. Iron overload might increase transplant-related mortality in haematopoietic stem cell transplantation. *Bone Marrow Transplant* 2002;29(12):987–9.

112. Majhail NS, DeFor T, Lazarus HM, Burns LJ. High prevalence of iron overload in adult allogeneic hematopoietic cell transplant survivors. *Biol Blood Marrow Transplant* 2008;14(7):790–4.

113. Alessandrino EP, Della Porta MG, Bacigalupo A, et al. Prognostic impact of pre-transplantation transfusion history and secondary iron overload in patients with myelodysplastic syndrome undergoing allogeneic stem cell transplantation: a GITMO study. *Haematologica* 95(3):476–84.

114. Lucarelli G, Angelucci E, Giardini C, et al. Fate of iron stores in thalassaemia after bone-marrow transplantation. *Lancet* 1993;342(8884):1388–91.

115. Kornreich L, Horev G, Yaniv I, Stein J, Grunebaum M, Zaizov R. Iron overload following bone marrow transplantation in children: MR findings. *Pediatr Radiol* 1997;27(11):869–72.

116. Li CK, Lai DH, Shing MM, Chik KW, Lee V, Yuen PM. Early iron reduction programme for thalassaemia patients after bone marrow transplantation. *Bone Marrow Transplant* 2000;25(6):653–6.

117. Moseley RH. Sepsis-associated cholestasis. *Gastroenterology* 1997;112(1):302–6.

118. Stanko RT, Nathan G, Mendelow H, Adibi SA. Development of hepatic cholestasis and fibrosis in patients with massive loss of intestine supported by prolonged parenteral nutrition. *Gastroenterology* 1987;92(1):197–202.

119. Amigues I, Cohen N, Chung D, et al. Hepatic safety of voriconazole after allogeneic hematopoietic stem cell transplantation. *Biol Blood Marrow Transplant* 2010;16(1):46–52.

120. Onozawa M, Hashino S, Haseyama Y, et al. Incidence and risk of postherpetic neuralgia after varicella zoster virus infection in hematopoietic cell transplantation recipients: Hokkaido Hematology Study Group. *Biol Blood Marrow Transplant* 2009;15(6):724–9.

121. Gruson D, Hilbert G, Le Bail B, et al. Fulminant hepatitis due to herpes simplex virus-type 2 in early phase of bone marrow transplantation. *Hematol Cell Ther* 1998;40(1):41–4.

122. Maeda Y, Teshima T, Yamada M, Harada M. Reactivation of human herpesviruses after allogeneic peripheral blood stem cell transplantation and bone marrow transplantation. *Leuk Lymphoma* 2000;39(3–4):229–39.

123. Norvell JP, Blei AT, Jovanovic BD, Levitsky J. Herpes simplex virus hepatitis: an analysis of the published literature and institutional cases. *Liver Transpl* 2007;13(10):1428–34.

124. Erard V, Wald A, Corey L, Leisenring WM, Boeckh M. Use of long-term suppressive acyclovir after hematopoietic stem-cell transplantation: impact on herpes simplex virus (HSV) disease and drug-resistant HSV disease. *J Infect Dis* 2007;196(2):266–70.

125. Boeckh M, Kim HW, Flowers ME, Meyers JD, Bowden RA. Long-term acyclovir for prevention of varicella zoster virus disease after allogeneic hematopoietic cell transplantation – a randomized double-blind placebo-controlled study. *Blood* 2006;107(5):1800–5.

126. David DS, Tegtmeier BR, O'Donnell MR, Paz IB, McCarty TM. Visceral varicella-zoster after bone marrow transplantation: report of a case series and review of the literature. *Am J Gastroenterol* 1998;93(5):810–13.

127. Leung TF, Chik KW, Li CK, et al. Incidence, risk factors and outcome of varicella-zoster virus infection in children after haematopoietic stem cell transplantation. *Bone Marrow Transplant* 2000;25(2):167–72.

128. Rogers SY, Irving W, Harris A, Russell NH. Visceral varicella zoster infection after bone marrow transplantation without skin involvement and the use of PCR for diagnosis. *Bone Marrow Transplant* 1995;15(5):805–7.

129. Morishita K, Kodo H, Asano S, Fujii H, Miwa S. Fulminant varicella hepatitis following bone marrow transplantation. *JAMA* 1985;253(4):511.

130. Hata A, Asanuma H, Rinki M, et al. Use of an inactivated varicella vaccine in recipients of hematopoietic-cell transplants. *N Engl J Med* 2002;347(1):26–34.

131. Hoshino Y, Kimura H, Tanaka N, et al. Prospective monitoring of the Epstein–Barr virus DNA by a real-time quantitative polymerase chain reaction after allogenic stem cell transplantation. *Br J Haematol* 2001;115(1):105–11.

132. Schonberger S, Meisel R, Adams O, et al. Prospective, comprehensive and effective viral monitoring in children undergoing allogeneic hematopoietic stem cell transplantation. *Biol Blood Marrow Transplant* 2010;16(10):1428–35.

133. Gruhn B, Meerbach A, Hafer R, Zell R, Wutzler P, Zintl F. Preemptive therapy with rituximab for prevention of Epstein–Barr virus-associated lymphoproliferative disease after hematopoietic stem cell transplantation. *Bone Marrow Transplant* 2003;31(11):1023–5.

134. van Esser JW, Niesters HG, van der Holt B, et al. Prevention of Epstein–Barr virus-lymphoproliferative disease by molecular monitoring and preemptive rituximab in high-risk patients after allogeneic stem cell transplantation. *Blood* 2002;99(12):4364–9.

135. Gustafsson A, Levitsky V, Zou JZ, et al. Epstein–Barr virus (EBV) load in bone marrow transplant recipients at risk to develop posttransplant lymphoproliferative disease: prophylactic infusion of EBV-specific cytotoxic T cells. *Blood* 2000;95(3):807–14.

136. Wakabayashi S, Ohashi K, Hanajiri R, et al. Rapidly progressive Epstein–Barr virus-associated lymphoproliferative disorder unpredictable by weekly viral load monitoring. *Intern Med* 2010;49(10):931–5.

137. Bowden RA, Slichter SJ, Sayers M, et al. A comparison of filtered leukocyte-reduced and cytomegalovirus (CMV) seronegative blood products for the prevention of transfusion-associated CMV infection after marrow transplant. *Blood* 1995;86(9):3598–603.

138. Ljungman P, de La Camara R, Milpied N, et al. Randomized study of valacyclovir as prophylaxis against cytomegalovirus reactivation in recipients of allogeneic bone marrow transplants. *Blood* 2002;99(8):3050–6.

139. Ljungman P, Lore K, Aschan J, et al. Use of a semi-quantitative PCR for cytomegalovirus DNA as a basis for pre-emptive antiviral therapy in allogeneic bone marrow transplant patients. *Bone Marrow Transplant* 1996;17(4):583–7.

140. Walter EA, Greenberg PD, Gilbert MJ, et al. Reconstitution of cellular immunity against cytomegalovirus in recipients of allogeneic bone marrow by transfer of T-cell clones from the donor. *N Engl J Med* 1995;333(16):1038–44.

141. Lau YL, Peiris M, Chan GC, Chan AC, Chiu D, Ha SY. Primary human herpes virus 6 infection transmitted from donor to recipient through bone marrow infusion. *Bone Marrow Transplant* 1998;21(10):1063–6.

142. Maeda Y, Teshima T, Yamada M, et al. Monitoring of human herpesviruses after allogeneic peripheral blood stem cell transplantation and bone marrow transplantation. *Br J Haematol* 1999;105(1):295–302.

143. Wang WH, Wang HL. Fulminant adenovirus hepatitis following bone marrow transplantation. A case report and brief review of the literature. *Arch Pathol Lab Med* 2003;127(5):e246–8.

144. Grigg AP, Brown M, Roberts AW, Szer J, Slavin MA. A pilot study of targeted itraconazole prophylaxis in patients with graft-versus-host disease at high risk of invasive mould infections following allogeneic stem cell transplantation. *Bone Marrow Transplant* 2004;34(5):447–53.

145. Wolff SN, Fay J, Stevens D, et al. Fluconazole vs low-dose amphotericin B for the prevention of fungal infections in patients undergoing bone marrow transplantation: a study of the North American Marrow Transplant Group. *Bone Marrow Transplant* 2000;25(8):853–9.

146. Ko CW, Murakami C, Sekijima JH, Kim MH, McDonald GB, Lee SP. Chemical composition of gallbladder sludge in patients after marrow transplantation. *Am J Gastroenterol* 1996;91(6):1207–10.

147. Murakami CS, Louie W, Chan GS, et al. Biliary obstruction in hematopoietic cell transplant recipients: an uncommon diagnosis with specific causes. *Bone Marrow Transplant* 1999;23(9):921–7.

148. Snover DC, Weisdorf S, Bloomer J, McGlave P, Weisdorf D. Nodular regenerative hyperplasia of the liver following bone marrow transplantation. *Hepatology* 1989;9(3):443–8.

149. Pezzullo L, Muretto P, De Rosa G, Picardi M, Lucania A, Rotoli B. Liver nodular regenerative hyperplasia after bone marrow transplant. *Haematologica* 2000;85(6):669–70.

Multiple choice questions

10.1 All of the following are considered risk factors for liver dysfunction following hematopoietic cell transplantation (HCT) except which one?

    a Donor HbsAg positivity.
    b Recipient HCV antibody positivity.
    c Abnormal donor or recipient liver aminotransferases.
    d Matched donor/recipient HCT.
    e High recipient ferritin level.

10.2 All of the following are important presenting features of sinusoidal obstruction syndrome (SOS) except which one?

    a Presence of weight gain and ascites.
    b Terminal hepatic venule occlusion on biopsy.
    c Elevated hepatic venous pressure gradient.
    d Hyperbilirubinemia.
    e Time period <21 days of HCT.

Answers to the multiple choice questions can be found in the Appendix at the end of the book.

These multiple choice questions are also available for you to complete online.
Visit http://www.schiffsdiseasesoftheliver.com/

CHAPTER 11
The Liver in Pregnancy

Yannick Bacq

Department of Hepatogastroenterology, Centre Hospitalier de Tours, Hôpital Trousseau, Tours, France

Key concepts

- During normal pregnancy, except for alkaline phosphatase, most values of serum liver tests remain below the upper normal limits established in nonpregnant women. Consequently, increased levels of aminotransferases, bilirubin, or serum bile acids usually indicate the presence of liver disease. By contrast, an increase in serum alkaline phosphatase in pregnancy is not specific for liver disease because it may be of placental origin.

- The liver disorders that occur in pregnancy can be divided into three groups: (i) liver diseases that are specifically pregnancy related; (ii) intercurrent liver diseases in pregnancy, i.e., acute liver disease occurring during pregnancy; and (iii) chronic liver diseases that may be revealed by pregnancy, or more often diagnosed fortuitously during pregnancy

- It is essential that liver disease in pregnancy is recognized and understood because certain disorders can threaten the lives of both mother and infant.

- Liver disorders unique to pregnancy include the exceptional primary hepatic pregnancy, liver dysfunction associated with hyperemesis gravidarum, intrahepatic cholestasis of pregnancy (ICP), liver disorders of preeclampsia including HELLP syndrome (hemolysis, elevated liver enzymes, and low platelets), and acute fatty liver of pregnancy (AFLP).

- ICP is a benign disease for the mother, but carries a risk for the baby because of the possibility of premature delivery and sudden fetal death. Generalized pruritus is the main symptom. Serum bile acid and aminotransferase levels are increased, although the γ-glutamyl transpeptidase levels may be normal or only slightly increased.

- AFLP is a form of hepatic failure associated with coagulopathy and occasionally encephalopathy and hypoglycemia. An association has been found between AFLP and a defect of long-chain 3-hydroxyacyl coenzyme A dehydrogenase (LCHAD) in the fetus. Women in whom AFLP develops and their offspring should undergo DNA testing for the main associated genetic mutation (c.1528G>C) in the gene coding for LCHAD.

- Certain liver diseases that can occur in anyone, pregnant or not, are more severe during pregnancy, for example, viral hepatitis E and herpes simplex hepatitis. Other disorders can be precipitated by pregnancy or during postpartum, such as cholelithiasis and Budd–Chiari syndrome.

- Pregnancy in patients with advanced chronic liver disease is rare, although patients with treatable liver diseases, such as autoimmune hepatitis and Wilson disease, may regain fertility and should be maintained on their treatment during gestation. By contrast, successful pregnancy in patients with mild chronic liver disease, such as viral hepatitis B or C, is common. Pregnancy after liver transplantation may be associated with prematurity and increased maternal complications, but not with teratogenicity.

Liver disease in a pregnant woman can make the consulting physician uneasy. Most gastroenterologists and hepatologists are unfamiliar with the pregnant state and the liver diseases associated with it, and pregnancy is rarely seen in patients with severe chronic liver disease. Also, the stakes are higher for these patients, given the presence of a second life in the form of the fetus. The distress on the part of the consultant is well founded because pregnancy is a state of altered, albeit normal, physiology. Certain disorders of the liver are unique to pregnancy and are not comparable with liver diseases in nonpregnant patients. Furthermore, some conditions that can affect anyone, pregnant or not, may follow an unusually severe course in the pregnant woman. Despite these problems, the care of these otherwise young and healthy women is gratifying, and most return to good health simply by being delivered. Recent advances in our understanding of liver diseases during pregnancy have rationalized the approach to these patients.

The liver in normal pregnancy

The changes involving the liver during normal pregnancy have been discussed in a review of the literature [1].

Schiff's Diseases of the Liver, Eleventh Edition. Edited by Eugene R. Schiff, Willis C. Maddrey and Michael F. Sorrell.
© 2012 John Wiley & Sons, Ltd. Published 2012 by John Wiley & Sons, Ltd.

Physical examination

Spider angiomata and palmar erythema are common during pregnancy and usually disappear after delivery. In late pregnancy, physical examination of the liver is difficult because of the expanding uterus.

Ultrasonographic examination

Ultrasonographic examination reveals no dilatation of the biliary tract, but increases in fasting gallbladder volume and residual volume after contraction are noted.

Pathology

Standard and ultrastructural examination of the liver during normal pregnancy reveals no or minimal abnormalities.

Hemodynamics

The plasma volume increases steadily between weeks 6 and 36 of gestation (by about 50%). The red cell volume also increases, but the increase is moderate (about 20%) and delayed. Consequently, the total blood volume increases with hemodilution reflected by a decrease in the hematocrit. It is necessary to bear this phenomenon of hemodilution in mind during an interpretation of serum concentrations during pregnancy. The plasma volume and red cell volume decrease rapidly after the termination of pregnancy, aided by the loss of blood at delivery. Cardiac output increases until the second trimester, then decreases and normalizes near term. Absolute hepatic blood flow remains unchanged, but the percentage of cardiac output to the liver decreases.

Serum protein and lipids

The serum albumin levels decrease during the first trimester, and this decrease becomes more accentuated as the pregnancy advances. However, the serum concentrations of some proteins increase, such as α_2-macroglobulin, ceruloplasmin, and fibrinogen. The serum cholesterol and triglyceride concentrations increase markedly during pregnancy, and measurement of these serum lipid concentrations is rarely useful during pregnancy. The prothrombin time is unchanged during pregnancy, and the fibrinogen level increases in late pregnancy.

Liver tests

A knowledge of the changes associated with normal pregnancies is necessary for the interpretation of liver test values and the management of liver diseases during pregnancy [2]. The serum alkaline phosphatase levels increase late in pregnancy, mainly during the third trimester, as a result of production of the placental isoenzyme and an increase in the bone isoenzyme. In the majority of published studies, the serum levels of alanine aminotransferase (ALT) and aspartate aminotransferase (AST) remain within normal limits during pregnancy. Serum γ-glutamyltransferase (GGT) activity decreases slightly during late pregnancy. The total and free bilirubin concentrations are lower than in nonpregnant controls during all three trimesters, as are the concentrations of conjugated bilirubin during the second and third trimesters. The serum 5'-nucleotidase activity is normal or slightly higher during the second and third trimesters than in nonpregnant women. Fasting serum total bile acid concentrations usually remain within normal limits, and their routine measurement remains useful for the diagnosis of cholestasis during pregnancy, especially when routine liver tests are still within normal limits. Thus, increased values of serum ALT and AST activity, serum bilirubin, and fasting total bile acid concentrations should be considered pathologic, as they are in nonpregnant women, and prompt further evaluation. The main changes in liver function tests during normal pregnancy compared to nonpregnant women are summarized in Box 11.1.

Liver diseases unique to pregnancy

The liver diseases unique to pregnancy include primary hepatic pregnancy, hyperemesis gravidarum, intrahepatic cholestasis of pregnancy (ICP), the liver disorders of preeclampsia with HELLP syndrome (hemolysis, elevated liver enzymes, and low platelets), and acute fatty liver of pregnancy (AFLP). The main factors of diagnosis

---

Box 11.1 Liver tests in normal pregnancy.

Tests not affected by pregnancy
- Serum aminotransferase levels (aspartate aminotransferase, alanine aminotransferase)
- Prothrombin time
- Serum concentration of total bile acids (fasting state)

Tests affected by pregnancy[a]
- Serum albumin levels (decreased from the first trimester)
- Alkaline phophatase levels (increased in the second and above all in the third trimester)
- Serum bilirubin levels (slightly decreased from the first trimester)
- 5' nucleotidase levels (slightly increased)
- γ-Glutamyltransferase levels (slightly decreased in late pregnancy)

[a]Increased or decreased in relation to values in nonpregnant women.

of liver disease in pregnancy are given in Box 11.2. Gestational age at the time of the onset of signs and symptoms can be helpful in the differential diagnosis. Hyperemesis gravidarum begins in the early part of the first trimester. ICP usually does not present until the second or third trimester. Preeclampsia is a disorder of the second half of pregnancy, and patients with HELLP syndrome usually present in the third trimester. Similarly, AFLP, which can be associated with preeclampsia, is usually a disorder of the third trimester of pregnancy. The main signs and symptoms of these liver diseases are given in Box 11.3.

Primary hepatic pregnancy

On exceedingly rare occasions, the inferior surface of the right lobe of the liver is the site of ectopic implantation. Such patients may present early in gestation with hemoperitoneum resulting from hepatic hemorrhage. If the pregnancy progresses toward term, the patient presents with a mass in the liver. Primary hepatic pregnancy can be diagnosed by ultrasound examination or computed tomography (CT) scan (Fig. 11.1) and termination of pregnancy by laparotomy is recommended in view of the risk of rupture.

Hyperemesis gravidarum

Nausea and vomiting are common symptoms of early pregnancy, occurring in up to 50% of all pregnancies and corresponding to "morning sickness." By contrast hyperemesis gravidarum occurs much less frequently, complicating about 0.5–1.5% of pregnancies [3,4]. There is no clear demarcation between common symptoms and severe forms, and thus there is no universally accepted definition. Hyperemesis gravidarum can be defined as persistent vomiting associated with weight loss greater than 5% of prepregnancy body weight, and large ketonuria [4]. Hyperemesis gravidarum leads to dehydration, and hospitalization is usually required. Liver involvement as described below is common in this condition [5].

Pathology

Liver biopsy is rarely needed to confirm this diagnosis, given its typical clinical presentation. When performed, it shows surprisingly little. There is no inflammation, but centrilobular vacuolization, necrosis with cell dropout, and rare bile plugs may be seen [6].

Clinical and biochemical findings

This disorder presents early in the first trimester of pregnancy, during weeks 4–10 of gestation, with intractable nausea and vomiting. As a rule, it resolves by the 20th week, regardless of therapy. It is more common during a first pregnancy than in multiparous women. In the modern era, liver disease is inconspicuous and jaundice is rare. This was not the case before the widespread use of intravenous fluids; for example, Charlotte Brontë, the author of *Jane Eyre*, died in 1855 with nausea, vomiting, and jaundice during the fourth month of her first pregnancy.

When the liver is involved, the most striking abnormality is the elevation of aminotransferase levels, with ALT levels exceeding AST levels as usual in nonalcoholic and noncirrhotic liver diseases. ALT levels are greatly variable and may be as high as 1,000 IU/L. Increases in bilirubin can occur. When the patient is treated with gut rest and

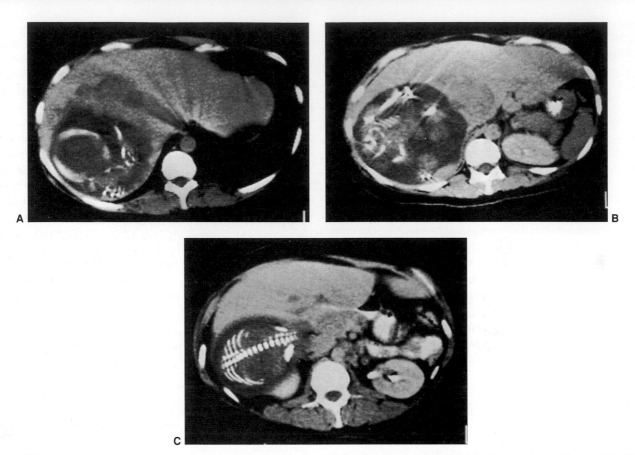

Figure 11.1 Intrahepatic pregnancy demonstrated by computed tomography. (A) A cut from below the dome of the liver showing skull bones of the fetus and the placenta invading the hepatic substance. (B, C) Lower cuts demonstrating fetal position with the spine protruding from the inferior surface of the liver. (Courtesy of Professor Caroline A. Riely.)

intravenous fluids, the abnormalities resolve. Pregnancies complicated by hyperemesis gravidarum have been associated with transient hyperthyroidism [7].

Affected patients may be thought to have hepatitis or gastric outlet obstruction resulting from peptic ulcer disease. Hepatitis serologies are always useful in the differential diagnosis. Abdominal pain is not a typical complaint.

Maternal and fetal outcome

Many affected patients respond to rehydration and a short period of gut rest followed by reintroduction of a diet rich in carbohydrates and low in fat. Thiamine supplementation is recommended especially for women who have vomited for several weeks to prevent Wernicke encephalopathy. Antiemetics including antihistamines (H1 receptor antagonists such as promethazine, cyclizine, doxylamine, and dimenhydrinate) and metoclopramide have a good safety during pregnancy and may be useful [8]. Ondesantron has also been proposed in this condition [9]. Intravenous corticosteroid treatment for hyperemesis gravidarum remains controversial and should be

reserved for more severe refractory cases [8]. Enteral nutrition via gastric or duodenal intubation is effective and preferable to the parenteral route [10]. Despite the severity of the illness and attendant weight loss, infants born following affected pregnancies usually do not differ in regard to birth weight, gestational age, and birth defects from infants born following pregnancies unaffected by hyperemesis gravidarum [3,11].

Pathophysiology

Hyperemesis gravidarum is a complex disease and the exact cause is unknown. Various associations, including infection with *Helicobacter pylori* and anatomic and hormonal factors, have been reported with this condition [8]. The pathogenesis of hyperemesis gravidarum is also unclear, but the liver involvement, like the thyroid involvement noted above, appears to be secondary to the disorder itself and not a causative factor.

Intrahepatic cholestasis of pregnancy

Intrahepatic cholestasis of pregnancy usually occurs during the second or third trimester and disappears spontaneously after delivery. The prevalence of ICP varies widely by country [12,13]. The highest frequencies have been reported in Bolivia and Chile. In Chile, the prevalence in 1974–1975 was reported to be 15.6%, ranging from 11.8% to 27.7% according to ethnic origin [14]. For unknown reasons, the prevalence has more recently appeared to decrease (to between 4.0% and 6.5%) [15,16]. In the United States, the prevalence has been estimated from 0.3% to 5.6% according to ethnic origin [17,18]. The prevalence is Europe is about 0.5–1.5% [13]. Generally, ICP is more common in twin pregnancies [19].

Pathology

Liver biopsy is rarely necessary for the diagnosis. Histopathology is characterized by pure cholestasis, sometimes with bile plugs in the hepatocytes and canaliculi, predominantly in zone 3. Inflammation and necrosis are not usually observed, and the portal tracts are unaffected [20].

Clinical and biochemical findings

Pruritus, which is the main symptom, is very uncomfortable and difficult to tolerate. It is often generalized but predominates on the palms and soles. It is more severe at night and disturbs sleep. Pruritus usually disappears within the first few days following delivery. The clinical examination findings are normal except for evidence of scratching. Fever, if present, is usually caused by an associated urinary tract infection. About 10% of patients have jaundice. The greater frequency of jaundice in some studies may be a consequence of concomitant urinary tract infection [21]. ICP with jaundice but without pruritus is rare [22]. Patients do not experience abdominal pain or encephalopathy. Ultrasonographic examination reveals no dilatation of the biliary tract, but may show gallstones.

Measurement of serum ALT activity is a sensitive test for the diagnosis of ICP. Patients with ICP frequently exhibit very significant increases in serum ALT activity that suggests acute viral hepatitis, which should be ruled out with suitable serologic tests [22]. Liver histology does not reveal necrotic lesions, and the ALT elevations may be secondary to an increase in membrane permeability. The serum GGT activity is normal or only slightly increased [22]. The serum bile acid concentrations are increased, and may be the first or only laboratory abnormality [22,23]. A relationship between maternal serum bile acid levels and fetal distress has been found [24], and evaluation of the serum bile acid concentration has been suggested as a mean of fetal assessment in patients with ICP [25]. At the present time, however, no consensus has been reached concerning the usefulness of evaluating the serum bile acid concentrations in the obstetric management of patients with ICP [26]. Little or no correlation

has been found between the serum total bile acid concentration and other liver test values [22]. The serum bile acid concentration and serum ALT activity decrease rapidly after delivery and, as a rule, normalize in a few weeks. Recently the measurement of serum glutathione-S-transferase, a maker of hepatocellular integrity, has been proposed to distinguish ICP from "benign pruritus gravidarum" [27]. The prothrombin time is usually normal. It may become abnormal in severe cholestasis with jaundice or in patients who have been treated with cholestyramine. The abnormality is caused by vitamin K deficiency, which should be anticipated and treated before delivery to prevent hemorrhage. Such therapy contributes to a good maternal prognosis.

Maternal and fetal outcome

Cholestasis frequently recurs in subsequent pregnancies. As a rule, the long-term maternal prognosis is good. However, a recent longitudinal retrospective population-based cohort study, from Finland, suggests reconsidering the long-term follow-up of patients suffering from ICP [28]. Patients with a history of ICP (10,504 women during the years 1972–2000) and 10,504 women with normal pregnancies (controls) were matched for age, time of delivery, and place of delivery. The results show an association of ICP with several liver diseases: hepatitis C, gallstones and cholecystitis, nonalcoholic pancreatitis, and nonalcoholic liver cirrhosis including cases of primary biliary cirrhosis [28].This large study questions the diagnosis of "true" ICP and confirms the importance of determining whether normalization of liver tests occurs after delivery in any woman suffering from cholestasis during pregnancy. This study confirms also the association between hepatitis C and ICP previously reported [29,30], and the importance of checking viral hepatitis serologies (especially hepatitis C) in any pregnant woman with elevated serum ALT.

ICP does carry a risk for the fetus [31]. The main complication of ICP is prematurity, which is more frequent in patients with ICP than in the general population [16]. The rate of prematurity varies greatly according to the study and may be increased because of the high rate of multiple pregnancies in patients with ICP [22]. The other complication of ICP is the risk of sudden fetal death. The prevalence is about 1% but varies according to studies. Sudden fetal death rarely occurs before the last month of pregnancy.

The administration of oral contraceptives to women with a history of ICP may rarely result in cholestasis, but ICP is not a contraindication for their use [22]. Oral contraception (either combined contraceptives with a low dose of estrogen, or progestin-only contraceptives) can be started after the liver test values have normalized. The patient should be informed of the possibility of cholestasis (abnormal liver tests with or without pruritus) during subsequent use of contraception.

Pathophysiology

The cause of ICP is unknown. The results of previous epidemiologic and clinical studies suggest that genetic, hormonal, and exogenous factors all play a role [32]. Genomic variants (mutations or polymorphisms) in genes coding for several hepatobiliary transporters were found in patients with ICP. The *ABCB4* gene encodes the multidrug resistance 3 P-glycoprotein (MDR3 P-glycoprotein) or ABCB4, which is the translocator of phosphatidylcholine across the canalicular membrane into bile. In the absence of phospholipids in bile, bile acids can injure the canalicular membrane, leading to cholestasis [33]. A non-sense mutation of the *ABCB4* gene has been found in a child with progressive familial intrahepatic cholestasis type 3 (PFIC3) and in three mothers suffering from cholestasis during pregnancy [34]. In this familial study, the infant with PFIC3 was homozygous for the ABCB4 mutations, whereas the mothers with ICP were heterozygous. Non-sense mutations in the *ABCB4* gene were then found in patients with ICP in a number of studies [35–38]. The prevalence of such mutations in Caucasian patients with a clearly defined phenotype of ICP was estimated to 16% [39]. Mutations in the *ABCB11* gene, which encodes the bile salt export pump (BSEP), have been found in only 1% of European patients with ICP [40]. However, one particular polymorphism in *ABCB11* (c.1331C>T, V444A) has been identified as a risk factor for ICP, suggesting a role for this gene in the pathogenesis of ICP [40]. Defects in the *ATP8B1* gene, which is associated with progressive familial intrahepatic cholestasis type 1 (PFIC1) and benign recurrent intrahepatic cholestasis (BRIC), have also been found in patients with ICP but it seems that this gene is not a major contributor to ICP [41].

A role of estrogens in ICP has been clearly established. Animal studies have shown that estrogens, in particular ethynyl estradiol, are cholestatic. Genetically determined abnormalities may lead to unique hepatic reactions to estrogens or to dysfunction of estrogen metabolism [32]. Progesterone metabolism is also involved in the pathophysiology. Abnormalities of progesterone metabolism, especially elevated levels of serum sulfated metabolites, have been found in women with ICP [42]. The formation of large amounts of sulfated progesterone metabolites, possibly related to greater 5α and 3α reduction, may in some genetically predisposed women result in a saturation of the hepatic transport system(s) involved in the biliary excretion of these compounds [43]. One study has shown that oral natural progesterone prescribed for threatened premature delivery can trigger ICP in predisposed women [22]. The intake of progesterone may place an additional load on the transport system of the sulfated metabolites. Progesterone treatment should therefore be avoided in pregnant women, especially late in pregnancy or when the patient has a history of ICP.

Some characteristics of ICP suggest that exogenous factors may be associated with an underlying genetic predisposition: (i) ICP recurs in only 60–70% of pregnancies in multiparous women; (ii) seasonal variability has been observed in several countries; and (iii) the prevalence of ICP has decreased in Chile. For example, a deficiency in selenium may be a factor involved in the pathophysiology of ICP [44].

Medical and obstetric Management

Hydroxyzine (25–50 mg/day) may alleviate the discomfort of pruritus. Cholestyramine (8–16 g/day) decreases the ileal absorption and increases the fecal excretion of bile salts. Its effect on pruritus is limited in patients with ICP. The efficacy of S-adenosyl-L-methionine is a matter of debate [15,45,46]. Currently, the most effective medical treatment is ursodeoxycholic acid [46–54]. Ursodeoxycholic acid relieves pruritus and improves liver function test values (Fig. 11.2). Ursodeoxycholic acid may also prevent prematurity. No side effects have been reported for mothers or babies [55]. Thus, ursodeoxycholic acid (usually 500 mg twice a day or 15 mg/kg/day) appears to be safe during late pregnancy and may be useful in improving liver tests and relieving cholestasis. The mechanism of the beneficial effect of ursodeoxycholic acid for the mother and the baby in ICP remains speculative. As in chronic liver diseases, ursodeoxycholic acid, which is a hydrophilic bile acid, may decrease signs of cholestasis in the mother by providing cytoprotection against the hepatotoxic effects of the hydrophobic bile acids, and by improving the hepatobiliary bile acid transport. In ICP, ursodeoxycholic acid may also have a specific effect by improving the transport of bile acid across the placenta.

It is often difficult to decide the best time for delivery and no consensus has been clearly established [56,57]; there are no randomized clinical trials to try and establish best obstetric management [58]. When cholestasis is severe (e.g., if the patient has clinical jaundice), delivery has been recommended at 36 weeks of gestation if the fetal lungs have matured, or as soon thereafter as possible [16].

Preeclampsia liver disorders

Liver disorders associated with preeclampsia are certainly the most frequent causes of liver abnormalities occurring during pregnancy [59]. Preeclampsia is a common complication of pregnancy (2–7% in healthy nulliparous women) and is a major cause of maternal and perinatal morbidities [60]. A variety of genetic and/or immunologic factors are suspected of playing a role in

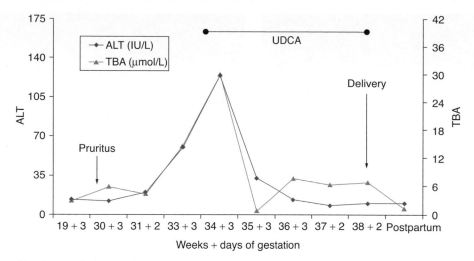

Figure 11.2 Treatment of intrahepatic cholestasis of pregnancy (ICP) with ursodeoxycholic acid (UDCA). This patient had experienced ICP during a previous pregnancy. Regular surveillance during the current pregnancy was proposed and once the diagnosis of recurrent ICP had been confirmed, treatment with UDCA was initiated. Serum total bile acid concentration (TBA, upper normal limit: 6 μmol/L) and serum alanine aminotransferase activity (ALT, upper normal limit: 35 IU/L) improved and the patient delivered at 38 weeks of gestation.

the mechanisms of this enigmatic disease [60–62]. The disease is thought to start early in pregnancy, with abnormal implantation of the trophoblast, which leads to restricted perfusion of the placenta. The fall in systemic vascular resistance typical of normal pregnancy does not occur in patients with preeclampsia; their sensitivity to vasospasm is enhanced, with resultant poor perfusion of and injury to a variety of organs, including the liver. Some risk factors for developing preeclampsia have been identified. In a systematic review of controlled studies, the most significant risk factors are a history of preeclampsia and the presence of antiphospholipid antibodies [63]. In the same study, the following factors clearly also increase the risk of preeclampsia: preexisting diabetes and prepregnancy body mass index (BMI) >35 kg/m^2, nulliparity, a family history of preeclampsia, a twin pregnancy, maternal age $\geq$40 years, booking BMI $\geq$35 kg/m^2, and hypertension (systolic blood pressure $\geq$130 mmHg) at the booking visit.

The typical presentation of preeclampsia is hypertension with proteinuria, presenting in the latter half of pregnancy. However, both conditions are not found in all patients with this multisystem disease. Patients may also have renal failure, seizures (eclampsia), pancreatitis, or pulmonary edema. Preeclampsia has long been known to affect the liver in a variety of ways including HELLP syndrome [64].

HELLP syndrome

The HELLP syndrome is defined as hemolysis (usually subclinical, with characteristic schistocytes and burr cells on a smear test), elevated liver enzymes (usually elevated aminotransferases), and low platelets [65]. Affected

women are less likely to be primiparous and tend to be older than the average woman with preeclampsia [64]. The hepatic histology is that of preeclamptic liver disease, with periportal hemorrhage and fibrin deposition. Little correlation is found between the degree of histologic aberration and the severity of the clinical findings. Fat may be seen, but as macrovesicular fat distributed in modest quantities throughout the liver lobule, not as the microvesicular centrizonal fat typical of AFLP [66]. Despite similar settings and occasional clinical overlap, these two conditions are histologically distinct [67].

The clinical presentation of HELLP varies markedly, with no symptom other than abdominal pain recorded in more than 50% of patients [68] The pain is usually located in the midepigastric, right upper quadrant, or substernal regions. Many patients have nausea, vomiting, and malaise, which suggest a diagnosis of viral hepatitis. Jaundice is present in about 5% of patients [68]. The majority of cases are diagnosed during the third trimester, although the condition may present postpartum. In a large series of 437 patients who had 442 pregnancies with HELLP syndrome, 70% of cases occurred before delivery and 30% after delivery; 11% developed before 27 weeks' gestation and 18% after 37 weeks [68]. Most, but not all, patients have the hypertension and proteinuria typical of preeclampsia. The diagnosis usually rests on clinical grounds, although imaging studies, particularly CT (Fig. 11.3) and magnetic resonance imaging (MRI), are useful in detecting the complications of hepatic infarct, hematoma, and rupture [69]. The outcome for mothers is generally good, but serious complications are relatively common. The maternal mortality rate was 1.1% in a large

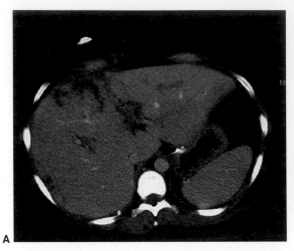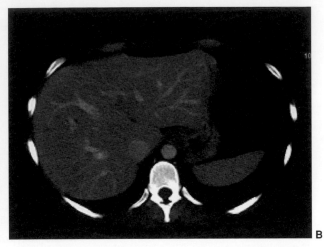

Figure 11.3 Hepatic involvement in a 24-year-old primipara with severe preeclampsia. (A) Abdominal computed tomography performed after delivery by cesarean section showing subcapsular ischemic lesions in the right lobe. (B) Follow-up image 7 months later showing complete recovery. (Courtesy of Dr Béatrice Scotto.)

series [68]. Rarely, patients may require liver transplantation [70]. The main risk for the fetus is prematurity.

Management is supportive and may include transfer to a medical intensive care unit, with ventilatory support and dialysis provided in severe cases. The cornerstone of therapy is early delivery, which is generally indicated, although temporizing management (24–48 hours) with intensive monitoring may be discussed before 34 weeks' gestation for some patients without fetal or maternal distress [64]. The condition starts to reverse with delivery. Long-term follow-up has shown an increased risk of obstetric complications in subsequent pregnancies, but no tendency for a repetition of the HELLP syndrome [71].

Hepatic hematoma and rupture

In rare pregnant patients, a hematoma develops beneath the Glisson capsule. This may remain contained, or rupture of the liver capsule may result in hemorrhage into the peritoneal cavity from multiple lacerations where the capsule has been lifted from the surface. Rupture usually occurs in the setting of the HELLP syndrome. Some patients do not have thrombocytopenia or typical preeclampsia [72]. Clinically, affected patients have abdominal pain and, when the liver has ruptured, swelling of the belly from hemoperitoneum, along with shock. The aminotransferase levels are usually slightly raised, but values in the range of 4,000–5,000 IU are seen occasionally [64]. CT or MRI of the body is more dependable than ultrasonography for detecting these lesions [69]. The management of a contained hematoma is supportive. If a rupture of hematoma is confirmed, transfusions, and radiological hemostatic measures or laparotomy are indicated. Liver transplantation has been used when the hemorrhage could not be contained [64]. Such patients are

thus best managed by a team experienced in liver surgery including liver transplantation [73]. Patients who survive have no hepatic sequelae and have been documented to have normal subsequent pregnancies [71].

Acute fatty liver of pregnancy

Acute fatty liver of pregnancy was distinguished as a specific clinical entity unique to pregnancy in 1940 [74]. Early diagnosis and prompt delivery have dramatically improved both maternal and fetal prognosis [75]. AFLP is a rare disease, and incidence has been evaluated at between 1 per 7,000 and 1 per 20,000 deliveries. The incidence was initially estimated to be 1 per 13,328 deliveries at the Los Angeles County University of Southern California Medical Center [76], and more recently to be 1 in 6,659 births in the same center [77]. The incidence was estimated to be 1 per 15,900 deliveries in Santiago, Chile [78]. In the United Kingdom, a large population-based study that included 1,132,964 pregnancies between 2005 and 2006 diagnosed 57 women with AFLP, i.e., about 1 case per 20,000 pregnancies [79].

Pathology

Liver biopsy is the best way to confirm the diagnosis of AFLP, but because it is invasive it is not always performed. Also, we can now take advantage of noninvasive procedures to demonstrate fat in the liver and exclude other liver diseases, such as viral hepatitis. Nevertheless, liver biopsy may be useful in atypical cases, especially if the appropriate treatment (delivery) is being delayed.

The overall architecture of the liver is not altered. The characteristic picture is a microvesicular fatty infiltration of the hepatocytes, which are swollen. The droplets are minute and surround centrally located nuclei, so that

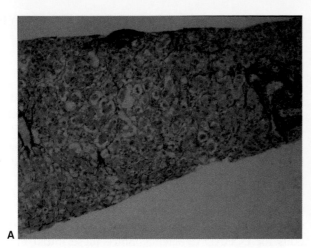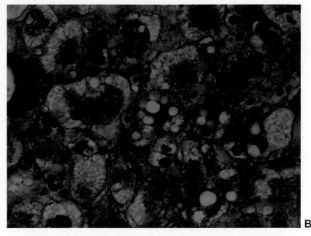

A   B

Figure 11.4 Acute fatty liver of pregnancy in a 24-year-old primipara. This woman had experienced nausea and vomiting, abdominal pains, and jaundice in late pregnancy. A transvenous liver biopsy was performed postpartum showing. (A) intact lobular architecture (hematoxylin and eosin, original ×200), and (B) typical microvesicular fatty infiltration in hepatocytes and features of cholestasis (original ×400). (Courtesy of Dr Anne de Muret.)

the cytoplasm has a foamy appearance (Fig. 11.4). In a few cases, rare, large fat vacuoles are associated with the microvesicular steatosis. The microvesicular fatty infiltration is most prominent in the pericentral zones and midzones (zones 2 and 3) and usually spares a rim of periportal cells. The droplets stain with oil red O, which is specific for fat. The histologic features of cholestasis (i.e., bile thrombi or bile deposits within hepatocytes) are common. Inflammation is not prominent but is also common [80]. The histologic features are not always evident, and cases of AFLP have been misdiagnosed as hepatitis. Necrosis with acidophilic bodies is inconspicuous, and massive panlobular hepatocellular necrosis, as in fulminant viral hepatitis, is not seen. Electron microscopy confirms the presence of fat droplets and has shown nonspecific changes in mitochondrial size and shape [81]. A stain specific for fat or electron microscopy is useful for pathologic confirmation of the diagnosis in patients with ballooning of the cytoplasm but no evident vacuolization. Therefore, whenever AFLP is suspected, a piece of the liver biopsy specimen should be reserved before paraffin embedding and processed appropriately with special stains to confirm the presence of fat in the hepatocytes. The pathologic changes normally reverse rapidly after delivery, and AFLP is not associated with progression to cirrhosis [82].

Clinical and biochemical findings

As a rule, AFLP is a disease of the third trimester that may occur during any gestation. However, some reports have detailed cases presenting at 22 weeks [83] or 26 weeks [84] of gestation. The onset of disease is never after delivery, but the diagnosis may be made after delivery. The frequency of twin gestations is increased among patients with AFLP (14–19%, vsersus ~1% in the general population) [79], and 7% of triplet pregnancies have been reported to be complicated by AFLP [85]. The most frequent initial symptoms are nausea or vomiting, abdominal pain (especially epigastric), anorexia, and jaundice. In the past, jaundice was almost always seen during the course of the disease, but because of earlier diagnosis, prompt delivery, and the diagnosis of milder cases, we now see affected patients without jaundice. The size of the liver is usually normal or small. Patients with AFLP rarely have pruritus but may have concurrent ICP [86]. About half of affected patients have high blood pressure or proteinuria, which are the main symptoms of preeclampsia [80] On the other hand, some affected patients do not have any of these signs. Patients may demonstrate asterixis and encephalopathy, with or without coma, and some have pancreatitis. Esophagitis and Mallory–Weiss syndrome related to severe vomiting have been reported. Gastrointestinal bleeding secondary to the esophageal lesions, in addition to gastric ulceration related to shock, have been reported. Genital bleeding is frequent. These hemorrhages are exacerbated by associated coagulation disorders. Ascites may be present and is partially related to portal hypertension. Polyuria and polydipsia have been noted in about 5% of patients with AFLP [80], and an association between transient diabetes insipidus and AFLP has been reported [87]. Pancreatitis is a rare but potentially severe complication [88].

The serum aminotransferase levels are raised, but usually the level is not as high as in acute viral hepatitis. The bilirubin level is almost always increased. Patients may demonstrate hypoglycemia. In severe cases, the prothrombin time is increased and the fibrinogen level decreased. These coagulation disorders are caused by hepatic insufficiency, disseminated intravascular coagulation, or both. A low platelet count is usual in AFLP and is not always associated with other signs of disseminated intravascular coagulation. Thrombocytopenia may be the most striking laboratory feature and normalizes spontaneously after delivery. The diagnosis of AFLP should always be considered when thrombocytopenia occurs during late pregnancy and should always prompt the performance of liver function tests, particularly determination of the aminotransferase levels. Renal failure (mainly functional) and hyperuricemia are usual. Ultrasonography of the liver may show increased echogenicity [89]. CT may be useful for the diagnosis, and a liver density that is lower than usual may be demonstrated by Hounsfield unit values in the liver that are equal to or lower than those in the spleen [90]. The findings on imaging studies may be normal, however; a study showed that the findings on CT, which is more sensitive than ultrasonography, were normal in half of patients with AFLP [91]. In clinical practice, these complementary examinations should not delay delivery, particularly in severe cases, which can usually be diagnosed on clinical grounds with routine biologic data.

Maternal and fetal outcome

The maternal mortality rate of AFLP was very high before 1970 (about 90%) [80]. The maternal prognosis is currently greatly improved, and maternal mortality is about 10% or less worldwide [92,93]. This improvement is related principally to early delivery, to advances in intensive care support for patients with severe forms, and also to the detection of patients with less severe forms. Most patients recover completely after delivery without sequelae. However, one patient remained in a prolonged coma after hemorrhagic shock [94], and cases of neurohypophyseal insufficiency have been reported associated in one case with definitive diabetes insipidus [95]. In a recent population-based study in the United Kingdom that included 57 women with AFLP, one patient died and one patient required liver transplantation [79].

AFLP may recur during subsequent pregnancies, although recurrence is not the rule. At least 25 cases without recurrence have been reported; 17 patients had a normal pregnancy, and four had two normal pregnancies following a pregnancy with AFLP. However, at least eight cases of recurrence have been reported since 1990 [96]. Mothers who have experienced AFLP should be informed of the risk for recurrence and closely followed during subsequent pregnancies. Follow-up should be both clinical and biologic (liver function tests, tests for uricemia, and platelet counts twice monthly during the third trimester).

Until 1985, fetal mortality was reported to be as high as 50% [82]. Early delivery has also resulted in an improved fetal prognosis, and the final outcome for infants delivered alive is usually considered to be good. However, in view of the possibility of congenital enzyme deficiency involving intramitochondrial β-oxidation of fatty acids,

these infants should be closely followed from birth (see below).

Pathophysiology

The cause of AFLP remains unknown, although good progress toward a better understanding of this disorder has recently been made. An association of inherited defects in the β-oxidation of fatty acids with AFLP was first suggested by Schoeman et al. [97] and Wilcken et al. [98] in 1991–1993. A case of long-chain 3-hydroxyacyl coenzyme A dehydrogenase (LCHAD) deficiency in a 4-month-old baby born to a mother who had had AFLP and HELLP syndrome at 36 weeks of pregnancy was then reported in 1994 [94]. Both parents were heterozygous for LCHAD deficiency. Since these initial reports, the association between AFLP and LCHAD deficiency has been confirmed by several studies. β-Oxidation of fatty acids, measured by the activity of LCHAD in skin fibroblast culture, was studied in 12 women who had had AFLP [99]. LCHAD activity was reduced in eight of them, consistent with heterozygosity for LCHAD deficiency. Four women had no deficiency. The eight heterozygous women had a total of nine pregnancies complicated by AFLP. Of the nine offspring delivered from these pregnancies, four were confirmed to be homozygous for LCHAD deficiency. Three other infants died with a clinical picture compatible with this diagnosis. The two other infants were healthy at 18 and 24 months of age and had LCHAD activity in the intermediate range. The five fathers tested were heterozygous [99]. These findings show that a deficiency in the β-oxidation enzyme in the fetus may lead to maternal hepatic steatosis in late pregnancy, if the mother is in the intermediate range for the deficiency.

Several mutations have been observed in the gene coding for LCHAD in three families with a child with LCHAD deficiency whose mothers had had AFLP or HELLP syndrome [100]. The mutation c.1528G>C (or p. E474Q, Glu474Gln) in the gene *HADHA* coding the α-subunit of LCHAD is the most common mutation in families with AFLP [101]. In the reported cases of AFLP where genetic screening was performed on the LCHAD-deficient offspring, all the fetuses were either homozygous for the c.1528G>C mutation or compound heterozygous with one c.1528G>C allele in combination with another mutation [102]. In other words, when a woman is heterozygous for a *HADHA* mutation, AFLP may occur regardless of her genotype if her fetus is deficient in LCHAD and carries at least one allele with the c.1528G>C mutation. It seems prudent, therefore, to screen all the offspring born to mothers suffering from AFLP for the mutation c.1528G>C [102]. Such screening can be life saving. Infants with a LCHAD deficiency can present with a metabolic crisis, or suffer a sudden unexpected death at a few months of age [102]. Therefore, screening in infants born to mothers with AFLP should be sought as soon as possible after delivery. In affected families, a prenatal diagnosis based on sampling of chorionic villi has proved both feasible and accurate [103]. These forms of AFLP associated with a genetic deficiency of β-oxidation have not been observed in all countries; the common mutation (c.1528G>C) was not found in 14 women with AFLP observed consecutively in a French hospital [104].

A deficiency of carnitine palmitoyltransferase I has also been associated with AFLP [105]. No familial cases (i.e., AFLP in mother and daughter) have been reported.

Medical and obstetric management

Acute fatty liver of pregnancy must be considered an obstetric emergency. AFLP does not usually resolve before delivery, and if delivery is delayed complications such as hemorrhage and intrauterine death may develop. Consequently, the primary therapy for AFLP is early delivery. The choice of the route of delivery remains the decision of the obstetrician and must be appropriate for the individual clinical situation. Generally speaking, if the patient is in labor and in good general condition and no sign of fetal distress is detected, then vaginal delivery may be attempted with careful monitoring of the mother and baby [106]. For patients with severe disease, urgent delivery must be considered, usually by cesarean section, after correction of the coagulation disorders, especially those related to the thrombocytopenia.

The etiology of AFLP is not known, and no specific medical treatment is available. Esophagitis should be treated with appropriate drugs to prevent bleeding. The blood sugar levels should be monitored and hypoglycemia treated by a continuous intravenous infusion of glucose. Patients with fulminant hepatic failure are best managed in an intensive care unit before and after delivery. Some patients with serious disease that continued after delivery were treated successfully by liver transplantation [79,107,108], and auxiliary transplantation has been used successfully in this setting [109]. Nevertheless, the role of liver transplantation in AFLP is probably limited. Early diagnosis and prompt delivery of a patient with AFLP should avoid the difficult decision about later liver transplantation.

Intercurrent liver disease in pregnancy

In addition to the disorders unique to pregnancy, pregnant women are susceptible to diseases that can affect anyone. Some common disorders can take a fulminant course in pregnant women, hepatitis E being the most frequently cited example. Furthermore, pregnancy predis-

poses a woman to the development of the usual liver diseases, such as cholelithiasis.

Acute viral hepatitis

The response of a pregnant woman to acute infection with the viruses that cause hepatitis varies depending on the type of virus.

Hepatitis A

Pregnant women who contract hepatitis A are not at increased risk of severe disease from this infection [110], although the risk for premature labor may be increased in women who are seriously ill during the third trimester [111,112].

Hepatitis B

In patients with documented acute hepatitis B, pregnancy is not associated with increased mortality or teratogenicity. Infection during gestation should not prompt termination of the pregnancy. Perinatal transmission of hepatitis B virus can occur, especially in women with acute infection during the third trimester. Such transmission should be prevented by immunoprophylaxis at birth. Women exposed to hepatitis B during gestation may be vaccinated without any reported increase in congenital anomalies.

Hepatitis E

Hepatitis E, caused by infection with hepatitis E virus, occurs both in epidemics and sporadically in endemic regions, e.g., India, Pakistan, northern Africa, and Mexico [113]. In nonendemic regions, until recently, autochthonous cases of hepatitis E were extremely uncommon. However, in the last few years, an increasing number of cases have been reported in nonendemic regions [113]. These cases appear related to zoonotic transmission from pigs or numerous wild species [113]. Women in the third trimester are more likely to have more severe disease than are other persons. The fatality rate in this group may be as high as 25% [114–116]. It is important to differentiate between acute hepatitis E and pregnancy-related acute liver disease to consider early delivery in AFLP or the HELLP syndrome. This differentiation may be difficult [115]; in this setting, the presence of ascites and hypertension is suggestive of pregnancy-related acute liver disease [117]. Women in the third trimester of pregnancy should carefully consider the risks associated with travel to areas where this disease is endemic. Hepatitis E virus can cause acute hepatitis in the newborn, and can be transmitted in utero to the fetus [114,116,118].

Hepatitis caused by herpes simplex virus

When it occurs in the third trimester of pregnancy, hepatitis resulting from a primary systemic infection with herpes simplex virus is likely to be severe. Most reported cases of fulminant herpetic hepatitis have occurred in pregnant women [119]. Affected patients may have a "viral" syndrome that includes fever and upper respiratory tract symptoms. Despite marked abnormalities in their aminotransferase levels (several thousands units per liter) and prothrombin time, these patients may be anicteric at presentation. A vesicular eruption is diagnostically useful but may not yet be visible at presentation. Cultures and histology of liver biopsy specimens are helpful in the differential diagnosis, which should include severe liver disorders associated with pregnancy, such as AFLP and the HELLP syndrome. Therapy with aciclovir is successful, and affected women need not be delivered early [119–121]. Why herpes simplex hepatitis is more severe and is associated with such increased hepatic injury in the third trimester of pregnancy is unclear. Herpes simplex hepatitis is known to be also more severe in certain immunocompromised states, such as chronic immunosuppression following transplantation [122].

Biliary tract disease and pancreatitis

Pregnancy decreases gallbladder motility and increases the lithogenicity of bile. Pregnancy has long been considered a risk factor for the development of gallstones; epidemiologic studies confirm an association with an increased risk for gallstones, but only for a 5-year period after pregnancy. Thereafter, the risk drops back to that of the never-pregnant population [123]. Ultrasonographic studies show that gallstones and biliary sludge may accumulate throughout gestation and then resolve with a return to nonpregnant physiology [124,125]. In a prospective study of 3,254 women, the cumulative incidence of new sludge, new stones, or progression of baseline sludge to stones was 10.2% by 4–6 weeks postpartum (versus 5.1% by the first trimester). In the same study, 28 women (0.8%) underwent cholecystectomy within the first year postpartum [126]. Higher BMI and serum leptin levels were independent risk factors for gallstones.

Acute cholecystitis may occur in pregnancy, and in many cases can be managed conservatively until delivery. Laparoscopic cholecystectomy by a skilled laparoscopic surgeon may be safely performed during pregnancy [127,128].

Acute pancreatitis may complicate pregnancy [129]. The serum amylase and lipase levels are normal during pregnancy, so abnormal values warrant attention [130]. Pancreatitis usually occurs in the setting of cholelithiasis [129], and gallstones should be sought in any affected patient. Patients with pancreatitis or symptomatic cholelithiasis during pregnancy may be managed by endoscopic retrograde cholangiopancreatography with sphincterotomy [131,132]. Pancreatitis complicating pregnancy may be associated etiologically with AFLP or preeclampsia. In rare cases, pancreatitis may occur in association with severe hyperemesis gravidarum, with familial hypertriglyceridemia, exacerbated by the physiologic hypertriglyceridemia of pregnancy [133], or with hyperparathyroidism [134,135].

A choledochal cyst may present during pregnancy, with abdominal pain, a mass, and jaundice [136]. Such presentations may represent cases of congenital choledochal cyst exacerbated by the effects of pregnancy on biliary motility. Spontaneous rupture of a choledochal cyst has been reported in pregnancy [137].

Budd–Chiari syndrome (hepatic vein thrombosis)

Reports from India suggest that Budd–Chiari syndrome is more common in pregnant women, usually occurring immediately after delivery [138,139]. The prognosis of such pregnant women has been considered as ominous. In a recent series of 43 women with Budd–Chiari syndrome, seven women (16%) presented with either liver disease during pregnancy (three women) or puerperium (four women), and all seven patients were alive after a median follow-up of 39 months (range 8 to 121 months) [140]. Two patients underwent transjugular intrahepatic portosystemic shunt (TIPS) and one orthotopic liver transplantation (OLT) within 2 months of delivery. Anticoagulation should be administered as soon as the diagnosis of Budd–Chiari syndrome is established. During pregnancy, oral anticoagulants are contraindicated, and low molecular weight heparin is preferred to unfractionated heparin [141]. Recurrence has been reported in a patient whose anticoagulants were stopped when she again became pregnant [142]. Several reports have linked acute Budd–Chiari syndrome during pregnancy in western women with an underlying procoagulant state, such as primary antiphospholipid [143], factor V Leiden mutation [144], thrombotic thrombocytopenic purpura [145], or myeloproliferative disease [140]. Among seven women with Budd–Chiari syndrome presenting during pregnancy or puerpuerium, at least one risk factor for hepatic vein obstruction (not including pregnancy) was found in six women, and several thrombotic risk factors were associated in some of the women [140]. So it is unlikely that pregnancy alone causes Budd–Chiari syndrome in the absence of other thrombotic risk factors [140].

Drug-induced hepatic injury

Because of concern about fetal teratogenicity, pregnant women in general take fewer drugs than those who are not pregnant. When they do take drugs, however, they run the same risks for adverse drug reactions as others. Drug-induced liver disease may occur during any trimester as well as during the postpartum period. Potentially fatal hepatotoxicity has been reported in pregnant women undergoing antiretroviral therapy for human immunodeficiency virus (HIV) infection [146]. Acetaminophen overdose leading to death has been reported [147]. α-Methyldopa, which is commonly used in the treatment of hypertension in pregnancy, rarely may induce acute severe hepatitis [148,149].

Malignant tumors of the liver

The liver is not palpable in normal pregnant women and thus hepatomegaly detected on physical examination requires immediate evaluation. Patients with extensive tumor invasion of the liver may present with abdominal or back pain, rupture of the liver, or hepatic failure. The usual source of metastasis is from a common tumor, such as carcinoma of the colon or pancreas. Gestational trophoblastic neoplasm (hydatidiform mole) can be a source of tumor spread to the liver. Breast cancer may also present with hepatomegaly during pregnancy. A patient presenting at 26 weeks' gestation with hypertension and thrombocytopenia, imitating HELLP syndrome, was found to have cholangiocarcinoma [150]. Severe epigastric pain may reveal ruptured hepatocellular carcinoma during pregnancy [151]. It is possible that the modest immunosuppressive state associated with pregnancy promotes extensive tumor spread and growth.

Other complicating illnesses

Sepsis, particularly urinary tract infections, may lead to cholestasis with or without jaundice in pregnant women as it can do in the nonpregnant state [152]. Echinococcal cysts of the liver have been reported during pregnancy [153]. While leptospirosis rarely occurs during pregnancy, a case without fever may mimic AFLP or HELLP syndrome in late pregnancy [154].

Pregnancy in women with chronic liver disease

Monitoring of liver disease is necessary when its presence is known before pregnancy, and this requires cooperation between the obstetric team and hepatologists. Most patients with severe liver disease are not women of childbearing age or they are infertile because of the associated anovulatory state. Nevertheless some of these women can become pregnant, and when they do some special problems arise. On the other hand, most young women with chronic but nonsevere liver disease can have full-term pregnancies without any particular risk. However, there is the question of the effect of liver disease or its treatment on the fetus. Certain drugs should not be stopped during pregnancy because of the risk of relapse of the liver disease due to withdrawal of treatment. This is the case, for example, with immunosuppressive treatment for chronic autoimmune hepatitis and with penicillamine used as a copper chelator in Wilson disease (see below). Other drugs, such as ribavirin used in the treatment of hepatitis C, are strictly contraindicated in pregnancy. In the case of ribavirin, the patient should be clearly informed of the need for effective contraception throughout treatment and during 6 months thereafter.

Cirrhosis and portal hypertension

Worsening jaundice with progressive liver failure, ascites, and hepatic coma have been reported during the course of pregnancy in women with cirrhosis. Whether the exacerbation of hepatic dysfunction is caused by gestation or is merely coincident with it is unclear. By contrast some women with cirrhosis can sustain pregnancy without any worsening of hepatic function. Published reports document an increased incidence of stillbirths, premature delivery, hypertension, and peripartum infection in women with cirrhosis, especially when ascites is present [155]. The fertility of women with noncirrhotic portal hypertension, as seen in congenital hepatic fibrosis or portal vein thrombosis, is not diminished; thus, pregnancy is encountered in this setting with some frequency [156,157]. A worsening of preexisting portal hypertension may be anticipated because of the marked increase in blood volume and azygos flow that occurs during normal pregnancy. Variceal hemorrhage during pregnancy or labor has been reported. It is not clear that the incidence of variceal hemorrhage in pregnant patients is higher than the incidence in nonpregnant patients with known varices. Sclerotherapy or endoscopic band ligation have been reported to be successful in pregnant women with variceal hemorrhage [156,158]. Prevention of hemorrhage due to esophageal varices in a woman with known cirrhosis who desires pregnancy is based on classic treatment with β-blockers and/or endoscopic ligature. In these patients, an upper endoscopy is therefore usually performed before pregnancy. Prophylaxis with β-blockers may be continued during pregnancy, but newborns should be monitored during the first days of life because of risks of hypoglycemia and bradycardia. Generally, vaginal delivery with early analgesics for the mother assisted by an extraction device is preferred to caesarean section, which must be reserved for obstetric indications [155].

Specific liver diseases

Alcoholic liver disease

Alcoholic liver disease is often associated with infertility. Most alcoholics do not have significant liver disease, however. Pregnancy in a fertile alcoholic woman can result in fetal alcohol syndrome in the infant, which includes typical facies, malformations, and developmental delay. For the most part, liver disease or its treatment is not teratogenic. The risk of prematurity is increased.

Chronic hepatitis B

In general, pregnancy is well tolerated by women who are chronic carriers of the hepatitis B virus (HBV) [159]; reactivation of the virus with exacerbation of disease during or after gestation is the exception rather than the rule [160]. The placenta forms an excellent barrier against transmission of this virus, and intrauterine infection with HBV is rare. The major problem for women who are chronic carriers of HBV is the risk of maternal-to-infant (vertical) transmission of infection at delivery. Transmission at birth is more likely if the mother is positive for hepatitis B e antigen (HBeAg) or has high circulating levels of HBV DNA [161]. The rate of transmission may be lower if the delivery is by cesarean section [162]. This is not indicated, however, because appropriate immunoprophylaxis for the newborn with both hepatitis B immunoglobulin (HBIg) and vaccine is very efficient in interrupting transmission. Routine prenatal screening of all pregnant women for hepatitis B surface antigen (HBsAg) is now the standard of care. A test for HBsAg screening should be ordered with other recommended screening tests, regardless of previous hepatitis B vaccination or previous negative HBsAg test results [163]. Infants born to infected mothers should be protected by the recommended combination of vaccine and HBIg at birth [164]. Infants born to carriers of the HBV precore mutant who are positive for antibody to HBeAg with high levels of HBV DNA in their serum are at risk for fulminant hepatitis B during the first 2–4 months following birth [165]. HBIg and vaccine should therefore be given to the infants of all mothers who are HBsAg-positive, regardless of their HBe status. In women with very high HBV DNA levels (as high as 9 $\log_{10}$ copies/mL), vertical transmission of HBV may occur despite vaccination of the child. In such women, treatment with lamivudine (100 or 150 mg/day) during the last months of pregnancy has been given to decrease the HBV DNA level and was associated with a reduction of the risk of HBV transmission [166–168]. Hepatitis D (delta) virus can also be transmitted from mother to infant at birth [169]. Breastfeeding is not contraindicated for infants born to HBsAg-positive mothers [170].

Chronic hepatitis C

Uneventful pregnancy without worsening disease or fetal complications has been reported in women with hepatitis C [171]. Several studies have demonstrated that aminotransferase levels decrease as the pregnancy progresses, whereas the hepatitis C virus (HCV) load increases during the course of gestation [172–174]. Early evidence suggests that the hepatic histopathology may worsen during gestation [175]. Whether or not pregnancy has any effect on the progression of this disease remains to be proved [176].

Transmission from mothers who are chronic carriers to their offspring may occur but appears to be much less efficient than the vertical transmission of hepatitis B. There are currently no interventions available to prevent vertical transmission of HCV [177], except successful antiviral treatment before the onset of pregnancy. Indeed, transmission of HCV occurs only when HCV RNA is detectable. Transmission may be related to higher levels, ranging from 4% to 7% per pregnancy [178]. No association with breastfeeding has been shown, and breastfeeding is not contraindicated [177–179]. It may be prudent for mothers who are HCV infected and who choose to breastfeed to consider abstaining from breastfeeding if their nipples are cracked and bleeding [179]. The rate of transmission is not lower in infants delivered by cesarean section and cesarean section is not recommended for women with chronic HCV infection alone [177,178]. Coinfection with HIV increases the rate of transmission [180]. HCV/HIV coinfected mothers should follow exiting HIV guidelines [177].

Testing a newborn can be misleading. Early after birth, antibodies acquired from the mother usually result in positivity for HCV, and transient viremia can be seen in infants who later test negative. Cord blood can be negative for HCV RNA, while the infant is subsequently shown to be HCV RNA-positive [172]. To reduce the number of tests, the minimum requirement to confirm or exclude infection would be an antibody test at 18 months of age, with a positive result confirming the presence of infection and a negative result confirming the absence of infection [177].

Autoimmune hepatitis

A distinctive clinical characteristic of autoimmune hepatitis is the rapid and complete (or nearly complete) remission that occurs in response to immunosuppression with corticosteroids, given either alone or in combination with azathioprine. The disorder presents frequently in young women, who become anovulatory in response to the active and severe hepatitis, which has sometimes progressed to cirrhosis by the time of diagnosis. Women appropriately treated for this disease with corticosteroids and azathioprine regain their fertility, and successful pregnancies without any increase in fatality have been reported [181]. The aminotransferase levels may decrease during the second and third trimesters of pregnancy, and some have advocated lowering doses of immunosuppressive drugs during gestation [182]. The conventional therapy should be reinstituted immediately before delivery [183]. Untreated patients may go into remission during pregnancy [184]. Worsening of the underlying disease or even initial presentation of autoimmune hepatitis have been reported during pregnancy [181]. The underlying disease may flare up after delivery, and women should be followed carefully for 3 months postpartum, particularly if the immunosuppressive dose has been decreased [181,185]. Azathioprine has been associated with congenital malformations in pregnant mice; however, it has not been reported to be teratogenic in humans in this setting of low-dose therapy, and seems to be safe for the mother and the baby [181,185,186]. Consequently, it is not usually recommended to stop azathioprine, either for conception or for the duration of pregnancy [187]. However, because the data concerning the safety of azathioprine in pregnant women remain limited, and because this drug is not essential in the management of autoimmune hepatitis, it may be prudent to substitute prednisone for azathioprine [183]. Successful treatment of infertility in these patients, with in vitro fertilization/embryo transfer, has been reported [188].

Primary biliary cirrhosis

The effects of pregnancy on women with this disease have been reported to be variable although studies are scarce. Pregnancy may be associated with an increase in cholestasis that resolves after delivery, regression of cholestasis, or progression of disease including the complications of portal hypertension [189–192]. Ursodeoxycholic acid has been used for ICP with no reports of adverse effects and can be used in patients with primary biliary cirrhosis at the very least during the second and third trimester. In a report of nine pregnancies in six women with ursodeoxycholic acid-treated primary biliary cirrhosis, pregnancy was associated with improvement of liver function tests [193].

Wilson disease

Women with ovulatory failure secondary to Wilson disease regain their fertility, often quite rapidly, when treated. Either they or their physicians may be tempted to discontinue therapy during gestation, but, as in nonpregnant patients with Wilson disease, cessation of therapy can have devastating effects and should not be attempted [194,195]. Successful pregnancies without teratogenicity have been reported in patients taking penicillamine or trientine [196–198]. Zinc treatment has also been successful during pregnancy [199]. Clearly, the major risk to the mother created by stopping therapy greatly outweighs the potential risk to the fetus, and therapy should be continued because successful pregnancy in treated women is the rule [195,196]. Doses of penicillamine or trientine may be reduced during the last trimester [195,196]. Women taking D-penicillamine should not breastfeed [195].

Benign liver tumors (hepatocellular adenoma, focal nodular hyperplasia, hemangioma)

Hepatocellular adenomas associated with the previous use of oral contraceptive agents have been reported to enlarge or rupture during subsequent pregnancy [200–203], and rupture is associated with high mortality [200]. Successful surgical resection of a large ($7 \times 9\,cm$) hepatocellular adenoma performed at 13 weeks' gestation has been reported; the patient complained of increasing epigastric pain and the tumor was in the left hepatic lobe [204].

A study of 216 women with focal nodular hyperplasia showed no association between oral contraceptive use and change in lesion size. Twelve women in this group became pregnant, with no change in lesion size or problems with pregnancy [205]. An enlargement of a focal nodular hyperplasia associated with the previous use of oral contraceptive was, however, reported in one pregnant woman [206].

The results of a prospective study of 94 women (with 181 hemangiomas) suggests that endogenous and exogenous female sex hormones may play a role in the pathogenesis of liver hemangiomas, although significant enlargement occurs only in a minority of patients [207]. These liver hemangiomas are rarely symptomatic and complications are exceptional.

Familial hyperbilirubinemia

The unconjugated hyperbilirubinemia of Gilbert syndrome is not exacerbated by pregnancy [208]. In Dubin–Johnson syndrome, however, the conjugated hyperbilirubinemia may worsen during gestation, but returns to prepregnancy levels after delivery [209]. Women with type II Crigler–Najjar syndrome have been reported to have uncomplicated pregnancies with or without phenobarbital therapy [210,211].

Porphyrias

These genetic disorders of heme metabolism, which may be exacerbated by estrogenic hormones, occasionally cause problems for affected women and their fetuses during pregnancy. Porphyria cutanea tarda has rarely been reported to present initially during pregnancy [212]. Acute attacks often complicate the course of pregnancy in patients with acute intermittent porphyria, variegate porphyria, or hereditary coproporphyria [213,214], and they may result in intrauterine growth retardation or, rarely, maternal death. On the other hand, many women with acute porphyria, particularly those with little clinical expression of the defect, weather pregnancy with no problems. Precipitation of an initial attack of acute intermittent porphyria by the nausea and vomiting of hyperemesis gravidarum, coupled with antiemetic therapy, has been reported [215].

Budd–Chiari syndrome

Women with Budd–Chiari syndrome have become pregnant after the syndrome has been treated and well controlled [216]. By contrast with a good maternal outcome, the fetal outcome remains relatively poor, possibly because of the underlying prothrombotic disorders. Patients should be fully informed of the persistent risk of such pregnancies [216].

Liver transplantation

Liver transplantation is now accepted as a treatment of both acute liver failure and end-stage chronic liver disease, with a 1-year survival exceeding 85%. Patients who have undergone transplantation regain their fertility promptly – within weeks or months of surgery [217]. Young women should be counseled about the risks of becoming pregnant and encouraged to use effective contraception, preferably barrier methods or intrauterine contraceptive devices, until their immunosuppressive regimen has been stabilized [218,219]. A review of 136 pregnancies after liver transplantation reported to the US National Transplantation Pregnancy Registry has shown that most are successful, with no birth defects in the offspring [220]. The number of premature infants was increased, and women whose renal function was compromised did not do as well. Ten episodes of acute rejection occurred during pregnancy in this study, and three women lost their grafts as a result. Seven of the women died, three within a year of the pregnancy [220]. The effects of prior transplantation on maternal and fetal outcomes were also analyzed in a US nationwide study [221]. Between 1993 and 2005, 146 deliveries among liver transplant recipients were identified and compared with a control group. There was no maternal mortality, but there was an increased fetal mortality and maternal and fetal complications, especially gestational hypertension and postpartum hemorrhage. The infants have an increased risk of prematurity, fetal distress, and growth restriction but not congenital anomalies [221]. The risk of teratogenicity with standard immunosuppressive agents, including prednisone, azathioprine, cyclosporine, and tacrolimus, is low [222,223]. It is preferable to delay pregnancy until the immunosuppressive regimen has been stabilized, i.e., 1 year after grafting [224]. Surveillance for infection, such as with cytomegalovirus, should be increased during gestation. If the results of liver tests become abnormal, then a liver biopsy should be performed to establish the nature of the dysfunction. Increased monitoring of the blood levels of cyclosporine and other immunosuppressive agents is necessary, both before and for several months after delivery [225]. Such pregnancies should be considered high risk and managed together with transplant hepatologists and experts in maternal–fetal medicine, and neonatologists when necessary [221]. Breastfeeding has been discouraged because of concerns about potential immunosuppression of the newborn, but many examples of successful breastfeeding without adverse effects have been reported [220].

Liver transplantation has been accomplished during pregnancy, with and without fetal wastage [220,226–228]. Livers from living related donors have also been transplanted during pregnancy [229]. Obviously, such heroic surgery must be considered with extreme care in this setting. If the condition prompting transplantation is caused by pregnancy (e.g., AFLP or HELLP syndrome), then prompt diagnosis, followed by termination of the pregnancy with maximum support for the mother, is the treatment of choice.

Further reading

Armenti VT, Herrine SK, Radomski JS, et al. Pregnancy after liver transplantation. *Liver Transpl* 2000;6:671–85.
A review of the complications and outcomes of 136 pregnancies after liver transplantation. Three stillbirths but no birth defects were recorded. Prematurity and low birth weight were common, as were preeclampsia and infection in the mothers. Such pregnancies should be considered high risk.

Arrese M, Macias RI, Briz O, et al. Molecular pathogenesis of intrahepatic cholestasis of pregnancy. *Expert Rev Mol Med* 2008;10:e9.
A comprehensive review that summarizes current knowledge on the potential mechanisms involved in intrahepatic cholestasis of pregnancy. Hormonal and genetic factors are important. Hormonal factors are well known and a genetic hypersensitivity to female hormones (estrogens and/or progesterone) is thought to impair bile secretary function. More recently data suggest that mutations of genes coding hepatobiliary transport proteins may predispose to intrahepatic cholestasis of pregnancy. Environmental factors may also influence the expression of this disease, but these factors have not been clearly identified

Bacq Y, Zarka O, Bréchot J-F, et al. Liver function tests in normal pregnancy: a prospective study of 103 pregnant women and 103 matched controls. *Hepatology* 1996;23:1030–4.
A prospective study of pregnant patients and matched controls. The results of standard liver tests in all three trimesters were considered. Levels of alkaline phosphatase rose in the third trimester. The total bile acid levels did not differ between the pregnant women and the controls. The levels of bilirubin and GGT were lower in the pregnant women than in the controls. AST and ALT values remained in normal limits.

Barton JR, Sibai BM. Gastrointestinal complications of pre-eclampsia. *Semin Perinatol* 2009;33:179–88.
A recent and comprehensive review on the hepatic and pancreatic complications of preeclampsia/eclampsia, with an emphasis on the HELLP syndrome. Clinical presentation, initial management, and management of hepatic complications of the HELLP syndrome are discussed.

Bottomley C, Bourne T. Management strategies for hyperemesis. *Best Pract Res Clin Obstet Gynaecol* 2009;23:549–64.
A comprehensive review on the pathogenesis, diagnosis, and management of this complex disorder unique to pregnancy. Treatment is supportive with intravenous rehydration, antiemetics, and correction of vitamin deficiency. This review discusses also the prevention, recognition, and treatment of serious complications associated with hyperemesis gravidarum such Wernicke encephalopathy, osmotic demyelinization syndrome (central pontine myelinolysis), and thromboembolism.

Castro MA, Fassett MJ, Reynolds TB, et al. Reversible peripartum liver failure: a new perspective on the diagnosis, treatment and cause of acute fatty liver of pregnancy, based on 28 consecutive cases. *Am J Obstet Gynecol* 1999;181:389–95.

A review of a large case series. The authors emphasize the high incidence of renal compromise and significant hypoglycemia, and plead that liver transplantation be avoided in those patients whose liver disease is reversible.

Gambarin-Gelwan M. Hepatitis B in pregnancy. *Clin Liver Dis* 2007; 11:945–63.

This article reviews in depth the consequences of HBV infection in pregnant women and discusses its management. Perinatal transmission of HBV from mother to infant is important and should be prevented by the administration of hepatitis B immunoglobulin and hepatitis B vaccine at birth. Even with such prevention, mother to infant transmission has been observed in some women with very high serum HBV DNA levels ($>8 \log_{10}$ IU/mL). In these women, antiviral therapy at the end of pregnancy (usually with lamivudine), in addition to immunoprophylaxis, has been proposed to decrease the risk of transmission. Breastfeeding is not contraindicated for infants born to HBsAg-positive mothers.

Heneghan MA, Norris SM, O'Grady JG, et al. Management and outcome of pregnancy in autoimmune hepatitis. *Gut* 2001;48:97–102.

A review of the King's College experience of 35 pregnancies in 18 women with autoimmune hepatitis. Two patients presented during pregnancy, and four had flares. No birth defects were noted despite azathioprine therapy in some.

Heneghan MA, Selzner M, Yoshida EM, Mullhaupt B. Pregnancy and sexual function in liver transplantation. *J Hepatol* 2008;49:507–19.

This article combines the opinion of several expert reviews on some relevant clinical questions related to the indications of transplantation during pregnancy and sexual function, contraception, and pregnancy after liver transplantation.

Ibdah JA, Bennett MH, Rinaldo P, et al. A fetal fatty acid oxidation disorder as a cause of liver disease in pregnant women. *N Engl J Med* 1999;340:1723–31.

A study of families affected by long-chain 3-hydroxyacyl coenzyme A dehydrogenase deficiency. The pregnancies of mothers of deficient fetuses carrying the Glu474Gln mutation were complicated by AFLP or HELLP, a unique example of maternal illness caused by deficiency in the fetus.

Ko CW, Beresford SA, Schulte SJ, Matsumoto AM, Lee SP. Incidence, natural history, and risk factors for biliary sludge and stones during pregnancy. *Hepatology* 2005;41:359–65.

A prospective study on biliary sludge and stones during pregnancy and postpartum in 3,254 women. Sludge or stones were found on at least one ultrasound study in 5.1% by the second trimester, 7.9% by the second trimester, and 10.2% by 4–6 weeks postpartum. Twenty-eight women (0.8%) underwent cholecystectomy within the first year postpartum. Prepregnancy body mass index and serum leptin were risk factors for gallbladder disease.

Kumar A, Beniwal M, Kar P, Sharma JB, Murthy NS. Hepatitis E in pregnancy. *Int J Gynaecol Obstet* 2004;85:240–4.

A prospective study of 62 pregnant women in India having jaundice in the third trimester. Twenty-eight patients (45.2%) had hepatitis E and 26.9% of these patients with hepatitis E infection died with fulminant hepatic failure (five patients died undelivered). Vertical transmission of hepatitis E virus was observed in 33.3% of cases. This study confirms the poor prognosis of hepatitis E during the third trimester of pregnancy.

Pembrey L, Newell ML, Tovo PA. The management of HCV infected pregnant women and their children. European Paediatric HCV Network. *J Hepatol* 2005;43:515–25.

A review with guidelines for the clinical management of HCV-infected pregnant women and their children. HCV infection is not a contraindication for pregnancy. The estimated risk of vertical transmission is 5%, ranging from 3% to 7%. There are currently no interventions available to prevent vertical transmission of HCV (except antiviral treatment with sustained virologic response before the pregnancy). Neither elective caesarean section nor

avoidance of breastfeeding should be recommended to prevent mother-to-child transmission of HCV. The minimum requirement to confirm or exclude infection in children born from HCV-infected mothers is an antibody test at 18 months of age, with a positive result confirming presence of infection and a negative result confirming absence of infection.

Rautou PE, Angermayr B, Garcia-Pagan JC, et al. Pregnancy in women with known and treated Budd–Chiari syndrome: maternal and fetal outcomes. *J Hepatol* 2009;51:47–54.

A retrospective study of 24 pregnancies in 16 women with Budd–Chiari syndrome that was known and treated before pregnancy. Anticoagulation was administered during 17 pregnancies. In two patients, symptomatic thrombosis recurred during pregnancy or postpartum. All patients were alive after a median follow-up of 34 months after the last delivery. By contrast, the prognosis of the babies was not so good. Seven fetuses were lost before gestation week 20 and there was one stillbirth. The prognosis of the 16 infants born alive was good although there was a high level of prematurity (12/16 cases). In the absence of obstetric indication for a caesarean, vaginal delivery should be encouraged in such patients.

Ropponen A, Sund R, Riikonen S, Ylikorkala O, Aittomaki K. Intrahepatic cholestasis of pregnancy as an indicator of liver and biliary diseases: a population-based study. *Hepatology* 2006;43:723–8.

This longitudinal retrospective population-based cohort study was designed to analyze the occurrence of liver and biliary diseases in women suffering from ICP in Finland. Patients with a history of ICP (10,504 women during the years 1972–2000) and 10,504 women with normal pregnancies (controls) were matched for age, time of delivery, and place of delivery. The results show an association of ICP with several liver diseases: hepatitis C (rate ratio (RR), 3.5; 95% CI, 1.6–7.6, P <0.001), gallstones and cholecystitis (RR, 3.7; 95% CI, 3.2–4.2;P <0.001), and nonalcoholic pancreatitis (RR, 3.2; 95% CI, 1.7–5.7; P <0.001). An association was also found with nonalcoholic liver cirrhosis including cases of primary biliary cirrhosis (RR, 8.2; 95% CI, 1.9–35.5; P <0.05). This last result suggests that the long-term follow-up of patient suffering from ICP may be reconsidered.

References

1. Bacq Y, Zarka O. Le foie au cours de la grossesse normale. *Gastroenterol Clin Biol* 1994;18:767–74.
2. Bacq Y, Zarka O, Brechot JF, et al. Liver function tests in normal pregnancy: a prospective study of 103 pregnant women and 103 matched controls. *Hepatology* 1996;23:1030–4.
3. Tsang IS, Katz VL, Wells SD. Maternal and fetal outcomes in hyperemesis gravidarum. *Int J Gynaecol Obstet* 1996;55:231–5.
4. Goodwin TM. Hyperemesis gravidarum. *Clin Obstet Gynecol* 1998;41:597–605.
5. Abell TL, Riely CA. Hyperemesis gravidarum. *Gastroenterol Clin North Am* 1992;21:835–49.
6. Larrey D, Rueff B, Feldmann G, et al. Recurrent jaundice caused by recurrent hyperemesis gravidarum. *Gut* 1984;25:1414–5.
7. Goodwin TM, Montoro M, Mestman JH. Transient hyperthyroidism and hyperemesis gravidarum: clinical aspects. *Am J Obstet Gynecol* 1992;167:648–52.
8. Bottomley C, Bourne T. Management strategies for hyperemesis. *Best Pract Res Clin Obstet Gynaecol* 2009;23:549–64.
9. Sullivan CA, Johnson CA, Roach H, et al. A pilot study of intravenous ondansetron for hyperemesis gravidarum. *Am J Obstet Gynecol* 1996;174:1565–8.
10. Hsu JJ, Clark-Glena R, Nelson DK, et al. Nasogastric enteral feeding in the management of hyperemesis gravidarum. *Obstet Gynecol* 1996;88:343–6.
11. Hallak M, Tsalamandris K, Dombrowski MP, et al. Hyperemesis gravidarum. Effects on fetal outcome. *J Reprod Med* 1996;41:871–4.
12. Bacq Y. Intrahepatic cholestasis of pregnancy. *Clin Liver Dis* 1999;3:1–13.

13. Geenes V, Williamson C. Intrahepatic cholestasis of pregnancy. *World J Gastroenterol* 2009;15:2049–66.

14. Reyes H, Gonzalez MC, Ribalta J, et al. Prevalence of intrahepatic cholestasis of pregnancy in Chile. *Ann Intern Med* 1978;88:487–93.

15. Ribalta J, Reyes H, Gonzalez MC, et al. *S*-adenosyl-L-methionine in the treatment of patients with intrahepatic cholestasis of pregnancy: a randomized, double-blind, placebo-controlled study with negative results. *Hepatology* 1991;13:1084–9.

16. Rioseco AJ, Ivankovic MB, Manzur A, et al. Intrahepatic cholestasis of pregnancy: a retrospective case–control study of perinatal outcome. *Am J Obstet Gynecol* 1994;170:890–5.

17. Laifer SA, Stiller RJ, Siddiqui DS, et al. Ursodeoxycholic acid for the treatment of intrahepatic cholestasis of pregnancy. *J Matern Fetal Med* 2001;10:131–5.

18. Lee RH, Goodwin TM, Greenspoon J, et al. The prevalence of intrahepatic cholestasis of pregnancy in a primarily Latina Los Angeles population. *J Perinatol* 2006;26:527–32.

19. Gonzalez MC, Reyes H, Arrese M, et al. Intrahepatic cholestasis of pregnancy in twin pregnancies. *J Hepatol* 1989;9:84–90.

20. Rolfes DB, Ishak KG. Liver disease in pregnancy. *Histopathology* 1986;10:555–70.

21. Reyes H. The spectrum of liver and gastrointestinal disease seen in cholestasis of pregnancy. *Gastroenterol Clin North Am* 1992;21:905–21.

22. Bacq Y, Sapey T, Brechot MC, et al. Intrahepatic cholestasis of pregnancy: a French prospective study. *Hepatology* 1997;26:358–64.

23. Favre N, Abergel A, Blanc P, et al. Unusual presentation of severe intrahepatic cholestasis of pregnancy leading to fetal death. *Obstet Gynecol* 2009;114:491–3.

24. Laatikainen T, Tulenheimo A. Maternal serum bile acid levels and fetal distress in cholestasis of pregnancy. *Int J Gynaecol Obstet* 1984;22:91–4.

25. Glantz A, Marschall HU, Mattsson LA. Intrahepatic cholestasis of pregnancy: relationships between bile acid levels and fetal complication rates. *Hepatology* 2004;40:467–74.

26. Egerman RS, Riely CA. Predicting fetal outcome in intrahepatic cholestasis of pregnancy: is the bile acid level sufficient? *Hepatology* 2004;40:287–8.

27. Dann AT, Kenyon AP, Seed PT, et al. Glutathione *S*-transferase and liver function in intrahepatic cholestasis of pregnancy and pruritus gravidarum. *Hepatology* 2004;40:1406–14.

28. Ropponen A, Sund R, Riikonen S, et al. Intrahepatic cholestasis of pregnancy as an indicator of liver and biliary diseases: a population-based study. *Hepatology* 2006;43:723–8.

29. Locatelli A, Roncaglia N, Arreghini A, et al. Hepatitis C virus infection is associated with a higher incidence of cholestasis of pregnancy. *Br J Obstet Gynaecol* 1999;106:498–500.

30. Paternoster DM, Fabris F, Palu G, et al. Intra-hepatic cholestasis of pregnancy in hepatitis C virus infection. *Acta Obstet Gynecol Scand* 2002;81:99–103.

31. Reyes H, Simon FR. Intrahepatic cholestasis of pregnancy: an estrogen-related disease. *Semin Liver Dis* 1993;13:289–301.

32. Arrese M, Macias RI, Briz O, et al. Molecular pathogenesis of intrahepatic cholestasis of pregnancy. *Expert Rev Mol Med* 2008;10:e9.

33. Oude Elferink RP, Paulusma CC. Function and pathophysiological importance of ABCB4 (MDR3 P-glycoprotein). *Pflugers Arch* 2007;453:601–10.

34. Jacquemin E, Cresteil D, Manouvrier S, et al. Heterozygous nonsense mutation of the MDR3 gene in familial intrahepatic cholestasis of pregnancy. *Lancet* 1999;353:210–11.

35. Dixon PH, Weerasekera N, Linton KJ, et al. Heterozygous MDR3 missense mutation associated with intrahepatic cholestasis of pregnancy: evidence for a defect in protein trafficking. *Hum Mol Genet* 2000;9:1209–17.

36. Mullenbach R, Linton KJ, Wiltshire S, et al. ABCB4 gene sequence variation in women with intrahepatic cholestasis of pregnancy. *J Med Genet* 2003;40:e70.

37. Pauli-Magnus C, Lang T, Meier Y, et al. Sequence analysis of bile salt export pump (ABCB11) and multidrug resistance p-glycoprotein 3 (ABCB4, MDR3) in patients with intrahepatic cholestasis of pregnancy. *Pharmacogenetics* 2004;14:91–102.

38. Floreani A, Carderi I, Paternoster D, et al. Hepatobiliary phospholipid transporter ABCB4, MDR3 gene variants in a large cohort of Italian women with intrahepatic cholestasis of pregnancy. *Dig Liver Dis* 2008;40:366–70.

39. Bacq Y, Gendrot C, Perrotin F, et al. ABCB4 gene mutations and single-nucleotide polymorphisms in women with intrahepatic cholestasis of pregnancy. *J Med Genet* 2009;46:711–15.

40. Dixon PH, van Mil SW, Chambers J, et al. Contribution of variant alleles of ABCB11 to susceptibility to intrahepatic cholestasis of pregnancy. *Gut* 2009;58:537–44.

41. Mullenbach R, Bennett A, Tetlow N, et al. ATP8B1 mutations in British cases with intrahepatic cholestasis of pregnancy. *Gut* 2005;54:829–34.

42. Meng LJ, Reyes H, Axelson M, et al. Progesterone metabolites and bile acids in serum of patients with intrahepatic cholestasis of pregnancy: effect of ursodeoxycholic acid therapy. *Hepatology* 1997;26:1573–9.

43. Reyes H, Sjovall J. Bile acids and progesterone metabolites in intrahepatic cholestasis of pregnancy. *Ann Med* 2000;32:94–106.

44. Reyes H, Baez ME, Gonzales MC, et al. Selenium, zinc and copper plasma levels in intrahepatic cholestasis of pregnancy, in normal pregnancies and in healthy individuals, in Chile. *J Hepatol* 2000;32:542–9.

45. Frezza M, Pozzato G, Chiesa L, et al. Reserval of intrahepatic cholestasis of pregnancy in women after high dose *S*-adenosyl-L-methionine administration. *Hepatology* 1984;4:274–8.

46. Floreani A, Paternoster D, Melis A, et al. *S*-adenosylmethionine versus ursodeoxycholic acid in the treatment of intrahepatic cholestasis of pregnancy: preliminary results of a controlled trial. *Eur J Obstet Gynecol Reprod Biol* 1996;67:109–13.

47. Diaferia A, Nicastri PL, Tartagni M, et al. Ursodeoxycholic acid therapy in pregnant women with cholestasis. *Int J Gynaecol Obstet* 1996;52:133–40.

48. Palma J, Reyes H, Ribalta J, et al. Ursodeoxycholic acid in the treatment of cholestasis of pregnancy: a randomized, double-blind study controlled with placebo. *J Hepatol* 1997;27:1022–8.

49. Nicastri PL, Diaferia A, Tartagni M, et al. A randomised placebo-controlled trial of ursodeoxycholic acid and *S*-adenosylmethionine in the treatment of intrahepatic cholestasis of pregnancy. *Br J Obstet Gynaecol* 1998;105:1205–7.

50. Roncaglia N, Locatelli A, Arreghini A, et al. A randomised controlled trial of ursodeoxycholic acid and *S*-adenosyl-l-methionine in the treatment of gestational cholestasis. *Br J Obstet Gynaecol* 2004;111:17–21.

51. Glantz A, Marschall HU, Lammert F, et al. Intrahepatic cholestasis of pregnancy: a randomized controlled trial comparing dexamethasone and ursodeoxycholic acid. *Hepatology* 2005;42:1399–405.

52. Kondrackiene J, Beuers U, Kupcinskas L. Efficacy and safety of ursodeoxycholic acid versus cholestyramine in intrahepatic cholestasis of pregnancy. *Gastroenterology* 2005;129:894–901.

53. Binder T, Salaj P, Zima T, et al. Randomized prospective comparative study of ursodeoxycholic acid and *S*-adenosyl-L-methionine in the treatment of intrahepatic cholestasis of pregnancy. *J Perinat Med* 2006;34:383–91.

54. Liu Y, Qiao F, Liu H, et al. Ursodeoxycholic acid in the treatment of intraheptic cholestasis of pregnancy. *J Huazhong Univ Sci Technolog Med Sci* 2006;26:350–2.

55. Zapata R, Sandoval L, Palma J, et al. Ursodeoxycholic acid in the treatment of intrahepatic cholestasis of pregnancy. A 12-year experience. *Liver Int* 2005;25:548–54.

56. Royal College of Obstetricians and Gynaecologists. Obstetric cholestasis. *R Coll Obstet Gynaecol Guidelines* 2006;43:1–10.

57. Sentilhes L, Bacq Y. La Cholestase Intrahépatique Gravidique. *J Gynecol Obstet Biol Reprod (Paris)* 2008;37:118–26.

58. Mays JK. The active management of intrahepatic cholestasis of pregnancy. *Curr Opin Obstet Gynecol* 2010;22:100–3.

59. Ch'ng CL, Morgan M, Hainsworth I, et al. Prospective study of liver dysfunction in pregnancy in southwest Wales. *Gut* 2002;51:876–80.

60. Sibai B, Dekker G, Kupferminc M. Pre-eclampsia. *Lancet* 2005; 365:785–99.

61. Roberts JM, Cooper DW. Pathogenesis and genetics of pre-eclampsia. *Lancet* 2001;357:53–6.

62. Serrano NC. Immunology and genetic of preeclampsia. *Clin Dev Immunol* 2006;13:197–201.

63. Duckitt K, Harrington D. Risk factors for pre-eclampsia at antenatal booking: systematic review of controlled studies. *Br Med J* 2005;330:565.

64. Barton JR, Sibai BM. Gastrointestinal complications of pre-eclampsia. *Semin Perinatol* 2009;33:179–88.

65. Weinstein L. Syndrome of hemolysis, elevated liver enzymes, and low platelet count: a severe consequence of hypertension in pregnancy. *Am J Obstet Gynecol* 1982;142:159–67.

66. Barton JR, Riely CA, Adamec TA, et al. Hepatic histopathologic condition does not correlate with laboratory abnormalities in HELLP syndrome (hemolysis, elevated liver enzymes, and low platelet count). *Am J Obstet Gynecol* 1992;167:1538–43.

67. Halim A, Kanayama N, El Maradny E, et al. Immunohistological study in cases of HELLP syndrome (hemolysis, elevated liver enzymes and low platelets) and acute fatty liver of pregnancy. *Gynecol Obstet Invest* 1996;41:106–12.

68. Sibai BM, Ramadan MK, Usta I, et al. Maternal morbidity and mortality in 442 pregnancies with hemolysis, elevated liver enzymes, and low platelets (HELLP syndrome). *Am J Obstet Gynecol* 1993;169:1000–6.

69. Barton JR, Sibai BM. Hepatic imaging in HELLP syndrome (hemolysis, elevated liver enzymes, and low platelet count). *Am J Obstet Gynecol* 1996;174:1820–5, discussion 5–7.

70. Zarrinpar A, Farmer DG, Ghobrial RM, et al. Liver transplantation for HELLP syndrome. *Am Surg* 2007;73:1013–16.

71. Sibai BM, Ramadan MK, Chari RS, et al. Pregnancies complicated by HELLP syndrome (hemolysis, elevated liver enzymes, and low platelets): subsequent pregnancy outcome and long-term prognosis. *Am J Obstet Gynecol* 1995;172:125–9.

72. Schwartz ML, Lien JM. Spontaneous liver hematoma in pregnancy not clearly associated with preeclampsia: a case presentation and literature review. *Am J Obstet Gynecol* 1997;176:1328–32, discussion 32–3.

73. Reck T, Bussenius-Kammerer M, Ott R, et al. Surgical treatment of HELLP syndrome-associated liver rupture – an update. *Eur J Obstet Gynecol Reprod Biol* 2001;99:57–65.

74. Sheehan HL. The pathology of acute yellow atrophy and delayed chloroform poisoning. *J Obstet Gynaecol* 1940;47:49–62.

75. Bernuau J, Degott C, Nouel O, et al. Non-fatal acute fatty liver of pregnancy. *Gut* 1983;24:340–4.

76. Pockros PJ, Peters RL, Reynolds TB. Idiopathic fatty liver of pregnancy: findings in ten cases. *Medicine (Baltimore)* 1984;63: 1–11.

77. Castro MA, Fassett MJ, Reynolds TB, et al. Reversible peripartum liver failure: a new perspective on the diagnosis, treatment, and cause of acute fatty liver of pregnancy, based on 28 consecutive cases. *Am J Obstet Gynecol* 1999;181:389–95.

78. Reyes H, Sandoval L, Wainstein A, et al. Acute fatty liver of pregnancy: a clinical study of 12 episodes in 11 patients. *Gut* 1994;35:101–6.

79. Knight M, Nelson-Piercy C, Kurinczuk JJ, et al. A prospective national study of acute fatty liver of pregnancy in the UK. *Gut* 2008;57:951–6.

80. Bacq Y, Constans T, Body G, et al. La stéatose hépatique aiguë gravidique. *J Gynecol Obstet Biol Reprod (Paris)* 1986;15: 851–61.

81. Rolfes DB, Ishak KG. Acute fatty liver of pregnancy: a clinicopathologic study of 35 cases. *Hepatology* 1985;5:1149–58.

82. Riely CA. Acute fatty liver of pregnancy. *Semin Liver Dis* 1987; 7:47–54.

83. Monga M, Katz AR. Acute fatty liver in the second trimester. *Obstet Gynecol* 1999;93:811–13.

84. Buytaert IM, Elewaut GP, Van Kets HE. Early occurrence of acute fatty liver in pregnancy. *Am J Gastroenterol* 1996;91:603–4.

85. Malone FD, Kaufman GE, Chelmow D, et al. Maternal morbidity associated with triplet pregnancy. *Am J Perinatol* 1998;15: 73–7.

86. Vanjak D, Moreau R, Roche-Sicot J, et al. Intrahepatic cholestasis of pregnancy and acute fatty liver of pregnancy. An unusual but favorable association? *Gastroenterology* 1991;100:1123–5.

87. Cammu H, Velkeniers B, Charels K, et al. Idiopathic acute fatty liver of pregnancy associated with transient diabetes insipidus. Case report. *Br J Obstet Gynaecol* 1987;94:173–8.

88. Moldenhauer JS, O'Brien J M, Barton JR, et al. Acute fatty liver of pregnancy associated with pancreatitis: a life-threatening complication. *Am J Obstet Gynecol* 2004;190:502–5.

89. Campillo B, Bernuau J, Witz MO, et al. Ultrasonography in acute fatty liver of pregnancy. *Ann Intern Med* 1986;105:383–4.

90. Goodacre RL, Hunter DJ, Millward S, et al. The diagnosis of acute fatty liver of pregnancy by computed tomography. *J Clin Gastroenterol* 1988;10:680–2.

91. Castro MA, Ouzounian JG, Colletti PM, et al. Radiologic studies in acute fatty liver of pregnancy. A review of the literature and 19 new cases. *J Reprod Med* 1996;41:839–43.

92. Fesenmeier MF, Coppage KH, Lambers DS, et al. Acute fatty liver of pregnancy in 3 tertiary care centers. *Am J Obstet Gynecol* 2005;192:1416–19.

93. Mjahed K, Charra B, Hamoudi D, et al. Acute fatty liver of pregnancy. *Arch Gynecol Obstet* 2006;274:349–53.

94. Treem WR, Rinaldo P, Hale DE, et al. Acute fatty liver of pregnancy and long-chain 3-hydroxyacyl-coenzyme A dehydrogenase deficiency. *Hepatology* 1994;19:339–45.

95. Piech JJ, Thieblot P, Haberer JP, et al. Grossesse gémellaire avec stéatose hépatique aiguë, puis insuffisance antéhypophysaire et diabète insipide. *Presse Med* 1985;14:1421–3.

96. Bacq Y, Assor P, Gendrot C, et al. Stéatose hépatique aiguë gravidique récidivante. *Gastroenterol Clin Biol* 2007;31:1135–8.

97. Schoeman MN, Batey RG, Wilcken B. Recurrent acute fatty liver of pregnancy associated with a fatty-acid oxidation defect in the offspring. *Gastroenterology* 1991;100:544–8.

98. Wilcken B, Leung KC, Hammond J, et al. Pregnancy and fetal long-chain 3-hydroxyacyl coenzyme A dehydrogenase deficiency. *Lancet* 1993;341:407–8.

99. Treem WR, Shoup ME, Hale DE, et al. Acute fatty liver of pregnancy, hemolysis, elevated liver enzymes, and low platelets syndrome, and long chain 3-hydroxyacyl-coenzyme A dehydrogenase deficiency. *Am J Gastroenterol* 1996;91:2293–300.

100. Sims HF, Brackett JC, Powell CK, et al. The molecular basis of pediatric long chain 3-hydroxyacyl-CoA dehydrogenase deficiency associated with maternal acute fatty liver of pregnancy. *Proc Natl Acad Sci USA* 1995;92:841–5.

101. Ibdah JA, Bennett MJ, Rinaldo P, et al. A fetal fatty-acid oxidation disorder as a cause of liver disease in pregnant women. *N Engl J Med* 1999;340:1723–31.

102. Ibdah JA. Role of genetic screening in identifying susceptibility to acute fatty liver of pregnancy. *Nat Clin Pract Gastroenterol Hepatol* 2005;2:494–5.

103. Ibdah JA, Zhao Y, Viola J, et al. Molecular prenatal diagnosis in families with fetal mitochondrial trifunctional protein mutations. *J Pediatr* 2001;138:396–9.

104. Mansouri A, Fromenty B, Durand F, et al. Assessment of the prevalence of genetic metabolic defects in acute fatty liver of pregnancy. *J Hepatol* 1996;25:781.

105. Innes AM, Seargeant LE, Balachandra K, et al. Hepatic carnitine palmitoyltransferase I deficiency presenting as maternal illness in pregnancy. *Pediatr Res* 2000;47:43–5.

106. Mabie WC. Acute fatty liver of pregnancy. *Gastroenterol Clin North Am* 1992;21:951–60.

107. Ockner SA, Brunt EM, Cohn SM, et al. Fulminant hepatic failure caused by acute fatty liver of pregnancy treated by orthotopic liver transplantation. *Hepatology* 1990;11:59–64.

108. Amon E, Allen SR, Petrie RH, et al. Acute fatty liver of pregnancy associated with preeclampsia: management of hepatic failure with postpartum liver transplantation. *Am J Perinatol* 1991;8:278–9.

109. Franco J, Newcomer J, Adams M, et al. Auxiliary liver transplant in acute fatty liver of pregnancy. *Obstet Gynecol* 2000;95:1042.

110. Tong MJ, el-Farra NS, Grew MI. Clinical manifestations of hepatitis A: recent experience in a community teaching hospital. *J Infect Dis* 1995;171(Suppl 1):S15–18.

111. Willner IR, Uhl MD, Howard SC, et al. Serious hepatitis A: an analysis of patients hospitalized during an urban epidemic in the United States. *Ann Intern Med* 1998;128:111–14.

112. Elinav E, Ben-Dov IZ, Shapira Y, et al. Acute hepatitis A infection in pregnancy is associated with high rates of gestational complications and preterm labor. *Gastroenterology* 2006;130:1129–34.

113. Aggarwal R, Naik S. Epidemiology of hepatitis E: current status. *J Gastroenterol Hepatol* 2009;24:1484–93.

114. Rab MA, Bile MK, Mubarik MM, et al. Water-borne hepatitis E virus epidemic in Islamabad, Pakistan: a common source outbreak traced to the malfunction of a modern water treatment plant. *Am J Trop Med Hyg* 1997;57:151–7.

115. Hamid SS, Jafri SMW, Khan H, et al. Fulminant hepatic failure in pregnant women: acute fatty liver or acute viral hepatitis. *J Hepatol* 1996;25:20–7.

116. Kumar A, Beniwal M, Kar P, et al. Hepatitis E in pregnancy. *Int J Gynaecol Obstet* 2004;85:240–4.

117. Devarbhavi H, Kremers WK, Dierkhising R, et al. Pregnancy-associated acute liver disease and acute viral hepatitis: differentiation, course and outcome. *J Hepatol* 2008;49:930–5.

118. Khuroo MS, Kamili S, Jameel S. Vertical transmission of hepatitis E virus. *Lancet* 1995;345:1025–6.

119. Klein NA, Mabie WC, Shaver DC, et al. Herpes simplex virus hepatitis in pregnancy. Two patients successfully treated with acyclovir. *Gastroenterology* 1991;100:239–44.

120. Pinna AD, Rakela J, Demetris AJ, et al. Five cases of fulminant hepatitis due to herpes simplex virus in adults. *Dig Dis Sci* 2002;47:750–4.

121. Jayanthi V, Udayakumar N. Acute liver failure in pregnancy: an overview. *Minerva Gastroenterol Dietol* 2008;54:75–84.

122. Norvell JP, Blei AT, Jovanovic BD, et al. Herpes simplex virus hepatitis: an analysis of the published literature and institutional cases. *Liver Transpl* 2007;13:1428–34.

123. Thijs C, Knipschild P, Leffers P. Pregnancy and gallstone disease: an empiric demonstration of the importance of specification of risk periods. *Am J Epidemiol* 1991;134:186–95.

124. Maringhini A, Marceno MP, Lanzarone F, et al. Sludge and stones in gallbladder after pregnancy. Prevalence and risk factors. *J Hepatol* 1987;5:218–23.

125. Tsimoyiannis EC, Antoniou NC, Tsaboulas C, et al. Cholelithiasis during pregnancy and lactation. Prospective study. *Eur J Surg* 1994;160:627–31.

126. Ko CW, Beresford SA, Schulte SJ, et al. Incidence, natural history, and risk factors for biliary sludge and stones during pregnancy. *Hepatology* 2005;41:359–65.

127. Date RS, Kaushal M, Ramesh A. A review of the management of gallstone disease and its complications in pregnancy. *Am J Surg* 2008;196:599–608.

128. Kuy S, Roman SA, Desai R, et al. Outcomes following cholecystectomy in pregnant and nonpregnant women. *Surgery* 2009;146:358–66.

129. Eddy JJ, Gideonsen MD, Song JY, et al. Pancreatitis in pregnancy. *Obstet Gynecol* 2008;112:1075–81.

130. Karsenti D, Bacq Y, Brechot JF, et al. Serum amylase and lipase activities in normal pregnancy: a prospective case–control study. *Am J Gastroenterol* 2001;96:697–9.

131. Tham TC, Vandervoort J, Wong RC, et al. Safety of ERCP during pregnancy. *Am J Gastroenterol* 2003;98:308–11.

132. European Association for the Study of the Liver. EASL Clinical Practice Guidelines. Management of cholestatic liver diseases. *J Hepatol* 2009;51:237–67.

133. De Chalain TM, Michell WL, Berger GM. Hyperlipidemia, pregnancy and pancreatitis. *Surg Gynecol Obstet* 1988;167:469–73.

134. Dahan M, Chang RJ. Pancreatitis secondary to hyperparathyroidism during pregnancy. *Obstet Gynecol* 2001;98:923–5.

135. Hong MK, Hsieh CT, Chen BH, et al. Primary hyperparathyroidism and acute pancreatitis during the third trimester of pregnancy. *J Matern Fetal Med* 2001;10:214–18.

136. Taylor TV, Brigg JK, Russell JG, et al. Choledochal cyst of pregnancy. *J R Coll Surg Edinb* 1977;22:424–7.

137. Jackson BT, Saunders P. Perforated choledochus cyst. *Br J Surg* 1971;58:38–42.

138. Khuroo MS, Datta DV. Budd–Chiari syndrome following pregnancy. Report of 16 cases, with roentgenologic, hemodynamic and histologic studies of the hepatic outflow tract. *Am J Med* 1980;68:113–21.

139. Singh V, Sinha SK, Nain CK, et al. Budd–Chiari syndrome: our experience of 71 patients. *J Gastroenterol Hepatol* 2000;15:550–4.

140. Rautou PE, Plessier A, Bernuau J, et al. Pregnancy: a risk factor for Budd–Chiari syndrome? *Gut* 2009;58:606–8.

141. James AH. Prevention and management of venous thromboembolism in pregnancy. *Am J Med* 2007;120:S26–34.

142. Ouwendijk RJ, Koster JC, Wilson JH, et al. Budd–Chiari syndrome in a young patient with anticardiolipin antibodies: need for prolonged anticoagulant treatment. *Gut* 1994;35:1004–6.

143. Segal S, Shenhav S, Segal O, et al. Budd–Chiari syndrome complicating severe preeclampsia in a parturient with primary antiphospholipid syndrome. *Eur J Obstet Gynecol Reprod Biol* 1996;68:227–9.

144. Deltenre P, Denninger MH, Hillaire S, et al. Factor V Leiden related Budd–Chiari syndrome. *Gut* 2001;48:264–8.

145. Hsu HW, Belfort MA, Vernino S, et al. Postpartum thrombotic thrombocytopenic purpura complicated by Budd–Chiari syndrome. *Obstet Gynecol* 1995;85:839–43.

146. Hill JB, Sheffield JS, Zeeman GG, et al. Hepatotoxicity with antiretroviral treatment of pregnant women. *Obstet Gynecol* 2001;98:909–11.

147. Wang PH, Yang MJ, Lee WL, et al. Acetaminophen poisoning in late pregnancy. A case report. *J Reprod Med* 1997;42:367–71.

148. Ali T, Srinivasan N, Le V, et al. Alpha-methyldopa hepatotoxicity in pregnancy. *J Coll Physicians Surg Pak* 2009;19:125–6.

149. Smith GN, Piercy WN. Methyldopa hepatotoxicity in pregnancy: a case report. *Am J Obstet Gynecol* 1995;172:222–4.

150. Balderston KD, Tewari K, Azizi F, et al. Intrahepatic cholangiocarcinoma masquerading as the HELLP syndrome (hemolysis, elevated liver enzymes, and low platelet count) in pregnancy: case report. *Am J Obstet Gynecol* 1998;179:823–4.

151. Hsu KL, Ko SF, Cheng YF, et al. Spontaneous rupture of hepatocellular carcinoma during pregnancy. *Obstet Gynecol* 2001;98:913–16.

152. Moseley RH. Sepsis and cholestasis. *Clin Liver Dis* 2004;8:83–94.

153. Rodrigues G, Seetharam P. Management of hydatid disease (echinococcosis) in pregnancy. *Obstet Gynecol Surv* 2008;63:116–23.

154. Gaspari R, Annetta MG, Cavaliere F, et al. Unusual presentation of leptospirosis in the late stage of pregnancy. *Minerva Anestesiol* 2007;73:429–32.

155. d'Alteroche L, Perarnau JM, Perrotin F, et al. Grossesse et hypertension portale. *Gastroenterol Clin Biol* 2008;32:541–6.

156. Kochhar R, Kumar S, Goel RC, et al. Pregnancy and its outcome in patients with noncirrhotic portal hypertension. *Dig Dis Sci* 1999;44:1356–61.

157. Aggarwal N, Sawhney H, Vasishta K, et al. Non-cirrhotic portal hypertension in pregnancy. *Int J Gynaecol Obstet* 2001;72:1–7.

158. Starkel P, Horsmans Y, Geubel A. Endoscopic band ligation: a safe technique to control bleeding esophageal varices in pregnancy. *Gastrointest Endosc* 1998;48:212–14.

159. Wong S, Chan LY, Yu V, et al. Hepatitis B carrier and perinatal outcome in singleton pregnancy. *Am J Perinatol* 1999;16:485–8.

160. Rawal BK, Parida S, Watkins RP, et al. Symptomatic reactivation of hepatitis B in pregnancy. *Lancet* 1991;337:364.

161. Wiseman E, Fraser MA, Holden S, et al. Perinatal transmission of hepatitis B virus: an Australian experience. *Med J Aust* 2009;190:489–92.

162. Lee SD, Lo KJ, Tsai YT, et al. Role of caesarean section in prevention of mother–infant transmission of hepatitis B virus. *Lancet* 1988;2:833–4.

163. US Preventive Services Task Force. Screening for hepatitis B virus infection in pregnancy: US Preventive Services Task Force reaffirmation recommendation statement. *Ann Intern Med* 2009;150:869–73, W154.

164. Kane M. Implementing universal vaccination programmes: USA. *Vaccine* 1995;13(Suppl 1):S75–6.

165. Terazawa S, Kojima M, Yamanaka T, et al. Hepatitis B virus mutants with precore-region defects in two babies with fulminant hepatitis and their mothers positive for antibody to hepatitis B e antigen. *Pediatr Res* 1991;29:5–9.

166. van Zonneveld M, van Nunen AB, Niesters HG, et al. Lamivudine treatment during pregnancy to prevent perinatal transmission of hepatitis B virus infection. *J Viral Hepat* 2003;10:294–7.

167. Xu WM, Cui YT, Wang L, et al. Lamivudine in late pregnancy to prevent perinatal transmission of hepatitis B virus infection: a multicentre, randomized, double-blind, placebo-controlled study. *J Viral Hepat* 2009;16:94–103.

168. Li XM, Yang YB, Hou HY, et al. Interruption of HBV intrauterine transmission: a clinical study. *World J Gastroenterol* 2003;9:1501–3.

169. Zanetti AR, Ferroni P, Magliano EM, et al. Perinatal transmission of the hepatitis B virus and of the HBV-associated delta agent from mothers to offspring in northern Italy. *J Med Virol* 1982;9:139–48.

170. Gambarin-Gelwan M. Hepatitis B in pregnancy. *Clin Liver Dis* 2007;11:945–63.

171. Floreani A, Paternoster D, Zappala F, et al. Hepatitis C virus infection in pregnancy. *Br J Obstet Gynaecol* 1996;103:325–9.

172. Conte D, Fraquelli M, Prati D, et al. Prevalence and clinical course of chronic hepatitis C virus (HCV) infection and rate of HCV vertical transmission in a cohort of 15,250 pregnant women. *Hepatology* 2000;31:751–5.

173. Gervais A, Bacq Y, Bernuau J, et al. Decrease in serum ALT and increase in serum HCV RNA during pregnancy in women with chronic hepatitis C. *J Hepatol* 2000;32:293–9.

174. Paternoster DM, Santarossa C, Grella P, et al. Viral load in HCV RNA-positive pregnant women. *Am J Gastroenterol* 2001;96:2751–4.

175. Fontaine H, Nalpas B, Carnot F, et al. Effect of pregnancy on chronic hepatitis C: a case–control study. *Lancet* 2000;356:1328–9.

176. Di Martino V, Lebray P, Myers RP, et al. Progression of liver fibrosis in women infected with hepatitis C: long-term benefit of estrogen exposure. *Hepatology* 2004;40:1426–33.

177. Pembrey L, Newell ML, Tovo PA. The management of HCV infected pregnant women and their children European paediatric HCV network. *J Hepatol* 2005;43:515–25.

178. Roberts EA, Yeung L. Maternal–infant transmission of hepatitis C virus infection. *Hepatology* 2002;36:S106–13.

179. Mast EE. Mother-to-infant hepatitis C virus transmission and breast-feeding. *Adv Exp Med Biol* 2004;554:211–16.

180. Marine-Barjoan E, Berrebi A, Giordanengo V, et al. HCV/HIV co-infection, HCV viral load and mode of delivery: risk factors for mother-to-child transmission of hepatitis C virus? *Aids* 2007;21:1811–15.

181. Heneghan MA, Norris SM, O'Grady JG, et al. Management and outcome of pregnancy in autoimmune hepatitis. *Gut* 2001;48:97–102.

182. Buchel E, Van Steenbergen W, Nevens F, et al. Improvement of autoimmune hepatitis during pregnancy followed by flare-up after delivery. *Am J Gastroenterol* 2002;97:3160–5.

183. Czaja AJ. Special clinical challenges in autoimmune hepatitis: the elderly, males, pregnancy, mild disease, fulminant onset, and non-white patients. *Semin Liver Dis* 2009;29:315–30.

184. Colle I, Hautekeete M. Remission of autoimmune hepatitis during pregnancy: a report of two cases. *Liver* 1999;19:55–7.

185. Werner M, Bjornsson E, Prytz H, et al. Autoimmune hepatitis among fertile women: strategies during pregnancy and breastfeeding? *Scand J Gastroenterol* 2007;42:986–91.

186. Manns MP, Czaja AJ, Gorham JD, et al. Diagnosis and management of autoimmune hepatitis. *Hepatology* 2010;51:2193–213.

187. Hirschfield GM, Kumagi T, Heathcote EJ. Preventative hepatology: minimising symptoms and optimising care. *Liver Int* 2008;28:922–34.

188. Powell EE, Molloy D. Successful in vitro fertilization and pregnancy in a patient with autoimmune chronic active hepatitis and cirrhosis. *J Gastroenterol Hepatol* 1995;10:233–5.

189. Rabinovitz M, Appasamy R, Finkelstein S. Primary biliary cirrhosis diagnosed during pregnancy. Does it have a different outcome? *Dig Dis Sci* 1995;40:571–4.

190. Olsson R, Loof L, Wallerstedt S. Pregnancy in patients with primary biliary cirrhosis – a case for dissuasion? The Swedish Internal Medicine Liver Club. *Liver* 1993;13:316–18.

191. Nir A, Sorokin Y, Abramovici H, et al. Pregnancy and primary biliary cirrhosis. *Int J Gynaecol Obstet* 1989;28:279–82.

192. Goh SK, Gull SE, Alexander GJ. Pregnancy in primary biliary cirrhosis complicated by portal hypertension: report of a case and review of the literature. *Br J Obstet Gynaecol* 2001;108:760–2.

193. Poupon R, Chretien Y, Chazouilleres O, et al. Pregnancy in women with ursodeoxycholic acid-treated primary biliary cirrhosis. *J Hepatol* 2005;42:418–19.

194. Shimono N, Ishibashi H, Ikematsu H, et al. Fulminant hepatic failure during perinatal period in a pregnant woman with Wilson's disease. *Gastroenterol Jpn* 1991;26:69–73.

195. Roberts EA, Schilsky ML. Diagnosis and treatment of Wilson disease: an update. *Hepatology* 2008;47:2089–111.

196. Sternlieb I. Wilson's disease and pregnancy. *Hepatology* 2000;31:531–2.

197. Walshe JM. The management of pregnancy in Wilson's disease treated with trientine. *Q J Med* 1986;58:81–7.

198. Devesa R, Alvarez A, de las Heras G, et al. Wilson's disease treated with trientine during pregnancy. *J Pediatr Gastroenterol Nutr* 1995;20:102–3.

199. Brewer GJ, Johnson VD, Dick RD, et al. Treatment of Wilson's disease with zinc. XVII: treatment during pregnancy. *Hepatology* 2000;31:364–70.

200. Kent DR, Nissen ED, Nissen SE, et al. Effect of pregnancy on liver tumor associated with oral contraceptives. *Obstet Gynecol* 1978;51:148–51.

201. Estebe JP, Malledant Y, Guillou YM, et al. [Spontaneous rupture of an adenoma of the liver during pregnancy.] *J Chir (Paris)* 1988;125:654–6.

202. Aulagnier G, Ramirez A, Delorme JM, et al. [Ruptured adenoma of the liver with severe pulmonary embolism discovered during a cesarean section.] *J Chir (Paris)* 1986;123:651–3.

203. Monks PL, Fryar BG, Biggs WW. Spontaneous rupture of an hepatic adenoma in pregnancy with survival of mother and fetus. *Aust NZ J Obstet Gynaecol* 1986;26:155–7.

204. Terkivatan T, de Wilt JH, de Man RA, et al. Management of hepatocellular adenoma during pregnancy. *Liver* 2000;20:186–7.

205. Mathieu D, Kobeiter H, Maison P, et al. Oral contraceptive use and focal nodular hyperplasia of the liver. *Gastroenterology* 2000;118:560–4.

206. Scott LD, Katz AR, Duke JH, et al. Oral contraceptives, pregnancy, and focal nodular hyperplasia of the liver. *JAMA* 1984;251:1461–3.

207. Glinkova V, Shevah O, Boaz M, et al. Hepatic haemangiomas: possible association with female sex hormones. *Gut* 2004;53:1352–5.

208. Friedlaender P, Osler M. Icterus and pregnancy. *Am J Obstet Gynecol* 1967;97:894–900.

209. Cohen L, Lewis C, Arias IM. Pregnancy, oral contraceptives, and chronic familial jaundice with predominantly conjugated hyperbilirubinemia (Dubin–Johnson syndrome). *Gastroenterology* 1972;62:1182–90.

210. Smith JF Jr, Baker JM. Crigler–Najjar disease in pregnancy. *Obstet Gynecol* 1994;84:670–2.

211. Ito T, Katagiri C, Ikeno S, et al. Phenobarbital following phototherapy for Crigler–Najjar syndrome type II with good fetal outcome: a case report. *J Obstet Gynaecol Res* 2001;27:33–5.

212. Rajka G. Pregnancy and porphyria cutanea tarda. *Acta Derm Venereol* 1984;64:444–5.

213. Brodie MJ, Moore MR, Thompson GG, et al. Pregnancy and the acute porphyrias. *Br J Obstet Gynaecol* 1977;84:726–31.

214. Kanaan C, Veille JC, Lakin M. Pregnancy and acute intermittent porphyria. *Obstet Gynecol Surv* 1989;44:244–9.

215. Milo R, Neuman M, Klein C, et al. Acute intermittent porphyria in pregnancy. *Obstet Gynecol* 1989;73:450–2.

216. Rautou PE, Angermayr B, Garcia-Pagan JC, et al. Pregnancy in women with known and treated Budd–Chiari syndrome: maternal and fetal outcomes. *J Hepatol* 2009;51:47–54.

217. Heneghan MA, Selzner M, Yoshida EM, et al. Pregnancy and sexual function in liver transplantation. *J Hepatol* 2008;49:507–19.

218. Laifer SA, Guido RS. Reproductive function and outcome of pregnancy after liver transplantation in women. *Mayo Clin Proc* 1995;70:388–94.

219. Mass K, Quint EH, Punch MR, et al. Gynecological and reproductive function after liver transplantation. *Transplantation* 1996;62:476–9.

220. Armenti VT, Herrine SK, Radomski JS, et al. Pregnancy after liver transplantation. *Liver Transpl* 2000;6:671–85.

221. Coffin CS, Shaheen AA, Burak KW, et al. Pregnancy outcomes among liver transplant recipients in the United States: a nationwide case–control analysis. *Liver Transpl* 2010;16:56–63.

222. Jain A, Venkataramanan R, Fung JJ, et al. Pregnancy after liver transplantation under tacrolimus. *Transplantation* 1997;64:559–65.

223. Kainz A, Harabacz I, Cowlrick IS, et al. Review of the course and outcome of 100 pregnancies in 84 women treated with tacrolimus. *Transplantation* 2000;70:1718–21.

224. Christopher V, Al-Chalabi T, Richardson PD, et al. Pregnancy outcome after liver transplantation: a single-center experience of 71 pregnancies in 45 recipients. *Liver Transpl* 2006;12:1138–43.

225. Roberts M, Brown AS, James OF, et al. Interpretation of cyclosporin A levels in pregnancy following orthoptic liver transplantation. *Br J Obstet Gynaecol* 1995;102:570–2.

226. Laifer SA, Darby MJ, Scantlebury VP, et al. Pregnancy and liver transplantation. *Obstet Gynecol* 1990;76:1083–8.

227. Merritt WT, Dickstein R, Beattie C, et al. Liver transplantation during pregnancy: anesthesia for two procedures in the same patient with successful outcome of pregnancy. *Transplant Proc* 1991;23:1996–7.

228. Friedman E, Moses B, Engelberg S, et al. Malignant insulinoma with hepatic failure complicating pregnancy. *South Med J* 1988;81:86–8.

229. Kato T, Nery JR, Morcos JJ, et al. Successful living related liver transplantation in an adult with fulminant hepatic failure. *Transplantation* 1997;64:415–17.

Multiple choice questions

11.1 **Which of the following items is not associated with intrahepatic cholestasis of pregnancy (ICP)?**

   a ICP is usually revealed by a generalized pruritus during the second or third trimester.
   b ICP recurs frequently during subsequent pregnancies (more than 50% of cases).
   c Ursodesoxycholic acid may be used in the treatment of ICP.
   d ICP is a cause of acute liver failure.
   e ICP may be responsible for intrauterine fetal death.

11.2 **Which of the following items is not associated with acute fatty liver of pregnancy (AFLP)?**

   a AFLP is the most frequent cause of liver disease unique to pregnancy.
   b AFLP is a cause of acute liver failure during the third trimester.
   c AFLP is an indication of prompt delivery.
   d AFLP may be associated with long-chain 3-hydroxyacyl-CoA dehydrogenase (LCHAD) deficiency.
   e AFLP may recur during subsequent pregnancies.

Answers to the multiple choice questions can be found in the Appendix at the end of the book.

These multiple choice questions are also available for you to complete online.
Visit http://www.schiffsdiseasesoftheliver.com/

CHAPTER 12
Hepatic Fibrosis

Scott L. Friedman

Mount Sinai School of Medicine, New York, NY, USA

Key concepts

- Hepatic fibrosis is a reversible wound-healing response characterized by the accumulation of extracellular matrix (ECM) or "scar;" it follows chronic, but not self-limited, liver disease. The ECM components in fibrotic liver are similar, regardless of the underlying cause.
- Activation of hepatic stellate cells is the central event in hepatic fibrosis. These perisinusoidal cells and related myofibroblasts from intra- and extrahepatic origins orchestrate an array of changes including degradation of the normal ECM of liver, deposition of scar molecules, vascular and organ contraction, and release of cytokines.

- Not only is hepatic fibrosis reversible, but it is also increasingly clear that cirrhosis may be reversible as well. The exact stage at which fibrosis/cirrhosis becomes truly irreversible, and its biologic determinants, are not known.
- Antifibrotic therapies have entered clinical trials. Emerging therapies will be targeted to those patients with reversible disease. The paradigm of stellate cell activation provides an important framework for defining therapeutic targets. Currently, the most significant impediment to drug development is the lack of robust noninvasive markers of fibrosis to accurately assess response to therapy.

Fibrosis is a reversible scarring response that occurs in almost all patients with chronic liver injury. Ultimately, hepatic fibrosis leads to cirrhosis, characterized by nodule formation and organ contraction. The causes of cirrhosis are multiple and include congenital, metabolic, inflammatory, and toxic liver diseases (Box 12.1).

It is essential to understand the molecular underpinnings of fibrosis because the fibrotic response underlies all the complications of end-stage liver disease, including portal hypertension, ascites, encephalopathy, synthetic dysfunction, and impaired metabolic capacity. Therefore, fibrosis is deleterious both by its direct effects on cellular function and by its mechanical contribution to increased portal resistance.

This chapter reviews the significant progress made toward elucidating the cellular basis of hepatic fibrosis and how these insights are leading to advances in the diagnosis and treatment of chronic liver disease.

Biologic basis of hepatic fibrosis

General principles

1 *Hepatic fibrosis is a wound-healing response* in which the damaged regions are encapsulated by extracellular matrix (ECM), or scar. In all circumstances, the composition of the hepatic scar is similar. The cells and soluble factors participating in this response in the liver are also similar to those involved in parenchymal injury to the kidney, lung, or skin. This understanding has helped to identify underlying mechanisms and will likely lead to new therapies for fibrotic diseases of many organs including the liver.

2 *Myofibroblast-like cells produce hepatic fibrosis regardless of the underlying cause.* As discussed in the subsequent text, the activated hepatic stellate cell is the key cellular source of these myofibroblasts, but additional origins of fibrogenic cells may include peribiliary fibroblasts, bone marrow, and even epithelial–mesenchymal transition (EMT) from epithelial cells. How stellate cells and related cells are activated in response to so large a variety of hepatic insults – from inborn metabolic defects to chronic viral hepatitis – is being increasingly revealed.

3 *Hepatic fibrosis follows chronic, not self-limited, injury.* For example, patients surviving fulminant hepatitis do not develop scarring despite an abundance of fibrogenic stimuli, unless chronic injury follows. Moreover, even fibrosis associated with sustained injury is often reversible. The reason for fibrosis reversibility, even in chronic liver disease, is not certain, but may be related to the relative activity of matrix-degrading enzymes and their inhibitors, as well as the relative extent of collagen cross-linking.

Schiff's Diseases of the Liver, Eleventh Edition. Edited by Eugene R. Schiff, Willis C. Maddrey and Michael F. Sorrell.
© 2012 John Wiley & Sons, Ltd. Published 2012 by John Wiley & Sons, Ltd.

Box 12.1 Causes of fibrosis and cirrhosis.

Presinusoidal fibrosis
- Schistosomiasis
- Idiopathic portal fibrosis

Parenchymal fibrosis
- Drugs and toxins:
  - Alcohol
  - Methotrexate
  - Isoniazid
  - Vitamin A
  - Amiodarone
  - Perhexiline maleate
  - α-Methyldopa
  - Oxyphenisatin
- Infections:
  - Chronic hepatitis B and C
  - Brucellosis
  - Echinococcosis
  - Congenital or tertiary syphilis
- Autoimmune disease:
  - Autoimmune hepatitis
- Vascular abnormalities:
  - Chronic passive congestion
  - Hereditary hemorrhagic telangiectasia
- Metabolic/genetic diseases:
  - Wilson disease
  - Genetic hemochromatosis
  - α_1-Antitrypsin deficiency
  - Carbohydrate metabolism disorders
  - Lipid metabolism disorders
  - Urea cycle defects
  - Porphyria
  - Amino acid metabolism disorders
  - Bile acid disorders
- Biliary obstruction:
  - Primary biliary cirrhosis
  - Secondary biliary cirrhosis
  - Cystic fibrosis
  - Biliary atresia/neonatal hepatitis
  - Congenital biliary cysts
- Idiopathic/miscellaneous:
  - Nonalcoholic steatohepatitis
  - Indian childhood cirrhosis
  - Granulomatous liver disease
  - Polycystic liver disease

Postsinusoidal fibrosis
- Sinusoidal obstruction syndrome (venoocclusive disease)

4 *Fibrosis occurs earliest in regions in which injury is most severe.* This is especially true in chronic inflammatory liver disease due to alcohol or viral infection. For example, pericentral injury is a hallmark of alcoholic hepatitis, and the development of pericentral fibrosis (also known as sclerosing hyaline necrosis or perivenular fibrosis) is an early marker of likely progression to panlobular cirrhosis.

Extracellular matrix composition of the normal liver and hepatic scars

Extracellular matrix refers to the array of macromolecules comprising the scaffolding of normal and fibrotic liver. The components of hepatic ECM include several families of structural and supporting molecules: collagens, non-collagen glycoproteins, matrix-bound growth factors, glycosaminoglycans, proteoglycans, and matricellular proteins. Of the 20 types of collagens characterized thus far, ten have been identified in the liver.

In the normal liver, so-called fibril-forming collagens (types I, III, V, and XI) are largely confined to the capsule, around large vessels, and in the portal triad, with only scattered fibrils containing types I and III collagen in the subendothelial space. Smaller amounts of other collagens, including types VI, XIV, and XVIII, can be found. Glycoproteins and matricellular proteins are also present, including subendothelial deposits of fibronectin, laminin, tenascin, secreted protein that is acidic and rich in cysteine (SPARC), and von Willebrand factor. Proteoglycans primarily consist of heparan sulfate proteoglycans including perlecan, as well as small amounts of decorin, biglycan, fibromodulin, aggrecan, glypican, syndecan, and lumican.

The fibrotic liver is characterized by both quantitative and qualitative differences in the matrix composition compared with the normal liver; as noted, these changes are similar regardless of the type of liver injury. Total collagen content increases 3–10-fold, although the collagen is not "abnormal" in sequence or structure. Overall, there is a marked increase in "interstitial matrix" that is typical of the healing wound, which includes fibril-forming collagens (types I, III, and V) and some nonfibril-forming collagens (types IV and VI), several glycoproteins (e.g., cellular fibronectin, laminin, SPARC, osteonectin, tenascin, and von Willebrand factor), a large number of proteoglycans and glycosaminoglycans (e.g., perlecan, decorin, aggrecan, lumican, and fibromodulin), and related receptors, including dystroglycan [1].

Biologic activity of extracellular matrix in the liver

Extracellular matrix is a dynamic regulator of cell function and not an inert "ground substance." Early, subendothelial matrix accumulation leading to "capillarization" of the subendothelial space of Disse is a key event and may be more important than overall increases in matrix content (Fig. 12.1). The basement membrane constituents within the subendothelial space may be essential for preserving the differentiated functions of hepatocytes,

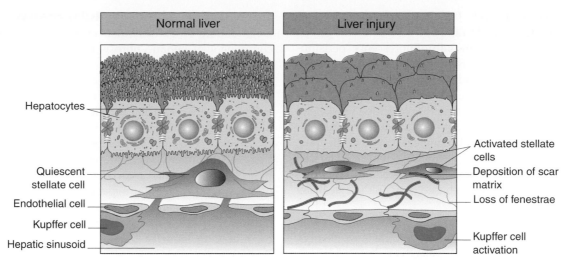

Figure 12.1 Matrix and cellular alterations in hepatic fibrosis. Changes in the subendothelial space of Disse as fibrosis develops in response to liver injury include alterations in both cellular responses and extracellular matrix composition. Stellate cell activation leads to an accumulation of scar (fibril forming) matrix This in turn contributes to the loss of hepatocyte microvilli and sinusoidal endothelial fenestrae, which results in the deterioration of hepatic function. Kupffer cell (macrophage) activation accompanies liver injury and contributes to the paracrine activation of stellate cells. (Reproduced from Friedman [168] with permission from American Society for Biochemistry and Molecular Biology.)

hepatic stellate cells, and endothelial cells. Replacement of the normally low-density matrix by interstitial matrix directly perturbs hepatocyte function and could explain the synthetic and metabolic dysfunction that is characteristic of more advanced fibrosis and cirrhosis. This high-density matrix also activates stellate cells and leads to a decrease in fenestrations of sinusoidal endothelial cells, which could impair the transport of solutes from the sinusoid to hepatocytes.

In liver injury, an increase in cellular fibronectin levels is among the first matrix alterations seen within this region. A consequence of this change is the activation of hepatic stellate cells and acceleration of fibrosis (see section below).

Altered cellular behavior induced by matrix alterations is typically mediated by cell membrane receptors. *Integrins*, a large family of homologous membrane linker proteins, are the best characterized type of ECM receptor. Integrins are noncovalent αβ-heterodimers that consist of a large extracellular domain, a membrane-spanning domain, and a cytoplasmic tail [2,3].

In addition to integrins, a growing number of other adhesion proteins and cell matrix receptors have been characterized, including cadherins and selectins, which mediate interactions between inflammatory cells and the endothelial wall. For example, upregulation of a tyrosine kinase receptor, discoidin domain receptor 2 (DDR2), has been identified during stellate cell activation, which signals in response to fibrillar collagens, leading to enhanced matrix metalloproteinase (MMP) expression and cell growth [4]. The DDR family is the only family of receptor tyrosine kinases whose ligands are ECM molecules rather than peptide ligands, and their upregulation could be a critical requirement to perpetuate liver fibrosis.

ECM can also indirectly affect cell function through the release of soluble growth factors (cytokines), which is in turn controlled by local metalloproteinases. These include platelet-derived growth factor (PDGF), hepatocyte growth factor (HGF), connective tissue growth factor (CTGF), tumor necrosis factor α (TNF-α), basic fibroblast growth factor (bFGF), and vascular endothelial cell growth factor (VEGF). Controlled release from ECM is a key mechanism for regulating cytokine activity because it provides a local, accessible source that is tightly regulatable through the actions of proteases and their inhibitors. In addition, ECM can regulate the activity of proteases through specific binding to collagens or fibronectins [1].

Cellular sources of extracellular matrix in normal and fibrotic liver

The identification of the cellular sources of ECM in hepatic fibrosis has been a significant advance that laid the groundwork for defining mechanisms of fibrosis and potential therapies. The *hepatic stellate cell* (previously called the lipocyte, Ito, fat-storing, or perisinusoidal cell) is the primary source of ECM in the normal and fibrotic liver. In addition, related mesenchymal cell types from a variety of sources may also make measurable contributions to total matrix accumulation, including classic portal fibroblasts (especially in biliary fibrosis) [5], bone marrow-derived cells [6], and fibroblast-derived EMT involving hedgehog signaling [7].

Hepatic stellate cells are resident perisinusoidal cells in the subendothelial space between hepatocytes and sinusoidal endothelial cells [8]. They are the primary sites for storing retinoids within the body. Stellate cells can be recognized by their vitamin A autofluorescence, perisinusoidal orientation, and expression of the cytoskeletal proteins desmin and glial acidic fibrillary protein. In strict terms, "stellate cells" may represent a heterogeneous population of mesenchymal cells with respect to cytoskeletal phenotype, vitamin A content, and localization, but collectively they are the key fibrogenic cell type in the liver. Moreover, the remarkable plasticity of the stellate cell phenotype has been documented in vivo and in culture, precluding a strict definition based only on the cytoskeletal phenotype.

Studies in situ in both animals and humans with progressive injury have defined a gradient of changes within stellate cells that are collectively termed *activation* (see subsequent text) [9]. Stellate cell activation refers to the transition from a quiescent vitamin A-rich cell to a highly fibrogenic cell characterized morphologically by the enlargement of rough endoplasmic reticulum, diminution of vitamin A droplets, ruffled nuclear membrane, appearance of contractile filaments, and proliferation. As noted in the preceding text, the proliferation of stellate cells occurs in regions of greatest injury, which is typically preceded by an influx of inflammatory cells and is associated with subsequent ECM accumulation.

Stellate cells have now been characterized in many human liver diseases. Alcoholic liver disease is the best studied example, with numerous reports documenting features of activation in situ; activation may occur even in the presence of steatosis alone without inflammation [10]. Activated stellate cells have also been observed in viral hepatitis [11]. In hepatocellular carcinoma, activated stellate cells contribute to the deposition of tumor stroma.

Remarkably, very few studies have defined the cellular or matrix composition of congenital hepatic fibrosis, an entity whose pathogenesis is not clear. Current theories suggest that as in adults, congenital hepatic fibrosis represents a final common pathway of fetal hepatic injury, whether from biliary malformations, viral infections (especially cytomegalovirus), or other insults, with the stellate cell playing a significant role. Very few studies have examined specific mediators, but stellate cells contribute to fibrosis in this disease as well [12]. It is unclear, however, why fibrosis develops in weeks to months in utero, whereas it requires months to years in adults (see "Fibrosis progression and reversibility" below).

ECM production by sinusoidal endothelial cells, although less than that by stellate cells, is nonetheless an important component of early fibrosis. After acute liver injury, increased expression of cellular isoforms of fibronectin by these cells is a key early event because their appearance creates a microenvironment that activates stellate cells [13].

Degradation of extracellular matrix

Degradation of extracellular matrix represents a key component of hepatic fibrosis for at least two reasons: (i) early disruption of the normal hepatic matrix by matrix proteases ("pathologic" matrix degradation) hastens its replacement by scar matrix, which in turn has deleterious effects on cell function (See "Biologic activity of extracellular matrix in the liver" above); and (ii) in established fibrosis in patients with chronic liver disease there is an urgent need to resorb the excess wound matrix ("therapeutic" matrix degradation) in the hope of arresting or reversing hepatic dysfunction and portal hypertension. Because fibrosis reflects a balance between matrix production and degradation, this balance must be shifted in favor of degradation for any antifibrotic therapy to succeed.

There has been significant progress in elucidating the fundamental mechanisms of matrix remodeling and how these apply to hepatic fibrosis. An enlarging family of MMPs (also known as matrixins) has been identified; they are calcium-dependent enzymes that specifically degrade collagens and noncollagenous substrates [14]. Broadly, these fall into five categories based on substrate specificity: (i) interstitial collagenases (MMP-1, -8, -13); (ii) gelatinases (MMP-2, -9) and fibroblast activation protein; (iii) stromelysins (MMP-3, -7, -10, -11); (iv) membrane-type MMPs (MMP-14, -15, -16, -17, -24, -25); and (v) a metalloelastase (MMP-12). Metalloproteinases are regulated at many levels to restrict their activity to discrete regions within the pericellular milieu. Inactive metalloproteinases can be activated through proteolytic cleavage by either membrane-type 1 matrix metalloproteinase (MT1-MMP) or plasmin, and inhibited by binding to specific inhibitors known as *tissue inhibitors of metalloproteinases* (TIMPs). The stoichiometry and molecular basis for these interactions has been greatly clarified. For example, MT1-MMP (MMP-14) and TIMP-2 form a ternary complex with MMP-2, possibly including $\alpha v \beta 3$ integrin, which is essential for optimal MMP-2 activity [15]. Similarly, plasmin activity is controlled by its activating enzyme, uroplasminogen activator, and a specific inhibitor, plasminogen activator inhibitor 1, and can be stimulated by active transforming growth factor $\beta 1$ (TGF-$\beta 1$). Therefore, net collagenase activity reflects the relative amounts of activated metalloproteinases and their inhibitors, especially TIMPs. In addition to TIMPs, other protease inhibitors may affect the net degradative activity, including α_2-macroglobulin.

In the liver, "pathologic" matrix degradation refers to the early disruption of the normal subendothelial matrix, which occurs through the actions of at least four enzymes: *MMP-2* (also called gelatinase A or 72 kDa type IV collagenase) and *MMP-9* (gelatinase B or 92 kDa type IV collagenase), which degrade type IV collagen;

membrane-type MMP-1 or -2, which activates latent MMP-2; and *stromelysin 1* (MMP-3), which degrades proteoglycans and glycoproteins and also activates latent collagenases. Stellate cells are a key source of MMP-2, MMP-13 in rodents, and stromelysin 1 [15]. Markedly increased expression of MMP-2 is characteristic of cirrhosis; yet, in experimental animals that lack MMP-2, fibrosis is worse than in normal animals after toxic liver injury [16], which suggests that MMP-2 may normally limit liver injury. These findings suggest that simple inhibition of metalloproteinases may not be an efficacious strategy to limit fibrosis.

Failure to degrade the increased interstitial or scar matrix is a major determinant of progressive fibrosis. MMP-1 is the main protease that can degrade type I collagen, the principal collagen in the fibrotic liver. However, the sources of this enzyme are not as clearly established as for the type IV collagenases. Progressive fibrosis is associated with marked increases in TIMP-1 and TIMP-2 [17], leading to a net decrease in protease activity and, there-

fore, more unopposed matrix accumulation. Stellate cells are the major source of these inhibitors [17]. Sustained TIMP-1 expression is emerging as a key reason for progressive fibrosis, and its diminution is an important prerequisite to allow for reversal of fibrosis (see below).

Stellate cell activation, the central event in hepatic fibrosis

It is useful to frame the pathophysiology of hepatic fibrosis around the mechanisms of hepatic stellate cell activation because this cell type is the major source of ECM. Activation consists of two major phases: *initiation* (also called a preinflammatory stage) and *perpetuation* (Fig. 12.2) [18]. Initiation refers to early changes in gene expression and phenotype, which render the cells responsive to other cytokines and stimuli, while perpetuation results from the effects of these stimuli on maintaining the activated phenotype and generating fibrosis. Initiation is largely due to paracrine stimulation, whereas perpetuation involves autocrine and paracrine loops.

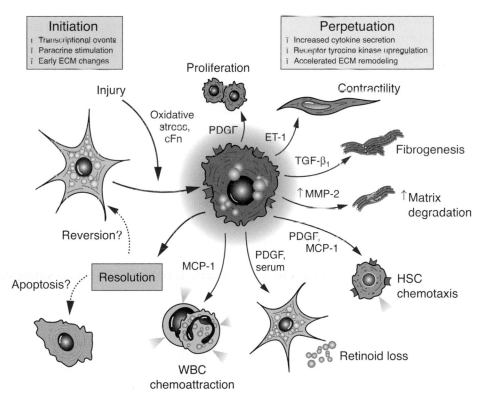

Figure 12.2 Phenotypic features of hepatic stellate cell activation during liver injury and resolution. Following liver injury, hepatic stellate cells undergo "activation," during which they are transformed from quiescent vitamin A-rich cells into proliferative, fibrogenic, and contractile myofibroblasts. The major phenotypic changes after activation include proliferation, contractility, fibrogenesis, matrix degradation, chemotaxis, retinoid loss, and white blood cell (WBC) chemoattraction. The key mediators underlying these effects are shown. The fate of activated stellate cells during the resolution of liver injury is uncertain but may include reversion to a quiescent phenotype or selective clearance by apoptosis. cFn, cellular fibronectin; ECM, extracellular matrix; ET-1, endothelin-1; HSC, hepatic stellate cell; MCP-1, monocyte chemoattractant protein 1; MMP-2, matrix metalloproteinase 2; PDGF, platelet-derived growth factor; TGF-β1, transforming growth factor β1. (Reproduced from Friedman [168] with permission from American Society for Biochemistry and Molecular Biology.)

Initiation of stellate cell activation

The earliest changes in stellate cells are likely to result from paracrine stimulation by all neighboring cell types, including sinusoidal endothelium, Kupffer cells, hepatocytes, and platelets. As noted in the preceding text, early injury to endothelial cells stimulates the production of cellular fibronectin, which has an activating effect on stellate cells [13]. On the other hand, resting endothelial cells may preserve stellate cell quiescence [19]. Sinusoidal endothelial cells, normally fenestrated to allow rapid bidirectional transport of solutes between sinusoidal blood and parenchymal cells, may rapidly lose their fenestrations following injury and express proinflammatory molecules including intercellular adhesion molecule 1 (ICAM-1), VEGF, and adhesion molecules. Together with stellate cells, they activate angiogenic pathways in response to hypoxia associated with local injury or malignancy [20].

Hepatic inflammation and Kupffer cell infiltration and activation also play prominent roles. An influx of Kupffer cells coincides with the appearance of stellate cell activation markers. Kupffer cells can stimulate matrix synthesis, cell proliferation, and the release of retinoids by stellate cells through the actions of cytokines (especially TGF-β1) and reactive oxygen intermediates/ lipid peroxides; they also secrete MMP-9, a type IV collagenase.

Early stimulation of stellate cells by oxidant stress in vivo may be important in many forms of liver fibrosis, particularly hepatitis C, nonalcoholic steatohepatitis (NASH), and iron overload [21]. Fibrosis is more likely among patients with NASH who are obese, which correlates with increased hepatic steatosis [22]. Because antioxidant levels are typically depleted in cirrhotic liver as fibrosis advances, their loss could further amplify the injurious effects of lipid peroxides.

Hepatocytes, as the most abundant cells in the liver, are a potent source of these fibrogenic lipid peroxides [21]. Steatosis in NASH and hepatitis C virus (HCV) correlates with increased stellate cell activation and fibrogenesis [23], possibly because fat represents an enhanced source of lipid peroxides. Whereas hepatocyte necrosis associated with lipid peroxidation is considered a classic inflammatory and fibrogenic stimulus, apoptosis, or programmed cell death, also stimulates the fibrogenic response associated with enhanced cell survival and upregulation of nicotinamide adenine dinucleotide phosphate (reduced form) (NADPH) oxidase, which further generates oxidant stress [24,25].

Platelets are often overlooked as a paracrine stimulus, but, in fact, they are a potent source of growth factors and are present within the injured liver. Potentially important platelet mediators include PDGF, TGF-β1, epidermal growth factor (EGF), and the chemokine ligand CXCL4 [26].

Perpetuation of stellate cell activation

Perpetuation of stellate cell activation involves at least seven discrete changes in cell behavior: (i) proliferation; (ii) chemotaxis; (iii) fibrogenesis; (iv) contractility; (v) matrix degradation; (vi) retinoid loss; (vii) chemokine, adipokine, and neuroendocrine signaling; and (viii) inflammatory and immune signaling. Either directly or indirectly, the net effect of these changes is to increase the accumulation of ECM. For example, proliferation and chemotaxis lead to increased numbers of collagen-producing cells, but there is also more matrix production per cell. Cytokine release by stellate cells can amplify the inflammatory and fibrogenic tissue responses, and matrix proteases may hasten the replacement of normal matrix with a matrix typical of the wound "scar."

Proliferation

Platelet-derived growth factor is the most potent stellate cell mitogen identified [27]. Induction of PDGF receptors early in stellate cell activation increases responsiveness to this mitogen. Downstream pathways of PDGF signaling have been carefully characterized in stellate cells and include PI3 kinase [28], and convergence with ephrin signaling [29], among others. Transgenic expression of PDGF-C in mice leads to both hepatic fibrosis and carcinoma [30]. Other mitogenic stimuli in stellate cells include VEGF [31], thrombin and its receptor EGF, TGF-α, and keratinocyte growth factor, among others [32].

Chemotaxis

Stellate cells can migrate towards cytokine chemoattractants, leading to their accumulation in zones of injury. Potent stellate cell chemoattractants include PDGF [33], MCP-1 [34], and CXCR3 [35]. PDGF-stimulated chemotaxis is associated with cell spreading at the tip, movement of the cell body towards the stimulant, and retraction of trailing protrusions associated with transient myosin phosphorylation [36]. In contrast, adenosine blunts chemotaxis and may immobilize cells once they reach the site of injury through reduced contractility [37].

Fibrogenesis

Stellate cells generate fibrosis not only by increased cell numbers, but also by increasing matrix production per cell. The best studied component of hepatic scar is collagen type I, the expression of which is regulated both transcriptionally and post-transcriptionally [38] in hepatic stellate cells by a growing number of stimuli and pathways.

The most potent stimulus for production of collagen I and other matrix constituents by stellate cells is TGF-β1, which is derived from both paracrine and autocrine sources [39]. Signals downstream of TGF-β1 include a family of bifunctional molecules known as Smads, upon which many extracellular and intracellular signals converge to fine-tune and enhance TGF-β's effects during fibrogenesis [39]. TGF-β1 also stimulates the production of other matrix components including cellular fibronectin and proteoglycans.

Connective tissue growth factor (CTGF/CCN2) is also a potent fibrogenic signal towards stellate cells [40] and may be upregulated by hyperglycemia and hyperinsulinemia [41]. While stimulation of CTGF production has traditionally been considered TGF-β dependent (42), there is also TGF-β-independent regulation [43].

Contractility

The collagenous bands typical of end-stage cirrhosis contain large numbers of activated stellate cells that contribute to contractility of both cells and the entire organ [44]. These bands impede portal blood flow by constricting individual sinusoids and by contracting the cirrhotic liver. Endothelin 1 and nitric oxide are major counterregulators controlling stellate cell contractility, in addition to a growing list of other mediators including angiotensinogen II, eicosanoids, atrial natriueretic peptide, somatostatin, and carbon monoxide, among others [44]. As stellate cells activate, the expression of the cytoskeletal protein α-smooth muscle actin (α-SMA) is increased, which confers increased contractile potential.

Another key contractile mediator in activated stellate cells is angiotensin II, which is synthesized by activated stellate cells in a NADPH-dependent pathway [45]. These findings are particularly relevant to human disease because antagonism of this pathway is an attractive antifibrotic therapy using a variety of safe, well-tolerated medications that are already available (see therapy section below) [46].

Matrix degradation

Quantitative and qualitative changes in matrix protease activity play an important role in the ECM remodeling that accompanies fibrosing liver injury (see "Degradation of extracellular matrix" above). Stellate cells express virtually all the key components required for pathologic matrix degradation and, therefore, play a key role not only in matrix production but also in matrix degradation.

Retinoid loss and nuclear receptor signaling

Activation of stellate cells is accompanied by the loss of the characteristic perinuclear retinoid (vitamin A) droplets. In culture, retinoid is stored as retinyl esters, whereas the form of retinoid released outside the cell during activation is retinol, suggesting that there is intracellular hydrolysis of esters prior to export [47]. Retinoid content and cellular activation may be linked through adipose differentiation-related protein (ADRP), which is increased as retinoids accumulate in stellate cells; its

knockdown by siRNA increases fibrogenesis in cultured stellate cells [48]. Interestingly, mice genetically deficient in lecithin:retinol acyltransferase (LRAT) lack lipid droplets in their stellate cells, but it is unknown what impact this has on their fibrogenic potential [49]. Thus, whether retinoid loss is required for the activation of stellate cells, or which retinoids might accelerate or prevent activation are not clarified.

Chemokine, adipokine, and neuroendocrine signaling

Chemokine signaling has been strongly implicated in the pathogenesis of hepatic fibrosis [50,51]. In particular, CCR1 and CCR5 are both fibrogenic, but they arise from distinct cellular sources [50]: CCR5 is derived from resident liver cells, whereas CCR1 is derived from bone marrow cells. Interestingly, sources of CCR2 evolve with progressive liver injury, and are initially derived from bone marrow cells but later derive from resident liver cells [51]. In contrast, activity of CXCL9 through its cognate receptor, CXCR3, is antifibrotic, and polymorphisms in CXCL9 may contribute to fibrosis progression risk in patients with chronic liver disease [52].

Pathways stimulated by adipokines, or polypeptides derived from adipose, are increasingly implicated in hepatic disease [53]. Whereas some adipokines are strictly derived from fat, others are also produced by resident liver cells. For example, leptin and adiponectin are both derived from hepatic stellate cells, among other sources, and their reciprocal dysregulation may drive fibrogenesis primarily through local paracrine signaling [54].

Neuroendocrine activity also contributes to hepatic fibrogenesis [55], especially cannabinoid signaling. Interruption of cannabinoid activity is an appealing therapeutic target, because CB1 receptor signaling is profibrogenic, and thus efforts to antagonize this molecule have met with significant success in animal models [56] and are being evaluated in human trials. Conversely, CB2 receptor signaling is antifibrogenic, and thus a strategy to agonize this receptor also shows promise [57]. On the other hand, CB2 agonists may amplify inflammation [58], suggesting that CB1 antagonism may be a more rational target than CB2. Similar to cannabinoids, data now also implicate neurotrophins [59,60], serotonin, and opioids in local fibrogenic signaling, and, like cannabinoids, divergent effects of these compounds in stellate cells may be elicited by different subtypes of their receptors [55].

Inflammatory and immune signaling

There has been tremendous progress in establishing a central role of stellate cells in inflammatory and immune signaling. Stellate cells are not only targets of immune mediators, but orchestrate immune responses as well. Recents studies have defined interactions not only with macrophages and traditional lymphocyte subsets (e.g., T and B cells), but also with natural killer (NK) cells, NK T cells [61,62], B cells [63], dendritic cells [64], and mast cells, as well as newly uncovered contributions by Toll-like receptors [65–68], nuclear factor κB (NF-κB) signaling [69], and the inflammasome [70]. Moreover, bidirectional interactions between stellate cells/myofibroblasts and immune cell subsets elicit specific cellular responses that modulate the composition of inflammatory infiltrates and the vigor of fibrogenesis [71,72]. In aggregate, these studies point to the liver as a major immunoregulatory organ, and underscore the critical contribution of immune cell subsets in modulating fibrosis as well as liver injury.

Gene regulation in hepatic stellate cells and myofibroblasts

The many advances in understanding gene regulation have benefited the study of hepatic stellate cell biology, including transcription factor activity, localization, and modification [73], as well as epigenetic regulation of gene expression by methylation [74,75], mRNA stabilization [76], and microRNA interactions [75,77,78]. Elucidating the precise molecular events underlying stellate cell activation and fibrogenesis is translating into fruitful new therapeutic approaches [69]. A growing repertoire of transcription factors cooperatively regulate gene expression through post-translational modification of regulatory proteins, particularly through phosphorylation. For example, stellate cell activation provokes phosphorylation of the RelA subunit of NF-κB at a specific serine residue (Ser^{536}) that leads to its nuclear import, resulting in increased NF-κB transcriptional activity [45], which increases survival of activated stellate cells. Treatment of either rodents with experimental fibrosis using an angiotensin-converting enzyme inhibitor, or humans with hepatitis C using an angiotensin receptor blocker, leads to reduced survival of activated stellate cells/myofibroblasts and regression of fibrosis by inhibiting this phosphorylation [45]. In an example of epigenetic regulation, myofibroblast activity can also be controlled by a microRNA, miR132, that releases a translational block on the methyl-CpG-binding protein, which in turn leads to repression of the peroxisome proliferator-activated receptor γ (PPARγ) transcription factor [75]. In a final example, phosphorylation of the transcription factor C/EBPb by the ribosomal S-6 kinase (RSK) is critical for stellate cell activation; this phosphorylation can be inhibited by cell-permeable peptides that block RSK and lead to cellular apoptosis [79].

Clinical aspects

Fibrosis progression and reversibility

There has been significant progress in our ability to predict the rate progression of fibrosis in an individual patient. Several general principles apply.

1 *Fibrosis usually requires at least several months to years of ongoing insult.* Three exceptions in adults are sinusoidal obstruction syndrome (SOS) (previously referred to as venoocclusive disease), subfulminant drug-induced liver injury, and mechanical biliary obstruction, in which fibrosis can progress more rapidly. In SOS, a dramatic deposition of ECM in pericentral zones associated with activated stellate cells can follow within weeks of myeloablative therapy, leading to rapid onset of ascites and possibly death [80]. In infants with neonatal obstruction, fibrosis can also develop in utero or within weeks of birth. Mechanisms underlying these examples of "fulminant fibrosis" remain obscure, but stellate cell activation and upregulation of fibrogenic cytokines accompany these fibrotic states as they do in more common forms of hepatic fibrosis.

2 *The severity of inflammation, necrosis, and injury usually correlate with the rate of progression*, as documented in studies of alcoholic liver disease and hepatitis C [81]. Indeed, patients with persistently normal alanine aminotransferase and HCV are less likely to progress [82], indicating decreased overall necroinflammation during the course of their disease.

3 *Concurrent hepatic insult by more than one agent is synergistic for the progression of fibrosis.* This has been especially well documented in patients with HCV infection who abuse large amounts of alcohol but is also true for those with viral coinfection, including hepatitis B virus (HBV) with either HCV or hepatitis delta virus (HDV) [83], as well as HCV with human immunodeficiency virus (HIV) [84]. In patients with HIV/HCV coinfection, direct effects of HIV proteins on stellate cells probably contribute to accelerated fibrosis [85].

Iron overload, whether primary or secondary, is also a risk factor for fibrosis progression [86]. In genetic hemochromatosis and rodent models of iron overload, a threshold iron concentration of 22,000 μg/g of dry weight has been identified. Higher iron content also correlates with increased inflammation and fibrosis, and synergizes inflammation. Increased steatosis is associated with increased fibrosis in patients infected with HCV or in those who have NASH. Other risk factors for fibrosis in patients with NASH include older age, obesity, and the presence of diabetes mellitus.

4 *Genetic risk is an important predictor of fibrosis progression, independent of other factors.* Fibrosis progression is strongly driven by genetic factors that can be identified by simple tests already available for clinicians. A large number of genetic markers have been uncovered that reportedly correlate with fibrosis progression rate, primarily in hepatitis C [52,87–89]. Among these, a seven-gene *cirrhosis risk score* (CRS), comprised of seven single nucleotide polymorphisms (SNPs) combined into a scoring system, is strongly

associated with fibrosis progression [90], and has been validated in two separate large prospective cohorts [91,92].

In addition to testing genetic markers in multiple populations, a key to establishing their relevance is to link these DNA sequence changes to altered pathways of disease pathogenesis, thereby providing a mechanism to explain the impact of the SNPs on fibrosis. At least two of the SNPs within the CRS have been linked to altered stellate cell activity [67,93], as well as several other SNPs [52,94,95].

5 *Environment and behavioral factors contribute to fibrosis risk.* In addition to genetic determinants, associations between environmental or behavioral risk factors and fibrosis progression have also been strengthened. For example, recent studies have demonstrated a protective effect of both coffee [96,97] and caffeine [98]. The profibrotic effect may be due to antagonism of adenosine receptor activity, which in animal models reduces the fibrogenic activity of stellate cells [99]. Moreover, while until recently there were no data linking specific viral factors with fibrosis progression, two recent studies have demonstrated that hepatitis B genotype C [100], and hepatitis C genotype 3 [101] are both associated with more rapid fibrosis progression. The findings complement the well-known impact of HIV on accelerating fibrosis progression due to hepatitis C coinfection, as underscored by a recent study based on repeated liver biopsies in coinfected patients [84].

6 *The exact moment when fibrosis becomes irreversible is not known,* in terms of either a histologic marker or a specific change in the matrix composition or content. Dense cirrhosis, with nodule formation and portal hypertension, is generally considered irreversible, but more intermediate lesions can show remarkable reversibility. It is important to consider the possibility that even advanced stages of fibrosis/cirrhosis might be reversible as clinical trials of antifibrotics emerge. Moreover, just as fibrosis may progress over decades, the reversal of fibrosis may also require many years, a fact that will influence the design of antifibrotic trials. Irreversibility may be conferred by the density and acellularity of the septal scars, leading to the loss of sources of interstitial collagenases.

Reversibility of cirrhosis has now been well documented in a number of diseases including HCV, HBV, HDV, and alcoholic liver disease [102,103]. More importantly, regression of fibrosis following clearance of HCV leads to improved clinical outcomes and reduced portal pressure in some patients [104–106].

Animal studies have also yielded significant insight into the mechanisms of fibrosis regression. Sustained experimental liver injury by carbon tetrachloride (CCl_4) leads to delayed reversibility because of thick collagen bands, high levels of TIMP-1, and significant collagen cross-linking by tissue transglutaminase [107] or lysl oxidase 2, whose expression is increased in activated stellate cells. A major activity of TIMP-1 is to inhibit the apoptosis of activated stellate cells, thereby allowing these fibrogenic cells to persist in the injured liver [108], associated with sustained NF-κB signaling that provides an intracellular signal to preserve this activated state [109]. Mice that overexpress TIMP-1 in the liver indeed have a delayed regression of experimental fibrosis [110], reinforcing its role in preventing reversibility. In addition, extracellular survival signals, some of which are bound to surrounding ECM, may further prevent apoptosis.

7 *Cirrhosis is more than a single stage, with a variable risk of decompensation.* Not all patients with cirrhosis have a comparable prognosis, as some will remain stable for up to 10 years while others may decompensate in a short interval [111]. These variable outcomes are not accurately predicted by either histologic staging systems or standard clinical parameters in patients with either a low model for end-stage liver disease (MELD) or Child–Pugh score. However, a recent large-scale analysis from the HALT-C low-dose interferon trial indicated that common clinical and laboratory features may be predictive in patients with more advanced disease [112]. Moreover, some, but not all studies suggest that transient elastography (see below) may identify patients with a higher likelihood of esophageal varices [113], or hepatocellular carcinoma [114].

Among the candidate modalities for predictive tests, hepatic venous pressure gradient (HVPG), while an invasive test requiring technical expertise, is remarkably accurate in addressing this need. For example, a long-term study of patients enrolled in a trial for β-blockers to prevent variceal hemorrhage demonstrated that patients with a baseline HVPG of ≤10 mmHg had only a ~15% chance of decompensation during a follow-up of 8 years, whereas those patients with a baseline HVPG of >10 mmHg had a ~70% risk of decompensation over the same interval [115]. Remarkably, simple pathologic features on liver biopsy may provide surrogates for these divergent outcomes, in that smaller nodule size and thicker septae both indicate a higher risk of decompensation, presumably because they reflect a higher HVPG [116]. Interestingly, these same features are also characteristic of more advanced experimental cirrhosis, and when fibrosis regresses in these models the smaller nodules begin to expand and thickened septae become thinner [117].

As underscored in a recent review [111], the increasingly refined view of cirrhosis as more than one stage demands a reassessment of staging systems to create better ways of predicting prognosis and anticipating complications.

Diagnosis and assessment

Accurate assessment of the extent of fibrosis is essential to guide management and predict prognosis in patients with chronic liver injury. Histologic assessment of a liver biopsy specimen remains the "gold standard" for quantifying fibrosis, with increasing interest in the use of noninvasive markers to allow more frequent sampling and avoid the risks of percutaneous biopsy.

Histologic and morphometric methods

Three methods of assessment of histologic fibrosis are in widest use: the Ishak score, the Metavir score, and the Desmet/Scheuer staging system [118]. Each relies on a progressive development of periportal fibrosis, then septal fibrosis, and finally nodule formation. The key distinguishing feature is the presence of two cirrhotic stages (5 and 6) in the Ishak system, and only one (F4) in the Metavir system. Interobserver variation is low in both systems, especially if pathologists have been "trained" before the use of these systems. However, sampling error may exceed 30%, as demonstrated by a study in which laparoscopic biopsies were obtained from both lobes of patients with HCV, yet 33% of the 124 patients had differences of at least one stage between the two lobes [119]. Two key features determining the accuracy of liver biopsy are length and width, with a minimum of 2.5 cm generally required to achieve reproducible sampling. In a study from Paris using the Metavir scoring system, 65% of biopsies 15 mm in length were categorized correctly, which increased to 75% for a 25 mm liver biopsy specimen [120]. This same study estimated, using "virtual" biopsy lengths, that only biopsy specimens 4 cm or greater in length would reliably avoid sampling error. This is not possible, of course, but it emphasizes that liver biopsy is unlikely to completely overcome the inherent problem of an uneven distribution of fibrosis in the liver. This, combined with inadequate sample size, is a problem amplified by increasing reliance on the use of radiologists to obtain liver biopsies using automated devices that are especially narrow. At best, a biopsy captures only 1/50,000th of the liver, and, therefore, some sampling error would seem inevitable. Morphometric and computerized systems may yield data that are continuous rather than discontinuous, but if the tissue sample is not adequate, or there is uneven distribution of fibrosis, then these quantitative methods will not enhance the quality of the data obtained.

Immunohistochemical and in situ mRNA hybridization methods to identify specific matrix components or α-smooth muscle actin (to reflect the extent of stellate cell activation), can be employed for experimental studies. These methods may have some clinical utility in assessing fibrosis progression [121]. Semiquantitative or real-time polymerase chain reaction can be used to measure mRNA transcripts for several cytokines and matrix components, for example PDGF and TGF-β1. This method has potential use for the analysis of liver biopsies because it may be more sensitive in assessing fibrogenesis than the evaluation of tissue sections stained for ECM. However, even when accurate, this method reflects mRNA levels and not protein levels, and the two may not always correlate.

Noninvasive methods

There is an urgent need for a noninvasive diagnostic procedure for liver fibrosis because this is currently the main limitation of drug testing in clinical trials. Assessment of fibrosis progression can be valuable in hepatitis C disease for at least four reasons:

1 The actual stage of fibrosis will indicate the likelihood of response to interferon-α or interferon-α/ribavirin because patients with advanced stages of fibrosis (Metavir F3 or F4) generally have a lower response rate to antiviral therapy.
2 If little fibrosis progression has occurred over a long interval, then treatment with antiviral therapy may be deemed as less urgent, and it may be safe to await more effective and/or better tolerated therapy.
3 The approximate time to the development of cirrhosis can be estimated.
4 As antiviral and antifibrotic therapies are refined, they will be most appropriately tested in "proof of principle" trials in patients who are at highest risk for progression in the absence of any treatment. This would not, however, indicate if/when clinical liver failure would eventuate, which may be delayed for up to a decade or more after the establishment of cirrhosis [115]. Accurate prediction of fibrosis progression will help identify those patients in whom the efficacy of an antifibrotic drug will be more easily uncovered in a controlled trial compared with placebo-treated control patients who have similar risk factors.

There has been a considerable effort to identify serum markers as noninvasive measures for the diagnosis of hepatic fibrosis. Although their accuracy and predictive value are improving, they have not yet supplanted direct analysis of the liver. The *ideal fibrosis marker* is one that is specific, biologically based, noninvasive, easily repeated in all patients, well correlated with disease severity and outcome, and not confounded by co-morbidities or drugs. Although this ideal has not yet been reached, progress can be anticipated on the basis of the advances to date and the intense interest in this area.

Serum markers of matrix molecules or modifying enzymes

There has been a major effort to identify serum markers as noninvasive measures of hepatic fibrosis. Although their accuracy and predictive value are improving, they cannot fully supplant direct analysis of liver. Thus far, no serum test has emerged as the perfect marker of fibrosis.

Serum markers have some limitations:

1 They typically reflect the rate of matrix turnover, not deposition, and therefore tend to be more elevated when there is high inflammatory activity. In contrast, extensive matrix deposition can go undetected if there is minimal inflammation.
2 None of the molecules are liver-specific, so extrahepatic sites of inflammation may contribute to elevated serum levels.
3 Serum levels are affected by clearance rates, which may be impaired because of either sinusoidal endothelial cell dysfunction or impaired biliary excretion.
4 They are surrogates, not biomarkers, of fibrosis.

Currently, two commercial serum marker systems have been extensively validated, the FibroTest® (marketed in the United States by Labcorp) [122,123] and the enhanced liver fibrosis (ELF) markers, utilizing a diagnostic algorithm and assays by Siemens Diagnostics [124]. In addition, a growing list of other noninvasive tests have been developed using a variety of standard serum hematologic or chemistry parameters in varying combinations [122,125].

To date there are only modest differences among the major serum assays, depending on the distribution of fibrosis severity and other factors [126,127], and their overall value can be summarized as follows:

1 The tests are extremely accurate (>95%) in determining the near absence (F0 or F1) of fibrosis in hepatitis C or the presence of cirrhosis, but are less accurate in intermediate stages of fibrosis. Therefore, in select clinical circumstances, the findings from these tests may obviate the need for biopsy, or may help guide decisions about treatment with antiviral combinations. Less is known about their value in patients with other forms of liver disease apart from hepatitis C, but data are beginning to emerge.
2 They suffer from a variable but significant number of indeterminate outcomes (up to 50% with the FibroTest).
3 There is no evidence yet that any test can discern changes in fibrosis content over time in an individual patient.
4 These tests are, however, proving valuable in cohort studies, in which mean changes in serum values among a group of patients correlate with changes in fibrosis. Moreover, they are more accurate than biopsy in predicting clinical outcomes [128,129], and show improvement when underlying HCV is cleared [130].

Overall, the serum assay approach is gaining value and appeal, in part because these tests may represent an "integrated" readout of liver activity rather than a minute sampling of the type obtained by conventional liver biopsy. Continued refinements are likely, and serum assays already have established an important niche, especially in patients who have a high risk of complications from liver biopsy or in those with liver disease not under the care of a hepatologist/gastroenterologist (e.g., patients coinfected with HCV/HIV). Their appeal also lies in the diminishing fraction of gastroenterologists and hepatologists who remain skilled in performing percutaneous liver biopsy.

Proteomics and glycomics

A different approach is the analysis of patterns of either protein or glycoprotein peaks, as assessed by mass spectroscopy of serum samples. These methods clearly represent "surrogate" markers and, in fact, the identities of the peaks are generally not known. None of these methods have yet reached the stage of widespread clinical testing and validation, however.

In summary, there remains for a need for improved noninvasive markers that accurately reflect the matrix content of the tissue and have better prognostic accuracy than standard clinical and laboratory indices such as the Child–Pugh or MELD classifications, which are only applicable to patients with cirrhosis.

Therapy

General considerations

The improved understanding of mechanisms underlying hepatic fibrosis makes effective antifibrotic therapy an emerging reality. However, treatment will remain a challenging task, and thus far no drugs have been approved as antifibrotic agents in humans. Therapies will have to be well tolerated over decades, with good targeting to the liver, and few adverse effects on other tissues. Combination therapies may prove synergistic rather than additive, but agents must first be tested individually to establish safety and "proof of principle." It is uncertain whether antifibrotic therapies will require intermittent or continuous administration. For putative agents, evidence of a direct antifibrotic effect must be established in experimental models rather than only an indirect effect by abrogating the injury. Candidate therapies must be effective in a liver that is already damaged – as in clinical liver disease – rather than only before the onset of injury. Antifibrotic therapies also carry the theoretical concern that inhibiting the scarring response will prevent the encapsulation of injured regions, leading to extension of tissue damage. In reality, however, antifibrotic therapies only need to downregulate the scar response to be effective, and in patients with cirrhosis it is the scarring, not injury, that usually leads to liver failure.

Antifibrotic therapies: rationale and specific agents

The paradigm of stellate cell activation provides an important framework to define sites of antifibrotic therapy (Box 12.2) [131,132]. The rationale is as follows: (i) cure the primary disease to prevent injury; (ii) reduce inflammation or the host response to avoid stimulating stellate cell activation; (iii) directly downregulate stellate cell activation; (iv) neutralize proliferative, fibrogenic, contractile, and/or proinflammatory responses of stellate cells; (v) stimulate apoptosis of stellate cells; and (vi) increase the degradation of scar matrix, either by stimulating cells that produce matrix proteases, downregulating their inhibitors, or by direct administration of matrix proteases.

We are still lacking a "proof of principle" trial that establishes the value of targeting fibrosis directly in the presence of ongoing liver disease. Despite this obstacle, the number of potential therapies is expanding rapidly, and the potential for antifibrotic therapies has been embraced by the pharmaceutical and biotech sectors, and by the public (reviewed in [131,133,134]). Moreover, exciting prospects for targeting either diagnostic agents or therapies directly to stellate cells may enhance efforts to improve both the diagnosis and treatment of hepatic fibrosis [135,136].

Primary disease cure

The most effective way to eliminate hepatic fibrosis is to clear the primary cause of liver disease. This includes abstinence in alcoholic liver disease, removal of excess iron or copper in precirrhotic genetic hemochromatosis or Wilson disease, clearance of HBV or HCV in chronic viral hepatitis, eradication of organisms in schistosomiasis, or decompression in mechanical bile duct obstruction. Not to be overlooked, weight loss through either diet and exercise, or bariatric surgery in patients with NASH [137], or even those with HCV who are overweight, may improve histology and is a simple recommendation. Eventual identification of the pathogenetic mechanisms underlying primary biliary cirrhosis and sclerosing cholangitis could lead to the elimination of bile duct injury and periductular fibrosis.

Reduction of inflammation and the immune response

Reduced fibrosis and improved clinical outcomes have been reported in patients with HCV successfully treated with pegylated interferon-α and ribavirin [105], presumably through its effect on viral replication and liver injury. Unfortunately, there was no long-term benefit on fibrosis or outcomes of low-dose maintenance interferon in the large multicenter HALT-C trial [138].

Box 12.2 Therapeutic strategies for hepatic fibrosis.

Reducing injury and inflammation
- Antiviral therapy for viral hepatitis
- Antihelminthic therapy for schistosomiasis
- Chelation/venesection, treatment of metabolic disease
- Angiotensin II type I receptor antagonists, ACE inhibitors
- Hepatoprotectants, e.g., HGF/HGF mimetics
- Corticosteroids for autoimmune disease
- Ursodeoxycholic acid for primary biliary cirrhosis

Attenuating stellate cell activation
- Antioxidants
- Vitamin E, PDTC
- Angiotensin II type I receptor antagonists
- Cytokine-directed therapy
- TGF-β antagonists
- Endothelin receptor antagonists
- HGF
- FXR agonists
- Aldosterone antagonists
- Pentoxyphylline

Inhibiting properties of activated stellate cells
- Antiproliferative
- PDGF and tyrosine kinase receptor antagonists
- Sodium exchange inhibitors
- Plasmin/thrombin receptor antagonists
- Anticontractile
- Endothelin/endothelin receptor antagonists
- Nitric oxide donors
- Antifibrogenic
- Collagen synthesis inhibitors
- TGF-β inhibitors (soluble receptors, neutralizing antibodies)
- HGF/HGF mimetics
- Angiotensin II type I receptor antagonists
- ACE inhibitors
- Integrin antagonists
- Smad 7 agonists
- Cannabinoid receptor 2 antagonists

Promoting specific apoptosis of hepatic stellate cells
- Gliotoxin
- Sulfasalazine
- Nerve growth factor agonists
- TIMP antagonists

Degrading scar matrix
- Direct collagenase administration
- Inhibitors of transglutaminase or collagen cross-linking
- TIMP antagonists
- TGF-β inhibitors

ACE, angiotensin-converting enzyme; FXR, farnesyl X receptor; HGF, hepatocyte growth factor; PDGF, platelet-derived growth factor; PDTC, pyrrolidine dithiocarbamate; TGF-β, transforming growth factor β; TIMP, tissue inhibitor of metalloproteinase.

A number of other agents have anti-inflammatory activity in vitro and in vivo, which may eliminate the stimuli for stellate cell activation. Corticosteroids have been used for decades to treat several types of liver disease, in particular autoimmune hepatitis. Their activity is solely as anti-inflammatory agents, with no direct antifibrotic effect on stellate cells. Antagonists to TNF-α or NF-κB modulators have some rationale, as do a growing number of biologically active agents currently used in other chronic inflammatory diseases, in particular inflammatory liver disease. Pentoxyphylline may exert its antifibrotic activity by downregulating TNF-α signaling, although an effect on renal blood flow seems more likely in patients with cirrhosis [139]. Other efforts to neutralize inflammatory cytokines include the use of integrin antagonists, which may limit injury and/or fibrogenesis [140].

The renin–angiotensin system may also amplify inflammation through the generation of oxidant stress, and therefore either angiotensin-converting enzyme antagonists and/or angiotensinogen II type I receptor antagonists may have anti-inflammatory and antifibrogenic activity [141,142].

A new class of drugs, broadly referred to as *hepatoprotectants*, are showing considerable promise in preclinical and clinical studies, including HGF, HGF deletion variants, and HGF synthetic mimetics [143]. HGF's antifibrotic activity is mediated at least in part through suppression of fibrogenic signaling [144]. Trials in large animals and humans are anticipated, with careful monitoring planned to screen for potential hepatocarcinogenesis because HGF is a hepatocyte mitogen.

Inhibition of stellate cell activation

Reducing the transformation of quiescent stellate cells to activated myofibroblasts is a particularly attractive target, given its central role in the fibrotic response. The most practical approach is to reduce oxidant stress, which is an important stimulus to activation. Antioxidants, including α-tocopherol (vitamin E), have recently shown benefit in a large multicenter trial among patients with NASH [145]. Other antioxidants can also reduce stellate cell activation in culture, which provides a rationale for antioxidant trials in humans, although more potent formulations than those currently available may be required.

Silymarin, a natural flavonoid component of the milk thistle *Silybum marianum*, has sparked interest as a potential antifibrotic therapy. The compound functions as an antioxidant and may decrease hepatic injury and fibrosis [146]. However, there is no conclusive evidence of antifibrotic efficacy from human clinical trials.

The cytokine interferon-γ has inhibitory effects on stellate cell activation in animal models of fibrosis. However, a clinical trial of interferon-γ did not show any antifibrotic benefit in patients with HCV [147].

PPARγ nuclear receptors are expressed in stellate cells, and synthetic PPARγ ligands (thiazolidinediones) downregulate stellate cell activation. Disappointingly, a recent clinical trial showed no antifibrotic benefit in patients with HCV [121]. Farnesoid X receptor (FXR) ligands appear to have similar effects and small molecule agonists are under study in preclinical models, with evidence of antifibrotic activity [148].

Leptin, produced by activated stellate cells, not only affects lipid metabolism but also directly stimulates wound healing. In fact, animals deficient in leptin have reduced hepatic injury and fibrosis [54]. On the basis of this finding, the discovery of adiponectin, a natural counterregulator to leptin, may lead to its use as an antifibrotic, particularly in patients with NASH [53].

Cannabinoid (CB1) receptor antagonists have consistently shown antifibrotic activity in animal models, and a human trial showed equal promise in patients with NASH [149,150]. However, the drug Rimonabant®, a CB1 receptor antagonist, was associated with high rates of depression that led to discontinuation of clinical trials. However, efforts are now underway to develop CB1 antagonists that do not cross the blood–brain barrier, which may prove highly effective in liver disease and will be better tolerated.

Progress in understanding transcriptional regulation has offered the opportunity to block stellate cell activation by inhibiting the activity of histone deacetylases (HDACs), enzymes critical for modifying chromatin during gene transcription. Highly specific HDAC inhibitors offer the potential for selectively blocking stellate cell activation with tolerable safety and good efficacy [151], but none has reached clinical use. Similarly, modulation of intracellular proteins including transcription factors remains an interesting but elusive target of antifibrotic therapy.

Herbal therapies and products derived from natural compounds that are commonly used in the Far East are increasingly being tested under controlled, scientifically rigorous conditions [152]. Some show promise of efficacy, in particular Sho-saiko-to, *Salvia miltiorrhiza*, and a green tea polyphenol.

Neutralization of proliferative, fibrogenic, contractile, and/or proinflammatory responses of stellate cells

Significant advances in growth factor biology will benefit the treatment of hepatic fibrosis through the development of antagonists to cytokines and their receptors. In particular, many proliferative cytokines including PDGF, FGF, and TGF-α signal through tyrosine kinase receptors, inhibitors of which are already undergoing clinical trials in other tissues [153,154].

Inhibition of matrix production has been the primary target of most antifibrotic therapies to date. This has been attempted directly by blocking matrix synthesis and processing, or indirectly by inhibiting the activity of TGF-β1, the major fibrogenic cytokine. Inhibitors of collagen synthesis such as HOE 077, which blocks the enzyme prolyl hydroxylase, were among the first antifibrotic compounds tested in liver diseases, but success with this agent has been modest. The emerging importance of translational regulation of collagen gene expression could lead to specific translational inhibitors with therapeutic value. Colchicine generated excitement at one time because of its apparent efficacy in a small group of patients; however, a more recent study of its use in alcoholic cirrhosis showed no benefit [155].

TGF-β antagonists are being extensively tested because neutralizing this potent cytokine would have the dual effect of inhibiting matrix production and accelerating its degradation Animal and culture studies using soluble TGF-β receptors or other means of neutralizing the cytokine, including monoclonal antibodies and protease inhibitors to block TGF-β activation, have established proof of principle [156]. There are concerns that inhibiting TGF-β may stimulate hepatocellular growth and enhance the risk of cancer, which could limit their utility. A number of even newer TGF-β antagonists are also being developed and may undergo testing soon. These could include recombinant Smad 7 [157], which antagonizes TGF-β activity in stellate cells, and integrin antagonists that block cell surface TGF-β activation [140].

Relaxin, a natural peptide hormone that mediates parturition, has been developed as an agent that decreases collagen synthesis by stellate cells and increases matrix degradation in vitro and in vivo. Stellate cells also express relaxin receptors which might represent an attractive target for antagonism [158,159].

Because endothelin-1 is an important regulator of wound contraction and blood flow regulation mediated by stellate cells, antagonists have been tested as both antifibrotic and portal hypotensive agents [160]. Bosentan, a mixed endothelin A and B receptor antagonist, has antifibrotic activity and reduces stellate cell activation in experimental hepatic fibrosis. This and other endothelin antagonists remain attractive drug development targets although some hepatotoxicity has been observed in clinical trials in patients with pulmonary disease.

Halofuginone, an anticoccidial compound, has antifibrotic activity by blocking collagen expression, and has been used in a number of models of tissue fibrosis, including the liver [161].

The potential utility of retinoids (vitamin A) as antifibrotic therapy has been limited by inadequate knowledge about their regulatory role in stellate cell activation, and by toxicity concerns. Although stellate cells export retinoid as they activate, it does not follow that restoration of cellular retinoid will prevent activation. In fact, some retinoids may accelerate fibrosis by augmenting membrane injury, for example in patients with hypervitaminosis A.

Stimulation of stellate cell apoptosis or senescence

Attention is increasingly focused on how liver fibrosis regresses, and in particular the fate of activated stellate cells as fibrosis recedes. Mounting evidence indicates that either reversal of the activated stellate cell phenotype or stellate cell senescence and apoptosis all occur in vivo [162,163]. In particular, as liver fibrosis is decreased, there is selective cell death of activated stellate cells. This exciting observation has led to animal studies using either gliotoxin or sulfasalazine, which provoke selective apoptosis of stellate cells in culture and in vivo, leading to reduced fibrosis [162,164]. A TIMP-1 neutralizing antibody has antifibrotic activity in experimental liver fibrosis [165], which also accelerates stellate cell apoptosis.

Degradation of scar matrix

This component of treatment is very important because antifibrotic therapy in human liver disease will need to provoke resorption of existing matrix, in addition to preventing the deposition of new scar. As noted in the preceding text, TGF-β antagonists have the advantage of stimulating matrix degradation by downregulating TIMPs and increasing net activity of interstitial collagenase. Retinoids may also stimulate matrix degradation but concerns over toxicity limit their utility. Relaxin can directly increase matrix degradation.

Direct expression of metalloproteinases in animal models of hepatic fibrosis has begun to confirm that matrix can be resorbed through the expression of exogenous enzymes [166]. Although this may seem impractical in humans, data have established the important proof of principle that hepatic ECM is responsive to degradation. Moreover, an experimental study has affirmed the importance of matrix degradation in the regression of hepatic fibrosis by demonstrating that a genetically altered mouse expressing mutant collagen resistant to degradation displayed delayed regression of fibrosis after liver injury [167].

Future prospects

Continued progress can be anticipated in unraveling the molecular regulation of fibrosis and its treatment. Rapid advances in gene therapy, tissue-specific targeting, and high-throughput small molecule screening of cytokine inhibitors are likely to benefit the diagnosis and therapy of hepatic fibrosis. New insights into the regulation of growth, apoptosis, and intracellular signaling by cytokines, adipokines, and hormones could have direct implications for stellate cell behavior in liver injury. Additionally, there is tremendous interest in herbal and natural antifibrotic remedies, particularly in the Far East, where many such compounds are undergoing clinical trials. Accelerating progress is certain once methods of noninvasive diagnosis are established that enable rapid assessment of fibrosis in clinical trials, and ultimately in clinical practice.

Supporting research grants

NIH: DK37340; NIH: DK56621; and NIH: AA017067.

References

1. Schuppan D, Ruehl M, Somasundaram R, Hahn EG. Matrix as modulator of stellate cell and hepatic fibrogenesis. *Semin Liver Dis* 2001;21(3):351–72.
2. McCall-Culbreath KD, Zutter MM. Collagen receptor integrins: rising to the challenge. *Curr Drug Targets* 2008;9(2):139–49.
3. Silva R, D'Amico G, Hodivala-Dilke KM, Reynolds LE. Integrins: the keys to unlocking angiogenesis. *Arterioscler Thromb Vasc Biol* 2008;28(10):1703–13.
4. Olaso E, Ikeda K, Eng FJ, et al. DDR2 receptor promotes MMP-2-mediated proliferation and invasion by hepatic stellate cells. *J Clin Invest* 2001;108(9):1369–78.
5. Dranoff JA, Wells RG. Portal fibroblasts: underappreciated mediators of biliary fibrosis. *Hepatology* 2010;51(4):1438–44.
6. Forbes SJ, Russo FP, Rey V, et al. A significant proportion of myofibroblasts are of bone marrow origin in human liver fibrosis. *Gastroenterology* 2004;126(4):955–63.
7. Choi SS, Diehl AM. Epithelial-to-mesenchymal transitions in the liver. *Hepatology* 2009;50(6):2007–13.
8. Friedman SL. Hepatic stellate cells – protean, multifunctional, and enigmatic cells of the liver. *Physiol Rev* 2008;88(1):125–72.
9. Friedman SL. Mechanisms of hepatic fibrogenesis. *Gastroenterology* 2008;134(6):1655–69.
10. Reeves HL, Burt AD, Wood S, Day CP. Hepatic stellate cell activation occurs in the absence of hepatitis in alcoholic liver disease and correlates with the severity of steatosis. *J Hepatol* 1996;25(5):677–83.
11. Gonzalez SA, Fiel MI, Sauk J, et al. Inverse association between hepatic stellate cell apoptosis and fibrosis in chronic hepatitis C virus infection. *J Viral Hepat* 2009;16(2):141–8.
12. Ramm GA, Shepherd RW, Hoskins AC, et al. Fibrogenesis in pediatric cholestatic liver disease: role of taurocholate and hepatocyte-derived monocyte chemotaxis protein-1 in hepatic stellate cell recruitment. *Hepatology* 2009;49(2):533–44.
13. Jarnagin WR, Rockey DC, Koteliansky VE, Wang SS, Bissell DM. Expression of variant fibronectins in wound healing: cellular source and biological activity of the EIIIA segment in rat hepatic fibrogenesis. *J Cell Biol* 1994;127(6):2037–48.
14. Consolo M, Amoroso A, Spandidos DA, Mazzarino MC. Matrix metalloproteinases and their inhibitors as markers of inflammation and fibrosis in chronic liver disease. *Int J Mol Med* 2009;24(2):143–52.
15. Benyon RC, Arthur MJ. Extracellular matrix degradation and the role of hepatic stellate cells. *Semin Liver Dis* 2001;21(3):373–84.
16. Radbill BD, Gupta R, Ramirez MC, et al. Loss of matrix metalloproteinase-2 amplifies murine toxin-induced liver fibrosis by upregulating collagen i expression. *Dig Dis Sci* 2011;56(2):406–16.
17. Iredale JP. Hepatic stellate cell behavior during resolution of liver injury. *Semin Liver Dis* 2001;21(3):427–36.
18. Friedman SL. Evolving challenges in hepatic fibrosis. *Nat Rev Gastroenterol Hepatol* 2010;7(8):425–36.
19. Deleve LD, Wang X, Guo Y. Sinusoidal endothelial cells prevent rat stellate cell activation and promote reversion to quiescence. *Hepatology* 2008;48(3):920–30.
20. Fernandez M, Semela D, Bruix J, Colle I, Pinzani M, Bosch J. Angiogenesis in liver disease. *J Hepatol* 2009;50(3):604–20.
21. Novo E, Parola M. Redox mechanisms in hepatic chronic wound healing and fibrogenesis. *Fibrogenesis Tissue Repair* 2008;1(1):5.
22. Cheung O, Sanyal AJ. Recent advances in nonalcoholic fatty liver disease. *Curr Opin Gastroenterol* 2009;25(3):230–7.
23. Clouston AD, Jonsson JR, Purdie DM, et al. Steatosis and chronic hepatitis C: analysis of fibrosis and stellate cell activation. *J Hepatol* 2001;34(2):314–20.
24. Zhan SS, Jiang JX, Wu J, et al. Phagocytosis of apoptotic bodies by hepatic stellate cells induces NADPH oxidase and is associated with liver fibrosis in vivo. *Hepatology* 2006;43(3):435–43.
25. Jiang JX, Mikami K, Venugopal S, Li Y, Torok NJ. Apoptotic body engulfment by hepatic stellate cells promotes their survival by the JAK/STAT and Akt/NF-kappaB-dependent pathways. *J Hepatol* 2009;51(1):139–48.
26. Zaldivar MM, Pauels K, von Hundelshausen P, et al. CXC chemokine ligand 4 (Cxcl4) is a platelet-derived mediator of experimental liver fibrosis. *Hepatology* 2010;51(4):1345–53.
27. Borkham-Kamphorst E, van Roeyen CR, Ostendorf T, Floege J, Gressner AM, Weiskirchen R. Pro-fibrogenic potential of PDGF-D in liver fibrosis. *J Hepatol* 2007;46(6):1064–74.
28. Lechuga CG, Hernandez-Nazara ZH, Hernandez E, et al. PI3K is involved in PDGF-beta receptor upregulation post-PDGF-BB treatment in mouse HSC. *Am J Physiol Gastrointest Liver Physiol* 2006;291(6):G1051–61.
29. Semela D, Das A, Langer D, Kang N, Leof E, Shah V. Platelet-derived growth factor signaling through ephrin-b2 regulates hepatic vascular structure and function. *Gastroenterology* 2008;135(2):671–9.
30. Campbell JS, Hughes SD, Gilbertson DG, et al. Platelet-derived growth factor C induces liver fibrosis, steatosis, and hepatocellular carcinoma. *Proc Natl Acad Sci USA* 2005;102(9):3389–94.
31. Yoshiji H, Kuriyama S, Yoshii J, et al. Vascular endothelial growth factor and receptor interaction is a prerequisite for murine hepatic fibrogenesis. *Gut* 2003;52(9):1347–54.
32. Pinzani M, Marra F. Cytokine receptors and signaling in hepatic stellate cells. *Semin Liver Dis* 2001;21(3):397–416.
33. Kinnman N, Hultcrantz R, Barbu V, et al. PDGF-mediated chemoattraction of hepatic stellate cells by bile duct segments in cholestatic liver injury. *Lab Invest* 2000;80(5):697–707.
34. Marra F, Romanelli RG, Giannini C, et al. Monocyte chemotactic protein-1 as a chemoattractant for human hepatic stellate cells. *Hepatology* 1999;29(1):140–8.
35. Bonacchi A, Romagnani P, Romanelli RG, et al. Signal transduction by the chemokine receptor CXCR3: activation of Ras/ERK, Src, and phosphatidylinositol 3-kinase/Akt controls cell migration and proliferation in human vascular pericytes. *J Biol Chem* 2001;276(13):9945–54.
36. Melton AC, Yee HF. Hepatic stellate cell protrusions couple platelet-derived growth factor-BB to chemotaxis. *Hepatology* 2007;45(6):1446–53.
37. Sohail MA, Hashmi AZ, Hakim W, et al. Adenosine induces loss of actin stress fibers and inhibits contraction in hepatic stellate cells via Rho inhibition. *Hepatology* 2009;49(1):185–94.

38. Kadler KE, Hill A, Canty-Laird EG. Collagen fibrillogenesis: fibronectin, integrins, and minor collagens as organizers and nucleators. *Curr Opin Cell Biol* 2008;20(5):495–501.

39. Inagaki Y, Okazaki I. Emerging insights into transforming growth factor beta Smad signal in hepatic fibrogenesis. *Gut* 2007;56(2):284–92.

40. Gao R, Brigstock DR. Connective tissue growth factor (CCN2) induces adhesion of rat activated hepatic stellate cells by binding of its C-terminal domain to integrin alpha(v)beta(3) and heparan sulfate proteoglycan. *J Biol Chem* 2004;279(10):8848–55.

41. Paradis V, Perlemuter G, Bonvoust F, et al. High glucose and hyperinsulinemia stimulate connective tissue growth factor expression: a potential mechanism involved in progression to fibrosis in nonalcoholic steatohepatitis. *Hepatology* 2001;34(4):738–44.

42. Grotendorst GR. Connective tissue growth factor: a mediator of TGF-beta action on fibroblasts. *Cytokine Growth Factor Rev* 1997;8(3):171–9.

43. Brigstock DR. The CCN family: a new stimulus package. *J Endocrinol* 2003;178(2):169–75.

44. Rockey DC. Vascular mediators in the injured liver. *Hepatology* 2003;37(1):4–12.

45. Oakley F, Teoh V, Ching ASG, et al. Angiotensin II activates I kappaB kinase phosphorylation of RelA at Ser 536 to promote myofibroblast survival and liver fibrosis. *Gastroenterology* 2009;136(7):2334–44, e1.

46. Bataller R, Sancho-Bru P, Gines P, Brenner DA. Liver fibrogenesis: a new role for the renin-angiotensin system. *Antioxid Redox Signal* 2005;7(9–10):1346–55.

47. Friedman SL, Wei S, Blaner WS. Retinol release by activated rat hepatic lipocytes: regulation by Kupffer cell-conditioned medium and PDGF. *Am J Physiol* 1993;264(5):G947–52.

48. Lee TF, Mak KM, Rackovsky O, et al. Downregulation of hepatic stellate cell activation by retinol and palmitate mediated by adipose differentiation-related protein (ADRP). *J Cell Physiol* 2010;223(3):648–57.

49. O'Byrne SM, Wongsiriroj N, Libien J, et al. Retinoid absorption and storage is impaired in mice lacking lecithin:retinol acyltransferase (LRAT). J Biol Chem 2005;280(42):35647–57.

50. Seki E, De Minicis S, Gwak GY, et al. CCR1 and CCR5 promote hepatic fibrosis in mice. *J Clin Invest* 2009;119(7):1858–70.

51. Seki E, de Minicis S, Inokuchi S, et al. CCR2 promotes hepatic fibrosis in mice. *Hepatology* 2009;50(1):185–97.

52. Wasmuth HE, Lammert F, Zaldivar MM, et al. Antifibrotic effects of CXCL9 and its receptor CXCR3 in livers of mice and humans. *Gastroenterology* 2009;137(1):309–19, e1–3.

53. Marra F, Bertolani C. Adipokines in liver diseases. *Hepatology* 2009;50(3):957–69.

54. Ikejima K, Okumura K, Kon K, Takei Y, Sato N. Role of adipocytokines in hepatic fibrosis. *J Gastroenterol Hepatol* 2007;22(Suppl 1):S87–92.

55. Ebrahimkhani MR, Elsharkawy AM, Mann DA. Wound healing and local neuroendocrine regulation in the injured liver. *Expert Rev Mol Med* 2008;10:e11.

56. Teixeira-Clerc F, Julien B, Grenard P, et al. CB1 cannabinoid receptor antagonism: a new strategy for the treatment of liver fibrosis. *Nat Med* 2006;12(6):671–6.

57. Munoz-Luque J, Ros J, Fernandez-Varo G, et al. Regression of fibrosis after chronic stimulation of cannabinoid CB2 receptor in cirrhotic rats. *J Pharmacol Exp Ther* 2008;324(2):475–83.

58. Deveaux V, Cadoudal T, Ichigotani Y, et al. Cannabinoid CB2 receptor potentiates obesity-associated inflammation, insulin resistance and hepatic steatosis. *PLoS One* 2009;4(6):e5844.

59. Passino MA, Adams RA, Sikorski SL, Akassoglou K. Regulation of hepatic stellate cell differentiation by the neurotrophin receptor p75NTR. *Science* 2007;315(5820):1853–6.

60. Kendall TJ, Hennedige S, Aucott RL, et al. p75 Neurotrophin receptor signaling regulates hepatic myofibroblast proliferation and apoptosis in recovery from rodent liver fibrosis. *Hepatology* 2009;49(3):901–10.

61. Gao B, Radaeva S, Park O. Liver natural killer and natural killer T cells: immunobiology and emerging roles in liver diseases. *J Leukoc Biol* 2009;86:513–28.

62. Notas G, Kisseleva T, Brenner D. NK and NKT cells in liver injury and fibrosis. *Clin Immunol* 2009;130(1):16–26.

63. Novobrantseva TI, Majeau GR, Amatucci A, et al. Attenuated liver fibrosis in the absence of B cells. *J Clin Invest* 2005;115(11):3072–82.

64. Connolly MK, Bedrosian AS, Mallen-St Clair J, et al. In liver fibrosis, dendritic cells govern hepatic inflammation in mice via TNF-alpha. *J Clin Invest* 2009;119(11):3213–25.

65. Seki E, De Minicis S, Osterreicher CH, et al. TLR4 enhances TGF-beta signaling and hepatic fibrosis. *Nat Med* 2007;13(11):1324–32.

66. Seki E, Brenner DA. Toll-like receptors and adaptor molecules in liver disease: update. *Hepatology* 2008;48(1):322–35.

67. Guo J, Loke J, Zheng F, et al. Functional linkage of cirrhosis-predictive single nucleotide polymorphisms of Toll-like receptor 4 to hepatic stellate cell responses. *Hepatology* 2009;49(3):960–8.

68. Mencin A, Kluwe J, Schwabe RF. Toll-like receptors as targets in chronic liver diseases. *Gut* 2009;58(5):704–20.

69. Chakraborty JB, Mann DA. NF-kappaB signalling: embracing complexity to achieve translation. *J Hepatol* 2010;52(2):285–91.

70. Watanabe A, Sohail MA, Gomes DA, et al. Inflammasome-mediated regulation of hepatic stellate cells. *Am J Physiol Gastrointest Liver Physiol* 2009;296(6):G1248–57.

71. Muhanna N, Doron S, Wald O, et al. Activation of hepatic stellate cells after phagocytosis of lymphocytes: a novel pathway of fibrogenesis. *Hepatology* 2008;48(3):963–77.

72. Holt AP, Haughton EL, Lalor PF, Filer A, Buckley CD, Adams DH. Liver myofibroblasts regulate infiltration and positioning of lymphocytes in human liver. *Gastroenterology* 2009;136(2):705–14.

73. Mann J, Mann DA. Transcriptional regulation of hepatic stellate cells. *Adv Drug Deliv Rev* 2009;61(7–8):497–512.

74. Mann J, Oakley F, Akiboye F, Elsharkawy A, Thorne AW, Mann DA. Regulation of myofibroblast transdifferentiation by DNA methylation and MeCP2: implications for wound healing and fibrogenesis. *Cell Death Differ* 2007;14(2):275–85.

75. Mann J, Chu DC, Maxwell A, et al. MeCP2 controls an epigenetic pathway that promotes myofibroblast transdifferentiation and fibrosis. *Gastroenterology* 2010;138(2):705–14, e1–4.

76. Fritz D, Stefanovic B. RNA-binding protein RBMS3 is expressed in activated hepatic stellate cells and liver fibrosis and increases expression of transcription factor Prx1. *J Mol Biol* 2007;371(3):585–95.

77. Guo CJ, Pan Q, Li DG, Sun H, Liu BW. miR-15b and miR-16 are implicated in activation of the rat hepatic stellate cell: an essential role for apoptosis. *J Hepatol* 2009;50(4):766–78.

78. Venugopal SK, Jiang J, Kim TH, et al. Liver fibrosis causes downregulation of miRNA-150 and miRNA-194 in hepatic stellate cells and their over-expression causes decreased stellate cell activation. *Am J Physiol Gastrointest Liver Physiol* 2009;298:G101–6.

79. Buck M, Chojkier M. A ribosomal S-6 kinase-mediated signal to C/EBP-beta is critical for the development of liver fibrosis. *PLoS One* 2007;2(12):e1372.

80. DeLeve LD, Shulman HM, McDonald GB. Toxic injury to hepatic sinusoids: sinusoidal obstruction syndrome (veno-occlusive disease). *Semin Liver Dis* 2002;22(1):27–42.

81. Shackel NA, McGuinness PH, Abbott CA, Gorrell MD, McCaughan GW. Insights into the pathobiology of hepatitis C virus-associated cirrhosis: analysis of intrahepatic differential gene expression. *Am J Pathol* 2002;160(2):641–54.

82. Hui CK, Belaye T, Montegrande K, Wright TL. A comparison in the progression of liver fibrosis in chronic hepatitis C between

persistently normal and elevated transaminase. *J Hepatol* 2003;38(4): 511–17.

83. Wilson LE, Torbenson M, Astemborski J, et al. Progression of liver fibrosis among injection drug users with chronic hepatitis C. *Hepatology* 2006;43(4):788–95.

84. Macias J, Berenguer J, Japon MA, et al. Fast fibrosis progression between repeated liver biopsies in patients coinfected with human immunodeficiency virus/hepatitis C virus. *Hepatology* 2009;50(4):1056–63.

85. Tuyama A, Hong F, Mosoian A, Schecter A, Klotman M, Bansal MB. HIV entry and replication in stellate cells promotes cellular activation and fibrogenesis: implications for hepatic fibrosis in HIV/HCV co-infection. *Hepatology* 2007;46(4):80A.

86. Bonkovsky HL, Naishadham D, Lambrecht RW, et al. Roles of iron and HFE mutations on severity and response to therapy during retreatment of advanced chronic hepatitis C. *Gastroenterology* 2006;131(5):1440–51.

87. Hold GL, Untiveros P, Saunders KA, El-Omar EM. Role of host genetics in fibrosis. *Fibrogenesis Tissue Repair* 2009;2(1):6.

88. Weber S, Gressner OA, Hall R, Grunhage F, Lammert F. Genetic determinants in hepatic fibrosis: from experimental models to fibrogenic gene signatures in humans. *Clin Liver Dis* 2008;12(4):747–57, vii.

89. Asselah T, Bieche I, Paradis V, Bedossa P, Vidaud M, Marcellin P. Genetics, genomics, and proteomics: implications for the diagnosis and the treatment of chronic hepatitis C. *Semin Liver Dis* 2007;27(1):13–27.

90. Huang H, Shiffman ML, Friedman S, et al. A 7 gene signature identifies the risk of developing cirrhosis in patients with chronic hepatitis C. *Hepatology* 2007;46(2):297–306.

91. Pradat P, Trepo E, Potthoff A, et al. The cirrhosis risk score predicts liver fibrosis progression in patients with initially mild chronic hepatitis C. *Hepatology* 2010;51(1):356–7.

92. Marcolongo M, Young B, Dal Pero F, et al. A seven-gene signature (cirrhosis risk score) predicts liver fibrosis progression in patients with initially mild chronic hepatitis C. *Hepatology* 2009;50(1):1038–44.

93. Guo J, Hong F, Loke J, et al. A DDX5 S480A polymorphism is associated with increased transcription of fibrogenic genes in hepatic stellate cells. *J Biol Chem* 2010;285(8):5428–37.

94. Wasmuth HE, Tag CG, Van de Leur E, et al. The Marburg I variant (G534E) of the factor VII-activating protease determines liver fibrosis in hepatitis C infection by reduced proteolysis of platelet-derived growth factor BB. *Hepatology* 2009;49(3):775–80.

95. Hung TM, Chang SC, Yu WH, et al. A novel nonsynonymous variant of matrix metalloproteinase-7 confers risk of liver cirrhosis. *Hepatology* 2009;50(4):1184–93.

96. Freedman ND, Everhart JE, Lindsay KL, et al. Coffee intake is associated with lower rates of liver disease progression in chronic hepatitis C. *Hepatology* 2009;50(5):1360–9.

97. Ruhl CE, Everhart JE. Coffee and tea consumption are associated with a lower incidence of chronic liver disease in the United States. *Gastroenterology* 2005;129(6):1928–36.

98. Modi AA, Feld JJ, Park Y, et al. Increased caffeine consumption is associated with reduced hepatic fibrosis. *Hepatology* 2010; 51(1):201–9.

99. Chan ES, Montesinos MC, Fernandez P, et al. Adenosine A(2A) receptors play a role in the pathogenesis of hepatic cirrhosis. *Br J Pharmacol* 2006;148(8):1144–55.

100. Chan HL, Wong GL, Tse CH, et al. Hepatitis B virus genotype C is associated with more severe liver fibrosis than genotype B. *Clin Gastroenterol Hepatol* 2009;7(12):1361–6.

101. Bochud PY, Cai T, Overbeck K, et al. Genotype 3 is associated with accelerated fibrosis progression in chronic hepatitis C. *J Hepatol* 2009;51(4):655–66.

102. Farci P, Roskams T, Chessa L, et al. Long-term benefit of interferon alpha therapy of chronic hepatitis D: regression of advanced hepatic fibrosis. *Gastroenterology* 2004;126(7):1740–9.

103. Pol S, Carnot F, Nalpas B, et al. Reversibility of hepatitis C virus-related cirrhosis. *Hum Pathol* 2004;35(1):107–12.

104. Roberts S, Gordon A, McLean C, et al. Effect of sustained viral response on hepatic venous pressure gradient in hepatitis C-related cirrhosis. *Clin Gastroenterol Hepatol* 2007;5(8):932–7.

105. Mallet V, Gilgenkrantz H, Serpaggi J, et al. Brief communication: the relationship of regression of cirrhosis to outcome in chronic hepatitis C. *Ann Intern Med* 2008;149(6):399–403.

106. Morgan TR, Ghany MG, Kim HY, et al. Outcome of sustained virological responders with histologically advanced chronic hepatitis C. *Hepatology* 2010;52(3):833–44.

107. Issa R, Zhou X, Constandinou CM, et al. Spontaneous recovery from micronodular cirrhosis: evidence for incomplete resolution associated with matrix cross-linking. *Gastroenterology* 2004;126(7):1795–808.

108. Murphy FR, Issa R, Zhou X, et al. Inhibition of apoptosis of activated hepatic stellate cells by tissue inhibitor of metalloproteinase-1 is mediated via effects on matrix metalloproteinase inhibition: implications for reversibility of liver fibrosis. *J Biol Chem* 2002;277(13):11069–76.

109. Watson MR, Wallace K, Gieling RG, et al. NF-kappaB is a critical regulator of the survival of rodent and human hepatic myofibroblasts. *J Hepatol* 2008;48(4):589–97.

110. Yoshiji H, Kuriyama S, Yoshii J, et al. Tissue inhibitor of metalloproteinases-1 attenuates spontaneous liver fibrosis resolution in the transgenic mouse. *Hepatology* 2002;36(4):850–60.

111. Garcia-Tsao G, Friedman S, Iredale J, Pinzani M. Now there are many (stages) where before there was one: in search of a pathophysiological classification of cirrhosis. *Hepatology* 2010;51(4): 1445–9.

112. Ghany MG, Lok AS, Everhart JE, et al. Predicting clinical and histologic outcomes based on standard laboratory tests in advanced chronic hepatitis C. *Gastroenterology* 2010;138:136–46.

113. Kazemi F, Kettaneh A, N'Kontchou G, et al. Liver stiffness measurement selects patients with cirrhosis at risk of bearing large oesophageal varices. *J Hepatol* 2006;45(2):230–5.

114. Masuzaki R, Tateishi R, Yoshida H, et al. Risk assessment of hepatocellular carcinoma in chronic hepatitis C patients by transient elastography. *J Clin Gastroenterol* 2008;42(7):839–43.

115. Ripoll C, Groszmann R, Garcia-Tsao G, et al. Hepatic venous pressure gradient predicts clinical decompensation in patients with compensated cirrhosis. *Gastroenterology* 2007;133(2):481–8.

116. Nagula S, Jain D, Groszmann RJ, Garcia-Tsao G. Histological-hemodynamic correlation in cirrhosis – a histological classification of the severity of cirrhosis. *J Hepatol* 2006;44(1):111–17.

117. Henderson NC, Iredale JP. Liver fibrosis: cellular mechanisms of progression and resolution. *Clin Sci (Lond)* 2007;112(5):265–80.

118. Goodman ZD. Grading and staging systems for inflammation and fibrosis in chronic liver diseases. *J Hepatol* 2007;47(4):598–607.

119. Regev A, Berho M, Jeffers LJ, et al. Sampling error and intraobserver variation in liver biopsy in patients with chronic HCV infection. *Am J Gastroenterol* 2002;97(10):2614–18.

120. Bedossa P, Dargere D, Paradis V. Sampling variability of liver fibrosis in chronic hepatitis C. *Hepatology* 2003;38(6):1449–57.

121. McHutchison J, Goodman Z, Patel K, et al. Farglitazar lacks antifibrotic activity in patients with chronic hepatitis C infection. *Gastroenterology* 2010;138(4):1365–73, e1–2.

122. Smith JO, Sterling RK. Systematic review: non-invasive methods of fibrosis analysis in chronic hepatitis C. *Aliment Pharmacol Ther* 2009;30(6):557–76.

123. Castera L, Vergniol J, Foucher J, et al. Prospective comparison of transient elastography, Fibrotest, APRI, and liver biopsy for

the assessment of fibrosis in chronic hepatitis C. *Gastroenterology* 2005;128(2):343–50.

124. Parkes J, Roderick P, Harris S, et al. Enhanced liver fibrosis test can predict clinical outcomes in patients with chronic liver disease. *Gut* 2010;59(9):1245–51.

125. Sebastiani G, Halfon P, Castera L, et al. SAFE biopsy: a validated method for large-scale staging of liver fibrosis in chronic hepatitis C. *Hepatology* 2009;49(6):1821–7.

126. Leroy V, Hilleret MN, Sturm N, et al. Prospective comparison of six non-invasive scores for the diagnosis of liver fibrosis in chronic hepatitis C. *J Hepatol* 2007;46(5):775–82.

127. Castera L, Sebastiani G, Le Bail B, de Ledinghen V, Couzigou P, Alberti A. Prospective comparison of two algorithms combining non-invasive methods for staging liver fibrosis in chronic hepatitis C. *J Hepatol* 2010;52(2):191–8.

128. Ngo Y, Munteanu M, Messous D, et al. A prospective analysis of the prognostic value of biomarkers (FibroTest) in patients with chronic hepatitis C. *Clin Chem* 2006;52(10):1887–96.

129. Mayo MJ, Parkes J, Adams-Huet B, et al. Prediction of clinical outcomes in primary biliary cirrhosis by serum enhanced liver fibrosis assay. *Hepatology* 2008;48(5):1549–57.

130. Fontana RJ, Bonkovsky HL, Naishadham D, et al. Serum fibrosis marker levels decrease after successful antiviral treatment in chronic hepatitis C patients with advanced fibrosis. *Clin Gastroenterol Hepatol* 2009;7(2):219–26.

131. Rockey DC. Current and future anti-fibrotic therapies for chronic liver disease. *Clin Liver Dis* 2008;12(4):939–62, xi.

132. Schuppan D, Popov Y. Rationale and targets for antifibrotic therapies. *Gastroenterol Clin Biol* 2009;33(10–11):949–57.

133. Schuppan D, Afdhal NH. Liver cirrhosis. *Lancet* 2008;371(9615): 838–51.

134. Ghiassi-Nejad Z, Friedman SL. Advances in antifibrotic therapy. *Expert Rev Gastroenterol Hepatol* 2008;2(6):803–16.

135. Friedman SL. Targeting siRNA to arrest fibrosis. *Nat Biotechnol* 2008;26(4):399–400.

136. Sato Y, Murase K, Kato J, et al. Resolution of liver cirrhosis using vitamin A-coupled liposomes to deliver siRNA against a collagen-specific chaperone. *Nat Biotechnol* 2008;26(4):431–42.

137. Klein S, Mittendorfer B, Eagon JC, et al. Gastric bypass surgery improves metabolic and hepatic abnormalities associated with non-alcoholic fatty liver disease. *Gastroenterology* 2006;130(6):1564–72.

138. Di Bisceglie AM, Shiffman ML, Everson GT, et al. Prolonged therapy of advanced chronic hepatitis C with low-dose peginterferon. *N Engl J Med* 2008;359(23):2429–41.

139. Lebrec D, Thabut D, Oberti F, et al. Pentoxifylline does not decrease short-term mortality but does reduce complications in patients with advanced cirrhosis. *Gastroenterology* 2010;138(5):1755–62.

140. Patsenker E, Popov Y, Stickel F, Jonczyk A, Goodman SL, Schuppan D. Inhibition of integrin alphavbeta6 on cholangiocytes blocks transforming growth factor-beta activation and retards biliary fibrosis progression. *Gastroenterology* 2008;135(2):660–70.

141. Moreno M, Gonzalo T, Kok RJ, et al. Reduction of advanced liver fibrosis by short-term targeted delivery of an angiotensin receptor blocker to hepatic stellate cells in rats. *Hepatology* 2009;51(3):942–52.

142. Colmenero J, Bataller R, Sancho-Bru P, et al. Effects of losartan on hepatic expression of non-phagocytic NADPH oxidase and fibrogenic genes in patients with chronic hepatitis C. *Am J Physiol Gastrointest Liver Physiol* 2009;297(4):G726–34.

143. Horiguchi K, Hirano T, Ueki T, Hirakawa K, Fujimoto J. Treating liver cirrhosis in dogs with hepatocyte growth factor gene therapy via the hepatic artery. *J Hepatobiliary Pancreat Surg* 2009;16(2):171–7.

144. Inagaki Y, Higashi K, Kushida M, et al. Hepatocyte growth factor suppresses profibrogenic signal transduction via nuclear export of Smad3 with galectin-7. *Gastroenterology* 2008;134(4):1180–90.

145. Sanyal AJ, Chalasani N, Kowdley KV, et al. Pioglitazone, vitamin E, or placebo for nonalcoholic steatohepatitis. *N Engl J Med* 2010;362(17):1–5.

146. Trappoliere M, Caligiuri A, Schmid M, et al. Silybin, a component of sylimarin, exerts anti-inflammatory and anti-fibrogenic effects on human hepatic stellate cells. *J Hepatol* 2009;50(6):1102–11.

147. Pockros PJ, Jeffers L, Afdhal N, et al. Final results of a double-blind, placebo-controlled trial of the antifibrotic efficacy of interferon-gamma1b in chronic hepatitis C patients with advanced fibrosis or cirrhosis. *Hepatology* 2007;45(3):569–78.

148. Fickert P, Fuchsbichler A, Moustafa T, et al. Farnesoid X receptor critically determines the fibrotic response in mice but is expressed to a low extent in human hepatic stellate cells and periductal myofibroblasts. *Am J Pathol* 2009;175(6):2392–405.

149. Gary-Bobo M, Elachouri G, Gallas JF, et al. Rimonabant reduces obesity-associated hepatic steatosis and features of metabolic syndrome in obese Zucker fa/fa rats. *Hepatology* 2007;46(1): 122–9.

150. Mallat A, Teixeira-Clerc F, Deveaux V, Lotersztajn S. Cannabinoid receptors as new targets of antifibrosing strategies during chronic liver diseases. *Expert Opin Ther Targets* 2007;11(3):403–9.

151. Niki T, Rombouts K, De Bleser P, et al. A histone deacetylase inhibitor, trichostatin A, suppresses myofibroblastic differentiation of rat hepatic stellate cells in primary culture. *Hepatology* 1999;29(3):858–67.

152. Kakizaki S, Takizawa D, Tojima H, Yamazaki Y, Mori M. Xenobiotic-sensing nuclear receptors CAR and PXR as drug targets in cholestatic liver disease. *Curr Drug Targets* 2009;10(11): 1156–63.

153. Wang Y, Gao J, Zhang D, Zhang J, Ma J, Jiang H. New insights into the antifibrotic effects of sorafenib on hepatic stellate cells and liver fibrosis. *J Hepatol* 2010;53(1):132–44.

154. Yoshiji H, Noguchi R, Kuriyama S, et al. Imatinib mesylate (STI-571) attenuates liver fibrosis development in rats. *Am J Physiol Gastrointest Liver Physiol* 2005;288(5):G907–13.

155. Cortez-Pinto H, Alexandrino P, Camilo ME, et al. Lack of effect of colchicine in alcoholic cirrhosis: final results of a double blind randomized trial. *Eur J Gastroenterol Hepatol* 2002;14(4):377–81.

156. Popov Y, Schuppan D. Targeting liver fibrosis: strategies for development and validation of antifibrotic therapies. *Hepatology* 2009;50(4):1294–306.

157. Dooley S, Hamzavi J, Breitkopf K, et al. Smad7 prevents activation of hepatic stellate cells and liver fibrosis in rats. *Gastroenterology* 2003;125(1):178–91.

158. Bennett RG, Dalton SR, Mahan KJ, Gentry-Nielsen MJ, Hamel FG, Tuma DJ. Relaxin receptors in hepatic stellate cells and cirrhotic liver. *Biochem Pharmacol* 2007;73(7):1033–40.

159. Bennett RG, Heimann DG, Tuma DJ. Relaxin reduces fibrosis in models of progressive and established hepatic fibrosis. *Ann NY Acad Sci* 2009;1160:348–9.

160. Feng HQ, Weymouth ND, Rockey DC. Endothelin antagonism in portal hypertensive mice: implications for endothelin receptor-specific signaling in liver disease. *Am J Physiol Gastrointest Liver Physiol* 2009;297(1):G27–33.

161. Gnainsky Y, Kushnirsky Z, Bilu G, et al. Gene expression during chemically induced liver fibrosis: effect of halofuginone on TGF-beta signaling. *Cell Tissue Res* 2007;328(1):153–66.

162. Oakley F, Meso M, Iredale JP, et al. Inhibition of inhibitor of kappaB kinases stimulates hepatic stellate cell apoptosis and accelerated recovery from rat liver fibrosis. *Gastroenterology* 2005;128(1): 108–20.

163. Krizhanovsky V, Yon M, Dickins RA, et al. Senescence of activated stellate cells limits liver fibrosis. *Cell* 2008;134(4):657–67.

164. Habens F, Srinivasan N, Oakley F, Mann DA, Ganesan A, Packham G. Novel sulfasalazine analogues with enhanced NF-kB inhibitory and apoptosis promoting activity. *Apoptosis* 2005;10(3):481–91.

165. Parsons CJ, Bradford BU, Pan CQ, et al. Antifibrotic effects of a tissue inhibitor of metalloproteinase-1 antibody on established liver fibrosis in rats. *Hepatology* 2004;40(5):1106–15.

166. Iimuro Y, Brenner DA. Matrix metalloproteinase gene delivery for liver fibrosis. *Pharm Res* 2008;25(2):249–58.

167. Issa R, Zhou X, Trim N, et al. Mutation in collagen-1 that confers resistance to the action of collagenase results in failure of recovery from CCl4-induced liver fibrosis, persistence of activated hepatic stellate cells, and diminished hepatocyte regeneration. *FASEB J* 2003;17(1):47–9.

168. Friedman SL. Molecular regulation of hepatic fibrosis, an integrated cellular response to tissue injury. *J Biol Chem* 2000;275: 2247–50.

CHAPTER 13

Preoperative Evaluation of the Patient with Liver Disease

Lawrence S. Friedman

Department of Medicine, Newton-Wellesley Hospital, Newton, MA, USA

Key concepts

- The diseased liver is particularly susceptible to the hemodynamic and hypoxic insults that may accompany anesthesia and surgery.
- Anesthesia, including spinal and epidural anesthesia, reduces hepatic blood flow and can precipitate hepatic decompensation in persons with liver disease. Certain anesthetic agents, particularly those that undergo little hepatic metabolism, are preferable in patients with liver disease.
- In general, elective surgery is contraindicated in patients with acute hepatitis, acute liver failure, or alcoholic hepatitis.

- In patients with cirrhosis, surgical risk has traditionally been predicted by the Child–Pugh class. The model for end-stage liver disease (MELD) score appears to provide a more precise estimate of surgical risk.
- Certain operations, particularly biliary tract surgery, cardiac surgery, and hepatic resection, as well as emergency surgery, pose particular risk in patients with cirrhosis.
- Careful preoperative preparation, including management of ascites, renal dysfunction, encephalopathy, coagulopathy, and malnutrition, and close postoperative monitoring are critical to successful outcomes in patients with liver disease who undergo surgery.

Surgery is performed in patients with liver disease more frequently now than in the past, in part because of the long-term survival of patients with cirrhosis since the advent of liver transplantation and new measures to treat the complications of portal hypertension. Hemodynamic instability in the perioperative period can worsen liver function in patients with liver disease, who are at risk of hepatic decompensation. Considerable progress has been made in estimating perioperative risk in patients with liver disease. Operative risk correlates with the severity of the underlying liver disease and the nature of the surgical procedure. Thorough preoperative evaluation is necessary prior to elective surgery to estimate the risk of surgery and attempt to reduce it. Surgery is contraindicated in patients with acute hepatitis, acute liver failure, and alcoholic hepatitis. The Child–Pugh classification (Child–Turcotte–Pugh score) and particularly the model for end-stage liver disease (MELD) score (see Chapter 14) provide reasonable estimations of perioperative mortality in patients with cirrhosis. However, they do not replace the need for clinical judgment as well as careful preoperative preparation and postoperative monitoring; early detection of complications is essential for improving outcomes. Medical therapy for specific manifestations of hepatic disease, including ascites, renal dysfunction, and encephalopathy, should be optimized preoperatively and, if necessary, administered in the postoperative period.

Consequences of reduced hepatic blood flow, hypoxemia, and altered drug metabolism

Liver disease, especially cirrhosis, causes a hyperdynamic circulation with increased cardiac output and decreased systemic vascular resistance. At baseline, hepatic arterial and portal-venous perfusion of the cirrhotic liver may be decreased: arterial blood flow can be decreased because of impaired autoregulation, and portal blood flow is reduced as a result of portal hypertension. Moreover, patients with liver disease may have alterations in the systemic circulation, including arteriovenous shunting and reduced splanchnic inflow to the liver. The decreased hepatic perfusion at baseline makes the diseased liver more susceptible to the consequences of hypotension and hypoxemia in the operating room [1]. Anesthetic agents,

Schiff's Diseases of the Liver, Eleventh Edition. Edited by Eugene R. Schiff, Willis C. Maddrey and Michael F. Sorrell.
© 2012 John Wiley & Sons, Ltd. Published 2012 by John Wiley & Sons, Ltd.

including spinal and epidural anesthesia, may reduce hepatic blood flow by 30–50% following induction and frequently lead to transient minor elevations in serum liver biochemical test levels in persons without liver disease [2]. Agents such as isoflurane, desflurane, and sevoflurane that cause less perturbation in hepatic arterial blood flow than other inhaled anesthetic agents are preferred in patients with liver disease. Propofol is another acceptable anesthetic agent in patients with liver disease; the elimination kinetic profile of propofol is similar in persons with and without cirrhosis, although recovery times are longer in those with cirrhosis [1].

Additional factors that may contribute to decreased hepatic blood flow perioperatively include hypotension, hemorrhage, and vasoactive drugs. Intermittent positive pressure ventilation and pneumoperitoneum during laparoscopic surgery mechanically decrease hepatic blood flow [3]. In addition, laparotomy with traction on the abdominal viscera may cause reflex dilatation of the splanchnic veins and thereby lower hepatic blood flow.

Risk factors for acute intraoperative hypoxemia in patients with liver disease include ascites, hepatic hydrothorax, hepatopulmonary syndrome (the triad of liver disease, an increased alveolar–arterial gradient, and intrapulmonary shunting), which is found in 5–32% of cirrhotic patients followed at transplant centers, and portopulmonary hypertension. Portopulmonary hypertension is found in up to 6% of patients with advanced liver disease and increases postoperative mortality after noncardiac surgery [4] (see Chapter 16). In general, ascites and hepatic hydrothorax should be treated preoperatively, and elective surgery should be avoided in patients with either hepatopulmonary syndrome or portopulmonary hypertension. During surgery, hypercarbia should be avoided in patients with liver disease because it initiates sympathetic stimulation of the splanchnic vasculature and thereby decreases portal blood flow.

The volume of distribution of nondepolarizing muscle relaxants is increased in patients with liver disease, and larger doses may therefore be required to achieve adequate neuromuscular blockade (see Chapter 28). Atracurium and cisatracurium are considered the preferred muscle relaxants in patients with liver disease because neither the liver nor the kidney are required for their elimination [1]. Vecuronium, rocuronium, and mivacurium are metabolized by the liver and must be used with caution in patients with liver disease. Doxacurium, which is metabolized by the kidney, is the preferred muscle relaxant for longer procedures such as liver transplantation. Sedatives and narcotics are generally tolerated in patients with compensated liver disease but must be used with caution in patients with hepatic dysfunction, because they may cause a prolonged depression of consciousness and precipitate hepatic encephalopa-

thy. In general, narcotics and benzodiazepines should be avoided in these patients; however, when necessary, remifentanil (and possibly sufentanil and fentanyl) and oxazepam are the preferred narcotic and sedative, respectively, because the metabolism of these agents is unaffected by liver disease. Morphine, meperidine, alfentanil, and dexmedetomidine (an α_2-adrenergic agonist with sedative and analgesic properties) should be used with caution in patients with advanced cirrhosis [1,2].

Operative risk in patients with liver disease

In a patient with liver disease, surgical risk depends on the severity of liver disease, nature of the surgical procedure, and presence of co-morbid conditions. A number of conditions related to liver disease are contraindications to elective surgery (Box 13.1). When these contraindications are absent, patients should undergo a thorough preoperative evaluation, and their conditions should be optimized prior to elective surgery. Patients found to have advanced liver disease may benefit from alternative nonsurgical therapies when available and appropriate.

Once liver disease is identified in a patient in need of surgery, an assessment of the severity of liver disease should be undertaken, as should an evaluation for other known risk factors for perioperative mortality (Box 13.2). Data from studies of patients with cirrhosis suggest that the severity of liver disease can best be assessed by the Child–Turcotte–Pugh (CTP) score (Child–Pugh, or Child, class) and MELD score (see later). The majority of published studies describing operative risk in patients with liver disease derive from single-center, retrospective cohorts and involve patients with cirrhosis. These data are susceptible to limitations, including small cohort size, selection bias, and lack of external validation. Despite these limitations, the results of studies describing operative risk in patients with liver disease have been remarkably consistent. As one might expect, operative morbidity and mortality increase with increasing severity of liver disease, whether measured

---

Box 13.1 Contraindications to elective surgery in patients with liver disease.

- Acute liver failure
- Acute kidney injury
- Acute viral hepatitis
- Alcoholic hepatitis
- Cardiomyopathy
- Hypoxemia
- Severe coagulopathy (despite treatment)

Box 13.2 Risk factors for mortality and morbidity in patients with cirrhosis who undergo surgery.

Patient characteristics
- Anemia
- Ascites
- Child–Pugh class (Child–Turcotte–Pugh score)
- Encephalopathy
- Hypoalbuminemia
- Hypoxemia
- Infection
- Malnutrition
- MELD score
- Portal hypertension
- Prolonged prothrombin time (>2.5 seconds) that does not correct with vitamin K

Type of surgery
- Cardiac surgery
- Emergency surgery
- Hepatic resection
- Open abdominal surgery (including biliary surgery)

MELD, model for end-stage liver disease.

by the Child–Pugh class or MELD score. In general, patients with compensated cirrhosis who have normal synthetic function have a low overall risk, and those with decompensated cirrhosis have a higher risk, which may be prohibitive in patients with severe hepatic decompensation.

Conditions for which elective surgery is generally contraindicated

Acute hepatitis

Patients with acute hepatitis of any cause have an increased operative risk [2] (see Chapters 23–25). This conclusion is based on data from older studies, in which operative mortality rates of 10–13% were reported among patients who underwent laparotomy to distinguish intrahepatic from extrahepatic causes of jaundice [5]. Although diagnostic and surgical techniques have improved since these studies were published, elective surgery is still considered contraindicated in patients with acute hepatitis. In most cases, acute hepatitis is either self-limited or treatable, and elective surgery can be undertaken after the patient improves clinically and biochemically.

Alcoholic hepatitis

Alcoholic hepatitis is a contraindication to elective surgery and greatly increases perioperative mortality

after surgery [6] (see Chapter 26). In one retrospective series of patients with alcoholic hepatitis, the mortality rate was 58% among the 12 patients who underwent open liver biopsy, compared with 10% among the 39 who underwent percutaneous liver biopsy. Because only one death in the former group was secondary to intra-abdominal hemorrhage, open abdominal surgery, rather than liver biopsy, is likely to have been responsible for the high mortality rate.

Acute liver failure

Patients with acute liver failure (defined as the development of jaundice, coagulopathy, and hepatic encephalopathy within 26 weeks in a patient with acute liver injury and without preexisting liver disease) are critically ill (see Chapter 19). All surgery other than liver transplantation is contraindicated in these patients.

Operative risk assessment in patients with cirrhosis

Surgical risk is increased in patients with cirrhosis. The magnitude of perioperative risk correlates with the degree of hepatic decompensation. Additional factors may affect surgical risk and perioperative management depending on the underlying cause of chronic liver disease (Box 13.3).

Stratification by Child–Pugh class

Since the 1970s, the standard for assessing perioperative morbidity and mortality in patients with cirrhosis has been the CTP scoring system, which is based on the patient's serum bilirubin and albumin levels, prothrombin time, and severity of encephalopathy and ascites [2] (see Chapter 14). The studies that led to this standard have all been retrospective and limited to a small number of highly selected patients, but the results have been remarkably consistent. Two of the most important studies, separated by 13 years, reported nearly identical results: mortality rates for patients undergoing surgery were 10% for those with Child–Pugh class A, 30% for those with Child–Pugh class B, and 76–82% for those with Child–Pugh class C cirrhosis [7,8]. In a third study of patients with cirrhosis undergoing abdominal operations published in 2010, mortality rates for patients with Child–Pugh class A, B, and C cirrhosis were 2%, 12%, and 12%, respectively, suggesting that mortality has declined with improvements in the overall care of critically ill patients in the past decade [9]. In addition to predicting perioperative mortality, the Child–Pugh class correlates with the frequency of postoperative complications, which include liver failure, worsening encephalopathy, bleeding, infection, renal failure, hypoxia, and intractable ascites.

Box 13.3 Perioperative considerations in patients with various causes of chronic liver disease.

Chronic viral hepatitis
- HBV and HCV carrier states per se do not affect surgical risk; risk correlates with biochemical and histologic severity of hepatitis
- Interruptions in antiviral therapy should be avoided, if possible

Autoimmune hepatitis
- Surgical risk correlates with biochemical and histologic severity of hepatitis
- "Stress" doses of glucocorticoids may be required in the perioperative period

Nonalcoholic fatty liver disease
- Mortality rate is increased (7–14%) following hepatic resection in patients with moderate to severe hepatic steatosis; whether steatohepatitis increases the risk further is unclear
- Additional surgical risk is associated with obesity and diabetes mellitus

Alcoholic liver disease
- Alcoholic hepatitis is a contraindication to elective surgery
- Alcoholic fatty liver per se is not associated with increased operative risk, but abstinence for 6–12 weeks before surgery is advised because of adverse effects of alcohol on drug metabolism (e.g., acetaminophen, halothane) and the risk of alcohol withdrawal in the postoperative period

Hemochromatosis
- Cardiomyopathy associated with hemochromatosis increases surgical risk
- Associated diabetes mellitus may increase surgical risk

Wilson disease
- Informed consent may be challenging in patients with neuropsychiatric disease
- Surgery may precipitate or aggravate neurologic disease
- The dose of D-penicillamine should be decreased in the perioperative period to reduce the risk of poor wound healing

Alpha-1 antitrypsin deficiency
- Associated pulmonary disease may increase surgical risk

Cirrhosis
- Surgical risk correlates with Child–Pugh class and MELD score (see text)

HBV, hepatitis B virus; HCV, hepatitis C virus; MELD, model for end-stage liver disease.

In patients with Child–Pugh class A cirrhosis, the risk of perioperative morbidity is increased when there is associated portal hypertension. Postoperative morbidity in patients with portal hypertension and Child–Pugh class A cirrhosis, and possibly with Child–Pugh class B

and C cirrhosis, has been reported to be reduced by preoperative placement of a transjugular intrahepatic portosystemic shunt (TIPS) [10–12].

Several other factors can increase the perioperative risk above and beyond the Child–Pugh class. Emergency surgery is associated with a higher mortality rate than that associated with nonemergency surgery, with comparative rates of 22% versus 10% for patients in Child–Pugh class A, 38% versus 30% for those in Child–Pugh class B, and 100% versus 82% for those in Child–Pugh class C in one study [8]. A diagnosis of chronic obstructive lung disease and surgery on the respiratory tract are also independent risk factors for perioperative mortality in patients with cirrhosis [13].

A general consensus is that elective surgery is well tolerated in patients with Child–Pugh class A cirrhosis, permissible with preoperative preparation in patients with Child–Pugh class B cirrhosis (except those undergoing cardiac surgery or extensive hepatic resection, see later), and contraindicated in patients with Child–Pugh class C cirrhosis.

Stratification by model for end-stage liver disease score

The MELD score was created to predict mortality after TIPS, then implemented to risk stratify patients awaiting liver transplantation, and more recently utilized to predict perioperative mortality [14]. The MELD score, a linear regression model based on a patient's serum bilirubin and creatinine levels and international normalized ratio (INR), has several distinct advantages over the Child–Pugh classification: it is objective, weights the variables, and does not rely on arbitrary cutoff values. Each 1-point increase in the MELD score makes an incremental contribution to operative risk, thereby suggesting that the MELD score increases precision in predicting postoperative mortality [15].

A number of studies have examined the MELD score as a predictor of surgical mortality in patients with cirrhosis. In a retrospective study of 140 patients with cirrhosis who underwent surgery, a 1% increase in mortality for each 1-point increase in the MELD score from 5 to 20 and a 2% increase in mortality for each 1-point increase in the MELD score above 20 was observed [16]. The largest study of the MELD score as a predictor of perioperative mortality (also retrospective), by Teh and colleagues [17], evaluated 772 patients with cirrhosis who underwent abdominal (other than laparoscopic cholecystectomy), orthopedic, and cardiovascular surgery. The patients' median preoperative MELD score was 8, and few had a MELD score greater than 15. In addition, most patients had a platelet count greater than 60,000 mm³/L and an INR of less than 1.5. In this selected cohort, patients with a MELD score of 7 or less had a mortality

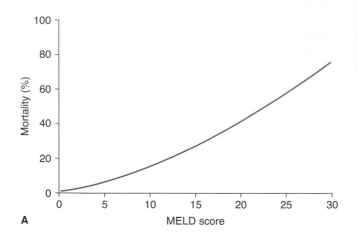

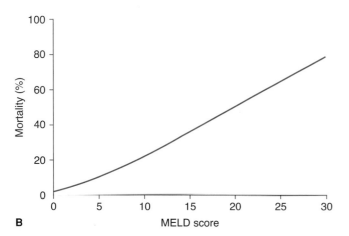

Figure 13.1 Relationship between operative mortality and model for end-stage liver disease (MELD) score in 772 patients with cirrhosis who underwent surgery in 1980–1990 and 1994–2004: (A) 30-day mortality; (B) 90-day mortality. For patients with a MELD score of >8, each 1-point increase in the MELD score was associated with a 14% increase in both 30-day and 90-day mortality rates. (Reproduced from Teh et al. [17] with permission from Elsevier.)

rate of 5.7%; patients with a MELD score of 8 to 11 had a mortality rate of 10.3%; and patients with a MELD score of 12 to 15 had a mortality rate of 25.4%. The increase in relative risk of death was nearly linear for MELD scores greater than 8 (Fig. 13.1).

In addition to the MELD score, an increasing American Society of Anesthesiologists (ASA) class (on a scale of I to V) and the age of the patient were shown by Teh et al. to contribute to the postoperative mortality risk (Box 13.4) [17]. Telem et al. [9] also found that an ASA class of more than III was a risk factor for morbidity and mortality. In the study by Teh et al. [17], an ASA class of IV added the equivalent of 5.5 MELD points to the mortality rate, whereas an ASA class of V was associated with a 100% mortality rate. The influence of the ASA class was

greatest in the first 7 days after surgery, after which the MELD score became the principal determinant of risk. In this study [17], no patient under 30 years old died, and an age greater than 70 years added the equivalent of 3 MELD points to the mortality rate. Unlike studies that evaluated the ability of the Child–Pugh class to predict surgical mortality, emergency surgery was not an independent predictor of mortality when the MELD score was considered, because patients who underwent emergency surgery had higher MELD scores than those who underwent elective surgery.

Based on the study of Teh et al. [17], a website (http://www.mayoclinic.org/meld/mayomodel9.html) was developed that can be used to calculate estimated 7-day, 30-day, 90-day, 1-year, and 5-year perioperative mortality rates based on a patient's age, ASA class, INR, and serum bilirubin and creatinine levels (the last three items constitute the MELD score). Use of the MELD score and Child–Pugh class are not mutually exclusive, however, and the two scoring systems appear to complement one another. The MELD score is probably the more precise predictor of perioperative mortality. The study by Telem et al. [9] has further suggested that in patients with a MELD score of 15 or more, a low serum albumin level (≤2.5 mg/dL) is associated with a particularly high mortality rate (60%) compared with the rate in patients with a serum albumin level of >2.5 mg/dL (14%).

Operative risk associated with specific types of surgery

In patients with cirrhosis, operative mortality is highest for biliary tract, cardiac, and hepatic resection surgery. The mortality rate is increased further when surgery is performed emergently. In patients with portal hypertension in particular, colectomy and gastric resection are also associated with a high operative risk.

Biliary tract surgery

Patients with cirrhosis are at increased risk of gallstone formation and associated complications when compared with noncirrhotic persons [18–21]. In a case–control study of patients who underwent laparoscopic cholecystectomy, a MELD score of ≥8 had a sensitivity of 91% and a specificity of 77% for predicting 90-day postoperative morbidity. In general, laparoscopic cholecystectomy is permissible for patients with Child-Pugh class A cirrhosis and selected patients with Child-Pugh class B cirrhosis without portal hypertension and is associated with lower rates of morbidity and blood transfusion and a reduced length of hospital stay compared with open cholecystectomy [20]. In contrast, in patients with Child–Pugh class C cirrhosis, cholecystostomy, rather than cholecystectomy, is recommended; when surgery is deemed the only option, an open rather than laparoscopic approach is recommended.

In patients with benign etiologies of obstructive jaundice or malignant causes that are not amenable to curative surgery, nonsurgical approaches to decompression via endoscopic retrograde cholangiopancreatography (ERCP) or percutaneous transhepatic cholangiography are preferred. Before ERCP was widely used, a study of patients with obstructive jaundice indentified three predictors of perioperative mortality: a hematocrit value less than 30%, an initial serum bilirubin level greater than 11 mg/dL (200 μmol/L), and a malignant cause of obstruction [22]. When all three factors were present, the mortality rate approached 60%; when none was present, the mortality rate was only 5%. Not surprisingly, malignant biliary obstruction carried a dramatically higher operative mortality rate (26.1%) than benign biliary obstruction (3.7%). In addition, patients with obstructive jaundice are at increased risk of infection, disseminated intravascular coagulation, gastrointestinal bleeding, delayed wound healing, wound dehiscence, incisional hernias, and renal failure. In patients undergoing surgery for cancer of the pancreatic head, routine preoperative decompression of an obstructed biliary tract (at least with plastic stents) does not appear to reduce subsequent operative mortality and may increase the rate of complications [23]. Preoperative relief of biliary obstruction is indicated, however, in patients with acute cholangitis and in those with severe pruritus in whom surgery is delayed.

Although endoscopic sphincterotomy is associated with an increased risk of bleeding in patients with cirrhosis, morbidity and mortality rates for this procedure are low even in patients with Child–Pugh class C cirrhosis. In patients with coagulopathy or thrombocytopenia, endoscopic papillary balloon dilation is associated with a lower risk of bleeding than standard sphincterotomy and is preferred despite a possibly higher risk of acute pancreatitis [24].

Cardiac surgery

Cardiac surgery and other procedures that require the use of cardiopulmonary bypass are associated with greater mortality in patients with cirrhosis than are most other surgical procedures. Risk factors for hepatic decompensation following cardiac surgery include the use of cardiac bypass, total time on bypass, use of nonpulsatile as opposed to pulsatile bypass flow, and need for perioperative vasopressor support. In retrospective series of patients who underwent surgery requiring cardiopulmonary bypass, relatively low mortality rates were observed in those with Child–Pugh class A cirrhosis (0–11%), but rates were markedly increased in those with Child–Pugh class B (18–50%) and C (67–100%) cirrhosis. In addition, more than 75% of Child–Pugh class B and C patients experienced hepatic decompensation following surgery [25–27]. Increased mortality following cardiac surgery is also predicted by an increased MELD score. A MELD score greater than 13 predicts a poor prognosis, although no "safe" cutoff score has been established. In general, a CTP score of 7 or less (Child–Pugh class A) or a low MELD score suggests that cardiopulmonary bypass can probably be accomplished safely in patients with cirrhosis.

In addition to an elevated CTP or MELD score, clinically significant portal hypertension is a contraindication to cardiothoracic surgery. Portal decompression with TIPS placement may make the risk acceptable if the CTP and MELD scores remain low [28]. However, elevated right-sided cardiac pressures from cardiac dysfunction and pulmonary hypertension are absolute contraindications to TIPS placement. Several centers have reported successful outcomes of combined liver transplantation and cardiac surgery (including heart transplantation) in selected patients with advanced liver disease and severe heart disease [29].

Hepatic resection

Mortality rates as high as 25% are reported following hepatic resection in patients with cirrhosis [30] (see Chapter 37). Risk stratification based on the Child–Pugh class and MELD score has allowed more appropriate selection of patients, thus leading to lower mortality rates. In an analysis of 82 cirrhotic patients who underwent hepatic resection for hepatocellular carcinoma, the perioperative mortality rate was 29% in patients with a MELD score ≥9 but 0% in those with a MELD score ≤8 [31]. Another study of 94 cirrhotic patients who underwent hepatic resection for hepatocellular carcinoma reported mortality rates of 15.3% and 0% in those with a MELD score ≥10 and ≤9, respectively [32]. On the other hand, one study [33] identified Child–Pugh class and ASA class, but not MELD score, as significant predictors of outcome following liver resection. In this study [33], the mean MELD score (6.5) was low, which likely limited the ability of the MELD score to discriminate between risk groups. In addition to predicting mortality, the MELD score can predict morbidity after liver resection. In one study [34], the frequency of post-liver resection liver failure was 0%, 3.6%, and 37.5% in patients with MELD scores of <9, 9–10, and >10, respectively. Additional predictors of mortality are the extent of hepatectomy and a low serum sodium concentration [35].

Post-resectional liver failure has been defined as a prothrombin time index (control prothrombin time divided by the patient's prothrombin time) of less than 50% (INR >1.7) and a serum bilirubin greater than 50 μmol/L (2.9 mg/dL), the so-called "50-50" criteria. When these criteria are met the postoperative mortality rate is 59%, compared with 1.2% in patients not meeting these criteria [36].

Endoscopic procedures

Endoscopy with moderate sedation is not contraindicated in patients with advanced cirrhosis, although coagulopathy may influence the approach to certain procedures such as polypectomy and sphincterotomy (see earlier). Variceal band ligation can be performed in patients with a high INR or thrombocytopenia. Gastrostomy tube placement should be avoided in patients with ascites, because of a high risk of leakage and infection, and in patients with visible abdominal wall collateral veins or enlarged intra-abdominal veins on imaging studies, because of the risk of bleeding.

Perioperative preparation

Every effort should be made to optimize the condition of a patient with liver disease prior to surgery. Ascites should be treated medically to avoid respiratory compromise, wound dehiscence, and abdominal wall herniation (see Chapter 17). In some cases, preoperative placement of a TIPS may be necessary. If abdominal surgery is undertaken, the ascites can be drained at surgery. The patient's volume status and renal function should be optimized to attempt to reduce the risk of hepatorenal syndrome in the postoperative period (see Chapter 15). Hepatic encephalopathy should be treated, but there is no evidence that prophylactic therapy in cirrhotic patients without encephalopathy in useful (see Chapter 18). In patients with cirrhosis, the INR correlates with impaired liver function but not with bleeding risk (see Chapters 12 and 14). Nevertheless, an attempt to improve coagulopathy with the administration of vitamin K, fresh frozen plasma, or both is often made. The use of recombinant factor VIIa in this setting is limited because of its high cost, transient effect, absence of data showing

improved outcomes, and associated risk of thromboembolism. Maintenance of a low central venous pressure during surgery may reduce intraoperative blood loss [37]. Finally, patients with advanced liver disease are likely to have protein–energy malnutrition, which contributes to mortality and morbidity, and may benefit from nutritional supplementation, preferably via the enteral route, before surgery.

Postoperative monitoring

Postoperatively, patients with cirrhosis need to be monitored for the development of signs of hepatic decompensation, including ascites, renal dysfunction, encephalopathy, coagulopathy, and worsening jaundice. The prothrombin time is the single best indicator of hepatic synthetic function. An elevated serum bilirubin can indicate worsening hepatic function but can be elevated for other reasons, including blood transfusions, resorption of extravasated blood, or infection. Renal function must be monitored closely. Hypoglycemia may occur in patients with decompensated cirrhosis or acute liver failure as a result of depleted hepatic glycogen stores and impaired gluconeogenesis. Serum glucose levels should be monitored closely when postoperative liver failure is suspected. Careful attention should be paid to the patient's intravascular volume, which is often difficult to assess in the setting of extravascular volume overload. Maintenance of intravascular volume minimizes the risk of hepatic and renal underperfusion. On the other hand, infusion of too much crystalloid may lead to acute hepatic congestion, increased venous oozing, and pulmonary edema and to postoperative ascites, peripheral edema, and wound dehiscence.

Further reading

Dixon JM, Armstrong CP, Duffy SW, et al. Factors affecting morbidity and mortality after surgery for obstructive jaundice: a review of 373 patients. Gut 1983;24:845–52.
A classic study demonstrating that major predictors of postoperative mortality in patients who undergo surgery for obstructive jaundice are a hematocrit value less than 30%, serum bilirubin level greater than 11 mg/dL, and malignant cause of biliary obstruction.

Garrison RN, Cryer HM, Howard DA, et al. Clarification of risk factors for abdominal operations in patients with hepatic cirrhosis. Ann Surg 1984;199:648–55.
A retrospective study of 100 patients with cirrhosis, predominantly alcoholic, in which 52 parameters were assessed in a multivariate analysis and the Child–Pugh class was found to be the best predictor of postoperative mortality and morbidity, with mortality rates of 10%, 31%, and 76% in patients with Child–Pugh class A, B, and C cirrhosis, respectively.

Gil A, Martinez-Regueira F, Hernandez-Lizoain JL, et al. The role of transjugular intrahepatic portosystemic shunt prior to abdominal tumoral surgery in cirrhotic patients with portal hypertension. Eur J Surg Oncol 2004;30:46–52.
One of several studies demonstrating that in patients with cirrhosis and portal hypertension, postoperative morbidity (e.g., ascites) is reduced by preoperative placement of a transjugular intrahepatic portosystemic shunt.

Harville DD, Summerskill WH. Surgery in acute hepatitis. Causes and effects. *JAMA* 1963;184:257–61.

A classic study that demonstrated a mortality rate of approximately 10% in patients with acute hepatitis who underwent laparotomy.

Mansour A, Watson W, Shayani V, et al. Abdominal operations in patients with cirrhosis: still a major surgical challenge. *Surgery* 1997;122:730–5.

A retrospective study of 100 patients with cirrhosis, 50% alcoholic and 50% viral, in which the Child–Pugh class was demonstrated, as in the study by Garrison et al., to be the best predictor of postoperative mortality, with rates of 10%, 30%, and 82% for Child–Pugh class A, B, and C cirrhosis, respectively.

O'Leary JG, Yachimski PS, Friedman LS. Surgery in the patient with liver disease. *Clin Liver Dis* 2009;13:211–31.

A detailed review of the effects of anesthesia and surgery on the liver, assessment of operative risk in patients with liver disease, operative risk associated with specific types of surgery, and perioperative preparation and care of the patient with liver disease.

Suman A, Barnes DS, Zein NN, et al. Predicting outcome after cardiac surgery in patients with cirrhosis: a comparison of Child–Pugh and MELD scores. *Clin Gastroenterol Hepatol* 2004;2:719–23.

A study showing that cardiac surgery can be performed safely in patients with Child–Pugh class A cirrhosis but carries a high risk in patients with Child class B or C cirrhosis or in those with a model for end-stage liver disease score greater than 13.

Teh SH, Christein J, Donohue J, et al. Hepatic resection of hepatocellular carcinoma in patients with cirrhosis: model of end-stage liver disease (MELD) score predicts perioperative mortality. *J Gastrointest Surg* 2005;9:1207–15.

A retrospective study of 82 patients with cirrhosis who underwent hepatic resection for hepatocellular carcinoma showing that the mortality rose substantially (to 29%) in those with a model of end-stage liver disease score of 9 or more.

Teh SH, Nagorney DM, Stevens SR, et al. Risk factors for mortality after surgery in patients with cirrhosis. *Gastroenterology* 2007;132:1261–9.

A retrospective study of 772 patients demonstrating that, in addition to the patient's age, the best predictor of 30-day and 90-day mortality in patients with cirrhosis who undergo surgery is the model for end-stage liver disease score. In the first postoperative week, the patient's preoperative American Society of Anesthesiologists class was a major predictor of mortality.

Telem DA, Schiano T, Goldstone R, et al. Factors that predict outcome of abdominal operations in patients with advanced cirrhosis. *Clin Gastroenterol Hepatol* 2010;8:451–7.

In this contemporary study of cirrhotic patients undergoing abdominal surgery, mortality rates were improved when compared with older studies. For patients with a model for end-stage liver disease score of ≥15, a preoperative serum albumin level of 2.5 mg/dL or less was associated with a high mortality rate (60%).

van den Broek MA, Olde Damink SW, Dejong CH, et al. Liver failure after partial hepatic resection: definition, pathophysiology, risk factors and treatment. *Liver Int* 2008;28:767–80.

Liver failure following partial hepatic resection for hepatocellular carcinoma in patients with cirrhosis is defined by the "50-50" criteria (a prothrombin time index of less than 50% (INR >1.7) and a serum bilirubin greater than 50 μmol/L (2.9 mg/dL)), which correlate with a postoperative mortality rate of 59%, compared with 1.2% in patients who do not meet these criteria.

van der Gaag NA, Rauws EA, van Eijck CH, et al. Preoperative biliary drainage for cancer of the head of the pancreas. *N Engl J Med* 2010;362:129–37.

One of several studies demonstrating that in the absence of cholangitis, routine preoperative decompression of an obstructed biliary tract does not reduce operative mortality in patients who undergo surgery for pancreatic cancer.

Ziser A, Plevak DJ, Wiesner RH, et al. Morbidity and mortality in cirrhotic patients undergoing anesthesia and surgery. *Anesthesiology* 1999;90:42–53.

Retrospective study demonstrating that chronic obstructive lung disease and surgery on the respiratory tract are independent risk factors for postoperative mortality in patients with cirrhosis.

References

1. Rothenberg DM, O'Connor CJ, Tuman KJ. Anesthesia and the hepatobiliary system. In: Miller RD, ed. *Miller's Anesthesia*, 7th edn Philadelphia: Churchill Livingstone Elsevier, 2010;2135–53.

2. O'Leary JG, Yachimski PS, Friedman LS. Surgery in the patient with liver disease. *Clin Liver Dis* 2009;13:211–31.

3. Sato K, Kawamura T, Wakusawa R. Hepatic blood flow and function in elderly patients undergoing laparoscopic cholecystectomy. *Anesth Analg* 2000;90:1198–202.

4. Lai HC, Wang KY, Lee WL, et al. Severe pulmonary hypertension complicates postoperative outcome of non-cardiac surgery. *Br J Anaesth* 2007;99:184–90.

5. Harville DD, Summerskill WH. Surgery in acute hepatitis. *Causes and effects.* JAMA 1963;184:257–61.

6. Greenwood SM, Leffler CT, Minkowitz S. The increased mortality rate of open liver biopsy in alcoholic hepatitis. *Surg Gynecol Obstet* 1972;134:600–4.

7. Garrison RN, Cryer HM, Howard DA, et al. Clarification of risk factors for abdominal operations in patients with hepatic cirrhosis. *Ann Surg* 1984;199:648–55.

8. Mansour A, Watson W, Shayani V, et al. Abdominal operations in patients with cirrhosis: still a major surgical challenge. *Surgery* 1997;122:730–5.

9. Telem DA, Schiano T, Goldstone R, et al. Factors that predict outcome of abdominal operations in patients with advanced cirrhosis. *Clin Gastroenterol Hepatol* 2010;8:451–7.

10. Gil A, Martinez-Regueira F, Hernandez-Lizoain JL, et al. The role of transjugular intrahepatic portosystemic shunt prior to abdominal tumoral surgery in cirrhotic patients with portal hypertension. *Eur J Surg Oncol* 2004;30:46–52.

11. Azoulay D, Buabse F, Damiano I, et al. Neoadjuvant transjugular intrahepatic portosystemic shunt: a solution for extrahepatic abdominal operation in cirrhotic patients with severe portal hypertension. *J Am Coll Surg* 2001;193:46–51.

12. Kim JJ, Dasika NL, Yu E, Fontana RJ. Cirrhotic patients with a transjugular intrahepatic portosystemic shunt undergoing major extrahepatic surgery. *J Clin Gastroenterol* 2009;43:574–9.

13. Ziser A, Plevak DJ, Wiesner RH, et al. Morbidity and mortality in cirrhotic patients undergoing anesthesia and surgery. *Anesthesiology* 1999;90:42–53.

14. Malinchoc M, Kamath PS, Gordon FD, et al. A model to predict poor survival in patients undergoing transjugular intrahepatic portosystemic shunts. *Hepatology* 2000;31:864–71.

15. O'Leary JG, Friedman LS. Predicting surgical risk in patients with cirrhosis: from art to science. *Gastroenterology* 2007;132:1609–11.

16. Northup PG, Wanamaker RC, Lee VD, et al. Model for end-stage liver disease (MELD) predicts nontransplant surgical mortality in patients with cirrhosis. *Ann Surg* 2005;242:244–51.

17. Teh SH, Nagorney DM, Stevens SR, et al. Risk factors for mortality after surgery in patients with cirrhosis. *Gastroenterology* 2007;132:1261–9.

18. Perkins L, Jeffries M, Patel T. Utility of preoperative scores for predicting morbidity after cholecystectomy in patients with cirrhosis. *Clin Gastroenterol Hepatol* 2004;2:1123–8.

19. Curro G, Baccarani U, Adani G, et al. Laparoscopic cholecystectomy in patients with mild cirrhosis and symptomatic cholelithiasis. *Transplant Proc* 2007;39:1471–3.

20. El-Awadi S, El-Nakeeb A, Youssef T, et al. Laparoscopic versus open cholecystectomy in cirrhotic patients: a prospective randomized study. *Int J Surg* 2009;7:66–9.

21. Yeh CN, Chen MF, Jan YY. Laparoscopic cholecystectomy in 226 cirrhotic patients. Experience of a single center in Taiwan. *Surg Endosc* 2002;16:1583–7.

22. Dixon JM, Armstrong CP, Duffy SW, et al. Factors affecting morbidity and mortality after surgery for obstructive jaundice: a review of 373 patients. *Gut* 1983;24:845–52.

23. van der Gaag NA, Rauws EA, van Eijck CH, et al. Preoperative biliary drainage for cancer of the head of the pancreas. *N Engl J Med* 2010;362:129–37.

24. Park DH, Kim MH, Lee SK, et al. Endoscopic sphincterotomy vs. endoscopic papillary balloon dilation for choledocholithiasis in patients with liver cirrhosis and coagulopathy. *Gastrointest Endosc* 2004;60:180–5.

25. Hayashida N, Shoujima T, Teshima H, et al. Clinical outcome after cardiac operations in patients with cirrhosis. *Ann Thorac Surg* 2004;77:500–5.

26. Suman A, Barnes DS, Zein NN, et al. Predicting outcome after cardiac surgery in patients with cirrhosis: a comparison of Child–Pugh and MELD scores. *Clin Gastroenterol Hepatol* 2004;2:719–23.

27. Filsoufi F, Salzberg SP, Rahmanian PB, et al. Early and late outcome of cardiac surgery in patients with liver cirrhosis. *Liver Transpl* 2007;13:990–5.

28. Semiz-Oysu A, Moustafa T, Cho KJ. Transjugular intrahepatic portosystemic shunt prior to cardiac surgery with cardiopulmonary bypass in patients with cirrhosis and portal hypertension. *Heart Lung Circ* 2007;16:465–8.

29. Ehtisham J, Altieri M, Salamé E, et al. Coronary artery disease in orthotopic liver transplantation: pretransplant assessment and management. *Liver Transpl* 2010;16:550–7.

30. Mullin EJ, Metcalfe MS, Maddern GJ. How much liver resection is too much? *Am J Surg* 2005;190:87–97.

31. Teh SH, Christein J, Donohue J, et al. Hepatic resection of hepatocellular carcinoma in patients with cirrhosis: model of end-stage liver disease (MELD) score predicts perioperative mortality. *J Gastrointest Surg* 2005;9:1207–15.

32. Delis SG, Bakoyiannis A, Dervenis C, Tassopoulos N. Perioperative risk assessment for hepatocellular carcinoma by using the MELD score. *J Gastrointest Surg* 2009;13:2268–75.

33. Schroeder RA, Marroquin CE, Bute BP, et al. Predictive indices of morbidity and mortality after liver resection. *Ann Surg* 2006;243:373–9.

34. Cucchetti A, Ercolani G, Vivarelli M, et al. Impact of model for end-stage liver disease (MELD) score on prognosis after hepatectomy for hepatocellular carcinoma on cirrhosis. *Liver Transpl* 2006;12:966–71.

35. Cescon M, Cucchetti A, Grazi GL, et al. Indication of the extent of hepatectomy for hepatocellular carcinoma on cirrhosis by a simple algorithm based on preoperative variables. *Arch Surg* 2009;144:57–63.

36. van den Broek MA, Olde Damink SW, Dejong CH, et al. Liver failure after partial hepatic resection: definition, pathophysiology, risk factors and treatment. *Liver Int* 2008;28:767–80.

37. Alkozai EM, Lisman T, Porte RJ. Bleeding in liver surgery: prevention and treatment. *Clin Liver Dis* 2009;13:145–54.

Multiple choice questions

13.1 A 45-year-old man sees his primary care physician (PCP) prior to an elective left inguinal hernia repair. He has no other medical problems but drinks two or three cocktails a day and more on weekends. Other than the hernia and a body mass index of $28\,kg/m^2$, the physical examination is unremarkable. Routine laboratory studies show a serum alanine aminotransferase level of 25 U/L and aspartate aminotransferase level of 142 U/L. The serum alkaline phosphatase level is 101 U/L, total bilirubin level 1.3 mg/dL, and albumin level 3.7 g/dL. The international normalized ratio (INR) is 1.3. Which of the following would you advise the PCP regarding the planned inguinal hernia repair?

    a Proceed with surgery if serologic markers for viral hepatitis are negative.
    b Proceed with surgery if a repeat INR is 1.0 after administration of vitamin K.
    c Proceed with surgery after excluding diabetes mellitus and hypertriglyceridemia.
    d Repeat the laboratory studies in 2 weeks; proceed with surgery if the results are stable.
    e Cancel the surgery.

13.2 In a patient with cirrhosis who undergoes hepatic resection for hepatocellular carcinoma, postoperative liver failure and mortality are predicted by the "50–50" rule. Which of the following defines the rule?

    a Resection of 50% of the liver.
    b Resection of 50% of the liver plus a serum bilirubin level of $>50\,\mu mol/L$.
    c A serum bilirubin level of $>50\,\mu mol/L$ plus a prothrombin time index of $<50\%$.
    d An increase in the serum bilirubin level of $50\,\mu mol/L$ and a decrease in the serum albumin level by 50% after surgery.
    e An increase in either the Child–Turcotte–Pugh score or the model for end-stage liver disease (MELD) score after surgery of 50%.

Answers to the multiple choice questions can be found in the Appendix at the end of the book.

These multiple choice questions are also available for you to complete online.
Visit http://www.schiffsdiseasesoftheliver.com/

CHAPTER 14

Portal Hypertension: Nonsurgical and Surgical Management

Hitoshi Maruyama[1] & Arun J. Sanyal[2]

[1]Department of Medicine and Clinical Oncology, Chiba University Graduate School of Medicine, Chiba, Japan
[2]Division of Gastroenterology and Hepatology, Virginia Commonwealth University, Richmond, VA, USA

Key concepts

- Portal hypertension is the most common and lethal complication of chronic liver diseases. It is responsible for the development of gastroesophageal varices, variceal hemorrhage, ascites, renal dysfunction, portosystemic encephalopathy, hypersplenism, and hepatopulmonary syndrome.

- Portal hypertension is defined by a pathologic increase in portal pressure, in which the pressure gradient between the portal vein and inferior vena cava (the portal pressure gradient (PPG)) is increased above the upper normal limit of 5 mmHg. Portal hypertension becomes clinically significant when the PPG increases above the threshold value of 10 mmHg (e.g., formation of varices) or 12 mmHg (e.g., variceal bleeding, ascites). PPG values between 6 and 10 mmHg represent subclinical portal hypertension.

- PPG is determined by the product of blood flow and vascular resistance within the portal-venous system. Portal hypertension is initiated by an increased resistance to portal blood flow and aggravated by an increased portal-venous inflow. The site of increased resistance to portal blood flow is the basis for the classification of portal hypertension: prehepatic (e.g., portal vein thrombosis), intrahepatic (e.g., cirrhosis), and posthepatic (e.g., hepatic vein thrombosis, heart disease).

- Increased resistance in cirrhosis represents not only disruption of the liver's vascular architecture by liver disease but also a dynamic component resulting from the active contraction of vascular smooth muscle cells, myofibroblasts, and hepatic stellate cells. Active contraction is caused by decreased production of vasodilators such as nitric oxide (NO) and by increased release of endogenous vasoconstrictors. Increased hepatic vascular tone is the basis for the use of vasodilators to treat portal hypertension in cirrhosis.

- Portal inflow is increased by splanchnic vasodilatation, which is caused by an increased release of local endothelial factors and humoral vasodilators. Splanchnic vasodilatation can be counteracted with vasoconstrictors and β-blockers, which is why these drugs are used to treat portal hypertension.

- Portal pressure is most commonly assessed clinically by measuring the hepatic venous pressure gradient (HVPG), which is the difference between the wedged hepatic venous pressure (WHVP) and free hepatic venous pressure (FHVP), at hepatic vein catheterization. The HVPG accurately reflects the portal pressure in both alcoholic and viral cirrhosis. HVPG has to be above 10 mmHg for varices to develop and above 12 mmHg for variceal bleeding. The threshold values define "clinically significant portal hypertension."

- Bleeding from ruptured esophageal or gastric varices is a major complication of portal hypertension and a frequent cause of death. Approximately 40% of patients with compensated cirrhosis have varices at the time of diagnosis. The rate of formation of varices is approximately 8% per year, so varices develop in most patients during long-term follow-up. The risk of bleeding increases as the pressure and size of the varices increase and as the thickness of the variceal wall decreases. These parameters determine the tension of the variceal wall; rupture and bleeding occur when wall tension increases above the elastic limit of the varices.

- Most drugs used to treat portal hypertension are splanchnic vasoconstrictors, which act primarily by reducing portal and collateral blood flow. This group includes vasopressin, terlipressin, the somatostatins, propranolol, nadolol, and other β-blockers.

- Vasodilators that decrease the portal pressure include isosorbide-5-mononitrate (IMN), which acts as an NO donor, and adrenergic antagonists, such as clonidine, prazosin, and carvedilol. A common problem with vasodilators is that they cause arterial hypotension, which in turn may enhance sodium retention and aggravate renal dysfunction in patients with cirrhosis and ascites.

- In combination therapy, a vasoconstrictor and a vasodilator are administered together. The combination prevents most of the adverse effects of the vasodilator and enhances the fall in portal pressure caused by the reduction in blood flow induced by the vasoconstrictor. Drug combinations with proven clinical efficacy are vasopressin plus nitroglycerin and propranolol or nadolol plus IMN.

Schiff's Diseases of the Liver, Eleventh Edition. Edited by Eugene R. Schiff, Willis C. Maddrey and Michael F. Sorrell.

- Either nonselective β-blockers or endoscopic variceal ligation are the treatments of choice for the primary prevention of variceal bleeding. They should be given to all patients with medium or high variceal bleeding risk (patients with medium or large varices or those with small varices and red color signs or with poor liver function – Child–Pugh class B and C) who have no contraindications to β-blockers. Therapy should be maintained indefinitely and is relatively well tolerated; the rate of discontinuation because of side effects or poor tolerance is 15%. Patients with high-risk varices and contraindications to β-blockers should be treated with endoscopic band ligation.
- During acute variceal hemorrhage, general supportive therapy including antibiotic prophylaxis of bacterial infections and a very conservative use of blood transfusion should be instituted. The prognosis is worse in patients with advanced liver failure or with early (first week) rebleeding. Terlipressin and somatostatin are drugs that have proved effective as a first-line treatment in arresting variceal bleeding and reducing mortality from variceal hemorrhage. Drug therapy has been shown to be as effective as and safer than emergency endoscopic therapy. Drug therapy should be started early on arrival at the emergency room or even during transfer to the hospital. Endoscopic band ligation is the endoscopic treatment of choice for acute esophageal variceal bleeding; however, endoscopic injection sclerotherapy can be used in the acute setting if endoscopic band ligation is technically difficult. Drug therapy is usually continued for 3–5 days even if the bleeding is apparently controlled by endoscopic therapy. Endoscopic variceal obturation with tissue adhesives is recommended for acute fundal gastric variceal bleeding.
- Failures of medical treatment should be managed aggressively with emergency surgery or a transjugular intrahepatic portosystemic shunt (TIPS), preferably using expanded polytetrafluoroethylene (ePTFE)

covered stents. Because of higher rates of morbidity and mortality, rescue derivative surgery should only be considered in low-risk patients (Child–Pugh score <8).
- A combination of β-blockers and band ligation is probably the best treatment option, especially in patients who have bleeding while under either therapy alone. Patients who rebleed despite combined endoscopic and pharmacologic treatment may be treated by transjugular intraheptic or surgical portosystemic shunting; TIPS is the only option in nonsurgical candidates. All Child–Pugh class C patients should be considered for liver transplantation.
- Patients who survive an episode of variceal bleeding are at high risk for rebleeding. Medical treatment with β-blockers ± isosorbide mononitrate is as effective as endoscopic band ligation in preventing rebleeding. The best results are obtained when the HVPG is reduced by at least 20% of the baseline value or below 12 mmHg. The combination of IMN and propranolol or nadolol significantly increases the number of patients in whom the target reduction in portal pressure is achieved.
- Variceal decompression is indicated for patients who fail primary therapy or who cannot undergo primary therapy. Decompression is performed with a transjugular intrahepatic portosystemic or surgical shunt.
- The occurrence of encephalopathy and liver failure after insertion of a shunt depends on the extent of liver disease and loss of portal perfusion.
- Devascularization procedures are a surgical alternative in the management of variceal bleeding in patients who cannot undergo shunting.
- Liver transplantation has significantly improved outcome among Child–Pugh class C patients with variceal bleeding, and is the only treatment that reliably prolongs life.

Anatomy and classification

The portal vein normally drains blood from the stomach, intestines, spleen, and pancreatic bed via the superior mesenteric, splenic, and left gastric veins (Fig. 14.1). The tributaries of the portal vein also communicate with veins draining into the systemic venous circulation with the following five portosystemic communications: (i) at the cardia via the intrinsic and extrinsic veins of the region; (ii) in the anal canal via anastomoses between the superior and middle hemorrhoidal veins; (iii) in the falciform ligament via recanalization of the paraumbilical veins and direction of flow to the veins draining the abdominal wall; (iv) in the splenic venous bed and the left renal vein; and (v) in the retroperitoneum. Among these communications, the gastroesophageal collaterals are of great clinical significance because they are associated with the development of gastroesophageal varices [1].

The veins draining the esophagus may be classified as intrinsic, extrinsic, and venae comitantes of the vagus nerve. The intrinsic veins include a subepithelial and submucosal plexus running along the length of the

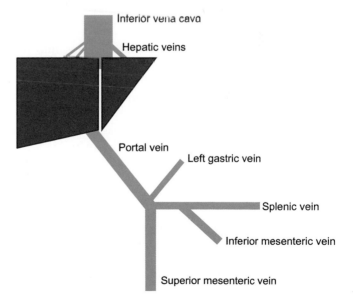

Figure 14.1 Anatomy of the portal-venous system. Although the flow direction of the portal vein, splenic vein, superior mesenteric vein, and inferior mesenteric vein is hepatopetal in normal subjects, it may change in cases of portal hypertension.

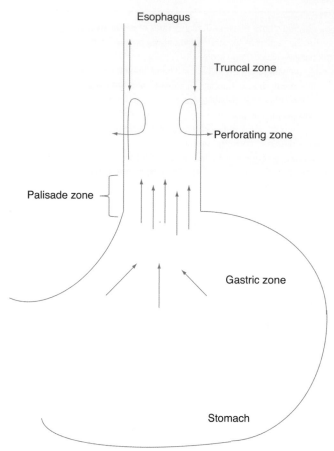

Figure 14.2 Venous anatomy of the gastroesophageal junction. There are four zones identified in this area: the gastric zone, palisade zone, perforating zone, and truncal zone. Increased venous blood flow in the palisade region causes varices.

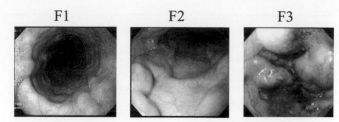

Figure 14.3 Endoscopic grade of esophageal varices, which are often graded by size, from F1 to F3. For details, see text.

esophagus. These drain via perforating veins into an extrinsic plexus of veins, which drain into the inferior thyroid and brachiocephalic veins in the neck, azygous veins in the thorax, and left gastric vein in the abdominal part of the esophagus.

The intrinsic veins of the gastroesophageal junction are divided into four well-defined zones (Fig. 14.2):

1 Gastric zone: this is a 2–3 cm zone with its upper border at the gastroesophageal junction and is composed of a radial band of veins in the submucosa and lamina propria.

2 Palisade zone: this commences at the gastroesophageal junction and extends cranially for 2–3 cm and is a direct extension of the veins of the gastric zone, which run in "palisades" or packs of longitudinally arrayed veins in the lamina propria. These veins are the primary site of communication between the portal bed and azygous bed.

3 Perforating zone: the intrinsic veins drain into the extrinsic veins primarily in this region via valved per-

forating veins, which only allow unidirectional flow normally. It extends 2–3 cm cranially from the palisade zone.

4 Truncal zone: an 8–10 cm zone extending upward from the perforating zone. The intrinsic veins are composed of three or four large venous trunks in the submucosa, which communicate with an irregular polygonal venous plexus in the submucosa. Flow direction in these veins is from a cranial to caudal direction and drains via the perforating veins into the extrinsic veins. In cases of portal hypertension, an adaptive increase in flow through the portasystemic communications occurs to return blood to the heart. The vessels involved, especially the intrinsic veins around the gastroesophageal (GE) junction dilate and become tortuous forming varicose veins.

Gastroesophageal varices show four basic patterns: (i) varices in the fundus of the stomach; (ii) gastric and palisade-zone varices; (iii) varices in the perforating zones; and (iv) paraesophageal varices, which involve the extrinsic esophageal veins. In contrast to normal individuals, the valves in the perforating veins become incompetent, thereby permitting reverse flow into the intrinsic plexus from the extrinsic veins. Clinically, GE varices are classified by location into esophageal and gastric varices.

Esophageal varices are often graded by size (Fig. 14.3). A common system is as follows:

• F1: small, straight varices.
• F2: enlarged, tortuous varices, occupying less than one third of the lumen.
• F3: large, coil-shaped varices, occupying more than one third of the lumen.

Gastric varices are classified primary by location. As agreed upon at the Baveno Consensus Conference, they are described as follows:

• Gastroesophageal varices (GOVs): gastric varices in continuity with esophageal varices:
  • type 1 (GOV1): along the lesser curve (usually 2–5 cm in length);
  • type 2 (GOV2): along the greater curve extending towards the fundus of the stomach.
• Isolated gastric varices (IGVs):
  • type 1 (IGV1): isolated cluster of varices in the fundus of the stomach;

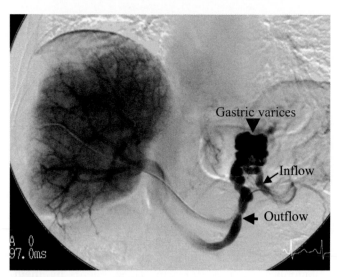

Figure 14.4 Angiographic feature of gastric varices. The portogram shows spontaneous collaterals from the splenic vein to the renal vein, feeding gastric varices. Thin arrow, inflow vessel; thick arrow, outflow route; arrow head, gastric varices.

- type 2 (IGV2): isolated gastric varices in other parts of the stomach.

GOV1 varices form when a branch of the left gastric vein penetrates the gastric wall (cardiac vein) and join the deep submucosal veins in the gastric zone; they are in direct continuity with those in the palisade zone and are usually associated with large esophageal varices. In contrast, large esophageal varices are present in only 50% of GOV2 varices. IGV1 are often associated with either segmental portal hypertension (splenic vein thrombosis) or the presence of spontaneous collaterals from the splenic vein to the renal vein, which feed these varices (Fig. 14.4). Almost half of cases with ectopic varices including IGV2 are associated with portal vein thrombosis.

Pathophysiology

The portal pressure is directly related to portal inflow and outflow resistance, expressed by the following formula:

$$\frac{\text{Portal}}{\text{pressure}} = \frac{\text{portal-venous}}{\text{inflow}} \times \frac{\text{outflow}}{\text{resistance}}$$

Sites and common causes of portal hypertension are presented in Box 14.1. Free hepatic venous pressure (FHVP) and wedged hepatic venous pressure (WHVP) are measured by hepatic venous catheterization, and the hepatic venous pressure gradient (HVPG) is calculated by folloing formula:

$$\text{HVPG} = \text{WHVP} - \text{FHVP}.$$

Box 14.1 Etiology of portal hypertension.

Prehepatic
- Splenic vein thrombosis
- Portal vein thrombosis
- Congenital stenosis of the portal vein
- Extrinsic compression of the portal vein
- Arteriovenous fistulae (splenic, aortomesenteric, aortoportal, and hepatic artery–portal vein)

Intrahepatic
- Partial nodular transformation
- Nodular regenerative hyperplasia
- Congenital hepatic fibrosis
- Peliosis hepatis
- Polycystic disease
- Idiopathic portal hypertension
- Hypervitaminosis A
- Arsenic, copper sulfate, and vinyl chloride monomer poisoning
- Sarcoidosis
- Tuberculosis
- Primary biliary cirrhosis
- Schistosomiasis
- Amyloidosis
- Mastocytosis
- Rendu–Osler–Weber syndrome
- Liver infiltration in hematologic diseases
- Acute fatty liver of pregnancy
- Severe acute viral hepatitis
- Chronic active hepatitis
- Hepatocellular carcinoma
- Hemochromatosis
- Wilson disease
- Hepatic porphyrias
- α_1-Antitrypsin deficiency
- Cyanamide toxicity
- Chronic biliary obstruction
- Cirrhosis from hepatitis B and C virus infection
- Alcoholic cirrhosis
- Alcoholic hepatitis
- Venoocclusive disease

Posthepatic
- Budd–Chiari syndrome
- Congenital malformations and thrombosis of the inferior vena cava
- Constrictive pericarditis
- Tricuspid valve diseases

WHVP reflects sinusoidal pressures, while FHVP corrects for the effects of intra-abdominal pressures.

Portal hypertension is initiated by an increase in outflow resistance from the portal-venous bed, and it is further worsened by splanchnic arterial dilatation, which increases portal-venous inflow in cirrhosis. Once portal hypertension occurs, a collateral circulation develops to return blood to the systemic circulation. For a given varice, the transmural pressure gradient is the product of flow and resistance: $P1 - P2 = Q \times R$, where $P1$ and $P2$ are the pressures within and outside the varices respectively, Q means the blood flow per unit time, and R means the resistance to flow through the varices.

Poiseuille's formula states that resistance to flow may be expressed as:

$$R = nl/\pi r^4,$$

where n is blood viscosity, and r and l are the length and radius of the vessel. The formula

$$\text{Wall tension} = [Q \times (nl/\pi r^4)] \times r/w$$

indicates variceal wall tension, which is determined by the transmural pressure, radius, and wall thickness (w) (Laplace's law). Variceal wall tension determines the probability of rupture. Based on this equation, long, large varices with high flow rates and thin walls are most likely to rupture and bleed. Conversely, by decreasing collateral flow, resistance to flow, or increasing wall thickness, the risk of variceal rupture should also be decreased. Most pharmacologic treatments are directed at decreasing collateral blood flow, which is usually achieved by decreasing portal pressure and/or increasing collateral resistance. However, the latter has complex effects on hemodynamics in collateral vessels by directly increasing wall tension and indirectly decreasing it by reducing collateral blood flow. This may explain some of the interindividual variability in hemodynamic response to pharmacologic treatment.

Vasoconstrictors and hepatic vascular bed

Endothelins (ETs) are a family of homologous 21-amino acid vasoactive peptides (ET-1, -2, and -3) that are thought to play a major role in modulating hepatic vascular tone in cirrhosis. The biologic properties of ETs are mediated essentially by two major ET receptors, ET-A and ET-B. The ET-A receptor shows a high affinity for ET-1, but not for ET-3, and mediates constriction; the ET-B receptor has equal affinity for ET-1 and ET-3. Activation of ET-B receptors located on the vascular smooth muscle cells promotes vasoconstriction, whereas activation of ET-B receptors located on endothelial cells promotes vasodilatation, which is mediated by enhanced nitric oxide (NO) and prostacyclin production by the endothelial cell.

Cirrhotic patients have increased circulating plasma levels of ET-1 and ET-3. The increase is greater and more consistently found in cirrhotic patients with ascites. A net release of ET-1 and ET-3 during splanchnic passage has been observed in cirrhotic patients but not in controls, suggesting an increased production of ET-1 and ET-3 in the splanchnic territory. Immunostaining and in situ hybridization studies have detected an increased expression of ET-1 in human cirrhotic livers; endothelial cells,

hepatic stellate cells (in their activated phenotype), and bile duct epithelial cells are the major intrahepatic sources of ET-1. A decreased clearance of ET-1 by the liver has also been demonstrated in cirrhotic rats.

ET-1 increases portal pressure by increasing intrahepatic resistance in isolated, perfused normal livers and carbon tetrachloride-induced cirrhotic livers. Although some experimental studies reported a slight reduction of portal pressure in cirrhotic animals after the administration of ET antagonists, this was not confirmed by other studies [2]. Therefore, the role of ETs in increasing the vascular tone in cirrhosis remains unsettled.

Norepinephrine is one of the vasoconstrictive factors, and is involved in the regulation of hepatic vascular tone. The increased resistance promoted by norepinephrine is completely blunted by the administration of α-adrenergic antagonists, such as prazosin. These agents by themselves markedly reduce hepatic resistance and portal pressure in cirrhotic patients. In contrast, the administration of α-adrenergic agonists, such as isoproterenol, reduces intrahepatic vascular resistance in perfused cirrhotic liver. These data suggest that adrenergic receptors may be involved in the regulation of intrahepatic resistance in cirrhosis and that α-adrenergic receptor blockers may decrease portal pressure in cirrhosis. In addition, the hepatic vascular bed of cirrhotic livers exhibits an exaggerated response to the α-adrenergic agonist methoxamine. This hyperresponse is associated with the overproduction of thromboxane A_2 (TXA_2) by cyclooxygenase 1 (COX-1) isoenzyme and is completely corrected by pretreating the livers with nonselective COX blockers, COX-1-selective blockers, or TXA_2 antagonists. Therefore, an increased production of TXA_2 markedly enhances the vasoconstrictive response of the cirrhotic hepatic vascular bed to methoxamine. Whether this effect is also shared by other vasoconstrictors has not been investigated so far. However, it is known that the coupling of different agonists to the membrane G-coupled receptors promotes the release of arachidonic acid from the plasma membrane, facilitating its metabolization to different prostanoids.

Angiotensin II is a powerful vasoconstrictor that may increase hepatic resistance. Strategies based on direct angiotensin II blockade by specific angiotensin II antagonists, inhibitors of the converting enzyme, or angiotensin II receptors blockers may reduce portal pressure but cause systemic hypotension.

Endothelial dysfunction

In normal conditions, the endothelium is able to generate vasodilator stimuli in response to increases in blood volume, blood pressure, or vasoconstrictor agents in an attempt to prevent or attenuate the concomitant increase in pressure. In several pathologic conditions, however, there is impairment in this endothelium-dependent vasodilatation, called endothelial dysfunction. Endothelial dysfunction is considered one of the main pathologic mechanisms involved in the increased vascular tone observed in several vascular disorders, such as arterial hypertension, diabetes, and atherosclerosis, and has been attributed to a diminished NO bioavailability or to an increased production of endothelial-derived contracting factors, such as prostaglandin H_2 (PGH_2)/TXA_2, ET, or anion superoxide [3].

The hepatic vascular bed in cirrhotic livers also exhibits endothelial dysfunction [4]. Indeed, studies performed both in cirrhotic patients and in experimental models have shown that, contrary to what happens in normal livers, the cirrhotic liver cannot accommodate the increased portal blood flow caused by the postprandial hyperemia, which determines an abrupt postprandial increase in portal pressure [5]. This is important because such repeated brisk increases in portal pressure and portal–collateral blood flow in response to meals and other physiologic stimuli are thought to be a major determinant of the progressive dilatation of the varices in patients with cirrhosis. In addition, endothelial dysfunction has been further characterized in experimental models of cirrhosis by showing that the cirrhotic liver exhibits an impaired response to the endothelium-dependent vasodilator acetylcholine [4,6]. This impaired response to acetylcholine was shown to be associated with an increased production of TXA_2 and completely prevented by selective COX-1 blockers and TXA_2 antagonists. These results suggest that an increased production of a COX-1-derived vasoconstrictor prostanoid, probably TXA_2, is, at least in part, responsible for endothelial dysfunction [6]. Acetylcholine coupling to the endothelial muscarinic M3 receptor has been shown to promote the stimulation of NO synthase and COX-1, with the subsequent release of NO and vasoconstrictor endoperoxides, respectively [3]. In physiologic states, a vasodilating response is the final balance between the interactions of these endothelial vasoactive mediators. However, in cirrhosis, as in other conditions such as hypertension, diabetes, and arteriosclerosis, there is a perturbation of this balance, resulting in endothelial dysfunction with a consequent impaired response to acetylcholine. All these findings suggest that there is an overactivation of the COX-1 pathway with an increased production of vasoconstrictor-derived compounds in cirrhotic livers.

Tetrahydrobiopterin, that is endothelial nitric oxide synthestase (eNOS) cofactor, increases eNOS activity and significantly improves the vasodilator response to acetylcholine in rats with cirrhosis [7]. Tetrahydrobiopterin supplementation may represent an additional treatment of portal hypertension by improving the endothelial dysfunction.

Recent studies suggest that statins decrease intrahepatic vascular reisitance and improve flow-mediated vasodilatation of liver vasculature in cirrhotic liver, due to an increase of NO production and improvement of hepatic endotherail dysfunction [8,9]. There is one clinical study showing the effectiveness of simvastatin to decrease HVPG [10].

Hepatic vasodilators

Nitric oxide

The role of NO in modulating intrahepatic vascular resistance is a subject of considerable interest. NO is a powerful endogenous vasodilator generated in several tissues by NO synthases from the amino acid L-arginine. It is the natural ligand for soluble guanylate cyclase and is responsible for an increase in the levels of cyclic guanosine monophosphate, the final agent responsible for the relaxation of the vascular wall through the extrusion of cytosolic Ca^{2+}.

NO blockade has been shown to increase portal pressure in isolated perfused rat livers. In addition, the hepatic response to norepinephrine is markedly enhanced after NO inhibition, suggesting a role for NO in modulating hepatic vascular tone in normal conditions [3]. In the cirrhotic liver, the synthesis of NO is insufficient to compensate for the activation of vasoconstrictor systems frequently associated with cirrhosis. This occurs despite a normal expression of eNOS mRNA and normal levels of eNOS protein [4], and the decreased activity of hepatic eNOS in cirrhosis is due in part to increased expression of caveolin [11]. This insufficient hepatic NO generation plays a major role in increasing intrahepatic vascular resistance in cirrhosis, thereby worsening portal hypertension. In accordance with this concept, the infusion of L-arginine, the precursor of NO biosynthesis, and the administration of nitrates (exogenous donors of NO) have been shown to decrease portal pressure. In addition, enhancement of the expression of NO synthase in liver cells, through the portal injection of adenovirus coupled with the gene encoding NO synthase, significantly reduces portal pressure. More recently, strategies aimed at increasing NO release by enhancing intrahepatic eNOS activity, on the basis of constitutively active *Akt* gene transfer, or by simvastatin administration have opened new perspectives with potential therapeutic implications [12,13]. NO also promotes hepatic stellate cell apoptosis through a signaling mechanism that involves mitochondria, is mediated by reactive oxygen species, and occurs independently of caspase activation [14]. This NO-dependent apoptosis, which may maintain sinusoidal homeostasis, is expected as a future treatment of portal hypertension.

Carbon monoxide

Carbon monoxide (CO) is a by-product of heme group oxidation by heme oxygenases, and is considered as an important modulator of intrahepatic vascular tone. CO, although less potent than NO, also activates guanylate cyclase and thereby promotes smooth muscle relaxation. The inhibition of CO production increases portal resistance in normal livers, and HO/CO system is activated in patients with liver cirrhosis, and this could contribute to the hyperdynamic circulatory syndrome observed in this condition [15]. Plasma CO levels directly correlated with cardiac output, and inversely with systemic vascular resistance and mean arterial pressure.

Splanchnic vasodilatation

An increased portal-venous inflow is characteristically observed in advanced stages of portal hypertension and is the result of marked arteriolar dilatation in the splanchnic organs draining into the portal vein. The increased blood flow contributes to the pathophysiology of portal hypertension [1].

Different mechanisms have been suggested to explain the observed hemodynamic abnormality, which likely represents a multifactorial phenomenon involving neurogenic, humoral, and local mechanisms. Initial studies focused on the potential role of increased levels of circulating vasodilators. Many candidate substances were proposed, most of them being vasodilators of splanchnic origin that undergo hepatic metabolism and accumulate in the systemic circulation when hepatic uptake is reduced in liver disease or during portosystemic shunting.

Glucagon

Glucagon is a humoral vasodilator that has a significant role in splanchnic hyperemia and portal hypertension. Plasma glucagon levels are elevated in cirrhotic patients and experimental models of portal hypertension, and hyperglucagonemia is caused, in part, by a decreased hepatic clearance of glucagon, but more importantly by an increased secretion of glucagon by pancreatic α cells. Normalizing circulating glucagon levels by administering glucagon antibodies or infusing somatostatin partially reverses the increase in splanchnic blood flow, and the response is specifically blocked by the concomitant infusion of glucagon in the portal hypertensive rat model. In addition, increasing circulating glucagon levels in normal rats to values similar to those observed in portal hypertension causes a significant increase in splanchnic blood flow. These findings suggest that hyperglucagonemia may account for approximately 30–40% of the splanchnic vasodilatation of chronic portal hypertension.

There are two estimated mechanisms for the vasodilatation effect by glucagons: relaxing the vascular smooth muscle and decreasing its sensitivity to endogenous vasoconstrictors, such as norepinephrine, angiotensin II, and vasopressin [16]. The role of glucagon in the splanchnic hyperemia of portal hypertension provides a rationale for the use of somatostatin and its synthetic analogs to reduce glucagon level, thereby treating portal hypertension [17].

Endocannabinoids

Recent data suggest that endocannabinoids have a significant role in the hyperdynamic circulation of portal hypertension [18]. Endogenous cannabinoid anandamide is increased in the monocyte fraction of blood from cirrhotic humans and rats, and expression of the cannabinoid 1 (CB1) receptors is increased in hepatic human endothelial cells. In addition, CB1 receptor blockade reduces portal blood flow and pressure and increases arterial pressure in cirrhotic rats. Although the mechanism of action is not well understood, it has been suggested that it could be due, at least in part, to an increased NO production, mediated by the activation of endothelial CB1 receptors.

Nitric oxide

Nitric oxide is involved in the regulation of splanchnic and systemic hemodynamics in portal hypertension. The splanchnic vasoconstrictive effect caused by NO inhibitors is significantly greater in portal hypertensive than in control animals, suggesting that an excessive production of NO may be responsible, at least in part, for the vasodilatation observed in portal hypertension [1]. In addition, NO inhibition has been shown to reverse the vascular hyporesponsiveness to vasoconstrictors that is characteristic of portal hypertension and is thought to contribute to systemic and splanchnic vasodilatation. Also, an overproduction of NO has been clearly demonstrated in vitro in perfused mesenteric artery preparations from portal hypertensive rats. The finding in cirrhotic patients of increased serum and urinary concentrations of nitrite and nitrate, which are products of NO oxidation, also supports a role for NO in the genesis of the circulatory disturbances of portal hypertension.

The increased production of NO is due both to an increased expression and an increased activity of eNOS. Factors likely to activate the constitutive NO synthase include shear stress, circulating vasoactive factors (e.g., ET, angiotensin II, vasopressin, and norepinephrine) and overexpression of the angiogenic factor vascular endothelial cell growth factor (VEGF) [19]. Recent study suggests that mild increases of portal pressure upregulates eNOS at the intestinal microcirculation through VEGF upregulation [20].

Prostaglandins

Prostacyclin is an endogenous vasodilator produced by vascular endothelial cells, showing a significant role in portal hemodynamics [21]. It causes vascular smooth muscle relaxation by activating adenylate cyclase and augmenting the intracellular level of cyclic adenosine monophosphate. Two different isoforms of COX are involved in the biosynthesis of prostacyclin. The constitutive isoform (COX-1) may be stimulated by factors similar to those that stimulate the constitutive isoform of NO synthase (eNOS). In addition, the inducible isoform (COX-2), like inducible NO synthase, can be expressed on stimulation with proinflammatory agents. Animal studies have shown a partial reversal of splanchnic vasodilatation after COX blockade. This effect is independent of that of NO. They have further shown that systemic levels of prostacyclin may be increased in patients with cirrhosis. In addition, the inhibition of prostaglandin biosynthesis by indomethacin reduces the hyperdynamic circulation and portal pressure in patients with cirrhosis and portal hypertension. Both isoenzymes COX-1 and COX-2 are involved in increased prostacyclin production by the mesenteric vascular bed of portal vein-ligated rats. The selective inhibition of COX-2, and to a lesser extent of COX-1, improve the endothelial-dependent vasodilatation in response to acetylcholine.

Carbon monoxide

An expression and activity of heme oxygenase is increased in splanchnic tissues in portal hypertensive rats [22]. The simultaneous inhibition of NO and heme oxygenase completely reverse the reduced vasoconstrictor response to potassium chloride in the mesenteric vascular bed. The splanchnic vasodilatation in portal hypertension is likely to be multifactorial in origin, being promoted in part by an excessive release of NO, CO, and other vasoactive mediators. When one of the vasoactive mediators is chronically inhibited, the enhancement of other vasoactive pathways may prevent the correction of splanchnic vasodilatation. Heme oxygenase also plays a detrimental role of stimulating VEGF production, contributing to the development of hyperdynamic splanchnic circulation, as well as a beneficial role of attenuating oxidative stress and inflammation in animal models [22]. Coupling of several vasoactive systems may cause the splanchnic vasodilatation seen in portal hypertensive states.

Portosystemic collateral circulation

The development of portal–collateral circulation is one of the hemodynamic features of portal hypertension. For-

mation of collaterals is a complex process involving the opening, dilatation, and hypertrophy of preexisting vascular channels. Collaterals develop in response to the increased portal pressure. A minimum HVPG threshold of 10 mmHg should be reached for the development of portosystemic collaterals and esophageal varices. In addition to the increased portal pressure, formation of portosystemic collateral vessels in portal hypertension is influenced by a VEGF-dependent angiogenic process and can be markedly attenuated by interfering with the VEGF/VEGF receptor 2 signaling pathway [19]. This finding suggests that manipulation of the VEGF may be of therapeutic value.

The collateral circulation may carry as much as 90% of the blood entering the portal system. In this circumstance, the vascular resistance of these vessels becomes a major component of the overall resistance to portal blood flow and, therefore, may be important in determining portal pressure. In addition, although it was traditionally thought that the hyperdynamic splanchnic circulatory state associated with portal hypertension was the consequence of active splanchnic vasodilatation, recent data suggest that the increased neovascularization in splanchnic organs plays an important role in allowing the increase in splanchnic blood inflow [19].

The elements that modulate collateral resistance are not well known. Studies performed in perfused portosystemic collateral beds suggest that NO may play a role in the control of portal–collateral vascular resistance. This may be the mechanism by which isosorbide-5-mononitrate (IMN) and nitroglycerin (NTG) reduce collateral resistance in patients with cirrhosis. These vessels are also probably hypersensitive to serotonin (5-HT), which markedly increases their vascular tone. In portal hypertensive animals, the administration of selective 5-HT_2 receptor blockers decreases portal pressure.

Hyperkinetic circulation

Splanchnic vasodilatation is typically associated with peripheral vasodilatation and a systemic hyperkinetic syndrome, which is characterized by reduced arterial pressure and peripheral resistance, and increased plasma volume and cardiac output. The pathophysiologic mechanisms involved in peripheral vasodilatation are similar to those previously described for splanchnic vasodilatation [1]. Peripheral vasodilatation plays a major role in the activation of endogenous neurohumoral systems that cause sodium retention and expansion of the plasma volume, followed by an increase in the cardiac index. Expansion of plasma volume is a necessary step to maintain an increased cardiac index, which in turn aggravates portal hypertension. This provides the rationale for using a low sodium diet and diuretics in the treatment of portal hypertension.

Pathophysiology-based therapy

The occurrence of clinical events due to portal hypertension is related to the hemodynamic changes observed during treatment, in cirrhotic patients who receive either placebo or long-term pharmacologic therapy. In other words, changes in the HVPG before and during maintenance therapy (or no treatment) are related to likelihood of the occurence of variceal bleeding or rebleeding [23]. HVPG response to treatment can be considered "good" when the HVPG decreases by at least 20% of the baseline value, indicating a very low risk for rebleeding (<10% at 2 years). The HVPG response is "optimal" when the HVPG decreases to 12 mmHg or below, in which case the risk for variceal bleeding is negligible [24]. An optimal response is also associated with a significant reduction of variceal size and a significantly longer survival. Therefore, decreasing the portal pressure below the critical threshold values for clinically significant portal hypertension make it possible to change the natural history of the portal hypertension with an improvement of prognosis. Thus, the goal of long-term pharmacologic therapy in patients with portal hypertension should be a reduction of the HVPG by at least 20% from baseline values, and preferably to below the threshold of 12 mmHg. The rational treatment of portal hypertension requires that the underlying alteration – the increase in HVPG – be modified. Such modification should be based on an understanding of the mechanisms that lead to increased portal pressure in liver disease.

Natural history and clinical manifestations

Esophageal varices

Approximately 8% of patients with cirrhosis without varices develop varices de novo each year. It is estimated that the majority of cirrhotic individuals will develop varices during their lifetimes. However, only about a third of all patients with esophageal varices will ever experience variceal bleeding. According to the cohort study in patients with hepatitis C, the risk of having esophageal varices increases with decreasing platelet counts, increasing bilirubin, and increasing international normalized ratio (INR) [25], and the development of varices is associated with patient race/ethnicity (Hispanic > Caucasian > African-American), lower baseline levels of albumin, and higher levels of hyaluronic acid [26]. Considering the approximately 20–30% mortality from each episode of variceal hemorrhage, it is important to be able to target those at greatest risk of bleeding. The follow-ing factors predict the risk of bleeding from esophageal varices:

1 *Portal pressure*: varices do not develop and therefore cannot bleed when the HVPG is under 12 mmHg. Varices are invariably associated with an HVPG >12 mmHg, but the risk of bleeding is not predicted by the absolute value of the HVPG above 12 mmHg.

2 *Size and location of varices*: the likelihood of variceal rupture is directly related to variceal diameter based on the effects of the radius in wall tension. Varices at the GE junction and palisade zone lie in the lamina propria and thus have a thinner coat and are most likely to bleed.

3 *Endoscopic features of varices*: although several endoscopic findings of esophageal varices have been shown to predict the risk of hemorrhage, so-called "red signs" are frequently applied.
   • Red wale marks: longitudinal red streaks on varices that resemble red corduroy wales.
   • Cherry red spots: discrete cherry-colored spots that are flat and overlie varices.
   • Hematocystic spots: raised, discrete red spots overlying varices, resembling "blood blisters."

4 *Degree of liver failure*: more advanced liver failure is a risk factor for variceal hemorrhage. The higher the bilirubin and prothrombin time and the lower the albumin levels, the more frequent the variceal bleeding.

5 *Presence of ascites*: tense ascites is an important risk factor for variceal hemorrhage.

These risk factors have been used to estimate the probability of variceal hemorrhage with relative precision. For example, in a patient with Child–Pugh class C cirrhosis, large varices, and red signs, the risk of hemorrhage is over 76% within 1 year, while another patient with Child–Pugh class A cirrhosis and small varices has a less than 10% likelihood of bleeding. The risk of bleeding also decreases over time from the time that varices are identified; most bleeding episodes occur within the first 2 years after identification of varices. Once bleeding occurs, spontaneous cessation of hemorrhage occurs in only 50% of individuals. Those with Child–Pugh class C cirrhosis and actively spurting varices are particularly prone to continue to bleed without active intervention.

Following cessation of active bleeding, there is a high risk of rebleeding for approximately 6 weeks. The risk of such early rebleeding is greatest within the first 48 hours and about 50% of all early rebleedign episodes occur during this period. The risk factors for early rebleeding are large varices, age >60 years, renal failure, and severe initial bleeding as defined by a hemoglobin <8 g/dL at admission. Also, overly aggressive volume replacement may cause rebound portal hypertension and precipitate early rebleeding. Survival during this acute phase depends not only on the control of active hemorrhage but also on the recurrence of bleeding. The long-term course after an index bleed is characterized by recurrent variceal hemorrhage, liver failure, and death. The risk of recurrent bleeding is related to the degree of liver failure, continued alcoholism, variceal size, renal failure, and the presence of a hepatoma. Overall, about 70% of untreated individuals rebleed and die within a year of their index bleed. In addition, patients with acute variceal haemorrhage and a model for end-stage liver disease (MELD) score of ≥18, requiring ≥4 units of packed red blood cells within the first 24 hours, or with active bleeding at endoscopy are at increased risk of dying within 6 weeks [27,28]. A MELD score of ≥18 is also a strong predictor of variceal rebleeding within the first 5 days.

Gastric varices

The likelihood of bleeding from gastric varices depends on their location [1]. Although GOV1 varices constitute over 70% of gastric varices, only 11% of gastroesophageal varices ever bleed. In contrast, about 80% of IGV1 varices experience hemorrhage even though they represent only 8% of all gastric varices. Bleeding from IGV1 varices is often associated with lower portal pressures than in non-bleeding subjects with esophageal varices. Furthermore, bleeding from such varices is more severe and the risk of encephalopathy is higher than in patients with bleeding esophageal varices. Overall, gastric varices bleed less frequently but more severely than esophageal varices. Endoscopic sclerotherapy for esophageal varices causes spontaneous obliteration of 60% of GOV1 varices. In those in whom GOV1 varices persist for more than 6 months after esophageal variceal obliteration, the risk for rebleeding is substantially greater than in those whose varices disappear (28 versus 2%). GOV2 varices are less affected by sclerotherapy for esophageal varices. Recently, the risk of bleeding from IGV1 varices was shown to correlate with the size of the varices (>10 mm), Child–Pugh class, and the presence of red spots on the varices. Based on these findings, the following prognostic index was calculated:

$$\text{Prognostic index} = 0.53 \times (\text{Child} - \text{Pugh class} + 0.78)$$
$$\times (\text{Varices size} + 0.72) \times (\text{Red spot}),$$

where Child–Pugh class A = 0, B = 1, and C = 2; the varices size is scored as small (<5 mm) = 0, medium (5–10 mm) = 1, or large (>10 mm) = 2; and red spot is scored as absent = 0 or present = 1. The risk of bleeding correlated directly with the prognostic index [29].

Portal hypertensive gastropathy and gastric antral vascular ectasia

Portal hypertensive gastropathy (PHG) is a gastric mucosal change associated with portal hypertension. The "mosaic pattern" and the "cherry red spots" are the most frequently observed elementary lesions in PHG. The former consists of multiple erythematous areas outlined by a white reticular network and is generally considered as "mild" PHG. The latter are round, red lesions, slightly raised over the surrounding hyperemic mucosa. These carry a higher bleeding risk and are considered to reflect "severe" PHG [30]. Reliability and the clinical relevance of this classification as mild or severe PHG has been recently validated [31]. The gastric mucosal changes of PHG are associated with increased gastric mucosal and submucosal perfusion and, therefore, are hyperemic – not "congestive" – changes. The term congestive gastropathy is not adequate and should not be used.

During the diagnosis of cirrhosis, the prevalence of PHG is approximately 30% and its incidence is approximately 12% per year [32]. However, patients with severe liver dysfunction and large esophageal varices are at higher risk of developing PHG, whereas large fundal varices may have a protective role, particularly when they are associated with spontaneous gastrorenal shunt [33]. Overall, during the course of cirrhosis, mild PHG may be observed in up to 50–70% of patients and severe PHG in 20–40% [32]. Endoscopic variceal sclerotherapy or banding is a risk factor for PHG.

The clinical course of PHG is characterized by overt or chronic gastric mucosal bleeding. The incidence of overt bleeding from any source in patients with mild PHG is approximately 5% per year, as compared to 15% for severe PHG. The source of bleeding is the gastric mucosa in most of these bleeding episodes. Overt bleeding from PHG is usually manifested by melena and has a far better prognosis than variceal bleeding, with less than 5% mortality per episode. Mortality is higher in patients with severe PHG, but this has been found to be dependent on the severity of liver dysfunction [32].

The incidence of minor mucosal blood loss, without overt bleeding, is approximately 8% per year in patients with mild PHG and up to 25% in those with severe PHG, in whom severe chronic iron deficiency anemia may result, requiring frequent hospital admissions and blood transfusions. It appears that the wide use of β-blockers in patients with cirrhosis is reducing both chronic and overt bleeding from PHG because it has been proved that β-blockers significantly reduce the rebleeding risk in patients who have bleeding from PHG [34].

PHG should be distinguished from gastric antral vascular ectasia (GAVE). This is a distinct entity that may be found in association with conditions other than cirrhosis, such as scleroderma or chronic gastritis. GAVE is characterized by aggregates of red spots, usually with a radial distribution from the pylorus in the antrum of the stomach (in this pattern it is also called *watermelon stomach*). The histology of GAVE is characterized by marked dilatation of capillaries and collecting venules in the gastric mucosa and submucosa, with areas of intimal thickening in fibromuscular hyperplasia, fibrohyalinosis, and thrombi. From a clinical point of view, GAVE behaves as severe PHG, but it may be less responsive to β-blocker treatment.

Imaging, interventional techniques, and surgical procedures

Ultrasound, computed tomography, and magnetic resonance imaging

The evaluation of patients with portal hypertension is based on the visualization of varices at endoscopy, definition of the portal–collateral anatomy by imaging modalities such as ultrasound, computed tomography (CT), magnetic resonance imaging (MRI), or angiography, and the measurement of portal pressure. There are also techniques to assess changes in pressure and blood flow in the collateral circulation. These have allowed a better understanding of the hemodynamic changes associated with portal hypertension, the mechanism of bleeding, and the effects of new forms of pharmacologic therapy.

Imaging techniques are useful in the initial evaluation of the patient with portal hypertension. Frequently, portal hypertension is first diagnosed when a dilated portal vein, portosystemic collaterals, ascites, or splenomegaly is detected. The patency of the portal vein or the presence of portal-venous thrombosis (PVT) should be investigated in every patient with portal hypertension. Portal venography obtained at the venous phase of splenic and mesenteric angiography is being replaced by noninvasive methods, such as Doppler ultrasonography, contrast-enhanced CT, or MRI. Retrograde wedged hepatic venography, performed with the use of carbon dioxide as a contrast medium during hepatic vein catheterization, is a safe technique that allows an adequate visualization of the portal vein.

Ultrasound, CT, and MRI are as accurate as angiography in detecting PVT. Ultrasonography is the preferred initial investigation because of its low cost and high accuracy. The use of Doppler ultrasound allows the determination of the presence, direction, and velocity of portal blood flow. Multiplying the portal flow velocity by the cross-sectional area of the portal vein provides an estimate of the portal blood flow. However, these estimates are subject to many errors and should be used with caution. Doppler ultrasound is also useful in the assessment of the patency of transjugular intrahepatic or surgical portacaval shunts and in the evaluation of the patency of arterial and venous anastomoses after orthotopic liver transplantation. A recent study has shown that liver stiffness measurement may represent a noninvasive tool for the identification of chronic liver disease patients with clinically significant or severe portal hypertension [35].

Endoscopy

Upper gastrointestinal endoscopy is mandatory in patients with cirrhosis or in those in whom portal hypertension is suspected to assess the number, appearance, and size of any esophageal varix and to note the presence of red color signs. Also, endoscopy should include a careful evaluation for the presence of gastric varices, and the presence, extent, and severity of PHG. Capsule endoscopy is now available for the examination of the upper gastrointestinal tract; initial studies suggest a high sensitivity in the detection of esophageal varices. It may be a possible substitute for conventional endoscopy in patients unable or unwilling to undergo endoscopy in the detection of varices [36].

Endoscopic band ligation

When performing band ligation, rubber rings are placed on the varices, which are sucked into a hollow cylinder attached to the tip of an endoscope (Fig. 14.5). An ischemic necrosis of the mucosa and submucosa occurs after the complete interruption of blood flow, and granulation takes place thereafter, with sloughing of the rubber rings and necrotic tissue. The whole process leaves shallow mucosal ulcerations that heal in 14–21 days [37]. Multiple shot devices allowing the placement of four to ten bands at a time have made the technique easier to perform than was possible with the one shot devices previously available. Application of the bands is started at the gastroesophageal junction and progresses upward in a helical arrangement for approximately 5–8 cm until four to eight bands have been applied. Band ligation sessions are repeated at 7–14-day intervals until the varices are obliterated, which usually requires two to four sessions.

Minor complications such as transient dysphagia and chest discomfort are relatively frequent. The shallow ulcers that develop at the site of ligation bleed less frequently than the ulcers that form after sclerotherapy [37]. Mechanical complications that follow use of the overtube (formerly required when only one shot devices were available) – which range from mucosal tears that cause bleeding to complete esophageal perforation – are less frequent now that multiple band ligating devices are coming into widespread use [38].

Endoscopic sclerotherapy

In endoscopic sclerotherapy, a substance that induces thrombosis in the vessel and inflammation of the surrounding tissue is injected into the variceal lumen (intravariceal technique) or adjacent to the varix (paravariceal technique) to obliterate the varix. The injection

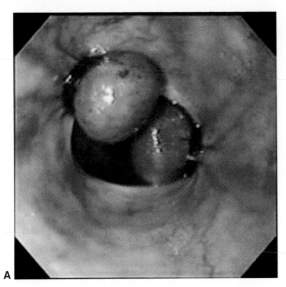
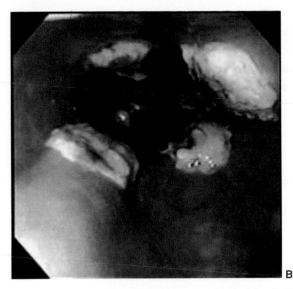

Figure 14.5 Endoscopic appearances of esophageal vaices after band ligation. (A) Esophageal varices just after band ligation with black bands. (B) Endoscopic findings 1 week after band ligation. Shallow mucosal ulcerations with ischemic necrosis of the mucosa are observed but the variceal appearance has almost disappeared.

needle is passed through a flexible endoscope. Injections are initiated at or just above the gastroesophageal junction and proceed upward. About 1–3 mL of sclerosant is injected at each site; the risk for complications increases as the volume of sclerosant injected increases. Variceal obliteration is usually achieved after a couple of sessions. After variceal obliteration, follow-up endoscopic procedures should be carried out at 3-month intervals for the first 6 months and at 12-month intervals thereafter to detect and treat recurrent varices. The most widely used sclerosing agents are 1–3% polidocanol, 5% ethanolamine oleate, 1–2% sodium tetradecyl sulfate, and 5% sodium morrhuate.

Complications of sclerotherapy are relatively frequent and sometimes severe enough to require treatment discontinuation (Table 14.1) [38]. Minor complications such as low-grade fever, retrosternal pain, transient dysphagia, and asymptomatic pleural effusions are common, occur within the first 24–48 hours, and do not require treatment. Asymptomatic transient bacteremia has been reported after treatment in 30–50% of cases. Esophageal ulcers occur in up to 90% of patients within 24–48 hours of injection and heal rapidly in most cases. The ulcers that follow sclerotherapy are frequently asymptomatic but may precipitate bleeding in up to 20% of patients. Esophageal ulcers hamper further injections, delay successful variceal obliteration, and prolong the risk for bleeding that is associated with varices. Sucralfate and omeprazole have been suggested as being potentially useful in healing esophageal ulcers, but convincing proof of such an effect is not available. Esophageal stenosis may

Table 14.1 Complications of sclerotherapy.

Local complications	Regional	Systemic	Complications to physician
Ulcers	Esophageal perforation	Sepsis	Sclerotherapist's eye
Bleeding	Mediastinitis	Aspiration	
Stricture	Pleural effusions	Spontaneous bacterial peritonitis and candidemia	
Esophageal dysmotility	Acute gastric dilatation	Ventilation–perfusion mismatch (hypoxia)	
Pain		Adult respiratory distress syndrome	
Odynophagia		Portal vein thrombosis	
Laceration			

occur in 2–10% of patients and frequently requires dilatation. Full-thickness esophageal wall necrosis resulting in esophageal perforation is rare but almost always fatal. PVT, seizures, and sepsis have also been reported. Altogether, the procedure-related mortality is approximately 1% in elective cases [38]. Morbidity and mortality are higher when the procedure is performed on an emergency basis in actively bleeding patients.

Measurement of portal pressure

The measurement of portal pressure is still the most important assessment of the severity of portal hypertension. Portal pressure should be expressed in terms of the pressure gradient (HVPG) between the porta and the inferior vena cava (IVC), which represents the perfusion pressure within the portal and hepatic circulation. Normal values of HVPG are up to 5 mmHg. Portal pressure expressed as HVPG is not affected by changes in the intra-abdominal pressure caused by tense ascites and total volume paracentesis. An increase in intra-abdominal pressure increases both the portal pressure and the IVC pressure but does not significantly affect the HVPG (except in the case of marked changes in the intra-abdominal pressure that are associated with changes in splanchnic and systemic hemodynamics).

The wide variations in HVPG response of individual patients to pharmacologic treatment suggests that it would be desirable to schedule follow-up measurements of the HVPG during long-term pharmacologic therapy, to determine whether the treatment is likely to offer adequate protection from the risk for bleeding [23]. An important concept that has been strongly substantiated in recent years is that the major factor in determining the development of complications and the clinical significance of portal hypertension is an increase in the HVPG above a critical threshold value. The threshold value of the HVPG for the formation of varices is 10 mmHg and that for the appearance of other complications, such as variceal bleeding, ascites, and PHG, is 12 mmHg [1]. Portal pressure can be assessed by direct or indirect methods.

Direct measurement

Direct measurements of portal pressure are invasive investigations based on surgical, percutaneous transhepatic, or transvenous (transjugular) catheterization of the portal vein. In these techniques, except for the transjugular approach, measurement of the IVC pressure requires the additional and simultaneous puncture of a hepatic vein to determine the HVPG. Because of this inconvenience and the associated surgical or hemorrhagic risk, direct measurements of portal pressure are rarely used. However, the percutaneous transhepatic approach is the preferred technique to measure portal pressure in case of presinusoidal portal hypertension [39]. The safety of percutaneous transhepatic catheterization of the portal vein can be increased by performing the procedure under ultrasonographic guidance. Although the hemorrhagic risk is greater in the percutaneous procedure, the risk can be reduced by using a thin needle. Transjugular

catheterization of the portal vein is the first step during a transjugular intrahepatic portosystemic shunt (TIPS) procedure.

Indirect measurement

The indirect measurement of portal pressure is achieved by hepatic vein catheterization, which provides the FHVP and WHVP utilizing a safe procedure. The former, measured when the tip of the catheter is maintained "free" in the hepatic vein, is close to the IVC pressure (maximal difference of 2 mmHg). The latter is measured by occluding the hepatic vein, either by inflating a balloon at the tip of the catheter (Fig. 14.6) or by advancing the catheter until it becomes "wedged" into a small branch of a hepatic vein. The balloon occlusion technique is preferred because it reflects the pressure of a greater hepatic area than does the "manual occlusion" technique. When blood flow in a hepatic vein is stopped by a "wedged" catheter or a balloon catheter, the static column of blood transmits the pressure to the preceding communicating vascular territory (the hepatic sinusoids). Therefore, the WHVP is a measurement of the hepatic sinusoidal pressure, not of the portal pressure itself. However, it is important to note that the WHVP adequately reflects the portal pressure in diseases causing "sinusoidal" portal hypertension, such as alcoholic liver diseases, nonalcoholic steatohepatitis, and cirrhosis due to hepatitis C virus or hepatitis B virus. The

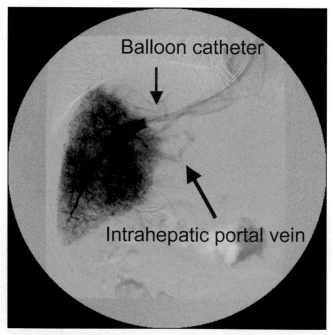

Figure 14.6 Hepatic vein catheterization. The hepatic veins were demonstrated by the injection of iodinated contrast material under balloon occlusion. Thin arrow, balloon catheter; thick arrow, intrahepatic portal vein, which was demonstrated by the inflow of contrast medium in a retrograde manner via hepatic sinuoids.

HVPG is the parameter most commonly used to report portal pressure in the medical literature. In the older literature, the HVPG was frequently referred to as corrected WHVP or corrected sinusoidal pressure.

A limitation of the HVPG is that it does not reflect the portal pressure in cases of portal hypertension with presinusoidal causes, such as PVT and some liver diseases predominantly affecting the portal tracts, including schistosomiasis, the initial stages of primary biliary cirrhosis, and idiopathic portal hypertension. In these cases, a direct measurement of the portal pressure may be preferred. On hepatic vein catheterization, in addition to measuring the HVPG, it is possible to obtain a wedged hepatic retrograde portography using carbon dioxide as a contrast agent. This demonstrates the portal vein in most instances, to the point that a failure to demonstrate the portal vein on carbon dioxide retrograde portography strongly suggests the presence of presinusoidal portal hypertension. An additional advantage of hepatic vein catheterization is that during the procedure (through a jugular vein), it is possible to obtain a liver biopsy specimen, which adds very little time, discomfort, and risk of complications. Furthermore, it is possible to measure the hepatic blood flow with indocyanine green; the intrinsic clearance of indocyanine green is a quantitative test of liver function that assesses overall hepatic metabolic activity.

Diseases causing a hepatic outflow block, classified as "postsinusoidal" or "posthepatic" portal hypertension, show increases in both WHVP and FHVP, with a normal range of HVPG. The main applications of hepatic vein catheterization are evaluation of portal hypertension, assessment of the response to pharmacologic therapy, preoperative evaluation of the risk of resection in patients with small hepatocellular carcinoma, prognostic evaluation during variceal bleeding and acute liver failure, and evaluation of the progression of chronic liver disease, especially severe chronic hepatitis C and alcoholic hepatitis, in which the HVPG may be a good index of the response to therapy [40]. A recent study showed that HVPG predicts clinical decompensation in patients with compensated cirrhosis, and patients with an HVPG of <10 mmHg have a 90% probability of not developing clinical decompensation in a median follow-up of 4 years [41].

The main advantages of the hepatic vein catheterization technique are its simplicity, reproducibility, and safety. Major complications have been limited to local injury to the femoral or jugular vein (e.g., arteriovenous fistulae, leakage, or rupture of venous introducers). Because of its many clinical applications, hepatic vein catheterization is becoming a routine test in many hospitals. Although it is easy and simple to perform, accurate measurements require specific training because the procedure differs from that used in cardiac catheterization laboratories and intensive care units.

Hepatic hemodynamics and its measurement

Under normal circumstances, the total hepatic blood flow represents approximately 25% of the cardiac output, and one third of this flow is contributed by the hepatic artery and the remainder by the portal vein. The methods described in this section are mainly research tools and their utility in routine clinical practice remains unclear.

Regulation of hepatic arterial flow

Hepatic arterial blood flow is regulated automatically, and a reduction in portal flow increases in hepatic arterial flow. Flow in the hepatic artery may increase up to 100% in response to a decrease in portal flow. Although the mechanism of this "hepatic artery buffer response" is not well known, it is considered that it may be mediated in part by adenosine release and washout in the vicinity of the portal tracts [42]. The "buffer response" is important when portal blood flow decreases dramatically, as in PVT and portacaval shunting. It has been suggested that after portacaval anastomosis, the prognosis correlates with the increase in arterial flow that follows the diversion of the portal blood flow. Arterial flow to the liver is not determined by oxygen demand. Under conditions of increased oxygen demand, oxygen extraction rather than arterial flow is augmented in the liver.

Portal-venous flow

The portal system is thought to be a passive vascular bed. The portal blood flow is composed of venous blood draining the stomach, intestines, pancreas, spleen, and omentum. Therefore, the factors that govern portal-venous flow are predominantly those that control the supply of blood to these organs, such as the ingestion of a meal. Contrary to the buffer response of the hepatic artery to decreases in portal blood flow, portal-venous hyperemia does not occur in response to a decrease in hepatic arterial flow, though the mechanism is still unclear.

Azygos blood flow

As most of gastroesophageal collaterals (including esophageal varices) drain into the azygos venous system, an increased azygos blood flow in patients with portal hypertension means the increase of outflow from collateral blood into the azygos vein [43]. However, in 25% of cases, the gastroesophageal collaterals drain into other thoracic veins (i.e., subclavian, innominate, and pulmonary). Therefore, a normal azygos blood flow does not necessarily indicate an absence of esophageal varices. Drainage into other thoracic veins may also be the reason why the azygos blood flow is not significantly correlated with the size of esophageal varices and the risk for bleeding.

The direct measurement of azygos blood flow requires retrograde catheterization of the azygos vein with a continuous thermal dilution catheter. This is a simple procedure performed in the course of routine hemodynamic investigations. Fick's principle is applied to measure blood flow by the thermodilution technique. Azygos blood flow is usually markedly increased in cases with portal hypertension. Values in healthy subjects range between 0.10 and 0.25 L/min, whereas these are increased on average to 0.65 L/min in cirrhotic patients with portal hypertension. The azygos blood flow is also increased in patients with noncirrhotic portal hypertension. Azygos blood flow is markedly reduced after surgical portacaval shunting, esophageal tamponade, and orthotopic liver transplantation.

The main application of measurements of azygos blood flow has been to monitor the effects of pharmacologic therapy in portal hypertension. The ability of the technique to detect changes in portal–collateral blood flow has increased the understanding of the beneficial effects of the vasoactive drugs currently used in the treatment of portal hypertension. It has been demonstrated that some splanchnic vasoconstrictors, such as propranolol, cause greater decreases in azygos blood flow than in portal pressure. On the other hand, equal falls in portal pressure can be associated with different effects on azygos blood flow. Obviously, a decrease in the HVPG and azygos blood flow, as obtained with propranolol, reflects a greater beneficial effect than a decrease only in the HVPG (as usually happens with vasodilator drugs). Azygos blood flow can also be measured noninvasively with phase-contrast magnetic resonance angiography [43].

Variceal blood pressure

The pressure in esophageal varices can be measured using endoscopy by direct puncture of the varices, with endoscopic pressure-sensitive gauges, or with an inflating–deflating balloon attached to the tip of the endoscope. The two latter techniques measure variceal pressure noninvasively, so that the risk for precipitating variceal hemorrhage is eliminated.

Noninvasive techniques are based on the assumption that because of their thin walls and lack of external tissue support, varices behave as elastic structures; therefore, the pressure needed to compress a varix (which can be sensed by a pressure gauge or directly visualized using a clear balloon) equals the pressure inside the varix. The endoscopic pressure gauge is the method used most commonly in prospective studies. A pressure-sensitive capsule, attached to the tip of an endoscope, consists of a small chamber covered by a thin latex membrane that is

continuously perfused with nitrogen. The perfusion pressure is continuously recorded by means of an electromagnetic pressure transducer. It is assumed that when the gauge is applied over a varix, the increase in pressure required to perfuse the gauge equals the pressure inside the varix. The difference between the pressure measured when the gauge is applied over a varix and when the gauge is free in the esophageal lumen equals the transmural variceal pressure, which is the value used to express results [44]. Although the intravenous administration of butyl scopolamine diminishes the artifacts caused by esophageal peristalsis without affecting variceal pressure measurements, endoscopic pressure measurement is not easy in small varices.

Variceal pressure is significantly lower than portal pressure, and this difference is thought to be a consequence of resistance to portal–collateral blood flow in the collaterals feeding the varices and indicates that measurements of variceal pressure cannot be used to estimate portal pressure. It has also been shown that variceal pressure is greater in patients whose varices have bled than in those whose varices have not bled, a finding that supports the concept that increased variceal pressure plays a key role in the mechanism of bleeding and suggests that measurements of variceal pressure may be of prognostic value in assessing the risk for bleeding. Repeated measurements of variceal pressure may detect acute and long-term changes in variceal pressure produced by the administration of pharmacologic agents, though they are difficult to apply for all patients. It has been demonstrated that drugs that decrease portal pressure cause equal or even greater falls in variceal pressure. A reduction of variceal pressure, after pharmacologic therapy, of at least 20% from baseline has been associated with a low actuarial probability of variceal bleeding on follow-up (7% at 3 years versus 46% in patients without this reduction) [45].

Variceal pressure measurement has only been performed in a few cases until now, and clinical significance of the data for the management of the patients is still controversial.

Endoscopic ultrasonography

Endoscopic ultrasonography (EUS) allows the visualization of esophageal and gastric varices, peri-/paraesophageal and peri-/paragastric collateral veins, the portal-venous system, and the azygos vein (Fig. 14.7). EUS, however, does not seem to add further important prognostic information about the risk for complications of portal hypertension in comparison with conventional endoscopy. The clinical use of EUS for gastroesophageal varices is in the diagnosis of gastric fundal varices when the results of endoscopy are doubtful and in the assessment of risk for recurrence after varices have been eradicated by endoscopic sclerotherapy or banding

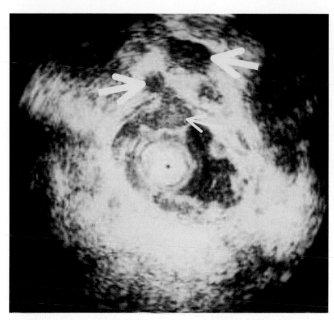

Figure 14.7 Endoscopic ultrasound images of esophageal varices. The images obtained by microprobe show cross-sectional findings of both esophageal varices (thin arrow) and peri- and paraesophageal collateral vessels (thick arrows).

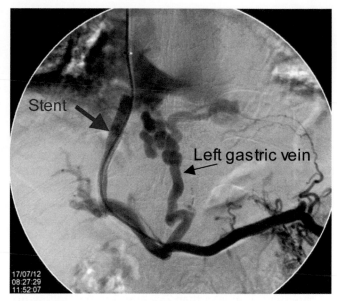

Figure 14.8 Angiogram after a TIPS procedure where the stent was successfully placed. Thin arrow, left gastric vein; thick arrow, stent.

ligation. In the latter situation, the finding of grossly dilated periesophageal veins or patent perforating veins below the gastroesophageal junction carries a high risk for the recurrence of varices. The combined use of EUS for an objective measurement of variceal diameter and endoscopy for the measurement of transmural variceal pressure allows a quantitative estimation of variceal wall tension, which is the relevant parameter in regard to risk for variceal bleeding.

Transjugular intrahepatic portosystemic shunt

A TIPS is an intrahepatic calibrated portosystemic shunt performed between an intrahepatic branch of the portal vein (usually the right) and one hepatic vein (usually the right) using vascular intervention radiologic techniques (Fig. 14.8). The HVPG decreases immediately after TIPS placement because of a marked decrease in absolute portal pressure and a slight increase in the IVC pressure. A reduction in the HVPG after TIPS placement is also associated with a marked reduction in portal–collateral blood flow.

The goal of transjugular intrahepatic portosystemic shunting is to reduce the HVPG below the threshold gradient of 12 mmHg, because complete protection from variceal bleeding is achieved when the HVPG decreases below 12 mmHg [46]. It is very effective where there is repeat variceal bleeding refractory to medical and endoscopic treatments. Despite the marked reduction in

HVPG observed after TIPS placement, the HVPG may increase again during follow-up because of thrombosis, stent retraction and kinking, stent stenosis, and development of right heart failure (Box 14.2). These events increase the HVPG above the 12 mmHg threshold (TIPS dysfunction) and patients reenter the bleeding risk zone again.

TIPS thrombosis usually occurs within the first month and is more likely to occur in moribund individuals. It usually develops in association with the presence of a biliary–TIPS fistula. It has been proposed that systemic anticoagulation can prevent TIPS thrombosis but that it increases the risk of inducing hemorrhage. Anticoagulation is not routinely used in North America. Both stent retraction into the parenchymal tissue tract and stent kinking can be avoided by careful attention to technique.

Box 14.2 Causes of gastrointestinal bleeding after transjugular intrahepatic portosystemic shunting.

- Continued variceal hemorrhage
- Stent dysfunction:
  Thrombosis
  Retraction
  Kinking
  Displacement
  Stenosis
- Hemobilia
- Persistent gastric varices:
  Associated with spontaneous splenorenal collaterals
  Associated with massive splenomegapy

The most common cause of recurrent portal hypertension is the ingrowth of the surrounding liver tissue into the stent lumen, with eventual occlusion. Such pseudointimal hyperplasia results from the proliferation and migration of mesenchymal cells of smooth muscle phenotype into the lumen, where they synthesize and secrete collagen. The majority of long-term survivors who have had a TIPS experience stent stenosis within the first 2 years, necessitating surveillance by either Doppler sonography or angiography. As the former technique is specific but somewhat insensitive, depending on the specific cutoffs used for the diagnosis of stent stenosis, angiography is the gold standard for the detection of stent stenosis and is required for its treatment. A commonly used regimen is angiography at 6 and 12 months after TIPS and annually thereafter for the first 3 years. The propensity for development of stent stenosis decreases after 4 years. Although the actuarial probability of TIPS dysfunction with the use of bare stents is greater than 75% after 1 year of follow-up, the introduction of ePTFE-covered stents has completely changed this scenario, with a reported 1-year actual rate of dysfunction as low as 10% [47].

There are some adverse effects related to TIPS procedures (Table 14.2). The most common event is hepatic encephalopathy, which occurs in about 30% of individuals. It manifests itself as altered mental status and usually appears about 2–3 weeks after TIPS placement. It is often precipitated by dietary indiscretion, constipation, urinary tract infections, or electrolyte imbalances. Most episodes are related to recurrent gastrointestinal bleeding 6 weeks after the procedure. Advanced age (>60 years), Child–Pugh class C, a prior history of encephalopathy, and shunt diameter are risk factors for encephalopathy.

Surgical procedures

Decompressive surgical shunts

Total portosystemic shunts

In the end-to-side portacaval shunt (Eck fistula) procedure, the liver end of the portal vein is ligated and the splanchnic end is anastomosed to the vena cava. As the hepatic sinusoids maintain their hypertension after this surgery, it does not relieve ascites. There are currently almost no indications for this surgery at present.

By contrast, side-to-side shunts decompress the portal hypertension both in the splanchnic bed and in the liver. The common factors n these shunts are that they are 10 mm or more in diameter and include side-to-side portacaval, mesocaval, and central splenorenal shunts. They may either be direct vein-to-vein anastomoses or incorporate prosthetic material. The pathophysiology of these shunts is associated with the portal vein acting as an outflow tract from the obstructed sinusoids, showing reversal of blood flow in the portal vein to the low-pressure shunt. Side-to-side shunts are excellent for controlling variceal bleeding and ascites but deprive the liver of prograde portal flow and increase the risks of progressive liver failure and encephalopathy [48]. The other major disadvantage of these shunts is that when prosthetic material is used as an interposition graft, there is increased risk of thrombosis. The indications for side-to-side shunts are at present relatively limited. A patient with massive continued bleeding who also has ascites can be treated with a side-to-side shunt, although TIPS achieves the same goal without surgery. The strongest advocates of emergency side-to-side portacaval shunts are Orloff et al. who in 1995 reported an extensive series with excellent outcome in a largely alcoholic group of patients [48].

Partial portosystemic shunts

Partial portosystemic shunts can be achieved by reducing the side-to-side portosystemic shunt diameter to 8 mm, which make it possible to maintain portal flow in 80% of patients, and to reduce portal pressure to 12 mmHg. A prospective, randomized controlled trial (RCT) showed a control of bleeding in 90% of patients [49]. The maintenance of some portal flow has been associated with a lower incidence of encephalopathy and liver failure than that with total portosystemic shunting. One randomized

Technique-related	Complications related to portosystemic shunting	Unique complications
Neck hematoma	Hepatic encephalopathy	TIPS-associated hemolysis
Cardiac arrhythmias	Increased susceptibility to bacteremia[a]	Infection of the stents
Perihepatic hematoma	Liver failure	
Rupture of liver capsule		
Extrahepatic puncture of portal vein		

[a]A hypothetical possibility, as yet unproven, that TIPS increases susceptibility to sepsis.

Table 14.2 Adverse effects of transjugular intrahepatic portosystemic shunting (TIPS).

trial compared the 8 mm portacaval surgical shunt to TIPS in a study population of 50% of patients with Child–Pugh class C cirrhosis and 63% of the patients with alcoholic liver disease. There was significantly better control of bleeding and lower need for transplantation in the surgical shunt group compared to the TIPS group, but survival was not significantly different [49].

Selective shunts

In selective variceal decompression, a different pathophysiologic concept is applied for the control of variceal bleeding. Varices are selectively decompressed, usually by a distal splenorenal shunt (DSRS) through the short gastric veins, spleen, and splenic vein to the left renal vein. Portal hypertension is maintained in the splanchnic and portal-venous system to maintain prograde portal flow to the cirrhotic liver. This surgery should be part of the repertoire of liver transplantation surgeons for patients who have refractory bleeding but still have good liver function.

Long-term patency of a DSRS is excellent with vein-to-vein anastomosis, and bleeding is controlled in more than 90% of patients [50]. Rebleeding is most frequent in the first 4–6 weeks while the short gastric and renal veins accommodate the increased flow from the enlarged spleen and varices. Maintenance of portal perfusion is achieved in 90% of patients in the short term. Long-term maintenance of portal perfusion has proved excellent in nonalcoholic patients, but 50% of alcoholic patients lose portal perfusion unless splenopancreatic disconnection is performed. This has resulted in the maintenance of portal flow in 84% of patients with alcoholic cirrhosis.

Studies in which the use of DSRS was compared with total shunts have shown almost equivalent control of bleeding. Recent multicenter trial comparing TIPS with distal splenirenal shunt showed similar rates of rebleeding, encephalopathy, and mortality in patients with Child–Pugh class A or B cirrhosis who had failed pharmacologic/endoscopic treatment, although reintervention was significantly greater with TIPS [51].

Devascularization procedures

Devascularization procedures include splenectomy, gastric and esophageal devascularization, and, in some situations, esophageal transection. The advantage of these procedures is that they maintain portal hypertension and portal flow to the cirrhotic liver and do not accelerate liver failure or encephalopathy. The disadvantage is that they have a higher rate of rebleeding, which probably depends on the extent of the surgical procedure. In patients who have extensive portal-venous thrombosis and in whom no vessels can be shunted, devascularization procedures are the only surgical option. When these patients do not have bleeding controlled by pharmacologic and endoscopic therapy, extensive devascularization may significantly reduce the risk of rebleeding. This is the major indication for devascularization procedures.

Liver transplantation

Liver transplantation has dramatically altered the outcome for patients with advanced liver disease, portal hypertension, and variceal bleeding. It is the one therapy that has significantly improved survival of patients with bleeding varices and Child–Pugh class C cirrhosis. The indication for liver transplantation, however, is end-stage liver disease rather than variceal bleeding.

Liver transplantation restores both hepatic function and relieves portal hypertension, making it the most effective shunt in the management of variceal bleeding. However, supply and demand dictates that transplantation cannot be the therapy for all cirrhotic patients with variceal bleeding. Nowadays, the sickest patients from the perspective of the severity of the liver disease receive priority, and variceal bleeding per se does not increase priority.

The outcome of liver transplantation has dramatically improved in the last decade. Currently, patients can anticipate an initial 6-month mortality of approximately 10%, with a continuing long-term risk of 2–5% per year for death or major morbidity. The major risk factors facing transplantation patients are recurrent disease (especially viral hepatitis), chronic rejection, and immunosuppression-related infection.

Liver transplantation is the most viable long-term treatment option for patients with variceal bleeding and end-stage disease. Timing is always a major issue, and with the increasing lengthening of waiting lists it becomes more problematic. Determining the correct "bridge" to transplantation is key, and the least therapy that can be used as a bridge, the better it is for the patient. However, when patients have bleeding refractory to endoscopic therapy, it may be appropriate to decompress the portal hypertension with TIPS. Surgical decompression is also an appropriate bridge for a patient who has a disease that may not necessitate transplantation for 5–10 years.

Treatment of portal hypertension

Primary prophylaxis of variceal hemorrhage

A key objective in the management of the cirrhotic patients is the primary prevention of variceal hemorrhage. The importance of primary prevention is underscored by the continuing high mortality from active hemorrhage as well as the progressive decline in survival following the index bleed (Table 14.3) [52–55].

Table 14.3 Primary prevention of variceal bleeding with pharmacologic and/or endoscopic treatment.

Treatment	N	Follow-up (months)	Bleeding (%)	Mortality (%)	Complications (%)	Reference
PL/EBL	44/45	14/13	43[a]/15[a]	11/11	36/18[b]	Sarin et al. [75]
			(Bleeding-related mortality, 9.1/6.7, NS)			
PL/EBL	31/31	11.8/18.1	12.9/0	12.9/0	6.5/17.9[c]	Jutabha et al. [78]
			(Bleeding-related mortality, 6.5/0, NS)			
PL/EBL	77/75	34.4	28.6/25.3	42.9/45.3	69/47	Schepke et al. [52]
			(Bleeding-related mortality, 10.4/12, NS)			
PL/EBL	31/31	12.3/16.8	9.7/6.5	9.7/9.7	16.1/6.5	Norberto et al. [57]
			(Bleeding-related mortality, 6.5/3.2, NS)			
NL/EBL	50/50	22.6/21.8	18/10	22/24	8/18	Lo et al. [53]
			(Bleeding-related mortality, 6/2, NS)			
NL+ISMN/	78/80	14.4/15.3	34.6/27.5	19.2/20	32/61[d]	García-Pagán et al. [127]
NL+ISMN+EBL			(Bleeding-related mortality, 10.3/6.25, NS)			
PL/ISMN/EBL	66/62/44	20.6/20.2/17.5	14/23/7[e]	25/27.3/22.6	45/42/2	Lui et al. [54]
			(Bleeding-related mortality, 6.1/3.2/2.3, NS)			
Cavediol/EBL	77/75	26.2/25.5	10/23	35/37	37.7/6.7[f]	Tripathi et al. [62]
			(Bleeding-related mortality, 3/2, NS)			

[a]Actuarial probability of first bleed at 18 months; P = 0.04.
[b]18%, transient retrosternal pain, which was the complication most frequently observed.
[c]17.9%, transient dysphagia.
[d]P <0.01.
[e]Intention-to-treat analysis.
[f]Per protocol analysis
EBL, endoscopic band ligation; ISMN, isosorbide mononitrate; NL, nadolol; NS, not significant; PL, propranolol.

Pharmacologic treatment

Nonselective β-blockers

An important determinant of portal pressure is the portal-venous inflow, which is dependent on mesenteric anteriolar resistance. α-Adrenergic agents constrict mesenteric arterioles, while β-adrenergic agents dilate these vessels. Conversely, β-adrenergic antagonists block the dilatory effects mediated via the β-receptors and allow unopposed α-adrenergic effects, resulting in mesenteric anteriolar constriction. Propranolol and nadolol are the two most studied β-adrenergic antagonists.

Pharmacodynamics

The HVPG decreases by 9–31% after either an oral or intravenous administration of propranolol. This decrease is primarily due to a decrease in hepatic wedge pressures, with a much lesser contribution from increased systemic venous pressures. In addition, decreases in heart rate and cardiac output contribute, to a lesser degree, to the portal hypotensive effects of these agents at higher doses.

Up to 50% of patients have failed to show a greater than 10% decrease in HVPG upon propranolol administration. The reason may be that a concomitant increase in collateral and/or hepatic sinusoidal resistance may negate the hypotensive effects of decreased portal inflow and/or a compensatory increase in hepatic arterial flow may maintain sinusoidal perfusion and maintain the increased wedge pressures. The site of portal obstruction, cause of cirrhosis, plasma propranolol levels, severity of liver failure, presence of ascites, basal hemodynamic values, and heart rate response to propranolol do not correlate with the portal hypotensive effects of propranolol.

In the long-term clinical course, the portal hypotensive effects are maintained in most patients. Tachyphylaxis does occur in some patients and is clinically important because only those with a sustained decrease in portal pressure may benefit from β-blockade. Four recent studies have shown that an acute hemodynamic response to β-blockers (intravenous propranolol, measured 20 minutes later) can be used to predict the long-term risk of first bleeding. An HVPG reduction of >10% from baseline is the best target to define response in primary prophylaxis [56].

Effects on portal hemodynamics

Propranolol has a highly lipophilic property and is almost completely absorbed after oral administration. It undergoes first-pass elimination to a variable degree, causing plasma levels to vary by up to 20-fold. With increasing doses, the relative hepatic extraction decreases, allowing plasma levels to rise. A sustained-release form of propranolol has also been developed that allows once-daily dosing. The clinical effects often do not correlate well with the plasma levels because of the formation of active metabolites, especially the (–) enantiomer, which are taken up by sympathetic nerve endings and then released slowly.

In contrast, nadolol is water soluble and only incompletely absorbed orally. Also, its interindividual pharmacokinetic variability is much less than that of propranolol. Although it does not cross the blood–brain barrier well due to its hydrophilic nature, clinical trials have not shown a significant decrease in the incidence of side effects in central nerve system compared to those of propranolol. Nadolol is excreted via the kidneys and its dose must be modified in response to renal insufficiency.

Adverse effects of β-blockade are numerous and there are multiple drug interactions. The most clinically important side effects involve bronchoconstriction, the development of heart failure, and impotence in cirrhosis. Despite the increase in activity and decrease in renal blood flow, renal dysfunction occurs only occasionally due to propranolol administration. The administration of β-blockers has not been shown to impair the hemodynamic response to acute blood loss.

The efficacy of nonselective β-blockers in the prevention of variceal rebleeding has been proved by many RCTs, and these drugs are now widely accepted as the first-line pharmacologic therapy in this setting [57,58]. Several meta-analyses of these studies consistently found a marked benefit from β-blockers. The rebleeding rate is reduced from 63% in controls to 42% in treated patients, with an absolute risk reduction (ARR) of –21% (95% CI, –30% to –13%) [59]. This means that the number of patients needed to treat (NNT) to prevent one rebleeding episode is 5. Mortality was significantly reduced, from 27% to 20% (ARR = –7%; 95% CI, –12% to –2%; NNT = 14) [59,60]. β-Blockers were compared with endoscopic sclerotherapy in ten RCTs including 862 patients. No significant differences were found between the two treatments, either for rebleeding (ARR = 7%; 95% CI, –2% to 17%) or for mortality (ARR = 2%; 95% CI, –5% to 8%). Side effects were significantly less frequent and less severe with β-blockers (ARR = –22%; 95% CI, –38% to –6%). The number of patients needed to be treated with β-blockers to prevent a harmful event, compared with sclerotherapy, is

four [59]. Meanwhile, an ineffective result of timolol has been reported in preventing varices in unselected patients with cirrhosis and portal hypertension, being associated with an increased number of adverse events. A recent study has shown that β2-AR gene polymorphisms influence the response to β-blockade, though HVPG reduction cannot be predicted from polymorphism analysis. Patients with the Gly16-Glu/Gln27 haplotypes may benefit from the association of hepatic vasodilators to propranolol therapy [61].

More recently, carvediol, a noncardioselective vasodilating β-blocker, has attracted attention because one study revealed that it is more effective in reducing portal pressure than propranolol [62]. Furthermore, the rate of first bleed was significantly lower in the carvediol group than in the band ligation group. It may become an option for primary prophylaxis in patients with high-risk varices.

Nitrosovasodilators

Pharmacodynamics

Nitric oxide is a potent vasodilator and an important mediator of the vasodilated state seen in cirrhosis. The "nitrosovasodilator" group of drugs acts via the NO pathway, producing vasodilatation in their target vascular beds. At usual pharmacologic doses, these agents are primarily venodilators and decrease cardiac output by decreasing venous return in those with normal myocardial length–tension relationships. Systemic venodilatation decreases postsinusoidal resistance and decreases portal pressure. At high doses of the drugs, arterial dilatation and systemic hypotension occur, causing reflex splanchnic vasoconstriction and further decreases in portal pressures. Also, nitrate-mediated baroreceptor reflexes in the pulmonary capillary bed trigger splanchnic vasoconstriction and contribute to the drugs' portal hypotensive action.

Nitrovasodilators such as NTG, isosorbide dinitrate (ISDN), and IMN, through their capacity to release NO, may compensate for the NO deficit within a cirrhotic liver and thereby reduce the intrahepatic vascular resistance. IMN, the most extensively studied nitrate, has been shown to reduce HVPG in cirrhotic patients without reducing the hepatic blood flow; its effect reflects a reduction in the hepatic vascular resistance. Although it is possible to determine the effect of pharmacologic agents on the individual factors that determine portal pressure (i.e., resistance and flow) in the experimental setting, it is not easy to do so in clinical studies. A further complication is the fact that the vasodilator action of these drugs is not limited to the hepatic and portal circulation but extends to the systemic circulation, where they cause arterial hypotension. This in turn may elicit reflex splanchnic vasoconstriction, with an ensuing reduction in portal blood flow. Vasodilators usually decrease the cardiac preload and hence the cardiac output, which may further decrease the splanchnic blood flow. Moreover, many vasodilators reduce the vascular resistance in the portal–collateral circulation. This represents another mechanism by which a vasodilator may reduce the HVPG, but at the expense of increased blood flow in the portosystemic collaterals and esophageal varices. In some instances, the beneficial effect of decreasing intrahepatic resistance by means of a vasodilator, in terms of a reduction in portal pressure, is offset by the splanchnic vasodilator effect of the drug, which increases the portal–collateral blood flow and prevents any decrease in portal pressure [63].

Another important limitation of vasodilators is that they may be dangerous in patients with advanced cirrhosis. These drugs, by enhancing preexisting peripheral vasodilatation, further decrease the arterial blood pressure and activate endogenous vasoactive systems, which may worsen sodium retention and ascites. However, it is reported that long-term treatment with IMN is safe when combined with β-blockade in patients with compensated cirrhosis [64]. Combined treatment, unlike treatment with IMN alone, does not cause adverse effects on renal function, sodium handling, or endogenous vasoactive systems. This is because the mild systemic vasoconstriction and suppression of renin release resulting from β-blockade oppose the adverse systemic and renal effects of IMN.

Another method to increase the intrahepatic production of NO is to administer agents that act preferentially in the liver [65–67]. Interest in this method has increased because of recent studies showing that in experimental models of cirrhosis the expression of NO synthase in liver cells can be enhanced by the portal injection of adenovirus transfected with the gene encoding neural NOS or eNOS, and that such treatment may significantly reduce portal pressure for some weeks [66]. Similarly, transfer of the constitutively active Akt results in enhanced eNOS activity and reduces portal pressure in carbon tetrachloride-induced cirrhotic rats [12]. Treatment with nitroflurbiprofen, an NO-releasing cyclooxygenase inhibitor, also improves portal hypertension without major adverse effects in thiacetamide-induced cirrhotic rats by attenuating intrahepatic vascular resistance, endothelial dysfunction, and hepatic hyperreactivity to vasoconstrictors [68].

Effects on portal hemodynamics

Acute administration of either isosorbide mononitrate (ISMN) or ISDN may cause up to a 40% decrease in HVPG, a 30% decrease in portal flow, and a 15% decrease in azygous flow. Plasma norepinephrine and renin activity increase, indicating increased sympathetic activity and an enhanced tendency to retain sodium. In the long term,

the degree of portal decompression is variable and the systemic hemodynamic effects become less pronounced. The effects of ISDN are less predictable than ISMN presumably due to their variable hepatic extraction in cirrhotic patients. Therefore, ISMN is the long-acting nitrate of choice for the treatment of portal hypertension.

A prospective randomized study including 118 patients to receive either ISMN (20 mg thrice daily) or propranolol (to the maximum tolerated dose) has shown no significant differences in either bleeding rates (18 versus 14%) or mortality (18 versus 15%) after a median follow-up of 29 months [69]. However, after 7 years, an increased mortality, especially in those over 51 years of age (72 versus 48%), were noted in those receiving ISMN. It is unclear whether these results reflect a beneficial effect of propranolol or an adverse effect of nitrates. Interpretation of the data is further confounded by the fact that about 50% of patients enrolled in each arm withdrew from the study. Another study shows that there was no benefit from ISMN in the prevention of first bleeding [70]. The combination of ISMN and β-blockers has also been compared with β-blockers alone in some RCTs, but the results do not support the use of combination therapy for the prevention of first variceal bleeding. At this time, the data do not support a role for nitrates as monotherapy for the primary prophylaxis of variceal hemorrhage.

Endoscopic treatment

Endoscopic sclerotherapy

Injection of sclerosant substances into varices results in the obliteration of varices and hemostasis of variceal bleeding. However, it requires a skilled endoscopist and is associated with serious complications in 10–20% of patients [59]. The clinical trials of sclerotherapy for primary prevention of variceal hemorrhage are difficult to compare because of the variability in patient populations and the use of sclerotherapy during episodes of active bleeding [71,72]. A large multicenter study found a significantly higher mortality in those treated with sclerotherapy despite a decrease in variceal hemorrhage in these patients [73]. β-Blockers alone are superior to sclerotherapy and equivalent to β-blocker plus sclerotherapy for this indication. Thus, sclerotherapy should not be used either alone or with β-blockers for primary prevention of variceal hemorrhage.

Endoscopic band ligation

Band ligation was compared with β-blockers in a numbers of RCTs [52,73–78]. Overall, they showed that band ligation is superior to no treatment, and that two meta-analyses of 12 trials comparing them showed that band ligation is associated with a small but significantly lower incidence of first variceal bleeding but without differences in mortality [79,80]. From the point of cost effectiveness, band ligation is more effective than β-blockers in the cost per quality-adjusted life-year [81]. The current American Association for the Study of Liver Diseases/American College of Gastroenterology (AASLD/ACG) practice guideline recommends either nonselective β-blockers or band ligation as an effective treatment to prevent first variceal bleeds, and that the appropriate therapy may be decided according to patient preferences and local resources.

Transjugular intrahepatic portosystemic shunt

Currently, no data exist to support a role for TIPS for primary prevention of variceal hemorrhage. In addition, TIPS does not improve the outcome following liver transplantation and in some cases may render the operation technically more difficult [82]. TIPS is thus not recommended for the primary prevention of variceal hemorrhage.

Surgical treatment

Four prospective randomized trials comparing surgical portacaval shunts with medical therapy were carried out over 25 years ago. They demonstrated that while surgery could effectively prevent variceal hemorrhage, the benefit was offset by sereve encephalopathy, which ensued in 30–60% of patients [72]. Moreover, as medically treated patients survived longer, the modality has been eliminated as an option for the primary prevention of variceal hemorrhage. Surgical procedures are not a recommended treatment for the primary prevention of variceal hemorrhage.

Clinical recommendations for primary prevention of variceal hemorrhage

All cirrhotic patients should undergo an endoscopic examination as part of their evaluation. Patients with

Child–Pugh class B or C cirrhosis with esophageal varices of any grade and those with Child–Pugh class A cirrhosis and large varices, especially with red signs, should be targeted for treatment. In those in whom varices are not present, endoscopy should be repeated at 2–3-year intervals.

Nonselective β-blockers or band ligation is the recommended treatment for the primary prevention of variceal hemorrhage in cirrhotic patients. No evaluable data currently exist for the clinical utility of β-blockers for the various types of gastric varices, although it appears to make intuitive sense to treat those at high risk for bleeding. Recent studies suggest that combined treatment with β-blockers and band ligation has little benefit for primary prophylaxis of variceal bleeding over monotherapy with band ligation (Table 14.4) [83,84].

It has been shown that patients who experience a 25% or greater drop in HVPG or an HVPG of <12 mmHg and maintain these changes over time, are most likely to remain free of bleeding. It has therefore been recommended that the HVPG be measured prior to initiation of therapy and after 1–3 months of treatment and that the dosage of the drug be changed appropriately to achieve the desired end-points. However, the cost effectiveness of this approach remains to be demonstrated. Moreover, HVPG measurement is not possible at many medical centers. Where such facilities are not available, the dose should be titrated to achieve a decrease in resting heart rate to 55–60 beats per minute.

Management of active variceal hemorrhage

Although active variceal hemorrhage accounted for about one third of all deaths realted to cirrhosis before the 1990s, recent studies have shown an improved survival of acute variceal hemorrhage due to current treatment strategies [85–87]. Recently, the Baveno V consensus meeting

Table 14.4 Primary prevention of variceal bleeding and the role of combined therapy with endoscopic and pharmacologic treatment.

Treatment	N	Follow-up (months)	Bleeding (%)	Mortality (%)	Complications (%)	Reference
EBL+PL/EBL	72/72	13.1/11.2	7/11[a]	8/15[a]	22[b]	Sarin et al. [83]
		(Bleeding-related mortality, NS)				
EBL+NL/NL	70/70	26/26.4	14/13	22.9/21.4	48/28[c]	Lo et al. [84]
		(Bleeding-related mortality, 1.4/2.9, NS)				

[a]Actuarial probability of first bleed/death at 20 months.
[b]Side effects due to propranolol were observed in 22% patients, and 8% patients quit treatment. The EBL group did not have any serious complications.
[c]Number of incidents, $P = 0.06$.
EBL, endoscopic band ligation; NL, nadolol; NS, not significant; PL, propranolol.

modified the Baveno IV consensus statement to define *"Failure to control bleeding"* as follows [88,89]:

1 The timeframe for the acute bleeding episode should be 120 hours (5 days).

2 Failure is defined as death or need to change therapy defined by one of the following criteria:

- Fresh hematemesis or nasogastric aspiration of $\geq$100 mL of fresh blood $\geq$2 hours after the start of a specific drug treatment or therapeutic endoscopy.
- Development of hypovolemic shock.
- A 3 g drop in hemoglobin (9% drop of hematocrit) within any 24-hour period if no transfusion is administered. This timeframe needs to be further validated.
- The potential value of an index of blood transfusion requires prospective validation.

Any bleeding occurring after initial hemostasis and more than 48 hours from time zero but less than 6 weeks after is considered to represent early rebleeding. There are three primary goals of management during the active bleeding episode. These include hemodynamic resuscitation, prevention and treatment of complications, and treatment of bleeding. All three need to be pursued simultaneously and often require coordinated critical care.

Hemodynamic resuscitation

The goal of resuscitation is to preserve tissue perfusion. Volume restitution should be initiated to restore and maintain hemodynamic stability [89]. Packed red blood cell transfusion should be done conservatively at a target hemoglobin level of between 7 and 8 g/dL, although transfusion policy in individual patients should also consider other factors such as comorbidities, age, hemodynamic status, and ongoing bleeding.

Although transfusion of platelets and fresh frozen plasma can be considered in patients with significant coagulopathy and/or thrombocytopenia, there are no available data to make a recommendation regarding management of them. Care should be taken to avoid overtransfusion with volume overload because of the risk of rebound portal hypertension and rebleeding. Also, in those receiving large volumes of blood products, the ionized $[Ca^{2+}]$ and platelet counts must be monitored and corrected as necessary.

Prevention and management of complications (Box 14.3)

Complications related to bleeding can lead to mortality from active hemorrhage. A severe complication with a frequently fatal outcome is aspiration pneumonia. All patients with altered mental status and active bleeding or those with massive hematemesis should be intubated for airway protection to avoid this complication. Also, renal function and fluid administration must be monitored to maintain a urine output of at least 50 mL/h. If renal failure develops, it must be evaluated quickly

---

Box 14.3 Clinical management for active variceal hemorrhage.

- Hemodynamic resuscitation:
    Packed cell transfusion
    Correction of coagulopathy
    Correction of thrombocytopenia
    Monitor for side effects of blood product administration
- Airway protection
- Prophylactic antibiotics
- Renal support:
    Maintain urine output >50 mL/h
    Avoid aminoglycosides
    Avoids nonsteroidal anti-inflammatory drugs (NSAIDs) for fever
- Neurologic support:
    Monitor mental status
- Avoid sedation
- Metabolic:
    Thiamine when indicated
    Monitor and treat delirium tremens
    Moonitor and treat acidosis or alkalosis
    Monitor phosphate levels, treat hypophosphatemia
    Monitor blood sugar

---

and managed appropriately. Lactulose should be given orally or by enema once bleeding is controlled to remove blood from the gastrointestinal tract and also to prevent encephalopathy.

Up to 20% of patients with bleeding have a bacterial infection at the time of hospital admission, and the risk of a nosocomial bacterial infection is nearly 50% in these patients compared to 5–7% of hospital-acquired infections in the general population [90]. Furthermore, bacterial infections significantly increase the risk of failure to control bleeding and increase the hospital mortality rate for patients with cirrhosis and gastrointestinal bleeding. The most frequent bacterial infections seen in patients with cirrhosis are urinary tract infection (12–29%, mostly *Escherichia coli* or *Klebsiella*), spontaneous bacterial peritonitis (7–23%, Gram-negative bacilli and aerobic Gram-positive cocci), respiratory tract infection (6–10%), and primary bacteremia (4–11%).

A recent meta-analysis including five RCTs (534 patients) has shown that antibiotic prophylaxis decreases the incidence of bacterial infections and increases the survival rate in patients admitted because of variceal bleeding [91]. An updated meta-analysis of the eight RCTs (789 patients) now available confirms a significant beneficial effect of antibiotic prophylaxis in decreasing both mortality (relative risk (RR) = 0.73; 95% CI, 0.55–0.95) and the incidence of bacterial infections (RR = 0.40; 95% CI, 0.32–0.51), bacteremia, pneumonia, spontaneous bacterial peritonitis, and urinary tract infection [92]. Decreased incidence of early rebleeding after receiving prophylactic antibiotics may be one of the reasons for improved survival [93].

The recommended antibiotics schedule is norfloxacin administered orally at a dose of 400 mg b.i.d. for 7 days [94]. Another study performed in patients with advanced cirrhosis and hemorrhage showed that intravenous (IV) ceftriaxone (1 g/day) was more effective than oral norfloxacin in preventing bacterial infections [95]. Following these studies, a recent consensus conference stated that antibiotic prophylaxis should be an integral part of the therapy for acute gastrointestinal bleeding in cirrhosis and should be instituted from admission [89].

Treatment of active hemorrhage

Pharmacological treatment

Vasopressin

Vasopressin directly constricts mesenteric arterioles and decreases portal-venous inflow, resulting in reduction of portal pressures. A recommended dose of vasopressin is a continuous IV infusion of 0.2–0.4 units/min, which can be increased to a maximal dose of 0.8 units/min. It should always be accompanied by IV nitroglycerin at a starting dose of 40 μg/min, which can be increased to a maximum of 400 μg/min, adjusted to maintain a systolic blood pressure of >90 mmHg. Vasopressin can achieve initial hemostasis in 60–80% of individuals but has only marginal effects on early rebleeding episodes. Also, vasopressin does not improve survival from active variceal hemorrhage. In fact, it may contribute to mortality owing to its coronary vasoconstrictive properties and the resultant myocardial, cerebral, and bowel ischemia. A fibrinolytic state induced by vasopressin, theoretically, can worsen the bleeding diathesis. Recent consensus shows that the portal hypotensive effect of vasopressin in non-bleeding cirrhosis is attenuated when variceal hemorrhage occurs.

Terlipressin

Terlipressin is a long-acting vasopressin derivative with much less severe side effects [63]. The effects of terlipressin are an increase in arterial pressure and splanchnic vasoconstriction. Compared with placebo or nonactive treatment, terlipressin significantly improves the rate of control of bleeding and survival, with one death prevented in every six patients treated [96]. Terlipressin is used in bolus IV injections at doses of 2 mg every 4–6 hours for up to 48 hours. After achieving an initial control of bleeding (a 24-hour bleeding-free period), the dose can be halved and the treatment maintained for 5 days to prevent early rebleeding. The more frequent side effects are relatively mild: abdominal cramps, diarrhea, bradycardia, and hypertension. Severe side effects (e.g., arrhythmias, angina, cerebrovascular accident, and limb ischemia) requiring discontinuation of the drug are in the order of 2–4% [96,97]. Terlipressin has been compared with vasopressin in some trials, and two studies com-

bined vasopressin with transdermal or sublingual NTG [59]. Overall, these studies did not show significant differences between the two drugs in the control of bleeding, rebleeding, or mortality, but side effects were significantly less frequent and less severe with terlipressin. The overall efficacy of terlipressin in controlling acute variceal bleeding is 75–80% across trials [96], and the results of terlipressin were similar to those of sclerotherapy in overall control rate, rebleeding, complications, and mortality [97]. There are two clinical studies regarding the control of variceal bleeding with terlipressin. One study showed that very early rebleeding (0% in terlipressin plus band ligation, 15% in terlipressin alone) and therapeutic failure (2% in terlipression plus band ligation, 24% in terlipressin alone) were less in terlipressin plus band ligation treatment than in terlipressin alone. The other study showed that hospital stay was significantly shorter in the terlipressin plus band ligation group than in the octreotide plus band ligation group (108 versus 126 days) [98,99].

Somatostatin and its analogs

Somatostatin is a 14-amino acid peptide named for its growth hormone-inhibiting properties. As somatostatin inhibits the release of vasodilator hormones (e.g., glucagon), it indirectly causes splanchnic vasoconstriction and a reduction of portal inflow. It disappears within minutes of a bolus infusion due to its very short half-life. Portal-venous inflow, portal pressures, azygous flow, and intravariceal pressures decrease within seconds after a bolus injection. Of these effects, the changes in portal pressure, as measured by wedged hepatic pressure, are most variable and the decrease in collateral flow (azygous flow) are those most consistently observed.

Somatostatin is usually administerd as a continuous IV infusion of 250 μg/h following an initial bolus of 250 μg. A recent study suggested that in high-risk patients (with active bleeding at the time of diagnostic endoscopy) it is wise to increase the infusion dose to 500 μg/h and to provide repeat 250 μg boluses during the initial hours of therapy [100]. Treatment may be maintained for up to 5 days. Side effects of somatostatin are usually mild, most frequently bradycardia, hyperglycemia, diarrhea, and abdominal cramps.

Several RCTs showed that somatostatin significantly improves the rate of control of bleeding compared with placebo or nonactive treatment. Although the results of these studies were heterogeneous, their meta-analysis showed that this heterogeneity was mainly due to one study with an unusually high rate of spontaneous bleeding cessation (83%, the highest ever reported) in the placebo-treated group [59]. However, despite the beneficial effect on the control of bleeding, somatostatin does not affect mortality. Compared with vasopressin, somatostatin is equivalent for mortality and control of bleeding but is associated with less frequent and less severe side effects than vasopressin.

Three studies compared somatostatin with terlipressin, including a total of 302 patients [59]. The two larger studies were double-blind placebo-controlled RCTs. Overall, no differences were found for failure to control bleeding, rebleeding, and mortality. Total side effects were 21% with somatostatin versus 29% with terlipressin (not significant), and major side effects requiring withdrawal of treatment or specific therapy were 4% in both treatment groups. Contrary to what has been shown for vasopressin, the addition of NTG to somatostatin does not improve therapeutic efficacy and induces more adverse effects.

Octreotide

Octreotide is a synthetic somatostatin analog with a longer half-life. Like somatostatin, bolus injections of octreotide cause a transient increase in mean arterial pressure and systemic vascular resistance, suggesting a systemic effect [101]. However, infusion of octreotide does not cause a sustained decrease in portal pressure or collateral blood flow at the doses generally used for variceal hemorrhage, or at even higher doses, and a rapid desensitization of the hemodynamic effects of octreotide after intravenous administration may be the reason [101]. Therefore, the hemodynamic effects of octreotide, the optimal dose, and the administration method have not been established.

Octreotide is usually used as a continuous IV infusion, at empiric dosages of 25–50 μg/h, in some instances after an initial IV bolus of 50 μg. Treatment duration was from 1 to 5 days. The efficacy of octreotide as a single therapy for variceal bleeding is controversial. Among four RCTs comparing octreotide with placebo, no benefit from octreotide was found in the only one using octreotide or placebo as the initial treatment, whereas in the three using sclerotherapy or ligation before or at the same time as octreotide administration, a significant benefit was found in two studies and was nearly significant in the third [59]. These results suggest that octreotide may improve the results of endoscopic therapy but has no or little effect if used alone. In addition, there is no benefit of octreotide on rebleeding or survival. When compared with other vasoactive drugs, octreotide was better than vasopressin for the control of bleeding in two RCTs and similar to terlipressin in another two, again suggesting a clinical value for the use of octreotide. However, the studies were not sized to test for equivalence. Side effects were less frequent and severe with octreotide than with either vasopressin or terlipressin, but the difference was significant only for vasopressin [59].

As summarized in a recent consensus conference, somatosatin appears to be more effective than placebo or vasopressin and has fewer side effects than vasopressin. It has therefore replaced vasopressin as the pharmacologic treatment of choice in the actively bleeding patient. Although the role of octreotide is less well established, it is the current drug of choice in the United States because of its easy availability as compared with somatostatin.

Endoscopic treatment

Endoscopic treatment is currently the definitive treatment of choice for active variceal hemorrhage. It can be performed at the same time as diagnostic endoscopy at the bedside by a trained gastroenterologist. Two forms of endoscopic treatment are available: endoscopic sclerotherapy and endoscopic variceal band ligation.

Endoscopic sclerotherapy

Endoscopic sclerotherapy had been widely used as a first-choice treatment because it is effective in about 80–90% of patients with variceal bleeding. Moreover, it allows the start of specific treatment for the prevention of long-term rebleeding at the time of diagnostic endoscopy. However, it requires a skilled endoscopist and is associated with serious complications in 10–20% of patients, with an overall mortality of 2% [59]. Furthermore, when compared with vasoactive drugs, sclerotherapy is similar to terlipressin, somatostatin, or octreotide as regards control of bleeding/early rebleeding or mortality (Tables 14.5 and 14.6) [97,102–105]. Nowadays, sclerotherapy is usually performed when band ligation is not possible.

Endoscopic band ligation

Endoscopic band ligation has been used worldwide because of its simple technique and effectiveness (Tables 14.7 and 14.8) [106–110]. A number of RCTs indicate significant benefit of band ligation in the initial control of bleeding compared to sclerotherapy. Sclerotherapy requires a skilled endoscopist and is associated with serious complications in 10–20% of patients, with an overall mortality of 2% [59]. Furtheremore, endoscopic sclerotherapy, not band ligation, causes a sustained increase in HVPG, which is followed by a higher rebleeding rate [111]. Although the choice of one or another procedure may depend on the expertise with each of these techniques, band ligation is a preferred treatment for acute variceal bleeding.

Combined endoscopic and pharmacologic therapy

The combination of endoscopic therapy (either sclerotherapy or banding) with pharmacologic therapy significantly improves initial control of bleeding and reduces the 5-day failure rate in terms of control of bleeding or rebleeding when compared with endoscopic therapy alone [112]. The use of band ligation instead of sclerotherapy added to somatostatin for the treatment of

Table 14.5 Comparison of the success rate for the initial control for variceal bleeding between pharmacologic treatment alone and endoscopic treatment alone.

Overall control rate				
Drug[a]	Sclerotherapy[a]	Liver disease	Study duration (days)	Reference
77% (somatostatin)	83%	Cirrhosis[b]	5	Shields et al. [102]
80% (somatostatin)	82.9%	Cirrhosis	2	Planas et al. [103]
85% (octreotide)	82%	Cirrhosis[b]	2	Jenkins et al. [104]
67% (terlipressin)	68%	Cirrhosis	2	Escorsell et al. [97]

[a]Not significant.
[b]The subject included heterogenous liver diseases other than cirrhosis.

Table 14.6 Comparison of the therapeutic results for variceal bleeding between pharmacologic treatment alone and endoscopic treatment alone.

Treatment	Rebleeding (%)	Complications (%)	Mortality (%)	Reference
Somatostatin/ endoscopic	23/17[a] (5 days)	13/29[a] (total)	30.7/19.5[a] (for 4 weeks)	Shields et al. [102]
Somatostain/ endoscopic	25/17.2[a] (2–5 days)	0/14.2[b] (major complications)	28.5/22.8[a] (for 6 weeks)	Planas et al. [103]
Octreotide/ endoscopic	15/18[a] (2 days)	26/19[a] (total)	31.5/16.9[a] (for 60 days)	Jenkins et al. [104]
Terlipressin/ endoscopic	43/44[a] (5 days)	20/30[a] (total)	24.8/16.7[a] (for 6 weeks)	Escorsell et al. [97]

[a]Not significant.
[b]P <0.05.

Table 14.7 Comparison of the success rate for the initial control of bleeding between sclerotherapy and band ligation.

Success rate			
Sclerotherapy[a]	Ligation[a]	Duration	Reference
77% (10/13)	86% (12/14)	8-hour control	Stiegmann GV [37]
92% (45/49)	91% (49/54)	12-hour control	Gimson et al. [106]
87.5% (14/16)	100% (20/20)	24-hour control	Hou et al. [107]
89% (8/9)	89% (8/9)	–	Laine et al. [132]
76% (26/34)	97% (36/37)	> 72-hour control	Lo et al. [109]

[a]Not significant.

acute variceal bleeding significantly improved efficacy and safety, and the 6-week survival probability without therapeutic failure was better with band ligation [113]. A recent study has shown that HVPG independently predicts short-term prognosis in patients with acute variceal bleeding treated with pharmacologic and endoscopic therapy [114].

Salvage therapy for patients with endoscopic treatment failure

Emergent endoscopic treatment fails to control bleeding in about 10–20% of patients. These patients are at high risk for exsanguination as well as all of the complications related to active bleeding. Usually by the time a diagnosis of failed endoscopic treatment is established, patients have already received a trial of pharmacologic treatment as well. In such patients, second attempts at endoscopic hemostasis may be made. However, if bleeding is not quickly and effectively stopped, more definitive therapy must be instituted immediately.

Table 14.8 Comparison of the therapeutic results for bleeding varices between sclerotherapy and band ligation.

Treatment	Rebleeding (%)	Complications (%)	Eradication (number)[a]	Mortality (%)	Reference
S/L	48/36[b]	22/2§[c]	5±2/4±2[b]	45/28* (a mean of 10 months)	Stiegmann et al. [38]
S/L	53/30*	57.1/66.7[bd]	4.9±3.5/3.4±2.2[†]	63/48[b]	Gimson et al. [106]
S/L	41.8/19.4[†]	22.4/4.5[†]	4.6±1.6/3.5±1.6§	16.4/21[b]	Hou et al. [107]
S/L	44/26[b]	56/24[†]	6.2/4.1§	15/11[b]	Laine et al. [132]
S/L	33/17[b]	29/5[†]	–/–	35/19[b] (1 month)	Lo et al. [109]

[a]Number of treatments needed to eradicate all varices.
[b]Not significant.
[c]Probabilities: *P <0.05, † P <0.01, ‡ P = 0.011; § P <0.001 (log-rank test).
[d]Esophageal ulcer.
S/L, sclerotherapy/ligation.

Balloon tamponade

Balloon tamponade is effective in achieving short-term hemostasis. However, it has a high risk of rebleeding following deflation of the balloon. Also, the airway must be protected in all patients receiving such treatment owing to their failure to clear oral secretions and the high risk of aspiration. The only role of such treatment is to temporarily stabilize the patient so that more definitive treatment can be instituted.

Variceal embolization

Variceal embolization using an angiographic technique is one of the options to control variceal bleeding. Percutaneous transhepatic embolization of gastroesophageal varices was proposed in the early 1970s, and was performed by catheterizing the gastric collaterals that supply blood to varices through the transhepatic route. However, it was practically abandoned because of its invasiveness and lesser effectiveness compared with sclerotherapy. Nowadays, variceal embolization is used as a complement to TIPS in patients with severe acute bleeding that is not controlled with endoscopic treatment, especially in patients with gastric varices.

Transjugular intrahepatic portosystemic shunt

A TIPS can stop bleeding in most patients with acute variceal hemorrhage [115]. Some centers use coil embolization of the vessels feeding the varices. The selection of patients with uncontrolled bleeding, many of them with advanced liver failure, probably accounts for the high 6-week mortality, ranging from 27% to 55%. One RCT showed that the best candidates for emergency TIPS for variceal bleeding are those with an HVPG of ≥20 mmHg in whom TIPS placement reduced the 6-week mortality from 38% to 17%, while the corresponding figure was 5% in patients with an HVPG of <20 mmHg

not so treated [116]. This result suggests that high-risk patients benefit from TIPS placement if applied soon. Whether other clinical risk indicators may be used in clinical practice instead of HVPG measurement should be assessed in future trials. Until such studies are available, given the very high proportion of patients in whom variceal bleeding is controlled by medical and/or endoscopic therapy, transjugular intrahepatic portosystemic shunting is confined to the rare patients (approximately 10% of cases) with uncontrollable variceal bleeding.

Surgery

Surgical intervention is rarely indicated for acute variceal bleeding. More than 90% of patients can be treated with pharmacologic and/or endoscopic therapy. In the small minority of cases in which this therapy fails, balloon tamponade with emergency decompression using TIPS in the next 24 hours is the best approach. An emergency portacaval shunting has been performed in limited facilities [48].

An algorithm for the management of active variceal hemorrhage (Fig. 14.9)

The initial management of active hemorrhage should include hemodynamic resuscitation, prevention of complications, and early endoscopy to establish the diagnosis and initiate specific treatment. Terlipressin, somatostatin, or octreotide (50 μg bolus followed by 50 μg/h by IV infusion) may be started in the emergency room in those at high risk for variceal hemorrhage. At diagnostic endoscopy, bleeding esophageal varices are usually treated by band ligation or sclerotherapy. If active bleeding persists or recurs within 48 hours, the application of TIPS or surgery should be considered. The choice of the definitive procedure depends on the patient's clinical condition and the expertise available. When bleeding occurs

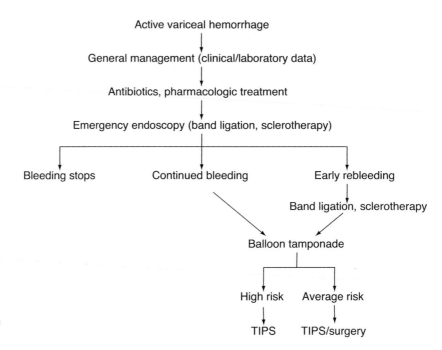

Figure 14.9 Algorithm for the clinical management of acute variceal bleeding.

more than 48 hours after initial endoscopic treatment, a second attempt at controlling hemorrhage by endoscopy is reasonable before proceeding to salvage therapy. The need for balloon tamponade prior to TIPS placement is important, because temporarily stabilizing the patients by balloon tamponade allows the procedure to be performed under more controlled circumstances without detracting the attention of the angiography personnel from the procedure.

Prevention of recurrent variceal hemorrhage

The natural history of an untreated patient who has survived an episode of variceal hemorrhage is characterized by recurrent hemorrhage with consequent liver failure, hepatic encephalopathy, and eventually death [117]. As the median rebleeding rate in untreated individuals is around 60% within 1–2 years of the index hemorrhage, with a mortality of 33%, it is imperative to prevent rebleeding.

Recently, the Baveno IV consensus statements were modified at Baveno V, and *"Failure of secondary prophylaxis"* was defined as follows [88,89]:

1 Failure to prevent rebleeding is defined as a single episode of clinically significant rebleeding from portal hypertensive sources after day 5.
2 Clinically significant rebleeding is recurrent melena or hematemesis resulting in any of the following:
 • Hospital admission.
 • Blood transfusion.
 • A 3 g drop in hemoglobin.
 • Death within 6 weeks.

Pharmacologic treatment

Nonselective β-blockers and combined pharmacologic treatment

The efficacy of nonselective β-blockers in the prevention of variceal rebleeding has been proved by many RCTs, and these drugs are now widely accepted as the first-line pharmacologic therapy in this setting (Table 14.9) [117]. Several meta-analyses of these studies consistently found a marked benefit from β-blockers. The rebleeding rate is reduced from 63% in controls to 42% in treated patients, with an ARR of −21% (95% CI, −30% to −13%) [67]. Nonselective β-blockers plus organic nitrates – the combined administration of propranolol or nadolol plus ISMN – was introduced after demonstrating that ISMN enhanced the portal pressure-reducing effect of nonselective β-blockers [118]. The combination of ISMN with propranolol or nadolol has been found to be superior to endoscopic sclerotherapy in one study [119]. However, there was no significance in the reduction of bleeding risk with combination pharmacologic therapy as compared with band ligation [120–122]. The heterogenous results in these studies may be explained by a different proportion of patients with large varices and/or different doses of medication.

Nowadays, there is a majority agreement that, as incorporated in the AASLD/ACG guidelines, the best approach in the prevention of recurrent esophageal variceal bleeding is the combination of nonselective β-blockers plus band ligation [123]. Two trials have shown the advantage of combined therapy over band ligation alone: 23% and 14% of rebleeding rate, respectively, for band ligation plus nadolol, compared to 47% and 38% for band ligation alone [124,125]. However,

Table 14.9 Secondary prophylaxis of variceal hemorrhage in cirrhotic patients with the use of pharmacologic and/or endoscopic treatment.

Treatment	N	Follow-up (months)	Rebleeding (%)	Mortality (%)	Complication (%)	Reference
NL+ISMN/EST	43/43	18/18	25.6/53.5[a]	9.3/20.9	16.3/37.2[b]	Villanueva et al. [119]
NL+ISMN/EBL	72/72	2022	33/49[b]	31.9/41.7	26/31	Villanueva et al. [120]
NL+ISMN/EBL	61/60	24/25	57/20	13.1/25	19/17	Lo et all. [122]
NL+EBL+SC/EBL	60/62	22/21	23.3/54.8	16.7/32.3	11.7/8.1	Lo et al. [124]
NL+EBL/EBL	43/37	17.5/15	14/38[c]	11.6/10.8	32.6/2.7	De la Peña et al. [125]
PL+ISMN+EBL/EBL	88/89	15/15	17/19	2/4	21/20	Kumar et al. [126]
NL+ISMN/NL +ISMN+EBL	78/80	14.4/15.3	34.6/27.5	19.2/20	32/61[c]	García-Pagán et al. [127]

[a]$P = 0.001$.

[b]$P < 0.05$.

[c]$P < 0.01$.

EBL, endoscopic band ligation; EST, endoscopic sclerotherapy; ISMN, isosorbide mononitrate; NL, nadolol; PL, propranolol; SC, sucralfate.

further discussion is necessary to establish the preferred treatment, because two recent papers showed negative results for this approach [126,127]. Compared with transjugular intrahepatic portosystemic shunting, the combination of IMN and propranolol is less effective for the prevention of rebleeding but is associated with significantly less encephalopathy, similar mortality, and much lower cost [128].

Monitoring the pharmacologic treatment response

Many studies, including RCTs and prospective consecutive series, have shown that the pharmacologic (or spontaneous) reduction of HVPG to less than 12 mmHg or by as much as or more than 20% of the baseline value virtually abolishes the risk of rebleeding [24,119–121,129,130]. When the results of these studies are combined in a meta-analysis, the odds ratio for rebleeding in patients achieving one of these hemodynamic targets compared with those not reaching any of them is 0.20 (95% CI, 0.08–0.47). Therefore, patients reaching one (or both) of these targets are considered hemodynamic responders to pharmacologic therapy. The evaluation of acute HVPG response to IV propranolol before initiating secondary prophylaxis for variceal bleeding is a useful tool in predicting the efficacy of nonselective β-blockers [131]. However, because it is still unclear whether patients with an insufficient hemodynamic response to pharmacologic therapy would benefit from alternative treatments, hemodynamic monitoring of pharmacologic therapy is presently recommended only in the setting of clinical research.

Endoscopic treatment

Endoscopic sclerotherapy

Endoscopic sclerotherapy had been extensively evaluated for the long-term prevention of recurrent variceal hemorrhage. However, the risk of variceal rebleeding is significantly reduced by band ligation when compared with sclerotherapy [110]. Furthermore, while there were no differences in mortality, complications were significantly less frequent and less severe with band ligation, and the number of endoscopic sessions needed to achieve eradication was significantly lower that with sclerotherapy. Also, sclerotherapy has no advantage over drug therapy and causes more frequent and severe side effects. Therefore, sclerotherapy may not be appropriate as a treatment of choice for secondary prophylaxis of variceal hemorrhage.

Endoscopic band ligation

Endoscopic band ligation has been developed as an alternate endoscopic treatment over the last 20 years [117]. Many studies have evaluated the relative efficacy of band ligation with sclerotherapy, showing that the former is associated with earlier variceal obliteration, less complications, and less rebleeding as well as improved survival when compared with the latter [110,132]. Because of this, band ligation has replaced sclerotherapy as the first-line treatment for the prevention of recurrent hemorrhage. However, as band ligation is associated with a greater risk of variceal recurrence and is technically difficult when varices are very small, sclerotherapy may be appropriate for such patients.

The meta-analysis comparing band ligation alone with combination endoscopic band ligation and sclerotherapy did not show any benefit either for rebleeding or for mortality. Furthermore, as complication rate was higher in combination endoscopic therapy, it is not a recommended therapy [110,133].

As described in the pharmacologic treatment section, there is majority agreement that the best approach in the prevention of recurrent esophageal variceal bleeding is the combination of nonselective β-blockers plus band ligation, as incorporated in AASLD/ACG guidelines.

Transjugular intrahepatic portosystemic shunt

A recent meta-analysis of 11 trials that compared TIPS with endoscopic treatment showed that hepatic encephalopathy occurred more frequently after TIPS placement with no difference of mortality between the two treatments, in spite of less frequent rebleeding with TIPS [134,135]. Although pharmacologic treatment, propranolol plus nitrates, was less effective than a TIPS in the prevention of rebleeding, it was associated with less hepatic encephalopathy, identical survival, and more frequent improvement of Child–Pugh class with lower costs than TIPS [128]. Therefore, despite the beneficial effects on bleeding, a TIPS procedure should not be used as first-line treatment but as a salvage therapy for those with recurrent bleeding. A major drawback of TIPS is the high rate of occlusion or dysfunction at 2 years, in the order of 60–80%. However, one recent multicenter randomized trial and two studies including consecutive patients with Budd–Chiari syndrome or cirrhosis reported much lower obstruction and reintervention rates with PTFE-covered stents and lower rates of recurrent bleeding or ascites, without an increased incidence of encephalopathy [47,58]. It is generally redommended that a coated stent be used for the TIPS procedure.

Surgery and orthotopic liver transplantation

There are several studies regarding the value of surgical treatment for the prevention of recurrent variceal hemorrhage. In general, surgical treatment may be considered to either achieve portal decompression or mechanically disconnect the varices. A complete shunt formation decompresses both the portal vein and hepatic sinusoids and converts the portal vein into an outflow tract. In contrast, the latter approach preserves some sinusoidal perfusion while decompressing the portal veins. Each particular operation has its proponents, but their data are not easily generalizable due to the failure of others to obtain similar results. Virtually all of the operations described are effective in arresting hemorrhage and preventing rebleeding. However, these procedures often do not provide any survival advantage over endoscopic treatment [72]. Recent multicenter trial comparing a TIPS with a distal splenorenal shunt showed similar rates of rebleeding, encephalopathy, and mortality in patients with Child–Pugh class A or B cirrhosis who had failed pharmacologic/endoscopic treatment, though reintervention was significantly greater with TIPS [51]. The choice between them may depend on available expertise and ability to monitor the shunt and reintervene when needed.

Orthotopic liver transplantation is the only treatment that not only effectively corrects the portal hypertension but also removes the cirrhotic liver and corrects liver failure. It is the only treatment that substantially improves the long-term outcome after variceal hemorrhage and must be considered in all patients who have survived an episode of variceal bleeding unless a contraindication exists.

Algorithm for the prevention of recurrent variceal hemorrhage

The goal of long-term treatment in patients with portal hypertension is the prevention of rebleeding, hepatic decompensation, and death. Orthotopic liver transplantation is the only treatment that reliably achieves all three objectives. Thus, all survivors of a variceal hemorrhage should be evaluated for liver transplantation. While those with Child–Pugh class B or C cirrhosis should be listed right away unless a contraindication exists, listing for those with Child–Pugh class A cirrhosis should be individualized. While patients are waiting for transplant, endoscopic band ligation is the initial treatment of choice in most cases. Some patients with Child–Pugh class A cirrhosis who are compliant with therapy may be treated with propranolol or nadolol. Selected patients with Child–Pugh class A cirrhosis may benefit from surgical portal decompression.

If bleeding recurs, the acute bleeding is managed by pharmacologic and endoscopic treatment, as described in the previous section. Those who continue to bleed or have bled despite adequate endoscopic band ligation combined with a nonselective β-blocker should be considered for salvage treatment with either TIPS or surgery. The choice of procedure should be individualized based on the patient's condition and operator expertise. Bleeding occurring after surgery or transjugular intrahepatic portosystemic shunting should lead to a workup for shunt thrombosis or stenosis. Angiography is the procedure of choice in such a patient because a patent Doppler sonogram does not exclude the possibility of TIPS stenosis.

Treatment of gastric varices, portal hypertensive gastropathy, and gastric antral vascular ectasia

Gastric varices

There are no specific measures or significant evidence for the prevention of first bleeding from gastric varices. It is conceivable that the results of pharmacologic therapy are similar to those achieved in the prevention of first bleeding from esophageal varices. Therefore, nonselective β-blockers should be given to patients with large gastric varices to prevent the first bleeding episode.

The usual initial treatment for bleeding gastric varices is a vasoactive drug, while balloon tamponade has been used with limited success. The tissue adhesive isobutyl-2-cyanoacrylate (bucrylate), mixed with lipiodol, has been found to be efficacious and superior to ethanolamine in nonrandomized studies, achieving hemostasis in 90% of patients. In a recent randomized trial, endoscopic obturation using cyanoacrylate proved more effective and safer than band ligation in the management of bleeding gastric varices [136]. However, cerebral embolism has been reported with the tissue adhesives, and interest is therefore focused on thrombin, which provides good hemostasis. Another randomized trial comparing *N*-butyl-2-cyanoacrylate with sclerotherapy in 37 patients had a subset of 17 patients with actively bleeding gastric varices [137]. Nonsignificant trends in favor of tissue adhesive were also seen in this small group, and variceal obliteration was significantly more common in the overall group (100% versus 44%). Because the rebleeding rate after endoscopic treatment is high, it is recommended that an early decision should be made for TIPS or surgery in patients rebleeding from gastric varices. A recent study has shown that cyanoacrylate therapy achieved better long-term morbidity than a TIPS procedure with similar results in the control and prevention of gastric variceal bleeding [138].

As no specific measures had been studied for the prevention of recurrent bleeding, nonselective β-blockers have been applied as first-line therapy in clinical practice. However, recently, a randomized controlled trial reported that cynanoacrylate injection was more effective than β-blockers for the prevention of gastric variceal rebleeding (GOV2 or IGV1) and improving survival [139]. In any event, TIPS or shunt surgery may be recommended as an additional treatment in case of failure after pharmacologic or endoscopic treatment. Over the past two decades, an interventional technique – the so-called "balloon-occluded retrograde transvenous obliteration (B-RTO)" – has been used in the treatment of gastric varices, and has shown more than 90% embolization effect with less recurrence [140]. However, as there is no randomized control study, clinical significance of this treatment remains unestablished.

Portal hypertensive gastropathy and gastric antral vascular ectasia

Acute bleeding from PHG should first be treated with the same vasoactive drugs as those for variceal bleeding, although there is no randomized control study specifically designed for PHG [141]. Oral propranolol may be used in hemodynamically stable patients, starting at 40 mg/day in two divided doses; the dosage may be then titrated up to the maximum tolerated amount. Recurrent bleeding from PHG should be prevented using nonselective β-blockers, at the same dosage as that used for treating esophageal varices [34]. Adequate iron supplementation may be useful to prevent or correct chronic iron deficiency anemia in patients with severe PHG. A TIPS may be considered as an alternative therapy for the rare patient who has repeated severe bleeding from PHG despite pharmacologic therapy. Portal decompres-

sive surgery is reserved for those who are not candidates for orthotopic liver transplantation. There is no indication supporting the primary prophylaxis of bleeding from PHG.

Patients bleeding from GAVE may benefit from endoscopic ablation by argon plasma coagulation, neodymium:yttrium-aluminum-garnet (Nd:YAG) laser, or heater probe. There is no proof that TIPS and β-blockers are effective in the prevention of recurrent bleeding from GAVE. For select patients with severe recurrent bleeding or uncontrollable acute bleeding from GAVE, an antrectomy with Billroth I anastomosis may be considered [141].

Management protocol of acute variceal bleeding

Day 0 (just after the arrival of the patient), general management
- Clinical and laboratory data to assess the severity of hemorrhage and liver disease:
  - Hemoglobin/hematocrit, white cell count, platelet count
  - Plasma urea and electrolytes, creatinine, prothrombin and partial thromboplastin times, baseline liver function tests
  - Routine cultures of blood, urine, and ascitic fluid
  - Chest X-ray and electrocardiogram
  - Blood gases (in decompensated patients and in those with chest problems?)

Day 0–1, initial therapy
- Correct hypovolemic shock to maintain hemodynamic stability:
  - Blood volume restitution: hemoglobin at approximately 8 g/dL
- Prevent complications associated with gastrointestinal bleeding:
  - Antibiotic prophylaxis against Gram-negative bacilli and Gram-positive cocci
- Achieve hemostasis at the bleeding site:
  - Give pharmacologic treatment immediately when variceal bleeding is suspected, before endoscopic confirmation of diagnosis:
    - terlipressin (in countries where it is available) is the first choice of treatment
    - somatostatin is an alternative to terlipressin
    - other drugs: octreotide and vasopressin (should be combined with nitroglycerin)
- Use emergent endoscopic therapy (preferably by banding ligation)
- Transjugular intrahepatic portosystemic shunting (TIPS) should be used in cases of failure of medical and endoscopic therapy
- Shunt surgery using interposition mesocaval graft shunts or traditional portacaval shunts may be an alternative to TIPS in Child–Pugh class A patients (preferably in nontransplantation candidates)

Days 2–5, general management
- Clinical and laboratory data to assess the severity of hemorrhage and liver disease and to confirm stability of general status
- Pharmacologic therapy should be maintained even after endoscopic therapy for 2–5 days

Further reading

D'Amico G, Garcia-Pagan JC, Luca A, et al. HVPG reduction and prevention of variceal bleeding in cirrhosis. A systematic review. *Gastroenterology* 2006;131:1611–24.
Investigators described that HVPG reduction to ≤12 mmHg or by ≥20% significantly reduces the risk of bleeding, and a reduction of ≥20% significantly reduces mortality based on the systematic review of available studies from the Cochrane Library and MEDLINE.

De Franchis R, on behalf of the Baveno V Faculty. Revising consensus in portal hypertension: report of the Baveno V consensus workshop on methodology of diagnosis and therapy in portal hypertension. *J Hepatol* 2010;53:762–8.
A summary of the international meeting held on May 21–22, 2010, to discuss current problems and provide accepted consensus. The main points discussed are the definition of key events concerning the bleeding episode and the therapeutic options in patients with portal hypertension.

Garcia-Tsao G, Bosch J. Management of varices and variceal hemorrhage in cirrhosis. *N Engl J Med* 2010;362:823–32.
This article shows a current concept of portal hypertension and provides an up-to-date treatment strategy for the management of variceal hemorrhage.

Garcia-Tsao G, Bosch J, Groszmann RJ. Portal hypertension and variceal bleeding – unresolved issues. Summary of an American Association for the Study of Liver Diseases and European Association for the Study of the Liver single-topic conference. *Hepatology* 2008;47:1764–72.
This article summarizes the results of conference on "Portal hypertension and variceal bleeding – unresolved issues" that took place in Atlanta, GA, June 4–6, 2007, and that was sponsored jointly by the American Association for the Study of Liver Diseases (AASLD) and the European Association for the Study of the Liver and constitutes the 6th international consensus conference in the area of varices and variceal hemorrhage.

Garcia-Tsao G, Sanyal AJ, Grace ND, et al. Prevention and management of gastroesophageal varices and variceal hemorrhage in cirrhosis. *Hepatology* 2007;46:922–38.
This updated practice guideline is based on the review of the randomized controlled trials and meta-analyses published in the last decade and has incorporated recommendations made by consensus. These recommendations provide a data-supported approach to the management of patients with varices and variceal hemorrhage, and are fully endorsed by the American Association for the Study of Liver Diseases and the American College of Gastroenterology.

Groszmann RJ, Garcia-Tsao G, Bosch J, et al. Beta-blockers to prevent gastroesophageal varices in patients with cirrhosis. *N Engl J Med* 2005;353:2254–61.
This clinical trial has shown that nonselective β-blockers are ineffective in preventing varices in unselected patients with cirrhosis and portal hypertension and are associated with an increased number of adverse events.

Sanyal AJ, Bosch J, Blei A, Arroyo V. Portal hypertension and its complications. *Gastroenterology* 2008;134:1715–28.
This review provides a comprehensive overview of the current understanding of the pathophysiology and treatment of portal hypertension.

References

1. Krawitt EL. *Medical Management of Liver Disease.* New York: Marcel Dekker, 1999.
2. Poo JL, Jimenez W, Maria MR, et al. Chronic blockade of endothelin receptors in cirrhotic rats: hepatic and hemodynamic effects. *Gastroenterology* 1999;116:161–7.
3. Wiest R, Groszmann RJ. Nitric oxide and portal hypertension: its role in the regulation of intrahepatic and splanchnic vascular resistance. *Semin Liver Dis* 1999;19:411–26.
4. Gupta TK, Toruner M, Chung MK, et al. Endothelial dysfunction and decreased production of nitric oxide in the intrahepatic microcirculation of cirrhotic rats. *Hepatology* 1998;28:926–31.
5. Bellis L, Berzigotti A, Abraldes JG, et al. Low doses of isosorbide mononitrate attenuate the postprandial increase in portal pressure in patients with cirrhosis. *Hepatology* 2003;37:378–84.
6. Graupera M, Garcia-Pagan JC, Pares M, et al. Cyclooxygenase-1 inhibition corrects endothelial dysfunction in cirrhotic rat livers. *J Hepatol* 2003;39:515–21.
7. Matei V, Rodríguez-Vilarrupla A, Deulofeu R, et al. Three-day tetrahydrobiopterin therapy increases in vivo hepatic NOS activity and reduces portal pressure in CCl4 cirrhotic rats. *J Hepatol* 2008;49:192–7.
8. Zafra C, Abraldes JG, Turnes J, et al. Simvastatin enhances hepatic nitric oxide production and decreases the hepatic vascular tone in patients with cirrhosis. *Gastroenterology* 2004;126:749–55.
9. Trebicka J, Hennenberg M, Laleman W, et al. Atorvastatin lowers portal pressure in cirrhotic rats by inhibition of RhoA/Rho-kinase and activation of endotherail nitric oxide synthase. *Hepatology* 2007;46:242–53.
10. Abraldes JG, Albillos A, Bañares R, et al. Simvastatin lowers portal pressure in patients with cirrhosis and portal hypertension: a randomized controlled trial. *Gastroenterology* 2009;136:1651–8.
11. García-Cardeña G, Martasek P, Masters BS, et al. Dissecting the interaction between nitric sxide synthase (NOS) and caveolin. Functional significance of the NOS caveolin binding domain in vivo. *J Biol Chem* 1997;272:25437–40.
12. Morales-Ruiz M, Cejudo-Martn P, Fernandez-Varo G, et al. Transduction of the liver with activated Akt normalizes portal pressure in cirrhotic rats. *Gastroenterology* 2003;125:522–31.
13. Zafra C, Abraldes JG, Turnes J, et al. Simvastatin enhances hepatic nitric oxide production and decreases the hepatic vascular tone in patients with cirrhosis. *Gastroenterology* 2004;126:749–55.
14. Langer DA, Das A, Semela D, et al. Nitric oxide promotes caspase-independent hepatic stellate cell apoptosis through the generation of reactive oxygen species. *Hepatology* 2008;47:1983–93.
15. Tarquini R, Masini E, La Villa G, et al. Increased plasma carbon monoxide in patients with viral cirrhosis and hyperdynamic circulation. *Am J Gastroenterol* 2009;104:891–7.
16. Wiest R, Tsai MH, Groszmann RJ. Octreotide potentiates PKC-dependent vasoconstrictors in portal-hypertensive and control rats. *Gastroenterology* 2001;120:975–83.
17. Garcia-Pagan JC, Escorsell A, Moitinho E, et al. Influence of pharmacological agents on portal hemodynamics: basis for its use in the treatment of portal hypertension. *Semin Liver Dis* 1999;19:427–38.
18. Batkai S, Jarai Z, Wagner JA, et al. Endocannabinoids acting at vascular CB1 receptors mediate the vasodilated state in advanced liver cirrhosis. *Nat Med* 2001;7:827–32.
19. Fernandez M, Mejias M, Angermayr B, et al. Inhibition of VEGF receptor-2 decreases the development of hyperdynamic splanchnic circulation and portal-systemic collateral vessels in portal hypertensive rats. *J Hepatol* 2005;43:98–103.
20. Abraldes JG, Iwakiri Y, Loureiro-Silva M, et al. Mild increases in portal pressure upregulate vascular endothelial growth factor and endothelial nitric oxide synthase in the intestinal microcirculatory bed, leading to a hyperdynamic state. *Am J Physiol Gastrointest Liver Physiol* 2006;290:G980–7.
21. Graupera M, Garcia-Pagan JC, Abraldes JG, et al. Cyclooxygenase-derived products modulate the increased intrahepatic resistance of cirrhotic rat livers. *Hepatology* 2003;37:172–81.
22. Angermayr B, Mejias M, Gracia-Sancho J, et al. Heme oxygenase attenuates oxidative stress and inflammation, and increases VEGF expression in portal hypertensive rats. *J Hepatol* 2006;44:1033–9.
23. Merkel C, Bolobnesi M, Berzigotti A, et al. Clinical significance of worsening portal hypertension during long-term medical treatment in patients with cirrhosis who had been classified as early good-responders on haemodynamic criteria. *J Hepatol* 2010;52:45–53.

24. Feu F, Garcia-Pagan JC, Bosch J, et al. Relation between portal pressure response to pharmacotherapy and risk of recurrent variceal haemorrhage in patients with cirrhosis. *Lancet* 1995;346:1056–9.

25. Sanyal AJ, Fontana RJ, Di Bisceglie AM, et al. The prevalence and risk factors associated with esophageal varices in subjects with hepatitis C and advanced fibrosis. *Gastrointest Endosc* 2006;64:855–64.

26. Fontana RJ, Sanyal AJ, Ghany MG, et al. Factors that determine the development and progression of gastroesophageal varices in patients with chronic hepatitis C. *Gastroenterology* 2010;138:2321–31.

27. Malinchoc M, Kamath PS, Gordon FD, et al. A model to predict poor survival in patients undergoing transjugular intrahepatic portosystemic shunts. *Hepatology* 2000;31:864–71.

28. Bambha K, Kim WR, Pedersen R, et al. Predictors of early rebleeding and mortality after acute variceal haemorrhage in patients with cirrhosis. *Gut* 2008;57:814–20.

29. Kim T, Shijo H, Kokawa H, et al. Risk factors for hemorrhage from gastric fundal varices. *Hepatology* 1997;25:307–12.

30. De Franchis R. Updating consensus in portal hypertension: report of the Baveno III consensus workshop on definitions, methodology and therapeutic strategies in portal hypertension. *J Hepatol* 2000;33:846–52.

31. Stewart CA, Sanyal AJ. Grading portal gastropathy: validation of a gastropathy scoring system. *Am J Gastroenterol* 2003;98:1758–65.

32. D'Amico G, Pagliaro L. The clinical course of portal hypertension in liver cirrhosis. In: Rossi P, ed. *Diagnostic Imaging and Imaging Guided Therapy*. Berlin: Springer-Verlag, 2000:15–24.

33. Fontana RJ, Sanyal AJ, Mehta S, et al. Portal hypertensive gastropathy in chronic hepatitis C patients with bridging fibrosis and compensated cirrhosis: results from the HALT-C trial. *Am J Gastroenterol* 2006;101:983–92.

34. Perez-Ayuso RM, Pique JM, Bosch J, et al. Propranolol in prevention of recurrent bleeding from severe portal hypertensive gastropathy in cirrhosis. *Lancet* 1991;337:1431–4.

35. Vizzutti F, Arena U, Romanelli RG, et al. Liver stiffness measurement predicts severe portal hypertension in patients with HCV-related cirrhosis. *Hepatology* 2007;45:1290–7.

36. Pena LR, Cox T, Koch AG, et al. Study comparing oesophageal capsule endoscopy versus EGD in the detection of varices. *Dig Liver Dis* 2008;40:216–23.

37. Stiegmann GV, Goff JS, Michaletz-Onody PA, et al. Endoscopic sclerotherapy as compared with endoscopic ligation for bleeding esophageal varices. *N Engl J Med* 1992;326:1527–32.

38. De Franchis R, Primignani M. Endoscopic treatments for portal hypertension. *Semin Liver Dis* 1999;19:439–55.

39. Pomier-Layrargues G, Kusielewicz D, Willems B, et al. Presinusoidal portal hypertension in non-alcoholic cirrhosis. *Hepatology* 1985;5:415–18.

40. Wadhawan M, Dubey S, Sharma BC, et al. Hepatic venous pressure gradient in cirrhosis: correlation with the size of varices, bleeding, ascites, and child's status. *Dig Dis Sci* 2006;51:2264–9.

41. Ripoll C, Groszmann R, Garcia-Tsao G, et al. Hepatic venous pressure gradient predicts clinical decompensation in patients with compensated cirrhosis. *Gastroenterology* 2007;133:481–8.

42. Lautt WW, Legare DJ, Ezzat WR. Quantitation of the hepatic arterial buffer response to graded changes in portal blood flow [see comments]. *Gastroenterology* 1990;98:1024–8.

43. Wu MT, Pan HB, Chen C, et al. Azygos blood flow in cirrhosis: measurement with MR imaging and correlation with variceal hemorrhage. *Radiology* 1996;198:457–62.

44. Nevens F, Sprengers D, Feu F, et al. Measurement of variceal pressure with an endoscopic pressure sensitive gauge: validation and effect of propranolol therapy in chronic conditions. *J Hepatol* 1996;24:66–73.

45. Escorsell A, Bordas JM, Castaneda B, et al. Predictive value of the variceal pressure response to continued pharmacological therapy in patients with cirrhosis and portal hypertension. *Hepatology* 2000;31:1061–7.

46. Casado M, Bosch J, Garcia-Pagan JC, et al. Clinical events after transjugular intrahepatic portosystemic shunt: correlation with hemodynamic findings. *Gastroenterology* 1998;114:1296–303.

47. Bureau C, Garcia-Pagan JC, Otal P, et al. Improved clinical outcome using polytetrafluoroethylene-coated stents for tips: results of a randomized study. *Gastroenterology* 2004;126:469–75.

48. Orloff MJ, Orloff MS, Orloff SL, et al. Three decades of experience with emergency portacaval shunt for acutely bleeding esophageal varices in 400 unselected patients with cirrhosis of the liver. *J Am Coll Surg* 1995;180:257–72.

49. Rosemurgy AS, Serofini FM, Zweibal BR, et al. TIPS versus small diameter prosthetic H-graft portacaval shunt: extended follow-up of an expanded randomized prospective trial. *J Gastrointest Surg* 2000;4:589–97.

50. Jenkins RL, Gedaly R, Pomposelli JJ, et al. Distal splenorenal shunt: role, indications, and utility in the era of liver transplantation. *Arch Surg* 1999;134:416–20.

51. Henderson JM, Boyer TD, Kutner MH, et al. Distal splenorenal shunt versus transjugular intrahepatic portal systematic shunt for variceal bleeding: a randomized trial. *Gastroenterology* 2006;130:1643–51.

52. Schepke M, Kleber G, Nurnberg D, et al. Ligation versus propranolol for the primary prophylaxis of variceal bleeding in cirrhosis. *Hepatology* 2004;40:65–72.

53. Lo GH, Chen WC, Chen MH, et al. Endoscopic ligation vs. nadolol in the prevention of first variceal bleeding in patients with cirrhosis. *Gastrointest Endosc* 2004;59:333–8.

54. Lui HF, Stanley AJ, Forrest EH, et al. Primary prophylaxis of variceal hemorrhage: a randomized controlled trial comparing ligation, propranolol, and isosorbide mononitrate. *Gastroenterology* 2002;123:735–44.

55. García-Pagán JC, Morillas R, Bañarres R, et al. Propranolol plus placebo versus propranolol plus isosorbide-5-mononitrate in the prevention of a first variceal bleed: a double-blind RCT. *Hepatology* 2003;37:1260–6.

56. Villanueva C, Aracil C, Colomo A, et al. Acute hemodynamic response to beta-blockers and prediction of long-term outcome in primary prophylaxis of variceal bleeding. *Gastroenerology* 2009;137:119–28.

57. Norberto L, Polese L, Cillo U, et al. A randomised study comparing ligation with propranolol for primary prophylaxis of variceal bleeding in candidates for liver transplantation. *Liver Transpl* 2007;13:1272–8.

58. Hernandez-Guerra M, Turnes J, Rubinstein P, et al. PTFE-covered stents improve TIPS patency in Budd–Chiari syndrome. *Hepatology* 2004;40:1197–202.

59. D'Amico G, Pagliaro L, Bosch J. Pharmacological treatment of portal hypertension: an evidence-based approach. *Semin Liver Dis* 1999;19:475–505.

60. Bernard B, Lebrec D, Mathurin P, et al. Beta-adrenergic antagonists in the prevention of gastrointestinal rebleeding in patients with cirrhosis: a meta-analysis. *Hepatology* 1997;25:63–70.

61. Turnes J, Hernández-Guerra M, Abraldes JG, et al. Influence of beta-2 adrenergic receptor gene polymorphism on the hemodynamic response to propranolol in patients with cirrhosis. *Hepatology* 2006;43:34–41.

62. Tripathi D, Ferguson JW, Kochar N, et al. Randomized controlled trial of carvediol versus variceal band ligation for the prevention of the first variceal bleed. *Hepatology* 2009;50:825–33.

63. Garcia-Pagan JC, Feu F, Luca A, et al. Nicardipine increases hepatic blood flow and the hepatic clearance of indocyanine green in patients with cirrhosis. *J Hepatol* 1994;20:792–6.

64. Morillas RM, Planas R, Cabre E, et al. Propranolol plus isosorbide-5-mononitrate for portal hypertension in cirrhosis: long-term hemodynamic and renal effects. *Hepatology* 1994;20:1502–8.

65. Albillos A, Lledo JL, Banares R, et al. Hemodynamic effects of alpha-adrenergic blockade with prazosin in cirrhotic patients with portal hypertension. *Hepatology* 1994;20:611–17.

66. Yu Q, Shao R, Qian HS, et al. Gene transfer of the neuronal NO synthase isoform to cirrhotic rat liver ameliorates portal hypertension. *J Clin Invest* 2000;105:741–8.

67. Abraldes JG, Zafra C, Bosch J. Possibilities of manipulating NO biosynthesis in the treatment of portal hypertension: statins. In: Groszmann RJ, Bosch J, eds. *Portal Hypertension in the 21st Century*. Dordrecht: Kluwer Academic Publishers, 2004:111–20.

68. Laleman W, Van Landeghem L, Van der Elst I, et al. Nitroflurbiprofen, a nitric oxide-releasing cyclooxygenase inhibitor, improves cirrhotic portal hypertension in rats. *Gastroenterology* 2007;132:709–19.

69. Angelico M, Carli L, Piat C, et al. Effects of isosorbide-5-mononitrate compared with propranolol on first bleeding and long-term survival in cirrhosis. *Gastroenterology* 1997;113:1632–9.

70. Garcia-Pagan JC, Villanueva C, Vila MC, et al. Isosorbide mononitrate in the prevention of first variceal bleed in patients who cannot receive beta blockers. *Gastroenterology* 2001;121:908–14.

71. Pagliaro L, D'Amico G, Sorensen TI, et al. Prevention of first bleeding in cirrhosis. A meta-analysis of randomized trials of nonsurgical treatment. *Ann Intern Med* 1992;117:59–70.

72. D'Amico G, Pagliaro L, Bosch J. The treatment of portal hypertension: a meta-analytic review. *Hepatology* 1995;22:332–54.

73. The Veterans Affairs Cooperative Variceal Sclerotherapy Group. Prophylactic sclerotherapy for esophageal varices in men with alcoholic liver disease. A randomized, single-blind, multicenter clinical trial. *N Engl J Med* 1991;324:1779–84.

74. Grace ND, Garcia-Pagan JC, Angelico M, et al. Primary prophylaxis for variceal bleeding. In: de Franchis R, ed. *Proceedings of the Fourth Baveno International Consensus Workshop on Definitions, Methodology and Therapeutic Strategies*. Oxford: Blackwell Science, 2005: 168–200.

75. Sarin SK, Lamba GS, Kumar M, et al. Comparison of endoscopic ligation and propranolol for the primary prevention of variceal bleeding. *N Engl J Med* 1999;340:988–93.

76. Lui HF, Stanley AJ, Forrest EH, et al. Primary prophylaxis of variceal hemorrhage: a randomized controlled trial comparing band ligation, propranolol, and isosorbide mononitrate. *Gastroenterology* 2002;123:735–44.

77. Thuluvath PJ, Maheshwari A, Jagannath S, et al. A randomized controlled trial of beta-blockers versus endoscopic band ligation for primary prophylaxis: a large sample size is required to show a difference in bleeding rates. *Dig Dis Sci* 2005;50:407–10.

78. Jutabha R, Jensen DM, Martin P, et al. Randomized study comparing banding and propranolol to prevent initial variceal hemorrhage in cirrhotics with high-risk esophageal varices. *Gastroenterology* 2005;128:870–81.

79. Khuroo MS, Khuroo NS, Farahat KL, et al. Meta-analysis: endoscopic variceal ligation for primary prophylaxis of oesophageal variceal bleeding. *Aliment Pharmacol Ther* 2005;21:347–61.

80. Garcia-Pagan JC, Bosch J. Endoscopic band ligation in the treatment of portal hypertension. *Nat Clin Pract Gastroenterol Hepatol* 2005;2:526–35.

81. Imperiale TF, Klein RW, Chalasani N. Cost-effectiveness analysis of variceal ligation vs. beta-blockers for primary prevention of variceal bleeding. *Hepatology* 2007;45:870–8.

82. Boyer TD, Haskal ZJ. The role of transjugular intrahepatic portosystemic shunt in the management of portal hypertension. *Hepatology* 2005;41:386–400.

83. Sarin SK, Wadhawan M, Agarwal SR, Tyagi P, Sharma BC. Endoscopic variceal ligation plus propranolol versus endoscopic variceal ligation alone in primary prophylaxis of variceal bleeding. *Am J Gastroenterol* 2005;100:797–804.

84. Lo GH, Chen WC, Wang HM, Lee CC. Controlled trial of ligation plus nadolol versus nadolol alone for the prevention of first variceal bleeding. *Hepatology* 2010;52:230–7.

85. D'Amico G, de Franchis R. Upper digestive bleeding in cirrhosis. Post-therapeutic outcome and prognostic indicators. *Hepatology* 2003;38:599–612.

86. Carbonell N, Pauwels A, Serfaty L, et al. Improved survival after variceal bleeding in patients with cirrhosis over the past two decades. *Hepatology* 2004;40:652–9.

87. Chalasani N, Kahi C, Francois F, et al. Improved patient survival after acute variceal bleeding: a multicenter, cohort study. *Am J Gastroenterol* 2003;98:653–9.

88. De Franchis R. Evolving consensus in portal hypertension: report of the Baveno IV consensus workshop on methodology of diagnosis and therapy in portal hypertension. *J Hepatol* 2005;43: 167–76.

89. De Franchis R, on behalf of the Baveno V Faculty. Revising consensus in portal hypertension: report of the Baveno V consensus workshop on methodology of diagnosis and therapy in portal hypertension. *J Hepatol* 2010;53:762–8.

90. Guarner C, Soriano G. Spontaneous bacterial peritonitis. *Semin Liver Dis* 2001;17:203–7.

91. Bernard B, Grange JD, Khac EN, et al. Antibiotic prophylaxis for the prevention of bacterial infections in cirrhotic patients with gastrointestinal bleeding: a meta-analysis. *Hepatology* 1999;29(6): 1655–61.

92. Soares-Weiser K, Brezis M, Tur-Kaspa R, et al. Antibiotic prophylaxis for cirrhotic patients with gastrointestinal bleeding. *Cochrane Database Syst Rev* 2002;2.CD002907.

93. Hou MC, Lin HC, Liu TT, et al. Antibiotic prophylaxis after endoscopic therapy prevents rebleeding in acute variceal hemorrhage: a randomized trial. *Hepatology* 2004;39:746–53.

94. Rimola A, Garcia-Tsao G, Navasa M, et al. Diagnosis, treatment and prophylaxis of spontaneous bacterial peritonitis: a consensus document. *J Hepatol* 2000;32:142–53.

95. Fernandez J, Ruiz del Arbol L, Gomez C, et al. Norfloxacin vs ceftriaxone in the prophylaxis of infections in patients with advanced cirrhosis and hemorrhage. *Gastroenterology* 2006;131:1049–56.

96. Ioannou G, Doust J, Rockey DC. Terlipressin for acute esophageal variceal hemorrhage (Cochrane review). *Cochrane Database Syst Rev* 2001;1:CD002147.

97. Escorsell A, Ruiz del Arbol L, Planas R, et al. Multicenter randomized controlled trial of terlipressin versus sclerotherapy in the treatment of acute variceal bleeding: the TEST study. *Hepatology* 2000;32:471–6.

98. Lo GH, Chen WC, Wang HM, et al. Low-dose terlipression plus banding ligation versus low-dose terlipressin alone in the prevention of very early rebleeding of oesophageal varices. *Gut* 2009;58: 1275–80.

99. Abid S, Jafri W, Hamid S, et al. Terlipressin vs. octreotide in bleeding esophageal varices as an adjuvant therapy with endoscopic band ligation: a randomized double-blind placebo-controlled trial. *Am J Gastroenterol* 2009;104:617–23.

100. Moitinho E, Planas R, Bañares R, et al. Multicenter randomized controlled trial comparing different schedules of somatostatin in the treatment of acute variceal bleeding. *J Hepatol* 2001;35:712–18.

101. Escorsell A, Bandi JC, Andreu V, et al. Desensitization to the effects of intravenous octreotide in cirrhotic patients with portal hypertension. *Gastroenterology* 2001;120:161–9.

102. Shields R, Jenkins SA, Baxter JN, et al. A prospective randomized controlled trial comparing the efficacy of somatostatin with injection sclerotherapy in the control of bleeding oesophageal varices. *J Hepatol* 1992;16:128–37.

103. Planas R, Quer JC, Boix J, et al. A prospective randomized trial comparing somatostatin and sclerotherapy in the treatment of acute variceal bleeding. *Hepatology* 1994;20:370–5.

104. Jenkins SA, Shields R, Davies M, et al. A multicentre randomized trial comparing octreotide and injection sclerotherapy in the management and outcome of acute variceal haemorrhage. *Gut* 1997;41:526–33.

105. D'Amico G, Pietrosi G, Tarantino I, et al. Emergency sclerotherapy versus vasoactive drugs for variceal bleeding in cirrhosis: a Cochrane meta-analysis. *Gastroenterology* 2003;124:1277–91.

106. Gimson AE, Ramage JK, Panos MZ, et al. Randomised trial of variceal banding ligation versus injection sclerotherapy for bleeding oesophageal varices. *Lancet* 1993;342:391–4.

107. Hou MC, Lin HC, Kuo BI, et al. Comparison of endoscopic variceal injection sclerotherapy and ligation for the treatment of esophageal variceal hemorrhage: a prospective randomized trial. *Hepatology* 1995;21:1517–22.

108. Laine L, Stein C, Sharma V. Randomized comparison of ligation versus ligation plus sclerotherapy in patients with bleeding esophageal varices. *Gastroenerology* 1996;110:529–33.

109. Lo GH, Lai KH, Cheng JS, et al. Emergency banding ligation versus sclerotherapy for the control of active bleeding from esophageal varices. *Hepatology* 1997;25:1101–4.

110. De Franchis R, Primignani M. Endoscopic treatments for portal hypertension. *Semin Liver Dis* 1999;19:439–55.

111. Avgernos A, Armonis A, Stefanidis G, et al. Sustained rise of portal pressure after sclerotherapy, but not band ligation, in acute variceal bleeding in cirrhosis. *Hepatology* 2004;39:1623–30.

112. Banares R, Albillos A, Rincon D, et al. Endoscopic treatment versus endoscopic plus pharmacologic treatment for acute variceal bleeding: a meta-analysis. *Hepatology* 2002;35:609–15.

113. Villanueva C, Piqueras M, Aracil C, et al. A randomized controlled trial comparing ligation and sclerotherapy as emergency endoscopic treatment added to somatostatin in acute variceal bleeding. *J Hepatol* 2006;45:560–7.

114. Abraldes JG, Villanueva C, Bañares R, et al. Hepatic venous pressure gradient and prognosis in patients with acute variceal bleeding treated with pharmacologic and endoscopic therapy. *J Hepatol* 2008;48:229–36

115. Burroughs AK, Patch D. Transjugular intrahepatic portosystemic shunt. *Semin Liver Dis* 1999;19:457–73.

116. Monescillo A, Martinez-Lagares F, Ruiz-del-Arbol L, et al. Influence of portal hypertension and its early decompression by TIPS placement on the outcome of variceal bleeding. *Hepatology* 2004;40: 793–801.

117. Bosch J, Garcia-Oagan JC. Prevention of variceal rebleeding. *Lancet* 2003;361:952–4.

118. Garcia-Pagan JC, Feu F, Bosch J, et al. Propranolol compared with propranolol plus isosorbide-5-mononitrate for portal hypertension in cirrhosis. A randomized controlled study. *Ann Intern Med* 1991;114:869–73.

119. Villanueva C, Balanzo J, Novella MT, et al. Nadolol plus isosorbide mononitrate compared with sclerotherapy for the prevention of variceal rebleeding. *N Engl J Med* 1996;334:1624–9.

120. Villanueva C, Minana J, Ortiz J, et al. Endoscopic ligation compared with combined treatment with nadolol and isosorbide mononitrate to prevent recurrent variceal bleeding. *N Engl J Med* 2001;345:647–55.

121. Patch D, Sabin CA, Goulis J, et al. A randomized, controlled trial of medical therapy versus endoscopic ligation for the prevention of variceal rebleeding in patients with cirrhosis. *Gastroenterology* 2002;123:1013–19.

122. Lo GH, Chen WC, Chen MH, et al. Banding ligation versus nadolol and isosorbide mononitrate for the prevention of esophageal variceal rebleeding. *Gastroenterology* 2002;123:728–34.

123. Ravipati M, Katragadda S, Swaminathan PD, et al. Pharmacotherapy plus endoscopic intervention is more effective than phar-

macotherapy or endoscopy alone in the secondary prevention of esophageal variceal bleeding: a meta-analysis of randomized, controlled trials. *Gastrointest Endosc* 2009;70:665–7.

124. Lo GH, Lai KH, Cheng JS, et al. Endoscopic variceal ligation plus nadolol and sucralfate compared with ligation alone for the prevention of variceal rebleeding: a prospective, randomized trial. *Hepatology* 2000;32:461–5.

125. De la Peña J, Brullet E, Sanchez-Hernandez E, et al. Variceal ligation plus nadolol compared with ligation for prophylaxis of variceal rebleeding: a multicenter trial. *Hepatology* 2005;41:572–8.

126. Kumar A, Jha SK, Shrma P, et al. Addition of propranolol and isosorbide mononitrate to endoscopic variceal ligation does not reduce variceal rebleeding incidence. *Gastroenterology* 2009;137: 892–901.

127. García-Pagán JC, Villanueva C, Albillos A, et al. Nadolol plus isosorbide mononitrate alone or associated with band ligation in the prevention of recurrent bleeding: a multicentre randomized controlled trial. *Gut* 2009;58:1144–50.

128. Escorsell A, Banares R, Garcia-Pagan JC, et al. TIPS versus drug therapy in preventing variceal rebleeding in advanced cirrhosis: a randomized controlled trial. *Hepatology* 2002;35:385–92.

129. Abraldes JG, Tarantino I, Turnes J, et al. Hemodynamic response to pharmacological treatment of portal hypertension and long-term prognosis of cirrhosis. *Hepatology* 2003;37:902–8.

130. Villanueva C, Lopez-Balaguer JM, Aracil C, et al. Maintenance of hemodynamic response to treatment for portal hypertension and influence on complications of cirrhosis. *J Hepatol* 2004;40: 757–65.

131. La Mura V, Abraldes JG, Raffa S, et al. Prognostic value of acute hemodynamic response to i.v. propranolol in patients with cirrhosis and portal hypertension. *J Hepatol* 2009;51:279–87.

132. Laine L, Cook D. Endoscopic ligation compared with sclerotherapy for treatment of esophageal variceal bleeding. A meta-analysis. *Ann Intern Med* 1995;123:280–7.

133. Karsan HA, Morton SC, Shekelle PG, et al. Combination endoscopic band ligation and sclerotherapy compared with endoscopic band ligation alone for the secondary prophylaxis of esophageal variceal hemorrhage: a meta-analysis. *Dig Dis Sci* 2005;50:399– 406.

134. Luca A, D'Amico G, LaGalla R, et al. TIPS for prevention of recurrent bleeding in patients with cirrhosis: meta-analysis of randomized clinical trials. *Radiology* 1999;212:411–21.

135. Papatheodoridis GV, Goulis J, Leandro G, et al. Transjugular intrahepatic portosystemic shunt compared with endoscopic treatment for prevention of variceal rebleeding. A meta-analysis. *Hepatology* 1999;30:612–22.

136. Lo GH, Lai KH, Cheng JS, et al. A prospective, randomized trial of butyl cyanoacrylate injection versus band ligation in the management of bleeding gastric varices. *Hepatology* 2001;33:1060–4.

137. Sarin SK, Jain AK, Jain M, et al. A randomized controlled trial of cyanoacrylate versus alcohol injection in patients with isolated fundic varices. *Am J Gastroenterol* 2002;97:1010–15.

138. Procaccini NJ, Al-Osami AM, Northup P, et al. Endoscopic cyanoacrylate versus transjugular intrahepatic portosystemic shunt for gastric variceal bleeding: a single-center US analysis. *Gastrointest Endosc* 2009;70:881–7.

139. Mishra SR, Chander Sharma B, Kumar A, Sarin SK. Endoscopic cyanoacrylate injection versus beta-blocker for secondary prophylaxis of gastric variceal bleed: a randomized controlled trial. *Gut* 2010;59:729–35.

140. Ryan BM, Stockbrugger RW, Ryan JM. A pathophysiologic, gastroenterologic, and radiologic approach to the management of gastric varices. *Gastroenterology* 2004;126:1175–89.

141. Garcia N, Sanyal AJ. Portal hypertensive gastropathy and gastric antral vascular ectasia. *Curr Treat Options Gastroenterol* 2001;4: 163–71.

Multiple choice questions

14.1 **What is the treatment that should not be chosen for actively bleeding esophageal varices in cirrhotic patients?**

   a Endoscopic sclerotherapy.
   b Endoscopic band ligation.
   c Nonselective β-blocker.
   d Terlipressin.
   e Somatostatin.

14.2 **Which of these has the lowest risk of bleeding?**

   a Small esophageal varices in Child–Pugh class A patients.
   b Esophageal varices with red signs.
   c Esophageal varices with large size.
   d Isolated gastric varices with large size.
   e Isolated gastric varices with red signs.

Answers to the multiple choice questions can be found in the Appendix at the end of the book.

These multiple choice questions are also available for you to complete online.
Visit http://www.schiffsdiseasesoftheliver.com/

CHAPTER 15

Renal Complications of Liver Disease and the Hepatorenal Syndrome

Florence Wong

Department of Medicine, University of Toronto and Toronto General Hospital, Toronto, Canada

---

Key concepts

- Renal impairment commonly occurs in patients with cirrhosis, and it can be due to structural damage in the kidneys or changes related to the renal circulation leading to impairment in renal function, so-called functional renal failure.
- Functional renal failure is usually related to a decreased renal blood flow, secondary to a decrease in the effective arterial blood volume. Cirrhotic patients with functional renal failure can respond to intravascular volume replacement with a reduction in serum creatinine. These patients are said to have prerenal renal failure.
- Cirrhotic patients with functional renal failure whose serum creatinine does not reduce with intravascular volume replacement are said to have hepatorenal syndrome. These patients tend to have a much worse prognosis.
- Acute kidney failure is a concept coined by nephrologists and is increasingly being used in hepatology literature. It encompasses all causes of acute kidney failure including causes that can produce structural damage in the kidneys such as glomerulonephritis or acute tubular necrosis. The acute cases of functional renal failure can be regarded as cases of acute kidney failure.
- Functional renal failure can be precipitated by various events that can cause either further arterial vasodilatation or further reduction of intravascular volume. These include bacterial infections, overdiuresis,

- gastrointestinal blood loss, vomiting or diarrhea, and large volume paracentesis without intravascular volume replacement.
- Drugs that compromise either the systemic circulation, by lowering the systemic blood pressure, or the renal circulation, such as nonsteroidal anti-inflammatory agents can also precipitate functional renal failure.
- It is imperative that clinicians caring for patients with advanced cirrhosis are vigilant for potential precipitating factors for functional renal failure, and to institute treatment as soon as possible.
- Treatment for functional renal failure, whether prerenal failure or hepatorenal syndrome, begins with intravascular volume replacement. Patients with hepatorenal syndrome will also need vasoconstrictor therapy. A transjugular intrahepatic portosystemic shunt may also be inserted in the appropriate patient with hepatorenal syndrome following vasoconstrictor therapy.
- Liver transplantation is the treatment of choice for patients with cirrhosis and hepatorenal syndrome, as it corrects many aspects of pathophysiology. Simultaneous liver–kidney transplant appears to yield worse outcomes for both patient and graft, and therefore is not recommended unless the patient has been waiting for more than 3 months on dialysis.
- Prevention is the best treatment for cirrhotic patients who are at risk for the development of functional renal disorder.

Renal dysfunction commonly occurs in patients with cirrhosis, especially in those with advanced cirrhosis with ascites. It has been estimated that chronic kidney disease occurs in approximately 1% of all hospitalized patients with cirrhosis, whereas acute kidney injury (AKI) occurs in up to 19% of cirrhotic patients admitted to hospital for whatever reason [1]. The prevalence of renal dysfunction in cirrhosis seems to be rising, due to an increasing number of patients worldwide affected by viral hepatitis, obesity, diabetes, and hypertension, and the propensity of these patients to develop various infections which are then complicated by renal failure [2].

The combination of liver disease and kidney dysfunction can occur as a result of systemic conditions that affect the liver and the kidney simultaneously, or the derangement of renal function can secondarily complicate primary disorders of the liver. In the latter scenario, the renal dysfunction can be related to intrinsic renal disorders, where there is structural renal damage. More often, the renal disorder is functional in nature, where no structural renal damage occurs. The most severe form of functional renal disorder complicating liver cirrhosis is the hepatorenal syndrome (HRS).

Structural renal disease in patients with liver disease

Simultaneous involvement of both the liver and the kidney occurs in many systemic conditions, causing both structural renal damage and liver injury. These include collagen vascular diseases, infiltrative disorders such as amyloidosis and sarcoidosis, inherited conditions such as polycystic disease, and acute fatty liver or toxemia of pregnancy.

Much more common are renal diseases that occur as a result of the liver disease (Table 15.1) [3]. Glomerulonephritis and polyarteritis nodosum are important extrahepatic manifestations of chronic hepatitis B virus (HBV) infection, related to the deposition of HBV antigen–antibody complexes in extrahepatic tissues. With the advent of effective antiviral therapy, the renal complications of HBV infection are rapidly becoming infrequent except in endemic areas. Hepatitis C virus infection-associated glomerulopathies, in contrast, are more commonly seen, possibly related to the frequent occurrence of cryoglobulinemia in these patients. Recent reports suggest that the hepatitis C virus itself may be involved directly in the pathogenesis of the various glomeru-

Table 15.1 Coexisting liver and kidney disorders

Liver disease	Associated renal disease
Hepatitis B virus infection	Membranoproliferative glomerulonephritis
	Membranous glomerulonephritis
	Polyarteritis nodosum
Hepatitis C virus infection	Cryoglobulinemia
	Membranoproliferative glomerulonephritis
	Membranous glomerulonephritis
Alcoholic cirrhosis	IgA nephropathy
	Renal tubular acidosis
Primary biliary cirrhosis	Interstitial nephritis
	Renal tubular acidosis
Autoimmune hepatitis	Renal tubular acidosis
Wilson disease	Renal tubular acidosis
Nonalcoholic fatty liver disease/ Steatohepatitis	Diabetic nephropathy
Drug-induced hepatic injuries (use of ACE inhibitors or angiotensin II receptor antagonists): cholestatic hepatitis hepatocellular damage	Chronic renal failure

ACE, angiotensin-converting enzyme.

lopathies as the viral RNA has been found along glomerular capillaries and in the mesangium. Alcoholic liver disease is uniquely linked to immunoglobulin A (IgA) nephropathy, a condition whereby circulating IgA immune complexes are deposited in renal glomeruli, due to their impaired clearance. Hematuria and proteinuria are common clinical features of IgA nephropathy, and patients can rarely present with nephrotic syndrome. Renal tubular acidosis, a syndrome associated with failure of the kidney to acidify the urine, can occasionally be seen in alcoholic hepatitis as well, although it is more often observed with autoimmune hepatitis, primary biliary cirrhosis, and Wilson disease.

An emerging combination of renal disease coexisting with liver disease is the presence of diabetic nephropathy in a patient with nonalcoholic fatty liver disease (NAFLD) or nonalcoholic steatohepatitis (NASH). A recent study showed that 31% of patients with NAFLD or NASH also had type 2 diabetes [4]. Both are part of the metabolic syndrome, and are linked to obesity. The key feature of the metabolic syndrome is insulin resistance; NAFLD and NASH are considered the hepatic manifestations of this syndrome, while type 2 diabetes is the direct result of insulin resistance. Hyperinsulinemia and poor glycemic control in type 2 diabetes is associated with an increased risk for diabetic microangiopathy, affecting the capillaries of the kidney, accounting for 41% of all cases of chronic renal failure [5]. With the incidence of obesity on the rise, the combination of diabetic nephropathy and NAFLD or NASH will become an important cause of simultaneous liver and renal dysfunction in the future.

Drug toxicity is also an important cause of combined renal and liver dysfunction. Exposure to toxins such as acetaminophen overdose is frequently associated with both liver and renal failure. The fluorinated anesthetic agents methoxyfluorane and fluroxene can occasionally cause both hepatic and renal damage. The patient with cirrhosis is susceptible to renal damage when prescribed certain classes of drugs such as the nonsteroidal anti-inflammatory drugs (NSAIDs) or aminoglycosides. NSAIDs inhibit the enzymes cyclooxygenase 1 and 2 that are responsible for renal prostaglandin synthesis, which cirrhotic patients depend on as renal vasodilators to maintain renal hemodynamics. There are numerous reports of renal failure following the use of NSAIDs. The recent development of cyclooxygenase type 2 inhibitors seems to be less renally toxic when given in the short term [6], whether long-term use of these agents is equally safe is unknown. Aminoglycosides can cause glomerular congestion, epithelial edema of proximal tubules, cellular desquamation, and ultimately glomerular atrophy and tubular necrosis. Awareness of susceptibility of cirrhotic patients to aminoglycoside toxicity has greatly reduced its use in the cirrhotic population. Therefore aminoglycoside nephrotoxicity is less of an issue amongst such patients in recent years.

Patients with diabetic nephropathy or hypertensive nephrosclerosis are frequently prescribed drugs that inhibit the renin–angiotensin pathway to provide either renal protection against proteinuria or for the control of their systemic hypertension. There are now an increasing number of post marketing reports of hepatotoxicity with these agents. Angiotensin-converting enzyme inhibitors mainly cause a cholestatic injury, which sometimes can be prolonged, and several members of this class of drugs – including ramipril, fosinopril, lisinopril, and enalapril – have been incriminated. Hepatotoxicity related to the use of angiotensin II receptor antagonists is less common; however, a clinical picture of acute hepatitis has been reported with losartan, valsartan, and candasartan. Therefore, it is important to consider hepatotoxicity when presented with a patient with hepatitis and chronic renal failure.

Functional renal disorders

Functional renal disorders, as opposed to intrinsic renal disorders as described above, occur much more frequently in patients with advanced liver cirrhosis, especially in those with ascites. Functional renal disorders are the results of hemodynamic changes that occur in advanced cirrhosis. A common presentation of functional renal disorder in cirrhosis is renal sodium retention, which starts at a very early stage of cirrhosis, even before the clinical appearance of ascites, and which becomes more avid as the cirrhosis progresses. Simultaneous to the progressive worsening of renal sodium retention is the development of renal vasoconstriction, which eventually leads to the development of functional renal failure (FRF) [7]. When the FRF is responsive to intravascular volume replacement with return of the renal function to a prefailure level, the patient is said to have prerenal renal failure. Hepatorenal syndrome is the most severe form of FRF and is not responsive to intravascular volume challenge. More recently, some investigators have recognized that episodes of FRF associated with bacterial infections seem to have a slightly different natural history and have subclassified those patients with infection-associated FRF as a separate group [8]. In a series of 263 cirrhotic patients with ascites admitted to two large tertiary centers in Barcelona for the management of ascites, 27.4% of patients developed prerenal renal failure, 14.1% developed infection-related FRF, and 7.6% developed HRS during a mean follow-up period of 41 months [8]. Interestingly, 7.6% of patients also developed renal failure due to structural renal diseases dur-

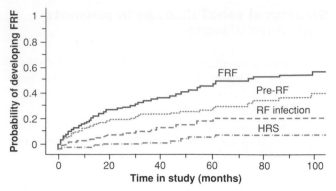

Figure 15.1 Actuarial probability of developing functional renal failure (FRF) in cirrhotic patients with ascites admitted into hospital. *P* <0.001 between the different subtypes. HRS, hepatorenal syndrome; RF, renal failure. (Adapted from Montoliu et al. [2] with permission from Elsevier.)

ing follow-up. The probability of developing the different types of FRF is depicted in Fig. 15.1 [8].

Definition of functional renal failure

Functional renal failure is defined as renal failure in which renal structure remains intact, and when the serum creatinine reaches above 1.5 mg/dL (133 μmol/L) [9]. The first mention of FRF occurred almost 70 years ago when the term hepatorenal syndrome was coined to describe acute renal failure following biliary surgery or hepatic trauma. Over the following decades, several key features of FRF were described. In the 1950s, Sherlock noted that the renal failure observed in patients with terminal stages of cirrhosis was associated with low urinary sodium and an absence of proteinuria [10]. Then later, Papper and his colleagues suggested that the pathogenesis of HRS was related to circulatory disturbance of an otherwise normal kidney [11]. This circulatory disturbance was found to be one of intense renal vasoconstriction, as demonstrated by Epstein in 1970 on a renal angiogram in a cirrhotic patient dying from renal failure. The same kidney at postmortem showed filling of all renal vessels to the periphery of the cortex, proving the functional nature of HRS [12]. Finally, in 1966, the International Ascites Club – an organization consisting of experts in hepatology as well as in renal physiology, hemodynamics, electrolyte disorders, cardiopulmonary function, and transplant medicine – set down the definition and diagnostic criteria of the most severe form of FRF, HRS [9], thereby allowing precise diagnosis that then helped develop treatment strategies.

In 2005, the International Ascites Club refined its previous definition and diagnostic criteria of HRS [12]. This occurred because treatment for HRS in the form of vasoconstrictor therapy was becoming available and HRS was no longer a universally fatal condition. Therefore, the group wanted to encourage early diagnosis of HRS,

Box 15.1 Diagnostic criteria of the hepatorenal syndrome.

- Cirrhosis with ascites
- Serum creatinine >1.5 mg/dL (133 μmol/L)
- No improvement of serum creatinine (decrease to a level of 1.5 mg/dL or less) after at least 2 days of diuretic withdrawal and volume expansion with albumin. The recommended dose of albumin is 1 g/kg of body weight per day up to a maximum of 100 g/day
- Absence of shock
- No current or recent treatment with nephrotoxic drugs
- Absence of parenchymal kidney disease as indicated by proteinuria of >500 mg/day, microhematuria (>50 red blood cells per high power field), and/or abnormal renal ultrasonography

Adapted from Salerno et al. [12].

to allow prompt institution of treatment. Furthermore, newer insights into the pathophysiology of HRS meant that the development of preventative measures was also becoming possible. The new definition of HRS [12] states that:

> HRS is a potentially reversible syndrome occurring in patients with cirrhosis, ascites, and liver failure. It is characterized by impaired renal function, marked alterations in the cardiovascular function and overactivity of the endogenous vasoactive systems. Marked vasoconstriction in the kidney causes low GFR, whereas in the systemic circulation, there is decreased vascular resistance due to splanchnic and peripheral arterial vasodilatation. A similar syndrome can also occur in acute liver failure and acute alcoholic hepatitis.

It is important to note that the definition of HRS also encompasses the hemodynamic changes that occur in a patient with cirrhosis and renal failure, emphasizing the functional nature of the condition, which is consequent upon abnormal hemodynamics.

Box 15.1 sets out the most recent criteria for the diagnosis of HRS, which continues to mandate a diagnosis of exclusion. The following changes from the earlier set of diagnostic criteria made the diagnosis of HRS much simpler:

- Creatinine clearance is removed because it is more complicated than simple serum creatinine for routine purposes, and it does not increase the accuracy of renal function estimation in cirrhotic patients
- Renal failure in the setting of an ongoing bacterial infection, but in the absence of septic shock, is considered as HRS. This enables the physician to start treatment of HRS without waiting for a complete infection recovery.
- Albumin replaces normal saline as the plasma volume expander of choice as saline is isotonic to serum and will mainly be transferred to the peritoneal cav-

ity as ascites without helping the systemic circulatory volume.
- Previous minor diagnostic criteria of HRS describing urinary findings are eliminated as they are not essential for the diagnosis.

Serum creatinine as an assessment of renal function: potential pitfalls

The current diagnosis of FRF requires a serum creatinine level of >1.5 mg/dL (133 μmol/L). However, deterioration of renal function in cirrhosis is not an all-or-none phenomenon, but rather a slow progression over time as the patient advances through the various stages of cirrhosis. The question is then raised as to whether a patient with cirrhosis and a serum creatinine of 1.3 mg/dL (114 μmol/L) is worthy of consideration for treatment of renal dysfunction, as recent literature has suggested that even small increases in serum creatinine are associated with a 2–6-fold increase in mortality risk in patients undergoing cardiothoracic surgery [13]. Furthermore, the measurement of serum creatinine is notoriously inaccurate in the diagnosis of renal dysfunction in cirrhosis; it is affected by gender, age, ethnicity, nutritional state, protein intake, and, importantly, liver disease [14]. Patients with cirrhosis of the liver often have low serum creatinine levels due to reduced production of creatinine from creatine in the liver, a greater volume of distribution due to increases in extracellular fluid, and significant muscle wasting. Furthermore, the serum creatinine measured by the Jaffe method can be artificially lowered in jaundiced patients as chromogens such as bilirubin can interfere with the assay by up to 25%. Conversely, the use of antibiotics such as the cephalosporins can artificially raise the serum creatinine levels as they positively interfere with the creatinine measurement using the Jaffe method. Therefore, a serum creatinine level within the laboratory's normal range may not represent normal renal function. In fact, it has been estimated that the baseline serum creatinine for the cirrhotic population should be 0.40–0.85 mg/dL (35–75 μmol/L) [3]. Consequently, using the rigid diagnostic criteria of a serum creatinine of >1.5 mg/dL will only diagnose patients in an advanced stage of renal failure. The measurement of renal function using creatinine clearance is similarly unreliable because of the falsely low serum creatinine in these patients. Furthermore, this requires a 24-hour urine collection, which is often incomplete, especially in an outpatient setting. Likewise, formulae such as the Cockcroft–Gault and "Modification of Diet in Renal Disease" that use serum creatinine to calculate the glomerular filtration rate (GFR) will tend to overestimate the GFR.

Therefore, until better measurements of GFR can be found, serum creatinine measurement still remains the most useful and widely accepted method for estimating renal function in clinical practice in patients with cirrhosis [15]. However, there is now interest in lowering the serum creatinine cutoff for the diagnosis of FRF, as a serum creatinine of 1 mg/dL (88 μmol/L) represents a GFR of 50 ml/min in a malnourished, wasted, cirrhotic patient [16]. Others have also advocated allowing smaller rises in serum creatinine such as 0.3 mg/dL (26.4 μmol/L), or a 50% increase in serum creatinine in a patient whose baseline creatinine level is within the normal laboratory range, to be diagnosed as having renal failure [2], especially in the setting of a precipitating event in a patient with severe cirrhosis and ascites.

Acute kidney injury in cirrhosis

Nephrologists have been defining acute kidney injury as a percentage rise rather an absolute increase in serum creatinine, as this seems to better represent the change in the patient's renal function. For example, a doubling of a patient's serum creatinine represents a significant deviation from the patient's normal renal function, even if the final creatinine level is still within the laboratory's normal range, and this may have implications for the patient's clinical outcome. Therefore, in 2004, the Acute Dialysis Quality Initiatives (ADQI) Workgroup developed a consensus definition and classification known as the RIFLE classification (R, renal risk; I, injury; F, failure; L, loss of kidney function; E, end-stage renal disease) for AKI, which stratified renal failure into grades of increasing severity based on changes in patients' serum creatinine or GFR and/or urine output (Fig. 15.2) [17]. Another col-

Table 15.2 Stages of acute kidney injury.

Stage	Serum creatinine criteria	Urine output criteria
1	↑ Serum creatinine of ≥0.3 mg/dL (≥26.4 μmol/L) or ≥150–200% (1.5–2-fold) from baseline	<0.5 mL/kg/hour for >6 hours
2	↑ Serum creatinine to >200% but ≤300% (>2–3-fold) from baseline	<0.5 mL/kg/h for >12 hours
3	↑ Serum creatinine to >300% (>3-fold) from baseline or serum creatinine of ≥4.0 mg/dL (≥354 μmol/L) with an acute increase of ≥0.5 mg/dL (44 μmol/L)	<0.3 mL/kg/h for 24 hours or anuria for 12 hours

Adapted from Francoz et al. [15].

laborative network consisting of members of the ADQI group and experts from several nephrology societies and intensive care medicine societies known as the Acute Kidney Injury Network (AKIN) further modified the RIFLE criteria [18], so that even smaller increases in serum creatinine than those considered in the RIFLE classification might be considered as AKI (Table 15.2), as patients with these minor increases in serum creatinine have been shown to have an adverse outcome [19]. It is interesting to note that both the ADQI and the AKIN groups do not reference the absolute level of the serum creatinine in the diagnosis of AKI except when renal failure sets in.

Both the RIFLE and AKIN diagnostic criteria address the issue of smaller increases in serum creatinine as being clinically significant. However, their direct applicability to the cirrhotic population is questionable. For example, cirrhotic patients with refractory ascites usually have a low urine output of approximately 500 mL/day because of their avid renal sodium and water retention even in the absence of AKI. A significant proportion of these patients will be regarded as having renal failure if these diagnostic criteria are used. The only accurate method of measuring GFR is to use clearance techniques employing exogenous markers such as inulin or iothalamate, but they are labor intensive and expensive and therefore cannot be used in routine clinical practice. All formulae that estimate the GFR tend to provide an overestimation of GFR in cirrhosis and therefore will underdiagnose renal failure. However, hepatologists are now beginning to embrace the concept of AKI [1,3], as this allows cirrhotic patients with renal dysfunction to be properly classified, thereby allowing appropriate studies to be conducted to define their prognosis and to devise treatment options. However, the hepatology community will need to tailor the AKI definitions to suit the cirrhotic population, and to validate such definitions in a large cohort of patients with cirrhosis.

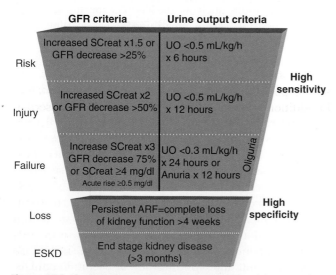

Figure 15.2 The RIFLE diagnostic criteria of acute kidney injury. A patient can fulfill the diagnostic criteria either through changes in serum creatinine or changes in urine output. ARF, acute renal failure; ESKD, end-stage kidney disease; GFR, glomerular filtration rate; SCreat, serum creatinine; UO, urine output. (Adapted from Bellomo et al. [17] with permission from Biomed Central Ltd.)

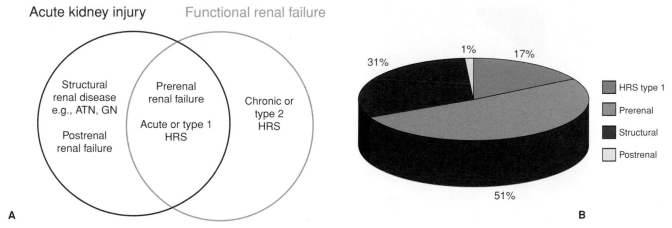

Figure 15.3 (A) Classification of the different types of renal dysfunction in cirrhosis. (B) Relative proportions of the different causes of acute kidney injury in cirrhosis. ATN, acute tubular necrosis; GN, glomerulonephritis; HRS, hepatorenal syndrome. (Data from references [1,16].)

One needs to be clear that AKI definitions describe acute renal failure from all causes, whether structural or functional renal diseases. Thus in this new classification of AKI, the entire spectrum of acute kidney failure is included. FRF, in contrast, only describes renal failure from functional changes in the kidneys related to hemodynamic changes in the systemic circulation and it can be acute or chronic (Fig. 15.3A). Acute or type 1 HRS only makes up a small proportion of patients with AKI (Fig. 15.3B). The common causes of AKI in cirrhosis are listed in Table 15.3, with the relative proportions of the different causes in hospitalized patients described in Figure 15.3B.

Table 15.3 Causes of acute kidney injury in cirrhosis.

Type	Disease entity
Functional renal failure, volume responsive	Prerenal renal failure: overdiuresis gastrointestinal bleeding vomiting and diarrhea infection
Functional renal failure, not volume responsive	Acute or type 1 hepatorenal syndrome
Structural	Acute glomerulonephritis Acute tubular necrosis: following type 1 hepatorenal syndrome following prerenal renal failure drug toxicity with aminoglycosides or nonsteroidal anti-inflammatory agents Osmotic tubulopathy from: contrast agents hydroxyethyl starch
Postrenal	Bladder neck obstruction

Pathophysiology of functional renal failure

Most intrarenal or postrenal causes of AKI in cirrhosis are related to structural abnormalities in either the kidneys or the lower urinary tract. In contrast, FRF, be it volume responsive or not, is a direct result of the hemodynamic derangement and cardiovascular changes of liver cirrhosis. The following is a summary of our understanding of the pathophysiology that has been implicated in the development of FRF, including HRS.

Portal hypertension as an initiator of hemodynamic changes in cirrhosis

The development of cirrhosis of the liver is associated with the laying down of fibrous tissues together with the formation of nodules, leading to a distortion of liver architecture. This results in alteration, compression, and sometime even obliteration of the hepatic vasculature, so the portal inflow is met with increased resistance. In addition, there is decreased production of vasodilators within the hepatic microcirculation, causing further increases in the resistance to portal inflow [20] and the development of portal hypertension. Changes in shear stress of the portal vessel wall lead to the production of various vasodilators such as nitric oxide, carbon monoxide, and endogeneous cannabinoids in the portal circulation [21–23]. As a result, portal-venous blood flow is increased and this contributes incrementally to the elevated portal pressure. It has been postulated that the increased flow to the splanchnic circulation can augment the shear stress on the splanchnic vasculature, causing further increased production of vasodilators such as nitric oxide. This portal-venous dilatation is eventually transferred to its tributaries, leading to splanchnic vasodilatation. Several other factors, including increased bacterial

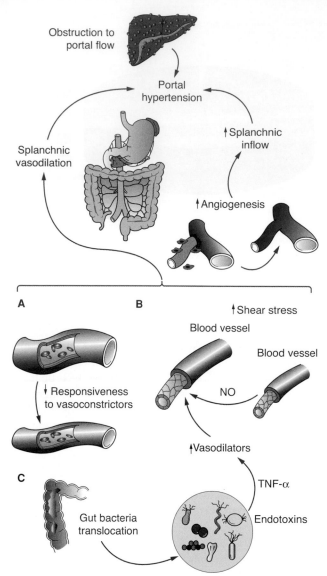

Figure 15.4 Portal hypertension as an initiator of hemodynamic changes in cirrhosis. There are three pathways that can lead to splanchnic vasodilatation: (a) decreased responsiveness to vasoconstrictors; (b) increased shear stress causing increased nitric oxide (NO) production, which in turn causes splanchnic vasodilatation; and (c) increased gut bacterial translocation leading to the production of bacterial products such as endotoxins and tumor necrosis factor α ((TNF-α), which are themselves vasodilators, causing splanchnic vasodilatation.

translocation, increased mesenteric angiogenesis, and hyporesponsiveness of the splanchnic vessels to vasoconstrictors, also contribute to the splanchnic vasodilatation and maintenance of the increased portal inflow (Fig. 15.4) [24].

Independent of the portal hypertension-related hemodynamic changes that occur in the splanchnic circulation and that eventually affect the systemic circulation, sinusoidal portal hypertension per se also has a direct effect

on the renal circulation. For example, the infusion of glutamine into the mesenteric vein – which enters the portal circulation, causing hepatocyte swelling that increases hepatic sinusoidal pressure, mimicking portal hypertension – has been shown to result in a reduction of GFR. The same glutamine, when infused into the jugular vein, has no effect on the renal circulation [25]. In cirrhotic patients who have a patent transjugular intrahepatic portosystemic stent (TIPS) shunt and therefore no portal hypertension, the placement and subsequent inflation of an angioplasty balloon into the TIPS tract instantly recreates portal hypertension, associated with an almost instantaneous reduction of renal blood flow. Deflation of the angioplasty balloon removes the portal hypertension and results in an immediate return of the renal blood flow to baseline levels [26]. Finally, lumbar sympathetic blockade in patients with HRS has been shown to increase renal blood flow, suggesting that the renal sympathetic activity is implicated in the efferent arm of this hepatorenal reflex [27].

Hemodynamic changes and circulatory dysfunction in cirrhosis

Although the splanchnic circulation is the major site of arterial vasodilatation in cirrhosis, the presence of portal hypertension can lead to the opening of portosystemic shunts, which divert some of the splanchnic blood to the systemic circulation. It is possible that excess vasodilators are being shunted from the splanchnic to the systemic circulation, causing either a direct vasodilatory effect on the systemic circulation or an increase in the release of nitric oxide, or both. The systemic circulation initially responds to the vasodilatation or reduction in systemic vascular resistance by increasing its cardiac output, and by improving the intravascular volume through renal sodium retention, thereby maintaining hemodynamic stability [28]. However, as the liver cirrhosis advances, arterial vasodilatation continues. In the splanchnic circulation, the increased portal inflow together with increased resistance to portal flow means that there is pooling of blood in this vascular bed. In the systemic circulation, the progressive arterial vasodilatation is compensated for by a further rise in cardiac output and more avid renal sodium retention. Therefore, the total blood volume is increased. However, the maldistribution of the blood volume to the splanchnic circulation means that there is effectively a subtraction of volume from the systemic circulation, despite no actual loss of total blood volume, akin to a splanchnic steal syndrome. This condition is known as a "reduction in the effective arterial blood volume." Therefore, the systemic circulation becomes more hyperdynamic and other compensatory mechanisms are recruited to maintain hemodynamic stability (Fig. 15.5).

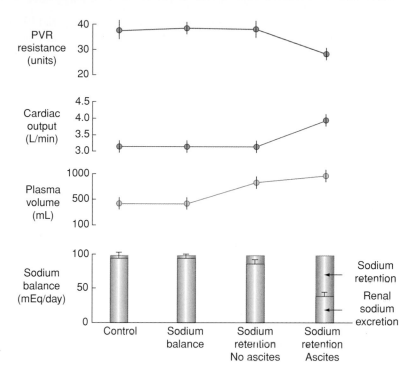

Figure 15.5 Schematic representation of hemodynamic changes and sodium retention during various stages in the natural history of cirrhosis. PVR, peripheral vascular resistance. (Adapted from Oliver and Verna [29].)

Excess renal vasoconstriction versus insufficient renal vasodilators

One of the consequences of a reduction in the effective arterial blood volume is the activation of various compensatory vasoconstrictor systems. These include the renin–angiotensin system, the sympathetic nervous system, and the nonosmotic release of vasopressin. Since the renal circulation is particularly sensitive to the effects of these vasoconstrictors, there is a decrease in renal blood flow with a consequent reduction in GFR. The relative renal ischemia from vasoconstriction of the renal artery also increases the production of various intrarenal vasoconstrictors such as angiotensin II, adenosine, and endothelin, causing further deterioration of renal hemodynamics and renal function. Normally, the kidneys maintain the renal circulation by increasing the production of renal vasodilators, which include nitric oxide, prostaglandins, and members of the natriuretic peptide family such as urodilatin. However, an overall reduction in the production of renal vasodilators in the presence of excess vasoconstrictors in advanced cirrhosis will render the cirrhotic patient susceptible to the development of renal failure. Any event that further disturbs this vasoconstrictor–vasodilator balance favoring the vasoconstrictors will precipitate renal failure [29].

Abnormal renal autoregulation in advanced cirrhosis

Acute renal failure in cirrhosis is not simply a case of too many vasoconstrictors versus too few vasodilators,

otherwise reducing the mismatch between the extent of arterial vasodilatation and the volume within the circulation by improving the effective arterial blood volume should reverse every case of renal failure in cirrhosis. It has been adequately shown in various treatment studies that albumin alone, which improves the intravascular volume, does not have any effect on the renal impairment in patients with HRS [30,31]. Changes in renal autoregulation in advanced cirrhosis also contribute to the further development of renal dysfunction in these patients. Renal autoregulation is the process whereby regulatory mechanisms ensure that the kidneys receive an approximately constant blood supply regardless of the day-to-day fluctuations in blood pressure. In healthy individuals, renal autoregulation is operational above a renal perfusion pressure of >65 mmHg. Below that level, renal perfusion falls in proportion to renal perfusion pressure. However, in cirrhosis, there is a shift of the autoregulation curve to the right [32]; the more severe the cirrhosis, the more the renal autoregulation curve moves to the right. That is, as the cirrhosis process advances, for every given level of renal perfusion pressure, the renal blood flow progressively falls. Therefore, in end-stage cirrhosis, despite a decent renal perfusion pressure, the renal blood flow is severely compromised (Fig. 15.6).

Abnormal cardiac function in cirrhosis

The hyperdynamic circulation observed in cirrhosis is thought to be a compensatory mechanism in response to the decreased systemic vascular resistance to maintain

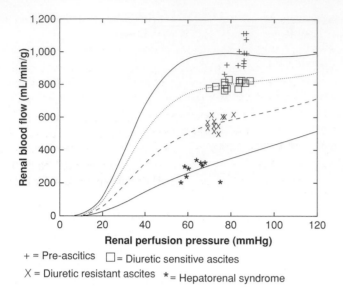

+ = Pre-ascitics   □ = Diuretic sensitive ascites

X = Diuretic resistant ascites   * = Hepatorenal syndrome

Figure 15.6 Changes in renal autoregulation with advancing stages of cirrhosis. (Adapted from Stadlbauer et al. [32] with permission from Nature Publishing Group.)

hemodynamic stability. This also means that patients with decompensated cirrhosis are encroaching on their cardiac reserve, and therefore any further reduction in the systemic vascular resistance may not be met with a similar increase in cardiac output. This is known as systolic incompetence, which can be brought out when there is further arterial vasodilatation such as during an episode of bacterial infection. When this happens, the circulation starts to fail, the blood pressure falls, and the renal circulation can be compromised and HRS can be precipitated. This systolic incompetence is now recognized as part of a syndrome known as cirrhotic cardiomyopathy, which also includes diastolic dysfunction and electrophysiologic abnormalities [33]. Indeed, in patients with cirrhosis and ascites, a relative low cardiac output and high plasma renin activity were significant predictors for the development of HRS [34]. A recent study indicated a correlation between low cardiac output, low mean arterial pressure, and low renal blood flow, supporting the role of cirrhotic cardiomyopathy in contributing to the development of renal failure in cirrhosis [35]. In a cohort of cirrhotic patients with ascites and spontaneous bacterial peritonitis, those who went on to develop HRS had significantly lower cardiac output at the time of infection resolution when compared to baseline, and also when compared to those who did not develop HRS at the time of infection resolution [36].

Factors that can precipitate functional renal failure in cirrhosis

Given the fact that one of the pathogenetic mechanisms for renal failure in cirrhosis is a reduction of effective arte-

rial blood volume secondary to systemic vasodilatation, any event that reduces the circulatory volume further, or increases the extent of arterial vasodilatation, will likely precipitate acute renal failure in these patients. Therefore events such as gastrointestinal bleed, overdiuresis, excess vomiting, or diarrhea can all cause intravascular volume contraction, and put the cirrhotic patient at risk for the development of acute renal failure.

However, bacterial infections are by far the commonest cause of acute renal failure in cirrhosis. In fact, renal failure occurs in approximately one third of patients with bacterial infections [37,38]. This is related to the fact that the proinflammatory response in a host with cirrhosis is significantly enhanced. The myriads of inflammatory cytokines, such as tumor necrosis factor α and interleukin 6, released by the bacteria can induce various changes in the microcirculation of many organs including the kidneys. These include impairment of capillary flow due to the development of microthrombi, endothelial dysfunction as a result of impairment in mitochondrial respiration related to nitric oxide overproduction, and increased capillary permeability leading to capillary leaks. The end result is decreased perfusion and cellular injury in the organs affected [39]. Since the renal circulation in cirrhosis is hypoperfused in advanced cirrhosis, further compromise of the renal circulation with bacterial infection places the patient at great risk for acute renal failure. The incidence of renal impairment is most significant among patients with a serum bilirubin level >4 mg/dL (68 μmol/L) and a serum creatinine level >1 mg/dL (88 μmol/L), that is, patients who have some degree of liver dysfunction and underlying renal impairment [40].

Various drugs can also precipitate acute renal failure in cirrhosis. NSAIDs inhibit the synthesis of prostaglandins and therefore put cirrhotic patients at risk for acute renal failure since renal prostaglandins are important in maintaining the intrarenal circulation. Cirrhotic patients who have coexisting diabetes are often given angiotensin II antagonists for renal protection. Since cirrhotic patients are dependent on the activated renin–angiotensin system to maintain systemic blood pressure, the use of these agents can result in arterial hypotension and renal failure in these patients.

Clinical presentation of functional renal failure

There are no specific clinical features that can identify a cirrhotic patient who is developing FRF. The patient is usually ill with severe cirrhosis and ascites with or without jaundice or hepatic encephalopathy. Laboratory tests usually reveal hyperbilirubinemia, hypoalbuminemia, anemia, coagulopathy, and thrombocytopenia. For those patients who are on diuretics, electrolyte abnormalities such as hyponatremia or hyperkalemia are common. Renal function can slowly deteriorate over weeks to months, due to the progressive hemodynamic changes that occur with advanced cirrhosis. When the serum creatinine reaches 1.5 mg/dL (133 μmol/L), the patient is said to have chronic or type 2 HRS [12] and this tends to follow a slowly downhill course. Occasionally, the renal function can spontaneously deteriorate rapidly, and this can be an episode that occurs in a patient whose serum creatinine suddenly rises from a normal level to higher than 1.5 mg/dL, or a patient who already has type 2 HRS suddenly shows an increase of serum creatinine to >2.5 mg/dL (220 μmol/L). More often, there is an event that precipitates a sudden worsening of renal function, and this is usually an episode of infection. Many of these episodes of acute renal failure are responsive to intravascular volume replacement, which can return the serum creatinine to baseline levels. Such episodes of acute renal failure are said to be episodes of prerenal renal failure. If the rise in serum creatinine reaches more than 2.5 mg/dL (220 μmol/L) in less than 2 weeks, associated with non-responsiveness to intravascular volume replacement, the patient is said to have acute or type 1 HRS [12].

Therefore, regular monitoring of renal function in patients with cirrhosis and ascites is of paramount importance, and the clinician caring for these patients has to be vigilant for potential clinical events that could precipitate acute deterioration in renal function. When a patient presents with a change in clinical state, whether it is the development of jaundice, excessive bruising, or hepatic encephalopathy, every effort should be made to exclude the development of acute renal failure and/or infection. The patient needs to be assessed for evidence of gastrointestinal blood loss, or dehydration from excess diuretic doses, or evidence of infection such as fever and tachycardia. Blood has to be taken for liver function and renal function tests. A full blood examination needs to be done to assess for leukocytosis or a fall in hemoglobin. A full septic workup including a chest X-ray, two sets of blood culture, ascitic fluid culture, and urine culture also need to be performed. An abdominal ultrasound and urinalysis, as well as a 24-hour urine collection, will need to be performed to exclude organic causes of renal failure (Table 15.4).

Management of functional renal failure including hepatorenal syndrome

General measures

Initial management of these patients requires the exclusion of reversible or treatable conditions. A diligent search

Table 15.4 Evaluation of patient who presents with acute deterioration of renal function

Type of evaluation	Investigations
Clinical assessment	Enquire about:
	excess diuretic doses
	excess fluid loss such as vomiting/diarrhea
	gastrointestinal bleeds
	potential nephrotoxic drugs
	fever, or symptoms to suggest infection
	Physical examination to look for:
	dehydration
	anemia
	evidence of infection
	worsening liver function
Laboratory tests	Liver function tests: INR, bilirubin, protein, albumin
	Liver enzymes: AST, ALT, ALP
	Renal function: daily serum creatinine and electrolytes
	Complete blood count: hemoglobin and white cell count
Full septic workup	Blood cultures × 2
	Urine culture
	Ascitic fluid cell count and culture
	Chest X-ray
Exclude other causes of renal failure	Abdominal ultrasound to assess kidney sizes and exclude bladder neck obstruction
	Urinalysis to assess for casts and sediments
	24-hour urine collection to assess for proteinuria

ALP, alkaline phosphatase; ALT, alanine transaminase; AST, aspartate transaminase; INR, international normalized ratio.

should be made for precipitating factors (infection, gastrointestinal bleeding) and treated accordingly (Fig. 15.7). Likewise nephrotoxic drugs should be removed. Cirrhotic patients with acute gastrointestinal bleed, poor liver function, and renal failure preferably should be managed in intensive care units to protect effective circulating blood volume and renal perfusion. Patients whose renal failure is due to hypovolemia from gastrointestinal bleeding should receive volume replacement in the form of blood or blood products. Arrangements should be made to perform endoscopies as soon as feasible.

Albumin as volume replacement therapy

Since one of the pathogenetic mechanisms for the development of FRF is a relative reduction in effective arterial blood volume, it stands to reason to replenish the intravascular volume. Albumin is preferred over normal saline as albumin is hypertonic to plasma and therefore able to maintain oncotic pressure better than saline, which can be easily transferred to the peritoneal cavity to

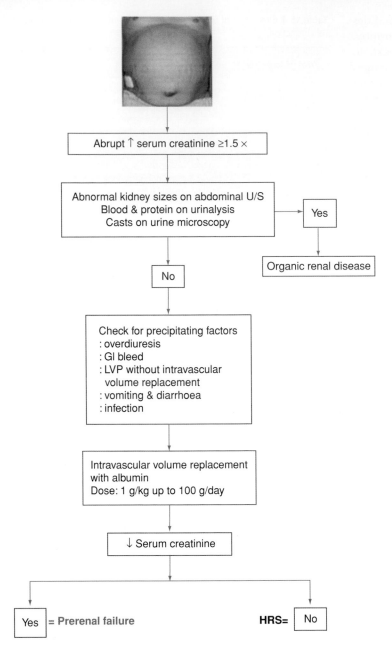

Abrupt ↑ serum creatinine ≥1.5 ×

Abnormal kidney sizes on abdominal U/S
Blood & protein on urinalysis
Casts on urine microscopy

Yes

Organic renal disease

No

Check for precipitating factors
: overdiuresis
: GI bleed
: LVP without intravascular
  volume replacement
: vomiting & diarrhoea
: infection

Intravascular volume replacement
with albumin
Dose: 1 g/kg up to 100 g/day

↓ Serum creatinine

Yes   = Prerenal failure   HRS=   No

Figure 15.7 Suggested algorithm to differentiate the various causes of renal failure in a cirrhotic patient with ascites who presents with an acute rise in serum creatinine. GI, gastrointestinal; HRS, hepatorenal syndrome; LVP, large volume paracentesis; U/S, ultrasound.

worsen the ascites. In addition, albumin is a negatively charged molecule, which has ligand-binding, antioxidant, and endothelial protective properties [41]. Therefore, albumin potentially can also reduce the extent of systemic arterial vasodilatation by binding various vasodilators. Patients with prerenal renal failure should respond to volume replacement with albumin, with a gradual reduction of serum creatinine back to baseline levels. The International Ascites Club recommends an albumin dose of 1 g/kg up to 100 g/day [12].

Hepatorenal syndrome by definition is a diagnosis of exclusion and, therefore, patients with HRS will not respond to volume replacement with albumin. It has

certainly been demonstrated that albumin alone is ineffective in the treatment of HRS [31]. There is some suggestion that albumin may not have any additional beneficial effects on renal function when used in combination with vasoconstrictors in the treatment of HRS. The largest retrospective study on the use of a vasoconstrictor, terlipressin, for HRS did not find any difference in the outcome of patients irrespective of whether albumin was added to terlipressin or not [42]. However, there is actually no study comparing vasoconstrictor therapy with or without albumin. Given the fact that there is no evidence that albumin actually does harm, it seems prudent to use albumin in the treatment of HRS. The International

Ascites Club recommends the use of 20–40 g of albumin per day in combination with vasoconstrictors, after an initial dose of 1 g/kg of body weight up to 100 g/day on the initial 2 days [12].

Treatment of hepatorenal syndrome

Vasoconstrictor therapy

The rationale of using systemic vasoconstrictors is to reduce the extent of the systemic vasodilatation. Their use should lead to a rise in the systemic arterial blood pressure, which in turn will improve the renal perfusion pressure. In addition, there will be a reduction in the difference between the vascular capacitance and the blood volume within in. The resultant improvement in the effective arterial blood volume will lead to a dampening of the activities of the various vasoconstrictors, thereby decreasing the renal vasoconstriction, with overall improvement in renal blood flow and glomerular filtration.

Terlipressin

Terlipressin is a vasopressin analog and has a similar mode of action as vasopressin but without many of the potential ischemic side effects. It is essentially a vasoconstrictor for both the systemic and splanchnic circulations. Its efficacy as a treatment for type 1 HRS has been reported in two large randomized controlled trials [31,43]. The infusion of terlipressin at a dose of 0.5–2 mg/4–6 hours intravenously for up to 15 days was associated with a reduction of serum creatinine to less than 1.5 mg/dL in 34–43% of patients. Treatment-related serious side effects were not excessive (9% and 22% in the two studies) and these included abdominal cramps and increased bowel movements, arrhythmia, and ischemia to the bowels, heart, and limbs. Upon withdrawal of terlipressin, the recurrence of HRS was infrequent. In those patients whose HRS recurred, retreatment with the same dose of terlipressin invariably led to the same favorable response [31,43]. There was no overall improvement in survival with terlipressin over placebo. However, in the subgroup of patients who responded to terlipressin with reversal of HRS, there was a significant increase in survival [43]. Recent meta-analyses of all the terlipressin studies have also not shown a significant improvement in survival with terlipressin [44,45]. However, when terlipressin was analyzed together with other vasoconstrictors used in the treatment of HRS, there was a slight improvement of survival favoring the vasoconstrictors [46]. It is not clear how much weight the terlipressin studies had on the outcome of the meta-analysis of all vasoconstrictors. However, if the outcome is even slightly improved, then the use of terlipressin may be sufficient to allow these patients to wait for a liver transplant. Predictors of response to terlipressin include a bilirubin level of <10 mg/dL and a rise in mean arterial pressure by >5 mmHg on day 3 of treatment [47]. In those patients who do not respond to terlipressin, the prognosis remains poor.

Terlipressin has also been used in a total of 43 patients with type 2 HRS with similar response rates [48–51]. However, the number of patients studied is too small to draw any firm conclusions on its use for type 2 HRS patients.

Norepinephrine

In a pilot study of 12 patients with cirrhosis, refractory ascites, and type 1 HRS, the use of intravenous norepinephrine (0.5–3 mg/h) in combination with albumin and intravenous furosemide resulted in the reversal of HRS in ten of the 12 patients after a median of 7 days [52]. In a follow-up study, comparing the efficacy of norepinephrine versus terlipressin in the treatment for both type 1 and type 2 HRS, norepinephrine resulted in a 70% complete response rate compared to that of ≥80% with terlipressin [50]. The response rate in this study is higher than expected, perhaps due to the large number of patients with type 2 HRS included in the study. Nonetheless, the results are very encouraging, especially since the patients receiving norepinephrine did not have significant ischemic side effects. Most of the patients in the study received a liver transplant within 1 month after completion of vasoconstrictor therapy, making it impossible to assess the role of improved renal function on ascites elimination and on survival.

In another head-to-head study comparing the efficacy of norepinephrine versus terlipressin in the management of type 1 HRS, 20 patients who received 0.5–3 mg/h of norepinephrine as a continuous infusion were compared to 20 patients who received 0.5–2 mg/4–6 hours of terlipressin as boluses [53]. There was no significant difference in terms of the response rate (ten patients in the norepinephrine group versus eight patients in the terlipressin group), associated with significant and similar reductions in plasma renin activity, suggesting that both drugs had induced a marked improvement in the effective arterial blood volume. The ischemic side effects were similar in both groups. The authors concluded that norepinephrine could be an effective and safe alternative to terlipressin as a treatment for HRS without the attendant high costs.

Midodrine and octreotide

Midodrine is an α-agonist that improves systemic blood pressure and hence improves renal perfusion pressure. Traditionally, it has been used in the management of postural hypotension. Despite this, midodrine alone has not been shown to be effective in patients with HRS [54]. Octreotide is a long-acting analog of somatostatin, which antagonizes the action of various splanchnic vasodilators and potentially can reduce the extent of splanchnic vasodilatation. The use of octreotide alone also has not been proven to be useful for patients with HRS [55]. However, when midodrine is combined with octreotide and plasma volume expansion with albumin, several studies, both prospective [56,57] and retrospective [58], have shown a significant reduction in serum creatinine, although renal function does not return to normal despite suppression of all measured neurohormonal systems to within their normal ranges. The systemic and renal hemodynamics, and urinary sodium excretion, all improve in patients with type 1 HRS but remain at subnormal levels. The doses used differed between the various studies. In general, the dose of midodrine was titrated to reach a mean arterial blood pressure of at least 90 mmHg, with a starting dose varying between 2.5 and 7.5 mg t.i.d. Likewise, octreotide can be given either subcutaneously at a dose of 100 µg t.i.d. or intravenously at 25 µg/h after an initial bolus of 25 µg. Recent retrospective data suggest that the combination can also improve short-term survival for up to 3 months [58,59]. Clearly, larger randomized controlled trials are needed to establish the combination as an effective treatment for type 1 HRS. Despite this, the combination is very popular in North America as a treatment for HRS because of the nonavailability of terlipressin. However, with the pharmaceutic industry actively trying to have terlipressin approved in North America, these randomized controlled trials may never be done.

Transjugular intrahepatic portosystemic stent shunt

Since sinusoidal portal hypertension is the initiator of the hemodynamic changes that lead to relative renal ischemia and hence decreased renal function, it makes physiologic sense to reduce the sinusoidal portal pressure with TIPS insertion. In addition, TIPS returns a significant portion of the splanchnic volume into the systemic circulation, leading to suppression of various vasoactive neurohormones and resulting in better renal perfusion.

To date, there are no controlled studies assessing the efficacy of TIPS for the management of HRS. Of the eight studies published so far [57,60–66], most have focused on patients with type 1 HRS, while two studies assessed a mixed population of type 1 and type 2 HRS patients [60,61], and one study only included type 2 HRS patients [62]. TIPS produced an improvement in renal function in all reported studies, associated with a significant suppression of the endogenous vasoactive systems [61]. The improvement was observed to last for up to 6 months in the study that had the longest duration of follow-up [61]. Despite the improvement in renal function, neither the GFR nor the renal plasma flow returned to normal in the studies where this was systematically examined [57,66]. Ascites was also reported to decrease significantly.

TIPS appears to confer a survival advantage over conventional medical treatment, with one study reporting an 18-month survival of 35% [61]. This may be related to the fact that TIPS can only be inserted in patients with relatively preserved hepatic function, thereby preselecting patients whose survival would have been expected to be reasonable even without TIPS. It is interesting to note that TIPS has not been cited in any recent publications on the treatment for HRS, suggesting that other treatment modalities may have supplanted its use. However, in the latest review on the clinical applications for TIPS, it has been suggested that it should be considered as a treatment for HRS in those patients whose liver function is relatively preserved, such as abstinent alcoholics, and/or patients who are candidates for liver transplantation [67].

Combined vasoconstrictor therapy and TIPS

The combination of vasoconstrictor therapy followed by TIPS effectively corrects different aspects of the pathophysiology of HRS, namely the elimination of portal hypertension and reduction of the extent of systemic arterial vasodilatation. Therefore, combination therapy should have an additive effect in improving renal function in patients with HRS. Midodrine, octreotide, and albumin were administered to 14 patients with type 1 HRS [57]. In those patients who responded to pharmacotherapy with improvement of renal function, TIPS insertion followed in those who were deemed suitable for such a procedure, and this normalized renal function over the course of 12 months and allowed the eventual elimination of ascites. The overall survival rate was 50%, with the longest patient surviving 30 months. In another study, 11 patients with type 2 HRS received terlipressin together with albumin, which maintained the central venous pressure to 10 cmH$_2$O [49]. TIPS placement was possible for nine of the 11 patients who showed a reduction in serum creatinine with terlipressin. The combination eventually brought the serum creatinine down to 1.36 ± 0.3 mg/dL at 1 month post TIPS. As expected, TIPS improved 24-hour urinary volume in all patients, leading to a lower postprocedure diuretic requirement. Ascites also significantly decreased in all patients and eventually disappeared from the second week onwards after TIPS [49,57].

Extracorporal albumin dialysis

Extracorporeal albumin dialysis is a procedure that uses a cell-free albumin-containing dialysate to remove albumin-bound substances, including bilirubin, bile acids, aromatic amino acids, medium chain fatty acids, and cytokines [68]. One such system is the molecular adsorbent recycling system or MARS. The rationale for using MARS to treat HRS is because some of the cytokines and bile acids are vasoactive substances. Therefore, they could be contributing to the vasodilatation and consequent reduction in effective arterial blood volume that is central to the pathogenesis of HRS. In a prospective, randomized controlled study, MARS improved clinical and biochemical parameters as well as survival in eight patients with type 1 HRS who were not candidates for TIPS insertion, when compared with a well-matched group of patients who were treated with volume expansion and standard dialysis [69]. In another study of eight patients with acute liver failure, five of whom had established HRS, the use of MARS also led to similar results [70]. In both studies, serum creatinine was used as a marker of renal function. Creatinine is a water-soluble compound, and therefore can be removed during dialysis with MARS treatment. In another study on MARS for HRS, renal function was assessed using inulin clearance as an index of GFR, while simultaneously measuring serum creatinine [71]. As expected, the serum creatinine decreased during the course of MARS treatment, while inulin clearance or GFR remained low and unchanged. Cessation of MARS treatment led to a prompt return of serum creatinine to the pretreatment elevated levels. Therefore, the seemingly beneficial effect of MARS on serum creatinine is transient and artificial. Furthermore, MARS is a very expensive therapy and is demanding on physician and nursing time. Based on the findings of the latest study, MARS may not be recommended for type 1 HRS in cirrhotic patients with refractory ascites.

Renal replacement therapy

Dialysis has been ineffective in the management of HRS [72,73]. The systemic hypotension induced by hemodialysis often compromises the patient's hemodynamic instability even further. However, in the patients who have potentially reversible liver damage due to toxins or sepsis, dialysis may have a role in supporting the patient over the critical period. In patients who are awaiting liver transplantation, dialysis may be life saving as a bridging therapy [74]. The use of continuous arteriovenous hemofiltration may prove to be more effective as the procedure induces less hypotension [75]. Careful maintenance of circulating blood volume and cardiac filling pressures is key to successful dialysis in suitably selected patients.

Liver transplantation

Liver transplantation is the definitive treatment for HRS. It corrects liver dysfunction and eliminates portal hypertension. The main limiting factor is the availability of donor organs, and many patients die while waiting for one. The model for end-stage liver disease (MELD) scoring system of organ allocation means that cirrhotic patients with severe liver dysfunction and renal failure are given preference for earlier transplantation [76]. Renal function improves in many patients with HRS after trans-

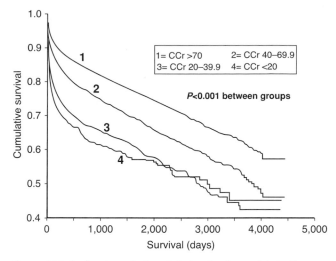

Figure 15.8 Pre liver transplant renal dysfunction is associated with a significantly reduced survival after transplant. CCr, creatinine clearance. (Adapted from Nair et al. [80] with permission from Plenum Publishers.)

plantation, associated with a reduction in plasma levels of vasoactive factors [77]. However, up to 40% of patients can remain dependent on dialysis after liver transplantation [78]. This may be related to the persistence of the hyperdynamic circulation with high cardiac output and high splanchnic blood flow after liver transplantation [79]. The presence of pretransplant renal dysfunction predicts a worse outcome after liver transplantation with a longer stay in intensive care units, longer hospitalization, more dialysis treatments, and reduced survival (Fig. 15.8) [80,81]. In addition, patients with HRS who are transplanted have a lower probability of both graft and patient survival after liver transplantation, compared with patients without HRS [82]. However, treatment of HRS with vasoconstrictors before liver transplant can improve the post-transplant outcome [83]. Longer follow-up is required to confirm that pretransplant normalization of renal function will improve post-transplant survival.

Because of the fact that not all patients with HRS will recover their renal function post transplant, there have been efforts to identify early those patients who will not do well after liver transplant and offer them a combined liver–kidney transplant (CLKT). Since the implementation of the MELD scoring system for the allocation of donor organs for liver transplantation, the number of patients who possibly need CLKT has risen significantly. Despite established guidelines, it is still difficult to separate those patients with structural renal disease from those with HRS, especially since HRS may evolve into acute tubular necrosis if the renal failure persists. The presence of alcoholic hepatitis, a need for pretransplant dialysis [78], as well as a duration of dialysis for more than 8 weeks pretransplant [84] have been found to be

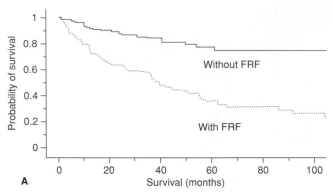
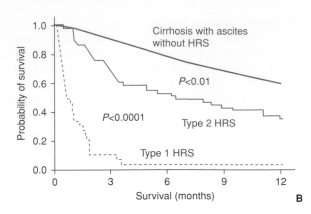

Figure 15.9 Actuarial probability of survival: (A) in patients with or without functional renal failure (FRF); and (B) in patients with hepatorenal syndrome (HRS). (Adapted from Montoliu et al. [2] with permission from Elsevier; Alessandria et al. [87] with permission from Plenum Publishers.)

predictors of poor renal recovery post transplant. Therefore, it has been proposed that patients who have had more than 8–12 weeks of pretransplant dialysis should be considered for CLKT [84,85]. However, recent data suggest that a wait-and-see approach is preferred, as patient and graft survivals are inferior for CLKT when compared to a liver transplant alone [86]. Therefore, there is merit in performing a liver transplant first and then considering a kidney transplant if there is no renal recovery after the first transplant.

Prognosis

The prognosis of patients with cirrhosis and FRF is poor [2]; this is in part related to the associated liver failure. Compared to patients with advanced cirrhosis but with-

out FRF, who have an 80% survival over 8 years, the 50% survival of these patients is reduced to 40 months (Fig. 15.9A). When HRS develops, survival without treatment is reduced even further (Fig. 15.9B) [87], with a median survival for type 1 HRS of 10 days. Predictive factors for the development of FRF in cirrhosis include advancing age, rising serum creatinine, and a high Child–Pugh score (Table 15.5) [2]. Once the patient has developed FRF, independent predictors of poor prognosis include advancing age, a high MELD score, a high Child–Pugh score, hyponatremia, and the presence of HRS [2,88]. If the patient has established type 1 HRS, a Child–Pugh score of >10, a MELD score of >20, and

Table 15.5 Predictive factors for the development of functional renal failure and for the survival of cirrhotic patients after the development of functional renal failure.

Condition	Predictors
Functional renal failure	Increasing age
	Increasing serum creatinine
	High Child–Pugh score
Poor survival after the development of functional renal failure	Increasing age
	High Child–Pugh score
	High MELD score
	Hyponatremia
	Presence of HRS
Poor survival after the development of type 1 HRS	Child–Pugh score >10
	MELD score >20
	Nonresponsiveness to treatment

HRS, hepatorenal syndrome; MELD, model for end-stage liver disease. Adapted from Montoliu et al. [2], Alessandria et al. [87], Schepke et al. [88], and Appenrodt et al. [89].

Table 15.6 Prevention of functional renal failure.

Condition	Action
Diuretic use	Frequent monitoring of electrolytes and serum creatinine
	Be willing to withdraw diuretics when there are electrolyte abnormalities or a rise in serum creatinine occurs
Gastrointestinal blood loss	Prompt replacement of intravascular blood volume
	Administer antibiotic prophylaxis to prevent infection
Bacterial infection	Administer albumin 20-40 mg/day in patients with a serum bilirubin level >4 mg/dL (68 μmol/L) and serum creatinine level >1 mg/dL (88 μmol/L)
Low ascitic fluid protein (<15 g/L), with poor liver renal functions [90]	Long-term norfloxacin 400 mg/day in patients with a serum bilirubin >3 mg/dL, Child–Pugh score >10, serum sodium <130 mmol/L, and serum creatinine >1.2 mg/dL to reduce the risk of infection
Nephrotoxic drugs	Do not administer nonsteroidal anti-inflammatory agents

failure to respond to treatment will predict an adverse outcome [87,89]. Therefore, to improve the overall prognosis of these patients, the treating clinician will need to be vigilant for tell-tale signs of impending liver failure and/or kidney failure, and to promptly correct any clinical or laboratory abnormalities to prevent the development of FRF (Table 15.6). The good news is that FRF used to be a condition with an almost certain fatal outcome, but is now rapidly becoming a treatable complication of liver cirrhosis.

Management protocol of functional renal failure in cirrhosis

A patient with cirrhosis and ascites presents with an acute increase in serum creatinine of 1.5 times baseline.

Initial assessment
- Enquire about:
  - Excess diuretic doses
  - Excess fluid loss such as vomiting/diarrhea
  - Gastrointestinal bleeds
  - Potential nephrotoxic drugs
  - Fever, or symptoms to suggest infection
- Physical examination for:
  - Dehydration
  - Anemia
  - Evidence of infection
  - Worsening liver function such as the development of jaundice or encephalopathy

Laboratory investigations
- Liver function tests: INR, bilirubin, protein, and albumin
- Liver enzymes: AST, ALT, and ALP
- Renal function: daily serum creatinine and electrolytes
- Complete blood count: hemoglobin and white cell count

Full septic workup
- Blood cultures ×2
- Urine culture
- Ascitic fluid cell count and culture
- Chest X-ray

Exclude other causes of renal failure
- Abdominal ultrasound to assess kidney sizes and exclude bladder neck obstruction
- Urinalysis to assess for casts and sediments
- 24-hour urine collection to assess for proteinuria

Initial management
- Intravascular volume expansion with albumin 1 g/kg up to a total dose of 100 g
- Empirical dose of an antibiotic such as a third generation cephalosporin until infection can be excluded. If infection is confirmed, change the antibiotic according to sensitivity testing
- If serum creatinine decreases with volume expansion, continue with daily albumin until the serum creatinine returns to baseline

- If serum creatinine does not change or increase despite volume expansion for 2 days, initiate treatment for hepatorenal syndrome

Treatment of hepatorenal syndrome
- Vasoconstrictor therapy:
  - Terlipressin as intravenous boluses 1–2 mg every 4–6 hours for 15 days, or
  - Norepinephrine 0.5–3 mg/h as a continuous infusion, or
  - Midodrine 2.5–7.5 mg orally t.i.d. plus octreotide either as 100 μg subcutaneous injections t.i.d. or as a continuous infusion of 25 μg/h after a 25 μg bolus
- A transjugular intrahepatic portosystemic stent shunt can be inserted either as a stand-alone treatment or following improvement of renal function with vasoconstrictor therapy in appropriate patients
- Renal replacement therapy is of no proven value unless patient is awaiting liver transplantation, and therefore needs dialysis as a bridge therapy

Liver transplantation
- Assessment should be initiated in all patients who do not have a contraindication for liver transplant
- Correction of renal function before transplant will significantly improve post-transplant survival

ALP, alkaline phosphatase; ALT, alanine transaminase; AST, aspartate transaminase; INR, international normalized ratio.

References

1. Garcia-Tsao G, Parikh CR, Viola A. Acute kidney injury in cirrhosis. *Hepatology* 2008;48:2064–77.
2. Montoliu S, Ballesté B, Planas R, et al. Incidence and prognosis of different types of functional renal failure in cirrhotic patients with ascites. *Clin Gastroenterol Hepatol* 2010;8:616–22.
3. Slack A, Yeoman A, Wendon J. Renal dysfunction in chronic liver disease. *Crit Care* 2010;14:214.
4. Neuschwander-Tetri BA, Clark JM, Bass NM, et al. Clinical, laboratory and histological associations in adults with nonalcoholic fatty liver disease. *Hepatology* 2010;52:913–24.
5. *Renal Data System. USRDS: 2006 Annual Data Report: atlas of end-stage renal disease in the United States.* Bethesda, MD: National Institute of Diabetes and Digestive and Kidney Disease, 2006.
6. Claria J, Kent JD, Lopez-Parra M, et al. Effects of celecoxib and naproxen on renal function in nonazotemic patients with cirrhosis and ascites. *Hepatology* 2005;41:579–87.
7. Blendis L, Wong F. The natural history and management of the hepatorenal disorders. From pre-ascites to hepatorenal syndrome. *Clin Med* 2003;3:154–9.
8. Arroyo V, Gines P, Gerbes AL, et al. Definition and diagnostic criteria of refractory ascites and hepatorenal syndrome in cirrhosis. *International Ascites Club.* Hepatology 1996;23:164–76.
9. Hecker R, Sherlock S. Electrolyte and circulatory changes in terminal liver failure. *Lancet* 1956;271:1121–5.
10. Papper S, Belsky JL, Bleifer KH. Renal failure in Laennec's cirrhosis of the liver. I. Description of clinical and laboratory features. *Ann Intern Med* 1959;51:759–73.
11. Epstein M, Berk DP, Hollenberg NK, et al. Renal failure in the patient with cirrhosis. The role of active vasoconstriction. *Am J Med* 1970;49:175–85.

12. Salerno F, Gerbes A, Gines P, et al. Diagnosis, prevention and treatment of hepatorenal syndrome in cirrhosis. *Gut* 2007;56: 1310–18.

13. Lassnigg A, Schmidlin D, Mouhieddine M, et al. Minimal changes of serum creatinine predict prognosis in patients after cardiothoracic surgery: a prospective cohort study. *J Am Soc Nephrol* 2004;15: 1597–605.

14. Caregaro L, Menon F, Angeli P, et al. Limitations of serum creatinine level and creatinine clearance as filtration markers in cirrhosis. *Arch Intern Med* 1994;154:201–5.

15. Francoz C, Glotz D, Moreau R, et al. The evaluation of renal function and disease in patients with cirrhosis. *J Hepatol* 2010;52:605–13.

16. Gines P, Guevara M, Arroyo V, et al. Hepatorenal syndrome. *Lancet* 2003;362:1819–27.

17. Bellomo R, Ronco C, Kellum JA, et al. Acute renal failure – definition, outcome measures, animal models, fluid therapy and information technology needs: the Second International Consensus Conference of the Acute Dialysis Quality Initiative (ADQI) Group. *Crit Care* 2004;8:R204–12.

18. Mehta RL, Kellum JA, Shah SV, et al. Acute Kidney Injury Network: report of an initiative to improve outcomes in acute kidney injury. *Crit Care* 2007;11:R31.

19. Praught ML, Shlipak MG. Are small changes in serum creatinine an important risk factor? *Curr Opin Nephro Hypertens* 2005;14:265–70.

20. Blendis L, Wong F. The hyperdynamic circulation in cirrhosis: an overview. *Pharmacol Ther* 2001;89:221–31.

21. Martin PY, Ginès P, Schrier RW. Nitric oxide as a mediator of hemodynamic abnormalities and sodium and water retention in cirrhosis. *N Engl J Med* 1998;339:533–41.

22. Van Landeghem L, Laleman W, Vander Elst I, et al. Carbon monoxide produced by intrasinusoidally located haem-oxygenase-1 regulates the vascular tone in cirrhotic rat liver. *Liver Int* 2009;29: 650–60.

23. Ros J, Clària J, To-Figueras J, et al. Endogenous cannabinoids: a new system involved in the homeostasis of arterial pressure in experimental cirrhosis in the rat. *Gastroenterology* 2002;122:85–93.

24. Colle I, Geerts AM, Van Steenkiste C, et al. Hemodynamic changes in splanchnic blood vessels in portal hypertension. *Anat Rec* 2008;291:699–713.

25. Lang F, Tschernko E, Schulze E, et al. Hepatorenal reflex regulating kidney function. *Hepatology* 1991;14:590–4.

26. Jalan R, Forrest EH, Redhead DN, et al. Reduction in renal blood flow following acute increase in the portal pressure: evidence for the existence of a hepatorenal reflex in man? *Gut* 1997;40:664–70.

27. Solis-Herruzo JA, Duran A, Favela V, et al. Effects of lumbar sympathetic block on kidney function in cirrhotic patients with hepatorenal syndrome. *J Hepatol* 1987;5:167–73.

28. Gines P, Schrier R. Renal failure in cirrhosis. *N Engl J Med* 2009; 361:1279–90.

29. Oliver JA, Verna EC. Afferent mechanisms of sodium retention in cirrhosis and hepatorenal syndrome. *Kidney Int* 2010;77:669–80.

30. Neri S, Pulvirenti D, Malaguarnera M, et al. Terlipressin and albumin in patients with cirrhosis and type I hepatorenal syndrome. *Dig Dis Sci* 2008;53:830–5.

31. Martín-Llahí M, Pépin MN, Guevara M, et al. Terlipressin and albumin vs. albumin in patients with cirrhosis and hepatorenal syndrome: a randomized study. *Gastroenterology* 2008;134:1352–9.

32. Stadlbauer V, Wright GA, Banaji M, et al. Relationship between activation of the sympathetic nervous system and renal blood flow autoregulation in cirrhosis. *Gastroenterology* 2008;134:111–19.

33. Wong F. Cirrhotic cardiomyopathy. *Hepatol Int* 2009;3:294–304.

34. Ruiz-del-Arbol L, Monescillo A, Arocena C, et al. Circulatory function and hepatorenal syndrome in cirrhosis. *Hepatology* 2005; 42:439–47.

35. Krag A, Bendtsen F, Henriksen JH, et al. Low cardiac output predicts development of hepatorenal syndrome and survival in patients with cirrhosis and ascites. *Gut* 2010;59:105–10.

36. Ruiz-del-Arbol L, Urman J, Fernandez J, et al. Systemic, renal, and hepatic hemodynamic derangement in cirrhotic patients with spontaneous bacterial peritonitis. *Hepatology* 2003;38:1210–18.

37. Follo A, Llovet JM, Navasa M, et al. Renal impairment after spontaneous bacterial peritonitis in cirrhosis: incidence, clinical course, predictive factors and prognosis. *Hepatology* 1994;20:1495–501.

38. Fasolato S, Angeli P, Dallagnese L, et al. Renal failure and bacterial infections in patients with cirrhosis: epidemiology and clinical features. *Hepatology* 2007;45:223–9.

39. Gustot T, Durand F, Lebrec D, et al. Severe sepsis in cirrhosis. *Hepatology* 2009;50:2022–33.

40. Sort P, Navasa M, Arroyo V, et al. Effect of intravenous albumin on renal impairment and mortality in patients with cirrhosis and spontaneous bacterial peritonitis. *N Engl J Med* 1999;341:403–9.

41. Peters T Jr. Serum albumin. *Adv Protein Chem* 1997;45:153–203.

42. Moreau R, Durand F, Poynard T, et al. Terlipressin in patients with cirrhosis and type 1 hepatorenal syndrome: a retrospective multicenter study. *Gastroenterology* 2002;122:923–30.

43. Sanyal AJ, Boyer T, Garcia-Tsao G, et al. A randomized, prospective, double-blind, placebo-controlled trial of terlipressin for type 1 hepatorenal syndrome. *Gastroenterology* 2008;134:1360–8.

44. Fabrizi F, Dixit V, Messa P, et al. Terlipressin for hepatorenal syndrome: a meta-analysis of randomized trials. *Int J Artif Organs* 2009;32:133–40.

45. Sagi SV, Mittal S, Kasturi KS, et al. Terlipressin therapy for reversal of type 1 hepatorenal syndrome: a meta-analysis of randomized controlled trials. *J Gastroenterol Hepatol* 2010;25:880–5.

46. Gluud LL, Christensen K, Christensen E, et al. Systematic review of randomized trials on vasoconstrictor drugs for hepatorenal syndrome. *Hepatology* 2010;51:576–84.

47. Nazar A, Pereira GH, Guevara M, et al. Predictors of response to therapy with terlipressin and albumin in patients with cirrhosis and type 1 hepatorenal syndrome. *Hepatology* 2010;51:219–26.

48. Ortega R, Gines P, Uriz J, et al. Terlipressin therapy with and without albumin for patients with hepatorenal syndrome: results of a prospective, nonrandomized study. *Hepatology* 2002;36: 941–8.

49. Alessandria C, Venon WD, Marzano A, et al. Renal failure in cirrhotic patients: role of terlipressin in clinical approach to hepatorenal syndrome type 2. *Eur J Gastroenterol Hepatol* 2002;14:1363–8.

50. Alessandria C, Ottobrelli A, Debernardi-Venon W, et al. Noradrenalin vs. terlipressin in patients with hepatorenal syndrome: a prospective, randomized, unblinded, pilot study. *J Hepatol* 2007;47: 499–50.

51. Testro AG, Wongseelashote S, Angus PW, et al. Long-term outcome of patients treated with terlipressin for types 1 and 2 hepatorenal syndrome. *J Gastroenterol Hepatol* 2008;23:1535–40.

52. Duvoux C, Zanditenas D, Hezode C, et al. Effects of noradrenalin and albumin in patients with type I hepatorenal syndrome: a pilot study. *Hepatology* 2002;36:374–80.

53. Sharma P, Kumar A, Shrama BC et al. An open label, pilot, randomized controlled trial of noradrenaline versus terlipressin in the treatment of type 1 hepatorenal syndrome and predictors of response. *Am J Gastroenterol* 2008;103:1689–97.

54. Angeli P, Volpin R, Piovan D, et al. Acute effects of the oral administration of midodrine, an α-adrenergic agonist, on renal hemodynamics and renal function in cirrhotic patients with ascites. *Hepatology* 1998;28:937–43.

55. Pomier-Layrargues G, Paquin SC, Hassoun Z, et al. Octreotide in hepatorenal syndrome: a randomized, double blind, placebo-controlled, crossover study. *Hepatology* 2003;38:238–43.

56. Angeli P, Volpin R, Gerunda G, et al. Reversal of type 1 hepatorenal syndrome with the administration of midodrine and octreotide. *Hepatology* 1999;29:1690–7.

57. Wong F, Pantea L, Sniderman K. The use of midodrine, octreotide and transjugular intrahepatic portosystemic stent shunt in the treatment of cirrhotic patients with ascites and renal dysfunction including hepatorenal syndrome. *Hepatology* 2004;40:55–64.

58. Skagen C, Einstein M, Lucey MR, et al. Combination treatment with octreotide, midodrine, and albumin improves survival in patients with type 1 and type 2 hepatorenal syndrome. *J Clin Gastroenterol* 2009;43:680–5.

59. Esrailian E, Pantangco ER, Kyulo NL, et al. Octreotide/midodrine therapy significantly improves renal function and 30-day survival in patients with type 1 hepatorenal syndrome. *Dig Dis Sci* 2007;52: 742–8.

60. Brensing KA, Textor J, Strunk H, et al. Transjugular intrahepatic portosystemic stent-shunt for hepatorenal syndrome. *Lancet* 1997; 349:697–8.

61. Brensing KA, Textor J, Perz J, et al. Long term outcome after transjugular intrahepatic portosystemic stent-shunt in non-transplant cirrhotics with hepatorenal syndrome: a phase II study. *Gut* 2000;47: 288–95.

62. Testino G, Ferro C, Sumberaz A, et al. Type-2 hepatorenal syndrome and refractory ascites: role of transjugular intrahepatic portosystemic stent-shunt in eighteen patients with advanced cirrhosis awaiting orthotopic liver transplantation. *Hepatogastroenterology* 2003;50:1753–5.

63. Spahr L, Fenyves D, Nguyen VV, et al. Improvement of hepatorenal syndrome by transjugular intrahepatic portosystemic shunt. *Am J Gastroenterol* 1995;90:1169–71.

64. Lake JR, Ring E, LaBerge J, et al. Transjugular intrahepatic portacaval stent shunts in patients with renal insufficiency. *Transplant Proc* 1993;25:1766–7.

65. Lerut J, Goffette P, Laterre PF, et al. Sequential treatment of hepatorenal syndrome and post hepatic cirrhosis by intrahepatic portosystemic shunt (TIPSS) and liver transplantation. *Hepatogastroenterology* 1995;42:985–7.

66. Guevara M, Gines P, Bandi JC, et al. Transjugular intrahepatic portosystemic shunt in hepatorenal syndrome: effects on renal function and vasoactive systems. *Hepatology* 1998;28.416 22.

67. Rossle M, Gerbes AL. TIPS for the treatment of refractory ascites, hepatorenal syndrome and hepatic hydrothorax: a critical update. *Gut* 2010;59:988–1000.

68. Stange J, Ramlow W, Mitzner S, et al. Dialysis against a recycled albumin solution enables the removal of albumin-bound toxins. *Artif Organs* 1993;17:809–13.

69. Mitzner SR, Stange J, Klammt S, et al. Improvement of hepatorenal syndrome with extracorporeal albumin dialysis MARS: results of a prospective, randomized, controlled clinical trial. *Liver Transpl* 2000;6:277–86.

70. Sen S, Davies NA, Mookerjee RP, et al. Pathophysiological effects of albumin dialysis in acute-on-chronic liver failure: a randomized controlled study. *Liver Transpl* 2004;10:1109–19.

71. Wong F, Raina N, Richardson R. Molecular adsorbent recirculating system is ineffective in the management of type 1 hepatorenal syndrome in patients with cirrhosis with ascites who have failed vasoconstrictor treatment. *Gut* 2010;59:381–6.

72. Perez GO, Golper TA, Epstein M, et al. Dialysis, hemofiltration and other extracorporeal techniques in the treatment of the renal complications of liver disease. In: Epstein M, ed. *The Kidney in Liver Disease*, 4th edn. Philadelphia: Hanley and Belfus 1996: 517–28.

73. Witzke O, Baumann M, Patschan D, et al. Which patients benefit from hemodialysis therapy in hepatorenal syndrome? *J Gastroenterolo Hepatol* 2004;19:1369–73.

74. Wong LP, Blackley MP, Andreoni KA, et al. Survival of liver transplant candidates with acute renal failure receiving renal replacement therapy. *Kidney Int* 2005;68:362–70.

75. Epstein M, Perez GO, Bedoya LA, et al. Continuous arterio-venous ultrafiltration in cirrhotic patients with ascites and renal failure. *Int J Artif Organs* 1986;9:253–6.

76. Wiesner R, Edwards E, Freeman R, et al. Model for end-stage liver disease (MELD) and allocation of donor livers. *Gastroenterology* 2003; 124:91–6.

77. Cassinello C, Moreno E, Gozalo A, et al. Effects of orthotopic liver transplantation on vasoactive systems and renal function in patients with advanced liver cirrhosis. *Digest Dis Sci* 2003;48:179–86.

78. Marik PE, Wood K, Starzl TE. The course of type 1 hepatorenal syndrome post liver transplantation. *Nephrol Dial Transplant* 2006;21:478–82.

79. Hadengue A, Lebrec D, Moreau R, et al. Persistence of systemic and splanchnic hyperkinetic circulation in liver transplant patients. *Hepatology* 1993;17:175–8.

80. Nair S, Verma S, Thuluvath PJ. Pre-transplant renal function predicts survival in patients undergoing orthotopic liver transplantation. *Hepatology* 2002;35:1179–85.

81. Weismuller TJ, Prokein J, Becker T, et al. Prediction of survival after liver transplantation by pre-transplant parameters. *Scand J Gastroenterol* 2008;43:736–46.

82. Gonwa TA, Klintmalm GB, Levy M, et al. Impact of pre-transplant renal function on survival after liver transplantation. *Transplantation* 1995;59:361–5.

83. Restuccia T, Ortega R, Guevara M, et al. Effects of treatment of hepatorenal syndrome before transplantation on post-transplantation outcome. A case–control study. *J Hepatol* 2004;40:140–6.

84. Davis CL, Feng S, Sung R, et al. Simultaneous liver–kidney transplantation: evaluation to decision making. *Am J Transplant* 2007;7:1702–9.

85. Papafragkakis H, Martin P, Akalin E. Combined liver and kidney transplantation. *Curr Opin Organ Transplant* 2010;15:263–8.

86. Locke JE, Warren DS, Singer AL, et al. Declining outcomes in simultaneous liver–kidney transplantation in the MELD era: ineffective usage of renal allografts. *Transplantation* 2008;85:935–42.

87. Alessandria C, Ozdogan O, Guevara M, et al. MELD score and clinical type predict prognosis in hepatorenal syndrome: relevance to liver transplantation. *Hepatology* 2005;41:1282–9.

88. Schepke M, Appenrodt B, Heller J, et al. Prognostic factors for patients with cirrhosis and kidney dysfunction in the era of MELD: results of a prospective study. *Liver Int* 2006;26:834–9.

89. Appenrodt B, Zielinski J, Brensing KA, et al. Degree of hepatic dysfunction and improvement of renal function predict survival in patients with HRS type I: a retrospective analysis. *Eur J Gastroenterol Hepatol* 2009;21:1428–32.

90. Fernández J, Navasa M, Planas R, et al. Primary prophylaxis of spontaneous bacterial peritonitis delays hepatorenal syndrome and improves survival in cirrhosis. *Gastroenterology* 2007;133:818–24.

Multiple choice questions

15.1 **Which of the following statements describes functional renal failure in cirrhosis?**

 a Renal failure where there is no structural damage in the kidneys.
 b Diagnosed when the serum creatinine is >2 mg/dL.
 c Acute renal failure that occurs in patients with cirrhosis.
 d The same as hepatorenal syndrome.

15.2 **Acute kidney failure in cirrhosis is which of the following?**

 a It is renal failure that occurs rapidly as a result of advanced cirrhosis.
 b It can include conditions such as glomerulonephritis in cirrhosis.
 c It requires an abnormal serum creatinine reading for diagnosis.
 d It is a widely accepted concept in the hepatology community.

15.3 **Which of the following statements applies in assessing a patient for a diagnosis of acute or type 1 hepatorenal syndrome?**

 a One should always look for a precipitating event as hepatorenal syndrome never occurs spontaneously.
 b The patient usually has signs to suggest a hyperdynamic circulation.
 c The rise in serum creatinine occurs within 48 hours.
 d The urinary sodium is always <10 mmol/day.

15.4 **Which of the following is true for the treatment for acute or type 1 hepatorenal syndrome?**

 a It should start as soon as all other cause of acute renal failure have been excluded.
 b It includes the empirical use of a broad-spectrum antibiotic.
 c It should continue for at least 15 days in order to determine whether the patient is likely to respond or not.
 d It could be either vasoconstrictor therapy or the insertion of a transjugular intrahepatic portosystemic stent shunt.

15.5 **Which of the following is true with regard to liver transplantation for patients with type 1 hepatorenal syndrome?**

 a The patient should receive a simultaneous kidney transplant.
 b The length of dialysis pre transplant has no impact on the decision regarding whether to perform a liver transplant alone or a combined liver–kidney transplant.
 c Since hepatorenal syndrome is a totally reversible condition, the presence of hepatorenal syndrome pre transplant does not have any effect on post-transplant graft and patient survival.
 d Correcting the renal failure pre transplant can significant improve patient survival post transplant.

Answers to the multiple choice questions can be found in the Appendix at the end of the book.

These multiple choice questions are also available for you to complete online.
Visit http://www.schiffsdiseasesoftheliver.com/

CHAPTER 16

Pulmonary Manifestations of Liver Disease

Rajan Kochar & Michael B. Fallon

Division of Gastroenterology, Hepatology and Nutrition, The University of Texas Health Science Center at Houston, Houston, TX, USA

Key concepts

- Liver disease, most commonly cirrhosis, is associated with unique pulmonary vascular abnormalities independent of intrinsic cardiopulmonary disease.
- About 15–30% of patients with cirrhosis develop hepatopulmonary syndrome (HPS), which results when vasodilatation in the pulmonary microvasculature leads to impaired gas exchange. The presence of HPS increases mortality in cirrhosis. Currently, liver transplantation is the only established therapy for HPS. However, when HPS is severe, the outcome of liver transplantation may be adversely affected.
- Portopulmonary hypertension (POPH) results when vasoconstriction and vascular remodeling increases pulmonary vascular resistance and elevates the mean pulmonary artery pressure. POPH occurs in 4–8% of patients with cirrhosis, and when moderate or severe prohibitively increases mortality after liver transplantation. Medical therapies can improve pressures but it is unclear whether liver transplantation reliably improves POPH.
- Screening for HPS and POPH is important in cirrhosis because the presence of these disorders influence survival and liver transplantation candidacy.

Dyspnea is common in patients with chronic liver disease, and an estimated 50–70% of patients with cirrhosis undergoing evaluation for liver transplantation complain of shortness of breath [1]. The differential diagnosis of dyspnea in chronic liver disease is broad and there a number of important causes to consider. The most common causes of these abnormalities are intrinsic cardiopulmonary disorders independent of liver disease (i.e., chronic obstructive pulmonary disease, interstitial lung disease, and congestive heart failure). Additionally, symptoms may result from general complications of cirrhosis such as patient deconditioning, muscular wasting, the presence of tense ascites, and/or hepatic hydrothorax (Chapter 17). Finally, certain liver diseases may be associated with specific pulmonary abnormalities such as panacinar emphysema in α_1-antitrypsin deficiency (Chapter 31) and fibrosing alveolitis, pulmonary hemorrhage, and granulomas in primary biliary cirrhosis (Chapter 21).

In a subset of patients though, two distinct pulmonary vascular complications of liver disease, the hepatopulmonary syndrome (HPS) and portopulmonary hypertension (POPH), are observed as important causes of pulmonary dysfunction. This chapter will review the epidemiology, clinical characteristics, and treatment of these disorders.

Hepatopulmonary syndrome

Definition

Hepatopulmonary syndrome is commonly defined as a widened age-corrected alveolar–arterial oxygen gradient ($AaPO_2$) on room air with or without hypoxemia that occurs as a result of intrapulmonary vasodilatation in the presence of hepatic dysfunction or portal hypertension [2,3].

Epidemiology, risk factors, and disease associations

Intrapulmonary vasodilatation is present in over 50% of cirrhotics evaluated for orthotopic liver transplantation (OLT). In addition, 15–30% of those with intrapulmonary shunting have impaired oxygenation leading to the diagnosis of HPS [4]. Prior definitions of HPS emphasized the need to exclude intrinsic cardiopulmonary disease in order to establish the diagnosis. However, recent data support the view that HPS may occur in the setting of other cardiopulmonary abnormalities [5,6].

Typically, HPS is diagnosed in subjects with cirrhosis and portal hypertension regardless of the underlying etiology of liver disease. However, cases of HPS have been described in patients with portal hypertension without cirrhosis (prehepatic portal hypertension, nodular regenerative hyperplasia, congenital hepatic fibrosis, and hepatic venous outflow obstruction [7–10]) and in patients with hepatic dysfunction in the absence of established portal hypertension (acute and chronic hepatitis [11–13]). These findings support that advanced liver disease is not required for HPS to develop. Controversy exists regarding whether HPS is more common or severe in patients with advanced cirrhosis, although a recent prospective multicenter study did not find an association between HPS and severity of liver disease in patients being evaluated for OLT [14].

Pathogenesis

The most important alteration in HPS is dilatation of the precapillary and postcapillary pulmonary vasculature [15], which leads to impaired oxygenation of venous blood as it passes through the lung [16,17].

Human studies have demonstrated increased pulmonary production of nitric oxide (NO), which may contribute to intrapulmonary vasodilatation. Exhaled NO levels are increased in cirrhotic HPS patients and normalize after liver transplantation [18–20], as HPS resolves. However, the increase in NO production is not unique

to HPS and inhibition of NO production or action does not reliably improve HPS [21–25].

In animal models, increased pulmonary production of NO appears to be a central event in the development of HPS through increased pulmonary vascular expression and activity of endothelial nitric oxide synthase (eNOS) [25–28]. Enhanced hepatic production and release of endothelin 1 (ET-1) and shear stress-mediated increase in pulmonary endothelial endothelin B (ET$_B$) receptor expression appear to be major contributors to the observed increase in eNOS [29–31]. These events lead to enhanced ET-1 activation of eNOS through the ET$_B$ receptor and are followed by the intravascular accumulation of macrophages and the production of inducible nitric oxide synthase (iNOS) [25,27,28] and heme oxygenase 1 (HO-1) [27,32] leading to increased NO and carbon monoxide production, respectively, which result in vasodilatation. In addition, a recent study has shown that angiogenesis is an important contributor to the development of experimental HPS and is associated with activation of the angiogenic pathways (such as vascular endothelial cell growth factor A (VEGF-A)), in part by intravascular monocytes [33]. Figure 16.1 summarizes the current understanding of mechanisms of pulmonary microvascular dilatation in experimental HPS. However, whether similar mechanisms are operative in human disease is unknown.

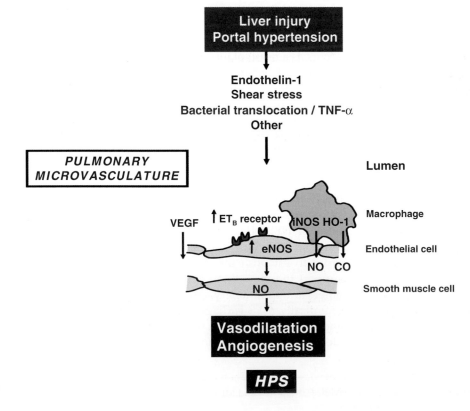

Figure 16.1 Proposed mechanisms of hepatopulmonary syndrome (HPS) based on findings in experimental models. Liver injury and/or portal hypertension trigger the production of cytokines and vasoactive mediators that increase vascular shear stress. Pulmonary microvascular dilatation is initiated by hepatic endothelin 1 production and release and endothelial nitric oxide synthase (eNOS)-derived nitric oxide (NO) production through an increased number of endothelial endothelin B (ET-B) receptors. Macrophage accumulate in the microvascular also contributes to vasodilatation by producing NO from inducible nitric oxide synthase (iNOS) and carbon monoxide (CO) from heme oxygenase 1 (HO-1). Activation of angiogenic pathways such as vascular endothelial growth factor A are also facilitated through intravascular mononuclear cells leading to angiogenesis. TNF-α, tumor necrosis factor α.

Clinical features

The diagnosis of HPS may be overlooked or delayed since many patients with HPS are asymptomatic or respiratory symptoms may be attributed to intrinsic lung disease, therefore a high index of suspicion is necessary to establish the diagnosis. In symptomatic patients, the insidious onset of dyspnea [1] is the most frequent complaint. Platypnea (increased dyspnea upon standing) and orthodeoxia (hypoxemia exacerbated in the upright position) are classic features of HPS. They are attributed to the predominance of vasodilatation in the lung bases and the increased "shunting" through these regions when upright leading to hypoxemia [34,35]. Spider angiomata, digital clubbing, and cyanosis are also commonly described in subjects with HPS and may increase the clinical suspicion for the diagnosis when present [35,36]. Chest radiographs are most commonly normal, but may reveal lower lobe interstitial changes that may be confused with interstitial lung disease [37]. Pulmonary function tests typically demonstrate well-preserved spirometry and lung volumes; however, the diffusing capacity for lung carbon monoxide (DLCO) is often significantly reduced. The DLCO is also commonly decreased in cirrhosis in the absence of HPS and the diagnostic utility of a reduced value has not been established [38].

Evaluation for hepatopulmonary syndrome

Pursuing the diagnosis of HPS is appropriate in patients complaining of dyspnea and/or in those who display digital clubbing or cyanosis. In patients being considered for liver transplantation, regardless of the presence of symptoms, screening is important as the presence of HPS may influence transplant candidacy and priority. Figure 16.2 summarizes one approach to the diagnosis of HPS.

The diagnosis of HPS is established by: (i) the presence of arterial gas exchange abnormalities; and (ii) documenting intrapulmonary vasodilatation. Gas exchange abnormalities, detected by arterial blood gas measurements, are defined as a widened $AaPO_2$ (>15–20 mmHg) with or without hypoxemia (PaO_2 <70 mmHg) [3]. Obtaining arterial blood gases in the sitting position may enhance the detection of hypoxemia in HPS due to the predominance of vasodilatation in the lower lung fields. Pulse oximetry is a noninvasive screening modality that indirectly measures oxygen saturation (SpO_2) and is a useful screening test for arterial hypoxemia and HPS [39]. From a clinical perspective, SpO_2 measurements can guide subsequent use of arterial blood gases and contrast echocardiography.

Two-dimensional transthoracic contrast echocardiography is the most sensitive and most commonly employed screening technique to detect intrapulmonary vasodi-latation (Fig. 16.3). It is performed by injecting agitated saline intravenously during normal transthoracic echocardiography, producing microbubbles that are visible on sonography. This bolus opacifies the right ventricle within seconds and in the absence of right-to-left shunting, bubbles are absorbed in the lungs. If an intracardiac shunt is present, contrast agent enters the left ventricle within three heartbeats (early shunting). If intrapulmonary shunting, characteristic of HPS, is present, the left ventricle opacifies at least three heartbeats after the right (delayed shunting).

Radionuclide lung perfusion scanning, using technetium-labeled macroaggregated albumin particles (^{99m}Tc-MAA scan), is another method for detecting intrapulmonary vasodilatation (Fig. 16.4). In this test, macroaggregated albumin particles 50–100 μm in size are injected intravenously. Normally, all the particles are trapped in the lung microvasculature. In HPS, some particles escape through dilated pulmonary capillaries and lodge in beds supplied by systemic arteries. Quantitative imaging of the lung and brain using a standardized methodology allows calculation of a shunt fraction [40]. The ^{99m}Tc-MAA scan offers one significant advantage over contrast echocardiography: a positive scan (shunt fraction >6%) is specific for the presence of HPS even in the setting of coexistent intrinsic lung disease [40]. It is valuable in determining the relative importance of intrapulmonary vasodilatation or the underlying pulmonary process as the major contributor for observed gas exchange abnormalities. However, as a screening test for intrapulmonary vasodilatation, ^{99m}Tc-MAA scanning is less sensitive than contrast echocardiography in adults.

Pulmonary angiography and high-resolution chest computerized tomography (CT) are other modalities to detect intrapulmonary vasodilatation that are more invasive and less sensitive compared with contrast echocardiography [41].

Prognosis and natural history

The natural history of HPS is incompletely characterized but available data indicate that most patients develop progressive intrapulmonary vasodilatation and worsening gas exchange over time and that spontaneous improvement is rare [42,43]. Mortality is significantly higher and quality of life is significantly lower in patients with HPS compared with cirrhotics without HPS [14]. The success of liver transplantation in reversing HPS and the policy of increasing priority for transplantation in HPS associated with significant hypoxemia, currently in place in the United States, may improve prognosis in this disorder.

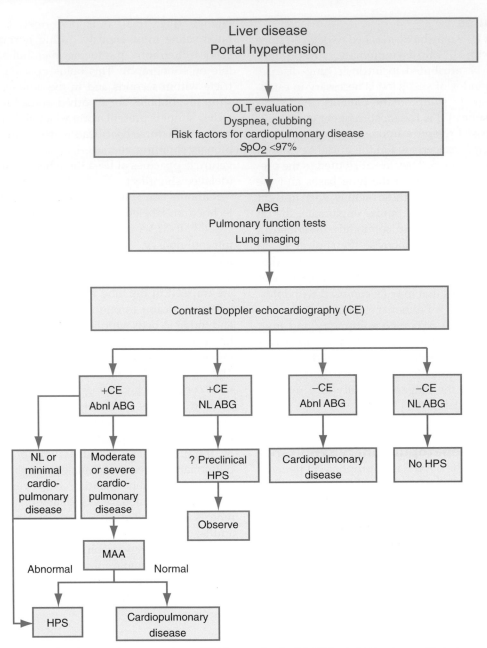

Figure 16.2 Diagnostic approach to hepatopulmonary syndrome (HPS) (see text for details). ABG, arterial blood gases; Abnl, abnormal; OLT, orthotopic liver transplantation; NL, normal; SpO_2, pulse oximetry oxygen saturation; MAA, technetium-labeled macroaggregated albumin scan.

Therapy

Case reports and small studies have suggested that a number of agents, including aspirin [44], garlic [45,46], norfloxacin [47], and inhaled nitro-L-arginine methyl ester (L-NAME) [48], might improve HPS. Recently, conflicting results were obtained from two small pilot studies using pentoxifylline in HPS. In a study that enrolled patients with more advanced liver disease and HPS, the drug was poorly tolerated, while benefit was found in those with mild disease [49]. However, no randomized trials have been performed. In patients with resting or exertional hypoxemia, supplemental oxygen therapy is appropriate although no studies have evaluated whether clinical benefit occurs. Portal decompression with transjugular intrahepatic portosystemic shunt (TIPS) has been attempted in a small number of cases. However, convincing evidence for sustained improvement is lacking and TIPS should be considered an experimental treatment. OLT is the only proven therapy for HPS based upon resolution or significant improvement in gas exchange

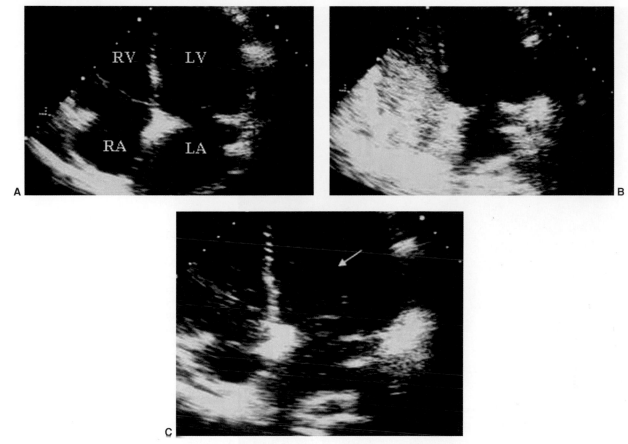

Figure 16.3 Contrast echocardiogram for detecting intrapulmonary vasodilatation. (A) Parasternal four-chamber view of the heart (LA, left atrium; LV, left ventricle; RA, right atrium; RV, right ventricle) prior to the administration of agitated saline contrast. (B) Four-chamber view immediately after the administration of demonstrating the presence of echogenic microbubbles in the right atrium and ventricle immediately after injection of agitated saline into the antecubital vein. (C) Visualization of echogenic microbubbles in the left atrium (arrow) and ventricle three cardiac cycles after visualization on the right due to intrapulmonary vasodilatation in a patient with hepatopulmonary syndrome. Intracardiac shunting results in immediate passage of microbubbles from the right to left chambers without a three cycle delay and can be excluded using this technique.

postoperatively in more than 85% of reported patients [8]. However, the length of time for resolution after transplantation varies and may be more than 1 year. In addition, mortality is increased after transplantation in HPS patients compared to subjects without HPS, particularly when hypoxemia is severe [50]. Currently, HPS patients with a PaO_2 <60 mmHg are eligible for increased priority for OLT (model for end-stage liver disease (MELD) exception), based on increased mortality and reduced survival after OLT with increased HPS severity. Therefore, screening for HPS and consideration of liver transplantation prior to the development of severe hypoxemia is appropriate.

Portopulmonary hypertension

Definition

Portopulmonary hypertension is defined by a mean pulmonary artery pressure (mPAP) >25 mmHg and a pulmonary capillary wedge pressure <15 mmHg occurring in the setting of portal hypertension [51]. An elevated transpulmonary gradient (mean pulmonary artery pressure – pulmonary capillary wedge pressure of >10 mmHg) and/or pulmonary vascular resistance (>120 dyne/s/cm^{5}) are additional criteria included in the definition of this syndrome.

Epidemiology, risk factors, and disease associations

Changes consistent with pulmonary hypertension were found in 0.7% of patients with cirrhosis compared to a prevalence of 0.1% in subjects without chronic liver disease in a series of 17,901 autopsies [52]. A subsequent prospective study of 507 patients who underwent right heart catheterization revealed a 2% prevalence of POPH [53]. More recently, retrospective studies in liver transplantation candidates have found a prevalence ranging from 3.5% to 16% [54–57]. To date, POPH has only been

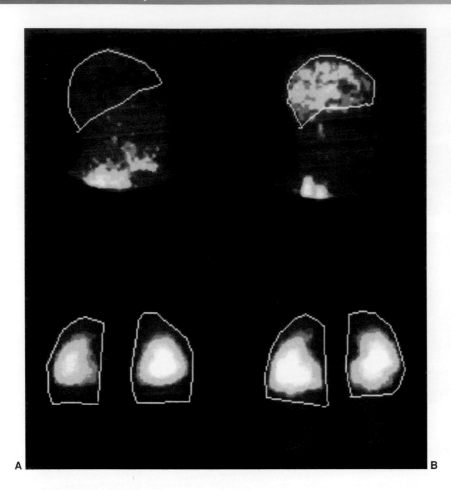

A   B

Figure 16.4 Technetium-labeled macroaggregated albumin (^{99m}Tc-MAA) scanning. (A) A normal ^{99m}Tc-MAA scan from a patient without hepatopulmonary syndrome with the regions of interest drawn around the lungs (below) and cerebrum (above). In the absence of intrapulmonary vasodilatation, there is a minimal passage of intravenously administered labeled albumin through the lungs and signal intensity is low in the cerebrum. Shunting is quantified by comparing the relative signal intensity in the lung and the brain. (B) A ^{99m}Tc-MAA scan in hepatopulmonary syndrome demonstrating significant cerebral uptake due to passage of labeled albumin through the dilated pulmonary microvasculature. (Reproduced from Abrams et al. [5] with permission from Elsevier.)

described in the presence of portal hypertension with or without cirrhosis. Although there are no definitive clinical predictors of POPH, a recent multicenter study found an increased risk of developing POPH in female patients and patients with autoimmune hepatitis; and a decreased risk in patients with hepatitis C as the etiology of liver disease [58]. Generally, the diagnosis of portal hypertension precedes the diagnosis of POPH by several years and data are controversial as to the relationship between severity of portal hypertension and risk or severity of POPH [57].

Pathology and pathogenesis

The histologic features of POPH are similar to those seen in primary pulmonary hypertension. These include smooth muscle hypertrophy and hyperplasia, concentric intimal fibrosis, plexogenic arteriopathy, and necrotizing vasculitis [15,51,59–61]. The underlying mechanisms in POPH remain incompletely understood and no animal models have been developed. Elevated portal pressure is critical for the development of pulmonary hypertension [53]. The hyperdynamic circulatory state, causing increased vascular shear stress, and portosystemic shunting, causing altered production or metabolism of vasoactive substances, have been hypoth-

esized to contribute to vascular changes in POPH [17]. Endothelial and circulating factors (endothelin 1, prostacyclin, and thromboxane) and polymorphisms in genes regulating estrogen signaling and cell growth regulators are associated with the risk of POPH. In addition, a recent study showed no association between serotonin transporter polymorphisms and POPH [62,63]. One hypothesis suggested that endothelial injury or dysfunction may be a key early event that contributes to vascular proliferation and inflammation leading to POPH (Fig. 16.5). In addition, HPS may coexist with POPH suggesting that these two entities may share underlying pathogenetic mechanisms. One emerging hypothesis is that the pulmonary endothelial response to alterations in liver disease and portal hypertension (NO overproduction and activation of angiogenic pathways in HPS versus dysfunction and injury in POPH) is important in determining whether HPS or POPH develops.

Clinical features

A majority of POPH patients may be asymptomatic [57]. The most common symptom described in POPH is dyspnea on exertion, with the development of progressive fatigue, dyspnea at rest, peripheral edema, syncope, and

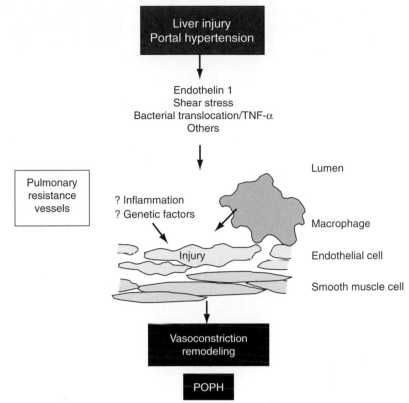

Figure 16.5 Proposed mechanisms of portopulmonary hypertension (POPH). Liver injury and/or portal hypertension trigger the production of cytokines and vasoactive mediators that increase vascular shear stress as is proposed for hepatopulmonary syndrome. In contrast, in the setting of POPH, modifying factors including inflammation and genetic factors may trigger endothelial injury resulting in smooth muscle proliferation and vascular remodeling. These events lead to pulmonary arterial hypertension. TNF-α, tumor necrosis factor α.

chest pain as severity increases [64]. Physical examination reveals jugular venous distention, a loud pulmonary component of the second heart sound, and a systolic murmur resulting from tricuspid regurgitation. Lower extremity edema is commonly noted. Electrocardiographic abnormalities are similar to those seen in primary pulmonary hypertension and include evidence of right atrial enlargement, right ventricular hypertrophy, right axis deviation, and/or right bundle branch block. Radiographic findings are generally subtle, but in advanced cases a prominent main pulmonary artery or cardiomegaly due to prominent right cardiac chambers may occur. Gas exchange abnormalities are generally mild and less severe than in HPS. An increased AaPO$_2$ with mild hypoxemia and hypocarbia may be seen, particularly in more severe disease [17,65].

Evaluation for portopulmonary hypertension

Patients with POPH are often asymptomatic and the diagnostic utility of various clinical features is low [55,66]. Therefore, the diagnosis of POPH requires a high index of suspicion (Fig. 16.6). Other causes of elevated pulmonary pressures and/or right heart failure, including left ventricular dysfunction, volume overload, and chronic obstructive lung disease, have to be excluded. In

general, in patients not being evaluated for liver transplantation, the presence of suggestive symptoms and signs – after exclusion of other cardiopulmonary diseases – makes it reasonable to screen for POPH. In all patients being evaluated for liver transplantation, regardless of signs or symptoms, screening is warranted because the presence of POPH may influence transplant candidacy [67].

Transthoracic Doppler echocardiography is the best noninvasive screening study. If combined with intravenous contrast injection, screening for HPS and POPH can be accomplished at the same time. The presence of pulmonary hypertension is suggested by an increased estimated pulmonary artery systolic pressure (derived from measuring the velocity of the tricuspid regurgitant jet), pulmonary valve insufficiency, right atrial enlargement, and/or right ventricular hypertrophy or dilatation. An estimated systolic pulmonary arterial pressure of >40–50 mmHg is used to define the need for direct measurement of pulmonary pressures by right heart catheterization. A mPAP of >25 mmHg with a pulmonary capillary wedge pressure of <15 mmHg confirms the diagnosis of pulmonary arterial hypertension. An elevated transpulmonary gradient (mean pulmonary artery pressure – pulmonary capillary wedge pressure of >10 mmHg) and pulmonary vascular resistance (>120 dyne/s/cm^5) are additional measurements used

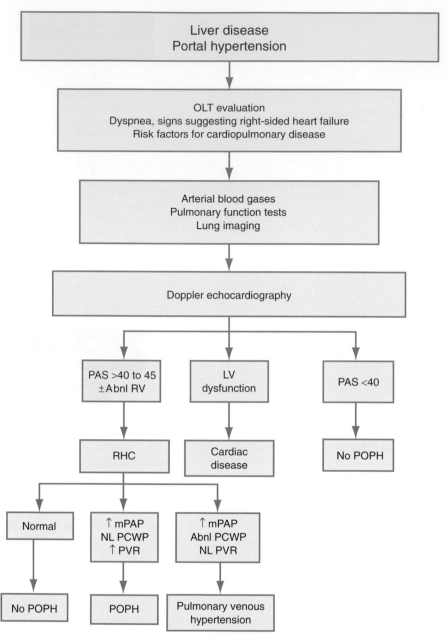

Figure 16.6 Diagnostic approach to portopulmonary hypertension (POPH) (see text for details). Abnl, abnormal; LV, left ventricle; mPAP, mean pulmonary artery pressure; NL, normal; OLT, orthotopic liver transplantation; PAS, estimated pulmonary artery systolic pressure; PCWP, pulmonary capillary wedge pressure; PVR, pulmonary vascular resistance; RHC, right heart catheterization; RV, right ventricle.

to distinguish pulmonary arterial hypertension from pulmonary venous hypertension that may be present due to the hyperdynamic circulation and volume overload that accompany cirrhosis.

Vasodilator responsiveness with a number of agents, most frequently nitric oxide and/or epoprostenol, may be undertaken in those with confirmed POPH in an effort to predict a favorable response to long-term vasodilator therapy [17]. However, the utility of vasodilator testing in the management of POPH has not been studied.

Prognosis and natural history

The major complication of POPH is the development of progressive right ventricular dysfunction and cor pulmonale. Survival in pulmonary hypertension correlates with the severity of right-sided cardiac dysfunction as assessed by the degree of elevation in the right-sided cardiac pressures and the degree of decline in the cardiac output [68]. Previous studies have suggested that survival in POPH was similar or even prolonged compared with primary pulmonary hypertension, possibly related to the beneficial effects of the hyperdynamic circulatory state [17]. Recent work has challenged this concept and found that mortality was higher in POPH relative to primary pulmonary hypertension despite a higher cardiac index and lower systemic and pulmonary vascular resistance [69]. To date, no studies have demonstrated that medical therapy for POPH improves survival. Liver transplantation in patients with mild POPH (<35 mmHg) appears to have comparable outcomes relative to patients without pulmonary hypertension although long-term follow-up has not been reported. At higher mean pulmonary artery pressures, perioperative mortality is increased, particularly in those with higher pulmonary vascular resistance values or lower cardiac output [67].

Therapy

Medical treatment for POPH is based largely on experience in primary pulmonary hypertension. However, anticoagulants and calcium channel blockers are not recommended due to their potential to increase bleeding and portal pressure, respectively. The use of β-adrenergic blockers for the prevention of variceal bleeding should be considered with caution given the potential for cardiac depression [70]. A number of medical therapies have been successfully used in POPH both as monotherapy or in combination. They include endothelin receptor antagonists (bosentan), phosphodiesterase V inhibitor (sildenafil), prostacyclin analogs (epoprostenol, treprostinil, iloprost), vasopressin analogs (terlipressin), and tyrosine kinase inhibitors (imatinib) [71,72]. However, most therapeutic interventions are described in case reports and retrospective analysis. No controlled trials have been undertaken, and whether medical therapy impacts survival is unknown. Bosentan has the potential for hepatotoxicity and its safety is uncertain in patients with advanced liver disease.

The safety and efficacy of OLT in patients with POPH is controversial. There are no well-designed, prospective studies to guide decision making, and the effect of OLT on the natural history of POPH is not well defined. Retrospective studies and case reports confirm that moderate to severe POPH (mPAP >35 mmHg), particularly if right ventricular dysfunction is present, is associated with substantial perioperative mortality and is a contraindication for transplantation [67]. Less severe POPH (mPAP <35 mmHg) is generally not considered a contraindication to OLT, but patients need to be evaluated individually to minimize risks. Several recent retrospective studies suggest that OLT may be feasible and beneficial in patients with moderate to severe POPH who are otherwise suitable OLT candidates if medical therapy lowers the mPAP to <35 mmHg [73,74]. Some guidelines recommend, and several United Network for Organ Sharing (UNOS) regions provide, MELD exception points for patients whose mPAP decreases below 35 mmHg on medical therapy [75]. However, the outcomes using such a strategy are unknown.

Summary and conclusions

Hepatopulmonary syndrome and POPH are unique pulmonary vascular complications of liver disease and/or portal hypertension that may cause significant morbidity and influence survival and liver transplant candidacy. HPS occurs in approximately 20% and POPH occurs in approximately 6% of patients with cirrhosis being evaluated for liver transplantation. Dilatation in the pulmonary microvasculature is an important event that leads to hypoxemia and symptoms in HPS. Vasoconstriction and remodeling in resistance vessels occur in POPH and may lead to right-sided cardiac dysfunction. The pathogenesis of pulmonary vascular abnormalities in HPS and POPH are areas of ongoing investigation and similar mechanisms may play a role in each syndrome. There are no effective medical therapies for HPS, but liver transplantation can reverse the syndrome in the majority of patients. In contrast, there are symptomatic medical therapies for POPH, but for many patients liver transplantation is currently contraindicated or controversial. Transplantation carries increased mortality in both severe HPS and POPH, underscoring the importance of screening for these disorders in patients undergoing liver transplantation evaluation.

Further reading

Arguedas M, Abrams GA, Krowka MJ, Fallon MB. Prospective evaluation of outcomes and predictors of mortality in patients with hepatopulmonary syndrome undergoing liver transplantation. *Hepatology* 2003;37:192–7.
The first prospective study that demonstrates that the outcome after liver transplantation in HPS is influenced by the severity of hypoxemia and intrapulmonary vasodilatation.

Fallon MB, Krowka MJ, Brown RS, et al.; Pulmonary Vascular Complications of Liver Disease Study Group. Impact of hepatopulmonary syndrome on quality of life and survival in liver transplant candidates. *Gastroenterology* 2008;135(4):1168–75.
Recent multicenter prospective study of a large group of liver transplant candidates demonstrating reduced quality of life and survival in patients with HPS.

Krowka M, Plevak D, Findlay J, Rosen C, Wiesner R, Krom R. Pulmonary hemodynamics and perioperative cardiopulmonary-related mortality in patients with portopulmonary hypertension undergoing liver transplantation. *Liver Transpl* 2000;6:443–50.
This retrospective study analyzes the outcomes of liver transplantation relative to the severity of POPH. It forms the basis for the practice of avoiding liver transplantation in moderate to severe POPH.

Roberts KE, Fallon MB, Krowka MJ, et al; Pulmonary Vascular Complications of Liver Disease Study Group. Genetic risk factors for portopulmonary hypertension in patients with advanced liver disease. *Am J Respir Crit Care Med* 2009;179(9):835–42.
The first study evaluating genetic risk factors for POPH using single nucleotide polymorphism analysis.

Rodríguez-Roisin R, Krowka MJ. Hepatopulmonary syndrome – a liver-induced lung vascular disorder. *N Engl J Med* 2008;358(22):2378–87.
Recent comprehensive review of HPS outlining epidemiology, pathogenesis, diagnosis, and current therapies.

Rodriguez-Roisin R, Krowka MJ, Herve P, Fallon MB, on behalf of the ERS Task Force Pulmonary–Hepatic Vascular Disorders (PHD) Scientific Committee. Pulmonary–hepatic vascular disorders (PHD). *Eur Respir J* 2004;24:861–80.
Recent comprehensive review of HPS and POPH outlining epidemiology, pathogenesis, diagnosis, and current therapies.

References

1. Sood G, Fallon MB, Niwas S, et al. Utility of a dyspnea-fatigue index for screening liver transplant candidates for hepatopulmonary syndrome [Abstract]. *Hepatology* 1998;28:2319.
2. Lange PA, Stoller JK. The hepatopulmonary syndrome. *Ann Intern Med* 1995;122:521–9.
3. Rodriguez-Roison R, Agusti AG, Roca J. The hepatopulmonary syndrome: new name, old complexities. *Thorax* 1992;47:897–902.
4. Abrams GA, Jaffe CC, Hoffer PB, et al. Diagnostic utility of contrast echocardiography and lung perfusion scan in patients with hepatopulmonary syndrome. *Gastroenterology* 1995;109:1283–8.
5. Abrams G, Nanda N, Dubovsky E, et al. Use of macroaggregated albumin lung perfusion scan to diagnose hepatopulmonary syndrome:a new approach. *Gastroenterology* 1998;114(2):305–10.
6. Martinez G, Barbera J, Navasa M, et al. Hepatopulmonary syndrome associated with cardiorespiratory disease. *J. Hepatol* 1999;30:882–9.
7. Dimand RJ, Heyman MB, Bass NM, et al. Hepatopulmonary syndrome: response to hepatic transplantation [Abstract]. *Hepatology* 1991;141(2):55A.
8. Abrams G, Fallon M. The hepatopulmonary syndrome. *Clin Liver Dis* 1997;1:185–200.
9. Binay K, Sen S, Biswas PK, et al. Hepatopulmonary syndrome in inferior vena cava obstruction responding to cavoplasty. Gastroenterology 2000;118:192–6.
10. Gupta D, Vijaya DR, Gupta R, et al. Prevalence of hepatopulmonary syndrome in cirrhosis and extrahepatic portal venous obstruction. *Am J Gastroenterol* 2001;96:3395–9.
11. Regev A, Yeshurun M, Rodriguez M, et al. Transient hepatopulmonary syndrome in a patient with acute hepatitis *Am J Viral Hep* 2001;8:83–6.
12. Teuber G, Teupe C, Dietrich C, et al. Pulmonary dysfunction in non-cirrhotic patients with chronic viral hepatitis. *Eur J Intern Med* 2002;13:311–18.
13. Fuhrmann V, Madl C, Mueller C, et al. Hepatopulmonary syndrome in patients with hypoxic hepatitis. *Gastroenterology* 2006;131:69–75.
14. Fallon M, Krowka M, Brown R, et al. Impact of hepatopulmonary syndrome on quality of life and survival in liver transplant candidates. *Gastroenterology* 2008;135(4):1168–75.
15. Schraufnagel D, Kay J. Structural and pathologic changes in the lung vasculature in chronic liver disease. *Clin Chest Med* 1996;17:1–15.
16. Herve P, Lebrec D, Brenot F, et al. Pulmonary vascular disorders in portal hypertension. *Eur Respir J* 1998;11:1153–66.
17. Budhiraja R, Hassoun PM. Portopulmonary hypertension: a tale of two circulations. *Chest* 2003;123:562–76.
18. Rolla G, Brussino L, Colagrande P, et al. Exhaled nitric oxide and oxygenation abnormalities in hepatic cirrhosis. *Hepatology* 1997;26:842–7.
19. Rolla G, Brussino L, Colagrande P. Exhaled nitric oxide and impaired oxygenation in cirrhotic patients before and after liver transplantation. *Ann Intern Med* 1998;129:375–8.
20. Cremona G, Higenbottam TW, Mayoral V, et al. Elevated exhaled nitric oxide in patients with hepatopulmonary syndrome. *Eur Respir J* 1995;8:1883–5.
21. Brussino L, Bucca C, Morello M, et al. Effect on dyspnoea and hypoxaemia of inhaled NG-nitro-L-arginine methyl ester in hepatopulmonary syndrome. *Lancet* 2003;362:43–4.
22. Rolla G, Bucca C, Brussino L. Methylene blue in the hepatopulmonary syndrome. *N Eng J Med* 1994;331:1098.
23. Schenk P, Madl C, Rezale-Majd S, et al. Methylene blue improves the hepatopulmonary syndrome. *Ann Intern Med* 2000;133:701–6.
24. Degano B, Mittaine M, Hervé P, **et al.** Nitric oxide production by the alveolar compartment of the lungs in cirrhotic patients. *Eur Respir J* 2009;34(1):138–44.
25. Fallon MB, Abrams GA, Luo B, et al. The role of endothelial nitric oxide synthase in the pathogenesis of a rat model of hepatopulmonary syndrome. *Gastroenterology* 1997;113:606–14.
26. Luo B, Abrams GA, Fallon MB. Endothelin-1 in the rat bile duct ligation model of hepatopulmonary syndrome: correlation with pulmonary dysfunction. *J Hepatol* 1998;29:571–8.
27. Zhang J, Ling Y, Luo B, et al. Analysis of pulmonary heme oxygenase-1 and nitric oxide synthase alterations in experimental hepatopulmonary syndrome. *Gastroenterology* 2003;125:1441–51.
28. Nunes H, Lebrec D, Mazmanian M, et al. Role of nitric oxide in hepatopulmonary syndrome in cirrhotic rats. *Am J Respir Crit Care Med* 2001;164:879–85.
29. Zhang M, Luo B, Chen SJ, et al. Endothelin-1 stimulation of endothelial nitric oxide synthase in the pathogenesis of hepatopulmonary syndrome. *Am J Physiol* 1999;277:G944–52.
30. Luo B, Liu L, Tang L,et al. Increased pulmonary vascular endothelin B receptor expression and responsiveness to endothelin-1 in cirrhotic and portal hypertensive rats: a potential mechanism in experimental hepatopulmonary syndrome. *J Hepatol* 2003;38:556–63.
31. Ling Y, Zhang J, Luo B, et al. The role of endothelin-1 and the endothelin B receptor in the pathogenesis of experimental hepatopulmonary syndrome. *Hepatology* 2004;39:1593–602.
32. Carter EP, Hartsfield CL, Miyazono M, et al. Regulation of heme oxygenase-1 by nitric oxide during hepatopulmonary syndrome. *Am J Physiol Lung Cellular Molec Physiol* 2002;283:L346–53.
33. Zhang J, Luo B, Tang L, et al. Pulmonary angiogenesis in a rat model of hepatopulmonary syndrome. *Gastroenterology* 2009;136:1070–80.
34. Robin ED, Laman D, Horn BR, et al. Platypnea related to orthodeoxia caused by true vascular lung shunts. *N Engl J Med* 1976;294:941–3.
35. Gomez F, Martinez-Palli G, Barbera J, et al. Gas exchange mechanism of orthodeoxia in hepatopulmonary syndrome. *Hepatology* 2004;40:660–6.
36. Martinez GP, Barbera JA, Visa J, et al. Hepatopulmonary syndrome in candidates for liver transplantation. *J Hepatol* 2001;34(5):651–7.
37. McAdams HP, Erasmus J, Crockett R, et al. The hepatopulmonary syndrome: radiologic findings in 10 patients. *Am J Roentgenol* 1996;166(6):1379–85.
38. Lima B, Franca A, Pazin-Filho A, et al. Frequency, clinical characteristics, and respiratory parameters of hepatopulmonary syndrome. *Mayo Clin Proc* 2004;79:42–8.
39. Abrams GA, Sanders MK, Fallon MB. Utility of pulse oximetry in the detection of arterial hypoxemia in liver transplant candidates. *Liver Transpl* 2002;8(4):391–6.
40. Abrams G, Nanda N, Dubovsky E, et al. Use of macroaggregated albumin lung perfusion scan to diagnose hepatopulmonary syndrome:a new approach. *Gastroenterology* 1998;114:305–10.
41. Lee KN, Lee HJ, Shin WW, et al. Hypoxemia and liver cirrhosis (hepatopulmonary syndrome) in eight patients: comparison of the central and peripheral pulmonary vasculature. *Radiology* 1999;211:549–53.
42. Krowka MJ, Dickson ER, Cortese DA. Hepatopulmonary syndrome. Clinical observations and lack of therapeutic response to somatostatin analogue. *Chest* 1993;104:515–21.

43. Swanson K, Wiesner R, Krowka M. Natural history of hepatopulmonary syndrome: impact of liver transplantation. *Hepatology* 2005; 41:1122–9.

44. Song JY, Choi JY, Ko JT, et al. Long-term aspirin therapy for hepatopulmonary syndrome. *Pediatrics* 1996;97(6):917–20.

45. Caldwell SH, Jeffers LJ, Narula OS, et al. Ancient remedies revisited: does *Allium sativum* (garlic) palliate the hepatopulmonary syndrome? *J Clin Gastroenterol* 1992;15:248–50.

46. Abrams GA, Fallon MB. Treatment of hepatopulmonary syndrome with *Allium sativum* L. (garlic): a pilot trial. *J Clin Gastroenterol* 1998; 27:232–5.

47. Anel RM, Sheagren JN. Novel presentation and approach to management of hepatopulmonary syndrome with use of antimicrobial agents. *Clin Infect Dis* 2001;32:E131–6.

48. Brussino L, Bucca C, Morello M, et al. Effect on dyspnoea and hypoxaemia of inhaled NG-nitro-L-arginine methyl ester in hepatopulmonary syndrome. *Lancet* 2003;362:43–4.

49. Tanikella R, Philips G, Faulk D, et al. Pilot study of pentoxifylline in hepatopulmonary syndrome. *Liver Transpl* 2008;14:1199–1203.

50. Arguedas M, Abrams GA, Krowka MJ, et al. Prospective evaluation of outcomes and predictors of mortality in patients with hepatopulmonary syndrome undergoing liver transplantation. *Hepatology* 2003;37:192–7.

51. Rich S, Dantzker D, Ayres S, et al. Primary pulmonary hypertension: a national prospective study. *Ann Intern Med* 1987;107:216–23.

52. McDonnell P, Toye P, Hutchins G. Primary pulmonary hypertension and cirrhosis: are they related? *Am Rev Respir Dis* 1983;127:437–41.

53. Hadengue A, Benhayoun M, Lebrec D, et al. Pulmonary hypertension complicating portal hypertension: prevalence and relation to splanchnic hemodynamics. *Gastroenterology* 1991;100:520–8.

54. Benjaminov FS, Prentice M, Sniderman KW, et al. Portopulmonary hypertension in decompensated cirrhosis with refractory ascites. *Gut* 2003;52:1355–62.

55. Kuo P, Plotkin J, Johnson L, et al. Distinctive clinical features of portopulmonary hypertension. *Chest* 1997;112:980–6.

56. Plevak D, Krowka M, Rettke S, et al. Successful liver transplantation in patients with mild to moderate pulmonary hypertension. *Transplant Proc* 1993;25:1840.

57. Colle I, Moreau R, Godinho E, et al. Portopulmonary hypertension in candidates for liver transplantation: diagnosis at evaluation comparing Doppler echocardiography with cardiac catheterization and incidence on the waiting list. *Hepatology* 2003;37:401–9.

58. Kawut S, Krowka M, Trotter J, et al. Clinical risk factors for portopulmonary hypertension. *Hepatology* 2008;48:196–203.

59. Edwards B, Weir E, Edwards W, et al. Coexistent pulmonary and portal hypertension: morphologic and clinical features. *J Am Coll Cardiol* 1987;10:1233–8.

60. Pietra G. Histopathology of primary pulmonary hypertension. *Chest* 1994;105:2S–6S.

61. Matsubara O, Nakamura T, Uehara T, et al. Histometrical investigation of the pulmonary artery in severe hepatic disease. *J Pathol* 1984;143:31–7.

62. Roberts KE, Fallon MB, Krowka MJ, et al. Genetic risk factors for portopulmonary hypertension in patients with advanced liver disease. *Am J Respir Crit Care Med* 2009;179(9):835–42.

63. Roberts KE, Fallon MB, Krowka MJ, et al. Serotonin transporter polymorphisms in patients with portopulmonary hypertension. *Chest.* 2009;135(6):1470–5.

64. Robalino B, Moodie D. Association between primary pulmonary hypertension and portal hypertension: analysis of its pathophysiology and clinical, laboratory and hemodynamic manifestations. *J Am Coll Cardiol* 1991;17:492–8.

65. Hoeper MM, Krowka MJ, Strassburg CP. Portopulmonary hypertension and hepatopulmonary syndrome. *Lancet* 2004;363:1461–8.

66. Pilatis N, Jacobs L, Rerkpattanapipat P, et al. Clinical predictors of pulmonary hypertension in patients undergoing liver transplant evaluation. *Liver Transpl* 2000;6:85–91.

67. Krowka M, Plevak D, Findlay J, et al. Pulmonary hemodynamics and perioperative cardiopulmonary-related mortality in patients with portopulmonary hypertension undergoing liver transplantation. *Liver Transpl* 2000;6:443–50.

68. D'Alonzo G, Barst R, Ayres S, et al. Survival in patients with primary pulmonary hypertension: results from a national prospective registry. *Ann Intern Med.* 1991;115:343–9.

69. Kawut SM, Taichman DB, Ahya VN, et al. Hemodynamics and survival of patients with portopulmonary hypertension. *Liver Transpl* 2005;11:1107–11.

70. Provencher S, Herve P, Jais X, et al. Deleterious effects of beta-blockers on exercise capacity and hemodynamics in patients with portopulmonary hypertension. *Gastroenterology* 2006;130(1):120–6.

71. Kalambokis G, Korantzopoulos P, Nikas S, et al. Significant improvement of portopulmonary hypertension after 1 week terlipressin treatment. *J Hepatol* 2009;48:678–80.

72. Tapper EB, Knowles D, Heffron T, et al. Portopulmonary hypertension: imatinib as a novel treatment and the emory experience with this condition. *Transplant Proc* 2009;41:1969–71.

73. Swanson KRH, Wiesner RSL, Nyberg S, et al. Survival in portopulmonary hypertension: Mayo Clinic experience categorized by treatment subgroups. *Am J Transpl* 2008;8:2445–53.

74. Ashfaq M, Chinnakotla S, Rogers L, et al. The impact of treatment of portopulmonary hypertension on survival following liver transplantation. *Am J Transpl* 2007;7:1258–1264.

75. Krowka MJ, Fallon MB, Mulligan DC, et al. Model for end-stage liver disease (MELD) exception for portopulmonary hypertension. *Liver Transpl* 2006;12:S114–16.

Multiple choice questions

16.1 A 65-year-old male with hepatitis C cirrhosis is seen in clinic for a follow-up visit. The patient complains of gradually worsening dyspnea on exertion over the past 3–4 months. He has no prior history of lung disease and quit smoking 20 years back with a cumulative 10-pack-year smoking history. He has ascites that is well controlled on diuretics. Physical examination reveals a nondistended abdomen, clear lungs, and no lower extremity edema. The chest X-ray and ECG are normal. Pulmonary function tests show normal spirometry and lung volumes, and the diffusion capacity of carbon monoxide is 43%. Lab results are: arterial blood gases – pH 7.43, PCO_2 36 mmHg, PO_2 62 mmHg; total bilirubin 1.6 mg/dL, AST : ALT 58 : 68, albumin 3.1 g/dL, and international normalized ratio (INR) 1.5. Which of the following is the most appropriate next step?

   a CT angiography of the chest.
   b Contrast Doppler echocardiography.
   c Start supplemental oxygen therapy.
   d Right heart catheterization.

16.2 A 54-year-old male with cryptogenic cirrhosis is being evaluated for liver transplantation. The patient has noticed decreased exercise tolerance gradually over the past 6 months and complains of fatigue. He has developed worsening ascites and marked lower extremity despite sodium restriction and the addition of spironolactone 100 mg per day and furosemide 40 mg per day. Physical examination reveals moderate ascites and 3+ pitting edema in the lower extremities. The chest X-ray and three-phase abdominal CT scan are unremarkable. Doppler cardiac echography reveals an estimated pulmonary artery systolic pressure of 50 mmHg, dilated right ventricle, and normal left ventricular function. Adenosine MIBI shows normal cardiac perfusion. Lab results are: total bilirubin 4.8 mg/dL, AST : ALT 70 : 84, albumin 2.8 g/dL, INR 2.0, BUN/Cr 21/1.4, Na 132, K +4.2, TSH 3.5, and MELD (model for end-stage liver disease) score 23. Which of the following is the most appropriate next step?

   a Increase diuretics, follow-up closely, and perform a repeat Doppler cardiac echogram.
   b List for liver transplantation.
   c Right heart catheterization.
   d Coronary angiography.

Answers to the multiple choice questions can be found in the Appendix at the end of the book.

These multiple choice questions are also available for you to complete online.
Visit http://www.schiffsdiseasesoftheliver.com/

CHAPTER 17

Ascites and Spontaneous Bacterial Peritonitis

Bruce A. Runyon

Division of Gastroenterology/Hepatology, Loma Linda University Medical Center, Loma Linda, CA, USA

Key concepts

- The most common cause of ascites, by a huge margin, is cirrhosis, followed by heart failure, malignancy, tuberculosis, and miscellaneous causes. A careful history, physical examination, ascitic fluid analysis, imaging, and special testing in unusual situations usually provide definitive diagnoses regarding the cause(s) of ascites and complications, such as spontaneous bacterial peritonitis.

- Treatment of patients with ascites is dependent on the cause(s) of fluid formation. For example, peritoneal carcinomatosis does not respond to diuretic therapy.

- Ascitic fluid forms in the setting of cirrhosis due to intrahepatic portal hypertension, splanchnic vasodilatation, and renal retention of sodium and water, in an effort to refill what is perceived as an underfilled intravascular space.

- A detailed history provides information regarding risk factors (alcohol, needle use, country of origin, obesity, etc.) as well as risk factors for heart failure, malignancy, and tuberculosis.

- Most patients with cirrhosis as the cause for ascites formation have physical findings that raise suspicion for liver disease, including vascular spiders, palmar erythema, and abdominal wall collaterals.

- Abdominal paracentesis with ascitic fluid analysis is crucial in detecting the cause of ascites formation and in detecting ascitic fluid infection. This simple, safe bedside or clinic procedure can be performed by an experienced operator, a person on the "procedure team," or an interventional radiologist. Despite coagulopathy in most patients, bleeding is rare. Patients with cirrhosis usually have a balanced deficiency of procoagulants and anticoagulants and normal global coagulation despite abnormal screening coagulation tests. Prophylactic transfusion of blood products is not data supported and is discouraged.

- The appearance of the fluid and the test results guide therapy. Patients with evidence of cirrhosis and a serum–ascites albumin gradient ≥1.1 g/dL should receive diet education regarding a 2000 mg/day sodium diet and dual diuretics. Patients with an elevated neutrophil count in the fluid should be pancultured and urgently started on an antibiotic that is known to penetrate the fluid in high enough concentrations to kill the bacteria. Cefotaxime 2 g intravenously every 8 hours is the most data-supported empirical antibiotic. Once susceptibility tests are available, a narrower spectrum drug can be chosen. Drugs with no data on ascitic fluid penetration should not be used.

- Ascitic fluid-specific leukocyte esterase strips or "dipsticks" are under investigation and should lead to a diagnosis of infection in 90–180 seconds. A delay in detection and treatment of infection worsens survival.

- Patients in specific subgroups benefit from selective intestinal decontamination with drugs such as norfloxacin to prevent recurrence of spontaneous bacterial peritonitis and ceftriaxone to prevent infection that regularly complicates gut hemorrhage in these patients.

- Diet combined with spironolactone and furosemide in single morning doses can control the fluid in >90% of compliant patients. Fluid restriction is unnecessary and not data supported. Treatment options for diuretic-resistant patients include therapeutic paracentesis every 2 weeks, transjugular intrahepatic portosystemic shunt (TIPS), and rarely peritoneovenous shunt. Liver transplantation is the ultimate solution to liver failure, but few organs are available and many of these patients have psychosocial contraindications to transplantation.

The patient with ascites is a common diagnostic and therapeutic challenge to the internist and gastroenterologist. Ascites due to cirrhosis is associated with significant morbidity and mortality, in part related to the severe underlying liver disease and in part due to the ascites per se. Approximately one half of patients in whom cirrhosis is detected prior to the development of "decompensation" (i.e., prior to development of ascites, jaundice,

encephalopathy, or gastrointestinal hemorrhage) develop ascites within 10 years [1]. Once ascites, or other evidence of decompensation is present, the expected mortality is ~50% in just 2 years [2].

The word "ascites" is of Greek derivation (*askos*) and refers to a bag or sack. The word is a noun, is singular, and is used to refer to the condition of pathologic fluid accumulation within the abdominal cavity. The adjective,

Schiff's Diseases of the Liver, Eleventh Edition. Edited by Eugene R. Schiff, Willis C. Maddrey and Michael F. Sorrell.
© 2012 John Wiley & Sons, Ltd. Published 2012 by John Wiley & Sons, Ltd.

ascitic, is used in conjunction with the word, fluid, to describe the liquid per se. The proper term is "ascitic fluid" not "ascites fluid."

Diagnosis and differential diagnosis

The most common setting in which ascites develops is in a patient with known cirrhosis or a patient with a risk factor for development of cirrhosis, e.g., alcohol abuse or chronic hepatitis C. As the patient develops jaundice or loses muscle mass, or deteriorates in another fashion, the abdomen swells, frequently as body weight increases. In this context, the diagnosis is readily suspected from the patient's history and is easily confirmed by the presence of shifting dullness on physical examination and by a successful abdominal paracentesis. Some patients are less cognizant of their physical appearance and weight; in this setting, when there is not a large volume of fluid, the diagnosis may be first detected on imaging. The presence of abdominal fullness and bulging flanks should lead to percussion of the flanks. If the amount of flank dullness is greater than usual – i.e., if the percussed air–fluid level is higher than normally found on the lateral aspect of the abdomen with the patient supine – then "shifting" of the dullness should be checked. If there is no flank dullness, there is no reason to check for shifting dullness. Approximately 1500 mL of fluid must be present before dullness is detected [3]. If no flank dullness is present, the patient has less than a 10% chance of having large volume ascites [3]. The fluid wave and "puddle sign" were found to be much less helpful in a study of physical findings in patients with small volume ascites [3].

A thick panniculus, gaseous distension of the bowel, and an ovarian mass can be confused with the presence of ascites. An obese abdomen may be diffusely dull to percussion, and an attempt at paracentesis (if there is significant suspicion of ascites) or abdominal ultrasound may be required to settle the question. Ultrasound or computerized tomography can detect as little as 100 mL of fluid in the abdomen. Gaseous distension should be apparent on percussion. Ovarian masses characteristically cause tympanitic flanks with central dullness.

Although parenchymal liver disease is the cause of ascites formation in most patients evaluated by internists and gastroenterologists, approximately 15% of patients have a cause other than liver disease (Table 17.1) [4]. Approximately 5% of patients with ascites have two causes of ascites formation, i.e., "mixed" ascites. Usually these patients have cirrhosis as well as one of the following: hepatocellular carcinoma, peritoneal carcinomatosis, or peritoneal tuberculosis (Table 17.1). Since tuberculosis is curable and potentially fatal, one must not assume that a patient has *only* liver disease as the cause of ascites

Table 17.1 Causes of ascites.

Cause	% of total number of patients
Parenchymal liver disease with or without infection:	84
"Mixed" ascites	5
Acute hepatitis with underlying cirrhosis	1
Chylous ascites due to cirrhosis	1
Fulminant hepatic failure	1
Heart failure	3
Malignancy	2.5
Tuberculosis	<1
Pancreatic	<1
Nephrogenous ("dialysis ascites")	<1
Chlamydia	<1
Nephrotic	<1
Miscellaneous	~5%

Based on a series of 901 paracenteses performed in a predominantly inpatient hepatology/general internal medicine setting [4].

formation, if the clinical situation is atypical. For example, if the ascitic fluid lymphocyte count is unusually high or there is persistent unexplained fever in the setting of cirrhosis, peritoneal tuberculosis may be present. Interpretation of ascitic fluid analysis is difficult in patients with mixed ascites but crucial to appropriate diagnosis and treatment (see below on ascitic fluid analysis). Additionally, not all patients with liver disease and ascites have cirrhosis. Ascites regularly develops in the setting of severe alcoholic hepatitis. Ascites along with hepatic coma can develop as manifestations of acute liver failure in viral hepatitis. However, because fulminant liver failure itself is quite uncommon, the total number of patients with ascites who have acute liver failure is quite small. One percent of the large series detailed in Table 17.1 involved acute liver failure, and 1% occurred in the setting of acute hepatitis superimposed on cirrhosis.

Cancer is an uncommon cause of ascites formation as seen by the hepatologist/general internist. Unfortunately, most patients with malignancy-related ascites (except ovarian cancer and lymphoma) only survive a few weeks after the onset of fluid retention [5]. If there is a delay in diagnosis because of confusion about the diagnosis, many of these patients will die during the hospitalization for which they presented with ascites. The physician's goal in treating this subgroup of patients with ascites should be to rapidly make a diagnosis and maximize the time that the patient can spend out of hospital. Not all malignancy-related ascites is due to peritoneal carcinomatosis; the characteristics of the ascitic fluid and the treatments vary depending on the pathophysiology of the ascites formation, e.g., peritoneal carcinomatosis versus massive liver metastases versus malignant lymph node obstruction with chylous ascites [5] (see also the section on ascitic fluid analysis).

In the past, heart failure was a common cause of ascites. Improved treatment of heart failure and a decreasing prevalence of heart disease have led to its decline to ~3% as a cause of ascites formation. Ascites is currently an uncommon complication of heart disease [6]. Meanwhile liver disease has increased dramatically as a cause of ascites.

In the United States, tuberculous peritonitis is a disease of immigrants and of patients with underlying cirrhosis, usually due to alcohol. More than 50% of patients with tuberculous peritonitis are found to have underlying cirrhosis, i.e., mixed ascites.

Pancreatitic ascites develops as a complication of severe acute pancreatitis or as a complication of chronic pancreatitis with pancreatic duct rupture or leakage from a pseudocyst. Patients with this form of ascites may also have underlying cirrhosis. Pancreatic ascites may be complicated by bacterial infection. This combination is frequently misdiagnosed and usually fatal.

Nephrogenous ascites is a poorly understood form of fluid overload that develops in patients undergoing hemodialysis [7]. On careful evaluation many of these patients are found to have underlying chronic liver disease or peritoneal disease. The presence of underlying liver disease may be the reason that they develop fluid overload more readily than dialysis patients who do not have liver disease.

In sexually active young women with fever and neutrocytic ascites, *Chlamydia* peritonitis should be placed near the top of the differential diagnosis. *Chlamydia* causes a Fitz-Hugh–Curtis syndrome [8]. This rapidly responds to doxycycline and is one of the few curable causes of ascites formation.

Although nephrotic syndrome used to be a common cause of ascites formation in children, it is quite rare in adults, causing <1% in the series reported in Table 17.1.

Some patients develop pathologic accumulations of fluid in the peritoneal cavity due to leakage from a ruptured viscus, e.g., "bile ascites" in the setting of a ruptured gallbladder [9]. The ascitic fluid analysis can be crucial to making a preoperative diagnosis of this condition (see below).

Conditions excluded from or not encountered in the series detailed in Table 17.1 include ambulatory peritoneal dialysis fluid, Budd–Chiari syndrome, myxedema ascites, ascites associated with benign ovarian disease, and ascites associated with connective tissue diseases. The iatrogenic form of ascites associated with peritoneal dialysis is usually under the management of nephrologists. Although Budd–Chiari syndrome is regularly (if not always) complicated by ascites, hepatic vein throm-

bosis itself is rare enough that it causes <1% (probably <0.1%) of cases of ascites. Ascites in patients with myxedema appears to be cardiac ascites, related to the subtle heart failure that these patients develop [10]. Treatment of the thyroid insufficiency cures the fluid retention. In recent years most ascites that is caused by ovarian disease involves peritoneal carcinomatosis [5]. Meigs syndrome (i.e., ascites and pleural effusion caused by benign ovarian neoplasms) is no longer a common cause of ascites formation. Serositis with ascites formation may complicate systemic lupus erythematosus [11].

Pathogenesis of ascites formation in liver disease

Simplistically, ascites forms in severe chronic and/or acute liver disease as a result of portal hypertension, baroreceptor activation, and neurohumorally mediated abnormalities in renal perfusion, with resulting sodium retention. The clinically apparent problem is that of intravascular and extravascular volume overload. The site of spillover of fluid is the peritoneal cavity because of the portal hypertension.

The questions that have puzzled investigators in this field are: (i) what is the *initial* event; and (ii) why is there neurohumoral excitation (which should be characteristic of volume depletion) in the setting of volume overload? Animals (including humans) have very sophisticated and duplicative systems for the detection and preservation of normal or near normal vascular perfusion pressures and intravascular osmolality. However, the animal's ability to sense abnormalities in intravascular *volume* status (especially volume overload) is limited and is linked largely to pressure receptors. This may partially explain the paradox of dramatic volume overload in the face of sympathetic nervous traffic and hormone levels that are indicative of intravascular volume depletion.

All current investigators in the field of the pathogenesis of ascites formation agree that patients are intravascularly volume overloaded once they reach the stage of large volume ascites. Now we recognize "compensated" and "decompensated" stages and that there is a spectrum of renal failure in patients with cirrhosis. Hepatorenal syndrome is the extreme end of the spectrum. The most recent theory – the peripheral arterial vasodilatation hypothesis – has proposed that both the older "underfill" and "overflow" theories of ascites formation are correct, but that each is operative at a different stage [12]. The first abnormality that eventually leads to fluid retention, according to this theory, is peripheral arterial vasodilatation that is mediated by nitric oxide. Intravascular underfilling occurs because the compartment enlarges. The vasodilatation hypothesis proposes that in the early compensated stage of cirrhosis (i.e., before fluid retention occurs), intravascular hypervolemia suppresses renin, aldosterone, vasopressin, and norepinephrine concentrations such that abnormally elevated levels of these hormones are usually not detected. Also, these patients usually have normal indices of renal function. As the state of vasodilatation worsens, renal function deteriorates and plasma levels of vasoconstrictor, sodium-retentive hormones increase; ascites develops, that is "decompensation" occurs. Hepatorenal syndrome is the extreme end of the spectrum.

Intrahepatic portal hypertension plays a crucial role in ascites formation. Patients with prehepatic portal hypertension (e.g., portal vein thrombosis) rarely develop ascites, usually in the setting of fluid resuscitation for gut hemorrhage. Only patients with high sinusoidal pressure regularly develop fluid retention. Patients or dogs with cirrhosis but normal portal pressures due to surgical decompression do not develop ascites [13].

The site of ascites formation is also dependent on the presence of portal hypertension. Theoretically, fluid could form from the surface of the liver or the gut. However, the data support the liver as the site of ascites formation. The hepatic sinusoid lacks a basement membrane and is therefore more permeable than the bowel. Lymph flow is linearly related to pressure. The large hydrostatic pressure gradient present in the portal hypertensive liver leads to loss of intravascular fluid across the hepatic sinusoids into the space of Disse, and weeping of the fluid from the liver surface as extravasated lymph. Older animal experiments confirm the liver as the source of ascites formation also. If the liver of a portal hypertensive dog is moved into the chest, the dog develops a pleural effusion rather than ascites [14]. If the liver is placed in a cellophane bag in situ, fluid forms within the bag [15].

In summary, in the early phase of ascites formation there is vasodilatation and renal retention of sodium with eventual overflow of fluid into the peritoneal cavity from the hepatic sinusoids. After ascites is formed, underfilling assumes a more prominent role. The sequestration of intravascular fluid in the abdomen in large quantities results in decreased "effective intravascular volume" and triggers: (i) increased non-osmotic secretion of antidiuretic hormone; (ii) renin and aldosterone release; (iii) further stimulation of sympathetic nervous system activity; and (v) further sodium and water retention. The cycle is self-perpetuating.

Evaluation of patients with ascites

History

Most ascites is due to cirrhosis. In the past most cirrhosis in the United States was caused by alcohol. Now many patients have chronic hepatitis C *and* excess alcohol use in the setting of obesity. Multiple insults are probably synergistic in causing cirrhosis. Patients who have a component of alcoholic liver disease and who intermittently reduce alcohol consumption may experience wet/dry cycles in terms of fluid retention. The cycles of ascites may be separated by years of normal sodium balance and tend to parallel their alcohol consumption. In contrast, patients who develop ascites with nonalcoholic liver disease tend to be persistently fluid overloaded, probably due to the late stage at which ascites forms in nonalcoholic liver disease and the lack of effective therapy other than liver transplantation. Cirrhosis due to reactivated hepatitis B is the exception here. These patients can also have a dramatic response to (non-interferon-based) antiviral therapy.

When the patient has a very long history of stable cirrhosis and then develops ascites, the possibility of hepatocellular carcinoma should be considered as the cause for decompensation.

Patients with ascites should also be questioned about risk factors for liver disease other than alcohol, e.g., intravenous drug use, homosexuality (a risk factor for hepatitis B), transfusions, acupuncture, tattoos, country of origin, etc. In the current obesity epidemic, nonalcoholic fatty liver disease (NAFLD) is also contributing to the development of cirrhosis, with or without other risk factors. Asking the patient about lifetime maximum body weight, diabetes, and number of years of being overweight/obese can provide a cause for cirrhosis that may have been thought to be "cryptogenic" [16].

Patients who have a history of cancer and develop ascites should be suspected of having malignancy-related ascites. Breast, colon, and pancreatic cancer are regularly complicated by ascites [5]. Patients with malignancy-related ascites frequently have abdominal pain, whereas ascites due to cirrhosis is usually not associated with abdominal pain unless there is superimposed bacterial peritonitis or alcoholic hepatitis.

Patients with cardiac ascites often have a past history of heart failure or restrictive lung disease. Alcoholics who develop ascites may have alcoholic cardiomyopathy or liver disease. The serum pro-BNP can help in the differential diagnosis of ascites due to heart failure from ascites due to cirrhosis [17] (see below).

Tuberculous peritonitis is usually manifested by fever and abdominal pain in a patient who has recently emigrated from an endemic area or a US resident with cirrhosis. More than one half of patients with tuberculous peritonitis have underlying cirrhosis as a second cause for ascites formation.

Patients who develop ascites and anasarca in the setting of longstanding diabetes should be suspected of having nephrotic ascites. Ascites developing in a patient with cold intolerance, lethargy, altered bowel motility, changes in the skin, etc. should prompt measurement of thyroid function tests. Serositis in connective tissue diseases may be complicated by ascites [11].

Physical examination

The details of the physical examination in detecting ascites are also discussed at the beginning of this chapter. The fluid wave has not been found to be of much value in the detection of ascites [3]. The puddle sign can detect 120 mL of fluid, but feeble patients cannot cooperate in the performance of this test; patients must remain in a hands-knees position during the examination. A simple ultrasound, which is available to many hepatologists now, can rule in ascites very rapidly, especially in the obese patient, where physical examination is difficult due to the thick panniculus.

The presence of palmar erythema or large pulsatile vascular spiders is very suggestive of the presence of cirrhosis. The presence of pathologically large abdominal wall collateral veins suggests that portal hypertension is present. The presence of large veins on the flanks and dorsum of the patient suggests inferior vena cava blockage by a fibrous caval web or malignant obstruction. A firm nodule in the umbilicus, the Sister Mary Joseph nodule, is very suggestive of peritoneal carcinomatosis – usually from a gastric primary. The neck veins of ascites patients should always be examined for distension in pursuit of a cardiac origin of ascites. Some patients with cardiac ascites will have bulging forehead veins that can be seen from across the room. Some will have no visible jugular venous distension. When patients with liver disease have peripheral edema, it is usually in the lower extremities and spares the arms. Patients with cardiac failure or nephrotic syndrome may have leg and arm edema, e.g., anasarca.

Ascites may be quantified using the following system:
- 1+: detectable only by careful examination.
- 2+: easily detected but of relatively small volume.
- 3+: obvious ascites but not tense.
- 4+: tense ascites.

This system works relatively well for patients with chronic ascites and flaccid abdominal wall muscles. However, patients with acute-onset ascites and good musculature, as in fulminant hepatic failure, may have a tense abdomen without a large volume of fluid.

Abdominal paracentesis

In the past many physicians avoided diagnostic paracentesis in the evaluation of patients with ascites, in part because of concern regarding complications of paracentesis. However, in view of the documented safety of this procedure and the frequency of ascitic fluid infection, paracentesis should: (i) be performed as a routine part of the evaluation of "new-onset" ascites; (ii) be repeated as part of the admission physical examination of patients hospitalized with ascites; and (iii) be repeated again in outpatients or during hospitalization if the patient develops any signs or symptoms suggestive of infection [18,19].

Choice of needle entry site and needle

In the past, the avascular midline was often chosen as the site for paracentesis. However, in the current obesity epidemic, the midline may be extremely thick. Also, many paracenteses these days are therapeutic. One cannot aspirate much fluid from the midline unless the patient is positioned such that the fluid is dependent. A recent prospective study has shown that the abdominal wall is thinner and the size of the pool of fluid is larger in the left lower quadrant [20]. The needle is inserted 3 cm cephalad and 3 cm medial to the anterior superior iliac spine. The left side is preferable to the right side to avoid appendectomy scars and to avoid a gas-filled cecum, common in patients taking lactulose.

Surgical scars pose a significant problem in the selection of a site for needle entry of the abdominal wall. Needles inserted near abdominal wall scars may enter the bowel, which may be adherent to the serosal surface of the abdomen [18]. The needle must be placed several centimeters from the scar.

If only a tiny amount is fluid is present, an image-guided tap by an interventional radiologist may be appropriate.

This author prefers to use standard metal 1.5 inch needles: 22-gauge for diagnostic taps and 16–18 gauge for therapeutic taps. Spinal needles (i.e., 3.5 inch needles) are needed if the abdominal wall is thick. Bare steel needles are preferable to plastic-sheathed cannulas because of the risk of the sheath shearing off into the peritoneal cavity and the tendency of the plastic sheath to kink. Metal needles do not puncture the bowel unless there is a surgical scar (tethering the bowel to the abdominal wall) or severe gaseous bowel distension. The steel needle can be left in the abdomen during a therapeutic tap for many minutes without injury, unless the needle is allowed to drift subcutaneously. Larger bore needles may speed drainage but leave larger defects if they inadvertently enter vessels or the bowel. A multihole disposable needle is now available.

Technique of diagnostic paracentesis

The skin is disinfected with an iodine solution. The skin and subcutaneous tissue should be infiltrated with a local anesthetic. Drapes, gown, hat, and mask are optional but sterile gloves should be used when actually obtaining the fluid. The sterile paper package insert in which the gloves are enclosed can be used as a sterile field on which to place syringes, needles, etc. If sterile gloves are not used there may be a high prevalence of skin contaminants growing from the cultures that are obtained.

The manner in which the needle is inserted is important in preventing continued leakage of fluid after the needle is withdrawn. Use of a "Z tract" minimizes leakage. To create a Z tract, the operator uses one gloved hand to move the skin ~2 cm caudad in relation to the deep abdominal wall and then inserts the paracentesis needle with the other hand. The key is to be able to manipulate the syringe with only one hand. The skin is not released until the needle has penetrated the peritoneum and fluid begins to flow. When the needle is removed, the skin slips back into its original position and seals the needle pathway. If the needle is inserted without a "Z", the fluid leaks out easily because its pathway is straight.

The needle should be advanced slowly in ~5 mm increments. If it is inserted in one rapid motion, vessels and bowel may be impaled by the needle. A slow insertion allows the operator to see a flash of blood if he enters a vessel; the needle can then be withdrawn before further damage is done. A slow insertion also allows the bowel to float away from the needle without needle penetration of it. The syringe that is attached to the needle should not be aspirated until there is fluid visible in the needle hub. If there is continuous suction on the needle during its insertion, bowel or omentum may be drawn to the end of the needle as soon as the needle enters the peritoneal cavity – giving the appearance of a "dry tap." Therefore, the needle should be inserted ~5 mm, then the syringe should be aspirated for a few seconds while the needle is stationary, then advanced, then aspirated, etc. until the peritoneum is entered and fluid is aspirated. A slow insertion also allows time for the elastic peritoneum to tent over and be pierced by the needle. Once fluid is flowing, the needle should be stabilized so that its position can be maintained in order to insure a steady flow. It is not unusual for flow to stop as bowel or omentum is suctioned over the bevel of the needle. When flow ceases, the syringe is removed from the needle, the needle is twisted 90° and then inserted in 1–2 mm increments until dripping of fluid from the needle hub is achieved. The syringe is then reattached and fluid is aspirated. Occasionally, fluid cannot be aspirated but it drips nicely from the needle hub. In this situation, as in a lumbar puncture, fluid is allowed to drip into a sterile container for collection.

Indications

Abdominal paracentesis is probably the most rapid and cost-effective method of diagnosing the cause of ascites and the only method of detecting ascitic fluid infection. In view of the relatively high prevalence of ascitic fluid infection at the time ascites patients are admitted to the hospital, a surveillance tap may detect unexpected infection at the time of hospitalization. Not all patients with

ascitic fluid infection are symptomatic, and the detection of infection at an early asymptomatic stage may reduce mortality [21]. Therefore, this investigator advocates sampling ascitic fluid in all inpatients and outpatients with *new-onset* ascites and in all patients admitted to hospital with ascites, i.e., a tap at the time of each hospitalization. Paracentesis should be *repeated* in outpatients and inpatients who develop signs or symptoms of infection. Signs, symptoms, and lab abnormalities suggestive of infection include hypotension, abdominal pain or tenderness, fever, encephalopathy, renal failure, acidosis, and peripheral leukocytosis.

Contraindications

Prospective studies regarding paracentesis complications in patients with ascites have documented its safety [18, 19,22]. Complications included 2/229 (0.9%) transfusion-requiring abdominal wall hematomas, and 2/229 (0.9%) small hematomas in one study [18]. No serious complications or death were reported in two of the studies [18,19]; the third study reported a bleeding rate of 1% and the death in two patients after a total of 515 paracenteses [22]. This study also reported the breakage of a plastic catheter into the peritoneum and other complications that cause the reader to be concerned about the attention to detail involved in the study [22]. The breakage of a plastic catheter confirms the wisdom of using steel needles (see above).

Most patients who undergo paracentesis have significant coagulopathy. In one series the international normalized ratio (INR) was as high as 8.7 and the platelet count was as low as 19,000 cells/mm^3, yet no one had a bleeding complication and no one received transfusions of blood products before or after paracentesis [19]. No study has showed a correlation of bleeding with INR [18,19,22], and none of the prospective studies gave prophylactic transfusions [18,19,22].

There are few contraindications to paracentesis. Coagulopathy is frequently viewed as a potential contraindication. Coagulopathy has only precluded this author from performing a paracentesis when there was clinically evident primary fibrinolysis or disseminated intravascular coagulation; these conditions occur less than once per 1,000 taps. There is no cutoff of coagulation parameters beyond which paracentesis should not be performed. Even patients with severe prolongation of prothrombin time usually have a trivial ascitic fluid red cell count after multiple paracenteses. Patients with cirrhosis and ascites but without clinically obvious coagulopathy do not bleed excessively from needle sticks unless a blood vessel is entered [18,19,22].

There is a common misconception that the INR correlates with bleeding risk. It is powerful in predicting death in the setting of cirrhosis, but is not a good predictor of bleeding risk. The liver makes most of the procoagulants and most of the anticoagulants. The INR measures only the absence of procoagulants [23]. When the liver is functioning poorly, there is usually a *balanced deficiency of both pro- as well as anticoagulants, such that global coagulation is normal* [23].

It is the policy of some physicians to give prophylactic blood products (fresh frozen plasma and/or platelets) routinely before paracentesis in patients with cirrhosis and coagulopathy. This practice is not supported by the data.

Differential diagnosis by ascitic fluid analysis

Gross appearance of the fluid

Most ascitic fluid is transparent and yellow-tinged. Deeply bile-stained ascitic fluid from jaundiced patients is less bile stained than paired serum. Fluid as dark as molasses usually indicates biliary perforation [9]. The opacity of most cloudy ascitic fluid specimens is caused by neutrophils. The presence of particulate matter, such as neutrophils, leads to a shimmering effect when a glass tube of the fluid is held in front of a bright light. Absolute neutrophil counts under $1,000/mm^3$ may be nearly clear. Counts over $5,000/mm^3$ are quite cloudy, and counts over $50,000/mm^3$ have a purulent consistency.

Ascitic fluid specimens are occasionally blood-tinged or frankly bloody. A red cell count of $10,000/mm^3$ is the threshold for a pink appearance; smaller concentrations result in clear or "turbid" fluid. Ascitic fluid with a red cell count $>20,000/mm^3$ is distinctly blood-tinged. Many ascitic fluid specimens are bloody due to a traumatic tap in the setting of cirrhosis; these specimens are heterogenously bloody and clot. In contrast, nontraumatic or remotely traumatic bloody ascitic fluid is homogenously pigmented and does not clot because it has already clotted and lysed. Some patients with portal hypertension have bloody hepatic lymph leading to bloody ascitic fluid, perhaps because of the rupture of high-pressure lymphatics. Greater than one half of samples from patients with hepatocellular carcinoma that this investigator has encountered are bloody, but only about 10% of samples from patients with peritoneal carcinomatosis have this appearance [5]. Overall only 22% of malignancy-related samples (including primary liver cancer) are bloody [5]. Although many physicians are of the opinion that tuberculosis (TB) results in bloody ascites, less than 5% of TB samples are hemorrhagic in this author's experience [24].

There is a spectrum of "milkiness" in ascitic fluid ranging from slightly cloudy "opalescent" fluid to completely opaque chylous fluid. The most opaque milky fluid has a triglyceride concentration $>200\,mg/dL$, usu-

ally $>1,000\,mg/dL$. Fluids that look like dilute skimmed milk usually have a concentration of between 100 and $200\,mg/dL$. A substantial minority of ascitic fluid samples are neither transparent nor frankly milky. Some physicians mistake this fluid for pus; it is not viscous enough to be pus. In this condition, which this author labels "opalescent" ascitic fluid, the cloudiness of the fluid has been found to be caused by a slightly elevated triglyceride concentration of $50–200\,mg/dL$ [25]. The lipid will usually layer out in the refrigerator over a 48–72-hour interval.

Pancreatic ascites may appear tea-colored due to the effect of pancreatic enzymes on ascitic fluid red cells. Such fluid may have to be centrifuged to spin the red cells down and reveal the discolored supernatant. In hemorrhagic pancreatitis, the fluid may be so darkly pigmented that it appears black. Malignant melanoma can also result in black ascites.

Ascitic fluid tests

Some physicians order every test that they can think of when analyzing ascitic fluid. This practice can be expensive and can be more confusing than helpful, especially when unexpectedly abnormal results are encountered. An algorithm approach to ascitic fluid analysis is more appropriate. Screening tests are performed on the initial specimen, and additional testing is performed (usually necessitating another paracentesis) based on the results of the screening tests. Most specimens will consist of uncomplicated ascites in the setting of cirrhosis. No further testing will usually be needed in this setting.

Based on cost analysis, this author has developed a list of routine, optional, unusual, and unhelpful tests (Box 17.1). The strategy used in this algorithm is discussed below.

Cell count

The cell count is the single most helpful ascitic fluid test. If only one drop of fluid is obtained, it should be sent for cell count. Only a few microliters are required for a standard manual hemocytometer count. The fluid should be submitted in an anticoagulant tube, i.e., ethylenediaminetetra-acetic acid (EDTA), to prevent clotting. Since the decision to begin empirical antibiotic treatment of suspected ascitic fluid infection is based largely on the rapidly available absolute neutrophil count rather than the not-so-rapidly available culture, the cell count is more important than the culture in the early approach to these patients with regard to ascitic fluid infection.

The mean total white blood cell count in uncomplicated ascites in the setting of cirrhosis is reported to be $281\pm25\,cells/mm^3$; the upper limit is said to be $500\,cells/mm^3$ [26]. However, during diuresis in patients with cirrhosis and ascites, the cells exit the peritoneal

Box 17.1 Ascitic fluid lab data that can be obtained on patients with ascites.

Routine
- Cell count
- Albumin

Optional
- Total protein
- Glucose
- Lactate dehydrogenase
- Amylase
- Culture in blood culture bottles
- Gram stain

Unusual
- Tuberculosis smear and culture
- Cytology
- Triglyceride
- Bilirubin

Unhelpful
- pH
- Lactate
- Cholesterol
- Fibronectin

cavity more slowly than the fluid and the mean ascitic fluid white cell count has been shown to increase to >1,000 cells/mm^3 [27]. This author has encountered several examples of end-of-diuresis white cell counts >3,000/mm^3 and one example of 7,000/mm^3. However, before a patient can be diagnosed as having a diuresis-related elevation of ascitic fluid white cell count, three criteria must be fulfilled: (i) a prediuresis count must be available and must be normal; (ii) there must be a predominance of lymphocytes; and (iii) there must be no unexplained clinical signs or symptoms, e.g., fever or abdominal pain.

The mean percentage of polymorphonuclear cells (PMNs) in uncomplicated ascites due to cirrhosis is $27 \pm 2\%$; the upper limit of the absolute PMN count in uncomplicated cirrhotic ascitic fluid is usually stated to be 250/mm^3 [21]. Fortunately, the short life expectancy of PMNs (hours only) results in a relative stability in the absolute PMN count during diuresis (42 to 68 cells/mm^3 from the beginning to end; difference not significant) [26]. Therefore, the 250 cells/mm^3 "cutoff" pertains even at the end of diuresis.

Leukocyte esterase strips or dipsticks have been proposed as useful tools in making a diagnosis of ascitic fluid infection in 90–180 seconds. However, the early studies used strips that were calibrated for urine and had a very high PMN threshold for positivity and therefore a low sensitivity in detecting spontaneous bacterial peritonitis (SBP). A more recent strip has been developed specifically

for ascitic fluid and has been shown to have 100% sensitivity in detecting a PMN count of 250 cells/mm^3 [27]. Use of such a strip permits the physician to write an order for a life-saving antibiotic before leaving the patient's ward. Too often the laboratory delays the availability of the cell count, and the physician may not follow through in looking up the cell count until the bacterial culture is reported positive the next day. The patient may have expired by that time.

Inflammation is the most common cause of an elevated ascitic fluid white cell count. SBP is the most common form of inflammation of ascitic fluid. In the setting of SBP, the total white cell count is elevated as well as the absolute PMN count; PMNs comprise more than 50% of the total white cells and usually more than 70%. Also, in tuberculous peritonitis and peritoneal carcinomatosis there is usually an elevated total white cell count but with a predominance of lymphocytes [5,24]. The white cell count of chylous ascites may be increased because of the leakage of lymphocytes from ruptured lymphatics.

Most bloody ascites is the result of a slightly traumatic tap in a patient with cirrhosis. If a tap is traumatic, white cells from peripheral blood enter the peritoneal cavity with the red cells, and the ascitic fluid white cell count usually increases because of this. Since neutrophils predominate the white cell differential in blood, the ascitic fluid differential may be altered by contamination of ascitic fluid with blood. To correct for this contamination one simply subtracts one PMN per 250 red cells [26]. If the leakage of blood is not recent, the PMNs will have lysed and the corrected PMN count will be a negative number. If the corrected PMN count in a bloody specimen is ≥250 cells/mm^3, the patient must be assumed to be infected until proven otherwise.

Serum–ascites albumin gradient

In the past, the ascitic fluid total protein concentration was used to classify ascites into exudates (≥2.5 g/dL) and transudates (<2.5 g/dL). Unfortunately this form of classification is an extrapolation from pleural fluid analysis that does not work well in ascitic fluid [4,28,29]. In fact these terms as applied to ascitic fluid were never carefully defined or validated. Similarly, analysis of lactate dehydrogenase (LDH) and serum : ascitic fluid ratios of LDH or protein have not been found to work well in classifying ascitic fluid into exudates and transudates [30]. The *serum–ascites albumin gradient* (SAAG) has been shown in multiple studies to categorize ascites better than the total protein concentration and better than other parameters [4,29–30]. The "gradient" is based on oncotic–hydrostatic balance. If there is an abnormally high hydrostatic pressure gradient between the portal bed and ascitic fluid (i.e., portal hypertension), there must be a commensurately

Box 17.2 Classification of ascites by the serum–ascites albumin concentration gradient.

Low gradient (<1.1 g/dL)

- Peritoneal carcinomatosis
- Tuberculous peritonitis
- Pancreatic ascites
- Biliary ascites
- Nephrotic syndrome
- Serositis in connective tissue diseases

High gradient (≥1.1 g/dL)

- Cirrhosis
- Alcoholic hepatitis
- Cardiac ascites
- Massive liver metastases
- Fulminant hepatic failure
- Budd–Chiari syndrome
- Portal vein thrombosis
- Venoocclusive disease
- Fatty liver of pregnancy
- Myxedema
- "Mixed" ascites

large difference between ascitic fluid and intravascular oncotic forces [29]. Albumin exerts more oncotic force per unit weight than other proteins. The difference between serum and ascitic fluid albumin concentration correlates directly with portal pressure [29].

It is this author's experience that some physicians try to make this simple concept more difficult to understand than it really is. The albumin gradient does not explain the pathogenesis of ascites formation. It does not explain where the albumin came from, i.e., liver or bowel. It simply gives the physician an accurate indirect index of portal pressure. Stated in another way, the higher the SAAG, the greater the portal pressure (Box 17.2). If the SAAG is ≥1.1 g/dL, the patient has portal hypertension with >95% accuracy [4,28–30]. Also, if the serum albumin-ascitic fluid *total protein* is ≥1.1 g/dL, the patient has portal hypertension, since ascitic fluid albumin cannot be greater than ascitic fluid total protein. Conversely, if the SAAG is <1.1 g/dL, the patient does not have portal hypertension. Calculating the SAAG involves measuring the albumin concentration of serum and ascitic fluid specimens and then simply *subtracting* the ascitic fluid value from the serum value. Again, there has been some confusion here. *It is a subtraction not a ratio.*

If the SAAG is obtained under the correct circumstances and performed properly, accuracy approaches 100%. In the largest series reported (involving 901 paired specimens), accuracy was 96.7% [4]. This test is accurate

despite SBP, diuresis, therapeutic paracentesis, albumin infusion (both serum and ascitic fluid albumin concentrations increase in parallel), and etiology of liver disease [29]. However, there are situations in which accuracy decreases. Specimens should be obtained relatively simultaneously. The ascitic fluid value from last week or last year cannot be subtracted from today's serum value; the state of hydration or nutrition of the patient may be different at different times. The specimens should be obtained on the same day – better yet, within the same hour. Both serum and ascitic fluid albumin concentrations change over time; however, the beauty of this test is that these values change in parallel such that the difference is stable. Another situation in which the test is potentially inaccurate is in the unstable (e.g., hypotensive) patient. If the arterial pressure is low, the portal pressure and albumin gradient may be lowered.

Accuracy of the albumin assay at low albumin concentrations, e.g. <1 g/dL, is important because many ascites patients have serum albumins in the 2.0–3.0 g/dL range and ascitic fluid albumins in the 0–1.0 g/dL range. Usually, the lab's albumin standards must be diluted to insure linearity of the assay at low range. Nephelometry is not appropriate for testing ascites. If the albumin assay is not accurate at a low range, errors will occur. Also, if a patient with cirrhosis has a serum albumin of <1.1 g/dL (this occurs in <1% of ascites patients), the gradient will be falsely low. In some labs lipid interferes with the albumin assay, therefore chylous ascites may have a falsely high albumin gradient.

A high serum globulin (>5 g/dL) is occasionally found in a patient with cirrhosis and ascites. A high serum globulin concentration leads to a high ascitic fluid globulin concentration and can narrow the albumin gradient by contributing to the oncotic forces. A narrowed gradient due to high globulin occurs in only ∼1% of ascitic fluid specimens. Correcting the gradient for high globulin increases accuracy of the gradient from ∼97% to ∼98% and explains some otherwise confusing cases. To correct the SAAG in the setting of a high serum globulin, the uncorrected SAAG is multiplied by (0.21 + (0.208 × serum globulin)) [31].

"High albumin gradient" and "low albumin gradient" should replace the terms "transudative" and "exudative" in the classification of ascites [4,28–30]. Another problem with the exudate/transudate system of classification is that it has no provision for patients with two causes for ascites formation, i.e., mixed ascites. Most of these patients have portal hypertension due to cirrhosis *plus* another cause for ascites formation, e.g., TB or peritoneal carcinomatosis [4]. Approximately 5% of ascites patients have mixed ascites (see Table 17.1) [4]. The presence of TB or peritoneal carcinomatosis would not be expected to lower the portal pressure. The albumin gradient remains high

($\geq$1.1 g/dL) in mixed ascites, as a reflection of the underlying portal hypertension.

Some physicians have the impression that a high albumin gradient is equivalent to a liver biopsy demonstrating cirrhosis and a low albumin gradient is equivalent to a peritoneal biopsy demonstrating carcinomatosis. However, the albumin gradient provides no histologic diagnosis; it is only an indirect measurement of portal pressure. Cirrhosis is the most common cause of a high albumin gradient, and peritoneal carcinomatosis is the most common cause of a low albumin gradient [4]. However, there are other causes of high and low gradients (see Box 17.2). The albumin gradient need only be performed on the first paracentesis in a given patient, it need not be repeated in subsequent specimens if the first value is definitive. If the first is borderline, e.g., 1.0 or 1.1 g/dL, a repeat paracentesis (performed at a time near when the blood is obtained) and analysis usually is definitive.

Culture

The most common bacterial infection of ascitic fluid is SBP [32]. The sensitivity of bacterial culture in detecting bacterial growth in neutrocytic ascites (i.e., ascitic fluid with a PMN count $\geq$250 cells/mm^3) varies dramatically depending on the method of culture used. In the studies that have been conducted, the older culture method has been found to detect bacterial growth in 42–43% of samples of neutrocytic ascites, whereas bedside inoculation of blood culture bottles with ascitic fluid detects growth in 91–93% [33,34]. In many hospitals, the sensitivity of older culture is only ~20–30% in this investigator's experience. The older method of culture consisted of inoculation of three agar plates and some culture broth with a few drops of fluid each, in the microbiology laboratory. At least one plate was designed to selectively support the growth of Gram-negative organisms and to suppress growth of other flora; the older method assumes that polymicrobial infection is the rule and that a large concentration of bacteria is common. However, SBP is essentially always a monomicrobial infection with a low colony count – very similar to bacteremia. Culturing ascitic fluid as if it is blood might be predicted to be superior to culturing the fluid as if it is urine or stool. In fact, multiple prospective studies have demonstrated the superiority of the blood culture bottle method; no study has demonstrated the superiority of the older method [33,34].

Some laboratories culture the centrifuged sediment of ~50 mL of fluid, presuming that this modification of the conventional method is superior to the older method of culture per se. Unfortunately, spinning the bacteria into the pelleted neutrophils results in a lower detection rate of bacteria than that of the conventional method, presumably because of the neutrophil-mediated killing of bacteria [33].

Box 17.3 Problems with the "exudate/transudate" system of ascites classification.

- Approximately two thirds of patients with cirrhosis develop total protein $\geq$2.5 g/dL during diuresis
- ~20% of patients with cirrhosis have ascitic fluid total protein $\geq$2.5 g/dL
- ~0% of SBP samples have ascitic fluid total protein $\geq$2.5 g/dL
- Exudate concept does not acknowledge "mixed" ascites
- Patients with massive liver metastases and hepatocellular carcinoma have ascitic fluid total protein <2.5 g/dL
- 100% of cardiac ascites samples have ascitic fluid total protein $\geq$2.5 g/dL
- 50% of tuberculous peritonitis patients have underlying cirrhosis and ascitic fluid total protein <2.5 g/dL

Some laboratories do not release blood culture bottles to the patient wards. Technicians bring the bottles with them when they draw blood for cultures. In this setting, bedside inoculation of the bottles would be difficult. However, bedside inoculation has been shown to be superior to delayed laboratory inoculation of blood culture bottles with ascitic fluid [35]. Laboratories should release the bottles to the physicians who are performing the paracenteses, so that bedside inoculation is possible.

Total protein

The old exudate/transudate system of ascitic fluid classification, which is based on ascitic fluid total protein concentration, is problematic (see above and Box 17.3). The protein concentration in ascites due to cirrhosis is entirely dependent on serum total protein concentration and portal pressure [29]. Therefore, a patient with a relatively high serum protein will have a relatively high ascitic fluid protein. Almost 20% of samples of uncomplicated ascites due to cirrhosis have >2.5 g/dL of protein [36]. During a 10 kg diuresis, ascitic fluid total protein increases from 1.4 to 2.9 g/dL; 67% of patients with ascites due to cirrhosis develop a protein >2.5 g/dL at the end of diuresis [26]. Ascitic fluid total protein concentration does not increase during SBP [37]. In fact, patients with the lowest protein ascites are the most prone to develop SBP [38]. Almost one third of patients with malignancy-related ascites have portal hypertension due to massive liver metastases or hepatocellular carcinoma as the cause of ascites formation; their fluid total protein is <2.5 g/dL [5]. Cardiac ascites protein concentration is always greater than 2.5 g/dL in this investigator's experience [6]. Therefore, cardiac ascites is classified in the exudate category while ascites due to cirrhosis is classified in the transudate category. A method of classification that categorizes cardiac and ascites due to cirrhosis in opposite groups is not very useful. In contrast, the albumin gradient classifies cardiac ascites in the high albumin gradient category, similar to cirrhosis with ascites. The high SAAG of cardiac ascites is presumably due to high right-sided heart pressures [6].

Measurement of ascitic fluid total protein, glucose, and LDH has been reported to be of value in distinguishing SBP from gut perforation into ascites [39]. Patients whose neutrocytic ascitic fluid meets two out of the following three criteria are likely to have surgical peritonitis and warrant immediate radiologic evaluation to determine if gut perforation into ascites has occurred: total protein >1 g/dL, glucose <50 mg/dL, and LDH above the upper limit of normal for serum [39,40]. A recent study has shown that these criteria and/or polymicrobial infection are 96% sensitive in detecting secondary bacterial peritonitis; 5% of patients in the series had secondary bacterial peritonitis [40].

Glucose

The ascitic fluid glucose concentration is similar to that of serum unless glucose is being consumed in the peritoneal cavity by white blood cells or bacteria [41]. However, the ascitic fluid glucose in early detected SBP is similar to that of sterile fluid [37]. If the gut perforates into ascitic fluid, e.g., perforated peptic ulcer or colonic diverticulum, the glucose usually drops to 0 mg/dL [39].

Lactate dehydrogenase

The ascitic fluid : serum (AF : S) ratio of LDH is 0.40 ± 0.20 in uncomplicated ascites due to cirrhosis; LDH is too large a molecule to readily enter the fluid from blood [37]. In SBP, the ascitic fluid LDH level rises because of neutrophil release of LDH, such that the mean ratio is 0.85 ± 0.29 [37].

Amylase

The ascitic fluid amylase concentration is 42 ± 44 IU/L and the AF : S ratio of amylase is 0.44 ± 0.33 in uncomplicated ascites due to cirrhosis [42]. The ascitic fluid amylase concentrations are markedly above these levels in patients with pancreatitis or gut perforation (with release of luminal amylase into the fluid). In pancreatic ascites, the ascitic fluid amylase concentration is $2,000 \pm 1,000$ IU/L and the AF:S ratio in pancreatic ascites 5 ± 0.0 [42].

Gram stain

A Gram stain of ascitic fluid for the detection of SBP is analogous to a Gram stain of blood in detecting bacteremia: it is only positive when there is an overwhelming infection present. The Gram stain of ascitic fluid is most helpful in ruling in or ruling out free perforation of the gut into ascites; sheets of multiple bacterial forms are found in gut perforation. In contrast, careful inspection of the centrifuged sediment of 50 mL of ascites is only 10% sensitive in visualizing bacteria in early-detected SBP [33]. Approximately 10,000 bacteria/mL are required for detection by Gram stain; the median concentration of bacteria in SBP is only 1 organism/mL [33].

Tests for tuberculosis

The direct smear of ascitic fluid for mycobacteria is almost never positive, for the same reason that the Gram stain is seldom positive in SBP [43,44]. This author has only seen one positive TB smear and that was a false positive. Although some older papers suggest the culture of a liter of fluid, most labs can only process 50 mL for TB culture [43,44]. The fluid is centrifuged and the pellet is cultured, but 50 mL centrifuge tubes and carriers are the largest commonly used. The sensitivity of peritoneoscopy, with histology and culture of peritoneal biopsies, in detecting tuberculous peritonitis approaches 100% [43]. Tuberculous peritonitis may mimic the culture-negative variant of SBP, but the predominance of cells is usually mononuclear in the setting of TB.

The ascitic fluid adenosine deaminase is helpful in detecting tuberculous peritonitis in endemic areas such as India [45]. However, in the United States >50% of patients with tuberculous peritonitis also have cirrhosis; in this setting adenosine deaminase is very insensitive [24]. DNA probes for TB are also available for body fluids and tissue [46].

Cytology

Cytology is reported to be only 58–75% sensitive in detecting "malignant ascites" [47,48]. However, these older studies did not compare cytology with a "gold standard" diagnosis such as autopsy or laparoscopy. Based on a study that did involve a gold standard diagnosis as to the location and type of tumor causing ascites formation, we now know that only about two thirds of patients with malignancy-related ascites have peritoneal carcinomatosis [5]. Essentially 100% of patients with peritoneal carcinomatosis have viable malignant cells exfoliating into their ascitic fluid and therefore have these cells detected in their ascitic fluid cytologies [5]. The remaining one third of patients with malignancy-related ascites have massive liver metastases, chylous ascites due to lymphoma, or hepatocellular carcinoma; these patients have negative cytologies [5]. The percentage of false-positive cytologies approaches zero [5,47,48]; this investigator has never encountered an example. Hepatomas rarely metastasize to the peritoneum, therefore cytology is almost never positive in patients with this tumor [5,48].

DNA cytometry has been shown to improve the sensitivity of effusion cell analysis to 95% [49].

Malignancy-related ascites may also have an elevated PMN count (16% of cases in one series) presumably because dying tumor cells may attract neutrophils into the fluid [5]. Usually, as in tuberculous peritonitis, there is a predominance of lymphocytes.

Triglyceride

If the ascitic fluid is opalescent or frankly milky, a triglyceride level should be obtained. Chylous ascites has a triglyceride concentration of >200 mg/dL and usually >1,000 mg/dL [50]. The sterile ascitic fluid specimens (in cirrhosis) that are slightly cloudy without an elevated cell count have an elevated triglyceride concentration: 64 ± 43 mg/dL compared to 18 ± 9 mg/dL for clear cirrhotic ascites [25].

Bilirubin

Ascitic fluid that is as brown as molasses should be tested for bilirubin concentration. An ascitic fluid bilirubin level greater than 6 mg/dL and greater than the serum level of bilirubin suggests biliary or upper gut perforation into ascites [9,39].

Tests that are seldom helpful

Ascitic fluid pH and lactate were proposed in the 1980s as helpful tests in the differential diagnosis of ascites, in particular in separating infected samples from uncomplicated ascites due to cirrhosis [51]. Unfortunately, the studies that attempted to validate the pH and lactate included only 6–18 infected patients per study, did not use optimal culture technique, and included an unusually high percentage (up to 67%) of surgical peritonitis patients. Surgical peritonitis patients have ascitic fluid that is at the extreme end of the spectrum of abnormality and would be predicted to have the lowest pH. Most series of peritonitis cases in the setting of ascites consist of ~95% SBP patients and ~5% secondary peritonitis patients [40]. In the two largest and most recent studies, which did not have some of the problems of the earlier studies, the ascitic fluid pH and lactate were not found to be helpful [52,53]. In one study the pH was found to be only about 40% sensitive in detecting infection, and the pH was found to remain normal (>7.35) until the PMN count rose over 2,000/mm^3 [52]. The pH was found to have no impact on decision making regarding the use of empirical antibiotics since patients were given antibiotics based on the PMN count even if the pH was normal. Measurement of arterial pH and pH gradient did not improve the sensitivity of the tests over that of ascitic fluid values alone and did not improve decision making [52]. Ascitic fluid pH appears to be simply an indirect measure of the presence of neutrophils. Why not just measure the neutrophils?

Measurement of carcinoembryonic antigen (CEA) in ascitic fluid has been proposed as a helpful test in detecting malignant ascites [54]. Patients with malignancy-related ascites were not subgrouped into those with and without peritoneal carcinomatosis in the only reported CEA study. Few patients were studied and no subsequent studies have been reported. Theoretically, this test should only be helpful in detecting the few tumors that make CEA. More studies, with subgrouping of patients and positive results, are required before CEA can be considered validated as a test of ascitic fluid.

Several ascitic fluid tests, such as fibronectin, cholesterol, α_1-antitrypsin, cyclic adenosine monophosphate (cAMP), and glycosaminoglycans, have been proposed as useful tests in detecting "malignant ascites." The large number of tests signifies that none of them is helpful enough to have been selected above the others. The basic premise of these studies is that the ascitic fluid cytology is too insensitive to be the only test used in detecting malignancy-related ascites. Unfortunately, most of these studies did not acknowledge that there are several subgroups of malignancy-related ascites and did not appreciate that the cytology would only be helpful in detecting peritoneal carcinomatosis. Also, appropriate control groups (patients with ascites caused by *conditions other than* cirrhosis or peritoneal carcinomatosis) were not included in these studies, and they had no provision for examples of mixed ascites. Other studies have demonstrated that the subgroup of patients with massive liver metastases do not have abnormally elevated ascitic fluid fibronectin or cholesterol concentrations [55,56]. Therefore, patients with negative cytologies also usually have negative "humoral tests of malignancy." In addition, patients with high protein ascites due to conditions other than cirrhosis essentially always have been reported to have false-positive "humoral tests of malignancy" [4,55,56]; these tests are more confusing than helpful.

Serum analysis

Measurement of serum albumin concentration is required to determine the albumin gradient. In patients with suspected SBP, blood should be cultured in addition to ascitic fluid, even if the patient is not febrile (only 67% of patients with SBP have fever) [32]. Profound peripheral hypoglycemia (as low as 5 mg/dL) can be found in patients with systemic bacterial infection and cirrhosis. If the ascitic fluid glucose is unusually low in a patient with neutrocytic ascites, measurement of serum glucose may explain the ascitic fluid hypoglycemia and lead to potentially life-saving emergency administration of glucose intravenously. Measurement of serum bilirubin or triglyceride concentration may be of value in comparison to the ascitic fluid concentrations. Measurement of serum α-fetoprotein (AFP) concentration (which is always higher in serum than in ascitic fluid) may be of value in detecting hepatocellular carcinoma as the explanation for the clinical deterioration of a patient with known cirrhosis [4].

The serum pro-BNP is a very useful test in separating ascites due to cirrhosis from ascites due to heart failure [17]. In the former, the median value is 166 pg/mL and the latter is 6,100 pg/mL, with complete separation of the data points [17]. Patients with cirrhosis *and* heart failure have values in the heart failure range. This test can be performed within ~20 minutes in the emergency department in a patient with alcohol abuse and ascites, to help determine whether alcoholic cirrhosis or alcoholic cardiomyopathy is present. This test can help direct the patient to the appropriate inpatient unit – the general medicine floor or the cardiac unit.

Complications of ascites

Infection

Ascitic fluid infection can be classified into five categories based on culture, PMN count, and the presence or absence of a surgical source of infection (Box 17.4). An abdominal paracentesis must be performed and ascitic fluid must be analyzed before a confident diagnosis of ascitic fluid infection can be made. A "clinical diagnosis" of infected ascitic fluid without a paracentesis is not enough.

Definitions

Of the three types of spontaneous ascitic fluid infection, the prototype form is spontaneous bacterial peritonitis (Box 17.4). This diagnosis is made when there is a positive ascitic fluid culture (essentially always a monomicrobial infection) and there is an elevated ascitic fluid absolute PMN count (i.e., ≥ 250 cells/mm^3) without an evident intra-abdominal source of infection that requires surgical treatment [32]. When Harold Conn coined the phrase

---

Box 17.4 Classification of ascitic fluid infection.[a]

Spontaneous ascitic fluid infection

- *Spontaneous bacterial peritonitis*
- *Monomicrobial nonneutrocytic bacterascites*
- *Culture-negative neutrocytic ascites*

Secondary bacterial peritonitis

- *Gut perforation*
- Nonperforation

Polymicrobial bacterascites

[a]The five main categories are emphasized in italic.

---

spontaneous bacterial peritonitis in 1975, his goal was to distinguish this form of infection from surgical peritonitis [57]. This author agrees with the importance of this distinction. Therefore, although many patients with SBP have a focus of infection, e.g., urinary tract infection or pneumonia, they are labeled as having SBP unless the focus requires surgical intervention, e.g., ruptured viscus [39,40].

The criteria for a diagnosis of monomicrobial non-neutrocytic bacterascites (MNB) include a positive ascitic fluid culture for a single organism, an ascitic fluid PMN count <250 cells/mm^3, and no evident intra-abdominal source of infection that requires surgical treatment [58]. The adjective "monomicrobial" is used to distinguish this form of ascitic fluid infection from polymicrobial bacterascites (see below). In the older literature this condition was either grouped with SBP or called asymptomatic bacterascites [59]. Since many patients with bacterascites have symptoms, the modifier "asymptomatic" does not seem appropriate [58]. The absence of PMNs in this variant has implications for prognosis as well as for understanding the pathogenesis and natural history of ascitic fluid infection (see below).

Culture-negative neutrocytic ascites (CNNA) is diagnosed when: (i) the ascitic fluid culture grows no bacteria; (ii) the ascitic fluid PMN count is ≥ 250 cells/cmm^3; (iii) no antibiotics have been given (even a single dose usually makes the culture negative); and (iv) there is no other explanation for an elevated PMN count (e.g., hemorrhage into ascites, peritoneal carcinomatosis, TB, or pancreatitis) [60]. This variant of ascitic fluid infection is seldom diagnosed when sensitive culture methods are used [33,34].

Secondary bacterial peritonitis is diagnosed when: (i) the ascitic fluid culture is positive (usually for multiple organisms); (ii) the PMN count is ≥ 250 cells/mm^3; and (iii) there is an identified intra-abdominal surgically treatable primary source of infection (e.g., perforated gut, perinephric abscess) [39,40]. The importance of distinguishing this variant from SBP is that secondary peritonitis is usually treated with antibiotics *and* surgery, whereas SBP is essentially always treated *only* with antibiotics [39,40]. Performing a laparotomy in the setting of SBP or treating secondary peritonitis with antibiotics and no surgical intervention usually results in the death of the patient.

Polymicrobial bacterascites is diagnosed when: (i) multiple organisms are cultured from ascitic fluid; and (ii) the PMN count is <250 cells/mm^3 [61]. This diagnosis should be suspected when: (i) the paracentesis is difficult because of ileus and/or it is traumatic; (ii) stool and/or air are aspirated into the paracentesis syringe; or (iii) multiple organisms but no PMNs are seen on Gram stain. Polymicrobial bacterascites is essentially diagnostic of inadvertent gut perforation by the paracentesis needle.

Setting

For all practical purposes the spontaneous variants of ascitic fluid infection, i.e., SBP, CNNA, and MNB, occur only in the setting of advanced liver disease. Spontaneous infection of ascites that is not due to cirrhosis is rare enough to be the subject of case reports [62–64]. Ninety-five percent of patients with SBP have an elevated serum bilirubin and 98% have an abnormal prothrombin time [32]. The liver disease is usually chronic, as in cirrhosis, but may be acute, as in fulminant hepatic failure, or subacute, as in alcoholic hepatitis. All forms of cirrhosis have been reported to be complicated by spontaneous ascitic fluid infection. Ascites is a prerequisite to the development of SBP; fluid is almost always clinically detectable at the time of infection. It is unlikely that SBP precedes the development of ascites. Usually this infection develops at the time of maximum ascites volume. Although nephrotic ascites was regularly complicated by SBP in the pre-antibiotic era, the use of diuretics and antibiotics have now made SBP uncommon in this setting.

About one half of SBP episodes are detected at the time of admission to hospital. The remainder develop during hospitalization [32].

Secondary bacterial peritonitis and polymicrobial bacterascites can develop in ascites of any type. The only prerequisite, in addition to the presence of ascites, for the development of the former infection is the presence of a surgical source of infection (e.g., ruptured viscus, perinephric abscess) [39,40]. The latter infection occurs due to needle entry of the bowel during attempted paracentesis [61].

Pathogenesis

In 1975 Harold Conn used the adjective "spontaneous" in describing bacterial peritonitis in the ascites patient to indicate that the infection appeared from nowhere [57]. Over the past 35 years the pathogenesis and natural history of the spontaneous forms of ascitic fluid infection have become more clear (Fig. 17.1; see Box 17.4). The enteric nature of most organisms that cause these infections implicates the gut as their source [32]. The pneumococcus is the only frequently isolated organism that does not reside in the gut. The body of currently available evidence suggests that SBP, CNNA, and MNB are probably the result of the colonization of susceptible ascitic fluid as a result of spontaneous bacteremia or the weeping of bacteria-laden lymph from the liver capsule as it forms ascitic fluid (Fig. 17.1). Although direct transmural migration of bacteria from the gut into ascites has been postulated as a route of colonization of ascitic fluid, this has been documented only after the loss of gut mucosal integrity [65]. If organisms could easily traverse the gut wall and directly enter the fluid, polymicrobial infections would be the rule rather the exception, and the flora of spontaneous ascitic fluid infections would be more representative of the flora of the gut. Although *Escherichia coli* and *Klebsiella pneumoniae* are present in the gut, they are outnumbered by 2–4 orders of magnitude by anaerobes and enterococci. Yet anaerobes and enterococci seldom cause spontaneous ascitic fluid infection [32].

Monomicrobial infections imply that the source of the infection is also monomicrobial, or that there is a filter mechanism or a series of filters between a polymicrobial source, such as the gut, and the ascitic fluid. Studies in rodents have demonstrated that under certain circumstances bacteria can "translocate" from the gut lumen across the mucosa into submucosal lymphatics and be detected in mesenteric lymph nodes [66]. Circumstances that promote translocation include bacterial overgrowth in the gut, chemotherapy-induced immunodeficiency, thermal burn, and hemorrhagic shock [66]. Translocation may explain how bacteria access the bloodstream in shock, leukemia, thermal burn, and multiple trauma. Patients with cirrhosis have altered gut flora, which would promote translocation. The inability of anaerobes to translocate is also of interest [66].

The gut mucosa is abnormally permeable in the setting of cirrhosis, leading to increased translocation of bacteria from the gut to the mesenteric lymph nodes and on to the peripheral blood (see Fig. 17.1). Bacteremia is common in patients with severe liver disease; more than 50% of patients with SBP have bacteremia documented at the time of diagnosis of peritoneal infection [32]. The flora of spontaneous bacteremia is similar to that of SBP and MNB and is also monomicrobial [32].

Complement is synthesized in the liver, and patients with severe enough liver disease to develop ascites usually have serum complement deficiency [67]. Neutrophil dysfunction and reticuloendothelial system dysfunction are also common in cirrhosis [68]. These defects in host defense against infection would be expected to lead to frequent and prolonged bacteremia.

Rats with cirrhosis and ascites have been shown to uniformly develop bacteremia after intratracheal exposure to pneumococci. These rats also have more prolonged bacteremia and more fatalities compared with rats without ascites and compared with normal rats [69].

Another animal model of cirrhosis and ascites has shown that the flora of the gut is altered as cirrhosis develops and that translocation of the overgrowing organism to mesenteric lymph nodes is common [70–72].

In summary, there is significant evidence favoring the gut as the source of most of the bacteria that cause spontaneous ascitic fluid infection. Translocation of bacteria from the gut to the mesenteric lymphatics of normal rodents is common under certain circumstances [66]. Translocation is more common in the setting of cirrhosis [71,72]. Seeding of ascitic fluid with gut-derived bacteria

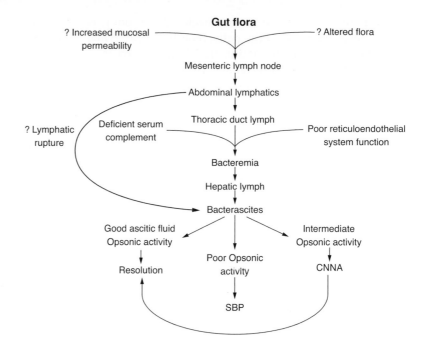

Figure 17.1 Pathogenesis of spontaneous ascitic fluid infection. CNNA, culture-negative neutrocytic ascites; SBP, spontaneous bacterial peritonitis.

could then be the result of at least two possible bacterial routes (see Fig. 17.1). Mesenteric lymphatic bacteria could (i) pass through lymph nodes, on to the thoracic duct, enter the bloodstream, and then leak across the sinusoids of the liver as ascites forms from the blood; or (ii) directly leak into ascitic fluid due to intra-abdominal lymphatic rupture.

Once bacteria enter the fluid in the abdomen, by whatever route, a battle ensues between the organism's virulence factors and the host's immune defenses. Several studies shed some light on the events that take place in this battle [37,38,58,71–73]. The protein concentration does not change with development of spontaneous infection [37]. Low protein concentration ascitic fluid, e.g., <1 g/dL, has been shown to be particularly prone to SBP [38]. The opsonic activity (endogenous antimicrobial activity) of human ascitic fluid correlates directly with the fluid's protein concentration [67]. Patients with deficient ascitic fluid opsonic activity have been shown to be predisposed to SBP [73]. Patients with detectable ascitic fluid opsonic activity are protected from SBP unless a particularly virulent organism, e.g., *Salmonella*, is involved [64,73].

Studies in both humans with cirrhosis and rats with experimental cirrhosis demonstrate that MNB is common [58,74]. In both humans and rats, most episodes (up to 62%) of bacterascites resolve without antibiotic treatment [58,74]. The fluid frequently becomes sterile without an evident PMN response. Apparently the host defense mechanisms are able to eradicate the invading bacteria on most occasions. Perhaps it is only when the defenses are particularly weak or the organism is particularly virulent

that uncontrolled fatal infection develops. Those patients with clinically apparent ascitic fluid infection may represent only the "tip of the iceberg." Bacterascites is probably much more common than SBP. Only frequent surveillance paracenteses would settle this question. Perhaps patients with ascites regularly have their ascitic fluid colonized by bacteria, and almost just as regularly these patients resolve the colonization. The entry of PMNs into the fluid likely signals failure of opsonins in combination with peritoneal macrophages to control the infection. As a rule MNB resolves spontaneously in rats and humans, whereas SBP is frequently fatal [58,70,74]. In summary, MNB probably represents an early stage of ascitic fluid infection that can resolve to sterile non-neutrocytic ascites or progress to SBP.

Most episodes of CNNA are diagnosed using insensitive culture methods where there are insufficient numbers of bacteria to reach the threshold of detectability [34,35]. Blood culture bottles can detect a single organism in the cultured aliquot of fluid, whereas the conventional method of culture probably requires at least 100 organisms/mL [35]. However, even when optimal culture methods are used, a small percentage of patients grow no bacteria in their neutrocytic ascitic fluid [60]. A study of rapid sequential paracenteses (before initiation of antibiotic treatment) in patients with CNNA demonstrated that in most cases the PMN count dropped spontaneously and the culture remained negative [74]. In the setting of sensitive culture technique, CNNA probably represents spontaneously resolving SBP in which the tap is performed after all bacteria have been killed by the host defenses but before the PMN count has normalized.

The pathogenesis of secondary bacterial peritonitis is no mystery compared to the pathogenesis of SBP. When the gut perforates into the ascitic fluid, billions of bacteria flood in. When there is secondary peritonitis without a frank perforation (e.g., a perinephric abscess or empyema of the gallbladder) bacteria cross inflamed tissue planes and enter ascites.

The pathogenesis of polymicrobial bacterascites is also apparent [61]. The paracentesis needle enters the bowel and the bowel contents are released. Fortunately, this event is rare. Even when needle puncture occurs, it usually resolves without antibiotic therapy, especially in high protein ascites [61].

Signs and symptoms

Although most patients with SBP are symptomatic at the time of diagnosis of infection, the symptoms or signs of infection may be very subtle or misinterpreted (Table 17.2) [32,58]. Minor changes in mental status that would only be detected by family members or a physician who is very familiar with the patient, may be the sole clinical evidence of infection. Unless such changes prompt paracentesis, the diagnosis and treatment of the ascitic fluid infection may be delayed.

Delays in the initiation of therapy regularly result in a fatal outcome. Survival decreases by 8% per hour of delay in the initiation of antibiotic treatment in one recent study of sepsis [75]. The signs and symptoms manifested in all five variants of ascitic fluid infection are listed in Table 17.2.

Prevalence

Prior to the 1980s abdominal paracentesis was not performed regularly because of the fear of complications of the procedure and because the utility of ascitic fluid analysis in the differential diagnosis of ascites was not fully recognized. Now that the complication rate is known to be usually <1% and the details of ascitic fluid analysis have been better defined, routine paracentesis is performed at the time of admission of many ascites patients [4,18,19,21,33,37,39]. Of patients with culture-positive ascitic fluid, about two thirds will have neutrocytic ascitic fluid, i.e., SBP, and one third will have monomicrobial bacterascites [58,74]. The prevalence of CNNA found amongst a series of neutrocytic ascitic fluid is largely dependent on culture technique [33,34]. Polymicrobial bacterascites is present in only about one per 1,000 patients [61]. Secondary bacterial peritonitis occurs in only 0–2% of ascites patients at the time of admission to hospital [21]. About 5% of patients that initially appear to have SBP will be shown to have secondary peritonitis; too often this diagnosis is made at autopsy [39,40].

Flora

Eshcerichia coli, streptococci (mostly pneumococci), and *Klebsiella* cause most episodes of SBP and MNB (Table 17.3). CNNA is by definition culture-negative. Polymicrobial bacterascites is by definition polymicrobial. The most apparent difference between the spontaneous forms of ascitic fluid infection and the nonspontaneous forms is that the former are nearly always monomicrobial and the latter are usually polymicrobial. Although older papers report ~6% of SBP cases to be caused by anaerobes, this is probably a reflection of the presence of unrecognized secondary bacterial peritonitis cases in series of purported SBP cases [21]. The high prevalence of polymicrobial infection among episodes of

Table 17.2 Signs and symptoms of ascitic fluid infection.[a]

Signs/symptoms	SBP	MNB	CNNA	2BP	Poly
Fever	68	57	50	33	10
Abdominal pain	49	32	72	67	10
Tender abdomen	39	32	44	50	10
Rebound	10	5	0	17	0
Decreased bowel sounds	12	2	28	83	0
Mental status	54	50	61	33	0

[a]Data presented as a percentage of the total number of patients in each of the five groups: SBP, spontaneous bacterial peritonitis; MNB, monomicrobial non-neutrocytic bacterascites; CNNA, culture-negative neutrocytic ascites; 2BP, secondary bacterial peritonitis; Poly, polymicrobial bacterascites.
Adapted from references [39,58,60,61].

Table 17.3 Flora of ascitic fluid infection.[a]

Organism	SBP	MNB	CNNA	2BP	Poly
Monomicrobial					
Escherichia coli	37	27	0	20	0
Klebsiella pneumoniae	17	11	0	7	0
Pneumococcus	12	9	0	0	0
Streptococcus viridans	9	2	0	0	0
Staphylococcus aureus	0	7	0	13	0
Misc. Gram-negative	10	14	0	7	0
Misc. Gram-positive	14	30	0	0	0
Polymicrobial	1	0	0	100	53

[a]Data presented as a percentage of the total number of patients in each of the five groups: SBP, spontaneous bacterial peritonitis; MNB, monomicrobial non-neutrocytic bacterascites; CNNA, culture-negative neutrocytic ascites; 2BP, secondary bacterial peritonitis; Poly, polymicrobial bacterascites.
Adapted from references [39,58,60,61].

anaerobic "SBP" further supports the contention that these represent misdiagnosed secondary peritonitis. Anaerobes cause ~1% of SBP [33,34,58]. The infrequency of anaerobic SBP is probably due to the relatively high PO_2 of ascites and the inability of anaerobes to translocate across the gut mucosa [66,72]. Fungi do not cause SBP. Fungal infection of ascitic fluid occurs only in the setting of disseminated systemic mycosis in the immunosuppressed patient or in secondary peritonitis with gut release of fungi into ascitic fluid [39,40].

Gram-negative organisms do not colonize the skin, and must be interpreted as pathogens, whereas Grampositive organisms are routine skin flora and must be considered to be contaminants in the absence of a PMN response. *Staphylococcus epidermidis* cannot be interpreted as a pathogen in ascitic fluid unless there is a foreign body (e.g., peritoneovenous shunt) present. α-Hemolytic streptococcus should also be considered a skin contaminant unless there is a PMN response or bacteremia with the same organism. Failure to use a sterile technique when performing a paracentesis or failure to sterilize the blood culture bottle tops with iodine before inoculation will increase the presence of contaminants in the cultures.

Risk factors

Patients with cirrhosis are unusually prone to bacterial infections because of multiple defects in their immune defense (see section on pathogenesis above). Two prospective studies have shown that up to 47% of patients with cirrhosis had a bacterial infection (ranging from asymptomatic urinary tract infections to fatal sepsis) during one hospitalization and 34% developed a bacterial infection during 1 year of follow-up [76,77]. Thirty-five percent of 87 women with primary biliary cirrhosis developed bacteriuria (70% E. coli, 7% *Klebsiella*, 6% streptococcal) during a 12-month period [78].

Some physicians have been taught that paracentesis itself poses a significant risk of causing ascitic fluid infection. This theoretical risk has not been substantiated in prospective studies of paracentesis complications [18,19]. In one study, SBP was statistically more likely to be diagnosed at the time of the first paracentesis compared to subsequent taps [18]. The most likely setting in which to expect iatrogenic peritonitis is when the paracentesis needle enters the bowel inadvertantly during attempted paracentesis [61]. Fortunately, this is very unusual. Skin flora, e.g. *Staphylococcus aureus*, would be expected to be isolated if poor paracentesis technique were the cause of many cases of SBP, yet skin flora are seldom isolated [33].

Gastrointestinal hemorrhage is temporally associated with the development of spontaneous bacteremia and SBP; prevention of infection with the use of antibiotics improves survival [79] (see below).

Diagnosis

An accurate and timely diagnosis of ascitic fluid infection requires a low threshold for performing a paracentesis and a high index of suspicion of infection. Clinical deterioration in a patient with ascites should always raise suspicion, especially if there is fever or abdominal pain. If the ascitic fluid PMN is elevated, the working diagnosis is ascitic fluid infection until proven otherwise.

Although peritoneal carcinomatosis, pancreatitis, hemorrhage into ascites, pancreatitis, and tuberculosis can lead to an elevated ascitic fluid PMN count, most cases of neutrocytic ascitic fluid are due to infection. A majority of PMNs in the white cell differential further lends credence to the diagnosis of infection. An elevated absolute ascitic fluid PMN count with a predominance of neutrophils in a clinical setting compatible with infection (e.g., a febrile patient with cirrhosis) should prompt empirical antibiotic therapy (see below).

Once the presumptive diagnosis of ascitic fluid infection is made, the next consideration should be whether there is a surgically treatable source of infection. Secondary peritonitis should be *considered* in any patient with neutrocytic ascites. However, because of the rarity of SBP in peritoneal carcinomatosis or cardiac ascites, a surgical source of peritonitis should be *presumed* in these conditions until proven otherwise. Surprisingly, even with free perforation of the colon into ascitic fluid, patients do not develop a classic surgical abdomen [39]. Peritoneal signs, such as rigid abdomen, require the contact of inflamed visceral and parietal peritoneal surfaces. This does not happen when there is a large volume of fluid present. Therefore, clinical signs and symptoms do not separate patients with secondary peritonitis from those with SBP [39,40]. Gut perforation can be suspected and pursued if neutrocytic ascitic fluid analysis meets two of the following three criteria: total protein >1 g/dL, glucose <50 mg/dL, or LDH >225 mU/mL (or more than the upper limit of normal for serum) [39,40]. Essentially all ascitic fluids culture multiple organisms in the setting of a perforated viscus [39,40]. If multiple organisms and PMNs are seen on Gram stain, the likehood of perforation is very high. Brown ascitic fluid with a bilirubin concentration >6 mg/dL (and greater than the serum level) is indicative of biliary or upper gut perforation into ascites [9].

The initial ascitic fluid analysis is very helpful in delineating which patients are likely to have a ruptured viscus. These patients need an emergent (within minutes) radiologic evaluation (usually computed tomography scan) to confirm and localize the site of rupture [39,40]. If perforation is documented, emergency intervention is mandatory to maximize survival; survivors have been reported. Antibiotic therapy without surgical intervention in the treatment of a ruptured viscus is predictably unsuccessful.

Patients with *nonperforation* secondary peritonitis tend *not* to have a diagnostic *initial* ascitic fluid analysis [39,40]. Fortunately, it is less urgent to make the diagnosis of secondary peritonitis in nonperforation peritonitis compared with perforation peritonitis. Therefore, there may be time to evaluate the response of the ascitic fluid culture and PMN count to treatment. These parameters have been shown to be helpful in distinguishing secondary from spontaneous peritonitis [39]. The best time to perform a single repeat paracentesis to assess response is after 48 hours of treatment; by 48 hours essentially every SBP patient who has been treated with an appropriate antibiotic will have a PMN count lower than the pretreatment value and the culture will be negative [39]. Prior to 48 hours of treatment, i.e., at 12 or 24 hours, the PMN count may higher than baseline even in SBP. Also, the culture remains positive in secondary peritonitis and becomes rapidly negative in SBP [39,40].

Treatment

Patients with ascitic fluid PMN counts ≥ 250 cells/mm^3 in a clinical setting compatible with ascitic fluid infection should receive empirical antibiotics [32]. Patients with hemorrhage into ascites, peritoneal carcinomatosis, pancreatic ascites, or tuberculous peritonitis may have an elevated PMN count that is not related to SBP. These patients usually do not require empirical treatment. However, if the situation is initially unclear, the physician should err on the side of overtreatment so long as non-nephrotoxic antibiotics are used. Usually patients with uninfected neutrocytic ascitic fluid (except those with hemorrhage) have a predominance of lymphocytes in their ascitic fluid differential. This helps distinguish them from patients with SBP, in which PMNs predominate. Patients with bloody ascites should have a "corrected" PMN count calculated (see "Cell count" above). Patients with bloody ascites do not need antibiotics unless their corrected PMN count is ≥ 250 cells/mm^3.

Patients with MNB are "special cases" regarding empirical antibiotic treatment. Many episodes resolve without treatment [58]. However, because of the hospitalization mortality associated with monomicrobial bacterascites, treatment appears to be warranted in many patients [58]. By definition, the PMN count is <250 cells/mm^3 in this variant of ascitic fluid infection. Because of this variant, the PMN count cannot be the only parameter upon which to hinge the decision about empirical therapy. Most of the patients with MNB who do not resolve the colonization and progress to SBP have signs or symptoms of infection [58]. Therefore, patients with cirrhosis, ascites, and *convincing signs or symptoms of infection* should receive treatment regardless of the PMN count in ascitic fluid. Empirical treatment can be discontinued after only 2–3 days if

the culture remains negative and suspicion of infection has diminished.

Patients with *asymptomatic* monomicrobial bacterascites should undergo a repeat paracentesis for cell count and culture, once it is known that the initial culture is growing bacteria. If the PMN count has risen above 250 cells/mm^3 in the follow-up ascitic fluid analysis, treatment should be started. Patients who have developed no PMN response or clinical evidence of infection do not require treatment [58]. These are the patients who have probably eradicated the colonization by their own immune defenses.

When initially faced with a patient who has CNNA, the physician does not know that the culture is destined to be "no growth." Therefore empirical treatment should be given. When the preliminary report demonstrates no growth, it is helpful to repeat the paracentesis to assess the response of the PMN count to therapy. A decline in PMN count confirms a response to treatment and probably warrants a few more days of therapy. A stable PMN count, especially if there is not a predominance of PMNs, indicates that a nonbacterial (or mycobacterial) cause of the neutrocytosis is present. Cytology and culture for TB may be appropriate. Because improper culture techniques result in negative cultures, one of the most important methods to reduce the prevalence of CNNA in a hospital that is still using the conventional method of culture is to convince the microbiology laboratory to convert to the optimal method of culture [33].

The ascitic fluid Gram stain is not very helpful in the choice of empirical antibiotic. This investigator has not found that the Gram stain allowed a narrowed spectrum of antibiotic coverage in even one patient out of ~300 with SBP. Only ~10% of Gram stains demonstrate organisms in early detected SBP [33]. The actual utility of the Gram stain is in assisting with the differential diagnosis of spontaneous versus nonspontaneous ascitic fluid infection [39,40]. Sheets of multiple different types of bacteria are found in gut perforation – this requires coverage of anaerobic flora in addition to aerobic and facultative anaerobic flora, as well as an emergency search for a source for the bacteria [39,40]. Therefore, a positive Gram stain may lead to broader spectrum coverage rather than narrower coverage. Choosing very narrow spectrum coverage, e.g., penicillin, based on a misinterpreted Gram stain may lead to the patient's death from uncontrolled infection before it is known that the isolated organism is resistant to the antibiotic that is in use. Patients with suspected ascitic fluid infection require relatively broad spectrum therapy until the results of susceptibility testing are available.

Cefotaxime, the first third-generation cephalosporin, is the most data-supported drug for the treatment of SBP [32,80–82]. This drug covers ~95% of flora and is usually the treatment of choice for suspected SBP. In contrast, ceftriaxone is highly protein bound and penetrates low protein ascites poorly. If it is used due to formulary issues, the minimum dose is 2 g daily. Ceftriaxone has a role in the prevention of bacterial infections in patients with cirrhosis and gut hemorrhage (see below).

Most drugs have not been tested for their ability to penetrate ascites. One cannot assume that just because a drug covers the flora that cause SBP, that it will treat this infection well. If it does not reach the ascites in a high concentration, it may not be efficacious.

For cefotaxime, 2 g intravenous doses are appropriate, and the dosing interval is 8–12 hours; 8 hours for a serum creatinine less than ~3 mg/dL and 12 hours for more severe renal failure [81]. The dosing interval does not *have* to be altered in renal failure because of the lack of toxicity of the drug. Ascitic fluid levels can exceed 300 μg/mL in the setting of renal failure and dosing every 8 hours [81]. Dosing more frequently than every 8 hours is not necessary because high ascitic fluid concentrations (>20-fold the minimal inhibitory concentrations of >90% of the flora) of the drug are attained after one dose and are sustained during every-8-hour dosing [81].

When susceptibility testing results are available, a more narrow spectrum drug can usually be substituted, e.g., pneumococci will usually be sensitive to penicillin and most *E. coli* species will usually be sensitive to ampicillin.

Many infectious disease experts treat life-threatening infections with 10–14 days of therapy. However, there are no data to support this duration of treatment of spontaneous ascitic fluid infection. The ascitic fluid cultures of culture-positive patients become sterile after one dose of cefotaxime in 86% of patients [39]. The ascitic fluid PMN count, in general, drops exponentially after treatment is started such that the PMN count after 48 hours of therapy is always less than the pretreatment value in patients with spontaneous ascitic fluid infection treated with appropriate antibiotics [39]. A randomized controlled trial involving 100 patients has demonstrated that 5 days of treatment is as efficacious as 10 days in the treatment of SBP and CNNA [82].

Bacterial infection further increases vasodilatation and can lead to impaired renal function and even death [83]. Intravenous albumin has been shown in a randomized trial to help prevent azotemia and to improve survival, presumably by "refilling the underfilled tank" related to this vasodilatation [83]. A dose of 1.5 g/kg body weight should be given within 6 hours of diagnosis of an elevated PMN count with a 1 g/kg dose at 72 hours [83]. This trial reports the lowest SBP hospitalization mortality ever: 10% [83].

Patients suspected of having secondary peritonitis require broader spectrum empirical antibiotic coverage than those with SBP, in addition to an emergency evaluation to assess the need for surgical intervention [39,40]. Cefotaxime plus metronidazole provide excellent initial empirical therapy of suspected secondary peritonitis while the radiologic workup is underway [39,40].

Surprisingly, needle perforation of the bowel (polymicrobial bacterascites) is relatively well tolerated. Only 10% (1/10) of patients with needle perforation of the gut into ascitic fluid developed peritonitis, and only 0.06% (1/1578) of paracenteses were documented to cause peritonitis in one large study [61]. The paracentesis-related peritonitis was not fatal. It appears that patients with low protein ascitic fluid are at most risk of developing a PMN response and clinical peritonitis related to needle perforation of the gut [61]. Most of the patients with high protein ascites (e.g., > 1g/dL) did not even receive antibiotics and yet did well. However, most physicians would probably feel uncomfortable withholding antibiotic treatment if needle perforation is suspected. If a decision to treat is made, anaerobic coverage should be included, e.g., cefotaxime and metronidazole. If a decision not to treat is made, follow-up paracentesis is helpful in following the PMN count and culture. If the number of organisms does not decrease and/or a PMN response occurs, antibiotic treatment should be initiated.

Prognosis

In the past, in spite of treatment, 48–95% of patients with spontaneous ascitic fluid infection died during the hospitalization in which the diagnosis was made [21,59]. The most recent series report the lowest mortality rates [82,83], some even as low as 10% hospitalization mortality [83]. This is a reflection of the earlier detection of infection as well as the avoidance of nephrotoxic antibiotics. In the older series about half of SBP patients died of the infection despite antibiotic treatment; now <5% of patients die of infection if timely and appropriate antibiotics are used [82,83]. However, because of the severity of the underlying liver disease, even now many patients are cured of their infection and yet die of liver and/or renal failure gastrointestinal bleeding, etc. Because spontaneous ascitic fluid infection is a marker of end-stage liver disease, it has been proposed as an indication for liver transplantation in a patient who is otherwise a candidate [21,32].

In the past a delay in diagnosis was, at least in part, responsible for the excessive mortality. If the physician waited until the patient developed convincing signs and symptoms of infection before performing a paracentesis, the infection was likely to be very advanced by the time the diagnosis is made. There have been no reported survivors of SBP in the absence of liver transplant when the diagnosis was made after the creatinine had risen above 4 mg/dL. In order to maximize survival, it is important to perform paracentesis on hospital admission so that infection can be diagnosed and treated early. In addition, paracentesis should be repeated during hospitalization if any deterioration occurs – including pain, fever, mental status change, renal failure, acidosis, peripheral leukocytosis, or gastrointestinal bleeding.

Early diagnosis and surgical intervention reduce the hospitalization mortality of secondary peritonitis into the same range as that of SBP [39,40]. Without surgical intervention, mortality approaches 100%.

Prevention

All series of patients with SBP report recurrences. The older series did not report a high rate, in part, because few patients survived the first episode. A prospective study reported in 1988 documented a 69% recurrence rate at 1 year [84]. An ascitic fluid protein concentration of <1.0 g/dL was the best predictor of recurrence. This impressive recurrence rate prompted studies of antibiotic prophylaxis. Norfloxacin 400 mg/day orally has been reported to successfully prevent recurrences of SBP with essentially no toxicity or superinfection (Table 17.4) [85]. In the United States norfloxacin is no longer being manufactured. If a generic company does not produce it, trimethoprim-sulfamethoxazole can be substituted at a dose of one double-strength tablet daily [32].

Antibiotic prevention of SBP (and other bacterial infections) in the setting of low protein ascites and gut hemorrhage has also been reported [86,87]. Norfloxacin is effective in the former situation and ceftriaxone intravenously in the latter [86,87]. There has been confusion regarding which patients with gut hemorrhage qualify. Any patient with cirrhosis (with or without ascites) who has a hemodynamically significant amount of bleeding (variceal or nonvariceal) warrants ceftriaxone [32,87]. It is ischemia/reperfusion of the gut and translocation of bacteria that lead to the high risk of bacterial infections. This investigator provides the intravenous drug during active

bleeding and converts to norfloxacin or trimethoprim-sulfamethoxazole twice daily once the patient begins to eat again – to complete a 7-day total course of antibiotics.

Primary prevention of SBP has been documented when norfloxacin is given to patients who meet a complicated number of inclusion criteria (Table 17.4) [88].

It is optimal to give these antibiotics only to patients who meet study inclusion criteria. Giving antibiotics more liberally can lead to selection of resistant flora and subsequent infection by these organisms, as well as fungal superinfection.

Tense ascites

Some patients with ascites do not seek medical attention until their intra-abdominal fluid exerts such pressure on their diaphragms that they can no longer breathe comfortably. The volume of fluid required before "tenseness" occurs is usually ~10 L. However, young patients with good muscle tone may develop a tense abdomen with only a few liters of fluid. Rapid accumulation of fluid (e.g., postoperatively in a patient with no prior fluid retention) does not give the abdominal wall time to stretch; these patients can also have small volume tense ascites.

Tense ascites requires urgent treatment – therapeutic paracentesis. Tense ascites can be drained without untoward hemodynamic effects [89]. "Total paracentesis" (i.e., removal of all mobilizable fluid) has recently been demonstrated to be safe [89]. Therapeutic paracentesis of ascites due to cirrhosis is less problematic than the textbooks and folklore of medicine would indicate. Many physicians were taught that large volume paracentesis leads to hemodynamic disasters. However, this concept was based on anecdotal observations in small numbers of patients and has been disproven by carefully conducted controlled trials [89].

Abdominal wall hernias

Abdominal wall hernias (usually umbilical or incisional, occasionally inguinal) are common in patients with ascites. Unfortunately, there is little published information available about these hernias. In one study, 17% of patients with cirrhosis and ascites were found to have umbilical hernias at the time of admission to the hospital [90]. The hernia recurs in 73% of patients who have ascites at the time of hernia repair but only in 14% of patients who have no ascites at the time of repair [91]. In general, patients with cirrhosis and ascites should avoid surgery and wear an abdominal binder. Hernias can be repaired electively during liver transplantation. If skin ulceration, crusting, or black discoloration develop surgery should be performed semiemergently. Emergent surgery should be performed for rupture or incarceration that is unresponsive to medical therapy [90]. Rupture, i.e., Flood syndrome (an eponym as well as a descriptive label), is the

Table 17.4 Prevention of spontaneous bacterial peritonitis.[a]

High-risk group	Drug	Duration
Prior SBP	Norfloxacin 400 mg daily or one trim-sulfa DS daily	Indefinitely
Ascitic fluid total protein <1.5 g/dL	Norfloxacin 400 mg daily	Duration of hospitalization
Gut hemorrhage	Ceftriaxone 1 g intravenously	7 days
Primary prophylaxis	Norfloxacin 400 mg daily	12 months

[a]Candidates for primary prophylaxis must meet the following criteria:
1) Cirrhosis with ascitic fluid total protein <1.5 g/dL.
2) Advanced liver failure with Child–Pugh score ≥9 and bilirubin ≥3 mg/dL, or impaired renal function with creatinine ≥1.2 mg/dL, or blood urea nitrogen ≥25 mg/dL, or serum sodium ≤130 mEq/L.
Trim-sulfa DS, trimethoprim-sulfamethoxazole double strength.
Adapted from references [85–88].

most feared complication of abdominal hernias. If surgical repair of Flood syndrome is delayed, fatal *Staphylococcus aureus* peritonitis usually develops.

Pleural effusions

Pleural effusions are common in patients with cirrhosis and ascites. They are usually unilateral and right-sided, but occasionally may be bilateral with the amount of fluid in the right being greater than that on the left. When there is a unilateral left-sided effusion, tuberculosis and pancreatitis should be high in the differential diagnosis.

When the effusion is large and obscures most of the right lung, it is referred to as hepatic hydrothorax [92]. Most carefully studied examples of hepatic hydrothorax have been shown to be due to a small defect in the right hemidiaphragm. Occasionally, a hydrothorax results in sudden shortness of breath as the abdomen decompresses. Occasionally, ascites is undetected in the face of a hepatic hydrothorax.

The predominant symptom associated with hepatic hydrothorax is shortness of breath. Infection of this fluid occurs, usually a result of SBP and transmission of bacteria across the diaphragm. Usually the fluid resembles ascites, but the total protein is higher (by 0.75–1.0 g/dL) in the pleural fluid than in ascites because the pleural fluid is subject to different pressures than those of the portal bed [92].

Treatment of hepatic hydrothorax is usually more difficult than anticipated [92]. These large right-sided effusions tend to occur in patients who are the least compliant or most refractory. Some authors have recommended tetracycline sclerosis using a chest tube. However, chest tube insertion with suction has been reported to lead to serious fluid and protein depletion and death [93]. Once a chest tube is inserted, usually it becomes very difficult to remove. Clamping the tube may lead to a leak of fluid around the tube's insertion site. Direct surgical repair of the defect can be considered, but typically these patients are very poor operative candidates. Medical therapy, i.e., sodium restriction and diuretics, is probably the safest and most effective form of therapy of hepatic hydrothorax. Transjugular intrahepatic portosystemic shunting (TIPS) or even liver transplantation can be performed when the fluid is unresponsive to medical therapy [92].

Treatment of ascites

Ascites is not always due to liver disease (see Table 17.1). Not all patients with ascites respond to routine salt restriction and diuretics. Therefore, an accurate diagnosis of the cause of ascites formation is important so that treatment can be tailored appropriately. The serum–ascites albumin gradient is helpful in therapeutic decision making. Patients with low SAAG ascites (except for those with nephrotic syndrome) usually do not respond to salt restriction and diuretics, whereas patients with a high SAAG usually are responsive.

Nonportal hypertension-related (low albumin gradient) ascites

The most common form of low albumin gradient ascites is peritoneal carcinomatosis [5]. Peripheral edema in these patients responds to diuretics, but the ascitic fluid usually does not; edema-free patients treated with diuretics lose only intravascular volume without loss of ascites. The cornerstone of treatment of peritoneal carcinomatosis is therapeutic paracentesis [5]. Patients with peritoneal carcinomatosis usually live only a matter of weeks, therefore the total number of taps required to minimize symptoms is not great. Patients with ovarian malignancy are an exception to this rule. They may have a good response to surgical debulking and chemotherapy.

Tuberculous peritonitis is cured by antituberculous therapy; there is no point in using diuretics unless the patient has concomitant portal hypertension from cirrhosis. Pancreatic ascites may resolve spontaneously or may require endoscopic stenting or operative intervention. *Chlamydia* peritonitis is cured by doxycycline therapy [8]. "Nephrogenous" ascites (dialysis ascites) may respond to vigorous dialysis [7].

Portal hypertension-related (high albumin gradient) ascites

The most common cause of portal hypertension-related ascites is cirrhosis, usually caused by chronic hepatitis C and/or alcohol abuse and/or obesity/nonalcoholic steatohepatitis (NASH). One of the most important steps in treating this form of ascites is to treat the underlying liver disease by convincing the patient to stop drinking alcohol. With time and healing of the reversible component of alcoholic liver disease, the ascites may resolve or at least convert from refractory to medical therapy to being nonrefractory to medical therapy. Patients with multiple causes for their cirrhosis can improve dramatically with abstinence from alcohol. Baclofen has been shown in a randomized trial to reduce alcohol craving and reduce alcohol consumption in patients with alcoholic liver disease; this drug works well in this regard in this author's experience [94]. Noninterferon-based antiviral treatment of decompensated cirrhosis due to hepatitis B can also lead to better control or loss of ascites.

Patients with autoimmune chronic active hepatitis, iron-storage disease, or Wilson disease should receive specific therapy for those diseases. This may improve their overall liver function and the management of their ascites. However, these diseases seem to be less reversible than alcoholic liver disease or chronic hepatitis B, and by the time ascites is present the patient may be a better candidate for liver transplantation than protracted medical therapy.

Patients who have ascites due to cirrhosis, based on history, physical examination, and ascitic fluid analysis, may require hospitalization for the diagnosis and management of their liver disease as well as their fluid overload, especially if the fluid retention is "new onset." Frequently, ascites formation is only part of the overall picture of decompensation of liver disease. Although outpatient treatment of ascites patients can be successful, frequently it fails and an intensive period of inpatient education and treatment is required. Once the patient realizes that the diet and diuretics are effective, he or she is frequently more compliant with the regimen.

Precipitating cause

In the initial management of the patient with ascites, it is usually of value to determine the precipitating cause of ascites formation. Frequently, ascites accumulates because of noncompliance either with the dietary sodium or diuretics, or ascites may accumulate because of the fluid resuscitation given in the treatment of variceal hemorrhage. Education regarding compliance may help prevent future hospitalizations for ascites. Ascites that is initiated by variceal hemorrhage may resolve after the bleeding is controlled without need for long-term diuretics.

Diet

In portal hypertension-related ascites, fluid loss and weight change are directly and predictably related to sodium balance. Dietary sodium restriction is essential, so the patient and the patient's cook (who is frequently not the patient) should be educated by a dietician in a salt-restricted diet. The more contact the dietician has with the patient and the cook, the better. A severe sodium-restricted diet, e.g., 500 mg or 22 mEq sodium per day, is feasible in an inpatient setting. However, this is an unrealistic diet for most outpatients as they will not follow a diet that contains less than 2 g/day (88 mEq/day) sodium. Such a diet is thus the preferred one [32] and the patient should be able to follow it at home. Using this diet in the hospital offers the opportunity to tailor a diuretic regimen that will match the salt intake in and out of the hospital.

Fluid restriction

Fluid restriction of all patients with ascites is inappropriate. There is no evidence that fluid restriction speeds weight loss. It is the sodium restriction that is important. Although rapidly developing hyponatremia (e.g., postoperative hyponatremia in a previously healthy patient) is associated with a high mortality, the chronic hyponatremia usually seen in cirrhotic ascites patients is far less morbid. Attempts to rapidly correct it can be much worse that the hyponatremia itself. The only indication for fluid restriction in the cirrhotic ascites patient is severe hyponatremia. This investigator does not restrict fluids in ascites patients unless their serum sodium drops below 120 mEq/L [32]. Patients with cirrhosis do not usually have symptoms from hyponatremia until the sodium is below 110 mEq/L or unless the decline in sodium is very rapid. To restrict fluids in patients with a serum sodium of >120 mEq/L serves only to alienate patients, nurses, and dieticians.

Urinary sodium concentration

Twenty-four hour urinary sodium measurements are useful in patients with portal hypertension-related ascites. Although a 24-hour collection is optimal, a random "spot" urinary sodium : potassium (Na : K) ratio is a satisfactory substitute in many cases. If the urine sodium is greater than the potassium in a random sample, the 24-hour urinary sodium excretion is usually enough to lead to weight loss [32].

If body weight is not declining satisfactorily, this may be due to inadequate natriuresis or failure to properly restrict sodium intake or both. Monitoring the random urine Na : K ratio and daily weight will usually clarify the problem. Since urinary excretion is the most important route of excretion of sodium in the absence of diarrhea or hyperthermia, dietary intake and urinary excretion should be equivalent (except for ~10 mEq/day of nonurinary losses) if the weight is stable. If 88 mEq are taken in with the diet and 10 mEq are lost by nonurinary routes, weight should be stable if urinary sodium excretion is >78 mEq/day. A random urine Na > K correlates with a 24-hour excretion of >78 mEq of sodium [32]. If the weight is increasing despite urine Na > K, one can assume that the patient is eating more than his/her allotted salt.

Diuretics

Spironolactone is the mainstay diuretic for treatment of patients with cirrhosis and ascites. The half-life of spironolactone in normal control patients is approximately 24 hours but is markedly prolonged in cirrhosis [32]. There is no reason to dose the drug multiple times per day in view of its long half-life. Single daily doses of pills are most appropriate and enhance compliance; 100 mg spironolactone pills are available. In general, spironolactone *and* furosemide are used together, starting with 100 mg/day spironolactone and 40 mg/day furosemide, then increasing both drugs simultaneously as needed. If weight loss is inadequate and urine Na is <K, diuretics are increased, usually in increments of

100 mg and 40 mg respectively, up to maximum doses of 400 mg/day spironolactone and 160 mg/day furosemide. The ratio of spironolactone and furosemide can be adjusted to correct serum potassium problems. Combined with a sodium-restricted diet, the spironoactone/furosemide regimen is effective in >90% of patients [32].

Intravenous furosemide causes an acute reduction in glomerular filtration rate in these patients and should be avoided. If rapid weight loss is desired, therapeutic paracenteses should be performed (see refractory ascites below). For patients who have massive edema, there is no limit to the daily weight loss; once the edema has resolved, 0.5 kg/24 hours is probably a reasonable maximum [32]. If patients develop encephalopathy, serum sodium is <120 mEq/L despite fluid restriction, or serum creatinine is >1.5 mg/dL, diuretics are usually stopped and then carefully reinstituted after the reason for discontinuation improves. The ratio of the doses of the diuretics is adjusted to maintain a normal serum potassium. Serious hyperkalemia despite adjustment of diuretics usually indicates intrinsic renal disease, e.g., diabetic nephropathy. Many of the patients who develop complications of diuretic treatment will be considered failures of first-line treatment and require second-line therapy.

Prostaglandin inhibitors, e.g., nonsteroidal anti-inflammatory drugs, should not be used in patients with ascites because they curtail diuresis, may promote renal failure, and cause gastrointestinal bleeding.

Complete removal of ascites may not always be achieved. However, a diuresis-mediated concentration of ascitic fluid increases the fluid's opsonic activity tenfold, and, theoretically, may be of value in attempting to prevent spontaneous ascitic fluid infection [32]. The maximum concentration of opsonins occurs at the end of diuresis. It is reasonable to attempt to achieve a dry abdomen in order to minimize the risk of infection and to decrease the risk of abdominal wall hernias and hepatic hydrothorax. However, the risks must be weighed against the benefits. Patients who become somewhat dehydrated may develop hepatic encephalopathy, dizziness, light-headedness, and may even fall. Dame Sheila Sherlock used to say "wet and wise or dry and demented" to describe the patient with fluid overload versus the patient with diuretic-induced dehydration.

Refractory ascites

A patient with refractory ascites is defined as fluid overload unresponsive to inpatient salt restriction and diuretic treatment. The failure may be manifested by minimal to no weight loss despite high-dose diuretics or the development of complications of diuretics. Randomized trials have shown that <10% of patients with cirrhosis and ascites are refractory to standard medical therapy [95].

Second-line therapy options include therapeutic paracenteses, TIPS, and liver transplantation. Peritoneovenous shunts are third-line options and are reserved for very special circumstances (see below).

Abdominal paracentesis is one of the oldest medical procedures. From the time of Celsus, who is credited with first describing the technique in ~20 BC, until the late 1940s, therapeutic paracentesis was essentially the only available therapy for ascites. This laborious procedure rapidly fell out of favor as a treatment option for patients with ascites. In the 1980s there was renewed interest in therapeutic paracentesis after randomized trials proved its safety [96]. However, no differences in morbidity or mortality could be demonstrated in this study [96]. Physically removing the fluid is predictably faster than diuretic treatment in achieving a dry abdomen. Some physicians have concluded from this study that therapeutic paracentesis should be first-line therapy for patients with tense cirrhotic ascites, but few physicians agree with this conclusion. In view of the ease and efficacy of diuretic therapy in >90% of patients, therapeutic paracentesis should probably be reserved for the treatment of tense ascites and ascites that is refractory to diuretic therapy [32]. Also, therapeutic paracentesis lacks the ascitic fluid opsonin-conserving advantage of diuresis; theoretically depletion of opsonins by paracentesis could predispose to spontaneous bacterial peritonitis.

One practical issue regarding therapeutic paracentesis is that of colloid replacement. In one study patients were randomized to receive albumin (10 g/L of fluid removed) versus no albumin after therapeutic paracentesis [97]. The group that received no albumin developed statistically significant greater (asymptomatic) changes in electrolytes, plasma renin, and serum creatinine than the albumin group, but no more clinical morbidity or mortality. The authors of this study recommend routine albumin infusion after therapeutic paracentesis. However, not all physicians agree with this recommendation. Albumin is very expensive. It is difficult to justify the expense of routine albumin infusion after every therapeutic paracentesis worldwide based on the data at hand [98]. Albumin infusion is not needed after the removal of <5 L of fluid; albumin infusion (6–8 g/L of fluid removed) is *optional* after the removal of a larger volume of fluid [32].

TIPS has become the main second-line option for the treatment of ascites due to cirrhosis [99]. Patients and their drivers (these patients are usually too ill to drive) get tired of therapeutic paracenteses after patients have undergone several. A TIPS is placed by an interventional radiologist. It is preferable to choose a radiologist who does a few TIPS per month. This is a technically challenging procedure. TIPS can convert diuretic-resistant ascites back to diuretic-sensitive ascites [99]. The main problem with this option is hepatic encephalopathy, which

Box 17.5 Criteria for TIPS.

- Age <65 years
- Caregiver in house to help monitor mental status and give more lactulose as needed
- Child–Pugh score ≤12 points
- MELD score <18
- No alcoholic hepatitis
- Cardiac ejection fraction ≥60%
- No severe spontaneous hepatic encephalopathy or other significant insult to the brain, e.g., prior subdural hematoma, stroke, or brain abscess

MELD, model for end-stage liver disease.

develops in ~25% of patients [99]. The model for end-stage liver disease (MELD) score was developed to assess risk of death within 90 days of TIPS insertion [100].

This author prefers to proceed with this procedure only when the patient meets the criteria detailed in Box 17.5. Although these criteria are not rigid, the risks of TIPS versus the benefits must be carefully weighed in each patient, involving the caregiver in the decision making as well. Patients who live alone should not undergo TIPS. There must be someone in the house to monitor the patient's mental status and provide extra lactulose as needed to avoid severe confusion.

A successful TIPS procedure can prevent the need for future therapeutic paracenteses. When patients have less ascitic fluid in their abdomens, they can eat better and actually gain weight. TIPS is perhaps the most important breakthrough in the treatment of ascites in the past two decades. Most of the published randomized trials of TIPS versus paracenteses used the obsolete uncovered stent. Trials of the covered stent are underway and will probably show a convincing survival advantage.

Orthotopic liver transplantation should be considered in the treatment options of a refractory ascites patient who is otherwise a transplant candidate. Unfortunately there are only ~6,000 transplants per year in the United States and it is estimated that there are 10 million patients with cirrhosis. There is less than one liver per 1,000 patients with cirrhosis. Transplant helps only a tiny percentage of patients with ascites in the United States and worldwide.

In the mid 1970s the peritoneovenous shunt was promoted as a new "physiologic" treatment in the management of ascites. The study that placed peritoneovenous shunts in the "third-line" category of options for the therapy of ascites due to cirrhosis was the Veterans Administration Cooperative Study [95]. This study documented: (i) no improved survival in shunted patients compared with medically treated patients; (ii) excessive infections in shunted patients; (iii) a continued need for sodium restric-

tion and diuretics despite a functional shunt; (iv) frequent shunt failure; and (v) most importantly *only ~10% failure of diuretic therapy* [95]. It is currently difficult to find a surgeon who has experience with and enthusiasm for these peritoneovenous shunts. At the present time peritoneovenous shunting is reserved for the very small group of patients who fail diuretic therapy and are not candidates for TIPS or transplant and have too many abdominal scars or too thick of an abdominal wall for paracentesis therapy. This does not happen very often.

Peritoneovenous shunts also have a role in the treatment of postoperative chylous ascites, e.g., after radical pelvic lymphadenectomy. This author has seen miraculous results in this setting. Once the ascites disappears, the shunt can be removed.

Summary of treatment of patients with cirrhosis and ascites

The mainstay of therapy of patients with cirrhosis and ascites is dietary sodium restriction and diuretics. Standard medical therapy is effective in >90% of patients. Therapeutic paracentesis should be performed to acutely treat tense ascites and as second-line chronic treatment of a portion of the 10% of patients who are refractory to medical therapy. Many patients who are refractory to medical therapy should be considered for TIPS (see Box 17.5). Patients who are liver transplant candidates and who develop refractory ascites should be prioritized for transplantation. Peritoneovenous shunting is third-line therapy and should be reserved for special circumstances, such as ascites due to surgical lymphatic tear that does not respond to medical therapy and for patients with ascites refractory to medical treatment and circumstances that preclude chronic therapeutic paracenteses, TIPS, or transplant.

Management protocol of patients with cirrhosis and ascites

Patients with new-onset ascites of large volume and patients with ascites and failure of outpatient management may require admission to the hospital for further evaluation and treatment.

Where to hospitalize?

If the patient is a possible liver transplant candidate, admission to a transplant center is appropriate. Candidates for transplant are usually <65 years old, nonsmokers (or ex-smokers), have no ongoing alcohol or drug abuse (with at least 6 months of being "clean and sober"), no malignancy within 5 years, no serious cardiopulmonary disease, compliance with clinic appointments and medications, and with a committed care giver. Nontransplant candidates should be admitted to hospitals where hepatologists or liver-focused gastroenterologists are available for consultation. These patients are very easily harmed by inappropriate treatments provided by well meaning, but inexperienced, physicians.

History and physical examination

A careful initial history and physical examination should provide evidence for or against the presence of cirrhosis. Body weight information should be sought. Many newly diagnosed patients with cirrhosis have nonalcoholic fatty liver disease as the cause of their cirrhosis. Most patients with cirrhosis and ascites will have palmar erythema, vascular spiders, and/or abdominal wall collaterals.

Initial laboratory testing and imaging

A complete blood count with platelet count, comprehensive metabolic panel, INR, serologic screening for causes for cirrhosis, α-fetoprotein, random urine Na/K, and liver and spleen ultrasound with Doppler should be obtained. If the α-fetoprotein or ultrasound suggest malignancy, a triphasic computed tomography scan should be obtained. If the estimated creatinine clearance is <30 mL/min, no contrast should be given unless a special protocol is used.

Paracentesis

A diagnostic paracentesis is performed on the day of admission and the tests detailed in Table 17.2 should be ordered. "The sun should not set on untapped ascites." If the patient has tense ascites, 4–5 L should be removed to relieve the pressure and prevent a leak.

Diet

The patient and their cook should be educated by a dietician in a 2 g/day sodium diet. Fluid restriction is not ordered unless the serum sodium is <120 mEq/L. This occurs in only 1% of patients with cirrhosis and ascites.

Diuretics

In general, daily doses of oral spironolactone (100 mg) and furosemide (40 mg) are ordered. If a patient has failed those doses, doubling the doses is appropriate.

Daily testing

Weights, basic metabolic panel, and urine Na/K should be followed daily. Diuretics should rapidly increase urine sodium. If urine Na is >K, the patient should be losing weight. If he/she is not, attention should be drawn to the diet. Many patients eat food brought in by friends or relatives.

Maintenance fluids

It is amazing to this author how often physicians infuse saline into patients with massive fluid overload. This is obviously counterproductive and should not happen unless the patient develops gut hemorrhage or azotemia. Albumin is usually given for azotemia rather than saline. Intravenous fluids should be avoided, even when patients are scheduled to be without food in preparation for endoscopy, etc. The massive buffer of fluid in the abdomen and tissues prevents dehydration for brief periods of time.

Follow-up

Approximately 90% of patients will lose fluid weight on this regimen. If the weight does not decrease and the urine Na is <K despite maximum tolerated doses of diuretics, second-line options should be considered. When the patient is discharged from the hospital, he/she should be seen in the clinic within 1–2 weeks to prevent rapid readmission due to volume depletion or further fluid overload.

References

1. Gines P, Quintero E, Arroyo V, et al. Compensated cirrhosis: natural history and prognostic factors. *Hepatology* 1987;7:12–18.
2. D'Amico G, Morabito A, Pagliaro L, et al. Survival and prognostic indicators in compensated and decompensated cirrhosis. *Dig Dis Sci* 1986;31:468–75.
3. Cattau EI, Benjamin SB, Knuff TE, et al. The accuracy of the physical exam in the diagnosis of suspected ascites. *JAMA* 1982;247:1164–6.
4. Runyon BA, Montano AA, Akriviadis EA, et al. The serum–ascites albumin gradient is superior to the exudates–transudate concept in the differential diagnosis of ascites. *Ann Intern Med* 1992;117:215–20.
5. Runyon BA, Hoefs JC, Morgan TR. Ascitic fluid analysis in malignancy-related ascites. *Hepatology* 1988;8:1104–9.
6. Runyon BA. Cardiac ascites: a characterization. *J Clin Gastroenterol* 1988;10:410–12.
7. Han S-HB, Reynolds TB, Fong T-L. Nephrogenic ascites. *Medicine* 1998;77:233–45.
8. Muller-Schoop JW, Wang SP, Munzinger J, et al. *Chlamydia trachomatosis* as possible cause of peritonitis and perihepatitis in young women. *Br Med J* 1978;1:1022–4.
9. Runyon BA. Ascitic fluid bilirubin concentration as a key to the diagnosis of choleperitoneum. *J Clin Gastroenterol* 1987;9:543–5.
10. Mauer K, Manzione NC. Usefullness of the serum–ascites albumin gradient in separating transudative from exudative ascites: another look. *Dig Dis Sci* 1988;33:1208–12.
11. Wilkins KW, Hoffman GS. Massive ascites in systemic lupus erythematosis. *J Rheumatol* 1985;12:571–4.
12. Schrier RW, Niederberger M, Weigert A, et al. Peripheral arterial vasodilation: a determinant of functional spectrum of cirrhosis. *Semin Liver Dis* 1994;14:14–22.
13. Unikowsky B, Wexler MJ, Levy M. Dogs with experimental cirrhosis of the liver but without intrahepatic hypertension do not retain sodium or form ascites. *J Clin Invest* 1983;72:1594–604.
14. Freeman S. Recent progress in the physiology and biochemistry of the liver. *Med Clin North Am* 1953;37:109–24.
15. Hyatt RE, Smith JR. The mechanism of ascites: a physiologic appraisal. *Am J Med* 1954;16:434–8.
16. Poonwala A, Nair SP, Thuluvath PJ. Prevalence of obesity and diabetes in cryptogenic cirrhosis. *Hepatology* 2000;32:689–92.
17. Sheer TA, Joo E, Runyon BA. Usefulness of serum N-terminal-pro BNP in distinguishing ascites due to cirrhosis from ascites due to heart failure. *J Clin Gastorenterol* 2010;44:e23–6.
18. Runyon BA. Paracentesis of ascitic fluid: a safe procedure. *Arch Intern Med* 1986;146:2259–61.
19. Grabau CM, Crago SF, Hoff LK, et al. Performance standards for therapeutic abdominal paracentesis. *Hepatology* 2004;40:484–8.
20. Sakai H, Sheer TA, Mendler M, et al. Choosing the location for non-image guided abdominal paracentesis. *Liver Internat* 2005;25:984–6.
21. Runyon BA. Spontaneous bacterial peritonitis: an explosion of information. *Hepatology* 1988;8:171–5.
22. de Gottardi A, Thevenot T, Spahr L, et al. Risk of complications after abdominal paracentesis in cirrhotic patients: a prospective study. *Clin Gastro Hep* 2009;7:906–9.
23. Mannucci PM. Abnormal hemostasis tests and bleeding in chronic liver disease: are they related? No. *J Thromb Haemost* 2006;4:721–3.
24. Hillebrand DJ, Runyon BA, Yasmineh WG, et al. Ascitic fluid adenosine deaminase insensitivity in detecting tuberculous peritonitis in the United States. *Hepatology* 1996;24:1408–12.
25. Runyon BA, Akriviadis EA, Keyser AJ. The opacity of portal hypertension-related ascites correlates with the fluid's triglyceride concentration. *Am J Clin Path* 1991;96:142–3.
26. Hoefs JC. Increase in ascites WBC and protein concentrations during diuresis in patients with chronic liver disease. *Hepatology* 1981;1:249–54.

27. Mendler MH, Agarwal A, Trimzi M, et al. A new highly sensitive point of care screen for spontaneous bacterial peritonitis using a leukocyte esterase method. *J Hepatol* 2010;53:477–83.

28. Pare P, Talbot J, Hoefs JC. Serum–ascites albumin concentration gradient: a physiologic approach to the differential diagnosis of ascites. *Gastroenterology* 1983;85:240–4.

29. Hoefs JC. Serum protein concentration and portal pressure determine the ascitic fluid protein concentration in patients with chronic liver disease. *J Lab Clin Med* 1983;102:260–73.

30. Runyon BA. Approach to the patient with ascites. In: Yamada T, Alpers DH, Kaplowitz N, Laine L, Owyang C, Powell DW, eds. *Textbook of Gastroenterology*, 4th edn. Philadelphia: Lippincott Williams and Wilkins, 2003:948–72.

31. Hoefs JC. Globulin correction of albumin gradient: correlation with measured serum to ascites colloid osmotic pressure gradients. *Hepatology* 1992;16:396–403.

32. Runyon BA. Management of adult patients with ascites due to cirrhosis: an update. *Hepatology* 2009;49:2087–107.

33. Runyon BA, Canawati HN, Akriviadis EA. Optimization of ascitic fluid culture technique. *Gastroenterology* 1988;95:1351–5.

34. Runyon BA, Umland ET, Merlin T. Inoculation of blood culture bottle with ascitic fluid: improved detection of spontaneous bacterial peritonitis. *Arch Intern Med* 1987;147:73–5.

35. Runyon BA, Antillon MR, Akriviadis EA, McHutchison JG. Bedside inoculation of blood culture bottles with ascitic fluid is superior to delayed inoculation in the detection of spontaneous bacterial peritonitis. *J Clin Microbiol* 1990;28:2811–12.

36. Sampliner RE, Iber FL. High protein ascites in patients with uncomplicated hepatic cirrhosis. *Am J Med Sci* 1974;256:275–9.

37. Runyon BA, Hoefs JC. Ascitic fluid analysis before, during, and after spontaneous bacterial peritonitis. *Hepatology* 1985;5:257–9.

38. Runyon BA. Low-protein-concentration ascitic fluid is predisposed to spontaneous bacterial peritonitis. *Gastroenterology* 1986;91:1343–6.

39. Akriviadis EA, Runyon BA. The value of an algorithm in differentiating spontaneous from secondary bacterial peritonitis. *Gastroenterology* 1990;98:127–33.

40. Soriano G, Castellote J, Alvarez C, et al. Secondary bacterial peritonitis in cirrhosis: a retrospective study of clinical and analytic characteristics, diagnosis and management. *J Hepatol* 2010;52:39–44.

41. Wilson JAP, Suguitan EA, Cassidy WA, et al. Characteristics of ascitic fluid in the alcoholic cirrhotic. *Dig Dis Sci* 1979;24:645–8.

42. Runyon BA. Amylase levels in ascitic fluid. *J Clin Gastroenterol* 1987;9:172–4.

43. Geake TMS, Spitaels JM, Moshel MG, et al. Peritoneoscopy in the diagnosis of tuberculous peritonitis. *Gastro Endosc* 1981;27:66–8.

44. Singh MM, Bhargava AN, Jain KP. Tuberculous peritonitis. *N Engl J Med* 1969;281:1091–4.

45. Bhargava DK, Gupta M, Nijhawan S, et al. Adenosine deaminase (ADA) in peritoneal tuberculosis: diagnostic value in ascitic fluid and serum. *Tubercle* 1990;71:121–6.

46. Altamirano M, Kelly MA, Wong A, et al. Characterization of a DNA probe for detection of *Mycobacterium* tuberculosis complex in clinical samples by polymerase chain reaction. *J Clin Microbiol* 1992;30:2173–6.

47. Johnson WD. The cytological diagnosis of cancer in serous effusions. *Acta Cytol* 1966;10:161–72.

48. Cardozo PL. A critical evaluation of 3000 cytologic analyses of pleural fluid, ascitic fluid, and pericardial fluid. *Acta Cytol* 1966;10:455–60.

49. Decker D, Stratmann H, Springer W, et al. Benign and malignant cells in effusions: diagnostic value of image DNA cytometry in comparison to cytological analysis. *Pathol Res Pract* 1998;194:791–5.

50. Press OW, Press NO, Kaufman SD. Evaluation and management of chylous ascites. *Ann Intern Med* 1982: 96:358–64.

51. Reynolds TB. Rapid presumptive diagnosis of spontaneous bacterial peritonitis. *Gastroenterology* 1986;90:1294–7.

52. Runyon BA, Antillon MR. Ascitic fluid pH and lactate: insensitive and nonspecific tests in detecting ascitic fluid infection. *Hepatology* 1991;13:929–35.

53. Albillos A, Cuervas-Mons V, Millan I, et al. Ascitic fluid polymorphonuclear cell count and serum to ascites albumin gradient in the diagnosis of bacterial peritonitis. *Gastroenterology* 1990;98:134–40.

54. Loewenstein MS, Rittgers RA, Feinerman AE, et al. CEA assay of ascites and detection of malignancy. *Ann Intern Med* 1978;88:635–8.

55. Runyon BA. Elevated ascitic fluid fibronectin: a non-specific finding. *J Hepatol* 1986;3:219–22.

56. Runyon BA. Ascitic fluid "humoral tests of malignancy." *Hepatology* 1986;6:1443–5.

57. Correia JP, Conn HO. Spontaneous bacterial peritonitis in cirrhosis: endemic or epidemic. *Med Clin North Am* 1975: 59:963–81.

58. Runyon BA. Monomicrobial nonneutrocytic bacterascites: a variant of spontaneous bacterial peritonitis. *Hepatology* 1990;12:710–15.

59. Conn HO, Fessel JM. Spontaneous bacterial peritonitis in cirrhosis: variations on a theme. *Medicine* 1971;50:161–97.

60. Runyon BA, Hoefs JC. Culture-negative neutrocytic ascites: a variant of spontaneous bacterial peritonitis. *Hepatology* 1984;4:1209–11.

61. Runyon BA, Canawati HN, Hoefs JC. Polymicrobial bacterascites: a unique entity in the spectrum of infected ascitic fluid. *Arch Intern Med* 1986;146:2173–5.

62. Runyon BA. Spontaneous bacterial peritonitis associated with cardiac ascites. *Am J Gastroenterol* 1984;79:796.

63. Kurtz RC, Bronzo RL. Does spontaneous bacterial peritonitis occur in malignant ascites? *Am J Gastroenterol* 1982;77:146–8.

64. Wolfe GM, Runyon BA. Spontaneous *Salmonella* infection of high protein non-cirrhotic ascites. *J Clin Gastroenterol* 1990;12:430–2.

65. Runyon BA. Fatal bacterial peritonitis secondary to nonobstructive colonic dilatation (Ogilvie's syndrome) in cirrhotic ascites. *J Clin Gastroenterol* 1986;8:687–9.

66. Berg RD, Garlington AW. Translocation of certain indigenous bacteria from the gastrointestinal tract to the mesenteric lymph nodes and other organs in a gnotobiotic mouse model. *Infect Immun* 1979;23:403–11.

67. Runyon BA, Morrissey R, Hoefs JC, et al. Opsonic activity of human ascitic fluid: a potentially important protective mechanism against spontaneous bacterial peritonitis. *Hepatology* 1985;5:634–7.

68. Runyon BA. Bacterial infections in patients with cirrhosis. *J Hepatol* 1993;18:271–2.

69. Mellencamp MA, Preheim LC. Pneumococcal pneumonia in a rat model of cirrhosis: effects of cirrhosis on pulmonary defense mechanisms against *Streptococcus pneumoniae*. *J Infec Dis* 1991;163: 102–8.

70. Runyon BA, Sugano S, Kanel G, et al. A rodent model of cirrhosis, ascites, and spontaneous bacterial peritonitis. *Gastroenterology* 1991;100:489–93.

71. Guarner C, Runyon BA, Young S, et al. Intestinal bacterial overgrowth and bacterial translocation in an experimental model of cirrhosis in rats. *J Hepatol* 1997;26:1372–8.

72. Runyon BA, Squier SU, Borzio M. Translocation of gut bacteria in rats with cirrhosis to mesenteric lymph nodes partially explains the pathogenesis of spontaneous bacterial peritonitis. *J Hepatol* 1994;21:792–6.

73. Runyon BA. Patients with deficient ascitic fluid opsonic activity are predisposed to spontaneous bacterial peritonitis. *Hepatology* 1988;8:632–5.

74. McHutchison JG, Runyon BA. Spontaneous bacterial peritonitis. In: Surawicz CM, Owen RL, eds. *Gastrointestinal and Hepatic Infections*. Philadelphia: WB Saunders, 1995:455–75.

75. Kumar A, Roberts D, Wood KE, et al. Duration of hypotension before initiation of effective antimicrobial therapy is the critical

determinant of survival in human septic shock. *Crit Care Med* 2006;34:89–96.

76. Caly WR, Strauss E. A prospective study of bacterial infections in patients with cirrhosis. *J Hepatol* 1993;18:353–8.

77. Borzio M, Salerno F, Piantoni L, et al. Bacterial infections in patients with advanced cirrhosis: a multicentre prospective study. *Dig Liver Dis* 2001;33:41–8.

78. Burroughs AK, Rosenstein IJ, Epstein O, et al. Bacteriuria and primary biliary cirrhosis. *Gut* 1984;25:133–7.

79. Bernard B, Grange J-D, Khac EN, et al. Antibiotic prophylaxis for the prevention of bacterial infections in cirrhotic patients with gastrointestinal bleeding: a meta-analysis. *Hepatology* 1999;29: 1655–61.

80. Felisart J, Rimola A, Arroyo V, et al. Randomized comparative study of efficacy and nephrotoxicity of ampicillin plus tobramycin versus cefotaxime in cirrhotics with severe infections. *Hepatology* 1985;5:457–62.

81. Runyon BA, Akriviadis FA, Sattler FR, et al. Ascitic fluid and serum cefotaxime levels in patients treated for spontaneous bacterial peritonitis. *Dig Dis Sci* 1991;36:1782–6.

82. Runyon BA, McHutchison JG, Antillon MR, et al. Short-course vs long-course antibiotic treatment of spontaneous bacterial peritonitis: randomized controlled trial. *Gastroenterology* 1991;100:1737–42.

83. Sort P, Navasa M, Arroyo V, et al. Effect of intravenous albumin on renal impairment and mortality in patients with cirrhosis and spontaneous bacterial peritonitis. *N Engl J Med* 1999;341:403–9.

84. Tito L, Rimola A, Gines P, et al. Recurrence of spontaneous bacterial peritonitis in cirrhosis: frequency and predictive factors. *Hepatology* 1988;8:27–31.

85. Gines P, Rimola A, Planas R, et al. Norfloxacin prevents spontaneous bacterial peritonitis recurrence in cirrhosis: results of a double-blind, placebo-controlled trial. *Hepatology* 1990;12:716–24.

86. Soriano G, Guarner C, Teixido M, et al. Selective intestinal decontamination prevents spontaneous bacterial peritonitis. *Gastroenterology* 1991;100:477–81.

87. Fernandez J, Ruis del Arbol L, Gomez C, et al. Norfloxacin vs ceftriaxone in the prophylaxis of infections in patients with advanced cirrhosis and hemorrhage. *Gastroenterology* 2006;131:1049–56.

88. Fernandez J, Navasa M, Planas R, et al. Primary prophylaxis of spontaneous bacterial peritonitis delays hepatorenal syndrome and improves survival in cirrhosis. *Gastroenterology* 2007;133: 818–24.

89. Tito L, Gines P, Arroyo V, et al. Total paracentesis associated with intravenous albumin management of patients with cirrhosis and ascites. *Gastroenterology* 1990;98:146–51.

90. Belghiti J, Durand F. Abdominal wall hernia in the setting of cirrhosis. *Semin Liver Dis* 1997;17:219–26.

91. Runyon BA, Juler GL. Natural history of umbilical hernias in patients with and without ascites. *Am J Gastroenterol* 1985;80:38–9.

92. Strauss RM, Boyer TD. Hepatic hydrothorax. *Semin Liver Dis* 1997;17:227–32.

93. Runyon BA, Greenblatt M, Ming RHC. Hepatic hydrothorax is a relative contraindication to chest tube insertion. *Am J Gastroenterol* 1986;81:566–7.

94. Addolorato G, Leggio L, Ferrulli A, et al. Effectiveness and safety of baclofen for maintenance of alcohol abstinence in alcohol-dependent patients with liver cirrhosis: randomized, double-blind controlled study. *Lancet* 2007;370:1915–22.

95. Stanley MM, Ochi S, Lee KK, et al. Peritoneovenous shunting as compared with medical treatment in patients with alcoholic cirrhosis and massive ascites. *N Engl J Med* 1989;321:1632–8.

96. Gines P, Arroyo V, Quintero E, et al. Comparison of paracentesis and diuretics in the treatment of cirrhotics with tense ascites: results of a randomized study. *Gastroenterology* 1987;93:234–41.

97. Gines P, Tito L, Arroyo V, et al. Randomized comparative study of therapeutic paracentesis with and without intravenous albumin in cirrhosis. *Gastroenterology* 1988;94:1493–502.

98. Runyon BA. Is albumin infusion necessary after large-volume paracentesis? Con – main arguments. *Liver Internat* 2009;29:638–40. (Con - rebuttal 2009,29:640 1.)

99. Boyer TD, Haskal ZJ. AASLD practice guidelines: the role of transjugular intrahepatic shunt (TIPS) in the management of portal hypertension. *Hepatology* 2010;51:1–16.

100. Malinchoc M, Kamath PS, Gordon FD, et al. A model to predict poor survival in patients undergoing transjugular intrahepatic portosystemic shunts. *Hepatology* 2000;31:864–71.

Multiple choice questions

17.1 First-line treatment of patients with cirrhosis and ascites includes 2 g/day sodium diet and which of the following?

    a Intravenous furosemide.
    b Oral furosemide.
    c Large volume paracentesis.
    d Oral spironolactone and furosemide.

17.2 Standard treatment of spontaneous bacterial peritonitis (SBP) includes which of the following?

    a Ampicillin and gentamicin.
    b Ceftriaxone 1 g intravenously daily for 5 days.
    c Cefotaxime 2 g intravenously every 8 hours for 5 days.
    d Cefotaxime and metronidazole.

Answers to the multiple choice questions can be found in the Appendix at the end of the book.

These multiple choice questions are also available for you to complete online.
Visit http://www.schiffsdiseasesoftheliver.com/

CHAPTER 18
Hepatic Encephalopathy

Ravi K. Prakash & Kevin D. Mullen

Division of Gastroenterology, MetroHealth Medical Center, Case Western Reserve University, Cleveland, OH, USA

Key concepts

- Hepatic encephalopathy (HE) is a serious complication of liver disease that encompasses a broad range of neurologic and neuropsychiatric abnormalities.
- HE is mainly classified into three types: type A is seen acute liver failure, type B is seen in subjects with large portosystemic shunts in the absence of intrinsic liver disease, and type C is the most common variety seen in cirrhosis.
- Overt HE is the clinical manifestation of HE where changes in consciousness and motor abnormalities are observed.
- Minimal HE is defined as patients with completely normal neurologic examination but who have cognitive deficits in specific domains which are detected by psychometric tests.
- Covert HE is a new term that has been proposed to encompass minimal HE and the mildest form of overt HE (stage I HE on the New Haven scale).
- Ammonia is still considered the most important factor in the pathogenesis of HE.

- Cerebral edema is seen in most patients with advanced liver disease, which can be explained by the entry of ammonia into astrocytes.
- Recent advances in a number of modalities of magnetic resonance imaging has shown cerebral edema mainly in the white matter in cirrhotics.
- The approach to treatment of HE is four pronged: supportive care of the patient, to identify and treat precipitating factors, to rule out other concomitant causes of encephalopathy, and to initiate empirical therapy.
- Lactulose, despite paucity of convincing randomized controlled trial data, is still considered the first-line therapeutic agent.
- Another therapeutic agent (nonabsorbable antibiotic, rifaximin) has been approved by the US FDA (Food and Drug Administration) for treatment of patients with recurrent episodes of overt HE.
- Rifaximin has also shown to improve driving skills in patients with minimal HE.

Hepatic encephalopathy (HE) is a term used to describe a broad range of neurologic and neuropsychiatric impairments seen in patients with significant underlying liver disease [1–4] Neurologic syndromes associated with liver disease were described as early as Hippocrates (460–370 BC), but the clinical syndrome of HE in chronic liver disease as we know it today was described by Adams and Foley (and Summerskill, Sherlock, and colleagues) in a series of papers published in the mid-twentieth century [1,3,5].

As this information was disseminated it became apparent to investigators like Gabuzda and others that they were encountering a similar syndrome in patients participating in clinical trials [6]. The study in particular was on resins to treat ascites associated with chronic liver disease which exchanged sodium for ammonia. It was noticed that these patients developed a neurologic syndrome similar to the one described by Foley and Adams. It was during this time that ammonia was implicated firmly in the

pathogenesis of HE [7]. However, in the ensuing decades there was some disenchantment about his theory as there was very little correlation between the levels of ammonia and the severity of HE. This in retrospect was due to unreliable ammonia assays [8]. Indeed, in that era there was only one report that showed good correlation between ammonia and HE [9,10]. As a result of this poor correlation a number of other theories were devised to explain the pathogenesis of HE, which will be discussing in the forthcoming sections.

The next major event in the understanding of hepatic encephalopathy came when it was realized that patients with both acute and chronic liver disease had cerebral edema [11,12]. It was already well known that patients with acute liver failure had pronounced cerebral edema and often developed intracranial hypertension. In contrast, a low grade of cerebral edema was identified in cirrhosis in the ensuing years [10,11]. What may have hidden this from view is the fact that some degree of cerebral atrophy is present in most patients with cirrhosis. Also, there are compensatory mechanisms to limit the degree of cerebral edema that operate in chronic liver disease states.

Nomenclature

The first significant effort to standardize the definitions of the different syndromes in HE was performed by the Hepatic Encephalopathy Consensus Group in 1998 at the World Congress of Gastroenterology meeting in Vienna. Prior to this "portosystemic encephalopathy" and "hepatic encephalopathy" were interchangeably used [2,13]. It was decided, with the permission of Dame Sheila Sherlock, to discard the term portosystemic encephalopathy, which indicated the influence of portosystemic shunts as being largely responsible for the development of changes in mental state. This is in fact rare in the absence of intrinsic liver disease. Therefore, hepatic encephalopathy was classified into three main categories as shown in Figure 18.1. As noted in this figure, type A is associated with acute liver failure, type B (B for bypass) is associated with portosystemic shunts without intrinsic liver disease, and type C is associated with chronic liver failure or cirrhosis. Type A HE, formerly known as alfa HE, is remarkably different from type B and type C. Some differences between type A and type C HE are shown in Table 18.1. Type C is the most commonly encountered clinical syndrome and is further subclassified into episodic, persistent, and minimal hepatic encephalopathy. This standardization of the nomenclature for HE has sucessfully enhanced communication throughout the world [14].

Table 18.1 Differences between type A (α) and type C hepatic encephalopathy (HE).

	Type A HE	Type C HE
Hepatic injury	Acute onset (<8 weeks)	Chronic (at least >6 months)
Animal model	Galactosamine in rabbits/rats	Bile duct ligation and/or carbon tetrachloride in rats
Pathology	Acute hepatocellular necrosis and hepatic insufficiency	Chronic hepatocellular injury, fibrosis, nodular regeneration, and circulatory bypass of liver
Clinical profile		
Onset	Acute	Variable: insidious versus acute
Precipitating factors	Uncommon	Common
Cerebral edema	High-grade edema present	Low-grade edema present
Nutritional state	Normal	Cachexia may be present
Ascites	Absent	Usually present
Portosystemic shunts	Absent	Present
Treatment.	Treat cause of liver failure. Usually need liver transplant	Treat precipitating cause along with empirical therapy
Immediate survival	Low without transplant	High
Persistent neuropsychiatric sequelae after acute episode	No	Prior overt HE patients have worse cognition

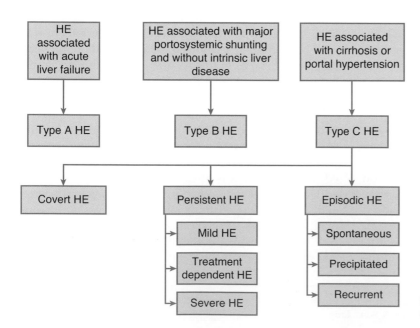

Figure 18.1 World Congress of Gastroenterology classification of hepatic encephalopathy (HE).

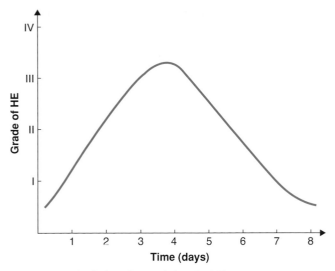

Figure 18.2 Episodic hepatic encephalopathy (HE).

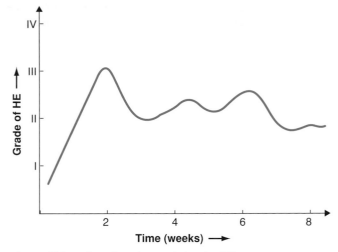

Figure 18.4 Persistent hepatic encephalopathy (HE).

Episodic HE is characterized by changes in the mental state that vary in severity and duration (Fig. 18.2). These episodes can be either secondary to a known precipitating factor, otherwise called precipitated HE, or can occur in the absence of any recognized precipitating factor, and called spontaneous HE. Recurrent HE is defined as occurring twice or more in 1 year (Fig. 18.3). Persistent HE is defined as the presence of cognitive impairment at baseline (lasting beyond 2 weeks) secondary to liver disease that negatively impacts on social and occupational functioning (Fig. 18.4).

The other term that perished during this time of terminology metamorphosis was "subclinical hepatic encephalopathy" [15]. Instead, the term "minimal hepatic encephalopathy" was introduced. This is defined as HE occurring in patients with liver disease who have com-

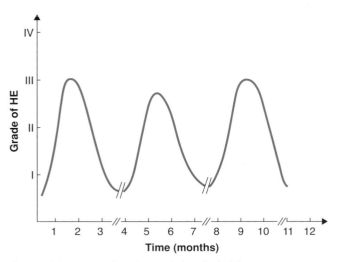

Figure 18.3 Recurrent hepatic encephalopathy (HE) (two or more episodes in 12 months).

pletely normal mental status and neurologic examination but who have cognitive deficits in specific neuropsychometric tests [2]. It is seen in a large proportion of cirrhotic subjects and has received a lot of attention by hepatic encephalopathy researchers over the last decade.

Overt HE is the clinical syndrome of HE, with varying degree of mental and neurologic changes, seen in patients with liver disease. Classification and semiquantification of the severity of overt HE was developed by Harold Conn in the 1970s and is well known as the West Haven criteria [16]. Table 18.2 illustrates the modified West Haven criteria along with the operative definition, which was proposed by Amodio et al. [17,18]. This has five stages ranging from stage 0, where the mental status is completely normal, to stage IV, where the patient is comatose. More recently it has been observed that there is a lot of variation amongst clinicians and researchers in the diagnosis of stage I HE. This is because the clinical criteria defining stage I are prone to a lot of subjective bias [19]. To eliminate this subjectivity and introduce an objective way of defining the various grades of HE, the International Society for Hepatic Encephalopathy and Nitrogen Metabolism (ISHEN) has proposed some further changes in terminology at the meeting held in Quebec, Canada in 2010. The term "covert HE" was introduced, which will encompass minimal HE and stage I HE (Fig. 18.5). Covert HE is diagnosed mainly by neuropsychiatric tests as most patients in stage I HE will have very subtle signs of mental status changes. This change in classification is very similar to the proposed low grade to high grade HE concept by Kircheis and Haussinger [19]. The spectrum of neurologic impairment in hepatic encephalopathy (SONIC) extends from patients with normal mental status at one end, to covert HE and various grades of overt HE on the other end (Fig. 18.6) [20].

Grade	Description	Operative definition
0	No abnormality detected	
Minimal HE	No neurologic symptoms Normal clinical examination Abnormal psychometric test performance	PHES >2 SD in two or more tests ICT >5 lures CF: critical frequency of 39 Hz or less
1	Trivial lack of awareness Euphoria or anxiety Shortened attention span Impairment of addition or subtraction	Naming ≤7 animals in 120 seconds Oriented in time and space

2	Lethargy or apathy
	Disorientation for time
	Obvious personality change
	Inappropriate behaviours
		Disoriented in time (≥3 items incorrect):
		    day of the week
		    day of the month
		    the month
		    the year
		Oriented in place

3	Somnolence to semistupor
	Responsive to stimuli
	Confused
	Gross disorientation
	Bizzare behaviour
		Disoriented in place (≥2 items incorrect):
		    state/country
		    region/country
		    city
		    place
		    floor/ward
		Disoriented in time, and reduction in
		    Glasgow coma scale(8–14)

4	Coma, unable to test mental state	Unresponsive to painful stimuli (Glasgow coma scale <8)

Table 18.2 Modified West Haven criteria for grading hepatic encephalopathy (HE) with operative definitions.

CF, critical frequency; ICT, inhibitory control test; PHES, psychometric hepatic encephalopathy score; SD, standard deviation.

Pathogenesis

The precise molecular mechanisms responsible for the pathogenesis of hepatic encephalopathy still remain largely unknown. There is an agreed principle that the

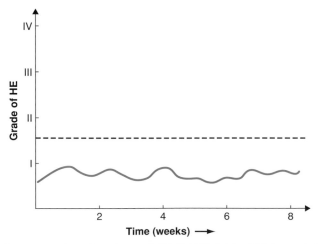

Figure 18.5 Covert hepatic encephalopathy (HE) (minimal HE plus grade I HE).

cause of HE is primarily due to gut-derived toxins (Fig. 18.7). This concept has largely stemmed from the observation that gut lavage and catharsis leads to the resolution of overt HE. In addition, as noted above, bouts of overt HE have been observed when ammonia-containing resins have been introduced into the gut [6]. In addition to ammonia quite a number of other putative toxins have been proposed as potential mediators of HE (Table 18.3) [21].

One interesting aspect of HE is the general lack of the syndrome in patients with major portosystemic shunting of blood but who do not have underlying liver disease. Many cases have been published that provide some exception to the rule that overt HE in this group is rarely seen [22]. Why the vast majority of patients with major portosystemic bypass and little intrinsic liver disease are largely free of overt HE is a bit of a mystery. Box 18.1 lists conditions that lead to this situation. It seems probable that quite a number of these patients may have evidence for minimal HE even though overt HE is rarely encountered.

Before discussing briefly some of the individual theories about the pathogenesis of HE, it is useful to think

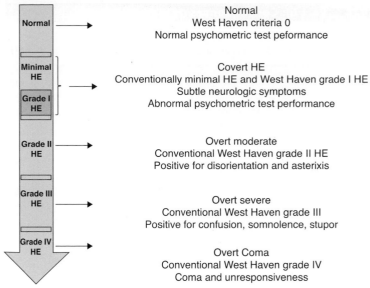

Normal
West Haven criteria 0
Normal psychometric test peformance

Covert HE
Conventionally minimal HE and West Haven grade I HE
Subtle neurologic symptoms
Abnormal psychometric test performance

Overt moderate
Conventional West Haven grade II HE
Positive for disorientation and asterixis

Overt severe
Conventional West Haven grade III
Positive for confusion, somnolence, stupor

Overt Coma
Conventional West Haven grade IV
Coma and unresponsiveness

Figure 18.6 Spectrum of neurologic impairment in cirrhosis. HE, hepatic encephalopathy.

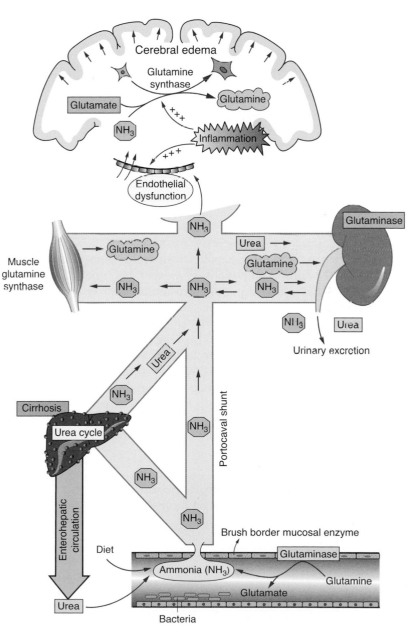

Figure 18.7 Pathogenesis of hepatic encephalopathy.

Table 18.3 Pathogenesis of hepatic encephalopathy.

Pathogenic factors	Some proposed mechanism
Ammonia	Combines with glutamate to form glutamine Intracelluar accumulation of glutamine causes astrocyte swelling and cerebral edema Involved in generation of reactive oxygen species(ROS)
Inflammation	Astrocytes and microglial cells release cytokines Cytokines affect the integrity of the blood–brain barrier and increase ammonia diffusion into the brain
Neurosteroids	Increased expression of protein 18 kDa stimulates neurosteroid synthesis Enhances GABAergic tone by a positive allosteric action on GABA-A receptor
Oxidative and nitrosative stress	Synthesized and released in response to ammonia, inflammatory mediators, hyponatremia, and benzodizepines Has a role in astrocyte swelling and tyrosine nitration of intracellular proteins
Manganese	Preferential accumulation in basal ganglia in cirrhotics with extensive portosystemic shunts Has role in formation of type II Alzheimer cells, stimulating neurosteroid synthesis and increasing GABAergic tone

GABA, γ-aminobutyric acid.

in broader terms. Assuming hepatic clearance of putative intestinal toxins is important to prevent HE, one can postulate that a lack of portal perfusion of the liver (because of spontaneous shunts or shunts formed after portal vein thrombosis) is usually not sufficient to cause hepatic encephalopathy on its own. Looking at it another way there may be compensatory mechanisms to make up for the loss of portal perfusion. Reasonably strong evidence exists that augmentation of hepatic arterial flow is seen in these patients that makes up for the lack of portal perfusion [23]. Other modulatory influences have been postulated to ameliorate the tendency to develop overt

Box 18.1 Causes of noncirrhotic portal hypertension with no intrinsic liver disease.
- Portal vein thrombosis/splanchnic vein thrombosis
- Congenital
- Hypercoagulable conditions
- Noncirrhotic portal fibrosis
- Large retroperitoneal and intrasplenic arteriovenous malformations
- Massive splenomegaly

HE with portosystemic shunting alone. Interestingly, any type of further manipulation of splanchnic venous circulation, such as proximal splenorenal shunts, can result in the onset of multiple bouts of overt HE, even though there still is minimal structural disease in these patients with noncirrhotic portal hypertension. Much more research on this issue of the modulation of the expression of HE is necessary.

Ammonia

There is a large body of information implicating ammonia as a major mediator of HE. During the period when many other theories were developed, few if any studies showed a correlation between the ammonia blood level and the severity of HE. As mentioned previously, this particular problem was presumably due to ammonia assay problems prevalent at that time. In the current quoted literature at least three studies show good correlation between ammonia levels and the severity of HE [8,10,24]. We will discuss in the next section on diagnosis the fact that these findings do not signify that ammonia levels are particularly useful in the diagnosis of HE.

Direct neurotoxicity of ammonia is clearly an issue when ammonia levels are extremely high, as seen in patients with urea cycle defects [25]. Seizures and florid cerebral edema are seen in acute liver failure with ammonia levels above established thresholds (over 200 μmol/L) [26]. However, in chronic liver failure seizures are rare and quite subtle cerebral edema is present. There are a lot of data indicating that ammonia is responsible for cerebral edema primarily through increasing intracerebral glutamine by combining with glutamate [27–30]. The mechanism for the effect of ammonia on the brain has been studied most extensively in astrocytes but it is assumed that the neurons are affected in a similar fashion (Fig. 18.8) [11,31,32]. The reason that brain swelling rarely results in intracranial hypertension in chronic liver disease patients is thought to be due to: (i) preexisting cerebral atrophy, especially in alcoholic liver disease patients; and (ii) compensatory extrusion of intracellular myoinositol in response to the intracellular osmolyte increases [33,34]. However, there are some rare cases of intracranial hypertension in chronic liver disease reported [35].

While there is a general acceptance of cerebral edema being present in the brain in chronic liver disease patients, the question remains as to how that specifically leads to the manifestation of overt HE [36]. Moreover, in all alcoholic patients whether they have no HE, minimal HE, or overt HE evidence exists for cerebral edema, especially in the white matter [37]. Successful liver transplantation removes all evidence of cerebral edema over time in parallel with the resolution of most of the neurologic problems existing pretransplant [12,38]. However,

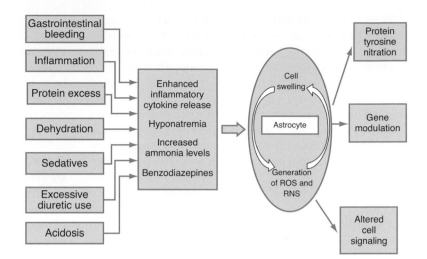

Figure 18.8 Astrocyte changes in the pathogenesis of hepatic encephalopathy. ROS, reactive oxygen species; RNS, reactive nitrogen species.

recently there have been a few reports suggesting that HE may not be totally reversible in all circumstances [39,40].

GABA/benzodiazepines

The original γ-aminobutyric acid (GABA) HE hypothesis was based on the observation of increased GABA receptors in brains in an animal model of HE [41]. This apparent increase in receptor density may have arisen from an effect of HE on the susceptibility of synaptosomes to solubilization in the assay used at that time [42,43]. There still remains evidence for increased GABA neurotransmission in some animal models of HE.

Experiments with a series of drugs active at the GABA/benzodiazepine receptor complex revealed that RO-15-1788 (a benzodiazepine receptor antagonist now called flumazenil) reversed HE in a rabbit model of liver failure [44]. The only plausible explanation for this observation was that there must be an accumulation of endogenous benzodiazepines in the brains of these animals [45]. The same phenomenon was noted in a rat model of HE, and the paper by Basile and Gammal identified benzodizepines in the brains of humans with HE [46]. Endogenous benzodiazepines have been identified in animals and plants for decades. However, the levels of these compounds are generally an order of magnitude less than required to cause "coma." Despite over 30% reversal of overt HE within minutes of administration of flumazenil, little attention has been paid to endogenous benzodiazepines in recent years [47]. Publications on the findings of these compounds in liver disease patients continue to appear [48]. One assumes more studies will arise in the coming years.

Endogenous opiates

There is quite strong evidence that the accumulation of endogenous opiates plays a major role in the pathogenesis of pruritis in cholestatic liver disease [49]. A number

of reports have indicated reversal of HE with naloxone in animal models. This reversal effect has not been easy to reproduce and may have a very specific dose-dependent therapeutic action. Anecdotal human reports of HE reversal have been published with opiate antagonists [50]. Ruling out occult narcotic intake prior to bouts of HE in these reports may have been ineffective.

Plasma amino acid imbalance/false neurotransmitter

The ratio of plasma branched chain amino acids to aromatic amino acids is greatly altered in cirrhotic patients. This imbalance led to the hypothesis that the accumulation of aromatic amino acids (phenylalanine, tyrosine and tryptophan) was occurring in the brains of patients with advanced liver disease because of the loss of normal competition between aromatic amino acids and branched chain amino acids (leucine, isoleucine, and valine) across the blood–brain barrier. It was proposed that these aromatic amino acids were leading to the production of intracerebral false neurotransmitters and serotonin [51]. This process was thought to be even further enhanced by the exchange of intracerebral glutamine across the blood–brain barrier [52].

This rather intricate hypothesis would have had more support if the proposed treatment to correct this plasma amino acid imbalance – with branched chain amino acid-enriched parenteral solutions – had been demonstrated to work, i.e., reversed HE [53]. A number of treatment trials were conducted without clear benefit. It is worth noting that at the time, and for nearly two decades after, barely any form of HE treatment was found to be effective. These trials were done in patients with very advanced liver disease, which made performing controlled trials nearly impossible [18]. Multiple precipitating factors and concomitant causes of encephalopathy may have been present in these patients, which may be why it was so difficult to prove therapies were effective. One can argue that the benefit of parenteral branched chain amino acid-enriched therapy may have been unfairly tested using the study design available at that time. In support of this therapeutic approach, it has been noted that oral branched chain amino acid supplements have been shown to be reasonably effective in reducing HE in a number of studies [54,55]. Another largely ignored aspect of branched chain amino acid therapy is the potential that this therapy may reduce HE by promoting maintenance or repletion of lean body mass. It may well transpire that this effect, especially noted with leucine, could be important in managing HE [56].

An additional point about branched chain amino acids is that hemoglobin is devoid of isoleucine. Since isoleucine is an essential amino acid, the tendency of patients to develop HE after major gastrointestinal hemorrhage can lead to the failure of whole-body protein synthesis and more pronounced hyperammonemia compared with the ingestion of other proteins [57]. Synthetic solutions simulating the amino acid composition of hemoglobin are now used as challenge tests to induce a worsening of HE in humans in a very controlled setting. These may simply reflect an oral ammonia challenge, but if the same solution with added isoleucine does not induce changes in HE (generally only covert or minimal HE is induced) there may be an incentive to explore this area of HE research further [58].

Role of systemic sepsis/inflammation

It has been noted for decades that infections in cirrhotic patients often precipitate bouts of overt HE. Indeed, the majority of very severe HE episodes are seen in septic patients. Severe infections in the absence of liver disease can cause an independent encephalopathy so perhaps the syndrome in septic patients is mediated by other mechanisms [59].

Many investigators now believe that sepsis or systemic inflammatory processes play a major role in modulating the expression of overt HE [60]. The same has been argued for covert or minimal HE, which has been reported to first appear once systemic inflammatory markers appear in the blood [61].

Various cytokines and standard markers of inflammation have been used in examining the role that inflammation may play in covert HE. The best illustration of this is the induction of hyperammonemia using an oral glutamine challenge [62]. The rapid breakdown of glutamine by intestinal glutaminase leads to a brisk 2–3-fold elevation of blood ammonia. By using a glutamine oral challenge test with sensitive psychometric tests, an important phenomenon has been reported. This challenge basically does not alter psychometric performance (e.g., the digit symbol test) in most patients unless systemic inflamma-

tory markers are raised. Whether this is mediated by the blood–brain barrier effects of inflammation or by some other mechanism, remains to be determined [63]. Binding of inflammatory cells or cytokines to cerebral endothelial cells allows it to bypass the normal exclusionary effect of the blood–brain barrier [64–66]. Whatever the mechanism, it is imperative to identify and treat infection as promptly as possible in the management of HE.

Overall concepts of the pathogenesis of hepatic encephalopathy

The literature on the possible mechanisms responsible for the pathogenesis of HE is enormous. Nonetheless, it is reasonable to propose multiple additive or synergistic processes that lead to HE [21]. Ammonia appears to be the key toxin involved in HE and a definitive connection between increased brain ammonia entry and cerebral edema has been established. Recent advances in nuclear magnetic resonance spectroscopy (H1-MRS) have allowed us to monitor alterations in brain chemistry during experimental induction of HE with ammonia elevations. Generally, increased intra-astrocytic glutamine levels are noted with reduced myoinositol levels. Astrocyte rather than neuronal edema has been demonstrated. Considerable edema in the white matter is also present. This usually low-grade cerebral edema in chronic liver disease is accentuated by hyponatremia, certain benzodiazepines, and other compounds [67]. Presumably, this major alteration in astrocyte cell function disrupts communication and/or the function of neuronal cells. An additional mechanism whereby swelling of the astrocyte may alter brain function is through the stimulation of neurosteroid production [68]. These compounds, rather like endogenous benzodiazepines, may enhance GABAergic neurotransmission. Peripheral benzodiazepine receptors (PBR) are expressed in astrocytes, and when upregulated by exposure to ammonia lead to increased neurosteroid production [69]. A whole array of other compounds may also be produced by PBR-upregulated astrocytes, which can lead to the activation of protein kinases and oxidative stress [70]. Ultimately, a very complex set of events are involved in the pathogenesis of HE. This brief overview deliberately does not comment much on other mechanisms proposed, which can be found in a number of excellent reviews by Butterworth, Cordoba, Haussinger, Norenberg, and their colleagues [70–75].

Diagnosis

Any change in mental status or prior performance in psychometric tests in patients with known or strongly suspected underlying cirrhosis should be considered to be due to hepatic encephalopathy unless proven otherwise.

Box 18.2 Concomitant causes of encephalopathy.

- Respiratory failure: hypoxia and hypercapnia
- Gross electrolyte abnormalities - potassium, magnesium, calcium
- Status epilepticus or postictal state
- Renal failure and uremia
- Cerebrovascular accident/stroke
- Hypoglycemia
- Central nervous system infections
- Intracerebral/intracranial hemorrhage
- Metabolic acidosis
- Drug intoxication
- Cerebral edema/intracranial hypertension
- Wenicke–Korsakoff syndrome
- Delirium tremens
- Pancreatic encephalopathy

Box 18.3 Causes of recurrent or intractable hepatic encephalopathy.

- Major portosystemic shunting
- Deep-seated abscess
- Occult medication use
- Underlying urea cycle disorder

Patients with decompensated cirrhosis are particularly prone to develop overt HE. However, advanced liver disease is also associated with other events (Box 18.2) that can cause changes in mental status. These need to be identified and treated, and technically the presence of other causes of encephalopathy makes it impossible to formally assign a diagnosis of HE. In reality often both the concomitant cause of encephalopathy and HE are diagnosed and treated at the same time. We have quite often encountered hypothyroidism occurring with HE [76].

As the term implies, to suspect HE one has to first identify the presence of underlying cirrhosis or, more rarely, portosystemic shunts without cirrhosis. Figure 18.9 illustrates the various clinical signs indicative of cirrhosis. When overt HE is encountered with well-preserved liver function (e.g., near-normal prothrombin time and albumin levels), one should look for large spontaneous portosystemic collaterals, a major septic focus, or occult intake of central nervous system active drugs (Box 18.3). Diabetes is reported to be associated with overt HE when liver function is still relatively well preserved. This may be related to motility disturbances in diabetics associated with small bowel bacterial overgrowth [77,78]. While these modulating factors may be encountered, most patients begin to experience bouts of overt HE once they develop more advanced cirrhosis(Child–Pugh class B and C). When biochemical evidence of loss of function of the liver is evident, then neurologic impairment is usually due to HE, especially when the classic signs of asterixis, confusion, and other prominent motor disturbances are detected. Box 18.4 shows the various tests employed for the diagnosis of hepatic encephalopathy .

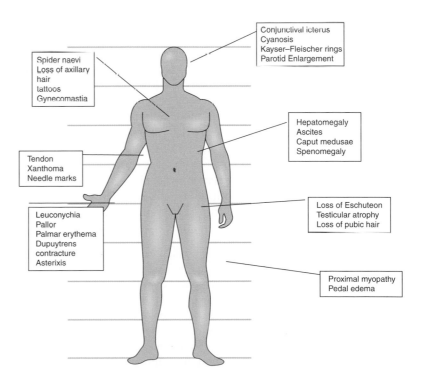

Figure 18.9 Physical signs seen in chronic liver disease.

Box 18.4 Diagnostic tests for hepatic encephalopathy.

Clinical diagnostic scales
- West Haven scale
- HESA (hepatic encephalopathy scoring algorithm)
- CHESS (clinical hepatic encephalopathy staging scale)

Laboratory diagnosis (see Box 18.5)

Psychometric tests
- Paper and pencil tests:
    PHES (psychometric hepatic encephalopathy score)
    RBANS (repeatable battery for assessment of neurological status)
- Computerized psychometric tests:
    ICT (inhibitory control test)
    CDR (cognitive drug research) test
    Neuropsychometric test: critical flicker frequency test

Electroencephalogram

Radiology

Neurologic assessment of patients with cirrhosis

Asterixis

Asterixis is defined as a tremor of the wrist when it is held in dorsiflexion, sometimes resembling a bird flapping its wings. "Asterixis" is derived from the Greek *a* (not) and *sterixis* (fixed position). It mainly denotes failure to actively maintain posture or position. It was first described by Foley and Adams in 1949 [1]. The classic method of eliciting it is by dorsiflexion of the hand with the forearm and fingers extended. The postural lapse that occurs consists of a series of rapid, involuntary, flexion–extension movements of the wrist; this has been called the "hepatic flap" [4]. Other places where asterixis could be elicited are tongue protrusion, dorsiflexion of the foot, fist clenching, and forced eye closure. The pathogenesis of asterixis is thought to be due to the abnormal function of the supraspinal motor centers. It is classically seen in grade II HE on the West Haven scale. However, it can be seen in other encephalopathies from renal failure, congestive heart failure, respiratory failure, frontal lobe tumors, and hypokalemia.

Other neurologic findings

Hypertonia, hyperreflexia, extensor plantar reflexia, and even transient decerebrate posturing may occur [79]. Very few studies have been done on the prevalence of neurologic abnormalities in patients with HE. The signs that can be elicited can be classified for convenience into three main categories: motor and coordination abnormalities, signs of progressive cerebral dysfunction or dementia, and those seen in metabolic encephalopathy. The disruption of smooth pursuit of eye movement (SPEM) is the most common motor abnormality seen in these patients [80]. There is evidence that this sign persists after a patient has an episode of HE whilst in remission [81]. Other signs include nystagmus, asterixis, hyperreflexia, ataxic heel-to-shin, ataxic finger-to-nose, and dysdiadakokinesia (slow alternating hand movement).

Clinical scales for the assessment of overt HE

West Haven criteria

Initially called the portosystemic encephalopathy index, this was the first attempt at objectively assessing the degree of hepatic encephalopathy. The scale is a semi-quantitative assessment of mental status and behavioral and neurologic function. It was devised by Professor Harold Conn in 1978 and has stood the test of time as it is still used in HE clinical trials [16,82,83]. The original scale has four grades ranging from grade I (trivial lack of awareness and euphoria) to grade IV (coma). In recent years, studies have shown that there is a lot of interobserver variability in assessing lower grades of HE, especially grade I [19]. In response to this, there were attempts to introduce objective scales that closely correlated with the different grades of the West Haven scale (see Table 18.2) [84]. Further studies are necessary to approve the widespread use of this version of the West Haven scale.

HESA (hepatic encephalopathy scoring algorithm)

In order to overcome the variability in assessment of lower grades of HE, this scale was devised by Hassanein et al. [85]. It incorporates simple neuropsychologic tests, along with clinical indicators for the classification of lower grades of HE (West Haven grade I/II). This scale was studied along with West Haven scale and Glasgow coma scale in a multicenter study that assessed the clinical utility of extracorporeal albumin dialysis as a treatment for HE [86]. It has shown early promise but, again, further studies are necessary for implementation of this scale in routine clinical use.

CHESS (clinical hepatic encephalopathy staging scale)

This scale was devised to simplify the characterization of HE into different stages. CHESS ranges from 0 to 9 depending on the subject's response to nine simple questions [87]. This has been shown to correlate well with the West Haven scale. Even though this scale has been used for lower grades of HE, it is not useful in the diagnosis of minimal HE.

Hepatic

Laboratory diagnosis

Laboratory testing adds limited value to diagnosing hepatic encephalopathy, especially in a cirrhotic patient with prior episodes of overt HE who presents with altered mental status. However, these tests can be judiciously deployed to rule out other causes of HE and the reason for precipitation of HE. There are four main aspects of laboratory testing (Box 18.5):

1 To confirm the presence of chronic liver disease.
2 To rule out other causes for metabolic/toxic encephalopathy.
3 To corroborate the diagnosis of HE.
4 To diagnose the cause for precipitation of HE.

Box 18.5 Laboratory testing for hepatic encephalopathy (HE).

Evidence for chronic liver disease
- Increased prothrombin time/INR
- Decreased serum albumin
- Pancytopenia/leucopenia/thrombocytopenia
- Hypergammaglobulinemia
- Hepatitis serology
- Autoimmune serology

Metabolic encephalopathies
- Hypoxia/hypercapnia:
    Arterial blood gas
    Clinical chemistry
    Pulmonary evaluation
- Hypoglycemia:
    Clinical chemistry
- Renal failure/azotemia:
    Blood chemistry
    Urine analysis
    Renal imaging
- Hyponatremia
    Blood chemistry
    Urine analysis
    Evaluate for chronic cardiac/renal/liver disease
- Diabetic coma (ketoacidosis/hyperosmolar):
    Arterial blood gas
    Clinical chemistry
    Urine analysis

Toxic encephalopathy
- Alcohol:
    Serum alcohol level
    Serum tylenol/salicyate level
    Blood/urine toxic screen
- Drugs (hypnotics, analgesics, heavy metals (lead/mercury/manganese)):
    Serum alcohol level
    Serum tylenol/salicyate level
    Blood/urine toxic screen

Diagnosing HE
- Serum ammonia (arterial/venous)
- CSF glutamine
- Plasma branched chain amino acid/aromatic amino acid ratio

Precipitation of HE
- Gastrointestinal bleeding:
    Complete blood count
    Coagulation profile
    Clinical chemistry
- Infection:
    Complete blood count with differential count
    Ascitic fluid studies
    CSF studies
    Microbiology studies: culture/Gram stain:
- Hypokalemia/alkalosis:
    Clinical chemistry
- Acute hepatic injury:
    Liver function tests
    Coagulation profile
    Toxic/metabolic/infectious/ischemic etiology workup
- Azotemia/diabetic coma:
    Clinical chemistry
    Arterial blood gas

CSF, cerebrospinal fluid; INR, international normalized ratio.

Serum ammonia

Altered mental status in a patient with chronic liver disease should be treated as HE unless proven otherwise. Hence, serum ammonia is not recommended routinely for the diagnosis of HE. However, it does help in very rare circumstances but for now is predominantly limited to use in the research setting. Also, a number of studies have shown a strong correlation between venous and arterial ammonia [8]. Box 18.6 depicts the appropriate way of testing for serum ammonia and Box 18.7 lists the most common causes for erroneous readings in serum ammonia levels.

Cerebrospinal fluid amino acids

In response to increased ammonia concentrations in the brain, glutamate is released from cellular stores and

Box 18.6 Serum ammonia testing.

- Blood should be collected from a stasis-free vein. Avoid clenching of fist or application of tourniquet, which can elevate ammonia levels due to release from skeletal muscle
- A lithium- or sodium heparin-containing vacutainer (green top vacutainer) should be used to collect blood. Heparin inhibits the release of ammonia from red cells
- Sample should be stored and transported in an ice bath within 20 minutes for assay

Box 18.7 Most common sources of laboratory error in ammonia assay.

- Prior exertional activity by patient (release of ammonia from skeletal muscle)
- Improper collection technique
- Delay in transportation
- Hemolysis or use of heparin lock during venipuncture

converted to glutamine, mainly in astrocytes. This amino acid is thought to spill over into the cerebrospinal fluid (CSF) causing increased concentrations. A number of experimental studies and postmortem human studies have demonstrated at least a two-fold rise in the CSF glutamine in subjects with HE [88]. The other amino acids that show a remarkable increase in HE are phenylalanine and tyrosine [89]. These biogenic amines are precursors of dopamine and norepinephrine, which could potentially alter monoaminergic function in the brain. The most predictable rise in amino acid level relating to the degree of neurologic deterioration was demonstrated by CSF alanine. It is thought to arise from the metabolism of glutamine, which incorporates into the Krebs cycle. These tests are currently employed only in research and have a long way before they have clinical applicability. Patients

presenting with HE are likely to have coagulation defects, therefore lumbar puncture is not performed unless absolutely necessary.

Psychometric tests

Minimal HE is a neurocognitive disorder wherein patients have abnormal performance in specific psychometric tests. It is generally associated with cirrhosis but can be seen in early stages of fibrosis and portosystemic shunts. This condition, recognized in the 1970s, was previously known as subclinical HE based on the performance of patients on the trail making and other cognitive tests [82,90]. The most comprehensive effort to understand the various neurocognitive domains impaired in this condition was performed by Hamster et al. [91]. He subjected 96 cirrhotic and 163 healthy age-matched controls to more than 30 different psychometric tests to assess cognitive domains ranging from premorbid intelligence levels and verbal abilities to visuomotor function and coordination. Using statistical discriminant analysis it was found that the line tracing test, peg board, aiming and steadiness of motor performance scale, and digit symbol test could effectively differentiate cirrhotic and noncirrhotic patients. It was these early efforts that paved the way for further standardization in the testing methods for what is now called minimal HE. Figure 18.10

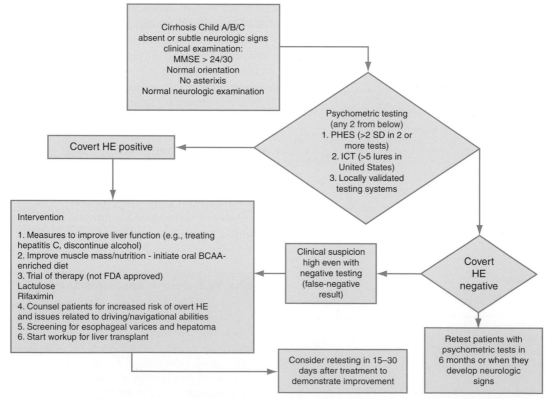

Figure 18.10 Algorithm for the diagnosis of covert or minimal hepatic encephalopathy (HE). BCAA, branched chain amino acid; FDA, Food and Drug Administration; ICT, inhibitory control test; MMSE, mini mental state examination; PHES, psychometric hepatic encephalopathy score.

illustrates the proposed algorithm for the diagnosis of covert or minimal HE.

Paper and pencil tests

PHES (Psychometric Hepatic Encephalopathy Score)

This test battery was devised by Weissenborn, Schomerus et al. based on the findings from the Hamster study [15]. The PHES includes the following tests: the number connection test A (NCT A), number connection test B (NCT B), digit symbol test (DST), line tracing test (LTT), and serial dotting test (SDT). This battery was employed on a large group of healthy volunteers in Germany to devise age-matched normative data and was further validated by testing on nonalcoholic cirrhotic patients. The domains tested were motor speed and accuracy, visual perception, visuospatial orientation, visual construction, concentration, attention, and to a lesser extent memory. In the subsequent World Congress of Gastroenterology meeting in Vienna, 1998, the Consensus Group for Hepatic Encephalopathy endorsed this as the temporary "gold standard" test for the diagnosis of minimal HE [2]. Further studies have shown that age and education have some influence on tests like the NCT A and NCT B [92]. This battery initially gained a lot of popularity and Italy, Spain, Mexico, and Great Britain have developed local normative data for it. Limited availability and copyright issues, along with difficulties experienced in administering and scoring this test, curtailed its popularity in the United States [93].

RBANS (Repeatable Battery for Assessment of Neuropsychological Status)

This is an established battery for the assessment of dementia and other neurocognitive disorders [94]. It is a paper and pencil test with four alternate forms (A, B, C, and D) and takes about 20–30 minutes to administer. It has extensive normative databases across the ages 20–89 years in the United States [92]. Preliminary studies done on patients waiting for liver transplantation showed close correlation between the model for end-stage liver disease (MELD) score and performance in RBANS [95]. Its main drawback is the remarkable learning effect shown by patients when tested at close intervals, which limits its utility in assessing response to treatment.

Computerized psychometric tests

Over the last few years a number of computerized test batteries have been validated to diagnose minimal HE [93]. These testing systems aim to circumvent some of the main problems encountered with the paper and pencil tests: availability, issues with administering the test,

and scoring. Most computerized tests are capable of generating age-matched results at the end of the testing session. These tests are available online and can be used free of charge or for a nominal fee. They also offer the convenience of being able to be administered in the outpatient setting. The most popular testing systems are the inhibitory control test (ICT) and cognitive drug research (CDR) test.

Inhibitory control test

This is an established test utilized mainly for determining deficits in attention and response inhibition in patients with attention deficit disorder, schizophrenia, and traumatic brain injury. Bajaj et al. validated this testing system for minimal HE diagnosis by comparing it with the standard psychometric test (a paper and pencil test) [96,97]. In this test the subject is shown several letters at 500 ms intervals on a computer screen. The subject is required to focus mainly on the X and Ys that are interspersed between these letters. They are instructed to respond (by pressing the space bar) when X is followed by Y or Y is followed by X, which is called "target," and to refrain from responding when X is followed by X or Y is followed by Y, which is called "lure." The subject has to go through six runs of 2 minutes each in addition to the training run at the beginning. They are graded based on their lure response, and more than five lures diagnoses minimal HE with 88% sensitivity. In the United States, this test has been mainly investigated and employed by a single investigator, Dr Bajaj, in two centers at Wisconsin and Virginia [98] (it is available online and can be downloaded free of charge from www.HEcme.TV). However, it did not perform consistently in Europe, making it less popular on the other side of the Atlantic [99].

Cognitive drug research test

This testing system was validated for the diagnosis of minimal HE by investigators in Newcastle, UK [100]. The CDR test is presented on a computer screen with patients responding with a "Yes/no" response box. The battery is composed of seven different tests. The scores are reported on a scale of performance in five different domains, which include power of attention, continuity of attention, quality of episodic memory, quality of working memory, and speed of memory. However, one of the limitations of this test is that patients need to undergo a practice session 1–7 days prior to the test date for familiarization.

Critical flicker fusion frequency test

Developed by Kircheis et al. in 2002 for the diagnosis of minimal HE, this is now a well-established neurophysiologic test based on the principle of hepatic retinopathy [101]. The Müller cells in the retina (which are glial cells) are thought to undergo changes similar to the astrocytes in the brain. This is, at least in part, thought to change the perception of light frequency by the retina. The test involves showing a patient light pulses, initially at high frequencies of 60 Hz, and then progressively reducing them by 0.1 Hz/s. At these high frequencies the subject perceives this as a single stream of light, but the critical frequency is when they first perceive it as discrete light pulses. A critical frequency of less than 39 Hz diagnoses minimal HE with high sensitivity and specificity, and positively correlates with paper and pencil psychometric tests. This test can be administered in inpatient and outpatient settings and takes about 15 minutes in total. Binocular vision is a prerequisite for optimal performance in this test. It is not influenced by education or occupation and only slightly influenced by age. It is widely used in therapeutic trials in hepatic encephalopathy due to it is ability to demonstrate improvement without any learning effect [102–104]. Limited availability is the main reason for its lack of popularity in the United States.

Electroencephalogram

Electroencephalograms (EEGs) help us study the neurophysiologic status of patients with cirrhosis [105–107]. It is commonly used in research and clinical settings. In the former it is used for the following:

- To monitor the effects of treatment (dietary or pharmacologic), portosystemic shunt insertion, or surgery or liver transplantation.
- To objectively quantify the degree of physiologic changes in the brain and to study its correlation with other tests employed to diagnose minimal HE.

In the clinical setting it is most commonly used as a diagnostic tool in cirrhotic patients with severely impaired consciousness

Some of the common findings on EEG are:

- Generalized slowing of the background EEG activity, which is objectively quantifiable but can be seen in other metabolic encephalopathies.
- A decrease in the amplitude of the waves.
- The presence of triphasic waves and bursts of slow activity in the theta and delta range.

Some studies report a sensitivity of about 83–100% for diagnosing overt HE and up to about 40% sensitivity diagnosing minimal HE patients. However, these are largely dependent of the technique used.

Some newer techniques have evolved:

- ANESS (artificial neural network expert system software).
- SEDACA (short epoch, dominant activity, cluster analysis).

These have helped to overcome some drawbacks although EEG still remains largely used in the research setting.

Brain imaging

Increasingly over the last couple of decades, cerebral edema has been demonstrated by a variety of magnetic resonance imaging techniques of the brain (Table 18.4) [37]. This is mainly seen in the white matter and in all grades of hepatic encephalopathy. A computerized tomographic scan of the brain is done routinely in patients with altered mental status, to rule out concomitant causes like intracranial hemorrhage and space-occupying lesions.

Treatment

The treatment of HE has empirically evolved over the decades primarily from data based on clinical observation. The current standard of care for management of overt HE consists of four main strategies (Fig. 18.11): (i) supportive care for the patient with altered mental status; (ii) concomitant causes for encephalopathy are sought and treated if possible; (iii) precipitating factors for bouts of HE are identified and corrected promptly; and (iv) empirical treatment is provided for HE. Until recently lactulose was the only approved therapy for HE in the United States. Now an alternative agent, rifaximin, is available to treat certain types of patients with recurrent HE [108].

Supportive care

The nasogastric tube delivery of overly large amounts of lactulose has become widespread in the treatment of HE [18]. As a consequence, aspiration is a significant risk for patients being treated in intensive care units. Most intensivists electively intubate patients with severe HE (e.g., stage III or IV, West Haven scale), which is certainly justified when major upper gastrointestinal bleeding is also an issue. Another supportive issue is the provision of nutrition to the unconscious patient. Data now exist to show that adequate nasogastric feeding can be delivered to patients as they emerge from bouts of severe HE. Generally, however, nutrient delivery is compromised in the first few days of hospitalization because of the frequency of tests and the need to lavage the gut to clear it of blood.

Other causes of encephalopathy

The second strategy of major importance in the management of HE is making sure that no other cause of encephalopathy is present in the unconscious patient diagnosed with overt HE (see Box 18.2). There are a number of issues that arise from this strategic point. The first is that technically, as mentioned previously, if a comatose patient has severe hypoglycemia or shock they cannot be labeled as having HE since other causes of encephalopathy need to be absent to make the diagnosis. In reality, HE and other causes of encephalopathy can occur

Table 18.4 Magnetic resonance imaging (MRI) in hepatic encephalopathy (HE).

Imaging modality	T1-weighted imaging	H1-magnetic resonance spectroscopy	MTI[a]	FLAIR imaging[b]	DWI[c]
MRI abnormality	Bilateral, symmetric, high signal intensity in the substantia nigra and globus pallidus	Increase in intracellular glutamate/glutamine signal. Concomitant decrease in myoinositol, taurine, and choline signals	Low magnetization transfer ratios (about10%) seen diffusely in the brain in normal-appearing white matter. This is not accompanied by any abnormalities in T1 or T2 signal intensities in that region	Diffuse white matter signal intensities involving the hemispheric white matter and the corticospinal tract on T2-weighted imaging	Increase in mean diffusivity in hemispheric white matter
Correlation with clinical severity of HE	No	No	Not established	Not established	Yes, and correlates with serum ammonia levels
Resolution of changes following liver transplantation	Yes (may take up to 1 year)	Yes (takes a few months)	Yes	Yes	Yes

[a]Magnetization transfer imaging (MTI) refers to the transfer of longitudinal magnetization between protons in water molecules that have been restricted in motion, such as those in the nuclei (bound to proteins), to those protons that are freely mobile, such as those in the cytoplasm. Low magnetization transfer is indicative of brain structures that are able to exchange magnetization with surrounding structures relatively easily, such as cell destruction and brain edema.

[b]FLAIR (fluid inversion attenuated recovery) imaging is used to suppress the effects of cerebrospinal fluid on the image and to enhance periventricular lesions.

[c]Diffusion-weighted imaging (DWI) can locate the compartment where there is a collection of water (intracellular or extracellular).

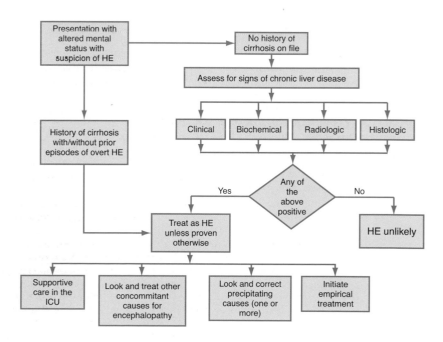

Figure 18.11 Algorithm for the management of hepatic encephalopathy (HE). ICU, intensive care unit.

simultaneously. Patients often will not recover unless these concomitant diseases are diagnosed and corrected. Vigilance is important in monitoring for the accidental induction of dehydration or other complication (e.g., hypomagnesaemia) of overly aggressive lactulose dosing.

Precipitating factors

The third strategy employed in the management of bouts of overt HE is extremely important. In advanced cirrhotic patients (Child–Pugh class C) most bouts of overt HE are precipitated by defined factors (Box 18.8). Prompt identification and correction of these factors is a very effective therapy for HE. Recovery rates of 80–90% have been reported with the correction of precipitating factors alone [109]. Because of overlap (e.g., lactulose used to clear gastrointestinal blood) it is sometimes difficult to know what actually reversed the HE episode. Complicating matters further, many patients have more than two simultaneous precipitating factors. These types of issues have made it very difficult to conduct randomized controlled trials in the treatment of overt HE. Multiple precipitating factors and additional concomitant causes of encephalopathy together make conducting a "controlled" trial well nigh impossible. In any event, seeking and treating precipitating factors is an effective treatment for overt HE. Patients with especially large spontaneous or surgically created portosystemic shunts tend to have more bouts of spontaneous HE [110].

Some additional comments are warranted on precipitating factors. One of the most dominant factors is likely sepsis. If a major focus of infection is not identified and treated successfully, recovery from bouts of HE can be very protracted or the patient may have recurrent bouts of overt HE [111]. When patients with cirrhosis develop severe HE, sepsis is the number one suspect. One issue

with sepsis is the fact that it is capable of inducing encephalopathy on its own [59]. This is another example of the difficulties in managing HE.

Upper gastrointestinal bleeding is a frequent precipitant for bouts of HE. It has been proposed that the digestion of blood in the gut generates an undue amount of ammonia that precipitates HE. The absence of the essential amino acid isoleucine from hemoglobin may make it more ammoniogenic than other forms of protein [57,112].

Gut lavage and catharsis are employed to clear the gut of blood and empirically one sees patients recovering from overt HE with this form of therapy. Because lactulose is a laxative it is difficult to know whether its unique action or the resulting purgative effect is responsible for the observed recovery from bouts of HE. Regardless, gut cleansing is a main stay of therapy. If constipation or ileus is present, clearing blood from the gut might not be achievable until gut motility is improved. It has been suggested that gastrointestinal motility is reduced by HE itself, perhaps generating a self-perpetuating mechanism for bouts of HE. In the setting of constipation, bowel obstruction, or ileus, the rectal administration of lactulose has shown to be effective for treatment of overt HE [113].

Hyponatremia, based on a number of papers, is clearly capable of aggravating or precipitating HE too [114]. Hyponatremia adds to the cerebral edema already present in patients with advanced cirrhosis [67]. Whether hyponatremia is a precipitating factor or a true pathogenetic factor for HE has not been clarified.

Drug therapy

Box 18.9 lists most of the empirical therapies employed at one point or another for the treatment of HE. We are going to confine most of our comments to the two approved agents for the treatment of HE, lactulose and rifaximin. Box 18.10 lists various therapies that have been utilized for the prophylaxis of hepatic encephalopathies. Figures 18.9 and 18.11 outline two detailed algorithms to clearly map out the possible therapeutic approaches to be taken in managing patients with minimal and overt HE, respectively.

Box 18.8 Precipitating factors for hepatic encephalopathy.

- Sepsis
- Gastrointestinal hemorrhage
- Electrolyte abnormalities (hypokalemia/alkalosis)
- Dehydration
- Central nervous system active drugs
- Constipation
- Dietary protein overload
- Poor compliance with lactulose therapy
- Uremia
- Ileus or bowel obstruction
- Prior anesthesia
- Superimposed hepatitis
- Development of hepatocellular carcinoma
- Portal decompression procedure/transjugular intrahepatic portosystemic shunt placement

---

Box 18.9 Empirical therapies for hepatic encephalopathy treatment.

- Lactulose 15–30 mL PO two to three times a day titrated to two to three soft bowel movements
- Rifaximin 550 mg PO twice daily
- Neomycin 500 mg PO four times daily (caution in renal failure and in high doses)
- Metronidazole 250 mg PO four times daily (only for short-term use)
- Vancomycin 250 mg PO four times daily
- Sodium benzoate 5 g PO twice daily
- Flumazenil 1–3 mg intravenous (short-lasting therapy)

Lactulose

This nonabsorbed disaccharide has been used for over 40 years to treat HE [16,115]. Like other drugs developed that long ago, there are concerns regarding the adequacy of data in support of its efficacy. There is little doubt in most physicians minds that lactulose is an effective treatment for HE. However, the published data in support of lactulose treatment for overt HE is not convincing [116]. Unfortunately, lactulose began to be believed to be a therapy that ethically could not be withheld from patients with overt HE. In particular, once that belief arose in the human investigation review boards in the United States, paradoxically neither lactulose nor any other therapy could be compared to placebo. Essentially, lactulose based on its original approval by the US Food and Drug Administration (FDA) in 1977 has continued to be used nearly exclusively for the treatment of HE. Some data have now been published showing that lactulose was superior to placebo in the treatment of covert or minimal HE [116–118].

One concern about the lack of data in support of lactulose treatment of overt HE relates to the mechanism of action of this drug. A variety of mechanisms have been reported that should limit the generation of ammonia in the gut and its subsequent absorption [119]. However, it is probable that simple laxatives could have the same effects with less cost and side effects. In some parts of the world, lactulose is no longer used because of lack of evidence-based data. It should be feasible now to get permission to conduct placebo-controlled trials against lactulose and formally establish its true efficacy. It is our opinion, based on data generated in the treatment of minimal HE, that lactulose clearly does have efficacy in treating HE [120]. The real question is how much it reverses HE compared with cheaper laxatives.

Rifaximin

This minimally absorbed broad spectrum antibiotic had previously been used in multiple HE treatment trials in Europe [121–124]. However, as with lactulose therapy, no placebo-controlled trials were performed. Instead rifaximin was compared with a variety of other agents (lactulose, lactitol, and other antibiotics) and consistently displayed similar efficacy [125,126]. Most studies were not sufficiently powered to verify therapeutic equivalence and this may explain the lack of use of rifaximin in Europe.

The publication of a recent, large ($n = 298$) rifaximin trial in the United States has provided data that clearly indicate that rifaximin reduces recurrent HE episodes in patients at high risk for these events (58% reduction) [108]. The study essentially showed that the prevention of HE episodes was largely in patients who had had lactulose treatment failure; 91% of the enrolled patients continued to take lactulose even though two or more overt episodes had already occurred while on lactulose. This is not to say that lactulose is totally ineffective as a treatment to prevent recurrent episodes of HE. The particular population recruited into this study had hardly any identifiable precipitating factors for their bouts of overt HE. More specifically, we do not know how many or how soon HE episodes would occur if lactulose therapy had been discontinued. Clearly, this could be identified in future studies. However, in the interim we know that rifaximin is effective in reducing recurrent episodes of HE in patients where lactulose has failed to do this.

The FDA approved rifaximin use for maintaining HE remission after recovery from previous bouts of overt HE. Already, the questions being raised is whether rifaximin can be used for shortening episodes of existing overt HE. There is no indication for this use at this time, but it is worth noting that designing and conducting a randomized controlled trial in patients with advanced liver disease with overt HE is a major challenge.

Other forms of treatment

Neomycin has been used to treat HE since the 1950s [127]. As with other agents for the treatment of HE there is not an abundance of evidence in support of its efficacy. Indeed a very well-conducted trial by Strauss and colleagues in Brazil essentially showed neomycin to be no more effective than placebo [109]. However, before dismissing neomycin totally based on that study it is worth pointing out a few of its features. One major aspect of study design was that patients in both arms of the study (e.g., neomycin versus placebo) had precipitating factors identified and corrected. This was associated with a 80–90% reversal of HE in both arms. The vast majority of studies never identify or treat precipitating factors, which based on this study can correct HE episodes in 90% of patients. Sufficient to say neomycin may have efficacy in treating HE but its toxicity has largely ended its use. Typically, antibiotics with activity in HE treatment have activity against anaerobic bacterial species [128]. Neomycin did not fit this profile but we now have an alternative mechanism for the action of neomycin. There is definite proof that it inhibits the intestinal mucosal enzyme glutaminase [129]. This particular enzyme is responsible for generating a large proportion of the blood ammonia contained in the portal vein. This may explain neomycin's apparent therapeutic effect in HE. Recently, it has been noted that differential gene inheritance for this glutaminase enzyme may modulate the expression of overt HE in patients [130]. More glutaminase inhibitor type drugs may be developed in the coming years.

Other antibiotics

Metronidazole [131], vancomycin [132], paramomycin [133], and some other antibiotics in various publications have been reported to reverse HE [124]. Possibly the major mechanism of action of antibiotics is exerted in the small intestine where bacterial overgrowth has been reported on a number of occasions [77]. It seems that intestinal motility reduction may play a role in small bowel bacterial overgrowth. One proposed advantage of rifaximin to treat small bowel bacterial overgrowth in cirrhotic patients and in other situations is its lack of a major effect on colonic bacterial flora. This should be formally proven but rifaximin is solubilized by bile salts in the small intestine and thus has very active antibiotic action. Once bile salts are reabsorbed across the intestinal wall, rifaximin is far less active and therefore does not suppress colonic flora to a major degree. Some action is still retained since rifaximin is known to have activity against *Clostridium difficile*. Future therapy in HE may use prokinetic and selected delivery antibiotics.

Other therapies

At the risk of omitting some interesting facts it is not feasible to address all the therapies ever applied to HE. The enthusiastic reader may want to delve into literature on urease immunization [134], colonic resection or bypass[135], arterialization of the portal vein stump [136], and other forms of therapy. Box 18.11 illustrates some important aspects of nutrition in patients with HE [137]. Because of their potential importance in the pathogenesis of HE, endogenous benzodiazepines are worth another brief mention [70,138]. Patients who have never taken benzodiazepine drugs are "awoken" by about 30% from severe HE by intravenous infusion of flumazenil. This phenomenon has been demonstrated in rat and rabbit models of HE. It has been argued that the "awakenings" from HE by flumazenil reflect benzodiazepine drug use in patients with HE. It is worth noting that animals, in which endogenous benzodiazepines have been found, do not have access to prescription drugs. In any event, when a 30% recovery from coma is reported from one short-

acting drug it would seem prudent to see if responders could be maintained out of coma by further dosing. This was actually reported upon once but never followed up with a formal study [139].

Box 18.11 Nutrition in patients with cirrhosis.

- Daily intake is 30–35 kcal/kg body weight:
    50–60% carbohydrate
    20–30% proteins (1–1.5 g/kg body weight)
    10–20% fat
- In patients with hepatic encephalopathy:
    There is little evidence for protein restriction
    If protein intolerant then change to vegetable-based protein
    Branched chain amino acid-enriched supplements
    Supplement with probiotics and prebiotics as they have
        ammonia-lowering properties
- Frequent small meals (4–6 times) with a light snack (carbohydrate) before bed time
- Screen for vitamins (A, D, E, and K) and mineral deficiencies (zinc, calcium, and magnesium) and supplement accordingly

---

Liver transplantation

When medical therapy fails to preserve adequate liver function for survival, liver transplantation is required. At present, liver transplantation is not usually performed because of recurrent or intractable HE. Instead, the priority is given using primarily the MELD score which has no component of HE [140]. Exceptions for severe HE are not granted, instead patients have to wait for liver transplant until their MELD score is sufficiently high to merit this intervention. The modification of the MELD score with the addition of hyponatremia may hasten transplant in some patients, which seems appropriate as hyponatremia is known to aggravate cerebral edema in cirrhotic patients [141]. Nonetheless, patients with persistent or frequently recurrent HE rapidly lose their muscle mass and become less fit for survival after liver transplantation.

The development of even more effective treatments to prevent or significantly delay the onset of HE would clearly be a major advance. Alternatively, earlier transplantation for patients before bouts of overt HE occur may improve neurologic outcomes [39,40,95,142].

Future directions

The decision to temporarily endorse PHES as the gold standard for the diagnosis of minimal HE by the World Congress Consensus Group had an important impact on

HE research. It largely, but not entirely, encouraged a standardized battery of psychometric tests to be used by all investigators. This quickly led to multiple publications all over the world on ninimal HE and its effect on driving ability[143–145], health-related quality of life [117,146,147], and the future prediction of patients at risk for developing overt HE. Treatment trials for various agents to reverse minimal HE have already commenced [118,148]. Placebo-controlled randomized controlled trials can now be undertaken for patients with minimal HE. As noted on a number of occasions in this chapter, attempting to conduct treatment trials in patients with overt HE and quite advanced liver disease is fraught with many uncontrolled issues. These are largely not a factor in minimal/covert HE trials. As we pursue even better systems for the detection and quantification of minimal HE, our ability to test drugs for treatment is enhanced. Truly a new era of therapeutics in HE has commenced.

We have until recently thought that overt HE is totally reversible. However, evidence is accumulating that this may not always be the case [98]. Indeed, a case can be made to intervene in the earliest stages of HE to prevent a loss of function in a number of domains of brain function. Liver transplantation outcomes in patients with bouts of overt HE have long been noted to demonstrate future reversal of all the effects of HE. This may eventually lead to transplantation being utilized earlier in the course of disease unless even more effective therapies can abolish the evolution from minimal to overt HE.

Finally, for a major paradigm shift to occur in the early detection of HE, i.e., minimal HE, a testing system needs to be developed available to all physicians.

References

1. Adams RD, Foley JM. The neurological changes in the more common types of severe liver disease. *Trans Am Neurol Assoc* 1949;74:217–19.
2. Ferenci P, Lockwood A, Mullen K, Tarter R, Weissenborn K, Blei AT. Hepatic encephalopathy – definition, nomenclature, diagnosis, and quantification: final report of the working party at the 11th World Congresses of Gastroenterology, Vienna, 1998. *Hepatology* 2002;35(3):716–21.
3. Adams RD, Foley JM. The neurological disorder associated with liver disease. *Proc Assoc Res Nerv Ment Dis* 1953;32:198–237.
4. Conn H, Lieberthal MM. The syndrome of portosystemic encephalopathy. In: Conn H, Lieberthal MM, eds. *The Hepatic Coma Syndrome and Lactulose*. Baltimore: Williams and Wilkins, 1978:189–219.
5. Summerskill WH, Davidson EA, Sherlock S, Steiner RE. The neuropsychiatric syndrome associated with hepatic cirrhosis and an extensive portal collateral circulation. *Q J Med* 1956;25(98): 245–66.
6. Gabuzda GJ Jr, Phillips GB, Davidson CS. Reversible toxic manifestations in patients with cirrhosis of the liver given cation-exchange resins. *N Engl J Med* 1952;246(4):124–30.
7. Phillips GB, Schwartz R, Gabuzda GJ, Jr., Davidson CS. The syndrome of impending hepatic coma in patients with cirrhosis of the liver given certain nitrogenous substances. *N Engl J Med* 1952;247(7):239–46.
8. Ong JP, Aggarwal A, Krieger D, et al. Correlation between ammonia levels and the severity of hepatic encephalopathy. *Am J Med* 2003;114(3):188–93.
9. Stahl J. Studies of the blood ammonia in liver disease. Its diagnostic, prognostic, and therapeutic significance. *Ann Intern Med* 1963;58:1–24.
10. Muting D, Kalk JF, Koussouris P, Motschenbacher MT, Rausche A. The role of protein metabolism in 204 liver cirrhotics with and without hepatic encephalopathy. I. Clinical and general biochemical findings. *Hepatogastroenterology* 1986;33(2):61–5.
11. Haussinger D, Kircheis G, Fischer R, Schliess F, vom Dahl S. Hepatic encephalopathy in chronic liver disease: a clinical manifestation of astrocyte swelling and low-grade cerebral edema? *J Hepatol* 2000;32(6):1035–8.
12. Cordoba J, Alonso J, Rovira A, et al. The development of low-grade cerebral edema in cirrhosis is supported by the evolution of (1)H-magnetic resonance abnormalities after liver transplantation. *J Hepatol* 2001;35(5):598–604.
13. Mullen KD. Terminology in hepatic encephalopathy: work in progress. In: Yurdaydin C, Bozkaya H, eds. *Advances in Hepatic Encephalopathy and Metabolism of Liver Disease*. Ankara: Ankara University Press, 2000.
14. Mullen KD. Review of the final report of the 1998 Working Party on definition, nomenclature and diagnosis of hepatic encephalopathy. *Aliment Pharmacol Ther* 2007;25(Suppl 1):11–16.
15. Weissenborn K, Ennen JC, Schomerus H, Ruckert N, Hecker H. Neuropsychological characterization of hepatic encephalopathy. *J Hepatol* 2001;34(5):768–73.
16. Conn HO, Leevy CM, Vlahcevic ZR, et al. Comparison of lactulose and neomycin in the treatment of chronic portal-systemic encephalopathy. A double blind controlled trial. *Gastroenterology* 1977;72(4 Pt 1):573–83.
17. Montagnese S, Amodio P, Morgan MY. Methods for diagnosing hepatic encephalopathy in patients with cirrhosis: a multidimensional approach. *Metab Brain Dis* 2004;19(3–4):281–312.
18. Mullen KD, Amodio P, Morgan MY. Therapeutic studies in hepatic encephalopathy. *Metab Brain Dis* 2007;22(3–4):407–23.
19. Kircheis G, Fleig WE, Gortelmeyer R, Grafe S, Haussinger D. Assessment of low-grade hepatic encephalopathy: a critical analysis. *J Hepatol* 2007;47(5):642–50.
20. Bajaj JS, Wade JB, Sanyal AJ. Spectrum of neurocognitive impairment in cirrhosis: implications for the assessment of hepatic encephalopathy. *Hepatology* 2009;50(6):2014–21.
21. Prakash R, Mullen KD. Mechanisms, diagnosis and management of hepatic encephalopathy. *Nat Rev Gastroenterol Hepatol* 2010;7(9):515–25.
22. Sarin SK, Nundy S. Subclinical encephalopathy after portosystemic shunts in patients with non-cirrhotic portal fibrosis. *Liver* 1985;5(3):142–6.
23. Mullen KD. Interplay of portal pressure, portal perfusion and hepatic arterial inflow in modulating expression of hepatic encephalopathy in patients with spontaneous or artificially created portosystemic shunts. *Indian J Gastroenterol* 2003;22(Suppl 2):S25–7.
24. Nicolao F, Efrati C, Masini A, Merli M, Attili AF, Riggio O. Role of determination of partial pressure of ammonia in cirrhotic patients with and without hepatic encephalopathy. *J Hepatol* 2003;38(4):441–6.
25. Burton BK. Urea cycle disorders. *Clin Liver Dis* 2000;4(4):815–30, vi.
26. Clemmesen JO, Larsen FS, Kondrup J, Hansen BA, Ott P. Cerebral herniation in patients with acute liver failure is correlated with arterial ammonia concentration. *Hepatology* 1999;29(3): 648–53.

27. Norenberg MD. Astrocytic-ammonia interactions in hepatic encephalopathy. *Semin Liver Dis* 1996;16(3):245–53.

28. Rama Rao KV, Jayakumar AR, Norenberg DM. Ammonia neurotoxicity: role of the mitochondrial permeability transition. *Metab Brain Dis* 2003;18(2):113–27.

29. Butterworth RF, Giguere JF, Michaud J, Lavoie J, Layrargues GP. Ammonia: key factor in the pathogenesis of hepatic encephalopathy. *Neurochem Pathol* 1987;6(1–2):1–12.

30. Albrecht J, Jones EA. Hepatic encephalopathy: molecular mechanisms underlying the clinical syndrome. *J Neurol Sci* 1999;170(2):138–46.

31. Lockwood AH, Ginsberg MD, Rhoades HM, Gutierrez MT. Cerebral glucose metabolism after portacaval shunting in the rat. Patterns of metabolism and implications for the pathogenesis of hepatic encephalopathy. *J Clin Invest* 1986;78(1):86–95.

32. Lockwood AH, Yap EW, Wong WH. Cerebral ammonia metabolism in patients with severe liver disease and minimal hepatic encephalopathy. *J Cereb Blood Flow Metab* 1991;11(2):337–41.

33. Shawcross DL, Balata S, Olde Damink SW, et al. Low myo-inositol and high glutamine levels in brain are associated with neuropsychological deterioration after induced hyperammonemia. *Am J Physiol Gastrointest Liver Physiol* 2004;287(3):G503–9.

34. Cordoba J, Sanpedro F, Alonso J, Rovira A. 1H magnetic resonance in the study of hepatic encephalopathy in humans. *Metab Brain Dis* 2002;17(4):415–29.

35. Donovan JP, Schafer DF, Shaw BW Jr, Sorrell MF. Cerebral oedema and increased intracranial pressure in chronic liver disease. *Lancet* 1998;351(9104):719–21.

36. Haussinger D. Low grade cerebral edema and the pathogenesis of hepatic encephalopathy in cirrhosis. *Hepatology* 2006;43(6):1187–90.

37. Rovira A, Alonso J, Cordoba J. MR imaging findings in hepatic encephalopathy. *AJNR Am J Neuroradiol* 2008;29(9):1612–21.

38. Rovira A, Cordoba J, Raguer N, Alonso J. Magnetic resonance imaging measurement of brain edema in patients with liver disease: resolution after transplantation. *Curr Opin Neurol* 2002;15(6):731–7.

39. Atluri DK, Asgeri M, Mullen KD. Reversibility of hepatic encephalopathy after liver transplantation. *Metab Brain Dis* 2010;25(1):111–13.

40. Garcia-Martinez R, Rovira A, Alonso J, et al. Hepatic encephalopathy is associated with posttransplant cognitive function and brain volume. *Liver Transpl* 2011;17(1):38–46.

41. Schafer DF, Jones EA. Hepatic encephalopathy and the gamma-aminobutyric-acid neurotransmitter system. *Lancet* 1982;1(8262):18–20.

42. Ferenci P, Ebner J, Zimmermann C, Kikuta C, Roth E, Haussinger D. Overestimation of serum concentrations of gamma-aminobutyric acid in patients with hepatic encephalopathy by the gamma-aminobutyric acid-radioreceptor assay. *Hepatology* 1988;8(1):69–72.

43. Rossle M, Mullen KD, Jones EA. Cortical benzodiazepine receptor binding in a rabbit model of hepatic encephalopathy: the effect of Triton X-100 on receptor solubilization. *Metab Brain Dis* 1989;4(3):203–12.

44. Bassett ML, Mullen KD, Skolnick P, Jones EA. Amelioration of hepatic encephalopathy by pharmacologic antagonism of the GABAA-benzodiazepine receptor complex in a rabbit model of fulminant hepatic failure. *Gastroenterology* 1987;93(5):1069–77.

45. Mullen KD, Martin JV, Mendelson WB, Bassett ML, Jones EA. Could an endogenous benzodiazepine ligand contribute to hepatic encephalopathy? *Lancet* 1988;1(8583):457–9.

46. Basile AS, Gammal SH. Evidence for the involvement of the benzodiazepine receptor complex in hepatic encephalopathy. Implications for treatment with benzodiazepine receptor antagonists. *Clin Neuropharmacol* 1988;11(5):401–22.

47. Barbaro G, Di Lorenzo G, Soldini M, et al. Flumazenil for hepatic coma in patients with liver cirrhosis: an Italian multicentre double-blind, placebo-controlled, crossover study. *Eur J Emerg Med* 1998;5(2):213–18.

48. Baraldi M, Avallone R, Corsi L, Venturini I, Baraldi C, Zeneroli ML. Natural endogenous ligands for benzodiazepine receptors in hepatic encephalopathy. *Metab Brain Dis* 2009;24(1):81–93.

49. Bergasa NV, Alling DW, Talbot TL, et al. Effects of naloxone infusions in patients with the pruritus of cholestasis. A double-blind, randomized, controlled trial. *Ann Intern Med* 1995;123(3):161–7.

50. Ozsoylu S, Kocak N. Naloxone in hepatic encephalopathy. *Am J Dis Child* 1985;139(8):749–50.

51. Fischer JE, Baldessarini RJ. False neurotransmitters and hepatic failure. *Lancet* 1971;2(7715):75–80.

52. James JH, Ziparo V, Jeppsson B, Fischer JE. Hyperammonaemia, plasma aminoacid imbalance, and blood–brain aminoacid transport: a unified theory of portal-systemic encephalopathy. *Lancet* 1979;2(8146):772–5.

53. Rossi-Fanelli F, Riggio O, Cangiano C, et al. Branched-chain amino acids vs lactulose in the treatment of hepatic coma: a controlled study. *Dig Dis Sci* 1982;27(10):929–35.

54. Horst D, Grace ND, Conn HO, et al. Comparison of dietary protein with an oral, branched chain-enriched amino acid supplement in chronic portal-systemic encephalopathy: a randomized controlled trial. *Hepatology* 1984;4(2):279–87.

55. Marchesini G, Bianchi G, Merli M, et al. Nutritional supplementation with branched-chain amino acids in advanced cirrhosis: a double-blind, randomized trial. *Gastroenterology* 2003;124(7):1792–801.

56. Vary TC, Lynch CJ. Nutrient signaling components controlling protein synthesis in striated muscle. *J Nutr* 2007;137(8):1835–43.

57. Olde Damink SW, Dejong CH, Deutz NE, van Berlo CL, Soeters PB. Upper gastrointestinal bleeding: an ammoniagenic and catabolic event due to the total absence of isoleucine in the haemoglobin molecule. *Med Hypotheses* 1999;52(6):515–19.

58. Olde Damink SW, Jalan R, Deutz NE, et al. Isoleucine infusion during "simulated" upper gastrointestinal bleeding improves liver and muscle protein synthesis in cirrhotic patients. *Hepatology* 2007;45(3):560–8.

59. Hasselgren PO, Fischer JE. Septic encephalopathy. Etiology and management. *Intensive Care Med* 1986;12(1):13–16.

60. Shawcross, Jalan R. The pathophysiologic basis of hepatic encephalopathy: central role for ammonia and inflammation. *Cell Mol Life Sci* 2005;62(19–20):2295–304.

61. Montoliu C, Piedrafita B, Serra MA, et al. IL-6 and IL-18 in blood may discriminate cirrhotic patients with and without minimal hepatic encephalopathy. *J Clin Gastroenterol* 2009;43(3):272–9.

62. Shawcross DL, Davies NA, Williams R, Jalan R. Systemic inflammatory response exacerbates the neuropsychological effects of induced hyperammonemia in cirrhosis. *J Hepatol* 2004;40(2):247–54.

63. Gorg B, Bidmon HJ, Keitel V, et al. Inflammatory cytokines induce protein tyrosine nitration in rat astrocytes. *Arch Biochem Biophys* 2006;449(1–2):104–14.

64. Shawcross DL, Shabbir SS, Taylor NJ, Hughes RD. Ammonia and the neutrophil in the pathogenesis of hepatic encephalopathy in cirrhosis. *Hepatology* 2010;51(3):1062–9.

65. Didier N, Romero IA, Creminon C, Wijkhuisen A, Grassi J, Mabondzo A. Secretion of interleukin-1beta by astrocytes mediates endothelin-1 and tumour necrosis factor-alpha effects on

human brain microvascular endothelial cell permeability. *J Neurochem* 2003;86(1):246–54.

66. Duchini A, Govindarajan S, Santucci M, Zampi G, Hofman FM. Effects of tumor necrosis factor-alpha and interleukin-6 on fluid-phase permeability and ammonia diffusion in CNS-derived endothelial cells. *J Investig Med* 1996;44(8):474–82.

67. Cordoba J, Garcia-Martinez R, Simon-Talero M. Hyponatremic and hepatic encephalopathies: similarities, differences and coexistence. *Metab Brain Dis* 2010;25(1):73–80.

68. Butterworth RF. Altered glial-neuronal crosstalk: cornerstone in the pathogenesis of hepatic encephalopathy. *Neurochem Int* 2010;57(4):383–8.

69. Panickar KS, Jayakumar AR, Rama Rao KV, Norenberg MD. Downregulation of the 18-kDa translocator protein: effects on the ammonia-induced mitochondrial permeability transition and cell swelling in cultured astrocytes. *Glia* 2007;55(16):1720–7.

70. Schliess F, Gorg B, Haussinger D. Pathogenetic interplay between osmotic and oxidative stress: the hepatic encephalopathy paradigm. *Biol Chem* 2006;387(10–11):1363–70.

71. Butterworth RF. Hepatic encephalopathy. *Alcohol Res Health* 2003;27(3):240–6.

72. Haussinger D, Gorg B. Interaction of oxidative stress, astrocyte swelling and cerebral ammonia toxicity. *Curr Opin Clin Nutr Metab Care* 2010;13(1):87–92.

73. Bemeur C, Desjardins P, Butterworth RF. Evidence for oxidative/nitrosative stress in the pathogenesis of hepatic encephalopathy. *Metab Brain Dis* 2010;l25(1):3–9.

74. Cordoba J, Minguez B. Hepatic encephalopathy. *Semin Liver Dis* 2008;28(1):70–80.

75. Albrecht J, Zielinska M, Norenberg MD. Glutamine as a mediator of ammonia neurotoxicity: a critical appraisal. *Biochem Pharmacol* 2010;80(9):1303–8.

76. Khairy RN, Mullen KD. Hypothyroidism as a mimic of liver failure in a patient with cirrhosis. *Ann Intern Med* 2007;146(4):315–16.

77. Gupta A, Dhiman RK, Kumari S, et al. Role of small intestinal bacterial overgrowth and delayed gastrointestinal transit time in cirrhotic patients with minimal hepatic encephalopathy. *J Hepatol* 2010;53(5):849–55.

78. Sigal SH, Stanca CM, Kontorinis N, Bodian C, Ryan E. Diabetes mellitus is associated with hepatic encephalopathy in patients with HCV cirrhosis. *Am J Gastroenterol* 2006;101(7):1490–6.

79. Sherlock S, Dooley J. Hepatic encephalopathy. In: Sherlock S, Dooley J, eds. Diseases of the Liver and Biliary System, 9th edn. Oxford. Blackwell Scientific, 1994:86–101.

80. Montagnese S, Gordon HM, Jackson C, et al. Disruption of smooth pursuit eye movements in cirrhosis: relationship to hepatic encephalopathy and its treatment. *Hepatology* 2005'42(4):772–81.

81. Krismer F, Roos JC, Schranz M, et al. Saccadic latency in hepatic encephalopathy: a pilot study. *Metab Brain Dis* 2010;25(3):285–95.

82. Conn HO. Trailmaking and number-connection tests in the assessment of mental state in portal systemic encephalopathy. *Am J Dig Dis* 1977;22(6):541–50.

83. Atterbury CE, Maddrey WC, Conn HO. Neomycin-sorbitol and lactulose in the treatment of acute portal-systemic encephalopathy. A controlled, double-blind clinical trial. *Am J Dig Dis* 1978;23(5):398–406.

84. Amodio P, Montagnese S, Gatta A, Morgan MY. Characteristics of minimal hepatic encephalopathy. *Metab Brain Dis* 2004;19(3–4):253–67.

85. Hassanein TI, Hilsabeck RC, Perry W. Introduction to the Hepatic Encephalopathy Scoring Algorithm (HESA). *Dig Dis Sci* 2008;53(2):529–38.

86. Hassanein T, Blei AT, Perry W, et al. Performance of the hepatic encephalopathy scoring algorithm in a clinical trial of patients with cirrhosis and severe hepatic encephalopathy. *Am J Gastroenterol* 2009;104(6):1392–400.

87. Ortiz M, Cordoba J, Doval E, et al. Development of a clinical hepatic encephalopathy staging scale. *Aliment Pharmacol Ther* 2007;26(6):859–67.

88. Therrien G, Butterworth RF. Cerebrospinal fluid amino acids in relation to neurological status in experimental portal-systemic encephalopathy. *Metab Brain Dis* 1991;6(2):65–74.

89. Butterworth J, Gregory CR, Aronson LR. Selective alterations of cerebrospinal fluid amino acids in dogs with congenital portosystemic shunts. *Metab Brain Dis* 1997;12(4):299–306.

90. Sood GK, Sarin SK, Mahaptra J, Broor SL. Comparative efficacy of psychometric tests in detection of subclinical hepatic encephalopathy in nonalcoholic cirrhotics: search for a rational approach. *Am J Gastroenterol* 1989;84(2):156–9.

91. Schomerus H, Hamster W. Neuropsychological aspects of portal-systemic encephalopathy. *Metab Brain Dis* 1998;13(4):361–77.

92. Randolph C, Hilsabeck R, Kato A, et al. Neuropsychological assessment of hepatic encephalopathy: ISHEN practice guidelines. *Liver Int* 2009;29(5):629–35.

93. Iduru S, Mullen KD. The demise of the pencil? New computer-assisted tests for minimal hepatic encephalopathy. *Gastroenterology* 2008;135(5):1455–6.

94. Randolph C. *The Repeatable Battery for the Assessment of Neuropsychological Status (RBANS)*. San Antonio: The Psychological Corporation, 1998.

95. Sotil EU, Gottstein J, Ayala E, Randolph C, Blei AT. Impact of preoperative overt hepatic encephalopathy on neurocognitive function after liver transplantation. *Liver Transpl* 2009;15(2):184–92.

96. Bajaj JS, Saeian K, Verber MD, et al. Inhibitory control test is a simple method to diagnose minimal hepatic encephalopathy and predict development of overt hepatic encephalopathy. *Am J Gastroenterol* 2007;102(4):754–60.

97. Bajaj JS, Hafeezullah M, Franco J, et al. Inhibitory control test for the diagnosis of minimal hepatic encephalopathy. *Gastroenterology* 2008;135(5):1591–600.

98. Bajaj JS, Schubert CM, Heuman DM, et al. Persistence of cognitive impairment after resolution of overt hepatic encephalopathy. *Gastroenterology* 2010;138(7):2332–40.

99. Amodio P, Ridola L, Schiff S, et al. Improving the inhibitory control task to detect minimal hepatic encephalopathy. *Gastroenterology* 2010;139(2):510–18.

100. Mardini H, Saxby BK, Record CO. Computerized psychometric testing in minimal encephalopathy and modulation by nitrogen challenge and liver transplant. *Gastroenterology* 2008;135(5):1582–90.

101. Kircheis G, Wettstein M, Timmermann L, Schnitzler A, Haussinger D. Critical flicker frequency for quantification of low-grade hepatic encephalopathy. *Hepatology* 2002;35(2):357–66.

102. Kircheis G, Bode JG, Hilger N, Kramer T, Schnitzler A, Haussinger D. Diagnostic and prognostic values of critical flicker frequency determination as new diagnostic tool for objective HE evaluation in patients undergoing TIPS implantation. *Eur J Gastroenterol Hepatol* 2009;21(12):1383–94.

103. Sharma P, Sharma BC, Sarin SK. Critical flicker frequency for diagnosis and assessment of recovery from minimal hepatic encephalopathy in patients with cirrhosis. *Hepatobiliary Pancreat Dis Int* 2010;9(1):27–32.

104. Schmid M, Peck-Radosavljevic M, Konig F, Mittermaier C, Gangl A, Ferenci P. A double-blind, randomized, placebo-controlled trial of intravenous L-ornithine-L-aspartate on postural control in patients with cirrhosis. *Liver Int* 2010;30(4):574–82.

105. Amodio P, Campagna F, Olianas S, et al. Detection of minimal hepatic encephalopathy: normalization and optimization of the Psychometric Hepatic Encephalopathy Score. A neuropsychological and quantified EEG study. *J Hepatol* 2008;49(3):346–53.

106. Amodio P, Orsato R, Marchetti P, et al. Electroencephalographic analysis for the assessment of hepatic encephalopathy: comparison of non-parametric and parametric spectral estimation techniques. *Neurophysiol Clin* 2009;39(2):107–15.

107. Guerit JM, Amantini A, Fischer C, et al. Neurophysiological investigations of hepatic encephalopathy: ISHEN practice guidelines. *Liver Int* 2009;29(6):789–96.

108. Bass NM, Mullen KD, Sanyal A, et al. Rifaximin treatment in hepatic encephalopathy. *N Engl J Med* 2010;362(12):1071–81.

109. Strauss E, Tramote R, Silva EP, et al. Double-blind randomized clinical trial comparing neomycin and placebo in the treatment of exogenous hepatic encephalopathy. *Hepatogastroenterology* 1992;39(6):542–5.

110. Riggio O, Efrati C, Catalano C, et al. High prevalence of spontaneous portal-systemic shunts in persistent hepatic encephalopathy: a case–control study. *Hepatology* 2005;42(5):1158–65.

111. Strauss E, da Costa MF. The importance of bacterial infections as precipating factors of chronic hepatic encephalopathy in cirrhosis. *Hepatogastroenterology* 1998;45(21):900–4.

112. Jalan R, Olde Damink SW, Lui HF, et al. Oral amino acid load mimicking hemoglobin results in reduced regional cerebral perfusion and deterioration in memory tests in patients with cirrhosis of the liver. *Metab Brain Dis* 2003;18(1):37–49.

113. Uribe M, Berthier JM, Lewis H, et al. Lactose enemas plus placebo tablets vs. neomycin tablets plus starch enemas in acute portal systemic encephalopathy. A double-blind randomized controlled study. *Gastroenterology* 1981;81(1):101–6.

114. Guevara M, Baccaro ME, Torre A, et al. Hyponatremia is a risk factor of hepatic encephalopathy in patients with cirrhosis: a prospective study with time-dependent analysis. *Am J Gastroenterol* 2009;104(6):1382–9.

115. Elkington SG, Floch MH, Conn HO. Lactulose in the treatment of chronic portal-systemic encephalopathy. A double-blind clinical trial. *N Engl J Med* 1969;281(8):408–12.

116. Als-Nielsen B, Gluud LL, Gluud C. Non-absorbable disaccharides for hepatic encephalopathy: systematic review of randomised trials. *Br Med J* 2004;328(7447):1046.

117. Prasad S, Dhiman RK, Duseja A, Chawla YK, Sharma A, Agarwal R. Lactulose improves cognitive functions and health-related quality of life in patients with cirrhosis who have minimal hepatic encephalopathy. *Hepatology* 2007;45(3):549–59.

118. Shukla S, Shukla A, Mehboob S, Guha S. Meta-analysis: the effects of gut flora modulation using prebiotics, probiotics and synbiotics on minimal hepatic encephalopathy. *Aliment Pharmacol Ther* 2011;33(6):662–71.

119. Conn HO. Lactulose: a drug in search of a modus operandi. *Gastroenterology* 1978;74(3):624–6.

120. Montgomery JY, Bajaj JS. Advances in the evaluation and management of minimal hepatic encephalopathy. *Curr Gastroenterol Rep* 2011;13(1):26–33.

121. Di Piazza S, Gabriella Filippazzo M, Valenza LM, et al. Rifaximine versus neomycin in the treatment of portosystemic encephalopathy. *Ital J Gastroenterol* 1991;23(7):403–7.

122. Bucci L, Palmieri GC. Double-blind, double-dummy comparison between treatment with rifaximin and lactulose in patients with medium to severe degree hepatic encephalopathy. *Curr Med Res Opin* 1993;13(2):109–18.

123. M iglio F, Valpiani D, Rossellini SR, Ferrieri A. Rifaximin, a non-absorbable rifamycin, for the treatment of hepatic encephalopathy. A double-blind, randomised trial. *Curr Med Res Opin* 1997;13(10):593–601.

124. Mullen K, Prakash R. Rifaximin for the treatment of hepatic encephalopathy. *Expert Rev Gastroenterol Hepatol* 2010;4(6):665–77.

125. Jiang Q, Jiang XH, Zheng MH, Jiang LM, Chen YP, Wang L. Rifaximin versus nonabsorbable disaccharides in the management of hepatic encephalopathy: a meta-analysis. *Eur J Gastroenterol Hepatol* 2008;20(11):1064–70.

126. Paik YH, Lee KS, Han KH, et al. Comparison of rifaximin and lactulose for the treatment of hepatic encephalopathy: a prospective randomized study. *Yonsei Med J* 2005;46(3):399–407.

127. Dawson AM, Mc Laren J, Sherlock S. Neomycin in the treatment of hepatic coma. *Lancet* 1957;273(7008):1262–8.

128. Rothenberg ME, Keeffe EB. Antibiotics in the management of hepatic encephalopathy: an evidence-based review. *Rev Gastroenterol Disord* 2005;5(Suppl 3):26–35.

129. Romero-Gomez M, Jover M, Galan JJ, Ruiz A. Gut ammonia production and its modulation. *Metab Brain Dis* 2009;24(1):147–57.

130. Romero-Gomez M, Jover M, Del Campo JA, et al. Variations in the promoter region of the glutaminase gene and the development of hepatic encephalopathy in patients with cirrhosis: a cohort study. *Ann Intern Med* 2010;153(5):281–8.

131. Morgan MH, Read AE, Speller DC. Treatment of hepatic encephalopathy with metronidazole. *Gut* 1982;23(1):1–7.

132. Tarao K, Ikeda T, Hayashi K, Sakurai A, et al. Successful use of vancomycin hydrochloride in the treatment of lactulose resistant chronic hepatic encephalopathy. *Gut* 1990;31(6):702–6.

133. Tromm A, Griga T, Greving I, et al. Orthograde whole gut irrigation with mannite versus paromomycine + lactulose as prophylaxis of hepatic encephalopathy in patients with cirrhosis and upper gastrointestinal bleeding: results of a controlled randomized trial. *Hepatogastroenterology* 2000;47(32):473–7.

134. LeVeen HH, LeVeen EG, LeVeen RF. Awakenings to the pathogenicity of urease and the requirement for continuous long term therapy. *Biomed Pharmacother* 1994;48(3–4):157–66.

135. Picone SB Jr, Donovan AJ, Yellin AE. Abdominal colectomy for chronic encephalopathy due to portal-systemic shunt. *Arch Surg* 1983;118(1):33–7.

136. Aldrete JS, Soyer MT, Han SY, Long term effects of arterialization of the portal vein stump in dogs with Eck's fistula. *Br J Surg* 1981;68(9):656–60.

137. Bemeur C, Desjardins P, Butterworth RF. Role of nutrition in the management of hepatic encephalopathy in end-stage liver failure. *J Nutr Metab* 2010 (Epub ahead of print, 489823).

138. Mullen KD, Jones EA, Natural benzodiazepines and hepatic encephalopathy. *Semin Liver Dis* 1996;16(3):255–64.

139. Ferenci P, Grimm G, Meryn S, Gangl A. Successful long-term treatment of portal-systemic encephalopathy by the benzodiazepine antagonist flumazenil. *Gastroenterology* 1989;96(1):240–3.

140. Thornton JG, Mullen KD. The role of hepatic encephalopathy in the era of MELD. *Liver Transpl* 2007;13(10):1364–5.

141. Lv XH, Liu HB, Wang Y, Wang BY, Song M, Sun MJ. Validation of model for end-stage liver disease score to serum sodium ratio index as a prognostic predictor in patients with cirrhosis. *J Gastroenterol Hepatol* 2009;24(9):1547–53.

142. Campagna F, Biancardi A, Cillo U, Gatta A, Amodio P. Neurocognitive-neurological complications of liver transplantation: a review. *Metab Brain Dis* 2010;25(1):115–24.

143. Bajaj JS, Hafeezullah M, Hoffmann RG, et al. Navigation skill impairment: another dimension of the driving difficulties in minimal hepatic encephalopathy. *Hepatology* 2008;47(2):596–604.

144. Kircheis G, Knoche A, Hilger N, et al. Hepatic encephalopathy and fitness to drive. *Gastroenterology* 2009;137(5):1706–15.

145. Bajaj JS, Heuman DM, Wade JB, et al. Rifaximin improves driving simulator performance in a randomized trial of patients with minimal hepatic encephalopathy. *Gastroenterology* 2010;140(2):478–87.

146. Sidhu SS, Goyal O, Mishra BP, Sood A, Chhina RS, Soni RK. Rifaximin improves psychometric performance and health-related quality of life in patients with minimal hepatic encephalopathy (the RIME trial). *Am J Gastroenterol* 2010;106(20):307–16.

147. Groeneweg M, Moerland W, Quero JC, Hop WC, Krabbe PF, Schalm SW. Screening of subclinical hepatic encephalopathy. *J Hepatol* 2000;32(5):748–53.

148. Dhiman RK, Chawla YK. Minimal hepatic encephalopathy: time to recognise and treat. *Trop Gastroenterol* 2008;29(1):6–12.

Multiple choice questions

18.1 A significant proportion of portal vein ammonia is generated by intestinal ammonia.

   a True.
   b False.

18.2 Hepatic encephalopathy (HE) primarily arises because of large portosystemic shunts.

   a True.
   b False.

18.3 Correction of precipitating factors for HE is effective therapy.

   a True.
   b False.

18.4 Prophylaxis with lactulose after transjugular intrahepatic portosystemic shunting has shown to reduce episodes of HE.

   a True.
   b False.

18.5 Decreased brain myoinositol levels on nuclear magnetic resonance spectroscopy support the presence of cerebral edema in HE.

   a True.
   b False.

18.6 The presence of minimal HE predicts the development of overt HE.

   a True.
   b False.

18.7 Blood ammonia level are useful for the diagnosis of HE.

   a True.
   b False.

18.8 Neomycin inhibits intestinal glutaminase activity.

   a True.
   b False.

18.9 Treatment of minimal HE is associated with improved driving ability.

   a True.
   b False.

18.10 Asterixis is highly specific for the diagnosis of HE:

   a True.
   b False.

Answers to the multiple choice questions can be found in the Appendix at the end of the book.

These multiple choice questions are also available for you to complete online.
Visit http://www.schiffsdiseasesoftheliver.com/

CHAPTER 19

Acute Liver Failure

Anne M. Larson

University of Texas Southwestern Medical Center, Dallas, TX, USA

Key concepts

- The syndrome of acute liver failure (ALF) is defined as an illness of less than 26 weeks' duration with coagulopathy (international normalized ratio ≥ 1.5) and any degree of hepatic encephalopathy in patients without preexisting liver disease or cirrhosis.
- There are many causes of ALF, which vary geographically and socioeconomically. Viral hepatitis remains the most common cause worldwide, while drug-induced ALF, particularly acetaminophen hepatotoxicity, predominates in the United States and many parts of Europe.
- The cause of ALF carries prognostic significance and directs specific treatment options where available.
- The clinical presentation of ALF is similar regardless of the cause. Depending upon the severity, it is associated with coagulopathy,

thrombocytopenia, hemodynamic instability, acid–base disturbances, renal insufficiency, metabolic derangements, electrolyte imbalance, infection and sepsis, and hepatic encephalopathy associated with cerebral edema.
- Management of ALF is complicated and requires a multidisciplinary approach, including transplant hepatologists, transplant surgeons, intensive care physicians, nephrologists, and neurosurgeons.
- Spontaneous survival ranges from 20% to 70% depending upon the cause. With the advent of liver transplantation as a treatment option in this setting, overall survival rates have improved to ~60%.
- Several prognostic models have been developed in an attempt to predict who will require transplantation and who will survive. None of these models can predict outcome with absolute certainty, however.

Acute liver failure (ALF) is a devastating multiorgan syndrome characterized by sudden and severe hepatocellular dysfunction (jaundice, coagulopathy, and encephalopathy) which develops in previously healthy individuals. This catastrophic illness can swiftly progress to coma and can result in death from cerebral edema and multiorgan system failure. ALF is associated with a variety of causes, including drug-induced liver injury and viral hepatitis, although in as many as 20% of cases no etiology can be found (indeterminate ALF) [1]. It may also be the presenting feature in certain chronic liver diseases, including Wilson disease and autoimmune hepatitis.

The clinical syndrome of ALF is the same, however, regardless of the cause. Complications include coagulopathy, hepatic encephalopathy, cerebral edema, brainstem herniation, infection, circulatory instability, renal failure, pulmonary failure, electrolyte disturbances, and acid–base disorders. Mortality ranges from 30% to 100% [1]. Aggressive multidisciplinary management and the judicious use of emergent orthotopic liver transplantation (OLT) have improved overall patient survival. However many patients are not candidates for OLT or will die before an organ becomes available [2–4]. There is

generally complete hepatic recovery if the patient survives without OLT (spontaneous survival).

Definitions

The syndrome of ALF was first described in the 1950s. Trey and Davidson in 1970 defined ALF as the onset of hepatic encephalopathy within 8 weeks of the first symptoms of illness in patients without preexisting liver disease [5]. ALF is described as a syndrome, rather than a specific disease, since it has multiple causes that vary in course and outcome. ALF is also variably called fulminant hepatic failure, fulminant liver failure, fulminant hepatic necrosis, or acute hepatic necrosis. The preferred terminology is acute liver failure or acute hepatic failure, since this encompasses all clinical presentations.

The clinical progression of ALF is a consequence of its etiology, predicting its eventual outcome. This fact has led some to suggest refinements to the basic definition [6,7]. O'Grady et al. proposed stratifying patients according to the time interval between the onset of jaundice and the development of encephalopathy into hyperacute (<7 days), acute (8–28 days), and subacute (28 days to 6 months) [6]. This classification system is currently used in the United Kingdom. A subcommittee of the International Association for the Study of the Liver (IASL) proposed two categories: acute liver failure, that which develops within 4 weeks of the onset of illness, and subacute liver failure, that developing 4 weeks to 6 months after the onset of symptoms. However, others have questioned the prognostic significance of these classifications independent of the etiology of the syndrome.

In general, the syndrome of ALF is currently described as an illness of less than 26 weeks' duration with coagulopathy (international normalized ratio (INR) ≥1.5) and any degree of hepatic encephalopathy in patients without preexisting liver disease or cirrhosis. Exceptions to this include Wilson disease, vertically acquired hepatitis B virus (HBV) infection, autoimmune hepatitis, or hepatitis D virus (HDV) superinfection in patients with chronic HBV infection, all of which may present with ALF despite the presence of unrecognized underlying chronic liver disease or cirrhosis.

Epidemiology

Acute liver failure affects about 2,000–2,800 persons annually in the United States [8,9]. It has been estimated that ALF accounts for about 0.1% of all deaths in the United States (3.5 deaths per million population) and 6% of all liver-related deaths. In addition, 5–6% of all US liver transplants are performed for acute liver failure [8,9].

Studies in the United States in the 1960s suggested that up to two thirds of ALF cases were due to viral hepatitis, with about 23% secondary to drug-induced liver injury (DILI) [10]. From the 1970s to the early 1980s, HBV emerged as a predominant cause [11]. In an equal number of patients, a cause could not be found (indeterminate cases). Drug-induced liver injury occurred in <20% and acetaminophen-induced ALF was not seen [11]. Case reports began to appear in the 1980s linking acetaminophen to cases of ALF. A 1983 to 1995 series from the University of Pittsburgh revealed that acetaminophen toxicity had emerged during that era as the cause for 19% of ALF cases. The incidence of HBV had decreased to 18% and 44% of cases were indeterminate [12]. The US Acute Liver Failure Study Group (ALFSG) retrospectively reviewed the causes of ALF between 1994 and 1996, revealing a 20% incidence of acetaminophen-induced ALF and a further decline in viral hepatitis (17%) [13]. In 1997, the ALFSG began to prospectively collect ALF patient data. Data collected on the first 308 cases enrolled between 1998 and 2001 revealed that over 50% of cases of ALF in the United States were secondary to medications, including herbal preparations (39% acetaminophen, 13% idiosyncratic drug reactions) [1]. Of those with acetaminophen-induced ALF, overdose was unintentional in 48% and most were consuming the medication for pain relief [14]. In this series, viral

Table 19.1 Clinical characteristics of ALF due to different etiology.

Cause of ALF						
Feature	**APAP** (*n* = 532)	**Drugs** (*n* = 133)	**Indeterminate** (*n* = 161)	**HAV** (*n* = 31)	**HBV** (*n* = 83)	**All others** (*n* = 207)
Age (years)[a]	37 (28–45)	46 (33–56)	38 (26–50)	47 (40–57)	42 (29–54)	42 (29–56)
Female sex	76%	67%	58%	45%	42%	76%
On presentation:						
HE grade ≥3	52%	38%	50%	55%	54%	41%
ALT (U/L)[a]	4,067 (2,138–6,731)	600 (260–1,537)	847 (396–2,111)	2404 (1,367–3,333)	1707 (745–2,815)	650 (172–1,867)
Bilirubin (mg/dL)[a]	4.5 (2.9–6.6)	20.2 (12.1–28.3)	23.0 (9.2–29.7)	11.9 (9.7–27.5)	19.7 (12.4–25.6)	15.3 (6.3–26.7)
Survival:						
Spontaneous	65%	29%	25%	58%	25%	34%
Transplantation	9%	41%	43%	29%	47%	33%
Death without transplantation	26%	31%	32%	13%	28%	33%

[a]Median and range.
APAP, acetaminophen; HAV, hepatitis A virus; HBV, hepatitis B virus; HE, hepatic encephalopathy.
Data from the ALFSG (William Lee, personal communication).

hepatitis accounted for only 12% of cases and a cause could not be found in 17% (indeterminate ALF). Acetaminophen overdose is now the commonest cause of ALF in both the United Kingdom and United States [13].

The majority of ALFSG patients in the United States are women (67–73%) and Caucasian (74%); however this varies with etiology (Table 19.1) [1,13]. Regardless of race, the groups are similar with regard to gender, years of education, age at presentation, and current alcohol or injection drug use. Acetaminophen appears to be the more common etiology among whites (52% whites, 28% blacks, 20% Asians). Asians are more likely to have viral hepatitis-induced ALF (8% whites, 19% blacks, 26% Asians) and blacks and Asians more likely to have drug-induced ALF than whites. There is no significant difference in overall mortality rate between racial groups; however, the odds of receiving liver transplantation are greater among Asians and Hispanics (and similar between whites and blacks).

ALF is less common in the United Kingdom. In contrast to the US data, acetaminophen overdose is the commonest cause, accounting for up to 70–75% of cases [15,16]. Other drugs are responsible for 5% of cases of ALF and viral hepatitis accounts for <5%. Most acetaminophen overdoses in the United Kingdom follow attempts at deliberate self-harm, rather than unintentionally consuming too much product. Following a surge in acetaminophen-induced cases of ALF in the United Kingdom, legislation was passed in 1998 aimed at restricting the quantity of acetaminophen which could be purchased [17]. This resulted in a decrease of approximately 30% in the number of hospital admissions, number of liver transplant listings, and deaths from acetaminophen poisoning [18].

Etiology

The causes of ALF are many and vary both geographically and socioeconomically (Box 19.1). Viral hepatitis remains the commonest cause worldwide, while drug-induced ALF, particularly acetaminophen, predominates in the United States and many parts of Europe [1,13–15,19]. Despite advances in diagnostic techniques, an etiology cannot be found (indeterminate ALF) in up to 20% of cases.

Viral hepatitis

Viral hepatitis is the leading cause of ALF worldwide, although ALF occurs in <5% of all viral hepatitis infections [10,20]. HBV accounts for the majority of these cases. Those with underlying liver disease or those who are older when infected appear to be at greater risk of developing ALF due to acute viral hepatitis [21].

Box 19.1 Etiologies of acute liver failure [324].

Viral
- Hepatitis A, B (±D), and E
- Hemorrhagic fever viruses
- Cytomegalovirus
- Herpes simplex viruses

Drugs/toxins
- Dose-related
  - Acetaminophen
  - Carbon tetrachloride
  - *Amanita* poisoning
  - *Bacillus cereus* emetic toxin
  - *Cyanobacteria microcystins*
- Idiosyncratic
  - Reye's syndrome (salicylic acid)
  - Herbal medications
  - Prescription medications (i.e., isoniazid, halothane, troglitazone, bromfenac)

Metabolic/genetic
- Galactosemia
- Fructose intolerance
- Tyrosinemia
- Neonatal iron storage disease
- Wilson disease
- α_1-Antitrypsin deficiency

Neoplastic
- Metastases: breast, melanoma, lung, lymphoma

Pregnancy-related
- Acute fatty liver of pregnancy
- HELLP syndrome (hemolysis, elevated liver function tests, low platelets)

Vascular
- Budd–Chiari syndrome
- Sinusoidal obstruction syndrome
- Ischemic (shock) liver

Miscellaneous
- Autoimmune hepatitis
- Heat stroke
- Primary graft nonfunction in liver transplant recipients

Indeterminate

Hepatitis A virus

The majority of acute hepatitis A virus (HAV) infections in children and adolescents are anicteric and asymptomatic, with symptoms becoming increasingly prevalent with increasing age. Acute liver failure occurs in 0.2–0.4% of cases of acute HAV; those over 40 years of age and those with preexisting liver disease are at higher risk [20,21].

It has been reported that patients with chronic hepatitis C virus (HCV) infection who are superinfected with HAV also have a greater risk of developing ALF [22], although this finding is not universal [1,23,24]. HAV accounts for 4–8% of cases of ALF in the United States, 5% in the United Kingdom, and 4% in France [1,13,25]. Approximately 40% of the US population is now immune to HAV, and the incidence of acute HAV, development of ALF, and mortality has dramatically declined [26–28]. Outbreaks, however, continue to occur.

Hepatitis B virus

Acute liver failure develops in 0.1–1.2% of patients with HBV infection, and women appear to be more susceptible than men. The percentage of HBV-ALF reflects the underlying prevalence of HBV in a particular population. In general, HBV-ALF is relatively more common in Asian and eastern European countries and is seen less frequently in the west. Superinfection with HDV must also be considered as a risk factor for ALF in the setting of chronic HBV.

The diagnosis of acute HBV in the setting of ALF is confirmed by the presence of serum immunoglobulin M (IgM) antibodies to the HBV core (anti-HBc) antigen. The hepatitis B surface antigen (HBsAg) may be absent in as many as 55% of cases of HBV-ALF. There have also been reports of HBV-ALF in the absence of all serologic markers, but this has not been confirmed in other series [29,30]. HBV-ALF may also occur in the setting of immunosuppression or chemotherapy whose withdrawal leads to viral reactivation [31–33].

ALF following acute HBV infection is related to a massive immunologic attack on the HBV-infected hepatocytes. This same exaggerated immune response may also be responsible for the ALF seen in chronically HBV-infected patients following the abrupt withdrawal of corticosteroids or chemotherapy. HBV-ALF patients who have more rapid viral clearance carry a more favorable outcome compared with patients who remain HBsAg-positive (mortality 53% versus 83%, respectively) [19]. In addition, those who clear virus also have a better outcome following liver transplantation.

Hepatitis C virus

It is generally believed that isolated acute HCV infection rarely, if ever, leads to ALF. Evidence of HCV infection in the setting of ALF is either not seen, or infrequently found [29,34,35]. HCV has been reported, however, as a coinfection or superinfection in cases of HBV-ALF [22,29]. It is of note that studies from Japan and Taiwan have shown that up to half of patients with non-A, non-B ALF have evidence of HCV infection [36]. There is also a single center report from the United States that reported detection of HCV-RNA in 60% of non-A, non-B ALF patients [37].

However, the causal role of HCV in this setting has not been established.

Hepatitis D virus

Hepatitis D virus (formerly delta virus), a defective viral particle, requires the presence of HBV for its replication. HDV is relatively uncommon in the west, is seen predominantly among injection drug users, and is associated with <5% of all cases of acute HBV infection in the United States [38]. It is endemic in the Mediterranean, however, including southern Italy and parts of Africa. In patients with HBV-ALF, HDV is seen in up to 40% [38,39]. HBV-HDV-ALF is also more severe than HBV-ALF alone, with a higher mortality [38].

Hepatitis E virus

Acute hepatitis E virus (HEV) infection presents with clinical features similar to those seen with acute HAV infection [40]. HEV-ALF is uncommon in western countries [29,34,35]. However, it accounts for sporadic and major epidemics of viral hepatitis in underdeveloped nations (e.g., India, Pakistan, Mexico, Central Asia, Southeast Asia, Russia, North Africa) and travelers returning from these areas [34]. The presence of anti-HEV IgM antibodies confirms the diagnosis. HEV infection has been reported to have a higher mortality rate among pregnant women, although this finding remains controversial [40,41].

Other viruses

Infection with several other viruses can lead to the development of ALF, including herpes simplex virus (HSV) types 1, 2, and 6, varicella zoster virus (VZV), cytomegalovirus (CMV), Epstein–Barr virus (EBV), parvovirus B19, human herpes virus 6 (HHV-6), Dengue virus, and yellow fever virus [42–45]. These viruses generally cause ALF in the setting of immune compromise or pregnancy, but cases in immunocompetent individuals have also been reported [42,46–49].

Drug- and toxin-induced liver injury

Numerous medications, toxins, and herbal remedies have been associated with liver injury; however the development of ALF is less common. DILI is divided into two broad categories. *Intrinsic (direct) hepatotoxins* predictably and reproducibly cause a dose-dependent hepatocellular necrosis with a brief period between exposure to the drug and development of liver toxicity (latent period). This is consistent from person to person and among animal models. In most cases, it is the compound itself, or one of its metabolites, that leads to the liver injury. *Idiosyncratic hepatotoxicity* is unpredictable. There is no constant relationship between the dose and the occurrence or severity of hepatotoxicity. The latent period is variable and unpredictable, and animal models are not consistently helpful. Idiosyncratic reactions present as either immune-mediated hypersensitivity or metabolic injury. While these reactions often occur within several weeks following initiation of the drug, they can occur after months to years of drug exposure or even after the drug has been discontinued.

Hepatotoxicity is the most common reason that medications and herbal products are removed from the market place (e.g., bromfenac, troglitazone), and many products have been associated with ALF [50–52]. DILI is the most frequent cause of ALF in the United States (>50% of cases) [1]. Acetaminophen is the most common offender (45–50% of all ALF cases) followed by idiosyncratic liver injury from other drugs and herbal products (11–15%) [1,14]. Those patients who develop ALF secondary to idiosyncratic drug toxicity carry a worse prognosis (25% survival) and a higher rate of liver transplantation (53%) than with many other causes of ALF [1].

Acetaminophen

Acetaminophen (N-acetyl-p-aminophenol or APAP), a mild non-narcotic analgesic and antipyretic agent, is widely used as a pain reliever and/or fever reducer. APAP was first introduced for prescription use in 1955, and subsequently approved by the US Food and Drug Administration (FDA) in 1960. APAP has been generally considered safe and effective when consumed as recommended (1–4 g/day). Its use has achieved great popularity, and it is available in hundreds of single ingredient and combination over-the-counter (OTC) products with over 1 billion tablets sold annually in the United States.

At supratherapeutic doses (generally >7–10 g/day), it is well documented that APAP causes severe or even fatal liver injury secondary to massive hepatic necrosis [14,53]. Hepatotoxicity has also been reported in patients taking therapeutic doses under certain conditions, such as chronic alcohol consumption or malnutrition [14,54–59]. It has recently been shown, however, that even normal individuals taking therapeutic doses of APAP can develop transient asymptomatic aminotransferase elevations [60,61]. This suggests that even at therapeutic dosing there may be some hepatotoxicity.

Metabolism

Following ingestion at therapeutic doses, about 2% of APAP is excreted in the urine unchanged [62,63]. Over 90% is metabolized via conjugation – two thirds via glucuronidation (urine diphosphate (UDP) glucuronosyltransferases) and one third through sulfation (sulfotransferases) [63]. The inactive nontoxic conjugates are largely excreted in the urine and bile. The remaining 5–9% undergoes oxidative conversion via several cytochromes (CYP1A2, CYP2A6, CYP2E1, CYP3A4) to the highly toxic metabolite N-acetyl-p-benzoquinone imine (NAPQI) [57,

63–65]. Cytochrome P450 2E1 (CYP2E1) conversion predominates, with minor contributions from CYP1A2, CYP2A6, and CYP3A4 [63]. NAPQI is a highly reactive two-electron species that can act as an electrophile or an oxidant. Normally, it is rapidly metabolized by conjugation to intracellular glutathione (GSH) forming a nontoxic APAP-GSH conjugate (3-(glutathione-S-yl)-APAP) [62,66]. Subsequent processing leads to its urinary excretion as mercapturic acid and cysteine conjugates [62,66]. APAP is also oxidized by myeloperoxidase and the peroxidase function of cyclooxygenase 1 (COX-1), the clinical significance of which is unknown.

Hepatotoxicity

Acetaminophen is an established dose-dependent hepatotoxin. Therapeutic doses of APAP result in small quantities of NAPQI that are easily detoxified by GSH. Excessive doses of APAP lead to the saturation of the glucuronic acid and/or sulfate pathways, shunting more APAP into the CYP system. Toxic doses are generally greater than 7–10 g/day in adults or 150 mg/kg in children, but there are reports of toxicity occurring with doses less than this [14,54,67,68]. Excessive CYP activation secondary to other medications or herbs may further drive APAP into the oxidative pathway, leading to increased free radical formation with the possibility of hepatocellular injury [69, 70]. Depletion of GSH stores via overdose, malnutrition, or alcohol ingestion results in the inability of the liver to detoxify many reactive metabolites and may increase the risk of APAP hepatotoxicity [57,59,71]. The importance of these latter mechanisms remains controversial [69,70,72].

The precise mechanism of hepatocyte death remains speculative. Glutathione stores within the liver are limited and may be depleted in an attempt to detoxify the increased NAPQI levels. When GSH stores are reduced by 70–80%, the detoxification capacity of the liver is exceeded and NAPQI accumulates, interacting with and destroying hepatocytes and other cells [62,73,74]. In the absence of GSH, covalent binding of NAPQI to the cysteine groups on hepatocyte macromolecules occurs, forming NAPQI–cysteine adducts [75–77]. This is the initial and irreversible step in the development of cell injury [62,78]. GSH depletion further contributes to cellular oxidant stress [79]. With NAPQI binding to critical cellular targets such as mitochondrial proteins, mitochondrial dysfunction and loss of cellular adenosine triphosphate (ATP) occurs [80,81]. Hepatocytes subsequently experience overall energy failure (cellular exhaustion). The ultimate result is alteration in calcium homeostasis, mitochondrial dysfunction with ATP depletion, DNA damage, and intracellular protein modification, leading to necrotic cell death [62,82].

Rodents models, however, suggest that the covalent binding of NAPQI to hepatic proteins in isolation does not cause hepatotoxicity. There is a growing body of evidence suggesting that inflammatory mediators (i.e., interferon γ (IFN-γ)) trigger the innate immune system, leading to an influx of natural killer/natural killer T cells, neutrophils, Kupffer cells, and macrophages that participate in the development and propagation of hepatocyte injury [83–86]. It has therefore been proposed that acetaminophen toxicity occurs in two phases: a metabolic phase and an oxidative phase.

Epidemiology

Acetaminophen hepatotoxicity usually is the direct result of acute deliberate self-poisoning (suicidal poisoning), accidental pediatric exposure, and repeated supratherapeutic ingestion (RSTI) [14,53,54,56,87,88]. In the 2006 Annual Report of the American Association of Poison Control Centers' National Poison Data System (NPDS), acetaminophen poisoning was mentioned in over 125,000 reports, of which over half were secondary to RSTI. Patients with RSTI often take combinations of products, generally for pain relief, each of which contains acetaminophen. Repeated supratherapeutic ingestion may lead to "accidental" or unintentional overdose [14,89–91]. Many of these patients are not aware that the products they are consuming may all contain acetaminophen [89–92].

The majority of patients with acetaminophen poisoning will recover without incident if treated early with the antidote N-acetylcysteine (NAC). Acute liver failure develops in only a few of these poisonings and death occurs in <1% of total exposures [93]. In the United Kingdom, the majority of cases of APAP overdose leading to ALF are secondary to intentional overdose (75%) with the deliberate intent to cause self-harm. Intentional overdose makes up a significant portion of APAP overdose in other western nations as well [14,87,88]. In the United States, however, unintentional (accidental) overdose makes up only about 50% of cases of APAP-ALF, with the remainder intentional [14,54].

Course of overdose

Acetaminophen-induced ALF follows a predictable course. Patients often have few signs or symptoms within the first 24 hours following an acute overdose (stage 1), but may develop nausea, vomiting, and malaise. Laboratory studies are usually normal during this period, and early symptoms may completely resolve. Clinical and laboratory evidence of hepatotoxicity appears from 24 to 72 hours after ingestion (stage 2). Patients may develop abdominal pain or liver tenderness and elevations in serum aminotransferases (aspartate aminotransferase (AST), alanine aminotransferase (ALT)), prothrombin time, and bilirubin. During stage 3 (72–96 hours), the most severe abnormalities occur – hepatic encephalopathy, coagulopathy, hyperbilirubinemia (median 4.5 mg/dL), renal dysfunction, and lactic acidosis. Marked aminotransferases elevations (median ~4,100 IU/L) are often seen and this degree of elevation is highly correlated with APAP poisoning [14,56]. During this stage, death most often occurs from cerebral herniation or from multiorgan system failure (MOSF). Once the signs of ALF (i.e., encephalopathy and coagulopathy) have developed, the risks of complications and death increase significantly, with overall mortality approaching 30% [1,14]. Patients who survive stage 3 enter the recovery phase, which is generally complete by 7–14 days after overdose. Hepatic recovery is generally complete, without development of chronic liver dysfunction. There appear to be no differences in presentation between intentional and unintentional overdose once the syndrome of ALF develops [14]. Acetaminophen-induced ALF has one of the best spontaneous survival rates (68%) and lowest rates of liver transplantation (6%) [14,54].

Mushroom poisoning

Amanita phalloides, responsible for the majority of mushroom poisoning deaths, is seen in areas where the mushroom is prevalent [94–99]. Two toxins are produced – phallotoxin and α-amanintin – and both are heat stable and not destroyed by cooking [95,100]. The phallotoxin causes damage to the enterocyte cell membrane [94]. The α-amanintin toxin (amatoxin) is dose dependent and responsible for hepatic injury by disrupting hepatocyte messenger RNA synthesis [94,95,100]. It is lethal at doses of as little as 0.1–0.3 mg/kg (50 g or two to three middle-sized mushrooms) [99].

Course of poisoning

Following ingestion, a 6–12-hour asymptomatic phase evolves into three clinical phases. The gastrointestinal phase (phase 1; 12–24 hours), consists of diarrhea, vomiting, and abdominal pain. During the hepatotoxic phase (phase 2: 24–48 hours) signs of liver damage occur and the disease may progress to the third clinical phase (4–7 days), during which ALF, hepatorenal syndrome, hemorrhage, convulsions, coma, and death occur [98]. Mortality approaches 10–30% [94,98,101,102].

Other direct hepatotoxins

Medications and chemicals that carry direct hepatotoxicity generally are recognized quickly and removed from use (i.e., carbon tetrachloride, chloroform, and tannic acid) [103]. Certain direct hepatotoxins have been allowed to remain in clinical use because their toxicity is well known and generally occurs only at high doses. Examples include APAP, iron sulfate, intravenous tetracycline, and phosphorus. Environmental toxins may also lead to ALF, including *Bacillus cereus* toxin, aflatoxin, cyanobacterial toxins, and yellow phosphorus (used in rat poison and fireworks) [104,105].

Idiosyncratic hepatotoxins

Overall, reactions to individual drugs are rare, occurring in 1 : 1,000 to 1 : 100,000 patients who receive a given medication. However, idiosyncratic drug reactions account for up to 20% of ALF cases, depending upon the geographic location [13,19].

Idiosyncratic hepatotoxins are believed to cause injury to susceptible individuals at least in part through the formation of neoantigens (i.e., drug–protein adducts), which either act as direct immunologic targets or they themselves directly interrupt normal cellular function. Neoantigens that interact with the immune system may lead to a *hypersensitivity (immune-mediated)* type of liver injury. These reactions are often accompanied by clinical and histologic evidence of hypersensitivity (i.e., rash, fever, eosinophilic leukocytosis, eosinophilic or granulomatous hepatic inflammation with hepatocyte necrosis and cholestasis) [103]. This type of liver injury is seen with medications such as phenytoin, amoxicillin-clavulanate, erythromycin, sulfonamides, halothane, dapsone, diclofenac, carbamazepine, and sulindac [106]. *Metabolic* idiosyncratic reactions show no hypersensitivity and are likely due to aberrant drug metabolism in susceptible individuals, who probably produce toxic metabolites to a greater degree than others. These reactions can occur at any time during the course of drug ingestion and can even occur up to several weeks after drug discontinuation. Examples include isoniazid, ketoconazole, disulfiram, valproate, troglitazone, and amiodarone [107].

The use of herbal and natural medications has increased significantly over the last few decades. These products are often considered safe simply because they are "natural." Many products have been associated with severe liver injury and acute liver failure, including chaparral, germander, comfrey, pennyroyal oil, Jin Bu Huan, Chinese herbs, black cohosh, kava kava, and the weight loss product Herbalife® [50,108–116]. Recreational drugs have also been reported to cause severe hepatic injury, particularly ecstasy (3,4,-methyledioxymetamphetamine) and cocaine (benzoylmethylecgonine) [117–119].

Indeterminate causes

Indeterminate causes account for up to 20% of ALF cases depending upon the country [13,19]. Despite significant advances in diagnostic techniques, an etiology for the ALF cannot be found.

Other causes

Pregnancy-associated acute liver failure

Acute fatty liver of pregnancy (AFLP) and the HELLP syndrome (hemolysis, elevated liver enzymes, and low platelets) are believed to represent a spectrum of the same disease process. ALF generally presents during the third trimester, but may rarely occur slightly earlier or shortly postpartum [120]. The incidence of AFLP ranges from one case per 7,000 to 20,000 deliveries, with no ethnic or geographic variation. Most women are young (16–39 years) primagravidas and hallmarks of preeclampsia (hypertension, proteinuria) may be present. The frequency of HELLP syndrome is about 1–2 per 1,000 pregnancies and it occurs in about 20% of women with severe preeclampsia. Ethnic variations exist, the risk being significantly higher in Caucasian and Chinese populations (relative risk of 2.2) when compared with East Indian populations. Risk is also higher in African-Americans when compared with Caucasians. The average maternal age of onset is about 25 years (14–40 years) with primagravidas constituting from 52% to 81%.

Fetal deficiencies in long-chain 3-hydroxyacyl-CoA dehydrogenase (LCHAD) have been identified, but are more commonly seen in the setting of AFLP [121,122]. The deficiencies in LCHAD may lead to poor processing of triglycerides and free fatty acids, which leads to the accumulation of medium- and long-chain fatty acids in the mother and deposition within the maternal hepatocytes. In addition, these patients develop increased vascular tone and platelet aggregation [123].

Patients with AFLP present with malaise, fatigue, anorexia, headache, right upper quadrant pain, nausea, vomiting, and occasionally pruritus. As the disease progresses, jaundice develops in nearly all patients. Within 1–2 weeks of symptom onset, and within days after the development of jaundice, patients may develop signs of ALF. Approximately 50% of cases will show evidence of preeclampsia (hypertension, proteinuria). Serum aminotransferases up to 1,000 IU/L and hyperbilirubinemia averaging 15 mg/dL are seen; however, bilirubin levels up to 30-40 mg/dL have been reported. Most HELLP syndrome patients will also present with abdominal pain, nausea, vomiting, and malaise; signs of preeclampsia are present in about 85% of cases. Serum aminotransferases and lactate dehydrogenase are usually less than 500 IU/L.

Clinical findings and laboratory studies suggest the diagnosis of AFLP or HELLP syndrome, and liver biopsy (the gold standard) is rarely needed. Histologically, the centrilobular and midzonal hepatocytes in AFLP are swollen with microvesicular fat globules. There may be sinusoidal compression but signs of hepatic necrosis and inflammation are often subtle. In the setting of the HELLP syndrome, there is often massive hepatic necrosis, marked steatosis, and necrotic vessels with intravascular thrombi.

Autoimmune hepatitis

Autoimmune hepatitis (AIH), most commonly viewed as a chronic illness, can present acutely in about a quarter of patients – some presenting with ALF [124–126]. AIH-ALF generally occurs in patients with unrecognized preexisting disease, and AIH represents the cause in about 5–6% of all US cases of ALF [1,13]. The presentation is identical to other causes of ALF, and there are no classic signs to suggest AIH as the etiology [127]. Exclusion of all other causes must be undertaken. Serum autoimmune antibodies may be absent, and in this situation liver biopsy may be helpful in establishing the diagnosis [125].

Wilson disease

Wilson disease is an autosomal recessive disorder of copper metabolism, with a prevalence of about 1 : 30,000 and a carrier frequency of about 1 : 90 [128]. The gene, located on chromosome 13q14.3, encodes a copper-transporting P-type ATPase (*ATP7B*) whose role is that of biliary copper excretion, and it is therefore expressed predominantly within the liver. Mutations lead to decreased hepatic copper excretion and its subsequent accumulation, particularly within the liver, brain, kidneys, and cornea. Most patients with Wilson disease or Wilson disease-induced ALF (WD-ALF) will present between the first and fourth decades, although both younger and older presentations have been reported.

WD-ALF accounts for <5% of all ALF cases [1]. It is usually seen in the setting of previously undiagnosed Wilson disease-induced cirrhosis, is clinically similar to all other cases of ALF, and is therefore considered classic ALF despite the presence of preexisting liver disease. The diagnosis of WD-ALF is crucial because it carries a nearly 100% mortality without liver transplantation [13,129]. In chronic Wilson disease, the diagnosis is based upon a low serum ceruloplasmin, the presence of Kayser–Fleischer rings, elevated hepatic copper, and increased urinary copper excretion. Diagnosis in the setting of ALF is more difficult, however, because these usual diagnostic studies lack sensitivity and specificity. Kayser–Fleischer rings are absent in up to 50%. Measures of copper metabolism are also of limited value since elevated urinary copper and alterations in serum copper can be seen in ALF due to other causes [130]. Serum ceruloplasmin is normal in up to 15% of WD-ALF cases, and low ceruloplasmin levels can be seen in ALF from other causes. However, WD-ALF is often accompanied by a Coombs-negative hemolytic anemia, severe hyperbilirubinemia, moderate elevations in aminotransferases (<500 IU/L), and high serum and urinary copper concentration [129]. WD-ALF should be strongly considered in the setting of a normal to low serum alkaline phosphatase level, an alkaline phosphatase to total bilirubin ratio of <2.0, or an AST to ALT ratio of >2.0–3.0 [130–134].

Cardiovascular diseases

Hepatic hypoxia, due to decreased hepatic blood flow, can lead to acute hepatic necrosis and at times ALF [13]. The most common form of hypoxic liver injury is hypoxic hepatopathy ("shock liver") seen after episodes of systemic hypotension or a low blood flow state [135,136]. Clinically, serum aminotransferases rapidly increase, sometimes to over 10,000 IU/L, followed by rapid resolution. Shock liver may be accompanied by mild coagulopathy and occurs in about 1% of critically ill patients [135]. The prognosis depends upon the patient's underlying disease state, and shock liver per se is rarely fatal. Severe vascular obstruction is more likely to lead to ALF and death. These conditions include Budd–Chiari syndrome, sinusoidal obstruction syndrome (venoocclusive disease) due to medications or herbs, and malignancies involving the liver (i.e., lymphoma) [137–142].

Pathogenesis

When parenchymal damage is so severe that the liver is no longer able to meet the metabolic demands of the body, the syndrome of ALF develops [143]. Unfortunately, significant hepatic damage has already occurred by the time the patient presents to medical care. Histologically, the most common picture is one of confluent necrosis with cellular dropout and parenchymal collapse, which may be either zonal or nonzonal in distribution (Fig. 19.1). Following the inciting event (i.e., toxin, viral,

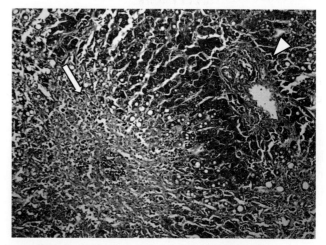

Figure 19.1 Hepatocellular injury secondary to acetaminophen hepatoxicity. The portal tract (arrowhead) shows very little injury and inflammation. There is marked centrilobular (zonal) necrosis, cellular loss, and parenchymal collapse (arrow). Original ×10. (Courtesy of Dr William M. Lee.)

ischemia), further injury may result from the activation of nonparenchymal cells within the liver and the release of cytokines. Other patterns of injury that may be seen in ALF include microvesicular steatosis (i.e., fatty liver of pregnancy, mitochondrial toxins, certain drugs) or malignant infiltration.

Depending upon the cause, one sees predominantly apoptosis (i.e., acetaminophen), necrosis (Wilson disease), or a combination of both [15,144,145]. Apoptosis is associated with nuclear shrinkage (pyknosis), followed by nuclear fragmentation, cytoplasmic shrinkage, and cell death. The cellular membrane is generally undisturbed, therefore minimal secondary inflammation is noted [143]. Apoptosis may be triggered either by the activation of hepatocyte receptors (extrinsic) or secondary to oxidative stress involving the mitochondria (intrinsic) [144]. Both the Fas ligand (FasL)/Fas receptor and tumor necrosis factor α (TNF-α)/TNF type I receptor apoptotic pathways have been implicated. Receptor activation triggers caspase cascades (cysteine proteases) leading to apoptosis and cellular death. The particular caspases activated depend upon the type of stimulus involved. Hepatocellular necrosis, on the other hand, is associated with the depletion of cellular ATP. This stress ultimately causes cellular swelling, cell lysis, and subsequent release of intracellular content resulting in secondary inflammation and further hepatocellular injury [5,144]. Cellular injury resulting in apoptosis may also precipitate necrosis if the mitochondria are severely damaged and ATP stores are sufficiently depleted [15,143]. Marked oxidative stress may also cause inhibition of the proapoptotic caspase cascade [15,144]. This may then result in progression from apoptotic cell death to necrosis [15,143,144]. Further products that mediate cellular death include antioxidants (i.e., glutathione), cellular nitric oxide, tyrosine kinases, transcription factors, pro- and anti-inflammatory cytokines, and chemokines [143].

The clinical result of this catastrophic injury is characterized by coagulopathy and hepatic encephalopathy, and is often associated with cerebral edema, hemodynamic changes, electrolyte disturbance, and renal failure. The exact relationship between hepatic injury and the syndrome of ALF is multifaceted, and our knowledge of the pathophysiology is limited by the lack of an adequate animal model of the disease.

Diagnosis

The early clinical features of ALF are nonspecific, including abdominal pain, fatigue, anorexia, malaise, and fever. This nonspecific phase often leads to significant delays in identification of the syndrome and the initiation of treatment. A high index of suspicion and recognition of the features characterizing the syndrome are crucial to a timely diagnosis. The presentation of ALF is similar regardless of the cause. Its hallmark is an altered mental status (hepatic encephalopathy) accompanied by jaundice and elevated serum aminotransferases and prothrombin time/INR in previously healthy individuals. The presence of moderate to severe hepatitis demands a careful mental status evaluation and measurement of the prothrombin time/INR. Family members and friends should be queried as to the presence of altered personality or mentation.

A careful history and physical examination will help establish ALF and suggest potential causes. Quickly identifying the specific etiology is vital to guide further management decisions, as several causes have specific treatments which may improve survival. One must pay particular attention to possible exposures (viral infections, drugs, or toxins). The details of dose ingested, amount and timing of last dose, duration of medication/herbal usage, and ingredients of nonprescription medications can be invaluable. An accurate history may be difficult or impossible to obtain from the encephalopathic patient; therefore family members or friends may be helpful in this setting.

A complete physical examination is a necessity, and mental status should be thoroughly and frequently assessed. A history of cirrhosis or the presence of its stigmata (i.e., spider angiomas, palmar erythema, or splenomegaly) suggests underlying chronic liver disease, which has a different course and prognosis. Abdominal tenderness may or may not be localized to the right upper quadrant. In the setting of infiltrative disease or hepatic outflow obstruction, hepatomegaly may be present. However, if there has been significant hepatocyte loss, the liver will not be palpable or percussable, which is an ominous prognostic sign. Jaundice may be absent until later in the course, particularly in the setting of microvesicular fatty injury. The initial laboratory evaluation should be extensive (Table 19.2) [146]. Markedly abnormal liver chemistries are usually seen on presentation, but may be normal early in the course of acetaminophen overdose. The arterial ammonia level may have prognostic implications, and an arterial blood gas and blood lactate can also help establish disease severity. Patients who present with a pH <7.3 often have a poor outcome, particularly in acetaminophen overdose, and immediate transfer to a transplant center should be considered [147].

The use of diagnostic liver biopsy remains controversial. Biopsy may be indicated if metastatic disease, lymphoma, or other infiltrative process is suspected. The presence of severe coagulopathy makes percutaneous biopsy impossible; therefore, tissue must be obtained via the transjugular route. It is rare, however, that a liver

Table 19.2 Laboratory evaluation in acute liver failure [146].

Test	Included tests
Serum chemistries	Sodium, potassium, chloride, bicarbonate, calcium, magnesium, phosphate, glucose, blood urea nitrogen, creatinine
Hepatic panel	AST, ALT, alkaline phosphatase, total bilirubin, albumin
Prothrombin time/INR	
Complete blood count	White blood cells, hemoglobin, hematocrit, platelets
Arterial blood gas	
Blood lactate level	
Acetaminophen level	
Toxicology screen	
Viral hepatitis serologies	Anti-HAV IgM, hepatitis B surface antigen, anti-HBc IgM, anti-HCV[a], anti-HEV (as indicated)
Autoimmune markers	Antinuclear antibody, antismooth muscle antibody, immunoglobulin G levels
Pregnancy test	
Ceruloplasmin level	If Wilson disease is suspected

[a]To identify underlying infection.
ALT, alanine aminotransferase; AST, aspartate aminotransferase; HAV, hepatitis A virus; HBc, hepatitis B core; HCV, hepatitis C virus; HEV, hepatitis E virus; IgM, immunoglobulin M; INR, international normalized ratio.

biopsy will help elucidate a diagnosis and the histologic findings do not generally alter the treatment course.

Clinical course and management

Patients suspected of having ALF should be swiftly evaluated for etiology and severity of liver injury. When the loss of hepatocyte mass becomes severe enough, hepatic function falls below a critical threshold. At this stage, multiorgan system failure is the rule, and death results from one of numerous complications [2,148]. The leading causes of death in ALF are cerebral edema with herniation and infection/sepsis [1,10,149].

Supportive measures

Immediate hospitalization is required for those with altered mental status and/or evidence of coagulopathy (prothrombin time prolonged by ≥4–6 seconds; INR ≥1.5), who by definition have ALF. ALF can progress rapidly from presentation to death, with patients worsening by the hour. Early transfer or direct admission to

the intensive care unit (ICU) for more intense monitoring is essential. Transfer to a transplant center, if appropriate, should be initiated early in the course, as specialized centers with experience in managing ALF will optimize care. Strong consideration should be given to moving the patient to a specialized unit if the INR exceeds 2.0 or the patient develops grade 2 or higher encephalopathy [150]. The development of complications requires immediate and aggressive treatment. Management is complicated and requires a multidisciplinary approach, including transplant hepatologists, transplant surgeons, intensive care physicians and nurses, nephrologists, and neurosurgeons. This group will make an urgent assessment as to the need and suitability for liver transplantation and coordinate the complicated medical care necessary to ensure the best patient outcome.

Hepatic encephalopathy and cerebral edema

Hepatic encephalopathy (HE) is a reversible neuropsychiatric syndrome of metabolic disturbance and depressed consciousness that develops following liver failure. Symptoms range from subclinical alterations to deep coma. The complete pathophysiology of HE remains poorly understood and is likely multifactorial. Accumulation of toxins in ALF, particularly ammonia, in the cerebrospinal fluid (CSF) has been postulated as the predominant mechanism of HE [151–154]. Serum accumulation of ammonia is further exacerbated by renal failure and impaired skeletal muscle function [155]. In addition, the disturbance of central pathways (i.e., glutamatergic, serotonergic, noradrenegeric), activation of γ-aminobutyric acid (GABA) receptors, production of false neurotransmitters, and altered cerebral energy metabolism likely contribute [154]. Disruption of the blood–brain barrier allows toxins to more freely enter the CSF [151,155]. There is also loss of cerebral autoregulation, such that the brain is more susceptible to changes in peripheral blood pressure, which compromises cerebral perfusion [151]. The development of the systemic inflammatory response syndrome (SIRS) is associated with progression of HE in ALF, as the weakened blood–brain barrier allows an influx of inflammatory cytokines [156,157].

ALF-induced hepatic encephalopathy is differentiated from that of cirrhosis by the development of elevated intracranial pressure (ICP) and cerebral edema. Hyperammonemia is considered a critical factor in the development of cerebral edema and herniation [158]. Cerebral detoxification of ammonia occurs predominantly within the astrocytes, which convert the ammonia to glutamine [159]. Ammonia-induced inhibition of α-ketoglutarate dehydrogenase leads to lactate accumulation, decreased tricarboxylic acid (Krebs) cycle activity, less efficient production of phosphate compounds (e.g., ATP), and ultimate swelling of the astrocytes [154,160,161]. Free radical formation within the astrocyte mitochondria further mediates cellular dysfunction [155,159]. Increasing evidence suggests that oxidative and nitrosative stress plays a significant role in the development of cerebral edema, although the precise cause is unclear [162]. There is a positive correlation between increases in brain ammonia and increased expression of heme oxygenase 1 (HO-1) and nitric oxide synthase (NOS) isoforms [162]. Both arterial ammonia and the partial pressure of ammonia (pNH_3) are independent predictors of intracranial hypertension. The pNH_3 correlates more closely with the clinical grade of HE than does the arterial ammonia [163]. In addition, the severity of multiorgan failure is also an independent predictor of intracranial hypertension in this setting [163].

Outcome worsens with increasing grades of HE – cerebral edema occurring in about 80% of patients who develop grade 4 HE [158,164]. The resultant increased intracranial hypertension compromises cerebral perfusion pressure (CPP), leading to ischemic brain damage or brainstem herniation, which accounts for up to half of ALF mortality. Electroencephalographic monitoring shows slowing of cortical activity in some patients with advanced encephalopathy, and ALF patients may undergo subclinical epileptiform activity due to excessive central nervous system glutamate [165]. Survivors may suffer from long-term neurologic deficits.

Treatment of HE in the setting of cirrhosis involves decreasing the production and absorption of these toxins. However, in the setting of ALF, these measures are less effective. Lactulose, a nonabsorbable disaccharide, has never been shown to improve overall survival in ALF [166]. It may help prolong survival, however, and could be used in the setting of grade 1 and 2 HE [148,166]. The risk of aspiration increases as the patient becomes more encephalopathic, therefore oral lactulose should not be used in these patients unless they are intubated [148]. The nonabsorbable antibiotics (i.e., rifaximin, neomycin) have not been tested in this setting.

Simple therapeutic measures that can be performed on all patients to minimize intracranial hypertension include elevation of the head of the bed to 30° and minimizing patient stimulation. Elective mechanical ventilation with sedation and/or paralysis can prevent patient movement and its associated increases in ICP. Acute hyperventilation fails to reduce the number of episodes of cerebral edema, and it does not delay the onset of herniation [167].

The development of an increased ICP is an ominous sign. Physical examination changes occur only after significant cerebral edema has developed; therefore they are generally not helpful in the diagnosis of cerebral edema. Head computed tomography (CT) is insensitive in the early stages of encephalopathy, but is recommended once stage 3–4 HE develops to rule out concurrent pathology

such as intracranial hemorrhage [148]. Advanced cerebral edema is associated with hyperventilation, systemic hypertension, pupillary abnormalities, decerebrate posturing, and ultimately uncal herniation and death. Arterial ammonia levels over 200 µg/dL have been strongly correlated with cerebral herniation and death [158]. Sustained ICPs of greater than 20 mmHg and CPPs of less than 50 mmHg for more than 2 hours are associated with irreversible brain injury [168].

ICP monitors may help to both diagnose intracranial hypertension and optimize its management, although their use remains contentious [168–171]. ICP monitors may be of significant value during the transplant operation, when fluctuations in ICP are common [172]. The placement of ICP monitors, however, carries risk in the patient with coagulopathy. Intracranial hemorrhage occurs in up to 10% of cases although fatality is rare. Nonrandomized trials have shown no survival advantage with ICP monitoring, and randomized controlled trials have not been performed [173].

ICP monitoring allows for more rapid recognition of fluctuations in ICP and potentially more rapid treatment [171]. Treatment is aimed at maintaining the CPP at >50 mmHg (the difference between the mean arterial pressure and the ICP), and the ICP at <20 mmHg [148,174,175]. If the CPP falls to <50 mmHg due to systemic hypotension, intravascular volume resuscitation and/or vasopressor support should be initiated. Mannitol (0.5 g/kg body weight) is the established first-line therapy in the setting of a sustained increased ICP (>20 mmHg), although its use may be limited in patients with concomitant renal failure [176,177]. Renal replacement therapy is required in this setting. Repeated mannitol dosing may be necessary. Other potential therapeutic measures proposed include thiopental or phenobarbital coma, phenytoin, and mild to moderate hypothermia (32–35°C) [157,165,169,178–181]. Small studies of hypothermia have shown promising results. Conflicting data exist regarding the use of prophylactic phenytoin [165,182]. Corticosteroids have no role in this setting [177].

Following transplantation, the elevated ICP and cerebral edema may persist for up to a day. It is therefore reasonable to maintain the therapies, including ICP monitoring, which were in place prior to and during the transplant, for at least 24 hours. As the patient awakens, these measures can be discontinued. If there is delayed graft function or primary nonfunction of the graft, these measures should be continued until hepatic recovery or retransplantation.

Hemodynamic abnormalities

Acute liver failure patients develop a hyperdynamic circulatory picture, characterized by splanchnic vasodilatation, low systemic and pulmonary vascular resistance, elevated cardiac output, increased metabolic rate, and systemic hypotension. These changes are most likely due to circulating endotoxin, cytokines (interleukins 6 and 8), and tumor necrosis factor, and are often exacerbated by the decreased oral intake and dehydration that accompanied the prodromal illness [183]. Abnormal peripheral oxygen transport and utilization frequently leads to lactic acidosis [184]. Clinically, these findings can be difficult to distinguish from sepsis.

The ideal resuscitative strategy in this setting is unknown. In general, hypovolemia should be corrected to achieve an adequate cardiovascular filling pressure [148]. Vasopressors may be required, and are indicated if the mean arterial pressure is consistently <50 mmHg in the setting of normal intravascular volume. Norepinephrine is often the recommended vasopressor, although dopamine may have a more beneficial effect on peripheral oxygen delivery [148]. Overuse of norepinephrine may exacerbate cerebral hyperemia. Small studies evaluating the use of the vasopressin prodrug, terlipressin, have shown conflicting results [185,186]. Corticosteroid insufficiency may contribute to hypotension in this setting, but is much less common than seen in other illness.

Coagulopathy and thrombocytopenia

Intact hepatic function is critical to the synthesis of protein products that are involved in both coagulation and thrombolysis. Multiple factors contribute to the coagulopathy associated with ALF, including decreased hepatic synthesis of both procoagulant and anticoagulant factors and low-grade disseminated intravascular coagulation [187]. Although hemostatic alterations are common in ALF, spontaneous hemorrhage or clinically significant bleeding are very rare (<5–10%) [188,189].

Coagulopathy, as measured by the prothrombin time/INR, develops following decreased hepatic synthesis of factors 2, 5, 7, and 10 [190]. Since this group of factors is vitamin K dependent, concomitant vitamin K deficiency must be excluded. Lack of improvement in the INR after vitamin K replenishment indicates decreased hepatic reserve. The prothrombin time/INR is one of the most sensitive liver function tests available in the setting of ALF and mirrors the prognosis and course of disease [147,191]. The tendency to spontaneously bleed is low despite marked elevations in the prothrombin time/INR, therefore fresh frozen plasma (FFP) should be used only for active bleeding or when needed to perform invasive procedures [192]. Prophylactic administration of FFP is not necessary, may contribute to volume overload, may worsen cerebral edema, and hinders the prognostic evaluation of the patient. Recombinant factor VII may be used with caution under certain conditions, such as prior to an invasive procedure [193,194].

The coagulopathy of ALF is balanced by decreased hepatic production of the procoagulant factors protein C, protein S, and antithrombin III [188,190]. In addition, there appears to be upregulation of factor VIII. Hypofibrinogenemia develops due to decreased hepatic synthesis and increased catabolism and contributes to diffuse mucosal and wound oozing [195]. It can be corrected with the administration of cryoprecipitate – generally if the fibrinogen level is <100 mg/dL and bleeding is evident.

There is also both quantitative and qualitative platelet dysfunction. The platelet count declines progressively over the course of the illness; reaching a nadir of <100,000 × 10^9/L in about 70% of ALF cases [187]. However, platelets rarely fall below 25,000 × 10^9/L or necessitate replacement [196].

Renal failure

Renal failure develops in up to 70% of ALF patients, particularly following acetaminophen overdose [197,198]. The cause is multifactorial, with contributions from direct medication nephrotoxicity (i.e., acetaminophen, nonsteroidal anti-inflammatories), depleted volume status from poor oral intake, hypotension secondary to the disease state itself, sepsis, and/or disseminated intravascular coagulation [197,199]. Hepatorenal syndrome may also contribute in the setting of high levels of renin and decreased renal blood flow [198,200]. The development of hepatorenal syndrome, however, does not appear to correlate with the severity of ALF [199,200]. The presence of SIRS predicts the development of renal dysfunction in nonacetaminophen-induced ALF [201].

Judicious intravenous fluid challenge should be attempted to exclude prerenal azotemia. Renal replacement therapy is often needed, particularly in the setting of acidosis, fluid overload, or cerebral edema requiring mannitol administration. Continuous forms (venoveno hemodiafiltration) are preferred as they minimize circulatory and cerebral fluctuations in pressure [202].

Infection and sepsis

Distinguishing sepsis from ALF-induced hemodynamic changes can be difficult, given the fact that many infected ALF patients may not develop leukocytosis or fever. Immune system function is impaired, with decreased complement and opsonization and impaired innate immunity. The risk of developing infection is greater in the setting of subacute ALF and increases with increasing time in the ICU [203,204]. The grade of hepatic encephalopathy on admission (grade >2) or a SIRS score >1 are independent predictors of bacteremia (odds ratio 1.6 and 2.7, respectively) [205]. Clinical or culture evidence of bacterial infection is seen in up to 90% of cases. The most common sites of infection are pulmonary (47%), blood (26%), and urine (23%) [16]. Gram-negative enteric bacteria (i.e., *Escherichia coli*) and staphylococcal or streptococcal species are the organisms usually identified. Bacterial infection is the cause of death in 10–37% of patients. Fungal infections, especially *Candida*, are seen in about 30%, occur later in the course of illness, particularly after the use of antibiotics or in the setting of renal dysfunction, and are often associated with bacterial infection [203]. The presence of infection worsens both HE and cerebral edema [156].

Infection can also trigger SIRS, thought to be the byproduct of multiple inflammatory pathways mediated by chemokine–cytokine responses. In acute liver failure, SIRS is linked to worsening hepatic encephalopathy, renal failure, adult respiratory distress syndrome, sepsis syndrome, and multiorgan system failure [12,156,201]. Prophylactic antibiotics have been shown to decrease the number of infections, but do not change the eventual outcome, and should be reserved for patients with advanced encephalopathy, renal failure, or awaiting transplantation [192]. Periodic surveillance cultures and frequent chest radiographs can help detect bacterial and fungal infections early. Proven infections should be vigorously treated.

Electrolyte and acid–base imbalance

Serum electrolyte abnormalities persist throughout the course of ALF. Decreased free water clearance is associated with renal sodium reabsorption and hyponatremia [206]. Serum and total body deficits of potassium follow. Hypophosphatemia, particularly common after acetaminophen overdose, is likely secondary to renal loss [207–210]. Mixed acid–base disturbances, including respiratory alkalosis and lactic acidosis, are common [184].

Pulmonary dysfunction

Acute lung injury can be seen in up to 40% of ALF patients, and significantly contributes to overall morbidity and mortality [211]. There is increased pulmonary vascular permeability, most likely secondary to endothelial damage, as well as structural alterations in the pulmonary vasculature [212]. Care should be taken with the use of protective ventilator strategies in the treatment of adult respiratory distress syndrome, as this may worsen cerebral edema.

Gastrointestinal bleeding

Acute liver failure patients are at increased risk of developing gastrointestinal bleeding. The use of intravenous antacids reduces both morbidity and mortality, and should be considered standard of care [148].

Hypoglycemia

Hepatic derangements lead to hypoglycemia in up to 45% of ALF patients. High serum levels of insulin are present.

In addition, the liver is unable to mobilize glycogen and gluconeogenesis is impaired. Frequent glucose monitoring is required and intravenous dextrose may be necessary to maintain normoglycemia.

Nutrition

Early consideration should be given to complete caloric replacement. ALF patients have significant nutritional and metabolic needs, with energy requirements up to 60% over baseline [213]. Hepatic glucose metabolism (glycogen storage, gluconeogenesis) is disordered, and energy must come from other sources, leading to depletion of muscle and fat stores [214]. In addition, decreased hepatic production of insulin-like growth factor 1 further contributes to protein breakdown [215]. Enteral nutrition is preferred in this setting since this has been shown to maintain gut integrity with decreased rates of bacterial translocation and potential infection [216]. The caloric requirements of ALF patients are as high as 50 kcal/kg/day, with protein needs of over 1 g/kg/day.

Specific therapies

There are several etiologies of ALF that have specific therapies which have been shown to improve outcome in many cases.

Acetaminophen overdose

Diagnosis

Prompt recognition of APAP intoxication is imperative to the management and prevention of hepatocellular injury, liver failure, and death. Identifying patients who have intentionally taken substantial amounts of APAP is often less challenging than identifying those with an unintentional overdose. The history of the amount of APAP ingested in both cases, however, is often unreliable. Patients may be unwilling or unable to admit to the amount or timing of the overdose. The vague or symptom-free latent phase may further confuse the clinical picture. Careful attention must be paid to the type of product ingested, quantity of APAP used, intent of the ingestion (intentional, unintentional), pattern of ingestion (single dose, repeated dosing), and other medications, drugs, herbs, or toxins consumed.

Ideally, plasma APAP levels should be obtained between 4 and 24 hours following ingestion. A negative value does not preclude a significant ingestion and false-positive levels have been seen in patients with hyperbilirubinemia ($>10\,\mu g/mL$) [217]. NAPQI–cysteine adducts are released into the circulation following hepatic injury and are detectable in both tissue and serum samples using high-pressure liquid chromatography with electrochemical detection (HPLD-EC) assay [218]. These APAP–cysteine adducts persist for an average of 7 days and decline in parallel with aminotransferase levels [75]. Adducts can be detected even in the setting of negative serum APAP levels. Since measurement of serum NAPQI–cysteine adducts reliably identifies acetaminophen toxicity, they may be a useful diagnostic test for cases lacking historical data or other clinical information [75]. Unfortunately, their measurement is not routinely available in most centers.

There is no correlation between the dose of APAP reportedly ingested and the serum APAP concentration measured [219]. Nor is there a correlation between dose ingested and outcome [220]. The most widely accepted approach to determine the risk of hepatotoxicity following acute single time-point ingestion is to plot the serum APAP concentration on the Rumack-Matthew nomogram [72,93]. Patients whose APAP concentration exceeds the lowest plotted line post-ingestion have a probable risk of hepatotoxicity. Following development of the nomogram, the FDA required that a more conservative measure be used to account for errors in plasma assays and estimated ingestion time [72,93]. This lower "safety" line is 25% lower than the original and patients with levels above this line are considered to be at "possible risk" for hepatotoxicity. This is the nomogram that is most commonly used in the United States [93]. Treatment is recommended if serum levels of APAP exceed this concentration.

The nomogram was developed for single time-point overdoses. It cannot be used to accurately predict risk of hepatotoxicity if patients have taken multiple large doses over time, the precise time of ingestion is unknown, or patients have been taking an extended-release product. There have been attempts to develop treatment algorithms in these settings, but none are used routinely [221,222].

Treatment

Data supporting the use of most poisoning interventions in the setting of APAP overdose are weak. Activated charcoal may be effective if administered within 1–2 hours following an acute ingestion [223]. Hepatotoxicity can be greatly attenuated if the antidote, N-acetylcysteine (NAC; Mucomyst® or Acetadote®), can be administered within 24 hours following an acute overdose, regardless of the initial APAP concentration [93,224–228]. Although often given up to 72 hours following overdose, the usefulness of administration of NAC more than 24 hours after an acute overdose has not been consistently shown [226].

NAC is a glutathione precursor and was first used for the treatment of APAP poisoning in 1977. Its mechanism of action is likely three-fold. First, it increases glutathione stores, acts as a glutathione substitute that binds with NAPQI, and enhances sulfate conjugation [62,229–231]. Second, it also has anti-inflammatory and antioxidant effects mediated via cytokines [226,227,232–235]. In addition, it has inotropic, and vasodilating effects that may further benefit the patient [226,227,232,233].

Adverse events following infusion of intravenous NAC range from 0.2% to 21% and include nausea, flushing, rash, pruritus, bronchospasm, rhinorrhea, hemolysis, fevers, chills, angioedema, hypotension, and anaphylaxis [236–238]. Many of these side effects occur when the drug is used endotracheally as a mucolytic [238]. Most of the reactions are mild and resolve with discontinuation of the infusion; however, occasionally, patients will require further treatment (i.e., antihistamine or epinephrine), and rare deaths have been reported [236,237]. Slowing the infusion rate of the initial dose does not decrease drug efficacy or lower the incidence of adverse events.

It is generally recommended that NAC be administered to all patients with ALF secondary to APAP overdose. Evidence has suggested that even late administration of NAC (up to 72 hours) is beneficial to patients who develop APAP-ALF, and progression to stage 3 or 4 encephalopathy is decreased in those ALF patients who receive NAC [226,227,232,233]. Intravenous NAC is preferred because it decreases risk of aspiration, results in higher serum concentrations, and has been shown to be beneficial in this setting [226,239]. The loading dose consists of 150 mg/kg over 60 minutes, followed by 12.5 mg/kg over the next 4 hours, then 6.25 mg/kg/h thereafter. NAC is continued until the serum acetaminophen level is unmeasurable and there is clear evidence of improvement in hepatic function (improving encephalopathy and resolution of coagulopathy (INR <1.5)), liver transplantation, or death [226,227, 232,233]. It should be emphasized that the duration of therapy in this setting is dictated by the clinical outcome, rather than an arbitrary time limit.

Concern has been raised regarding the extended use of NAC in the setting of ALF [227]. Recent animal data have suggested that the prolonged use of NAC impairs liver regenerative capacity [240]. These findings have not been supported by others [241]. Therefore, the appropriate duration of NAC therapy in this setting remains uncertain.

Pregnancy-related acute liver failure

Acute fatty liver of pregnancy and the HELLP syndrome are medical and obstetric emergencies. Patients should be promptly admitted to a liver failure unit, since it is impossible to predict which patients will worsen. Following aggressive maternal care and stabilization, delivery should be attempted as soon as reasonably possible. With early diagnosis and management, the severity of disease and need for liver transplantation can be minimized. Maternal mortality, historically up to 50%, can be lowered to 15% with early delivery. Fetal death occurs in 42–49% with only minimal improvement with early delivery (36%). Patients will slowly improve following delivery – full recovery often takes up to a month, and there are no hepatic sequelae. HELLP syndrome may be complicated by hepatic infarction or hepatic rupture.

Autoimmune hepatitis

It is well established that the treatment response to corticosteroids is the only predictor of outcome in the setting of chronic AIH. There are no prospective trials outlining the role of corticosteroid or immunosuppressant therapy in the setting of AIH-ALF; therefore, their use in this setting has not been firmly established [125,242,243]. AIH-ALF patients in the ALFSG study who were treated with corticosteroids had a higher rate of spontaneous recovery compared with those who were not treated. In general, AIH-ALF patients who worsen, or whose serum aminotransferases and bilirubin fail to improve within 2 weeks of initiating treatment, carry a 100% mortality without OLT [244].

Wilson disease

d-Penicillamine, trientene, and zinc are often ineffective in the setting of WD-ALF [245,246]. Plasmapheresis may help to bridge the patient to OLT, but itself carries no survival benefit [246,247]. Mortality approaches 100% so listing for transplant should be considered early in the course of disease [130,245].

Mushroom poisoning

Randomized controlled trials of therapy for *Amanita* poisoning do not exist. Severe cases often require transplantation. Silibinin (20–50 mg/kg/day) or penicillin G (250 mg/kg/day) may be effective if administered early following ingestion, although this remains controversial [98,248–252]. Overall mortality following *Amanita* poisoning ranges between 10% and 40% [13].

Hepatitis B virus

The usefulness of antiviral medications in the setting of HBV-ALF remains uncertain. Several small series using foscarnet, lamivudine, or entecavir have suggested benefit with rapid viral suppression. A small randomized trial using lamivudine in 71 patients failed to show any benefit [253]. A more recent randomized trial of 80 patients, however, showed that treatment of HBV-ALF patients with lamivudine therapy was an independent predictor of survival [254]. It is, therefore, probably reasonable to consider antiviral medication in this setting.

Herpes simplex virus

The diagnosis of HSV-induced ALF is often made late in the course of illness because characteristic vesicles are often absent. If HSV is suspected, intravenous aciclovir is both safe and has proven benefit [255]. Unless treatment is initiated early, HSV-induced ALF has a very poor prognosis [43,49].

Nonspecific therapies

Nonspecific therapies that have shown no benefit in the setting of ALF include corticosteroids, heparin, insulin and glucagon, and prostaglandin E1. Other therapies that have been evaluated show promise, but in general prospective randomized trials are lacking.

Drug-induced liver injury

There is currently no standard therapy in the setting of DILI except discontinuation of the offending agent. However, establishing causality in cases of idiosyncratic DILI remains challenging, particularly in the setting of ingestion of multiple products. Numerous medications have been implicated, but some of the more commonly reported offenders include antituberculous drugs, sulfonamides, phenytoin, antibiotics, and herbal and dietary supplements.

N-acetylcysteine for non-acetaminophen acute liver failure

A recent prospective, randomized, double-blind, placebo-controlled trial in the setting of ALF not due to acetaminophen showed a significant improvement in transplant-free survival in patients with early-stage encephalopathy (stage 1–2) who received NAC [256]. There was no difference in overall survival in the entire group (all stages of encephalopathy). Thus, NAC use early in the course of ALF may prevent progression to deeper encephalopathy with its associated complications. It has been suggested that in this setting NAC also exerts renal protective effects and is beneficial to the hemodynamics of multisystem organ failure.

Hypothermia

Mild to moderate hypothermia (33–35°C) has been shown to both delay progression of hepatic encephalopathy and consistently lower intracranial pressures, and thus decrease the likelihood of cerebral edema [157,257,258]. Hypothermia normalizes cerebral blood flow, attenuates increases in brain concentrations of ammonia, and decreases brain extracellular glutamate, as well as reducing brain levels of nitrites/nitrates [162,259]. Nitrite/nitrate reduction leads to a decrease in cellular oxidative/nitrosative stress, and could in part explain the beneficial effects described when hypothermia is used in the management of ALF [181,257]. However, the clinical benefits of hypothermia remain to be confirmed in large randomized clinical trials, and complications of hypothermia itself remain a concern [259].

Liver assist therapies

The goal of liver assist therapies has been to either support the patient until the native liver has had time to recover, or to bridge the patient to liver transplantation. Liver support therapies can be broadly divided into either artificial or bioartificial. Artificial therapies provide detoxification support without the use of biologic (cellular) material. Bioartificial support systems utilize cellular material and, in theory, provide not only detoxification, but also assume some of the synthetic function of the failing liver.

Artificial liver support

There has to date been no evidence that any artificial therapy reliably reduces mortality in the setting of ALF. Plasmapheresis has been shown to decrease ammonia levels, improve cerebral blood flow, improve cerebral perfusion pressures, improve hepatic encephalopathy, and to improve systemic hemodynamic parameters. However, its benefit on survival remains unproven. The molecular absorbent recirculation system (MARS) was introduced in the 1990s and first used clinically in 1999 (Fig. 19.2) [260]. MARS is a two-circuit system, which allows albumin-bound toxins to be removed. The blood circuit, a high flux dialyzer, passes the patient's blood over an albumin impermeable membrane, allowing the efflux of small- to medium-sized molecular weight molecules. The secondary circuit, a low flux dialysis, comprised of exogenous human albumin dialysate, provides detoxification over adsorbent columns (an anion exchange resin and activated charcoal column) [261]. A meta-analysis of studies using MARS failed to show a significant survival benefit in ALF patients [262]. The

Prometheus® albumin dialysis system was introduced clinically in 1999 [263]. This system uses a membrane that is permeable to albumin and albumin-bound proteins; therefore the secondary circuit utilizes the patient's own albumin for detoxification [264]. The system functions similarly to MARS, but appears to carry a greater risk of clotting [264]. There exist even fewer data on the survival benefit of this system.

Bioartificial support

Given the outcome data with artificial support systems, many experts believe the focus of artificial support for ALF should be cell-based. Bioartificial liver support would ideally incorporate human hepatocytes, which would provide both detoxification and synthetic functions of the liver (Fig. 19.3). The use of normal human hepatocytes is limited, however, by both their poor capacity to grow in vitro as well as their decreased biologic function when cultured [265]. Therefore, bioartificial liver support systems have utilized immortalized cell lines (C3A human hepatoblastoma) [266,267]. Using potentially oncogenic cells has raised safety concerns, although there have been no reports of cellular transmission in this setting. Porcine hepatocytes have also been utilized and are more readily available than human hepatocytes. Despite the lack of evidence that these cells may spread zoonotic disease, this concern remains.

Five systems have been tested clinically: HepatAssist® (Arbios, formerly Circe, Waltham, MA), extracorporeal liver support device (ELAD®, Vital Therapies, San Diego, CA), modular extracorporeal liver support system (MELS®, Charité, Berlin, Germany), bioartificial liver support system (BLSS®, Excorp Medical, Minneapolis, MN), and the Amsterdam Medical Center bioartificial liver (AMC-BAL®, AMC, Amsterdam) [268–272]. HepatAssist was the first cell-based liver assist device tested, and in a small randomized trial showed a survival advantage in patients with ALF and subacute liver failure [268]. Despite this, the FDA did not approve the device and

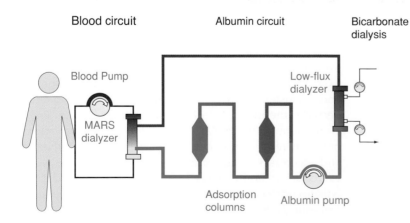

Blood circuit   Albumin circuit   Bicarbonate dialysis

Blood Pump

Low-flux dialyzer

MARS dialyzer

Adsorption columns

Albumin pump

Figure 19.2 Schematic diagram of the molecular adsorbent recirculation system (MARS) circuit. (Reproduced from Mitzner et al. [325] with permission from Wiley-Blackwell.)

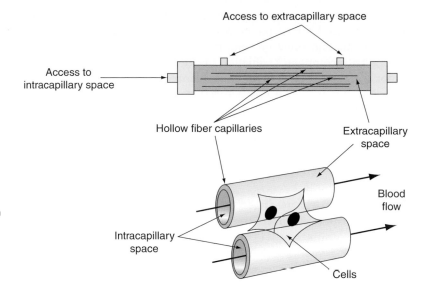

Figure 19.3 Diagram of a hollow fiber cartridge, on which the bioartificial liver (BAL) and extracorporeal liver assist device (ELAD) are based. The close-up view shows cells attached to the external surface of the hollow fibers. (Reproduced from Ellis et al. [326] with permission from Cambridge University Press.)

recommended further testing in patients with ALF. Small series using ELAD in the setting of ALF have suggested benefit, however there have been no large, randomized trials [267,273]. Phase I studies in small numbers of ALF patients have demonstrated safety and efficacy using MELS, BLSS, and AMC-BAL [270–272]. Larger scale data for these devices are lacking.

Liver transplantation

Advances in critical care medicine have improved the spontaneous survival in ALF patients from 10–20% to about 40% [1]. However, orthotopic liver transplantation remains the only treatment modality that improves survival in those who will not recover. With the advent of OLT as a treatment option in this setting, overall survival rates have further improved to ~60%. Thus, liver transplantation has been recommended for the treatment of ALF since the early 1980s. Candidacy for transplantation must be determined quickly, given the rapid pace of the syndrome. Acute liver failure is one of the very few conditions for which a patient can be listed as a United Network for Organ Sharing (UNOS) status 1A (urgent) patient in the United States and "super urgent" in the UK. Although about half of ALF patients undergo liver transplantation, ALF accounts for less than 10% of US transplants and approximately 11% in Europe [274].

Overall, the 1-year survival following OLT for ALF is less (60–80%) than that seen in patients who have been transplanted for chronic liver failure (80–90%) [1,3, 274,275]. The majority of these deaths occur in the first 2–3 months following the transplantation, usually due to neurologic complications or sepsis. However, by 1–4 years following transplantation this trend has reversed,

and ALF patients have a better survival than those transplanted for chronic liver disease. Poorer outcomes are seen in centers performing less than 25 liver transplants per year and less than 20 split-liver grafts per year for those doing living donor liver transplantation [276].

In addition to whole-organ deceased donor liver transplantation, various others types of liver transplantation may be utilized depending on the situation: living donor liver transplants (LDLTs), incompatible ABO status transplants, and auxiliary liver transplants. In the setting of organ shortage, the risk of mortality while waiting for an organ must be weighed against the risk of complications or failure using an alternative graft.

Living donor liver transplant

The use of LDLT in this setting remains controversial [277–280]. Between January 1, 1988 and March 31, 2010, LDLTs accounted for approximately 2% of transplants for ALF (based on Organ Procurement and Transplantation Network (OPTN) data as of July 5, 2010). It is important to consider the need for an adequately sized graft for the recipient with sufficient residual mass for the donor. Grafts in excess of 40% of standard liver volume are necessary in the setting of ALF, and outcomes are better with a graft-to-recipient weight ratio greater than 0.8, with 1.0 (whole organ) being ideal [281]. LDLT is associated with potential recipient complications, such as biliary complications (in 15–65%) [282–284]. The graft is at risk of small-for-size syndrome. A graft of less than 40% of standard liver weight is at risk for the development of portal hypertension following reperfusion leading to sinusoidal damage and graft injury [285]. Nevertheless, right lobe LDLT improves survival of patients with acute liver failure, and the 1-year survival rate following LDLT is approximately 75% [280].

Unique ethical issues exist in the setting of LDLT. Given the urgent need for an organ in the setting of ALF, the donor evaluation must be compressed. This carries the risk of an incomplete evaluation and the possibility of donor coercion. The donor and transplant team must consider the fact that LDLT is associated with significant donor complications, including death in 0.2% [282,283]. In regions where cadaveric organs are not as readily available, the risk of the recipient's death while waiting for a cadaveric organ must be weighed against the risk to the living donor.

ABO-incompatible liver transplant

Although ABO identical grafts are preferable, ABO-compatible grafts (e.g., O graft, A recipient) have a comparable 1-year survival following OLT for ALF. Alternatively, ABO-incompatible grafts (e.g., A graft, B recipient) show less favorable outcome (30% 1-year graft survival). A Canadian group reported overall 5-year graft survival rates of 54–60% and 5-year patient survival rates of 61–77%, although the number of study subjects was small [286]. At present, survival of the graft is generally seen in up to 60% of ABO-incompatible transplants, likely related to intensive management (use of quadruple immunosuppression, plasmapheresis, splenectomy, methylprednisolone, or prostaglandin E1). Use of an ABO identical graft is still preferred.

Auxiliary liver transplant

Auxiliary OLT leaves the recipient's liver in place, using a partial left or right lobe from the donor which acts as temporary support for the recipient's injured liver. Ideally, in this setting, immunosuppression may be withdrawn following native liver recovery allowing the graft to atrophy naturally or it is surgically removed [287]. The partial graft is placed below the native liver (heterotopic auxiliary transplantation) or replaces a resected right or left native liver lobe (auxiliary partial liver transplantation). While easier to perform, implantation of the heterotopic graft onto the infrahepatic vena cava may lead to venous outflow obstruction, resulting in slower hepatocyte regeneration, presumably due to cytokine release from residual necrotic liver tissue. There is an increased incidence of primary graft nonfunction and portal vein thrombosis with heterotopic auxiliary transplantation compared with auxiliary partial or whole graft OLT. Unique complications may develop following auxiliary transplantation. Portal blood flow is partially diverted from the native liver to the graft, thus regeneration of the native liver may be impaired and graft function may be impaired. Moreover, due to the smaller mass of the transplanted liver, cerebral edema and neurologic dysfunction may continue to progress [287]. In addition, leaving the necrotic graft in situ following immunosuppression withdrawal may lead to the development of multisystem organ failure, or, over time, cirrhosis in the native liver [288,289].

The best outcomes with auxiliary transplantation are in young patients with hyperacute presentations due to a viral or autoimmune disorder [4,290]. Overall survival rate for auxiliary transplantation is reported to be between 60% and 65%, and immunosuppression has successfully been withdrawn in 65–85% of these patients by 1-year post-transplant [280,287,290,291].

Prognosis and prognostic models

It is critical to quickly and accurately identify those patients most likely to benefit from emergent OLT. To minimize the risk of unnecessarily committing individuals to lifelong immunosuppression, one must balance the desire to delay transplantation to allow for the potential of spontaneous recovery against the risk of death with that delay and the risk of the surgery itself. Of patients listed for transplantation, 37% will recover spontaneously without the need for OLT and it is estimated that as many as 20% of ALF patients may be transplanted needlessly. Once listed, a significant number of ALF patients will progress and die awaiting OLT. In the United Kingdom, ~30% of patients initially considered for OLT ultimately become untransplantable following the development of complications (i.e., cerebral edema, sepsis, hemodynamic abnormalities, multiorgan system failure) [292]. In the US ALFSG, 44% of patients were listed for OLT, yet only 25% of the entire cohort received a transplant. Additionally, many patients have medical or psychosocial contraindications to transplantation, including irreversible brain injury, underlying cardiovascular disease, infection/sepsis, alcohol or drug abuse, poorly controlled psychiatric disease, or inadequate family support [293]. Therefore, it is important to identify and even delist patients who are too ill to benefit from OLT.

It is, therefore, crucial that reliable predictive models of survival and need for liver transplantation be developed. Successfully predicting outcome would allow more judicious use of scarce organs and spare those who will ultimately recover anyway the necessity of transplantation and lifelong immunosuppression. The varying causes of ALF, with wide variability in patient survival, and the unpredictability of subsequent complications makes it very difficult to determine who will survive without OLT. There are at present no standardized criteria to predict who should be listed for OLT with ALF.

Clinical predictors

Clinical predictors of death may help determine which patients are more likely to die; however these are generally unreliable. The degree of serum aminotransferase elevation and the rate of its recovery do not predict prognosis. In fact, improvement of aminotransferase levels in conjunction with worsening bilirubin, encephalopathy, and coagulopathy (INR) signals complete liver failure and is an ominous sign. The criteria most commonly used to exclude a patient from OLT vary between transplant centers but generally include: age older than 70 years, the presences of certain malignancies outside the liver, severe cardiac, lung, or multiple organ failure, severe infection, uncontrolled septic shock, and brain death.

Etiology

The etiology of ALF is one of the more important predictors of outcome [1]. In the past, mortality from ALF approached 100%. However, with the epidemiologic shift to more benign causes (e.g., acetaminophen), the advent of improved clinical management, and selected utilization of liver transplantation, the overall mortality now ranges between 30% and 40%. The lowest mortality is seen with ALF due to acetaminophen hepatotoxicity (~30%), hepatitis A virus infection (~50%), shock liver, and pregnancy-related ALF [1,14,25]. In contrast, the mortality for the remainder of causes is abysmal (80–100%) [1].

Multiorgan failure

The severity of multiorgan failure at the time of OLT is also a predictor of post-transplant survival. Decreased renal function is associated with worse spontaneous survival in non-APAP-induced liver injury. In a multivariate analysis of UNOS data (1988–2003), four risk factors predicting post-transplant survival were identified: pretransplant use of life support, recipient age >50 years, recipient body mass index $\geq 30 \text{ kg/m}^2$, and serum creatinine >2 mg/dL. If an individual had all of these risk factors, the 5-year post-transplant survival was only 44–47%. Whereas, if none of these features were present, the 5-year post-transplant survival was 82–83% [275].

Hepatic encephalopathy

Mortality rates also appear to correlate with the severity of hepatic encephalopathy, with 30% morality for those who reach grade 2 HE, 45–50% for grade 3 HE, and 80–90% for grade 4 HE [20]. Paradoxically, those with more rapid development of hepatic encephalopathy (i.e., acetaminophen induced) appear to have a better outcome compared with those with a longer interval between the development of symptoms and encephalopathy (i.e., DILI) [6,19,147].

Graft quality

The quality of the graft impacts post-transplant outcome [294]. Graft steatosis, reduced graft size, and ABO-incompatible grafts have all been shown in multivariate analyses to lead to decreased patient and graft survival [292,294]. Unfortunately, graft quality must be weighed against transplant urgency, since patients may deteriorate while waiting for optimal grafts, sometimes to the point when they are no longer feasible candidates. Suboptimal grafts may fail, however, leading to the need for retransplantation.

Prognostic models

Multiple prognostic models have been proposed to help determine the likelihood of spontaneous survival [7,147,156,191,295–302]. However, many of these models are methodologically flawed and subject to bias. In addition, many equate liver transplantation with death, which falsely elevates the positive predictive value of these prognostic systems [303,304].

King's College Hospital criteria

The most widely applied prognostic system is that using the King's College Hospital criteria (Kings criteria), developed from a retrospective cohort of nearly 600 patients (Table 19.3) [147,305]. The Kings criteria incorporate both the etiology of ALF and the clinical parameters of disease. When applied to ALF patients in the United Kingdom, these criteria have a positive predictive value for death from APAP-ALF of 84%, and 82% in all other causes, and a negative predictive value of 86% and 82%, respectively [147]. In a meta-analysis of studies using the Kings criteria, the pooled sensitivity and specificity were 69% and

Table 19.3 King's College Hospital criteria for predicting death or need for transplantation in acute liver failure (ALF) [147,305].

Acetaminophen ALF	Non-acetaminophen ALF
Strongly consider OLT listing if arterial lactate >3.5 mmol/L after early fluid resuscitation	List for OLT if: INR >6.5 irrespective of degree of hepatic encephalopathy
List for OLT if: pH <7.3 *or* Arterial lactate >3.0 mmol/L after adequate fluid resuscitation	*or any three of the following*: Age <10 or >40 years Jaundice for >7 days before encephalopathy INR >3.5 Bilirubin >17 mg/dL
List for OLT if all three of the following occur within a 24-hour period: Presence of grade 3 or 4 hepatic encephalopathy INR >6.5 Creatinine >3.4 mg/dL	*Or* Unfavorable etiology, such as: Wilson disease Idiosyncratic drug reaction Halothane Seronegative hepatitis

INR, international normalized ratio; OLT, orthotopic liver transplantation.

92%, respectively [304]. However, patients who do not meet these criteria may ultimately still require transplantation. In general, the predictive accuracy of these criteria appear to be less when applied to patients from other regions and countries [40,306–309]. Following the finding that the arterial lactate improved the sensitivity of the model in APAP-ALF, the Kings criteria have been recently refined [19,207,305].

Clichy criteria

The French Clichy criteria were developed in a cohort of patients with acute hepatitis B virus infection [297]. These criteria suggested that a serum factor V level of <20% in patients younger than 30 years or <30% in any patient with grade 3–4 HE has validity as a marker of mortality. The criteria predicted a poor outcome with a sensitivity and specificity of 86% and 76%, respectively [297,298,310]. Factor V level measurements are less readily available than the measures in the Kings criteria, meaning this prognostic model is not commonly utilized [306,310]. In addition, this model has not been validated in the non-HBV population.

Serum α-fetoprotein

Serum α-fetoprotein (AFP) is a marker of hepatocyte turnover, generally considered indicative of hepatocellular regeneration. No correlation is seen between the absolute AFP level and outcome in ALF [311]. However, an increasing AFP level is strongly associated with a favorable outcome [296,311]. In one study, on the day of peak ALT levels, AFP values were significantly higher in survivors than in nonsurvivors [312]. A threshold AFP of ≤3.9 µg/L 24 hours after the peak ALT identified nonsurvivors with a sensitivity of 100%, a specificity of 74%, a positive predictive value of 45%, and a negative predictive value of 100%. A second study showed that a rising level of AFP between day 1 and day 3 frequently indicated survival without transplantation (71%), whereas a decreasing level was seen in 80% of those who succumbed [311].

Gc-globulin

The Gc-globulin (group-specific component) scavenges monomeric actin and, together with gelsolin, constitutes the extracellular actin scavenger system. The level of Gc-globulin is markedly reduced in all forms of tissue injury. This marker has not been shown to reliably predict survival in those with APAP-induced ALF. In non-APAP-ALF, however, using a cutoff value of ≤80 mg/L, the Gc-globulin level carried a positive predictive value of 74% and a negative predictive value of 81% [296].

Arterial ammonia

An elevated arterial ammonia increases the risk of developing intracranial hypertension, and a level of >150 µmol/L predicts the development of intracranial hypertension with a sensitivity of 60% and a specificity of 84% [163]. Concentrations of >100–150 µmol/L have also been correlated with cerebral herniation [151, 152,158,313]. Patients with renal and circulatory insufficiency are at risk of intracranial hypertension at even lower ammonia levels [151].

Other models

The model for end-stage liver disease (MELD) score carries a specificity and sensitivity of <75% in predicting outcome in both APAP-ALF and non-APAP-ALF [151,314,315]. The acute physiology and chronic health evaluation (APACHE) scoring system is also ineffective in predicting who will survive without transplantation, since many patients who do not meet the severity criteria will ultimately die of subsequent complications. A factor V <10% has been shown to predict a poor outcome with a sensitivity of 91% and a specificity of 100%; while a factor VIII : V ratio of >30 similarly predicts outcome (91% sensitivity, 91% specificity) [295]. Persistently elevated phosphate levels may be associated with a poorer prognosis in the setting of acetaminophen-induced ALF [207,208]. A serum phosphate level >1.2 mmol/L on day 2 or 3 following APAP overdose carries a sensitivity of 89% and a specificity of 100% for poor outcome [208,209]. A liver volume of <1,000 mL on CT imaging is also associated with a high mortality rate [302]. Liver biopsy has also been proposed to determine the severity of liver damage, with greater than 70% hepatic necrosis associated with a transplant-free survival of <10% in one analysis [316]. However, there is a great degree of sampling error, and more recently a multivariate analysis of 97 consecutive patients showed that the amount of necrosis was not predictive of mortality [317].

Based upon the available data, the current prognostic scoring systems have not consistently demonstrated reliable accuracy in predicting outcome from ALF and the subsequent need for OLT. Therefore, the American Association for the Study of Liver Diseases does not recommend sole reliance on any one of these systems.

Outcomes

There are unique postoperative issues that plague ALF patients. Despite transplantation, elevated ICP and cerebral edema can persist for up to a day or more. In ALF patients who die post-OLT, as many as 13% succumbed to brain death [275]. Protective strategies, such as continued ICP monitoring, may be helpful through this period of risk. Although renal function often improves dramatically, patients may require renal replacement therapy for many weeks post-OLT, particularly in the setting of APAP-ALF. This author and others have adopted immunosuppressive strategies that attempt to minimize nephrotoxic agents, such as calcineurin inhibitors, in this critical recovery period. Nearly one third of post-OLT deaths in this setting are from bacterial or fungal infections [275].

Long-term clinical outcomes in ALF patients have not been well described [318,319]. Life-altering complications that may occur include permanent neurologic injury secondary to cerebral edema or persistent or recurrent disease following recovery [318,319]. There exist very few data on long-term neurologic impairment and its consequences. Rapidly recurrent disease in the newly transplanted liver is generally less common. It has been noted in the setting of autoimmune hepatitis, acute HAV, and acute HBV infections [320,321].

Following spontaneous recovery, patients with psychiatric illness who had taken a deliberate APAP overdose are at risk of repeated overdoses [292]. However, risk of repeated overdose appears to be less common in this group if they have been transplanted, perhaps due to the intensity of postoperative care. In two series from the United Kingdom, APAP-ALF patients who underwent OLT showed similar long-term survival (median 5 years and 9 years) compared with patients transplanted for chronic liver disease [322,323]. Less than 5% of those transplanted for APAP overdose reattempted overdose. There was a worse 30-day mortality for the APAP-ALF patients, and a greater probability of post-OLT medical nonadherence and adverse events in those who had taken APAP for deliberate self-harm compared with both non-APAP-ALF patients and chronic liver disease patients [323].

Conclusions

ALF is a rare but rapidly fatal disorder leading to jaundice, coagulopathy, hepatic encephalopathy, and multisystem organ failure. Idiosyncratic drug-induced hepatotoxicity and acetaminophen overdose remain the most common causes identified in the United States. The early recognition of ALF requires a high index of suspicion and thorough evaluation. Despite improvements in care, these patients remain medically challenging and mortality is high. Early intervention is crucial, and involvement of an experienced multidisciplinary team and transfer to a specialty center will maximize survival. Cerebral edema with intracranial hypertension and infections remain the leading causes of death. Liver transplantation remains the

treatment of choice in those who are not recovering and its use has markedly improved overall survival. Optimal prognostic survival models are lacking and many patients will ultimately die without transplantation.

References

1. Ostapowicz G, Fontana RJ, Schiodt FV, et al. Results of a prospective study of acute liver failure at 17 tertiary care centers in the United States. *Ann Intern Med* 2002;137:947–54.
2. O'Grady J. Modern management of acute liver failure. *Clin Liver Dis* 2007;11:291–303.
3. Farmer DG, Anselmo DM, Ghobrial RM, et al. Liver transplantation for fulminant hepatic failure: experience with more than 200 patients over a 17-year period. *Ann Surg* 2003;237:666–75.
4. Brandsaeter B, Hockerstedt K, Friman S, et al. Fulminant hepatic failure: outcome after listing for highly urgent liver transplantation – 12 years experience in the Nordic countries. *Liver Transpl* 2002;8.1055–62.
5. Trey C, Davidson CS. The management of fulminant hepatic failure. In: Popper H, Schaffner F, eds. *Progress in Liver Diseases*. New York: Grune and Stratton; 1970:282–98.
6. O'Grady JG, Schalm SW, Williams R. Acute liver failure: redefining the syndromes. *Lancet* 1993;342:273–5.
7. Bernuau J. Selection for emergency liver transplantation. *J Hepatol* 1993;19:486–7.
8. Khashab M, Tector AJ, Kwo PY. Epidemiology of acute liver failure. *Curr Gastroenterol Rep* 2007;9:66–73.
9. Bower WA, Johns M, Margolis HS, et al. Population-based surveillance for acute liver failure. *Am J Gastroenterol* 2007;102:2459–63.
10. Ritt DJ, Whelan G, Werner DJ, et al. Acute hepatic necrosis with stupor or coma. An analysis of thirty-one patients. *Medicine (Baltimore)* 1969;48:151–72.
11. Rakela J, Mosley JW, Edwards VM, et al. A double-blinded, randomized trial of hydrocortisone in acute hepatic failure. The Acute Hepatic Failure Study Group. *Dig Dis Sci* 1991;36:1223–8.
12. Shakil AO, Kramer D, Mazariegos GV, et al. Acute liver failure: clinical features, outcome analysis, and applicability of prognostic criteria. *Liver Transpl* 2000;6:163–9.
13. Schiodt FV, Atillasoy E, Shakil AO, et al. Etiology and outcome for 295 patients with acute liver failure in the United States. *Liver Transpl Surg* 1999;5:29–34.
14. Larson AM, Polson J, Fontana RJ, et al. Acetaminophen-induced acute liver failure: results of a United States multicenter, prospective study. *Hepatology* 2005;42:1364–72.
15. Khan SA, Shah N, Williams R, Jalan R. Acute liver failure: a review. *Clin Liver Dis* 2006;10:255–66.
16. Bernal W. Changing patterns of causation and the use of transplantation in the United Kingdom. *Semin Liver Dis* 2003;23:227–37.
17. Hawton K, Simkin S, Deeks J, et al. UK legislation on analgesic packs: before and after study of long term effect on poisonings. *Br Med J* 2004;329:1076.
18. Hughes B, Durran A, Langford NJ, Mutimer D. Paracetamol poisoning – impact of pack size restrictions. *J Clin Pharm Ther* 2003;28:307–10.
19. Bernuau J, Rueff B, Benhamou JP. Fulminant and subfulminant liver failure: definitions and causes. *Semin Liver Dis* 1986;6:97–106.
20. Hoofnagle JH, Carithers RL Jr, Shapiro C, Ascher N. Fulminant hepatic failure: summary of a workshop. *Hepatology* 1995;21:240–52.
21. Lefilliatre P, Villeneuve JP. Fulminant hepatitis A in patients with chronic liver disease. *Can J Public Health* 2000;91:168–70.
22. Vento S, Garofano T, Renzini C, et al. Fulminant hepatitis associated with hepatitis A virus superinfection in patients with chronic hepatitis C. *N Engl J Med* 1998;338:286–90.

23. Bianco E, Stroffolini T, Spada E, et al. Case fatality rate of acute viral hepatitis in Italy: 1995–2000. An update. *Dig Liver Dis* 2003;35:404–8.

24. Sagnelli E, Stroffolini T, Almasio P, et al. Exposure to HAV infection in patients with chronic liver disease in Italy, a multicentre study. *J Viral Hepat* 2006;13:67–71.

25. Schiodt FV, Davern TJ, Shakil AO, et al. Viral hepatitis-related acute liver failure. *Am J Gastroenterol* 2003;98:448–53.

26. Taylor RM, Davern T, Munoz S, et al. Fulminant hepatitis A virus infection in the United States: incidence, prognosis, and outcomes. *Hepatology* 2006;44:1589–97.

27. Alter MJ, Mast EE. The epidemiology of viral hepatitis in the United States. *Gastroenterol Clin North Am* 1994;23:437–55.

28. Vogt TM, Wise ME, Bell BP, Finelli L. Declining hepatitis A mortality in the United States during the era of hepatitis A vaccination. *J Infect Dis* 2008;197:1282–8.

29. Feray C, Gigou M, Samuel D, et al. Hepatitis C virus RNA and hepatitis B virus DNA in serum and liver of patients with fulminant hepatitis. *Gastroenterology* 1993;104:549–55.

30. Wright TL, Mamish D, Combs C, et al. Hepatitis B virus and apparent fulminant non-A, non-B hepatitis. *Lancet* 1992;339:952–5.

31. Kim TW, Kim MN, Kwon JW, et al. Risk of hepatitis B virus reactivation in patients with asthma or chronic obstructive pulmonary disease treated with corticosteroids. *Respirology* 2010;15:1092–7.

32. Matsue K, Kimura SI, Takanashi Y, et al. Reactivation of hepatitis B virus after rituximab-containing treatment in patients with CD20-positive B-cell lymphoma. *Cancer* 2010;116:4769–76.

33. Lubel JS, Angus PW. Hepatitis B reactivation in patients receiving cytotoxic chemotherapy: diagnosis and management. *J Gastroenterol Hepatol* 2010;25:864–71.

34. Kuwada SK, Patel VM, Hollinger FB, et al. Non-A, non-B fulminant hepatitis is also non-E and non-C. *Am J Gastroenterol* 1994;89:57–61.

35. Sallie R, Silva AE, Purdy M, et al. Hepatitis C and E in non-A non-B fulminant hepatic failure: a polymerase chain reaction and serological study. *J Hepatol* 1994;20:580–8.

36. Yoshiba M, Dehara K, Inoue K, et al. Contribution of hepatitis C virus to non-A, non-B fulminant hepatitis in Japan. *Hepatology* 1994;19:829–35.

37. Villamil FG, Hu KQ, Yu CH, et al. Detection of hepatitis C virus with RNA polymerase chain reaction in fulminant hepatic failure. *Hepatology* 1995;22:1379–86.

38. Govindarajan S, Chin KP, Redeker AG, Peters RL. Fulminant B viral hepatitis: role of delta agent. *Gastroenterology* 1984;86:1417–20.

39. Smedile A, Farci P, Verme G, et al. Influence of delta infection on severity of hepatitis B. *Lancet* 1982;2:945–7.

40. Acharya SK, Dasarathy S, Kumer TL, et al. Fulminant hepatitis in a tropical population: clinical course, cause, and early predictors of outcome. *Hepatology* 1996;23:1448–55.

41. Hamid SS, Jafri SM, Khan H, et al. Fulminant hepatic failure in pregnant women: acute fatty liver or acute viral hepatitis? *J Hepatol* 1996;25:20–7.

42. Norvell JP, Blei AT, Jovanovic BD, Levitsky J. Herpes simplex virus hepatitis: an analysis of the published literature and institutional cases. *Liver Transpl* 2007;13:1428–34.

43. Harma M, Hockerstedt K, Krogerus L, Lautenschlager I. Pretransplant human herpesvirus 6 infection of patients with acute liver failure is a risk factor for posttransplant human herpesvirus 6 infection of the liver. *Transplantation* 2006;81:367–72.

44. Poovorawan Y, Hutagalung Y, Chongsrisawat V, et al. Dengue virus infection: a major cause of acute hepatic failure in Thai children. *Ann Trop Paediatr* 2006;26:17–23.

45. Palanduz A, Yildirmak Y, Telhan L, et al. Fulminant hepatic failure and autoimmune hemolytic anemia associated with Epstein–Barr virus infection. *J Infect* 2002;45:96–8.

46. Abbo L, Alcaide ML, Pano JR, et al. Fulminant hepatitis from herpes simplex virus type 2 in an immunocompetent adult. *Transpl Infect Dis* 2007;9:323–6.

47. Rodriguez-Moreno A, Sanchez-Fructuoso AI, Calvo N, et al. Varicella infection in adult renal allograft recipients: experience at one center. *Transplant Proc* 2006;38:2416–18.

48. Anderson DR, Schwartz J, Hunter NJ, et al. Varicella hepatitis: a fatal case in a previously healthy, immunocompetent adult. Report of a case, autopsy, and review of the literature. *Arch Intern Med* 1994;154:2101–6.

49. Ichai P, Roque Afonso AM, Sebagh M, et al. Herpes simplex virus-associated acute liver failure: a difficult diagnosis with a poor prognosis. *Liver Transpl* 2005;11:1550–5.

50. Food and Drug Administration. Kava-containing dietary supplements may be associated with severe liver injury. Food and Drug Administration, 2002 (cited November 26). Available from www.cfsan.fda.gov/~dms/addskava.html.

51. Fontana RJ, McCashland TM, Benner KG, et al. Acute liver failure associated with prolonged use of bromfenac leading to liver transplantation. The Acute Liver Failure Study Group. *Liver Transpl Surg* 1999;5:480–4.

52. Murphy EJ, Davern TJ, Shakil AO, et al. Troglitazone-induced fulminant hepatic failure. Acute Liver Failure Study Group. *Dig Dis Sci* 2000;45:549–53.

53. Larsen FS, Kirkegaard P, Rasmussen A, Hansen BA. The Danish liver transplantation program and patients with serious acetaminophen intoxication. *Transplant Proc* 1995;27:3519–20.

54. Schiodt FV, Rochling FA, Casey DL, Lee WM. Acetaminophen toxicity in an urban county hospital. *N Engl J Med* 1997;337:1112–17.

55. Slattery JT, Nelson SD, Thummel KE. The complex interaction between ethanol and acetaminophen. *Clin Pharmacol Ther* 1996;60:241–6.

56. Zimmerman HJ, Maddrey WC. Acetaminophen (paracetamol) hepatotoxicity with regular intake of alcohol: analysis of instances of therapeutic misadventure. *Hepatology* 1995;22:767–73.

57. Whitcomb DC, Block GD. Association of acetaminophen hepatotoxicity with fasting and ethanol use. *JAMA* 1994;272:1845–50.

58. Seeff LB, Cuccherini BA, Zimmerman HJ, et al. Acetaminophen hepatotoxicity in alcoholics. A therapeutic misadventure. *Ann Intern Med* 1986;104:399–404.

59. Maddrey WC. Hepatic effects of acetaminophen. Enhanced toxicity in alcoholics. *J Clin Gastroenterol* 1987;9:180–5.

60. Watkins PB, Kaplowitz N, Slattery JT, et al. Aminotransferase elevations in healthy adults receiving 4 grams of acetaminophen daily: a randomized controlled trial. *JAMA* 2006;296:87–93.

61. Kuffner EK, Temple AR, Cooper KM, et al. Retrospective analysis of transient elevations in alanine aminotransferase during long-term treatment with acetaminophen in osteoarthritis clinical trials. *Curr Med Res Opin* 2006;22:2137–48.

62. Mitchell JR, Thorgeirsson SS, Potter WZ, et al. Acetaminophen-induced hepatic injury: protective role of glutathione in man and rationale for therapy. *Clin Pharmacol Ther* 1974;16:676–84.

63. Manyike PT, Kharasch ED, Kalhorn TF, Slattery JT. Contribution of CYP2E1 and CYP3A to acetaminophen reactive metabolite formation. *Clin Pharmacol Ther* 2000;67:275–82.

64. Chen W, Koenigs LL, Thompson SJ, et al. Oxidation of acetaminophen to its toxic quinone imine and nontoxic catechol metabolites by baculovirus-expressed and purified human cytochromes P450 2E1 and 2A6. *Chem Res Toxicol* 1998;11:295–301.

65. Thummel KE, Lee CA, Kunze KL, et al. Oxidation of acetaminophen to N-acetyl-p-aminobenzoquinone imine by human CYP3A4. *Biochem Pharmacol* 1993;45:1563–9.

66. Kaplowitz N. Acetaminophen hepatoxicity: what do we know, what don't we know, and what do we do next? *Hepatology* 2004;40:23–6.

67. Eriksson LS, Broome U, Kalin M, Lindholm M. Hepatotoxicity due to repeated intake of low doses of paracetamol. *J Intern Med* 1992;231:567–70.

68. Moling O, Cairon E, Rimenti G, et al. Severe hepatotoxicity after therapeutic doses of acetaminophen. *Clin Ther* 2006;28:755–60.

69. Bray GP, Harrison PM, O'Grady JG, et al. Long-term anticonvulsant therapy worsens outcome in paracetamol-induced fulminant hepatic failure. *Hum Exp Toxicol* 1992;11:265–70.

70. Mutlib AE, Goosen TC, Bauman JN, et al. Kinetics of acetaminophen glucuronidation by UDP-glucuronosyltransferases 1A1, 1A6, 1A9 and 2B15. Potential implications in acetaminophen-induced hepatotoxicity. *Chem Res Toxicol* 2006;19:701–9.

71. McClain CJ, Kromhout JP, Peterson FJ, Holtzman JL. Potentiation of acetaminophen hepatotoxicity by alcohol. *JAMA* 1980;244:251–3.

72. Rumack BH. Acetaminophen hepatotoxicity: the first 35 years. *J Toxicol Clin Toxicol* 2002;40:3–20.

73. Prescott LF. Paracetamol overdosage. Pharmacological considerations and clinical management. *Drugs* 1983;25:290–314.

74. Linden CH, Rumack BH. Acetaminophen overdose. *Emerg Med Clin North Am* 1984;2:103–19.

75. Davern TJ, James LP, Hinson JA, et al. Measurement of serum acetaminophen–protein adducts in patients with acute liver failure. *Gastroenterology* 2006;130:687–94.

76. James LP, Mayeux PR, Hinson JA. Acetaminophen-induced hepatotoxicity. *Drug Metab Dispos* 2003;31:1499–506.

77. Roberts DW, Pumford NR, Potter DW, et al. A sensitive immunochemical assay for acetaminophen–protein adducts. *J Pharmacol Exp Ther* 1987;241:527–33.

78. Pumford NR, Hinson JA, Benson RW, Roberts DW. Immunoblot analysis of protein containing 3-(cystein-S-yl)acetaminophen adducts in serum and subcellular liver fractions from acetaminophen-treated mice. *Toxicol Appl Pharmacol* 1990;104:521–32.

79. Roberts LJ, Morrow JD. Analgesic-antipyretic and antiinflammatory agents and drugs employed in the treatment of gout. In: Brunton L, Lazo J, Parker K, eds. *Goodman and Gilman's the Pharmacological Basis of Therapeutics*, 10th edn. New York: McGraw-Hill, 2001:687–731.

80. Harman AW, Kyle ME, Serroni A, Farber JL. The killing of cultured hepatocytes by N-acetyl-p-benzoquinone imine (NAPQI) as a model of the cytotoxicity of acetaminophen. *Biochem Pharmacol* 1991;41:1111–17.

81. Jaeschke H, Knight TR, Bajt ML. The role of oxidant stress and reactive nitrogen species in acetaminophen hepatotoxicity. *Toxicol Lett* 2003;144:279–88.

82. Jaeschke H, Bajt ML. Intracellular signaling mechanisms of acetaminophen-induced liver cell death. *Toxicol Sci* 2006;89:31–41.

83. Blazka ME, Wilmer JL, Holladay SD, et al. Role of proinflammatory cytokines in acetaminophen hepatotoxicity. *Toxicol Appl Pharmacol* 1995;133:43–52.

84. Liu ZX, Govindarajan S, Kaplowitz N. Innate immune system plays a critical role in determining the progression and severity of acetaminophen hepatotoxicity. *Gastroenterology* 2004;127:1760–74.

85. Liu ZX, Kaplowitz N. Role of innate immunity in acetaminophen-induced hepatotoxicity. *Expert Opin Drug Metab Toxicol* 2006;2:493–503.

86. Ishida Y, Kondo T, Ohshima T, et al. A pivotal involvement of IFN-gamma in the pathogenesis of acetaminophen-induced acute liver injury. *FASEB J* 2002;16:1227–36.

87. Gow PJ, Jones RM, Dobson JL, Angus PW. Etiology and outcome of fulminant hepatic failure managed at an Australian liver transplant unit. *J Gastroenterol Hepatol* 2004;19:154–9.

88. Gow PJ, Smallwood RA, Angus PW. Paracetamol overdose in a liver transplantation centre: an 8-year experience. *J Gastroenterol Hepatol* 1999;14:817–21.

89. Heard K, Sloss D, Weber S, Dart RC. Overuse of over-the-counter analgesics by emergency department patients. *Ann Emerg Med* 2006;48:315–18.

90. Cham E, Hall L, Ernst AA, Weiss SJ. Awareness and use of over-the-counter pain medications: a survey of emergency department patients. *South Med J* 2002;95:529–35.

91. Myers RP, Shaheen AA, Li B, et al. Impact of liver disease, alcohol abuse, and unintentional ingestions on the outcomes of acetaminophen overdose. *Clin Gastroenterol Hepatol* 2008;6:918–25.

92. Fosnocht D, Taylor JR, Caravati EM. Emergency department patient knowledge concerning acetaminophen (paracetamol) in over-the-counter and prescription analgesics. *Emerg Med J* 2008;25:213–16.

93. Smilkstein MJ, Knapp GL, Kulig KW, Rumack BH. Efficacy of oral N-acetylcysteine in the treatment of acetaminophen overdose. Analysis of the national multicenter study (1976 to 1985). *N Engl J Med* 1988;319:1557–62.

94. Escudie L, Francoz C, Vinel JP, et al. *Amanita phalloides* poisoning: reassessment of prognostic factors and indications for emergency liver transplantation. *J Hepatol* 2007;46:466–73.

95. Erguven M, Yilmaz O, Deveci M, et al. Mushroom poisoning. *Indian J Pediatr* 2007;74:847–52.

96. Joshi A, Awale P, Shrestha A, Lee M. Acute mushroom poisoning: a report of 41 cases. *J Nepal Med Assoc* 2007;46:7–12.

97. Diaz JH. Evolving global epidemiology, syndromic classification, general management, and prevention of unknown mushroom poisonings. *Crit Care Med* 2005;33:419–26.

98. Enjalbert F, Rapior S, Nouguier-Soule J, et al. Treatment of amatoxin poisoning: 20-year retrospective analysis. *J Toxicol Clin Toxicol* 2002;40:715–57.

99. Larrey D, Pageaux GP. Hepatotoxicity of herbal remedies and mushrooms. *Semin Liver Dis* 1995;15:183–8.

100. Scheurlen C, Spannbrucker N, Spengler U, et al. *Amanita phalloides* intoxications in a family of russian immigrants. Case reports and review of the literature with a focus on orthotopic liver transplantation. *Z Gastroenterol* 1994;32:399–404.

101. Ganzert M, Felgenhauer N, Zilker T. Reassessment of predictors of fatal outcome in amatoxin poisoning: some critical comments. *J Hepatol* 2007;47:424–5.

102. Ganzert M, Felgenhauer N, Zilker T. Indication of liver transplantation following amatoxin intoxication. *J Hepatol* 2005;42:202–9.

103. Zimmerman HJ. Drug-induced liver disease. In: Schiff E, Sorrell M, Maddrey W, eds. *Schiff's Diseases of the Liver*. Philadelphia, PA: Lippincott-Raven, 1999:973.

104. Jochimsen EM, Carmichael WW, An JS, et al. Liver failure and death after exposure to microcystins at a hemodialysis center in Brazil. *N Engl J Med* 1998;338:873–8.

105. Mahler H, Pasi A, Kramer JM, et al. Fulminant liver failure in association with the emetic toxin of *Bacillus cereus*. *N Engl J Med* 1997;336:1142–8.

106. Gomez-Lechon MJ, Carrasquer J, Berenguer J, Castell JV. Evidence of antibodies to erythromycin in serum of a patient following an episode of acute drug-induced hepatitis. *Clin Exp Allergy* 1996;26:590–6.

107. Lewis JH. Medication-related and other forms of toxic liver injury. In: Brandt LJ, ed. *Clinical Practice of Gastroenterology*. Philadelphia, PA: Churchill Livingstone, 1998:855.

108. Horowitz RS, Feldhaus K, Dart RC, et al. The clinical spectrum of Jin Bu Huan toxicity. *Arch Intern Med* 1996;156:899–903.

109. Katz M, Saibil F. Herbal hepatitis: subacute hepatic necrosis secondary to chaparral leaf. *J Clin Gastroenterol* 1990;12:203–6.

110. Batchelor WB, Heathcote J, Wanless IR. Chaparral-induced hepatic injury. *Am J Gastroenterol* 1995;90:831–3.

111. Larrey D, Vial T, Pauwels A, et al. Hepatitis after germander (*Teucrium chamaedrys*) administration: another instance

of herbal medicine hepatotoxicity. *Ann Intern Med* 1992;117: 129–32.

112. Gow PJ, Connelly NJ, Hill RL, et al. Fatal fulminant hepatic failure induced by a natural therapy containing kava. *Med J Aust* 2003;178:442–3.

113. Lontos S, Jones RM, Angus PW, Gow PJ. Acute liver failure associated with the use of herbal preparations containing black cohosh. *Med J Aust* 2003;179:390–1.

114. Yoshida EM, McLean CA, Cheng ES, et al. Chinese herbal medicine, fulminant hepatitis, and liver transplantation. *Am J Gastroenterol* 1996;91:2647–8.

115. Anderson IB, Mullen WH, Meeker JE, et al. Pennyroyal toxicity: measurement of toxic metabolite levels in two cases and review of the literature. *Ann Intern Med* 1996;124:726–34.

116. Schoepfer AM, Engel A, Fattinger K, et al. Herbal does not mean innocuous: ten cases of severe hepatotoxicity associated with dietary supplements from Herbalife products. *J Hepatol* 2007;47:521–6.

117. Andreu V, Mas A, Bruguera M, et al. Ecstasy: a common cause of severe acute hepatotoxicity. *J Hepatol* 1998;29:394–7.

118. Brauer RB, Heidecke CD, Nathrath W, et al. Liver transplantation for the treatment of fulminant hepatic failure induced by the ingestion of ecstasy. *Transpl Int* 1997;10:229–33.

119. Kanel GC, Cassidy W, Shuster L, Reynolds TB. Cocaine-induced liver cell injury: comparison of morphological features in man and in experimental models. *Hepatology* 1990;11:646–51.

120. Sibai BM, Ramadan MK, Usta I, et al. Maternal morbidity and mortality in 442 pregnancies with hemolysis, elevated liver enzymes, and low platelets (HELLP syndrome). *Am J Obstet Gynecol* 1993;169:1000–6.

121. Wilcken B, Leung KC, Hammond J, et al. Pregnancy and fetal long-chain 3-hydroxyacyl coenzyme A dehydrogenase deficiency. *Lancet* 1993;341:407–8.

122. Treem WR, Rinaldo P, Hale DE, et al. Acute fatty liver of pregnancy and long-chain 3-hydroxyacyl-coenzyme A dehydrogenase deficiency. *Hepatology* 1994;19:339–45.

123. Rahman TM, Wendon J. Severe hepatic dysfunction in pregnancy. *Q J Med* 2002;95:343–57.

124. Santos RG, Alissa F, Reyes J, et al. Fulminant hepatic failure: Wilson's disease or autoimmune hepatitis? Implications for transplantation. *Pediatr Transplant* 2005;9:112–16.

125. Kessler WR, Cummings OW, Eckert G, et al. Fulminant hepatic failure as the initial presentation of acute autoimmune hepatitis. *Clin Gastroenterol Hepatol* 2004;2:625–31.

126. Ferrari R, Pappas G, Agostinelli D, et al. Type 1 autoimmune hepatitis: patterns of clinical presentation and differential diagnosis of the 'acute' type. *Q J Med* 2004;97:407–12.

127. Krawitt EL. Autoimmune hepatitis. *N Engl J Med* 2006;354:54–66.

128. Ala A, Schilsky ML. Wilson disease: pathophysiology, diagnosis, treatment, and screening. *Clin Liver Dis* 2004;8:787–805, viii.

129. McCullough AJ, Fleming CR, Thistle JL, et al. Diagnosis of Wilson's disease presenting as fulminant hepatic failure. *Gastroenterology* 1983;84:161–7.

130. Eisenbach C, Sieg O, Stremmel W, et al. Diagnostic criteria for acute liver failure due to Wilson disease. *World J Gastroenterol* 2007;13:1711–14.

131. Emre S, Atillasoy EO, Ozdemir S, et al. Orthotopic liver transplantation for Wilson's disease: a single-center experience. *Transplantation* 2001;72:1232–6.

132. Sallie R, Katsiyiannakis L, Baldwin D, et al. Failure of simple biochemical indexes to reliably differentiate fulminant Wilson's disease from other causes of fulminant liver failure. *Hepatology* 1992;16:1206–11.

133. Shaver WA, Bhatt H, Combes B. Low serum alkaline phosphatase activity in Wilson's disease. *Hepatology* 1986;6:859–63.

134. Korman JD, Volenberg I, Balko J, et al. Screening for Wilson disease in acute liver failure: a comparison of currently available diagnostic tests. *Hepatology* 2008;48:1167–74.

135. Henrion J. Hypoxic hepatitis: the point of view of the clinician. *Acta Gastroenterol Belg* 2007;70:214–16.

136. Birrer R, Takuda Y, Takara T. Hypoxic hepatopathy: pathophysiology and prognosis. *Intern Med* 2007;46:1063–70.

137. Segev DL, Nguyen GC, Locke JE, et al. Twenty years of liver transplantation for Budd–Chiari syndrome: a national registry analysis. *Liver Transpl* 2007;13:1285–94.

138. Dellon ES, Morris SR, Tang W, et al. Acute liver failure due to natural killer-like T-cell leukemia/lymphoma: a case report and review of the literature. *World J Gastroenterol* 2006;12:4089–92.

139. El-Sayed MH, El-Haddad A, Fahmy OA, et al. Liver disease is a major cause of mortality following allogeneic bone-marrow transplantation. *Eur J Gastroenterol Hepatol* 2004;16:1347–54.

140. Stillman AS, Huxtable R, Consroe P, et al. Hepatic veno-occlusive disease due to pyrrolizidine (*Senecio*) poisoning in Arizona. *Gastroenterology* 1977;73:349–52.

141. McDonald GB, Hinds MS, Fisher LD, et al. Veno-occlusive disease of the liver and multiorgan failure after bone marrow transplantation: a cohort study of 355 patients. *Ann Intern Med* 1993;118: 255–67.

142. Rowbotham D, Wendon J, Williams R. Acute liver failure secondary to hepatic infiltration: a single centre experience of 18 cases. *Gut* 1998;42:576–80.

143. Riordan SM, Williams R. Mechanisms of hepatocyte injury, multiorgan failure, and prognostic criteria in acute liver failure. *Semin Liver Dis* 2003;23:203–15.

144. Kaplowitz N. Mechanisms of liver cell injury. *J Hepatol* 2000; 32(Suppl 1):39–47.

145. Strand S, Hofmann WJ, Grambihler A, et al. Hepatic failure and liver cell damage in acute Wilson's disease involve CD95 (APO-1/Fas) mediated apoptosis. *Nat Med* 1998;4:588–93.

146. Larson AM. Acute liver failure. *Dis Mon* 2008;54:457–85.

147. O'Grady JG, Alexander GJ, Hayllar KM, Williams R. Early indicators of prognosis in fulminant hepatic failure. *Gastroenterology* 1989;97:439–45.

148. Stravitz RT, Kramer AH, Davern T, et al. Intensive care of patients with acute liver failure: recommendations of the US Acute Liver Failure Study Group. *Crit Care Med* 2007;35:2498–508.

149. Wade J, Rolando N, Philpott-Howard J, Wendon J. Timing and aetiology of bacterial infections in a liver intensive care unit. *J Hosp Infect* 2003;53:144–6.

150. Stravitz RT, Kramer DJ. Management of acute liver failure. *Nat Rev Gastroenterol Hepatol* 2009;6:542–53.

151. Bernal W, Hall C, Karvellas CJ, et al. Arterial ammonia and clinical risk factors for encephalopathy and intracranial hypertension in acute liver failure. *Hepatology* 2007;46:1844–52.

152. Bhatia V, Singh R, Acharya SK. Predictive value of arterial ammonia for complications and outcome in acute liver failure. *Gut* 2006;55:98–104.

153. Belanger M, Butterworth RF. Acute liver failure: a critical appraisal of available animal models. *Metab Brain Dis* 2005;20: 409–3.

154. Butterworth RF. Pathophysiology of hepatic encephalopathy: a new look at ammonia. *Metab Brain Dis* 2002;17:221–7.

155. Wendon J, Lee W. Encephalopathy and cerebral edema in the setting of acute liver failure: pathogenesis and management. *Neurocrit Care* 2008;9:97–102.

156. Rolando N, Wade J, Davalos M, et al. The systemic inflammatory response syndrome in acute liver failure. *Hepatology* 2000; 32(4):734–9.

157. Jalan R, Rose C. Hypothermia in acute liver failure. *Metab Brain Dis* 2004;19:215–21.

158. Clemmesen JO, Larsen FS, Kondrup J, et al. Cerebral herniation in patients with acute liver failure is correlated with arterial ammonia concentration. *Hepatology* 1999;29:648–53.

159. Norenberg MD, Jayakumar AR, Rama Rao KV, Panickar KS. New concepts in the mechanism of ammonia-induced astrocyte swelling. *Metab Brain Dis* 2007;22:219–34.

160. Haussinger D, Kircheis G, Fischer R, et al. Hepatic encephalopathy in chronic liver disease: a clinical manifestation of astrocyte swelling and low-grade cerebral edema? *J Hepatol* 2000;32:1035–8.

161. Ranjan P, Mishra AM, Kale R, et al. Cytotoxic edema is responsible for raised intracranial pressure in fulminant hepatic failure: in vivo demonstration using diffusion-weighted MRI in human subjects. *Metab Brain Dis* 2005;20:181–92.

162. Jiang W, Desjardins P, Butterworth RF. Hypothermia attenuates oxidative/nitrosative stress, encephalopathy and brain edema in acute (ischemic) liver failure. *Neurochem Int* 2009;55:124–8.

163. Kitzberger R, Funk GC, Holzinger U, et al. Severity of organ failure is an independent predictor of intracranial hypertension in acute liver failure. *Clin Gastroenterol Hepatol* 2009;7:1000–6.

164. Jalan R, Olde Damink SW, Hayes PC, et al. Pathogenesis of intracranial hypertension in acute liver failure: inflammation, ammonia and cerebral blood flow. *J Hepatol* 2004;41:613–20.

165. Ellis AJ, Wendon JA, Williams R. Subclinical seizure activity and prophylactic phenytoin infusion in acute liver failure: a controlled clinical trial. *Hepatology* 2000;32:536–41.

166. Alba L, Hay J, Angelo P, Lee WM. Lactulose therapy in acute liver failure (Abstract). *J Hepatol* 2002;36:33A.

167. Ede RJ, Gimson AE, Bihari D, Williams R. Controlled hyperventilation in the prevention of cerebral oedema in fulminant hepatic failure. *J Hepatol* 1986;2:43–51.

168. Bass NM. Monitoring and treatment of intracranial hypertension. *Liver Transpl* 2000;6(4 Suppl 1):S21–6.

169. Stravitz RT, Larsen FS. Therapeutic hypothermia for acute liver failure. *Crit Care Med* 2009;37(Suppl7):S258–64.

170. Bernuau J, Durand F. Intracranial pressure monitoring in patients with acute liver failure: a questionable invasive surveillance. *Hepatology* 2006;44:502–4.

171. Keays RT, Alexander GJ, Williams R. The safety and value of extradural intracranial pressure monitors in fulminant hepatic failure. *J Hepatol* 1993;18:205–9.

172. Philips BJ, Armstrong IR, Pollock A, Lee A. Cerebral blood flow and metabolism in patients with chronic liver disease undergoing orthotopic liver transplantation. *Hepatology* 1998;27:369–76.

173. Gasco J, Rangel-Castilla L, Franklin B, et al. State-of-the-art management and monitoring of brain edema and intracranial hypertension in fulminant hepatic failure. A proposed algorithm. *Acta Neurochir Suppl* 2010;106:311–14.

174. Lidofsky SD, Bass NM, Prager MC, et al. Intracranial pressure monitoring and liver transplantation for fulminant hepatic failure. *Hepatology* 1992;16:1–7.

175. Munoz SJ, Moritz MJ, Martin P, et al. Relationship between cerebral perfusion pressure and systemic hemodynamics in fulminant hepatic failure. *Transplant Proc* 1993;25:1776–8.

176. Wendon JA, Harrison PM, Keays R, Williams R. Cerebral blood flow and metabolism in fulminant liver failure. *Hepatology* 1994;19:1407–13.

177. Canalese J, Gimson AE, Davis C, et al. Controlled trial of dexamethasone and mannitol for the cerebral oedema of fulminant hepatic failure. *Gut* 1982;23:625–9.

178. Forbes A, Alexander GJ, O'Grady JG, et al. Thiopental infusion in the treatment of intracranial hypertension complicating fulminant hepatic failure. *Hepatology* 1989;10:306–10.

179. Murphy N, Auzinger G, Bernel W, Wendon J. The effect of hypertonic sodium chloride on intracranial pressure in patients with acute liver failure. *Hepatology* 2004;39:464–70.

180. Dmello D, Cruz-Flores S, Matuschak GM. Moderate hypothermia with intracranial pressure monitoring as a therapeutic paradigm for the management of acute liver failure: a systematic review. *Intensive Care Med* 2010;36:210–13.

181. Vaquero J, Belanger M, James L, et al. Mild hypothermia attenuates liver injury and improves survival in mice with acetaminophen toxicity. *Gastroenterology* 2007;132:372–83.

182. Bhatia V, Batra Y, Acharya SK. Prophylactic phenytoin does not improve cerebral edema or survival in acute liver failure – a controlled clinical trial. *J Hepatol* 2004;41:89–96.

183. Wilkinson SP, Arroyo V, Gazzard BG, et al. Relation of renal impairment and haemorrhagic diathesis to endotoxaemia in fulminant hepatic failure. *Lancet* 1974;1:521–4.

184. Bihari D, Gimson AE, Lindridge J, Williams R. Lactic acidosis in fulminant hepatic failure. Some aspects of pathogenesis and prognosis. *J Hepatol* 1985;1:405–16.

185. Shawcross DL, Davies NA, Mookerjee RP, et al. Worsening of cerebral hyperemia by the administration of terlipressin in acute liver failure with severe encephalopathy. *Hepatology* 2004;39:471–5.

186. Eefsen M, Dethloff T, Frederiksen HJ, et al. Comparison of terlipressin and noradrenalin on cerebral perfusion, intracranial pressure and cerebral extracellular concentrations of lactate and pyruvate in patients with acute liver failure in need of inotropic support. *J Hepatol* 2007;47:381–6.

187. O'Grady JG, Langley PG, Isola LM, et al. Coagulopathy of fulminant hepatic failure. *Semin Liver Dis* 1986;6:159–63.

188. Lisman T, Leebeek FW. Hemostatic alterations in liver disease: a review on pathophysiology, clinical consequences, and treatment. *Dig Surg* 2007;24:250–8.

189. Munoz SJ, Rajender RK, Lee W. The coagulopathy of acute liver failure and implications for intracranial pressure monitoring. *Neurocrit Care* 2008;9:103–7.

190. Kerr R, Newsome P, Germain L, et al. Effects of acute liver injury on blood coagulation. *J Thromb Haemost* 2003;1:754–9.

191. Harrison PM, O'Grady JG, Keays RT, et al. Serial prothrombin time as prognostic indicator in paracetamol induced fulminant hepatic failure. *Br Med J* 1990;301:964–6.

192. Stravitz RT. Critical management decisions in patients with acute liver failure. *Chest* 2008;134:1092–102.

193. Fontana RJ. Acute liver failure including acetaminophen overdose. *Med Clin North Am* 2008;92:761–94, viii.

194. Shami VM, Caldwell SH, Hespenheide EE, et al. Recombinant activated factor VII for coagulopathy in fulminant hepatic failure compared with conventional therapy. *Liver Transpl* 2003;9:138–43.

195. Pernambuco JR, Langley PG, Hughes RD, et al. Activation of the fibrinolytic system in patients with fulminant liver failure. *Hepatology* 1993;18:1350–6.

196. Schiodt FV, Balko J, Schilsky M, Harrison ME, Thornton A, Lee WM. Thrombopoietin in acute liver failure. *Hepatology* 2003;37:558–61.

197. Wilkinson SP, Moodie H, Arroyo VA, Williams R. Frequency of renal impairment in paracetamol overdose compared with other causes of acute liver damage. *J Clin Pathol* 1977;30:141–3.

198. Ring-Larsen H, Palazzo U. Renal failure in fulminant hepatic failure and terminal cirrhosis: a comparison between incidence, types, and prognosis. *Gut* 1981;22:585–91.

199. Wilkinson SP, Portmann B, Hurst D, Williams R. Pathogenesis of renal failure in cirrhosis and fulminant hepatic failure. *Postgrad Med J* 1975;51:503–5.

200. Guarner F, Hughes RD, Gimson AE, Williams R. Renal function in fulminant hepatic failure: haemodynamics and renal prostaglandins. *Gut* 1987;28:1643–7.

201. Leithead JA, Ferguson JW, Bates CM, et al. The systemic inflammatory response syndrome is predictive of renal dysfunction in patients with non-paracetamol-induced acute liver failure. *Gut* 2009;58:443–9.

202. Davenport A, Will EJ, Davidson AM. Improved cardiovascular stability during continuous modes of renal replacement therapy in critically ill patients with acute hepatic and renal failure. *Crit Care Med* 1993;21:328–38.

203. Rolando N, Harvey F, Brahm J, et al. Fungal infection: a common, unrecognised complication of acute liver failure. *J Hepatol* 1991;12:1–9.

204. Salmeron JM, Tito L, Rimola A, et al. Selective intestinal decontamination in the prevention of bacterial infection in patients with acute liver failure. *J Hepatol* 1992;14:280–5.

205. Karvellas CJ, Pink F, McPhail M, et al. Predictors of bacteraemia and mortality in patients with acute liver failure. *Intensive Care Med* 2009;35:1390–6.

206. Wilkinson SP, Arroyo VA, Moodie H, et al. Abnormalities of sodium excretion and other disorders of renal function in fulminant hepatic failure. *Gut* 1976;17:501–5.

207. Macquillan GC, Seyam MS, Nightingale P, et al. Blood lactate but not serum phosphate levels can predict patient outcome in fulminant hepatic failure. *Liver Transpl* 2005;11:1073–9.

208. Schmidt LE, Dalhoff K. Serum phosphate is an early predictor of outcome in severe acetaminophen-induced hepatotoxicity. *Hepatology* 2002;36:659–65.

209. Chung PY, Sitrin MD, Te HS. Serum phosphorus levels predict clinical outcome in fulminant hepatic failure. *Liver Transpl* 2003;9:248–53.

210. Baquerizo A, Anselmo D, Shackleton C, et al. Phosphorus as an early predictive factor in patients with acute liver failure. *Transplantation* 2003;75:2007–14.

211. Trewby PN, Warren R, Contini S, et al. Incidence and pathophysiology of pulmonary edema in fulminant hepatic failure. *Gastroenterology* 1978;74:859–65.

212. Williams A, Trewby P, Williams R, Reid L. Structural alterations to the pulmonary circulation in fulminant hepatic failure. *Thorax* 1979;34:447–53.

213. Walsh TS, Wigmore SJ, Hopton P, et al. Energy expenditure in acetaminophen-induced fulminant hepatic failure. *Crit Care Med* 2000;28:649–54.

214. McCullough AJ, Tavill AS. Disordered energy and protein metabolism in liver disease. *Semin Liver Dis* 1991;11:265–77.

215. Fryburg DA, Jahn LA, Hill SA, et al. Insulin and insulin-like growth factor-I enhance human skeletal muscle protein anabolism during hyperaminoacidemia by different mechanisms. J Clin Invest 1995;96:1722–9.

216. Qiu JG, Delany HM, Teh EL, et al. Contrasting effects of identical nutrients given parenterally or enterally after 70% hepatectomy: bacterial translocation. *Nutrition* 1997;13:431–7.

217. Polson J, Wians FH Jr, Orsulak P, et al. False positive acetaminophen concentrations in patients with liver injury. *Clin Chim Acta* 2008;391:24–30.

218. Muldrew KL, James LP, Coop L, et al. Determination of acetaminophen–protein adducts in mouse liver and serum and human serum after hepatotoxic doses of acetaminophen using high-performance liquid chromatography with electrochemical detection. *Drug Metab Dispos* 2002;30:446–51.

219. Ambre J, Alexander M. Liver toxicity after acetaminophen ingestion. Inadequacy of the dose estimate as an index of risk. *JAMA* 1977;238:500–1.

220. Gregory B, Larson AM, Reisch J, Lee WM. Acetaminophen dose does not predict outcome in acetaminophen-induced acute liver failure. *J Investig Med* 2010;58:707–10.

221. Daly FF, O'Malley GF, Heard K, et al. Prospective evaluation of repeated supratherapeutic acetaminophen (paracetamol) ingestion. *Ann Emerg Med* 2004;44:393–8.

222. Sivilotti ML, Yarema MC, Juurlink DN, et al. A risk quantification instrument for acute acetaminophen overdose patients treated with N-acetylcysteine. *Ann Emerg Med* 2005;46:263–71.

223. McNamara RM, Aaron CK, Gemborys M, Davidheiser S. Efficacy of charcoal cathartic versus ipecac in reducing serum acetaminophen in a simulated overdose. *Ann Emerg Med* 1989;18:934–8.

224. Heard KJ. Acetylcysteine for acetaminophen poisoning. *N Engl J Med* 2008;359:285–92.

225. Prescott LF, Illingworth RN, Critchley JA, Proudfoot AT. Intravenous N-acetylcysteine: still the treatment of choice for paracetamol poisoning. *Br Med J* 1980;280:46–7.

226. Keays R, Harrison PM, Wendon JA, et al. Intravenous acetylcysteine in paracetamol induced fulminant hepatic failure: a prospective controlled trial. *Br Med J* 1991;303:1026–9.

227. Jones AL. Mechanism of action and value of N-acetylcysteine in the treatment of early and late acetaminophen poisoning: a critical review. *J Toxicol Clin Toxicol* 1998;36:277–85.

228. Burkhart KK, Janco N, Kulig KW, Rumack BH. Cimetidine as adjunctive treatment for acetaminophen overdose. *Hum Exp Toxicol* 1995;14:299–304.

229. Lin JH, Levy G. Sulfate depletion after acetaminophen administration and replenishment by infusion of sodium sulfate or N-acetylcysteine in rats. *Biochem Pharmacol* 1981;30:2723–5.

230. Corcoran GB, Todd EL, Racz WJ, et al. Effects of N-acetylcysteine on the disposition and metabolism of acetaminophen in mice. *J Pharmacol Exp Ther* 1985;232:857–63.

231. Slattery JT, Wilson JM, Kalhorn TF, Nelson SD. Dose-dependent pharmacokinetics of acetaminophen: evidence of glutathione depletion in humans. *Clin Pharmacol Ther* 1987;41:413–18.

232. Harrison PM, Keays R, Bray GP, et al. Improved outcome of paracetamol-induced fulminant hepatic failure by late administration of acetylcysteine. *Lancet* 1990;335:1572–3.

233. Harrison PM, Wendon JA, Gimson AE, et al. Improvement by acetylcysteine of hemodynamics and oxygen transport in fulminant hepatic failure. *N Engl J Med* 1991;324:1852–7.

234. Dambach DM, Durham SK, Laskin JD, Laskin DL. Distinct roles of NF-kappaB p50 in the regulation of acetaminophen-induced inflammatory mediator production and hepatotoxicity. *Toxicol Appl Pharmacol* 2006;211:157–65.

235. Gardner CR, Laskin JD, Dambach DM, et al. Exaggerated hepatotoxicity of acetaminophen in mice lacking tumor necrosis factor receptor-1. Potential role of inflammatory mediators. *Toxicol Appl Pharmacol* 2003;192:119–30.

236. Mant TG, Tempowski JH, Volans GN, Talbot JC. Adverse reactions to acetylcysteine and effects of overdose. *Br Med J (Clin Res Ed)* 1984;289:217–19.

237. Dawson AH, Henry DA, McEwen J. Adverse reactions to N-acetylcysteine during treatment for paracetamol poisoning. *Med J Aust* 1989;150:329–31.

238. Bailey B, McGuigan MA. Management of anaphylactoid reactions to intravenous N-acetylcysteine. *Ann Emerg Med* 1998;31:710–15.

239. Kanter MZ. Comparison of oral and i.v. acetylcysteine in the treatment of acetaminophen poisoning. *Am J Health Syst Pharm* 2006;63:1821–7.

240. Yang R, Miki K, He X, et al. Prolonged treatment with N-acetylcysteine delays liver recovery from acetaminophen hepatotoxicity. *Crit Care* 2009;13:R55.

241. Manov I, Hirsh M, Iancu TC. N-acetylcysteine does not protect HepG2 cells against acetaminophen-induced apoptosis. *Basic Clin Pharmacol Toxicol* 2004;94:213–25.

242. Ichai P, Duclos-Vallee JC, Guettier C, et al. Usefulness of corticosteroids for the treatment of severe and fulminant forms of autoimmune hepatitis. *Liver Transpl* 2007;13:996–1003.

243. Viruet EJ, Torres EA. Steroid therapy in fulminant hepatic failure secondary to autoimmune hepatitis. *P R Health Sci J* 1998;17:297–300.

244. Czaja AJ. Corticosteroids or not in severe acute or fulminant autoimmune hepatitis: therapeutic brinksmanship and the point beyond salvation. *Liver Transpl* 2007;13:953–5.

245. Bellary S, Hassanein T, Van Thiel DH. Liver transplantation for Wilson's disease. *J Hepatol* 1995;23:373–81.

246. Rodriguez FE, Tremosa LG, Xiol Q, et al. D-penicillamine and plasmapheresis in acute liver failure secondary to Wilson's disease. *Rev Esp Enferm Dig* 2003;95:60–5.

247. Asfaha S, Almansori M, Qarni U, Gutfreund KS. Plasmapheresis for hemolytic crisis and impending acute liver failure in Wilson disease. *J Clin Apher* 2007;22:295–8.

248. Broussard CN, Aggarwal A, Lacey SR, et al. Mushroom poisoning – from diarrhea to liver transplantation. *Am J Gastroenterol* 2001;96:3195–8.

249. Magdalan J, Ostrowska A, Piotrowska A, et al. Failure of benzylpenicillin, *N*-acetylcysteine and silibinin to reduce alpha-amanitin hepatotoxicity. *In Vivo* 2009;23:393–9.

250. Tong TC, Hernandez M, Richardson WH III, et al. Comparative treatment of alpha-amanitin poisoning with *N*-acetylcysteine, benzylpenicillin, cimetidine, thioctic acid, and silybin in a murine model. *Ann Emerg Med* 2007;50:282–8.

251. Hruby K, Csomos G, Fuhrmann M, Thaler H. Chemotherapy of *Amanita phalloides* poisoning with intravenous silibinin. *Hum Toxicol* 1983;2:183–95.

252. Wellington K, Jarvis B. Silymarin: a review of its clinical properties in the management of hepatic disorders. *BioDrugs* 2001;15:465–89.

253. Kumar M, Satapathy S, Monga R, et al. A randomized controlled trial of lamivudine to treat acute hepatitis B. *Hepatology* 2007;45:97–101.

254. Yu JW, Sun LJ, Zhao YH, et al. The study of efficacy of lamivudine in patients with severe acute hepatitis B. *Dig Dis Sci* 2010;55:775–83.

255. Levitsky J, Duddempudi AT, Lakeman FD, et al. Detection and diagnosis of herpes simplex virus infection in adults with acute liver failure. *Liver Transpl* 2008;14:1498–504.

256. Lee WM, Hynan LS, Rossaro L, et al. Intravenous *N*-acetylcysteine improves transplant-free survival in early stage non-acetaminophen acute liver failure. *Gastroenterology* 2009;137:856–64.

257. Jalan R, Shawcross D, Davies N. The molecular pathogenesis of hepatic encephalopathy. *Int J Biochem Cell Biol* 2003;35:1175–81.

258. Stravitz RT, Lee WM, Kramer AH, et al. Therapeutic hypothermia for acute liver failure: toward a randomized, controlled trial in patients with advanced hepatic encephalopathy. *Neurocrit Care* 2008;9:90–6.

259. Vaquero J, Rose C, Butterworth RF. Keeping cool in acute liver failure: rationale for the use of mild hypothermia. *J Hepatol* 2005;43:1067–77.

260. Stange J, Mitzner SR, Risler T, et al. Molecular adsorbent recycling system (MARS): clinical results of a new membrane-based blood purification system for bioartificial liver support. *Artif Organs* 1999;23:319–30.

261. Steiner C, Sen S, Stange J, et al. Binding of bilirubin and bromosulphthalein to albumin: implications for understanding the pathophysiology of liver failure and its management. *Liver Transpl* 2004;10:1531–8.

262. Khuroo MS, Khuroo MS, Farahat KL. Molecular adsorbent recirculating system for acute and acute-on-chronic liver failure: a meta-analysis. *Liver Transpl* 2004;10:1099–106.

263. Falkenhagen D, Strobl W, Vogt G, et al. Fractionated plasma separation and adsorption system: a novel system for blood purification to remove albumin bound substances. *Artif Organs* 1999;23:81–6.

264. Rifai K, Manns MP. Review article: clinical experience with Prometheus. *Ther Apher Dial* 2006;10:132–7.

265. Allen JW, Hassanein T, Bhatia SN. Advances in bioartificial liver devices. *Hepatology* 2001;34:447–55.

266. Ellis AJ, Hughes RD, Nicholl D, et al. Temporary extracorporeal liver support for severe acute alcoholic hepatitis using the BioLogic-DT. *Int J Artif Organs* 1999;22:27–34.

267. Ellis AJ, Hughes RD, Wendon JA, et al. Pilot-controlled trial of the extracorporeal liver assist device in acute liver failure. *Hepatology* 1996;24:1446–51.

268. Demetriou AA, Brown RS Jr, Busuttil RW, et al. Prospective, randomized, multicenter, controlled trial of a bioartificial liver in treating acute liver failure. *Ann Surg* 2004;239:660–7.

269. Millis JM, Losanoff JE. Technology insight: liver support systems. *Nat Clin Pract Gastroenterol Hepatol* 2005;2:398–405.

270. Sauer IM, Kardassis D, Zeillinger K, et al. Clinical extracorporeal hybrid liver support – phase I study with primary porcine liver cells. *Xenotransplantation* 2003;10:460–9.

271. Patzer JF, Lopez RC, Aggarwal S. Intracranial pressure observations in a canine model of acute liver failure supported by a bioartificial liver support system. *Artif Organs* 2007;31:834–9.

272. Sosef MN, Abrahamse LS, van de Kerkhove MP, et al. Assessment of the AMC-bioartificial liver in the anhepatic pig. *Transplantation* 2002;73:204–9.

273. Millis JM, Cronin DC, Johnson R, et al. Initial experience with the modified extracorporeal liver-assist device for patients with fulminant hepatic failure: system modifications and clinical impact. *Transplantation* 2002;74:1735–46.

274. Freeman RB Jr, Steffick DE, Guidinger MK, et al. Liver and intestine transplantation in the United States, 1997–2006. *Am J Transplant* 2008;8:958–76.

275. Barshes NR, Lee TC, Balkrishnan R, et al. Risk stratification of adult patients undergoing orthotopic liver transplantation for fulminant hepatic failure. *Transplantation* 2006;81:195–201.

276. Adam R, Cailliez V, Majno P, et al. Normalised intrinsic mortality risk in liver transplantation: European Liver Transplant Registry study. *Lancet* 2000;356:621–7.

277. Uemoto S, Inomata Y, Sukarai T. Living donor liver transplantation for fulminant hepatic failure. *Transplantation* 2000;70:152–7.

278. Liu CL, Fan ST, Lo CM, et al. Right-lobe live donor liver transplantation improves survival of patients with acute liver failure. *Br J Surg* 2002;89:317–22.

279. Nishizaki T, Hiroshige S, Ikegami T, et al. Living-donor liver transplantation for fulminant hepatic failure in adult patients with a left-lobe graft. *Surgery* 2002;131:S182–9.

280. Campsen J, Blei AT, Emond JC, et al. Outcomes of living donor liver transplantation for acute liver failure: the adult-to-adult living donor liver transplantation cohort study. *Liver Transpl* 2008;14:1273–80.

281. Kiuchi T, Kasahara M, Uryuhara K. Impact of graft size mismatching on graft prognosis in liver transplantation from living donors. *Transplantation* 1999;67:321–7.

282. Yasutomi M, Uemoto S, Inomata Y, Tanaka K. Liver failure following living donor liver transplantation for fulminant hepatic failure. *Transplant Proc* 2000;32:2133.

283. Ghobrial RM, Freise CE, Trotter JF, et al. Donor morbidity after living donation for liver transplantation. *Gastroenterology* 2008;135:468–76.

284. Fan ST, Lo CM, Liu CL, et al. Biliary reconstruction and complications of right lobe live donor liver transplantation. *Ann Surg* 2002;236:676–83.

285. Man K, Fan ST, Lo CM, et al. Graft injury in relation to graft size in right lobe live donor liver transplantation: a study of hepatic sinusoidal injury in correlation with portal hemodynamics and intragraft gene expression. *Ann Surg* 2003;237:256–64.

286. Toso C, Al-Qahtani M, Alsaif FA. ABO-incompatible liver transplantation for critically ill adult patients. *Transplant Int* 2007;20:675–81.

287. Van Hoek B, de Boer J, Boudjema K, et al. Auxiliary versus orthotopic liver transplantation for acute liver failure. EURALT Study Group. European Auxiliary Liver Transplant Registry. *J Hepatol* 1999;30:699–705.

288. Villamil F, Yantorno SET, Kremers W. MELD is superior to King's College and Clichy criteria to assess prognosis in fulminant hepatic failure. *Liver Transpl* 2007;13:822–8.

289. Wigg AJ, Gunson BK, Mutimer DJ. Outcomes following liver transplantation for seronegative acute liver failure: experience during a 12-year period with more than 100 patients. *Liver Transpl* 2005;11:27–34.

290. Chenard-Neu MP, Boudjema K, Bernuau J, et al. Auxiliary liver transplantation: regeneration of the native liver and outcome in 30 patients with fulminant hepatic failure – a multicenter European study. *Hepatology* 1996;23:1119–27.

291. Boudjema K, Bachellier P, Wolf P, et al. Auxiliary liver transplantation and bioartificial bridging procedures in treatment of acute liver failure. *World J Surg* 2002;26:264–74.

292. Bernal W, Wendon J, Rela M, et al. Use and outcome of liver transplantation in acetaminophen-induced acute liver failure. *Hepatology* 1998;27:1050–5.

293. Simpson KJ, Bates CM, Henderson NC, et al. The utilization of liver transplantation in the management of acute liver failure: comparison between acetaminophen and non-acetaminophen etiologies. *Liver Transpl* 2009;15:600–9.

294. Bismuth H, Samuel D, Castaing D, et al. Orthotopic liver transplantation in fulminant and subfulminant hepatitis. The Paul Brousse experience. *Ann Surg* 1995;222:109–19.

295. Pereira LM, Langley PG, Hayllar KM, et al. Coagulation factor V and VIII/V ratio as predictors of outcome in paracetamol induced fulminant hepatic failure: relation to other prognostic indicators. *Gut* 1992;33:98–102.

296. Schiodt FV, Rossaro L, Stravitz RT, et al. Gc-globulin and prognosis in acute liver failure. *Liver Transpl* 2005;11:1223–7.

297. Bernuau J, Goudeau A, Poynard T, et al. Multivariate analysis of prognostic factors in fulminant hepatitis B. *Hepatology* 1986;6:648–51.

298. Bernuau J, Samuel D, Durand F. Criteria for emergency liver transplantation in patients with acute viral hepatitis and factor V below 50% of normal: a prospective study (Abstract). *Hepatology* 1991;14:abstract 49A.

299. Antoniades CG, Berry PA, Bruce M, et al. Actin-free Gc globulin: a rapidly assessed biomarker of organ dysfunction in acute liver failure and cirrhosis. *Liver Transpl* 2007;13:1254–61.

300. Itai Y, Sekiyama K, Ahmadi T, et al. Fulminant hepatic failure: observation with serial CT. *Radiology* 1997;202:379–82.

301. Van Thiel DH. When should a decision to proceed with transplantation actually be made in cases of fulminant or subfulminant hepatic failure: at admission to hospital or when a donor organ is made available? *J Hepatol* 1993;17:1–2.

302. Shakil AO, Jones BC, Lee RG, et al. Prognostic value of abdominal CT scanning and hepatic histopathology in patients with acute liver failure. *Dig Dis Sci* 2000;45:334–9.

303. Craig DG, Ford AC, Hayes PC, Simpson KJ. Systematic review: prognostic tests of paracetamol-induced acute liver failure. *Aliment Pharmacol Ther* 2010;31:1064–76.

304. Bailey B, Amre DK, Gaudreault P. Fulminant hepatic failure secondary to acetaminophen poisoning: a systematic review and meta-analysis of prognostic criteria determining the need for liver transplantation. *Crit Care Med* 2003;31:299–305.

305. Bernal W, Donaldson N, Wyncoll D, Wendon J. Blood lactate as an early predictor of outcome in paracetamol-induced acute liver failure: a cohort study. *Lancet* 2002;359:558–63.

306. Pauwels A, Mostefa-Kara N, Florent C, Levy VG. Emergency liver transplantation for acute liver failure. Evaluation of London and Clichy criteria. *J Hepatol* 1993;17:124–7.

307. Anand AC, Nightingale P, Neuberger JM. Early indicators of prognosis in fulminant hepatic failure: an assessment of the King's criteria. *J Hepatol* 1997;26:62–8.

308. Renner EL. How to decide when to list a patient with acute liver failure for liver transplantation? Clichy or King's College criteria, or something else? *J Hepatol* 2007;46:554–7.

309. Schmidt LE, Larsen FS. Prognostic implications of hyperlactatemia, multiple organ failure, and systemic inflammatory response syndrome in patients with acetaminophen-induced acute liver failure. *Crit Care Med* 2006;34:337–43.

310. Izumi S, Langley PG, Wendon J, et al. Coagulation factor V levels as a prognostic indicator in fulminant hepatic failure. *Hepatology* 1996;23:1507–11.

311. Schiodt FV, Ostapowicz G, Murray N, et al. Alpha-fetoprotein and prognosis in acute liver failure. *Liver Transpl* 2006;12:1776–81.

312. Schmidt LE, Dalhoff K. Alpha-fetoprotein is a predictor of outcome in acetaminophen-induced liver injury. *Hepatology* 2005;41:26–31.

313. Tofteng F, Hauerberg J, Hansen BA, et al. Persistent arterial hyperammonemia increases the concentration of glutamine and alanine in the brain and correlates with intracranial pressure in patients with fulminant hepatic failure. *J Cereb Blood Flow Metab* 2006;26:21–7.

314. Schmidt LE, Larsen FS. MELD score as a predictor of liver failure and death in patients with acetaminophen-induced liver injury. *Hepatology* 2007;45:789–96.

315. Dhiman RK, Jain S, Maheshwari U, et al. Early indicators of prognosis in fulminant hepatic failure: an assessment of the Model for End-Stage Liver Disease (MELD) and King's College Hospital criteria. *Liver Transpl* 2007;13:814–21.

316. Scotto J, Opolon P, Eteve J, et al. Liver biopsy and prognosis in acute liver failure. *Gut* 1973;14:927–33.

317. Voigt M, Onwuameze O, LaBrecque D. Liver biopsy to predict mortality in fulminant hepatic failure. *Hepatology* 2007;46:499A.

318. Alper G, Jarjour IT, Reyes JD, et al. Outcome of children with cerebral edema caused by fulminant hepatic failure. *Pediatr Neurol* 1998;18:299–304.

319. Jackson EW, Zacks S, Zinn S, et al. Delayed neuropsychologic dysfunction after liver transplantation for acute liver failure: a matched, case-controlled study. *Liver Transpl* 2002;8:932–6.

320. Mohamed R, Hubscher SG, Mirza DF, et al. Posttransplantation chronic hepatitis in fulminant hepatic failure. *Hepatology* 1997;25:1003–7.

321. Eisenbach C, Sauer P, Mehrabi A, et al. Prevention of hepatitis B virus recurrence after liver transplantation. *Clin Transplant* 2006;20:111–16.

322. Karvellas CJ, Safinia N, Auzinger G, et al. Medical and psychiatric outcomes for patients transplanted for acetaminophen-induced acute liver failure: a case–control study. *Liver Int* 2010;30:826–33.

323. Cooper SC, Aldridge RC, Shah T, et al. Outcomes of liver transplantation for paracetamol (acetaminophen)-induced hepatic failure. *Liver Transpl* 2009;15:1351–7.

324. Ostapowicz G, Lee WM. Acute hepatic failure: a Western perspective. *J Gastroenterol Hepatol* 2000;15:480–8.

325. Mitzner SR, Stange J, Klammt S, et al. Improvement of hepatorenal syndrome with extracorporeal albumin dialysis MARS: results of a prospective, randomized, controlled clinical trial. *Liver Transpl* 2000;6:277–86.

326. Ellis AJ, Sussman NL, Kelly JH, Williams R. Clinical experience with an extracorporeal liver assist device. In: Lee WM, Williams R, eds. *Acute Liver Failure*. Cambridge, UK: Cambridge University Press, 1997:255–66.

Multiple choice questions

19.1 The use of *N*-acetylcysteine (NAC) in the setting of acute liver failure (ALF) not due to acetaminophen has been shown to improve transplant-free survival if given prior to the development of stage 1–2 hepatic encephalopathy.

    a False.
    b True.

19.2 The most common cause of death in the setting of acute liver failure is which of the following?

    a Fungal infection.
    b Cerebral edema and brainstem herniation.
    c Electrolyte imbalance.
    d Renal failure.

19.3 The most common cause of ALF worldwide is which of the following?

    a Drug-induced liver injury.
    b Viral hepatitis.
    c Autoimmune hepatitis.
    d Ischemic hepatitis.

Answers to the multiple choice questions can be found in the Appendix at the end of the book.

These multiple choice questions are also available for you to complete online.
Visit http://www.schiffsdiseasesoftheliver.com/

PART IV
Cholestatic Disorders

CHAPTER 20
Primary Sclerosing Cholangitis

Douglas L. Nguyen, Nicholas F. LaRusso, & Konstantinos N. Lazaridis

Center for Basic Research in Digestive Diseases, Division of Gastroenterology and Hepatology, Mayo Clinic College of Medicine, Rochester, MN, USA

Key concepts

- Primary sclerosing cholangitis (PSC) is a progressive, cholestatic liver disease that is characterized by diffuse chronic inflammation and fibrosis of the biliary tree.
- PSC affects primarily young to middle-aged men and is frequently associated with inflammatory bowel disease, most often chronic ulcerative colitis.
- The cause of PSC remains unknown, although the interaction between exogenous factors with the genetically predisposed individual is likely critical in disease pathogenesis.

- PSC patients are at increased risk for the development of cholangiocarcinoma and colon cancer.
- Currently, no medical therapy has been of proven benefit.
- Liver transplantation is the best available treatment option for patients with advanced PSC; however, the disease can recur in about 20% of recipients after successful transplantation.

Primary sclerosing cholangitis (PSC) is a chronic cholestatic liver disease of unknown etiology, characterized by diffuse inflammation and fibrosis of the biliary tree, resulting in ductal obliteration, biliary cirrhosis, and hepatic failure. PSC was first described by Delbet in 1924 [1]. Before the widespread availability of endoscopic retrograde cholangiopancreatography (ERCP) in the mid-1970s, PSC was considered a rare disease [2]. It remains unclear whether the prevalence of the disease has truly increased in recent decades or merely that an enhanced frequency of PSC diagnosis has occurred with the greater availability of ERCP and magnetic resonance cholangiopancreatography (MRCP). Though we have a better understanding of the natural course of PSC, the etiology for disease development and an effective medical therapy remain elusive.

Epidemiology

Two epidemiological studies from the United States and United Kingdom described the incidence and prevalence of PSC in the community setting. The first study from Olmsted county, Minnesota, estimated the age-adjusted incidence of PSC to be 0.9 per 100,000 individuals with point prevalence of 13.6 per 100,000 persons in 2000 [3].

Specifically, the age-adjusted incidence was 1.25 and 0.54 per 100,000 men and women, respectively. The estimated prevalence was 20.9 per 100,000 for males and 6.3 per 100,000 females [3]. Based on this study, it was projected that approximately 29,000 cases of PSC exist in the white US population. Moreover, the median age at PSC diagnosis was 40 years; 68% (15/22) of the patients were males and 73% (16/22) of the patients had concurrent IBD [3].

The second study from Swansea, Wales, reported an annual incidence of 0.91 per 100,000 and a point prevalence of 12.7 per 100,000 individuals [4]. The median age at PSC onset was 52 years, 62% (33/53) of the patients were men, and 62% (33/53) of the patients had coexisting IBD [4]. These two studies have shed light on the epidemiology of the disease, but additional population-based studies are required to better define the prevalence and natural history of PSC.

Pathogenesis

Although a number of avenues have been explored in the past three decades, the exact pathogenesis of PSC is unknown. A consensus pathogenesis postulates that PSC develops as the result of acquired exotoxins, infections,

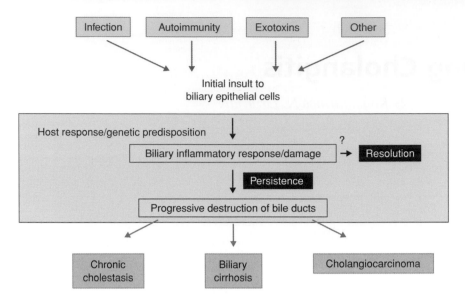

Figure 20.1 Proposed pathogenesis of primary sclerosing cholangitis.

or other agents interacting with predisposing host factors (Fig. 20.1). It is proposed that this interplay leads to an initial damage of cholangiocytes, the target epithelial cells that line the bile ducts. Subsequently, a biliary inflammatory response takes place but most individuals recover without consequences. Perhaps, the genetic predisposition of the host and other unknown mechanisms may contribute to persistance of inflammation of the bile ducts resulting in progressive biliary destruction, chronic cholestasis, biliary cirrhosis, and, in some cases, cholangiocarcinoma (Fig. 20.1).

Genetic factors

Prior studies have documented familial PSC cases and a significantly higher prevalence of PSC among first-degree relatives of affected patients [5,6], supporting the presence of inherited elements in disease pathogenesis. In addition, several case–control studies have demonstrated the genetic predisposition to PSC development by identifying genetic variants associated with patients compared to controls. Chapman et al. first reported the human leu-

cocyte antigen B8 (HLA-B8) frequency to be significantly higher in patients with PSC (60%) compared with controls (25%) ($P < 0.001$) [7]. Subsequently, Donaldson et al. demonstrated an association of PSC with the HLA-A1, -B8, -DR3 haplotype (40% in cases versus 12% in controls, $P < 0.0005$) [8].

In recent years, genetic polymorphisms associated with susceptibility to PSC have been reported, including: (i) the promoter region of the tumor necrosis factor α (TNF-α) receptor [9]; (ii) stromelysin (i.e., matrix metalloproteinase 3) [10]; (iii) the *MICA* gene (i.e., major histocompatibility complex class I related MIC gene family) [11]; (iv) the CCR5-delta 32 mutation [12]; and (v) intracellular adhesion molecule 1 (ICAM-1) [13] (Table 20.1). From a theoretical standpoint, the variety of susceptibility genes interacting with environmental factors likely explain the heterogeneity of PSC phenotype as this relates to disease development, progression, and complications. It is expected that many genetic variants (i.e., susceptibility alleles) predispose to disease, each of which contribute a small effect on the PSC phenotype. To this end, large association (i.e., case–control) and familial studies are needed

Table 20.1 Susceptibility genes in primary sclerosing cholangitis.

Gene	Type	Variaton	Reference
TNF-α	Cytokine	G/A, substitution	Mitchell et al. 2001 [9]
Stromelysin	Matrix metalloproteinase	5A/6A alleles	Satsangi et al. 2001 [10]
MICA	MHC	*002/*008 alleles	Norris et al. 2001 [11]
CCR5-delta32	Chemokine	32 base pair deletion	Eri et al. 2004 [11]
ICAM-1	Adhesion molecule	K469E	Yang et al. 2004 [12]

CCR5, chemokine, CC motif receptor 5; ICAM-1, intracellular adhesion molecule 1; MICA, major histocompataibility complex class I-related MIC gene family; TNF-α, tumor necrosis factor α.

to better dissect the genetic susceptibility of PSC. Such results will aid in the development of novel diagnostic tools and intervening therapies.

Abnormalities in humoral and cellular immunity

Abnormalities of the humoral immune system in PSC include the presence of: (i) hypergammaglobulinemia, particularly elevated immunoglobulin M levels; (ii) circulating immune complexes; and (iii) activated complement [14]. Moreover, PSC patients have serum positivity for several autoantibodies including antineutrophil cytoplasmic antibodies (ANCA), anticardiolipin antibodies, and antinuclear antibodies (53%) [15]. In addition, the cellular immune system in PSC can be abnormal, as indicated by a decrease in the total number of circulating T cells due to a decline in CD8 (suppressor/cytotoxic cells) and an increase in circulating B cells. Furthermore, the documented aberrant expression of HLA class II antigens on the biliary epithelial cells may serve to target an immune response against the biliary cells [16,17], while the presence of ICAM-1, which serves as a ligand for the leukocyte function-associated antigen 1 (LFA-1), may help form connections between T lymphocytes and antigen-presenting cells. Indeed, increased levels of ICAM-1 have been found in both the bile duct epithelial cells and serum [17–19]. LFA-1 also appears to be overexpressed by intrahepatic lymphocytes, but this expression may simply be induced by proinflammatory cytokines [20]. Despite all these observations, the documented altered immune status may simply be an epiphenomenon and yet not linked directly to PSC pathogenesis.

Other proposed hypotheses of pathogenesis

Due to the strong clinical association between IBD and PSC, much interest has been paid to the potential role of an inflamed colon in causing the liver disease [21]. It was proposed that inflammation of the colon may increase the colonic permeability to various intraluminal products leading to liver injury. To this extent, bacteria or bacterial toxins have been considered but have not been convincingly demonstrated to play a pathogenetic role in PSC [22]. In addition, abnormal bile acids generated by bacterial action in the diseased colon and directly absorbed through the colonic mucosa into the portal system have been suggested as a possible etiology of PSC. Nevertheless, no direct evidence in support of this theory has been forthcoming.

In an animal model, inflammatory bacterial peptides led to portal inflammation and histologic changes suggestive of PSC [23,24]. In this model, a variety of agents were useful in blocking this response, including an inhibitor of TNF. However, when pentoxifylline, a TNF inhibitor, was used in patients with PSC, no clinical benefit was found [25]. Furthermore, the finding that PSC can develop in approximately 25% of patients without concurrent IBD, the lack of association between the severity of colonic inflammation and the likelihood of PSC development, and the fact that proctocolectomy for chronic ulcerative colitis (CUC) does not alter the natural history of PSC [26] speak against the role of the inflamed colon in the development of liver disease.

At present, there is no convincing evidence of a virus or other microorganism causing PSC. The usual hepatotrophic viruses (i.e., hepatitis A, B, and C virus) have been excluded. Cytomegalovirus can produce changes suggestive of PSC in patients with acquired immunodeficiency states, but in immunocompetent patients no evidence of cytomegalovirus infection has been found [27]. Reovirus type 3 was considered a possible causative agent but further work excluded it as an etiology for PSC [28].

Clinical features

Primary sclerosing cholangitis affects men almost twice as commonly as it does women and the average age at diagnosis is the early forties [3]. In the past two decades, a frequent clinical scenario of diagnosis includes asymptomatic patients who come to medical attention solely because of abnormal liver function tests. Physical examination may be unrevealing, but splenomegaly, hyperpigmentation, and skin excoriation can be found. Symtoms of advanced PSC such as jaundice, pruritus, fever, or portal hypertension on initial presentation are uncommon. Health-related quality of life is significantly impaired among patients with PSC relative to the healthy population [29,30].

PSC usually affects the entire biliary tree. Approximately 20% of patients have involvement of the intrahepatic bile ducts alone and 5% have disease involving the interlobular and septal bile ducts (i.e., small duct PSC) seen only on liver biopsy, while the ERCP is normal [31–34]. Up to 15% of patients can have involvement of the cystic duct and gallbladder [35]. Another clinical entity is the overlap syndrome, in which PSC and autoimmune hepatitis coexist and occurs in about 5% of adult patients [31–33]. Rarely, PSC can afflict children and in this population the disease will often have features of autoimmune hepatitis [36].

Natural history

Primary sclerosing cholangitis is usually a progressive disease. In a retrospective study with 174 PSC patients

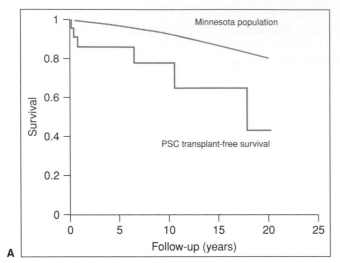
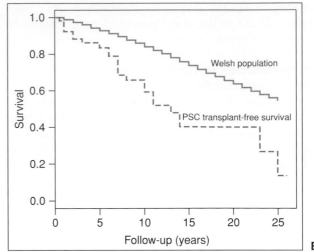

Figure 20.2 Transplant-free survival of primary sclerosing cholangitis (PSC) patients compard with age- and sex-matched population controls from the corresponding counties of Olmsted, Minnesota (A) and Swansea, Wales (B). (Reproduced from Bambha et al. [3] and Kingham et al. [4] with permission from Elsevier.)

from the United States, the median survival rate from the time of diagnosis was approximately 12 years, which was less than that for an age-matched population [37]. In another study from Norway, investigators estimated the median survival time of PSC patients to be 17 years [38,39].

Recent population-based epidemiologic data also reported that PSC is a progressive disease and shortens life expectancy. Studies from Olmsted County, Minnesota and Swansea, Wales indicated that the liver transplantation-free survival was 65% at 10 years after the diagnosis of PSC and significantly less than the age- and sex-matched populations (Fig. 20.2) [3,4].

Given these natural history studies, prognostic models have been developed to more accurately forecast an individual patient's disease progression, and thus define the best timing for liver transplantation. The variables for these prognostic models were created using Cox multivariable regression analysis [38,40–42]. The revised Mayo PSC natural history model employs five independent and reproducible parameters (age, total bilirubin, albumin, aspartate aminotransferase, and history of variceal bleeding) to estimate the survival of patients [40]. Recently, the model of end-stage liver disease (MELD) score has been widely used to prioritize liver transplantation in PSC patients with end-stage liver disease [43].

Small duct PSC is associated with a better long-term prognosis compared with large duct PSC [44]. In a comparative study, small duct PSC appeared to have significantly longer transplantation-free survival than large duct PSC, and cholangiocarcinoma did not seem to occur in patients with small duct PSC unless the disease pro-

gressed to large duct PSC. Small duct PSC can progress to large duct PSC over a course of approximately 7 years in an estimated 22.9% of cases [44,45]. Finally, secondary sclerosing cholangitis has a poorer long-term outcome when compared with PSC, with a signficantly shorter survival free of liver transplantation [46].

Associated diseases

The close association of PSC with IBD, particularly CUC, is now widely recognized. This association is found in 70–80% of patients with PSC. Crohn disease has been reported as the cause of colitis in 10–15% of patients with PSC [21,47]. There is no clear temporal association between the diagnosis of PSC and IBD, although the diagnosis of IBD is usually established before the liver disease is clinically apparent. Nevertheless, there are well-documented cases of IBD occurring years after the diagnosis of PSC. Additionally, patients can develop PSC many years after proctocolectomy for colitis [26]. In patients with PSC and colitis, the bowel disease is one of relatively quiescent disease. However, the risk of development of colon cancer in patients with coexisting PSC and CUC appears to be substantially greater than if patients did not have PSC. There has been no association between the severity of bowel disease and the severity of liver disease, and therapy for the bowel disease, including proctocolectomy, does not affect the liver disease [26].

Aside from IBD, a variety of diseases have been reported to occur with PSC (Box 20.1). It is unclear, however, whether these associations are true, and thus share a pathogenetic mechanism, or coexist by chance.

Box 20.1 Diseases associated with primary sclerosing cholangitis.

- Inflammatory bowel disease
- Autoimmune hepatitis
- Chronic pancreatitis
- Celiac disease
- Rheumatoid arthritis
- Retroperitoneal fibrosis
- Peyronie disease
- Riedel thyroiditis
- Bronchiectasis
- Sjögren disease
- Glomerulonephritis
- Systemic lupus erythematosus
- Pseudotumor of the orbit
- Vasculitis
- Autoimmune hemolytic anemia
- Immune thrombocytopenic purpura
- Angioimmunoblastic lymphadenopathy
- Histiocytosis X
- Cystic fibrosis
- Sarcoidosis
- Systemic mastocytosis
- Polymyositis
- Alopecia universalis
- Thymoma
- Ankylosing spondylitis

Laboratory findings

Biochemical testing

The biochemical findings of PSC patients are nonspecific. Nevertheless, chronic biochemical cholestasis is typically apparent. Alkaline phosphatase is the most commonly elevated liver enzyme although patients with well-documented PSC and normal alkaline phosphatase levels have occasionally been described [48]. Aminotransferase levels are frequently elevated, but the degree of elevation is only modest except in patients with overlap syndrome where levels can be markedly increased. Serum bilirubin is typically normal but in advanced disease can be very high.

Imaging studies

Visualization of the biliary tree is essential for establishing the diagnosis of PSC. ERCP has been the diagnostic procedure of choice, although MRCP is equally sensitive and specific for detection of the disease [49] and may be more cost effective [50–52]. A percutaneous transhepatic cholangiogram (PTC) can be used, but because of the frequently sclerotic intrahepatic biliary system gaining access via the percutaneous route can be challenging.

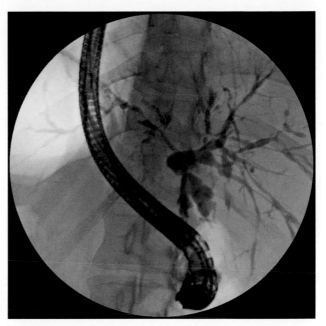

Figure 20.3 ERCP of a patient with primary sclerosing cholangitis. Extensive extrahepatic and intrahepatic biliary disease is evident.

Typical cholangiographic findings of PSC include multifocal stricturing and beading, usually involving both the intra- and extrahepatic biliary system (Fig. 20.3). Often the strictures are diffusely distributed, short in length, and annular. During cholangiography, the presence of polypoid masses should raise the suspicion of cholangiocarcinoma, although the diagnosis of the latter can be very difficult to establish.

Histology

Liver biopsy findings alone are generally nondiagnostic of PSC. The classic onion-skin fibrosis is seen in fewer than 10% of biopsy specimens, but when present is almost pathognomonic (Fig. 20.4) [53]. The histologic grading

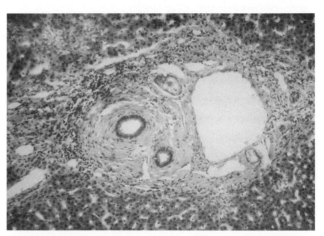

Figure 20.4 This characteristic onion-skin lesion is not typically found in liver biopsy specimens from patients with primary sclerosing cholangitis.

Box 20.2 Histologic staging of primary sclerosing cholangitis.

Portal stage (stage I)
- Portal edema, inflammation, ductal proliferation; abnormalities do not extend beyond the limiting plate

Periportal stage (stage II)
- Periportal fibrosis, inflammation with or without ductular proliferation; piecemeal necrosis may be present

Septal stage (stage III)
- Septal fibrosis or bridging necrosis can be identified

Cirrhotic stage (stage IV)
- Biliary cirrhosis

system, proposed by Ludwig et al. [53], has four stages: stage 1, portal; stage 2, periportal; stage 3, septal; and stage 4, cirrhosis (Box 20.2). Intrestingly, the histologic changes seem to be quite variable in different segments of the same liver, and therefore histologic staging has been avoided as a component of current PSC survival models [38,40–42].

Diagnostic criteria and differential diagnosis

The current diagnostic criteria for PSC include: (i) typical cholangiographic abnormalities involving any part of the biliary tree; (ii) compatible clinical and biochemical findings (i.e., cholestasis for more than 6 months); and (iii) exclusion of other causes of secondary sclerosing cholangitis (Box 20.3). Liver biopsy has been used in the past to

Box 20.3 Diagnostic criteria for primary sclerosing cholangitis (PSC).

- Typical cholangiographic abnormalities involving any part of the biliary tree
- Compatible clinical (cholestatic symptoms, history of inflammatory bowel disease) and biochemical (2–3-fold increase in serum alkaline phosphatase level for longer than 6 months) findings
- Exclusion of identifiable causes of secondary sclerosing cholangitis:
    AIDS (acquired immune deficiency syndrome) cholangiopathy
    Bile duct neoplasm (unless diagnosis of PSC has been previously established)
    Biliary tract surgery, trauma
    Choledocholithiasis
    Congenital abnormalities of biliary tract
    Caustic sclerosing cholangitis
    Ischemic stricturing of bile ducts
    Toxicity or stricturing of bile ducts related to intra-arterial infusion of floxuridine

help confirm the diagnosis, although the specificity and sensitivity of the biopsy have come under question. Nevertheless, liver biopsy may be useful to diagnose small duct PSC in a patient with normal cholangiography and in the setting of a patient with overlap syndrome. The differential diagnosis of PSC is outlined in Box 20.3.

Finally, PSC predisposes to the development of colon cancer and cholangiocarcinoma (see below). Patients with PSC and CUC have a significantly greater risk of developing colon cancer compared with patients having CUC only [54]. Therefore, PSC patients should undergo surveillance colonoscopies annually.

Management

The complications of PSC include: (i) advanced stage liver disease (i.e., portal hypertension, decompensated cirrhosis, and hepatic failure); (ii) chronic cholestasis; and (iii) the underlying disease (i.e., specific for PSC). The management of complications of portal hypertension, decompensated cirrhosis, and hepatic failure are discussed in Chapters 11, 12, and 33. The management of complications related to chronic cholestasis and those specific for PSC are discussed below.

Complications of chronic cholestasis

Pruritus

Although not common, pruritus can be disabling and associated with a diminished quality of life. The pathogenesis of pruritus in cholestasis is unknown, although endogenous opioids and retention of factors usually excreted in the bile have been considered [55,56]. The severity of the pruritus does not seem to parallel the severity of the liver disease, and pruritus may diminish as the liver disease progresses. Cholestyramine, antihistamines, rifampin, and opiate receptor antagonists have been used with varying results to treat patients with cholestatic pruritus [57,58]. The usual doses of these medications are shown in Box 20.4. It is important to remember that rifampin is associated with a reversible hepatotoxicity in 15% of cases. Therefore, it is important to monitor the liver function tests closely if this drug is used.

Box 20.4 Medications used for the management of pruritus.

- Ursodiol: 15–30 mg/kg/day orally
- Cholestyramine: 4 g 3–4 times per day orally
- Naltrexone: 50 mg/day orally
- Rifampin: 150–300 mg twice per day orally

Box 20.5 Vitamin replacement therapy for primary sclerosing cholangitis.

- Vitamin A: 25,000–50,000 units 2–3 times per week orally
- Vitamin D: 25,000–50,000 units 2–3 times per week orally
- Vitamin E: 100 units/day orally
- Vitamin K: 5–10 mg/day orally

Fat-soluble vitamin deficiency

Fat-soluble vitamin deficiency is relatively common among patients with PSC, particularly as the patient progresses towards liver transplantation [59]. Up to 40% of patients have vitamin A deficiency, and vitamin D and E deficiencies have been found among 14% and 2% of patients, respectively [59]. Vitamin K deficiency is uncommon. If this condition is suspected, a short trial of 10 mg water-soluble vitamin K can be considered. If the prothrombin time responds after a few doses, long-term therapy should be recommended. Vitamin E deficiency is rare and unfortunately once established can be very difficult to correct with replacement therapy. The usual fat-soluble doses of vitamin replacement therapy are shown in Box 20.5.

Metabolic bone disease

Metabolic bone disease, usually caused by osteoporosis rather than osteomalacia, is relatively common and an important complication among PSC patients [60]. The glucocorticoids used to treat the accompanying IBD aggravate osteoporosis. Unfortunately, there is no proven therapy that can help these patients. Use of estrogen replacement therapy by women can be considered, but it is not of proven benefit. Calcitonin does not appear to be useful to patients with osteoporosis associated with PBC, but it has not been tested in the treatment of PSC patients. Bisphosphonates have been used with varying results to treat patients with PBC, but have not been tested in the care of patients with PSC [61]. Patients with PSC and IBD, undergoing long-term glucocorticoid therapy for the latter, may benefit from the oral administration of vitamin D and calcium, particularly those with a bone density in the range of osteopenia or osteoporosis.

Steatorrhea

Steatorrhea can occur in patients with PSC secondary to a diminished delivery of bile acids to the intestine either from coexisting chronic pancreatitis or celiac disease. These conditions should be considered in the evaluation of patients with steatorrhea in the setting of PSC [62] before treatment is recommended. If steatorrhea in patients with PSC is primary, a low-fat diet and the substitution of medium-chain triglycerides for long-chain ones may be benificial.

Specific complications of primary sclerosing cholangitis

Gallstones, choledocholithiasis, and gallbladder polyps

Stones involving the gallbladder or bile ducts (i.e., choledocholithiasis) occur in approximately one third of patients with PSC. Chronic cholestasis predisposes to the formation of cholesterol gallstones and bile stasis, with bacterial cholangitis leading to the formation of pigment stones of the bile ducts. In PSC patients, choledocholithiasis may present with acute deterioration of liver function, worsening jaundice, or bacterial cholangitis if the bile duct becomes obstructed, but can be treated endoscopically once the diagnosis is established. Additionally, recent case series have reported a high incidence of adenocarcinoma in polypoid lesions of the gallbladder in PSC patients, even in polyps of less than 1 cm diameter, and elective cholecystectomy may be justified once these lesions are detected [63].

Biliary strictures

In the largest series to date, dominant biliary strictures occurred in only 7% of patients whose cases were followed for up to 10 years. These dominant strictures are usually in the extrahepatic biliary system and may be associated with jaundice, pruritus, or relapsing bacterial cholangitis. If any of these symptoms occur in PSC patients, cholangiography should be strongly considered. Any evidence of dominant stricture(s) requires brush cytologic specimens for standard cytology, fluorescence in situ hybridization (FISH), and digitized image analysis (DIA) to exclude cholangiocarcinoma (see below). Often, bile duct strictures can be dilated endoscopically with a balloon catheter. Short-term biliary stenting has been shown to improve the prognosis of liver disease in some studies, whereas others have shown that patients with biliary stents are at increased risk of complications [64]. Direct surgical intervention for biliary strictures is seldom used and may predispose patients to recurrent bacterial cholangitis because of the widely patent surgical anastomosis, and may make future liver transplantation more technically demanding.

Prophylaxis for bacterial cholangitis should be considered in the care of patients with PSC undergoing biliary manipulation. The Mayo Clinic experience suggests that PSC patients have a much higher risk for cholangitis than patients without PSC (4% versus 0.2%, $P < 0.0002$), while the risks for other complications of pancreatitis, perforation, and bleeding are similar in PSC and non-PSC patients [65]. Ciprofloxacin or other broad-spectrum antibiotics with high biliary excretion are frequently administered both immediately before and 1 or 2 days after the procedure.

Cholangiocarcinoma

Cholangiocarcinoma (CCA) is the most feared complication among patients with PSC. CCA may occur in 7–15% of patients with PSC at an annual incidence of 0.5–1% [66–69]. Interestingly, the development of CCA does not correlate with the severity of PSC. Chronic inflammation of the bile ducts and cholestasis are likely predisposing factors associated with the development of CCA in PSC. Smoking and the presence of IBD have been suggested as predisposing conditions although they remain controversial. The diagnosis of CCA in PSC patients can often be difficult to establish because it is not easy to differentiate between benign and malignant dominant biliary stricture(s). Furthermore, conventional imaging of computed tomography and ultrasound have poor sensitivity for the detection of CCA. A recent study suggested that dynamic positron emission tomography (PET) may be more useful for screening CCA compared with conventional modalities, but more studies are necessary to define the role and routine use of PET in PSC patients [70].

Serum markers for the early detection of CCA in PSC have not been helpful. As a screening test, carbohydrate antigen 19-9 (CA 19-9) does not appear to be sensitive enough, and the specificity is limited. For instance, CA 19-9 levels may be elevated due to bacterial cholangitis secondary to benign strictures, thus limiting the specificity of the test [71]. Nevertheless, in a patient with PSC, sudden and unexpected clinical deterioration – which is associated with a progressive elevation of alkaline phosphatase and serum CA 19-9 (>100 U/mL) – in the absence of bacterial cholangitis indicates a probable development of CCA.

New diagnostic methods such as DIA and FISH offer promise in evaluating bile duct lesions for cellular aneuploidy and chromosomal aberrations [71]. To perform DIA and FISH assays, bile duct brushings are collected at the time of ERCP or PTC. DIA allows DNA content quantification, assessment of chromatin distribution, and nuclear morphology. In one study, DIA was found to be significantly more sensitive (39.3%) than standard cytology (17.9%, $P = 0.014$) [72].

The biliary FISH assay uses fluorescently labeled DNA-based probes to detect chromosomal aberrations in brushings of bile duct cells. A FISH assay is declared positive when five or more cells display gains of two or more chromosomes, or ten or more cells demonstrate a gain of a single chromosome (Fig. 20.5) [71]. A recent study of nearly 500 patients demonstrated that the sensitivity of polysomy FISH for carcinoma (42.9%) was significantly higher than standard cytology (20.1%), while maintaining identical specificity (99.6%) ($P < 0.001$) [73]. Multivariable modeling using standard cytology and FISH findings, age, and PSC status may be used to estimate the probability of carcinoma in individual patients [73].

Overall, in a patient with PSC, the diagnosis of CCA is usually made by combining the clinical examination, biochemical results, and imaging procedures. In medical practice, it is not uncommon to make the diagnosis of CCA based on clinical grounds and imaging studies without tissue-proven evidence of tumor. Physicians who evaluate PSC patients should be highly suspicious for the development of CCA when these patients present with sudden clinical deterioration. Because we lack methods of

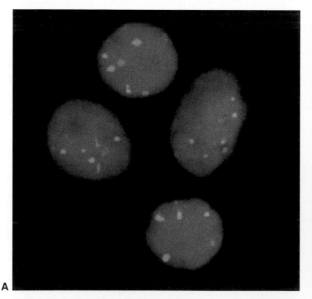
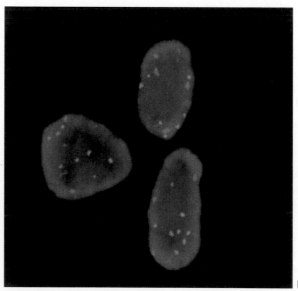

Figure 20.5 FISH of normal (A) and maligant (B) bile duct cells. Normal cells display duplicate color for each chromosomal probe while malignant cells reveal multiple gains of chromosomes (i.e., polysomy). (Reproduced from Lazaridis and Gores [71] with permission from Elsevier.)

early CCA detection in PSC, the outcome of these patients is poor. Nevertheless, early diagnosis of CCA in PSC can be successfully treated by liver transplantation in selected medical centers [74].

Peristomal varices

Peristomal varices can occur in patients with ileostomy after proctocolectomy for underlying IBD [75]. The bleeding of peristomal varices can be severe and refractory to local measures, including ileostomy revision and injection of sclerosants. A transjugular intrahepatic portosystemic shunt or portacaval shunt can be considered, although many of these patients with bleeding peristomal varices have severe underlying liver disease with portal hypertension and thus should be considered for liver transplantation.

Specific management

Medical therapy

A variety of drugs have been tested as therapeutic agents for PSC, but none have been found to be disease modifying. Randomized, placebo-controlled trials of penicillamine, colchicine, methotrexate, and ursodeoxycholic acid (UDCA) (13–15 mg/kg/day) have all been ineffective [76–80]. Small-scale studies using nicotine, pirfenidone, pentoxifylline, and budesonide have not demonstrated clinical benefit [25,81–84]. Pilot studies using high-dose UDCA (20–30 mg/kg/day) initially appeared to have improvement in survival probability, with trends toward Ludwig histologic stabilization/improvement [85,86]. Unfortunately, larger randomized, placebo-control trials failed to demonstrate an improvement in symptoms, quality of life, survival, and risk for cholangiocarcionoma with higher doses of UDCA [76,77]. Specifically, over the course of a 5-year longitudinal follow-up, patients randomized to the high-dose UDCA group had a greater than two-fold increased risk for serious adverse events, death, or transplantation compared with the placebo group [77]. Interestingly, UDCA has been shown to decrease the prevalence of colonic dysplasia in patients with PSC and CUC [78]. Nevertheless, we need prospective studies to confirm the chemopreventive effect of UDCA in patients with coexisting PSC and CUC before its implementation as routine prophylactic therapy.

Surgical therapy

Surgical therapy other than liver transplantation is seldom warranted for PSC. Biliary reconstruction has been suggested to be helpful [79], but this aggressive approach has not been validated in prospective controlled studies.

Liver transplantation

The most pressing need of patients with PSC is for effective medical therapy for the underlying disease. Until this therapy is found, liver transplantation is the only option for patients with advanced PSC. The results of liver transplantation for patients with PSC have steadily improved: the 1- and 5-year survival rates are now reported to be 90–97% and 85–88%, respectively [80,87]. Nevertheless, PSC can recur after liver transplantation, and as the follow-up period lengthens the risk of recurrence seems to increase, although the recurrent disease is typically mild [88,89]. Patients with PSC and CUC who have undergone liver transplantation seem to be at particularly high risk of colon cancer if they have an intact colon. These patients need screening with annual colonoscopy and surveillance biopsies [90].

Conclusions

Primary sclerosing cholangitis is a progressive, chronic cholestatic liver disease of unknown cause. A number of complications can occur and should be considered in the treatment of these patients, the most important being the development of cholangiocarcinoma. Unfortunately, no medical therapy has been of proven benefit for the underlying liver disease. Currently, liver transplantation is the only effective, life-extending option for patients with advanced PSC. Additional basic and clinical research studies are necessary to understand the pathogenesis of PSC in order to develop better medical therapies for this devastating disease.

Further reading

Aoki C, Bowlus C, Gershwin M. The immunobiology of primary sclerosing cholangitis. *Autoimmune Rev* 2005;4:137–43.
A recent review about the immunobiology of PSC.

Bambha K, Kim W, Talwalkar J, et al. Incidence, clinical spectrum, and outcomes of primary sclerosing cholangitis in a United States community. *Gastroenterology* 2003;125:1364–9.
A population-based study about the prevalence and incidence of PSC.

Bergquist A, Lindberg G, Saarinen S, Broome U. Increased prevalence of primary sclerosing cholangitis among first-degree relatives. *J Hepatol* 2005;42:252–6.
An interesting paper about the increased prevelance of PSC among family members of affected individuals.

McFaul G, Chapman R. Sclerosing cholangitis. *Curr Opin Gastroenterol* 2005;21:348–53.
An excellent recent review of PSC.

References

1. Delbet P. Retrecissement du choledoque cholecystoduodenostomie. *Bull Mem Soc Chir Paris* 1924;50:1144–6.
2. Brantigan CO, Brantigan OC. Primary sclerosing cholangitis: case report and review of the literature. *Am Surg* 1973;39:191–8.

3. Bambha K, Kim WR, Talwalkar J, et al. Incidence, clinical spectrum, and outcomes of primary sclerosing cholangitis in a United States community. *Gastroenterology* 2003;125:1364–9.

4. Kingham JG, Kochar N, Gravenor MB. Incidence, clinical patterns, and outcomes of primary sclerosing cholangitis in South Wales, United Kingdom. *Gastroenterology* 2004;126:1929–30.

5. Bergquist A, Lindberg G, Saarinen S, Broome U. Increased prevalence of primary sclerosing cholangitis among first-degree relatives. *J Hepatol* 2005;42:252–6.

6. Bergquist A, Montgomery SM, Bahmanyar S, et al. Increased risk of primary sclerosing cholangitis and ulcerative colitis in first-degree relatives of patients with primary sclerosing cholangitis. *Clin Gastroenterol Hepatol* 2008;6:939–43.

7. Chapman RW, Varghese Z, Gaul R, Patel G, Kokinon N, Sherlock S. Association of primary sclerosing cholangitis with HLA-B8. *Gut* 1983;24:38–41.

8. Donaldson PT, Doherty DG, Hayllar KM, McFarlane IG, Johnson PJ, Williams R. Susceptibility to autoimmune chronic active hepatitis: human leukocyte antigens DR4 and A1-B8-DR3 are independent risk factors. *Hepatology* 1991;13:701–6.

9. Mitchell SA, Grove J, Spurkland A, et al. Association of the tumour necrosis factor alpha -308 but not the interleukin 10-627 promoter polymorphism with genetic susceptibility to primary sclerosing cholangitis. *Gut* 2001;49:288–94.

10. Satsangi J, Chapman RW, Haldar N, et al. A functional polymorphism of the stromelysin gene (MMP-3) influences susceptibility to primary sclerosing cholangitis. *Gastroenterology* 2001;121:124–30.

11. Norris S, Kondeatis E, Collins R, et al. Mapping MHC-encoded susceptibility and resistance in primary sclerosing cholangitis: the role of MICA polymorphism. *Gastroenterology* 2001;120:1475–82.

12. Eri R, Jonsson JR, Pandeya N, et al. CCR5-Delta32 mutation is strongly associated with primary sclerosing cholangitis. *Genes Immun* 2004;5:444–50.

13. Yang X, Cullen SN, Li JH, Chapman RW, Jewell DP. Susceptibility to primary sclerosing cholangitis is associated with polymorphisms of intercellular adhesion molecule-1. *J Hepatol* 2004;40:375–9.

14. Mandal A, Dasgupta A, Jeffers L, et al. Autoantibodies in sclerosing cholangitis against a shared peptide in biliary and colon epithelium. *Gastroenterology* 1994;106:185–92.

15. Angulo P, Peter JB, Gershwin ME, et al. Serum autoantibodies in patients with primary sclerosing cholangitis. *J Hepatol* 2000;32:182–7.

16. Broome U, Glaumann H, Hultcrantz R, Forsum U. Distribution of HLA-DR, HLA-DP, and HLA-DQ antigens in liver tissue from patients with primary sclerosing cholangitis. *Scand J Gastroenterol* 1990;25:54–8.

17. Van Milligen de Wit AWM, van Deventer SJH, Tytgat GNJ. Immunogenetic aspects of primary sclerosing cholangitis: implications for therapeutic strategies. *Am J Gastroenterol* 1995;90:893–900.

18. Adams DH, Hubscher SG, Shaw J, et al. Increased expression of intercellular adhesion molecule 1 on bile ducts in primary biliary cirrhosis and primary sclerosing cholangitis. *Hepatology* 1991;14:426–31.

19. Bloom S, Fleming K, Chapman R. Adhesion molecule expression in primary sclerosing cholangitis and primary biliary cirrhosis. *Gut* 1995;36:604–9.

20. Broome U, Hultcrantz R, Scheynius A. Lack of concomitant expression of ICAM-1 and HLA-DR on bile duct cells from patients with primary sclerosing cholangitis and primary biliary cirrhosis. *Scand J Gastroenterol* 1993;28:126–30.

21. Fausa O, Schrumpf E, Elgjo K. Relationship of inflammatory bowel disease and primary sclerosing cholangitis. *Semin Liver Dis* 1991;11:31–9.

22. Palmer KR, Duerden BJ, Holdworth CD. Bacteriological and endotoxin studies in cases of ulcerative colitis submitted to surgery. *Gut* 1980;21:851–4.

23. Hobson CH, Butt TJ, Ferry DM, Hunter J, Chadwick VS, Broom MF. Enterohepatic circulation of bacterial chemotactic peptide in rats with experimental colitis. *Gastroenterology* 1988;94:1006–13.

24. Lichtman SN, Sartor RB, Keku J, Schwab JH. Hepatic inflammation in rats with experimental small intestinal bacterial overgrowth. *Gastroenterology* 1990;98:414–23.

25. Bharucha AE, Jorgensen R, Lichtman SN, LaRusso NF, Lindor KD. A pilot study of pentoxifylline for the treatment of primary sclerosing cholangitis. *Am J Gastroenterol* 2000;95:2338–42.

26. Cangemi JR, Wiesner RH, Beaver SJ, et al. Effect of proctocolectomy for chronic ulcerative colitis on the natural history of primary sclerosing cholangitis. *Gastroenterology* 1989;96:790–4.

27. Mehal WZ, Hattersley AT, Chapman RW, Fleming KA. A survey of cytomegalovirus (CMV) DNA in primary sclerosing cholangitis (PSC) liver tissues using a sensitive polymerase chain reaction (PCR) based assay. *J Hepatol* 1992;15:396–9.

28. Minuk GY, Rascanin N, Paul RW, Lee PW, Buchan K, Kelly JK. Reovirus type 3 infection in patients with primary biliary cirrhosis and primary sclerosing cholangitis. *J Hepatol* 1987;5:8–13.

29. Kim WR, Lindor KD, Malinchoc M, Petz JL, Jorgensen R, Dickson ER. Reliability and validity of the NIDDK-QA instrument in the assessment of quality of life in ambulatory patients with cholestatic liver disease. *Hepatology* 2000;32:924–9.

30. Younossi ZM, Boparai N, Price LL, Kiwi ML, McCormick M, Guyatt G. Health-related quality of life in chronic liver disease: the impact of type and severity of disease. *Am J Gastroenterol* 2001;96:2199–205.

31. McNair AN, Moloney M, Portmann BC, Williams R, McFarlane IG. Autoimmune hepatitis overlapping with primary sclerosing cholangitis in five cases. *Am J Gastroenterol* 1998;93:777–84.

32. Kaya M, Angulo P, Lindor KD. Overlap of autoimmune hepatitis and primary sclerosing cholangitis: an evaluation of a modified scoring system. *J Hepatol* 2000;33:537–42.

33. Van Buuren HR, van Hoogstraten HJE, Terkivatan T, Schalm SW, Vleggaar FP. High prevalence of autoimmune hepatitis among patients with primary sclerosing cholangitis. *J Hepatol* 2000;33:543–8.

34. Angulo P, Maor-Kendler Y, Lindor KD. Small-duct primary sclerosing cholangitis: a long-term follow-up study. *Hepatology* 2002;35:1494–500.

35. Brandt DJ, MacCarty RL, Charboneau JW, LaRusso NF, Wiesner RH, Ludwig J. Gallbladder disease in patients with primary sclerosing cholangitis. *AJR Am J Roentgenol* 1988;150:571–4.

36. Feldstein AE, Perrault J, El-Youssif M, Lindor KD, Freese DK, Angulo P. Primary sclerosing cholangitis in children: a long-term follow-up study. *Hepatology* 2003;38:210–17.

37. Wiesner RH, Grambsch PM, Dickson ER, et al. Primary sclerosing cholangitis: natural history, prognostic factors, and survival analysis. *Hepatology* 1989;10:430–6.

38. Broome U, Olsson R, Loof L, et al. Natural history and prognostic factors in 305 Swedish patients with primary sclerosing cholangitis. *Gut* 1996;38:610–15.

39. Okolicsanyi L, Fabris L, Viaggi S, Carulli N, Podda M, Ricci G. Primary sclerosing cholangitis: clinical presentation, natural history and prognostic variables: an Italian multicentre study. *Eur J Gastroenterol Hepatol* 1996;8:685–91.

40. Kim WR, Therneau TM, Wiesner RH, et al. A revised natural history model for primary scleroising cholangitis. *Mayo Clin Proc* 2000;75:688–94.

41. Farrant JM, Hayllar KM, Wilkinson ML, et al. Natural history and prognostic variables in primary sclerosing cholangitis. *Gastroenterology* 1991;100:1710–17.

42. Shetty K, Rybicki L, Carey WD. The Child–Pugh classification as a prognostic indicator for survival in primary sclerosing cholangitis. *Hepatology* 1997;25:1049–53.

43. Kamath PS, Wiesner RH, Malinchoc M, et al. A model to predict survival in patients with end-stage liver disease. *Hepatology* 2001;33:464–70.

44. Bjornsson E, Olsson R, Bergquist A, et al. The natural history of small-duct primary sclerosing cholangitis. *Gastroenterology* 2008;134: 975–80.

45. Angulo P, Maor-Kendler Y, Donlinger JJ. Small-duct primary sclerosing cholangitis: prevalance and natural history. *Gastroenterology* 2000;118:A902.

46. Gossard AA, Angulo P, Lindor KD. Secondary sclerosing cholangitis: a comparison to primary sclerosing cholangitis. *Am J Gastroenterol* 2005;100:1330–3.

47. Loftus EV Jr, Sandborn WJ, Lindor KD. Interactions between chronic liver disease and inflammatory bowel disease. *Inflamm Bowel Dis* 1997;3:288–302.

48. Balasubramaniam K, Grambsch PM, Wiesner RH, et al. Diminished survival and asymptomatic primary biliary cirrhosis, a prospective study. *Gastroenterology* 1990;98:1567–71.

49. Berstad AE, Aabakken L, Smith HJ, Aasen S, Boberg KM, Schrumpf E. Diagnostic accuracy of magnetic resonance and endoscopic retrograde cholangiography in primary sclerosing cholangitis. *Clin Gastroenterol Hepatol* 2006;4:514–20.

50. Soto JA, Barish MA, Yucel EK, Siegenberg D, Ferrucci JT, Chuttani R. Magnetic resonance cholangiography: comparison with endoscopic retrograde cholangiopancreatography. *Gastroenterology* 1996;110:589–97.

51. Angulo P, Pearce DH, Johnson CD, et al. Magnetic resonance cholangiography in patients with biliary disease: its role in primary sclerosing cholangitis. *J Hepatol* 2000;33:520–7.

52. Talwalkar JA, Angulo P, Johnson CD, Petersen BT, Lindor KD. Cost-minimization analysis of MRC versus ERCP for the diagnosis of primary sclerosing cholangitis. *Hepatology* 2004;40:39–45.

53. Ludwig J, Barham SS, LaRusso NF, Elveback LR, Wiesner RH, McCall JT. Morphologic features of chronic hepatitis associated with primary sclerosing cholangitis or chronic ulcerative colitis. *Hepatology* 1981;1:632–40.

54. Claessen MM, Vleggaar FP, Tytgat KM, Siersema PD, van Buuren HR. High lifetime risk of cancer in primary sclerosing cholangitis. *J Hepatol* 2009;50:158–64.

55. Spivey JR, Jorgensen RA, Gores GJ, Lindor KD. Methionine-enkephalin concentrations correlate with stage of disease but not pruritus in patients with primary biliary cirrhosis. *Am J Gastroenterol* 1994;89:2028–32.

56. Jones EA, Bergasa NV. The pruritus of cholestasis. *Hepatology* 1999;29:1003–6.

57. Bachs L, Pares A, Elena M, Piera C, Rodes J. Effects of long-term rifampicin administration in primary biliary cirrhosis. *Gastroenterology* 1992;102:2077–80.

58. Wolfhagen FHJ, Sternieri E, Hop WCJ, Vitale G, Bertolotti M, Van Buuren HR. Oral naltrexone treatment for cholestatic pruritus: a double-blind, placebo-controlled study. *Gastroenterology* 1997;113:1264–9.

59. Jorgensen RA, Lindor KD, Sartin JS, LaRusso NF, Wiesner RH. Serum lipid and fat-soluble vitamin levels in primary sclerosing cholangitis. *J Clin Gastroenterol* 1995;20:215–19.

60. Hay JE, Lindor KD, Wiesner RH, Dickson ER, Krom RAF, LaRusso NF. The metabolic bone disease of primary sclerosing cholangitis. *Hepatology* 1991;14:257–61.

61. Guanabens N, Pares A, Ros I, et al. Alendronate is more effective than etidronate for increasing bone mass in osteopenic patients with primary biliary cirrhosis. *Hepatology* 1999;30:472A.

62. Lanspa SJ, Chan ATH, Bell JS III, Go VLW, Dickson ER, DiMagno EP. Pathogenesis of steatorrhea in primary biliary cirrhosis. *Hepatology* 1985;5:837–42.

63. Karlsen TH, Schrumpf E, Boberg KM. Gallbladder polyps in primary sclerosing cholangitis: not so benign. *Curr Opin Gastroenterol* 2008;24:395–9.

64. Ponsioen CY, Lam K, van Milligen de Wit AW, Huibregtse K, Tytgat GN. Four years experience with short term stenting in primary sclerosing cholangitis. *Am J Gastroenterol* 1999;94: 2403–7.

65. Bangarulingam SY, Gossard AA, Petersen BT, Ott BJ, Lindor KD. Complications of endoscopic retrograde cholangiopancreatography in primary sclerosing cholangitis. *Am J Gastroenterol* 2009;104: 855–60.

66. Kornfeld D, Ekbom A, Ihre T. Survival and risk of cholangiocarcinoma in patients with primary sclerosing cholangitis. A population-based study. *Scand J Gastroenterol* 1997;32:1042–5.

67. Kaya M, de Groen PC, Angulo P, et al. Treatment of cholangiocarcinoma complicating primary sclerosing cholangitis: the Mayo Clinic experience. *Am J Gastroenterol* 2001;96:1164–9.

68. Chalasani N, Baluyut A, Ismail A, et al. Cholangiocarcinoma in patients with primary sclerosing cholangitis: a multicenter case–control study. *Hepatology* 2000;31.7–11.

69. De Groen PC, Gores GJ, LaRusso NF, Gunderson LL, Nagorney DM. Biliary tract cancers. *N Engl J Med* 1999;341:1368–78.

70. Prytz H, Keiding S, Bjornsson E, Broome U, Almer S, Castedal M, Munk OL. Dynamic FDG-PET is useful for detection of cholangiocarcinoma in patients with PSC listed for liver transplantation. *Hepatology* 2006;44:1572–80.

71. Lazaridis KN, Gores GJ. Cholangiocarcinoma. *Gastroenterology* 2005;128:1655–67.

72. Baron TH, Harewood GC, Rumalla A, et al. A prospective comparison of digital image analysis and routine cytology for the identification of malignancy in biliary tract strictures. *Clin Gastroenterol Hepatol* 2004;2:214–19.

73. Fritcher EG, Kipp BR, Halling KC, et al. A multivariable model using advanced cytologic methods for the evaluation of indeterminate pancreatobiliary strictures. *Gastroenterology* 2009;136:2180–6.

74. Heimbach JK, Haddock MG, Alberts SR, et al. Transplantation for hilar cholangiocarcinoma. *Liver Transpl* 2004;10:S65–8.

75. Wiesner RH, LaRusso NF, Dozois RR, Beaver SJ. Peristomal varices after proctocolectomy in patients with primary sclerosing cholangitis. *Gastroenterology* 1986;90:316–22.

76. Olsson R, Boberg KM, de Muckadell OS, et al. High-dose ursodeoxycholic acid in primary sclerosing cholangitis: a 5-year multicenter, randomized, controlled study. *Gastroenterology* 2005;129: 1464–72.

77. Lindor KD, Kowdley KV, Luketic VA, et al. High-dose ursodeoxycholic acid for the treatment of primary sclerosing cholangitis. *Hepatology* 2009;50:808–14.

78. Tung BY, Emond MJ, Haggitt RC, et al. Ursodiol use is associated with lower prevalence of colonic neoplasia in patients with ulcerative colitis and primary sclerosing cholangitis. *Ann Intern Med* 2001;134:89–95.

79. Cameron JL, Pitt HA, Zinner MJ, et al. Resection of hepatic duct bifurcation and transhepatic stenting for sclerosing cholangitis. *Ann Surg* 1988;207:614–20.

80. Narumi S, Roberts JP, Emond JC, Lake J, Ascher NL. Liver transplantation for sclerosing cholangitis. *Hepatology* 1995;22:451–7.

81. Angulo P, Bharucha AE, Jorgensen RA, et al. Oral nicotine in treatment of primary sclerosing cholangitis: a pilot study. *Dig Dis Sci* 1999;44:602–7.

82. Angulo P, MacCarty RL, Sylvestre PB, et al. Pirfenidone in the treatment of primary sclerosing cholangitis. *Dig Dis Sci* 2002;47: 157–61.

83. Van Hoogstraten HJ, Vleggaar FP, Boland GJ, et al. Budesonide or prednisone in combination with ursodeoxycholic acid in

primary sclerosing cholangitis: a randomized double-blind pilot study. Belgian–Dutch PSC Study Group. *Am J Gastroenterol* 2000;95: 2015–22.

84. Angulo P, Batts KP, Jorgensen RA, LaRusso NA, Lindor KD. Oral budesonide in the treatment of primary sclerosing cholangitis. *Am J Gastroenterol* 2000;95:2333–7.

85. Mitchell SA, Bansi DS, Hunt N, Von Bergmann K, Fleming KA, Chapman RW. A preliminary trial of high-dose ursodeoxycholic acid in primary sclerosing cholangitis. *Gastroenterology* 2001;121: 900–7.

86. Cullen SN, Rust C, Fleming K, Edwards C, Beuers U, Chapman RW. High dose ursodeoxycholic acid for the treatment of primary sclerosing cholangitis is safe and effective. *J Hepatol* 2008;48:792–800.

87. Goss JA, Shackleton CR, Farmer DG,et al. Orthotopic liver transplantation for primary sclerosing cholangitis. A 12-year single center experience. *Ann Surg* 1997;225:472–81.

88. Sheng R, Campbell WL, Zajko AB, Baron RL. Cholangiographic features of biliary strictures after liver transplantation for primary sclerosing cholangitis: evidence of recurrent disease. *AJR Am J Roentgenol* 1996;166:1109–13.

89. Graziadei IW, Wiesner RH, Marotta PJ, et al. Long-term results of patients undergoing liver transplantation for primary sclerosing cholangitis. *Hepatology* 1999;30:1121–7.

90. Knechtle SJ, D'Allesandro AM, Harms BA, Pirsch JD, Belzer FO, Kalayoglu M. Relationships between sclerosing cholangitis, inflammatory bowel disease, and cancer in patients undergoing liver transplantation. *Surgery* 1995;118:615–20.

Multiple choice questions

20.1 There is a strong association between inflammatory bowel disease (IBD) and primary sclerosing cholangitis (PSC). According to the current knowledge, which of the following statements about IBD in PSC patients is true?

    a Crohn disease is the predominant form of IBD in PSC patients.
    b Approximately 20% of patients with PSC will have concomittant IBD.
    c Treatment for underlying IBD will improve the natural history of liver disease.
    d Generally, IBD is diagnosed prior to liver disease.
    e Patients with PSC and concomittant IBD are at lower risk for developing colon cancer than patients with IBD alone.

20.2 Which of the following therapies have been consistently shown to improve outcomes in patients with PSC?

    a Ursodeoxycholic acid at 13–15 mg/kg/day.
    b Ursodeoxycholic acid at 20–30 mg/kg/day.
    c Liver transplantation.
    d Pentoxifylline.
    e Corticosteroids.

Answers to the multiple choice questions can be found in the Appendix at the end of the book.

These multiple choice questions are also available for you to complete online.
Visit http://www.schiffsdiseasesoftheliver.com/

CHAPTER 21
Primary Biliary Cirrhosis

Stephen P. James

Division of Digestive Diseases and Nutrition, National Institute of Diabetes and Digestive and Kidney Diseases, National Institutes of Health, Bethesda, MD, USA

Key concepts

- Primary biliary cirrhosis (PBC) is an uncommon condition that primarily affects middle-aged women throughout the world.
- Most patients are identified in an asymptomatic phase, but they gradually develop symptoms of pruritus, fatigue, and symptoms of associated syndromes or end-stage liver disease.
- Typical laboratory findings are elevations of alkaline phosphatase levels, modest elevations of aspartate aminotransferase (AST) and alanine aminotransferase (ALT) levels, increases in total cholesterol level, and positive antimitochondrial antibody test results.
- The characteristic pathologic features of PBC are destruction and dropout of intrahepatic bile ducts, chronic portal tract inflammation,

cholestasis, and progressive fibrosis, cirrhosis, and portal hypertension.
- About one half of patients have associated autoimmune syndromes, most commonly sicca syndrome, thyroid disease, arthritis, and scleroderma or CREST syndrome (calcinosis, Raynaud phenomenon, esophageal motility disorders, sclerodactyly, and telangiectasia).
- Treatment options include ursodeoxycholic acid (UDCA), cholestyramine, replacement of fat-soluble vitamins, management of complications of portal hypertension, and liver transplantation for end-stage disease.

Primary biliary cirrhosis (PBC) is a chronic, progressive disease of unknown etiology characterized by necrosis of the intrahepatic bile ducts that leads to chronic cholestasis, portal fibrosis, and cirrhosis. The disease is characterized by female predominance, characteristic antimitochondrial antibodies (AMAs), associated autoimmune syndromes, and chronic inflammatory histologic features that have led to its classification as an autoimmune syndrome. Although the first descriptions of PBC appeared in the 19th century [1], wider recognition of the disease did not occur until the publication of reviews in the 20th century that clarified the clinical characteristics of this distinct syndrome [2,3]. Other important developments were the discovery of AMAs [4], which led not only to an important diagnostic test but also to research into the pathogenesis of PBC that continues to the present time. Another advance was the introduction of cholestyramine to treat intractable pruritus and, more recently, ursodeoxycholic acid (UDCA) treatment to improve the biochemical features and to retard the progression of disease. PBC is now frequently recognized in asymptomatic patients, who may have a slow and insidious disease course. Nonetheless, most patients ultimately develop symptoms and have progressive disease. For those who

develop end-stage liver disease, liver transplantation is the only therapeutic option.

Epidemiology

Primary biliary cirrhosis appears to occur throughout the world and in all races; however, there is uneven geographic distribution (Box 21.1). Studies of the epidemiology of PBC are hampered by methodologic problems, including variation in case definition and ascertainment and absence of noninvasive markers of high sensitivity and specificity. The estimates of incidence and prevalence vary widely, from 2 to 24 per million and 19 to 240 per million population, respectively, with the highest incidence and prevalence reported in northern Europe [5–8]. Here the prevalence appears to be increasing, although the relative contributions of methodologic differences, increased awareness, or a true increase in prevalence are uncertain. The median age of diagnosis is approximately 50 years, with a broad range of diagnosis from approximately 20 to 90 years, and 90% of patients are women. Within regions of high prevalence, clustering of cases has been observed, suggesting a contribution of environmental factors to the

Box 21.1 Epidemiology and genetics of primary biliary cirrhosis.

- Incidence: 2–24/1,000,000
- Prevalence: 19–240/1,000,000
- Median age (range): 50 years (20–90 years)
- Female: 90%
- Environmental risk factors: Smoking, environmental toxins?
- Associated autoimmune syndromes: 50%
- Familial clustering: 1–2%
- Twin concordance rate: Monozygotic 0.63/dizygotic 0.0
- Genome-wide association study: HLA class II, IL12A, IL12RB2

HLA, human leucocyte antigen.

pathogenesis [7]. Clustering of cases near superfund toxic waste sites in the United States suggests a role for environmental toxins [9]. Case–control studies have searched for risk factors with inconsistent results: In the United Kingdom, an association with smoking was found, while in the United States an association with non-PBC autoimmune disease, genitourinary tract infections, and previous tonsillectomy was identified [10].

Genetics

There are multiple lines of evidence indicating that genetic susceptibility plays a role in the pathogenesis of PBC (Box 24.1). This evidence includes striking female predominance, familial clustering, association with other autoimmune syndromes, concordance in twin studies, and the results of genome-wide association studies [11–13]. The striking female predominance of PBC obviously links the pathogenesis of the disease to the genetic basis of sex determination, as for many other autoimmune diseases. However, the specific causal mechanisms are currently unclear. Among candidate mechanisms are direct effects of female hormones, immunologic differences between males and females, and increased monosomy X in women with PBC. A commonly recognized feature of diseases that are thought to have an autoimmune basis is that different autoimmune diseases tend to occur with increased frequency within families, which forms the basis for the hypothesis that the tendency to autoimmunity is based in part on shared genetic traits. PBC has long been associated with a variety of autoimmune syndromes both in individual patients and within families of patients with PBC (see subsequent text). One recent population-based study confirmed that autoimmune conditions are found in approximately one half

of patients and that the prevalence of autoimmune disease in first-degree family members is 14% [14], consistent with the thesis that PBC shares common genetic susceptibility traits with other autoimmune conditions. Many case series and epidemiologic studies have noted the familial tendency of PBC, which although uncommon, appears to be increased compared to the general population. The estimates of familial prevalence have ranged from approximately 1% to a high of 6.4%, with estimates in the largest studies being in the 1–2% range. These estimates are similar in different geographic regions, including England, the United States, Sweden, Italy, and Japan. The familial occurrence of PBC also supports a genetic basis, although, of course, environmental etiologies also cause familial clustering.

One of the important traditional methods to evaluate the heritability of disease is to determine concordance rates in twins. In two older reports of single twin pairs, one was reported to be concordant and the other discordant. More recently, an international study evaluated 16 twin pairs with PBC, of whom eight were confirmed to be monozygotic [13]. The concordance rate was 0.63 in monozygotic twins and 0.0 in dizygotic twins. The concordance rates were potentially subject to bias because cases were collected from referral centers and the internet, which differs from traditional population-based twin registry studies. Nonetheless, the high concordance rate for monozygotic twins suggests an important contribution of genetic susceptibility to PBC.

The first genome-wide association study of PBC performed in 536 Canadian and US subjects using a 373,400 single nucleotide polymorphism (SNP) platform identified significant associations in loci in the human leucocyte antigen (HLA) class II region and the interleukin 12A (IL12A) and IL12RB2 regions, as well as lower statistical significance for an association with two other loci implicated in immunologic processes, STAT4 and CTLA4 [12]. The association of PBC with HLA class II alleles confirms and clarifies earlier candidate gene studies, and is consistent with the general association of autoimmune diseases with the HLA class II region. The unexpected association with IL12A and IL12RB2 suggests that abnormal signaling through the IL12 cytokine pathway may play a role in pathogenesis. These observations are particularly intriguing because other lines of evidence implicate the IL12 pathway in autoimmunity and host defense. IL12 represents a potential pathway that could be a target of therapy.

Symptoms

In the past, patients were frequently diagnosed with initial symptoms of fatigue, pruritus, and jaundice, and

---

Box 21.2 Symptoms and physical findings in primary biliary cirrhosis.

Symptoms
- Asymptomatic (most common)
- Fatigue
- Pruritus
- Symptoms of associated syndromes (e.g., sicca, arthritis, Raynaud disease)

Physical findings
- Hepatomegaly
- Splenomegaly
- Jaundice
- Xanthoma
- Increased skin pigmentation, excoriations
- End stage: ascites, edema, wasting, encephalopathy

---

physical findings such as hepatomegaly. However, currently, most patients are diagnosed with PBC at an early stage of disease before the onset of any specific symptoms or physical findings (Box 21.2). The reasons for the shift to early, asymptomatic diagnosis include the widespread use of screening laboratory studies including serum alkaline phosphatase, increased physician awareness of the features of the disease, the ready availability of AMA tests, and, finally, recognition that the disease does in fact have a long, presymptomatic phase in which a specific diagnosis is readily accomplished [15,16]. Most patients, if followed up long enough, eventually develop symptoms that are attributed to the disease.

In order of frequency, the most common symptoms of PBC are fatigue, pruritus, and jaundice. Occasionally, patients have right upper quadrant abdominal pain. Many other symptoms may be present, including that of associated syndromes, such as dry mouth and eyes, Raynaud phenomenon, and arthralgias. Occasionally, patients are brought to attention because of xanthoma, xanthelasma, increasing skin pigmentation, or fracture. Much less commonly, the presenting symptoms may be due to decompensated liver disease, including ascites, edema, bleeding, or encephalopathy.

Fatigue may have an insidious onset and is often the dominant symptom, significantly diminishing the quality of life of patients [17]. It is not uncommon for patients to be initially misdiagnosed with other conditions in which fatigue is prominent, including depression, chronic fatigue syndrome, fibromyalgia, or thyroid disease, which may be associated with PBC. The cause of fatigue in PBC is unclear, but it has been suggested to have a central etiology [18], although other causes might exist, such as mechanisms related to chronic inflammation. Pruritus is also a significant, sometimes debilitating,

symptom in PBC, occurring much earlier in the course of the disease than in other more common forms of liver disease, in which it is commonly associated with hepatic decompensation. As in other cholestatic liver diseases, the pathogenic mechanisms of pruritus are unknown [19].

Physical findings

Early in the course of the disease, physical abnormalities are often completely absent. As the disease progresses, the most common physical findings are hepatomegaly, splenomegaly, excoriations, skin hyperpigmentation, jaundice, and xanthelasma [20]. Late in the course of the disease, physical findings of decompensated liver disease may be present, including ascites, edema, palmar erythema, spider nevi, muscle wasting, and signs of encephalopathy. Uncommonly, patients have physical findings of associated syndromes such as xerophthalmia and xerostomia. Very rarely, patients have Kayser–Fleischer rings because of copper retention.

Routine laboratory tests

The routine laboratory abnormalities in PBC are typical of chronic cholestatic syndromes and chronic liver disease (Box 21.3). Almost invariably, the serum alkaline phosphatase and γ-glutamyltransferase levels are elevated, typically approximately 2–2.5 times the upper limit of normal at the time of diagnosis [21]. Serum alkaline phosphatase levels often remain relatively stable and do not closely correlate with the stage or progression of disease. Rarely, patients have been identified with normal alkaline

---

Box 21.3 Characteristic laboratory abnormalities in primary biliary cirrhosis.

• Alkaline phosphatase:	2–2.5 times upper limit of normal
• AST, ALT:	<5 times upper limit of normal
• Bilirubin:	Normal in early phase, progressive rise late phase
• Cholesterol, HDL cholesterol:	Elevated
• Serum IgM:	Elevated
• Antimitochondrial antibodies:	Present titer >1:40 in 95% of patients
• Other autoantibodies:	ANA, RF, SMA, and others commonly found

ALT, alanine aminotransferase; ANA, antinuclear antibody; AST, aspartate aminotransferase; HDL, high-density lipoprotein; IgM, immunoglobulin M; RF, rheumatoid factor; SMA, smooth muscle antibody.

phosphatase levels on the basis of positive serum AMAs and typical liver histologic abnormalities, presumably at a very early stage of disease [22]. Serum alanine aminotransferase (ALT) and aspartate aminotransferase (AST) levels are only modestly elevated, usually less than five times the upper limit of normal, and their levels also do not correlate with stage of disease. Serum bilirubin levels are typically normal early in disease and rise with disease progression. Serum bilirubin is a major component of the prognostic indices for end-stage PBC [23]. In common with other cholestatic syndromes, serum lipid levels are abnormal in PBC. Patients occasionally have striking hypercholesterolemia, which correlates with the physical finding of xanthomas. However, there is a corresponding increase in high-density lipoprotein cholesterol, which may explain why patients with PBC seem to have only an average risk for cardiovascular complications [24]. In addition, although low-density lipoprotein (LDL) levels are also increased, a subfraction, lipoprotein X, is present that may inhibit the atherogenic properties of LDL lipoproteins [25]. Late in the course of disease serum cholesterol levels may decline along with other synthetic functions during end-stage liver failure, including a fall in serum albumin level and rise in prothrombin time, which may be exacerbated by malabsorption of fat-soluble vitamins such as vitamin K. Because of the overwhelming fatigue experienced by some patients, concern may arise because of anemia in patients with PBC, which is similar to the anemia of chronic disease. Rarely patients are identified with autoimmune Coombs-positive hemolytic anemia [26], which may confound the interpretation of serum bilirubin levels, or pernicious anemia [27]. Thrombocytopenia, if present, is usually a manifestation of portal hypertension, although rare cases of idiopathic thrombocytopenic purpura have been associated with PBC. PBC, like other cholestatic syndromes, leads to copper retention, resulting in raised urinary copper and serum ceruloplasmin levels [28]. Other laboratory abnormalities may be present as a result of associated autoimmune syndromes. Patients with PBC typically have elevated serum immunoglobulin M (IgM), sometimes to striking levels [3], some of which may be monomeric rather than pentameric [29].

Autoantibodies

The presence of autoantibodies, particularly AMAs, is a clinical hallmark and important diagnostic feature of PBC, first reported as a distinguishing characteristic compared with other forms of chronic cholestasis by Doniach et al. in 1966 [4]. Since that time, extensive studies have refined diagnostic testing for AMAs, which are found in up to 95% of patients [30]. Furthermore, AMAs have been

a major theme in research on the pathogenesis of PBC. Initial studies defined AMAs by indirect tissue immunofluorescence. Subsequent studies showed that serum autoantibodies react with trypsin-sensitive components of the inner mitochondrial membrane, the so-called M2 antigen, in a nontissue-specific manner with broad cross-reactivity to antigens present in many species, including both eukaryotes and prokaryotes such as *Escherichia coli* [31,32]. Other mitochondrial antigens, arbitrarily designated M1 to M9 [33], have been previously described as the target of PBC autoantibodies. Some, such as M1, represent anticardiolipin of syphilis and are unrelated to PBC. Others, such as M4, M8, and M9, were previously described as being PBC specific; however, the specificity of these antigens has been questioned and they are not routinely used for diagnosis [34].

Cloning and characterization of the M2 autoantigens recognized by PBC sera has led to the identification of four major components of a family of mitochondrial antigens that contain lipoic acid and are members of the 2-oxoacid dehydrogenase (2-OAD) multimeric enzyme complexes [35,36]. These include the pyruvate dehydrogenase complex (PDC), 2-oxoglutarate dehydrogenase complex (OGDC), and branched-chain 2-oxoacid dehydrogenase complex (BCOADC). All the members of this family play important roles in cellular metabolism. Approximately 95% of sera of patients with PBC react with both the PDC core dihydrolipoamide acetyl transferase (E2) structure and the E3-binding protein (E3BP) by immunoblot or enzyme-linked immunosorbent assay (ELISA), these two subunits being completely cross-reactive. PBC sera also react, at a much lower frequency, with other components of PDC, including the E1α and E1β subunits. Sera also react with the E2 subunits of OGDC and BCOADC with a frequency of 90% and 50%, respectively. Considerable information is available on the B-cell epitopes, and they all appear to be defined by conformational structures contained within the lipoic acid-binding domains. AMAs block the enzymatic activity of 2-OAD complexes in vitro [37,38]; however, it is not known whether PBC autoantibodies have in vivo activity against these enzymes.

Even though serum IgM may be elevated to striking levels, AMAs are present in all three immunoglobulin classes, including secretory IgA, and no consistent clinical correlations have been reported with different immunoglobulin classes of reactivity.

Although there has been considerable progress in the definition of AMAs in PBC, the literature consistently contains patients who are negative for AMAs but otherwise have the same typical clinical, biochemical, and liver histologic features of the disease [39,40]. Some patients are found to be positive for AMAs when the more sensitive and specific tests available in research laboratories are used [41]. Some studies have reported a high frequency of antinuclear antibodies (ANAs) in this group of patients and have referred to this condition as autoimmune cholangiopathy [39,42]. However, because the clinical features of the two conditions overlap considerably [43], it is unclear whether these are separate conditions or variants of the same condition with differing autoantibody patterns. The views on these conditions are more than semantic. The absence of AMAs in patients with PBC-like syndromes has been used as an argument that AMAs are only an epiphenomenon, rather than pathogenic. However, this argument would be dismissed if future research on "autoimmune cholangiopathy" identifies a different etiologic basis compared to AMA-positive PBC.

Other autoantibodies are frequently found in patients with PBC. Approximately 25% of patients have ANAs with a "nuclear rim" and "multiple nuclear dots," which correlate with autoantibodies recognizing gp210, nucleoporin 62, and nuclear body protein sp100. These ANAs are relatively specific for PBC [44]. Other autoantibodies that have been reported in patients with PBC include those connected with associated autoimmune syndromes (see below) such as antithyroid autoantibodies, rheumatoid factor, and antibodies found in Sjögren syndrome, as well as a long list of other antibodies of unknown significance, including antilymphocytotoxic antibodies, anti-acetylcholine receptor antibodies, antiplatelet antibodies, antihistone antibodies, anticentromere antibodies, and antibodies against carbonic anhydrase II, α-enolase, lactoferrin, and smooth muscles.

Historically, AMA has been detected by indirect immunofluorescence on rat tissue sections showing a cytoplasmic granular pattern of the mitochondria. False-positive reactions may occur because of the presence of other serologic cross-reactions, such as those with anticardiolipin [45]. AMAs may be detected by immunoblot of submitochondrial particle preparations such as antigens or by ELISA using recombinant antigens for PDC-E2, BCOADC-E2, and OADC-E2. It appears that immunoblot and ELISA methods have higher sensitivity and specificity for PBC than immunofluorescence tests. Currently, clinical AMA testing is usually performed by ELISA directed against E2 antigens. AMAs may be found in patients with other syndromes, particularly overlap syndromes and autoimmune hepatitis (AIH), but also occasionally in primary sclerosing cholangitis (PSC) and drug-induced liver disease.

Pathology

The gross pathologic features of PBC are not specific for the disease and include bile staining of the liver, enlarge-

ment, fine nodularity, and, eventually, a grossly cirrhotic appearance. The extrahepatic biliary system is normal, with the exception of an increased prevalence of gallstones. Enlarged lymph nodes may be found in the porta hepatis, along with other intra-abdominal sites, and these do not have any characteristic features other than the occasional appearance of granulomas. Enlargement of the spleen, along with other pathologic features of portal hypertension, appear later in the course of the disease.

Characteristic microscopic hepatic abnormalities include portal inflammation with the destruction and disappearance of intrahepatic bile ducts, abnormal bile duct proliferation, fibrosis, and cirrhosis (Fig. 21.1). Although, overall, the disease is characterized by progressive destruction and loss of bile ducts with portal fibrosis progressing to cirrhosis, in the early and intermediate stages of the disease the process is not uniformly distributed throughout the liver. There is therefore potential for significant sampling error when performing needle biopsy of the liver. Two similar staging systems, as proposed by Ludwig et al. [46] and Scheuer [47], have been widely adopted to describe the liver histologic lesions. Because of the focal nature of the lesions, multiple stages – sometimes all four histologic stages – of lesions have occasionally been identified in the same liver.

In stage 1, which is thought to represent the earliest pathologic lesions of the disease, there is destruction of the intrahepatic septal and interlobular bile ducts, which can range in size up to 100 μm in diameter. This stage has been called the *portal stage* in the Ludwig system and the *florid duct lesion stage* in the Scheuer system. Portal lesions are characterized by damage to the bile ducts, which may be associated with vacuolated or pyknotic biliary epithelial cells and even frank rupture or disappearance of portions of the duct. The duct is typically surrounded by a dense lymphocytic infiltrate, which may also include histiocytes, plasma cells, eosinophils, and, occasionally, true epithelioid giant cells. Neutrophils are absent or infrequent, and periductular fibrosis, as found in PSC and biliary obstruction, is absent. Inflammation does not extend beyond the portal tracts, and hepatocyte injury is minimal.

The second stage of the disease is characterized by the appearance of abnormal proliferating bile ductules without duct lumens, the disappearance of normal bile ducts, and extension of the portal inflammation into the hepatic parenchyma. Typically, there is limited piecemeal necrosis of periportal hepatocytes with surrounding foamy macrophages and limited fibrosis confined to the portal tract.

In stage 3, there is a substantial increase in fibrosis, and fibrous septa may link portal tracts. Lymphocytic infiltrates remain in the portal tracts, but bile ducts may be difficult to identify or completely absent.

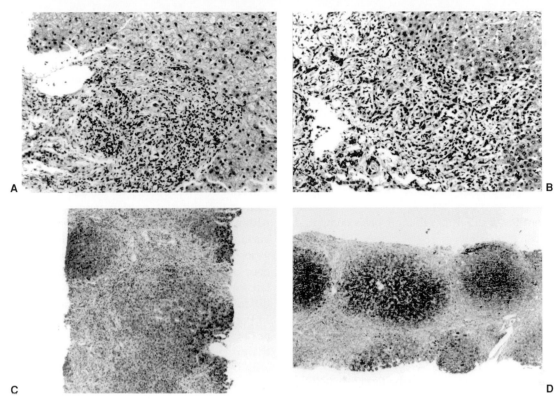

Figure 21.1 Liver histologic abnormalities in primary biliary cirrhosis. (A) Stage 1: a damaged bile duct is surrounded by chronic inflammatory cells. (B) Stage 2: proliferation of abnormal bile ductules and chronic inflammation of portal tract. (C) Stage 3: portal fibrosis. (D) Stage 4: cirrhosis.

Stage 4 is characterized by frank cirrhosis with regenerative nodules.

Other histologic abnormalities may be found that are not specific for PBC, including Mallory bodies and deposition of copper, which are found in other cholestatic liver diseases.

Immunologic techniques have been used to further define the histologic lesions of PBC [35,48,49]. The lymphocytic portal infiltrates primarily contain CD4+ T cells, although CD8+ T cells predominate in areas of piecemeal necrosis, and their levels may be increased in early stages of the disease. The infiltrating CD4+ T cells have a CD45RO high phenotype characteristic of memory T cells. The bile duct epithelium contains small numbers of intraepithelial lymphocytes, potentially analogous to those found in the intestinal epithelium, that are predominantly CD8+ T cells and are found in PBC bile duct lesions. Natural killer T (NKT) cells represent only approximately 5% of lymphoid cells in liver infiltrates. Infiltrates also contain B cells, plasma cells, eosinophils, macrophages, and dendritic cells. The cytokine profile of PBC tissue is predominantly characterized by expression of interferon-γ, but interleukins IL2, IL5, IL6, and transforming growth factor-β (TGF-β) are also expressed, so that PBC does not have a clear T_H1 or T_H2 profile.

A number of bile duct abnormalities have been defined using immunologic techniques. Bile ducts in patients with PBC have aberrant expression of the AMA antigen PDC-E2 on the cell surface [50]. In addition, major histocompatibility complex (MHC) class II antigens, which are usually not expressed on normal bile ducts, have increased expression on bile ducts in PBC. Other molecules have also been noted to have increased expression on bile duct cells in PBC, including intercellular adhesion molecule 1 (ICAM-1), vascular cell adhesion molecule 1 (VCAM-1), the cytokines IL6 and tumor necrosis factor-α (TNF-α), and the chemotactic molecule fractalkine [51].

Associated syndromes

Numerous case reports and descriptions of patient cohorts have noted the association of PBC with other diseases, particularly autoimmune syndromes (Box 21.4). There are no extensive epidemiologic studies with case–controls to evaluate the true prevalence of autoimmune syndromes in PBC, and many of the reports are likely subject to referral and reporting bias. In one study of a geographically based PBC cohort, the most commonly identified associated conditions were Sjögren syndrome (25%), Raynaud phenomenon (24%), autoimmune

Box 21.4 Associated syndromes of primary biliary cirrhosis.[a]

- Sjögren syndrome
- Raynaud phenomenon
- Thyroid disease
- Rheumatoid arthritis
- Scleroderma and CREST
- Systemic lupus erythematosus
- Glomerulonephritis
- Type 1 diabetes
- Polymyositis
- Myasthenia gravis
- Autoimmune thrombocytopenic purpura
- Pernicious anemia
- Addison disease
- Celiac disease
- Skin diseases (e.g., lichen planus, pemphigoid, dermatomyositis)

[a] Listed in approximate order of decreasing frequency.
CREST, calcinosis, Raynaud phenomenon, esophageal motility disorders, sclerodactyly, and telangiectasia.

thyroid disease (23%), rheumatoid arthritis (17%), CREST syndrome (scleroderma and calcinosis, Raynaud phenomenon, esophageal motility disorders, sclerodactyly, and telangiectasia) (8%), and pernicious anemia (4%) [52]. The overall prevalence of autoimmune conditions in patients with PBC was 53% in this study. The association with Sjögren syndrome, arthritis, Raynaud phenomenon, and autoimmune thyroid disease is the most commonly reported associated syndrome in other reports on autoimmunity in PBC [53–56]. The most common thyroid disease is Hashimoto thyroiditis, but rarely Graves disease or hyperthyroidism is found. Antithyroid antibodies are frequently found in patients with PBC without clinical evidence of thyroid dysfunction. Sicca symptoms are relatively common in PBC, but only a minority of patients have anti-Ro or anti-La antibodies typical of primary Sjögren syndrome. Similarly, although arthralgia is common in PBC patients, only a minority fulfill American Rheumatism Association criteria for definite or probable rheumatoid arthritis. Patients having manifestations of scleroderma most often have the limited CREST variant of this disease. Among patients with PBC who have one autoimmune condition, most also have a second one.

Overlap syndromes

Patients with PBC may have features that overlap significantly with those of AIH [57,58]. Positive AMAs, high serum alkaline phosphatase levels, and histologic bile duct lesions are sometimes found in patients with oth-

erwise typical features of AIH. Conversely, patients with PBC may have significant hepatocyte injury and high titer positive ANAs. Additional heterogeneity is represented by patients with typical clinical features of PBC except for the absence of AMAs, and some of these patients have high ANA levels. This latter syndrome has been called *autoimmune cholangiopathy* and is otherwise indistinguishable from PBC. Individual reports have indicated the presence of features of AIH in 2–19% of patients with PBC. Overlap features may be present at the time of initial diagnosis or appear subsequently. Different scoring systems have been proposed for the diagnosis of overlap, but further definition of overlap syndromes will depend on new specific information on the etiopathogenesis of these various conditions to differentiate whether overlap represents a spectrum of one disease or the simultaneous presence of two different conditions. The diagnosis of overlap syndrome is not purely academic because there are different treatment recommendations for AIH and PBC. In patients with significant features of AIH in addition to PBC, a treatment trial with corticosteroids and/or azathioprine should be entertained in addition to treatment with UDCA [59] (see below).

Complications

The early course of most patients with PBC who are not asymptomatic is marked by fatigue, pruritus, and, occasionally, symptoms or complications of associated conditions; however, patients often continue to have a good functional status. Sometimes, the symptoms of pruritus and fatigue may be quite disabling and emotionally disturbing to patients. Interestingly, depression does not seem to be a common diagnosis in PBC because there are alternative explanations for mood alterations. One small trial of an antidepressant in patients with fatigue found no benefit [60].

Late in the course of the disease, the major complications are related to chronic cholestasis, portal hypertension, and cirrhosis (Box 21.5). Chronic cholestasis is

Box 21.5 Complications of primary biliary cirrhosis.

- Emotional disturbance: debilitating pruritus and fatigue
- Metabolic bone disease
- Portal hypertension: ascites, edema, encephalopathy, varices
- Malabsorption: fat-soluble vitamins
- Hyperlipidemia
- Hepatocellular carcinoma
- Asymptomatic urinary tract infection
- Distal renal tubular acidosis

associated with metabolic bone disease [61], which may cause painful fractures. The etiology of bone disease appears to be primarily the direct effects of cholestasis on bone, rather than malabsorption of vitamin D. The full spectrum of complications of portal hypertension is found in patients with PBC, often before the appearance of stage IV cirrhosis on liver biopsy specimens [62]. Historically, complications due to portal hypertension were common either as presenting symptoms or shortly after diagnosis, but these are now uncommon. There do not seem to be any unique features related to variceal bleeding, ascites, edema, encephalopathy, or wasting due to end-stage liver disease, with the possible exception of the additional contribution of malabsorption due to chronic cholestasis. Hyperlipidemia is a manifestation of chronic cholestasis, although the specific lipid abnormalities do not provide independent additional risk factors for cardiovascular disease. Although hepatocellular carcinoma has been reported in PBC, it may not be as common as other forms of cirrhosis [63,64]. There have been reports of an increase in breast cancer in women with PBC, but this has not been confirmed by others. An increased frequency of asymptomatic urinary tract infection has been reported in PBC, however the significance of this finding is unclear. Distal renal tubular acidosis has been reported in 30–60% of patients with PBC.

Pathogenesis

The etiology and pathogenesis of PBC are unknown. A variety of etiologies have been postulated, including infectious causes; however, the most common view is that the disease falls within the category of autoimmune diseases [35]. The rationale for this thesis is that multiple features of PBC support a primary autoimmune pathogenesis, including: (i) the histologic features of bile duct lesions; (ii) characteristic autoantibodies; (iii) strong female predominance; (iv) an association, although weak, with MHC class II genes; (v) the frequent association with other autoimmune syndromes; and (vi) the presence of similar bile duct lesions in other immunologically mediated diseases, namely, graft-versus-host disease (GVHD), both in humans and animal models, and the recurrence of PBC in liver allografts. One feature that unfortunately sets PBC apart from other autoimmune diseases is the apparent lack of benefit of immunosuppressive therapies. Until recently, the lack of robust animal models for the disease has impaired rapid exploration of novel hypotheses, and patient-based research is hindered by the indolent and slowly progressive nature of the disease. Much current research into the pathogenesis of PBC parallels that of other autoimmune diseases, including a search for environmental triggers, a genetic basis of susceptibility, and

details about the effector mechanisms responsible for the primary bile duct lesions. This will hopefully lead to the identification of new therapeutic targets.

AMAs are the most distinctive specific immunologic characteristic of PBC and, not surprisingly, have been the focus of numerous studies. As noted in the preceding text, AMAs can inhibit the enzymatic activity of their target antigens in vitro, but it is not known whether this occurs in vivo. Autoantibodies may potentially cause tissue injury, regardless of whether they alter the function of their target antigen; therefore, this particular issue does not resolve the question of the pathogenicity of AMAs. AMAs fix complement, although remarkably little attention has been directed at determining whether there is specific deposition of AMAs at sites of tissue injury in the liver. An intriguing piece of evidence suggesting a potential pathogenic role for AMAs in liver disease is the association of neonatal hepatitis in two cases with the presence of AMAs of maternal origin, which resolved on disappearance of the AMAs [65]. Another observation is that patients with GVHD have histologic lesions of chronic nonsuppurative destructive cholangitis [66] that has features similar to those of PBC. This disease is mediated by the recognition of alloantigens by T cells, and the disease can be recapitulated in animal models, including the production of bile duct lesions [67]. Although this model is useful in elucidating the specific immunologic mechanisms present in GVHD, it is as yet unknown whether the lessons learned extend to PBC. PBC may recur [68] in approximately 20–30% of patients within 10 years of orthotopic liver transplantation, characterized by typical bile duct lesions and persistence of AMAs. Recurrent PBC following liver transplantation potentially affords an opportunity to study pathogenic mechanisms in the liver prospectively from the onset of disease. However, the mechanisms of recurrence per se are no less complicated to dissect than the primary disease itself, and as yet no new insights into pathogenesis have emerged from studies of recurrent PBC.

Considerable information has emerged to define the nature of both the B-cell and T-cell responses to the autoantigens recognized by AMAs. There is overlap between epitopes recognized by B cells and both CD4+ T cells and CD8+ T cells, and there is enrichment for specific antigen-reactive clones within the liver [69]. Cytokines produced in liver infiltrates are dominated by T_H1 cytokines but also contain T_H2 cytokines, providing a mixed picture. Furthermore, the expression of adhesion molecules and chemokines, such as fractalkine, by biliary epithelial cells provides further details on potential mediators involved in the formation of inflammatory lesions within the liver. However, the precise sequence of events and specific effector mechanisms contributing to bile duct injury are as yet undefined, and the possibility that the inflammatory lesions are entirely secondary in nature has not been eliminated.

Recently there has been progress in developing animal models to study the pathogenesis of PBC. These models include completely unrelated, genetically modified strains with systemic diseases that were created for other purposes, which spontaneously developed liver injury, and animals that have been immunized with PBC relevant antigens with the intent of inducing liver injury. Among the former models, mice with modified TGF-β signaling [70], specific modified strains of the nonobese diabetic (NOD) mouse [71], the Scurfy mouse, and Ae2$_{a,b}$-deficient mice lacking the CL$^-$/HCO3$^-$ anion exchanger [72] have all been observed to have a number of features of PBC. These features include serum AMA, portal lymphoid infiltrates, and bile duct injury. Some of these animals have widespread systemic immunologically mediated injury and autoimmunity, including injury to the gut. By analogy with animal research in the field of inflammatory bowel disease, although animals with spontaneous PBC-like abnormalities may or may not provide insight into the genetic or environmental causes of PBC, they may be extremely useful in studying detailed pathologic pathways and mechanisms in PBC that could lead to new targets for diagnosis and treatment. In contrast to the spontaneous models, there have been many previous attempts to purposefully immunize animals to produce specific liver diseases, including PBC. Recently, immunization approaches using lipoic acid, the cofactor of PDC-E2, have produced histologic lesions and AMA [73], lending support to the hypothesis that specific xenobiotics could trigger PBC.

The mechanisms that trigger the immunologic abnormalities observed in PBC remain a matter of speculation. The highly conserved sequences in antigens are recognized by AMAs across species, including prokaryotes, suggesting that molecular mimicry could play a role in triggering autoimmune responses. Multiple microbes have been identified with sequence homology, including *E. coli*, *Neurospora crassa*, *Pseudomonas putida*, *Novosphingobium aromaticivorans*, and others [74]. It has also suggested that xenobiotics might trigger immune recognition of self-antigens; however, other than lipoic acid, no specific candidates have emerged in PBC.

Another theory for the pathogenesis of PBC is that it is the direct result of an infection. In the search for a transmissible agent, filtrates of lymph nodes from patients with PBC were shown to induce the expression of PDC-E2 in biliary epithelial cell cultures [75]. Further studies identified viral particles in biliary epithelial cultures and tissues from patients with PBC, and were able to clone exogenous retroviral sequences from cultured biliary cells, which were identified as a β-retrovirus related to murine mammary tumor virus (MMTV) [76]. How-

ever, others have not been able to verify the presence of MMTV-related retrovirus in PBC [77]. In an uncontrolled pilot study, combination therapy using lamivudine and zidovudine in a small number of patients showed improvement in liver histology and biochemical abnormalities. This suggests the possibility that antiviral therapy might be of benefit, but validation of this approach would require further controlled trials [78].

Diagnosis

The diagnosis of PBC is based on the presence of typical clinical features, routine laboratory tests, AMAs, liver biopsy specimen abnormalities, and the absence of other conditions that could resemble PBC [20,79]. PBC should be suspected in patients with symptoms such as profound fatigue, pruritus, abdominal pain, or hepatomegaly and with routine laboratory test results consistent with cholestasis – that is, an elevated alkaline phosphatase level with minimal or modest elevation of serum transaminase levels (less than five times the upper limit of normal). Other typical features are hypercholesterolemia and a high serum IgM level. As noted in the preceding text, most patients are now diagnosed because of abnormal liver biochemical test results obtained on screening examinations in the absence of any symptoms. Occasionally, patients are diagnosed during the evaluation of symptoms of an associated syndrome, such as sicca syndrome, thyroid disease, or arthritis. The most important confirmatory laboratory test is the detection of serum AMA. The sensitivity and specificity of AMAs are both approximately 95%, but there is variation in the literature, depending on case definition and the test used [80]. Approximately 0.5% of the general population is AMA-positive, but the great majority of these individuals do not develop PBC. Approximately 5% of patients are AMA-negative, and some of these patients have other autoantibodies, particularly ANAs. These latter patients are sometimes referred to as having autoimmune cholangitis; however, their clinical syndrome is not clearly distinguishable from PBC. Rarely, patients have been identified with normal serum alkaline phosphatase levels and positive AMAs, with typical liver biopsy findings.

Although, historically, a liver biopsy was considered mandatory to make a specific diagnosis of PBC and to provide prognostic information on the basis of histologic stage, a recent study has suggested that most patients do not need a liver biopsy for diagnosis [81]. On the basis of a retrospective analysis of a large sample of patients who had undergone liver biopsy, AMA level determination, and serum biochemical tests, the combination of positive AMAs, alkaline phosphatase levels greater than 1.5 times the upper limit of normal, and AST levels less than five times the upper limit of normal (found in 112 of 131 patients; 85% of patients reviewed) had a positive predictive value of 98.2% for the diagnosis of PBC. Although other studies confirming this analysis have not been done, patients falling within this profile probably do not need a liver biopsy unless other clinical features raise the possibility of a different diagnosis. A liver biopsy to confirm the diagnosis should certainly be entertained in the approximately 15% of patients who do not meet the above criteria. An additional rationale for restricting the use of liver biopsy in patients suspected of having PBC is that valid prognostic information can be obtained from indices based on noninvasive testing, and that histologic stage as determined by liver biopsy is not needed for clinical decisions.

Imaging studies are important in the evaluation of patients with cholestatic liver disease. In patients with typical clinical features of PBC, imaging studies may not be necessary. However, as the differential diagnosis of PBC includes other hepatobiliary diseases with overlapping clinical features, cholangiography may be indicated to exclude stones, strictures, tumors, PSC, or other uncommon conditions affecting the biliary system. The imaging procedure of choice is magnetic resonance cholangiography; endoscopic retrograde cholangiopancreatography (ERCP) is generally indicated only when therapeutic intervention is required. Magnetic resonance imaging may be indicated in the detection of advanced fibrosis, cirrhosis, or hepatocellular carcinoma, but is generally not indicated for interval evaluation. The utility of other noninvasive methods, such as elastography, has not been conclusively established for PBC [82].

The differential diagnosis of cholestatic syndromes includes: extrahepatic biliary obstruction due to stones, strictures, or tumors; PSC; drug-induced cholestasis; cholestatic viral hepatitis; sarcoidosis; idiopathic granulomatous hepatitis; AIH; and idiopathic adulthood ductopenia (Box 21.6). Other conditions that cause injury

to bile ducts should be straightforward to differentiate and include GVHD, hepatic allograft rejection, ischemic cholangitis, and infectious cholangitis in immunosuppressed patients. Finally, clinical features of PBC may coexist with features of AIH in an overlap syndrome. PSC should be suspected in patients with inflammatory bowel disease. AMAs are only occasionally positive in patients with PSC. The diagnostic procedure of choice for PSC is cholangiography because the specific liver biopsy specimen lesions of PBC and PSC are each found in only a minority of their respective conditions, and nonspecific liver biopsy specimen features may be similar. The use of drugs known to cause chronic cholestasis could cause difficulty in diagnosis, particularly because some drugs also induce autoantibody production. Patients with viral hepatitis occasionally have a chronic cholestatic syndrome and bile duct lesions on liver biopsy specimens; however, AMAs are negative and serologic tests for viral hepatitis are positive. Occasionally, differentiation of PBC from hepatic sarcoidosis presents a difficult diagnostic problem [83]. AMAs are typically negative in sarcoidosis, and the presence of typical extrahepatic manifestations is necessary to make the diagnosis of sarcoidosis. In about one fourth of patients with AIH, AMAs are positive, usually in low titer, and bile duct lesions may be found on liver biopsy specimens. Idiopathic adulthood ductopenia is a somewhat recently described condition in adults characterized by paucity of bile ducts, chronic cholestasis, and, by definition, the absence of any defining characteristics of other ductopenic diseases, including inflammatory liver histologic lesions, autoantibodies, or associated conditions such as IBD [84].

Treatment

Medical treatments of PBC have included primary therapies aimed at the underlying disease processes and at preventing or delaying progression, therapies for symptoms such as fatigue and pruritus to improve quality of life, and therapies directed at complications, including osteoporosis, fat-soluble vitamin deficiency, and complications of portal hypertension (such as ascites, edema, variceal bleeding, and hepatic encephalopathy) (Table 21.1). Comprehensive practice guidelines have been published, representing a consensus of expert opinion for the management of PBC [85]. There are no specific treatments for complications related to portal hypertension in PBC that differ from other causes of end-stage liver disease, and they will not be discussed here. Therapy may also be needed for associated syndromes, such as thyroid disease, arthritis, or Sjögren syndrome, and they will also not be discussed here. In evaluating treatment trials for PBC, it should be kept in mind that this is a difficult disease to

---

Box 21.6 Differential diagnosis of primary biliary cirrhosis.

- Extrahepatic biliary obstruction (e.g., stone, stricture, tumor)
- Primary sclerosing cholangitis
- Drug-induced cholestasis
- Cholestatic viral hepatitis
- Sarcoidosis
- Idiopathic granulomatous hepatitis
- Autoimmune hepatitis
- Idiopathic adulthood ductopenia
- Special situations with bile duct injury: graft-versus-host disease, liver allograft rejection, ischemic cholangitis, infectious cholangitis in immunocompromised host

Table 21.1 Treatment therapies for primary biliary cirrhosis.

Therapy	Drug	Dose
Primary therapy	Ursodeoxycholic acid	13–15 mg/kg/day
Therapies for pruritus	Cholestyramine or colestipol	Up to 16 g/day in divided doses[a]
	Alternatives: rifampin, phenobarbital, opioid antagonists, plasmapheresis	
Therapies for complications:		
Metabolic bone disease	Calcium, vitamin D	
Malabsorption	Water-soluble forms of vitamins A, D, E, and K	
Sicca	Artificial tears, dental hygiene	
Portal hypertension complications	As indicated	
Other associated syndromes	As indicated	

[a]May interfere with drug absorption; do not administer with other drugs.

study because of many factors, including the indolent and variable natural history of the disease, sampling error in liver biopsy, and the absence of robust biomarkers for the early stages of the disease, in which therapeutic interventions might be expected to have the greatest benefit.

Ursodeoxycholic acid, the only US Food and Drug Administration (FDA)-approved medical therapy for PBC, is generally agreed to ameliorate serum biochemical abnormalities and to potentially delay progression of disease to death or need for transplantation [86]. A number of mechanisms have been proposed by which UDCA is therapeutic in PBC, including anticholestatic effects and antiapoptotic actions. However, the precise mechanisms are unclear and may not involve the primary abnormalities that lead to autoimmune destruction of the bile ducts. Numerous treatment trials of PBC with UDCA alone, or in combination with other agents, have been conducted using varying numbers of patients and trial designs, and these are summarized in detail elsewhere [87,88]. In the largest reported trial – a Canadian multicenter double-blinded, placebo-controlled study of 222 patients – treatment with UDCA at a dosage of 13–15 mg/kg/day resulted in improvement in transaminases, alkaline phosphatase, total cholesterol, and IgM levels and prevention of a rise in serum bilirubin level. However, no improvement in symptoms, liver biopsy results, or need for liver transplantation was noted. In a subsequent meta-analysis of 11 randomized trials involving 1,272 patients, improvements in biochemical studies were found, but no difference between placebo and UDCA was found for progression of liver histology or the need for liver transplantation [89]. In contrast, a meta-analysis of the five studies [90–94] that included data obtained from open-label long-term follow-up periods reached a different conclusion, showing a significant reduction in risk of death or liver transplantation (odds ratio, 0.68 (95% CI, 0.48 to 0.95)) equiv-

alent to a 32% reduction in patients treated with UDCA [95]. Because UDCA consistently ameliorates serum biochemistry abnormalities, concern has been raised that predictive models for PBC might underestimate progression of disease. However, models such as the Mayo risk score still accurately predict the clinical course in patients with PBC who are receiving UDCA [96]. Studies have also reported a delay in progression of liver fibrosis [97]. A subsequent analysis of histologic data from four large placebo-controlled trials demonstrated that UDCA therapy had a beneficial effect in stage 1 or 2 disease, reducing periportal inflammation and ductular proliferation [98]. Continuing analyses of open-label follow-up of patients have provided conflicting interpretations of the benefits of UDCA. In one randomized study in which patients received UDCA or placebo for 2 years, followed by open-label treatment in 112 patients for a subsequent 2 years, no differences were found in death or the need for liver transplantation [99]. In another study of long-term UDCA treatment comparing treated and nontreated patients for a mean of 5.8 years, there was amelioration of serum biochemical abnormalities in treated patients; however, there was no significant difference in death, need for transplantation, symptoms, or complications. It should be noted that this study did not evolve from a randomized trial, and required data analyses taking into account baseline differences and prognostic models [100]. Another analysis of 262 treated patients followed up for a mean of 8 years, using a Markov model and the updated Mayo model for control predictions, found that treatment with UDCA normalized survival rate (for death or transplantation) for patients with stage 1 or 2 disease who were treated, whereas those with more advanced stages had significantly worse survival [101]. A more recent long-term follow-up study demonstrated that patients with early PBC who were treated with UDCA have a prognosis similar to that of the general population, and those with advanced PBC who had a biochemical response to UDCA had a better prognosis than nonresponders [102]. In summary the weight of evidence supports the use of UCDA as primary therapy for PBC at all stages of disease.

Fortunately, UDCA is relatively well tolerated, the main side effect being diarrhea, and therapy appears to have no significant long-term complications. The currently recommended dosage is 13–15 mg/kg/day, although higher dosage regimens have been investigated. If cholestyramine is used concurrently to treat pruritus, there should be a 4-hour delay between the administration of cholestyramine and UDCA. Multiple other agents have been tested as therapies for PBC, including azathioprine [103], methotrexate [104,105], prednisolone [106], chlorambucil [107], cyclosporin A [108], and D-penicillamine [109]. There is no clear overall benefit of most of these therapies, and some, such as systemic corticosteroids, are associated with significant bone complications [3]. Although one prospective double-blind trial of colchicine showed improved survival after 4 years in one study, subsequent studies have shown much less benefit and no improvement in survival [20].

UDCA has also been used in combination with other drugs, including prednisolone, budesonide, azathioprine, methotrexate, and colchicines – drugs that individually have not shown consistent benefit for the disease in multiple trials. The results of these trials can be summarized as showing benefits no different from UDCA alone, and sometimes with more side effects [110]. Small pilot studies have been undertaken with other agents, including mycophenolate mofetil, silymarin, and bezafibrate, but results of these studies are at best preliminary. At present, there is no strong evidence for any combination therapy using UDCA [85,110].

Pruritus is a distressing, and sometimes disabling, symptom of PBC. Although antihistamines are frequently used because they are well tolerated, most patients do not show an adequate response. UDCA treatment is associated with a reduction of this symptom in some patients, but overall results of randomized trials do not demonstrate a significant improvement. Cholestyramine has been the mainstay of therapy for decades [111]. There are no randomized controlled trials of the anion exchange resins cholestyramine and colestipol, although there is extensive clinical experience supporting their efficacy. Most patients have improvement in response to symptoms within about 2 weeks of initiating therapy. Typically, the drug is administered as 4 g doses, up to four times per day. These drugs are typically not well tolerated because of unpleasant taste, abdominal discomfort, and constipation. Anion exchange resins may contribute to malabsorption and may interfere with the absorption of other medications, including UDCA, thyroxin, digoxin, and oral contraceptives. Phenobarbital has been used occasionally and may be helpful. Rifampin has been used to treat pruritus at a dosage of 300–600 mg/day in divided doses [112,113]. Although well tolerated, its use has occasionally been associated with hepatotoxicity and bone marrow aplasia. On the basis of the theory that pruritus occurs because of endogenous opioids, opioid antagonists have been used to treat PBC [114]. Two randomized controlled trials of intravenous naloxone demonstrated benefit for intractable pruritus [115,116], and subsequent studies with oral naltrexone and oral nalmefene have also shown benefit [117,118]. Symptoms of opioid withdrawal may occur as a side effect during the initiation of opioid antagonist therapy. It has been suggested that the serotonin system may also be involved in pruritus [114], and drugs such as ondansetron and sertraline have been shown to beneficial in patients with PBC in small trials [119]. Plasmapheresis has been used as a therapy in intractable patients.

Metabolic bone disease, osteopenia, and osteoporosis may present a significant problem in patients with PBC. The pathogenesis is complex and may involve, among other factors, malabsorption of fat-soluble vitamins and, more importantly, direct effects of cholestasis on bone metabolism. Although their efficacy is uncertain, calcium and vitamin D supplementation are routinely provided for patients with PBC [120,121], calcium at 1.5 g/day and vitamin D at 800 IU/day. Two studies of etidronate provided mixed results on the benefits for patients with PBC [122,123]; however, a more recent study with alendronate demonstrated favorable effects on bone mass [124]. The role of hormone replacement therapy in women with PBC is unclear, given recent results in other conditions that question its efficacy in relation to the increased risk of cancer and vascular disease. Insufficient data are available to recommend calcitonin or sodium fluoride as therapy for bone disease in PBC.

Fat-soluble vitamin deficiencies may secondarily contribute to morbidity in PBC, including night blindness, bone disease, bleeding disorders or, rarely, neurologic symptoms of vitamin E deficiency. Deficiencies have been documented for vitamins A, D, K, and E, in decreasing order of frequency, with approximately one third of patients being deficient in vitamin A [125,126]. Deficiencies correlate with advanced-stage disease and higher risk scores. Vitamin A supplementation should be based on serum retinol levels because excessive vitamin A may be hepatotoxic. Since zinc is necessary for the function of retinols, zinc repletion may be necessary for the correction of vitamin A deficiency in patients with concurrent zinc deficiency. Although the evidence base for the effectiveness of therapy is limited, it has been recommended that patients with hyperbilirubinemia be treated with water-soluble forms of vitamins A, D, E, and K, and patients with prolonged prothrombin times can be treated with parenteral vitamin K with a 10 mg/month dosage [84].

Hyperlipidemia and xanthomas are common manifestations of PBC and cholestasis, although patients with PBC may be relatively protected from the adverse effects of hyperlipidemia [24]. Cholestyramine or colestipol (Colestid®) is used to treat pruritus and UDCA because primary therapy may improve hypercholesterolemia. Nonetheless, additional therapy may be warranted in patients with other risk factors for cardiovascular disease. Clofibrate has been found to cause a paradoxical elevation of serum cholesterol level in two small studies [127,128]. In other studies, 3-hydroxy-3-methylglutaryl coenzyme A (HMG-CoA) reductase inhibitors (statins) have been shown to improve lipid levels without causing evident hepatotoxicity [129].

Additional medical therapy considerations should include treatment for sicca syndrome, with artificial tears, dental hygiene, antireflux measures, and vaginal lubricants, and treatment of thyroid disease when present.

Liver transplantation

Liver transplantation is the only option for patients with PBC with life-threatening end-stage liver disease and its complications or severe intractable symptoms. PBC is a relatively common indication for liver transplantation, representing 12% of patients in the European Liver Transplant Registry, which includes results for 3,357 patients with PBC undergoing transplantation between 1988 and 2003 [130]. However, recently there has been a decline in the number of transplants performed yearly for PBC. In general, patients with PBC are good candidates for transplantation and have a better long-term prognosis compared with those with other common indications for transplantation such as viral hepatitis or alcoholic liver disease, with 1-, 5-, and 10-year survival of 84%, 78%, and 69%, respectively [130]; similar results have been obtained in the United States. Most experience is based on cadaveric transplantation, but living related donor transplantation has also been performed successfully for PBC. The indications for liver transplantation in PBC include symptoms and signs of end-stage liver disease and its complications. In addition, patients have been considered for transplantation because of intractable severe pruritus, profound fatigue, and severe bone disease. Patients are typically considered for transplantation when their predicted survival is 1 year or less. The Mayo risk score has been validated as a reliable prognostic index for patients with PBC. This index was derived from analyses of large datasets, and is calculated from easily obtained clinical information: age, serum bilirubin, albumin, prothrombin time, and presence of edema. The prognostic value

of the Mayo risk score has been validated for patients treated with UDCA, which improves serum biochemical values in many patients. More recently, the allocation of cadaveric organs in the United States is based on the model for end-stage liver disease (MELD) score [131]. Both the Mayo risk score and the MELD score contain multiple factors, with serum bilirubin level being the major component of both. A serum bilirubin level greater than 8.5 mg/dL generally correlates with Mayo and MELD scores that are indicative of a need for liver transplantation.

PBC recurs in approximately 20–30% of patients 10 years after orthotopic liver transplantation [78,132], characterized by typical bile duct lesions and the persistence of AMAs. The diagnosis is based on liver biopsy and cannot be made on clinical features alone because of the overlap with features of transplant rejection and drug toxicity. There has been interest in the possibility that transplantation immunosuppressive regimens may alter the natural history of the recurrent disease and, in particular, that some regimens may retard progression better than others. However, the recurrent disease does not appear to be of major clinical consequence in most patients, and there is too little information available to select transplantation regimens on the basis of disease recurrence [133]. There have only been rare cases of retransplantation for recurrent PBC [78].

Natural history and prognosis

The initial descriptions of PBC were based on observations in patients diagnosed at a relatively late symptomatic stage of disease, with relatively rapid progression to liver failure and death in approximately 6 years [2,3]. The full clinical spectrum of PBC and its natural history are now much better defined. The disease has a variable spectrum but appears to be invariably progressive, whether presenting in asymptomatic or symptomatic patients. Multiple publications (with data largely from the pre-UDCA treatment era) have indicated that overall survival to death or transplantation is better in asymptomatic patients, approximately 10–15 years [134–136], although significantly worse than in control populations. One large study of 770 patients found that the symptom status had little effect on overall mortality from all causes, with a median survival of 9.6 versus 8.0 years in asymptomatic versus symptomatic patients, respectively [21]. However, in the latter study, less than one third of deaths among asymptomatic patients with PBC were attributable to liver disease. In asymptomatic patients with a recent diagnosis (i.e., patients presumably in the early stages of the disease), it is difficult to predict the ultimate course on the basis of serum biochemical or

AMA titer, or liver histology. In considering the limited medical therapies currently available that may change the underlying disease (e.g., UDCA), management decisions should not depend on a precise definition of where the patient may be along the course of the natural history of the disease. Considerably more is known about defining the late stages of the disease, which is important in considering the optimal timing for liver transplantation. A rising serum bilirubin level is an ominous prognostic sign in PBC [137]. Multivariate analysis of survival in PBC as a function of multiple different parameters has resulted in the Mayo index, which has been validated in many subsequent analyses [138]. More recently, the timing of transplantation has been supplanted by the use of the MELD score for prioritization for organ allocation. The MELD score is based on serum bilirubin level, creatinine level, international normalized ratio (INR) for prothrombin time, and etiology of liver disease, and it has been validated for prediction of death within 3 months for patients with PBC [139]. Further progress in developing better treatment approaches will depend on the identification of better biomarkers and surrogate markers, particularly for patients with early stages of PBC, as suggested by approaches using multiple serum biochemical measurements [140].

Further reading

Kaplan MM, Gershwin ME. Primary biliary cirrhosis. N Engl J Med 2005;353:1261–73.
This is an excellent review of the clinical features of primary biliary cirrhosis.

Kuiper EM, Hansen BE, deVries RA, et al. Improved prognosis of patients with primary biliary cirrhosis that have a biochemical response to ursodeoxycholic acid. Gastroenterology 2009;136:1281–7.
The long-term follow-up of patients treated with UDCA shows improved prognosis, similar to that of the general population in early-stage PBC and improved in biochemical responders with late-stage disease.

Lindor KD, Gershwin ME, Poupon R, et al. Primary biliary cirrhosis. Hepatology 2009;50:291–308.
Management guidelines for primary biliary cirrhosis from the American Association for the Study of Liver Diseases.

References

1. Addison T, Gull W. On a certain affection of the skin-vitiligoidea-α-plana-β-tuberosa. Guys Hosp Rep 1851;7:265–72.
2. Ahrens EH, Rayne MA, Kunkel HG, et al. Primary biliary cirrhosis. Medicine 1950;29:299–364. (Reproduced in Medicine (Baltimore) 1994;73:264–78.)
3. Sherlock S, Scheuer PJ. The presentation and diagnosis of 100 patients with primary biliary cirrhosis. N Engl J Med 1973;289:674–8.
4. Doniach D, Roitt IM, Walker JG, et al. Tissue antibodies in primary biliary cirrhosis, active chronic (lupoid) hepatitis, cryptogenic cirrhosis and other liver diseases and their clinical implications. Clin Exp Immunol 1966;1:237–62.
5. Metcalf J, James O. The geoepidemiology of primary biliary cirrhosis. Semin Liver Dis 1997;17:13–22.
6. Kim WR, Lindor KD, Locke GR III, et al. Epidemiology and natural history of primary biliary cirrhosis in a US community. Gastroenterology 2000;119:1631–6.
7. Prince MI, Chetwynd A, Diggle P, et al. The geographical distribution of primary biliary cirrhosis in a well-defined cohort. Hepatology 2001;34:1083–8.
8. Selmi C, Invernizzi P, Keefe EB, et al. Epidemiology and pathogenesis of primary biliary cirrhosis. J Clin Gastroenterol 2004;38:264–71.
9. Ala A, Stanca CM, Bu-Chanim et al. Increased incidence of primary biliary cirrhosis near superfund toxic waste sites. Hepatology 2006;43:525–31.
10. Parikh-Patel A, Gold EB, Worman H, et al. Risk factors for primary biliary cirrhosis in a cohort of patients from the United States. Hepatology 2001;33:16–21.
11. Jones DEJ, Donaldson PT. Genetic factors in the pathogenesis of primary biliary cirrhosis. Clin Liver Dis 2003;7:841–64.
12. Hirschfield GM, Liu X, Xu C, et al. Primary biliary cirrhosis associated with HLA, IL12A, and IL12RB2 variants. N Engl J Med 2009;360:2544–55.
13. Selmi C, Mayo MJ, Bach N, et al. Primary biliary cirrhosis in monozygotic and dizygotic twins: genetics, epigenetics, and environment. Gastroenterology 2004;127:485–92.
14. Watt FE, James OFW, Jones DEJ. Patterns of autoimmunity in primary biliary cirrhosis patients and their families: a population-based cohort study. Q J Med 2004;97:396–406.
15. Prince M, Chetwynd A, Newman W, et al. Survival and symptom progression in a geographically based cohort of patients with primary biliary cirrhosis: follow-up for up to 28 years. Gastroenterology 2002;123:1044–51.
16. Kurtovic J, Riordan SM, Williams R. The natural history of asymptomatic primary biliary cirrhosis. Q J Med 2005;98:331–6.
17. Stanca CM, Bach N, Krause C, et al. Evaluation of fatigue in US patients with primary biliary cirrhosis. Am J Gastroenterol 2005;100:1104–9.
18. Abbas G, Jorgensen RA, Lindor KD. Fatigue in primary biliary cirrhosis. Nat Rev Gastroenterol Hepatol 2010;6:13–19.
19. Bergasa NV. Pruritus in primary biliary cirrhosis: pathogenesis and therapy. Clin Liver Dis 2008;12:385–406.
20. Kaplan MM, Gershwin ME. Primary biliary cirrhosis. N Engl J Med 2005;353:1261–73.
21. Prince MI, Chetwynd A, Craig WL, et al. Asymptomatic primary biliary cirrhosis: clinical features, prognosis, and symptom progression in a large population based cohort. Gut 2004;53:865–70.
22. Caldwell SH. Primary biliary cirrhosis [Letter]. N Engl J Med 1997;336:1387–8.
23. Dickson ER, Grambsch PM, Fleming TR, et al. Prognosis in primary biliary cirrhosis: model for decision making. Hepatology 1989;10:1–7.
24. Longo M, Crosignani A, Battezzati PM, et al. Hyperlipidaemic state and cardiovascular risk in primary biliary cirrhosis. Gut 2002;51:265–9.
25. Chang PY, Lu SC, Su TC, et al. Lipoprotein-X reduces LDL atherogenicity in primary biliary cirrhosis by preventing LDL oxidation. J Lipid Res 2004;45:2116–22.
26. Fuller SJ, Kumar P, Weltman M, et al. Autoimmune hemolysis associated with primary biliary cirrhosis responding to ursodeoxycholic acid as sole treatment. Am J Hematol 2003;72:31–3.
27. Aoyama H, Sakugawa H, Nakasone H, et al. A rare association of primary biliary cirrhosis and pernicious anemia. J Gastroenterol 2002;37:560–3.
28. Ritland S, Steinnes E, Skrede S. Hepatic copper content, urinary copper excretion, and serum ceruloplasmin in liver disease. Scand J Gastroenterol 1977;12:81–8.
29. Roberts-Thomson PJ, Shepherd K. Low molecular weight IgM in primary biliary cirrhosis. Gut 1990;31:88–91.
30. Talwalkar JA, Lindor KD. Primary biliary cirrhosis. Lancet 2003;362:53–61.

31. Berg PA, Doniach D, Roitt IM. Mitochondrial antibodies in primary biliary cirrhosis. I. Localization of the antigen to mitochondrial membranes. *J Exp Med* 1967;126:277–90.

32. Lindenborn-Fotinos J, Baum H, Berg PA. Mitochondrial antibodies in primary biliary cirrhosis: species and nonspecies specific determinants of M2 antigen. *Hepatology* 1985;5:763–9.

33. Berg PA, Klein R, Lindenborn-Fotinos J. Antimitochondrial antibodies in primary biliary cirrhosis. *J Hepatol* 1986;2:123–31.

34. Palmer JM, Yeaman SJ, Bassendine MF, et al. M4 and M9 autoantigens in primary biliary cirrhosis – a negative study. *J Hepatol* 1993;18:251–4.

35. Gershwin ME, Ansari AA, Mackay IR, et al. Primary biliary cirrhosis: an orchestrated immune response against epithelial cells. *Immunol Res* 2000;174:210–25.

36. Yeaman SJ, Kirby JA, Jones DE. Autoreactive responses to pyruvate dehydrogenase complex in the pathogenesis of primary biliary cirrhosis. *Immunol Rev* 2000;174:238–49.

37. Van de Water J, Fregeau D, Davis P, et al. Autoantibodies of primary biliary cirrhosis recognize dihydrolipoamide acetyltransferase and inhibit enzyme function. *J Immunol* 1988;141:2321–4.

38. Rowley MJ, McNeilage LJ, Armstrong JM, et al. Inhibitory autoantibody to a conformational epitope of the pyruvate dehydrogenase complex, the major autoantigen in primary biliary cirrhosis. *Clin Immunol Immunopathol* 1991;60:356–70.

39. Goodman ZD, McNally PR, Davis DR, et al. Autoimmune cholangitis, a variant of primary biliary cirrhosis. Clinicopathologic and serologic correlations in 200 cases. *Dig Dis Sci* 1995;40: 1232–42.

40. Lacerda MA, Ludwig J, Dickson ER, et al. Antimitochondrial antibody-negative primary biliary cirrhosis. *Am J Gastroenterol* 1995;90:247–9.

41. Muratori P, Muratori L, Gershwin ME, et al. "True" antimitochondrial antibody-negative primary biliary cirrhosis, low sensitivity of the routine assays or both? *Clin Exp Immunol* 2004;135:154–8.

42. Muratori P, Muratori L, Ferrari R, et al. Characterization and clinical impact of antinuclear antibodies in primary biliary cirrhosis. *Am J Gastroenterol* 2003;98:431–7.

43. Watanabe S, Deguchi A, Uchida N, et al. Histopathologic comparison of anti-mitochondrial antibody-positive primary biliary cirrhosis and autoimmune cholangiopathy. *Hepatol Res* 2001;19:41–51.

44. Worman HJ, Courvalin JC. Antinuclear antibodies specific for primary biliary cirrhosis. *Autoimmun Rev* 2003;2:211–17.

45. Meroni PL, Harris EN, Brucato A, et al. Anti-mitochondrial type M5 and anti-cardiolipin antibodies in autoimmune disorders: studies on their association and cross-reactivity. *Clin Exp Immunol* 1987;67:484–91.

46. Ludwig J, Dickson ER, McDonald GSA. Staging of chronic non-suppurative destructive cholangitis (syndrome of primary biliary cirrhosis). *Virchows Arch* 1978;379:103–12.

47. Scheuer PJ. Primary biliary cirrhosis. *Proc R Soc Med* 1967;60:1257–60.

48. Hashimoto E, Lindor KD, Homburger HA, et al. Immunohistochemical characterization of hepatic lymphocytes in primary biliary cirrhosis in comparison with primary sclerosing cholangitis and autoimmune chronic active hepatitis. *Mayo Clin Proc* 1993;68:1049–55.

49. Bjorkland A, Festin R, Mendel-Hartvig I, et al. Blood and liver-infiltrating lymphocytes in primary biliary cirrhosis: increase in activated T and natural killer cells and recruitment of primed memory T cells. *Hepatology* 1991;13:1106–11.

50. Joplin R, Wallace LL, Johnson GD, et al. Subcellular localization of pyruvate dehydrogenase dihydrolipoamide acetyltransferase in human intrahepatic biliary epithelial cells. *J Pathol* 1995;176: 381–90.

51. Isse K, Harada K, Zen Y, et al. Fractalkine and CX3CR1 are involved in the recruitment of intraepithelial lymphocytes of intrahepatic bile ducts. *Hepatology* 2005;41:506–16.

52. Watt FE, James OFW, Jones DEJ. Patterns of autoimmunity in primary biliary cirrhosis patients and their families: a population-based cohort study. *Q J Med* 2004;97:397–406.

53. Golding PL, Smith M, Williams R. Multisystem involvement in chronic liver disease. *Am J Med* 1973;55:772–82.

54. Clarke AK, Galbraith GM, Hamilton EBD, et al. Rheumatic disorders in primary biliary cirrhosis. *Ann Rheum Dis* 1978;37:42–7.

55. Culp KS, Fleming CR, Duffy J, et al. Autoimmune associations in primary biliary cirrhosis. *Mayo Clin Proc* 1982;57:365–70.

56. Crowe JP, Christensen E, Bulter J, et al. Primary biliary cirrhosis: the prevalence of hypothyroidism and its relationship to thyroid autoantibodies and sicca syndrome. *Gastroenterology* 1980;78:1437–41.

57. Schramm C, Lohse AW. Overlap syndromes of cholestatic liver diseases and auto-immune hepatitis. *Clin Rev Allergy Immunol* 2005;28:105–14.

58. Kuiper EM, Zondervan PE, van Buuren HR. Paris criteria are effective in diagnosis of primary biliary cirrhosis and autoimmune hepatitis overlap syndrome. *Clin Gastroenterol Hepatol* 2010;8: 530–4.

59. Czaja AJ, Muratori P, Muratori L, et al. Diagnostic and therapeutic implications of bile duct injury in autoimmune hepatitis. *Liver Int* 2004;24:322–9.

60. Ter Borg PC, van Os E, van den Broek WW, et al. Fluvoxamine for fatigue in primary biliary cirrhosis and primary sclerosing cholangitis: a randomised controlled trial. *BMC Gastroenterol* 2004;4:13.

61. Newton J, Francis R, Prince M, et al. Osteoporosis in primary biliary cirrhosis revisited. *Gut* 2001;49:282–7.

62. Colina F, Pinedo F, Solis JA, et al. Nodular regenerative hyperplasia of the liver in early histological stages of primary biliary cirrhosis. *Gastroenterology* 1992;102:1319–24.

63. Howel D, Metcalf JV, Gray J, et al. Cancer risk in primary biliary cirrhosis: a study in northern England. *Gut* 1999;45:756–60.

64. Shibuya A, Tanaka K, Miyakawa H, et al. Hepatocellular carcinoma and survival in patients with primary biliary cirrhosis. *Hepatology* 2002;35:1172–8.

65. Hannam S, Bogdanos DP, Davies ET, et al. Neonatal liver disease associated with placental transfer of anti-mitochondrial antibodies. *Autoimmunity* 2002;35:545–50.

66. Shulman HM, Sharma P, Amos D, et al. A coded histologic study of hepatic graft-versus-host disease alter human bone marrow transplantation. *Hepatology* 1988;8:463–70.

67. Howell CD, Li J, Chen W. Role of intercellular adhesion molecule-1 and lymphocyte function-associated antigen-1 during nonsuppurative destructive cholangitis in a mouse graft-versus-host disease model. *Hepatology* 1999;29:766–76.

68. Neuberger J. Recurrent primary biliary cirrhosis. *Liver Transpl* 2003;9(6):539–46.

69. Ichiki Y, Selmi C, Shimoda S, et al. Mitochondrial antigens as targets of cellular and humoral auto-immunity in primary biliary cirrhosis. *Clin Rev Allergy Immunol* 2005;28:83–91.

70. Oertelt S, Lian Z-X, Cheng C-M, et. al. Anti-mitochondrial antibodies and primary biliary cirrhosis in TGF-α receptor II dominant-negative mice. *J Immunol* 2006;177:1655–60.

71. Irie J, Wu Y, Wicker LS, et al. NOD.c3c4 congenic mice develop autoimmune biliary disease that serologically and pathogenetically models human primary biliary cirrhosis. *J Exp Med* 2006;203:1209–19.

72. Salas JT, Banales JM, Sarvide S, et al. Ae2$_{a,b}$-deficient mice develop antimitochondrial antibodies and other features resembling primary biliary cirrhosis. *Gastroenterology* 2008;134:1482–93.

73. Wakabayashi K, Lian ZX, Leung PS, et. al. Loss of tolerance in C56BL/6 mice to the autoantigen E2 subunit of pyruvate dehydrogenase by a xenobiotic with ensuing biliary ductular disease. *Hepatology* 2008;48:531–40.

74. Selmi C, Ichiki Y, Invernizzi P, et al. The enigma of primary biliary cirrhosis. *Clin Rev Allergy Immunol* 2005;28:73–81.

75. Sadamoto T, Joplin R, Keogh A, et al. Expression of pyruvate-dehydrogenase complex PDC-E2 on biliary epithelial cells induced by lymph nodes from primary biliary cirrhosis. *Lancet* 1998;352:1595–6.

76. Xu L, Shen Z, Guo L, et al. Does a betaretrovirus infection trigger primary biliary cirrhosis? *Proc Natl Acad Sci USA* 2003;100:8454–9.

77. Selmi C, Ross SR, Ansari AA, et al. Lack of immunological or molecular evidence for a role of mouse mammary tumor retrovirus in primary biliary cirrhosis. *Gastroenterology* 2004;127:493–501.

78. Mason AL, Farr GH, Xu L, et al. Pilot studies of single and combination antiretroviral therapy in patients with primary biliary cirrhosis. *Am J Gastroenterol* 2004;99:2348–55.

79. Kim WR, Ludwig J, Lindor KD. Variant forms of cholestatic diseases involving small bile ducts in adults. *Am J Gastroenterol* 2000;95:1130–8.

80. Heseltine L, Turner IB, Fussey SP, et al. Primary biliary cirrhosis. Quantitation of autoantibodies to purified mitochondrial enzymes and correlation with disease progression. *Gastroenterology* 1990;99:1786–92.

81. Zein CO, Angulo P, Lindor KD. When is liver biopsy needed in the diagnosis of primary biliary cirrhosis? *Clin Gastroenterology Hepatol* 2003;1:89–95.

82. Friedrich-Rust M, Muller C, Winckler A, et al. Assessment of liver fibrosis and steatosis in primary biliary cirrhosis with Fibro Scan, MRI, MR-spectroscopy and serum markers. *J Clin Gastroenterol* 2010;44:58–65.

83. Ishak KG. Sarcoidosis of the liver and bile ducts. *Mayo Clin Proc* 1998;73:467–72.

84. Ludwig J. Idiopathic adulthood ductopenia: an update. *Mayo Clin Proc* 1998;73:285–91.

85. Lindor KD, Gershwin ME, Poupon R, et al. Primary biliary cirrhosis. *Hepatology* 2009;50:291–308.

86. Lindor K. Ursodeoxycholic acid for the treatment of primary biliary cirrhosis. *N Engl J Med* 2007;357:1524–9.

87. Gluud C, Christensen E. Ursodeoxycholic acid for primary biliary cirrhosis. *Cochrane Database Syst Rev* 2002;1:CD000551.

88. Levy C, Lindor KD. Current management of primary biliary cirrhosis and primary sclerosing cholangitis. *J Hepatol* 2003;38:S24–37.

89. Goulis J, Leandro G, Burroughs AK. Randomised controlled trials of ursodeoxycholic-acid therapy for primary biliary cirrhosis: a meta analysis. *Lancet* 1999;354:1053–60.

90. Heathcote EJ, Cauch-Dudek K, Walker V, et al. The Canadian multicenter double-blind randomized controlled trial of ursodeoxycholic acid in primary biliary cirrhosis. *Hepatology* 1994;19:1149–56.

91. Poupon R, Balkau B, Eschwege E, et al. A multicenter, controlled trial of ursodiol for the treatment of primary biliary cirrhosis. UDCA-PBC Study Group. *N Engl J Med* 1991;324:1548–54.

92. Lindor K, Dickson R, Baldus W, et al. Ursodeoxycholic acid in the treatment of primary biliary cirrhosis. *Gastroenterology* 1994;106:1284–90.

93. Combes B, Carithers R, Maddrey W, et al. A randomized double-blind placebo controlled trial of ursodeoxycholic acid in primary biliary cirrhosis. *Hepatology* 1995;22:759–66.

94. Erickson L, Olsson R, Glauman H, et al. Ursodeoxycholic acid treatment in patients with primary biliary cirrhosis. A Swedish multicentre, double-blind, randomized controlled study. *Scand J Gastroenterol* 1997;32:179–86.

95. Lindor K, Poupon R, Poupon R, et al. Ursodeoxycholic acid for primary biliary cirrhosis. *Lancet* 2000;355:657–8.

96. Angulo P, Lindor KD, Therneau TM, et al. Utilization of the Mayo risk score in patients with primary biliary cirrhosis receiving ursodeoxycholic acid. *Liver* 1999;12:115–21.

97. Corpechot C, Carrat F, Bonnand A, et al. The effect of ursodeoxycholic acid therapy on liver fibrosis progression in primary biliary cirrhosis. *Hepatology* 2000;32:1196–9.

98. Poupon RE, Lindor KD, Pares A, et al. Combined analysis of the effect of treatment with ursodeoxycholic acid on histologic progression in primary biliary cirrhosis. *J Hepatol* 2003;39:12–16.

99. Combes B, Luketic VA, Peters MG, et al. Prolonged follow-up of patients in the US multicenter trial of ursodeoxycholic acid for primary biliary cirrhosis. *Am J Gastroenterol* 2004;99:264–8.

100. Chan CW, Gunsar F, Feudjo M, et al. Long-term ursodeoxycholic acid therapy for primary biliary cirrhosis: a follow-up to 12 years. *Aliment Pharmacol Ther* 2005;21:217–26.

101. Corpechot C, Carrat F, Bahr A, et al. The effect of ursodeoxycholic acid therapy on the natural course of primary biliary cirrhosis. *Gastroenterology* 2005;128:297.

102. Kuiper EM, Hansen BE, deVries, et al. Improved prognosis of patients with primary biliary cirrhosis that have a biochemical response to ursodeoxycholic acid. *Gastroenterology* 2009;136:1281–7.

103. Christensen E, Neuberger J, Crowe J, et al. Beneficial effect of azathioprine and prediction of prognosis in primary biliary cirrhosis: final results of an international trial. *Gastroenterology* 1985;89:1084–91.

104. Bonis PA, Kaplan M. Methotrexate improves biochemical tests in patients with primary biliary cirrhosis who respond incompletely to ursodiol. *Gastroenterology* 1999;117:395–9.

105. Hendrickse MT, Rigney E, Giaffer MH, et al. Low-dose methotrexate is ineffective in primary biliary cirrhosis: long-term results of a placebo-controlled trial. *Gastroenterology* 1999;117:400–7.

106. Mitchison HC, Palmer JM, Bassendine MF, et al. A controlled trial of prednisolone treatment in primary biliary cirrhosis. Three year results. *J Hepatol* 1992;15:336–44.

107. Hoofnagle JH, Davis GL, Schafer DF, et al. Randomized trial of chlorambucil for primary biliary cirrhosis. *Gastroenterology* 1986;91:1327–34.

108. Lombard M, Portmann B, Neuberger J, et al. Cyclosporine A treatment in primary biliary cirrhosis: results of a long-term placebo controlled trial. *Gastroenterology* 1993;104:519–26.

109. Dickson ER, Fleming TR, Wiesner RH, et al. Trial of penicillamine in advanced primary biliary cirrhosis. *N Engl J Med* 1985;312:1011–15.

110. Poupon R. Primary biliary cirrhosis: a 2010 update. *J Hepatol* 2010;52:745–58. .

111. Van Itallie TB, Hashim SA, Crampton RS, et al. The treatment of pruritus and hypercholesteremia of primary biliary cirrhosis with cholestyramine. *N Engl J Med* 1961;265:469–74.

112. Talwalkar JA, Souto E, Jorgensen RA, et al. Natural history of pruritus in primary biliary cirrhosis. *Clin Gastroenterol Hepatol* 2003;4:297–302.

113. Bachs L, Pares A, Elena M, et al. Effects of long-term rifampicin administration in primary biliary cirrhosis. *Gastroenterology* 1992;102:2077–80.

114. Bergasa NV. Pruritus and fatigue in primary biliary cirrhosis. *Clin Liver Dis* 2003;4:879–900.

115. Bergasa NV, Talbot TL, Alling DW, et al. A controlled trial of naloxone infusions for the pruritus of chronic cholestasis. *Gastroenterology* 1992;102:544–9.

116. Bergasa NV, Alling DW, Talbot TL, et al. Effects of naloxone infusions in patients with the pruritus of cholestasis. A double-blind, randomized, controlled trial. *Ann Intern Med* 1995;123:161–7.

117. Wolfhagen FH, Sternieri E, Hop WC, et al. Oral naltrexone treatment for cholestatic pruritus: a double-blind, placebo-controlled study. *Gastroenterology* 1997;113:1264–9.

118. Bergasa NV, Alling DW, Talbot TL, et al. Oral nalmefene therapy reduces scratching activity due to the pruritus of cholestasis: a controlled study. *J Am Acad Dermatol* 1999;41:431–4.

119. Mayo MJ, Handem I, Saldana S, et. al. Sertraline as a first-line treatment for cholestatic pruritus. *Hepatology* 2007;45:666–74.

120. Pusl T, Beuers U. Extrahepatic manifestations of cholestatic liver diseases: pathogenesis and therapy. *Clin Rev Allergy Immunol* 2005;28:147–57.

121. Levy C, Lindor KD. Management of osteoporosis, fat-soluble vitamin deficiencies, and hyperlipidemia in primary biliary cirrhosis. *Clin Liver Dis* 2003;7:901–10.

122. Wolfhagen FH, van Buuren HR, den Ouden JW, et al. Cyclical etidronate in the prevention of bone loss in corticosteroid-treated primary biliary cirrhosis. A prospective, controlled pilot study. *J Hepatol* 1997;26:325–30.

123. Guanabens N, Pares A, Monegal A, et al. Etidronate versus fluoride for treatment of osteopenia in primary biliary cirrhosis: preliminary results after 2 years. *Gastroenterology* 1997;113:219–24.

124. Guanabens N, Pares A, Ros I, et al. Alendronate is more effective than etidronate for increasing bone mass in osteopenic patients with primary biliary cirrhosis. *Am J Gastroenterol* 2003;98:2268–74.

125. Phillips J, Angulo P, Petterson T, et al. Fat-soluble vitamin levels in patients with primary biliary cirrhosis. *Am J Gastroenterol* 2001;96:2745–50.

126. Kaplan MM, Elta GH, Furie B, et al. Fat-soluble vitamin nutriture in primary biliary cirrhosis. *Gastroenterology* 1988;95:787–92.

127. Schaffner F. Paradoxical elevation of serum cholesterol by clofibrate in patients with primary biliary cirrhosis. *Gastroenterology* 1965;57:253–5.

128. Summerfield JA, Elias E, Sherlock S. Effects of clofibrate in primary biliary cirrhosis hypercholesterolemia and gallstones. *Gastroenterology* 1975;69:998–1000.

129. Abu Rajab M, Kaplan MM. Statins in primary biliary cirrhosis: are they safe? *Dig Dis Sci* 2010;55:2086–8.

130. *European Liver Transplant Registry*. Registry of the European Liver Transplant Association, available online at www.eltr.org.

131. Combes JM, Trotter JF. Development of the allocation system for deceased donor liver transplantation. *Clin Med Res* 2005;3: 87–92.

132. Silveira MG, Talwalkar JA, Lindor KD, Wiesner RH. Recurrent primary biliary cirrhosis after liver transplantation. *Am J Transplant* 2010;10:720–6.

133. Jacob DA, Neumann UP, Bahra M, et al. Liver transplantation for primary biliary cirrhosis: influence of primary immunosuppression on survival. *Transplant Proc* 2005;37:1691–2.

134. Mahl TC, Shockcor W, Boyer JL. Primary biliary cirrhosis: survival of a large cohort of symptomatic and asymptomatic patients followed for 24 years. *J Hepatol* 1994;20:707–13.

135. Balasubramaniam K, Grambsch PM, Wiesner RH, et al. Diminished survival in asymptomatic primary biliary cirrhosis: a prospective study. *Gastroenterology* 1990;98:1567–71.

136. Springer J, Cauch-Dudek K, O'Rourke K, et al. Asymptomatic primary biliary cirrhosis: a study of its natural history and progression. *Am J Gastroenterol* 1999;94:47–53.

137. Shapiro JM, Smith H, Schaffner F. Serum bilirubin: a prognostic factor in primary biliary cirrhosis. *Gut* 1979;20:137–40.

138. Dickson E, Grambsch PM, Felming TR, et al. Prognosis in primary biliary cirrhosis: model for decision making. *Hepatology* 1989;10:1–7.

139. Kamath PS, Wiesner RH, Malinchoc M, et al. A model to predict survival in patients with end-stage liver disease. *Hepatology* 2001;33:464–70.

140. Mayo MJ, Parkes J, Adams-Huet B, et. al. Prediction of clinical outcomes in primary biliary cirrhosis by serum enhanced fibrosis assay. *Hepatology* 2008;48:1549–57.

Multiple choice questions

21.1 **What is the most specific diagnostic test for primary biliary cirrhosis?**

    a Magnetic resonance (MR) image of the liver.
    b MR cholangiography.
    c Serum antimitochondrial antibody.
    d Percutaneous liver biopsy.

21.2 **Which therapy for primary biliary cirrhosis improves the natural history compared with an age-matched general population?**

    a Oral budesonide.
    b Colchicine.
    c Ursodeoxycholic acid.
    d Azathioprine.
    e Liver transplantation.

Answers to the multiple choice questions can be found in the Appendix at the end of the book.

These multiple choice questions are also available for you to complete online.
Visit http://www.schiffsdiseasesoftheliver.com/

CHAPTER 22
Autoimmune Hepatitis

Edward L. Krawitt

Department of Medicine, University of Vermont, Burlington, VT, USA

Key concepts

- Autoimmune hepatitis is a chronic hepatitis characterized by immune and autoimmune features.
- The pathogenesis of autoimmune hepatitis involves a loss of tolerance to self-antigens, but the tolerogenic mechanisms are incompletely understood.
- The predominant genetic factor in autoimmune hepatitis is a human leukocyte antigen (HLA) association, with variable expression in different ethnic groups.
- An autoantibody classification of types 1 and 2 is commonly applied.
- Other autoimmune diseases are frequently seen in patients with autoimmune hepatitis and/or their family members.
- The histologic severity in autoimmune hepatitis extends from mild chronic hepatitis to active cirrhosis.
- The biopsy finding of interface hepatitis with an abundance of plasma cells in the infiltrate is characteristic of autoimmune hepatitis

- Because of asymptomatic periods and a fluctuating course, cirrhosis is often present at the time of the initial biopsy.
- Despite the disappearance of symptoms and normalization of laboratory abnormalities once treatment has been instituted, continuing activity may be evident histologically.
- Circulating hyperglobulinemia, in particular hypergammaglobulinemia, and circulating autoantibodies occur frequently in autoimmune hepatitis but their presence is not unique to, nor specific to, autoimmune hepatitis.
- Patients usually respond to anti-inflammatory/immunosuppressive therapy, but life-long treatment may be required, particularly in children and in adults who present with cirrhosis.
- Liver transplantation has been successful in patients who do not respond to medical treatment, but post-transplantation hepatitis may occur.

Pathogenesis

Autoimmune hepatitis is a chronic hepatitis characterized by immunologic and autoimmunologic features that generally responds to immunospuppresive therapy [1,2]. One paradigm for the pathogenesis of autoimmune hepatitis embraces the concept that an environmental agent triggers an autoimmune process in a genetically predisposed individual, resulting in a diminution or loss of tolerance to self-antigens. However, the precise relationships between the genes and the autoimmune process remain largely undefined and speculative [3]. Infectious agents, immunizations, herbs, and drugs have been suggested as triggering agents, but in most cases no specific inducer of autoimmunity is identified when autoimmune hepatitis appears. Potential mechanisms of induction include molecular mimicry, exposure of a sequestered antigen, alterations of a self-antigen, or the formation of a neoantigen by the combination of a foreign determinant and a self-antigen [4]. There is some evidence implicating hepatitis viruses, herpes simplex virus, varicella zoster virus, cytomegalovirus, Epstein–Barr virus, and measles virus as initiators of disease, perhaps involving a long latency period after infection. Immunizations for hepatitis A and B, among others, as well as a variety of herbs and drugs, have been proposed as triggers.

Drug-induced hepatocellular injury that resembles autoimmune hepatitis has been recognized over many years from drugs including oxyphenisatin, methyldopa, nitrofurantoin, diclofenac, and minocycline [5]. Although circulating autoantibodies and hyperglobulinemia occur in so-called drug-induced autoimmune hepatitis, there is no unequivocal evidence that a self-perpetuating injury exists after discontinuation of the drug, nor has there been evidence of a drug or metabolite producing a relevant neoantigen for autoimmune hepatitis. The administration of interferon may unmask or induce a variety of autoimmune diseases, including autoimmune hepatitis.

The search for genetic predisposing factors has for many years been largely directed at genes of the

Schiff's Diseases of the Liver, Eleventh Edition. Edited by Eugene R. Schiff, Willis C. Maddrey and Michael F. Sorrell.
© 2012 John Wiley & Sons, Ltd. Published 2012 by John Wiley & Sons, Ltd.

immunoglobulin superfamily, which includes those encoding human leukocyte antigens (HLA) located in the major histocompatibility complex (MHC), immunoglobulins, and T-cell receptor molecules [2,3,6]. It is likely that multiple genes are involved but that MHC genes account for much of the susceptibility.

In Caucasians, type 1 disease is strongly associated with the HLA-DR3 serotype (which is found in linkage disequilibrium with HLA-B8 and HLA-A1) and with HLA-DR4. DRB1*0301 and DRB3*0101 are common genotypes in North America; in South America DRB1*1301 is common. Additional associations have been found in Mexico, Brazil, and Argentina where mixed ethnicity is common. In Japan, where HLA-DR3 is rare, there is a primary association with the HLA-DR4 serotype, genotype DRB1*0405, and genotype DQB1*0401. Type 2 disease is associated with HLA-DRB1*07, HLA-DRB1*03, and DQB1*0201 alleles.

How the HLA alleles confer susceptibility to autoimmune hepatitis is not well understood. One theory designates a common susceptibility determinant in the HLA class II-binding groove crucial to antigen recognition that is carried by the DRB1*0301, DRB3*0101, and DRB1*0401 alleles in Caucasians [3,6]. There may be weaker associations with HLA class I MICA genes, the promoter region of tumor necrosis factor α (TNF-α), and complement genes (class III). Associations with TNF promoter polymorphisms appear to reflect an extended DRB1*0301 haplotype.

A genome-wide association study in 81 Japanese patients looking for weaker associations than those that occur at HLA loci found 26 candidate susceptibility regions in DR4-positive patients [7]. Understanding the weaker associations in autoimmune hepatitis will require genome-wide association analysis of large numbers of patients and/or other advanced modalities to insure statistical validity.

Based upon the character of the hepatic inflammatory infiltrate from patients with autoimmune hepatitis, and experimental findings from patients and animal models, the ongoing necroinflammatory process in autoimmune hepatitis appears to be mediated by CD4+ T cells. Clonal analyses of the T-cell receptor (TCR) chain variable region repertoires in liver-infiltrating lymphocytes have demonstrated oligoclonality for CDR region 3. Polyclonal T-cell responses to CYP2D6 appear to be involved in type 2 autoimmune hepatitis [8]. Despite the abundance of circulating autoantibodies found in autoimmune hepatitis, there is little evidence for direct antibody-induced liver damage, although abnormalities in B-cell function may yet prove to be important in the pathogenic process.

Implicit in the hypothesis of an immunoregulatory effect is an escape from tolerogenic mechanisms, probably involving suppression of self-reactive T cells. Early studies of immune regulation, based primarily upon in vitro observations, supported the hypothesis of a defect in the downregulation of the immune response, presumably mediated by CD8 suppressor T cells; the defect was reversed in autoimmune hepatitis patients with corticosteroid treatment [9–11]. The concept of suppressor T-cell function specifically mediated by CD8+ lymphocytes, came into question but the hypothesis of escape from suppressive mechanisms remains viable and is supported by studies of CD4+, CD25+ regulatory T cells (Tregs) that express CTLA-4, and the forkhead transcription factor Foxp3. Defects in expansion, generation, and function of Tregs have been discovered [3,12,13].The precise roles of CTLA-4 and Foxp3 and their relationship to Th 17 cells and CTLA-4 polymorphisms awaits further experimentation.

Histopathology and differential diagnosis

The histologic appearance of autoimmune hepatitis is that of chronic hepatitis, and is crucial to the diagnosis of autoimmune hepatitis. Although certain changes are characteristic, there are no findings specific to the disease [14]. The histologic differential diagnosis of chronic hepatitis is provided in Box 22.1. Based on advances in virologic studies and refinements of cholangiographic methods to exclude other entities, diagnosis has become easier.

The inflammatory component is characterized by a mononuclear cell infiltrate, which invades the sharply

---

Box 22.1 Histologic differential diagnosis of chronic hepatitis.

- Autoimmune liver disease:
    Autoimmune hepatitis
    Primary biliary cirrhosis
    Primary sclerosing cholangitis
    Variant syndromes
- Chronic viral hepatitis:
    Chronic hepatitis B
    Chronic hepatitis C
    Chronic hepatitis delta
    Chronic hepatitis due to other viruses
- Chronic drug-induced hepatitis
- Alpha$_1$-antitrypsin deficiency
- Wilson disease
- Granulomatous hepatitis
- Systemic lupus erythematosus
- Graft-versus-host disease
- Alcoholic steatohepatitis
- Nonalcoholic steatohepatitis

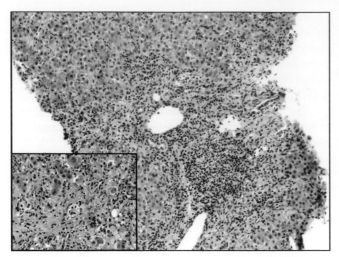

Figure 22.1 Interface and lobular hepatitis with a mixed inflammatory infiltrate composed of plasma cells, lymphocytes, and eosinophils, accompanied by ballooning degeneration and stage 2 fibrosis in a biopsy from a 56-year-old woman who presented with acute onset autoimmune hepatitis. Hematoxylin and eosin (H&E).

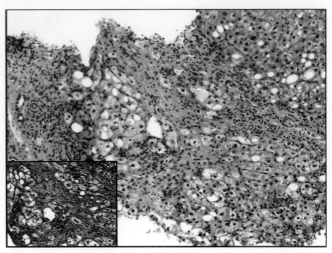

Figure 22.3 Significant lymphoplasmacytic inflammatory infiltrate accompanied by bridging fibrosis, regenerative nodules, ballooning degeneration, steatosis, and perisinusoidal and pericentral fibrosis characteristic of autoimmune hepatitis with nonalcoholic steatohepatitis in a biopsy obtained from a 53-year-old woman with diabetes mellitus. H&E; insert trichrome.

demarcated hepatocyte boundary (limiting plate) surrounding the portal triad and permeates the surrounding parenchyma (periportal infiltrate, piecemeal necrosis, and interface hepatitis) and beyond (lobular hepatitis). It may include an abundance of plasma cells and/or eosinophils, but the portal lesion generally spares the biliary tree. A dense plasma cell infiltrate is characteristic; in the past this led to the use of the term "plasma cell hepatitis" (Figs 22.1–22.3). In all but the mildest forms, fibrosis is present. In advanced disease fibrosis is extensive (bridging fibrosis) and, with distortion of the hepatic lobule and

appearance of regenerative nodules, cirrhosis occurs [14]. On occasion, pericentral necrosis may be present [15].

Steatosis in autoimmune hepatitis patients not treated with corticosteroids has been thought to be uncommon, but given the increasing prevalence of diabetes, dyslipidemia, and obesity in many parts of the world, nonalcoholic fatty liver disease (NAFLD) may be seen more often accompanying autoimmune hepatitis (Fig. 22.3). Whether the co-morbidity of steatosis and steatohepatitis accelerate the progression of disease in autoimmune hepatitis is unknown. The discovery of portal inflammatory changes in NAFLD [16], particularly in children, and the prevalence of autoantibodies in NAFLD, however, emphasizes the diagnostic difficulties of differentiating these disorders.

The prevalence of cirrhosis in patients ≥60 years at presentation was found to be higher than that in patients ≤30 years; when comparing groups of patients ≥60 years with those <60 years, however, no differences were found [17,18]. In patients with a spontaneous or pharmacologically induced remission, histologic findings may revert to normal; inflammation may be confined to portal areas; cirrhosis may become inactive; and fibrosis may regress or disappear [19] (Fig. 22.4).

The histologic findings differ somewhat when comparing patients with acute-onset autoimmune hepatitis to those with an insidious presentation. Patients presenting with fulminant hepatic failure have more interface and lobular hepatitis, lobular disarray, hepatocyte necrosis, central necrosis, and submassive necrosis, but less fibrosis and cirrhosis compared with patients presenting with a more chronic course [17].

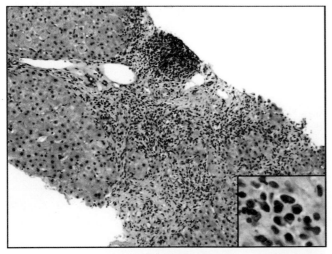

Figure 22.2 Marked interface and lobular activity with an abundance of plasma cells accompanied by bridging fibrosis and early regenerative nodules in a biopsy from a 64-year-old asymptomatic man. H&E.

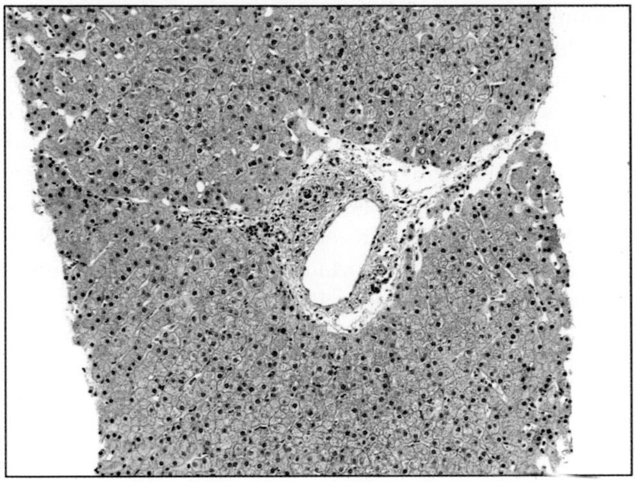

Figure 22.4 No histologic abnormalities were present in a follow-up biopsy obtained 3 years later when the patient described in Fig. 22.1 was in clinical remission on maintenance therapy. H&E.

Although the histologic appearance of autoimmune hepatitis is characteristic, it is not specific to the disease. Fulminant Wilson disease is difficult to distinguish from severe autoimmune hepatitis. Many of the features seen in autoimmune hepatitis are common to chronic viral hepatitis. Cholestatic autoimmune diseases may at times be indistinguishable from autoimmune hepatitis but are commonly characterized by a paucity of bile ducts and/or bile duct inflammation, fibrosis, and damage [14].

Autoantibody classification

Since the first descriptions of autoimmune hepatitis in the twentieth century, it has been known by a variety of terms; autoimmune hepatitis is now accepted as the most appropriate and least redundant term. Its heterogeneity is underscored by a variety of clinical manifestations, histologic findings, immunogenetic phenotypes, and serologic abnormalities. Thus, classification can be based on a number of features. Since 1987, when Jean-Claude Homberg and his colleagues described a second type of autoimmune hepatitis [20], an autoantibody-based classification has been in common usage with type 1 and type 2 designations based on differing circulating autoantibody patterns (Box 22.2).

In type 1 autoimmune hepatitis, the main circulating autoantibodies, although not specific for the disease, are antinuclear antibody (ANA), smooth muscle antibody (SMA), and anti-F actin antibody (AAA) (Box 22.2). Although AAAs may be more specific for type 1 autoimmune hepatitis, until recently they have not generally been measured in clinical laboratories. Antiactin antibodies (immunoglobulin G (IgG) anti-F actin) measured by enzyme-linked immunosorbent assay (ELISA) [21] have now become more readily available, and in some laboratories have replaced SMA in autoantibody profiles. This may require using equivalence of levels when utilizing the recently published, simplified criteria [22] for the diagnosis of autoimmune hepatitis (see below).

Soluble liver antigen antibodies (anti-SLAs) have been found in approximately 10–30% of adult patients with type 1 autoimmune hepatitis but are more common in children with type 1 and type 2 disease. Anti-SLA was found to be identical to an antibody to a liver–pancreas (LP) antigen, which had been described in a subset of patients with autoimmune hepatitis, accounting for the term anti-SLA/LP. SLA is also known as SEPSECS (Sep (O-phosphoserine) tRNA synthase), a selenocysteine synthase. Sometimes anti-SLA may be the only circulating antibody found in autoimmune hepatitis patients [1].

Atypical p-antineutrophil cytoplasmic antibody (pANCA), sometimes referred to as peripheral antineutrophil nuclear antibody (pANNA), recognizes neutrophil nuclear lamina proteins and is frequently present in type 1 autoimmune hepatitis. It is also common in primary sclerosing cholangitis and in inflammatory bowel disease.

Although not frequently sought, antibodies to double-stranded DNA, which are most commonly associated with systemic lupus erythematosus, and single-stranded DNA can occur in autoimmune hepatitis. Antimitochondrial antibodies (AMAs), although more specific and sensitive for primary biliary cirrhosis, can also be seen

Box 22.2 Autoantibody classification of autoimmune hepatitis.

Type 1 (classic)

- Antinuclear antibody (ANA)
- Smooth muscle antibody (SMA)
- Anti-F actin antibody (AAA)
- Antisoluable liver/liver–pancreas antigen (SLA, SLA/LP, SEPSECS)
- Atypical perinuclear antineutrophil cytoplasmic antibody (pANCA, pANNA)
- Antimitochondrial antibody (AMA)[a]

Type 2

- Antiliver–kidney microsome-1 (ALKM-1)
- Antiliver cytosol-1 (ALC-1)
- UDP–glucuronosyl transferases (UGT1A, ALKM-3)[b]

[a] Occurs infrequently in association with other characteristic autoantibodies. It may be the sole antibody present in AMA-negative autoimmune hepatitis.
[b] Occurs rarely.
pANCA, p-antineutrophil cytoplasmic antibody; pANNA, peripheral antineutrophil nuclear antibody; UDP, uridine diphosphate.

in type 1 autoimmune hepatitis, generally with ANA and/or SMA and rarely as the only autoantibody [23]. The frequency of these autoantibodies in autoimmune hepatitis varies significantly in different reports but is generally in the 5–20% range. Variations are probably in part due to the definitions of variant/overlap syndromes used [24,25].

In type 2 autoimmune hepatitis, a disease that occurs predominantly in girls and young women, antiliver–kidney microsome-1 (ALKM-1) antibodies and anti-cytosol-1 (ALC-1) antibodies are the major circulating autoantibodies (see Box 22.2). ALKM-1 antibodies, which are directed at the cytochrome P450 enzyme CYP2D6, are also found in approximately 5% of patients with chronic hepatitis C and 25% of those with halothane-induced hepatitis. ACL-1 antibody, which recognizes formiminotransferase cyclodeaminase (FTCD), a liver-specific 58 kDa metabolic enzyme, generally occurs in conjunction with ALKM-1 antibody, but may be the sole circulating autoantibody [26]. Antibodies to ALKM-3 rarely occur in type 2 disease [1].

Variant syndromes

Autoimmune hepatitis–primary biliary cirrhosis overlap patients have characteristic clinical, histologic, and immunologic findings of both diseases [25,27,28]. Patients with autoimmune hepatitis–primary sclerosing cholangitis overlaps (referred to in children as autoimmune sclerosing cholangitis) have serologic and histologic features of autoimmune hepatitis with cholangiographic abnormalities characteristic of primary sclerosing cholangitis (Table 22.1) [25,29].

Table 22.1 Autoimmune hepatitis variant syndromes.

	AIH-PBC	AIH-PSC
Antinuclear antibody	Often present	Often present
Smooth muscle antibody	Often present	Often present
Antimitochondrial antibody	Present	Absent
Biochemical cholestasis	Present	Present
Histologic evidence of bile duct abnormalities	Present	Sometimes present
Cholangiographic abnormalities	Absent	Present
Responsiveness to immunosupression	Variable	Variable

AIH-PBC, autoimmune hepatitis–primary biliary cirrhosis; AIH-PSC, autoimmune hepatitis–primary sclerosing cholangitis

Some authors recognize additional overlap syndromes including "autoimmune hepatitis–cryptogenic hepatitis," "autoimmune hepatitis–sarcoidosis," and "autoimmune hepatitis–chronic hepatitis C." However, the existence of these disorders as distinct overlap syndromes is less clear.

The list of recognized IgG4-associated diseases continues to grow, and IgG4-associated pancreatitis and IgG4-associated cholangitis are now well-established entities. Whether or not IgG4-associated autoimmune hepatitis is a distinct entity is not clear [30,31]. Documentation of its existence awaits a more extensive description of clinical and immune-histologic features.

Clinical features

Although there is a female predominance, autoimmune hepatitis occurs in children and adults of both sexes in diverse ethnic groups. Type 2 disease, which is seen predominantly in children and young women, is rare in North America. Although autoimmune hepatitis was previously thought to be a disease of the young or middle aged, it is now clear that it also occurs in the elderly, generally defined as ≥60 years of age [17,18].

The heterogeneous, sometimes fluctuating, nature of autoimmune hepatitis leads to marked variability in clinical manifestations. Presentation may be asymptomatic or insidious, with mild nonspecific symptoms only, or may mimic acute viral hepatitis, sometimes presenting as fulminant hepatic failure [17,18,24]. Patients with occult disease may have undetected cirrhosis. The group of patients now labeled as cryptogenic cirrhosis, includes some patients without detectable standard autoantibodies. Measurement of other autoantibodies may be helpful in clarifying a diagnosis of autoimmune liver disease (Fig. 22.5).

Many patients with an acute presentation have histologic evidence of chronic disease indicating that they have had antecedent subclinical disease, although the duration of the subclinical anicteric course is generally difficult to ascertain. In retrospect, a fluctuating course, which had been thought to reflect some other disease, can be identified. Long periods of subclinical disease may also ensue after presentation. Surveys of pregnancy in autoimmune hepatitis indicate that the initial presentations may occur not only during pregnancy but in the early postpartum period. A variety of putative autoimmune diseases, including the gastrointestinal immune-mediated disorders of inflammatory bowel disease and celiac disease, occur in conjunction with both type 1 and 2 disease. Arthralgia, commonly involving small joints, is common; inflammatory arthritis may be particularly troublesome even after immune suppression has been successful in quieting the hepatitis.

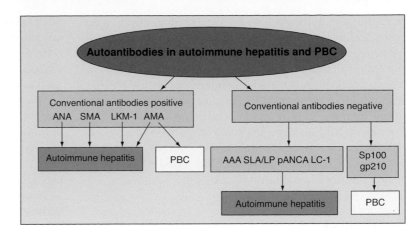

Figure 22.5 The use of conventional and other serum antibodies as an aid in diagnosing autoimmune hepatitis. AAA, anti-F actin antibody; ALC-1, anticytosol-1; ALKM-1, antiliver–kidney microsome-1; AMA, antimitochondrial antibody; ANA, antinuclear antibody; anti-SLA/LP, soluble liver antigen/liver–pancreas antigen antibody; SMA, smooth muscle antibody; pANCA, p-antineutrophil cytoplasmic antibody; Sp 100 and gp 210, multinuclear dot ANAs.

Complications of autoimmune hepatitis are those seen in any progressive liver disease and primary hepatocellular carcinoma is an expected, although uncommon, consequence [32,33]. There are no established guidelines for hepatocellular carcinoma screening in cirrhosis, but a reasonable approach is surveillance with abdominal ultrasonography and α-fetoprotein every 6–12 months.

Diagnosis

In the presence of a compatible histologic picture, the diagnosis of autoimmune hepatitis is based on characteristic clinical and biochemical findings, circulating autoantibodies, and abnormalities of serum globulins. A scoring system, proposed and subsequently revised by the International Autoimmune Hepatitis Group [34], to standardize diagnosis for clinical trials and population studies, has been adapted by clinicians but found to be problematic when applied to individual patients, especially children. The International Autoimmune Hepatitis Group has devised a less complicated system [22] for application in individual patients, which uses serum autoantibodies measured by immunofluorescence, serum IgG levels, histologic findings, and the absence of viral hepatitis (Table 22.2) as follows:

- *Autoantibodies*: assign 1 point if the ANA or SMA are 1 : 40 *or* assign 2 points if the ANA or SMA are ≥1 : 80 (*or* if the ALKM-1 is ≥1 : 40 *or* if the anti-SLA is positive).
- *IgG*: assign 1 point if the IgG is greater than the upper limit of normal (ULN) *or* assign 2 points if the IgG is >1.1 times the ULN.
- *Liver histology* (evidence of hepatitis is a mandatory condition): assign 1 point if the histologic features are compatible with autoimmune hepatitis *or* 2 points if the histologic features are typical of autoimmune hepatitis.
- *Absence of viral hepatitis*: assign 2 points if viral hepatitis has been excluded. In the validation study, patients were mainly tested for hepatitis B and C.

A probable diagnosis of autoimmune hepatitis is made if the total is 6 points, while a definite diagnosis is made if the total points are ≥7 (Table 22.2).

A scoring system for a "strictly" defined autoimmune hepatitis–primary biliary cirrhosis variant has been devised by Chazouilleres et al. [27,28], requiring at least two of three accepted criteria for each diasease. Primary biliary cirrhosis criteria are: (i) alkaline phosphatase levels at least two times the ULN or γ-glutamyl transpeptidase levels five times the ULN; (ii) a positive AMA; and (iii) a liver biopsy specimen showing florid duct lesions. Autoimmune hepatitis criteria are: (i) serum alanine aminotransferase levels more than five times the ULN; (ii) serum IgG levels at least two times the ULN or a positive SMA; and (iii) a liver biopsy specimen showing moderate or severe periportal hepatitis.

Autoimmune sclerosing cholangitis should be suspected in all children being evaluated for autoimmune

Table 22.2 Simplified diagnostic criteria for autoimmune hepatitis.[a]

Variable	1 point	2 points
ANA or SMA ≥1 : 40	1	–
ANA or SMA ≥1 : 80	–	2
or LKM ≥1 : 40	–	2
or SLA-positive	–	2
IgG > upper normal limit	1	–
IgG > 1.1 times upper normal limit	–	2
Liver histology compatible with AIH[b]	1	–
Liver histology typical AIH[b]	–	2
Absence of viral hepatitis	–	2

[a]Points achieved for autoantibodies: maximum 2 points. Probable autoimmune hepatitis: 6 points. Definite autoimmune hepatitis: ≥7 points.
[b]Evidence of hepatitis is a necessary condition.
ANA, antinuclear antibody; IgG, immunoglobulin G; LKM, liver–kidney microsome; SLA, soluble liver antigen; SMA, smooth muscle antibody.

liver disease. It should also be suspected in adults who have clinical and serologic features of autoimmune hepatitis as well as: pruritus, chronic ulcerative colitis, bile duct abnormalities by biopsy, serum cholestatic biochemical changes of an elevated alkaline phosphatase and/or γ-glutamyl transpeptidase, poor response to corticosteroid therapy, and/or an abnormal cholangiogram. The overlap should also be suspected in patients diagnosed with primary sclerosing cholangitis who have high levels of IgG, circulating ANAs or SMAs, and moderate to severe interface hepatitis on liver biopsy.

Treatment

Despite the striking heterogeneity and our incomplete understanding of its pathogenesis, autoimmune hepatitis is in general a "steroid-responsive" condition. Appropriate management can improve quality of life, mitigate inflammation and fibrosis, prolong survival, and delay the need for liver transplantation. The life expectancy of treated patients is similar to age- and gender-matched controls in patients who have been followed for up to 20 years [35].

Standard medications for initial and maintenance regimens are still considered to be prednisone (or prednisolone) alone or in combination with azathioprine (or 6-mercaptopurine) (Table 22.3) [1,36].

Progress in nonstandard treatment for patients with inadequate responses or intolerance to therapy with glucocorticosteroids alone or in combination with azathioprine or 6-mercaptopurine has been slow [1,36]. In view

of the paucity of trials with nonstandard forms of therapy most decisions must be based on data obtained from case reports and series of small numbers of patients. Cyclosporine, which has been used successfully in children to induce remission [36], and tacrolimus are used on occasion to treat adults. Off-label use of mycophenolate mofetil has become more frequently employed in intolerant or nonresponsive adults [37–40] and is considered a promising agent [1]. In children it has proved to be effective in autoimmune hepatitis but not in autoimmune cholangitis [40].

The role of budesonide in treating autoimmune hepatitis has not been extensively studied. A recent investigation suggests that it may be as effective in noncirrhotic patients and may serve as an alternative to prednisone or prednisolone [41].

One issue of concern is toxicity and/or intolerance to 6-mercaptopurine and its prodrug azathioprine. The methylation of 6-mercaptopurine and 6-thioguanosine 5′-monophosphate is catalyzed by thiopurine methyltransferase (TPMT). The genes encoding TPMT are highly polymorphic. Homozygosity and heterozygosity for mutations in TPMT genes occur in Caucasian and other populations, and these patients may accumulate high levels of thioguanine nucleotides in bone marrow cells. Patients who are homozygous for a mutation of TPMT are at high risk for severe toxicity, including death. Patients who are heterozygous for the TMPT mutation probably have an intermediate risk of toxicity. These findings have led to the suggestion that prior to placing patients on azathioprine or 6-mercaptopurine, TPMT genotyping may be appropriate. Despite reliable methods

Table 22.3 Suggested regimens for the treatment of autoimmune hepatitis.

Regimen	Single-drug therapy	Combination therapy
Adults		
Initial	Prednisone 20–40 mg daily[a]	Prednisone 10–30 mg daily *and* azathioprine 50–100 mg daily *or* 6-mercaptopurine 25–50 mg daily
Maintenance	Prednisone 5–15 mg daily *or* azathioprine 100–200 mg daily *or* 6-mercaptopurine 50–100 mg daily	Prednisone 5-10 mg daily *and* azathioprine, 50–150 mg daily *or* 6-mercaptopurine 25–75 mg daily
Children		
Initial	Prednisone 1–2 mg/kg of body weight daily (up to 60 mg/day)	Prednisone 1–2 mg/kg of body weight daily (up to 60 mg/day) *and* azathioprine 1–2 mg/kg of body weight daily
Maintenance	Prednisone 0.1–0.2 mg/kg of body weight daily *or* 5 mg daily *or* azathioprine 1–2 mg/kg of body weight daily	Prednisone 0.1–0.2 mg/kg of body weight daily *or* 5 mg daily *and* azathioprine 1 mg/kg of body weight daily

[a]Prednisolone may be used as well.

for TMPT genotyping and measurement of levels of 6-mercaptopurine metabolites, their assessment in the clinical management of autoimmune hepatitis is not established and must be evaluated in the context of severity of disease, as advanced fibrosis has been shown to predict azathioprine toxicity [42].

Glucocorticoid-related side effects must be considered in treatment and may influence the decision or timing of treatment and the choice of medications, particularly in patients with brittle diabetes, osteoporosis, emotional lability or a history of psychosis, or poorly controlled hypertension. These conditions are not necessarily contraindications for the use of glucocorticoids, but their presence may require special precautions and monitoring. Budesonide may have an impact on decisions regarding the treatment of patients with these conditions. A recent retrospective analysis of corticosteroid treatment in patients with severe and fulminant autoimmune hepatitis, suggested that steroids did not obviate the need for transplantation and may have promoted septic complications [43].

A subset of patients with cirrhosis with inactive disease, characterized by the absence of inflammatory cells on liver biopsy and normal or near-normal serum aminotransferases, were included in a group of patients considered to have cryptogenic cirrhosis. This group is now presumed to have autoimmune hepatitis based upon the clinical setting, the presence of serologic markers, and the absence of other causes of liver disease. They may be at increased risk for the development of glucocorticoid-related side effects, while the benefit of treatment is uncertain.

Cessation of therapy during pregnancy has been associated with the relapse of autoimmune hepatitis and such patients need to be monitored carefully during pregnancy and several months postpartum because of the risk of flares in disease activity.

In the rare instances in which autoimmune hepatitis is accompanied by chronic hepatitis C virus infection, treatment should first be directed toward autoimmune hepatitis because of the danger of exacerbating autoimmune hepatitis with interferon. Although this approach may result in raising circulating levels of hepatitis C virus, it is the safer initial strategy.

The initial approach to therapy in autoimmune hepatitis depends in part upon histologic findings. The decision to treat patients with only mild hepatitis is often based on symptoms. Asymptomatic patients with mild inflammation may be observed without institution of treatment, but their clinical status should be monitored carefully, including performance of repeat liver biopsies at appropriate intervals for evidence of disease progression, so that therapy can be instituted if indicated. Treatment should not be withheld from patients with decom-

pensated cirrhosis who have active disease. The response may be excellent even in those who have already experienced bleeding from esophageal varices or who have significant ascites.

Since autoimmune hepatitis tends to be more severe in children compared to adults, possibly because of a delay in diagnosis, treatment is generally recommended in children at the time of diagnosis, except in those with inactive cirrhosis (Table 22.3) [1,36].

There are no trials on which to base the treatment of autoimmune hepatitis variant/overlap syndromes. Patients who have AMA-positive autoimmune hepatitis should be treated and followed as for patients with type 1 autoimmune hepatitis as they are generally steroid-responsive [23]. In the overlap syndrome defined by Chazouilleres and colleagues, a combination of glucocorticosteroids and ursodeoxycholate is recommended [27,28]. Reports of therapy for the autoimmune hepatitis–primary sclerosing cholangitis overlap syndrome have been limited to small case series using a variety of regimens, often combining ursodeoxycholic acid with immunosupression [25,44]. For children with autoimmune sclerosing cholangitis, ursodeoxycholic acid is usually added to corticosteroids and azathioprine [1,36].

Although some patients will remain in remission when drug treatment is withdrawn, the majority require long-term maintenance therapy. In general, the response is better with milder disease. Adults with active cirrhosis at the time of initial biopsy and children, particularly those with type 2 disease, rarely stay in remission when treatment is withdrawn and almost always require life-long maintenance therapy.

No firm guidelines exist for decisions regarding the withdrawal of medications because histologic changes may lag behind biochemical responses. A quiescent histologic appearance and normal biochemical findings while patients are still receiving therapy are not necessarily predictive of continued remission once therapy is withdrawn. Although, in the past, aminotransferase levels less than two times normal were proposed as a guideline to reducing medication, relapse has been shown to be less likely in patients who achieve normal transaminase and γ-globulin (or IgG) levels [45]. The utilization of transaminase levels also should include consideration of gender-based differences, which may not be reflected in a laboratory's normal values, and variability in ULN levels among different laboratories.

A reasonable approach following a relapse is to resume drug therapy at initial induction doses and then to attempt drug withdrawal once clinical remission is achieved again. Patients who continue to relapse can be treated with the lowest dose of either azathioprine, 6-mercaptopurine, or prednisone that controls symptoms and laboratory test results. These strategies are effective in controlling the disease in the majority of patients. The decision involves weighing the long-term side effects of the medications used.

Patients who are refractory to or intolerant of therapy may develop decompensated cirrhosis and require liver transplantation. Five-year patient survival rates are in the 70–90% range [46,47]. As in other autoimmune liver diseases, recurrence of chronic hepatitis may occur after transplantation and mandate modifications of the post-transplant immunosuppressive regimens [48]. So-called de novo autoimmune hepatitis, also referred to as post-transplant immune hepatitis, plasma cell hepatitis, or graft dysfunction mimicking autoimmune hepatitis, occurs after liver transplantation for diseases other than autoimmune hepatitis in both adults and children, and may require changes in post-transplant therapy as well [49,50].

Acknowledgments

I am indebted to Ms Margo Mertz for editorial assistance, to Ms Laura Krawitt for preparing Fig. 22.5, and to Dr Rebecca Wilcox for her advice and expertise preparing the histologic images.

References

1. Manns MP, Czaja AJ, Gorham JD, et al. Diagnosis and management of autoimmune hepatitis. *Hepatology* 2010;51:2193–213.
2. Krawitt EL, Autoimmune hepatitis. *N Engl J Med* 2006;354:54–66.
3. Vergani D, Mieli-Vergani G. Aetiopathogenesis of autoimmune hepatitis. *World J Gastroenterol* 2008;14:3306–312.
4. Rose NR. Fundamental concepts of autoimmunity and autoimmune disease. In: Krawitt EL, Wiesner RH, Nishioka M, eds. *Autoimmune Liver Diseases*, 2nd edn. Amsterdam: Elsevier Science Publishers BV, 1998:1–20.
5. Bjornsson E, Talwalker J, Treeprasertsuk, et al. Drug-induced autoimmune hepatitis: clinical characteristics and prognosis. *Hepatology* 2010;51:2040–8.
6. Donaldson PT. Genetics of autoimmune and viral liver diseases; understanding the issues. *J Hepatol* 2004;41:327–32.
7. Yokosawa S, Yoshizawa K, Ota M, et al. A genomewide DNA microsatellite association study of Japanese patients with autoimmune hepatitis type 1. *Hepatology* 2007;45:384–90.
8. Ma Y, Bogdanos DP, Hussain MJ, et al. Polyclonal T-cell responses to cytochrome P450IID6 are associated with disease activity in autoimmune hepatitis type 2. *Gastroenterology* 2006;130:868–82.
9. Hodgson HJ, Wands JR, Isselbacher KJ. Alteration in supressor cell activity in chronic active hepatitis. *Proc Natl Acad Sci USA* 1978;75:1549–53.
10. Krawitt El, Kilby AE, Albertini RJ, et al. An immunogenetic study of suppressor cell activity in autoimmune chronic active hepatitis. *Clin Immunol Immunopathol* 1988;46:249–57.
11. Nouri-Aria KT, Hegarty JE, Alexander GJM, et al. Effect of corticosteroids on suppressor-cell activity in "autoimmune" and viral chronic active hepatitis. *N Engl J Med* 1982;307:1301–4.
12. Longhi, MS, Meda, F, Wang, P, et al. Expansion and de novo generation of potentially therapeutic regulatory T cells in patients with autoimmune hepatitis. *Hepatology* 2008;47:581–91.
13. Longhi, MS, Mitry, RR, Samyn M, et al. Vigorous activation of monocytes in juvenile autoimmune liver disease escapes the control of regulatory T-cells. *Hepatology* 2009;50:130–42.
14. Batts KJ, Ludwig J. Histopathology of autoimmune hepatitis, primary biliary cirrhosis and primary sclerosing cholangitis. In: Krawitt EL, Wiesner RS, Nishioka M, eds. *Autoimmune Liver Diseases*, 2nd edn. Amsterdam: Elsevier, 1998:115–40.
15. Pratt DS, Fawaz KA, Rabson A, et al. A novel histological lesion in glucocorticoid-responsive chronic hepatitis. *Gastroenterology* 1997;113:664–8.
16. Brunt EM, Kleiner DE, Wilson LA, et al. Portal chronic inflammation in nonalcoholic fatty liver disease (NAFLD): a histologic marker of advanced NAFLD. *Hepatology* 2009;49:809–20.
17. Al-Chalabi T, Boccato S, Portman BC, et al. Autoimmune hepatitis (AIH) in the elderly: a systematic retrospective analysis of a large group of consecutive patients with definite AIH followed at a tertiary referral centre. *J Hepatol* 2006;45:575–83.
18. Czaja AJ, Carpenter HA. Distinctive clinical phenotypes and treatment outcome of type 1 autoimmune hepatitis in the elderly. *Hepatology* 2006;43:532–8.
19. Czaja AJ, Carpenter HA. Decreased fibrosis during corticosteroid therapy of autoimmune hepatitis. *J Hepatol* 2004;40:646–52.
20. Homberg J-C, Abuaf N, Bernard O, et al. Chronic active hepatitis associated with antiliver/kidney microsome antibody type 1: a second type of "autoimmune" hepatitis. *Hepatology* 1987;7:1333–9.
21. Frenzel C, Herkel J, Luth S, et al. Evaluation of F-actin ELISA for the disagnosis of autoimmune hepatitis. *Am J Gastroenterol* 2006;101:2731–6.
22. Hennes EM, Zeniya M, Czaja AJ, et al. Simplified criteria for the diagnosis of autoimmune hepatitis. *Hepatology* 2008;48:169–76.
23. O'Brien C, Joshi S, Feld JJ, et al. Long-term follow-up of antimitochondrial antibody-positive autoimmune hepatitis. *Hepatology* 2008;48:550–6.
24. Muratori P, Granito A, Quarneti C, et al. Autoimmune hepatitis in Italy: the Bologna experience. *J Hepatol* 2009;50:1210–18.
25. Rust C, Beuers U. Overlap syndromes amoung autoimmune liver diseases. *World J Gastroenterol* 2008;14:3368–73.
26. Bridoux-Henno L, Maggiore G, Johanet C, et al. Features and outcome of autoimmune hepatitis type 2 presentng with isolated positivity for anti-liver cytosol antibody. *Clin Gastroenterol Hepatol* 2004;2:825–30.
27. Chazouilleres O, Wendum D, Serfaty L, et al. Primary biliary cirrhosis-autoimmune hepatitis overlap syndrome: clinical features and response to therapy. *Hepatology* 1998;28:296–301.
28. Chazouilleres O, Wendum D, Serfaty L, et al. Long-term outcome and response to therapy of primary biliary cirrhosis – autoimmune hepatitis overlap syndrome. *J Hepatol* 2006;44:400–6.
29. Gregorio GV, Portmann B, Karani J, et al. Autoimmune hepatitis/sclerosing cholangitis overlap syndrome in childhood: a 16-year prospective study. *Hepatology* 2001;33:544–53.
30. Umemura T, Zen Y, Hanano H, et al. Immunoglobin G4-hepatopathy: association of immunoglobin G4-bearing plasma cells in liver with autoimmune pancreatitis. *Hepatology* 2007;46:463–71.
31. Umemura T, Zen Y, Nakanuma Y, et al. Another cause of autoimmune hepatitis. *Hepatology* 2010;52:389–90.
32. Yeoman AD, Al-Chalabi T, Karani JB, et al. Evaluation of risk factors in the development of hepatocellular carcinoma in autoimmune hepatitis: implication for follow-up and screening. *Hepatology* 2008;48:863–70.
33. Werner M, Almer S, Prytz H, et al. Hepatic and extrahepatic malignancies in autoimmune hepatitis. A long-term follow-up in 473 Swedish patients. *J Hepatol* 2009;50:388–93.
34. Alvarez F, Berg PA, Bianchi FB, et al. International Autoimmune Hepatitis Group report: review of criteria for diagnosis of autoimmune hepatitis. *J Hepatol* 1999;31:929–38.

35. Roberts SK, Therneau TM, Czaja AJ. Prognosis of histological cirrhosis in type 1 autoimmune hepatitis. *Gastroenterology* 1996;110: 848–57.

36. Mieli-Vergani G, Heller S, Jara P, et al. Autoimmune hepatitis. *J Pediatr Gastroenterol Nutr* 2009;49:158–60.

37. Inductivo-Yu I, Adams A, Gish RG, et al. Mycophenolate mofetil in autoimmune hepatitis patients not responsive or intolerant to standard immunosuppressive therapy. *Clin Gastro Hepatol* 2007: 799–802.

38. Hlivko JT, Shiffman ML, Stravitz RT, et al. A single center review of the use of mycophenolate mofetil in the treatment of autoimmune hepatitis. *Clin Gastro Hepatol* 2008;6:1036–40.

39. Hennes EM, Oo YH, Schramm C, et al. Mycophenolate mofetil as a second line therapy in autoimmune hepatitis? *Am J Gastroenterol* 2008;103:3063–70.

40. Aw MM, Dhawan A, Samyn M, et al. Mycophenolate mofetil as rescue treatment for autoimmune liver disease in children: a 5-year follow-up. *J Hepatol* 2009;51:156–60.

41. Manns MP, Woynarowski M, Kreisel W, et al. Azathioprine with budesonide induces remission more effectively than with prednisone in patients with autoimmune hepatitis. *Gastroenterology* 2010;139:1198–206.

42. Heneghan MA, Allan JL, Bornstien JD, et al. Utility of thiopurine methyltransferase genotyping and phenotyping, and measurement of azathioprine metabolites in the management of patients with autoimmune hepatitis. *J Hepatology* 2006;45:584–91.

43. Ichai P, Dulcos-Vallee JC, Guettier C, et al. Usefulness of corticosteroids for the treatment of severe and fulminant forms of autoimmune hepatitis. *Liver Transpl* 2007;13:996–1003.

44. Luth S, Kanzler S, Frenzel C, et al. Characteristics of long-term prognosis of the autoimmune hepatitis/primary sclerosing cholangitis overlap syndrome. *J Clin Gastroenterol* 2009;43:75–80.

45. Montano-Loza AJ, Carpenter HA, Czaja AJ. Improving the end point of corticosteroid therapy in type 1 autoimmune hepatitis to reduce the frequency of relapse. *Am J Gastroenterol* 2007;102:1005–12.

46. Campsen J, Zimmerman MA, Trotter JF, et al. Liver transplantation for autoimmune hepatitis and the success of aggressive corticosteroid withdrawal. *Liver Transpl* 2008;14:1281–6.

47. Schramm C, Bubheim M, Adam R, et al. Primary liver transplantation for autoimmune hepatitis: a comparative analysis of the European liver transplant registry *Liver Transpl* 2010;16:461–9.

48. Montano-Loza AJ, Mason AL, Ma M, et al. Risk factors for recurrence of autoimmune hepatitis after liver transplantation. *Liver Transpl* 2009;15:1254–61.

49 Salcedo M, Rodriguez-Mahou M, Rodriguez-Sainz C, et al. Risk factors for developing *de novo* autoimmune hepatitis associated with anti-glutathione *S*-transferase T1 antibodies after liver transplantation. *Liver Transpl* 2009;15:530–9.

50. Ward SC, Schiano TD, Thung SN, et al. Plasma cell hepatitis in hepatitis C virus patients post-liver transplantation: case–control study showing poor outcome and predictive features in the liver explant. *Liver Transpl* 2009;15:1826–33.

PART V
Viral Hepatitis

Overview

Eugene R. Schiff

We are entering an era when the prevention and successful treatment of viral hepatitis is rapidly escalating. Universal vaccination against hepatitis A in 1–2-year-old babies is highly effective in controlling transmission to children but also through herd immunity to adults as well. Hepatitis A vaccine is effective in postexposure settings within 14 days of exposure and may be preferable to immunoglobulin since active immunization provides long-term immunity. Hepatitis B vaccine prevents infection and hepatocellular carcinoma. Universal hepatitis B vaccination is actively progressing, particularly in endemic areas in Southeast Asia. Inability to prevent intrauterine infection leads to vaccine failure in some newborns of hepatitis B virus (HBV) infected mothers, particularly in those mothers with high HBV DNA levels. Nucleos(t)ide analogs are safe during the third trimester and have been known to reduce the rate of perinatal transmission in mothers with HBV DNA levels >10^8 IU/mL. An effective hepatitis E vaccine has been developed but is not widely available.

Treatment of hepatitis B patients with nucleos(t)ide analogs that have high genetic barriers to resistance (i.e., entecavir and tenofovir) is becoming the norm. These first-line antivirals have proven to be effective in safely sustaining HBV DNA negativity, the normalization of aminotransferases, and the amelioration of hepatic necroinflammation and fibrosis. However, long-term therapy is the rule, with the exception of those undergoing hepatitis B surface antigen (HBsAg) seroconversion. HBeAg seroconversion and long-term HBV DNA suppression is not sufficient to confidently predict the durability of disease remission. Treatment of immunotolerant patients is controversial and requires research in clinical trials. These relatively young patients with very high HBV DNA levels and relatively little or no histologic injury often will become inactive carriers over time and if treated will require long-term indefinite treatment. Nevertheless, a subgroup will be undergoing malignant transformation at a molecular level and if identified would certainly be candidates for early treatment. It has become apparent in recent years that prior to treatment with cancer chemotherapy patients should be screened for HBsAg and anti-hepatitis B core (HBc). This is done to identify those patients to be treated prophylactically with antiviral therapy to prevent the reactivation of hepatitis B that can evolve into severe hepatic failure.

Protease inhibitors of hepatitis C virus (HCV) will be licensed and a spectrum of other direct antiviral agents (DAAs) targeting NS3/4A protease, NS5B polymerase, NS5A, NS5B, and NS4B should be forthcoming over the next 3–5 years. The ultimate goal is an interferon-free regimen with a high sustained virologic response (SVR) rate and with a relatively low side effect profile. SVR rates have proven to be durable and equate with a cure. Response-guided therapy should permit shorter durations of treatment in those achieving HCV RNA negativity by 4 weeks (rapid virologic response (RVR)). Individualized therapy will undoubtedly relate to the earliest time point of HCV RNA negativity. Rapid escape from host responses by resistant mutants will have to be monitored to develop antiviral strategies. HCV resistance is likely to become an important issue in clinical practice. Interleukin 28B (IL28B) polymorphism, a gene on chromosome 19, is the most powerful host factor in determining interferon responsiveness. How useful this parameter will be with the use of DAAs is being studied. Hepatic steatosis and insulin resistance are common in patients infected with HCV and are associated with disease progression and reduced response to antiviral therapy. Low serum levels of vitamin D are related to low responsiveness to interferon-based therapy, and vitamin D supplementation has been associated with higher SVR rates but the mechanism for this phenomenon is unknown. One of the biggest unmet needs is successful treatment in transplant recipients with recurrent hepatitis C. Drug–drug interaction will undoubtedly modify antiviral regimens. Treatment of coinfected patients with human immunodeficiency virus (HIV) presents a similar challenge.

Studies with therapeutic vaccines are designed to improve SVR rates by enhancing cellular immune response.

Interferon is the only effective therapy for hepatitis D. It has become apparent that hepatitis E may evolve into chronic hepatitis among solid organ transplant patients and interferon may also be effective in clearing hepatitis E virus (HEV) in chronic hepatitis.

These major advances in the management of viral hepatitis will eventually change the spectrum of candidates for liver transplantation. However, the aging cohort of hepatitis C patients are increasingly at advanced stages of liver disease where successful antiviral therapy will have little impact on decompensated cirrhosis and the risk for hepatocellular carcinoma.

CHAPTER 23

Hepatitis A and E

Joshua Watson & Maria H. Sjogren

Gastroenterology Service, Department of Medicine, Walter Reed Army Medical Center, Washington, DC, USA

Key concepts

- Hepatitis A and E viruses (HAV and HEV) are worldwide infections that cause outbreaks or sporadic, self-contained infections.
- The precise mechanism of hepatic uptake in human liver is unknown for both viruses, but once infection occurs HAV or HEV is distributed throughout the liver.
- Infection with HAV or HEV does not result in chronic disease in immunocompetent hosts. HAV rarely can have a prolonged course or a relapsing course, and profound cholestasis can occasionally occur.

- Mortality rate is low in previously healthy persons; however, HEV has a reported mortality of 15–25% in pregnant women.
- Acute hepatitis A and hepatitis E are clinically indistinguishable from other forms of viral hepatitis. A diagnosis requires serologic confirmation.
- Hepatitis A vaccine is widely available and is approved for subjects over the age of 1 year. An HEV vaccine has successfully completed a phase III trial, but it is not commercially available.

Experimental work in humans led to the clinical recognition that viruses were etiologic agents of hepatitis A (infectious hepatitis) and hepatitis B (serum hepatitis) [1,2]. Later, the existence of two distinct hepatitis viruses was demonstrated: hepatitis A virus (HAV) and hepatitis B virus (HBV) [3]. HAV was first characterized in 1973 when scientists detected the virus in stools from human volunteers who were infected with HAV [4]. The ensuing development of sensitive and specific serologic assays for the diagnosis of HAV infection and the isolation of HAV in cell culture [5] were important advances that permitted the understanding of the epidemiology of HAV infection and, ultimately, control of the disease.

With the accurate diagnosis of hepatitis A and hepatitis B, it became apparent that at least two non-A, non-B infectious agents existed. One was similar to hepatitis B, mainly transmitted parenterally, and another was similar to hepatitis A, transmitted by the fecal–oral route. In the 1980s, two seminal discoveries correctly identified the first one as hepatitis C [6], and the second one became known as hepatitis E [7].

Since then, hepatitis E virus (HEV) has been recognized as the agent responsible for enterically transmitted non-A, non-B hepatitis. Research to understand the epidemiology, viral characteristics, and immunity against this viral agent was propelled by the work of Balayan et al. [7] and subsequently by cloning the virus [8], which allowed the development of diagnostic assays, better understand-ing of its epidemiology, and development of vaccine candidates.

Virology

Hepatitis A virus

In 1982, HAV was classified as an enterovirus type 72 belonging to the Picornaviridae family. Subsequent determination of the sequence of HAV nucleotides and amino acids led to questioning of this classification, and a new genus, hepatovirus, was created for HAV [9]. HAV has an icosahedral shape and is a nonenveloped virus. It measures 27–28 nm in diameter, has a buoyant density of 1.33–1.34 g/cm [3] in cesium chloride, and has a sedimentation coefficient of 156–160S by ultracentrifugation. HAV survives exposure to ether and an acid environment at pH 3. It also survives heat exposure at 60°C for 60 minutes but is inactivated at 85°C for 1 minute. HAV is capable of surviving in seawater (4% survival rate), dried feces at room temperature for 4 weeks (17% survival), or live oysters for 5 days (12% survival) [10].

Only one serotype of HAV is known, and there is no antigenic cross-reactivity with the hepatitis B, C, D, E, or G agents. The HAV genome consists of a positive-sense RNA that is 7.48 kb long, single stranded, and linear. HAV RNA has a sedimentation coefficient of 32–33S and a molecular weight of 2.8×10^4 daltons. The HAV RNA

Schiff's Diseases of the Liver, Eleventh Edition. Edited by Eugene R. Schiff, Willis C. Maddrey and Michael F. Sorrell.
© 2012 John Wiley & Sons, Ltd. Published 2012 by John Wiley & Sons, Ltd.

has a long open reading frame (ORF) of 6,681 nucleotides and is covalently linked to a 5' terminal protein and a 3' terminal polyadenosine tract.

The onset of HAV replication in cell culture systems takes from weeks to months. Primate cells, including African green monkey kidney cells, primary human fibroblasts, human diploid cells (MRC-5), and fetal rhesus kidney cells, are favored for the cultivation of HAV in vitro. The virus is not cytopathic, and persistent infection in the cell cultures is the rule. Two conditions control the outcome of HAV replication in cell culture [11]. First, the genetic make-up of the virus is important; HAV strains mutate in distinct regions of the viral genome as they become cell culture adapted. The second condition is the metabolic activity of the host cell at the time of infection. Cells in culture, although infected simultaneously, initiate HAV replication in an asynchronous manner. This asynchronicity may be caused by differences in the metabolic activity of individual cells, but there is no definitive evidence of cell-cycle dependence of HAV replication [12].

An initial step in the life cycle of a virus is its attachment to a cell surface receptor. The location and function of these receptors determines tissue tropism. Little is known about the mechanism of entry of HAV into cells. Some work has suggested that HAV could infect cells by a surrogate receptor-binding mechanism (by a nonspecified serum protein). HAV infectivity in tissue culture has been shown to require calcium and to be inhibited by the treatment of the cells with trypsin, phospholipases, and β-galactosidase [13]. A surface glycoprotein (HAVcr-1) on African green monkey kidney cells has been identified as a receptor for HAV. Blocking of HAVcr-1 with specific monoclonal antibodies prevents infection of otherwise susceptible cells. Experimental data suggest that HAVcr-1 not only serves as an attachment receptor, but may also facilitate the uncoating of HAV and its entry into hepatocytes [14].

Whatever the entry mechanism, once HAV enters a cell, the viral RNA is uncoated, cell host ribosomes bind to viral RNA, and polysomes are formed. HAV is translated into a large polyprotein of 2,227 amino acids. This polyprotein is organized into three regions: P1, P2, and P3. The P1 region encodes the structural proteins VP1, VP2, VP3, and a putative VP4. The P2 and P3 regions encode nonstructural proteins associated with viral replication.

The HAV RNA polymerase copies the plus RNA strand. The RNA transcript, in turn, is used for translation into proteins, which are used for assembly into mature virions. It appears that downregulation of HAV RNA synthesis occurs as defective HAV particles appear [15]. In addition, a group of specific RNA-binding proteins have been observed during persistent infection [16]. The origin

and nature of these proteins is unknown, but they exert activity on the RNA template and are believed to play a regulatory role in the replication of HAV [17].

Numerous strains of HAV exist with considerable nucleotide sequence variability (15–25% difference within the P1 region of the genome). Human HAV strains can be grouped into four different genotypes (I, II, III, and VII), whereas simian strains of HAV belong to genotypes IV, V, and VI [18]. Despite the nucleotide sequence heterogeneity, the antigenic structure of human HAV is highly conserved among strains.

The HAV VP1/2A and 2C genes are thought to be responsible for viral virulence on the basis of experiments in which recombinant HAV caused acute hepatitis in animals following the construction of 14 chimeric virus genomes from two infectious complementary DNA clones that encoded a virulent and an attenuated HAV isolate (HM175 strain). Using this method, the genotype and phenotype of each virus were then compared [19].

Among the many strains of HAV, the HM175 and CR326 human HAV strains were used for the production of commercially available vaccines. Strain HM175 was isolated in 1978 from the human feces of Australian patients in a small outbreak of hepatitis A. CR326 was isolated from Costa Rican patients infected with HAV. The nucleotide and amino acid sequences showed 95% identity between the two strains. Vaccines prepared from these strains are thought to provide protection against all relevant human strains of HAV.

Variations in the HAV genome are thought to play a role in the development of acute liver failure (ALF) during acute HAV infection. The 5' untranslated region of the HAV genome was sequenced in serum samples from 84 patients with HAV infection, including 12 with ALF [20]. The investigators observed relatively fewer nucleotide substitutions in the HAV genome of patients with ALF than in those without ALF ($P < 0.001$). The differences were most prominent between nucleotides 200 and 500, suggesting that nucleotide variation in the central portion of the 5' untranslated region influences the clinical severity of HAV infection.

Hepatitis E virus

Hepatitis E virus was first visualized in 1983 when it was transmitted to a human volunteer and subsequently to an experimental animal model, thereby establishing its role as the etiologic agent of hepatitis E [7]. HEV is a spherical nonenveloped virus 32–34 nm in size with spikes and indentations on its surface. It was recently classified into the separate genus *Hepevirus*, which is the only member of the family Hepeviridae [21]. The genome of the virus is a positive single-stranded polyadenylated RNA of approximately 7.5 kb. It consists of three overlapping ORFs and short untranslated regions at the 5' and

Table 23.1 Geographic distribution of hepatitis E virus genotypes [22,23].

Genotypes	Isolates
Genotype 1	Throughout Asia
	North Africa
Genotype 2	Mexico
	Central and western Africa (e.g., Chad, Nigeria)
Genotype 3 (found in humans and swine)	North America
	South America
	Europe (e.g., United Kingdom, France, Netherlands, Spain, Austria, Greece, Italy)
	Japan
	Australia
	New Zealand
Genotype 4	East and Southeast Asia (e.g., China, Japan, Taiwan, Vietnam)
Genotype 5	Avian isolates (appears to be a separate genus)
Heterogeneous	Europe
	Argentina

3′ termini. ORF1 is located at the 5′ end and consists of the nonstructural genes, while the 3′ end ORF2 represents one or more structural or capsid proteins. ORF2 contains important epitopes that can induce neutralizing antibodies and is the prime genomic area selected for vaccine development [22]. The function of ORF3 has not been elucidated.

Although there is no consensus on genotype classification, it is generally accepted that – on the basis of viruses having nucleotide divergence of not more than 20% of the nucleotides in the ORF2 region – five major HEV genotypes exist (Table 23.1). Genotypes 1 and 2 are strictly human pathogens. Genotypes 3 and 4 are likely from swine origin, but also infect humans. Genotype 5 is an avian strain common among chicken flocks that is considered unlikely to infect humans [23]. In addition, genetically heterogeneous isolates from several European countries have been designated as new genotypes, but this concept is not widely accepted. Similarly, two novel HEV genotypes have been described from Argentina [22]. Despite the diversity of HEV genotype, it is accepted that HEV exists as a single serotype [24], a concept that makes possible the development of a broadly protective vaccine.

In 1990, the genome of HEV was cloned from infectious experimental animal bile. These experiments established that the clone ET1.1 represented a genuine portion of the HEV genome [8]. Such advances permitted the development of sensitive and accurate assays that allow the diagnosis of the infection, better understanding of its epidemiology, and development of candidate vaccines.

Epidemiology

Hepatitis A virus

Acute hepatitis A is a reportable infectious disease in the United States with a 90% decline in incidence since 1995. In 2006, there were 3,579 reported cases of HAV infection, corresponding to a rate of infection of 1.2 per 100,000, which was down from 4 per 100,000 in 2001. With the underreporting of cases and the occurrence of asymptomatic infections taken into consideration, the true number HAV infections in 2006 was calculated to be 32,000, which was down from 93,000 in 2001 [25,26]. The greatest rates of decline have been among children from states where routine vaccination of children has been recommended since 1999. The highest rate of reported disease has historically been among children aged 5–14 years. However, due to the rapid rate of decline in children, rates are similar among different age groups, with adults aged 20–44 years holding the highest rate of disease in 2006 [27].

The epidemiologic risk factors for HAV infection reported for the US population in 2006 were as follows: unknown, 65%; international travel, 15%; sexual or household contact with a patient who has hepatitis A, 10%; other contact with hepatitis A patient, 12%; male homosexual activity, 9%; food or water borne outbreak, 8%; child or employee in a daycare center, 4%; contact with a daycare child or employee, 4%; and injection drug use, 2% [27].

HAV infection generally follows one of three epidemiologic patterns [28]. In countries where sanitary conditions are poor, most children are infected at an early age. Although earlier seroepidemiologic studies routinely showed that 100% of preschool children in these countries had detectable antibody to HAV (anti-HAV) in serum, presumably reflecting previous subclinical infection, subsequent studies have shown that the average age of infection has increased rapidly to 5 years and above, when symptomatic infection is more likely. For example, 82% of 1,393 Bolivian school children were shown to have detectable anti-HAV. When they were stratified into two groups according to family income, a significant difference was found between the groups: 95% of children from low-income families had detectable anti-HAV versus 56% of children from high-income families [29]. The second epidemiologic pattern is seen in industrialized countries, where the prevalence of HAV infection is low among children and young adults. In the United States, the prevalence of anti-HAV is approximately 10% in children but 37% in adults [30]. The third epidemiologic pattern is observed in closed or semiclosed communities, such as some isolated communities in the South Pacific, where HAV is capable (through epidemics) of infecting the entire population, which then becomes immune.

Table 23.2 Detection of hepatitis A virus (HAV) and infectivity of human secretions or excretions.

Secretion/excretion	Comment	Reference
Stool	Main source of infection. HAV is detectable during the incubation period and for several weeks after the onset of disease. After the onset of symptoms, HAV is detectable in 45% and 11% of fecal specimens from the first and second week, respectively, whereas HAV RNA (by a polymerase chain reaction assay) is detectable for 4–5 months	Coulepis et al. [35]; Rosenblum et al. [36]
Blood	Viremia is present during the incubation period. Blood collected 3 and 11 days before the onset of symptoms caused post-transfusion infection in donors. Chronic viremia does not occur	Francis et al. [37]; Harden et al. [38]
Bile	HAV has been detected in the bile of chimpanzees infected with HAV	Schulman et al. [39]
Urine	HAV is detected in low titer during the viremic phase. A urine sample infected one of 12 subjects after oral inoculation. Urine contaminated with blood was also infectious	Giles et al. [40]; Findlay [41]
Nasopharyngeal	Unknown in humans. HAV has been identified in the oropharynx of experimentally infected chimpanzees	Cohen et al. [42]
Semen, vaginal fluid	Uncertain. HAV may be detectable during the viremic phase	Berge et al. [43]

Thereafter, newborns remain susceptible until the virus is reintroduced into the community.

Whatever the epidemiologic pattern, the primary route of transmission of HAV is the fecal–oral route, by either person-to-person contact or ingestion of contaminated food or water. Although rare, transmission of HAV by a parenteral route has been documented following blood transfusion [31,32] or use of blood products [33]. Cyclic outbreaks among users of injection and noninjection drugs and among men who have sex with men (up to 10% may become infected in outbreak years) have been reported [34]. Table 23.2 provides information about the detection of HAV and its infectivity in human body fluids [35–43].

Approximately 11–22% of patients with acute hepatitis A require hospitalization with an average length of stay of 4.6 days costing, on average, US$7,926 per patient in 2004 [44]. In one outbreak involving 43 persons, the total cost was approximately $800,000 [45]. On average, 27 workdays are lost per adult case of hepatitis A. In adolescents and adults, the combined direct and indirect costs associated with HAV infection in the United States totaled approximately $488.8 million in 1997 compared with $93 million in 2006 [44]. This is a direct result of the dramatic reduction in infections seen since the introduction of the HAV vaccine combined with the US HAV vaccination policies [46].

Hepatitis E virus

Like HAV, the primary route of transmission of HEV is the fecal–oral route, most often via contaminated water. HEV causes outbreaks of acute hepatitis or is a source of sporadic, self-contained infections. The massive water-borne outbreaks of acute hepatitis in New Delhi in the 1955–1956 period [47] were diagnosed as "classic" waterborne hepatitis A. However, serologic testing of the available specimens in 1980 ruled out acute hepatitis A and acute hepatitis B allowing the recognition of the infection as non-A, non-B hepatitis [48]. Since then, at least 17 HEV outbreaks have occurred in India [49] and more than 50 in Asia, Africa, and the American continents [22]. In 1975, sporadic cases from Costa Rica were reported in which the illnesses were neither hepatitis A nor hepatitis B [50]. In 1986 and 1987, outbreaks of acute hepatitis occurred in two rural villages in Mexico; 223 cases were diagnosed as non-A, non-B hepatitis, and stool samples from some cases yielded viral particles 32–34 nm in size, similar to the enterically transmitted non-A, non-B hepatitis from Asia [51].

Hepatitis E has been detected among US travelers to endemic regions as well [52]; however, a unique HEV whose genome is significantly different from the Burmese or Mexican strains has been described in the United States in humans and swine [53]. In 2004, approximately 4,000 suspected cases of hepatitis E were reported by health clinics in Darfur, Sudan. Thousands of possible cases were also reported among refugees in Chad and Iraq [54]. Hepatitis E is a common disease in many areas of the world, and it is recognized as a frequent cause of sporadic hepatitis in Asia. It is the second leading cause (behind hepatitis B) of acute clinical hepatitis in adults in North Africa and the Middle East, and is the most common cause in Nepal, India, and throughout Central and Southeast Asia [55,56]. Table 23.3 shows the percentage of clinical viral hepatitis attributable to each of the viral hepatitides in selected regions.

Table 23.3 Etiologies of clinical viral hepatitides among adults in selected regions [56].

Location	Etiology						
	A (%)	B (%)	C (%)	D (%)	E (%)	Non A–E (%)	Mulitple (%)
United States: all ages (sentinel counties)	49.0	34.0	15.0	NR	NR	2.0	NR
Egypt (Cairo)	1.4	40.5	8.4	5.6	21.7	11.9	10.5
Saudi Arabia (Jedda, Mecca)	5.1	46.1	13.8	4.1	17.5	13.4	NR
India (New Delhi)	5.3	10.7	8.0	NR	53.3	22.7	NR

NR, not reported.
Adapted from Purcell and Emerson [56].

Anti-HEV has been detected in many areas of the world, including industrialized countries where no defined epidemics have been reported. Some species of animals (swine, rodents, monkeys, etc.) have been found to have detectable anti-HEV [57], raising the possibility of HEV being a zoonotic disease that can be acquired from animals; however, there is no confirmation of such transmission. Other possible zoonotic reservoirs include wild boars, cows, sheep, goats, and deer [55]. In areas where sporadic cases of HEV due to genotypes 3 and 4 occur in humans, swine have been found to have detectable HEV from the same genotypes [58].

Each genotype of HEV that infects humans has a distinct geographic distribution (see Table 23.1 and Fig. 23.1). Genotype 1 is found in most parts of Asia and in northern Africa. Genotype 2 was initially identified in an epidemic in Mexico in the 1980s, but it has also been found in western Africa. Genotype 3 mostly causes sporadic cases in nonendemic areas such as the United States, Europe, South America, and Japan. Genotype 4 also causes sporadic cases in nonendemic regions and has been isolated from cases in Taiwan, China, Japan, and Vietnam [23,56].

The prevalence of antibody to HEV varies in different regions of the world, showing differing patterns even among areas where the disease is endemic. For instance, in a highly endemic area like India, the prevalence of anti-HEV would be expected to mirror that of other enterically transmitted viruses, such as HAV, where nearly all of the population is exposed at a young age. However, the prevalence of anti-HEV in India does not appear to have a substantial increase until the second decade of life, when it levels out at a prevalence of around 40% thereafter. The prevalence of anti-HEV in Egypt, however, where no water-borne epidemics have been reported, more closely resembles that of anti-HAV in developing countries with close to 90% of the population developing the antibody within the first decade of life. In industrialized countries, like the United States, where clinical cases of HEV are rare, the prevalence of anti-HEV is much higher than expected and is even higher than that of anti-HAV in some areas (Fig. 23.2). The highest prevalence of anti-HEV in the United States has been found in states that are large producers of swine, leading to the conclusion that zoonotic transmission of attenuated strains of HEV

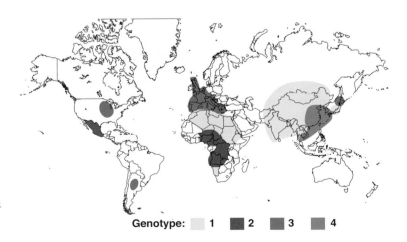

Figure 23.1 Geographic distribution of human hepatitis E virus genotypes. (Reproduced from Purcell and Emerson [56] with permission from Elsevier.)

Genotype: ☐ 1 ■ 2 ■ 3 ☐ 4

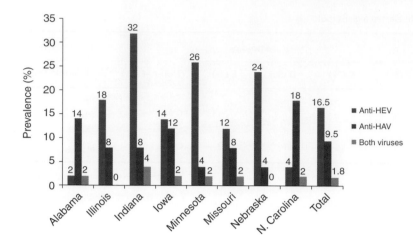

Figure 23.2 Prevalence of anti-hepatitis A virus (anti-HAV) and anti-hepatitis E virus (anti-HEV) in 400 US blood donors from eight states in 2000. (Adapted from Purcell and Emerson [56].)

(likely genotypes 3 and 4) may be the cause of this finding [56]. Supporting this conclusion is the observation that the seroprevalence rate of anti-HEV in Indonesia is ten-fold higher in Hindus than Muslims, which indicates a possible role of consuming pork [55,59]. The meaning of such high prevalences in low endemic areas is still a source of uncertainty. In addition to representing true HEV infection, some scientists attribute the high prevalence to the nonspecificity of the serologic assays, whereas others believe that it may be a cross-reaction with another infectious agent.

Recent reports have also shown that HEV is a cause of graft hepatitis in solid-organ transplant recipients, even in low endemic areas [60–63]. While HEV is typically a self-limited infection, it appears to cause chronic liver disease in some of these immunosuppressed individuals. A French group reported the largest case series to date describing 14 solid-organ transplant recipients receiving immunosuppressive drugs who had an early onset of elevated transaminase levels and were found to have detectable HEV RNA [60]. Eight of these 14 patients had persistent HEV viremia and liver enzyme elevation at follow-ups of 10–24 months, which would indicate evolution to chronic hepatitis. Liver biopsies in some of these patients with chronic hepatitis E showed dense lymphocytic infiltrate of the portal areas with variable degrees of piecemeal necrosis and fibrosis. Of note, the patients who developed chronic hepatitis E had a significantly shorter time between transplantation and development of HEV infection; therefore, their CD2, CD3, and CD4 lymphocyte counts were lower than those of patients whose HEV infection resolved [23]. To date, all reports of chronic hepatitis E infection in solid-organ transplant recipients have been infections with genotype 3, which is the genotype found commonly in domesticated livestock. The persistence of HEV infection in this population could be a phenomenon similar to that seen with other generally self-limited viral agents, such as Epstein–Barr virus

and cytomegalovirus, which are also known to cause persistent infections in immunocompromised hosts. Further studies are needed to determine if genotype 1 can also cause persistent infection, as this genotype is responsible for the majority of human HEV infections worldwide.

Pathogenesis

Hepatitis A virus

Once HAV is ingested and survives gastric acid, it traverses the small intestine mucosa and reaches the liver through the portal vein. The precise mechanism of hepatic uptake in humans is unknown (see earlier). In an experimental model on African green monkey kidney cells, the putative cellular receptor for HAV has been identified as a surface glycoprotein [14]. Once the virus reaches the hepatocyte, it starts replicating in the cytoplasm, where it is seen on electron microscopy as a fine granular pattern; however it is not present in the nucleus. HAV is distributed throughout the liver. Although HAV antigen has been detected in other organs (lymph nodes, spleen, kidney), the virus appears to replicate exclusively in hepatocytes. Once the virus is mature, it reaches the systemic circulation through the hepatic sinusoids and is released into the biliary tree through the bile canaliculi, passed into the small intestine, and eventually excreted in the feces.

The pathogenesis of HAV-associated hepatocyte injury is not completely defined. The lack of injury to cells in cell culture systems suggests that HAV is not cytopathic. Immunologically mediated cell damage is more likely. The emergence of anti-HAV could result in hepatic necrosis during the immunologically mediated elimination of HAV.

Hepatitis E virus

Studies in human volunteers and animal models have permitted the characterization of the pathogenesis of

HEV. In humans, abnormal levels of aminotransferases were detected 4–5 weeks after the ingestion of contaminated material, and they remained abnormal for 1–3 months [7,64]. Viral particles were excreted in stool approximately 4 weeks after ingestion of the inoculum, and the shedding lasted approximately 2 weeks when tested by immune electron microscopy. Using molecular biology techniques, shedding of viral particles has been observed close to 2 months after the ingestion. Immunoglobulin M (IgM) antibody to HEV parallels the rise of aminotransferase levels and declines in titer quickly, disappearing in a few weeks, although some patients may have detectable IgM anti-HEV for a few months. The IgG anti-HEV level rises slowly and remains detectable for months, probably years, after the infection.

Little is known about what happens once the virus is ingested. It is likely that the virus traverses through the small intestine and reaches the liver through the portal vein. The precise mechanism of hepatic uptake in humans is not known. Histopathologic features of HEV infection include necroinflammatory processes seen in acute viral hepatitis and cholestatic hepatitis. HEV antigen was observed in the cytoplasm of infected hepatocytes as soon as 10 days after experimental intravenous inoculation and persisted for approximately 3 weeks [65]. Interestingly, in some outbreaks, the cholestatic hepatitis has been described as a gland like transformation of hepatocytes with bile stasis. The pathogenesis of HEV-associated hepatocyte injury is not completely defined.

Clinical features

Hepatitis A virus

Infection with HAV does not result in chronic disease, but in an acute, self-limited episode of hepatitis. Rarely, acute hepatitis A can have a prolonged or a relapsing course, and profound cholestasis can occasionally occur. Commonly, the incubation period is 2–4 weeks, rarely up to 6 weeks. The mortality rate is low in previously healthy persons. Morbidity can be significant in adults and older children.

The clinical characteristics of cases of hepatitis A reported in 2007 in the United States were similar to those in previous years, with a slight preponderance of cases in men of all age groups. Overall, 73% of patients manifested jaundice, 35% required hospitalization, and 0.8% died. The need for hospitalization increased with age, from 21% among children less than 5 years old to 53% among persons 60 years of age or older [66].

HAV infection usually presents in one of five different clinical patterns: (i) asymptomatic without jaundice; (ii) symptomatic with jaundice and self-limited for approximately 8 weeks; (iii) cholestatic with jaundice lasting 10 weeks or more; (iv) relapsing with two or more bouts of acute HAV infection occurring over a 6–10-week period; and (v) acute liver failure.

Children aged between 2 and 5 years of age are usually asymptomatic, and jaundice develops in only 20% of cases. On the other hand, symptoms develop in 80% of children aged 5 years or older. A high rate of symptoms occurs in adolescents and adults as well. HAV infection with prolonged cholestasis is also a rare variant. The clinical and laboratory findings in this setting can resemble pancreatic cancer, which occasionally leads to invasive diagnostic procedures (inappropriately) because the diagnosis of acute hepatitis may not be readily accepted in patients with jaundice for several months, even in the presence of detectable anti-HAV of the IgM class [67]. A relapsing course is observed in approximately 10% of patients with acute hepatitis A. Shedding of HAV in stool has been documented during the relapse phase. This variant is benign, and the infection ultimately resolves [68]. Neither the cholestatic variant nor relapsing hepatitis A is associated with increased mortality, though the cholestatic variant can prove fatal in the elderly. In all cases, treatment is symptomatic. Acute hepatitis A, unlike hepatitis E, is not associated with an increased mortality rate in pregnant women.

Prodromal symptoms in patients with acute hepatitis A include fatigue, weakness, anorexia, nausea, vomiting, and abdominal pain. Less common symptoms include fever, headache, arthralgias, myalgias, and diarrhea. Dark urine precedes other symptoms in approximately 90% of infected persons; this symptom occurs within 1–2 weeks of the onset of prodromal symptoms. Symptoms of hepatitis may last from a few days to 2 weeks and usually decrease with the onset of clinical jaundice. Right upper quadrant tenderness and mild liver enlargement are present on physical examination in 85% of patients; splenomegaly and cervical lymphadenopathy are each present in 15%. Complete clinical recovery is achieved in 60% of affected persons within 2 months and in almost everyone by 6 months. The overall prognosis of acute hepatitis A in otherwise healthy adults is excellent. Potentially fatal complications (e.g., ALF) develop in a few patients (see below).

Acute HAV infection must be differentiated from other causes of acute viral hepatitis, autoimmune hepatitis, and other causes of acute hepatitis by appropriate serologic testing. However, in some cases, the diagnosis may be difficult to make because the patient may harbor more than one viral infection, such as chronic hepatitis B or chronic hepatitis C, with superimposed acute HAV infection.

Hepatitis E virus

The clinical features of HEV are difficult to differentiate from those of other types of viral hepatitis. The incubation period ranges between 15 and 60 days, usually becoming symptomatic 40 days after exposure. Adults appear to be at a greater risk of developing symptoms than adolescents and children. Most patients experience malaise, lack of appetite, nausea, and vomiting. A third of infected patients experience fever or abdominal pain. Few patients experience diarrhea, arthralgias, or skin rash. Serum tests show abnormal levels of aminotransferases and hyperbilirubinemia. Most patients do well, and because there are no chronic sequelae, they recover fully. However, acute liver failure is associated with HEV more often than with any other viral hepatitis [69], particularly among pregnant women. Case fatality rates among HEV-infected pregnant women have been reported of between 15% and 25% [70,71]; however, work with experimental pregnant animals failed to show differences in severity of HEV infection when compared with nonpregnant animals [72].

Acute liver failure with hepatitis A and E

Hepatitis A virus

Acute liver failure caused by HAV is rarely seen in children, adolescents, or young adults. However, the case fatality rate in people over 49 years of age with acute hepatitis A is reported to be 1.8%, which is much higher than the overall rate of 0.3% in persons of all ages. Hepatic failure caused by hepatitis A becomes manifest in the first week of illness in approximately 55% of affected patients and during the first 4 weeks in 90%; ALF is rarely seen after 4 weeks [73]. The contribution of HAV to ALF has been reported to be increased in populations classified as hyperendemic for HAV. In a report from India, where 276 patients with ALF were seen between 1994 and 1997, 10.6% of the cases among adults were caused by HAV. HAV had been responsible for only 3.5% of cases among 206 patients with ALF seen in the same community from 1978 to 1981 [74].

Certain populations have increased morbidity and a high risk of ALF from HAV infection. Among these groups are the elderly [75] and persons with chronic liver disease. A 1998 report described the clinical outcome of 256 persons hospitalized for acute hepatitis A in Tennessee from January 1994 through December 1995 [76]. On admission, 89% had experienced prolonged nausea or vomiting, and 26% had a prolonged prothrombin time (>3 seconds); 39 had serious complications (19 were hepatobiliary in nature and 20 were extrahepatic complications), and five (2%) died. Morbidity and mortality correlated with age. Twenty-five percent of patients aged 40 and above had at least one complication as compared with 11% of patients younger than 40 years of age ($P = 0.014$).

Although two reports since the late 1990s have described a decline in the number of cases of acute viral hepatitis among patients with ALF in the United States [77,78], this decline is attributable principally to the control of hepatitis B. The contribution of HAV infection to ALF has remained unchanged since the 1970s, despite the availability of highly efficacious vaccines.

Hepatitis E virus

Acute liver failure resulting in death or liver transplant due to HEV has been observed as well. Unlike HAV, there is not a clear age-dependent severity seen with HEV. Also, the reported case fatality rate of HEV (0.5–4%) is considerably higher than that of HAV. This higher mortality rate with HEV may reflect selection bias as much of the data have been obtained from hospitalized cases that may represent more severe disease [23]. Indeed, in population studies during outbreaks of HEV in India and China, mortality rates have been much lower, ranging from 0.07% to 0.6% [79,80].

The HEV genotype appears to play a role in the severity of illness. ALF has been reported with all genotypes with the possible exception of genotype 2 [81]. Genotype 1, which is the most common subtype in endemic areas, is more pathogenic in humans, whereas genotypes 3 and 4, which can be passed via zoonotic transmission, appear to be less pathogenic in humans [82].

Interestingly, the case fatality rate of HEV infection is much higher in pregnant women, ranging anywhere from 15% to 25%. The reasons for this increased mortality during pregnancy are unclear. Differences in immune and hormonal factors that occur during pregnancy as well as genetic and environmental factors have been postulated [82]. Also, some data have suggested that severe fetal infections and fetal death may lead to more severe maternal outcomes through the production of toxins that overwhelm the maternal circulation [83].

The increased mortality in pregnancy varies across geographic regions as well. In a recent study from a tertiary care center in northern India, hepatitis E infection accounted for 60% of viral hepatitis among pregnant females admitted to the hospital with jaundice. Of these pregnant females with hepatitis E, 55% (73/132) developed ALF [84]. In contrast, no cases of severe acute viral hepatitis from HEV have been reported in Egypt where the prevalence of anti-HEV is high in rural communities. In one recent cohort study of 2,428 pregnant women in the Nile delta, the anti-HEV prevalence was 84.3%; however, no cases of severe acute viral hepatitis were reported [85]. The reasons for this geographic difference are unclear. It could be related to differences in virulence of HEV strains in the different areas, or it could be related to the age of exposure to HEV in different regions and subsequent development of long-lasting immunity or modification of responses to later exposures.

Diagnosis

Hepatitis A virus

Acute hepatitis A is clinically indistinguishable from other forms of viral hepatitis. The diagnosis of infection is based on the detection of specific antibodies against HAV (anti-HAV) in serum. A diagnosis of acute hepatitis A requires the demonstration of IgM anti-HAV in serum. The test is positive from the onset of symptoms [86] and usually remains positive for approximately 4 months [87]. Some patients may have low levels of detectable IgM anti-HAV for more than 1 year after the initial infection [86]. IgG anti-HAV is also detectable at the onset of the disease, remains present usually for life, and is interpreted as a marker of previous HAV infection following clinical recovery. Figure 23.3 shows the typical serological profile seen with acute HAV infection.

Testing for HAV RNA is limited to research laboratories. HAV RNA has been detected in serum, stool, and liver tissue. Viral RNA can be amplified by polymerase chain reaction (PCR) methodology [33]. With a PCR assay, HAV RNA has been documented in human sera for up to 21 days after the onset of illness [88]. The use of HAV RNA testing has been described in a report of 76 French patients with acute HAV infection seen between January 1987 and April 2000; 19 of them had ALF [89]. Ten patients required liver transplantation, and one patient died while awaiting liver transplantation. The HAV RNA status was determined in 39 of the 50 patients in whom sera and clinical data were available, including the 19 with ALF. HAV RNA was detected in 36 of these 50 patients (72%). The likelihood that HAV RNA was undetectable was greater in patients with ALF than in those without ALF ($P < 0.02$). When HAV RNA was detectable, titers were lower in patients with encephalopathy than in patients without ALF (3.6 log versus 4.4 log, $P = 0.02$). These data suggest that the detection of IgM anti-HAV and undetectable or low-titer HAV RNA in patients with severe acute hepatitis may signal an ominous prognosis and the need for early referral for liver transplantation. As in other studies, HAV genotype did not seem to play a role in the severity of clinical manifestations [90].

Hepatitis E virus

For HEV, the development of modern diagnostic tests was possible in part because of cloning of the virus [8] and the development of four recombinant viral antigens representing two distinct antigenic domains from two HEV strains [91]. Before this advance, scientists relied on immune electron microscopy to detect viral particles in stool with the consequent limitations of intensive labor and reduced sensitivity. Enzyme immunoassays are available to detect antibodies against HEV IgM or IgG classes of antibodies [91]. These tests have an 80–100% probability of detecting the markers of acute infection (e.g., IgM anti-HEV). Data are limited to evaluate the longevity of IgG anti-HEV. Some studies have shown that IgG anti-HEV persists for at least 1 year after an acute infection [92]; others have found that it may last longer. When 53 children from the outbreak in Mexico in the period 1986–1987 [51] were tested for anti-HEV 9 years later, 70% were found to have detectable IgG antibody [93]. Figure 23.4 shows the typical serological profile seen with acute HEV infection.

Prevention and treatment

Hepatitis A virus

Recommendations concerning immunoprophylaxis against HAV were published in December 1999 by the Advisory Committee on Immunization Practices (ACIP)

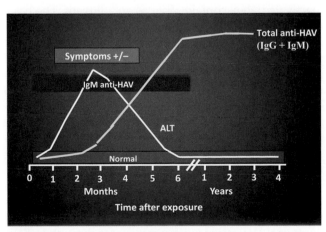

Figure 23.3 Typical serologic profile of acute hepatitis A virus (HAV) infection. ALT, alanine aminotransferase; IgG, IgM, immunoglobulin G and M.

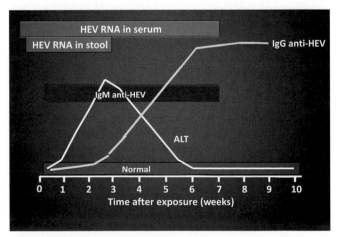

Figure 23.4 Typical serologic profile of acute hepatitis E virus (HEV) infection. ALT, alanine aminotransferase; IgG, immunoglobulin G.

Box 23.1 Groups at high risk of hepatitis A virus infection.

- Healthy persons who travel to endemic areas, work in occupations for which the likelihood of exposure is high, are family members of infected patients, or adopt infants or children from endemic areas
- Persons with chronic liver disease
- Persons who have tested positive for human immunodeficiency virus
- Men who have sex with men
- Users of injection and noninjection illicit drugs
- Persons with clotting factor disorders

[34]. The overall strategy was to protect persons from disease and to lower the incidence of HAV infection in the United States. The available monovalent vaccines were licensed for use in children older than 2 years of age but became licensed for use after 12 months of age [34,94]. In accordance with the 1999 ACIP guidelines, high-risk populations were targeted for immunization. After achieving a dramatic reduction in incidence rates, a universal childhood vaccination policy was enacted in 2006 with the hope of eventually eliminating indigenous HAV transmission in the United States. The decline in rates has intuitively been greater in children than in adults, effectively removing children as a high-risk population and potentially removing the virus's primary reservoir in the United States [27,44]. Currently, all children should receive hepatitis A vaccine at age 1 year or older; high-risk populations are targeted for immunization and are listed in Box 23.1.

There are no specific medications to treat acute hepatitis A; symptomatic treatment is the rule. Attention to sanitation and administration of serum immunoglobulin have been the mainstays of preventing HAV infection. The availability of excellent HAV vaccines has rendered the use of immunoglobulin for preexposure prophylaxis unnecessary. Furthermore, in June 2007, the HAV vaccine was granted approval for postexposure prophylaxis in immunocompetent individuals 12 months to 40 years of age without chronic liver disease [97]. This change was made following the results of a study comparing the efficacy of the vaccine to immunoglobulin in postexposure prophylaxis. There were low rates of clinical infection in both groups: 4.4% of individuals in the vaccine group developed clinical hepatitis A compared with 3.3% in the immunoglobulin group [96]. This study, however, likely excluded asymptomatic infections. In the vaccine group, 162 individuals with positive HAV IgM antibodies were excluded compared with 50 individuals in the immunoglobulin group either due to a lack of symptoms and/or because they did not have an elevated alanine aminotransferase (ALT) more than two times the normal limit. Indeed, it is possible that within this group there existed a number of asymptomatic hepatitis A infections that still posed an infectious risk to others.

The ACIP discussed the findings and limitations of the HAV vaccine versus immunoglobulin noninferiority study taking into account data from Canada and the United Kingdom, countries that have been using the vaccine as postexposure prophylaxis for more than 5 years. They concluded the vaccine is safe and comparable to immunoglobulin in protecting against clinical disease. ACIP guidelines allow for persons who have recently been exposed to HAV and who have not been vaccinated previously to be administered a single dose of single-antigen hepatitis A vaccine or immunoglobulin (0.02 mL/kg) as soon as possible within 2 weeks after exposure. Some of the benefits of the vaccine include long-term immunity if the second dose is received in accordance with the standard vaccine schedule (Table 23.4), cost savings, and a wide availability when compared with immunoglobulin [95]. Although immunoglobulin is considered safe, there is a perceived health risk as it is a blood derived product. Immunoglobulin can cause fever and myalgias just as the vaccine can, but pain at the injection site is usually more pronounced. Postexposure prophylaxis with immunoglobulin can be given safely at the same time as initiation of active immunization with the vaccine [97].

The HAV vaccine was first licensed in the United States in 1995; two inactivated HAV vaccines are commercially available. Extensive use of the vaccines in clinical trials and postmarketing surveillance support the safety and efficacy of these products. Havrix® is manufactured by SmithKline Biologicals (Rixensart, Belgium) and Vaqta® by Merck Sharp and Dohme (West Point, Pennsylvania). Both vaccines are derived from HAV grown in cell culture. The final products are purified and formalin-inactivated; they contain alum as an adjuvant. The basic difference between the two commercially available vaccines is the HAV strain used for preparation. Havrix is prepared with the HM175 strain, whereas Vaqta is prepared with the CR326 strain [98,99]. The difference is of little practical importance because both vaccines are safe and immunogenic. The doses and schedule of immunization are shown in Table 23.4. After vaccination with Havrix, anti-HAV is estimated to remain detectable in serum for approximately 20 years; immunity may last longer [100].

From the time the HAV vaccine was licensed in the United States through to 2005, more than 50 million doses were administered. Worldwide, more than 188 million doses of HAV vaccine were administered through to 2005. Among adults, the most common local side effects were soreness at the injection site (56%), headache (14%), and malaise (7%). In children, the most common side effects were soreness at the injection site (15%), feeding problems (8%), headache (4%), and injection site induration (4%) [44].

In the United States through to 2005, the national Vaccine Adverse Event Reporting System received 6,136 reports of unexplained adverse events after immunization with the HAV vaccine alone or in combination with other vaccines. Of the 6,136 reports, 871 were considered serious and included Guillian–Barré syndrome, idiopathic thrombocytopenic purpura, elevated liver transaminases, and seizures in children [44]. However, no reported serious event could be attributed definitively to the HAV vaccine, and the reported rates did not exceed the expected background rates. For example, the general population incidence of Guillain–Barré syndrome ranges from 0.5 to 2.4 cases per 100,000 person-years, and among adult HAV vaccine recipients the incidence of Guillain–Barré was 0.2 cases per 100,000 person-years [44].

A combined formulation of hepatitis A and B vaccines (Twinrix®) is available and has an excellent record of efficacy and safety [101]. Although there have been some long-term studies that show antibody persistence in children and adolescents, there is evidence of lower seroconversion rates in children 1–6 years of age when compared with the standard monovalent vaccines [102]. It is therefore currently only Food and Drug Administration (FDA) approved for individuals 18 years of age and older.

As a result of the reduction in endemic cases of hepatitis A in the United States, the largest proportion of patients being infected are nonimmune adults traveling abroad to endemic areas. Even if medical advice is sought prior to travel there is usually insufficient time to complete the standard immunization schedule. Havrix and Vaqta share an FDA-approved accelerated vaccination schedule for this purpose. If given at least 2 weeks prior to travel, a single dose of either monovalent vaccine results in appropriate protective serum antibody titers [95]. On March 28, 2008 the FDA approved an accelerated vaccination schedule for Twinrix that can be completed within 30 days with a booster at 12 months, after studies showed equivalent protection compared with standard and alternate scheduled individual monovalent vaccine doses. After 1 year, HAV seroconversion rates were 100%, and HBV seroconversion rates were 96.4–100% [103,104]. The Twinrix accelerated schedule is being discussed for use in US correctional facilities for new convicts where high-risk activities place them at risk for both hepatitis A outbreaks and hepatitis B infections [105]. The dosing schedules are shown in Table 23.4.

Hepatitis E virus

For acute HEV infection, no defined antiviral therapy exists, so treatment is mainly supportive. In cases of acute liver failure from HEV, liver transplantation should be considered. Some investigators have evaluated the efficacy of pre- or postexposure to serum immunoglobulins as prophylaxis to prevent acute HEV hepatitis. Unfortunately, even when using serum immunoglobulins from

Table 23.4 Recommended regimens for hepatitis A vaccination (intramuscular injection in deltoid).

Vaccine	Age (years)	Dose	Volume (mL)	Dosing schedule
Havrix:	1–18	720 ELU	0.5	0 and 6–12 months
	>18	1440 ELU	1.0	0 and 6–12 months
Accelerated schedule	1+	One age-appropriate dose	Age appropriate	≥2 weeks prior to travel[a]
Postexposure prophylaxis[b]	1+	One age-appropriate dose	Age appropriate	<2 weeks after exposure[a]
Vaqta:	1–18	25 units	0.5	0 and 6–18 months
	>18	50 units	1.0	0 and 6–18 months
Accelerated schedule	1+	One age-appropriate dose	Age appropriate	≥2 weeks prior to travel[a]
Postexposure prophylaxis[b]	1+	One age-appropriate dose	Age appropriate	<2 weeks after exposure[a]
Twinrix:	≥18	720 ELU HAV, 20 mg HBV	1.0	0, 1, and 6 months
Accelerated schedule	≥18	720 ELU HAV, 20 mg HBV	1.0	0, 7, and 21–30 days[a]
Postexposure prophylaxis				Not FDA approved

[a]Boosters necessary for long-term protection: Vaqta at 6 months; Havrix between 6 and 12 months, and Twinrix at 12 months (not FDA approved).
[b]For individuals exposed to HAV who were not previously immunized against HAV.
ELU, enzyme-linked immunoassay (ELISA) units; FDA, Food and Drug Administration; HAV, hepatitis A virus; HBV, hepatitis B virus.

Table 23.5 Status of hepatitis E vaccines.

Type	Pharmaceutical company or research group	Clinical stage
56 kDa ORF-2 protein VLPs (baculovirus)	GlaxoSmithKline/US Army/US National Institutes of Health	Phase II/III
50 kDa ORF-2 protein VLPs (*Escherichia coli*)	Beijing Wantai Biological Pharmacy Enterprise Company/China National Institute of Diagnostics and Vaccine Development in Infectious Diseases	Phase II/III
DNA vaccine (ORF-2)	US Navy	Preclinical
Live swine virus vaccine	US National Institutes of Health	Preclinical

DNA, deoxyribonucleic acid; ORF, open reading frame; VLP, virus-like particle.
Adapted and updated from World Health Organization [107].

endemic regions (e.g., India), no clinical benefit was observed [106]. Prevention against HEV infection is associated with hygienic measures and clean water. No vaccine for human use is commercially available yet, but several recombinant HEV proteins have been evaluated as vaccine candidates. Table 23.5 shows some of these vaccines [107].

GlaxoSmithKline (GSK) Biologicals has worked on the development of a hepatitis E vaccine to protect adolescents and adults. The vaccine is a 56 kDa recombinant product expressed in insect cells from a baculovirus vector. It was initially developed at the National Institutes of Health (NIH) in the United States and subjected to successful phase I studies [108]. Recently, a blinded, placebo-controlled study was conducted in Nepal involving 2,000 adults from the Royal Nepalese Army. The study was a collaboration between GSK, the US Army, the Royal Nepalese Army, and the US NIH. The vaccine was administered as three injectable doses at 0, 1, and 6 months, and it was shown to be safe and immunogenic. The vaccine efficacy was calculated to be 97% among vaccine recipients because only three subjects among the 898 who were fully immunized developed acute HEV, while 66 of the 896 placebo recipients had acute HEV [109].

While promising, this study had several limitations. First, the subjects were overwhelmingly young men (mean age 25 years). Further study is therefore needed to determine if the vaccine is safe and effective for women of child-bearing age, children, and other populations at high risk, including those with chronic liver disease. Also, the study looked at clinical disease rate and not HEV infection rate, so no inference can be made about the vaccine's effectiveness at reducing transmission of the virus within a community. Finally, the anti-HEV antibody titers were significantly decreased in a large percentage of the study subjects by the end of the follow-up period, so the duration of protection from the vaccine needs to be

further studied [23]. According to a recent *Vaccine* conference report, the vaccine "needs 4–5 years' more work and further investment of at least US$ 50 million for research and development to reach a licensing stage" [55].

A Chinese scientific group has been developing another HEV vaccine named HEV 239. Like the GSK vaccine, this vaccine is produced with truncated structural proteins but is more extensively truncated, consists of 23 nm virus-like particles, and is expressed in *Escherichia coli*. In a randomized, controlled phase II clinical trial of the vaccine it was administered as either two or three injectable doses at 0 and 6 months, or at 0, 1, and 6 months. The study showed that vaccination with two or three doses induced protective antibodies in 98% or 100% of subjects, respectively. New HEV infections (inferred by asymptomatic seroconversion or rise in antibody titers) occurred less often in vaccine recipients than in control subjects, thereby indicating that the vaccine was protective [110]. A phase III trial of this vaccine was recently completed as well. The study included over 100,000 participants, of whom 48,693 received three doses of the vaccine. Fifteen of 48,663 participants in the placebo group developed hepatitis E compared with none in the vaccine group during a follow-up period of 12 months. The vaccine was therefore considered 100% effective after three doses [111]. The duration of protection as well as the safety and efficacy in high-risk populations (i.e., pregnant women, infants, and chronic liver disease patients) remains unknown.

Antiviral therapy for chronic HEV has been considered and attempted. A recent report detailed treatment for chronic HEV in two immunocompromised patients. Both subjects received daily oral ribavirin 12 mg/kg for 12 weeks. At the end of therapy and during an 8–12-week follow-up, the patients stopped shedding HEV, their liver tests normalized, and the HEV RNA remained undetectable. Ribavirin was considered potentially effective in patients with chronic HEV [112].

Immunization against hepatitis A virus in patients with chronic liver disease

Persons with chronic liver disease are at increased risk of HAV- and HEV-related morbidity and mortality if they become infected with one of these viruses. Therefore, preexposure prophylaxis with the HAV vaccine has been recommended for patients with chronic liver disease who are susceptible to HAV [113]. This recommendation should be extended to pre- and postliver transplant recipients, although the immunogenicity of the HAV vaccine is reduced in these persons [114,115].

An episode of acute hepatitis in a patient with underlying chronic liver disease poses the risk of considerable morbidity and mortality. Although the current guidelines recommend immunization against HAV for all patients with chronic liver disease [34], the results of several cost-effective analyses have been conflicting. A report published in 2000 found that saving the life of one patient with HCV infection by HAV vaccination would cost 23 million Canadian dollars [116]; however, some of the assumptions in this report have been challenged [117]. Two other studies of patients with chronic hepatitis C showed a decided benefit to immunization against HAV [118]. The methods used in these studies were dissimilar, and some analyses may have been insensitive to the incidence of HAV or may have underestimated the economic and societal costs of a case of ALF. Universal immunization against HAV during childhood before the possible occurrence of chronic liver disease offers the promise of preventing HAV infection [119].

References

1. MacCallum FO, McFarlan AM, Miles JAR, et al., eds. *Infective Hepatitis: studies in East Anglia during the period 1943–1947.* Medical Research Council, Special Report No. 273. London: HMSO, 1951.
2. Havens WP, Paul JR. Infectious hepatitis and serum hepatitis. In: Rivers TM, Horsfall F, eds. *Viral and Rickettsial Infections of Man*, 3rd edn, Vol. 261. Philadelphia, PA: JB Lippincott, 1959:729–34.
3. Krugman S, Ward R, Giles JP, et al. Infectious hepatitis: detection of virus during the incubation period and in clinically inapparent infections. *N Engl J Med* 1959;261:729–34.
4. Feinstone SM, Kapikian AZ, Purcell RH. Hepatitis a: detection by immune electron microscopy of a viruslike antigen associated with acute illness. *Science* 1973;182:1026–8.
5. Provost PJ, Hilleman MR. An inactivated hepatitis A virus vaccine prepared from infected marmoset liver. *Proc Soc Exp Biol Med* 1978;159:201–3.
6. Choo QL, Kuo G, Weiner AJ, et al. isolation of a cDNA clone derived from a blood-borne non-A, non-B viral hepatitis. *Science* 1989;244:359.
7. Balayan MS, Andjaparaidze AG, Savinskaya SS, et al. Evidence for a virus in non-A, non-B hepatitis transmitted via the fecal–oral route. *Interviroloogy* 1983;20:23–31.
8. Reyes GR, Purdy MA, Kim JP, et al. Isolation of a cDNA from the virus responsible for enterically transmitted non-A, non-B hepatitis. *Science* 1990;247:1335–9.
9. Minor PD. Picornaviridae. Classification and nomenclature of viruses. Fifth report of the International Committee on Taxonomy of Viruses. *Arch Virol Suppl* 1991;2:320–6.
10. Sobsey MD, Shields PA, Hauchman FS, et al. Survival and persistence of hepatitis A virus in environmental samples. In: Zuckerman AJ, ed. *Viral Hepatitis and Liver Disease*. New York: Alan R Liss, 1988:121–4.
11. Siegl G. Replication of hepatitis A virus and processing of proteins. *Vaccine* 1992;10:S32–5.
12. Harmon SA, Summers DF, Ehrenfeld E. Detection of hepatitis A virus RNA and capsid antigen in individual cells. *Virus Res* 1989;12:361–9.
13. Seganti L, Superti F, Orsi N, et al. Study of the chemical nature of Frp/3 cell recognition units for hepatitis A virus. *Med Microbiol Immunol* 1987;176:21–6.
14. Kaplan G, Totsuka A, Thompson P, et al. Identification of a surface glycoprotein on African green monkey kidney cells as a receptor for hepatitis A virus. *EMBO J* 1996;15:4282–96.
15. Siegl G, Nüesch JPF, de Chastonay J. DI-particles of hepatitis A virus in cell culture and clinical specimens. In: Brinton MA, Heinz FX, eds. *New Aspects of Positive Strand RNA Viruses*. Washington: American Society for Microbiology, 1990:102–7.
16. Nüesch JPF, Weitz M, Siegl G. Proteins specifically binding to the 3′ untranslated region of hepatitis A virus RNA in persistently infected cells. *Arch Virol* 1993;128:65–79.
17. Robertson BH, Jansen RW, Khanna B, et al. Genetic relatedness of hepatitis A virus strains recovered from different geographic regions. *J Gen Virol* 1992;73:1365–77.
18. Mathiesen LR, Feinstone SM, Purcell RH, et al. Detection of hepatitis A antigen by immunofluorescence. *Infect Immun* 1977;18:524–30.
19. Emerson SU, Huang YK, Nguyen H, et al. Identification of VP1/2A and 2C as a virulence genes of hepatitis A virus and demonstration of genetic instability of 2C. *J Virol* 2002;76:8551–9.
20. Fujiwara K, Yokosuka O, Ehata T, et al. Association between severity of type A hepatitis and nucleotide variations in the 5′ non-translated region of hepatitis A virus RNA: strains from fulminant hepatitis have fewer nucleotide substitutions. *Gut* 2002;51:82–8.
21. Emerson SU, Anderson D, Arankalle A, et al. Hepevirus. In: Fauquet CM, Mayo MA, Maniloff J, et al., eds. *Virus Taxonomy*, VIIIth Report of the ICTV. London: Elsevier/Academic Press, 2005:853–7.
22. Wang L, Zhuang H. Hepatitis E: an overview and recent advances in vaccine research. *World J Gastroenterol* 2004;10:2157–62.
23. Aggarwal R, Naik S. Epidemiology of hepatitis E: current status. *J Gastroenterol Hepatol* 2009;24:1484–93.
24. Schlauder GG, Mushahwar IK. Genetic heterogeneity of hepatitis E virus. *J Med Virol* 2001;65:282–92.
25. Centers for Disease Control and Prevention (CDC). Summary of notifiable diseases United States 2006. *MMWR* 2008;55(53):1–92.
26. Centers for Disease Control and Prevention (CDC). Summary of notifiable diseases United States 2001. *MMWR* 2001;50(53):1–108.
27. Centers for Disease Control and Prevention (CDC). Surveillance for acute viral hepatitis United States 2006. *MMWR Survill Summ* 2008;57(2):1–24.
28. Gust ID. Epidemiological patterns of hepatitis A in different parts of the world. *Vaccine* 1992;10:S56–8.
29. Gandolfo GM, Ferri GM, Conti L, et al. Prevalence of infections by hepatitis A, B, C and E viruses in two different socioeconomic groups of children from Santa Cruz, Bolivia. *Med Clin (Barc)* 2003;120:725–7.
30. Centers for Disease Control and Prevention (CDC). Prevention of hepatitis A through active or passive immunization: recommendations of the Advisory Committee on Immunization Practices (ACIP). *MMWR* 1996;45(RR-15):1–30.
31. Skidmore SJ, Boxall EH, Ala F. A case report of post-transfusion hepatitis A. *J Med Virol* 1982;10:223.

32. Hollinger FB, Khan NC, Oefinger PE, et al. Posttransfusion hepatitis type A. *JAMA* 1983;250:2313–17.

33. Mannucci PM, Gdovin S, Gringeri A, et al. Transmission of hepatitis A to patients with hemophilia by factor VIII concentrates treated with organic solvent and detergent to inactivate viruses. *Ann Intern Med* 1994;120:1–7.

34. Centers for Disease Control and Prevention (CDC). Prevention of hepatitis A through active or passive immunization: recommendations of the Advisory Committee on Immunization Practices (ACIP). *MMWR* 1999: 48(RR-12):1–37.

35. Coulepis AG, Locarnini SA, Lehmann NI, et al. Detection of HAV in feces. *J Infect Dis* 1980;141:151–6.

36. Rosenblum LS, Villarino ME, Nainan OV, et al. Hepatitis A outbreak in a neonatal intensive care unit: risk factors for transmission and evidence of prolonged viral excretion among preterm infants. *J Infect Dis* 1991;164:476–82.

37. Francis T Jr, Frisch AW, Quilligan JJ. Demonstration of infectious hepatitis virus in presymptomatic period after transfer by transfusion. *Proc Soc Exp Biol Med* 1946;61:276–80.

38. Harden AG, Barondess JA, Parker B. Transmission of infectious hepatitis by transfusion of whole blood. *N Engl J Med* 1955;253: 923–5.

39. Schulman AN, Dienstag JL, Jackson DR, et al. Hepatitis A antigen particles in liver, bile and stool of chimpanzees. *J Infect Dis* 1976;134:80–4.

40. Giles JP, Liebhaber H, Krugman S, et al. Early viremia and viruria in infectious hepatitis. *Virology* 1964;24:107–8.

41. Findlay GM. Infective hepatitis in West Africa: 1. *Mon Bull Ministry Health* 1948;7:2–11.

42. Cohen JI, Feinstone S, Purcell RH. Hepatitis A virus infection in a chimpanzee: duration of viremia and detection of virus in saliva and throat swabs. *J Infect Dis* 1989;160:887–90.

43. Berge JJ, Drennan D, Jacobs J, et al. The cost of hepatitis A infections in American adolescents and adults in 1997. *Hepatology* 2000;31:469–73.

44. Centers for Disease Control and Prevention (CDC). Prevention of hepatitis A through active or passive immunization: recommendations of the Advisory Committee on Immunization Practices (ACIP). *MMWR* 2006: 55(RR-7):1–23.

45. Dalton CB, Haddix A, Hoffman RE, Mast EE. The cost of a foodborne outbreak of hepatitis A in Denver, Colo. *Arch Intern Med* 1996;156:1013–16.

46. Koslap-Petraco MB, Shub M, Judelsohn R. Hepatitis A: disease burden and current childhood vaccination strategies in the United States. *J Pediatr Health Care* 2008;22:3–11.

47. Viswanathan R, Sidhu AS. Infectious hepatitis: clinical findings. *Indian J Med Res* 1957;45(Suppl):49–58.

48. Wong DC, Purcell RH, Sreenivasam MA, et al. Epidemic and endemic hepatitis in India. Evidence for a non-A, non-B hepatitis. *Lancet* 1980;2:876–9.

49. Arankalle VA, Chadha MS, Tsarev SA, et al. Seroepidemiology of water-borne hepatitis in India and evidence for a third enterically transmitted hepatitis agent. *Proc Natl Acad Sci* 1994;91:3428–32.

50. Villarejos VM, Kirsten PH, Visona MS, et al. Evidence for viral hepatitis other than type A or type B among persons in Costa Rica. *N Engl J Med* 1975;293:1350–2.

51. Velazquez O, Stetler HC, Avila C, et al. Epidemic transmission of enterically transmitted non-A, non-B hepatitis in Mexico, 1986–1987. *JAMA* 1990;263:3281–5.

52. Centers for Disease Control and Prevention (CDC). Hepatitis E among US travelers 1989–92. *MMWR* 1993;42:1–4.

53. Meng XJ, Purcell RH, Halbur PG, et al. A novel virus in swine is closely related to the human hepatitis E virus. *Proc Natl Acad Sci* 1997;94:9860–5.

54. Emerson SU, Purcell RH. Running like water – the omnipresence of hepatitis E. *N Engl J Med* 2004;351:2367–8.

55. FitzSimons D, Hendrickx G, Vorsters A, Van Damme P. Hepatitis A and E: update on prevention and epidemiology. *Vaccine* 2010;28:583–8.

56. Purcell RH, Emerson SU. Hepatitis E: an emerging awareness of an old disease. *J Hepatol* 2008;48:494–503.

57. Vander Poel WHM, Verschoor F, Van der Heide R. Hepatitis E virus sequences in swine related to sequences in humans, the Netherlands. *Emerg Infect Dis* 2001;7:970–6.

58. Shukla P, Chauhan UK, Naik S, Anderson D, Aggarwal R. Hepatitis E virus infection among animals in northern India: an unlikely source of human disease. *J Viral Hepat* 2007;14:295–7.

59. Surya IG, Kornia K, Suwardewa TG, et al. Serological markers of hepatitis B, C, and E viruses and human immunodeficiency virus type-1 infections in pregnant women in Bali, Indonesia. *J Med Virol* 2005;75:499–503.

60. Kamar N, Selves J, Mansuy JM, et al. Hepatitis E virus and chronic hepatitis in organ-transplant recipients. *N Engl J Med* 2008;358:811–17.

61. Gerolami R, Moal V, Colson P. Chronic hepatitis E with cirrhosis in a kidney-transplant recipient. *N Engl J Med* 2008;358:859–60.

62. Haagsma EB, van den Berg AP, Porte RJ, et al. Chronic hepatitis E virus infection in liver transplant recipients. *Liver Transpl* 2008;14:547–53.

63. Pischke S, Suneetha PV, Baechlein C, et al. Hepatitis E virus infection as a cause of graft hepatitis in liver transplant recipients. *Liver Transpl* 2010;16:74–82.

64. Chauhan A, Jameel S, Dilaware JB, et al. Hepatitis E virus transmission to a volunteer. *Lancet* 1993;341:149–50.

65. Krawczynski K, Bradley DW. Enterically transmitted non-A, non-B hepatitis: identification of virus-associated antigen in experimentally infected cynomologous macaques. *J Infect Dis* 1989;159: 1041–9.

66. Centers for Disease Control and Prevention (CDC). Surveillance for acute viral hepatitis – United States, 2007. *MMWR* 2009;58: 1–27.

67. Gordon SC, Reddy KR, Schiff ER. Prolonged intrahepatic cholestasis secondary to acute hepatitis A. *Ann Intern Med* 1984;101:635–7.

68. Sjogren MH, Tanno H, Fay O, et al. Hepatitis A virus in stool during clinical relapse. *Ann Intern Med* 1987;106:221–6.

69. Nanda SK, Yalenkaya K, Panigrahi AK, et al. Etiological role of hepatitis E virus in sporadic fulminant hepatitis. *J med Virol* 1994;42:133–7.

70. Khuroo MS, Teli MR, Skidmore S, et al. Incidence and severity of viral hepatitis in pregnancy. *Am J Med* 1981;70:252–5.

71. Tsega E, Hanson BG, Krawczynski K, et al. Acute sporadic viral hepatitis in Ethiopia: causes, risk factors, and effect on pregnancy. *Clin Infect Dis* 1992;14:961–5.

72. Tsarev SA, Tsareva TS, Emerson SU, et al. Experimental hepatitis E in pregnant rhesus monkeys: failure to transmit hepatitis E to offspring and evidence of naturally acquired antibodies to HEV. *J Infect Dis* 1995;172:31–7.

73. William R. Classification, etiology and considerations of outcome in acute liver failure. *Semin Liver Dis* 1996;16:343–8.

74. Chadha MS, Walimbe AM, Chobe LP, et al. Comparison of etiology of sporadic acute and fulminant viral hepatitis in hospitalized patients in Pune, India during 1978–81 and 1994–97. *Indian J Gastroenterol* 2003;22(1):11–15.

75. Brown GR, Persley K. Hepatitis A epidemic in the elderly. *South Med J* 2002;95:826–33.

76. Willner IR, Mark DU, Howard SC, et al. Serious hepatitis A: an analysis of patients hospitalized during an urban epidemic in the United States. *Ann Intern Med* 1998;128:111–14.

77. Ostapowicz G, Fontana R, Schiedt FV, et al. Results of a prospective study of acute liver failure at 17 tertiary care centers in the United States. *Ann Intern Med* 2002;137:947–54.

78. Schiodt FV, Atillasoy E, Shakill AO, et al. Etiology and outcome for 295 patients with acute liver failure in the United States. *Liver Transpl Surg* 1999;5:29–34.

79. Naik SR, Aggarwal R, Salunke PN, Mehrotra NN. A large water-borne viral hepatitis E epidemic in Kanpur, India. *Bull WHO* 1992;70:597–604.

80. Zhuang H, Cao X-Y, Liu C-B, Wang G-M. Enterically transmitted non-A, non-B hepatitis in China. In: Shikata T, Purcell RH, Uchida T, eds. *Viral Hepatitis C, D, and E.* Amsterdam: Excerpta Medica, 1991:277–85.

81. Okamoto H. Genetic variability and evolution of hepatitis E virus. *Virus Res* 2007;127:216–28.

82. Navaneethan U, Al Mohajer M, Shata MT. Hepatitis E and pregnancy: understanding the pathogenesis. *Liver Int* 2008;28:1190–9.

83. Khuroo MS, Khuroo MS. Hepatitis E virus. *Curr Opin Infect Dis* 2008;21:539–43.

84. Patra S, Kumar A, Trivedi SS, et al. Maternal and fetal outcomes in pregnant women with acute hepatitis E virus infection. *Ann Intern Med* 2007;147:28–33.

85. Stoszek SK, Abdel-Hamid M, Saleh DA, et al. High prevalence of hepatitis E antibodies in pregnant Egyptian women. *Trans R Soc Trop Med Hyg* 2006;100:95–101.

86. Liaw YF, Yang CY, Chu CM, et al. Appearance and persistence of hepatitis A IgM antibody in acute clinical hepatitis A observed in an outbreak. *Infection* 1986;14:156–8.

87. Kao HW, Ashcavai M, Redeker AG. The persistence of hepatitis A IgM antibody after acute clinical hepatitis A. *Hepatology* 1984;4:933–6.

88. Yotsuyanagi H, Iino S, Koike K, et al. Duration of viremia in human hepatitis A viral infection as determined by polymerase chain reaction. *J Med Virol* 1993;40:35–8.

89. Rezende G, Roque-Alsonso M, Samuel D, et al. Viral and clinical factors associated with fulminant course of hepatitis A infection. *Hepatology* 2003;38:613–18.

90. Fujiwara K, Yokosuka O, Imazeki F, et al. Analysis of the genotype-determining region of hepatitis A viral RNA in relation to disease severities. *Hepatol Res* 2003;25:124–34.

91. Dawson GJ, Chau KH, Cabal CM, et al. Solid phase enzyme linked immunosorbent assay for hepatitis E virus IgG and IgM utilizing recombinant antigens and synthetic peptides. *J Virol Methods* 1992;38:175–86.

92. Koshy A, Grover S, Hyams KC. Short term IgM and IgG antibody responses to hepatitis E infection. *Scand J Infect Dis* 1996;28:439–41.

93. Sjogren MH, Siegl G. Advances in hepatitis A and hepatitis E. In: Rizzetto M, Purcell RH, Gerin JL, et al., eds. *Viral Hepatitis and Liver Diseases*, Turin, Italy: Minerva Medica, 1997:903–5.

94. Centers for Disease Control and Prevention (CDC). Advisory Committee on Immunization Practices recommends Tdap vaccine for health care workers. *MMWR* 2006;55(RR07):1–23.

95. Centers for Disease Control and Prevention (CDC). Prevention of hepatitis A after exposure to hepatitis A virus and in international travelers. *MMWR* 2007: 56(41); 1080–4.

96. Victor JC, Monto AS, Surdina TY, et al. Hepatitis A vaccine versus immune globulin for postexposure prophylaxis. *N Engl J Med* 2007;357:1685–94.

97. Leentvaar-Kuijpers A, Coutinho RA, Brulein V, et al. Simultaneous passive and active immunization against hepatitis A. *Vaccine* 1992;10:S138–41.

98. Andre FE, D'Hondt E, Delem A, et al. Clinical assessment of the safety and efficacy of an inactivated hepatitis A vaccine. *Vaccine* 1992;10(Suppl 1):S160–8.

99. Provost PJ, Hughes JN, Miller WJ, et al. An inactivated hepatitis A viral vaccine of cell culture origin. *J Med Virol* 1986;19:23–31.

100. Van Damme P, Thoelen S, Cramm K, et al. Inactivated hepatitis A vaccine: reactogenicity, immunogenicity, and long-term antibody persistence. *J Med Virol* 1994;44:446–51.

101. Centers for Disease Control and Prevention (CDC). FDA approval for a combined hepatitis A and B vaccine. *MMWR* 2001;50(37):806–7.

102. Diaz-Mitoma F, Law B, Subramanya A, Hoet B. Long-term antibody persistence induced by a combined hepatitis A and B vaccine in children and adolescents. *Vaccine* 2008;26(14):1759–63.

103. Northdurft HD, Dietrich M, Zuckerman JN, et al. A new accelerated vaccination schedule for rapid protection against hepatitis A and B. *Vaccine* 2002;20:1157–62.

104. Connor BA, Blatter MM, Beran J, et al. Rapid and sustained immune response against hepatitis A and B achieved with combined vaccine using an accelerated administration schedule. *J Travel Med* 2007;14:9–15.

105. Centers for Disease Control and Prevention (CDC). Prevention and control of infections with hepatitis viruses in correctional settings. *MMWR* 2003;52(RR-01):1–33.

106. Khuroo MS, Dar MY. Hepatitis E: evidence for person-to-person transmission and inability of low dose immune serum globulin from an Indian source to prevent it. *Indian J Gastroenterol* 1992;11:113–16.

107. World Health Organization. *New Vaccines against Infectious Diseases: research and development status.* April 2005 (updated February 2006), www.who.int/vaccine.

108. Purcell RH, Nguyen H, Shapiro M, et al. Pre-clinical immunogenicity and efficacy trial of a recombinant hepatitis E vaccine. *Vaccine* 2003;21:2607–15.

109. Shrestha MP, Scott RM, Joshi DM, et al. Safety and efficacy of a recombinant hepatitis E vaccine. *N Engl J Med* 2007;356:895–903.

110. Zhang J, Liu CB, Li RC, et al. Randomized-controlled phase II clinical trial of a bacterially expressed recombinant hepatitis E vaccine. *Vaccine* 2009;27:1869–74.

111. Zhu F, Zhang J, Zhang X, et al. Efficacy and safety of a recombinant hepatitis E vaccine in healthy adults: a large-scale, randomised, double-blind placebo-controlled, phase 3 trial. *Lancet* 2010;376:895–902.

112. Mallet V, Nicand E, Sultanik P, et al. Brief communication: case reports of ribavirin treatment for chronic hepatitis E. *Ann Intern Med* 2010;153:85–9.

113. Reiss G, Keefe EB. Review article: hepatitis vaccination in patients with chronic liver disease. *Aliment Pharmacol Ther* 2004;19:715–27.

114. Aeslan M, Wiesner RH, Poterucha JJ, et al. Safety and efficacy of hepatitis A vaccination in liver transplantation recipients. *Transplantation* 2001;72:272–6.

115. Myers RP, Gregor JC, Marotta P. The cost-effectiveness of hepatitis A vaccination in patients with chronic hepatitis C. *Hepatology* 2000;31:834–9.

116. Jacobs RJ, Koff, RS. Cost-effectiveness of hepatitis A vaccination in patients with chronic hepatitis C. *Hepatology* 2000;32:873–4.

117. Jacobs RJ, Koff RS, Meyerhoff AS. The cost-effectiveness of vaccinating chronic hepatitis C patients against hepatitis A *Am J Gastroenterol* 2002;97:427–34.

118. Arguedas MR, Heudebert GR, Fallon MB, et al. The cost-effectiveness of hepatitis A vaccination in patients with chronic hepatitis C viral infection in the United States. *Am J Gastroenterol* 2002;97:721–8.

119. Rosenthal P. Cost-effectiveness of hepatitis A vaccination in children, adolescents and adults. *Hepatology* 2003;37:44–51.

Multiple choice questions

23.1 What is the gold standard to diagnose acute hepatitis A?

a A history of recent ingestion of raw oysters.
b Alanine aminotransferase >1,000 U/L.
c Detectable IgM anti-HAV.
d Detectable total anti-HAV (IgG and IgM).

23.2 If after 3 years of receiving full immunization against HAV, the antibody is no longer detectable, which of the following should the patient do?

a Be immunized again.
b Retest for anti-HAV.
c Be told that immunologic memory exists despite absence of anti-HAV.
d Await newer vaccines.

Answers to the multiple choice questions can be found in the Appendix at the end of the book.

These multiple choice questions are also available for you to complete online.
Visit http://www.schiffsdiseasesoftheliver.com/

CHAPTER 24

Hepatitis B and D

Anna S. F. Lok[1] & Francesco Negro[2]

[1]Division of Gastroenterology, University of Michigan Medical Center, Ann Arbor, MI, USA
[2]Departments of Internal Medicine, and of Pathology and Immunology, University of Geneva Medical Center, Geneva, Switzerland

Key concepts

- There are approximately 350 million hepatitis B carriers worldwide and 1 million carriers in the United States. The prevalence of hepatitis B virus (HBV) infection is related to the predominant mode of transmission and the age at infection.
- Acute HBV infection may manifest as subclinical hepatitis, icteric hepatitis, or acute liver failure. Chronic HBV infection may manifest as inactive carrier state, chronic hepatitis, cirrhosis, or hepatocellular carcinoma (HCC).
- HBV vaccination has been shown to prevent HBV infection as well as HBV-related HCC.

- The aims of antiviral treatment of chronic hepatitis B are to suppress HBV replication, induce remission in liver disease, and prevent the development of cirrhosis and HCC.
- Approved treatments of chronic hepatitis B include interferon-α (standard and pegylated), lamivudine, adefovir, entecavir, telbivudine, and tenofovir.
- Hepatitis D virus is dependent on HBV. Hepatitis D occurs as coinfection with HBV or superinfection in persons with chronic HBV infection. Interferon-α is the only effective treatment for chronic hepatitis D.

Hepatitis B

Epidemiology

Hepatitis B infection is a global public health problem. It is estimated there are approximately 350 million hepatitis B virus (HBV) carriers in the world, of whom over 600,000 die annually from hepatitis B-associated liver disease [1]. In the United States, an estimated 0.8–1.4 million individuals are chronically infected with HBV [2].

Prevalence

The prevalence of HBV infection varies in different geographic areas (Table 24.1). The wide range in carrier rate is related to differences in the predominant mode of transmission and the age at infection. In low prevalence areas such as the United States, western Europe, Australia, and New Zealand, the hepatitis B surface antigen (HBsAg) carrier rate is approximately 0.1–2%. In intermediate prevalence areas like the Mediterranean countries, Japan, India, and Singapore, the carrier rate is approximately 3–5%. In high prevalence areas such as Southeast Asia and sub-Saharan Africa, the carrier rate is 8–20%. The prevalence of current and past HBV infection is estimated to be 5% in the United States and more than 50% among adults in Southeast Asia and Africa. In general, there is an increasing prevalence of HBV infection with age. Within the United States, the prevalence of HBV infection is higher among African-Americans, Hispanics, and Asians than in the white population.

In most high prevalence areas such as China, perinatal transmission is the major mode of spread, accounting for 40–50% of chronic HBV infection. However, horizontal spread during the first 2 years of life is the major mode of transmission in other endemic areas including Africa and the Middle East. The exact reason for the preponderance of perinatal transmission among Orientals is not clear but is at least in part related to the high prevalence of hepatitis B e antigen (HBeAg) among Asian carriers of reproductive age – 40–50% versus 10–20% among African carriers of the same age group [3,4]. In intermediate prevalence areas, transmission occurs among all age groups but early childhood infection accounts for most cases of chronic infection. In low prevalence areas, most infections are acquired in early adult life through unprotected sexual intercourse or intravenous drug use. The age at infection has a significant impact on the clinical outcome because chronic infection occurs in approximately 90% of infants infected at birth, in 25–50% of children infected between the age of 1 and 5 years, and in less than 5% of those infected during adult life [5–8].

Schiff's Diseases of the Liver, Eleventh Edition. Edited by Eugene R. Schiff, Willis C. Maddrey and Michael F. Sorrell.

Table 24.1 Patterns of hepatitis B virus infection.

	Prevalence		
	High	**Intermediate**	**Low**
Carrier rate	8–20%	3–7%	0.1–2%
Geographic distribution	Southeast Asia	Mediterranean basin	United States and Canada
	China	Eastern Europe	Western Europe
	Pacific Islands	Central Asia	Australia
	Sub-Saharan Africa	Japan	New Zealand
	Alaska (Eskimos)	Latin and South America	
		Middle East	
Predominant age at infection	Perinatal and early childhood	Early childhood	Adult
Predominant mode of transmission	Maternal–infant	Sexual	Sexual
	Percutaneous	Percutaneous	Percutaneous

Mode of transmission

Transfusion

The exclusion of paid donors and the application of hepatitis B serologic screening in the 1970s dramatically reduced the incidence of post-transfusion HBV infection. In the United States, both HBsAg and hepatitis B core antibody (anti-HBc) are used for blood donor screening. Anti-HBc was initially used as a surrogate marker for non-A, non-B hepatitis virus. Anti-HBc has been retained after the implementation of hepatitis C testing to detect donors who are in the window phase during recovery from acute hepatitis B or who have low level chronic HBV infection. The residual risk of transfusion-related hepatitis B in the United States is approximately 1 in 300,000 [9], while the residual risk of transfusion-related hepatitis B in China, where HBV infection is endemic and blood donors are screened for HBsAg only, is 1 in 17,500 [10].

Recently, there have been debates on the role of nucleic acid testing (NAT) of blood donors. One review concluded that NAT for HBV will probably detect only a few more donor units that may be associated with risk of transmitting HBV infection compared with serologic screening for HBsAg and anti-HBc [11]. With the current estimated 13 million donations per year in the United States and 1.8 transfused components per donation, the introduction of NAT would be expected to prevent 30–35 HBV-containing transfusions per year. NAT has a higher yield and may be more cost-effective in high prevalence areas where additional screening for anti-HBc is not practical.

Percutaneous transmission

Percutaneous inoculation of blood or body fluids plays a major role in the transmission of hepatitis B infection. Needle sharing by intravenous drug users is an impor-

tant route of transmission of hepatitis B. The reuse of contaminated needles for tattoos, acupuncture, and ear piercing also provides opportunities for percutaneous transmission.

Sexual transmission

In the United States and many developed countries, sexual transmission is the most important mode of spread of HBV. The Centers for Disease Control and Prevention reported that sexual transmission accounted for almost 50% of acute HBV infection among individuals in whom data on risk factors were available [12]. A high prevalence of chronic HBV infection has been reported in men who have sex with men as well as in heterosexuals with multiple sex partners. The annual incidence of new HBV infections among homosexual men decreased significantly in the 1980s as a result of education on safe sex practice to prevent human immunodeficiency virus (HIV) infection [13]. However, recent reports in the United States suggest that both heterosexual transmission and transmission among homosexual men are again on the rise [12]. The risk of sexual transmission of HBV infection is associated with the number of lifetime sex partners, low education level, paid sex, and history of sexually transmitted diseases.

Perinatal transmission

Perinatal transmission of HBV infection is rare in countries where universal vaccination of newborns is implemented. The risk of maternal–infant transmission is related to the HBV replicative status of the mother. The risk is 85–90% for infants born to HBeAg-positive mothers and 30% for infants born to HBeAg-negative mothers [14]. More recent studies have demonstrated that maternal serum HBV DNA levels correlate better with the risk of transmission [15]. Maternal–infant transmission takes place at the time of delivery by maternal–fetal transfusion or exposure to maternal blood during passage through the birth canal and postnatally through intimate mother–baby contact. Intrauterine transmission is uncommon. This explains why passive–active immunization at birth has an efficacy rate of more than 90% in the prevention of HBV infection [16]. Cesarean section has not been shown to eliminate the risk of perinatally acquired HBV infection [17] and should not be routinely recommended for carrier mothers. Although HBsAg can be detected in breast milk, there is no evidence that HBV infection can be transmitted by breastfeeding [18]; infants born to carrier mothers may be breastfed if they have been vaccinated. The risk of transmission during amniocentesis is also low [19]. Universal vaccination of all newborns and the additional administration of hepatitis B immunoglobulin (HBIg) to those who are born to carrier mothers were initiated in many Southeast Asian countries in the 1980s. These programs have led to a significant reduction in HBsAg carrier rate as well as a decrease in the incidence of hepatocellular carcinoma (HCC) among children [20]. As of 2008, 92% of the countries in the world have integrated HBV vaccination into their childhood immunization programs.

Health care environment

Hepatitis B virus is the most commonly transmitted blood-borne virus in the health care setting [21]. Transmission generally occurs from patient to patient or from patient to health care personnel via contaminated instruments or accidental needlestick injury. Despite the implementation of universal precautions, outbreaks of HBV infection continue to occur in health care settings even in developed countries. A review of cases of viral hepatitis in the United States from 1998 to 2008 in health care settings outside hospitals revealed 18 outbreaks with 173 persons with new/acute HBV infection. These outbreaks occurred mainly in outpatient clinics or ambulatory hemodialysis centers due to lapses in infection control measures like syringe reuse, contamination of injectable medications or flush solutions, and the reuse of fingerstick devices meant only for single use [22]. Transmission of HBV infection from health care workers to patients is rare. One outbreak was traced to a cardiothoracic surgeon despite no identified flaws in precautions on infection control during surgeries [23]. Nosocomial transmission can be prevented by screening of blood and blood products, use of disposable needles and equipment, proper sterilization of surgical instruments, enforcement of infection control measures, and vaccination of health care workers.

In many developed countries, guidelines have been established to define the parameters within which health care workers with hepatitis B can practice. The Society for Healthcare Epidemiology of America recommended that HBsAg-positive health care providers with serum HBV DNA $>10^4$ genome equivalents/mL should routinely use double-gloving for all instances in which gloving is recommended, and that these providers should not perform activities identified as associated with a risk for provider-to-patient HBV transmission [24]. Similar recommendations were made by a European consortium [25]. It has been proposed that health care workers with high HBV DNA levels receive antiviral therapy to enable them to return to work without risking nosocomial infection. These workers will need to be monitored to insure that serum HBV DNA levels remain suppressed.

Hemodialysis patients

Patients with renal failure on hemodialysis may be infected through blood transfusions, contamination of dialysis machines or equipment, as well as interpersonal horizontal transmission in the dialysis units. Improved infection control and the availability of vaccines have reduced the annual incidence of HBV infection among hemodialysis patients from 3% in 1980 to 0.1% in 1993 in the United States and has remained stable in the past decade [26]. However, dialysis patients have impaired antibody response to vaccines. Therefore, vigilance is still needed to prevent outbreaks.

In a recent survey of all US chronic hemodialysis centers [26], the percent of patients vaccinated against HBV infection increased from 47% to 56% and the percent of staff vaccinated increased from 87% to 90% between 1997 and 2002. A possible contributing factor for continued transmission of HBV infection in adult hemodialysis units appears to be the presence of occult HBV infection (serum HBsAg-negative but HBV DNA-positive). In a study of 241 adult hemodialysis patients in a North American urban center [27], only two patients (0.8%) were HBsAg-positive but nine (4%) HBsAg-negative patients were HBV DNA-positive. Another study of 585 Italian dialysis patients found that 1.9% were HBsAg-positive and 36% anti-HBc-positive, none of the anti-HBc-positive patients had detectable serum HBV DNA [28].

Transplantation

Organ donors are routinely screened for HBsAg. Transmission of HBV infection has been reported after transplantation of extrahepatic organs such as kidneys from HBsAg-positive donors. This may be related to residual blood in the vascular pedicles due to inadequate flushing. The transmission of HBV infection has also been reported after transplantation of avascular tissues such as corneas [29] but this is believed to be rare.

The role of anti-HBc testing in organ donor screening is uncertain because of the possibility of false-positive results, the potential loss of up to 5% of donors even in low endemic areas [30], and the uncertainty about the infectivity of organs from donors who are HBsAg-negative, anti-HBc positive [31]. The incidence of HBV infection from donors with isolated anti-HBc is very low (0–2%) in heart and kidney recipients but varies from 0% to 78% in liver recipients [30,32–34]. A recent study found that the estimated probability of undetected hepatitis B viremia is higher among tissue donors compared with first-time blood donors and the addition of NAT to the screening of tissue donors is expected to reduce the risk of HBV infection [35].

Other transmission routes

In endemic areas, horizontal transmission among children may result from close bodily contact leading to the transfer of virus across minor skin breaks and mucous membranes. Blood-feeding insects like mosquitoes have been demonstrated to serve as vectors for HBV transmission in animal models but firm evidence for this mode of transmission in humans is lacking. Various body secretions have been reported to test positive for HBsAg but only semen and saliva have been consistently shown to harbor infectious virions. Although HBV DNA has been detected in the saliva of some hepatitis B carriers, there is no convincing evidence that hepatitis B can be transmitted orally [36,37]. As HBV survives for a long time outside the human body, transmission via contaminated environmental surfaces and daily articles such as toothbrushes, razors, eating utensils, or even toys may also be possible.

High-risk groups

Health care workers have a higher hepatitis B carrier rate than the general population. The prevalence is particularly high among surgeons, pathologists, and physicians working in hemodialysis and oncology units. Apparent skin breaks, minor cuts, and accidental needlestick injuries serve as portals of entry. Other health care workers having increased risk of HBV infection include dentists and laboratory personnel who have contact with serum. Institutionalized mentally handicapped persons as well as their attendants and family members also have a high rate of hepatitis B infection. Despite screening of blood products, patients requiring frequent transfusion of blood or blood products have an increased risk of contracting hepatitis B infection. Other high-risk groups include intravenous drug users, particularly those who share syringes, men who have sex with men and promiscuous heterosexuals, immigrants from HBV endemic countries, and spouses, sexual partners, and household members of HBV carriers.

Changing epidemiology

The worldwide incidence of HBV infection is decreasing [1]. Mass vaccination of newborns and catch-up vaccination of children and adolescents have played a major role in reducing HBV infection among infants and children. Increased public awareness of hepatitis, educational campaigns to prevent HIV infection leading to modification of high-risk sexual behavior, and reduction of syringe sharing among intravenous drug users have contributed to the decrease in HBV infection among adults.

In the United States, the incidence of acute hepatitis B has significantly declined over the past decade. According to the Centers for Disease Control and Prevention, there has been an 82% decline in the incidence of acute hepatitis B between 1990 and 2007 [38]; the most significant decline was seen among children aged <15 years. Sexual transmission among susceptible individuals remains a significant risk factor for hepatitis B transmission in the United States. This is in part related to lack of resources and infrastructure for vaccination of adults as well as missed opportunities. Another important aspect of HBV epidemiology is that in many developed countries, immigrants from countries that are endemic for HBV infection now constitute an increasing proportion of those with chronic HBV infection [39]. These studies suggest that screening and immunization of susceptible adults, along with immunization of children (especially if they were born in countries where universal vaccination is not in place) whose parents immigrated from HBV endemic countries, is important in controlling HBV infection in developed countries.

Vaccination against hepatitis B

Indications

Vaccination against hepatitis B remains the mainstay of prevention. Universal vaccination of all newborns or at least newborns of all HBV-infected mothers is currently practiced in most countries throughout the world. The World Health Organization (WHO) has recommended that a combination of hepatitis B and childhood vaccines be used where possible, to reduce the logistic costs of vaccine delivery, especially in areas where it is most needed. In some developed countries, where universal vaccination of all newborns is not in place, vaccination of adolescents to prevent sexual transmission is implemented. The vaccination of adults is recommended for high-risk groups including health care workers, men who have sex with men, persons with multiple sex partners, injection drug users, sex partners, and household members of HBV carriers, public safety workers, institutionalized patients, and patients on chronic hemodialysis (Box 24.1) [39,40].

Administration schedule

There are two types of hepatitis B vaccines, plasma-derived and recombinant; the latter is currently used in most countries. Recombinant HBV vaccines consist of

Box 24.1 Indications for hepatitis B vaccine.

- All newborns[a]
- All children and adolescents not vaccinated at birth
- High-risk adults:
    Men who have sex with men
    Persons with multiple sexual partners
    Injection drug users
    Patients on hemodialysis
    Institutionalized patients
    Health care workers and public safety workers
    Spouse, sexual partners, and household members of hepatitis B
      virus carriers

[a]For infants born to carrier mothers, hepatitis B immune globulin (HBIg) is also administered at birth.

HBV small S protein (HBsAg) produced by yeast or mammalian cells. Hepatitis B vaccine has been successfully combined with hepatitis A vaccine and with diphtheria, tetanus, and acellular pertussis and inactivated poliovirus vaccine without reducing its efficacy. These combination vaccines facilitate the integration of HBV vaccination into routine childhood immunization, reducing the number of injections and increasing the rate of compliance. Hepatitis B vaccine is usually administered intramuscularly in three doses at 0, 1, and 6 months, the dose being 10–20 μg in adults and 5–10 μg in children (Table 24.2). For adults, the injections are given in the deltoid muscle, whereas in newborns and young children the recommended site is the anterolateral thigh. In patients with hemophilia, it is recommended to administer the vaccine subcutaneously.

For infants born to HBsAg-negative mothers and unvaccinated children/adolescents up to 19 years of age, three doses (at 0, 1, and 6 months) of vaccine at half strength should be administered. For adults 20 years and older, the same regimen is implemented using full doses

Table 24.2 Hepatitis B vaccines and dosage recommendations.

Vaccine brand[a]	Age group (years)	Dose (μg)	Volume (mL)	Number of doses
Engerix-B	0–19	10	0.5	3
	≥20	20	1.0	3
Recombivax HB	0–19	5	0.5	3
	≥20	10	1.0	3
(Optional two doses)	11–15	10	1.0	2

[a]For hemodialysis patients, the recommended dose is 40 μg with each dose (Engerix-B 40 μg/2.0 mL and Recombivax HB dialysis formulation 40 μg/1.0 mL).

(10 μg of Recombivax HB® or 20 μg of Engerix-B®). An alternative two-dose schedule had been approved for adolescents.

For newborns of HBsAg carrier mothers, HBIg 0.5 mL and the first dose of vaccine should be administered within 12 hours of birth, using different sites. A combination of HBIg and hepatitis B vaccine has been shown to be 95% efficacious in preventing perinatal transmission of HBV infection [16,41,42].

For patients on hemodialysis or immunocompromised patients, higher doses of vaccine are needed: 40 μg of Recombivax HB or Engerix-B. Hepatitis B surface antibody (anti-HBs) titers should be monitored annually, and booster doses administered when the anti-HBs titer falls below 10 IU/L.

Follow-up testing for protective antibodies is recommended for individuals who continue to be at risk, including infants born to HBsAg-positive mothers, health care workers, hemodialysis patients, and sexual partners of HBsAg carriers. Some vaccines have also incorporated pre-S1 (large S) and/or pre-S2 (middle S) proteins to increase the immunogenicity but these vaccines are not available in most countries.

Efficacy

A protective response – defined as an anti-HBs titer of more than 10 IU/L – is achieved in approximately 95% of vaccine recipients. Several studies have shown that vaccination is effective in inducing protective immunity and in preventing HBV infection in men who have sex with men [43–45], and in newborns of carrier mothers [16,41,46]. In countries where the prevalence of HBeAg among carrier mothers is low, it has been shown that vaccine alone has similar efficacy as a combination of vaccine and HBIg in preventing perinatal infection [46]. Although this approach can be cost saving, it may not be adequate in countries where the prevalence of HBeAg among carrier mothers is high or in countries where a high percent of HBeAg-negative mothers have high serum HBV DNA levels.

Factors associated with nonresponse and the management of vaccine nonresponders

Approximately 2.5–10% of vaccine recipients fail to respond with adequate anti-HBs titers after one course of HBV vaccine. The reasons for nonresponse are several and include older age, obesity, chronic medical illnesses (such as renal failure, diabetes, and cirrhosis), immunosuppression (such as in patients with HIV infection or organ transplantation), and technical problems (such as intragluteal injection and inadvertent freezing of the vaccines). Nonresponse to HBV vaccine has been reported to be associated with impaired lymphocyte activation as well as genetic factors, including certain human leukocyte antigen (HLA) class II genes such as HLA-DRB1*0301 and cytokine gene polymorphisms [47,48].

For individuals who fail to respond after a full course of vaccination, the recommendation is to repeat another course of vaccine. If a person still remains a nonresponder, further vaccination is usually not effective but most of these individuals can mount an adequate immune response upon infection because exposure to HBV stimulates both T- and B-cell responses to HBsAg as well as hepatitis B core antigen (HBcAg). Nonresponders to two courses of vaccine should be tested for HBsAg as some may be undiagnosed carriers.

Durability of vaccine response and need for boosters

Several studies have shown that 30–66% of individuals had protective levels of anti-HBs ($\geq$10 IU/L) for 15 years or more after receiving HBV vaccines and 90% had an anamnestic response after booster vaccination [49–52]. Breakthrough infections are rare and appear to occur mostly among those who did not have an initial response to vaccination. A recent study suggested that anamnestic responses may wane over time. In this study, 105 young adults vaccinated at birth with no detectable anti-HBs were revaccinated and only 48% had an anamnestic response [53]. The need for booster vaccinations among young adults who were vaccinated at birth is controversial.

Impact of vaccination

Hepatitis B virus vaccination has been shown to reduce the incidence of acute HBV infection and HCC, and the prevalence of chronic HBV infection [20,54–56]. HBV vaccine is the first vaccine that has been shown to prevent cancer (HCC) in humans. After the implementation of a nationwide vaccination program for newborns and children in 1984, the carrier rate among children in Taiwan decreased from 10% to 1.2% and the incidence of childhood HCC decreased by 70% [20]. In the United States, universal vaccination of all newborns was implemented in 1991 and it was expanded to include vaccination of all adolescents aged 11–12 years in 1995, and children aged less than 18 years, who had not been vaccinated previously, in 1999. This has resulted in a 90% reduction of acute hepatitis B in children and adolescents.

Safety of vaccines

The safety of HBV vaccines has been well established. The most common adverse reaction is soreness over the injection site. Other adverse reactions include low-grade fever, malaise, headache, arthralgia, and myalgia. Hepatitis B vaccines have no teratogenic effects and can be administered during pregnancy [57,58].

There has been concern about the possibility of hepatitis B vaccine leading to the development of demyelinating central nervous system diseases including multiple sclerosis and Guillain–Barré syndrome. However, many studies have failed to show a statistically significant temporal or causal association between HBV vaccine and these neurologic or immunologic conditions [59–62]. Because of concerns about mercury exposures, current preparations of HBV vaccines do not contain thimerosal as a preservative.

Special settings

Individuals with isolated hepatitis B core antibody

The presence of an isolated anti-HBc does not always denote prior exposure to HBV infection. HBV vaccination has been recommended to differentiate those who have had prior exposure from those with false-positive anti-HBc test results [63]. With improved specificity of anti-HBc assays, most individuals with isolated anti-HBc have genuinely positive test results and do not need to be vaccinated but there is no harm if vaccine is administered.

Patients on chronic hemodialysis

All patients on chronic hemodialysis should be vaccinated. Because response to HBV vaccine is impaired in patients with renal failure and dialysis patients have an increased risk of HBV infection, anti-HBs titer should be monitored annually and a booster vaccination administered if the anti-HBs titer decreases to <10 IU/L.

Patients with chronic liver disease

Hepatitis B vaccination, along with vaccination against hepatitis A, is recommended for all patients with underlying chronic liver disease. Acute hepatitis B superimposed on chronic hepatitis C has been reported to be associated with increased risk of liver failure [64]. The immune response to HBV vaccines among patients with chronic liver disease is similar to healthy subjects with no liver disease, but response rates are decreased in patients with cirrhosis and may be <50% in patients with decompensated cirrhosis awaiting liver transplantation [65,66]. Therefore, it is recommended that HBV vaccination should be administered early, before a patient develops cirrhosis.

Patients with human immunodeficiency virus infection

Several reports have suggested that patients with HIV infection have a blunted response to HBV vaccine compared to HIV-negative individuals. A large, randomized, double-blind study of two doses of recombinant HBV vaccine [67] showed that a response was seen in 34% and 47% in the standard and double dose groups, respectively.

Response rates were higher in those with a high CD4 count and low HIV RNA level. Anti-HBs titers should be checked 1 month after completion of the vaccine series to document response. Revaccination can be considered in those with no immune response. Among responders, anti-HBs titers drop more rapidly than in immunocompetent persons and breakthrough infections have been reported when anti-HBs titers decrease to <10 IU/L.

Novel methods of vaccine administration

In an effort to reduce the number of injections and to increase compliance, several combination vaccines have been developed. They include combinations of hepatitis A and B vaccine for adults and children, and a hexavalent vaccine against diphtheria, pertussis, tetanus, polio, *Haemophilus*, and hepatitis B for children. These combined vaccines have been shown to be safe and to have similar immunogenicity as the monovalent vaccines [68,69].

Various strategies have been examined to improve immunogenicity of HBV vaccines. One approach is to use more potent adjuvants [70,71]; another is to activate mucosal T cells through nasal vaccination [72]. Other approaches include intradermal administration, coadministration with interleukin 2, and incorporation of pre-S1 and/or pre-S2 antigens [73–75].

Diagnosis

The diagnosis of hepatitis B was revolutionized by the discovery of Australia antigen, now called HBsAg, by Blumberg in 1965 (76). During the ensuing decade, serologic assays for HBsAg and anti-HBs with increasing sensitivity and specificity were developed. In the 1970s, additional HBV antigens and antibodies were identified and serologic assays for their detection established. Advances in molecular biology techniques led to the development of assays for the direct determination of virus replication, and polymerase chain reaction (PCR) assays currently in use can detect as little as 10 IU of HBV DNA per mL of serum. The diagnosis of HBV infection can also be made by the detection of HBsAg or HBcAg in liver tissues by immunohistochemical staining and of HBV DNA by Southern hybridization, in situ hybridization, or PCR.

Serologic diagnosis

Hepatitis B surface antigen and hepatitis B surface antibody

Hepatitis B surface antigen is the serologic hallmark of HBV infection. HBsAg appears in serum 1–10 weeks after an acute exposure to HBV, approximately 2–6 weeks before the onset of hepatitis symptoms or elevation of alanine aminotransferase (ALT). In patients who subsequently recover, HBsAg usually becomes undetectable

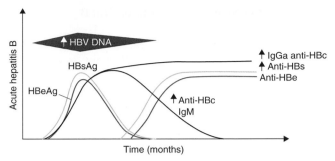

Figure 24.1 Serologic markers during acute hepatitis B virus infection. anti-HBc, hepatitis B core antibody; anti-HBe, hepatitis B e antibody; anti-HBs, hepatitis B surface antibody; HBeAg, hepatitis B e antigen; HBsAg, hepatitis B surface antigen; HBV, hepatitis B virus; IgG, immunoglobulin G; IgM, immunoglobulin M.

after 4–6 months. Persistence of HBsAg for more than 6 months implies chronic infection. The disappearance of HBsAg is followed by the appearance of anti-HBs. Although anti-HBs is produced early in the course of acute infection in individuals who subsequently recover, it is frequently not detectable until after a window period of several weeks to months when neither HBsAg nor anti-HBs can be detected (Fig. 24.1). The appearance of anti-HBs marks the recovery from hepatitis B. In most patients, the presence of anti-HBs persists for life, thereby conferring long-term immunity. Anti-HBs is the only protective antibody induced by most of the currently available vaccines, which consist of recombinant HBsAg only.

HBV can be classified into nine genotypes [77,78] and four major serotypes. All HBV serotypes share one common antigenic determinant, "a," which is a conformational epitope located in the HBsAg. There are two additional pairs of mutually exclusive subtypic determinants "d" or "y" and "w" or "r" constituting the four major serotypes: adr, ayr, adw, and ayw. Antibodies to the "a" determinant confer protection to all HBV serotypes [79]. At least 50% of the anti-HBs that develops after recovery from acute hepatitis B or immunization with hepatitis B vaccines is directed against the "a" determinant, providing cross-protection against other serotypes of HBV.

Coexistence of HBsAg and anti-HBs has been reported in approximately 24% of HBsAg-positive individuals [80]. In most instances, the antibodies are directed against one of the subtypic determinants and not the common "a" determinant and are unable to neutralize the circulating virions. These individuals should therefore be regarded as carriers.

Pre-S1 and pre-S2 antigens have been detected in patients infected with HBV. In general, the presence of these antigens correlates with the detection of HBV DNA and virus replication [81]. During recovery from acute hepatitis B, antibodies to pre-S1 and pre-S2 antigens appear early [82], prior to the detection of anti-HBs.

Hepatitis B core antigen and hepatitis B core antibody

Hepatitis B core antigen is an intracellular antigen that is expressed in infected hepatocytes. It is not detectable in serum. Its antibody – anti-HBc – however, can be detected throughout the course of HBV infection. During acute HBV infection, anti-HBc is predominantly immunoglobulin M (IgM) class. IgM anti-HBc is the first antibody to be detected (Fig. 24.1). It usually appears within 1 month after the appearance of HBsAg. It is the sole marker of HBV infection during the window period, that is, the time gap between the disappearance of HBsAg and the appearance of anti-HBs [83]. During convalescence, the titer of IgM anti-HBc declines while the titer of IgG anti-HBc increases. Therefore, the detection of IgM anti-HBc is usually taken as an indication of acute HBV infection. However, in 20% of patients, IgM anti-HBc may remain detectable up to 2 years after the acute infection. In addition, low-titer IgM anti-HBc persists in most patients with chronic HBV infection. Therefore, the reliability of IgM anti-HBc in the differentiation of acute from chronic HBV infection depends on the cutoff level in the assay. Even in assays with high cutoff values, IgM anti-HBc can be detected in patients with chronic HBV infection during exacerbations [84]. This may lead to misdiagnosis of acute hepatitis B in patients who are not previously known to have had chronic HBV infection. Studies in endemic areas demonstrated that many patients presenting with acute hepatitis who test positive for HBsAg have exacerbations of chronic hepatitis B and not acute hepatitis B, and that less than 1% of immunocompetent adult patients with genuine acute hepatitis B progress to chronic infection [8,85].

IgM anti-HBc titers have been reported to correlate with ALT and serum HBV DNA levels in patients with chronic hepatitis B, especially during exacerbations [86]. IgG anti-HBc persists along with anti-HBs in patients who recover from acute hepatitis B and in association with HBsAg in those who progress to chronic HBV infection.

An isolated presence of anti-HBc in the absence of HBsAg and anti-HBs has been reported in 0.4–1.7% of blood donors in low prevalence areas [87,88] and in 10–20% of the population in endemic countries [63,89]. An isolated detection of anti-HBc may occur during the window period of acute hepatitis B when the anti-HBc is predominantly IgM class, many years after recovery from acute hepatitis B when anti-HBs has fallen to undetectable levels, or after many years of chronic HBV infection when the HBsAg titer has decreased below the level for detection. The clinical significance of isolated anti-HBc is complex. Although HBV DNA has been detected in the serum of individuals with isolated anti-HBc, the frequency of detection varies from 0% to 20% [90,91]. Transmission of HBV infection has been reported from blood

and organ donors with isolated anti-HBc but the incidence ranged from 0.4% to 78% [33,90,92], the risk being highest when livers from anti-HBc-positive donors are transplanted into seronegative recipients. Several studies found that 50–70% of asymptomatic individuals with isolated anti-HBc had false-positive test results [63,93]; the false-positive rate has decreased with improved anti-HBc assays. The evaluation of individuals with isolated anti-HBc should include repeat testing for anti-HBc, HBsAg, anti-HBs, and hepatitis B e antibody (anti-HBe). Individuals with evidence of chronic liver disease and those with HIV infection should be tested for HBV DNA to exclude low-level chronic HBV infection.

Hepatitis B e antigen and hepatitis B e antibody

Hepatitis B e antigen is a secretory protein that is processed from the precore protein. It is generally considered to be a marker of HBV replication and infectivity. Its presence is usually associated with high levels of HBV DNA in serum. Epidemiologic studies reported significantly higher rates of transmission of HBV infection from HBeAg-positive carrier mothers to their babies [94,95] and from HBeAg-positive patients to health care workers who sustain needlestick injuries [96].

During acute HBV infection, HBeAg appears shortly after the appearance of HBsAg. In patients who recover, HBeAg to anti-HBe seroconversion precedes that of HBsAg to anti-HBs seroconversion (see Fig. 24.1). Anti-HBe may persist for many years after the resolution of acute hepatitis B. In patients with chronic HBV infection, HBeAg may persist for years to decades (Fig. 24.2). During the HBeAg-positive phase, most patients have high levels of HBV DNA in serum and active liver disease. In patients with perinatally acquired HBV infection, there may be an immune tolerant phase with normal ALT levels and minimal inflammation in the liver. Seroconversion from HBeAg to anti-HBe is usually associated with a marked decrease in serum HBV DNA level and remission of liver disease. However, some

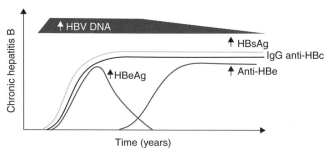

Figure 24.2 Serologic markers during chronic hepatitis B virus infection. anti-HBc, hepatitis B core antibody; anti-HBe, hepatitis B e antibody; HBeAg, hepatitis B e antigen; HBsAg, hepatitis B surface antigen; HBV, hepatitis B virus.

Table 24.3 Diagnosis of hepatitis B virus (HBV) infection.

	HBsAg	HBeAg	IgM anti-HBc	IgG anti-HBc	Anti-HBs	Anti-HBe	HBV DNA	Interpretation
Acute	+	+	+	−	−	−	+++	Early phase
HBV	−	−	+	−	−	+	+	Window phase
infection	−	−	−	+	+	+	±	Recovery phase
Chronic	+	+	−	+	−	−	+++	HBeAg+ chronic hepatitis
HBV	+	−	−	+	−	+	±	Inactive carrier state
infection	+	−	−	+	−	+	++	HBeAg- chronic hepatitis

anti-HBc, hepatitis B core antibody; anti-HBe, hepatitis B e antibody; anti-HBs, hepatitis B surface antibody; HBeAg, hepatitis B e antigen; HBsAg, hepatitis B surface antigen; IgG, immunoglobulin G; IgM, immunoglobulin M.

anti-HBe-positive patients continue to have active liver disease and detectable HBV DNA in serum. This may be due to low levels of wild-type HBV or the presence of precore HBV variants.

Tests for hepatitis B virus DNA in serum

Quantification of HBV DNA in serum is important in determining the phase of chronic HBV infection, in predicting risks of clinical outcomes, and in monitoring response to treatment. Currently, most diagnostic laboratories use real-time PCR assays that have a lower limit of detection of 10–50 IU/mL and a range of linearity up to 8–9 $\log_{10}$ IU/mL. It should be noted that fluctuating HBV DNA levels are common in patients with chronic HBV infection; therefore, the HBV DNA level on a single occasion may not be accurate in assessing HBV replicative status and the need for antiviral therapy. With PCR assays, HBV DNA can be detected up to 2–3 weeks before the appearance of HBsAg in patients with acute HBV infection. Recovery from acute hepatitis B is accompanied by a rapid decrease in serum HBV DNA level but HBV DNA may remain detectable for many years [97].

In patients with chronic HBV infection, spontaneous or treatment-induced HBeAg seroconversion is usually accompanied by a marked decrease in serum HBV DNA level but HBV DNA frequently remains detectable except in patients who have lost HBsAg. The major role of serum HBV DNA assays in patients with chronic HBV infection is to assess HBV replication and candidacy for antiviral therapy and to monitor response to antiviral treatment.

Rarely, tests for HBV DNA in serum help to identify HBV as the etiology of liver disease in HBsAg-negative patients. This is especially important in patients with acute liver failure, who may have cleared HBsAg by the time they present [98]. Most patients with chronic liver disease due to occult HBV infection have low levels of HBV, whereas a small percent may be infected with HBV variants that downregulate the production of HBsAg or produce aberrant HBsAg that cannot be detected in conventional serologic assays [99].

Diagnostic algorithm

The diagnosis of acute hepatitis B is based on the detection of HBsAg and IgM anti-HBc (Table 24.3). During the initial phase of infection, markers of HBV replication, HBeAg and HBV DNA, are present. Recovery is accompanied by the disappearance of HBV DNA, HBeAg to anti-HBe seroconversion, and subsequently HBsAg to anti-HBs seroconversion. Rarely, patients may have entered the window period at the time of presentation and IgM anti-HBc is the sole marker of acute HBV infection in these patients. This situation is more common in patients with acute liver failure where virus clearance tends to be more rapid.

Past HBV infection is diagnosed by the detection of anti-HBs and anti-HBc (IgG). Immunity to HBV infection after vaccination is indicated by the presence of anti-HBs only.

The diagnosis of chronic HBV infection is based on the detection of HBsAg and IgG anti-HBc (Table 24.3). Additional tests for HBV replication, HBeAg and serum HBV DNA, should be performed to determine if the patient should be considered for antiviral therapy. Tests for hepatitis C and hepatitis D should also be performed to rule out superinfection with other hepatitis virus(es).

Clinical manifestations

The spectrum of HBV infection varies from subclinical hepatitis, anicteric hepatitis, and icteric hepatitis to acute liver failure during the acute phase; and from inactive carrier state to chronic hepatitis, cirrhosis, and HCC during the chronic phase. The clinical manifestations and outcome of HBV infection depend on the age at infection, the level of HBV replication, and the immune status of the host. Perinatal or childhood infection is usually associated with few or no symptoms but a high risk of chronicity, whereas adult-acquired infection is usually associated with symptomatic hepatitis but a low risk of chronicity.

Acute hepatitis B virus infection

Approximately 70% of patients have subclinical or anicteric hepatitis during acute HBV infection; only 30% have icteric hepatitis. Symptomatic hepatitis is rare in neonates and it occurs in approximately 10% of children less than 4 years old and in approximately 30% of adults.

Symptoms and signs

The incubation period of acute HBV infection lasts 1–4 months. This period may be shorter in patients who have been exposed to a large inoculum. During the prodromal period, a serum sickness-like syndrome may develop. This is followed by an insidious onset of constitutional symptoms including malaise, anorexia, nausea, and occasionally vomiting, low-grade fever, myalgia, and easy fatigability. Patients may have altered gustatory acuity and smell sensation. Some patients may experience right upper quadrant or midepigastric pain. In patients with icteric hepatitis, jaundice usually begins within 10 days after the onset of constitutional symptoms. Constitutional symptoms generally subside as jaundice develops. Clinical symptoms and jaundice usually disappear after 1–3 months but some patients may have persistent fatigue even after the ALT levels have returned to normal.

Physical examination can be unrevealing in many patients. The most common findings include low-grade fever, clinical icterus, and soft, mildly tender hepatomegaly. Splenomegaly may be found in approximately 5–15% of patients. Rarely, palmar erythema or spider nevi can be detected. Patients with acute liver failure may present with features of hepatic encephalopathy, progressive decrease in liver span, and ascites.

Laboratory findings

The elevation of liver enzymes – ALT and aspartate aminotransferase (AST) – is the hallmark of acute hepatitis. Values of 1,000–2,000 IU/L are typically seen during the acute phase. An increase in liver enzymes may precede the onset of symptoms. In patients with icteric hepatitis, the increase in bilirubin levels usually lags behind the increase in ALT levels. Although the peak ALT level reflects the degree of hepatocellular injury, it has no correlation with prognosis. Prothrombin time is the best indicator of prognosis in patients with acute hepatitis. In patients who recover, ALT levels usually return to normal values after 1–4 months, followed by normalization in bilirubin levels. An elevation of ALT levels for more

than 6 months suggests chronic liver injury and persistent infection.

Histologic findings

Liver biopsy is seldom indicated in acute hepatitis. Histologic changes of acute hepatitis include lobular disarray, acidophilic degeneration of hepatocytes, focal lobular necrosis, disruption of bile canaliculi with cholestasis, portal and parenchymal infiltration of inflammatory cells, as well as hypertrophy and hyperplasia of Kupffer cells and macrophages. Inflammatory infiltrates are predominantly lymphocytes and macrophages. In patients with severe hepatitis, hepatocyte necrosis is more extensive leading to bridging.

Sequelae

The risk of chronicity is inversely proportional to the age at infection. Less than 5% of immunocompetent adults with acute HBV infection progress to chronic infection, but up to 90% of those infected during infancy will develop chronic infection [5–8]. Acute liver failure due to HBV has declined in the last decade but HBV remains the most common viral cause of acute liver failure [100]. It is estimated that only 0.1–0.5% of acute hepatitis B runs a fulminant course. Mortality from acute liver failure is high, approaching 80%, unless liver transplantation can be performed. Contrary to transplantation for HBV cirrhosis, reinfection after liver transplantation for acute liver failure is uncommon.

Chronic hepatitis B virus infection

Symptoms and signs

In areas of low or intermediate prevalence, approximately 30–50% of patients with chronic HBV infection have a history of classic acute hepatitis that progressed to chronic infection. The remaining 50–70% of patients with chronic HBV infection in these areas and most of those in high prevalence areas (predominantly perinatal infection) have no prior history of acute hepatitis. Many patients with chronic HBV infection are asymptomatic, while others have nonspecific symptoms such as fatigue. Occasionally mild, right upper quadrant pain may be present. Patients with chronic HBV infection may experience exacerbations that may be asymptomatic or mimic acute hepatitis with fatigue and jaundice and in rare instances hepatic decompensation.

Physical examination may be unrevealing or there may be stigmata of chronic liver disease such as spider angioma and palmar erythema, and a mild hepatomegaly. In patients with cirrhosis, additional findings such as splenomegaly may be present. As the liver disease advances, hepatic decompensation may develop manifesting as variceal bleeding, ascites, peripheral edema, jaundice, and hepatic encephalopathy.

Laboratory findings

Laboratory tests can be entirely normal even in patients with cirrhosis. Mild to moderate AST and ALT elevation may be the only biochemical abnormality in many patients with chronic hepatitis B. ALT levels may range from normal to five-fold elevated. Very high ALT levels, more than 1,000 IU/L, may be seen during exacerbations. Markers of impaired hepatic synthetic function may be observed during the exacerbations, especially in patients with underlying cirrhosis. In addition, an increase in α-fetoprotein (AFP) levels, up to 1,000 ng/mL, may be present [101]. In these cases, the AFP levels tend to parallel or follow the ALT levels. Progression to cirrhosis is suspected when the platelet count is decreased, when there is hypoalbuminemia, hyperbilirubinemia, prolongation in prothrombin time, and when the AST : ALT ratio is greater than 1. It has been suggested that the upper limit of normal for ALT in most diagnostic laboratories is too high and the true normal is closer to 20–30 IU/L [102,103].

Histologic findings

Liver biopsy is useful in assessing the severity of liver damage, in predicting prognosis, and in monitoring response to treatment. However, liver histology can improve significantly in patients who have a sustained response to antiviral therapy or spontaneous HBeAg seroconversion and it can worsen rapidly during exacerbations of hepatitis B.

The predominant histologic findings include inflammatory cell infiltration in the portal tracts and periportal necrosis. The inflammatory infiltrate consists mainly of mononuclear cells. Periportal necrosis may be mild or severe leading to disruption of the limiting plate (piecemeal necrosis or interface hepatitis). As the liver damage progresses, fibrous tissue is deposited initially within the portal tracts, later extending into the centrilobular (zone 3) areas and adjacent portal tracts, forming bridging fibrosis and eventually cirrhosis. In some patients, ground glass hepatocytes that stain positive for HBsAg can be found. Recent studies showed that these cells are found in association with the retention of HBsAg [104]. To provide a more objective assessment of liver injury, several numeric scoring systems have been established to permit statistical comparisons of necroinflammatory activity and fibrosis [105–107]. An international panel recommended that the histologic diagnosis should include the etiology of hepatitis, the grade of necroinflammatory activity, and the stage (extent of fibrosis) of the liver disease [108].

Immunohistochemical staining reveals the presence of HBsAg in patients with chronic HBV infection. The distribution of HBsAg can be either membranous or cytoplasmic. In patients with high levels of HBV replication, HBcAg can also be demonstrated. The distribution of HBcAg is usually nuclear but the distribution is shifted to the cytoplasm in patients with exacerbations or active liver disease [109].

Extrahepatic manifestations

Extrahepatic manifestations have been reported in patients with both acute and chronic HBV infection. Extrahepatic manifestations are more commonly associated with acute hepatitis B than other forms of acute viral hepatitis and may be present in approximately 10–20% of patients with chronic HBV infection. They are believed to be mediated by circulating immune complexes, the formation of which is favored by high levels of HBV replication.

Serum sickness

Acute hepatitis B is sometimes heralded by a serum sickness-like syndrome manifested as fever, skin rash, polyarthralgia, and arthritis. Skin and joint manifestations usually subside rapidly with the onset of jaundice.

Polyarteritis nodosa

Approximately 10–50% of patients with polyarteritis nodosa (PAN) are found to be HBsAg-positive. The decline in HBV infection over the past decade, especially in developed countries, has also been associated with a decrease in frequency of HBV-related PAN [110]. Immune complexes involving HBV antigens and antibodies are believed to trigger the vascular injury. Vasculitis may affect large, medium, and small-sized vessels in multiple organs, including cardiovascular (pericarditis, hypertension, cardiac failure), renal (hematuria, proteinuria), gastrointestinal (abdominal pain, mesenteric vasculitis), musculoskeletal (arthralgia, arthritis), neurologic (mononeuritis, central nervous system involvement), and dermatologic (rashes) systems. A review of 348 patients with PAN seen over a 42-year period found that 35% were HBV related [111]. The fact that HBV-related PAN is related to virus-mediated immune complexes suggests that therapy should be directed against HBV itself. Case reports and case series have suggested a possible role of interferon (IFN) therapy as well as nucleos(t)ide analogs (NUCs) alone or in combination with plasma exchange [112–115]. One study found that HBeAg seroconversion was associated with the complete remission of PAN [115].

Glomerulonephritis

Hepatitis B virus-related glomerulonephritis is more often found in children and the incidence has been declining since the implementation of HBV vaccination programs. Membranous glomerulonephritis is most common, especially among children, but membranopro-liferative glomerulonephritis, mesangiocapillary and focal glomerulonephritis, minimal change disease, and IgA nephropathy have also been reported [116]. Immune complexes of hepatitis B surface, core, and e antigens and antibodies together with complement components have been demonstrated in glomerular basement membrane and mesangium [117]. The severity of the renal disease does not correlate with the severity of the liver disease.

Approximately 30–60% of children with HBV-related membranous glomerulonephritis undergo spontaneous remission. A substantial proportion of adults (30%) may progress to renal failure. IFN has been reported to induce remission of HBV-related renal disease in small clinical trials, especially among patients with membranous glomerulonephritis [118,119]. An improvement of renal disease has also been reported with lamivudine [120]. A meta-analysis found that HBeAg clearance was associated with remission of nephrotic syndrome [121].

Essential mixed cryoglobulinemia
Mixed cryoglobulinemia is a systemic disease involving mainly small vessels presenting as glomerulonephritis, arthritis, and purpura. HBsAg, anti-HBs, and HBV-like particles have been demonstrated in cryoprecipitates [122] but recent studies questioned the association between chronic HBV infection and essential mixed cryoglobulinemia.

Papular acrodermatitis (Gianotti–Crosti disease)
Papular acrodermatitis is strongly associated with HBs antigenemia in children, particularly among those under the age of 4 years [123,124]. Circulating HBsAg and anti-HBs immune complexes are thought to play a role in the pathogenesis [123]. It manifests as symmetric, erythematous, maculopapular, nonitchy (or nonpruritic) eruptions over the face, buttocks, limbs, and occasionally the trunk, lasting for 15–20 days. Evidence of acute hepatitis may coincide with the onset of the skin eruption or, more commonly, begins as the dermatitis starts to wane.

Aplastic anemia
Isolated cases of severe aplastic anemia occurring in the early phase of acute hepatitis have been reported [125]. However, one study suggested that most cases of hepatitis-associated aplastic anemia are not related to hepatitis viruses but are mediated by immunopathologic mechanisms [126].

Special patient groups

Pediatric patients
Acute HBV infection has been estimated to account for 10–25% of all cases of childhood acute hepatitis. Extra-

hepatic manifestations including arthralgia, arthritis, skin rash, and Gianotti papular acrodermatitis are common and have been reported in 25% of patients.

Despite the availability of HBV vaccines, HBV infection remains the most important cause of chronic hepatitis in pediatric patients. The clinical manifestation of chronic HBV infection in children is dependent on the age at infection. Perinatal HBV infection results in a high rate (90%) of chronic infection and a prolonged replicative phase. Children with perinatally acquired HBV infection are usually asymptomatic with normal ALT values despite high serum HBV DNA levels. The progression of liver disease may occur over time, particularly in those who remain HBeAg-positive and in those with other etiologies of liver disease such as hepatitis C virus (HCV) coinfection and alcoholism [127,128]. Cirrhosis is uncommon in children and appears to be more frequent in boys and in those with a history of acute hepatitis [129]. HCC has also been reported among children with chronic HBV infection [127,130]. It is more common among Asian children, and in children with cirrhosis or a family history of HCC. HBV-related acute liver failure is extremely rare in children. Most reported cases occurred in infants born to HBeAg-negative mothers [131].

Immunocompromised patients
The clinical manifestations and natural course of chronic HBV infection in immunocompromised patients may be different from that in immunocompetent patients because of enhanced HBV replication and impaired immune response. Immunosuppressive therapy can increase HBV replication directly by stimulating the glucocorticoid responsive element in the enhancer region of the HBV genome [132] or indirectly by diminishing the immune response. Abrupt withdrawal of immunosuppressive therapy, as in cyclical chemotherapy or a rapid tapering of steroid treatment, has been reported to be associated with exacerbations of liver disease in HBsAg carriers as well as in persons with past HBV infection [133, 134]. These exacerbations are believed to be due to massive lysis of infected hepatocytes as the immune system recovers. Although most of the exacerbations are asymptomatic, fatal hepatic decompensation has been reported [133,135]. Prophylactic antiviral therapy has been shown to reduce the incidence of hepatitis flares associated with HBV reactivation [136].

Patients with chronic renal failure on hemodialysis have an increased risk of HBV infection. Dialysis patients are usually HBeAg- and serum HBV DNA-positive but have no symptoms, normal ALT levels, and minimal liver damage on liver biopsies [137]. The clinical course of postrenal transplantation is, however, very different, with exacerbations, rapid progression to cirrhosis, and an increased risk of HCC and death from liver failure

[138–141]. Recent reports showed that preemptive treatment with lamivudine decreased the risk of reactivation of hepatitis B post transplantation [142,143]. In addition, lamivudine has been reported to be effective in treating hepatitic flares and hepatic decompensation due to reactivation of hepatitis B after renal transplantation. The American Society of Transplantation and the American Society of Transplant Surgeons Clinical Practice Guidelines for the care of renal transplant recipients recommend that all HBsAg-positive renal transplant recipients receive antiviral prophylaxis, preferably with tenofovir or entecavir or lamivudine. Additionally, the guidelines recommend that patients who have developed resistance to lamivudine should be treated with tenofovir or adefovir, and that HBsAg-negative patients who have an anti-HBs titer of <10 IU/L should receive a booster vaccination [144].

Patients with HIV infection have a high prevalence of HBV infection. This is probably related to the similarities in the mode of transmission of HBV and HIV. In western countries, 6–10% of patients with HIV infection are coinfected with HBV and both viruses are acquired in adult life. In countries where HBV is endemic, 10–25% of patients with HIV infection are coinfected with HBV; most of the coinfected patients develop chronic HBV infection as infants and then acquire HIV as adults. Patients who are coinfected with HBV and HIV tend to have higher serum HBV DNA levels, lower ALT levels, lower rates of spontaneous as well as treatment-related HBeAg seroconversion, and a higher risk of cirrhosis [145–148]. Reactivation of HBV replication has been described in association with HIV infection [149] and may lead to an acceleration of liver disease progression [150,151]. In contrast, HBV coinfection does not appear to have any significant effect on the rate of progression of HIV disease [147,152]. Flares of hepatitis B and deaths due to liver failure have also been reported in patients receiving highly active antiretroviral therapy (HAART). The exacerbations are felt to be related to "immune reconstitution" with subsequent immune-mediated injury directed against infected hepatocytes [153]. Several studies have shown that patients coinfected with HIV and HBV have an increased risk of liver-related mortality compared to those with HIV or HBV monoinfection [154,155].

Natural history
The natural course of HBV infection is determined by the interplay between the virus (HBV replication, HBV genotype, and viral variants), host (age, gender, race/ethnicity, genetic make-up, and immune response), and environment (alcohol, concomitant infection with other viruses – HCV, hepatitis D virus (HDV), and HIV – and carcinogens such as aflatoxin).

Progression from acute to chronic hepatitis B virus infection
The overall rate of progression from acute to chronic (persisting for >6 months) HBV infection has been estimated to be 5–10%. The risk is inversely proportional to the age at infection: 90% for perinatal infection, 20% for childhood infection, and less than 5% for adult infection [5–8]. Careful analyses of patients presenting with "acute hepatitis B" found that the risk of progression to chronic HBV infection among immunocompetent adults was less than 1% after the exclusion of patients who had acute exacerbations of chronic HBV infection.

Hepatitis B virus infection is a life-long infection
The advent of sensitive molecular virology assays has revolutionized the concept of viral clearance and recovery from HBV infection. Many studies found that HBV DNA and a vigorous immune response to HBV antigens can be detected more than 10 years after recovery from acute HBV infection, that is, HBsAg to anti-HBs seroconversion [156,157]. These findings indicate that HBV persists but is contained by the host immune response. This accounts for reports of chemotherapy-induced reactivation of HBV replication in patients with "recovered" HBV infection [133].

The likelihood of spontaneous viral clearance in patients with chronic HBV infection is very low because of the presence of extrahepatic reservoirs of HBV, the integration of HBV DNA into the host genome, and the presence of an intracellular conversion pathway whereby newly replicated HBV DNA reenters the hepatocyte nuclei and is used to amplify covalently closed circular HBV DNA (cccDNA) [158]. This intracellular pathway enables the establishment of a pool of transcriptional templates in the hepatocyte without the need for multiple rounds of reinfection.

Clinical course of chronic hepatitis B virus infection
The natural course of chronic HBV infection is characterized by fluctuations in the level of HBV replication and activity of liver disease. The clinical course of chronic HBV infection can be considered as comprising four phases (Fig. 24.3), although not all patients go through every phase.

Immune tolerant phase
In patients with perinatally acquired HBV infection, the initial phase is characterized by high levels of HBV replication: the presence of HBeAg and high levels of HBV DNA in serum (10^6–10^{10} IU/mL), normal ALT, and minimal changes on liver biopsy [159–161]. A mild degree of liver injury despite high levels of HBV replication is believed to be due to immune tolerance to HBV. The

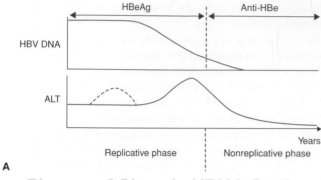

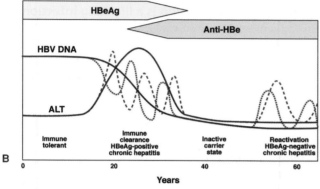

Figure 24.3 Natural history of chronic hepatitis B virus (HBV) infection. ALT, alanine aminotransferase; anti-HBe, hepatitis B e antibody; HBeAg, hepatitis B e antigen.

exact mechanism(s) for immune tolerance is unknown. Experiments in mice suggest that transplacental transfer of maternal HBeAg may induce a specific unresponsiveness of helper T cells to HBeAg [162]. Because HBeAg and HBcAg are cross-reactive at the T-cell level, deletion of the T-helper cell response to HBeAg results in an ineffective cytotoxic T-cell response to HBcAg.

During the immune tolerant phase, which lasts one to four decades, there is a very low rate of spontaneous HBeAg clearance. The cumulative rate of spontaneous HBeAg clearance is estimated to be approximately 2% during the first 3 years [163] and only 15% after 20 years of infection [164]. The persistence of high levels of viremia in adolescents and young adults accounts for the high frequency of maternal–infant transmission of HBV in Asia. The lack of assistance from immune-mediated viral clearance also contributes to a low rate of treatment-related HBeAg seroconversion.

A study from Taiwan that followed 240 adult patients who presented in the immune tolerant phase found that only 5% progressed to cirrhosis and none to HCC during a mean follow-up of 10.5 years [165], confirming that there is very little liver injury during this phase. In patients with childhood or adult-acquired HBV infection, the immune tolerant phase is short-lived or absent.

Immune clearance phase/HBeAg-positive chronic hepatitis

This phase is characterized by the presence of HBeAg, high levels of serum HBV DNA, and active liver disease (elevated ALT and necroinflammation on liver biopsy). In patients with perinatally acquired HBV infection, transition from the immune tolerant to the immune clearance phase usually occurs during the second to fourth decades of life. Most patients with childhood or adult-acquired HBV infection are already in the immune clearance phase at presentation.

During this phase, spontaneous HBeAg clearance occurs at an annual rate of 10–20% (Fig. 24.3) [164, 165]. HBeAg seroconversion is frequently but not always accompanied by biochemical exacerbations [164,166]. These exacerbations are believed to be due to a sudden increase in immune-mediated lysis of infected hepatocytes, and are often preceded by an increase in serum HBV DNA level and a change in the distribution of HBcAg from nuclear to cytoplasmic localization in the hepatocytes.

Most exacerbations are asymptomatic but some are accompanied by symptoms of acute hepatitis. Occasionally, IgM anti-HBc may be detected leading to misdiagnosis of acute hepatitis B in previously unrecognized carriers. Exacerbations may be associated with increase in AFP levels [101]. In approximately 2.5% of patients (especially those with preexisting cirrhosis), exacerbations may result in hepatic decompensation and rarely death from hepatic failure [167].

Not all exacerbations lead to HBeAg seroconversion [164,168,169]. Some patients have abortive immune clearance. These patients may develop recurrent exacerbations with intermittently undetectable serum HBV DNA with or without transient loss of HBeAg. Repeated episodes of necroinflammation may increase the risk of cirrhosis and HCC. Exacerbations are more commonly observed in men than in women [169] and may account for a higher incidence of HBV-related cirrhosis and HCC among men.

An important outcome of the immune clearance phase is HBeAg to anti-HBe seroconversion. Factors associated with higher rates of spontaneous HBeAg seroconversion include older age, higher ALT levels, and HBV genotype B (compared to genotype C) [164,170,171]. High ALT levels are believed to be a reflection of a vigorous host immune response, accounting for its strong correlation with spontaneous as well as treatment-related HBeAg seroconversion. A study of 483 patients who had no evidence of cirrhosis or HCC at the time of HBeAg seroconversion found that the 15-year cumulative risk of HBeAg-negative hepatitis, cirrhosis, and HCC was 31.2%, 3.7%, and 2.1% for those who seroconverted before the age of 30 years and 66.7%, 42.9%, and 7.7%, respectively, for those who seroconverted after the age of 40. This indicates that earlier HBeAg seroconversion is associated with better prognosis [172].

Inactive carrier phase

This phase is characterized by the absence of HBeAg, presence of anti-HBe, persistently normal ALT levels, and low or undetectable serum HBV DNA (usually $<10^3$ IU/mL) (see Fig. 24.3). Liver biopsy generally shows mild hepatitis and minimal fibrosis but inactive cirrhosis may be observed in patients who had accrued substantial liver injury during the preceding immune clearance phase.

The inactive carrier phase may persist indefinitely, in which case the prognosis is generally favorable, especially if this phase is reached early. This is supported by the finding of comparable survival between HBsAg-positive blood donors (almost all were HBeAg-negative and had normal ALT at baseline) and uninfected controls over a 30-year period [173]. However, inactive carriers are still at risk of HCC and liver-related death. A study of 20,069 subjects in Taiwan including 1,932 inactive HBsAg carriers followed for a mean of 13.1 years found that the annual incidence of HCC and liver-related death was 0.06% and 0.04%, respectively, among the inactive carriers and 0.02% and 0.02% among the HBsAg-negative controls [174].

Some patients in the inactive carrier phase eventually clear HBsAg. The annual rate of HBsAg clearance has been estimated to be 0.5–2% [171,175] but HBsAg clearance does not occur at a linear rate, being very uncommon during the early stages and increasing over time [175]. HBsAg clearance is generally accompanied by undetectable serum HBV DNA, normalization of ALT, and improved liver histology [176]. However, low levels of HBV DNA may be detectable in some patients, more so in the liver than serum. The prognosis of patients who have cleared HBsAg is excellent but HCC has been observed in patients who cleared HBsAg after the age of 50 years or after progression to cirrhosis as well as in those with HCV coinfection [177,178].

Some inactive carriers have reactivation of HBV replication later in life. Reactivation may occur spontaneously or as a result of immunosuppression, and may be due to wild-type HBV or HBV variants that abolish or downregulate HBeAg production. In one study of 283 Chinese patients followed for a median of 8.6 years after spontaneous HBeAg seroconversion, 67% had sustained remission, 4% had HBeAg reversion, and 24% had HBeAg-negative chronic hepatitis [179]. Cirrhosis developed in 8% and HCC in 2%, the risk being higher in those who had active hepatitis after HBeAg seroconversion.

Reactivation of hepatitis B virus replication/HBeAg-negative chronic hepatitis

This phase is characterized by the absence of HBeAg, presence of anti-HBe, detectable serum HBV DNA, elevated ALT, and chronic inflammation ± fibrosis on biopsy (see Fig. 24.3). Patients in this phase are usually older and have more advanced liver disease because this represents a later phase in the course of chronic HBV infection. Serum HBV DNA levels are lower than in HBeAg-positive patients but may reach 10^8–10^9 IU/mL.

The hallmark of this phase is its fluctuating course. In one study where patients were monitored at monthly intervals, 36% had persistently elevated ALT, 20% had fluctuating abnormal ALT, and 44% had fluctuating ALT with intermittently normal values [180]. Several investigators have attempted to define cutoff HBV DNA levels that would differentiate patients with HBeAg-negative chronic hepatitis from inactive carriers; because of the fluctuating course, serial testing is more reliable than any single HBV DNA level in verifying the inactive carrier state [181,182].

HBeAg-negative chronic hepatitis was originally reported in Mediterranean countries. It has now been reported in all parts of the world. The geographic variations in the prevalence of HBeAg-negative chronic hepatitis are related to the predominant HBV genotype in that region. Recent studies in Europe, Asia, and the United States have all reported an increased prevalence of HBeAg-negative and a decreased prevalence of HBeAg-positive chronic hepatitis [183,184]. This may be related to increased awareness of HBeAg-negative chronic hepatitis, a decrease in new HBV infections due to vaccination, and a progression of the existing pool of HBV carriers to later stages of chronic HBV infection.

Latent/occult hepatitis B virus infection

Occult HBV infection is defined as the detection of HBV DNA in persons who are HBsAg-negative [99,185]. HBV DNA is more often detected in liver than in serum. The prevalence of occult HBV infection is higher in countries that are endemic for HBV, in individuals with serologic markers of previous HBV infection, and in those with HIV or HCV infection. Occult HBV infection is more common among patients with cirrhosis or HCC [99,186]. Many of these patients probably had chronic HBV infection for decades leading to liver damage but HBsAg is no longer detectable when cirrhosis or HCC is diagnosed. Low levels of HBV may also be a cofactor of liver disease in patients with chronic HCV infection or other causes of chronic liver disease.

Sequelae of chronic hepatitis B virus infection

The sequelae of chronic HBV infection vary from inactive carrier state to chronic hepatitis, cirrhosis, hepatic decompensation, HCC, and death. The clinical outcome of patients with chronic HBV infection depends on the severity of liver damage prior to sustained HBeAg seroconversion and the durability of the inactive carrier phase.

The annual rate of progression from chronic hepatitis to cirrhosis has been estimated to be 2–5% for HBeAg-positive and 3–10% for HBeAg-negative patients [187]; the higher rate in HBeAg-negative patients is related to older age and more advanced liver disease at presentation. Factors that have been reported to be associated with an increased rate of progression to cirrhosis include: host (older age, male), virus (persistent high levels of HBV replication, HBV genotype (C > B), coinfection with HCV, HDV, and HIV), and environment (alcohol and, more recently, obesity) [187,188].

The annual rate of progression from compensated cirrhosis to hepatic decompensation has been estimated to be 3–5% [187]. Survival after the development of compensated cirrhosis is favorable initially (85% at 5 years) but decreases dramatically after the onset of decompensation to 55–70% at 1 year and 14–35% at 5 years [187]. The lifetime risk of a liver-related death has been estimated to be 40–50% for men and 15% for women among patients with perinatally acquired chronic HBV infection [189].

The annual rate of HCC development has been estimated to be 0.5–1.0% for noncirrhotic carriers and 2–3% for patients with cirrhosis [187]. Risk factors for HCC include: host (older age, male, being Asian, having first-degree relatives with HCC), virus (high levels of HBV replication, HBV genotype (C > B), core promoter mutations, coinfection with HCV), and environment (alcohol, aflatoxin, and, more recently smoking, obesity, and diabetes) [187,188]. It is important to note that although HCC is more common among patients with cirrhosis, 30–50% of HCC associated with HBV occurs in the absence of cirrhosis.

There is overwhelming evidence that high serum HBV DNA levels, delayed HBeAg seroconversion, and HBV reactivation with or without seroreversion after HBeAg loss are associated with increased risk of cirrhosis, HCC, and liver-related mortality [171,172,190–194]. One of the largest studies, including more than 3,500 HBsAg-positive Chinese adults aged 30–65 years, followed for a mean of 11 years, found that compared to carriers with serum HBV DNA $<4 \log_{10}$ copies/mL, those who had serum HBV DNA $>6 \log_{10}$ copies/mL at entry had an adjusted relative risk of 6.5 for cirrhosis and 6.1 for HCC [193,194].

Several studies from Asia reported that genotype C is associated with more rapid progression to cirrhosis and an increased risk of HCC compared with genotype B [191,195–197]. These findings may be related to observations that patients with genotype C undergo spontaneous

HBeAg seroconversion later and have a higher frequency of core promoter mutations [170,183].

Coinfection of hepatitis B virus and hepatitis C virus

Acute coinfection of HBV and HCV has been reported in transfused patients as well as in intravenous drug users. Coinfection with HCV may delay the onset and shorten the duration of HBs antigenemia as well as lowering the peak ALT levels compared with acute HBV infection alone [198]. These findings suggest that HCV coinfection may interfere with the replication of HBV leading to attenuation of liver damage. However, acute coinfection of HCV and HBV has been reported to increase the risk of fulminant hepatic failure [199]. HCV superinfection in HBsAg carriers typically manifests as acute icteric hepatitis and is associated with a high risk of hepatic decompensation and death from hepatic failure [200]. HCV superinfection has also been reported to decrease HBV DNA levels and to be associated with earlier HBsAg clearance [201,202]. Patients coinfected with HCV and HBV have higher risks of cirrhosis and HCC compared to patients infected with either virus alone [203,204].

Hepatitis B virus and hepatocellular carcinoma

Worldwide, HCC is the third most common cause of cancer deaths, accounting for approximately 500,000 deaths each year. The vast majority (85%) of HCC is concentrated in eastern and southeastern Asia and sub-Saharan Africa where HBV infection is endemic. Several lines of evidence support an etiologic association between chronic HBV infection and HCC. There is a close correlation between the geographic distribution of HBsAg carriers and the occurrence of HCC [205]. Long-term follow-up studies of HBsAg carriers showed a marked increase in risk of HCC. One study of 22,707 Taiwanese men followed for a mean of 8.9 years found that the incidence of HCC was 495/100,000 per year for HBsAg-positive and 5/100,000 per year for HBsAg-negative men, with a relative risk of 98 [189]. HBV vaccination and antiviral therapy have both been shown to reduce the incidence of HCC [20,206].

Mechanisms of hepatocarcinogenesis

Chronic HBV infection can induce HCC directly by activating cellular oncogenes or by inactivating tumor suppressor genes, or indirectly through chronic liver injury, inflammation, and regeneration [207].

Integrated HBV DNA is frequently found in neoplastic as well as non-neoplastic liver tissue of patients with HBV-related HCC. Integration of HBV DNA may activate cellular protooncogenes or suppress growth-regulating genes. Integration of HBV DNA can also induce carcinogenesis via transactivation. Integration of the intact or truncated versions of the *X* gene is found in most HCCs. The HBx protein has been shown to be a potent and promiscuous transactivator of viral as well as cellular enhancers and promoters and may play an important role in carcinogenesis [208]. The integration of HBV DNA can also cause cancers indirectly via chromosomal deletions or translocations.

An alternate path by which chronic HBV infection leads to HCC is through the induction of liver injury. Chronic liver cell injury initiates a cascade of events characterized by increased rates of cellular DNA synthesis and impaired cellular repair, thereby setting the scene for acquired mutations. During regeneration, transformed cells that have a growth advantage are selected resulting in clonal expansion and eventually tumor formation. Clinical studies demonstrate that long durations of high levels of HBV replication and active hepatitis increase the risk of HCC.

Hepatitis B virus genotypes and variants

The HBV genome consists of four partially overlapping open reading frames: the *pre-S/S* gene that codes for the envelope proteins, the *pre-C/C* gene that codes for the e antigen and core protein, the *P* gene that codes for the DNA polymerase and reverse transcriptase, and the *X* gene that codes for a protein of unclear significance. Although HBV is a DNA virus, it is prone to mutations with a rate of nucleotide substitutions estimated at 1×10^{-5} to 3×10^{-5}/site per year [209]. This is related to the reverse transcription of an RNA intermediate during the replication cycle of HBV.

Hepatitis B virus genotypes

Hepatitis B virus can be classified into nine genotypes designated A to I [77,78,210]. The geographic distribution of HBV genotypes is summarized in Table 24.4. There is an association between HBV genotypes and precore and core promoter variants. The most common precore variant ($G_{1896}A$) is predominantly found in patients with HBV genotypes B, C, and D and rarely in patients with geno-

type A [183,211,212]. This accounts for the high prevalence of HBeAg-negative chronic hepatitis and the precore stop codon variant ($G_{1896}A$) in Asia and the Mediterranean basin and their low prevalence in the United States and northern Europe. The most common core promoter variant ($A_{1762}T$, $G_{1764}A$) is more frequently found in patients with HBV genotypes A, C, and D [183].

Several studies suggest that HBV genotypes may be related to the rate of recovery or likelihood of a fulminant course during acute infection; these studies involved small numbers of patients and the data need to be confirmed.

Studies in Asia where genotypes B and C are predominant found that genotype B is associated with a lower prevalence of HBeAg, earlier HBeAg seroconversion, higher likelihood of sustained remission after HBeAg seroconversion, and less active liver disease compared with genotype C [170,213–215]. HBV genotype B is also associated with a slower rate of progression to cirrhosis and HCC [195–197,216–218]. One study in Taiwan found that the incidence of HCC among carriers with genotype C infection was more than double those with genotype B infection, 786 versus 306 per 100,000 person-years [197]. Data on the relation between other HBV genotypes and HBV replication and liver disease are scanty. Available data suggest that genotype A is associated with a higher likelihood of sustained virologic and biochemical remission after HBeAg seroconversion than genotype D [219]. A study in Alaska confirmed that genotype C is associated with a lower rate of HBeAg seroconversion compared with other genotypes and that genotype F is associated with a high incidence of HCC [220,221].

HBV genotype may also affect the response to IFN therapy. Several studies reported that HBeAg-positive patients with genotypes A and B have higher rates of HBeAg loss than those with genotypes C and D after IFN therapy [222–224]. Patients with genotype A also have higher rates of HBsAg loss [225]. NUCs appear to be equally effective in virus suppression across all HBV genotypes [226].

Table 24.4 Geographic distribution of hepatitis B virus (HBV) genotypes.

HBV genotypes	Distribution areas
A	Northwest Europe, North America, Central Africa
B	China, Japan, Indonesia, Vietnam
C	China, Japan, East Asia, Korea, Vietnam, Polynesia
D	Mediterranean basin, Middle East, India
E	Africa
F	American natives, Polynesia
G	United States, France
H	Mexico, Latin America

Precore variants

Among the naturally occurring HBV mutations, mutations in the precore region have been most extensively studied (Fig. 24.4). The precore region consists of 87 nucleotides (29 amino acids) that precede the core region. The *preC/C* gene codes for two 3.5 kb RNA transcripts. The precore mRNA is slightly longer and codes for the precore/core protein that is processed to a smaller secretory protein – HBeAg [227]. The pregenomic RNA serves as a template for reverse transcription into the (–) strand HBV DNA. It also serves as an mRNA for translation into the core protein and polymerase protein.

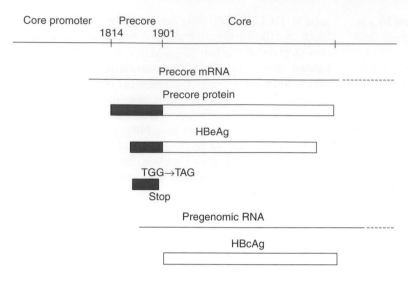

Figure 24.4 Transcription and translation of precore/core open reading frame. Precore mRNA is translated into precore protein, which is processed at the N and C terminal ends to hepatitis B e antigen (HBeAg). Mutation of nucleotide 1896 from G to A converts codon 28 in the precore region from tryptophan to a stop codon, thereby preventing production of HBeAg. Pregenomic RNA is translated into core and polymerase protein and reverse transcribed into hepatitis B virus DNA. HBcAg, hepatitis B core antigen.

The predominant mutation in the precore region is a G-A change at nucleotide 1896, creating a stop codon at codon 28 (Box 24.2) [228]. This mutation leads to premature termination of the precore/core protein, thereby preventing the production of HBeAg.

Initial reports of the $G_{1896}A$ variant came from the Mediterranean countries and Japan. This variant has been detected in diverse geographic areas [183,229]. A recent study found that the precore variant can be found in up to 30% patients with chronic HBV infection in the United States [183]. The variability in the prevalence of the $G_{1896}A$ variant in different countries is related to the predominant HBV genotype. The $G_{1896}A$ variant is replication competent and transmission has been documented in humans as well as in chimpanzee experiments [230–232]. However, infection with precore HBV variant is less likely to progress to chronic infection, possibly due to the lack of the tolerogenic effect of HBeAg.

The $G_{1896}A$ variant is usually found in HBeAg-negative patients but may be present as a mixture with wild-type virus in HBeAg-positive patients. It has been observed to emerge or become selected around the time of HBeAg seroconversion [233,234]. The $G_{1896}A$ variant was initially thought to cause more severe liver disease because it was found in patients with severe chronic hepatitis or acute liver failure [230,231,235,236] but it has also been detected in anti-HBe-positive asymptomatic carriers [237]. Therefore, the $G_{1896}A$ mutation alone may have no direct pathogenic role; instead host immune response and mutations in other regions of the HBV genome may be more important in determining the severity of liver disease.

Core promoter mutations

Mutations in the core promoter region can also decrease HBeAg production by downregulating the transcription of the precore mRNA. The most common core promoter variant has dual mutations involving A to T change at nucleotide 1762 and G to A change at nucleotide 1764 ($A_{1762}T$, $G_{1764}A$) (Box 24.2). These two changes result in amino acid substitutions in codons 130 and 131 of the overlapping X gene. Unlike precore variants, core promoter variants can be detected in similar proportions of HBeAg-negative and HBeAg-positive patients. Core

---

Box 24.2 Common forms of hepatitis B virus (HBV) variants.

HBeAg-negative phenotype

Precore region

• G-A at nt 1896, tryptophan stop at codon 28 (G1896A, eW28X)

Core promoter region

• A-T at nt 1762 and G-A at nt 1764 (A1762T, G1764A, ×K130M, ×V131I)

HBIg/HBV vaccine escape

S gene

• Glycine–arginine at codon 145 (sG145R)

Antiviral resistance (primary resistance mutations)

P gene (reverse transcriptase/polymerase region)

• Lamivudine	A181V/T, M204V/I
• Adefovir	A181V/T, N236T
• Entecavir	T184G, S202G/I, M250V
• Telbivudine	M204I
• Tenofovir	A181V/T, A194T, N236T
• A181V/T	Alanine–valine or threonine at codon 181
• T184G	Threonine–glycine at codon 184
• A194T	Alanine–threonine at codon 194
• S202G/I	Serine–glycine or isoleucine at codon 202
• M204V/I	Methionine–valine or isoleucine at codon 204
• N236T	Asparagine–threonine at codon 236
• M250V	Methionine–valine at codon 250

HBeAg, hepatitis B e antigen; HBIg, hepatitis B immune globulin; nt, nucleotide.

promoter variants were reported to be more common in patients with acute liver failure [238,239] and have been shown in many studies to be associated with HCC [240, 241]. A cohort study in Taiwan found that the multivariate adjusted hazard ratios of developing HCC were 1.76 for genotype C versus B, 1.73 for core promoter mutations versus wild-type core promoter sequence, and 0.34 for precore mutations versus wild-type precore sequence [197].

S gene mutations

Vaccinees

Mutations in the S gene have been described in infants born to carrier mothers despite adequate anti-HBs response after vaccination [242–244]. The most common mutation involves a glycine to arginine substitution at codon 145 (G145R) in the "a" determinant (Box 24.2). This mutation has been shown to exhibit decreased binding to monoclonal anti-"a" antibodies thereby allowing the virus to escape neutralization. Chimpanzee experiments demonstrated that the G145R variant is infectious [245], raising concerns about the possibility of widespread dissemination of vaccine escape variants. One study from Taiwan found that the prevalence of vaccine escape variants among HBsAg-positive children increased after the introduction of universal vaccination, from 7.8% in 1984 to 23% in 1999 [246] but the carrier rate decreased from 9.8% to 0.7% during the same period [247]. Another study among 784 preschool children in four Pacific Island countries, who received HBV vaccine, failed to detect any "a" determinant mutation [248]. These data suggest that the emergence of vaccine escape mutants occurs rarely and has not diminished the efficacy of HBV vaccines. Apart from G145R, other mutations in the "a" determinant have also been reported. Some of these variants may yield false-negative results in serology assays that rely on monoclonal antibodies but practically all the S variants can be detected in HBsAg assays that utilize polyclonal anti-HBs for capture and/or detection.

Liver transplant recipients

Mutations in the HBV S gene have also been reported in liver transplant recipients who developed HBV reinfection despite prophylaxis with monoclonal or polyclonal anti-HBs (HBIg) [249–251]. Most of the mutations are located in the "a" determinant, the most common being the G145R mutation. Prophylaxis with a combination of HBIg and NUC decreases the risk of immune escape and rate of reinfection [252].

Pre-S mutations

Deletions and mutations in the pre-S1 and pre-S2 regions have also been described and are more commonly seen in patients with progressive liver disease or HCC [253].

P gene mutations

Naturally occurring HBV polymerase gene mutations are rarely reported. The most common P gene mutations have been found in association with the use of NUCs for the treatment of chronic HBV infection (see Box 24.2).

Treatment

The main goal of treatment of chronic hepatitis B is to prevent cirrhosis, hepatic decompensation, and HCC. This goal is best achieved by eradicating HBV before there is irreversible liver damage. However, it is not possible to eradicate HBV because of the presence of extrahepatic reservoirs of HBV, the integration of HBV DNA into the host genome, and the presence of an intracellular conversion pathway that replenishes the pool of transcriptional templates (cccDNA) in the hepatocyte nucleus without the need for reinfection [158]. Parameters used to assess response include normalization of serum ALT, decrease in serum HBV DNA level, loss of HBeAg with or without detection of anti-HBe (for HBeAg-positive patients), loss of HBsAg, and improvement in liver histology.

Currently, there are seven approved treatments for hepatitis B: standard and pegylated IFN-α, and five NUCs lamivudine, adefovir, entecavir, telbivudine, and tenofovir. Responses to these treatment in phase III trials are summarized in Table 24.5.

IFNs are administered for predefined durations while NUCs are usually administered until a specific endpoint is achieved. The difference in approach is related to the observation that HBeAg seroconversion frequently occurs a few months after cessation of IFN treatment, presumably because of the lag between immune priming and decrease in expression of viral protein, whereas viral relapse is inevitable if NUCs are withdrawn prior to achieving the therapeutic endpoint. For HBeAg-positive patients, virus suppression can be sustained in 50–90% patients if NUC treatment is stopped after HBeAg seroconversion is achieved and at least 6 months of consolidation therapy is administered. For HBeAg-negative patients, relapse is frequent even when HBV DNA has been suppressed to undetectable levels for more than a year.

IFNs have antiviral, antiproliferative, and immunomodulatory effects. The antiviral effects of IFN depend on its binding to specific receptors, which then triggers a series of intracellular events including activation of 2′,5′-oligoadenylate synthetase (2′5′-AS). IFNs also have immunomodulatory functions that may be important in eradicating virus infections.

Table 24.5 Responses to 48–52 weeks of approved treatments of hepatitis B in treatment-naïve patients.

Response	No treatment (%)	Pegylated IFN ± lamivudine (%)[a]	Lamivudine (%)	Adefovir (%)	Entecavir (%)	Telbivudine (%)	Tenofovir (%)
HBeAg-positive patients							
Undetectable HBV DNA	0–17	69/25	36–44	21	67	60	76
HBeAg seroconversion	4–6	22/27	16–21	12–21	21	22	21
Loss of HBsAg	0–1	3/3	~1	0	2	0	3
Normalization of ALT	7–24	46/39	41–75	48–61	68	77	68
Histologic improvement	NA	41/38[b]	49–56	53	72	65	74
Genotypic resistance	0	4/0	15–30	0	0	11	0
HBeAg-negative patients							
Undetectable HBV DNA	0–20	87/63	60–73	51	90	88	93
Loss of HBsAg	<1	2/3	<1	0	<1	<1	0
Normalization of ALT	10–29	49/38	62–78	72	78	74	76
Histologic improvement	33	38/48[b]	61–66	64–69	70	67	72
Genotypic resistance	0	0	10–25	0	0	5	0

[a]Responses in patients who received pegIFN monotherapy/pegIFN + lamivudine.
[b]Assessed at week 72 (24 weeks after discontinuation of treatment).
ALT, alanine aminotransferase; HBeAg, hepatitis B e antigen; HBsAg, hepatitis B surface antigen; HBV, hepatitis B virus; IFN, interferon; NA, not available.

Standard interferon-α

Efficacy

1 *HBeAg-positive chronic hepatitis.* Several meta-analyses confirmed a beneficial effect of IFN therapy in HBV DNA suppression, ALT normalization, and HBeAg loss [254,255].

2 *HBeAg-negative chronic hepatitis.* Results of randomized controlled trials showed that treated patients were more likely than controls to have viral suppression but most patients relapsed when treatment was stopped. One study found a higher rate (30%) of sustained response after 24 months of IFN-α therapy compared with 15–20% rates reported in other studies that administered IFN-α for 12 months [256] suggesting that a longer duration of treatment may increase the rate of sustained response.

3 *HBV DNA-positive clinical cirrhosis.* Patients with histologic cirrhosis but no evidence of hepatic decompensation appeared to tolerate IFN-α treatment. However, IFN-α even when administered in very low doses is associated with a high risk of serious infections and severe exacerbations leading to hepatic failure in patients with clinically evident cirrhosis [257,258].

Role of prednisone priming

Steroid withdrawal has been observed to be frequently accompanied by a flare in serum ALT levels and HBeAg seroconversion. Prednisone priming followed by IFN-α treatment had very little additional beneficial effect compared with IFN-α alone [259] and there is a risk of fatal exacerbation in patients with underlying cirrhosis.

Long-term outcome of therapy with interferon-α
Hepatitis B e antigen-positive patients
Most HBeAg-positive patients who responded to IFN-α therapy are able to maintain their response. Relapses usually occur within 1 year of cessation of treatment, but delayed reactivation can occur. Among the sustained responders, an increasing proportion cleared HBsAg during the course of follow-up. The percent of sustained responders who cleared HBsAg within 5 years of HBeAg clearance varied from 65% in one US study [260], to 19–24% in European studies [261–263], to 0–9% in two studies from Asia [264,265] despite similar durations of follow-up. A sustained antiviral response, especially in those who clear both HBeAg and HBsAg, is almost invariably accompanied by normalization of ALT levels and a decrease in necroinflammation but residual liver damage may be present. Follow-up of 101 male patients who participated in a controlled trial of IFN-α therapy in Taiwan for 8 years found that treated patients had a lower incidence of HCC (1.5% versus 12%, $P = 0.04$) and a higher survival rate (98% versus 57%, $P = 0.02$) compared to controls but there was no difference in the rate of new onset of cirrhosis [265]. Clinical benefits were not observed in a study from Hong Kong [266]. IFN-α has not been shown

to decrease the incidence of HCC in European or North American patients, probably because of the low rate of HCC in untreated patients. However, studies comparing the outcome of responders versus nonresponders found that patients who cleared HBeAg had better overall survival and survival free of hepatic decompensation and a clinical benefit was most evident among patients with cirrhosis [255,261,262,267,268].

Hepatitis B e antigen-negative patients

Relapse after cessation of IFN-α treatment is frequent, with sustained response rates of only 15–30% [269,270]. Among the long-term responders, approximately 20% cleared HBsAg after 5 years of follow-up [271]. IFN-α therapy did not have any overall effect on survival, complication-free survival, or HCC, but patients with sustained response had significantly lower rates of hepatic decompensation [270,271].

Dose regimen

IFN-α is administered as subcutaneous injections. The recommended dose for adults is 5 MU daily or 10 MU thrice weekly and for children is 6 MU/m² thrice weekly to a maximum of 10 MU. The recommended duration of treatment for patients with HBeAg positive chronic hepatitis B is 16–24 weeks. Patients with HBeAg-negative chronic hepatitis B should be treated for at least 12 months; one study suggested that higher rates of sustained response can be achieved with 24 months of treatment [256].

Pegylated interferon-α

The attachment of polyethylene glycol to a protein (pegylation) reduces its renal clearance, and decreases immunogenicity of the protein, with a resultant increase in the half-life of the pegylated protein. Clinical trials suggest that efficacy of pegylated IFN-α (pegIFN-α) is similar to or slightly better than standard IFN-α. PegIFN-α has the advantage of more convenient administration and more sustained virus suppression and has largely replaced standard IFN-α.

Efficacy

1 *HBeAg-positive chronic hepatitis.* In one phase II trial, 194 patients were randomized to receive 90, 180, or 270 μg pegIFN-α2a weekly or 4.5 MU standard IFN-α2a thrice weekly for 24 weeks. A higher percent of patients who received pegIFN-α had HBeAg seroconversion: 32% versus 25% of those who received standard IFN-α [272]. In a subsequent phase III trial, 814 patients were randomized to receive pegIFN-α2a 180 μg weekly, pegIFN-α2a 180 μg weekly + lamivudine 100 mg daily, or lamivudine 100 mg daily for 48

weeks. At the end of treatment, virus suppression was most marked in the group that received the combination therapy: mean HBV DNA reduction in the three groups was 4.5, 7.2, and 5.8 log₁₀ copies/mL, respectively [273]. HBeAg seroconversion was similar in the three groups at the end of treatment (27%, 24%, and 20%, respectively), but significantly higher in the two groups that received pegIFN-α when response was assessed 24 weeks after treatment was stopped (32%, 27%, and 19%, respectively) (Table 24.5). These data indicate that pegIFN-α2a monotherapy was superior to lamivudine monotherapy in inducing HBeAg seroconversion, and comparable to the combination therapy of pegIFN-α2a and lamivudine. Similar results were reported in two trials, in which pegIFN-α2b was administered in tapering doses (100 → 50 μg) for 52 weeks or 1.5 μg/kg for 32 weeks. Twenty-four weeks after treatment was stopped, one study reported identical rates (29%) of HBeAg seroconversion in patients who received pegIFN-α2b monotherapy with and without lamivudine [274], whereas the other study reported a significantly higher rate of HBeAg seroconversion in those who received a combination of pegIFN-α2b and lamivudine versus those who received lamivudine only, 36% versus 14% [275].

Follow-up of patients in one study of pegIFN-α2b for a mean of 3.5 years after completion of pegIFN + lamivudine found that 37% had lost HBeAg and 11% had lost HBsAg [225]. The rate of HBsAg loss was significantly higher in patients with genotype A infection: 28% compared to 3% in those with non-A genotypes. Among the initial responders, 81% had durable HBeAg loss and 30% had HBsAg loss.

2 *HBeAg-negative chronic hepatitis.* In a phase III trial of pegIFN-α in HBeAg-negative patients, 552 patients were randomized to receive 48 weeks of pegIFN-α2a 180 μg weekly, a combination of pegIFN-α2a 180 μg weekly + lamivudine 100 mg daily, or lamivudine 100 mg daily. Virus suppression was most marked in the group that received combination therapy: the mean HBV DNA reduction at week 48 in the three groups was 4.1, 5.0, and 4.2 log₁₀ copies/mL, respectively [276]. However, the sustained response (HBV DNA undetectable by PCR and normalization of ALT at week 72) was comparable in the groups that received pegIFN-α2a alone or in combination with lamivudine, and superior to the group that received lamivudine monotherapy: 15%, 16%, and 6%, respectively (Table 24.5). Three years after completion of treatment, a serum HBV DNA of <10,000 copies/mL was maintained in 22.6% versus 9.4%, ALT normalization in 31.3% versus 18.9%, and HBsAg loss in 8.7% versus 0% of patients who received pegIFN ± lamivudine versus lamivudine alone, respectively [277].

Dose regimen

The recommended dose of pegIFN-α2a for both HBeAg-positive and HBeAg-negative hepatitis is 180 μg weekly for 48 weeks. The optimal dose and duration of pegIFN-α2b for hepatitis B is unclear.

Adverse effects of standard and pegylated interferon-α therapy

Interferon-α therapy is associated with a broad spectrum of side effects. The most common side effect is an initial influenza-like illness: fever, chills, headache, malaise, and myalgia. Other common side effects include fatigue, anorexia, weight loss, and mild increase in hair loss. IFN-α has myelosuppressive effects, but significant neutropenia ($<1,000/\text{mm}^3$) or thrombocytopenia ($<60,000/\text{mm}^3$) requiring dose reduction or premature termination are uncommon except in patients who have decreased cell counts prior to treatment. The most troublesome side effect of IFN-α is emotional lability: anxiety, irritability, depression, and even suicidal tendency. These symptoms can occur in the absence of a prior history of emotional problems. IFN-α has been reported to induce the development of a variety of autoantibodies. In most instances, this is not accompanied by clinical illness. However, both hyper- and hypothyroidism that require treatment have been reported. In addition, there have been reports of worsening liver disease as a result of IFN-α-induced exacerbation of an underlying autoimmune hepatitis. Rarely, retinal changes and even impaired vision have been reported.

Predictors of response to standard and pegylated interferon-α

Predictors of response to standard and pegIFN-α are similar. The strongest predictor of response in HBeAg-positive patients is the pretreatment ALT level [278,279]. Other factors that have been identified to be associated with a higher rate of IFN-related HBeAg seroconversion include high histologic activity index, low HBV DNA level, and HBV genotypes A and B versus C and D [223,224]. Retrospective analyses found that patients who experienced a greater decline in HBeAg or HBsAg titer during treatment were more likely to undergo HBeAg seroconversion [280].

Factors associated with a higher rate of sustained response in HBeAg-negative patients include low pretreatment HBV DNA level, undetectable HBV DNA at the end of 48 weeks of treatment, and HBV genotype B or C versus D [281]. Two studies showed that patients who experienced a greater decline in HBsAg titer during treatment and those who had a lower HBsAg titer at the end of treatment were more likely to have sustained virologic response during post-treatment follow-up [282,283].

Lamivudine

Lamivudine is the (–) enantiomer of 2′,3′-dideoxy-3′-thiacytidine. It is phosphorylated to the triphosphate (3TC-TP), which competes with deoxycytidine triphosphate (dCTP) for incorporation into growing DNA chains causing chain termination.

Efficacy

Lamivudine monotherapy is effective in suppressing HBV replication and in ameliorating liver disease.

1 *HBeAg-positive chronic hepatitis B.* Randomized clinical trials of patients who received lamivudine for 1 year reported that HBeAg seroconversion occurred in 16–21% of treated patients compared to 4–6% of untreated controls (see Table 24.5) [284–286]. Histologic improvement, defined as a reduction in necroinflammatory score of ≥2 points, was observed in 49–56% of treated patients and in 23–25% controls. HBeAg seroconversion rates increased with the duration of treatment to approximately 50% at 5 years [287].

   Experience with lamivudine in children is limited. One controlled trial involved 286 children with elevated ALT randomized to receive lamivudine (3 mg/kg/day up to 100 mg/day) or placebo for 52 weeks. A significantly higher proportion of treated children developed HBeAg seroconversion compared to placebo controls, 22% versus 13% [288]. Lamivudine was well tolerated but lamivudine resistance mutations were detected in 19% after 1 year and in 64% after 3 years of treatment [289].

2 *HBeAg-negative chronic hepatitis B.* In one placebo-controlled study, virologic and biochemical response was achieved in 34 of 54 (63%) patients who received 24 weeks of lamivudine therapy versus 3 of 53 (6%) patients on placebo ($P <0.001$) [290]. Several studies have shown that HBV DNA is suppressed to undetectable levels in 60–73% patients after 1 year of treatment (see Table 24.5) [291,292]. However, the vast majority (~90%) of patients relapsed when treatment was stopped. Extending the duration of treatment results in progressively lower rates of maintained response due to the selection of drug-resistance mutations [293].

3 *Nonresponders to IFN-α treatment.* In a multicenter trial on IFN-α nonresponders, 238 HBeAg-positive patients were randomized to receive lamivudine monotherapy for 52 weeks, a combination of 24 weeks lamivudine and 16 weeks of standard IFN-α, or no treatment. Patients who received lamivudine monotherapy had the highest HBeAg seroconversion rate: 18% compared to 12% and 13%, respectively in the other groups [294]. These data suggest that patients who failed IFN-α treatment have similar responses to lamivudine as treatment-naïve patients and retreatment with a

combination of standard IFN-α and lamivudine did not confer any added benefit compared to retreatment with lamivudine monotherapy.

4 *Advanced liver disease.* Lamivudine has been shown to delay clinical progression in patients with advanced fibrosis or cirrhosis. In a double-blind, randomized, placebo-controlled trial, 651 Asian patients who were HBeAg-positive or had detectable HBV DNA by branched DNA assay (>700,000 genome equivalents/mL), and bridging fibrosis or cirrhosis on liver biopsy, were randomized to receive lamivudine or placebo. After a median duration of 32 months, a statistically significant difference was observed between the two groups for overall disease progression (increase in Child–Pugh score, hepatic decompensation, or HCC) – 7.8% versus 17.7% – as well as in HCC development – 3.9% versus 7.4% [206]. The benefit was observed mainly among those patients who did not have virologic breakthrough. These data indicate that antiviral therapy can improve clinical outcome in patients who have maintained virus suppression.

5 *HBV DNA-positive clinical cirrhosis.* Studies of lamivudine in patients with decompensated cirrhosis have shown that lamivudine treatment is well tolerated and can stabilize or improve liver function, thereby obviating or delaying the need for liver transplantation. However, these studies showed that clinical benefit takes 3–6 months, and that HCC can occur even among patients with clinical improvement [295–298]. Furthermore, hepatitis flares secondary to drug resistance can lead to a rapid worsening of liver failure.

Predictors of response

Pretreatment serum ALT is the strongest predictor of response among HBeAg-positive patients. Pooled data from four studies with a total of 406 patients who received lamivudine for 1 year found that HBeAg seroconversion occurred in 2%, 9%, 21%, and 47% patients with pretreatment ALT levels within normal, one to two times normal, two to five times normal, and more than five times normal, respectively. The corresponding figures for 196 patients in the placebo group were 0%, 5%, 11%, and 14%, respectively [279]. There are no data on predictors of response to lamivudine treatment of HBeAg-negative patients.

Durability of response

Durability of HBeAg seroconversion has been reported to vary from 50% to 80%. In a follow-up report of patients in the United States and Europe, who completed 1 year of lamivudine treatment, 30 of 39 (77%) patients with HBeAg seroconversion had a durable response after a median follow-up of 37 months (range 5 to 46 months) [299]. In addition, eight (20%) patients developed HBsAg

seroconversion. Some studies reported lower rates of durability [300–303]. Several factors have been identified as being associated with increased durability of HBeAg seroconversion, including longer duration of consolidation treatment (continued treatment after HBeAg seroconversion), younger age, lower HBV DNA level at the time treatment was stopped, and genotype B versus C; the most consistent factor appears to be duration of consolidation treatment [300,302,304]. Although there are no good direct comparison data, it appears that durability of lamivudine-induced HBeAg seroconversion is less than that for IFN.

Among HBeAg-negative patients, durability of virus suppression after 1 year of lamivudine treatment is less than 10%. One study reported that durability of virologic response can be improved to 50% in patients who have completed 2 years treatment [305].

Lamivudine resistance

The selection of lamivudine resistance mutations is the main concern with lamivudine treatment. The most common mutation affects the YMDD motif of the HBV DNA polymerase (methionine to valine or isoleucine M204V/I) [306]. Alanine to threonine or valine substitution at position 181 (A181T/V) has also been shown to be associated with lamivudine resistance but is far less common than the M204V/I mutation. Genotypic resistance can be detected in 14–32% of HBeAg-positive patients after 1 year of lamivudine treatment [284–286] and increases with the duration of treatment to 60–70% after 5 years of treatment [287]. The rates of lamivudine resistance in patients treated for HBeAg-negative chronic hepatitis B varies from 10% to 56% at 2 years [290,292,307]. In vitro studies showed that the M204V/I mutation decreases replication fitness of HBV [308,309], but that compensatory mutations such as leucine to methionine substitution (L180M), valine to leucine substitution (V173L), and changes at L80 selected during continued treatment can restore replication fitness. Therefore, over time, serum HBV DNA levels continue to increase and virologic breakthrough is usually followed by biochemical breakthrough and in some instances hepatitis flares and hepatic decompensation. The frequency of hepatitis flares increases with the duration of lamivudine resistance, from 43% in year 1 to greater than 80% after 3 years [287].

Long-term outcome of lamivudine-treated patients

Follow-up of patients receiving continued lamivudine treatment showed that the rates of maintained virologic and biochemical response decrease with time due to the selection of drug-resistance mutations. As a group, liver histology after 3 years of treatment is improved compared to baseline but histologic benefit after the first year of treatment is negated among patients with virologic breakthrough [299]. Despite increasing rates of breakthrough infection, two studies with a median follow-up of 2–4 years reported that lamivudine treatment decreased the overall rate of hepatic decompensation as well as liver-related mortality [310,311].

Adverse events

In general, lamivudine is very well tolerated. Various adverse events, including a mild (two- to three-fold) increase in ALT level have been reported in patients receiving lamivudine, but these events occurred with the same frequency among the controls.

Dose regimen

The recommended dose for adults with normal renal function and no HIV infection is 100 mg daily PO. Dose reduction is necessary for patients with renal insufficiency. Patients with HIV coinfection should be treated with 150 mg b.i.d. doses in addition to other antiretroviral therapies. The recommended dose for children is 3 mg/kg/day with a maximum dose of 100 mg/day.

Adefovir dipivoxil

Adefovir is a nucleotide analog of adenosine monophosphate. It can inhibit reverse transcriptase as well as DNA polymerase activity. In vitro and clinical studies showed that it is effective in suppressing wild-type as well as lamivudine-resistant HBV.

Efficacy

1 *HBeAg-positive chronic hepatitis.* A phase III clinical trial included 515 patients with compensated liver disease randomized to receive two doses of adefovir (30 or 10 mg daily) or placebo (see Table 24.5) [312]. After 48 weeks of treatment, histologic improvement was observed in 59%, 53%, and 25%, respectively. The proportion of patients with undetectable HBV DNA was 39%, 21%, and 0%, respectively. Normalization of ALT was observed in 55%, 48%, and 16%, whereas HBeAg seroconversion occurred in 14%, 12%, and 6%, respectively. All assessments of response showed a statistical difference between the two treatment groups and the placebo group, and a trend indicating superiority of the 30 mg dose. However, 8% of patients in the 30 mg dose group had nephrotoxicity defined as a reproducible increase in serum creatinine by ≥ 0.5 mg/dL. Cumulative HBeAg seroconversion was estimated to be 48% after 5 years of treatment [313].

2 *HBeAg-negative chronic hepatitis.* A phase III clinical trial included 185 patients with compensated liver disease randomized to receive adefovir 10 mg daily or placebo [314]. After 48 weeks of treatment, patients who received adefovir were more likely to have improve-

ment in liver histology (77% versus 33%), undetectable HBV DNA (51% versus 0%), and normalization of ALT (72% versus 29%) (see Table 24.5). A follow-up report of 70 patients who completed 5 years of continued adefovir treatment showed that serum HBV DNA was undetectable in 53% and ALT normalized in 59% [315].

3 *Lamivudine-resistant HBV.* Clinical trials confirmed that adefovir is effective in suppressing lamivudine-resistant HBV [316,317]. Although adefovir monotherapy has similar antiviral efficacy to combination therapy of adefovir and lamivudine, sequential monotherapy increases the risk of adefovir resistance. In patients with decompensated liver disease, the addition of adefovir has been shown to result in clinical improvement, reduction in risk of recurrent hepatitis B postliver transplant, and possibly increased survival [318,319]. One study included 128 pre- and 196 post-transplant patients [318]. Among the patients who received 48 weeks treatment, 81% of the pre- and 34% of the post-transplant patients had undetectable HBV DNA, and 76% and 49%, respectively, had normalization of ALT. The Child–Turcotte–Pugh score improved in more than 90% of patients in both groups, and 1-year survival was 84% for the pre- and 93% for the post-transplant patients. Follow-up of 226 pretransplant patients showed that viral suppression was maintained in 65% of patients [320].

Predictors of response

Retrospective analyses of data from the two phase III clinical trials showed that HBV DNA reduction was comparable across the four major HBV genotypes (A to D) [226], but an association between adefovir-related HBeAg seroconversion or durability of response and HBV genotypes could not be analyzed because of the small number of responders.

Durability of response and long-term outcome of adefovir-treated patients

Follow-up of 45 patients for a median of 150 weeks off treatment found that HBeAg seroconversion was maintained in 41 (91%) patients. The high rate of durability may be related to a long duration of consolidation treatment [321].

Among HBeAg-negative patients, viral suppression was sustained in only 8% of patients who stopped adefovir after 1 year of treatment [322]. Most patients who continued treatment up to 5 years maintained their response and HBsAg loss was observed in 5% of patients after 4–5 years of continued treatment [315]. Long-term treatment was also associated with a decrease in fibrosis score but HCC developed in 3% of patients. A preliminary report of 33 patients who had received adefovir for

4–5 years and had been followed for up to 5 years after cessation of treatment showed that all patients had virologic relapse initially but 18 patients subsequently had virologic and biochemical remission and nine of these patients later lost HBsAg [323].

Dose regimen

The approved dose of adefovir for adults is 10 mg daily PO. Dose adjustment is necessary in patients with impaired renal function. Although higher doses appeared to have more potent antiviral effect, concerns for nephrotoxicity limit their use in clinical practice. Adefovir at the approved dose of 10 mg daily is ineffective in inhibiting HIV replication.

Adverse events

Adefovir is in general well tolerated. The most worrisome adverse event is nephrotoxicity – an increase in serum creatinine and/or renal tubular defects manifested as hypophosphatemia and Fanconi syndrome. Nephrotoxicity has been reported in 3% of patients with compensated liver disease after 4–5 years of continued adefovir therapy [315], and in 6% of patients on the transplant waiting list, 47% of patients who underwent liver transplantation during the study, and 21% of post-transplant patients after a median of 39–99 weeks of treatment [320]. Concomitant nephrotoxic medications or hepatorenal syndrome may contribute to the higher frequency of nephrotoxicity in post-transplant patients and in patients with decompensated liver disease. Renal function should be monitored in all patients receiving adefovir and dosing intervals should be adjusted in patients with an estimated creatinine clearance of less than 50 mL/min.

Adefovir resistance

Resistance to adefovir was not seen in clinical trials of nucleoside-naïve patients who received 48 weeks of treatment [324]. However, mutations conferring resistance to adefovir (asparagine to threonine substitution N236T and A181V/T substitution) have been described [325,326]. Follow-up of 67 HBeAg-negative patients who participated in the phase III trial found that the cumulative rate of resistance increased from 0% at 1 year to 29% after 5 years of treatment [315]. Risk factors for adefovir resistance include suboptimal virus suppression and sequential monotherapy.

In vitro and human studies showed that adefovir-resistant HBV variants are susceptible to lamivudine, telbivudine, and entecavir. However, in patients with prior lamivudine resistance, a reemergence of lamivudine resistance mutations has been reported shortly after the reintroduction of lamivudine [327].

Entecavir

Entecavir is an orally administered cyclopentyl guanosine analog. In vitro studies showed that entecavir is effective in suppressing lamivudine-resistant HBV but susceptibility is reduced compared to wild-type HBV. Entecavir has also been found to be effective in suppressing adefovir-resistant HBV in in vitro studies.

Efficacy

1 *HBeAg-positive patients.* In a phase III clinical trial 715 patients with compensated liver disease were randomized to receive entecavir 0.5 mg or lamivudine 100 mg daily (see Table 24.5). At week 48, entecavir resulted in statistically higher rates of histologic (72% versus 62%), virologic (67% versus 36%), and biochemical (68% versus 60%) responses compared to lamivudine [328]. However, despite more potent viral suppression (6.9 versus 5.4 $\log_{10}$ copies/mL), HBeAg seroconversion rates were similar in the two groups: 21% versus 18%. In a follow-up report of 146 patients who received entecavir for up to 5 years, the percent of patients with undetectable serum HBV DNA increased from 55% at the end of year 1 to 83% at the end of year 2 and 94% at the end of year 5 [329]. ALT normalization was maintained in 85% of patients at year 5. At the end of year 2, HBeAg seroconversion was observed in 31% and HBsAg loss in 5% of the original cohort of 354 patients. Among the 141 patients who remained HBeAg-positive at the end of year 2, 33 underwent HBeAg seroconversion and two lost HBsAg by year 5 [329]. It should be noted that in this long-term treatment study, a higher dose of entecavir (1.0 mg daily) was used after year 2. A trial of 69 patients found that entecavir resulted in more marked viral suppression than adefovir [330]. Another trial of 139 patients showed that entecavir and telbivudine resulted in a similar decline in serum HBV DNA after 24 weeks of therapy [331].

2 *HBeAg-negative patients.* In a phase III clinical trial, 648 patients with compensated liver disease were randomized to receive entecavir 0.5 mg or lamivudine 100 mg daily. At week 48, entecavir resulted in statistically higher rates of histologic (70% versus 61%), virologic (90% versus 72%), and biochemical (78% versus 71%) responses compared to lamivudine (see Table 24.5) [332].

3 *Decompensated cirrhosis.* Entecavir has been shown to be effective in suppressing HBV replication and in improving the Child–Turcotte–Pugh score and model for endstage liver disease (MELD) score in patients with decompensated cirrhosis [333].

4 *Lamivudine-refractory HBV.* In one study 286 patients, who had persistent viremia while on lamivudine with or without confirmed lamivudine-resistance mutations, were randomized to receive entecavir 1.0 mg or

lamivudine 100 mg daily. At week 48, entecavir resulted in statistically higher rates of histologic (55% versus 28%), virologic (19% versus 1%), and biochemical (61% versus 15%) responses compared to lamivudine, and a nonstatistical difference in rate of HBeAg seroconversion [334]. During continued treatment, genotypic resistance to entecavir increased from 6% in year 1 to 51% in year 5 [335] indicating that entecavir is not an optimal treatment for patients with lamivudine resistance.

Predictors of response

Entecavir appears to be equally effective in decreasing the serum HBV DNA level and in inducing histologic improvement in Asians and whites, and across HBV genotypes A to D. Among HBeAg-positive patients, response rates are lower in patients with minimally elevated ALT. Retrospective analysis of the phase III trial in HBeAg-positive patients found that patients with pretreatment ALT <2 times normal had lower rates of HBeAg seroconversion (8% versus 23%), undetectable serum HBV DNA (48% versus 73%), and normal ALT (55% versus 73%) compared with those with pretreatment ALT >2 times normal [336]. Predictors of response in HBeAg-negative patients have not been determined.

Durability of response

Of the 74 HBeAg-positive patients who lost HBeAg during the first year and who discontinued treatment at week 48, suppression of serum HBV DNA to undetectable levels, normalization of ALT, and HBeAg seroconversion was sustained in 39%, 79%, and 77%, respectively after 24 weeks of follow-up [337]. It should be noted that most of these patients had no or a very short duration of consolidation therapy. Viral suppression was sustained in only 3% of HBeAg-negative patients who stopped treatment at week 48 [338].

Dose regimen

The approved dose for nucleoside-naïve patients is 0.5 mg daily PO and for lamivudine-refractory patients is 1.0 mg daily PO. Doses should be adjusted for patients with an estimated creatinine clearance of less than 50 mL/min.

Adverse events

Entecavir had a similar safety profile including on-treatment ALT flares as lamivudine in clinical trials. Studies in rodents exposed to doses 3–40 times those in humans found an increased incidence of lung adenomas, liver cancers, and brain gliomas [339]. Long-term follow-up studies are ongoing to determine if these observations have relevance to humans. Lactic acidosis has been reported in one case series of patients receiving entecavir for liver failure [340], but lactic acidosis has not been observed in other studies of entecavir in patients with decompensated liver disease and may be a class effect of NUCs.

Entecavir resistance

Resistance to entecavir occurs through a two-hit mechanism with an initial selection of M204V/I mutation followed by amino acid substitutions at rtT184, 202, or 250. In vitro studies showed that mutations at these positions on their own have a minimal effect on susceptibility to entecavir, but susceptibility to entecavir is greatly decreased when one of these mutations is present with M204V/I mutation [341]. Resistance to entecavir is rare in nucleos(t)ide-naïve patients. A report of 108 patients found that only 1.2% of nucleos(t)ide-naïve patients had entecavir resistance after 5 years of treatment [335]; however, it should be noted that the number of patients studied is small and a higher dose (1.0 mg) of entecavir was used during years 3–5. Follow-up of 33 lamivudine-refractory patients found that 51% of patients had evidence of entecavir resistance after 5 years of high-dose (1.0 mg) entecavir treatment [335]. These data are not surprising because the preexisting presence of the M204V/I mutation decreases the barrier to entecavir resistance.

Emtricitabine

Emtricitabine is a potent inhibitor of HBV replication. It selects for the same resistance mutations as lamivudine. In one phase II trial, emtricitabine 200 mg daily resulted in a significantly higher rate of histologic (62% versus 25%), virologic (54% versus 2%), and biochemical (65% versus 25%) responses at week 48 but HBeAg seroconversion rates were identical – 12% in the two groups [342]. Antiviral resistance mutations were detected in 13% of patients who received emtricitabine.

Tenofovir

Tenofovir disoproxil fumarate is a nucleotide analog. It is approved for treatment of HBV infection as Viread® (tenofovir only) and also approved for treatment of HIV infection as Viread or Truvada® (tenofovir + emtricitabine as a single pill). Tenofovir is structurally similar to adefovir. In vitro studies showed that tenofovir and adefovir are equipotent. Because tenofovir appears to be less nephrotoxic, the approved dose is much higher than that of adefovir, 300 mg versus 10 mg daily. This may explain why tenofovir has more potent antiviral activity in clinical studies.

Efficacy

Two phase III trials of tenofovir were conducted, one in HBeAg-positive ($n = 266$) and one in HBeAg-negative ($n = 375$) patients with compensated liver disease. Patients were randomized to receive tenofovir 300 mg or adefovir 10 mg daily in a 2:1 ratio. At week 48, patients in the adefovir group were rolled over to tenofovir treatment. At week 72, patients in both groups with detectable serum HBV DNA received additional treatment with emtricitabine.

1 *HBeAg-positive patients.* At week 48, tenofovir resulted in a significantly higher proportion of patients with undetectable serum HBV DNA (76% versus 13%), ALT normalization (68% versus 54%), and HBsAg loss (3% versus 0%), and similar rates of histologic response (74% versus 68%) and HBeAg seroconversion (21% versus 18%) compared with adefovir (see Table 24.5) [343]. At week 144, 71% of the patients had undetectable serum HBV DNA, 26% had HBeAg seroconversion, and an estimated 8% had HBsAg loss [344].

2 *HBeAg-negative patients.* At week 48, tenofovir resulted in significantly more patients with undetectable serum HBV DNA (93% versus 63%) [343]. ALT normalization (76% versus 77%) and histologic response (72% versus 69%) were similar in the two groups (see Table 24.5). At week 144, 87% of the patients had undetectable serum HBV DNA but none of the patients lost HBsAg [345].

3 *Lamivudine-refractory HBV.* Studies of patients who had previously received treatment with lamivudine showed that tenofovir is effective in suppressing lamivudine-resistant HBV. Case series and retrospective studies suggest that switching from lamivudine to tenofovir monotherapy is sufficient in suppressing lamivudine-resistant HBV [346,347], but larger studies are needed to determine whether resistance to tenofovir will emerge with longer duration of follow-up.

4 *Adefovir-resistant HBV.* In vitro studies showed that adefovir resistance mutations N246T and A181V/T are associated with a three to four-fold decrease in response to tenofovir. Available data indicate that tenofovir is effective in suppressing serum HBV DNA levels in patients with adefovir resistance but viral suppression is less marked compared with nucleos(t)ide-naïve patients and adefovir resistance mutations persist [346,348]. These data indicate that tenofovir is not an appropriate treatment for adefovir-resistant HBV.

Dose regimen

The approved dose of tenofovir is 300 mg orally once daily. The dose should be reduced in patients with an estimated creatinine clearance of <50 mL/min.

Adverse events

Tenofovir is less nephrotoxic than adefovir. However, tenofovir has been occasionally reported to cause Fanconi syndrome and renal insufficiency [352–354]. Almost all of these adverse events occurred in patients with HIV coinfection receiving antiretroviral therapy. A decrease in bone density has also been reported and may be related to increased loss of phosphate through the kidneys [355]. Although the effect appears to be mild and short-lived, the effect on bones is more prominent in children and tenofovir should not be used in children. In the two phase III clinical trials, serum creatinine remained stable over 3 years. Only two patients experienced an increase in serum creatinine ≥ 0.5 mg/dL and four patients (<1%) experienced a reduction in serum phosphorus <2 mg/dL which resolved on continued tenofovir therapy [343].

Tenofovir resistance

Tenofovir-resistant HIV mutations had been reported in patients who received tenofovir for HIV monoinfection. However, there is no corresponding site in the HBV genome. One study reported virologic breakthrough and alanine to threonine substitution (rtA194T) in two patients with HIV/HBV coinfection who had prior lamivudine resistance [349], but the association between this mutation and tenofovir resistance is controversial [350,351]. In vitro and in vivo data indicate that rtA181V/T and rtN236T mutations are associated with a decreased response to tenofovir.

In the two phase III clinical trials, virologic breakthroughs were observed in 2.3% of patients during the first year but tenofovir resistance HBV mutations were not detected in any of these patients [343]. Continued surveillance for up to 3 years did not identify any patient with tenofovir resistance mutations, but patients at the highest risk of antiviral resistance, those in whom serum HBV DNA remained detectable at week 72, received additional treatment with emtricitabine. Therefore, data on resistance to entecavir monotherapy beyond 72 weeks cannot be determined.

Telbivudine

Telbivudine is a nucleoside analog with potent antiviral effects against HBV. However, it is associated with a high rate of drug resistance and selects for the same mutations as lamivudine.

Efficacy

1 *HBeAg-positive patients.* A phase III clinical trial of 921 patients showed that a significantly higher percent of patients who received telbivudine had undetectable HBV DNA compared with those who received lamivudine: 60% versus 40% and 56% versus 39% after 1 and 2 years treatment, respectively (see Table 24.5) [356,357]. Telbivudine also resulted in a significantly higher percent of patients with normalization of ALT: 70% versus 62% at 2 years; but HBeAg seroconversion was similar, 35% versus 29% at 2 years.

2 *HBeAg-negative patients.* In a phase III trial of 446 HBeAg-negative patients, telbivudine resulted in a

higher percent of patients with undetectable HBV DNA compared with those who received lamivudine: 88% versus 71%, and 82% versus 57%, after 1 and 2 years treatment, respectively (see Table 24.5) [356,357]. ALT normalization was observed in a similar percent of patients at 1 and 2 years.

Predictors of response

Patients with undetectable serum HBV DNA by 24 weeks of treatment had significantly higher rates of response and significantly lower rates of antiviral resistance at week 96 compared to patients with HBV DNA $\geq 4 \log_{10}$ copies/mL at week 24. However, a small percent of these rapid responders were noted to have virologic rebound due to drug resistance by week 96 [358].

Dose regimen

The approved dose of telbivudine is 600 mg daily. Doses should be reduced for patients with an estimated creatinine clearance of <50 mL/min.

Adverse events

Telbivudine is well tolerated when used as monotherapy and has a safety profile similar to lamivudine. However, cases of myopathy and peripheral neuropathy have been reported. In the phase III trials, an asymptomatic grade 3 or 4 increase in creatine kinase was observed in 12.9% versus 4.1% of patients after 1 year of telbivudine and lamivudine, respectively [356]. During continued treatment up to year 4, a grade 3 or 4 increase in creatine kinase was observed in 16% and myositis in 0.5% [359]. Telbivudine in combination with pegIFN was associated with a higher rate and an earlier onset of peripheral neuropathy compared with telbivudine monotherapy.

Telbivudine resistance

Mutations associated with telbivudine resistance (rtM204I and rtA181V/T) are similar to those associated with resistance to lamivudine except that rtM204V has not been observed. Telbivudine is associated with a high rate of drug resistance. In the phase III trials, genotypic resistance after 2 years of treatment was observed in 25% of HBeAg-positive and in 11% of HBeAg-negative patients [357].

Clevudine

Clevudine is a pyrimidine nucleoside analog that is effective in inhibiting HBV replication. Clinical trials showed that clevudine in doses of 30 mg daily for up to 24 weeks was well tolerated. Serum HBV DNA became undetectable in 59% of HBeAg-positive and in 92% of HBeAg-negative patients [360,361]. A unique feature of clevudine is the durability of viral suppression, persisting for up to 24 weeks after withdrawal of treatment in some patients. Clevudine selects for the same resistance mutations as lamivudine, rtM204V/I and rtA181V/T. A major problem with clevudine is the occurrence of myopathy, which is related to mitochondrial toxicity, in patients who received treatment for longer than 24 weeks [362,363]. The onset of symptoms has been reported to occur as early as 8 months and usually manifests as proximal muscle weakness, although involvement of the bulbar muscles has also been observed. Global clinical trials and the development of clevudine have been terminated.

Combination therapies

The potential advantages of combination therapies are additive or synergistic antiviral effects, and diminished or delayed resistance. The potential disadvantages of combination therapies are added costs, increased toxicity, and drug interactions. To date, none of the combination therapies evaluated have been proven to be superior to monotherapy in inducing a higher rate of sustained response. Although several combination therapies have been shown to reduce the rate of lamivudine resistance compared with lamivudine monotherapy, there are as yet no data to support the suggestion that combination therapies will reduce the rate of resistance to antiviral agents that have a high genetic barrier to resistance such as entecavir or tenofovir.

Standard or pegylated interferon-α and lamivudine

The combination of IFN-α and lamivudine seems logical because monotherapy with each agent is effective, and IFN-α and lamivudine have different mechanisms of action.

1 *Treatment-naïve patients*. Five large trials (one using standard IFN-α and four using pegIFN-α, four in HBeAg-positive patients and one in HBeAg-negative patients) were conducted comparing a combination of IFN-α and lamivudine to lamivudine alone and/or IFN-α alone [273–276,286]. All studies found that combination therapy had greater on-treatment virus suppression but there was no difference in the sustained off-treatment virologic response compared to IFN-α alone. All studies showed that combination therapy resulted in higher rates of sustained off-treatment response compared to lamivudine alone. Although combination therapy was associated with lower rates of lamivudine resistance compared with lamivudine monotherapy, a low rate of lamivudine resistance was encountered compared to none in patients who received IFN-α alone.

2 *Interferon-α nonresponders*. Combination therapy of standard IFN-α and lamivudine is not more effective than lamivudine alone in the retreatment of IFN-α nonresponders [294].

Lamivudine and adefovir

1 *Nucleosid(t)e naïve patients.* One trial included 115 HBeAg-positive patients randomized to receive a combination of lamivudine and adefovir or lamivudine alone. At week 104, serum HBV DNA was undetectable in 26% versus 14%, ALT normalization in 45% versus 34%, and HBeAg seroconversion in 13% vsersus 20% in patients who received combination therapy and lamivudine monotherapy, respectively (*P* was not significant for all responses) [364]. Genotypic resistance was less common in the patients who received combination therapy, 15%, versus 43% in the patients who received lamivudine monotherapy. These data indicate that a combination of lamivudine and adefovir as de novo therapy does not have additive or synergistic antiviral activity and resistance to lamivudine is decreased but not completely prevented.

2 *Patients with lamivudine-resistance.* One small trial in patients with compensated liver disease showed that a combination of adefovir and lamivudine was not superior to adefovir alone in decreasing serum HBV DNA levels [316]. However, hepatitis flares were less frequent during the transition period in the combination therapy group. Several studies showed that adding adefovir is superior to switching to adefovir for patients with lamivudine-resistant HBV [365,366]. Preliminary data suggest that switching to tenofovir monotherapy may be sufficient in suppressing lamivudine-resistant HBV [346], possibly because it has more potent antiviral activity than adefovir, but long-term efficacy needs to be confirmed.

Lamivudine and telbivudine

One trial conducted in nucleoside-naïve HBeAg-positive patients demonstrated that a combination of lamivudine and telbivudine had no advantage over telbivudine alone [367]. In fact, the combination group showed a trend toward an inferior result in all parameters: virus suppression, ALT normalization, HBeAg seroconversion, and mutations in the YMDD motif. These data suggest that lamivudine and telbivudine, both being L-nucleosides, may antagonize each other by competing for the same binding site on the HBV reverse transcriptase.

Immunomodulatory therapy

Nonspecific immunomodulation is largely ineffective in clearing HBV infection.

Thymosin

Thymic-derived peptides can stimulate T-cell function. Thymosin is well tolerated but data on efficacy are conflicting [368–371]. A meta-analysis that included five controlled trials with a total of 353 patients concluded that patients treated with thymosin were significantly more likely than controls to have a virologic response [372]. The maximal rate of response was not seen until 12 months after discontinuing therapy. Thymosin is approved for the treatment of hepatitis B in some countries, mainly in Asia.

Hepatitis B virus-specific immunomodulation

S and pre-S antigen vaccines

Several uncontrolled trials have reported that vaccines with HBV S with or without pre-S antigens used for the prevention of HBV infection were effective in inducing an anti-HBs response and in decreasing serum HBV DNA levels in patients with chronic hepatitis B [373,374]. These data need to be confirmed in controlled clinical trials.

Deoxyribonucleic acid vaccination

Unlike peptide vaccines, vaccination with plasmid DNA that expresses viral proteins in situ can stimulate not only a B-cell but also a T-cell (both helper and cytotoxic) response. In addition, DNA vaccines lead to more prolonged expression of viral proteins [375]. One pilot study reported that DNA vaccination was effective in activating T-cell response and in decreasing serum HBV DNA levels in patients with chronic HBV infection [376].

T-cell vaccines

Patients with chronic HBV infection have been demonstrated to have an impaired cytotoxic T-lymphocyte (CTL) response to HBV antigens, resulting in ineffective virus clearance. One phase II study showed that CTL response can be stimulated in patients with chronic HBV infection who were inoculated with a vaccine that contained an HLA restricted HBcAg CTL epitope, but the antiviral effect was weak [377].

Recommendations for the treatment of chronic hepatitis B

Current therapy of chronic hepatitis B has limited long-term efficacy. Therefore a, careful balance of patient's age, severity of liver disease, likelihood of response, and potential adverse events is needed before treatment is initiated. Guidelines and recommendations for treatment have been developed by professional societies and at an National Institutes of Health Consensus Conference [378–381]. Table 24.6 summarizes current recommendations on whom to treat and when to start treatment. Because of the fluctuating nature of chronic HBV infection, the risk of liver-related morbidity and mortality and the likelihood of response may vary as a patient progresses through the course of chronic HBV infection. Therefore, continued monitoring is essential for risk assesment.

Table 24.6 Recommended strategies for patients with chronic hepatitis B.

HBeAg	HBV DNA (IU/mL)	ALT[a]	Recommended strategy
+	>20,000	≤2 × ULN	Monitor ALT and HBV DNA levels every 3–6 months Consider biopsy in persons >40 years, ALT 1–2 x ULN, or with family history of HCC Consider treatment if biopsy shows moderate inflammation or advanced fibrosis
+	>20,000	>2 × ULN	Observe for 3–6 months, treat if no spontaneous HBeAg loss Immediate treatment if jaundice or clinical decompensation Duration of treatment: pegIFN, 48 weeks; NUC, until 12 months after HBeAg seroconversion
−	<2,000 2,000–20,000	≤ ULN 1 to >2x ULN	Monitor ALT and HBV DNA every 3–6 months for 1 year, then every 6–12 months Consider biopsy in persons >40 years, ALT > ULN, or with family history of HCC Consider treatment if biopsy shows moderate inflammation or advanced fibrosis
−	>20,000	> ULN	Initiate treatment Duration of treatment: pegIFN, 48 weeks; NUC, until HBsAg loss
+/−		Compensated cirrhosis	HBV DNA <2,000: initiate treatment if ALT elevated HBV DNA >2,000: initiate treatment regardless of ALT Duration of treatment: indefinite or until HBsAg loss
+/−		Decompensated cirrhosis	Refer for liver transplant HBV DNA detectable: initiate treatment regardless of HBV DNA/ALT level

ALT, alanine aminotransferase; HBeAg, hepatitis B e antigen; HBV, hepatitis B virus; HCC, hepatocellular carcinoma; NUC, nucleos(t)ide analog; pegIFN, pegylated interferon; ULN, upper limit of normal.
Adapted from Lok and McMahon [40].

In choosing which antiviral agent to use as initial therapy, consideration should be given to the safety and efficacy of the treatment, duration of treatment needed to achieve the desired response, risks of drug resistance, costs of the treatment, as well as patient preference, and for women – when and whether they plan to start a family. IFN-α is contraindicated in patients with acute liver failure, decompensated cirrhosis, or severe exacerbation of chronic hepatitis B and in patients with medical or psychiatric conditions that may be exacerbated by IFN-α. Other patients may be treated with either IFN-α or NUCs. The advantages of IFN-α treatment include a finite duration of treatment, higher rates of HBeAg and HBsAg loss, and lack of drug resistance, while the disadvantage is the frequent occurrence of adverse events. PegIFN-α is administered for 48 weeks in both HBeAg-positive and HBeAg-negative patients. The advantages of NUCs is the ease of administration and the rare occurrence of adverse events, allowing them to be used in patients with decompensated cirrhosis, severe exacerbations of chronic hepatitis B, or acute liver failure. The disadvantages of NUCs include the risk of drug resistance and the need for long durations of treatment. NUCs are administered indefinitely in patients with cirrhosis. In precirrhotic patients, NUCs are admin-istered until 12 months after HBeAg seroconversion in HBeAg-positive patients and indefinitely or until HBsAg loss in HBeAg-negative patients. Among the approved NUCs, tenofovir and entecavir are preferred because of their potency and high genetic barrier to resistance (low resistance rate).

Patients who failed to respond to IFN may be retreated with NUCs. Patients who failed with NUCs should be tested for antiviral drug resistance mutations, particularly if the patient failed with more than one NUC, to confirm that treatment failure is related to genotypic resistance and to guide selection of rescue therapy. Virologic breakthrough defined as >1 log increase in serum HBV DNA from nadir or redetection of HBV DNA in serum after its initial disappearance, is the first manifestation of antiviral drug resistance and may precede biochemical breakthrough (elevation of ALT after initial normalization) by months to years. Genotypic resistance is defined as the detection of signature antiviral resistance mutations. Rescue therapy should be initiated early, once virologic breakthrough or genotypic resistance is confirmed. Rescue therapy is less effective if treatment is initiated when serum HBV DNA levels are high and compensatory mutations have been selected. Table 24.7 lists the options for rescue therapy.

Table 24.7 Rescue therapy options for antiviral-resistant hepatitis B virus.

Type of resistance	Preferred rescue therapy	Other options
Lamivudine or telbivudine resistance	Tenofovir – add or switch	Add adefovir Switch to tenofovir + emtricitabine
Adefovir	Entecavir – add or switch	Switch to tenofovir + emtricitabine Add lamivudine or telbivudine (if no prior resistance to these two drugs)
Entecavir	Tenofovir – add or switch	Add adefovir

Hepatitis D

Hepatitis D is caused by a defective virus: the hepatitis D virus. Although HDV is often referred to as hepatitis delta virus, the term hepatitis D virus is preferred. HDV can replicate autonomously [382] but the simultaneous presence of HBV is required for complete virion assembly and secretion.

Hepatitis D virus structure and replication

The HDV virion comprises an RNA genome, a single HDV encoded antigen, and a lipoprotein envelope provided by HBV and consisting of the same proteins found in the envelope of the HBV virion. The HDV genome is a small single-stranded circular RNA (1676–1683 nucleotides in size) with structural analogies to plant viroids and a high degree of self-complementarity causing the molecule to collapse into a rod-like structure [383]. Significant sequence heterogeneity exists among HDV isolates and a classification into eight clades has been proposed [384]. The only antigen associated with HDV, the hepatitis D antigen (HDAg), is a structural component of the virion: about 70 molecules of HDAg are complexed with the HDV RNA genome to form a ribonucleoprotein structure (Fig. 24.5) [385]. Hepatocytes are the only host cells where HDV replicates at very high levels [386]. HDV

replicates via transcription into a full-length complementary RNA (antigenomic HDV RNA) [383]. HDV virion assembly and release is dependent on the simultaneous presence of HBV, which provides the envelope proteins.

Patterns of hepatitis D virus infection

Due to its dependence upon HBV, HDV infection always occurs in association with HBV infection. The clinical and laboratory findings vary with the type of infection. *Coinfection of HBV and HDV* in an individual susceptible to HBV infection results in an acute hepatitis clinically indistinguishable from classic acute hepatitis B and is usually self-limited, although a fulminant course has been frequently reported among injection drug users [387]. The rate of progression to chronic infection is similar to that observed after HBV monoinfection [388]. *HDV superinfection* of a chronic HBsAg carrier may present as a severe acute hepatitis in a HBV carrier, or as an exacerbation of preexisting chronic hepatitis B. Progression to persistent HDV infection is typical [389].

Epidemiology

Data on HDV epidemiology have mostly been gathered in HBV carriers superinfected with HDV. It was estimated that approximately 5% of the HBV carriers worldwide may be infected with HDV [390]. However, substantial changes in HDV epidemiology have occurred in the past decades. Improvements in socioeconomic conditions, an increased awareness of the risk of transmitting infectious diseases fostered by AIDS prevention policy, and aggressive vaccination campaigns against HBV have all contributed to a dramatic decrease in the incidence of HBV infection and the spread of HDV infection [391–394]. HDV prevalence, however, stopped decreasing at the end of the 1990s, at least in Europe, where it has remained mostly stable [395]. This is partly due to an increased immigration from endemic regions (such as eastern Europe or the Middle East), although intravenous drug use, high-risk sexual practices, and body modification procedures may also play a role. In general, although HDV infection is dependent on HBV infection, the geographic distribution of HDV infection does not parallel

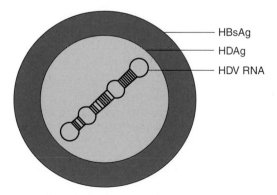

Figure 24.5 Schematic representation of the hepatitis D virus (HDV) virion with extensive intramolecular base pairing of the HDV RNA genome. HBsAg, hepatitis B surface antigen; HDAg, hepatitis D antigen.

HBsAg
HDAg
HDV RNA

that of HBV, as areas endemic for HBV may be almost HDV-free. The level of HDV endemicity is only partially related to the route of transmission. Sexual transmission of HDV is less frequent than in the case of HBV infection, especially among male homosexuals [396].

Diagnosis

Hepatitis D antigen elicits a specific immune response consisting of antibodies of the IgM and IgG class (anti-HDV). In HDV-infected individuals, the timing of appearance and level of HDV RNA, HDAg, and anti-HDV in serum, together with the pattern of HBV markers, allow three HDV-related clinical entities to be identified: acute HBV/HDV coinfection, acute HDV superinfection of a chronic HBV carrier, and chronic HDV infection (Table 24.8). Due to the dependence of HDV on HBV, the presence of HBsAg is necessary for the diagnosis of HDV infection. The additional presence of IgM antibody to hepatitis B core antigen (IgM anti-HBc) is necessary for the diagnosis of acute HBV/HDV coinfection.

In acute HDV infection, serum HDAg appears early and is short-lived and may escape detection [397]. Total anti-HDV antibody appears late in acute infection, and repeated testing is recommended since anti-HDV seroconversion may be the only way to diagnose acute HDV infection in the absence of other markers of HDV infection [397,398]. Anti-HDV of the IgM class is transient and delayed if the course of acute hepatitis D is self-limited, but is of high titer and long-lasting if HDV infection progresses to chronicity. Although it may be the only serum marker of acute HDV infection [397], anti-HDV IgM lacks specificity since it is usually found at high titers in chronic hepatitis D. As discussed above, differentiation between HBV/HDV coinfection and HDV superinfection in an HBV carrier depends on the detection of high-titer IgM anti-HBc, found only in patients with coinfection.

The development of anti-HDV hampers the detection of HDAg further along the course of infection, due to the formation of immune complexes. The most sensitive way to diagnose active HDV infection is the detection of HDV

RNA in serum by reverse transcriptase-polymerase chain reaction (RT-PCR) [399,400]. HDV RNA is an early and sensitive marker of HDV replication in acute hepatitis D [401] and confirms infection in chronic hepatitis D. Furthermore, quantitative determination of HDV RNA is the test of choice for measuring HDV replication in patients undergoing antiviral treatment [402]. Although the detection of intrahepatic HDAg by immunohistochemistry was formerly proposed as the gold standard for the diagnosis of ongoing HDV infection [403], the detection of HDV RNA in serum by RT-PCR is more sensitive, especially during late stages of the disease.

In summary, HDV coinfection should be suspected in patients with acute hepatitis B at high risk of blood-borne infection, such as in intravenous drug users, in persons from HDV endemic countries, or in those presenting a severe course. Coinfected patients have high-titer IgM anti-HBc. Markers of HBV replication may precede or follow those of HDV. Occasionally, patients may have already seroconverted to anti-HBs, e.g., at the time of the second phase of a biphasic hepatitis. These patients should still be positive for IgM anti-HBc. Serum HDV RNA is usually positive at presentation, but if this assay is not available total anti-HDV should be repeatedly tested to document seroconversion.

In acute hepatitis of undetermined origin in an HBV carrier, tests for HDV should be considered to rule out HDV superinfection. Since HDV superinfection may occur in previously unrecognized HBV carriers, distinguishing between this condition and acute HBV/HDV coinfection may be difficult.

Testing for HDV should also be carried out in patients with chronic hepatitis B, who live or have lived in HDV endemic countries or who are at high risk of HDV infection, to rule out simultaneous chronic HDV infection. This is best achieved by screening for total anti-HDV antibody and then confirmed by staining for HDAg in liver tissues and/or measurement of serum HDV RNA. In chronic HDV infection, HBV replication is usually suppressed, and patients are typically anti-HBe-positive.

Table 24.8 Diagnosis of hepatitis D virus (HDV) infection.

	Acute HDV/HBV coinfection	HDV superinfection of HBV carrier	Chronic HDV infection
HDAg	Early and short-lived	Early, but soon masked by anti-HDV	Undetectable (masked by antibodies)
Anti-HDV, IgM	Transient and delayed	High titer and long-lasting	High titer
Anti-HDV, IgG	Late, increasing titers	Late, increasing titers	High titer
HDV RNA	Early and sensitive marker	Early and sensitive marker	Usually high level
IgM anti-HBc	Positive	Negative	Negative

anti-HBc, hepatitis B core antibody; HBV, hepatitis B virus; HDAg, hepatitis D antigen; IgG, immunoglobulin G; IgM, immunoglobulin M.

Pathogenesis and natural history

The mechanisms by which HDV induces liver damage (referred to as hepatitis D) are unknown, but are largely thought to be due to the host immune response [383].

The clinical sequelae of HDV infection encompass a spectrum of manifestations from fulminant liver failure to an asymptomatic carrier state. In general, HDV super-infection has been associated with an accelerated progression of liver disease, with an increased risk of HCC [404].

Overall, the degree of expression of HDV-related liver disease depends on the interplay of HDV-associated (such as HDV genotype), host-associated (such as immune response), and helper virus-associated (such as HBV genotype and replication level) factors. The HDV genotype seems important since infection with genotype 3, which is predominant in South America, induces a particularly severe acute hepatitis with high risk of liver failure [405]. On the other hand, genotype 2, which prevails in the Far East, is infrequently associated with a fulminant course; likewise, chronic hepatitis D with this genotype seems less progressive [406]. The HBV genotype has been shown to affect HDV RNA levels and to correlate with outcome [407,408]. Finally, high levels of HBV replication are associated with more severe liver damage in persons coinfected with HDV [409].

Treatment

The primary endpoint of treatment is the suppression of HDV replication, which is accompanied by normalization of ALT level and amelioration of hepatic necroinflammatory activity. Undetectable HDV RNA in serum and HDAg in the liver document the suppression of HDV replication. A secondary, albeit rarely observed, endpoint is the eradication of HBV infection, with HBsAg to anti-HBs seroconversion.

The only drug effective in the treatment of chronic hepatitis D is IFN-α. The mechanism of action of IFN-α in hepatitis D is unclear. In vitro studies showed that IFN-α does not have antiviral activity against HDV [410,411]. HDV directly interferes with the early steps of the IFN-α signaling pathway [412]. Thus, the efficacy of IFN-α in patients with chronic hepatitis D may depend on its antiviral activity on HBV or on immune modulatory effects. The total number of chronic hepatitis D patients who have been treated with IFN-α (both standard and pegylated) and reported in the literature is small. Thus, it is difficult to draw firm conclusions on the efficacy, optimal dose regimen, and factors predictive of response to IFN-α.

In early clinical trials using standard IFN-α, the results were rather disappointing. In a large multicenter study, 61 Italian patients with chronic hepatitis D were randomly assigned to receive IFN-α in doses of 5 MU/m^2 body surface area three times a week (t.i.w.) for 4 months, followed by 3 MU/m^2 t.i.w. for an additional 8 months, or placebo [413]. At the end of follow-up, the proportion of patients with undetectable HDV RNA was similar in the two groups (45% versus 33%). Likewise, liver histology also improved with similar frequency in the two groups (57% versus 36%; P, not significant). In another study, 42 patients with chronic hepatitis D were randomly assigned to receive two different doses (9 MU versus 3 MU t.i.w.) of IFN-α for 48 weeks or placebo [414]. Complete response (normal ALT level and undetectable serum HDV RNA at the end of treatment) was more frequent in the 9 MU group (50%, 21%, and 0% in the three arms, respectively). Treatment with 9 MU doses of IFN-α was associated with a marked improvement in liver histology. However, none of the patients had sustained clearance of HDV RNA. A follow-up report found that ALT normalization correlated with improved hepatic function [415]. Compared to treatment with low-dose IFN-α or placebo, those who received high dose IFN-α were more likely to have a sustained decrease in serum HDV RNA levels, and some patients had HDV clearance. Patients in the high-dose group were also more likely to have improvement in histologic activity and fibrosis and survival.

More recent work has evaluated the efficacy of pegIFN-α. Response rates seem more encouraging in comparison with standard IFN-α. One study found that some nonresponders to standard IFN-α cleared HDV RNA when retreated with a 6-month course of pegIFN-α [416]. Nonetheless, pegIFN-α is still insufficient to cure most chronic hepatitis D patients. In a prospective trial from Italy, 38 patients received 48 weeks of pegIFN-α2b (1.5 μg/kg/week) with or without ribavirin, followed by another 24 weeks of pegIFN-α alone. At the end of follow-up, only 21% of patients had undetectable HDV RNA and 26% had a biochemical response [417]. In a small trial from France, a sustained virologic response was achieved in six of 14 patients (43%) treated for 12 months with pegIFN-α2b (1.5 μg/kg/week) [402]. Another small study from Germany showed a sustained virologic response in merely two of 12 patients (17%) [418]. This work suggested also a treatment futility rule for patients with a less than 3 log decrease of serum HDV RNA after 6 months of treatment. A negative pre-treatment predictor of response seems to be the presence of cirrhosis. A recent large trial compared 32 patients who received pegIFN-α2a plus adefovir, 29 patients who received pegIFN-α2a plus placebo, and 30 patients who received adefovir alone for 48 weeks [419]. At week 48, HDV RNA was undetectable in 23%, 24%, and 0%, in these three groups, respectively. The efficacy of pegIFN was sustained for 24 weeks after treatment; HDV RNA was undetectable in 28% of patients who received pegIFN with or without adefovir and none of those who received adefovir alone.

These data confirmed the efficacy of pegIFN in suppressing HDV replication. NUCs active against HBV replication have no effect on HDV replication and do not have additive effects when combined with pegIFN [419, 420,421].

Prevention

The mainstay of prevention of HDV infection is vaccination against its helper virus, HBV. Anti-HBs-positive chimpanzees have been successfully vaccinated against experimental HDV infection [422]. However, passive prophylaxis with HBIg has not completely prevented reinfection of transplanted livers by HDV.

Annotated references

Beasley RP. Hepatitis B virus. The major etiology of hepatocellular carcinoma. *Cancer* 1988;61:1942–56.
Elegant review article providing convincing evidence of the etiologic association between chronic HBV infection and HCC.

Beasley RP, Hwang LY, Lee GC, et al. Prevention of perinatally transmitted hepatitis B virus infections with hepatitis B immune globulin and hepatitis B vaccine. *Lancet* 1983;2:1099–102.
Seminal study demonstrating the efficacy of HBV vaccine and HBIg in preventing perinatal transmission of HBV infection.

Chang MH, Chen CJ, Lai MS, et al. Universal hepatitis B vaccination in Taiwan and the incidence of hepatocellular carcinoma in children. Taiwan Childhood Hepatoma Study Group. *N Engl J Med* 1997;336:1855–9.
Study demonstrating the efficacy of HBV vaccine in preventing HCC.

Chang TT, Gish R, de Man R, et al. A comparison of entecavir and lamivudine for HBeAg-positive chronic hepatitis B. *N Engl J Med* 2006;354:1001–10.
Phase III trial comparing the responses to 48 weeks of entecavir versus lamivudine therapy in patients with HBeAg-positive chronic hepatitis B.

Chen CJ, Yang HI, Su J, et al. Risk of hepatocellular carcinoma across a biological gradient of serum hepatitis B virus DNA level. *JAMA* 2006;295:65–73.
Cohort study demonstrating the association between serum HBV DNA level and risk of HCC.

Fattovich G, Bortolotti F, Donato F. Natural history of chronic hepatitis B: special emphasis on disease progression and prognostic factors. *J Hepatol* 2008;48:335–52.
Comprehensive review of the natural history of chronic HBV infection.

Lai CL, Shouval D, Lok AS, et al. Entecavir versus lamivudine for patients with HBeAg-negative chronic hepatitis B. *N Engl J Med* 2006;354:1011–20.
Phase III trial comparing the responses to 48 weeks of entecavir versus lamivudine therapy in patients with HBeAg-negative chronic hepatitis B.

Lau GK, Piratvisuth T, Luo KX, et al. Peginterferon alfa-2a, lamivudine, and the combination for HBeAg-positive chronic hepatitis B. *N Engl J Med* 2005;352(26):2682–95.
Phase III trial comparing responses to a 48-week course of pegylated interferon + lamivudine to pegylated interferon monotherapy and lamivudine monotherapy for the treatment of HBeAg-positive chronic hepatitis B.

Liaw YF, Sung JJ, Chow WC, et al. Lamivudine for patients with chronic hepatitis B and advanced liver disease. *N Engl J Med* 2004;351:1521–31.
Seminal study demonstrating the efficacy of antiviral therapy in preventing clinical outcomes in patients with advanced chronic hepatitis B.

Lok AS, McMahon BJ. Chronic hepatitis B. *Hepatology* 2007;45:507–39.
American Association for the Study of Liver Diseases guidelines for the management of hepatitis B.

Marcellin P, Heathcote EJ, Buti M, et al. Tenofovir disoproxil fumarate versus adefovir dipivoxil for chronic hepatitis B. *N Engl J Med* 2008;359:2442–55.
Phase III clinical trial comparing responses to 48-week treatment of tenofovir versus adefovir in HBeAg-positive and in HBeAg-negative patients.

Marcellin P, Lau GK, Bonino F, et al. Peginterferon alfa-2a alone, lamivudine alone, and the two in combination in patients with HBeAg-negative chronic hepatitis B. *N Engl JMed* 2004;351(12):1206–17.
Phase III trial comparing the responses to a 48-week course of pegylated interferon + lamivudine to pegylated interferon monotherapy and lamivudine monotherapy for the treatment of HBeAg-negative chronic hepatitis B.

Mast EE, Margolis HS, Fiore AE, et al. A comprehensive immunization strategy to eliminate transmission of hepatitis B virus infection in the United States: recommendations of the Advisory Committee on Immunization Practices (ACIP) Part 1: immunization of infants, children, and adolescents. *MMWR Recomm Rep* 2005;54:1–31.
Centers for Disease Control and Prevention recommendations on HBV vaccination.

Mast EE, Weinbaum CM, Fiore AE, et al. A comprehensive immunization strategy to eliminate transmission of hepatitis B virus infection in the United States: recommendations of the Advisory Committee on Immunization Practices (ACIP) Part II: immunization of adults. *MMWR Recomm Rep* 2006;55:1–33.
Centers for Disease Control and Prevention recommendations on HBV vaccination.

Yim HJ, Lok AS. Natural history of chronic hepatitis B virus infection: what we knew in 1981 and what we know in 2005. *Hepatology* 2006;43:S173–81.
Comprehensive review of the natural history of chronic HBV infection.

References

1. Lavanchy D. Chronic viral hepatitis as a public health issue in the world. *Best Pract Res Clin Gastroenterol* 2008;22:991–1008.
2. Centers for Disease Control and Prevention, http://www.cdc.gov/hepatitis/statistics.htm, accessed July 2010.
3. Lok AS, Lai CL, Wu PC, et al. Hepatitis B virus infection in Chinese families in Hong Kong. *Am J Epidemiol* 1987;126:492–9.
4. Botha JF, Ritchie MJ, Dusheiko GM, et al. Hepatitis B virus carrier state in black children in Ovamboland: role of perinatal and horizontal infection. *Lancet* 1984;1:1210–12.
5. Stevens CE, Beasley RP, Tsui J, et al. Vertical transmission of hepatitis B antigen in Taiwan. *N Engl J Med* 1975;292:771–4.
6. Beasley RP, Hwang LY, Lin CC, et al. Incidence of hepatitis B virus infections in preschool children in Taiwan. *J Infect Dis* 1982;146:198–204.
7. Coursaget P, Yvonnet B, Chotard J, et al. Age- and sex-related study of hepatitis B virus chronic carrier state in infants from an endemic area (Senegal). *J Med Virol* 1987;22:1–5.
8. Tassopoulos NC, Papaevangelou GJ, Sjogren MH, et al. Natural history of acute hepatitis B surface antigen-positive hepatitis in Greek adults. *Gastroenterology* 1987;92:1844–50.
9. Zou S, Stramer SL, Notari EP, et al. Current incidence and residual risk of hepatitis B infection among blood donors in the United States. *Transfusion* 2009;49:1609–20.
10. Shang G, Seed CR, Wang F, et al. Residual risk of transfusion-transmitted viral infections in Shenzhen, China, 2001 through 2004. *Transfusion* 2007;47:529–39.
11. Busch MP. Should HBV DNA NAT replace HBsAg and/or anti-HBc screening of blood donors? *Transfus Clin Biol* 2004;11:26–32.
12. Incidence of acute hepatitis B – United States, 1990–2002. *MMWR* 2004;52:1252–4.

13. Alter MJ, Hadler SC, Margolis HS, et al. The changing epidemiology of hepatitis B in the United States. Need for alternative vaccination strategies. *JAMA* 1990;263:1218–22.

14. Stevens CE, Toy PT, Tong MJ, et al. Perinatal hepatitis B virus transmission in the United States. Prevention by passive–active immunization. *JAMA* 1985;253:1740–5.

15. Wiseman E, Fraser MA, Holden S, et al. Perinatal transmission of hepatitis B virus: an Australian experience. *Med J Aust* 2009;190:489–92.

16. Wong VC, Ip HM, Reesink HW, et al. Prevention of the HBsAg carrier state in newborn infants of mothers who are chronic carriers of HBsAg and HBeAg by administration of hepatitis-B vaccine and hepatitis-B immunoglobulin. Double-blind randomised placebo-controlled study. *Lancet* 1984;1:921–6.

17. Giraud P, Drouet J, Dupuy JM. Hepatitis-B virus infection of children born to mothes with severe hepatitis [Letter]. *Lancet* 1975;2:1088–9.

18. Beasley RP, Stevens CE, Shiao IS, et al. Evidence against breast-feeding as a mechanism for vertical transmission of hepatitis B. *Lancet* 1975;2:740–1.

19. Towers CV, Asrat T, Rumney P. The presence of hepatitis B surface antigen and deoxyribonucleic acid in amniotic fluid and cord blood. *Am J Obstet Gyn* 2001;184:1514–18; discussion 1518–20.

20. Chang M, You S, Chen C, et al. Decreased incidence of hepatocellular carcinoma in hepatitis B vaccinees: a 20-year follow-up study. *J Natl Cancer Inst* 2009;101:1348–55.

21. Gerberding JL. The infected health care provider [Letter; comment]. *N Engl J Med* 1996;334:594–5.

22. Thompson ND, Perz JF, Moorman AC, et al. Nonhospital health care-associated hepatitis B and C virus transmission: United States, 1998–2008. *Ann Intern Med* 2009;150:33–9.

23. Harpaz R, Von Seidlein L, Averhoff FM, et al. Transmission of hepatitis B virus to multiple patients from a surgeon without evidence of inadequate infection control. *N Engl J Med* 1996;334:549–54 (see comments).

24. Henderson DK, Dembry L, Fishman NO, et al. SHEA guideline for management of healthcare workers who are infected with hepatitis B virus, hepatitis C virus, and/or human immunodeficiency virus. *Infect Control Hosp Epidemiol* 2010;31:203–32.

25. Gunson RN, Shouval D, Roggendorf M, et al. Hepatitis B virus (HBV) and hepatitis C virus (HCV) infections in health care workers (HCWs): guidelines for prevention of transmission of HBV and HCV from HCW to patients. *J Clin Virol* 2003;27: 213–30.

26. Finelli L, Miller JT, Tokars JI, et al. National surveillance of dialysis-associated diseases in the United States, 2002. *Semin Dial* 2005;18:52–61.

27. Minuk GY, Sun DF, Greenberg R, et al. Occult hepatitis B virus infection in a North American adult hemodialysis patient population. *Hepatology* 2004;40:1072–7.

28. Fabrizi F, Messa PG, Lunghi G, et al. Occult hepatitis B virus infection in dialysis patients: a multicentre survey. *Aliment Pharmacol Ther* 2005;21:1341–7.

29. Hoft RH, Pflugfelder SC, Forster RK, et al. Clinical evidence for hepatitis B transmission resulting from corneal transplantation. *Cornea* 1997;16:132–7 (see comments).

30. Turner DP, Zuckerman M, Alexander GJ, et al. Risk of inappropriate exclusion of organ donors by introduction of hepatitis B core antibody testing. *Transplantation* 1997;63:775–7.

31. Caldwell SH. Hard times and imperfect organs. *Liver Trans Surg* 1997;3:181–4.

32. Wachs ME, Amend WJ, Ascher NL, et al. The risk of transmission of hepatitis B from HBsAg(–), HBcAb(+), HBIgM(–) organ donors. *Transplantation* 1995;59:230–4.

33. Dickson RC, Everhart JE, Lake JR, et al. Transmission of hepatitis B by transplantation of livers from donors positive for antibody to hepatitis B core antigen. The National Institute of Diabetes and Digestive and Kidney Diseases Liver Transplantation Database. *Gastroenterology* 1997;113:1668–74.

34. Douglas DD, Rakela J, Wright TL, et al. The clinical course of transplantation-associated de novo hepatitis B infection in the liver transplant recipient. *Liver Trans Surg* 1997;3:105–11.

35. Zou S, Dodd RY, Stramer SL, et al. Probability of viremia with HBV, HCV, HIV, and HTLV among tissue donors in the United States. *N Engl J Med* 2004;351:751–9.

36. Scott RM, Snitbhan R, Bancroft WH, et al. Experimental transmission of hepatitis B virus by semen and saliva. *J Infect Dis* 1980;142:67–71.

37. Bancroft WH, Snitbhan R, Scott RM, et al. Transmission of hepatitis B virus to gibbons by exposure to human saliva containing hepatitis B surface antigen. *J Infect Dis* 1977;135:79–85.

38. Daniels D, Grytdal S, Wasley A. Surveillance for acute viral hepatitis – United States, 2007. *MMWR Surveill Summ* 2009;58:1–27.

39. Mast EE, Weinbaum CM, Fiore AE, et al. A comprehensive immunization strategy to eliminate transmission of hepatitis B virus infection in the United States: recommendations of the Advisory Committee on Immunization Practices (ACIP) Part II: immunization of adults. *MMWR Recomm Rep* 2006;55:1–33.

40. Lok AS, McMahon BJ. Practice Guidelines: chronic hepatitis B. *Hepatology* 2007;45:507–39.

41. Beasley RP, Hwang LY, Lee GC, et al. Prevention of perinatally transmitted hepatitis B virus infections with hepatitis B virus infections with hepatitis B immune globulin and hepatitis B vaccine. *Lancet* 1983;2:1099–102.

42. Mast EE, Margolis HS, Fiore AE, et al. A comprehensive immunization strategy to eliminate transmission of hepatitis B virus infection in the United States: recommendations of the Advisory Committee on Immunization Practices (ACIP) Part 1: immunization of infants, children, and adolescents. *MMWR Recomm Rep* 2005;54:1–31.

43. Szmuness W, Stevens CE, Harley EJ, et al. Hepatitis B vaccine: demonstration of efficacy in a controlled clinical trial in a high-risk population in the United States. *N Engl J Med* 1980;303:833–41.

44. Francis DP, Hadler SC, Thompson SE, et al. The prevention of hepatitis B with vaccine. Report of the centers for disease control multi-center efficacy trial among homosexual men. *Ann Intern Med* 1982;97:362–6.

45. Goilav C, Piot P. Vaccination against hepatitis B in homosexual men. A review. *Am J Med* 1989;87:S21–5.

46. Poovorawan Y, Sanpavat S, Pongpunlert W, et al. Comparison of a recombinant DNA hepatitis B vaccine alone or in combination with hepatitis B immune globulin for the prevention of perinatal acquisition of hepatitis B carriage. *Vaccine* 1990;8(Suppl):S56–9; discussion S60–2.

47. Alper CA, Kruskall MS, Marcus-Bagley D, et al. Genetic prediction of nonresponse to hepatitis B vaccine. *N Engl J Med* 1989;321:708–12 (see comments).

48. Godkin A, Davenport M, Hill AV. Molecular analysis of HLA class II associations with hepatitis B virus clearance and vaccine nonresponsiveness. *Hepatology* 2005;41:1383–90.

49. Floreani A, Baldo V, Cristofoletti M, et al. Long-term persistence of anti-HBs after vaccination against HBV: an 18 year experience in health care workers. *Vaccine* 2004;22:607–10.

50. Lu CY, Chiang BL, Chi WK, et al. Waning immunity to plasma-derived hepatitis B vaccine and the need for boosters 15 years after neonatal vaccination. *Hepatology* 2004;40:1415–20.

51. McMahon BJ, Bruden DL, Petersen KM, et al. Antibody levels and protection after hepatitis B vaccination: results of a 15-year follow-up. *Ann Intern Med* 2005;142:333–41.

52. Boxall EH, Sira A, El-Shuhkri N, et al. Long-term persistence of immunity to hepatitis B after vaccination during infancy in a country where endemicity is low. *J Infect Dis* 2004;190:1264–9.

53. Jan CF, Huang KC, Chien YC, et al. Determination of immune memory to hepatitis B vaccination through early booster response in college students. *Hepatology* 2010;51:1547–54.

54. Salleras L, Dominguez A, Bruguera M, et al. Dramatic decline in acute hepatitis B infection and disease incidence rates among adolescents and young people after 12 years of a mass hepatitis B vaccination programme of pre-adolescents in the schools of Catalonia (Spain). *Vaccine* 2005;23:2181–4.

55. Chang MH, Chen CJ, Lai MS, et al. Universal hepatitis B vaccination in Taiwan and the incidence of hepatocellular carcinoma in children. *Taiwan Childhood Hepatoma Study Group. N Engl J Med* 1997;336:1855–9 (see comments).

56. Ni YH, Huang LM, Chang MH, et al. Two decades of universal hepatitis B vaccination in Taiwan: impact and implication for future strategies. *Gastroenterology* 2007;132:1287–93.

57. Ayoola EA, Johnson AO. Hepatitis B vaccine in pregnancy: immunogenicity, safety and transfer of antibodies to infants. *Int J Gynaecol Obstet* 1987;25:297–301.

58. Levy M, Koren G. Hepatitis B vaccine in pregnancy: maternal and fetal safety. *Am J Perinatol* 1991;8:227–32.

59. McMahon BJ, Helminiak C, Wainwright RB, et al. Frequency of adverse reactions to hepatitis B vaccine in 43,618 persons. *Am J Med* 1992;92:254–6.

60. Niu MT, Davis DM, Ellenberg S. Recombinant hepatitis B vaccination of neonates and infants: emerging safety data from the Vaccine Adverse Event Reporting System. *Ped Infect Dis J* 1996;15:771–6.

61. Ascherio A, Zhang SM, Hernan MA, et al. Hepatitis B vaccination and the risk of multiple sclerosis. *N Engl J Med* 2001;344:327–32 (see comments).

62. Confavreux C, Suissa S, Saddier P, et al. Vaccinations and the risk of relapse in multiple sclerosis. Vaccines in Multiple Sclerosis Study Group. *N Engl J Med* 2001;344:319–26 (see comments).

63. Lok AS, Lai CL, Wu PC. Prevalence of isolated antibody to hepatitis B core antigen in an area endemic for hepatitis B virus infection: implications in hepatitis B vaccination programs. *Hepatology* 1988;8:766–70.

64. Reiss G, Keeffe EB. Review article: hepatitis vaccination in patients with chronic liver disease. *Aliment Pharmacol Ther* 2004;19: 715–27.

65. Chalasani N, Smallwood G, Halcomb J, et al. Is vaccination against hepatitis B infection indicated in patients waiting for or after orthotopic liver transplantation? *Liver Trans Surg* 1998;4:128–32.

66. Dominguez M, Barcena R, Garcia M, et al. Vaccination against hepatitis B virus in cirrhotic patients on liver transplant waiting list. *Liver Transpl* 2000;6:440–2.

67. Fonseca MO, Pang LW, de Paula Cavalheiro N, et al. Randomized trial of recombinant hepatitis B vaccine in HIV-infected adult patients comparing a standard dose to a double dose. *Vaccine* 2005;23:2902–8.

68. Mallet E, Belohradsky BH, Lagos R, et al. A liquid hexavalent combined vaccine against diphtheria, tetanus, pertussis, poliomyelitis, *Haemophilus influenzae* type B and hepatitis B: review of immunogenicity and safety. *Vaccine* 2004;22:1343–57.

69. Zepp F, Knuf M, Heininger U, et al. Safety, reactogenicity and immunogenicity of a combined hexavalent tetanus, diphtheria, acellular pertussis, hepatitis B, inactivated poliovirus vaccine and *Haemophilus influenzae* type b conjugate vaccine, for primary immunization of infants. *Vaccine* 2004;22:2226–33.

70. Traquina P, Morandi M, Contorni M, et al. MF59 adjuvant enhances the antibody response to recombinant hepatitis B surface antigen vaccine in primates. *J Infect Dis* 1996;174:1168–75.

71. Vandepapeliere P, Rehermann B, Koutsoukos M, et al. Potent enhancement of cellular and humoral immune responses against recombinant hepatitis B antigens using AS02A adjuvant in healthy adults. *Vaccine* 2005;23:2591–601.

72. Aguilar JC, Lobaina Y, Muzio V, et al. Development of a nasal vaccine for chronic hepatitis B infection that uses the ability of hepatitis B core antigen to stimulate a strong Th1 response against hepatitis B surface antigen. *Immunol Cell Biol* 2004;82: 539–46.

73. Raz R, Dagan R, Gallil A, et al. Safety and immunogenicity of a novel mammalian cell-derived recombinant hepatitis B vaccine containing Pre-S1 and Pre-S2 antigens in children. *Vaccine* 1996;14:207–11.

74. Zuckerman JN, Zuckerman AJ, Symington I, et al. Evaluation of a new hepatitis B triple-antigen vaccine in inadequate responders to current vaccines. *Hepatology* 2001;34:798–802.

75. Rahman F, Dahmen A, Herzog-Hauff S, et al. Cellular and humoral immune responses induced by intradermal or intramuscular vaccination with the major hepatitis B surface antigen. *Hepatology* 2000;31:521–7.

76. Blumberg BS, Alter HJ, Visnich S. A "new" antigen in leukemia sera. *JAMA* 1965;191:541–6.

77. Norder H, Courouce AM, Magnius LO. Complete genomes, phylogenetic relatedness, and structural proteins of six strains of the hepatitis B virus, four of which represent two new genotypes. *Virology* 1994;198:489–503.

78. Schaefer S, Magnius L, Norder H. Under construction: classification of hepatitis B virus genotypes and subgenotypes. *Intervirology* 2009;52:323–5.

79. Szmuness W, Stevens CE, Harley EJ, et al. Hepatitis B vaccine in medical staff of hemodialysis units: efficacy and subtype cross-protection. *N Engl J Med* 1982;307:1481–6.

80. Tsang TK, Blei AT, O'Reilly DJ, et al. Clinical significance of concurrent hepatitis B surface antigen and antibody positivity. *Dig Dis Sci* 1986;31:620–4.

81. Theilmann L, Klinkert MQ, Gmelin K, et al. Detection of pre-S1 proteins in serum and liver of HBsAg-positive patients: a new marker for hepatitis B virus infection. *Hepatology* 1986;6:186–90.

82. Budkowska A, Dubreuil P, Capel F, et al. Hepatitis B virus pre-S gene-encoded antigenic specificity and anti-pre-S antibody: relationship between anti-pre-S response and recovery. *Hepatology* 1986;6:360–8.

83. Perrillo RP, Chau KH, Overby LR, et al. Anti-hepatitis B core immunoglobulin M in the serologic evaluation of hepatitis B virus infection and simultaneous infection with type B, delta agent, and non-A, non-B viruses. *Gastroenterology* 1983;85:163–7.

84. Maruyama T, Schodel F, Iino S, et al. Distinguishing between acute and symptomatic chronic hepatitis B virus infection. *Gastroenterology* 1994;106:1006–15.

85. Chu CM, Liaw YF, Pao CC, et al. The etiology of acute hepatitis superimposed upon previously unrecognized asymptomatic HBsAg carriers. *Hepatology* 1989;9:452–6.

86. Sjogren M, Hoofnagle JH. Immunoglobulin M antibody to hepatitis B core antigen in patients with chronic type B hepatitis. *Gastroenterology* 1985;89:252–8.

87. Hadler SC, Murphy BL, Schable CA, et al. Epidemiological analysis of the significance of low-positive test results for antibody to hepatitis B surface and core antigens. *J Clin Microbiol* 1984;19: 521–5.

88. Joller-Jemelka HI, Wicki AN, Grob PJ. Detection of HBs antigen in "anti-HBc alone" positive sera. *J Hepatol* 1994;21:269–72.

89. Feret E, Larouze B, Diop B, et al. Epidemiology of hepatitis B virus infection in the rural community of Tip, Senegal. *Am J Epidemiol* 1987;125:140–9.

90. Chung HT, Lee JS, Lok AS. Prevention of posttransfusion hepatitis B and C by screening for antibody to hepatitis C virus and antibody to HBcAg. *Hepatology* 1993;18:1045–9.

91. Mosley JW, Stevens CE, Aach RD, et al. Donor screening for antibody to hepatitis B core antigen and hepatitis B virus infection in transfusion recipients. *Transfusion* 1995;35:5–12.

92. Hoofnagle JH, Seefe LB, Bales ZB, et al. Type B hepatitis after transfusion with blood containing antibody to hepatitis B core antigen. *N Engl J Med* 1978;298:1379–83.

93. McMahon BJ, Parkinson AJ, Helminiak C, et al. Response to hepatitis B vaccine of persons positive for antibody to hepatitis B core antigen. *Gastroenterology* 1992;103:590–4 (see comments).

94. Okada K, Kamiyama I, Inomata M, et al. e antigen and anti-e in the serum of asymptomatic carrier mothers as indicators of positive and negative transmission of hepatitis B virus to their infants. *N Engl J Med* 1976;294:746–9.

95. Beasley RP, Trepo C, Stevens CE, et al. The e antigen and vertical transmission of hepatitis B surface antigen. *Am J Epidemiol* 1977;105:94–8.

96. Alter HJ, Seeff LB, Kaplan PM, et al. Type B hepatitis: the infectivity of blood positive for e antigen and DNA polymerase after accidental needlestick exposure. *N Engl J Med* 1976;295:909–13.

97. Michalak TI, Pasquinelli C, Guilhot S, et al. Hepatitis B virus persistence after recovery from acute viral hepatitis. *J Clin Invest* 1994;93:230–9 (erratum appears in *J Clin Invest* 1994;94(2):following 905).

98. Wright TL, Mamish D, Combs C, et al. Hepatitis B virus and apparent fulminant non-A, non-B hepatitis. *Lancet* 1992;339:952–5 (see comments).

99. Raimondo G, Allain JP, Brunetto MR, et al. Statements from the Taormina expert meeting on occult hepatitis B virus infection. *J Hepatol* 2008;49:652–7.

100. Lee WM. Etiologies of acute liver failure. *Semin Liver Dis* 2008;28:142–52.

101. Lok AS, Lai CL. Alpha-fetoprotein monitoring in Chinese patients with chronic hepatitis B virus infection: role in the early detection of hepatocellular carcinoma. *Hepatology* 1989;9:110–15 (see comments).

102. Prati D, Taioli E, Zanella A, et al. Updated definitions of healthy ranges for serum alanine aminotransferase levels. *Ann Intern Med* 2002;137:1–10.

103. Lee JK, Shim JH, Lee HC, et al. Estimation of the healthy upper limits for serum alanine aminotransferase in Asian populations with normal liver histology. *Hepatology* 2010;51:1577–83.

104. Wang HC, Wu HC, Chen CF, et al. Different types of ground glass hepatocytes in chronic hepatitis B virus infection contain specific pre-S mutants that may induce endoplasmic reticulum stress. *Am J Pathol* 2003;163:2441–9.

105. Ishak K, Baptista A, Bianchi L, et al. Histological grading and staging of chronic hepatitis. *J Hepatol* 1995;22:696–9.

106. Knodell RG, Ishak KG, Black WC, et al. Formulation and application of a numerical scoring system for assessing histological activity in asymptomatic chronic active hepatitis. *Hepatology* 1981;1:431–5.

107. Bedossa P, Poynard T. An algorithm for the grading of activity in chronic hepatitis C. The METAVIR Cooperative Study Group. *Hepatology* 1996;24:289–93.

108. Desmet VJ, Gerber M, Hoofnagle JH, et al. Classification of chronic hepatitis: diagnosis, grading and staging. *Hepatology* 1994;19:1513–20.

109. Hsu HC, Su IJ, Lai MY, et al. Biologic and prognostic significance of hepatocyte hepatitis B core antigen expressions in the natural course of chronic hepatitis B virus infection. *J Hepatol* 1987;5:45–50.

110. Guillevin L, Lhote F, Cohen P, et al. Polyarteritis nodosa related to hepatitis B virus. A prospective study with long-term observation of 41 patients. *Medicine* 1995;74:238–53.

111. Pagnoux C, Seror R, Henegar C, et al. Clinical features and outcomes in 348 patients with polyarteritis nodosa: a systematic retrospective study of patients diagnosed between 1963 and 2005 and entered into the French Vasculitis Study Group Database. *Arthritis Rheum* 2010;62:616–26.

112. Guillevin L, Lhote F, Sauvaget F, et al. Treatment of polyarteritis nodosa related to hepatitis B virus with interferon-alpha and plasma exchanges. *Ann Rheum Dis* 1994;53:334–7.

113. Simsek H, Telatar H. Successful treatment of hepatitis B virus-associated polyarteritis nodosa by interferon alpha alone. *J Clin Gastroenterol* 1995;20:263–5.

114. Wicki J, Olivieri J, Pizzolato G, et al. Successful treatment of polyarteritis nodosa related to hepatitis B virus with a combination of lamivudine and interferon alpha. *Rheumatology (Oxford)* 1999;38:183–5.

115. Guillevin L, Mahr A, Callard P, et al. Hepatitis B virus-associated polyarteritis nodosa: clinical characteristics, outcome, and impact of treatment in 115 patients. *Medicine* 2005;84:313–22.

116. Lai KN, Lai FM, Tam JS, et al. Strong association between IgA nephropathy and hepatitis B surface antigenemia in endemic areas. *Clin Nephrol* 1988;29:229–34.

117. Lai KN, Lai FM, Tam JS. Comparison of polyclonal and monoclonal antibodies in determination of glomerular deposits of hepatitis B virus antigens in hepatitis B virus-associated glomerulonephritides. *Am J Clin Pathol* 1989;92:159–65.

118. Lisker-Melman M, Webb D, Di Bisceglie AM, et al. Glomerulonephritis caused by chronic hepatitis B virus infection: treatment with recombinant human alpha-interferon. *Ann Intern Med* 1989;111:479–83.

119. Conjeevaram HS, Hoofnagle JH, Austin HA, et al. Long-term outcome of hepatitis B virus-related glomerulonephritis after therapy with interferon alfa. *Gastroenterology* 1995;109:540–6.

120. Connor FL, Rosenberg AR, Kennedy SE, et al. HBV associated nephrotic syndrome: resolution with oral lamivudine. *Arch Dis Child* 2003;88:446–9.

121. Fabrizi F, Dixit V, Martin P. Meta-analysis: anti-viral therapy of hepatitis B virus-associated glomerulonephritis. *Aliment Pharmacol Ther* 2006;24:781–8.

122. Levo Y, Gorevic PD, Kassab HJ, et al. Association between hepatitis B virus and essential mixed cryoglobulinemia. *N Engl J Med* 1977;296:1501–4.

123. Ishimaru Y, Ishimaru H, Toda G, et al. An epidemic of infantile papular acrodermatitis (Gianotti's disease) in Japan associated with hepatitis-B surface antigen subtype ayw. *Lancet* 1976;1:707–9.

124. Caputo R, Gelmetti C, Ermacora E, et al. Gianotti–Crosti syndrome: a retrospective analysis of 308 cases. *J Am Acad Dermatol* 1992;26:207–10.

125. Casciato DA, Klein CA, Kaplowitz N, et al. Aplastic anemia associated with type B viral hepatitis. *Arch Intern Med* 1978;138:1557–8.

126. Brown KE, Tisdale J, Barrett AJ, et al. Hepatitis-associated aplastic anemia. *N Engl J Med* 1997;336:1059–64 (see comments).

127. Conjeevaram HS, Di Bisceglie AM. Management of chronic viral hepatitis in children. *J Pediatr Gastroenterol Nutr* 1995;20:365–75.

128. Bortolotti F, Guido M, Bartolacci S, et al. Chronic hepatitis B in children after e antigen seroclearance: final report of a 29-year longitudinal study. *Hepatology* 2006;43:556–62.

129. Bortolotti F, Calzia R, Cadrobbi P, et al. Liver cirrhosis associated with chronic hepatitis B virus infection in childhood. *J Pediatr* 1986;108:224–7.

130. Wu TC, Tong MJ, Hwang B, et al. Primary hepatocellular carcinoma and hepatitis B infection during childhood. *Hepatology* 1987;7:46–8.

131. Beath SV, Boxall EH, Watson RM, et al. Fulminant hepatitis B in infants born to anti-HBe hepatitis B carrier mothers. *Br Med J* 1992;304:1169–70 (see comments).

132. Tur-Kaspa R, Burk RD, Shaul Y, et al. Hepatitis B virus DNA contains a glucocorticoid-responsive element. *Proc Natl Acad Sci USA* 1986;83:1627–31.

133. Lok AS, Liang RH, Chiu EK, et al. Reactivation of hepatitis B virus replication in patients receiving cytotoxic therapy. Report of a prospective study. *Gastroenterology* 1991;100:182–8.

134. Hoofnagle JH. Reactivation of hepatitis B. *Hepatology* 2009;49:S156–65.

135. Lau JY, Lai CL, Lin HJ, et al. Fatal reactivation of chronic hepatitis B virus infection following withdrawal of chemotherapy in lymphoma patients. *Q J Med* 1989;73:911–17.

136. Loomba R, Rowley A, Wesley R, et al. Systematic review: the effect of preventive lamivudine on hepatitis B reactivation during chemotherapy. *Ann Intern Med* 2008;148:519–28.

137. Degott C, Degos F, Jungers P, et al. Relationship between liver histopathological changes and HBsAg in 111 patients treated by long-term hemodialysis. *Liver* 1983;3:377–84.

138. Degos F, Lugassy C, Degott C, et al. Hepatitis B virus and hepatitis B-related viral infection in renal transplant recipients. A prospective study of 90 patients. *Gastroenterology* 1988;94:151–6.

139. Lee WC, Shu KH, Cheng CH, et al. Long-term impact of hepatitis B, C virus infection on renal transplantation. *Am J Nephrol* 2001;21:300–6.

140. Mathurin P, Mouquet C, Poynard T, et al. Impact of hepatitis B and C virus on kidney transplantation outcome. *Hepatology* 1999;29:257–63 (see comments).

141. Fabrizi F, Martin P, Dixit V, et al. HBsAg seropositive status and survival after renal transplantation: meta-analysis of observational studies. *Am J Transplant* 2005;5:2913–21.

142. Han DJ, Kim TH, Park SK, et al. Results on preemptive or prophylactic treatment of lamivudine in HBsAg (+) renal allograft recipients: comparison with salvage treatment after hepatic dysfunction with HBV recurrence. *Transplantation* 2001;71:387–94.

143. Chan TM, Fang GX, Tang CS, et al. Preemptive lamivudine therapy based on HBV DNA level in HBsAg-positive kidney allograft recipients. *Hepatology* 2002;36:1246–52.

144. KDIGO clinical practice guideline for the care of kidney transplant recipients. *Am J Transplant* 2009;9(Suppl 3):S1–155.

145. Housset C, Pol S, Carnot F, et al. Interactions between human immunodeficiency virus-1, hepatitis delta virus and hepatitis B virus infections in 260 chronic carriers of hepatitis B virus. *Hepatology* 1992;15:578–83.

146. Bodsworth N, Donovan B, Nightingale BN. The effect of concurrent human immunodeficiency virus infection on chronic hepatitis B: a study of 150 homosexual men. *J Infect Dis* 1989;160:577–82.

147. Gilson RJ, Hawkins AE, Beecham MR, et al. Interactions between HIV and hepatitis B virus in homosexual men: effects on the natural history of infection. *AIDS* 1997;11:597–606 (see comments).

148. Colin JF, Cazals-Hatem D, Loriot MA, et al. Influence of human immunodeficiency virus infection on chronic hepatitis B in homosexual men. *Hepatology* 1999: 1306–10.

149. Vento S, di Perri G, Luzzati R, et al. Clinical reactivation of hepatitis B in anti-HBs-positive patients with AIDS. *Lancet* 1989;1:332–3.

150. Koziel MJ, Peters MG. Viral hepatitis in HIV infection. *N Engl J Med* 2007;356:1445.

151. Thio CL, Seaberg EC, Skolasky R Jr, et al. HIV-1, hepatitis B virus, and risk of liver-related mortality in the Multicenter Cohort Study (MACS). *Lancet* 2002;360:1921–6.

152. Sinicco A, Raiteri R, Sciandra M, et al. Coinfection and superinfection of hepatitis B virus in patients infected with human immunodeficiency virus: no evidence of faster progression to AIDS. *Scand J Infect Dis* 1997;29:111–15.

153. Carr A, Cooper DA. Restoration of immunity to chronic hepatitis B infection in HIV-infected patient on protease inhibitor. *Lancet* 1997;349:995–6.

154. Sheng WH, Chen MY, Hsieh SM, et al. Impact of chronic hepatitis B virus (HBV) infection on outcomes of patients infected with HIV in an area where HBV infection is hyperendemic. *Clin Infect Dis* 2004;38:1471–7.

155. Hoffmann CJ, Seaberg EC, Young S, et al. Hepatitis B and long-term HIV outcomes in coinfected HAART recipients. *AIDS* 2009;23:1881–9.

156. Blackberg J, Kidd-Ljunggren K. Occult hepatitis B virus after acute self-limited infection persisting for 30 years without sequence variation. *J Hepatol* 2000;33:992–7.

157. Rehermann B, Ferrari C, Pasquinelli C, et al. The hepatitis B virus persists for decades after patients' recovery from acute viral hepatitis despite active maintenance of a cytotoxic T-lymphocyte response. *Nature Med* 1996;2:1104–8.

158. Lenhoff RJ, Summers J. Coordinate regulation of replication and virus assembly by the large envelope protein of an avian hepadnavirus. *J Virol* 1994;68:4565–71.

159. Lok AS, Lai CL. A longitudinal follow-up of asymptomatic hepatitis B surface antigen-positive Chinese children. *Hepatology* 1988;8:1130–3.

160. Chang MH, Hwang LY, Hsu HC, et al. Prospective study of asymptomatic HBsAg carrier children infected in the perinatal period: clinical and liver histologic studies. *Hepatology* 1988;8:374–7.

161. Chu CM, Karayiannis P, Fowler MJ, et al. Natural history of chronic hepatitis B virus infection in Taiwan: studies of hepatitis B virus DNA in serum. *Hepatology* 1985;5:431–4.

162. Milich DR, Jones JE, Hughes JL, et al. Is a function of the secreted hepatitis B e antigen to induce immunologic tolerance in utero? *Proc Natl Acad Sci USA* 1990;87:6599–603.

163. Chang MH, Hsu HY, Hsu HC, et al. The significance of spontaneous hepatitis B e antigen seroconversion in childhood: with special emphasis on the clearance of hepatitis B e antigen before 3 years of age. *Hepatology* 1995;22:1387–92.

164. Lok AS, Lai CL, Wu PC, et al. Spontaneous hepatitis B e antigen to antibody seroconversion and reversion in Chinese patients with chronic hepatitis B virus infection. *Gastroenterology* 1987;92:1839–43.

165. Chu CM, Hung SJ, Lin J, et al. Natural history of hepatitis B e antigen to antibody seroconversion in patients with normal serum aminotransferase levels. *Am J Med* 2004;116:829–34.

166. Liaw YF, Chu CM, Su IJ, et al. Clinical and histological events preceding hepatitis B e antigen seroconversion in chronic type B hepatitis. *Gastroenterology* 1983;84:216–19.

167. Sheen IS, Liaw YF, Tai DI, et al. Hepatic decompensation associated with hepatitis B e antigen clearance in chronic type B hepatitis. *Gastroenterology* 1985;89:732–5.

168. Liaw YF, Tai DI, Chu CM, et al. Acute exacerbation in chronic type B hepatitis: comparison between HBeAg and antibody-positive patients. *Hepatology* 1987;7:20–3.

169. Lok AS, Lai CL. Acute exacerbations in Chinese patients with chronic hepatitis B virus (HBV) infection. Incidence, predisposing factors and etiology. *J Hepatol* 1990;10:29–34.

170. Chu CJ, Hussain M, Lok AS. Hepatitis B virus genotype B is associated with earlier HBeAg seroconversion compared with hepatitis B virus genotype C. *Gastroenterology* 2002;122:1756–62.

171. McMahon BJ, Holck P, Bulkow L, et al. Serologic and clinical outcomes of 1536 Alaska Natives chronically infected with hepatitis B virus. *Ann Intern Med* 2001;135:759–68.

172. Chen YC, Chu CM, Liaw YF. Age-specific prognosis following spontaneous hepatitis B e antigen seroconversion in chronic hepatitis B. *Hepatology* 2010;51:435–44.

173. Manno M, Camma C, Schepis F, et al. Natural history of chronic HBV carriers in northern Italy: morbidity and mortality after 30 years. *Gastroenterology* 2004;127:756–63.

174. Chen JD, Yang HI, Iloeje UH, et al. Carriers of inactive hepatitis B virus are still at risk for hepatocellular carcinoma and liver-related death. *Gastroenterology* 2010;138:1747–54.

175. Chu CM, Liaw YF. HBsAg seroclearance in asymptomatic carriers of high endemic areas: appreciably high rates during a long-term follow-up. *Hepatology* 2007;45:1187–92.

176. Ahn SH, Park YN, Park JY, et al. Long-term clinical and histological outcomes in patients with spontaneous hepatitis B surface antigen seroclearance. *J Hepatol* 2005;42:188–94.

177. Yuen MF, Wong DK, Fung J, et al. HBsAg seroclearance in chronic hepatitis B in Asian patients: replicative level and risk of hepatocellular carcinoma. *Gastroenterology* 2008;135:1192–9.

178. Chen YC, Sheen IS, Chu CM, et al. Prognosis following spontaneous HBsAg seroclearance in chronic hepatitis B patients with or without concurrent infection. *Gastroenterology* 2002;123:1084–9.

179. Hsu YS, Chien RN, Yeh CT, et al. Long-term outcome after spontaneous HBeAg seroconversion in patients with chronic hepatitis B. *Hepatology* 2002;35:1522–7.

180. Brunetto MR, Oliveri F, Coco B, et al. Outcome of anti-HBe positive chronic hepatitis B in alpha-interferon treated and untreated patients. a long term cohort study. *J Hepatol* 2002;36: 263–70.

181. Manesis EK, Papatheodoridis GV, Sevastianos V, et al. Significance of hepatitis B viremia levels determined by a quantitative polymerase chain reaction assay in patients with hepatitis B e antigen-negative chronic hepatitis B virus infection. *Am J Gastroenterol* 2003;98:2261–7.

182. Chu CJ, Hussain M, Lok AS. Quantitative serum HBV DNA levels during different stages of chronic hepatitis B infection. *Hepatology* 2002;36:1408–15.

183. Chu CJ, Keeffe EB, Han SH, et al. Prevalence of HBV precore/core promoter variants in the United States. *Hepatology* 2003;38: 619–28.

184. Sagnelli E, Stroffolini T, Mele A, et al. Chronic hepatitis B in Italy: new features of an old disease – approaching the universal prevalence of hepatitis B e antigen-negative cases and the eradication of hepatitis D infection. *Clin Infect Dis* 2008;46:110–13.

185. Conjeevaram HS, Lok AS. Occult hepatitis B virus infection: a hidden menace? *Hepatology* 2001;34:204–6.

186. Marrero JA, Lok AS. Occult hepatitis B virus infection in patients with hepatocellular carcinoma: innocent bystander, cofactor, or culprit? *Gastroenterology* 2004;126:347–50.

187. Fattovich G, Bortolotti F, Donato F. Natural history of chronic hepatitis B: special emphasis on disease progression and prognostic factors. *J Hepatol* 2008;48:335–52.

188. Yim HJ, Lok AS. Natural history of chronic hepatitis B virus infection: what we knew in 1981 and what we know in 2005. *Hepatology* 2006;43:S173–81.

189. Beasley RP. Hepatitis B virus. The major etiology of hepatocellular carcinoma. *Cancer* 1988;61:1942–56.

190. Yang HI, Lu SN, Liaw YF, et al. Hepatitis B e antigen and the risk of hepatocellular carcinoma. *N Engl J Med* 2002;347:168–74.

191. Yu MW, Yeh SH, Chen PJ, et al. Hepatitis B virus genotype and DNA level and hepatocellular carcinoma: a prospective study in men. *J Natl Cancer Inst* 2005;97:265–72.

192. Chu CM, Liaw YF. Incidence and risk factors of progression to cirrhosis in inactive carriers of hepatitis B virus. *Am J Gastroenterol* 2009;104:1693–9.

193. Iloeje U, Yang H, Su J, et al. Predicting cirrhosis risk based on the level of circulating hepatitis B viral load. *Gastroenterology* 2006;130:678–86.

194. Chen CJ, Yang HI, Su J, et al. Risk of hepatocellular carcinoma across a biological gradient of serum hepatitis B virus DNA level. *JAMA* 2006;295:65–73.

195. Kao JH, Chen PJ, Lai MY, et al. Hepatitis B genotypes correlate with clinical outcomes in patients with chronic hepatitis B. *Gastroenterology* 2000;118:554–9.

196. Sumi H, Yokosuka O, Seki N, et al. Influence of hepatitis B virus genotypes on the progression of chronic type B liver disease. *Hepatology* 2003;37:19–26.

197. Yang HI, Yeh SH, Chen PJ, et al. Associations between hepatitis B virus genotype and mutants and the risk of hepatocellular carcinoma. *J Natl Cancer Inst* 2008;100:1134–43.

198. Mimms LT, Mosley JW, Hollinger FB, et al. Effect of concurrent acute infection with hepatitis C virus on acute hepatitis B virus infection. *Br Med J* 1993;307:1095–7 (see comments).

199. Feray C, Gigou M, Samuel D, et al. Hepatitis C virus RNA and hepatitis B virus DNA in serum and liver of patients with fulminant hepatitis. *Gastroenterology* 1993;104:549–55 (see comments).

200. Liaw YF, Chen YC, Sheen IS, et al. Impact of acute hepatitis C virus superinfection in patients with chronic hepatitis B virus infection. *Gastroenterology* 2004;126:1024–9.

201. Pontisso P, Ruvoletto MG, Fattovich G, et al. Clinical and virological profiles in patients with multiple hepatitis virus infections. *Gastroenterology* 1993;105:1529–33 (see comments).

202. Liaw YF, Tsai SL, Chang JJ, et al. Displacement of hepatitis B virus by hepatitis C virus as the cause of continuing chronic hepatitis. *Gastroenterology* 1994;106:1048–53.

203. Benvegnu L, Fattovich G, Noventa F, et al. Concurrent hepatitis B and C virus infection and risk of hepatocellular carcinoma in cirrhosis. A prospective study. *Cancer* 1994;74:2442–8.

204. Yu MW, You SL, Chang AS, et al. Association between hepatitis C virus antibodies and hepatocellular carcinoma in Taiwan. *Cancer Res* 1991;51:5621–5.

205. Parkin DM, Bray F, Ferlay J, et al. Global cancer statistics, 2002. *CA Cancer J Clin* 2005;55:74–108.

206. Liaw YF, Sung JJ, Chow WC, et al. Lamivudine for patients with chronic hepatitis B and advanced liver disease. *N Engl J Med* 2004;351:1521–31.

207. Brechot C. Pathogenesis of hepatitis B virus-related hepatocellular carcinoma: old and new paradigms. *Gastroenterology* 2004;127:S56–61.

208. Koike K. Hepatitis B virus X gene is implicated in liver carcinogenesis. *Cancer Lett* 2009;286:60–8.

209. Okamoto H, Imai M, Kametani M, et al. Genomic heterogeneity of hepatitis B virus in a 54-year-old woman who contracted the infection through materno-fetal transmission. *Jpn J Exp Med* 1987;57:231–6.

210. Kurbanov F, Tanaka Y, Mizokami M. Geographical and genetic diversity of the human hepatitis B virus. *Hepatol Res* 2010;40:14–30.

211. Rodriguez-Frias F, Buti M, Jardi R, et al. Hepatitis B virus infection: precore mutants and its relation to viral genotypes and core mutations. *Hepatology* 1995;22:1641–7.

212. Lindh M, Andersson AS, Gusdal A. Genotypes, nt 1858 variants, and geographic origin of hepatitis B virus – large-scale analysis using a new genotyping method. *J Infect Dis* 1997;175:1285–93.

213. Fung SK, Lok AS. Hepatitis B virus genotypes: do they play a role in the outcome of HBV infection? *Hepatology* 2004;40:790–2.

214. Shiina S, Fujino H, Kawabe T, et al. Relationship of HBsAg subtypes with HBeAg/anti-HBe status and chronic liver disease. Part II: evaluation of epidemiological factors and suspected risk factors of liver dysfunction. *Am J Gastroenterol* 1991;86:872–5.

215. Lindh M, Hannoun C, Dhillon AP, et al. Core promoter mutations and genotypes in relation to viral replication and liver damage in East Asian hepatitis B virus carriers. *J Infect Dis* 1999;179:775–82.

216. Orito E, Mizokami M, Sakugawa H, et al. A case–control study for clinical and molecular biological differences between hepatitis B viruses of genotypes B and C. Japan HBV Genotype Research Group. *Hepatology* 2001;34:218–23.

217. Chan HL, Hui AY, Wong ML, et al. Genotype C hepatitis B virus infection is associated with an increased risk of hepatocellular carcinoma. *Gut* 2004;53:1494–8.

218. Fujie H, Moriya K, Shintani Y, et al. Hepatitis B virus genotypes and hepatocellular carcinoma in Japan. *Gastroenterology* 2001;120:1564–5.

219. Sanchez-Tapias JM, Costa J, Mas A, et al. Influence of hepatitis B virus genotype on the long-term outcome of chronic hepatitis B in western patients. *Gastroenterology* 2002;123:1848–56.

220. Livingston SE, Simonetti JP, Bulkow LR, et al. Clearance of hepatitis B e antigen in patients with chronic hepatitis B and genotypes A, B, C, D, and F. *Gastroenterology* 2007;133:1452–7.

221. Livingston SE, Simonetti JP, McMahon BJ, et al. Hepatitis B virus genotypes in Alaska Native people with hepatocellular carcinoma: preponderance of genotype F. *J Infect Dis* 2007;195:5–11.

222. Kao JH, Wu NH, Chen PJ, et al. Hepatitis B genotypes and the response to interferon therapy. *J Hepatol* 2000;33:998–1002.

223. Wai CT, Chu CJ, Hussain M, et al. HBV genotype B is associated with better response to interferon therapy in HBeAg(+) chronic hepatitis than genotype C. *Hepatology* 2002;36:1425–30.

224. Flink H, van Zonneveld M, Hansen B, et al. Treatment with peg-interferon alpha-2b for HBeAg-positive chronic hepatitis B: HBsAg loss is associated with HBV genotype. *Am J Gastroenterol* 2006;101:297–303.

225. Buster EH, Flink HJ, Cakaloglu Y, et al. Sustained HBeAg and HBsAg loss after long-term follow-up of HBeAg-positive patients treated with peginterferon a-2b. *Gastroenterology* 2008;135:459–67.

226. Westland C, Delaney WE IV, Yang H, et al. Hepatitis B virus genotypes and virologic response in 694 patients in phase III studies of adefovir dipivoxil1. *Gastroenterology* 2003;125:107–16.

227. Ou JH, Laub O, Rutter WJ. Hepatitis B virus gene function: the precore region targets the core antigen to cellular membranes and causes the secretion of the e antigen. *Proc Natl Acad Sci USA* 1986;83:1578–82.

228. Carman WF, Hadziyannis S, McGarvey MJ, et al. Mutation preventing formation of hepatitis B e antigen in patients with chronic hepatitis B infection. *Lancet* 1989;2(8663):588–91.

229. Funk ML, Rosenberg DM, Lok AS. World-wide epidemiology of HBeAg-negative chronic hepatitis B and associated precore and core promoter variants. *J Viral Hepatitis*. 2002;9:52–61.

230. Omata M, Ehata T, Yokosuka O, et al. Mutations in the precore region of hepatitis B virus DNA in patients with fulminant and severe hepatitis. *N Engl J Med* 1991;324:1699–704 (see comments).

231. Ogata N, Miller RH, Ishak KG, et al. The complete nucleotide sequence of a pre-core mutant of hepatitis B virus implicated in fulminant hepatitis and its biological characterization in chimpanzees. *Virology* 1993;194:263–76.

232. Liang TJ, Hasegawa K, Rimon N, et al. A hepatitis B virus mutant associated with an epidemic of fulminant hepatitis. *N Engl J Med* 1991;324:1705–9 (see comments).

233. Okamoto H, Yotsumoto S, Akahane Y, et al. Hepatitis B viruses with precore region defects prevail in persistently infected hosts along with seroconversion to the antibody against e antigen. *J Virol* 1990;64:1298–303.

234. Lok AS, Akarca US, Greene S. Predictive value of precore hepatitis B virus mutations in spontaneous and interferon-induced hepatitis B e antigen clearance. *Hepatology* 1995;21:19–24.

235. Carman WF, Jacyna MR, Hadziyannis S, et al. Mutation preventing formation of hepatitis B e antigen in patients with chronic hepatitis B infection. *Lancet* 1989;2:588–91.

236. Brunetto MR, Giarin MM, Oliveri F, et al. Wild-type and e antigen-minus hepatitis B viruses and course of chronic hepatitis. *Proc Natl Acad Sci USA* 1991;88:4186–90.

237. Akarca US, Greene S, Lok AS. Detection of precore hepatitis B virus mutants in asymptomatic HBsAg-positive family members. *Hepatology* 1994;19:1366–70.

238. Okamoto H, Tsuda F, Akahane Y, et al. Hepatitis B virus with mutations in the core promoter for an e antigen-negative phenotype in carriers with antibody to e antigen. *J Virol* 1994;68:8102–10.

239. Baumert TF, Rogers SA, Hasegawa K, et al. Two core promotor mutations identified in a hepatitis B virus strain associated with fulminant hepatitis result in enhanced viral replication. *J Clin Invest* 1996;98:2268–76.

240. Baptista M, Kramvis A, Kew MC. High prevalence of 1762(T) 1764(A) mutations in the basic core promoter of hepatitis B virus isolated from black Africans with hepatocellular carcinoma compared with asymptomatic carriers. *Hepatology* 1999;29:946–53.

241. Fang ZL, Ling R, Wang SS, et al. HBV core promoter mutations prevail in patients with hepatocellular carcinoma from Guangxi, China. *J Med Virol* 1998;56:18–24.

242. Carman WF, Zanetti AR, Karayiannis P, et al. Vaccine-induced escape mutant of hepatitis B virus. *Lancet* 1990;336:325–9.

243. Harrison TJ, Hopes EA, Oon CJ, et al. Independent emergence of a vaccine-induced escape mutant of hepatitis B virus. *J Hepatol* 1991;13(Suppl 4):S105–7.

244. Lee PI, Chang LY, Lee CY, et al. Detection of hepatitis B surface gene mutation in carrier children with or without immunoprophylaxis at birth. *J Infect Dis* 1997;176:427–30.

245. Ogata N, Zanetti AR, Yu M, et al. Infectivity and pathogenicity in chimpanzees of a surface gene mutant of hepatitis B virus that emerged in a vaccinated infant. *J Infect Dis* 1997;175:511–23.

246. Chang MH. Breakthrough HBV infection in vaccinated children in Taiwan: surveillance for HBV mutants. *Antivir Ther* 2010;15:463–9.

247. Ni YH, Chang MH, Huang LM, et al. Hepatitis B virus infection in children and adolescents in a hyperendemic area: 15 years after mass hepatitis B vaccination. *Ann Intern Med* 2001;135:796–800.

248. Basuni AA, Butterworth L, Cooksley G, et al. Prevalence of HBsAg mutants and impact of hepatitis B infant immunisation in four Pacific Island countries. *Vaccine* 2004;22:2791–9.

249. Carman WF, Trautwein C, van Deursen FJ, et al. Hepatitis B virus envelope variation after transplantation with and without hepatitis B immune globulin prophylaxis. *Hepatology* 1996;24:489–93.

250. McMahon G, Ehrlich PH, Moustafa ZA, et al. Genetic alterations in the gene encoding the major HBsAg: DNA and immunological analysis of recurrent HBsAg derived from monoclonal antibody-treated liver transplant patients. *Hepatology* 1992;15:757–66.

251. Ghany MG, Ayola B, Villamil FG, et al. Hepatitis B virus S mutants in liver transplant recipients who were reinfected despite hepatitis B immune globulin prophylaxis. *Hepatology* 1998;27:213–22.

252. Degertekin B, Han SH, Keeffe EB, et al. Impact of virologic breakthrough and HBIG regimen on hepatitis B recurrence after liver transplantation. *Am J Transplant* 2010;10:1823–33.

253. Chen BF, Liu CJ, Jow GM, et al. High prevalence and mapping of pre-S deletion in hepatitis B virus carriers with progressive liver diseases. *Gastroenterology* 2006;130:1153–68.

254. Wong DK, Cheung AM, O'Rourke K, et al. Effect of alpha-interferon treatment in patients with hepatitis B e antigen-positive chronic hepatitis B. A meta-analysis. *Ann Intern Med* 1993;119:312–23 (see comments).

255. Craxi A, Di Bona D, Camma C. Interferon-alpha for HBeAg-positive chronic hepatitis B. *J Hepatol* 2003;39(Suppl 1):S99–105.

256. Lampertico P, Del Ninno E, Manzin A, et al. A randomized, controlled trial of a 24-month course of interferon alfa 2b in patients

with chronic hepatitis B who had hepatitis B virus DNA without hepatitis B e antigen in serum. *Hepatology* 1997;26:1621–5.

257. Hoofnagle JH, Di Bisceglie AM, Waggoner JG, et al. Interferon alfa for patients with clinically apparent cirrhosis due to chronic hepatitis B. *Gastroenterology* 1993;104:1116–21.

258. Perrillo R, Tamburro C, Regenstein F, et al. Low-dose, titratable interferon alfa in decompensated liver disease caused by chronic infection with hepatitis B virus. *Gastroenterology* 1995;109:908–16.

259. Cohard M, Poynard T, Mathurin P, et al. Prednisone-interferon combination in the treatment of chronic hepatitis B: direct and indirect metanalysis. *Hepatology* 1994;20:1390–8.

260. Korenman J, Baker B, Waggoner J, et al. Long-term remission of chronic hepatitis B after alpha-interferon therapy. *Ann Intern Med* 1991;114:629–34.

261. Fattovich G, Giustina G, Realdi G, et al. Long-term outcome of hepatitis B e antigen-positive patients with compensated cirrhosis treated with interferon alfa. European Concerted Action on Viral Hepatitis (EUROHEP). *Hepatology* 1997;26:1338–42.

262. Niederau C, Heintges T, Lange S, et al. Long-term follow-up of HBeAg-positive patients treated with interferon alfa for chronic hepatitis B. *N Engl J Med* 1996;334:1422–7.

263. Krogsgaard K. The long-term effect of treatment with interferon-alpha 2a in chronic hepatitis B. The Long-Term Follow-up Investigator Group. The European Study Group on Viral Hepatitis (EUROHEP). Executive Team on Anti-Viral Treatment. *J Viral Hepat* 1998;5:389–97.

264. Lok AS, Chung HT, Liu VW, et al. Long-term follow-up of chronic hepatitis B patients treated with interferon alfa. *Gastroenterology* 1993;105:1833–8.

265. Lin SM, Sheen IS, Chien RN, et al. Long-term beneficial effect of interferon therapy in patients with chronic hepatitis B virus infection. *Hepatology* 1999;29:971–5.

266. Yuen MF, Hui CK, Cheng CC, et al. Long term follow up of interferon alfa treatment in Chinese patients with chronic hepatitis B infection: the effect on hepatitis B e antigen seroconversion and the development of cirrhosis-related complications. *Hepatology* 2001;34:139–45.

267. Lau DT, Everhart J, Kleiner DE, et al. Long-term follow-up of patients with chronic hepatitis B treated with interferon alfa. *Gastroenterology* 1997;113:1660–7.

268. van Zonneveld M, Honkoop P, Hansen BE, et al. Long-term follow-up of alpha-interferon treatment of patients with chronic hepatitis B. *Hepatology* 2004;39:804–10.

269. Manesis EK, Hadziyannis SJ. Interferon alpha treatment and retreatment of hepatitis B e antigen-negative chronic hepatitis B. *Gastroenterology* 2001;121:101–9.

270. Papatheodoridis GV, Manesis E, Hadziyannis SJ. The long-term outcome of interferon-alpha treated and untreated patients with HBeAg-negative chronic hepatitis B. *J Hepatol* 2001;34:306–13.

271. Lampertico P, Del Ninno E, Vigano M, et al. Long-term suppression of hepatitis B e antigen-negative chronic hepatitis B by 24-month interferon therapy. *Hepatology* 2003;37:756–63.

272. Cooksley WG, Piratvisuth T, Lee SD, et al. Peginterferon alpha-2a (40 kDa): an advance in the treatment of hepatitis B e antigen-positive chronic hepatitis B. *J Viral Hepat* 2003;10:298–305.

273. Lau GK, Piratvisuth T, Luo KX, et al. Peginterferon Alfa-2a, lamivudine, and the combination for HBeAg-positive chronic hepatitis B. *N Engl J Med* 2005;352:2682–95.

274. Janssen HL, van Zonneveld M, Senturk H, et al. Pegylated interferon alfa-2b alone or in combination with lamivudine for HBeAg-positive chronic hepatitis B: a randomised trial. *Lancet* 2005;365:123–9.

275. Chan HL, Leung NW, Hui AY, et al. A randomized, controlled trial of combination therapy for chronic hepatitis B: comparing pegy-lated interferon-alpha2b and lamivudine with lamivudine alone. *Ann Intern Med* 2005;142:240–50.

276. Marcellin P, Lau GK, Bonino F, et al. Peginterferon alfa-2a alone, lamivudine alone, and the two in combination in patients with HBeAg-negative chronic hepatitis B. *N Engl J Med* 2004;351:1206–17.

277. Marcellin P, Bonino F, Lau GK, et al. Sustained response of hepatitis B e antigen-negative patients 3 years after treatment with peginterferon alpha-2a. *Gastroenterology* 2009;136:2169–79, e1–4.

278. Lok AS, Wu PC, Lai CL, et al. A controlled trial of interferon with or without prednisone priming for chronic hepatitis B. *Gastroenterology* 1992;102:2091–7.

279. Perrillo RP, Lai CL, Liaw YF, et al. Predictors of HBeAg loss after lamivudine treatment for chronic hepatitis B. *Hepatology* 2002;36:186–94.

280. Fried MW, Piratvisuth T, Lau GK, et al. HBeAg and hepatitis B virus DNA as outcome predictors during therapy with peginterferon alfa-2a for HBeAg-positive chronic hepatitis B. *Hepatology* 2008;47:428–34.

281. Bonino F, Marcellin P, Lau GK, et al. Predicting response to peginterferon alpha-2a, lamivudine and the two combined for HBeAg-negative chronic hepatitis B. *Gut* 2007;56:699–705.

282. Moucari R, Mackiewicz V, Lada O, et al. Early serum HBsAg drop: a strong predictor of sustained virological response to pegylated interferon alfa-2a in HBeAg-negative patients. *Hepatology* 2009;49:1151–7.

283. Brunetto MR, Moriconi F, Bonino F, et al. Hepatitis B virus surface antigen levels: a guide to sustained response to peginterferon alfa-2a in HBeAg-negative chronic hepatitis B. *Hepatology* 2009;49:1141–50.

284. Dienstag JL, Schiff ER, Wright TL, et al. Lamivudine as initial treatment for chronic hepatitis B in the United States. *N Engl J Med* 1999;341:1256–63.

285. Lai CL, Chien R, Tsung N, et al. A one-year trial of lamivudine for chronic hepatitis B. Asia Hepatitis Lamivudine Study Group. *N Engl J Med* 1998;339:61–8.

286. Schalm SW, Heathcote J, Cianciara J, et al. Lamivudine and alpha interferon combination treatment of patients with chronic hepatitis B infection: a randomised trial. *Gut* 2000;46:562–8 (see comments).

287. Lok AS, Lai CL, Leung N, et al. Long-term safety of lamivudine treatment in patients with chronic hepatitis B. *Gastroenterology* 2003;125:1714–22.

288. Jonas MM, Kelley DA, Mizerski J, et al. Clinical trial of lamivudine in children with chronic hepatitis B. *N Engl J Med* 2002;346:1706–13.

289. Sokal EM, Kelly DA, Mizerski J, et al. Long-term lamivudine therapy for children with HBeAg-positive chronic hepatitis B. *Hepatology* 2006;43:225–32.

290. Tassopoulos NC, Volpes R, Pastore G, et al. Efficacy of lamivudine in patients with hepatitis B e antigen-negative/hepatitis B virus DNA-positive (precore mutant) chronic hepatitis B. Lamivudine Precore Mutant Study Group. *Hepatology* 1999;29:889–96.

291. Hadziyannis SJ, Papatheodoridis GV, Dimou E, et al. Efficacy of long-term lamivudine monotherapy in patients with hepatitis B e antigen-negative chronic hepatitis B. *Hepatology* 2000;32:847–51.

292. Rizzetto M, Tassopoulos NC, Goldin RD, et al. Extended lamivudine treatment in patients with HBeAg-negative chronic hepatitis B. *J Hepatol* 2005;42:173–9.

293. Papatheodoridis GV, Dimou E, Laras A, et al. Course of virologic breakthroughs under long-term lamivudine in HBeAg-negative precore mutant HBV liver disease. *Hepatology* 2002;36:219–26.

294. Schiff ER, Dienstag JL, Karayalcin S, et al. Lamivudine and 24 weeks of lamivudine/interferon combination therapy for hepatitis B e antigen-positive chronic hepatitis B in interferon nonresponders. *J Hepatol* 2003;38:818–26.

295. Villeneuve JP, Condreay LD, Willems B, et al. Lamivudine treatment for decompensated cirrhosis resulting from chronic hepatitis B. *Hepatology* 2000;31:207–10.

296. Fontana RJ, Hann HW, Perrillo RP, et al. Determinants of early mortality in patients with decompensated chronic hepatitis B treated with antiviral therapy. *Gastroenterology* 2002;123:719–27.

297. Yao FY, Bass NM. Lamivudine treatment in patients with severely decompensated cirrhosis due to replicating hepatitis B infection. *J Hepatol* 2000;33:301–7 (see comments).

298. Perrillo RP, Wright T, Rakela J, et al. A multicenter United States–Canadian trial to assess lamivudine monotherapy before and after liver transplantation for chronic hepatitis B. *Hepatology* 2001;33:424–32.

299. Dienstag JL, Cianciara J, Karayalcin S, et al. Durability of serologic response after lamivudine treatment of chronic hepatitis B. *Hepatology* 2003;37:748–55.

300. Chien RN, Yeh CT, Tsai SL, et al. Determinants for sustained HBeAg response to lamivudine therapy. *Hepatology* 2003;38:1267–73.

301. Song BC, Suh DJ, Lee HC, et al. Hepatitis B e antigen seroconversion after lamivudine therapy is not durable in patients with chronic hepatitis B in Korea. *Hepatology* 2000;32:803–6.

302. Lee HC, Suh DJ, Ryu SH, et al. Quantitative polymerase chain reaction assay for serum hepatitis B virus DNA as a predictive factor for post-treatment relapse after lamivudine induced hepatitis B e antigen loss or seroconversion. *Gut* 2003;52:1779–83.

303. Reijnders JG, Perquin MJ, Zhang N, et al. Nucleos(t)ide analogues only induce temporary hepatitis B e antigen seroconversion in most patients with chronic hepatitis B. *Gastroenterology* 2010;139:491–8.

304. Lee HW, Lee HJ, Hwang JS, et al. Lamivudine maintenance beyond one year after HBeAg seroconversion is a major factor for sustained virologic response in HBeAg-positive chronic hepatitis B. *Hepatology* 2010;51:415–21.

305. Fung SK, Wong F, Hussain M, et al. Sustained response after a 2-year course of lamivudine treatment of hepatitis B e antigen-negative chronic hepatitis B. *J Viral Hepat* 2004;11:432–8.

306. Allen MI, Deslauriers M, Andrews CW, et al. Identification and characterisation of mutations in hepatitis B virus resistant to lamivudine. *Lamivudine Clinical Investigation Group.* Hepatology 1998;27:1670–7.

307. Lau DT, Khokhar MF, Doo E, et al. Long-term therapy of chronic hepatitis B with lamivudine. *Hepatology* 2000;32:828–34.

308. Melegari M, Scaglioni PP, Wands JR. Hepatitis B virus mutants associated with 3TC and famciclovir administration are replication defective. *Hepatology* 1998;27:628–33.

309. Ono-Nita SK, Kato N, Shiratori Y, et al. YMDD motif in hepatitis B virus DNA polymerase influences on replication and lamivudine resistance: a study by in vitro full-length viral DNA transfection. *Hepatology* 1999;29:939–45.

310. Papatheodoridis GV, Dimou E, Dimakopoulos K, et al. Outcome of hepatitis B e antigen-negative chronic hepatitis B on long-term nucleos(t)ide analog therapy starting with lamivudine. *Hepatology* 2005;42:121–9.

311. Di Marco V, Marzano A, Lampertico P, et al. Clinical outcome of HBeAg-negative chronic hepatitis B in relation to virological response to lamivudine. *Hepatology* 2004;40:883–91.

312. Marcellin P, Chang T, Lim SG, et al. Adefovir dipivoxil for the treatment of hepatitis B e antigen-positive chronic hepatitis B. *N Engl J Med* 2003;348:808–16.

313. Marcellin P, Chang TT, Lim SG, et al. Long-term efficacy and safety of adefovir dipivoxil for the treatment of hepatitis B e antigen-positive chronic hepatitis B. *Hepatology* 2008;48:750–8.

314. Hadziyannis SJ, Tassopoulos NC, Heathcote EJ, et al. Adefovir dipivoxil for the treatment of hepatitis B e antigen-negative chronic hepatitis B. *N Engl J Med* 2003;348:800–7.

315. Hadziyannis S, Tassopoulos N, Heathcote E, et al. Long-term therapy with adefovir dipivoxil for HBeAg-negative chronic hepatitis B for up to 5 years. *Gastroenterology* 2006;131:1743–51.

316. Peters MG, Hann H, Martin P, et al. Adefovir dipivoxil alone or in combination with lamivudine in patients with lamivudine-resistant chronic hepatitis B. *Gastroenterology* 2004;126:91–101.

317. Perrillo R, Hann HW, Mutimer D, et al. Adefovir dipivoxil added to ongoing lamivudine in chronic hepatitis B with YMDD mutant hepatitis B virus. *Gastroenterology* 2004;126:81–90.

318. Schiff ER, Lai CL, Hadziyannis S, et al. Adefovir dipivoxil therapy for lamivudine-resistant hepatitis B in pre- and post-liver transplantation patients. *Hepatology* 2003;38:1419–27.

319. Marzano A, Lampertico P, Mazzaferro V, et al. Prophylaxis of hepatitis B virus recurrence after liver transplantation in carriers of lamivudine-resistant mutants. *Liver Transpl* 2005;11:532–8.

320. Schiff E, Lai CL, Hadziyannis S, et al. Adefovir dipivoxil for wait-listed and post-liver transplantation patients with lamivudine-resistant hepatitis B: final long-term results. *Liver Transpl* 2007;13:349–60.

321. Wu IC, Shiffman ML, Tong MJ, et al. Sustained hepatitis B e antigen seroconversion in patients with chronic hepatitis B after adefovir dipivoxil treatment: analysis of precore and basal core promoter mutants. *Clin Infect Dis* 2008;47:1305–11.

322. Hadziyannis S, Tassopoulos N, Heathcote EJ, et al. Long-term (3-year) therapy with adefovir dipivoxil for the treatment of hepatitis B e antigen negative chronic hepatitis B. *N Engl J Med* 2005;352:2673–81.

323. Hadziyannis S, Sevastianos V, Rapti I. Outcome of HBeAg-negative chronic hepatitis B (CHB) 5 years after discontinuation of long term adefovir dipivoxil (ADV) treatment. *J Hepatol* 2009;50:S9, abstract 18.

324. Westland C, Yang H, Delaney WE IV, et al. Week 48 resistance surveillance in two phase 3 clinical studies of adefovir dipivoxil for chronic hepatitis B. *Hepatology* 2003;38:96–103.

325. Angus P, Vaughan R, Xiong S, et al. Resistance to adefovir dipivoxil therapy associated with the selection of a novel mutation in the HBV polymerase. *Gastroenterology* 2003;125:292–7.

326. Villeneuve JP, Durantel D, Durantel S, et al. Selection of a hepatitis B virus strain resistant to adefovir in a liver transplantation patient. *J Hepatol* 2003;39:1085–9.

327. Yim HJ, Hussain M, Liu Y, et al. Evolution of multi-drug resistant hepatitis B virus during sequential therapy. *Hepatology* 2006;44:703–12.

328. Chang TT, Gish RG, de Man R, et al. A comparison of entecavir and lamivudine for HBeAg-positive chronic hepatitis B. *N Engl J Med* 2006;354:1001–10.

329. Chang TT, Lai CL, Kew Yoon S, et al. Entecavir treatment for up to 5 years in patients with hepatitis B e antigen-positive chronic hepatitis B. *Hepatology* 2010;51:422–30.

330. Leung N, Peng CY, Hann HW, et al. Early hepatitis B virus DNA reduction in hepatitis B e antigen-positive patients with chronic hepatitis B: a randomized international study of entecavir versus adefovir. *Hepatology* 2009;49:72–9.

331. Zheng MH, Shi KQ, Dai ZJ, et al. A 24-week, parallel-group, open-label, randomized clinical trial comparing the early antiviral efficacy of telbivudine and entecavir in the treatment of hepatitis B e antigen-positive chronic hepatitis B virus infection in adult Chinese patients. *Clin Ther* 2010;32:649–58.

332. Lai CL, Shouval D, Lok AS, et al. Entecavir versus lamivudine for patients with HBeAg-negative chronic hepatitis B. *N Engl J Med* 2006;354:1011–20.

333. Shim JH, Lee HC, Kim KM, et al. Efficacy of entecavir in treatment-naive patients with hepatitis B virus-related decompensated cirrhosis. *J Hepatol* 2010;52:176–82.

334. Sherman M, Yurdaydin C, Sollano J, et al. Entecavir for treatment of lamivudine-refractory, HBeAg-positive chronic hepatitis B. *Gastroenterology* 2006;130:2039–49.

335. Tenney DJ, Rose RE, Baldick CJ, et al. Long-term monitoring shows hepatitis B virus resistance to entecavir in nucleoside-naive patients is rare through 5 years of therapy. *Hepatology* 2009;49:1503–14.

336. Wu IC, Lai CL, Han SH, et al. Efficacy of entecavir in chronic hepatitis B patients with mildly elevated alanine aminotransferase and biopsy-proven histological damage. *Hepatology* 2010;51:1185–9.

337. Gish RG, Lok AS, Chang TT, et al. Entecavir therapy for up to 96 weeks in patients with HBeAg-positive chronic hepatitis B. *Gastroenterology* 2007;133:1437–44.

338. Shouval D, Lai CL, Chang TT, et al. Relapse of hepatitis B in HBeAg-negative chronic hepatitis B patients who discontinued successful entecavir treatment: the case for continuous antiviral therapy. *J Hepatol* 2009;50:289–95.

339. FDA. FDA Drug Advisory Committee Meeting on Entecavir. http://www.fda.gov/ohrms/dockets/ac/05/slides/2005-4094S1 _02_01-BMS-Entecavir_files/frame.htm#slide1504.htm, 2005.

340. Lange CM, Bojunga J, Hofmann WP, et al. Severe lactic acidosis during treatment of chronic hepatitis B with entecavir in patients with impaired liver function. *Hepatology* 2009;50:2001–6.

341. Tenney DJ, Levine SM, Rose RE, et al. Clinical emergence of entecavir-resistant hepatitis B virus requires additional substitutions in virus already resistant to lamivudine. *Antimicrob Agents Chemother* 2004;48:3498–507.

342. Lim SG, Ng TM, Kung N, et al. A double-blind placebo-controlled study of emtricitabine in chronic hepatitis B. *Arch Intern Med* 2006;166:49–56.

343. Marcellin P, Heathcote EJ, Buti M, et al. Tenofovir disoproxil fumarate versus adefovir dipivoxil for chronic hepatitis B. *N Engl J Med* 2008;359:2442–55.

344. Heathcote EJ, Gane EJ, De Man RA, et al. Three years of tenofovir disoproxil (TDF) treatment in HBeAg-positive patients (HBeAg+) with chronic hepatitis B (Study 103), preliminary analysis (abstract 483). *Hepatology* 2009;50:533A–4A.

345. Marcellin P, Buti M, Krastev Z, et al. Three years of tenofovir disoproxil fumarate (TDF) treatment in HBeAg-negative patients with chronic hepatitis B (Study 102); preliminary analysis (abstract 481). *Hepatology* 2009;50:532A–3A.

346. van Bommel F, de Man RA, Wedemeyer H, et al. Long-term efficacy of tenofovir monotherapy for hepatitis B virus-monoinfected patients after failure of nucleoside/nucleotide analogues. *Hepatology* 2010;51:73–80.

347. Kuo A, Dienstag JL, Chung RT. Tenofovir disoproxil fumarate for the treatment of lamivudine-resistant hepatitis B. *Clin Gastroenterol Hepatol* 2004;2:266–72.

348. Tan J, Degertekin B, Wong SN, et al. Tenofovir monotherapy is effective in hepatitis B patients with antiviral treatment failure to adefovir in the absence of adefovir-resistant mutations. *J Hepatol* 2008;48:391–8.

349. Sheldon J, Camino N, Rodes B, et al. Selection of hepatitis B virus polymerase mutations in HIV-coinfected patients treated with tenofovir. *Antivir Ther* 2005;10:727–34.

350. Delaney WE, Ray AS, Yang H, et al. Intracellular metabolism and in vitro activity of tenofovir against hepatitis B virus. *Antimicrob Agents Chemother* 2006;50:2471–7.

351. Amini-Bavil-Olyaee S, Herbers U, Sheldon J, et al. The rtA194T polymerase mutation impacts viral replication and susceptibility to tenofovir in hepatitis B e antigen-positive and hepatitis B e antigen-negative hepatitis B virus strains. *Hepatology* 2009;49:1158–65.

352. Verhelst D, Monge M, Meynard JL, et al. Fanconi syndrome and renal failure induced by tenofovir: a first case report. *Am J Kidney Dis* 2002;40:1331–3.

353. Malik A, Abraham P, Malik N. Acute renal failure and Fanconi syndrome in an AIDS patient on tenofovir treatment – case report and review of literature. *J Infect* 2005;51:E61–5.

354. Antoniou T, Raboud J, Chirhin S, et al. Incidence of and risk factors for tenofovir-induced nephrotoxicity: a retrospective cohort study. *HIV Med* 2005;6:284–90.

355. Purdy JB, Gafni RI, Reynolds JC, et al. Decreased bone mineral density with off-label use of tenofovir in children and adolescents infected with human immunodeficiency virus. *J Pediatr* 2008;152:582–4.

356. Lai CL, Gane E, Liaw YF, et al. Telbivudine versus lamivudine in patients with chronic hepatitis B. *N Engl J Med* 2007;357:2576–88.

357. Liaw YF, Gane E, Leung N, et al. 2-Year GLOBE trial results: telbivudine is superior to lamivudine in patients with chronic hepatitis B. *Gastroenterology* 2009;136:486–95.

358. Zeuzem S, Gane E, Liaw YF, et al. Baseline characteristics and early on-treatment response predict the outcomes of 2 years of telbivudine treatment of chronic hepatitis B. *J Hepatol* 2009;51:11–20.

359. Wang Y, Thongsawat S, Gane EJ, et al. Efficacy and safety outcomes after 4 years of telbivudine treatment in patients with chronic hepatitis B (CHB) – abstract 482. *Hepatology* 2009;50:533A.

360. Yoo BC, Kim JH, Chung YH, et al. Twenty-four-week clevudine therapy showed potent and sustained antiviral activity in HBeAg-positive chronic hepatitis B. *Hepatology* 2007;45:1172–8.

361. Yoo BC, Kim JH, Kim TH, et al. Clevudine is highly efficacious in hepatitis B e antigen-negative chronic hepatitis B with durable off-therapy viral suppression. *Hepatology* 2007;46:1041–8.

362. Seok JI, Lee DK, Lee CH, et al. Long-term therapy with clevudine for chronic hepatitis B can be associated with myopathy characterized by depletion of mitochondrial DNA. *Hepatology* 2009;49:2080–6.

363. Tak WY, Park SY, Cho CM, et al. Clinical, biochemical, and pathological characteristics of clevudine-associated myopathy. *J Hepatol* 2010;53:261–6.

364. Sung JJ, Lai JY, Zeuzem S, et al. Lamivudine compared with lamivudine and adefovir dipivoxil for the treatment of HBeAg-positive chronic hepatitis B. *J Hepatol* 2008;48:728–35.

365. Lampertico P, Vigano M, Manenti E, et al. Low resistance to adefovir combined with lamivudine: a 3-year study of 145 lamivudine-resistant hepatitis B patients. *Gastroenterology* 2007;133:1445–51.

366. Rapti I, Dimou E, Mitsoula P, et al. Adding-on versus switching-to adefovir therapy in lamivudine-resistant HBeAg-negative chronic hepatitis B. *Hepatology* 2007;45:307–13.

367. Lai CL, Leung N, Teo EK, et al. A 1-year trial of telbivudine, lamivudine, and the combination in patients with hepatitis B e antigen-positive chronic hepatitis B. *Gastroenterology* 2005;129:528–36.

368. Chien RN, Liaw YF, Chen TC, et al. Efficacy of thymosin alpha1 in patients with chronic hepatitis B: a randomized, controlled trial. *Hepatology* 1998;27:1383–7.

369. Mutchnick MG, Lindsay KL, Schiff ER, et al. Thymosin alpha1 treatment of chronic hepatitis B: results of a phase III multicentre, randomized, double-blind and placebo-controlled study. *J Viral Hepat* 1999;6:397–403.

370. Fattovich G, Giustina G, Alberti A, et al. A randomized controlled trial of thymopentin therapy in patients with chronic hepatitis B. *J Hepatol* 1994;21:361–6.

371. Andreone P, Cursaro C, Gramenzi A, et al. A randomized controlled trial of thymosin-alpha1 versus interferon alfa treatment in patients with hepatitis B e antigen antibody – and hepatitis B virus DNA-positive chronic hepatitis B. *Hepatology* 1996;24:774–7.

372. Chan HL, Tang JL, Tam W, et al. The efficacy of thymosin in the treatment of chronic hepatitis B virus infection: a meta-analysis. *Aliment Pharmacol Ther* 2001;15:1899–905.

373. Pol S, Driss F, Carnot F, et al. [Efficacy of immunotherapy with vaccination against hepatitis B virus on virus B multiplication.] *C R Acad Sci III* 1993;316:688–91.

374. Couillin I, Pol S, Mancini M, et al. Specific vaccine therapy in chronic hepatitis B: induction of T cell proliferative responses specific for envelope antigens. *J Infect Dis* 1999;180:15–26 (erratum appears in *J Infect Dis* 1999;180(5):1756).

375. Whalen RG, Leclerc C, Deriaud E, et al. DNA-mediated immunization to the hepatitis B surface antigen. Activation and entrainment of the immune response. *Ann NY Acad Sci* 1995;772:64–76.

376. Mancini-Bourgine M, Fontaine H, Scott-Algara D, et al. Induction or expansion of T-cell responses by a hepatitis B DNA vaccine administered to chronic HBV carriers. *Hepatology* 2004;40:874–82.

377. Heathcote J, McHutchison J, Lee S, et al. A pilot study of the CY-1899 T-cell vaccine in subjects chronically infected with hepatitis B virus. The CY1899 T Cell Vaccine Study Group. *Hepatology* 1999;30:531–6 (see comments).

378. Lok AS, McMahon BJ. Chronic hepatitis B: update 2009. *Hepatology* 2009;50:661–2.

379. EASL Clinical Practice Guidelines: management of chronic hepatitis B. *J Hepatol* 2009;50:227–42.

380. Liaw YF, Leung N, Kao JH, et al. Asian–Pacific consensus statement on the management of chronic hepatitis B: a 2008 update. *Hepatol Int* 2008;2:263–83.

381. Sorrell MF, Belongia EA, Costa J, et al. National Institutes of Health Consensus Development Conference Statement: management of hepatitis B. *Ann Intern Med* 2009;150:104–10.

382. Bichko V, Netter HJ, Wu TT, et al. Pathogenesis associated with replication of hepatitis delta virus. *Infect Agents Dis* 1994;3:94–7.

383. Taylor J, Negro F, Rizzetto M. Hepatitis delta virus: from structure to disease expression. *Rev Med Virol* 1992;2:161–7.

384. Le Gal F, Gault E, Ripault MP, et al. Eighth major clade for hepatitis delta virus. *Emerg Infect Dis* 2006;12:1447–50.

385. Ryu WS, Netter HJ, Bayer M, et al. Ribonucleoprotein complexes of hepatitis delta virus. *J Virol* 1993;67:3281–7.

386. Gowans EJ, Baroudy BM, Negro F, et al. Evidence for replication of hepatitis delta virus RNA in hepatocyte nuclei after in vivo infection. *Virology* 1988;167:274–8.

387. Smedile A, Farci P, Verme G, et al. Influence of delta infection on severity of hepatitis B. *Lancet* 1982;2:945–7.

388. Caredda F, d'Arminio Monforte A, Rossi E, et al. Prospective study of epidemic delta infection in drug addicts. *Prog Clin Biol Res* 1983;143:245–50.

389. Smedile A, Dentico P, Zanetti A, et al. Infection with the delta agent in chronic HBsAg carriers. *Gastroenterology* 1981;81:992–7.

390. Rizzetto M, Durazzo M. Hepatitis delta virus (HDV) infections. Epidemiological and clinical heterogeneity. *J Hepatol* 1991;13(Suppl 4):S116–18.

391. Grigorescu M, Pascu O, Acalovschi M, et al. What is the real prevalence of the D virus infection in chronic hepatitis and liver cirrhosis in Romania? *Rom J Gastroenterol* 2003;12:179–82.

392. Kao JH, Chen PJ, Lai MY, et al. Hepatitis D virus genotypes in intravenous drug users in Taiwan: decreasing prevalence and lack of correlation with hepatitis B virus genotypes. *J Clin Microbiol* 2002;40:3047–9.

393. Gaeta GB, Stroffolini T, Chiaramonte M, et al. Chronic hepatitis D: a vanishing disease? An Italian multicenter study. *Hepatology* 2000;32:824–7.

394. Stroffolini T, Ferrigno L, Cialdea L, et al. Incidence and risk factors of acute delta hepatitis in Italy: results from a national surveillance system. *SEIEVA Collaborating Group.* J Hepatol 1994;21:1123–6.

395. Le Gal F, Castelneau C, Gault E, et al. Hepatitis D virus infection – not a vanishing disease in Europe! – Reply. *Hepatology* 2007;45:1332–3.

396. Weisfuse IB, Hadler SC, Fields HA, et al. Delta hepatitis in homosexual men in the United States. *Hepatology* 1989;9:872–4.

397. Aragona M, Macagno S, Caredda F, et al. Serological response to the hepatitis delta virus in hepatitis D. *Lancet* 1987;1:478–80.

398. Buti M, Esteban R, Jardi R, et al. Serological diagnosis of acute delta hepatitis. *J Med Virol* 1986;18:81–5.

399. Mederacke I, Bremer B, Heidrich B, et al. Establishment of a novel quantitative hepatitis D virus (HDV) RNA assay using the Cobas TaqMan platform to study HDV RNA kinetics. *J Clin Microbiol* 2010;48:2022–9.

400. Schaper M, Rodriguez-Frias F, Jardi R, et al. Quantitative longitudinal evaluations of hepatitis delta virus RNA and hepatitis B virus DNA shows a dynamic, complex replicative profile in chronic hepatitis B and D. *J Hepatol* 2010;52:658–64.

401. Buti M, Esteban R, Roggendorf M, et al. Hepatitis D virus RNA in acute delta infection: serological profile and correlation with other markers of hepatitis D virus infection. *Hepatology* 1988;8:1125–9.

402. Castelnau C, Le Gal F, Ripault MP, et al. Efficacy of peginterferon alpha-2b in chronic hepatitis delta: relevance of quantitative RT-PCR for follow-up. *Hepatology* 2006;44:728–35.

403. Di Bisceglie AM, Negro F. Diagnosis of hepatitis delta virus infection. *Hepatology* 1989;10:1014–16.

404. Fattovich G, Giustina G, Christensen E, et al. Influence of hepatitis delta virus infection on morbidity and mortality in compensated cirrhosis type B. The European Concerted Action on Viral Hepatitis (Eurohep). *Gut* 2000;46:420–6.

405. Casey JL, Brown TL, Colan EJ, et al. A genotype of hepatitis D virus that occurs in northern South America. *Proc Natl Acad Sci USA* 1993;90:9016–20.

406. Wu JC, Choo KB, Chen CM, et al. Genotyping of hepatitis D virus by restriction-fragment length polymorphism and relation to outcome of hepatitis D. *Lancet* 1995;346:939–41.

407. Kiesslich D, Crispim MA, Santos C, et al. Influence of hepatitis B virus (HBV) genotype on the clinical course of disease in patients coinfected with HBV and hepatitis delta virus. *J Infect Dis* 2009;199:1608–11.

408. Su CW, Huang YH, Huo TI, et al. Genotypes and viremia of hepatitis B and D viruses are associated with outcomes of chronic hepatitis D patients. *Gastroenterology* 2006;130:1625–35.

409. Smedile A, Rosina F, Saracco G, et al. Hepatitis B virus replication modulates pathogenesis of hepatitis D virus in chronic hepatitis D. *Hepatology* 1991;13:413–16.

410. Ilan Y, Klein A, Taylor J, et al. Resistance of hepatitis delta virus replication to interferon-alpha treatment in transfected human cells. *J Infect Dis* 1992;166:1164–6.

411. McNair AN, Cheng D, Monjardino J, et al. Hepatitis delta virus replication in vitro is not affected by interferon-alpha or -gamma despite intact cellular responses to interferon and dsRNA. *J Gen Virol* 1994;75(6):1371–8.

412. Pugnale P, Pazienza V, Guilloux K, et al. Hepatitis delta virus inhibits alpha interferon signaling. *Hepatology* 2009;49:398–406.

413. Rosina F, Pintus C, Meschievitz C, et al. A randomized controlled trial of a 12-month course of recombinant human interferon-alpha in chronic delta (type D) hepatitis: a multicenter Italian study. *Hepatology* 1991;13:1052–6.

414. Farci P MA, Coiana A, Lai ME, et al. Treatment of chronic hepatitis D with interferon alfa-2a. *N Engl J Med* 1994: 88–94.

415. Farci P, Roskams T, Chessa L, et al. Long-term benefit of interferon alpha therapy of chronic hepatitis D: regression of advanced hepatic fibrosis. *Gastroenterology* 2004;126:1740–9.

416. Ferenci P, Formann E, Romeo R. Successful treatment of chronic hepatitis D with a short course of peginterferon alfa-2a. *Am J Gastroenterol* 2005;100:1626–7.

417. Niro G, Ciancio A, Gaeta GB, et al. Pegylated interferon alpha-2b as monotherapy or in combination with ribavirin in chronic hepatitis delta. *Hepatology* 2006;44:713–20.

418. Erhardt A, Gerlich W, Starke C, et al. Treatment of chronic hepatitis delta with pegylated interferon-alpha2b. *Liver Int* 2006;26:805–10.

419. Wedemeyer H, Yurdaydìn C, Dalekos GN, Erhardt A, Çakaloğlu Y, Değertekin H, Gürel S, Zeuzem S, Zachou K, Bozkaya H, Koch A, Bock T, Dienes HP, Manns MP; HIDIT Study Group.Peginterferon plus adefovir versus either drug alone for hepatitis delta. *N Engl J Med* 2011;364:322-31.

420. Lau DT, Doo E, Park Y, et al. Lamivudine for chronic delta hepatitis. *Hepatology* 1999;30:546–9.

421. Wolters LM, van Nunen AB, Honkoop P, et al. Lamivudine-high dose interferon combination therapy for chronic hepatitis B patients co-infected with the hepatitis D virus. *J Viral Hepat* 2000;7:428–34.

422. Rizzetto M, Canese MG, Gerin JL, et al. Transmission of the hepatitis B virus-associated delta antigen to chimpanzees. *J Infect Dis* 1980;141:590–602.

CHAPTER 25
Hepatitis C

Jama M. Darling, Stanley M. Lemon, & Michael W. Fried

UNC Liver Center, University of North Carolina at Chapel Hill, Chapel Hill, NC, USA

Key concepts

- Hepatitis C infection is a leading cause of morbidity and mortality with a global prevalence of approximately 3%.
- Diagnosis of chronic hepatitis C relies on establishing the presence of risk factors or evidence of liver disease and testing patients with sensitive and specific serologic and virologic assays.
- Hepatitis C virus (HCV) is a single-stranded RNA virus with one open reading frame that encodes a large polyprotein. Viral proteases are required for protein processing and viral replication. Replication can be profoundly inhibited by drugs that target these enzymes, which is the rational for the newest generation of HCV therapeutics.

- Hepatitis C is a heterogeneous virus with multiple genotypes that have important implications for therapeutic response.
- Pegylated interferon (pegIFN) and ribavirin achieve sustained virologic response in 45–80% of patients, depending upon genotype.
- Response-guided therapy utilizes the change in hepatitis C viremia during treatment to modify the treatment course or the choice of therapeutic regimens.
- Small molecules, such as protease inhibitors, combined with pegIFN and ribavirin will further enhance treatment response and minimize the emergence of viral resistance. Additional side effects may occur in these triple therapy combinations.

A discovery that changed the practice of hepatology

When sensitive serologic tests for hepatitis A virus (HAV) and hepatitis B virus (HBV) infection became available in the mid-1970s, it became clear that most cases of post-transfusion hepatitis could not be attributed to either virus [1,2]. This led to the description of a new disease entity termed "non-A, non-B" (NANB) hepatitis, and prompted a fierce search for a new, previously unrecognized hepatitis virus. Post-transfusion and community-acquired NANB hepatitis were increasingly recognized as potential causes of cirrhosis and hepatocellular carcinoma [3,4]. An early breakthrough in identifying the virus came with the demonstration that chimpanzees (*Pan troglodytes*) were susceptible to NANB infection when inoculated with blood products from affected patients [5,6]. This proved that the disease was due to an infectious agent, which was then shown to be susceptible to lipid solvents and capable of passing though a 50–80 nm filter, and thus likely to be a small, enveloped virus [7,8]. The responsible agent, hepatitis C (HCV), was subsequently identified by a group of scientists led by Michael Houghton, who screened a λ-phage complemen-

tary DNA (cDNA) expression library derived from chimpanzee material for reactivity with serum antibodies from patients with chronic NANB hepatitis [9,10]. Antigen expressed by a single molecular clone, 5-1-1, was recognized only by serum antibodies from patients with well-documented NANB hepatitis, setting the stage for all future work on HCV [11]. Arguably, the discovery of HCV was the most important discovery in modern hepatology, leading to an explosion of research in the virology, epidemiology, and therapeutics of this disease, which is now curable in many patients.

Hepatitis C virus virology

Classification and genome organization

Hepatitis C virus is classified in the genus *Hepacivirus* of the family Flaviviridae. It is an enveloped, hepatotropic virus with a positive-sense, single-stranded RNA genome about 9.6 kb in length (for a detailed review, see [12]). The genome is organized to include untranslated RNA segments (UTRs) at both ends and a single large open reading frame encoding a giant 327 kD polyprotein that is processed by cellular and virally encoded proteases into ten

Schiff's Diseases of the Liver, Eleventh Edition. Edited by Eugene R. Schiff, Willis C. Maddrey and Michael F. Sorrell.
© 2012 John Wiley & Sons, Ltd. Published 2012 by John Wiley & Sons, Ltd.

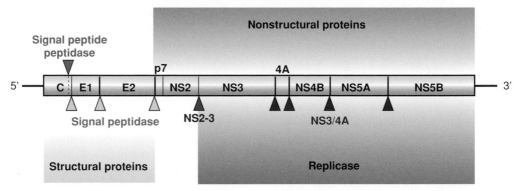

Figure 25.1 Genomic organization of hepatitis C virus. (Reproduced from Lemon [59] with permission from American Society for Biochemistry and Molecular Biology.)

mature viral proteins (Fig. 25.1). The viral RNA lacks the 5′ methylated cap structure typical of cellular mRNAs, and contains a highly conserved internal ribosomal entry site (IRES) within the 5′ UTR that directs cap-independent initiation of translation. There are six well-defined genotypes of HCV, which differ in nucleotide sequence at ~30% of base positions [13].

Untranslated RNA segments

The 5′ and 3′ UTRs are highly conserved in sequence and adopt conserved secondary and tertiary RNA folds that recruit cellular and viral factors required for translation of the polyprotein and replication of the RNA [12,14]. Phylogenetic, biochemical, and mutational analyses suggest that the 342 nucleotide-long 5′ UTR is comprised of four distinct structural domains, designated stem loops I–IV [15,16]. The 5′ 125 nucleotides constitute domains I and II, which are essential for RNA replication [17]. Within this region of the RNA, between stem loops I and II, are two sites that bind the cellular microRNA, miR-122, an interaction that is critically important for viral translation and genome amplification [18,19]. Downstream, the IRES is formed by nucleotides 45–342 (domains II–IV), and thus partially overlaps the RNA replication signals at the extreme 5′ terminus of the genome. Its folded structure has high affinity for the 40S ribosomal subunit, and directs the cap-independent assembly of a 48S ribosomal complex on the viral RNA [20,21]. The IRES also binds eukaryotic initiation factor, eIF-3, and initiates translation without a requirement for other canonical cellular transcriptional factors [20,21].

The 3′ UTR is 200–235 nucleotides in length and consists of three distinct regions: a variable region, a poly-U/UC tract, and an absolutely conserved 98 nucleotide-long "3′ X" region [22]. The 3′ X region folds into conserved stem-loop structures that are involved in RNA–RNA and RNA–protein interactions essential for efficient replication of the viral RNA [23,24].

Structural proteins

The amino terminus of the polyprotein is proteolytically processed by the endoplasmic reticulum (ER) resident signal peptidase to produce a series of structural proteins that are components of the infectious virus particle (Fig. 25.1). These include the ~23 kD, 191-amino-acid-residue-long core protein [25], which is further processed by another cellular membrane-resident protease, signal peptide peptidase, removing the C-terminal signal sequence to yield the ~21 kD mature core protein [26–29].

The core protein has been implicated in a variety of interactions with a wide array of host cell proteins, leading potentially to pleiotropic effects on the cell [30]. Important host factors that putatively interact with the core protein include those involved in cell signaling, transcription, apoptosis, lipid metabolism, immunomodulation, oxidative stress, cell cycle regulation, and carcinogenesis (reviewed in [30–33]).

The HCV genome encodes for two envelope glycoproteins, E1 and E2, which are processed from the polyprotein by cellular signal peptidase. Both the glycoproteins are embedded in the viral envelope, which is derived from host membranes, as noncovalent heterodimers [34] due to charged residues within the transmembrane domains [35]. They appear to interact with the core protein, as well as NS2 (see below). The E2 glycoprotein plays a major role in viral entry as it binds to the HCV co-receptor CD81, a member of the tetraspanin family of proteins that is central to HCV entry and that is expressed on the surface of the hepatocytes, and scavenger receptor B1 (SR-B1) [36–38].

Nonstructural proteins

Downstream of the envelope proteins within the polyprotein are p7 and NS2 (see Fig. 25.1). p7 is a viroporin, a membrane-embedded ion channel that prevents the acidification of intracellular vessicles [39]. p7 is essential for HCV infectivity in the chimpanzee model [40] and plays a crucial role in the assembly and release of infectious virions from infected cells by protecting nascent viral particles from an acidic environment [39,41].

NS2 plays a dual role in viral replication, contributing both to processing of the polyprotein and assembly of the viral particle. It is a membrane-bound protein that is cleaved from the polyprotein at its N-terminus by signal peptidase [42]. Its C-terminus is processed by an autocatalytic proteinase activity residing in the C-terminal domain of NS2 and the N-terminal domain of NS3 [43–45]. The NS2-3 protease is an unusual enzyme as it is a dimeric structure with two composite active sites, in which the active site residues within each site are derived from both members of the dimer [46]. Thus two copies of the polyprotein must be expressed and capable of interacting with each other prior to processing beyond the NS2–3 junction. Although NS2 is not required for viral RNA synthesis and genome amplification [47], recent data suggest that NS2, but not its protease activity, plays a crucial role in viral assembly [48–50]. It acts as a scaffold, bridging the envelope proteins to NS5A and other nonstructural proteins in an early step in particle assembly, and also participates in a late stage of virus assembly that confers and/or enhances infectivity [51,52].

The nonstructural proteins NS3–5B are both necessary and sufficient for robust replication of the genome in cultured hepatoma cells [47]. All of these proteins are associated with intracellular membranes, and serve as components of the membrane-bound replicase complex (sometimes referred to as the "membranous web") that is responsible for viral RNA synthesis. Most if not all of these proteins are multifunctional, a common attribute of small RNA viruses such as HCV that have limited genetic coding capacity. The NS3 protein contains two distinct, independently folding structural domains, an amino terminal serine protease, and a carboxy terminal helicase [53]. The protease comprises the first 180 amino acids of the protein.

The chymotrypsin-like NS3/4A serine protease [54] is the major protease activity expressed by HCV. It is responsible for cleavage at the NS3–4A junction and other sites downstream within the polyprotein, thereby generating the remaining nonstructural proteins: NS4A, NS4B, NS5A, and NS5B (see Fig. 25.1) [55]. It also cleaves at least two cellular proteins – mitochondrial antiviral signaling protein (MAVS, also known as IPS-1, Cardif, or VISA) [56] and Toll-like receptor (TLR)/interleukin 1 (IL1) receptor domain-containing adaptor-inducing interferon-β (TRIF, otherwise known as TICAM-1) [56–58] – both of which are signaling adaptor proteins involved in the induction of interferon synthesis in virus-infected cells [59].

The carboxy terminal two thirds of NS3 is a superfamily-2 helicase with nucleoside triphosphatase (NTPase), RNA translocase, and unwindase activity [60].

It is indispensable for viral replication [61,62]. The NS3 helicase domain plays a central role during an early step in virion assembly [63–65].

NS4A is a cofactor for the NS3 serine protease, as described above. Since it is a membrane-bound protein, it is likely to mediate the membrane association of NS3 [66]. NS4B is an integral membrane protein that induces formation of the "membranous web" [67,68], the probable site of HCV RNA replication within cells [69]. It contains a guanosine triphosphatase (GTPase) activity and associates with the early endosome Rab5 protein [70,71].

The NS5A protein is unique, with no known human or viral homologs other than NS5A in the closely related GB virus B (GBV-B). It appears to have multiple functions in the virus life cycle and to interact with numerous viral and host proteins [72], but it is poorly understood at a mechanistic level. It is a phosphoprotein [73–75], and the phosphorylation status of NS5A may regulate various aspects of genome replication and virus assembly [76,77]. NS5A possesses three distinct domains, which are separated by segments of the protein that are relatively disordered. The N-terminal domain (domain I) contains a zinc-binding motif, and is essential for viral RNA replication [78]. The middle domain of NS5A is involved in antagonizing innate immune responses, while the C-terminal domain III of NS5A is poorly conserved between different viral genotypes and has been considered to be relatively unstructured [79]. NS5A appears to play an important role in the assembly of infectious particles, as it interacts with NS2 and is also recruited to the surface of cytoplasmic lipid droplets decorated with the viral core protein [52,80,81]. NS5A, in association with NS2, is also likely to act at a later step in virus production, following intracellular particle assembly but prior to the release of infectious virus [51].

NS5B, the viral RNA-dependent RNA polymerase (RdRp), is the catalytic core of the replicase complex that directs the synthesis of new RNA genomes. It is anchored to cellular membranes via its carboxy terminal hydrophobic tail [82]. Although NS5B can catalyze both primer-independent and primer-dependent RNA synthesis in vitro, the available evidence supports primer-independent, de novo RNA synthesis regulated by a conformational change in the polymerase [83–85]. Like all RdRps, NS5B lacks proofreading capability, and has a relatively high rate of base mis-incorporation. The error-prone nature of HCV RNA synthesis, coupled with selective immune pressure, generates extensive sequence diversity and quasispecies heterogeneity [86].

Replication cycle

It is not possible to culture wild-type strains of HCV efficiently in cell culture, and this has impeded the elucidation of the viral life cycle. However, much has been learned from the development of RNA replicons, in which the segment of the HCV genome encoding the core NS2 proteins is replaced by a sequence encoding a selectable marker (for example, neomycin phosphotransferase) and translation of the downstream nonstructural proteins (NS3–5B) is initiated by a heterologous, picornaviral IRES [47]. These RNAs replicate efficiently in Huh7 human hepatoma cells, and appear to do so by a process that is similar if not identical to RNA replication in HCV-infected cells. Some replicons have been engineered to express the entire viral polyprotein, or easily quantifiable reporter enzymes such as firefly luciferase. Beginning about 2005, however, it became possible to generate infectious virus and study the entire virus life cycle in cell culture using an unusual genotype 2a cDNA clone. This clone was isolated from a Japanese patient with a rare case of fulminant hepatitis C, designated as JFH-1 (Japanese fulminant hepatitis 1) [87,88]. The JFH-1 clone has been used as the backbone for a number of chimeric viral RNAs that are also capable of producing infectious virus when transfected into Huh7 cells [50,89, 90]. A highly cell-culture-adapted genotype 1a genome containing five adaptive mutations (H77S) has also been shown to produce virus when transfected into Huh7 cells, but does so with less efficiency than JFH-1 RNA [91,92]. Virus produced in vitro by transfection of either JFH-1 or H77S RNA is infectious for the chimpanzee.

Viral entry into the hepatocyte is a complex process that is initiated by interactions of the envelope glycoproteins with glycosaminoglycans on the cell surface [93–95]. This is followed by specific receptor interactions leading to clathrin-mediated endocytosis [96], and delivery of the viral RNA to the cytoplasm via an organized, stepwise process [36,97,98]. Early steps in this process include the engagement of the CD81 and SR-B1 co-receptors, both of which have been shown to bind to the E2 glycoprotein and to mediate infectious virus entry [99]. Subsequent steps in entry involve cellular proteins associated with tight junctions – claudin-1 [100] and occludin [101] – but it is not clear that these proteins engage in direct interactions with the viral envelope.

Following entry and uncoating of the viral genome [102], the IRES directs initiation of polyprotein translation. This, like all subsequent steps in the life cycle, occurs within the cytoplasm. The nascent polyprotein is cotranslationally processed by cellular and viral proteases, as described above, giving rise to the seven nonstructural and four structural viral proteins described in the preceding section. These proteins are involved in the formation of membrane-associated replication complexes, and the assembly of new viral particles [12]. As with other positive-strand RNA viruses, replication proceeds in an asymmetric fashion with a single copy of negative-strand RNA producing multiple copies of positive-strand genomes, leading to a 10–100-fold excess of positive- over negative-strand molecules. Importantly, only a small proportion of the nonstructural proteins produced by the virus appear to be engaged in this process of RNA synthesis [103]. Finally, newly synthesized viral genomes and structural proteins (core, E1, and E2) are assembled as virions, in a process that is facilitated by multiple nonstructural proteins, as described above, in association with lipid droplets. Mature viral particles appear to be released from infected cells via an unusual mechanism that usurps some components of the very low density lipoprotein (VLDL) secretory pathway [104,105]. This may account for the very low density of mature virions [106] and their association with host ApoE lipoprotein [107–109].

Innate immune response to HCV

Most persons with acute HCV infection fail to clear the virus and progress to chronic hepatitis C (reviewed in [59]). Virus-specific T-cell immunity is important in determining the infection outcome. While the mechanisms that underlie the failure of adaptive T-cell responses to clear infection remain undefined, there is growing evidence that early innate cytokine and chemokine responses play a fundamental role in shaping later adaptive immunity, and that these early responses to virus infections are critical to successful antigen-specific B- and T-cell immunity [110–113]. There has thus been increasing interest in how HCV infection is sensed by the innate immune system in the liver, and how the virus may have evolved to overcome these early host responses, including the antiviral effects of interferon (IFN). Current evidence suggests that HCV disrupts IFN responses at three levels: (i) the induction of IFN synthesis following sensing of the infection by retinoic acid-inducible gene I (RIG-I) and Toll-like receptor 3 (TLR3), pathogen-associated molecular pattern (PAMP) receptors that recognize double-stranded viral RNA (dsRNA) in cytosolic and extracellular compartments, respectively; (ii) IFN-induced signaling through the Janus kinase and signal transducer and activator of transcription (Jak-STAT) pathway following binding of type I IFNs to their receptor; and (iii) the effector function of some interferon-stimulated genes (ISGs), such as protein kinase R (PKR) (reviewed in [59]).

Innate immune sensing of hepatitis C virus infection

Interferon regulatory factor 3 (IRF-3) is a highly regulated transcription factor constitutively expressed in the cytoplasm in a latent, inactive form. It plays a key role in the induction of IFN synthesis [114]. Infections with RNA viruses such as HCV are associated with the

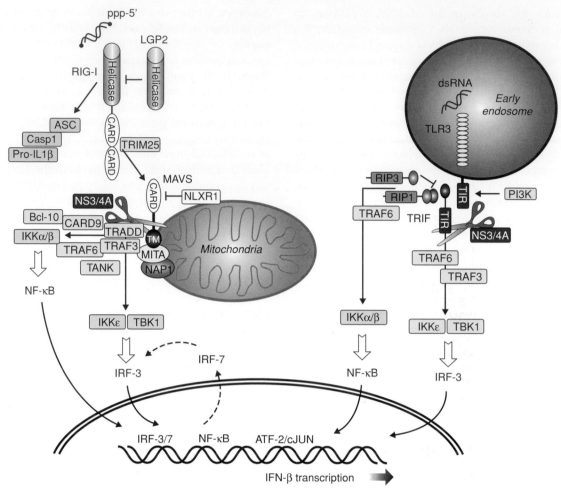

Figure 25.2 Retinoic acid-inducible gene I (RIG-I) and Toll-like receptor 3 (TLR3) sensing of viral RNAs. IFN, interferon; IRF, interferon regulatory factor; MAVS, mitochondrial antiviral signaling; NF-κB, nuclear factor κB; TRIF, TLR/IL-1 receptor domain-containing adaptor-inducing interferon-β. (Reproduced from Lemon [59] with permission from American Society for Biochemistry and Molecular Biology.)

production of dsRNA, an essential replication intermediate. This RNA is distinct from cellular RNAs and is sensed by and activates signaling pathways leading to C-terminal phosphorylation of IRF-3. This results in the dimerization and nuclear transport of IRF-3, where in coordination with nuclear factor κB (NF-κB) and activating transcription factor 2 (ATF-2)/c-Jun, it activates the IFN-β promoter, leading to the synthesis of type I IFN-α/β [115]. IRF-3 can be activated through several distinct signaling pathways initiated by different sensors (Fig. 25.2). RIG-I, a DExD helicase family member, senses HCV RNA in the cytosol [116–118]. TLR3, which is expressed in an early endosomal compartment, senses HCV dsRNA in a luminal compartment [119]. Both pathways culminate in IRF-3 activation and type I IFN synthesis, and, when activated, both partially restrict HCV replication [116,119]. A third, potentially important, sensor is TLR7, which signals through the related IRF, IRF-7. Little is known about its role in the induction of IFN

responses to HCV in the liver, but recent studies suggest its potential importance [120]. Although they act to some extent redundantly, these sensors differ in terms of: (i) the PAMPs they sense; (ii) the cell types in which they are expressed; and (iii) the adaptor proteins they utilize and signaling pathways they activate (reviewed in [59]).

RIG-I signaling

RIG-I (DDX58) is a DExD-box helicase expressed within the cytoplasm of hepatocytes. It senses short non-self double-stranded (ds) and single-stranded (ss) RNAs with free 5′ triphosphates [121–123]. Once engaged by its RNA ligand, RIG-I undergoes a conformational change [124], promoting its self-association as well as interactions with its adaptor protein, MAVS, through shared caspase recruitment domains (CARDs) [57,125,126]. This leads to the assembly of a signaling complex on the mitochondrial surface, where MAVS is located, that activates downstream noncanonical kinases of the IkappaB kinase

4 Chapter 25: Hepatitis C 587

(IKK) complex that in turn direct the phosphorylation of IRF-3 [127]. A large number of other signaling partners participate in the formation of this complex, which is both positively and negatively regulated (reviewed in [59]). RIG-I has been shown to sense HCV infection in Huh7 hepatoma cells, leading to transient nuclear translocation of IRF-3 and activation of the IFN-β promoter [128]. Injection of large amounts of synthetic HCV RNA into the tail vein of mice delivers the RNA directly to the liver, resulting in activation of RIG-I signaling [117]. Studies using this system suggest that a conserved poly-(U/C) sequence within the 3′ UTR of HCV is a PAMP that is specifically recognized by RIG-I.

NS3/4A, the major protease expressed by HCV, inhibits activation of the IFN-β promoter in cells containing HCV replicons [129]. This is due to NS3/4A-mediated cleavage of the RIG-I adaptor protein MAVS [57,58]. Proteolysis occurs close to the C-terminus of MAVS, releasing it from the mitochondrial membrane and eliminating its capacity to signal. Although RIG-I initially senses HCV infection in hepatoma cells, signaling is shut down as infection progresses, NS3/4A accumulates, and MAVS is degraded [116]. The NS3/4A-mediated shutdown of RIG-I signaling can be reversed by small molecule NS3/4A protease inhibitors, but such reversal appears to occur only at concentrations far exceeding the effective antiviral concentration of drugs (EC$_{50}$) [130]. Why higher drug concentrations are required to restore signaling and IFN synthesis is unknown. The fact that restoration of RIG-I signaling is only observed at high drug concentrations suggests that protease inhibitors are unlikely to provide any therapeutic advantage over other small molecule antivirals based on this mechanism [130].

There is good clinical evidence that HCV functionally disrupts RIG-I signaling by targeting MAVS for cleavage by NS3/4A, as immunoblots show MAVS to be cleaved in liver biopsies from some patients with chronic hepatitis C [116]. Despite this, intrahepatic IFN-stimulated gene responses are observed in many patients, particularly those who are refractory to treatment with pegylated interferon (pegIFN) and ribavirin [131]. These responses are likely induced through alternative signaling pathways, or may originate in newly infected cells that have yet to accumulate sufficient NS3/4A to ablate signaling.

TLR3 signaling

In addition to the cytosolic RIG-I-like receptors, membrane-bound TLRs also sense RNA virus infections and are equally, if not more, important in activation of T-cell responses [113]. HCV disruption of these sensing pathways could thus be very important for persistence. TLR3 is expressed within an early endosomal compartment where it senses extracellular dsRNA molecules greater than 40–50 base pairs in length [132,133]. Struc-

tural models suggest that the dsRNA binds sites at opposite ends of a horseshoe-shaped TLR3 ectodomain and that this results in its dimerization [134]. Dimerization leads to signaling through its cytosolic, Toll–interleukin 1 receptor homology (TIR) domain, resulting in recruitment of the adaptor protein, TRIF (see Fig. 25.2) [135,136]. Although many details remain uncertain, TRIF then relocates to distinct punctate cytoplasmic bodies to which tumor necrosis factor (TNF) receptor-associated factor 6 (TRAF6), TRAF3, and TANK-binding kinase 1 (TBK-1) are recruited [133]. This leads to phosphorylation of IRF-3 and subsequent activation of the IFN-β promoter, providing a pathway to induction of IFN synthesis that operates in parallel to the RIG-I pathway [135,137]. TLR3 ligation of dsRNA also strongly induces NF-κB activity and proinflammatory cytokine synthesis via interactions of TRIF with receptor-interacting protein 1 (RIP-1) kinase [135,138].

Both TLR3 and TRIF are expressed in human hepatocytes, and primary human hepatocyte cultures induce a robust IFN response when stimulated with poly-(I:C), a dsRNA surrogate that acts as a TLR3 ligand [119,139]. These responses are blocked by the HCV NS3/4A protease, which is capable of cleaving TRIF [56,140]. The amino acid sequence of TRIF at the site of NS3–4A cleavage is closely related to the sequence at the NS4B–5A junction in the HCV polyprotein, representing a remarkable example of molecular mimicry. TRIF is absolutely required for TLR3-mediated IFN responses [136,141], and TRIF expression and TLR3 signaling were ablated in HeLa cells containing an HCV replicon [56]. Signaling was restored by treating the cells with a protease inhibitor [56].

TLR7 signaling

Plasmacytoid dendritic cells (pDCs) are professional IFN-producing cells that are recruited to sites of viral infection and play a central role in effective antiviral host responses [25]. pDCs express TLR7 and TLR8, which sense guanosine- or uridine-rich ssRNA molecules associated with RNA virus infections. In response to these ligands, pDCs secrete enormous quantities of types I and III IFN-α/β/λ, producing as much as 1–2 units/cell/24 h [25]. pDCs are the source of most IFN produced in response to many types of RNA virus infections in mice. pDCs are activated when viral RNA is sensed by TLR7, which, like TLR3, is expressed in an endosomal location. Autophagy appears to play a key role in this process [44]. TLR7 signals through a third, widely utilized adaptor protein, myeloid differentiation response gene 88 (MyD88), directly activating IRF-7, which is expressed at high abundance in pDCs. While there is no widely-accepted evidence that HCV replicates in pDCs, co-cultivation of human pDCs with Huh7 cells infected with the JFH-1 strain of HCV results in abundant secretion of IFN-α, while exposure of pDCs to purified virus does not [120]. While the mechanism is not clear, the infected Huh7 cells in some way "present" viral ssRNA to the pDCs, thereby inducing IFN production through the TLR7 pathway. Such a hypothesis is consistent with infiltration of abundant BDCA2+ (blood dendritic cell antigen 2) pDCs in the liver of patients with hepatitis C [142]. Furthermore, this could explain the source of the IFN driving ISG expression in the liver of many patients with chronic hepatitis C [131], despite disruption of TLR3 and RIG-I signaling. TLR7 may also be expressed at low levels in hepatocytes, as a potent TLR7 agonist has been shown to induce an antiviral response in Huh7 cells containing an HCV replicon [143]. It is not known whether HCV inhibits TLR7 signaling.

Hepatitis C virus and interferon resistance

In addition to its ability to disrupt signaling pathways involved in the induction of IFN synthesis, HCV may also block the antiviral actions of IFN. Activated IRF-3 induces the synthesis of IFN-α/β, as described above. It also controls transcription of type III IFNs, including IFN-λ3 (otherwise known as IL28B) [144], which recent genome-wide association studies show to be of crucial importance both in resolution of acute HCV infection and in response to therapy [145,146].

Once its synthesis is induced through any of the pathways described above, IFN-β is secreted from the cell. It then binds the type I IFN-α/β receptor (IFNAR), resulting in autocrine/paracrine activation of the Jak-STAT pathway. This leads in turn to expression of many dozens of ISGs controlled by promoters containing IFN response elements (ISREs). Among the genes induced are the α-IFNs as well as IRF-7; the latter forms heterodimers with IRF-3 and acts to amplify the induction of ISGs [147]. IFN-l binds a distinct heterodimeric receptor comprised of IL10R2 and IFN-LR1 subunits, but utilizes the same Jak-STAT signaling pathway downstream to activate ISG transcription [148]. Thus it induces the same complex of ISGs. Activated IRF-3 also directly mediates the transcription of a subset of ISGs, some of which (like ISG56) have direct antiviral activity against HCV [149,150]. Despite this elaborate orchestration of antiviral gene expression, many HCV-infected patients fail to mount an effective antiviral response to either endogenous IFN or exogenous pegIFN and ribavirin therapy.

Recent studies in both patients and HCV-infected chimpanzees have begun to provide some mechanistic insights concerning this lack of response to IFN [131,151]. Poor therapeutic responses to pegIFN were found to be associated with high intrahepatic transcription of ISGs prior to treatment. In contrast, patients who experienced a rapid virologic response (RVR: negative serum HCV RNA after 4 weeks of treatment) to pegIFN had little ISG expression in the liver before therapy, but demonstrated impressive upregulation of ISGs when treated [131]. Importantly, the ISG response to pegIFN in RVR patients did not exceed that found before treatment in nonresponder patients. The preactivation of ISGs was confined largely to the liver, and was not present in peripheral blood mononuclear cells (PBMCs) (highlighting the need to characterize IFN responses in liver, not PBMCs) [131]. These seminal observations indicate that some patients do not induce an IFN response despite being infected with HCV, while the virus persists in others in the face of a robust IFN-mediated antiviral response.

These observations raise two important questions. The first relates to the source of the IFN driving the ISG response in some infected patients. As mentioned above, it may be produced by newly infected hepatocytes through RIG-I or TLR3 sensing of viral RNA prior to the expression of sufficient NS3/4A to shut down signaling [116]. Or, alternatively, IFN might be produced by uninfected hepatocytes that sense dsRNA in the extracellular environment through TLR3-mediated signaling [119]. Yet another possibility is that HCV infection might be sensed by TLR7 in infiltrating pDCs [120]. An equally important question is how the virus survives despite robust ISG expression. This may be due to viral evasion of the antiviral actions of specific ISGs, such as PKR, which is antagonized by NS5A [152]. Alternatively, given the diversity of antiviral ISGs potentially induced by IFN-α, HCV may disrupt Jak-STAT signaling downstream of the IFNAR to escape the antiviral actions of IFN.

While Jak-STAT signaling is not completely disrupted, recent studies have directly documented that it is impaired in HCV-infected human liver tissue ex vivo [153]. Several mechanisms have been proposed to account for this (Fig. 25.3) (reviewed in [59]). Core protein may inhibit Jak-STAT signaling by interacting directly with STAT1, leading to reduced phospho-STAT1 [154,155]. In addition, protein phosphatase 2A (PP2A) is upregulated in transgenic mice expressing core protein [156]. This leads to reduced methylation of STAT1 due to inhibition of protein arginine methyl transferase 1 (PRMT1), which promotes its association with protein inhibitor of activated STAT1 (PIAS1), a negative regulator of STAT1 gene transcription [153,157,158]. Other data suggest that poor treatment outcome may be related to enhanced hepatic expression of suppressor of cytokine signaling 3 (SOCS3), which impedes Jak-STAT signaling [155,159].

Poor responses to pegIFN therapy are also associated with increased expression of ubiquitin-specific peptidase 18 (USP18, or UBP43) [131,160]. USP18 interacts with

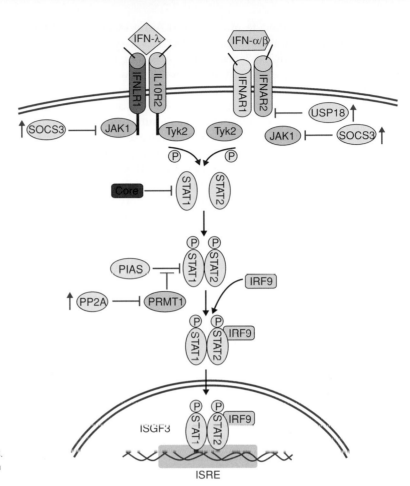

Figure 25.3 Interferon-induced Jak–STAT signaling in hepatitis C. IFN, interferon; IERS, interferon response elements. (Reproduced from Lemon [59] with permission from American Society for Biochemistry and Molecular Biology.)

the IFNAR2 subunit of IFNAR, and may thus suppress Jak-STAT signaling induced by type I IFNs [161]. USP18 also possesses ISG15 deconjugase activity, and silencing its expression in cell culture potentiates the antiviral activity of IFN-α against HCV [162]. Like Jak-STAT signaling induced by type I IFN, IFN-l-induced signaling is subject to suppression by PP2A and SOCS3, but would not be affected by the interaction of USP18 with IFNAR2 [161]. This is an interesting observation given the potent influence of *IL28B* polymorphisms near the IFN-λ3 gene, both in natural clearance of HCV infection and in the response of HCV to pegIFN therapy (discussed further below) [145,146].

Interactions of hepatitis C virus with host immune cells

Hepatitis C virus–host interactions commence immediately with infection as HCV interacts with elements of the innate immune system and modifies cellular antiviral components. These interactions may influence the development of acquired immunity, which is essential for HCV clearance. Conventional dendritic cells (cDCs) are highly specialized antigen-presenting cells (APCs)

that can activate both primary and secondary immune responses through the presentation of antigens mediated by major histocompatibility complex (MHC) class I or class II molecules. Maturation and functional differentiation of cDCs in HCV infection are altered with decreased IL12 and increased IL10 production [163,164]. Furthermore, cDCs obtained from HCV-infected patients may exhibit impaired proliferation and stimulatory activity [164–166]. None the less, there does not seem to be a global impairment of cDC function in chronic HCV. Deficient function of cDCs at critical times early in infection may lead to impaired T-cell priming and contribute to delayed cellular responses.

Natural killer (NK) cells are part of the innate immune system and provide a first-line defense against viral infections because they require no priming to trigger cytotoxic activity and produce IFN-γ. The normal liver has a unique group of resident lymphocytes with up to 65% being NK cells, γ/δ T cells, or NK-like T cells, compared with less than 20% in peripheral blood [167]. The role of NK cells in the control of HCV infection remains undefined but they may play a role in viral clearance. Genetic factors determine the responsiveness of NK cells via human leukocyte antigens (HLAs) and killer-cell immunoglobulin-like receptors (KIR). Homozygosity for HLA-C1 and KIR2DL3 resulted in a higher rate of spontaneous clearance of HCV infection with low inoculums [168]. This KIR/HLA pair delivered a lower inhibition signal, which translated into easier activation of NK cells with viral stimulation. This is supported by faster NK-cell degranulation and IFN-γ release in vitro [169]. Interestingly, the inflammatory environment in the HCV liver may alter NK responses from IFN-γ production towards cytotoxicity, resulting in ongoing liver damage [170,171]. This polarized NK-cell phenotype correlates with alanine aminotransferase (ALT) levels, suggesting participation of virus-induced effector NK cells in liver necroinflammation [170,171]. The HCV protein E2 binds to human CD81 on NK cells and directly inhibits NK-cell function in vitro but this inhibition does not occur when E2 is part of an infectious virion [172,173]. NK cells are potent activators of cDCs and, conversely, cDCs may stimulate NK-cell activity. In chronic HCV infection, NK cells isolated from patients are impaired in their ability to activate cDCs owing to overexpression of the inhibitory receptor CD94/NKG2a as well as production of TGF-β and IL10, which blunt the adaptive response [174].

Adaptive immune responses against hepatitis C virus

The key to development of vaccines and novel immunotherapies to combat HCV lies in careful study of the cellular immune responses of those who successfully clear virus. Most work in humans is done either retrospectively or in incidental patients who present with symptomatic acute infection or with needlestick injuries. Although there is currently no small animal model of HCV infection, the common chimpanzee *Pan troglodytes* is a faithful, replicative model of HCV infection and provides an opportunity to carefully dissect components of immune responses to HCV in a controlled, prospective manner.

CD4+ T-cell responses

CD4+ T cells are specifically activated when their receptors engage complexes of peptides and MHC class II molecules. Their responses are typically characterized by proliferation and/or cytokine production following incubation with recombinant viral proteins or overlapping peptides. Differential cytokine production underpins the specific types of T helper (Th) induced immune responses. CD4+ T cells are absolutely essential for successful immune responses against HCV. The appearance of HCV-specific T cells in the peripheral blood and liver in acute infection precisely coincides with a drop in viral load [175]. A vigorous and multispecific CD4+ T-cell pro-

liferative response against HCV antigens in acute infection correlates with successful clearance [176–178] and this response must be sustained or viral recrudescence will occur [179–181]. This proliferative response is accompanied by IFN-γ and IL2 production [182,183]. The evolution of this multispecific CD4+ T-cell response initially targets a limited number of dominant epitopes and then spreads to additional targets once viremia is better controlled [184].

In resolved infection, HCV-specific CD4+ T memory cells are maintained in the absence of virus; they are expandable in vitro with antigen stimulation and mediate appropriate effector functions [185–187]. When HCV-specific CD4+ T cells from the peripheral blood of recovered versus chronically infected patients are evaluated for cytokine production, responses are predominantly of the Th1 type [185,187,188] and are ten times more frequent in resolvers than chronics and four times more broad [187]. The strength of HCV-specific T-cell responses correlates inversely with viral loads in chronic disease [185,187]. Loss of virus-specific CD4+ T cells may be epitope dependent, with cells specific for core antigen being more readily detectable [189,190].

Since HCV-specific CD4+ T-cell responses in the peripheral blood are generally weak or absent using functional assays, MHC class II peptide tetramers have been used to directly analyze the phenotypes of circulating HCV memory cells in resolved infection. HCV-specific CD4+ T cells were not detected in the peripheral blood in chronically infected patients using class II tetramers. The majority of HCV-specific CD4+ T cells analyzed had a central memory phenotype [191]. These cells, when exposed to antigen, can rapidly proliferate and produce IL2 [192] and are critical for the expansion of memory cytotoxic T lymphocytes (CTLs) [193–195]. As is seen in class I tetramer-based analyses of HCV-specific CD8+ T cells from resolvers [196], the class II tetramer-positive population is polyclonal, utilizing multiple TCR Vβ chains [191]. Using this method of detection, HCV-specific CD4+ memory T cells are 10–100 times less frequent in peripheral blood than their CD8+ counterparts.

CD8+ T-cell responses

CD8+ T cells recognize viral peptides presented by MHC class I molecules on the surface of infected cells. Activation of CD8+ T cells by peptide–MHC complexes can lead to cytolytic and noncytolytic viral control and eradication. HCV-specific T cells appear 5–9 weeks post exposure [180, 197]. As illustrated in Fig. 25.4, a multispecific (targeting multiple viral proteins) and polyclonal (using multiple T-cell receptors) CD8+ T-cell response in the first weeks of acute HCV infection correlates with successful clearance of virus [180,181,197,198]. Frequencies of HCV-specific CTLs at specific epitopes in acute infection may exceed

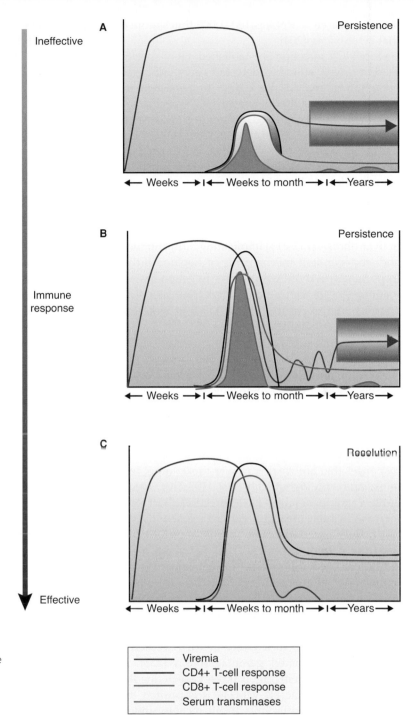

Figure 25.4 Viral and T-cell kinetics with serum transaminases in acute HCV infection. (A–C) Three possible patterns are represented depending upon the strength and durability of the T-cell response including viral persistence due to lack of T-cell response, viral persistence due to lack of durability of T-cell response, and viral clearance with robust and sustained T-cell response. (Reproduced from Bowen and Walker [734] with permission from Nature.)

3–4%. If these robust CD4+ or CD8+ T-cell responses are delayed, transient, or too narrowly focused, viral persistence will ensue. Early in acute infection when ALT levels are elevated, HCV-specific CD8+ T cells exhibit impaired proliferation and cytotoxicity and produce limited amounts of IFN-γ [180,199]. This "restrained phenotype" of CTL is seen in other viral infections and is consistent with high antigen exposure and elevated levels

of programmed death 1 (PD-1) [200–202]. Interestingly, in those who clear infection, this dysfunction resolves when HCV-specific CD4+ T-cell responses develop and viremia ceases [180,182]. During acute infection, a broadly targeted CTL response in the liver may be seen in the absence of biochemical liver disease, which may be secondary to noncytolytic effector functions similar to those seen in HBV infection [181,203]. IFN-γ-mediated inhibition of HCV RNA is 100–1,000 times more effective that cytotoxicity [204].

Once HCV infection is established, HCV-specific CD8+ T cells may still be detected in peripheral blood by tetramer analysis [205–208]. In persistent infection, there are a lower frequency of HCV-specific CTLs and fewer epitopes recognized, although some responses can approximate resolved infection [209]. When compared with CTLs from resolved infection, HCV-specific CD8+ T cells in chronic infection show impaired function, as discussed below [208]. Although most virus-specific CTLs are concentrated in the liver [205], they have not been consistently associated with disease severity [210,211]. Proinflammatory cytokines have been correlated with severity of liver fibrosis [212,213] implicating both antigen-specific and -independent mechanisms of hepatocellular injury. Importantly, in those who resolve infection, HCV-specific memory T cells can be recovered from blood and liver decades after exposure [214,215] and provide some protection against reinfection.

B-cell responses

A role for antibodies in HCV protection or clearance has been difficult to define. Resolution of HCV infection in patients deficient in B cells (agammaglobulinemia) argues that antibodies are not essential for successful HCV immunity [216,217]. Humans and chimpanzees who resolve HCV infection appear to exhibit antibody responses that are weaker (lower titer), target fewer proteins, and may be quickly lost [197,218]. Neutralizing antibodies appear late in HCV infection (8–20 weeks), and increase in titer, breadth, and cross-reactivity over time [219]. They are often isolate specific and difficult to identify from patient to patient [220]. Likewise, neutralizing antibodies exert immune selection pressure, particularly in the hypervariable region of E2 and contribute to quasispecies development [220,221]. In a cohort of chimpanzees challenged with HCV, viral clearance was not associated with anti-E1 or anti-E2 antibodies [222]. Similar findings were reported in a group of Irish women infected by HCV-contaminated gammaglobulin [223]. Nonspecific immunoglobulins (IgG) and IgG-secreting B cells are increased in chronic HCV [224]. It is posited that HCV may stimulate B cells in a B-cell receptor-independent manner resulting in enhanced conversion to Ig-secreting cells [224]. Clonal expansion of B cells is seen within the liver, bone marrow, and peripheral blood in chronic HCV infection and is associated with mixed cryoglobulinemia and non-Hodgkin lymphoma [224,225]. These are further discussed in the HCV natural history section below.

Strategies for viral persistence

A striking feature of HCV infection is the rapidity of viral spread after a percutaneous exposure, which often reaches maximum titers weeks before immune responses are detectable [180]. The ability of HCV to outpace the CD8+ T-cell response or to subvert early innate responses may contribute to its propensity to develop chronic infection. Discussed below are several strategies which HCV may employ to evade T-cell responses.

T-cell anergy

HCV-specific T cells from patients with chronic infection are functionally impaired or "anergic." Over time, these virus-specific T cells become progressively impaired to the point that only weak IFN-γ production remains as a readout [180,198,208,226]. This is not a universal phenomenon in chronic viral infections [206]. HCV-specific CD8+ T cells may be impaired even after viral clearance, which makes their role in viral persistence less clear [206]. These functionally impaired HCV-specific CD8+ T cells are associated with a weak CD4+ T-cell response to HCV antigens [208]. In murine and human systems, maintenance of effective CTL responses in chronic viral infections is dependent upon virus-specific CD4+ T cells that may develop decreased proliferation with repeated antigen exposure [227,228]. Dysfunctional HCV-specific T cells express PD-1 secondary to chronic antigen stimulation [229]. In general, T cells that undergo chronic antigen stimulation lose function over time until only IFN-γ secretion remains [230], as can be seen in chronic HCV infection. PD-1 ligand is highly expressed in liver and its interaction with PD-1-expressing T cells results in apoptosis [231]. Impaired CD8+ T-cell effector function in chronic HCV infection may also be a result of direct interaction with HCV proteins. Extracellular (nonvirion-associated) core protein can bind to the complement receptor gC1qR on T cells [232] and inhibit T-cell proliferation and IFN-γ production [233]. In chronic HCV infection, cellular immune responses are present and may play a role in controlling viremia but lack the fortitude to eliminate virus. Restoring CD8+ T cells to functional competence appears dependent upon the presence of functional CD4 help and appropriate antigen concentrations.

Mutational escape

Hepatitis C virus has a high propagation rate and replicates via an RNA-dependent RNA polymerase that lacks a proofreading mechanism. Each infected individual has their own signature virus made up of quasispecies that result from the error-prone replication process in conjunction with host pressures on the virus [234]. HCV prolifically generates minor viral variants with the potential to avoid immune recognition. Both T and B cells (discussed earlier) provide immune selection pressure on the virus. Based on full-length HCV sequencing studies, HCV escape mutants are selected on a population level in the context of the prevailing HLA haplotypes. When

HCV is transmitted to a person with a different HLA type, it reverts to the original sequence, which is indirect evidence of HLA-restricted selection pressure [235, 236]. Mutations at targeted MHC class I-restricted epitopes were first demonstrated in the chimpanzee model, with human studies characterizing acute infection or single source outbreaks soon to follow [235,237–239]. The highest level of CD8+ T-cell-mediated selection pressure occurs during acute infection and decreases with chronicity [237,240]. Importantly, loss of CD4+ T-cell help during acute infection leads to CD8+ T-cell escape mutations and viral persistence [241]. Viral epitopes may be lost due to amino acid substitutions, which result in proteasomal destruction [235], altered binding to MHC molecules [235,242], or poor recognition by CD8+ [237,242] or CD4+ T cells [243]. While mutational escape can occur at class II-restricted epitopes, this is rare when compared with class I-restricted sites [244]. Altered peptide ligands may also downregulate T-cell responses against wild-type virus or decrease the priming of new T cells [242]. T-cell receptor (TCR) diversity can influence escape mutations as one or a few TCRs recognizing an epitope are less able to constrain the emergence of escape mutations [245]. Some of the more successful T-cell responses in HCV are against epitopes which do not "allow" sequence changes due to high viral replication fitness cost [246]. While no single mechanism fully explains how HCV evades the adaptive immune response, a lack of CD4+ helper T cells during critical times in infection may strongly contribute to viral escape mutations and T-cell anergy.

Regulatory T cells

A subset of HCV-specific CD8+ T cells derived from the liver of a chronically infected patient were noted to produce the immunosuppressive cytokine IL10 [247]. This was the first MHC class I-restricted T-cell population with the potential to modulate antiviral T cells. HCV-specific T cells that preferentially produce IL10 can be expanded from liver, and suppress IFN-γ production and proliferation of HCV-specific T cells in vitro [248]. IL10 levels are elevated in chronic HCV infection and may be able to attenuate necroinflammatory changes in the liver [249,250]. In addition to a group of intrahepatic regulatory CD8+ T cells, there is another group of CD4+ T cells found in HCV patients that may have immune modulating features.

Immunoregulatory CD4+CD25+ T cells (T regs) mediate T-cell suppression through cell–cell interactions and have been implicated in the development of self-tolerance [251]. Repetitive stimulation with immature dendritic cells can induce the formation of T regs in vitro [252]. Patients with chronic HCV infection have an increased frequency of T regs in the peripheral blood when compared with normal or recovered controls, and these cells

can directly suppress IFN-γ production by HCV-specific CD8+ T cells, thereby rendering them less effective [187,253,254]. Depletion of these CD25+ T cells resulted in increased responsiveness of HCV-specific T cells in vitro, but suppression extended to other antiviral T cells such as Epstein–Barr virus (EBV) [253,255]. Likewise, T reg-mediated suppression did not differ between those who cleared HCV infection and those who developed persistent disease [256]. This implies that T regs may be a generalized "brake" for the cellular immune response in the setting of chronic inflammatory stimuli like HCV.

Immune responses with antiviral therapy

Studying successful immune responses against HCV secondary to antiviral therapy increases our understanding of the complex interplay between virus and host in chronic infection. The mechanisms by which IFN-α and ribavirin aid in the clearance of HCV are not completely understood. IFN-α has antiviral effects through ISGs as well as immunomodulatory effects [257], and ribavirin augments the induction of critical ISGs [258] and interferes with viral replication efficacy [257,259]. Immunomodulatory actions of IFN-α include the promotion of memory T-cell proliferation and the prevention of T cell apoptosis as well as the stimulation of NK-cell activation and cDC maturation [260]. IFN-α promotes antiviral Th1 cytokines and upregulates class I and II which increases antigen presentation. Likewise, by decreasing viral load, IFN-α may improve the function of downregulated HCV-specific T cells that have been under constant antigen stimulation.

T-cell analyses during treatment-induced clearance have yielded differing results. Patients who develop a strong proliferative CD4+ T-cell response to multiple HCV antigens early in treatment and maintain this response successfully, clear the virus [188,261]. Sustained virologic response and histologic improvement was more likely to occur in patients with a vigorous, multispecific CD4+ T-cell response that persisted during and after treatment. Transient responses resulted in viral recurrence [188]. Limited studies examining common class I-restricted CD8+ T-cell epitopes have found that successful clearance on therapy is associated with increased frequency of HCV-specific CTLs [262] and conversion from a monoclonal to a polyclonal CTL response [196].

Others have found that the breath and frequency of HCV-specific CTL responses in acute infection decrease on IFN-α treatment and that patients with viral breakthrough may also exhibit a strong HCV-specific response [183,263,264]. Part of the discrepancy may be due to which functional studies are utilized as well as from which compartment these HCV-specific T cells are obtained. Most of the analyses are from T cells in the peripheral blood although IFN-α exerts much of its effects in the liver. After liver transplant, recurrent HCV infection develops in virtually all newly transplanted livers and liver biopsies are commonly used to assess recurrent disease severity. Despite immunosuppression, transplant patients with recurrent HCV infection can develop an early, multispecific CD4+ T-cell response against HCV antigens in the liver [265], and those who are able to sustain their CD4+ T-cell response with IFN-α therapy are able to successfully clear virus [266]. This argues that compartmentalization effects of IFN-α may exist. Likewise, administration of IFN-α therapy early in acute HCV infection results in a rapid decline in HCV-specific T cells likely due to the sudden departure of short-lived effector T cells and not memory T cells [264]. Interestingly, antiviral therapy in acute infection is able to "rescue" a small subset of polyfuctional HCV-specific memory T cells [267]. Capitalizing on this population of T cells may be important in the design of therapeutic vaccines.

Direct acting antiviral agents including protease and polymerase inhibitors are being added to the HCV antiviral armamentarium. Areas in the HCV NS3 protease and NS5b polymerase are under both HLA-driven pressures as well as drug selection [268], meaning that viral escape mutants may predate treatment. As noted earlier in this section, maximally upregulated intrahepatic ISGs before treatment predict failure to respond to pegIFN-α and ribavirin [131]. Secretion of IFN-γ by intrahepatic CTLs and NK cells also contribute to ISG expression [269]. The chronic activation of innate immune responses in chronic HCV correlates with increased interferon-γ-inducible protein 10 (IP-10) levels and treatment failure [270]. Similarly, chronic stimulation of HCV-specific CTLs identified by elevated levels of PD-1 also predict failure to respond [271]. Diminishing the effects of chronic immune stimulation by the virus may aid in the development of future therapies.

Correlates of protective immunity against hepatitis C virus

Unlike infection with hepatitis B where neutralizing antibodies against surface antigen exist, the role for antibodies in clearance and/or protection in HCV infection has been difficult to prove. Successful resolution of acute HCV infection in chimpanzees is associated with a robust HCV-specific CD8+ T-cell response but a weak and short-lived antibody response to multiple HCV antigens [197]. HCV-specific memory T cells were found in the peripheral blood of recovered patients exposed two decades earlier, while 42% had no detectable antibody response [214]. Also, HCV-specific CTLs have been cloned from the livers of recovered chimpanzees and humans years after infection [215]. These HCV-specific memory T cells appear to protect recovered chim-

panzees against reinfection with homologous, heterologous, and cross-genotype HCV [272–274]. Previously recovered chimpanzees rechallenged with HCV have an attenuated course compared with primary infection with lower viral titers and ALT levels and more rapid resolution of viremia, indicating that a degree of protective (but not sterilizing) immunity exists against HCV [272, 274,275]. Immune protection can be lost if chimpanzees are challenged multiple times with HCV [276], similar to that observed in multiply transfused patients [277]. When injection drug users were followed prospectively for HCV viremia, those who had been previously exposed to HCV and had cleared infection (HCV antibody-positive and RNA-negative) were 12 times less likely to develop persistent HCV infection than those infected for the first time [278]. Taken together, these data argue that an HCV-specific memory immune response exists and provides some protection against reinfection.

To dissect the essential components of the recall immune response against HCV, recovered chimpanzees were rechallenged with homologous strain virus. The duration and peak of viremia diminished after the second infection and was associated with rapid and robust expansion of functional memory helper and cytotoxic T cells [215,272]. The rapid control of the second challenge was seen prior to an increased anti-HCV antibody titer [215], substantiating the claim that the humoral component is not necessary for protection against HCV persistence. The CD8+ T-cell responses trailed the HCV-specific CD4+ responses, and functionally active CD8+ T cells were associated with a phenotypic change to effector memory cells [272]. Antibody depletion of CD8+ T cells prior to the third infection greatly prolonged viremia, and infection was not terminated until memory CD8+ T cells recovered [215]. To further elucidate the essential components of protective HCV immunity, two additional recovered chimpanzees were depleted of CD4+ T cells prior to homologous rechallenge [241]. Despite the detection of strong HCV-specific CD8+ T-cell responses in the liver, HCV RNA persisted at low levels for >300 days indicating that CD8+ memory T cells alone were not sufficient for HCV resolution without CD4+ T-cell support. These experiments demonstrate that CD8+ T cells are essential for viral clearance and that their success rests on the adequacy of CD4+ T-cell help.

Vaccine strategies

As previously discussed, spontaneous clearance of HCV leads to long-lived memory T cells that control and rapidly clear HCV on repeat exposure. There are three types of HCV vaccines which are being pursued. The first prevents initial infection (sterilizing immunity), the second prevents viral persistence in those who become infected (enhances the clearance rate above the background level of spontaneous clearance), and the third increases the rate of sustained virologic response in those who are chronically infected (therapeutic vaccine). Since much of the morbidity of HCV is associated with chronic disease, a prophylactic vaccine that prevents persistent infection rather than sterilizing immunity is a reasonable approach. Unfortunately, there is still no immunocompetent, small animal model for HCV infection so the chimpanzee remains the only model in which vaccines can be tested.

Choosing the correct target antigens in HCV is difficult due to high genetic diversity and the potential to escape from the vaccine-induced immune response. Inducing cross-neutralizing antibodies by targeting the envelope region remains a possibility [279] but there is intense variation in this region. Despite conflicting data, antibodies against surface glycoproteins have been shown to "control" viremia in vivo [280–282]. The most comprehensive prophylactic vaccine studies have used an oil/water adjuvanted HCV envelope gpE1/gpE2 vaccine designed to induce neutralizing antibodies and focused T-cell responses [283,284]. Another successful approach used DNA plasmid to induce anti-E1E2 immune responses and found modified infection and rapid clearance of HCV associated with high anti-envelope antibody titers [285]. T-cell vaccines have been the primary focus of prophylactic and therapeutic vaccines due to the importance of the HCV-specific T-cell response in viral clearance. T-cell vaccines are also able to target the more conserved areas of the virus, including nonstructural proteins. Different approaches have been used to generate T-cell responses against HCV antigens, including the use of virus-like particles and defective or attenuated viral vectors with or without priming of the immune system with DNA plasmids [286,287].

There are at least a dozen chimpanzee studies published that evaluate prophylactic HCV vaccines (reviewed in [288]). Prophylactic vaccine goals include the induction of neutralizing antibodies, the stimulation of HCV-specific T cells, or both. Prophylactic vaccines have been moderately successful at inducing a response similar to natural infection. In vaccinated animals, peak titers were lower and the virus was controlled more quickly, similar to rechallenged animals. A summary of the published studies evaluating prophylactic HCV vaccines reveal a 61.9% chronicity rate among naïve animals, 28.3% among vaccinated animals, and 16.7% in rechallenged animals [288]. Those vaccines that include nonstructural proteins alone generate a strong T-cell response but still have a high rate of persistence, whereas structural proteins (core/E1/E2) have a chroncity rate of 13.8%, similar to natural infection [288]. Qualitative differences in T-cell responses may result depending upon the type of antigen utilized. Inclusion of envelope proteins with the nonstructural targets may have a beneficial effect on vaccine-induced T-cell responses.

There are multiple different therapeutic vaccines under development, which are being tested in patients with chronic HCV or healthy controls [288]. Most focus on boosting the HCV-specific T-cell responses against nonstructural proteins via a variety of delivery methods. All appear to decrease viral load to some degree and strengthen T-cell immunity but the effects are short lived. Immune escape from the vaccine-induced T-cell responses is a concern, hence therapeutic vaccines may be most effective if given with additional antiviral therapy. Likewise, delivery of co-stimulatory molecules to aid in T-cell performance is also being explored.

Epidemiology

It is estimated that between 2% and 3% of the global population is infected with hepatitis C, corresponding to approximately 130–170 million individuals (Fig. 25.5) [289–293]. However, it is acknowledged that prevalence data are incomplete from many areas of the world so that the true prevalence may be underestimated. HCV prevalence varies among different global regions as reported by the World Health Organization (WHO) [289,294,295]. The highest estimated prevalence of HCV infection is in Africa (5.3%) followed by the eastern Mediterranean region (4.6%), western Pacific region (3.9%), Southeast Asia (2.2%), and Europe (1%) [289]. Within these regions, prevalence of hepatitis C is also variable and may reflect unique circumstances or local practices that foster HCV transmission (discussed further below). Thus, the prevalence of HCV infection in southern European countries such as Spain, Italy, and Greece ranges between 2.5% and 3.5%, compared to a prevalence of <1% in northern European regions such as the United Kingdom and Scandinavia [289,290]. Similarly, one of the highest rates of HCV infection is noted in Egypt where the prevalence is estimated at 11–14%.

Chronic hepatitis C is the most common cause of liver disease in the United States and is responsible for 12,000 deaths annually, although the morbidity and mortality associated with HCV infection will continue to increase over the next few decades [290,296,297]. A report by the Institute of Medicine concluded that the current surveillance system for viral hepatitis in the United States is not optimal and provided specific recommendations to improve state and federal surveillance programs in order to provide accurate and timely representations of the burden of viral hepatitis in the United States [298]. Despite these perceived limitations, the Sentinel Counties Study of Viral Hepatitis conducted by the Centers for Disease Control and the third National Health and Nutrition

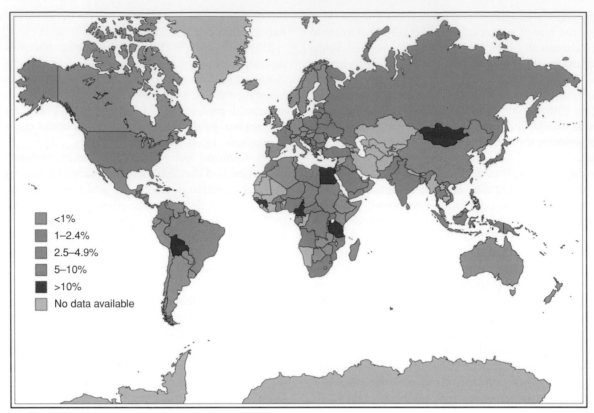

Figure 25.5 Global epidemiology of hepatitis C infection. (Reproduced from Cohen [293] with permission from American Association for the Advancement of Science.)

Survey (NHANES III) provided important epidemiologic data regarding the incidence and prevalence of hepatitis C in the United States and also served as the basis for projections regarding the future burden of this disease [291,299–301]. Modeling of the trends in HCV infection in the United States suggest that infection with HCV was uncommon in the early 1960s (45 infections per 100,000 persons) and peaked in the late 1980s (80–200 infections per 100,000 persons) with an estimate of 200,000 to as many as 500,000 new infections annually during this period [295,300]. By the early 1990s there was an 85% decrease in reported new HCV infections, likely due to a sharp decrease in intravenous drug use, with an estimated current annual incidence of less than 18,000–20,000 cases [302,303].

Utilizing serum samples from participants in the most recent NHANES study, the prevalence of antibody to HCV (anti-HCV) was 1.6% (95% CI, 1.3–1.9%), which corresponds to an estimated 4.1 million people (95% CI, 3.4–4.9 million) in the United States [292,301]. Chronic infection characterized by detectable HCV RNA was found in 1.3% of the participants (3.2 million persons; 95% CI, 2.7–3.9 million). These prevalence data are likely underestimates of the true prevalence of HCV infection in the United States since they did not include partici-

pants who were institutionalized, incarcerated, or homeless – all populations with a high rate of HCV infection [292,301].

The prevalence of HCV in the United States also shows marked gender and racial disparities. Age-adjusted prevalence estimates indicate that the majority of HCV-infected persons were born between 1945 and 1964, now roughly corresponding to them being between 50 and 60 years of age [301]. The prevalence of anti-HCV by race, age, and gender is shown in Fig. 25.6. Among all male participants, a peak prevalence of 6% occurred between the ages of 40 and 49 (at the time of the survey) while the prevalence in females was ~2%. The highest prevalence of HCV infection, ~14%, was found in male, non-Hispanic, black participants between the ages of 40 and 49 years, compared with approximately 6% of male, non-Hispanic, white participants in the same age group (Fig. 25.5) [301].

Risk factors

Several risk factors account for the majority of cases of transmission of hepatitis C, including intravenous drug use, blood transfusions from unscreened donors, and

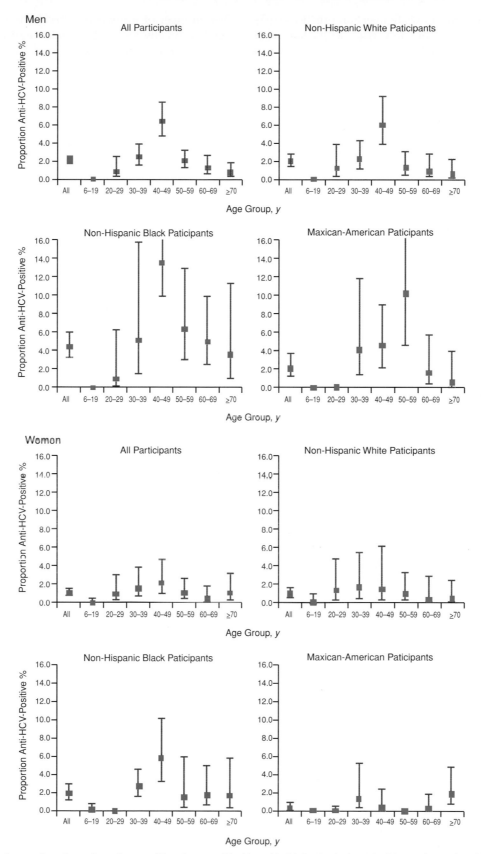

Figure 25.6 Age- and race-adjusted prevalence for men (A) and women (B) of hepatitis C infection in the United States. (Reproduced from Armstrong et al. [301] with permission from American College of Physicians.)

iatrogenic exposure from unsafe injection practices [295]. The relative importance of these risk factors may vary by country and developed nation status. Other risk factors such as sexual transmission, perinatal exposure, and health care occupational exposures occur infrequently.

Intravenous drug use

Intravenous drug use is the most common risk factor for acquiring hepatitis C in developed countries such as the United States, the European continent, and Australia, among others [290,295,299,304,305]. From the NHANES study, the prevalence of anti-HCV was found to be 48% in those between the ages of 20 and 59 years who had ever injected illicit drugs and it is estimated that up to 80% of current infections are due to a past history of injection drug use [301]. Among long-term injection drug users the prevalence of hepatitis C infection has been reported to be as high as 94%. The prevalence of anti-HCV among persons who had engaged in intravenous drug use for less than 1 year was already 65%, indicating that this activity is a highly efficient mode of HCV transmission [306]. Although sharing syringes has been most frequently implicated in the transmission of HCV, the shared use of other drug preparation equipment may have contributed to infection in an estimated 37% of recent HCV infections [307].

Illicit drug use other than marijuana has also been linked to higher rates of HCV infection [301]. In particular, the extent of the risk of intranasal cocaine has been debated [308–311]. A systematic review found the prevalence of HCV infection among noninjecting drug users to range between 2.3% and 35.3%, suggesting that other routes of transmission besides purely percutaneous exposures may occur [312]. However, inconsistent methodologies and case ascertainment in these studies have prevented firm conclusions about this controversial issue such that the risk of noninjecting drug use remains unsettled.

Unsafe therapeutic injection practices

In developing countries, unsafe therapeutic injection practices, where syringes or needles may be reused without sterilization, continues to contribute to incident cases of hepatitis C and remains a major transmission risk for blood-borne infections [294,295,313]. WHO estimates that 30% of hepatitis C infection, or 2–4 million annual cases, can be attributed to unsafe injection practices in low-income countries. Perhaps the most compelling story of unsafe injection practices resulting in tragic consequences is derived from a nationwide campaign in Egypt to eradicate schistosomiasis [314,315]. Millions of Egyptians were administered intravenous tartar emetic over a 30-year period beginning in the 1950s and ending in the 1980s when effective oral therapies became available.

The number of intravenous injections administered correlated directly with the prevalence of HCV infection in Egypt and soon surpassed schistosomiasis as the leading cause of liver disease in that country. Furthermore, the increasing incidence of hepatocellular carcinoma is now being driven by advanced liver disease due to hepatitis C. Similarly, parenteral therapy for trypanosomiasis has been implicated in HCV transmission in equatorial Africa [316]. In Asia, folk remedies that involve skin piercing have been shown to contribute to high rates of HCV infection in certain regions [317]. Programs to promote safe injection practices have been implemented by WHO in recognition of the gravity of this problem.

The failure of aseptic techniques during medical procedures is rare in developed countries. Nevertheless, a recent outbreak at a Las Vegas endoscopy center in which ten patients were infected after the reuse of multidose anesthetic vials [318], as well as numerous other case reports of similar types of exposures, underscores the importance of continued vigilance and strict adherence to infection control measures [319].

Blood transfusions

Post-transfusion hepatitis develops in approximately 10% of individuals and subsequent serologic testing has indicated that at least 85% of cases were due to hepatitis C [295,301]. Patients who received blood transfusions prior to 1992 are considered to be at risk for hepatitis C infection with an odds ratio of 2.6 compared with individuals who did not receive transfusions, and older patients are more likely to have acquired HCV infection as a result of blood transfusions [301]. Overall, it has been estimated that past blood transfusions account for about 10% of cases of chronic hepatitis C.

Rates of non-A, non-B post-transfusion hepatitis were markedly decreased as efforts to improve the safety of the blood supply were sequentially implemented. These included the use of all-volunteer donors, screening of donors for surrogate markers of NANB hepatitis (such as serum ALT activity and markers of hepatitis B infection), testing for human immunodeficiency virus (HIV), and eliciting a history of risk factors for blood-borne infections [295]. Nevertheless, a background rate of transfusion-associated hepatitis remained until 1990 when anti-HCV antibody testing was implemented in the United States, shortly after the discovery of the hepatitis C virus [295]. Later generation antibody assays, more sensitive and specific for hepatitis C, were utilized and eventually screening also included nucleic acid testing which virtually assured the safety of the United States' blood supply [320].

Certain populations of patients requiring multiple transfusions were placed at extraordinary risk for hepatitis C infection prior to adequate donor screening procedures. The estimated prevalence of anti-HCV among patients with thalassemia ranges between 4.4% and 85%. In a thalassemia registry from North America, 35% of registrants had evidence of hepatitis C infection [321]. Similarly, among patient with sickle cell disease, the prevalence of HCV infection, estimated to be between 10% and 20%, is related to the number of transfusions received [322,323].

The greatest burden of hepatitis C infection is found in patients with hemophilia who received factor concentrates prior to the mid-1980s. Coagulation factor concentrates were derived from pooled plasma, often from thousands of donors, which led to a large number of patients with hemophilia being infected with HIV and HCV. It has been estimated that in the United States 80% of persons with hemophilia during that time period became infected with hepatitis C [324,325]. Viral inactivation procedures such as solvent detergent exposure, nanofiltration, and heat treatment dramatically diminished the risk, while the subsequent availability of recombinant factors has virtually eliminated the threat of blood-borne infections for younger persons with hemophilia [324]. Nevertheless, infection with hepatitis C and progression to advanced liver disease is a leading cause of morbidity and mortality among persons with hemophilia [325–327]. A study from Italy analyzing mortality among a population of patients with hemophilia between 1990 and 2007 attributed 13% of overall deaths to complications related to hepatitis C [328]. Furthermore, the predominant causes of mortality have shifted with the advent of effective therapies for HIV infection. Between 2000 and 2007, more patients with hemophilia died from HCV-related complications than from acquired immune deficiency syndrome (AIDS), underscoring the importance of antiviral therapy for this population [328]. Patients with hemophilia and hepatitis C respond in a similar manner to nonhemophilic populations when treated with interferon-based therapies [329–331].

Sexual transmission

Sexual transmission of hepatitis C occurs rarely and usually is associated with specific cofactors. Early epidemiologic studies demonstrated that individuals with an increased number of lifetime sexual partners (>10) have an increased prevalence of anti-HCV antibody [310]. HCV RNA sequences have been inconsistently isolated from biologic specimens such as semen and vaginal secretions, although direct infection from these sources in humans has not been demonstrated [332,333]. Cases of transmission to heterosexual partners have been reported and HCV phylogenetic analyses have suggested the potential for sexual transmission [334,335]. However, a comprehensive review critically evaluated 80 published studies related to sexual transmission of hepatitis C and

concluded that sexual transmission was extremely rare and usually occurred only under special circumstances [336]. Among longitudinal studies of HIV-negative heterosexual couples where the index partner was infected with hepatitis C, there was no increased risk of transmission to partners even after a decade of follow-up [336]. In the few instances of potential sexual transmission, other common source exposures could not be completely excluded. Preexisting sexually transmitted infection, such as herpes simplex type II and trichomonas, appears to increase the risk of HCV acquisition among heterosexual partners [336].

The presence of HIV infection, on the other hand, has regularly been associated with a higher likelihood of sexual transmission of HCV in both heterosexuals and among men who have sex with men (MSM) [336–339]. Recent case reports of acute HCV infection among MSM from Europe suggest that the incidence is increasing [337]. The increased rate of acquisition and transmission of HCV in MSM may be due to higher HCV viral loads associated with HIV infection or other factors such as concomitant high-risk sexual activity [336,338].

Perinatal transmission

Transmission of hepatitis to a neonate from an HCV-infected mother has been extensively investigated in retrospective and prospective studies and has been reviewed [339,340]. The perinatal transmission rate from HCV RNA-positive mothers is estimated to range between 4% and 10% [341]. The rate increases substantially to between 6% and 23% when the mother is coinfected with HIV. An increased risk of perinatal transmission appears to be associated with higher levels of maternal HCV RNA, and this may be the mechanism by which vertical transmission is increased in HIV-positive mothers, although conflicting data have been reported [340,341]. HCV genotype is not associated with differences in the vertical transmission of HCV.

Obstetric procedures such as amniocentesis and invasive monitoring with fetal scalp electrodes have been associated with an increased risk of neonatal transmission, although no specific recommendations regarding these procedures exist due to the limited data [339,340]. There are no randomized trials evaluating the impact of mode of delivery, vaginal versus cesarean, with neonatal infection [342]. However, most observational studies have not shown differences in the rate of perinatal transmission for women with only HCV infection. The European Paediatric Hepatitis C Network enrolled a total of 1,474 HCV-infected women of whom 35% were also infected with HIV [343,344]. In HIV-negative mothers, no effect on mode of delivery or breastfeeding was identified. However, in HIV-coinfected mothers, cesarean section decreased perinatal transmission by 60% and those breastfeeding were four times more likely to transmit HCV to their child.

Recent recommendations by the Centers for Disease Control [341] established that for women with chronic hepatitis C infection who are uninfected with HIV, no changes to routine delivery and breastfeeding are required. However, for mothers coinfected with HCV and HIV, scheduled cesarean delivery and proscription of breastfeeding (when safe infant formula is available) are recommended in order to diminish the risk of neonatal transmission.

Occupational exposure in health care providers

The prevalence of hepatitis C infection in health care providers is similar to that in the general population in the United States, indicating that occupational exposure is not a major risk factor for transmission [345,346]. The likelihood of acquiring hepatitis C from a needlestick injury from an HCV-infected patient is estimated to be approximately 2%. Rare cases of blood splash exposure have been reported. A larger inoculum is associated with a higher risk of transmission, and injuries with hollow-bore needles transmit HCV more frequently than solid instruments. Similarly, higher levels of viremia of $>10^6$ copies/mL are also associated with an 11-fold higher risk of transmission compared with levels of $<10^4$ copies/mL [346]. Health care workers who sustain a needlestick injury from an index case with hepatitis C should be reassured about the low rate of infection. There is no role for postexposure prophylaxis [347]. Baseline liver enzymes and anti-HCV antibody should be obtained immediately and follow-up testing performed at 1, 3, and 6 months [348,349]. The absence of HCV RNA in the needlestick recipient using a sensitive polymerase chain reaction (PCR)-based assay at 4 and 8 weeks of exposure can further reduce the anxiety associated with accidental exposure [348–350]. Patients with evidence of acute infection should be followed to determine if spontaneous resolution will occur or be treated within 12–16 weeks after infection in order to maximize the chances of cure (see the section on acute hepatitis C).

Diagnosis and testing

The clinical validation of the first anti-HCV antibody assay was reported by Harvey Alter and colleagues in 1989 [351]. All patients with post-transfusion chronic NANB hepatitis seroconverted for anti-HCV with a mean delay of 22 weeks after transfusion. The anti-HCV antibody was detected in 88% of the donor serum implicated in the transmission of NANB hepatitis in these patients, while surrogate markers for blood-borne

pathogens used for blood donor screening at the time – elevated serum ALT activity and anti-hepatitis B core (anti-HBc) antibody – were detectable in only about 50% of donors. Numerous seroepidemiologic studies confirmed that anti-HCV was an important diagnostic marker for hepatitis C infection and transmissibility of infected blood products [291,352,353].

A positive anti-HCV antibody is a marker of past or current infection with hepatitis C. A single fusion polypeptide, designated C-100, derived from the NS4 nonstructural region of HCV formed the basis for the first-generation anti-HCV enzyme-linked immunosorbent assay (ELISA), which was licensed in 1990 [353,354]. The reliance on only one target antigen produced false-negative and false-positive results. Subsequent generations of assays have incorporated antigens from additional regions of the HCV genome, including NS3 and NS5, which improved the sensitivity and specificity of the anti-HCV antibody assay [355]. Furthermore, these refinements shortened the duration from exposure to detection of anti-HCV seroconversion to less than 3 weeks [356]. Therefore, the anti-HCV antibody by enzyme immunoassay (EIA) remains the best screening test for the diagnosis of hepatitis C, and current assays have a specificity of >99% [354].

False-negative anti-HCV antibody testing may rarely occur in severely immunosuppressed patients, patients with agammaglobulinemia, and patients on hemodialysis [296]. Nucleic acid testing for HCV RNA should be performed in these populations when patients have unexplained aminotransferase abnormalities with a negative anti-HCV. Despite an excellent specificity, false-positive EIA results may also occur, particularly among populations with a low prevalence of HCV infection such as volunteer blood donors. Signal to cutoff ratios of >4.0 are highly associated with true exposure to hepatitis C infection and additional serologic testing is not routinely recommended, although nucleic acid testing to demonstrate viremia is important [354]. When signal to cutoff ratios are low, supplemental testing with a recombinant immunoblot assay (RIBA), which assesses the reaction of a patient's sera to multiple HCV antigens, may assist with diagnosis. A positive anti-HCV antibody supplemented with a positive RIBA (positive reaction to two or more HCV antigens) indicates a true past or present infection with HCV. A negative RIBA indicates a false-positive anti-HCV antibody test without HCV infection and the patient may be reassured without further evaluation of HCV [354]. An indeterminate RIBA may occur in the earliest stages of infection or in association with a false-positive screening antibody. Patients with an indeterminate RIBA should have another serologic test performed at least 1 month later, along with consideration of nucleic acid testing for HCV RNA (Table 25.1).

Table 25.1 Interpretation of diagnostic tests for hepatitis C infection.

Anti-HCV	RIBA	HCV RNA	Interpretation	Action
+	+	Detectable	Current HCV infection	Evaluate for chronic liver disease, test HCV genotype
+	+	Undetectable	Past HCV infection with spontaneous or treatment-induced viral clearance	Repeat HCV RNA testing in 3–6 months to confirm absence of viremia
+	–	Undetectable	False-positive anti-HCV	No further follow-up for HCV required
+	Indeterminate	Undetectable	Likely false-positive anti-HCV, particularly in patients without risk factors	Repeat HCV RNA testing in 3–6 months to confirm absence of viremia

HCV, hepatitis C virus; RIBA, recombinant immunoblot assay.

Nucleic acid testing for hepatitis C using highly sensitive assays is of critical importance for confirming persistent viremia in chronic infection and for assessing the response to antiviral therapy. Qualitative assays detect only the presence or absence of HCV RNA in plasma or serum, while quantitative assays provide a measurement of the amount of virus per unit of volume. Historically, HCV RNA assays were inconsistent in their results, with widely varying sensitivities and specificities leading to false-positive and -negative results [357]. Clinical specimens also require careful sample handling to avoid degradation of HCV RNA. The WHO developed guidelines and standards for HCV RNA assays that included utilizing the international unit per milliliter as the only recognized unit of measurement, incorporating an internal standard or external validation method into commercial assays, and defining acceptable levels of sensitivity and reproducibility of results [358]. These requirements enabled greater confidence in the results of commercial assays for diagnostic and therapeutic purposes and greatly advanced the management of patients with chronic hepatitis C.

HCV nucleic acid analysis relies on either amplification of the detection signal or amplification of the nucleic acid target [358]. The branched DNA method of signal amplification detects HCV RNA with a lower limit of quantification of 615 IU/mL [358,359]. This level of sensitivity is generally inadequate for measuring response to antiviral therapy where the goal is viral eradication. Thus, the most frequently utilized commercial qualitative and quantitative assays rely on target amplification, either by transcription-mediated amplification (TMA) or by reverse transcription polymerase chain reaction (RT-PCR), which provides a much higher sensitivity and a broad dynamic range [358]. One qualitative TMA assay (Versant®, Siemens) provides the lowest level of HCV RNA detection of 10 IU/mL. Other qualitative assays using RT-PCR methods have a lower limit of detection of 50 IU/ml (Amplicor v2.0® and Cobas v2.0®, Roche).

Any of these are adequate for determining the presence or absence of HCV RNA in untreated hepatitis C infection.

Early quantitative assays were substantially less sensitive than qualitative assays for detecting viral nucleic acid, and at times a combination of both types of assays were required to determine sustained virologic response. However, technologic advances have obviated the need for multiple assays, although limitations still exist regarding precise quantitation at high viral levels or with certain genotypes [360,361]. There are several important features of quantitative assays to consider, particularly with response-guided treatment algorithms (discussed below). The dynamic range of quantification defines the lower and upper limits of quantification for the assay. A broader dynamic range allows for better quantification of HCV RNA at the highest levels of viremia prior to initiation of treatment. The broadest dynamic ranges are seen in assays using real-time RT-PCR methodology (COBAS TaqMan®, Roche; and Abbott) where the upper limit of quantification is 10^7 IU/mL [358]. More important is defining the lowest level at which HCV RNA is measured. The lower limit of quantification (LLQ) refers to the lowest level of HCV RNA that can be confidently, reproducibly quantified by the assay. The lower limit of detection (LLD) is the lowest level at which an assay will detect the presence of any viral nucleic acid, although below the threshold for which assignment of a numeric value is possible. Assays should have similar thresholds of LLQ and LLD. Real-time RT-PCR assays provide the best LLQs (ranging between 12 and 43 IU/mL) and LLDs (12–15 IU/mL). There is ongoing debate about the relevance of LLQs versus LLDs in the era of direct acting antiviral agents and their clinical significance for treatment response requires further study [362].

Hepatitis C is a heterogeneous virus with at least six major genotype and multiple subtypes that have a varied geographic distribution (Fig. 25.7) [363]. Genotype 1 is the

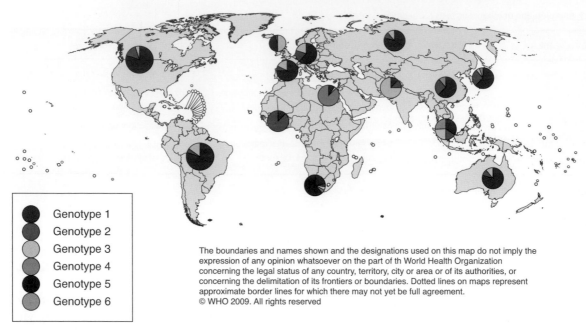

Genotype 1
Genotype 2
Genotype 3
Genotype 4
Genotype 5
Genotype 6

The boundaries and names shown and the designations used on this map do not imply the expression of any opinion whatsoever on the part of th World Health Organization concerning the legal status of any country, territory, city or area or of its authorities, or concerning the delimitation of its frontiers or boundaries. Dotted lines on maps represent approximate border lines for which there may not yet be full agreement.

Figure 25.7 Geographic distribution of HCV genotypes. (Reproduced from WHO 2009 with permission.)

most common genotype around the world and accounts for approximately 75% of infections in the United States [364]. The remaining infections in the United States are usually genotype 2 (14%) or genotype 3 (8%) [364]. Recently, a high prevalence of genotype 3a has been identified in injecting drug users in Europe although genotype 3 is also an important infection in Pakistan. Genotype 4 is most common in the Middle East, particularly in Egypt. Genotypes 5 and 6 are most prevalent in South Africa and Southeast Asia, respectively [363].

The HCV genotype forms the basis for recommendations regarding the duration of treatment with pegIFN and ribavirin, and correct classification has important prognostic implications for therapy. The gold standard for HCV genotyping is direct sequencing of an HCV genomic region, such as NS5B or core/E1 [359,365]. While considered to be the most accurate method and the most precise for subtyping, direct sequencing is labor intensive and requires a high degree of technical expertise such that it is not practical for clinical use. Several commercial genotyping assays are available that focus on the highly conserved 5′ UTR of the HCV genome. The line probe reverse hybridization assay (Versant HCV LiPA®, Bayer) is the most widely used method for HCV genotyping. PCR products from amplification of the 5′ UTR are hybridized to a membrane containing genotype-specific probes and the pattern of hybridization bands determines the HCV genotype [365]. Early versions of this assay could not reliably differentiate genotype 1 from genotype 6, nor provide accurate differentiation of the most common sub-

types. A second generation LiPA assay adds sequences from the HCV core region to improve differentiation of genotypes and subtypes. TRUGENE® 5′ NC genotyping is a sequenced-based assay directed at the 5′ UTR and results correlate well with LiPA and other assays that utilize the 5′ UTR region [365]. Accurate subtyping (1a versus 1b) will become more important with direct-acting antiviral agents since the development of viral variants to protease inhibitors appears to be more frequent in genotype 1a than in 1b.

Since most patients with chronic hepatitis C are asymptomatic, the diagnosis and management of hepatitis C relies on applying the aforementioned serologic and nucleic acid tests to individuals with risk factors for HCV or evidence of chronic liver disease [366]. Thus, health care providers should routinely inquire about potential risk factors for the acquisition of hepatitis C and test their patients accordingly. Epidemiologic studies in the United States have demonstrated that the majority of people infected with hepatitis C (~85%) had at least one of three characteristics noted: abnormal serum ALT activity, a history of intravenous drug use, or a history of blood transfusion. Targeting any of these risk factors would identify most cases of hepatitis C infection (Table 25.2) [301].

When patients with HCV infection are identified, health care providers should counsel patients about measures to decrease the risk of HCV transmission [296]. Persons infected with hepatitis C should avoid sharing toothbrushes or shaving equipment and keep bleeding

Table 25.2 Recommendations for testing for hepatitis C virus (HCV) infection.

Testing required	Testing not routinely required
Persons who have at any time injected illegal drugs regardless of number of events	Health care, emergency medical, or public safety workers
Persons who received a transfusion or organ transplant before July 1992	Pregnant women
Persons who received clotting factor concentrates before 1987	Household contacts
Persons who were at any time on long-term hemodialysis	General population
Persons with persistently abnormal alanine aminotransferase levels	
Persons with needlestick, sharp, or splash exposure to HCV-positive blood	
Children born to an HCV-positive mother	
Sexual partners of HCV-infected patients	

wounds covered to prevent others from contact with their blood. HCV-infected patients should not donate blood, body organs, other tissues, or semen. Patients should be reassured that the risk of sexual transmission is low and modifying sexual practices within monogamous relationships is not required [296].

Natural history

Acute hepatitis C virus infection

Acute infection with HCV is asymptomatic in the majority of individuals, with only a minority seeking medical attention. HCV RNA in the serum is the first evidence of infection and is usually detectable 7–21 days after exposure [367]. The titer of the HCV inoculum is negatively associated with time to detection of virus in the serum [368]. HCV-specific antibodies are detectable 20–150 days postexposure (average 50 days) even when using the third generation assays [369,370]. If there is a high clinical index of suspicion for acute HCV infection, an HCV RNA should be obtained in the absence of detactable anti-HCV antibody. Serum aminotransferases increase 4–12 weeks postexposure and can range from mildly elevated to >1,000 U/L. Jaundice occurs in less than 20% but this clinical sign may be associated with higher rates of spontaneous clearance [369,371]. Symptoms of acute HCV infection are similar to other forms of viral hepatitis and include malaise, fatigue, myalgias, nausea, and right upper quadrant pain. This clinical syndrome can persist from days up to 12 weeks, especially with acute icteric disease [372]. Fulminant presentation is rare in acute hepatitis C infection unless other underlying chronic liver disease is present. HCV RNA levels may fluctuate dramatically during acute infection, ranging from very high to undetectable. Following successful therapy for acute hepatitis C infection, a marked decline in anti-HCV antibodies is seen post-treatment [373]. In those who spontaneously clear HCV, one study found that 42% had no detectable anti-HCV antibodies two decades postexpo-

sure although HCV-specific memory T cells were recoverable from the peripheral blood [214].

While spontaneous clearance of HCV is possible, the risk of developing chronic infection is the highest for any hepatotropic viral infection. The mechanism by which the virus evades immune recognition and establishes a foothold is further discussed in the section on HCV pathogenesis. In earlier cohort studies of blood donors, transfusion recipients, and injection drug users, chronicity rates of 76–86% were reported, although selected populations may have lower rates of chronicity [374–376]. Children who received infected blood products developed chronicity in 55–71% of cases [377,378]. Likewise, only 55% of young women who received HCV-contaminated anti-rhesus D immunoglobulin in Ireland and Germany developed chronic infection [379,380]. Female injection drug users also have higher rates of spontaneous clearance when compared with males [381]. Therefore, gender and age at the time of acquisition of HCV are important factors associated with chronicity versus clearance.

Host, viral, and environmental factors have been associated with the likelihood of viral resolution or chronicity. Selected polymorphisms near the *IL28B* gene, which encodes for interferon-λ3, are strongly tied to both spontaneous and treatment-induced viral clearance [145,146,382]. In one study, the presence of the CC haplotype at rs12979860 was associated with a spontaneous clearance rate of approximately 55% compared with only 16–20% in those with the TT haplotype [146]. The frequency of spontaneous HCV clearance varies markedly across ethnic groups [383] and may be partly explained by the differences of allele frequency of this *IL28B* polymorphism among different populations. The global frequency of the favorable allele for HCV clearance is highest in East Asia, intermediate in Europe, and lowest in Africa [145, 146]. This likely explains at least part of the discrepancy in spontaneous clearance rates observed between Caucasians at 36.4% and African-Americans at 9.3% in a large, US-based study of injection drug users [376].

The association with *IL28B* genotype, clinical presentation, and viral clearance was further refined by evaluating German women who had been exposed to HCV genotype 1b through contaminated anti-D immunoglobulin [384]. The spontaneous clearance rate in women with the CC genotype was 64.2% and was not significantly associated with jaundice. Interestingly, of those with the CT genotype, 50% with jaundice cleared infection spontaneously while <20% did so in the absence of jaundice. The clearance rate in the TT group was low regardless of clinical presentation [384]. This study suggests that the association between jaundice and viral clearance in acute infection differs according to *IL28B* genotype. A more vigorous innate immune response in those with the CC genotype may enable viral clearance without the cell-mediated injury associated with jaundice in acute HCV infection. Other immunologic factors associated with spontaneous viral clearance included carriage of the class I HLA B57 allele as well as the class II alleles HLA DRB1 and DQB1 [385–387]. Spontaneous viral clearance at low infectious doses has also been tied to low inhibitory NK-cell responses associated with homozygosity for HLA-C1 and KIR2DL3 [168]. When injection drug users were followed prospectively for HCV viremia, those who had been previously exposed to HCV and cleared infection (HCV antibody-positive and RNA-negative) were 12 times less likely to develop persistent HCV infection than those infected for the first time [278].

Viral coinfection and alcohol consumption are additional factors that influence spontaneous viral clearance. In one study conducted in US Veterans, alcohol and HIV coinfection negatively impacted spontaneous HCV clearance during primary infection, while HBV coinfection was positively associated with HCV clearance [388]. Patients with HIV coinfection are less likely to spontaneously clear acute HCV infection, as are those with heavy alcohol use [371,376,388]. Size of inoculum, mode of acquisition, and viral genotype have not been consistently linked to viral clearance although genotype 3 may have a higher spontaneous clearance rate [389].

Chronic hepatitis C virus infection

Most patients who present with chronic HCV infection are completely asymptomatic [390]. The most common but least specific complaint is fatigue and this may improve with successful treatment of HCV [390–392]. Other symptoms include myalgias, arthralgias, nausea, anorexia, and decreased concentration [390,391]. In one study, patients with histologically mild HCV infection were noted to have cognitive impairment and specifically decreased concentration and speed of working memory when compared with patients who had cleared HCV infection [393]. This was independent of depression or drug abuse history. Several studies have noted lower quality of life scores with the diagnosis of chronic HCV that are independent of disease severity [394–397]. Longitudinal studies reassessing these parameters following successful treatment have not been conducted. Symptoms related to extrahepatic manifestations of chronic HCV infection can occur and are discussed in a separate section. Once cirrhosis develops, patients may have more overt symptoms including worsening fatigue, fluid retention, confusion from encephalopathy, or gastrointestinal bleeding [390].

Serum aminotransferases fluctuate over time in patients with chronic HCV and up to one third will have a persistently normal ALT activity [398]. Most have levels 1.5–3 times the upper limit of normal, rarely more than ten-fold elevated. Unfortunately, aminotransferase levels do not serve as an accurate surrogate for liver histology [399–401]. Patients with persistently normal activity may have evidence of inflammation and fibrosis on liver biopsy although it may be milder with attenuated progression [372]. Markedly elevated ALT (more than ten-fold) correlates with piecemeal necrosis on biopsy and an aspartate aminotransferase (AST):ALT ratio of >1 may correlate with histologic cirrhosis [399,402,403]. Likewise, during chronic HCV infection, viral load fluctuations of about 1 log are common but viral load does not correlate with disease severity in immunocompetent hosts. Hence, liver biopsy remains the most accurate measurement of disease activity and severity in chronic HCV (see histology section).

In those who develop chronic HCV infection, disease progression is quite variable, with only a portion developing serious complications including cirrhosis or hepatocellular carcinoma (HCC). Natural history studies of HCV are tempered by which population is studied and for how long. Few studies go beyond 20 years and most are cross-sectional. Unfortunately, the onset of hepatitis C infection is usually silent and its course prolonged, making natural history studies difficult. Likewise, multiple host and environmental factors affect HCV progression rates (discussed below).

Cirrhosis estimates over a 20-year period vary from 4% to 24% depending upon the group evaluated. Healthy blood donors found to have HCV developed cirrhosis at a rate of about 4% (95% CI, 1–7%) over 20 years, while a post-transfusion cohort had a 24% (95% CI, 11–37%) rate of cirrhosis development over the same period. Similarly, a community-based series had a 20-year cirrhosis rate of 7% (4–10%) while patients referred to liver clinics had a mean frequency of cirrhosis of 22% (18–26%) [404,405]. A systematic review of 111 studies evaluating the natural history of HCV estimated the cirrhosis prevalence at 16% after 20 years of infection [406]. While cross-sectional analyses may provide an estimate of fibrosis progression in chronic HCV infection, paired biopsy studies are the most accurate way to assess fibrosis progression. In five paired biopsy studies, progression of at least one fibrosis stage was seen in 27–41% with average follow-up periods of 2.2–6.5 years [407–411]. These data support the practice of considering a repeat staging biopsy at various intervals in the setting of chronic HCV infection.

The development of cirrhosis is often clinically silent but physical examination and laboratory values may be helpful in diagnosing this stage of disease [412]. Spider angiomata, palmer erythema, and splenomegaly may be present on exam with blood tests revealing decreased albumin, elevated bilirubin, or decreased platelet count from portal hypertension [413]. Unlike in chronic hepatitis B infection, only chronic HCV patients with advanced fibrosis or cirrhosis are at increased risk of developing HCC. The risk for the development of HCC in the setting of chronic HCV infection is about 3% per year (1–7%) [414–416]. Older age, male sex, African-American race, and obesity as well as steatosis and diabetes are independent risk factors for HCC development in the setting of HCV cirrhosis [417–422]. Screening for HCC using abdominal imaging should be instituted in all HCV patients with advanced fibrosis or cirrhosis [423]. α-Fetoprotein (AFP) is used to assist in the diagnosis of HCC but is a poor screening test for the detection of HCC in the setting of chronic HCV. In a large cohort of American patients with chronic HCV who had advanced fibrosis or cirrhosis, baseline AFP levels were >20 ng/mL in 16.6% in the absence of HCC [424]. Higher AFP levels were seen in cirrhotics, women, and African-Americans [424]. Serum AFP levels correlated strongly with serum ALT, AST, and the degree of hepatic inflammation on liver biopsy, suggesting that AFP production is enhanced in the presence of injury, possibly resulting from increased hepatocyte turnover. Also, a third of the patients in this study who developed HCC did not have an AFP level >20 ng/mL.

Once a patient with chronic HCV has developed cirrhosis, the risk of decompensation of their liver disease is about 4% per year. The most common decompensation events include the development of ascites, followed by variceal bleeding and encephalopathy [425]. This is based on a study of 384 patients with compensated cirrhosis from HCV infection who were followed over time. From this same cohort, the 3-, 5-, and 10-year survival rates of compensated HCV cirrhosis were 96%, 91%, and 79%, respectively. Unfortunately, once a patient has developed decompensation, the 5-year survival falls to around 50% without liver transplant (Fig. 25.8) [425,426]. For this reason, patients with cirrhosis should be referred for

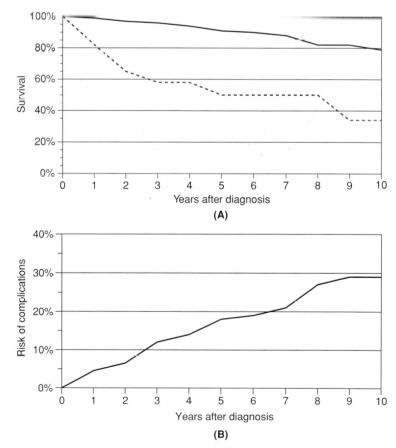

Figure 25.8 (A) Survival in patients with cirrhosis due to chronic hepatitis C. Effect of complications and decompensation. Solid line, compensated cirrhosis; dashed line, decompensated cirrhosis. (B) Risk of developing decompensated liver disease among patients with stable cirrhosis due to chronic hepatitis C. (Reproduced from Fattovich et al. [425] with permission from Elsevier.)

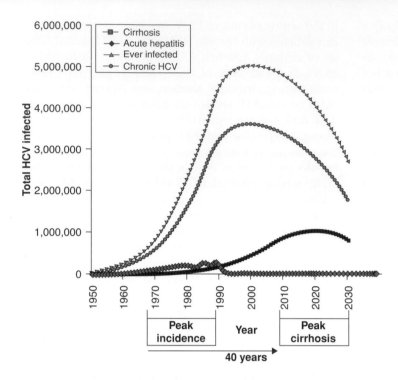

Figure 25.9 Estimates by year of prevalent cases of cirrhosis, acute hepatitis, and chronic hepatitis C virus (HCV), and ever infected cases. Peak prevalence of HCV infection was in 2001 while the highest prevalence of cirrhosis is projected between 2010 and 2030. (Reproduced from Davis et al. [297] with permission from Elsevier.)

transplantation when they experience their first major complication of cirrhosis (ascites, variceal bleeding, or hepatic encephalopathy) or when they develop evidence of hepatic dysfunction (Child–Pugh score >7 or model for end-stage liver disease (MELD) score >10) [427]. HCV cirrhosis is currently the leading cause for liver transplantation in the United States. While recurrent HCV in the graft is universal unless the patient has a treatment-induced cure prior to transplant, long-term outcomes are similar to other etiologies [428]. The majority of patients transplanted for HCV-related cirrhosis or HCC will have minimal injury with HCV recurrence, but up to 30% will have progressive disease leading to cirrhosis by 5 years post-transplant [429]. Also, less than 5% will have severe recurrence of HCV associated with cholestasis and aggressive fibrosis (whose features are described in the histology section). Recurrent HCV post liver transplant and risk factors for progressive disease are further discussed elsewhere in this volume.

Death certificate data indicate that HCV-related mortality has increased substantially since 1995, especially in persons 45 years and older, with the most significant increases in males and non-Hispanic blacks [430]. It has now become an important cause of premature mortality due to the relatively young ages of those dying from HCV-related deaths [430]. As previously mentioned, few natural history studies go beyond 20 years and modeling is the best way to assess the long-term impact of HCV infection. A multicohort natural history model of HCV infection published in 2010 projected that the propor-

tion of US patients with cirrhosis from chronic HCV will peak at around 1 million in 2020 and reach 45% of those infected by 2030 (Fig. 25.9) [297]. Hepatic decompensation and HCC will continue to increase over the next decade with those older than 60 years being most affected. The projected peak for HCV-related HCC is 2019, at about 14,000 cases. Interestingly, the authors noted that antiviral therapy could significantly alter disease end-points from a population perspective. Based on their model, treatment of all infected patients in 2010 could reduce the risk of liver-related deaths by 36% in 2020, reinforcing the need for more aggressive HCV diagnosis and treatment [297].

Factors linked to disease progression

Host, viral, and environmental factors are associated with progressive fibrosis and cirrhosis. Acquisition of HCV infection after the age of 40 is associated with more rapid progression of liver injury [404,431]. In addition, duration of infection and advancing age are risk factors for cirrhosis, perhaps due to decreased regenerative capacity and waning immunity in an older liver [432]. Fibrosis progression is not linear and some models suggest that the risk of fibrosis progression increases with age [433]. Males are 2.5 times more likely to develop cirrhosis and HCC when compared with females [431]. Since this risk is independent of alcohol consumption and body mass index, estrogens may have some protective affects against fibrosis development [434,435]. Interestingly, African-Americans have a three times higher risk of developing HCC when compared with Caucasians [436], yet other studies have found a slower histologic progression rate and lower ALT levels [437,438]. The cause of this discrepancy is unclear. Several studies have found an association between the degree of inflammation on liver biopsy and the rate of fibrosis progression over time [439,440]. Patients who have moderate to severe inflammation on biopsy may have an accelerated rate of fibrosis [432].

Liver iron accumulation is a common finding on biopsy in chronic HCV regardless of HFE genotype (see histology section below) [441]. Both iron storage and HFE mutations have been associated with fibrosis and, more specifically, risk for severe fibrosis [442–445]. For those without HFE mutations, iron accumulation is usually mild and is reflected by elevated serum ferritin levels [446]. Increased hepatic iron may also contribute to increased inflammatory activity and progressive fibrosis in HCV infection [446,447] including observations from a small longitudinal study [448]. An improvement in histologic activity index (HAI) and reduction in aminotransferase levels have been observed after phlebotomy in patients with chronic HCV [449,450]. Hepatic iron may play a part in hepatic injury via the production of oxygen-derived free radicals. Lower responses to interferon therapy have also been correlated to increased stainable iron in the liver, but unfortunately phlebotomy pretreatment has minimal effect on antiviral response [449,451,452].

As discussed in the histology section, steatosis is a common finding on liver biopsy in patients with chronic HCV, with the majority having at least mild steatosis (<30%) [453]. This feature is important from both an etiologic stand point as well as for its clinical significance. Patients with genotype 3 HCV have virally associated steatosis that correlates with HCV titers and resolves with successful antiviral therapy [454]. Steatosis in patients with genotype 1 infection is associated with components of the metabolic syndrome. Obesity, diabetes, and insulin resistance (as well as excess alcohol intake) have all been linked to hepatic steatosis in patients with chronic HCV. Interestingly, African-American patients with HCV geno-

type 1 infection have a lower prevalence of hepatic steatosis than Caucasians in a large US-based study [455].

Hepatic steatosis as well as superimposed steatohepatitis are important risk factors for fibrosis progression in chronic HCV infection [456–459]. Metabolic steatosis appears to be a common cofactor for increasing liver necroinflammatory activity and accelerating fibrosis in chronic HCV infection [457]. Steatosis negatively impacts on response to antiviral therapy and increases the risk of developing HCC by 2.8-fold [421,460]. Obesity is also a metabolic risk factor for the development of HCC in the setting of chronic HCV infection. In a study of 1,431 HCV patients followed for up to 10 years, the risk of HCC increased in proportion to body mass index with obese patients (hazard ratio 3.10) being at higher risk than overweight patients (hazard ratio 1.86) [418]. Likewise, insulin resistance is associated with steatosis in genotype 1 infection even in the absence of overt diabetes [461]. Diabetes and insulin resistance are strongly associated with advanced fibrosis in genotype 1 infection. One group demonstrated that diabetic patients were twice as likely to have advanced fibrosis (60%) compared to those with insulin resistance without overt diabetes (30%) [462]. In population-based studies, diabetes carries a two to threefold increased risk of HCC independent of other factors [422] and this has been confirmed in patients with chronic HCV infection [420].

While viral factors such as genotype, viral load, and quasispecies have not been consistently linked to outcome, coinfection with other viruses or parasites may influence disease course in chronic HCV infection (Table 25.3). Dual infection with hepatitis B can result in faster progression to cirrhosis although one virus usually predominates [463,464]. Coinfection with schistosomiasis and HCV, which is common in Egypt, is associated with more aggressive fibrosis than HCV infection alone [465]. In the era of highly active antiretroviral therapy (HAART), end-stage liver disease has emerged as a serious cause of morbidity and mortality in patients with HIV, with chronic HCV being the causal agent in the

Table 25.3 Factors associated with increased disease progression in chronic hepatitis C infection.

Host factors	Viral factors	Environmental factors
Older age at acquisition	Coinfection with HBV	Alcohol intake >50 g/day
Duration of infection	Coinfection with HIV	Regular marijuana use
Male gender		
Obesity		
Hepatic steatosis		
Insulin resistance		
Hepatic iron overload		

HBV, hepatitis B virus; HIV, human immunodeficiency virus.

majority [466]. Coinfection with HIV in the setting of chronic HCV may have markedly elevated HCV RNA levels and carries a two to five-fold increased risk of advanced fibrosis or cirrhosis [467–469]. In one study, the median time to cirrhosis for HCV/HIV coinfected patients was 26 years (95% CI, 22–34 years), while a matched cohort of HCV-monoinfected patients had a mean time to cirrhosis of 38 years (95% CI, 32–47 years) [470]. The severity of HIV disease may also identify patients with the highest risk of HCV progression, such as those with low CD4 counts or detectable HIV viral load [471–473]. Most data regarding accelerated fibrosis in the setting of HIV were collected pre-HAART. Multiple studies have now shown a beneficial effect of HAART on progression of liver disease in the setting of HCV/HIV coinfection, including a decrease in liver-related mortality [470,474,475].

Heavy alcohol consumption (>50 g/day) is clearly associated with accelerated fibrosis and cirrhosis in chronic HCV patients. In a meta-analysis evaluating more than 15,000 people with chronic HCV infection, the pooled relative risk of cirrhosis development with heavy alcohol intake was 2.33 (95% CI, 1.67–3.26) [476]. In this study, heavy alcohol use was defined as 210–560 g/week or 2.3–5.6 drink equivalents per day. Interestingly, the effects of HCV and alcohol intake at 50 g/day appear to be additive in their profibrogenic effects on the liver, but at >125 g of alcohol per day the effects on the liver are synergistic [477]. Light or moderate alcohol intake and its effect on HCV fibrosis is more controversial. In a study of 800 HCV patients undergoing liver biopsy, alcohol intake was evaluated as none, light, moderate, or heavy. Only a consumption of >50 g/day had an association with fibrosis, not lesser amounts [478]. As there continues to be a paucity of conclusive information linking light or moderate alcohol use with accelerated fibrosis in HCV, it is recommended that those with HCV either abstain from alcohol or limit alcohol intake to two drinks per day for men or one drink per day for women [479]. In addition to alcohol consumption, other external factors may play a role in fibrosis progression in the setting of chronic HCV. Daily marijuana use has been associated with more rapid hepatic scarring [480,481], while daily coffee consumption may decrease risk of fibrosis progression [482,483].

Extrahepatic manifestations
While HCV infection is most often thought of as a liver disease, some have advocated that it should be considered a systemic disease. Chronic HCV has been associated with numerous extrahepatic manifestations [484]. The list of possible associations is long, but those strongly associated with HCV have been proven based on pathogenic and epidemiologic data. Small studies with inadequate controls or selection bias are often misleading. For those

complications where the pathogenesis is virally mediated, HCV therapy is the treatment of choice to alleviate symptoms (see HCV treatment section below).

B-cell lymphoproliferative disorders, which include essential mixed cryoglobulinemia and non-Hodgkin lymphoma (NHL) are the best studied of the extrahepatic HCV disorders. Cryoglobulins found in patients with chronic HCV are primarily mixed cryoglobulins type II or III. The key components in this form of cryoprecipitate are monoclonal or polyclonal IgM rheumatoid factor and polyclonal IgG directed against HCV viral antigens [485]. While cryoglobulins can be detected in up to 50% of chronic HCV patients [486], only about 5–10% manifest symptoms consistent with a small- to medium-vessel vasculitis. The hallmark of mixed cryoglobulinemia syndrome is the clinical triad of weakness, arthralgias, and palpable purpura, which usually involve the lower extremities [487]. Peripheral neuropathy is also commonly seen as well as Raynaud phenomenon, sicca syndrome, and membranoproliferative glomerulonephritis. All patients with chronic HCV should be questioned about symptoms of mixed cryoglobulinemia, and if present cryocrit, rheumatoid factor, and urinalysis should be performed.

Sequencing of the antigen recognition region of the immunoglobulin heavy chain on B cells from liver, peripheral blood, and bone marrow from patients with chronic HCV infection has shown that oligoclonal expansion of B cells, specifically within the liver, is highly associated with mixed cryoglobulinemia [488]. It is likely that B-cell clones begin expanding in the liver and circulate to other compartments. Since mixed cryoglobulinemia syndrome is clearly virally mediated, a trial of HCV treatment is usually warranted unless multiorgan involvement precludes it. Mixed cryoglobulinemia can also be associated with a bcl-2 rearrangement and may evolve into a frank B-cell NHL in 8–10% [489]. Interestingly, B cells harboring this mutation regress after successful viral clearance [490]. Sustained activation of B cells through host and viral mechanisms may lead to successive mutational events eventually driving the lymphoproliferative disorder towards independence from viral stimulation.

Even in the absence of overt mixed cryoglobulinemia, HCV infection has been associated with the development of B-cell NHL [491–493] as well as primary hepatic lymphoma [494]. A meta-analysis of 48 studies found the prevalence of NHL in HCV patients was 15% compared with about 1.5% in the general population [491]. For low-grade lymphomas, a trial of antiviral therapy is often indicated. Monoclonal gammopathy, usually monoclonal gammopathy of undetermined significance (MGUS), is another HCV-associated lymphoproliferative disorder most often seen with genotype 2 in patients over the age of 60 years [495,496].

There are several dermatologic conditions associated with HCV including leukocytoclastic vasculitis, which is by far the most common manifestation of mixed cryoglobulinemia (Fig. 25.10A). Porphyria cutanea tarda (PCT) is a skin disorder associated with decreased levels of hepatic uroporphyrinogen decarboylase activity (Fig. 25.10B). Clinically, it is characterized by photosensitivity, skin fragility, and vesicles or bullae that are often hemorrhagic. There is a strong association between the sporadic form of PCT and chronic HCV infection [497]. PCT can be "triggered" by HCV infection in genetically predisposed individuals but does not appear to be a direct result of the virus. Iron overload also plays an important role in the pathogenesis of PCT and iron levels should be checked in these patients. Likewise, phlebotomy should be undertaken prior to antiviral treatment as many symptoms improve with iron depletion alone and can be made worse with ribavirin-induced hemolysis [498]. Lichen planus is a mucocutaneous disease with a predominance of CD4+ T cells on biopsy. Up to 27% of oral lichen planus patients are HCV-positive and HCV RNA has been isolated from mucous membrane biopsies supporting this association (499) [499,500]. Lichen planus may actually worsen on interferon therapy, possibly due to increased stimulation of cell-mediated immunity. Necrolytic acral erythema results in pruritic, psoriasis-like skin lesions in an acral distribution on the dorsal side of hands and feet. HCV antibodies were found in all 30 patients who presented with this disorder in one series [501]. Some reports confirm improvement with antiviral therapy as well as with the treatment of zinc deficiency [502].

A high prevalence of type 2 diabetes mellitus has been observed in patients with chronic HCV independent of liver disease [503,504]. While risk factors such as older age, obesity, advanced fibrosis, and family history may play a role [504], this association has been somewhat difficult to reconcile with the virus. Insulin resistance without overt diabetes has been associated with fibrosis progression and high HCV RNA [505,506]. The most compelling argument for a viral association is that the risk of diabetes development decreases with successful response to antiviral therapy [507,508].

Histology

Liver biopsy remains an important part of the evaluation of patients with chronic HCV infection. It provides confirmation of diagnosis based on characteristic features, exclusion of other liver diseases, and assessment of grade and stage of disease. Histologic features beyond the stage of fibrosis such as steatosis or iron deposition may also have predictive value in disease progression and efficacy of antiviral therapy. Assessment of these should be routinely requested as part of the staging liver biopsy pathology report.

Of all the histologic features of chronic HCV, the most characteristic are prominent lymphoid aggregates, steatosis, and bile duct damage. While these features may be seen in chronic hepatitis B or autoimmune hepatitis, they are more frequently observed in biopsies from patients with chronic HCV [453]. Lymphoid follicles are seen in about 60% of liver biopsies from chronic HCV patients [453]. Immunohistochemical studies have shown that these lymphoid follicles are comprised of B cells surrounded by a T-cell zone [509]. There is growing evidence that these lymphoid follicles contain true germinal centers where B cells are activated and undergo differentiation, clonal selection, and proliferation, presumably in response to local antigens [510, 511]. Oligoclonal expansion of B cells, specifically within the liver, is highly associated with mixed cryoglobulinemia [488].

Steatosis is seen in approximately 55% (40–70%) of biopsies taken for HCV staging [441]. It is usually

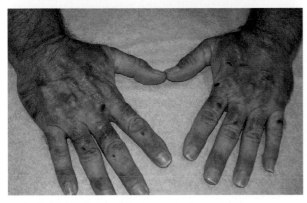

A © ACR

B

Figure 25.10 Clinical findings of leukocytoclastic vasculitis in cryoglobulinemia and porphyria cutanea tarda: (A) cryoglobulin-associated vasculitis, and (B) characteristic changes of porphyira cutanea tarda. (From DermAtlas 2001, http://dermatlas.med.jhmi.edu/derm/IndexDisplay .cfm?ImageID=543456724.

macrovesicular and graded as mild to moderate (<30%), although the percent of affected hepatocytes differs with varied grading systems. The distribution of steatosis in HCV may be zonal (with increased fat in acinar zone 1 or 3), panacinar, or focal [441]. Infection with genotype 3 as well as high body mass index have been consistently associated with the degree of steatosis in multivariate analyses [458,512,513]. Viral steatosis associated with genotype 3 infection diminishes following successful antiviral therapy [460,513] and may be associated with HCV core protein [514]. Concomitant steatohepatitis is seen in about 5% of HCV biopsies [441] and is associated with more aggressive fibrosis in both alcoholic and nonalcoholic disease [456,515]. Histologic features of steatohepatitis – including zone 3 injury, ballooning hepatocytes, Mallory bodies, and perisinusoidal fibrosis – are further discussed elsewhere in this textbook. The presence of metabolic steatosis on biopsy has also been associated with resistance to interferon-based therapy [460].

About 25% of HCV biopsies will have bile duct damage consisting of swelling, vacuolization, and nuclear irregularity of biliary epithelial cells [453]; predominantly lymphocytes, but sometimes plasma cells or neutrophils, will infiltrate the duct. In contrast to primary biliary cirrhosis, which can result in ductopenia, the ducts are not destroyed in chronic HCV.

Multiple staging systems have been proposed for chronic HCV with slightly different definitions and scoring but the principles are the same. In general, *grading* of a liver biopsy reflects inflammatory disease activity. *Staging* focuses on fibrosis assessment ranging from none to cirrhosis. Once cirrhosis is reached, clinical scales such as MELD or Child–Pugh must be used to further characterize HCV disease. While noninvasive techniques continue to be developed for determining the degree of fibrosis, liver biopsy remains the gold standard for determining fibrosis stage in the noncirrhotic liver.

Table 25.4 outlines various staging systems, allowing comparison between the different systems regarding spectrum of fibrosis. The extent of fibrosis affects both the natural history of HCV as well as the response to interferon-based therapy [460,516]. The Metavir system is the most widely used in clinical practice today [517]. It is the simplest but the accuracy of grading and staging relies heavily on the adequacy of the specimen and the experience of the pathologist reading the liver biopsies [518]. Biopsies of less than 2 cm may lead to underscoring of fibrosis [519,520]. The Ishak scale subdivides cirrhosis into incomplete and definite cirrhosis, which may be useful in clinical trials [521].

Most systems divide inflammation into portal, periportal (interface hepatitis), lobular, and focal components. An evaluation of hepatocyte or confluent necrosis is also made [441]. The HAI of Knodell [522] and the modified HAI of Ishak [521] are most frequently used to assess inflammation and fibrosis semiquantitatively in clinical trials. Most patients have mild inflammation but moderate or severe grades of inflammation have been associated with accelerated fibrosis [439,440]. Therapeutic interventions often have the greatest effect on inflammatory activity (grading) but successful antiviral therapy is associated with improvement in fibrosis score (staging). A large treatment study with paired liver biopsies found that successful viral clearance was associated with fibrosis stability/improvement in 88% and cirrhosis regression in 64% [523].

Increased iron staining is a common finding in chronic HCV and is seen in about 40% of liver biopsies regardless of HFE genotype [441,447]. Increased hepatic iron may also contribute to necroinflammatory changes (higher grading) and progressive fibrosis in HCV infection [446, 447]. Stainable iron is also appreciated more often with cirrhosis. Improvement in HAI has been observed with phlebotomy in patients with chronic HCV, especially males [449,450]. Lower responses to interferon therapy have been correlated to increased stainable iron in the liver, particularly within the reticuloendothelial system [524]. In addition to iron staining, some pathologists

Table 25.4 Staging systems for evaluating hepatic histology in chronic hepatitis C.

Score	Knodell	Ishak	Scheuer	Metavir
0	None	None	None	None
1	Portal	Portal	Portal	Portal
2		Periportal	Periportal	Septae
3	Bridging fibrosis	Focal bridging	Architectural distortion without cirrhosis	Bridging fibrosis
4	Cirrhosis	Diffuse bridging	Cirrhosis	Cirrhosis
5		Extensive bridging		
6		Cirrhosis		

routinely perform periodic acid–Schiff diastase (PAS/D) staining on liver biopsies. The majority of patients with PAS/D-staining globules have an undetected α_1-antitrypsin (AAT) abnormality [525]. In the setting of chronic HCV, even patients with heterozygous AAT deficiency (PI*Z) may develop a more progressive liver injury [526,527].

Fibrosing cholestatic hepatitis (FCH) is a particularly aggressive form of recurrent HCV seen post liver transplant in a minority of patients. Although uncommon, it has a high morbidity and mortality as well as histologic features that are different from those seen in chronic HCV. The histologic features of FCH include marked cholestasis, ballooning of hepatocytes, and pericellular fibrosis [528]. It is important to recognize the early features of FCH as this may be the only time to intervene prior to graft loss. The first abnormality appears to be recurrent HCV with cholestasis but fibrosis develops soon after (within several weeks), and both continue to worsen [529]. Early fibrosis consists of delicate pericellular bands that gradually extend until the classic fibrosis pattern becomes discernable. FCH is usually evident in the late-stage form, but the subtle features of cholestasis and early sinusoidal fibrosis can easily be overlooked. A novel sinusoidal fibrosis scoring system and cholestasis scoring system have been proposed to aid in the diagnosis of this entity (529).

The proportion and distribution of infected hepatocytes in chronic hepatitis C has been difficult to determine using conventional immunohistochemistry and in situ hybridization methods. Using two-photon microscopy with fluorescent, semiconductor quantum dot probes, Liang and colleagues were able to visualize core and NS3 proteins as well as dsRNA from patient liver samples [530]. Interestingly, between 7% and 20% of hepatocytes were infected in patients with HCV RNA levels

of 10^5 IU/mL or greater. Infected cells were in clusters, which suggested spread of the virus from cell to cell. dsRNA, a product of viral replication, was abundant within cells at the center of the clusters, but was often sparse in cells at the periphery, consistent with more recent infection of cells at the periphery.

Therapy

Rapid progress has been made in establishing effective therapy for chronic hepatitis C since the virus was discovered in 1989. Sustained virologic response rates (SVRs) have increased from 5–10% with standard interferon therapy to over 40% when standard interferon is combined with ribavirin. Modification of interferon (pegylation) to improve its pharmacokinetics further has increased rates of SVR. Finally, combining these agents with direct-acting antiviral agents has now pushed SVR rates to over 70% for patients with genotype 1 infection. The path to maximizing SVR with novel therapeutic regimens is described below.

Assessing response to antiviral therapy

Patterns of response to antiviral therapy are shown in Fig. 25.11. The goal of antiviral therapy of chronic hepatitis C is sustained virologic response defined as undetectable HCV RNA in the serum when measured 6 months after the end of treatment. Patients who remain with undetectable HCV RNA at this time point have an extremely durable response such that the relapse rate when evaluated up to 7 years after treatment is less than 1% [531]. Indeed, the persistent inability to detect HCV RNA in serum or in hepatic tissue using sensitive molecular techniques implies that permanent viral eradication has occurred and that SVR is analogous to "cure" of

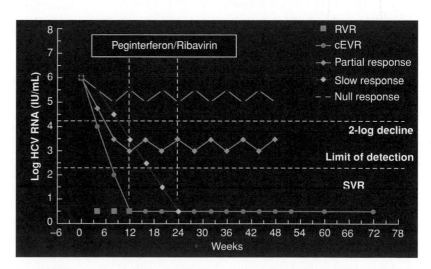

Figure 25.11 Patterns of response to antiviral therapy. cEVR, complete early virologic response; HCV, hepatitis C virus; RVR, rapid virologic response; SVR, sustained virologic response.

Table 25.5 Definitions of treatment milestones and their implications for response-guided therapy.

Response	Time to assess	Definition	Implication
RVR: rapid virologic response	4 week	HCV RNA undetectable	Best positive predictor for SVR; may respond as well with only 24 weeks of treatment
pEVR: partial early virologic response	12 week	HCV RNA decreased by ≥2 logs from baseline	Failure to achieve EVR associated with almost no chance of SVR and treatment can usually be stopped
cEVR: complete early virologic response	12 week	HC RNA undetectable	cEVR associated with higher chance of SVR
ETR	End of treatment	HCV RNA undetectable	On treatment response; observe for SVR or relapse
SVR: slow virologic response	24 weeks after treatment	HCV RNA undetectable by PCR or TMA	Eradication of virus

ETR, end-of-treatment response; HCV, hepatitis C virus; PCR, polymerase chain reaction; TMA, transcription-mediated amplification.

this chronic viral infection [532,533]. However, some conflicting and controversial evidence exists whereby HCV viral sequences have been detected in peripheral blood mononuclear cells even in patients with SVR, although no clinical sequelae have been shown in these patients [534,535]. Nevertheless, patients who achieve a SVR have consistent improvement in several parameters of hepatic disease and also demonstrate long-term clinical benefits. Serum ALT activity usually decreases into the low normal range and hepatic histology shows marked decrease in necroinflammatory activity. Improvement in hepatic fibrosis may also occur [533,536,537]. Importantly, patients who have achieved a SVR as a result of antiviral therapy have lower rates of subsequent hepatic decompensation and hepatocellular carcinoma compared with treatment failures [538–540]. A study of 21,000 US Veterans suggested that SVRs after antiviral therapy were associated with a significant decrease in all-cause mortality compared with treated patients who did not achieve SVRs [541].

Definition of nonresponse and relapse

Patients who remain with detectable HCV RNA throughout a course of therapy are considered to be nonresponders. Within the nonresponder category, null responders achieve the least reduction in HCV RNA, usually less than a 1 log decrease in HCV levels by 12 weeks of treatment, and are considered the most refractory to pegIFN and ribavirin therapy. Partial responders may have multiple log-fold decreases in HCV RNA in serum but always have detectable viremia during treatment (see Fig. 25.11) [542,543].

In contrast, relapsers are those who do achieve undetectable HCV RNA during treatment, as measured by a sensitive standardized assay, but then recur with HCV

RNA measurable in the serum after the end of a prescribed treatment regimen. Relapsers can be further categorized based upon the time point at which they cleared virus for the first time (Table 25.5). Rapid virologic responders achieve undetectable viremia by week 4 of treatment. Patients who achieve undetectable viremia for the first time at week 12 have had a complete early virologic response (cEVR), whereas those whose HCV RNA decreased by at least 2 logs at this point but remained detectable are considered to have had only a partial early virologic response (pEVR). Patients with a pEVR who then become undetectable by week 24 are considered to have a slow virologic response (Table 25.5) [542]. Accurate characterization of virologic response during treatment may influence decisions regarding retreatment of patients with new triple therapy combinations, as will be discussed below.

Interferon and ribavirin

Interferon is effective treatment for chronic hepatitis C

In 1986, several years before the discovery of the hepatitis C virus, the first report of successful treatment for NANB hepatitis was published by Hoofnagle and colleagues from the National Institutes of Health (544). Ten patients received recombinant human α-interferon (IFN-α) at doses between 0.5 million and 5 million IU for 4–12 months. Serum aminotransferases rapidly decreased during therapy in most patients and remained normal in those with prolonged therapy. Hepatic histology also demonstrated improvement in some patients. This uncontrolled series suggested that interferon could achieve clinical improvement in patients with NANB hepatitis and provided a rationale for more comprehensive studies of interferon for chronic hepatitis C.

Davis and colleagues [545] published a large placebo-controlled trial that randomized patients to 6 months of therapy with IFN-α-2b at either 1 or 3 million IU thrice weekly or placebo. Normalization of ALT was achieved in 46% of those treated with 3 million IU, compared with only 28% treated with the lower dose. A significant reduction in periportal and lobular inflammation was also observed in liver biopsy specimens. However, 51% of patients with an initial biochemical response relapsed once treatment was discontinued. This landmark study confirmed that patients with chronic hepatitis C could benefit from treatment with interferon, although the high frequency of relapse was a harbinger of challenges that we continue to face today. A smaller placebo-controlled trial by Di Bisceglie and colleagues published simultaneously demonstrated nearly identical results [546].

Another early controlled trial of IFN-α-2b for NANB hepatitis included 252 patients with anti-HCV antibody [547]. Patients were treated for 6 months with IFN-α-2b at 3 million IU and then randomized to either stop therapy, continue for an additional 12 months, or continue a lower dose for an additional 12 months. In those treated for a total of 18 months with the higher dose of interferon, 22% maintained normalization of serum ALT after discontinuation of therapy, compared with only about 10% in those with shorter treatment duration group or receiving lower doses of interferon. As with most studies of this era, the protocol was initiated prior to the availability of routine HCV RNA testing and this was not a prospective end-point. Retrospective analysis of a small subset of patients for whom frozen sera was available indicated that HCV RNA could be eradicated in some patients. Again, this study provided insights into themes that would become important as attempts were made to optimize treatment with interferon-based regimens; longer duration of therapy with interferon improved response rates and decreased the likelihood of relapse.

A flurry of subsequent studies utilizing interferon further supported the importance of this agent for the treatment of hepatitis C [548]. However, biochemical response rates remained fairly constant despite attempts to further manipulate dosing and treatment duration. Lindsay and colleagues [549] treated patients with 3, 5, or 10 million IU thrice daily for the first 12 weeks of therapy to determine if higher initial doses improved biochemical response rates. Higher doses of interferon did not increase the likelihood of sustained biochemical response, which overall was quite low and ranged between 8% and 17%. Furthermore, dose escalation in patients who had not had a biochemical response by week 12 did not improve the rate of sustained normalization of serum ALT activity once treatment was discontinued. This study also demonstrated that patients with genotype 1 were less likely to be responsive to treatment than those with genotypes 2 and 3 [549].

By 1999, approximately 76 randomized controlled trials of interferon for the treatment of chronic hepatitis C had been performed as reported in a meta-analysis [550]. Importantly, later studies included in this analysis had begun to measure HCV RNA in serum, the sustained clearance of which would become the definitive, desired outcome for antiviral therapy. In aggregate, these trials indicated that 17% of patients treated with interferon remained HCV RNA-negative for at least 6 months after therapy was discontinued, indicating sustained virologic response. This meta-analysis also suggested that longer duration of therapy and higher doses of interferon were associated with a better rate of sustained virologic response [550].

The road to ribavirin combination therapy

The greatest incremental advance in the treatment of hepatitis C was the recognition that ribavirin, a relatively obscure medication with antiviral activity against a broad range of RNA and DNA viruses including Flaviviridae, could dramatically increase the rate of SVR when it was combined with IFN-α-2b [551]. Ribavirin is a guanosine nucleoside analog approved initially for the treatment of respiratory syncytial virus in neonates [552]. Several postulated mechanisms of action of ribavirin for the treatment of hepatitis C have been proposed since its clinical utility for this disease was recognized. These theories and supportive evidence have been detailed in excellent reviews by Feld, Hoofnagle, and Chung et al. [257,553]:

1 Ribavirin may directly inhibit hepatitis C virus replication by acting as a chain terminator when ribavirin triphosphate is incorporated into viral RNA by viral RNA polymerases. However, high concentrations of ribavirin, not achieved in clinical settings, were required to demonstrate this activity [554].
2 Ribavirin may act as an inhibitor of inosine monophosphate dehydrogenase (IMPDH). Depletion of guanosine triphosphate in this manner will prevent viral RNA synthesis. Interestingly, this concept has been tested clinically in patients treated with pegIFN and ribavirin combined with mycophenolate mofetil, an IMPDH inhibitor used as an immunosuppressant in transplantation. No additive effects on viral suppression were noted with mycophenylate [555].
3 Ribavirin may increase the rate of naturally occurring mutations leading to defective HCV RNA that decreases the ability of HCV RNA to replicate. Studies of the frequency of mutations in patients with hepatitis C treated with ribavirin have yielded conflicting results [257,553].
4 Ribavirin may have immunomodulatory activity by altering the balance between different types of CD4+

T-cell responses, perhaps favoring sustained virologic clearance [257,553].

5 A recent, intriguing proposed mechanism of ribavirin action suggests that ribavirin augments the regulation of interferon-signaling genes. Feld and colleagues [556] measured mRNA expression in hepatic tissue obtained from patients after an injection of pegIFN. Those who had been pretreated with ribavirin had upregulation of interferon signaling genes compared with those who had not received ribavirin. A subsequent study demonstrated that ribavirin improved early viral kinetics in patients who demonstrated an initial response to pegIFN and that this also correlated with measures of enhanced interferon signaling gene expression [557].

Ribavirin monotherapy improves serum alanine aminotransferase activity

The availability of ribavirin with its broad, albeit poorly understood, antiviral activity led to several studies to evaluate ribavirin as a single agent for the treatment of chronic hepatitis C. In two studies that treated patients only with ribavirin 1,200 mg daily for 12 months, serum aminotransferases decreased to normal or near normal in about 35–40% of patients. Concomitant improvement in necroinflammatory activity was also found in liver biopsies obtained at the end of treatment [558,559]. These results were rarely sustained, however, and once ribavirin was discontinued serum ALT activity returned to baseline values in most patients. In these early studies, HCV RNA levels remained unchanged despite the other measures of clinical improvement. Prolonged therapy with ribavirin in patients who did not respond to interferon and ribavirin yielded similar results [560]. Among patients who remained HCV RNA-positive after 24 weeks of interferon and ribavirin, those randomized to continue ribavirin monotherapy for an additional 48 weeks had improvement in serum aminotransferases and hepatic histology, with no effect on HCV RNA levels in serum. These studies demonstrated that there is no role for ribavirin monotherapy for the treatment of chronic hepatitis C.

Combining ribavirin with interferon substantially improves antiviral response

With essentially negative results from the ribavirin monotherapy trials, it was unexpected that combining ribavirin with interferon would provide such dramatic improvement in outcomes compared to interferon alone. Indeed, combination therapy of interferon and ribavirin has remained the cornerstone of treatment for chronic hepatitis C. The first suggestion that ribavirin enhanced outcomes was reported in a small pilot study by Brillanti and colleagues in 1994 [551]. Twenty patients who had not responded to interferon previously were randomly assigned to retreatment with interferon plus ribavirin or interferon alone. Remarkably, 40% of patients treated with combination interferon and ribavirin had undetectable HCV RNA when measured 9 months after treatment discontinuation, compared with none in the interferon-only group [551].

Two seminal studies published in 1998 confirmed this initial report and established combination therapy as the standard of care for all patients with chronic hepatitis C [561]. McHutchison and colleagues [561] randomized over 900 patients to treatment with IFN-α-2b alone or IFN-α-2b plus ribavirin (1,000–1,200 mg/day) for 24 or 48 weeks. The SVR for those treated with combination therapy was 31% and 38% (24 and 48 weeks, respectively) compared with only 6% and 13% for those treated with interferon monotherapy. Genotype 1 patients had a substantially lower rate of SVR even when treated with combination therapy: 28% and 16% with 24 or 48 weeks of treatment, respectively. Nearly 70% of patients with genotype 2 or 3 had a SVR, regardless of treatment duration [561]. In a separate study, the rate of SVR was 43% for those treated with interferon and ribavirin for 48 weeks [562]. Several independent factors (genotype 2 or 3, HCV RNA <2 million copies/mL, age less than 40 years, minimal fibrosis stage, and female gender) were associated with a higher likelihood of SVR.

Modification of interferon with pegylation improves pharmacokinetics

Standard recombinant alpha interferons utilized in the past to treat chronic hepatitis C have short half-lives of approximately 6 hours which necessitated dosing several times per week [563,564]. These unmodified forms of interferon administered subcutaneously were characterized by rapid absorption with high peak levels of interferon concentration achieved within hours, followed by rapid disappearance from the serum, without attainment of steady state concentrations. Combining an inactive polyethylene glycol (PEG) moiety with a native protein to improve pharmacokinetic parameters has been applied to a number of therapeutic agents, including epoetin-α and chemotherapeutic agents [565]. Peginterferon-α-2b (PEG-Intron®, Merck), approved by the US Food and Drug Administration (FDA) in 2001, consists of a 12 kD linear PEG molecule attached covalently to the IFN-α-2b molecule; while peginterferon-α-2a, approved in 2002 (Pegasys, Hoffman La-Roche), links a 40 kD branched PEG molecule to IFN-α-2a [564]. These enhancements diminish clearance of both interferons and prolong the half-lives to approximately 24 hours and 65 hours, respectively, which allows for once-weekly administration [563, 564,566]. PegIFN-α-2b is predominantly excreted through the kidney while pegIFN-α-2a is hepatically metabolized. The size and structure of the PEG moiety also impacts upon other parameters such as volume of distribution, rate of absorption, and biologic activity although, as discussed below, clinical outcomes with either pegIFN combined with ribavirin is similar [563,567].

Peginterferon combined with ribavirin improves rates of sustained virologic response

Pivotal clinical trials of pegIFN-α-2b and -2a were reported in 2001 and 2002, respectively [568,569]. Manns et al. [569] randomized over 1,500 patients to treatment for 48 weeks with either: (i) pegIFN-α-2b 1.5 μg/kg/week; (ii) pegIFN-α-2b 1.5 μg/kg/week for 4 weeks then decreased to 0.5 μg/kg/week; (iii) or IFN-α-2b 3 MU subcutaneously three times per week. All patients received ribavirin 1,000–1,200 mg/day. Overall, SVR rates (54%, 47%, and 47%, respectively) demonstrated that the higher dose pegIFN was significantly more effective. Among genotype 1 patients, rates of SVR were 42% for the higher dose pegIFN compared with 34% for the lower dose pegIFN and 33% for the standard interferon arm. Genotype 2 or 3 patients, as expected, fared better with SVR rates as high as 82% with higher dose pegIFN. Several pretreatment characteristics were associated with SVR, including non-1 genotype, lower baseline viral load, lighter weight, younger age, and the absence of cirrhosis. Logistic regression analysis indicated that the dose of ribavirin on a mg/kg basis was an important factor in determining treatment outcome. Thus, patients who received more than 10.6 mg/kg/day of ribavirin had higher rates of SVR for all dose groups and genotypes [569].

Fried and colleagues [568] compared the efficacy of three treatment regimens: pegIFN-α-2a 180 μg/week alone or in combination with ribavirin 1,000–1,200 mg/day, or standard interferon and ribavirin. The best rate of overall SVR, 56%, was achieved in those treated with pegIFN-α-2a and ribavirin compared with 44% of those treated with standard interferon and ribavirin and only 29% with pegIFN alone. Genotype 1 patients had SVR rates of 46%, 36%, and 21%, respectively, while patients with genotype 2 or 3 achieved a SVR in 76% of those treated with pegIFN-α-2a and ribavirin. Three factors, non-1 genotype, age less than 40 years, and body weight of 75 kg or less were independently associated with virologic response [568].

Refining treatment regimens to optimize response

The above registration trials established the superior efficacy of peginterferons combined with ribavirin for the treatment of chronic hepatitis C. Subsequent analyses of these data and additional studies sought to further refine the treatment algorithm in order to maximize the chances of response while minimizing exposure to medications with a substantial burden of side effects. Hadziyannis et al. [570] randomized over 1,300 patients to four arms of treatment with pegIFN-α-2a 180 μg/week plus ribavirin at doses of either 1,000–1,200 mg/day or 800 mg/day for either 24 or 48 weeks' duration. The factorial study design that included patients with genotypes 1, 2, and 3 allowed for several comparisons between ribavirin dosing and treatment duration across genotypes. The results confirmed that genotype 1 patients required higher doses of ribavirin (1,000–1,200mg/day) for 48 weeks. Those treated for 24 weeks or with only 800 mg/day of ribavirin had a higher chance of relapse once therapy was discontinued. In contrast, patients with genotypes 2 or 3 did equally well regardless of duration or ribavirin dosing suggesting that 24 weeks of treatment with only 800 mg/day of ribavirin was sufficient [570].

In aggregate, these studies provided the rationale for FDA approval of the two pegIFN preparations and the general recommendations for the treatment of chronic hepatitis C, which are based upon HCV genotype, as shown in Table 25.6. PegIFN-α-2b is administered subcutaneously once weekly as a weight-based dose (1.5 μg/kg/week) while pegIFN-α-2a is administered as a fixed weekly dose of 180 μg/week. Both drugs must be combined with ribavirin for maximal efficacy, although with modest differences in ribavirin dosing recommendations. In general, a 48-week course of treatment is recommended for patients with genotype 1 or 4 utilizing

Table 25.6 Standard recommendations for dosing and duration of treatment of peginterferon (PEG) and ribavirin according to viral genotype.

Genotype	PEG dose (per week)	Ribavirin dose (mg/day)	Duration (weeks)	SVR (%)
1	180 μg PEG-α-2a or 1.5 μg/kg PEG-α-2b	800–1,400 (weight based)	48	41–42
2	180 μg PEG-α-2a or 1.5 μg/kg PEG-α-2b	800	24	60–84
3	180 μg PEG-α-2a or 1.5 μg/kg PEG-α-2b	800	24	60–84
4	180 μg PEG-α-2a or 1.5 μg/kg PEG-α-2b	1,000–1,200	48	55
5	180 μg PEG-α-2a or 1.5 μg/kg PEG-α-2b	1,000–1,200	48	64
6	180 μg PEG-α-2a or 1.5 μg/kg PEG-α-2b	1,000–1,200	48	63

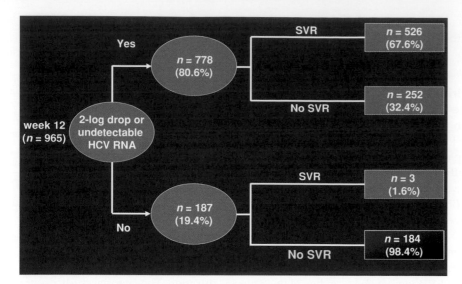

Figure 25.12 Absence of early virologic response is associated with treatment failure with pegIFN and ribavirin. HCV, hepatitis C virus; SVR, sustained virologic response. (Reproduced from Davis [571] with permission from Plenum.)

higher doses of ribavirin. Treatment termination is recommended when patients fail to achieve undetectable viremia by week 24 of a planned 48-week course of therapy for patients with genotype 1. Patients with genotypes 2 or 3 may be treated for 24 weeks with only 800 mg of ribavirin. Recommendations for other genotypes are based on sparse data but follow similar recommendations as for genotype 1.

Response-guided therapy

The standardized treatment recommendations described above solely rely on differences in viral genotypes to dictate a course of therapy. In practice, there is ongoing assessment of virologic response to determine the advisability of continuing therapy when SVR is unlikely. This is to guide whether a prolonged course of pegIFN and ribavirin may be warranted to decrease the chance of relapse in slow virologic responders, and also to determine whether therapy can be successfully shortened without sacrificing the chances for SVR among those who rapidly respond to pegIFN and ribavirin. As will be discussed in detail below, response-guided therapy will form the basis of treatment recommendations for triple therapy combinations of pegIFN and ribavirin combined with a hepatitis C protease inhibitor or other direct-acting antiviral agents in the future.

Viral kinetics is associated with the likelihood of sustained virologic response

The rapidity with which a patient clears HCV RNA during therapy has important implications for subsequent treatment outcome [542]. The earliest studies of pegIFN and ribavirin combination therapy retrospectively evaluated the kinetics of viral response to determine when treatment failure was all but assured. Absence of an early

virologic response (EVR) has the best negative predictive value for treatment outcome [568,571]. Thus, patients who failed to achieve an EVR (either complete or partial) had a vanishingly small chance of ultimately achieving SVR, and stopping futile therapy at week 12 of treatment was considered on an individual basis (Fig. 25.12). Conversely, patients who achieve a RVR have the highest chance of achieving a SVR (over 90%) during the initial course of therapy [572,573]. In a retrospective analysis of patients with genotypes 1–4 treated with pegIFN-α-2a and ribavirin, RVR was attained in only 16% of individuals with genotype 1 and in 60–71% of those with genotype 2 or 3. However, among those with RVR, the rate of SVR was high across all genotypes ranging from 88% to 100% (Fig. 25.13). Baseline factors predictive of RVR included genotype non-1, lower initial viral load, higher ALT levels, absence of advanced fibrosis, and younger age. Notably, the presence of RVR was most predictive of SVR when compared with baseline characteristics regardless of HCV genotype, although the *IL28B* genotype was not included in this analysis [572]. Taken to the extreme, several investigators have also suggested that viral declines within the first 24–72 hours of treatment initiation are also highly predictive of subsequent outcome [574]. However, these observations have not been clinically embraced to alter therapeutic regimens.

Utilizing rapid virologic response to shorten treatment in genotype 1

As mentioned previously, 48 weeks of treatment for genotype 1 patients yields a better rate of SVR than a shorter 24-week treatment duration due to a lower relapse rate (the difference between end-of-treatment virologic response and sustained virologic response). However, the recognition that patients with RVR, present in about 15%

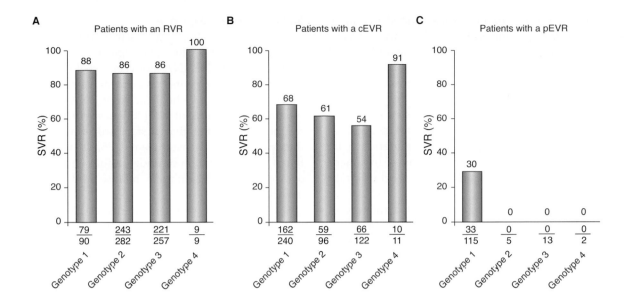

Figure 25.13 Likelihood of achieving sustained virologic response (SVR) related to achieving rapid virologic response (RVR), complete early virologic response (cEVR), or partial early virologic response (pEVR) across all genotypes with treatment with pegIFN and ribavirin. (Reproduced from Fried et al. [572] with permission from Elsevier.)

of patients treated with pegIFN and ribavirin, had the highest chance of SVR led to retrospective and prospective studies to determine whether a treatment duration shorter than the recommended 48 weeks would be effective for this subgroup with the highest likelihood of success. Indeed, interrogation of large databases that included patients with genotype 1 treated for only 24 weeks with pegIFN and ribavirin demonstrated that the rates of SVR among those who had first achieved RVR were comparable to those treated for 48 weeks [575]. Baseline viral loads of less than 600,000 IU/mL were most highly associated with this response.

Several trials have prospectively treated patients with genotype 1 and RVR for only 24 weeks [576]. In a single-arm study of patients with a pretreatment viral load of <600,000 IU/mL, Zeuzem and colleagues treated those who had first achieved an RVR with pegIFN-α-2b and ribavirin for a total of 24 weeks and found an SVR rate of 89% [577]. The PREDICT study utilized a response-guided algorithm to treat RVR patients with genotype 1 and a low viral load for 24 weeks [578]. This study yielded an SVR of 88% for the short treatment duration, adding support to the assertion that 24 weeks of treatment was sufficient for those with RVR. Other studies that prospectively embedded a 24-week treatment arm for patients who achieved RVR within a response-guided protocol also found similar results – that patients with RVR with low baseline viral loads received maximal benefit from only 24 weeks of treatment with pegIFN and ribavirin [579–581]. Common to all these studies was the diminished rate of relapse when RVR was attained, which was only approximately 10% [581].

These data led to the recommendation incorporated into European practice to truncate therapy to 24 weeks for patients with genotype 1 and a low baseline viral load who had achieved RVR. It should be noted that all of these studies on shortened duration of therapy in genotype 1 patients have been performed in populations outside the United States in whom therapeutic responses are generally more favorable for a variety of reasons, including race (and, by inference, attendant *IL28B* genotype) and differences in body mass index, among others features. Therefore, the application of shortened duration of therapy to US populations who achieve RVR may be considered but approached with caution, particularly in patients with multiple factors associated with poor treatment outcomes.

Utilizing rapid virologic response to shorten treatment in genotype 2 or 3

Patients infected with genotype 2 or 3 have the highest rates of SVR compared with other genotypes. Although the recommended treatment duration is already shorter than that of genotype 1 (24 weeks versus 48 weeks), a number of studies have also investigated whether treatment duration times as short as 12 weeks can be utilized in this population without compromising SVR [576]. Mangia and colleagues [582] randomized genotype 2 or 3 patients to treatment with a standard 24-week regimen of pegIFN-α-2b and weight-based ribavirin

(1,000–1,200 mg/day) or to a response-guided treatment whereby patients achieving RVR received only 12 weeks of treatment and non-RVR participants completed 24 weeks of therapy. Similar overall rates of SVR were achieved in both the fixed 24-week duration and the RVR-guided regimen (76% and 77%, respectively). Numeric differences in SVR among those who achieved RVR (91% versus 85%) were not statistically significant, suggesting that the shorter treatment regimen was not inferior to the fixed 24-week regimen. However, the end-of-treatment relapse rate was noted to be higher in the short duration treatment arm despite a RVR.

The largest study to investigate truncated therapy in genotypes 2 and 3 was performed by Shiffman et al. [583]. Nearly 1,500 patients were randomized a priori to either 16 weeks or 24 weeks of treatment with pegIFN-α-2a plus ribavirin 800 mg/day. In this study, a response-guided algorithm was not prospectively incorporated but post hoc analyses provided important information. The overall SVR rate was significantly lower in the 16-week treatment arm compared with the standard 24-week treatment regimen (62% versus 70%, respectively). An increase in relapse was evident among patients treated for 16 weeks (31% versus 18%). Multivariate analysis suggested that treatment response was positively associated viral genotype 2 versus genotype 3, low viral load at baseline (<400,000 IU/mL), age <45 years, weight <80 kg, higher serum ALT activity, the absence of advanced fibrosis, and longer treatment duration [583]. Patients with lower pretreatment HCV RNA had similar rates of SVR with either treatment duration (~80%). Even among patients who achieved RVR, the rate of SVR was still lower in those treated for a shorter duration (79% versus 85%). Strikingly, among non-RVR patients the SVR rate was low regardless of duration of therapy: 26% (16 weeks) and 45% (24 weeks) [583].

The interpretation of these multiple studies regarding shortening therapy for genotypes 2 and 3 is hampered by differences in treatment duration, variability in prospective randomization based upon RVR, and also differences in the dosing of ribavirin. Numerically lower response rates and higher relapse rates for patients treated with 12–16 weeks of therapy appear to be a consistent theme, which has been analyzed in a recent meta-analysis [584]. Thus, these data suggest that 24 weeks remains the optimal treatment duration for most patients with genotypes 2 or 3, although an ideal patient with a low viral level <400,000 IU/mL who achieves RVR may be considered for shortened duration of treatment. However, the impact of negative prognostic factors such as African-American race, HIV coinfection, cirrhosis, and obesity has been incompletely characterized and thus shortened therapy should only be selectively considered [576].

Slow virologic response

Approximately 15% of patients treated with pegIFN and ribavirin exhibit a slow virologic response defined as undetectable HCV RNA between weeks 12 and 24 of therapy. These patients have lower rates of SVR compared with patients who clear HCV RNA earlier in their treatment. Modeling of viral kinetics with slow virologic response suggested that a standard 48-week course of therapy would be insufficient [585]. It was postulated that a longer duration of undetectable viremia of at least 36 weeks would minimize relapse and maximize the chances of SVR [585].

Several studies have contributed to the body of evidence suggesting that prolonging treatment with pegIFN and ribavirin for slow virologic responders may be beneficial [576]. Berg and colleagues [586] performed one of the earliest studies to evaluate whether extended therapy with pegIFN and ribavirin would enhance rates of SVR. Patients with genotype 1 were randomized to treatment with pegIFN-α-2a and ribavirin 800 mg/day for either 48 or 72 weeks. SVR rates for both groups were almost identical. However, post hoc analysis demonstrated that slow virologic responders had a significantly higher rate of SVR (29% versus 17%) and a lower relapse rate (40% versus 64%) when treated for 72 weeks. The TeraVic-4 study focused on patients who failed to achieve a RVR and prospectively randomized them to 48 weeks or 72 weeks of therapy with pegIFN-α-2a and ribavirin 800 mg/day. Again, significant improvement was seen in SVR with prolonged treatment (44% versus 28%) along with diminished relapse rates [586].

Pearlman and colleagues [587] performed the most relevant study on this topic for clinicians in the United States. This single-center study of genotype 1 patients included a representative population with numerous treatment-resistant characteristics such as African-American race, high baseline levels of HCV RNA, and advanced fibrosis. Slow virologic responders treated with pegIFN-α-2b and ribavirin 800–1,400 mg/day for 72 weeks had a significantly higher rate of SVR compared with those who received a standard 48-week regimen (38% versus 18%). Relapse rates were also lower with the extended treatment duration [587].

Interestingly, a multicenter study performed in Europe did not support the concept that prolonged therapy was beneficial in patients with slow virologic response. The SUCCESS trial also randomized slow virologic responders to pegIFN-α-2b and weight-based ribavirin for either 48 weeks or 72 weeks [588]. In the intention-to-treat analysis SVR rates were similar for the extended duration treatment (48%) to those treated for only 48 weeks (43%). However, the study did show that relapse rates were ~14% lower with prolonged therapy, although this was not statistically significant.

Furthermore, in post hoc analyses of adherent patients and those who completed treatment, a numeric but statistically insignificant advantage for prolonged therapy was also evident [588].

A meta-analysis examined all randomized controlled trials to date that have evaluated extended duration of therapy for patients with a non-RVR [589]. Despite heterogeneity in the trials regarding type of interferon, ribavirin dosing, criteria for randomization, and populations studied, the authors concluded that prolonged therapy with pegIFN and ribavirin in slow virologic responders provided about a 15% higher chance to achieve SVR (95% CI, 4–26%) along with a similar decline in the chance for relapse, which likely was the contributing factor to improved SVR [589].

Importance of ribavirin, side effects, and management

Ribavirin is critical to the success of pegIFN combination therapies, including direct-acting antiviral regimens, in spite of controversy over its mechanism of action. The critical threshold for ribavirin dosing is approximately 11 mg/kg/day and doses below that level are associated with lower rates of response for patients with genotype 1 [569]. From modeling studies of ribavirin exposure versus response, higher doses of ribavirin (up to 15 mg/kg/day) are also found to be associated with higher rates of anemia and SVR [590,591]. Thus, ribavirin dosing in the range of 13–15 mg/kg appears to be the best balance between optimized efficacy and intolerable hemolytic anemia that develops at higher doses. Indeed, an informative pilot study of ten patients whose ribavirin dosing was increased until target serum levels were achieved demonstrated an impressive rate of SVR but with severe anemia requiring growth factor supplementation and, in some cases, blood transfusion [592].

Lack of adherence to ribavirin throughout a course of therapy is highly predictive of treatment failure and patients that maintain the highest levels of treatment adherence, greater than 80% of their prescribed medications, have the best rates of SVR [593]. Retrospective analyses indicate that modest dose reductions of ribavirin have a minimal impact on rates of sustained response. However, dose reductions to less than 60%, usually associated with temporary or permanent discontinuation of ribavirin, will significantly decrease the likelihood of SVR [594]. This was underscored in a clinical trial that randomized patients, already negative for HCV RNA at week 24, to either discontinue ribavirin (while maintaining pegIFN dosing) or continue combination therapy with pegIFN and ribavirin for the remaining 24 weeks of treatment [595]. Lower rates of SVR and significantly higher relapse rates were seen in patients who discontinued ribavirin early.

Ribavirin is highly concentrated in erythrocytes through a nucleoside es transporter and induces an extravascular hemolysis in essentially all patients [596]. The mechanism of hemolysis is related to depletion of erythrocyte adenosine triphosphate stores and increased susceptibility to oxidative damage to red blood cell membranes [597]. Peginterferon also contributes to anemia through its effect on bone marrow suppression. The average decrease in hemoglobin during combination therapy is approximately 2.5 g/dL, although the range is quite wide and severe anemia (hemoglobin <10 g/dL) may develop in up to 25% of patients [568,569,598]. Interestingly, the presence of severe anemia with standard dosing of ribavirin may also be a pharmacodynamic marker for adequacy of ribavirin dosing and is associated with higher SVR [599]. Severe anemia contributes to the fatigue, malaise, and diminished quality of life while on combination antiviral therapy.

Stepwise dose reduction by 200 mg decrements is the cornerstone of management for ribavirin-induced anemia. Ribavirin achieves steady-state concentrations in serum between weeks 4 and 6 of treatment, coinciding with the development of early and sometimes severe anemia. Product labeling recommends dose reduction of ribavirin when hemoglobin falls to <10 g/dL. However, the slope of hemoglobin reduction may also provide clues as to who will be at greatest risk for severe anemia. A decrease in hemoglobin of 1.5 g/dL at week 2 of therapy has been associated with the risk of severe anemia and treatment interruption at later time points [600]. Thus, close monitoring of hemoglobin early during the course of treatment, and modest dose reduction when severe anemia is likely to develop, may obviate the need for dose interruption or the addition of growth factors.

Epoetin-α (EPO) is effective for mitigating the anemia of ribavirin-induced hemolysis and also improves quality of life for those who have developed severe anemia [601,602]. The use of erythropoietic-stimulating agents due to the development of early-onset anemia (within 8 weeks of starting HCV treatment) was retrospectively associated with improved rates of SVR and less treatment discontinuation [599]. For anemia that developed later during combination antiviral treatment, the addition of EPO had no impact on these parameters. Few studies have prospectively evaluated the impact of EPO on SVR rates. EPO use was associated with improved rate of SVR when higher doses of ribavirin (~15 mg/kg/day, 1,000–1,600 mg/day) were initiated but had no impact on SVR with standard ribavirin dosing [602]. Whether modest dose reductions would have accomplished similar results could not be ascertained from this study. A recent study that randomized genotype 1 anemic patients during pegIFN and ribavirin treatment demonstrated an improvement in sustained response with EPO administration (SVR = 60%) compared to management with dose reductions of 200–400 mg/day (SVR = 34%) [603].

While selected patients with severe anemia may potentially benefit from adjunctive therapy with EPO, these agents are not approved by regulatory authorities for the treatment of ribavirin-induced anemia. Furthermore, enthusiasm for the use of erythropoietic growth factors has been tempered by the occurrence of the rare complication of red cell aplasia, as well as the concern for thrombosis risk when hemoglobin values increase to over 12 g/dL as a result of EPO administration [604].

A genome-wide association study, confirmed in a second independent dataset, of patients treated with pegIFN and ribavirin has identified variants in the gene for inosine triphosphatase that appear to protect patients from ribavirin-induced hemolysis [605,606]. Patients with two polymorphisms associated with inosine triphosphatase deficiency had lower rates of anemia and lower rates of anemia related to ribavirin dose reductions. The protective mechanism of these variants remains speculative but may involve competition between the accumulation of inosine triphosphate and ribavirin triphosphate within red blood cells. The role of inosine triphosphatase (ITPA)-variant genetic testing in clinical practice remains to be defined.

Alternatives to ribavirin with similar efficacy and fewer adverse events would be of great potential benefit. Taribavirin is an oral prodrug of ribavirin with a distinct structure that diminishes the ability of this agent to enter erythrocytes, thus resulting in less anemia [607]. Phase III clinical trials confirmed the lower incidence of anemia, however they failed to meet the end-point of SVR rates seen with ribavirin [608,609]. A recent phase II study utilizing weight-based doses of taribavirin demonstrated comparable rates of SVR and diminished anemia compared to standard ribavirin. At the highest doses of taribavirin (30 mg/kg/day) a stepwise increase of anemia was noted suggesting that increasing the taribavirin dose above this level would mitigate its advantage over standard ribavirin.

IL28B genotype and treatment response

Numerous host, environmental, and virologic factors have been associated with outcomes of interferon-based therapies. Ge and colleagues identified the single most important pretreatment host factor from an elegant genome-wide association study of over 1,100 patients treated with pegIFN and ribavirin in the IDEAL study [145,567]. Investigators identified a single nucleotide polymorphism (SNP) (rs12979860) on chromosome 19, 3 kb upstream of the *IL28B* gene encoding IFN-λ3, which was strongly associated with SVR. Patients with the favorable CC genotype were twice as likely to have a SVR as patients with the TT or CT genotypes (Fig. 25.14). The SVR rate among European-Americans with the CC allele was ~80%, while for those with genotype CT or TT the SVR rates were ~40% and ~35%, respectively. The influence of the *IL28B* genotype remained the strongest predictor of outcome when it was compared with other pretreatment factors known to be associated with treatment

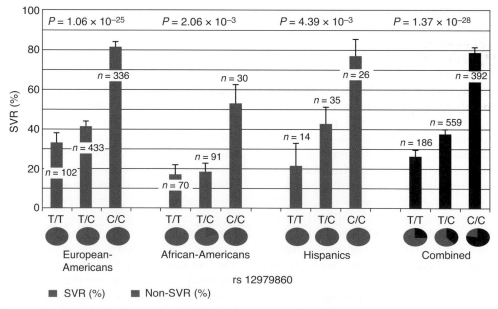

Figure 25.14 *IL28B* genotype and likelihood of sustained virologic response (SVR) CC genotype is the most favorable for treatment response. (Reproduced from Ge et al. [145] with permission from Nature.)

response, such as baseline viral load, extent of hepatic fibrosis, and race.

Interestingly, the same relative association was identified in African-American patients; however, the absolute rates of SVR remained lower among African-Americans even in those with the favorable CC genotype when compared with European-Americans. Further analyses in this study demonstrated that the frequency of the C allele varied across different racial groups. African-Americans were least likely to harbor the C allele, while East Asians had the highest frequency. Thus, it appears that the *IL28B* genotype accounts for a significant proportion, estimated to be ~50%, of the racial disparity in response to interferon-based therapies although other factors remain to be elucidated [145].

A flurry of studies confirmed and expanded these initial findings in global populations from Asia, Australia, and Europe, and additional cohorts in the United States [382,610–612]. Although methodologies were different and several additional SNPs, such as rs8099917 – some of whom were in linkage disequilibrium with rs12979860 – were identified, the robust association of SVR with SNPs in the IL28B region was unequivocal [611]. The association was evident as well in HIV/HCV coinfected patients [382].

The impact of *IL28B* on viral kinetics was also investigated [613]. In genotype 1 patients, the *IL28B* CC genotype was associated with a steeper decline in HCV RNA during the first phase of viral clearance, with CC genotype having a median reduction of viral load of $-2.6 \log_{10}$ IU/mL, compared to less than $-1 \log_{10}$ IU/mL decrease for other genotypes at week 2 of therapy. RVR (undetectable HCV RNA at week 4) was also significantly more frequent in patients with the CC genotype, compared to the CT or TT genotypes (28% versus 5% and 5%, respectively) [613]. Among patients with HCV genotype 2 and 3, where the overall response rate is high, there was only a modest but significant relationship between SVR and *IL28B* genotype. The greatest impact of the *IL28B* genotype was in patients who did not achieve RVR, in whom SVR rates for CC, CT, and TT genotypes were 87%, 67%, and 29%, respectively [614].

The mechanism associated with *IL28B* genotype and therapeutic response remains largely speculative, as discussed above and reviewed previously [610,611]. Several studies have evaluated the relationship between *IL28B* with interferon signaling gene (ISG) expression in liver tissue and peripheral blood mononuclear cells [615,616]. Elevated ISG expression prior to antiviral therapy is associated with diminished therapeutic response [131,556]. Interestingly, intrahepatic expression of ISGs was shown to correlate with *IL28B* genotype, whereby patients with a favorable responder *IL28B* genotype had lower baseline expression of ISG and, thus, presumably, a better

chance of responding to antiviral therapy. Expression of *IL28B* mRNA in liver tissue was not associated with *IL28B* genotype. In contrast, another study that evaluated intrahepatic ISG expression concluded that *IL28B* polymorphisms and intrahepatic ISG expression appeared to be independent predictors of antiviral response [617]. Additional insights into the relationship between *IL28B* and ISG is provided in a study by Darling and colleagues [618] that demonstrated that serum interferon-γ-inducible protein (IP-10), a marker of responsiveness to interferon-based therapies, significantly enhanced the predictability of *IL28B* genotype, particularly for patients with non-CC genotypes. IP-10 levels in this study were also independent of *IL28B* genotype [618].

IL28B genotyping assays are now available commercially, although their role in clinical practice remains to be clearly defined. Certainly, the absence of a favorable genotype should not be used to exclude an otherwise suitable candidate for treatment since a large proportion of patients with an unfavorable *IL28B* genotype will still respond to pegIFN and ribavirin. However, individual genotype data may be used to counsel patients about their pretreatment likelihood of response and allow them to make informed choices about beginning treatment with pegIFN and ribavirin or waiting until triple therapy regimens are available. The impact of *IL28B* genotype with triple therapies is not known at this time. Preliminary data suggest that the potent antiviral activity of protease inhibitors will ameliorate to a large extent the negative effects of an unfavorable *IL28B* genotype, although final results from retrospective analyses and prospective clinical trials are still pending.

Patient selection for therapy

According to the National Institutes of Health Consensus Statement on Management of Hepatitis C, all patients are potential candidates for antiviral therapy [350]. In practice, various issues must be considered prior to embarking on treatment with pegIFN and ribavirin, specifically assessing the risks and benefits of treatment for an individual patient. There are few absolute contraindications to treatment with pegIFN and ribavirin. However, female patients who are pregnant, considering pregnancy within 6 months of completing a course of ribavirin, or unwilling to use adequate contraception (including female partners of male patients) should not be treated due to the teratogenic risk of ribavirin. Ribavirin-induced hemolytic anemia may also exacerbate symptomatic coronary artery disease. Poorly controlled psychiatric diseases, including recent suicide attempts, are also absolute contraindications to therapy due to the frequent neuropsychiatric side effects of pegIFN [296].

Numerous other relative contraindications or cautions are listed in the product inserts of pegIFN preparations, including the presence of autoimmune diseases that can be exacerbated by the immunomodulatory actions of pegIFN, hemoglobinopathies such as sickle cell anemia or major thalassemia that will be worsened by ribavirin, end-stage kidney disease in whom ribavirin clearance is diminished resulting in intractable anemia, and decompensated cirrhosis where treatment has been associated with fatal outcomes. Decisions about treating patients with any of these conditions, and others not listed here, must be carefully considered on an individual basis [296]. Furthermore, treatment decisions should also weigh other factors such as severity of liver disease, likelihood of treatment success, likelihood of tolerating treatment with pegIFN and ribavirin, and patient motivation.

Side effects of therapy

Clinicians must counsel patients about the natural history of hepatitis C, expected outcomes, and the potential side effects of treatment, all tailored to the specific clinical situation of the individual patient in order to arrive at an informed decision about treatment. Quality of life, in all its dimensions, is diminished during treatment with pegIFN and ribavirin as measured by standardized instruments such as SF-36, Health-Related Quality of Life Questionnaire, Hepatitis Quality of Life Questionnaire, and the Sexual Health, and Work Productivity and Impairment Index [619,620]. The side effects of pegIFN and ribavirin are well known and have been reviewed in detail in a number of publications [598]. Influenza-like symptoms (low-grade fever, myalgia, arthralgia) are most common during the first few weeks of combination antiviral therapy and can be managed successfully with analgesics and antipyretics. Insomnia, headache, and gastrointestinal symptoms of nausea, vomiting, and diarrhea are also common and may be symptomatically managed. Injection site reactions, usually mild, may occur with pegIFN preparations. Skin rash from ribavirin, manifested usually as a maculopapular eruption, occurs in less than 10% of patients and may be managed with topical or systemic antihistamines [621]. Continued treatment is warranted provided the skin manifestations are not progressive. Laboratory abnormalities (anemia and thrombocytopenia) are the most frequent indications for dose reduction (either temporary or permanent), which occurs in up to 25% of patients. In the registration trials of pegIFN-α-2a and pegIFN-α-2b, combined with ribavirin, 10–14% of patients prematurely discontinued therapy due to adverse events.

Hematologic abnormalities

Ribavirin-induced anemia has been discussed previously. PegIFN causes neutropenia and thrombocytopenia due to its suppressive effects on the bone marrow. Dose reductions of pegIFN are recommended in the product insert when neutrophil counts fall below 750 cells/cm^3. However, retrospective analysis in several studies has not identified an association between neutropenia and increased risk for infections. Thus, a more liberal dose reduction criterion (<500 absolute neutrophils x10^6/L) has been adopted prospectively in some studies without an increase in adverse events [622]. Therefore, the use of granulocyte colony-stimulating factors should be reserved only for the most severe neutropenia not responsive initially to dose reduction of pegIFN. The incidence of clinically significant thrombocytopenia is low and usually responds to dose reduction to maintain platelet counts above 50,000 × 10^6/L. Only 3% of patients discontinued treatment due to thrombocytopenia [598].

Interferon-associated depression

A high proportion of individuals with chronic hepatitis C have psychiatric co-morbidities, including substance abuse, that complicate antiviral therapy [623]. Up to 75% of patients referred for evaluation may be initially deferred from treatment due to these concurrent issues [624]. Prior to starting interferon-based therapy at a tertiary referral center, a remarkable 47% reported a past history of depression and 14% reported anxiety [625]. The frequency of preexisting psychiatric disease and the incidence of interferon-associated neuropsychiatric adverse events is variable and somewhat dependent on the method of ascertaining the diagnosis [626].

In registration trials of pegIFN and ribavirin, the most common reason for withdrawal of therapy was interferon-associated depression, which occured by self-report in 20–30% of patients [568,569,598]. In the VIRAHEP-C cohort, a study of African-American and Caucasian-American patients treated with pegIFN-α-2a and ribavirin, depression as defined by a screening instrument was present at baseline in 12% of patients [627]. These patients were more likely to have psychiatric adverse events, to begin antidepressants during treatment, or to have earlier treatment discontinuation, although their SVR rate was not significantly different from those without baseline depression. New-onset depression developed in 26% of patients, usually during the first 12 weeks of combination antiviral therapy. One third of patients started antidepressants during the course of the study. Interestingly, patients with new-onset depression were less likely to discontinue treatment (6% versus 15%) and had similar SVR rates compared with those who did not develop depression (47% versus 38%). There was no difference in the rates of depression before or during treatment between the African-American and the Caucasian-American participants [627].

Specific questions about depressive symptoms and past history of depression, treatment with antidepressants, suicide attempts, or psychiatric hospitalizations suggest significant psychiatric disease that may be a contraindication to interferon-based therapies. Those with poorly controlled mood disorders or who have had treatment-limiting depression during prior interferon treatment warrant evaluation by mental health professionals. Patients with stable depression, including those on pharmacologic therapy, with access to mental health providers may be treated with interferon-based therapies albeit with close monitoring for exacerbation.

Studies that have evaluated prophylactic selective serotonin reuptake inhibitor (SSRI) antidepressants have not demonstrated consistent benefit in decreasing the rate of major depression, although the severity of depressive symptoms during treatment has been reduced in those with elevated depressive symptoms at baseline [628]. Patients who experienced major depression during an earlier course of interferon have lower depression scores during retreatment when preemptively started on an SSRI [629]. Thus, selective use of pretreatment antidepressants appears warranted in those at highest risk for interferon-associated depression. In all others, symptom-directed management when depressive symptoms occur may be the best strategy. Depression first manifested during antiviral therapy can usually be managed with antidepressants, such as an SSRI, that have been shown to ameliorate symptoms and allow for completion of antiviral therapy [630]. Selecting the best agent for an individual patient should involve weighing the benefits against the potential for adverse events and drug–drug interactions [626]. Pharmacologic therapy, close monitoring, and regular follow-up with mental health providers will maximize the chances of successful antiviral treatment.

Uncommon side effects

Package inserts for both pegIFN preparations list numerous uncommon side effects that clinicians should be aware of and should consider in their differential diagnosis of symptoms during pegIFN and ribavirin therapy.

Thyroid dysfunction may develop in approximately 10% of patients treated with interferon-based regimens. Risk factors include female gender and the presence of pretreatment thyroid autoantibodies, although these are not measured routinely [631]. Patients should be monitored clinically and for changes in thyroid-stimulating hormone approximately every 12 weeks during therapy and during 6 months of post-treatment follow-up. Hypothyroidism can usually be managed with thyroid hormone replacement while continuing pegIFN and ribavirin. Mild hyperthyroidism may be managed symptomatically while still on therapy although progressive or severe hyperthyroidism may require discontinuation of antiviral therapy as well as thyroid ablative regimens. Thyroid abnormalities may spontaneously resolve in the majority of patients once pegIFN is discontinued.

Ocular abnormalities include cotton wool spots, retinal hemorrhage, and retinal vein thrombosis [632,633]. Patients with risk factors for diabetic or hypertensive retinopathy should undergo baseline fundoscopic examination as part of their routine medical follow-up. Cotton wool spots are frequently evanescent and rarely prompt discontinuation of therapy. Retinal hemorrhage has been reported in patients undergoing routine ophthalmologic examination with or without visual symptoms and may also resolve with continued treatment. Visual loss from retinal vein thrombosis and retinal detachment has also been reported and should prompt discontinuation of treatment. Patients with visual disturbances during pegIFN and ribavirin therapy require close ophthalmologic follow-up.

Interstitial pneumonitis is another extremely rare complication of interferon-based therapies with fewer than 100 reported cases in the literature [634]. However, interstitial pneumonitis may progress to respiratory failure and death and, thus, must be differentiated from other pulmonary processes such as bacterial/viral pneumonia, interferon-induced sarcoidosis, or the benign, dry cough that may be seen with ribavirin administration. Pneumonitis is usually characterized by fever, dyspnea, and characteristic findings on chest X-ray or high-resolution chest computed tomography. Prompt recognition and immediate discontinuation of pegIFN may prevent progression, although severe cases may require steroid therapy.

Treatment of hepatitis C virus in special populations

Cirrhosis and decompensated cirrhosis

Many patients present to medical attention for the first time with evidence of cirrhosis and portal hypertension due to the asymptomatic nature of hepatitis C infection. Patients with decompensated cirrhosis are not candidates for treatment with pegIFN and ribavirin due to the high rate of morbidity and mortality. However, patients with well-compensated cirrhosis may be treated with these agents although rates of SVR are somewhat lower than for earlier stages of liver disease [568,569,635]. Hepatic decompensation as a result of interferon-based therapy has been rarely reported so careful selection of treatment candidates and regular monitoring for adverse events and hepatic dysfunction is warranted. Patients with cirrhosis and portal hypertension may have lower levels of platelets and neutrophils at baseline, which further complicates the management of this population. Patients with cirrhosis who achieve a SVR have diminished complications of liver disease during long-term follow-up and may remain free of HCV infection after liver transplantation [635–638]. There is still a risk for hepatocellular carcinoma in the presence of cirrhosis so that appropriate surveillance is indicated despite the resolution of HCV infection [637].

African-Americans and Latinos

Racial disparity exists in the response to pegIFN and ribavirin for chronic hepatitis C [639,640]. The VIRAHEP-C study treated more than 400 African-American and Caucasian-American patients with pegIFN-α-2a and ribavirin at conventional doses [622]. SVR was 28% in African-American and 52% in Caucasian-American participants. As discussed above, a large proportion of the racial disparity can be attributed to the prevalence of the unfavorable *IL28B* genotype in African-Americans, although other factors as yet unidentified contribute to differences in therapeutic response. A study of Latino patients also demonstrated a diminished rate of SVR compared with non-Latino white patients: 34% versus 49%, respectively [641]. Reasons for ethnic disparities in this group remain speculative.

Coinfection with human immunodeficiency virus

Patients with chronic hepatitis C who are coinfected with HIV represent unique challenges for the management of hepatitis C. The natural history of hepatitis C with HIV coinfection appears to be truncated, with patients progressing more rapidly to cirrhosis compared with hepatitis C infection alone. As antiretroviral therapy has become more effective with more patients living with HIV infection, the incidence of HCC is one of the non-AIDS defining cancers that has increased in the last decade in the United States and is a leading cause of liver-related mortality among HIV/HCV coinfected patients in a report from France [642–644]. Furthermore, HIV patients with chronic hepatitis C may have a higher incidence of hepatotoxicity from antiretroviral therapy, which can complicate management of HIV infection [645]. Thus, HCV viral eradication is warranted in an attempt to prevent complications and improve outcomes in this population.

Drug–drug interactions, particularly with ribavirin, must be evaluated and HIV treatment regimens potentially altered to minimize the risk of added toxicities. The use of didanosine (DDI) is prohibited during HCV therapy due to the increased risk of mitochondrial toxicity and lactic acidosis. Increased anemia has been observed in patients treated with azidothymidine (AZT) and ribavirin [644]. Abacavir, another guanosine analog that may compete with ribavirin for intracellular phosphorylation, has been associated with diminished antiviral response to pegIFN and ribavirin, although another study has recently challenged this assertion [646,647]. A recent study suggested that laboratory evidence of mitochondrial toxicity, itself associated with higher dosage of ribavirin, was also associated with higher rates of SVR [648].

Patients with HIV infection under adequate control with CD4 counts above 200 are generally considered good candidates for HCV therapy provided they have no additional contraindications to pegIFN and ribavirin. Guidelines for monitoring treatment response utilizing a response-guided approach, importance of ribavirin exposure, and management of adverse events are similar to those for the HCV monoinfected population. Several studies have evaluated both pegIFN preparations combined with ribavirin for the treatment of HCV/HIV coinfected patients. Unfortunately, SVR rates are consistently lower in the HIV-positive population, ranging from 29% to 36% for genotype 1 disease and 55% to 60% for genotypes 2 and 3 [649]. Several studies have investigated *IL28B* genotype and treatment response in the coinfected population. Although the overall SVR rates are substantially lower, the relationship between favorable CC and unfavorable CT or TT genotypes is still evident in this group [650,651].

Early studies utilized lower doses of ribavirin due to concerns related to drug–drug interactions and adverse events [652–654]. A recent multicenter study randomized over 400 genotype 1 patients to pegIFN-α-2a and ribavirin at doses of either 800 mg/day (FDA-approved labeling) or conventional doses of 1,000–1,200 mg/day based on body weight [655]. SVR rates for both arms were similar and disappointing, 19% versus 22%, respectively. The suboptimal treatment responses to current therapies coupled with the unfavorable natural history among HCV/HIV coinfected populations underscores the critical need for more effective therapies. Triple therapy combinations with pegIFN, ribavirin, and protease inhibitors remain under investigation although no preliminary data are currently available in the HIV-positive population.

Hepatitis C in renal disease and dialysis

Testing for hepatitis C is routinely recommended for patients on hemodialysis. In the United States, approximately 15% of these patients have evidence of hepatitis C infection, although the prevalence varies around the world with prevalence rates of 2.6% and 22.9% reported in the United Kingdom and Spain, respectively [296]. While most patients on hemodialysis have independent risk factors for HCV infection, such as blood transfusion or intravenous drug use, a measurable rate of de novo acquired hepatitis C has been reported and can be traced to a breakdown of universal precautions during the dialysis procedure [296,656,657]. The hemodialysis machine and dialysis membranes themselves are not considered sources of HCV infection and patients do not need to be dialyzed on dedicated machines.

Higher mortality rates have been reported in dialysis patients with hepatitis C infection compared with noninfected patients. Similarly, studies of patients who underwent kidney transplantation indicate that survival for HCV-positive recipients and their grafts diverge from observed outcomes in the HCV-negative transplant population during long-term follow-up [658,659].

Treatment for hepatitis C in patients with chronic kidney disease is associated with generally lower response rates and higher rates of adverse events [660,661]. Treatment must be modified according to the severity of renal impairment. For patients with intact glomerular filtration rate, treatment with pegIFN and ribavirin can be managed according to published guidelines. Standard interferon or pegIFN at reduced doses (pegIFN-α-2a 135 μg/week and pegIFN-α-2b 1.0 μg/kg/week) can be administered to patients on hemodialysis. Interestingly, SVR rates utilizing interferon-based monotherapy are higher in those on dialysis (SVR $\sim$30%) than historically reported from other populations treated with interferon alone [296,661]. Extreme caution is required with the use of ribavirin in the setting of hemodialysis since this medication is not dialyzed and hemolytic anemia will worsen. Ribavirin is contraindicated when the glomerular filtration rate falls below 50 cm^3/min although several small studies have utilized low-dose weekly dosing, or dosing titrated to blood ribavirin levels in an attempt to improve SVR and minimize adverse events [661].

Treatment of chronic hepatitis C in patients following kidney transplantation has not been routinely recommended due to concerns of renal graft dysfunction and rejection, which has been reported in the majority of participants in small clinical trials of interferon-based treatment [662]. The notable exception are those patients who develop fibrosing cholestatic hepatitis, a rapidly progressive, frequently fatal, liver injury reported in several types of solid organ transplantation [663]. Interferon-based therapy may improve liver injury due to fibrosing cholestatic hepatitis even in the absence of SVR [296,664].

Cryoglobulinemia and glomerulonephritis

The pathogenesis of cryoglobulinemia has been discussed above. The clinical manifestations of cryoglobulinemia associated with hepatitis C infection are quite variable but may include purpuric skin rash due to a leukocytoclastic vasculitis usually on the lower extremities, glomerulonephritis with potential to progress to chronic kidney disease, and peripheral neuropathy [665,666]. In a large study from Italy nearly 50% of 343 consecutively evaluated patients with chronic hepatitis C had measurable cryoglobulins [667]. However, few had cryoglobulinemic syndromes or signs of vasculitis. The presence of cryoglobulins in this large prospective cohort did not impact upon the development of cirrhosis, overall survival, or the response to interferon-based treatments.

Treatment with pegIFN and ribavirin can be considered for patients with hepatitis C and mild manifestations of cryoglobulinemia. When patients have progressive vasculitis and organ damage, therapy is focused on gaining immediate control of the vasculitis utilizing therapies such as corticosteroids, plasma exchange, cyclophosphamide, or rituximab, which has been shown to exert its effect through the suppression of cryoglobulin-producing B cells [666]. Once stable, definitive treatment with pegIFN and ribavirin can be considered.

Membranoproliferative glomerulonephritis, usually in association with cryoglobulinemia, is the most common form of kidney disease associated with hepatitis C [657]. Treatment with interferon and ribavirin resulting in SVR has been associated with improvement in proteinuria and kidney function.

Acute hepatitis C

Clinicians rarely identify acute hepatitis C since the majority of infections are asymptomatic. Approximately 50% of patients with acute hepatitis C will spontaneously resolve the acute infection without treatment [668,669]. Thus, patients should be followed initially with serial quantitative HCV RNA determinations to determine whether spontaneous resolution may occur. Within the first 12 weeks of presentation, persistently high levels of viremia with failure to demonstrate log-folds of decline in viremia as a prelude to undetectable HCV RNA suggests that spontaneous resolution is unlikely and treatment should be instituted, if possible. Delaying therapy beyond 12–16 weeks appears to be associated with diminished treatment response approaching the expected rates of SVR for chronic HCV.

Numerous studies have evaluated a variety of treatment regimens for acute hepatitis C utilizing either standard interferon or pegIFN monotherapy for treatment durations ranging between 4 and 24 weeks [668,670–672]. Impressive therapeutic responses for patients treated in the acute phase of HCV infection are seen with rates of SVR usually greater than 80%. These results are significantly higher than historical studies of chronic HCV infection, emphasizing the importance of early diagnosis and treatment of acute HCV once spontaneous clearance is excluded. The best treatment regimen remains controversial, although treatment for between 12 and 24 weeks of treatment is likely the optimal duration as currently recommended. One study evaluated 8, 12, or 24 weeks of treatment with pegIFN-α-2b and attained a SVR in 68%, 82%, and 91% of patients, respectively [673]. Genotypes 2, 3, and 4, and those with a rapid virologic response did well with shorter duration of therapy, while genotype 1 patients did best with 24 weeks of treatment in the acute setting. Thus, consideration can be given to individualizing therapy based upon virologic response, however this must be weighed against the risk of relapse for an individual patient. Combination therapy with ribavirin has been used to treat acute HCV [674]. SVR rates have also been uniformly excellent, although the contribution of ribavirin compared with pegIFN monotherapy cannot be ascertained from the currently available data.

Treatment-experienced patients

The decision to embark on a repeated course of therapy must be individualized for each patient by considering the potential benefits when options are limited and the chances for success are quite low [543,675]. The likelihood of SVR during a second course of treatment with pegIFN and ribavirin is associated with the prior response achieved during their first course of combination therapy. Prior null and partial responders are least likely to benefit from another course of treatment with pegIFN and ribavirin, with SVR rates rarely surpassing 15% [676]. Success rates may be even lower when there are multiple unfavorable treatment factors. Previous pegIFN/ribavirin nonresponders with a constellation of unfavorable treatment characteristics, such as advanced fibrosis and high viral load, had only a modest response when treated with consensus interferon. The SVR rate was 7% and 11% when patients were treated with either 9 or 15 µg of consensus interferon daily, respectively, combined with ribavirin [677]. SVR rates were higher (32%) if patients had demonstrated at least a 2-log decrease in viremia during their previous course of pegIFN/ribavirin.

Prior relapsers have a better chance of achieving SVR during a second course of treatment. Poynard and colleagues [678] retreated over 2,300 prior nonresponders and relapsers (all with advanced fibrosis) with pegIFN-α-2b and ribavirin (800–1,400 mg/day) for 48 weeks. The SVR rate was 38% among prior relapsers but only 14% among prior nonresponders. This marked difference in success rates between relapsers and nonresponders further emphasizes the importance of accurately characterizing prior treatment response. Genotype non-1, HCV RNA <600,00 IU/mL, and lower fibrosis stage were associated with improved treatment response. Patients who failed to clear HCV RNA by week 12 of retreatment had no chance of SVR, suggesting that a short trial of retreatment incorporating firm stopping rules could minimize futile therapy.

Modifying a treatment course to improve response

Intensifying treatment regimens with higher doses of pegIFN, higher doses of ribavirin, or extended duration of therapy in these patients has met with only limited success. Extending therapy to 72 weeks has been shown to decrease relapse rates among genotype 1 slow virologic responders. A four-arm study compared 12 weeks of

higher dose induction of pegIFN with standard doses in combination with ribavirin for either 48 or 72 weeks [679]. Similar rates of SVR were attained in the induction dose (16%) or standard dose group (14%) treated for 72 weeks. These were higher than the 48-week treatment regimens, suggesting that the duration of therapy rather than the induction dose of pegIFN was of greater importance in prior treatment failures.

Role of maintenance therapy

Prolonged treatment with pegIFN alone has been investigated in an attempt to decrease adverse clinical outcomes among patients with advanced fibrosis. The HALT-C study treated a large cohort of these patients with a low dose of pegIFN-α-2a for 3.5 years to determine if maintenance therapy, without viral eradication, would decrease the rates of fibrosis progression, hepatic decompensation, and HCC [680]. In a rigorously controlled trial, there were no differences in the rates of these events between the treated group and an observational control group. A preliminary report from this study suggested that the incidence of HCC was decreased in the treated population, which only became evident after year 6 of follow-up [681]. The CO-PILOT study treated 555 patients with advanced fibrosis with low-dose pegIFN-α-2b or colchicine for up to 4 years. In both intention-to-treat (ITT) and per-protocol analyses, the rates of clinical end-points (death, liver transplant, HCC, or worsening Child–Pugh score) were similar between the two groups [682]. In a subset of patients with portal hypertension, those treated with maintenance pegIFN had a lower incidence of variceal hemorrhage. Nearly 50% of patients discontinued treatment prematurely during the study. At this point, maintenance therapy cannot be endorsed for prior nonresponders to therapy.

For all of these strategies that utilize intensified/modified treatment regimens, one must consider the costs and side effects against the marginal benefit gained by treatment-experienced patients. Furthermore, new direct-acting antiviral agents, in triple combination therapy with pegIFN and ribavirin, will provide many patients with additional therapeutic options and a greater chance of success.

Direct-acting antiviral agents

The treatment of chronic hepatitis C will be transformed with the availability of direct-acting antiviral agents that specifically target critical enzymes in the replication of HCV. As described above, several HCV proteins possess well-defined enzymatic activities, including NS2 (a *cis*-acting protease), NS3/4A (serine protease-helicase), NS4B (GTPase), and NS5B (RNA-dependent RNA polymerase) that serve as targets for HCV therapy (Fig. 25.15).

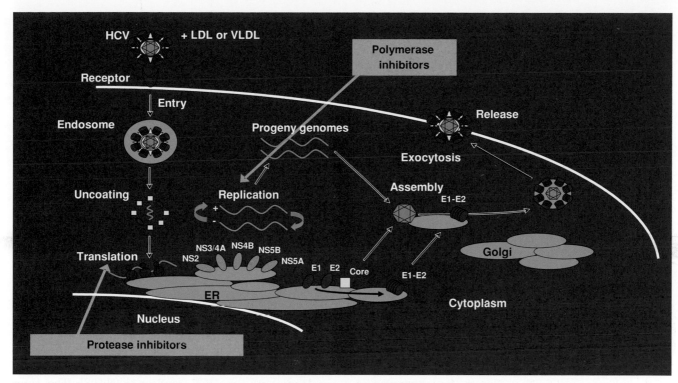

Figure 25.15 Targets for small molecule antiviral therapy. (Reproduced from Racanelli and Rehermann [732] with permission from Elsevier.)

The NS3/4A protease and NS5B polymerase have proven to be particularly promising targets for developing antiviral drugs against HCV. Inhibition of NS3/4A protease activity, because of its essential role in polyprotein processing, ablates virus replication. Inhibitors of the NS5B polymerase also block replication of the virus by preventing synthesis of the viral RNA. In a departure from prior antiviral drug discovery efforts, however, recent work has proven that HCV proteins that lack defined enzymatic activity (e.g., NS5A) also may be exceptionally good targets for antiviral drug development.

A major generic issue with the use of most small molecule antivirals against HCV is the relatively rapid selection of drug-resistant virus. This is fueled in part by the error-prone nature of HCV RNA replication, coupled with high-level replication of the virus in the typical infected individual [683]. In clinical practice, this will be countered by the use of these novel therapeutics as a component of combination therapy, at first together with pegIFN/ribavirin and eventually all-small-molecule combinations.

NS3/4A protease inhibitors

The NS3/4A protease plays a central role in processing the HCV polyprotein, and is distinct structurally from cel-

lular proteases. Early studies demonstrated that the protease is subject to inhibition by short peptide sequences representing the carboxy terminal NS3 sequence [684]. Although the substrate-binding cleft is otherwise unusually broad and shallow for a viral protease, it has been possible to design peptidomimetic compounds with substantial inhibitory activity. Such compounds fall into two general classes: linear peptidomimetics (e.g., telaprevir and boceprevir) and macrocyclic compounds (e.g., ciluprevir (BILN2061), danoprevir (ITMN-191), and TMC434350). While protease inhibitors also block HCV-induced MAVS and TRIF cleavage, there are no data suggesting that the resulting rescue of endogenous IFN responses contributes to their antiviral effect in infected persons. As with many small molecule antivirals, protease inhibitors present a relatively low barrier to resistance, with resistant virus emerging rapidly in many patients placed on monotherapy with these compounds [685,686].

NS5B polymerase inhibitors

A large number of small molecule inhibitors of the NS5B polymerase have been identified. These fall into two general types: nucleoside analogs that bind into the active site, and non-nucleoside inhibitors (NNIs) derived from a variety of chemical backbones including benzimidazoles, benzothiadiazines, and thiophene 2-carboxylic acids [687–689]. Nucleoside analogs typically demonstrate potent inhibition of polymerase activity; they undergo phosphorylation within the cell and generally act by competing with other nucleotide triphosphates as well as by chain termination of nascent RNA strands. Available evidence suggests that the nucleoside analogs provide a high barrier to resistance, as mutations within the active site that confer resistance to these inhibitors typically result in virus with very low replication fitness [690]. Non-nucleoside polymerase inhibitors appear to inhibit only the initiation of RNA synthesis, not elongation [691]. NNIs are typically less potent than the nucleoside analogs, and present a much lower barrier to resistance with treatment leading to relatively rapid selection of resistant virus mutants with good replication fitness.

Nonenzymatic polyprotein targets

Potent inhibitors of HCV replication directed against NS5A, a nonstructural protein with no known enzymatic function, have been identified in high-throughput, cell-based screens for chemical compounds that inhibit HCV replicon amplification. Exactly how these NS5A inhibitors function is not known, but they may be interacting with dimeric NS5A and possibly blocking its ability to participate in replicase assembly or function. Consistent with the in vitro potency observed with these compounds, a single dose of BMS-790052 produced a 3.6 $\log_{10}$ decline in plasma virus load [692]. Recent clinical data suggest that these compounds, like the protease inhibitors and allosteric inhibitors of NS5B, may present a relatively low barrier to resistance, especially for genotype 1 virus. Other nonenzymatic targets exist for the development of antiviral agents, including the interaction of miR-122 with the 5' UTR of the HCV genomic RNA [693] and an interaction of NS4B with viral RNA [694].

Protease inhibitors

The landmark study of BILN-2061, a macrocyclic NS3 protease inhibitor, was published in 2003 and demonstrated dramatic viral inhibition of HCV RNA in patients with genotype 1. After only 48 hours of treatment with a twice-daily oral solution of BILN-2061, most patients had HCV RNA levels below the limit of quantitation, corresponding to a decrease of approximately 3-logs of HCV RNA [695]. Viremia gradually returned to pretreatment levels within 1 week of cessation of therapy. Subsequent short-term studies in more patients confirmed these impressive virologic responses [696]. However, optimism for this compound was arrested when animal toxicology studies demonstrated cardiac toxicity over a 4-week dos-

ing period, which led to permanent discontinuation of the development of BILN-2061. Nevertheless, proof of concept had been established that an NS3 protease inhibitor could be a potent treatment for chronic hepatitis C. This discovery led to an intensive period of drug development, continuing today, of multiple classes of drugs targeting different aspects of HCV replication. Dozens of direct-acting antiviral agents have been synthesized and are being tested in human studies with varying degrees of success; some agents are proceeding along the pathway toward approval and clinical use while many others have failed due to efficacy or safety issues.

Telaprevir and boceprevir, also protease inhibitors, have successfully completed phase III clinical trials and are expected to be approved by the US FDA in 2011. The development of these agents has provided important insights into the promises and perils of direct-acting antiviral therapy and has provided a roadmap for exciting new therapies.

Telaprevir in treatment-naïve patients

Telaprevir is a selective, covalent NS3/NS4 protease inhibitor active against the protease of genotypes 1–4 in studies of the HCV replicon [697,698]. The short half-life of telaprevir, approximately 4–5 hours, necessitates frequent dosing and current studies have utilized telaprevir 750 mg administered every 8 hours, although higher doses administered every 12 hours are under investigation.

A phase Ib study treated patients with three different regimens of telaprevir monotherapy or placebo for a total of only 14 days [699]. Remarkably, all patients treated with telaprevir 750 mg administered every 8 hours achieved at least a 3-log reduction in HCV RNA with a median maximal decrease of –4.77 $\log_{10}$ from baseline. This dose appeared to be optimal for subsequent phase II and phase III studies. However, this study also confirmed that telaprevir monotherapy was not viable for the treatment of chronic hepatitis since virologic breakthrough and viral variants with reduced sensitivity to telaprevir were identified in patients [700].

Studies of utilizing replicons demonstrated that NS3 variants expected with telaprevir remained sensitive to interferon, and clinical studies, fortunately, confirmed that the combination of telaprevir with pegIFN and ribavirin mitigated the impact of viral resistance [701–703]. Kieffer and colleagues [702] performed a detailed analysis of viral resistance and the impact of pegIFN on subsequent virologic response. Patients who developed virologic rebound during telaprevir monotherapy had multiple resistant variants at the end of a 14-day course of treatment. When these patients were then treated only with pegIFN and ribavirin, HCV RNA became

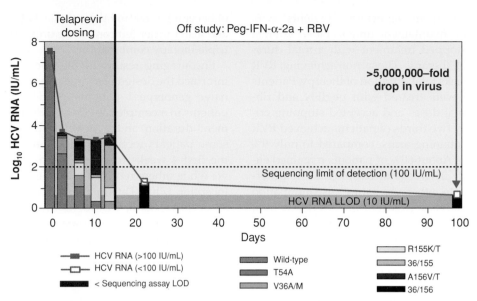

Figure 25.16 Resistance virus is selected with telaprevir alone but declines with pegylated interferon-α-2a (pegIFN-α-2a) and ribavirin (RBV). HCV, hepatitis C virus; LLOD, lower limit of detection; LOD, limit of detection. (Reproduced from Kieffer et al [702] with permission from Plenum.)

undetectable (Fig. 25.16). A separate small cohort of patients who were initially treated with telaprevir and pegIFN demonstrated a more consistent decline in HCV RNA with only rare resistant mutations detected during the initial 14 days of treatment. Furthermore, subsequent therapy with only pegIFN and ribavirin maintained patients with undetectable viremia [702]. This important study provided the rationale for triple combination therapy as a way to prevent the selection of telaprevir resistant variants. A detailed discussion of viral variant-associated protease inhibitors will be provided below.

The encouraging results from phase I studies provided impetus for a series of phase II trials that incrementally contributed to our understanding of the clinical utility of telaprevir. In a study designated PROVE1, noncirrhotic genotype 1 patients were randomized to 12 weeks of treatment with telaprevir 850 mg every 8 hours + pegIFN and ribavirin [704]. Two arms of the study extended treatment with pegIFN and ribavirin only for an additional 12 weeks (24 weeks total treatment) or for 36 weeks (48 weeks total treatment). In order to qualify for a shorter duration of therapy, patients were required to have a RVR (undetectable HCV RNA at week 4). RVR was achieved in 81% of patients in both arms and SVR rates were 61% and 67%, respectively. A small number of patients in an exploratory regimen were treated with triple therapy for only 12 weeks without any additional pegIFN/ribavirin and achieved an SVR of 35%, while in the pegIFN and ribavirin control group, the rate of SVR was 41%. Virologic breakthrough was seen in 7% of patients treated with telaprevir. Adverse events were more frequent in the

telaprevir-containing arms and the most common reason for treatment discontinuation was skin rash (7%). Thus, triple therapy for 12 weeks followed by pegIFN and ribavirin significantly improved the rate of SVR over pegIFN and ribavirin alone. Total treatment duration of 48 weeks did not appear to increase SVR compared with the 24-week telaprevir regimen [704].

PROVE2 sought to investigate whether ribavirin contributed to SVR in the presence of telaprevir and also to further investigate the feasibility of shortening the duration of therapy in a population of European patients with genotype 1 [705]. The study design included two arms treated for only 12 weeks with either triple therapy or pegIFN and telaprevir (no ribavirin). SVR in these arms was 60% and 36% and, importantly, demonstrated that the absence of ribavirin impaired antiviral response by permitting more virologic breakthrough and relapse [705]. The study also confirmed that SVR for a complete course of only 12 weeks of triple therapy (60%) was, again, numerically, inferior to 12 weeks of triple therapy plus 12 weeks of pegIFN and ribavirin (69%), although the SVR rate was higher than that seen in PROVE1 for the same treatment regimen (60% versus 35%, respectively).

The foregoing studies informed the plans for phase III trials that have recently been reported [706]. The study design for ADVANCE is shown below. Patients ($n = 1,088$) were randomized to therapy with telaprevir plus pegIFN-α-2a 180 μg/week and ribavirin 1,000–1,200 mg/day for either 8 weeks or 12 weeks, both of which were followed with pegIFN and ribavirin only for an additional 12 weeks. Using a response-guided treatment algorithm, patients who achieved RVR and maintained undetectable viremia through week 12 stopped treatment with a total duration of 24 weeks of therapy. Those not achieving RVR received up to 48 weeks total duration of therapy. Patients in the control arm were treated with pegIFN and ribavirin at conventional doses and accepted stopping criteria. Approximately two thirds of patients achieved RVR in the telaprevir-containing arms, compared to only 9% in the control group. About 60% of patients remained eligible to receive only 24 weeks of treatment. The difference was attributed to either premature discontinuation of telaprevir due to adverse events or the development of virogical breakthrough. SVR rates in the 12-week and 8-week triple therapy arms were 75% and 69%, respectively, both significantly greater than the control arm of 44%. Of note, the virologic failure rate was lower in the 12-week triple therapy arm compared with the 8-week regimen (5% versus 10%, respectively) [706].

ILLUMINATE was another phase III trial with a noninferiority design to compare a 24-week regimen to a 48-week regimen in patients with a RVR [707]. All patients received an initial 12 weeks of triple therapy with telaprevir. Those who achieved undetectable viremia at weeks 4 and 12 were randomized to either an additional 12 weeks or 36 weeks of dual combination therapy with pegIFN and ribavirin. Approximately 60% of patients were eligible for randomization having achieved and maintained RVR during the first 12 weeks of triple therapy treatment. Among these RVR patients, 92% treated for only 24 weeks achieved a SVR compared with 88% of those treated for 48 weeks. The difference in response indicated that 24 weeks was noninferior to 48 weeks of treatment [707].

Boceprevir

Boceprevir is another peptiometic, ketoamide NS3 protease inhibitor that has demonstrated potent efficacy in patients with genotype 1 infection. A phase Ib study in prior interferon nonresponders assigned noncirrhotic patients to treatment sequentially with boceprevir monotherapy for 7 days, followed by pegIFN-α-2b for 14 days, and then boceprevir combination therapy for 14 days [708]. The sequence of treatment was altered and two different doses of boceprevir (200 or 400 mg three times daily) were used, yielding a six-arm study design. The study demonstrated that the mean maximal decrease in HCV RNA in the higher boceprevir monotherapy dosing group was $-1.61\log_{10}$ after 1 week while the combination of boceprevir and pegIFN yielded a greater mean maximal change of $-2.48\log_{10}$ during the same period. The combination treatment was well tolerated with few serious adverse events [708]. A subsequent phase II study in a difficult-to-treat null responder population, defined as failure to achieve an EVR, suggested that a higher dose

of boceprevir (800 mg three times daily) would be optimal and also further reinforced the importance of ribavirin in triple therapy combinations [709].

Encouraging results in the nonresponder population informed the design of a large phase II study in treatment-naïve genotype 1 patients. SPRINT-1 randomized 595 patients in a complex seven-arm design to evaluate treatment duration and a novel lead-in strategy, whereby some patients received pegIFN and ribavirin alone for the first 4 weeks followed by the addition of boceprevir while others received all three drugs from treatment inception [710]. Thus, patients received a total of either 28 or 48 weeks of treatment. The results indicated that all four boceprevir-containing regimens had significantly better rates of SVR (ranging between 54% and 75%) compared to the pegIFN and ribavirin control arm (38%). RVR rates for those treated with boceprevir during the initial 4 weeks of treatment were also higher. Overall, attainment of RVR was associated with the best rates of SVR, ranging between 74% and 94%. Furthermore, relapse rates were lowest in the patients treated for 48 weeks with boceprevir (3–11%), either with or without the pegIFN/ribavirin lead-in phase, compared with shorter duration of therapy (24–30%) [710].

The inclusion of a lead-in phase in this study also demonstrated that the lowest rates of virologic breakthrough (4%) occurred in patients who received pegIFN and ribavirin alone, before initiation of boceprevir, compared with those receiving triple therapy with treatment initiaition (9%) [710]. Population sequencing confirmed the presence of viral mutants resistant to boceprevir. A viral kinetic analysis evaluating the likelihood of SVR with the change in HCV RNA during the first 4 weeks of the lead-in phase suggested that patients who had an initial decline of HCV RNA of at least $1.5\log_{10}$ had comparable rates of SVR with the 28-week regimen (SVR = 73%) or the 48-week regimen (SVR = 80%).

This study also included one treatment arm using a lower dose of ribavirin to determine if the addition of boceprevir could allow for ribavirin-sparing regimens. For all efficacy parameters, lower dose ribavirin was suboptimal with lower rates of SVR, and higher rates of relapse and virologic breakthrough confirming the ongoing importance of adequate ribavirin dosing even with triple therapy combinations.

The phase III study of boceprevir, SPRINT-2, was recently presented [711]. Two cohorts of patients, non-black ($n = 938$) and black ($n = 159$), were prospectively included and analyzed separately. Patients were randomized to treatment with pegIFN-α-2b 1.5 μg/kg/week and ribavirin 800–1,400 mg/day as a lead-in during the first 4 weeks of treatment. Boceprevir 800 mg t.i.d. was added after 4 weeks and patients were treated for another 44 weeks with triple therapy (fixed duration of 48 weeks) or for a total of 28 weeks utilizing a response-guided algorithm, whereby patients were required to achieve RVR and maintain undetectable viremia through week 20. Approximately 47% of patients were eligible for the shorter treatment duration based upon the favorable viral knetic response. SVR rates in both the fixed duration and the response-guided algorithm boceprevir arms among non-black patients were significantly better than the pegIFN and ribavirin control arm: 68% and 67% versus 40%, respectively. Similarly, although SVR rates were substantially lower for black participants, the same benefit of boceprevir was evident with SVR rates of 53% for the fixed duration and 42% for the response-guided algorithm arms, compared with 23% in the control group. Resistance-associated variants were developed most commonly among patients with the least decrease in HCV RNA ($<1 \log_{10}$) during the 4-week lead-in phase [711].

In aggregate, these series of phase II and phase III studies demonstrated several important points related to protease inhibitor therapy with telaprevir and boceprevir:

1 Teleprevir and boceprevir are potent protease inhibitors that must be used in combination with pegIFN and ribavirin to minimize viral resistance.
2 Ribavirin remains a critical component of triple therapy combination in order to further diminish viral resistance and prevent relapse.
3 Triple therapy combination with protease inhibitors significantly improves rates of SVR compared with combination therapy with pegIFN and ribavirin alone.
4 The recommended treatment algorithms differ between telaprevir and boceprevir. Telaprevir treatment should incorporate triple therapy beginning with treatment inception while boceprevir regimens should utilize a 4-week lead-in with pegIFN and ribavirin alone before adding boceprevir. Both regimens should incorporate response-guided algorithms to determine the duration of therapy and to guide when protease inhibitors and/or all drugs should be discontinued in order to minimize viral resistance and exposure of patients to futile therapy.
5 The rate of RVR is substantially increased with triple therapy and many patients will be eligible for a shortened treatment regimen of 24–28 weeks total duration based on a response-guided treatment algorithm.

Adverse events of telaprevir and boceprevir

The majority of adverse events associated with triple therapy combinations can be ascribed to the well-known side effects of pegIFN and ribavirin. Nevertheless, some adverse events are accentuated with the addition of a protease inhibitor and new treatment emergent events, unique to this class, have also been described. In the phase III telaprevir studies, the rate of treatment discon-

tinuation with all study medications during the period of triple therapy treatment was low and ranged between 7% and 8% compared to 4% in the control arm [706,707]. In the ILLUMINATE study intention-to-treat population, 17% of patients ultimately discontinued all study drugs due to adverse events during the entire duration of the study. Up to 12% of patients discontinued only telaprevir for any adverse event, most frequently skin rash (7%) of patients treated with telaprevir for 12 weeks [707]. The skin rash was predominantly eczematous and resolved when telaprevir therapy was discontinued, as recommended for moderate or severe progressive skin rash. Mild to moderate rash was managed with topical agents and/or oral antihistamines. Pruritus, in the absence of rash, and gastrointestinal disturbance were also more frequent with telaprevir.

Anemia was also more common in regimens including telaprevir, inducing an additional 1 g/dL decline of hemoglobin in excess of that with pegIFN and ribavirin alone. In the ADVANCE study, up to 40% of patients treated with telaprevir had hemoglobin <10 g/dL compared to 14% in the control arm. Anemia was managed with ribavirin dose reduction and hematopoietic growth agents were prohibited [706].

In the boceprevir SPRINT-2 study, treatment discontinuations due to adverse events were similar in the fixed duration boceprevir regimens and the control group (16% in each), while slightly lower in the response guided algorithm arm (12%) [711]. Treatment with boceprevir was associated with increased anemia; 49% of patients developed anemia during boceprevir treatment compared with only 29% in the control arm. Erythropoietic-stimulating agents were allowed to be prescribed in this study and over 40% of patients received epoetin-α for anemia management during boceprevir treatment, compared with 23% of controls. Dysgeusia, abnormal taste, was also more frequent with boceprevir therapy.

Triple therapy in treatment-experienced patients

Treatment-experienced patients with genotype 1 who do not achieve a sustained virologic response to pegIFN and ribavirin will benefit from the availability of direct-acting antiviral agents [543].

Telaprevir for treatment-experienced patients: phase II results

PROVE3 treated both nonresponders (~60%) and relapsers (~40%) with telaprevir [712]. The study evaluated the impact of different durations of triple therapy, different total treatment duration, and the importance of ribavirin. In an effort to minimize the development of viral resistance, treatment was discontinued if HCV RNA remained detectable at week 4. Among prior relapsers, SVR was achieved in 76% of those treated for a total duration of 48 weeks (24 weeks of telaprevir triple therapy followed by 24 weeks of dual pegIFN and ribavirin). The SVR rate in patients treated with only 24 weeks' total duration (12 weeks of triple therapy and an additional 12 weeks of dual combination therapy) was 69%. Prior nonresponders had substantially lower rates of SVR, although nearly 40% achieved SVR with these regimens [712]. Interestingly, when telaprevir and pegIFN were used without ribavirin, the rate of SVR was substantially diminished, emphasizing the importance of ribavirin in triple therapy combinations. The risk of virologic breakthrough, defined as an increase of HCV RNA of more than 1 log from baseline or to more than 100 IU/mL if previously undetectable, was more frequent in previous nonresponders than previous relapsers. By week 24 of treatment, up to 13% of prior relapsers and 45% of prior nonresponders had evidence of virologic breakthrough [543,712].

Telaprevir for treatment-experienced patients: phase III results

The study design of the phase III REALIZE trial, reported only in preliminary form [713], included triple therapy with pegIFN, ribavirin, and telaprevir for 12 weeks begun simultaneously or with a prior lead-in of pegIFN and ribavirin, followed by pegIFN and ribavirin for a total of 48 weeks. In previous relapsers, the SVR rate was 86% in the combined telaprevir arms and 57% in partial responders. The SVR rate in previous null responders was only 31%, confirming the differential response based upon prior experience with dual combination therapy. Only 24% of prior relapsers, 15% of prior partial responders, and 5% of prior null responders achieved SVR when retreated with pegIFN and ribavirin.

Boceprevir for treatment-experienced patients

RESPOND-2 is a phase III trial reported only in preliminary form that included nonresponders and relapsers treated with boceprevir [714]. The three-arm study, in which null responders were excluded, compared a response-guided regimen including boceprevir with a fixed duration 48-week triple regimen versus 48 weeks of pegIFN and ribavirin. Top-line results indicate that 75% of prior relapsers and 52% of prior nonresponders treated with a fixed triple therapy boceprevir regimen achieved SVR. Relapsers and nonresponders in the response-guided treatment arm also had substantial SVR rates of 69% and 40%, respectively [714].

Protease inhibitor resistance

As these small molecule inhibitors of the NS3/4A protease are likely to be licensed for clinical use in the near future, it is appropriate to focus on the special issues posed by the emergence of resistance to these drugs. The

highly replicative nature of HCV infection coupled with the error-prone nature of viral RNA synthesis sets the stage for a rapid emergence of resistance to almost any small molecule inhibitor used as monotherapy. As many as 1×10^{12} virus particles are produced each day in a typical, chronically infected individual [715]. The NS5B RNA-dependent RNA polymerase lacks a proof-reading mechanism, and the base misincorporation rate is as high as 10^{-3} to 10^{-4} per nucleotide. Since the genome is only $\sim 10^4$ nucleotides in length, each of the 10^{12} newly synthesized copies of the RNA genome produced each day in the typical patient is likely to contain one or more base substitutions. While many, perhaps most, of these base substitutions are detrimental to viral fitness, others may allow for escape from a particular virus-neutralizing antibody, cytotoxic T-cell clone, or small molecule therapeutic.

All possible single, most double, and many triple nucleotide substitutions are likely to be present in the viral quasispecies prior to the initiation of protease inhibitor therapy [716]. In one study that examined treatment-naïve patients for preexisting resistance mutations, 44.4% of genotype 1b patients had at least one identifiable mutation at sites associated with resistance to one of 27 small molecule antivirals targeting NS3 or NS5B (i.e., protease inhibitors, nucleosides, and non-nucleoside polymerase inhibitors) and 2.7% had mutations in both NS3 and NS5B [268]. A greater frequency of preexisting mutations would undoubtedly be found with more extensive sequencing. Most resistant mutants are present at relatively low frequencies in pretreatment quasispecies, because they are less fit and do not replicate as efficiently as the wild type, but they rapidly become dominant when replication of wild-type virus is suppressed with an antiviral. The emergence of resistance is thus due most often to selection of preexisting variants and not de novo mutations in the virus.

Two general structural classes of HCV protease inhibitors have been developed thus far. Boceprevir and teleprevir are both linear peptidomimetic ketoamides [717,718]. Several other inhibitors now in phase I/II development (i.e., ITMN191, TMC435, and MK7009) [719–721] and are macrocyclic compounds. A variety of amino acid substitutions near the NS3 protease active site can result in resistance to both classes of inhibitors, with the specific responsible mutations dependent on the chemical class and compound (Fig. 25.17). In general, mutations involving Val36 and Thr54 are associated with resistance against the linear ketoamides, while mutations at Asp168 cause resistance to the macrocyclics. However, there is a great deal of overlap, and mutations at Arg155 and Ala156 typically cause high-level cross-resistance to drugs in both groups (Fig. 25.17). Clinical experience in dealing with these mutant viruses is limited. Some may still respond

NS3 residue	Linear peptidomimetic		Macrocyclic			
	VX-950 Telaprevir	SCH503034 Boceprevir	ITMN191 Danoprevir	TMC435	BILN2061 Clluprevir	MK7009 Vaniprevir
V36	A,G,L,M	A,L,M				
Q41		R	R	R		
F43		C,S	S	I,S,V		
T54	A,S	A				
V55		A				
Q80				H,K,R	R	
R109				K		
S138			T			
R155	G,I,K,M,S,T	K,M,Q,T		K	Q	E,G,K,M,N,Q,S,T
A156	I,S,T,V	S,T,V	S,T,V	G,T,V	T,V	T,V
D168			A,E,G,H,N,V	A,E,H,I,N,T,V,Y	A,V	E,G,V,Y
V170		A,T				
S489			R			

Figure 25.17 Resistance profiles of protease inhibitors.

to continued inhibitor therapy to some extent, while others may not. Most will be replaced over time by wild-type virus when the drug is discontinued, but how long this will take and how complete this replacement will be is uncertain. Also uncertain is the extent to which prior emergence of resistance to one protease inhibitor will render a patient not likely to benefit from treatment with another – i.e., class resistance.

Many of the mutations have a significant negative impact on viral fitness (replication capacity), both in cell culture and in infected humans. For example, a common resistance mutation (A156T) lowers the capacity of RNA replicons to undergo autonomous amplification in cell culture [722,723]. However, replicons containing drug-resistance mutations are not universally impaired in their ability to replicate as RNA, as those with V36A, Q41R, T54A, A156S, or I170A mutations appear to replicate at least as well as wild-type virus [724–728]. A subset of mutations has also been shown to impair the assembly of infectious viral particles [729].

In general, the first protease inhibitors to be licensed will be restricted in their activity to genotype 1 viruses due to intergenotypic sequence variation at the NS3/4A active site. Newer, second-generation protease inhibitors now under development may provide broader genotype coverage, and also may have increased activity against resistant variants emerging during therapy to first-generation inhibitors. It is too early to predict whether these second-generation inhibitors will be of clinical use in treating these resistant viruses, however.

Since protease inhibitor resistance mutations occur within the NS3 protein, they have no effect on the susceptibility of the virus to polymerase (NS5B) or NS5A inhibitors. The reverse is also true, but both of these classes of antiviral drugs have their own sets of resistant mutants that they select. Resistance to any of these antivi-rals has no known impact on the susceptibility of virus to pegIFN/ribavirin.

Progress towards interferon-free regimens

It is evident that triple therapy combinations will be the next therapeutic innovation that clearly enhances rates of SVR. However, clinicians and patients would welcome all oral therapies without injectable pegIFN in an attempt to minimize adverse events and extend treatment to populations who are not candidates for interferon-based regimens. As discussed earlier, knowledge of hepatitis C replication pathways and novel drug development strategies have provided numerous potential targets for HCV treatment that are in early stages of exploration.

The INFORM-1 study demonstrated proof-of-concept that combining two classes of direct-acting antiviral agents in a short-term study, without pegIFN or ribavirin, could induce viral suppression without the development of viral resistance [730]. The two drugs used in this study have complementary profiles. RG7128 is a nucleoside NS5B polymerase with a high genetic barrier that is predominantly excreted through the kidneys. Danoprevir is an NS3 protease inhibitor with a typical-for-class lower genetic barrier that is predominantly metabolized in the liver. Genotype 1 patients ($n = 88$) were randomly assigned to treatment for 13 days with different dosages of RG7128 combined with danoprevir. Among treatment-naïve patients, the median change in HCV RNA compared with baseline was $-5.1 \log_{10}$. Remarkably, among prior null responders also included in this study, the median decrease of HCV RNA was $-4.9 \log_{10}$. Importantly, all patients had a continuous decline in HCV RNA that was maintained throughout the short dosing interval. Viral sequencing of the protease and polymerase domains in patients with detectable HCV RNA at the end of treatment did not demonstrate any resistant mutations [730].

These promising data have enabled other short-term clinical studies to test the efficacy of combining various classes of drugs without interferon. These have only been reported in preliminary form to date and success rates have varied. In one study of a protease inhibitor and a non-nucleoside polymerase inhibitor, the absence of ribavirin resulted in substantially lower rates of virologic response and higher rates of viral breakthrough and resistant mutations, suggesting that, once again, ribavirin may be indispensable even in interferon-free regimens [731]. Much debate surrounds the feasibility of curing hepatitis C without interferon as well as defining the optimal duration of therapy and which drugs/classes of drugs would be most efficacious, particularly among patients with unfavorable treatment characteristics. A small proof-of-principle study treated prior null-responder patients with only an oral combination of BMS-790052 (NS5A inhibitor) and BMS-650032 (NS3 protease inhibitor) for 24 weeks. Four of 11 patients (36%) achieved sustained virological response with oral combination, demonstrating for the first time that human HCV infection could be eradicated in the absence of interferon or ribavirin [732]. These exciting results will likely lead to a rapid acceleration of development of interferon-free, oral combination regimens to treat chronic hepatitis C.

References

1. Prince A, Grady G, Hazzi C, et al. Long-incubation post-transfusion hepatitis without serological evidence of exposure to hepatitis-B virus. *Lancet* 1974:241–6.
2. Feinstone SM, Kapikian AZ, Purcell RH, Alter HJ, Holland PV. Transfusion-associated hepatitis not due to viral hepatitis type A or B. *N Engl J Med* 1975;292:767–70.
3. Berman M, Alter HJ, Ishak KG, Purcell RH, Jones EA. The chronic sequelae of non-A, non-B hepatitis. *Ann Intern Med* 1979;91: 1–6.
4. Kiyosawa K, Sodeyama T, Tanaka E, et al. Interrelationship of blood transfusion, non-A, non-B hepatitis and hepatocellular carcinoma: analysis by detection of antibody to hepatitis C virus. *Hepatology* 1990;12:671–5.
5. Alter HJ, Tabor E, Meryman HT, et al. Transmission of hepatitis B virus infection by transfusion of frozen-deglycerolized red blood cells. *N Engl J Med* 1978;298:637–42.
6. Hollinger FB, Gitnick GL, Aach RD, et al. Non-A, non-B hepatitis transmission in chimpanzees: a project of the Transfusion-Transmitted Viruses Study Group. *Intervirology* 1978;10:60–8.
7. Bradley DW, McCaustland KA, Cook EH, Schable CA, Ebert JW, Maynard JE. Posttransfusion non-A, non-B hepatitis in chimpanzees: physicochemical evidence that the tubule-forming agent is a small, enveloped virus. *Gastroenterology* 1985;88:773–9.
8. Feinstone SM, Mihalik KB, Kamimura T, Alter HJ, London WT, Purcell RH. Inactivation of hepatitis B virus and non-A, non-B hepatitis by chloroform. *Infect Immun* 1983;41:816–21.
9. Choo QL, Kuo G, Weiner AJ, Overby LR, Bradley DW, Houghton M. Isolation of a cDNA clone derived from a blood-borne non-A, non-B viral hepatitis genome. *Science* 1989;244:359–62.
10. Houghton M. The long and winding road leading to the identification of the hepatitis C virus. *J Hepatol* 2009;51:939–48.
11. Kuo G, Choo QL, Alter HJ, et al. An assay for circulating antibodies to a major etiologic virus of human non-A, non-B hepatitis. *Science* 1989;244:362–4.
12. Lemon SM, Walker C, Alter MJ, et al. Hepatitis C virus. In: DM Knipe and PM Howley (Eds.) *Fields Virology*, 5th edn. Philadelphia, PA: Lippincott Williams and Wilkins, 2007:1253–304.
13. Simmonds P, Bukh J, Combet C, et al. Consensus proposals for a unified system of nomenclature of hepatitis C virus genotypes. *Hepatology* 2005;42:962–73.
14. Bartenschlager R, Frese M, Pietschmann T. Novel insights into hepatitis C virus replication and persistence. *Adv Virus Res* 2004;63:71–180.
15. Honda M, Beard MR, Ping LH, Lemon SM. A phylogenetically conserved stem-loop structure at the 5′ border of the internal ribosome entry site of hepatitis C virus is required for cap-independent viral translation. *J Virol* 1999;73:1165–74.
16. Lukavsky PJ, Kim I, Otto GA, Puglisi JD. Structure of HCV IRES domain II determined by NMR. *Nat Struct Biol* 2003;10:1033–8.
17. Friebe P, Lohmann V, Krieger N, Bartenschlager R. Sequences in the 5′ nontranslated region of hepatitis C virus required for RNA replication. *J Virol* 2001;75:12047–57.
18. Jopling CL, Schutz S, Sarnow P. Position-dependent function for a tandem microRNA miR-122-binding site located in the hepatitis C virus RNA genome. *Cell Host Microbe* 2008;4:77–85.
19. Jangra RK, Yi M, Lemon SM. miR-122 regulation of hepatitis C virus translation and infectious virus production. *J Virol* 2010;84:6615–25.
20. Pestova TV, Shatsky IN, Fletcher SP, Jackson RJ, Hellen CU. A prokaryotic-like mode of cytoplasmic eukaryotic ribosome binding to the initiation codon during internal translation initiation of hepatitis C and classical swine fever virus RNAs. *Genes Dev* 1998;12:67–83.
21. Lukavsky PJ. Structure and function of HCV IRES domains. *Virus Res* 2009;139:166–71.
22. Kolykhalov AA, Feinstone SM, Rice CM. Identification of a highly conserved sequence element at the 3′ terminus of hepatitis C virus genome RNA. *J Virol* 1996;70:3363–71.
23. Yi M, Lemon SM. 3′ nontranslated RNA signals required for replication of hepatitis C virus RNA. *J Virol* 2003;77:3557–68.
24. Yi M, Lemon SM. Structure–function analysis of the 3′ stem-loop of hepatitis C virus genomic RNA and its role in viral RNA replication. *RNA* 2003;9:331–45.
25. Hijikata M, Kato N, Ootsuyama Y, Nakagawa M, Shimotohno K. Gene mapping of the putative structural region of the hepatitis C virus genome by in vitro processing analysis. *Proc Natl Acad Sci USA* 1991;88:5547–51.
26. Yasui K, Wakita T, Tsukiyama-Kohara K, et al. The native form and maturation process of hepatitis C virus core protein. *J Virol* 1998;72:6048–55.
27. Santolini E, Migliaccio G, La Monica N. Biosynthesis and biochemical properties of the hepatitis C virus core protein. *J Virol* 1994;68:3631–41.
28. Boulant S, Vanbelle C, Ebel C, Penin F, Lavergne J-P. Hepatitis C virus core protein is a dimeric alpha-helical protein exhibiting membrane protein features. *J Virol* 2005;79:11353–65.
29. McLauchlan J, Lemberg MK, Hope G, Martoglio B. Intramembrane proteolysis promotes trafficking of hepatitis C virus core protein to lipid droplets. *EMBO J* 2002;21:3980–8.
30. McLauchlan J. Properties of the hepatitis C virus core protein: a structural protein that modulates cellular processes. *J Viral Hepat* 2000;7:2–14.
31. Lai MM, Ware CF. Hepatitis C virus core protein: possible roles in viral pathogenesis. *Curr Top Microbiol Immunol* 2000;242:117–34.
32. Ray RB, Ray R. Hepatitis C virus core protein: intriguing properties and functional relevance. *FEMS Microbiol Lett* 2001;202:149–56.

33. Irshad M, Dhar I. Hepatitis C virus core protein: an update on its molecular biology, cellular functions and clinical implications. *Med Princ Pract* 2006;15:405–16.

34. Deleersnyder V, Pillez A, Wychowski C, et al. Formation of native hepatitis C virus glycoprotein complexes. *J Virol* 1997;71:697–704.

35. Cocquerel L, Wychowski C, Minner F, Penin F, Dubuisson J. Charged residues in the transmembrane domains of hepatitis C virus glycoproteins play a major role in the processing, subcellular localization, and assembly of these envelope proteins. *J Virol* 2000;74:3623–33.

36. Dubuisson J, Helle F, Cocquerel L. Early steps of the hepatitis C virus life cycle. *Cell Microbiol* 2008;10:821–7.

37. Pileri P, Uematsu Y, Campagnoli S, et al. Binding of hepatitis C virus to CD81. *Science* 1998;282:938–41.

38. Bartosch B, Vitelli A, Granier C, et al. Cell entry of hepatitis C virus requires a set of co-receptors that include the CD81 tetraspanin and the SR-B1 scavenger receptor. *J Biol Chem* 2003;278:41624–30.

39. Wozniak AL, Griffin S, Rowlands D, et al. Intracellular proton conductance of the hepatitis C virus p7 protein and its contribution to infectious virus production. *PLoS Pathog* 2010;6:e1001087.

40. Sakai A, Claire MS, Faulk K, et al. The p7 polypeptide of hepatitis C virus is critical for infectivity and contains functionally important genotype-specific sequences. *Proc Natl Acad Sci USA* 2003;100:11646–51.

41. Steinmann E, Penin F, Kallis S, Patel AH, Bartenschlager R, Pietschmann T. Hepatitis C virus p7 protein is crucial for assembly and release of infectious virions. *PLoS Pathog* 2007;3:e103.

42. Selby MJ, Glazer E, Masiarz F, Houghton M. Complex processing and protein:protein interactions in the E2:NS2 region of HCV. *Virology* 1994;204:114–22.

43. Reed KE, Grakoui A, Rice CM. Hepatitis C virus-encoded NS2-3 protease: cleavage site mutagenesis and requirements for bimolecular cleavage. *J Virol* 1995;69:4127–36.

44. Hijikata M, Mizushima H, Akagi T, et al. Two distinct proteinase activities required for the processing of a putative nonstructural precursor protein of hepatitis C virus. *J Virol* 1993;67:4665–75.

45. Pallaoro M, Lahm A, Biasiol G, et al. Characterization of the hepatitis C virus NS2/3 processing reaction by using a purified precursor protein. *J Virol* 2001;75:9939–46.

46. Lorenz IC, Marcotrigiano J, Dentzer TG, Rice CM. Structure of the catalytic domain of the hepatitis C virus NS2-3 protease. *Nature* 2006;442:831–5.

47. Lohmann V, Korner F, Koch J, Herian U, Theilmann L, Bartenschlager R. Replication of subgenomic hepatitis C virus RNAs in a hepatoma cell line. *Science* 1999;285:110–13.

48. Steinmann E, Brohm C, Kallis S, Bartenschlager R, Pietschmann T. Efficient trans-encapsidation of hepatitis C virus RNAs into infectious virus-like particles. *J Virol* 2008;82:7034–46.

49. Jirasko V, Montserret R, Appel N, et al. Structural and functional characterization of nonstructural protein 2 for its role in hepatitis C virus assembly. *J Biol Chem* 2008;283:28546–62.

50. Yi M, Ma Y, Yates J, Lemon SM. Compensatory mutations in E1, p7, NS2 and NS3 enhance yields of cell culture-infectious intergenotypic chimeric hepatitis C virus. *J Virol* 2007;81:629–38.

51. Yi M, Ma Y, Yates J, Lemon SM. Trans-complementation of an NS2 defect in a late step in hepatitis C virus (HCV) particle assembly and maturation. *PLoS Pathog* 2009;5:e1000403.

52. Ma Y, Anantpadma M, Timpe JM, et al. Hepatitis C virus NS2 protein serves as a scaffold for virus assembly by interacting with both structural and nonstructural proteins. *J Virol* 2011;85:86–97.

53. Yao N, Reichert P, Taremi SS, Prosise WW, Weber PC. Molecular views of viral polyprotein processing revealed by the crystal structure of the hepatitis C virus bifunctional protease-helicase. *Structure Fold Des* 1999;7:1353–63.

54. Kim JL, Morgenstern KA, Lin C, et al. Crystal structure of the hepatitis C virus NS3 protease domain complexed with a synthetic NS4A cofactor peptide. *Cell* 1996;87:343–55.

55. Bartenschlager R. The NS3/4A proteinase of the hepatitis C virus: unravelling structure and function of an unusual enzyme and a prime target for antiviral therapy. *J Viral Hepat* 1999;6:165–81.

56. Li K, Foy E, Ferreon JC, et al. Immune evasion by hepatitis C virus NS3/4A protease-mediated cleavage of the TLR3 adaptor protein TRIF. *Proc Natl Acad Sci USA* 2005;102:2992–7.

57. Meylan E, Curran J, Hofmann K, et al. Cardif is an adaptor protein in the RIG-I antiviral pathway and is targeted by hepatitis C virus. *Nature* 2005;437:1167–72.

58. Li XD, Sun L, Seth RB, Pineda G, Chen ZJ. Hepatitis C virus protease NS3/4A cleaves mitochondrial antiviral signaling protein off the mitochondria to evade innate immunity. *Proc Natl Acad Sci USA* 2005;102:17717–22.

59. Lemon SM. Induction and evasion of innate antiviral responses by hepatitis C virus. *J Biol Chem* 2010;285:22741–7.

60. Dumont S, Cheng W, Serebrov V, et al. RNA translocation and unwinding mechanism of HCV NS3 helicase and its coordination by ATP. *Nature* 2006;439:105–8.

61. Lam AM, Frick DN. Hepatitis C virus subgenomic replicon requires an active NS3 RNA helicase. *J Virol* 2006;80:404–11.

62. Kolykhalov AA, Mihalik K, Feinstone SM, Rice CM. Hepatitis C virus-encoded enzymatic activities and conserved RNA elements in the 3′ nontranslated region are essential for virus replication in vivo. *J Virol* 2000;74:2046–51.

63. Ma Y, Yates J, Liang Y, Lemon SM, Yi M. NS3 helicase domains involved in infectious intracellular hepatitis C virus particle assembly. *J Virol* 2008;82:7624–39.

64. Han Q, Xu C, Wu C, Zhu W, Yang R, Chen X. Compensatory mutations in NS3 and NS5A proteins enhance the virus production capability of hepatitis C reporter virus. *Virus Res* 2009;145:63–73.

65. Phan T, Beran RK, Peters C, Lorenz IC, Lindenbach BD. Hepatitis C virus NS2 protein contributes to virus particle assembly via opposing epistatic interactions with the E1-E2 glycoprotein and NS3-NS4A enzyme complexes. *J Virol* 2009;83:8379–95.

66. Hamill P, Jean F. Enzymatic characterization of membrane-associated hepatitis C virus NS3-4A heterocomplex serine protease activity expressed in human cells. *Biochemistry* 2005;44:6586–96.

67. Elazar M, Liu P, Rice CM, Glenn JS. An N terminal amphipathic helix in hepatitis C virus (HCV) NS4B mediates membrane association, correct localization of replication complex proteins, and HCV RNA replication. *J Virol* 2004;78:11393–400.

68. Egger D, Wolk B, Gosert R, et al. Expression of hepatitis C virus proteins induces distinct membrane alterations including a candidate viral replication complex. *J Virol* 2002;76:5974–84.

69. Gosert R, Egger D, Lohmann V, et al. Identification of the hepatitis C virus RNA replication complex in Huh-7 cells harboring subgenomic replicons. *J Virol* 2003;77:5487–92.

70. Stone M, Jia S, Heo WD, Meyer T, Konan KV. Participation of rab5, an early endosome protein, in hepatitis C virus RNA replication machinery. *J Virol* 2007;81:4551–63.

71. Einav S, Elazar M, Danieli T, Glenn JS. A nucleotide binding motif in hepatitis C virus (HCV) NS4B mediates HCV RNA replication. *J Virol* 2004;78:11288–95.

72. Tellinghuisen TL, Rice CM. Interaction between hepatitis C virus proteins and host cell factors. *Curr Opin Microbiol* 2002;5:419–27.

73. Huang Y, Staschke K, De Francesco R, Tan SL. Phosphorylation of hepatitis C virus NS5A nonstructural protein: a new paradigm for phosphorylation-dependent viral RNA replication? *Virology* 2007;364:1–9.

74. Kaneko T, Tanji Y, Satoh S, et al. Production of two phosphoproteins from the NS5A region of the hepatitis C viral genome. *Biochem Biophys Res Commun* 1994;205:320–6.

75. Tanji Y, Kaneko T, Satoh S, Shimotohno K. Phosphorylation of hepatitis C virus-encoded nonstructural protein NS5A. *J Virol* 1995;69:3980–6.

76. Evans MJ, Rice CM, Goff SP. Phosphorylation of hepatitis C virus nonstructural protein 5A modulates its protein interactions and viral RNA replication. *Proc Natl Acad Sci USA* 2004;101:13038–43.

77. Gao L, Aizaki H, He JW, Lai MM. Interactions between viral nonstructural proteins and host protein hVAP-33 mediate the formation of hepatitis C virus RNA replication complex on lipid raft. *J Virol* 2004;78:3480–8.

78. Tellinghuisen TL, Marcotrigiano J, Gorbalenya AE, Rice CM. The NS5A protein of hepatitis C virus is a zinc metalloprotein. *J Biol Chem* 2004;279:48576–87.

79. Hanoulle X, Verdegem D, Badillo A, Wieruszeski JM, Penin F, Lippens G. Domain 3 of non-structural protein 5A from hepatitis C virus is natively unfolded. *Biochem Biophys Res Commun* 2009;381:634–8.

80. Miyanari Y, Atsuzawa K, Usuda N, et al. The lipid droplet is an important organelle for hepatitis C virus production. *Nat Cell Biol* 2007;9:1089–97.

81. Boulant S, Targett-Adams P, McLauchlan J. Disrupting the association of hepatitis C virus core protein with lipid droplets correlates with a loss in production of infectious virus. *J Gen Virol* 2007;88:2204–13.

82. Yamashita T, Kaneko S, Shirota Y, et al. RNA-dependent RNA polymerase activity of the soluble recombinant hepatitis C virus NS5B protein truncated at the C-terminal region. *J Biol Chem* 1998;273:15479–86.

83. Ranjith-Kumar CT, Kim YC, Gutshall L, et al. Mechanism of de novo initiation by the hepatitis C virus RNA-dependent RNA polymerase: role of divalent metals. *J Virol* 2002;76:12513–25.

84. Chinnaswamy S, Yarbrough I, Palaninathan S, et al. A locking mechanism regulates RNA synthesis and host protein interaction by the hepatitis C virus polymerase. *J Biol Chem* 2008;283:20535–46.

85. Oh JW, Ito T, Lai MM. A recombinant hepatitis C virus RNA-dependent RNA polymerase capable of copying the full-length viral RNA. *J Virol* 1999;73:7694–702.

86. Simmonds P. Genetic diversity and evolution of hepatitis C virus – 15 years on. *J Gen Virol* 2004;85:3173–88.

87. Wakita T, Pietschmann T, Kato T, et al. Production of infectious hepatitis C virus in tissue culture from a cloned viral genome. *Nature Med* 2005;11:791–6.

88. Zhong J, Gastaminza P, Cheng G, et al. Robust hepatitis C virus infection in vitro. *Proc Natl Acad Sci USA* 2005;102:9294–9.

89. Lindenbach BD, Evans MJ, Syder AJ, et al. Complete replication of hepatitis C virus in cell culture. *Science* 2005;309:623–6.

90. Pietschmann T, Kaul A, Koutsoudakis G, et al. Construction and characterization of infectious intragenotypic and intergenotypic hepatitis C virus chimeras. *Proc Natl Acad Sci USA* 2006;103:7408–13.

91. Yi M, Villanueva RA, Thomas DL, Wakita T, Lemon SM. Production of infectious genotype 1a hepatitis C virus (Hutchinson strain) in cultured human hepatoma cells. *Proc Natl Acad Sci USA* 2006;103:2310–15.

92. Shimakami T, Welsch C, Yamane D, et al. Protease inhibitor-resistant hepatitis C virus mutants with reduced fitness from impaired production of infectious rirus. *Gastroenterology* 2011;140:667–75. Epub 2010 Nov 4.

93. Germi R, Crance JM, Garin D, et al. Cellular glycosaminoglycans and low density lipoprotein receptor are involved in hepatitis C virus adsorption. *J Med Virol* 2002;68:206–15.

94. Barth H, Schafer C, Adah MI, et al. Cellular binding of hepatitis C virus envelope glycoprotein E2 requires cell surface heparan sulfate. *J Biol Chem* 2003;278:41003–12.

95. Basu A, Kanda T, Beyene A, Saito K, Meyer K, Ray R. Sulfated homologues of heparin inhibit hepatitis C virus entry into mammalian cells. *J Virol* 2007;81:3933–41.

96. Blanchard E, Belouzard S, Goueslain L, et al. Hepatitis C virus entry depends on clathrin-mediated endocytosis. *J Virol* 2006;80:6964–72.

97. Sabahi A. Hepatitis C virus entry: the early steps in the viral replication cycle. *Virol J* 2009;6:117.

98. von Hahn T, Rice CM. Hepatitis C virus entry. *J Biol Chem* 2008;283:3689–93.

99. Zeisel MB, Koutsoudakis G, Schnober EK, et al. Scavenger receptor class B type I is a key host factor for hepatitis C virus infection required for an entry step closely linked to CD81. *Hepatology* 2007;46:1722–31.

100. Evans MJ, von Hahn T, Tscherne DM, et al. Claudin-1 is a hepatitis C virus co-receptor required for a late step in entry. *Nature* 2007;446:801–5.

101. Ploss A, Evans MJ, Gaysinskaya VA, et al. Human occludin is a hepatitis C virus entry factor required for infection of mouse cells. *Nature* 2009;457:882–6.

102. Tscherne DM, Jones CT, Evans MJ, Lindenbach BD, McKeating JA, Rice CM. Time- and temperature-dependent activation of hepatitis C virus for low-pH-triggered entry. *J Virol* 2006;80:1734–41.

103. Quinkert D, Bartenschlager R, Lohmann V. Quantitative analysis of the hepatitis C virus replication complex. *J Virol* 2005;79:13594–605.

104. Jones DM, McLauchlan J. Hepatitis C virus: assembly and release of virus particles. *J Biol Chem* 2010;285:22733–9.

105. Gastaminza P, Cheng G, Wieland S, Zhong J, Liao W, Chisari FV. Cellular determinants of hepatitis C virus assembly, maturation, degradation and secretion. *J Virol* 2008;82:2241–9.

106. Lindenbach BD, Meuleman P, Ploss A, et al. Cell culture-grown hepatitis C virus is infectious in vivo and can be recultured in vitro. *Proc Natl Acad Sci USA* 2006;103:3805–9.

107. Nielsen SU, Bassendine MF, Burt AD, Martin C, Pumeechockchai W, Toms GL. Association between hepatitis C virus and very-low-density lipoprotein (VLDL)/LDL analyzed in iodixanol density gradients. *J Virol* 2006;80:2418–28.

108. Shimizu Y, Hishiki T, Sugiyama K, et al. Lipoprotein lipase and hepatic triglyceride lipase reduce the infectivity of hepatitis C virus (HCV) through their catalytic activities on HCV-associated lipoproteins. *Virology* 2010;407:152–9.

109. Jiang J, Luo G. Apolipoprotein E but not B is required for the formation of infectious hepatitis C virus particles. *J Virol* 2009;83:12680–91.

110. Kabelitz D, Medzhitov R. Innate immunity – cross-talk with adaptive immunity through pattern recognition receptors and cytokines. *Curr Opin Immunol* 2007;19:1–3.

111. Lang KS, Georgiev P, Recher M, et al. Immunoprivileged status of the liver is controlled by Toll-like receptor 3 signaling. *J Clin Invest* 2006;116:2456–63.

112. Schulz O, Diebold SS, Chen M, et al. Toll-like receptor 3 promotes cross-priming to virus-infected cells. *Nature* 2005;433:887–92.

113. Iwasaki A, Medzhitov R. Regulation of adaptive immunity by the innate immune system. *Science* 2010;327:291–5.

114. Hiscott J. Triggering the innate antiviral response through IRF-3 activation. *J Biol Chem* 2007;282:15325–9.

115. Panne D, Maniatis T, Harrison SC. Crystal structure of ATF-2/c-Jun and IRF-3 bound to the interferon-beta enhancer. *EMBO J* 2004;23:4384–93.

116. Loo YM, Owen DM, Li K, et al. Viral and therapeutic control of interferon beta promoter stimulator 1 during hepatitis C virus infection. *Proc Natl Acad Sci USA* 2006;103:6001–6.

117. Saito T, Owen DM, Jiang F, Marcotrigiano J, Gale M Jr. Innate immunity induced by composition-dependent RIG-I recognition of hepatitis C virus RNA. *Nature* 2008;454:523–7.

118. Sumpter R Jr, Loo MY, Foy E, et al. Regulating intracellular antiviral defense and permissiveness to hepatitis C virus RNA replication through a cellular RNA helicase, RIG-I. *J Virol* 2005;79: 2689–99.

119. Wang N, Liang Y, Devaraj S, Wang J, Lemon SM, Li K. Toll-like receptor 3 mediates establishment of an antiviral state against hepatitis C virus in hepatoma cells. *J Virol* 2009;83:9824–34.

120. Takahashi K, Asabe S, Wieland S, et al. Plasmacytoid dendritic cells sense hepatitis C virus-infected cells, produce interferon, and inhibit infection. *Proc Natl Acad Sci USA* 2010;107:7431-6.

121. Yoneyama M, Kikuchi M, Natsukawa T, et al. The RNA helicase RIG-I has an essential function in double-stranded RNA-induced innate antiviral responses. *Nat Immunol* 2004;5:730–7.

122. Pichlmair A, Schulz O, Tan CP, et al. RIG-I-mediated antiviral responses to single-stranded RNA bearing 5′ phosphates. *Science* 2006;314:999–1001.

123. Hornung V, Ellegast J, Kim S, et al. 5′-Triphosphate RNA is the ligand for RIG-I. *Science* 2006:314;994–7.

124. Saito T, Hirai R, Loo YM, et al. Regulation of innate antiviral defenses through a shared repressor domain in RIG-I and LGP2. *Proc Natl Acad Sci USA* 2007;104:582–7.

125. Seth RB, Sun L, Ea CK, Chen ZJ. Identification and characterization of MAVS, a mitochondrial antiviral signaling protein that activates NF-kappaB and IRF 3. *Cell* 2005;122:669–82.

126. Kawai T, Takahashi K, Sato S, et al. IPS-1, an adaptor triggering RIG-I- and Mda5-mediated type I interferon induction. *Nat Immunol* 2005;6:981–8.

127. Fitzgerald KA, McWhirter SM, Faia KL, et al. IKKepsilon and TBK1 are essential components of the IRF3 signaling pathway. *Nat Immunol* 2003;4:491–6.

128. Loo YM, Gale M Jr. Viral regulation and evasion of the host response. *Curr Top Microbiol Immunol* 2007;316:295–313.

129. Foy E, Li K, Wang C, et al. Regulation of interferon regulatory factor-3 by the hepatitis C virus serine protease. *Science* 2003;300:1145–8.

130. Liang Y, Ishida H, Lenz O, et al. Antiviral suppression vs restoration of RIG-I signaling by hepatitis C protease and polymerase inhibitors. *Gastroenterology* 2008;135:1710–18.

131. Sarasin Filipowicz M, Oakeley EJ, Duong FH, et al. Interferon signaling and treatment outcome in chronic hepatitis C. *Proc Natl Acad Sci USA* 2008;105:7034–9.

132. Matsumoto M, Funami K, Tanabe M, et al. Subcellular localization of Toll-like receptor 3 in human dendritic cells. *J Immunol* 2003;171:3154–62.

133. Funami K, Sasai M, Ohba Y, Oshiumi H, Seya T, Matsumoto M. Spatiotemporal mobilization of Toll/IL-1 receptor domain-containing adaptor molecule-1 in response to dsRNA. *J Immunol* 2007;179:6867–72.

134. Liu L, Botos I, Wang Y, et al. Structural basis of toll-like receptor 3 signaling with double-stranded RNA. *Science* 2008;320:379–81.

135. Sato S, Sugiyama M, Yamamoto M, et al. Toll/IL-1 receptor domain-containing adaptor inducing IFN-beta (TRIF) associates with TNF receptor-associated factor 6 and TANK-binding kinase 1, and activates two distinct transcription factors, NF-kappaB and IFN-regulatory factor-3, in the Toll-like receptor signaling. *J Immunol* 2003;171:4304–10.

136. Oshiumi H, Matsumoto M, Funami K, Akazawa T, Seya T. TICAM-1, an adaptor molecule that participates in Toll-like receptor 3-mediated interferon-beta induction. *Nat Immunol* 2003;4:161–7.

137. Hacker H, Redecke V, Blagoev B, et al. Specificity in Toll-like receptor signalling through distinct effector functions of TRAF3 and TRAF6. *Nature* 2006;439:204–7.

138. Meylan E, Burns K, Hofmann K, et al. RIP1 is an essential mediator of Toll-like receptor 3-induced NF-kB activation. *Nat Immunol* 2004;5:503–7.

139. Jouan L, Melancon P, Rodrigue-Gervais I, et al. Distinct antiviral signaling pathways in primary human hepatocytes and their differential disruption by HCV NS3 protease. *J Hepatology* 2010;52: 167–75.

140. Ferreon JC, Ferreon ACM, Li K, Lemon SM. Molecular determinants involved in TRIF proteolysis by the hepatitis C virus NS3/4A protease. *J Biol Chem* 2005;280:20483–92.

141. Yamamoto M, Sato S, Mori K, et al. Cutting edge: a novel Toll/IL-1 receptor domain-containing adapter that preferentially activates the IFN-beta promoter in the Toll-like receptor signaling. *J Immunol* 2002;169:6668–72.

142. Lau DT, Fish PM, Sinha M, Owen DM, Lemon SM, Gale M Jr. Interferon regulatory factor-3 activation, hepatic interferon-stimulated gene expression, and immune cell infiltration in hepatitis C virus patients. *Hepatology* 2008;47:799–809.

143. Lee J, Wu CC, Lee KJ, et al. Activation of anti-hepatitis C virus responses via Toll-like receptor 7. *Proc Natl Acad Sci USA* 2006;103: 1828–33.

144. Onoguchi K, Yoneyama M, Takemura A, et al. Viral infections activate types I and III interferon genes through a common mechanism. *J Biol Chem* 2007;282:7576–81.

145. Ge D, Fellay J, Thompson AJ, et al. Genetic variation in IL28B predicts hepatitis C treatment-induced viral clearance. *Nature* 2009;461:399–401.

146. Thomas DL, Thio CL, Martin MP, et al. Genetic variation in IL28B and spontaneous clearance of hepatitis C virus. *Nature* 2009;461:798–801.

147. Sato M, Suemori H, Hata N, et al. Distinct and essential roles of transcription factors IRF-3 and IRF-7 in response to viruses for IFN-alpha/beta gene induction. *Immunity* 2000:13:539–48.

148. Uze G, Monneron D. IL-28 and IL-29: newcomers to the interferon family. *Biochimie* 2007;89:729–34.

149. Grandvaux N, Servant MJ, tenOever B, et al. Transcriptional profiling of interferon regulatory factor 3 target genes: direct involvement in the regulation of interferon-stimulated genes. *J Virol* 2002;76:5532–9.

150. Wang C, Pflugheber J, Sumpter R Jr, et al. Alpha interferon induces distinct translational control programs to suppress hepatitis C virus RNA replication. *J Virol* 2003;77:3898–912.

151. Lanford RE, Guerra B, Bigger CB, Lee H, Chavez D, Brasky KM. Lack of response to exogenous interferon-alpha in the liver of chimpanzees chronically infected with hepatitis C virus. *Hepatology* 2007;46:999–1008.

152. Pflugheber J, Fredericksen B, Sumpter R Jr, et al. Regulation of PKR and IRF-1 during hepatitis C virus RNA replication. *Proc Natl Acad Sci USA* 2002;99:4650–5.

153. Duong FH, Filipowicz M, Tripodi M, La Monica N, Heim MH. Hepatitis C virus inhibits interferon signaling through up-regulation of protein phosphatase 2A. *Gastroenterology* 2004;126:263–77.

154. Lin W, Kim SS, Yeung E, et al. Hepatitis C virus core protein blocks interferon signaling by interaction with the STAT1 SH2 domain. *J Virol* 2006;80:9226–35.

155. Bode JG, Ludwig S, Ehrhardt C, et al. IFN-alpha antagonistic activity of HCV core protein involves induction of suppressor of cytokine signaling-3. *FASEB J* 2003;17:488–90.

156. Blindenbacher A, Duong FH, Hunziker L, et al. Expression of hepatitis c virus proteins inhibits interferon alpha signaling in the liver of transgenic mice. *Gastroenterology* 2003;124:1465–75.

157. Christen V, Treves S, Duong FH, Heim MH. Activation of endoplasmic reticulum stress response by hepatitis viruses up–regulates protein phosphatase 2A. *Hepatology* 2007;46:558–65.

158. Duong FH, Christen V, Filipowicz M, Heim MH. S-Adenosylmethionine and betaine correct hepatitis C virus induced inhibition of interferon signaling in vitro. *Hepatology* 2006;43:796–806.

159. Kim KA, Lin W, Tai AW, et al. Hepatic SOCS3 expression is strongly associated with non-response to therapy and race in HCV and HCV/HIV infection. *J Hepatol* 2009;50:705–11.

160. Chen L, Borozan I, Feld J, et al. Hepatic gene expression discriminates responders and nonresponders in treatment of chronic hepatitis C viral infection. *Gastroenterology* 2005;128:1437–44.

161. Malakhova OA, Kim KI, Luo JK, et al. UBP43 is a novel regulator of interferon signaling independent of its ISG15 isopeptidase activity. *EMBO J* 2006;25:2358–67.

162. Randall G, Chen L, Panis M, et al. Silencing of USP18 potentiates the antiviral activity of interferon against hepatitis C virus infection. *Gastroenterology* 2006;131:1584–91.

163. Dolganiuc A, Kodys K, Kopasz A, et al. Hepatitis C virus core and nonstructural protein 3 proteins induce pro- and anti-inflammatory cytokines and inhibit dendritic cell differentiation. *J Immunol* 2003;170:5615–24.

164. Auffermann-Gretzinger S, Keeffe EB, Levy S. Impaired dendritic cell maturation in patients with chronic, but not resolved, hepatitis C virus infection. *Blood* 2001;97:3171–6.

165. Kanto T, Hayashi N, Takehara T, et al. Impaired allostimulatory capacity of peripheral blood dendritic cells recovered from hepatitis C virus-infected individuals. *J Immunol* 1999;162:5584–91.

166. Bain C, Fatmi A, Zoulim F, Zarski JP, Trepo C, Inchauspe G. Impaired allostimulatory function of dendritic cells in chronic hepatitis C infection. *Gastroenterology* 2001;120:512–24.

167. Doherty DG, O'Farrelly C. Innate and adaptive lymphoid cells in the human liver. *Immunol Rev* 2000;174:5–20.

168. Khakoo SI, Thio CL, Martin MP, et al. HLA and NK cell inhibitory receptor genes in resolving hepatitis C virus infection. *Science* 2004;305:872–4.

169. Ahlenstiel G, Martin MP, Gao X, Carrington M, Rehermann B. Distinct KIR/HLA compound genotypes affect the kinetics of human antiviral natural killer cell responses. *J Clin Invest* 2008;118:1017–26.

170. Ahlenstiel G, Titerence RH, Koh C, et al. Natural killer cells are polarized toward cytotoxicity in chronic hepatitis C in an interferon-alfa-dependent manner. *Gastroenterology* 138:325–35,e321–2.

171. Oliviero B, Varchetta S, Paudice E, et al. Natural killer cell functional dichotomy in chronic hepatitis B and chronic hepatitis C virus infections. *Gastroenterology* 2009;137:1151–60,e1151–7.

172. Crotta S, Stilla A, Wack A, et al. Inhibition of natural killer cells through engagement of CD81 by the major hepatitis C virus envelope protein. *J Exp Med* 2002;195:35–41.

173. Tseng CT, Klimpel GR. Binding of the hepatitis C virus envelope protein E2 to CD81 inhibits natural killer cell functions. *J Exp Med* 2002;195:43–9.

174. Jinushi M, Takehara T, Tatsumi T, et al. Negative regulation of NK cell activities by inhibitory receptor CD94/NKG2A leads to altered NK cell-induced modulation of dendritic cell functions in chronic hepatitis C virus infection. *J Immunol* 2004;173:6072–81.

175. Shin EC, Seifert U, Kato T, et al. Virus-induced type I IFN stimulates generation of immunoproteasomes at the site of infection. *J Clin Invest* 2006;116:3006–14.

176. Missale G, Bertoni R, Lamonaca V, et al. Different clinical behaviors of acute hepatitis C virus infection are associated with different vigor of the anti-viral cell-mediated immune response. *J Clin Invest* 1996;98:706–14.

177. Gruner NH, Gerlach TJ, Jung MC, et al. Association of hepatitis C virus-specific CD8+ T cells with viral clearance in acute hepatitis C. *J Infect Dis* 2000;181:1528–36.

178. Cucchiarini M, Kammer AR, Grabscheid B, et al. Vigorous peripheral blood cytotoxic T cell response during the acute phase of hepatitis C virus infection. *Cell Immunol* 2000;203:111–23.

179. Gerlach JT, Diepolder HM, Jung MC, et al. Recurrence of hepatitis C virus after loss of virus-specific CD4(+) T-cell response in acute hepatitis C. *Gastroenterology* 1999;117:933–41.

180. Thimme R, Oldach D, Chang KM, Steiger C, Ray SC, Chisari FV. Determinants of viral clearance and persistence during acute hepatitis C virus infection. *J Exp Med* 2001;194:1395–406.

181. Thimme R, Bukh J, Spangenberg HC, et al. Viral and immunological determinants of hepatitis C virus clearance, persistence, and disease. *Proc Natl Acad Sci USA* 2002;99:15661–8.

182. Urbani S, Amadei B, Fisicaro P, et al. Outcome of acute hepatitis C is related to virus-specific CD4 function and maturation of antiviral memory CD8 responses. *Hepatology* 2006;44:126–39.

183. Kaplan DE, Sugimoto K, Newton K, et al. Discordant role of CD4 T-cell response relative to neutralizing antibody and CD8 T-cell responses in acute hepatitis C. *Gastroenterology* 2007;132:654–66.

184. Shoukry NH, Sidney J, Sette A, Walker CM. Conserved hierarchy of helper T cell responses in a chimpanzee during primary and secondary hepatitis C virus infections. *J Immunol* 2004;172:483–92.

185. Rosen HR, Miner C, Sasaki AW, et al. Frequencies of HCV-specific effector CD4+ T cells by flow cytometry: correlation with clinical disease stages. *Hepatology* 2002;35:190–8.

186. Day CL, Lauer GM, Robbins GK, et al. Broad specificity of virus-specific CD4+ T-helper-cell responses in resolved hepatitis C virus infection. *J Virol* 2002;76:12584–95.

187. Sugimoto K, Ikeda F, Stadanlick J, Nunes FA, Alter HJ, Chang KM. Suppression of HCV-specific T cells without differential hierarchy demonstrated ex vivo in persistent HCV infection. *Hepatology* 2003;38:1437–48.

188. Kamal SM, Fehr J, Roesler B, Peters T, Rasenack JW. Peginterferon alone or with ribavirin enhances HCV-specific CD4 T-helper 1 responses in patients with chronic hepatitis C. *Gastroenterology* 2002;123:1070–83.

189. MacDonald AJ, Duffy M, Brady MT, et al. CD4 T helper type 1 and regulatory T cells induced against the same epitopes on the core protein in hepatitis C virus-infected persons. *J Infect Dis* 2002;185:720–7.

190. Semmo N, Day CL, Ward SM, et al. Preferential loss of IL-2-secreting CD4+ T helper cells in chronic HCV infection. *Hepatology* 2005;41:1019–28.

191. Day CL, Seth NP, Lucas M, et al. Ex vivo analysis of human memory CD4 T cells specific for hepatitis C virus using MHC class II tetramers. *J Clin Invest* 2003;112:831–42.

192. Sallusto F, Lenig D, Forster R, Lipp M, Lanzavecchia A. Two subsets of memory T lymphocytes with distinct homing potentials and effector functions. *Nature* 1999;401:708–12.

193. Shedlock DJ, Shen H. Requirement for CD4 T cell help in generating functional CD8 T cell memory. *Science* 2003;300:337–9.

194. Sun JC, Bevan MJ. Defective CD8 T cell memory following acute infection without CD4 T cell help. *Science* 2003;300:339–42.

195. Janssen EM, Lemmens EE, Wolfe T, Christen U, von Herrath MG, Schoenberger SP. CD4+ T cells are required for secondary expansion and memory in CD8+ T lymphocytes. *Nature* 2003;421:852–6.

196. Darling JM, Erickson AL, Kanistanon D, et al. Analysis of CD8+ T cell receptor (TCR) diversity to an NS3 epitope in spontaneously cleared and chronic HCV infection: plasticity of TCR may influence outcome of HCV infection. *Hepatology* 2002;36:263A.

197. Cooper S, Erickson AL, Adams EJ, et al. Analysis of a successful immune response against hepatitis C virus. *Immunity* 1999;10:439–49.

198. Lechner F, Wong DK, Dunbar PR, et al. Analysis of successful immune responses in persons infected with hepatitis C virus. *J Exp Med* 2000;191:1499–512.

199. Lechner F, Gruener NH, Urbani S, et al. CD8+ T lymphocyte responses are induced during acute hepatitis C virus infection but are not sustained. *Eur J Immunol* 2000;30:2479–87.

200. Shankar P, Russo M, Harnisch B, Patterson M, Skolnik P, Lieberman J. Impaired function of circulating HIV-specific CD8(+) T cells in chronic human immunodeficiency virus infection. *Blood* 2000;96:3094–101.

201. Dalod M, Dupuis M, Deschemin JC, et al. Weak anti-HIV CD8(+) T-cell effector activity in HIV primary infection. *J Clin Invest* 1999;104:1431–9.

202. Kasprowicz V, Schulze Zur Wiesch J, Kuntzen T, et al. High level of PD-1 expression on hepatitis C virus (HCV)-specific CD8+ and CD4+ T cells during acute HCV infection, irrespective of clinical outcome. *J Virol* 2008;82:3154–60.

203. Guidotti LG, Ishikawa T, Hobbs MV, Matzke B, Schreiber R, Chisari FV. Intracellular inactivation of the hepatitis B virus by cytotoxic T lymphocytes. *Immunity* 1996;4:25–36.

204. Jo J, Aichele U, Kersting N, et al. Analysis of CD8+ T-cell-mediated inhibition of hepatitis C virus replication using a novel immunological model. *Gastroenterology* 2009;136:1391–401.

205. He XS, Rehermann B, Lopez-Labrador FX, et al. Quantitative analysis of hepatitis C virus-specific CD8(+) T cells in peripheral blood and liver using peptide-MHC tetramers. *Proc Natl Acad Sci USA* 1999;96:5692–7.

206. Gruener NH, Lechner F, Jung MC, et al. Sustained dysfunction of antiviral CD8+ T lymphocytes after infection with hepatitis C virus. *J Virol* 2001;75:5550–8.

207. Grabowska AM, Lechner F, Klenerman P, et al. Direct ex vivo comparison of the breadth and specificity of the T cells in the liver and peripheral blood of patients with chronic HCV infection. *Eur J Immunol* 2001;31:2388–94.

208. Wedemeyer H, He XS, Nascimbeni M, et al. Impaired effector function of hepatitis C virus-specific CD8+ T cells in chronic hepatitis C virus infection. *J Immunol* 2002;169:3447–58.

209. Urbani S, Amadei B, Fisicaro P, et al. Heterologous T cell immunity in severe hepatitis C virus infection. *J Exp Med* 2005;201:675–80.

210. Nelson DR, Marousis CG, Davis GL, et al. The role of hepatitis C virus-specific cytotoxic T lymphocytes in chronic hepatitis. *J Immunol* 1997;158:1473–81.

211. Freeman AJ, Pan Y, Harvey CE, et al. The presence of an intrahepatic cytotoxic T lymphocyte response is associated with low viral load in patients with chronic hepatitis C virus infection. *J Hepatol* 2003;38:349–56.

212. Napoli J, Bishop GA, McGuinness PH, Painter DM, McCaughan GW. Progressive liver injury in chronic hepatitis C infection correlates with increased intrahepatic expression of Th1-associated cytokines. *Hepatology* 1996;24:759–65.

213. McGuinness PH, Painter D, Davies S, McCaughan GW. Increases in intrahepatic CD68 positive cells, MAC387 positive cells, and proinflammatory cytokines (particularly interleukin 18) in chronic hepatitis C infection. *Gut* 2000;46:260–9.

214. Takaki A, Wiese M, Maertens G, et al. Cellular immune responses persist and humoral responses decrease two decades after recovery from a single-source outbreak of hepatitis C. *Nat Med* 2000;6:578–82.

215. Shoukry NH, Grakoui A, Houghton M, et al. Memory CD8+ T cells are required for protection from persistent hepatitis C virus infection. *J Exp Med* 2003;197:1645–55.

216. Adams G, Kuntz S, Rabalais G, Bratcher D, Tamburro CH, Kotwal GJ. Natural recovery from acute hepatitis C virus infection by agammaglobulinemic twin children. *Pediatr Infect Dis J* 1997;16:533–4.

217. Semmo N, Lucas M, Krashias G, Lauer G, Chapel H, Klenerman P. Maintenance of HCV-specific T-cell responses in antibody-deficient patients a decade after early therapy. *Blood* 2006;107:4570–1.

218. Beld M, Penning M, van Putten M, et al. Quantitative antibody responses to structural (core) and nonstructural (NS3, NS4, and NS5) hepatitis C virus proteins among seroconverting injecting drug users: impact of epitope variation and relationship to detection of HCV RNA in blood. *Hepatology* 1999;29:1288–98.

219. Logvinoff C, Major ME, Oldach D, et al. Neutralizing antibody response during acute and chronic hepatitis C virus infection. *Proc Natl Acad Sci USA* 2004;101:10149–54.

220. Dowd KA, Netski DM, Wang XH, Cox AL, Ray SC. Selection pressure from neutralizing antibodies drives sequence evolution during acute infection with hepatitis C virus. *Gastroenterology* 2009;136:2377–86.

221. Farci P, Shimoda A, Coiana A, et al. The outcome of acute hepatitis C predicted by the evolution of the viral quasispecies. *Science* 2000;288:339–44.

222. Bassett S, Brasky KM, Lanford RE. Analysis of hepatitis C virus-inoculated chimpanzees reveals unexpected clinical profiles. *J Virol* 1998;72:2589–99.

223. Grellier L, Brown D, Power J, Dusheiko G. Absence of anti-envelope antibodies and clearance of hepatitis C virus in a cohort of Irish women infected in 1977. *J Viral Hepat* 1997;4:379–81.

224. Racanelli V, Frassanito MA, Leone P, et al. Antibody production and in vitro behavior of CD27-defined B-cell subsets: persistent hepatitis C virus infection changes the rules. *J Virol* 2006;80:3923–34.

225. Dammacco F, Sansonno D, Piccoli C, Racanelli V, D'Amore FP, Lauletta G. The lymphoid system in hepatitis C virus infection: autoimmunity, mixed cryoglobulinemia, and overt B-cell malignancy. *Semin Liver Dis* 2000;20:143–57.

226. Urbani S, Boni C, Missale G, et al. Virus-specific CD8+ lymphocytes share the same effector-memory phenotype but exhibit functional differences in acute hepatitis B and C. *J Virol* 2002;76:12423–34.

227. Zajac AJ, Blattman JN, Murali-Krishna K, et al. Viral immune evasion due to persistence of activated T cells without effector function. *J Exp Med* 1998;188:2205–13.

228. Younes SA, Yassine-Diab B, Dumont AR, et al. HIV-1 viremia prevents the establishment of interleukin 2-producing HIV-specific memory CD4+ T cells endowed with proliferative capacity. *J Exp Med* 2003;198:1909–22.

229. Rutebemberwa A, Ray SC, Astemborski J, et al. High-programmed death-1 levels on hepatitis C virus-specific T cells during acute infection are associated with viral persistence and require preservation of cognate antigen during chronic infection. *J Immunol* 2008;181:8215–25.

230. Wherry EJ, Blattman JN, Murali-Krishna K, van der Most R, Ahmed R. Viral persistence alters CD8 T-cell immunodominance and tissue distribution and results in distinct stages of functional impairment. *J Virol* 2003;77:4911–27.

231. Radziewicz H, Ibegbu CC, Hon H, et al. Impaired hepatitis C virus (HCV)-specific effector CD8+ T cells undergo massive apoptosis in the peripheral blood during acute HCV infection and in the liver during the chronic phase of infection. *J Virol* 2008;82:9808–22.

232. Kittlesen DJ, Chianese-Bullock KA, Yao ZQ, Braciale TJ, Hahn YS. Interaction between complement receptor gC1qR and hepatitis C virus core protein inhibits T-lymphocyte proliferation. *J Clin Invest* 2000;106:1239–49.

233. Yao ZQ, Nguyen DT, Hiotellis AI, Hahn YS. Hepatitis C virus core protein inhibits human T lymphocyte responses by a complement-dependent regulatory pathway. *J Immunol* 2001;167:5264–72.

234. Marrone A, Sallie R. Genetic heterogeneity of hepatitis C virus. The clinical significance of genotypes and quasispecies behavior. *Clin Lab Med* 1996;16:429–49.

235. Timm J, Lauer GM, Kavanagh DG, et al. CD8 epitope escape and reversion in acute HCV infection. *J Exp Med* 2004;200:1593–604.

236. Ray SC, Fanning L, Wang XH, Netski DM, Kenny-Walsh E, Thomas DL. Divergent and convergent evolution after a common-source outbreak of hepatitis C virus. *J Exp Med* 2005;201:1753–9.

237. Erickson AL, Kimura Y, Igarashi S, et al. The outcome of hepatitis C virus infection is predicted by escape mutations in epitopes targeted by cytotoxic T lymphocytes. *Immunity* 2001;15:883–95.

238. Cox AL, Mosbruger T, Mao Q, et al. Cellular immune selection with hepatitis C virus persistence in humans. *J Exp Med* 2005;201:1741–52.

239. Tester I, Smyk-Pearson S, Wang P, et al. Immune evasion versus recovery after acute hepatitis C virus infection from a shared source. *J Exp Med* 2005;201:1725–31.

240. Fernandez J, Taylor D, Morhardt DR, et al. Long-term persistence of infection in chimpanzees inoculated with an infectious hepatitis C virus clone is associated with a decrease in the viral amino acid substitution rate and low levels of heterogeneity. *J Virol* 2004;78:9782–9.

241. Grakoui A, Shoukry NH, Woollard DJ, et al. HCV persistence and immune evasion in the absence of memory T cell help. *Science* 2003;302:659–62.

242. Chang KM, Rehermann B, McHutchison JG, et al. Immunological significance of cytotoxic T lymphocyte epitope variants in patients chronically infected by the hepatitis C virus. *J Clin Invest* 1997;100:2376–85.

243. von Hahn T, Yoon JC, Alter H, et al. Hepatitis C virus continuously escapes from neutralizing antibody and T–cell responses during chronic infection in vivo. *Gastroenterology* 2007;132:667–78.

244. Fuller MJ, Shoukry NH, Gushima T, et al. Selection-driven immune escape is not a significant factor in the failure of CD4 T cell responses in persistent hepatitis C virus infection. *Hepatology* 2010;51:378–87.

245. Meyer-Olson D, Shoukry NH, Brady KW, et al. Limited T cell receptor diversity of HCV-specific T cell responses is associated with CTL escape. *J Exp Med* 2004;200:307–19.

246. Uebelhoer L, Han JH, Callendret B, et al. Stable cytotoxic T cell escape mutation in hepatitis C virus is linked to maintenance of viral fitness. *PLoS Pathog* 2008;4:e1000143.

247. Koziel MJ, Dudley D, Afdhal N, et al. HLA class I-restricted cytotoxic T lymphocytes specific for hepatitis C virus: identification of multiple epitopes and characterization of patterns of cytokine release. *J Clin Invest* 1995;96:2311–21.

248. Accapezzato D, Francavilla V, Paroli M, et al. Hepatic expansion of a virus-specific regulatory CD8(+) T cell population in chronic hepatitis C virus infection. *J Clin Invest* 2004;113:963–72.

249. Piazzolla G, Tortorella C, Schiraldi O, Antonaci S. Relationship between interferon-gamma, interleukin-10, and interleukin-12 production in chronic hepatitis C and in vitro effects of interferon-alpha. *J Clin Immunol* 2000;20:54–61.

250. Abel M, Sene D, Pol S, et al. Intrahepatic virus-specific IL-10-producing CD8 T cells prevent liver damage during chronic hepatitis C virus infection. *Hepatology* 2006;44:1607–16.

251. D'Ambrosio D, Sinigaglia F, Adorini L. Special attractions for suppressor T cells. *Trends Immunol* 2003;24:122–6.

252. Jonuleit H, Schmitt E, Schuler G, Knop J, Enk AH. Induction of interleukin 10-producing, nonproliferating CD4(+) T cells with regulatory properties by repetitive stimulation with allogeneic immature human dendritic cells. *J Exp Med* 2000;192:1213–22.

253. Boettler T, Spangenberg HC, Neumann-Haefelin C, et al. T cells with a CD4+CD25+ regulatory phenotype suppress in vitro proliferation of virus-specific CD8+ T cells during chronic hepatitis C virus infection. *J Virol* 2005;79:7860–7.

254. Cabrera R, Tu Z, Xu Y, et al. An immunomodulatory role for CD4(+)CD25(+) regulatory T lymphocytes in hepatitis C virus infection. *Hepatology* 2004;40:1062–71.

255. Rushbrook SM, Ward SM, Unitt E, et al. Regulatory T cells suppress in vitro proliferation of virus-specific CD8+ T cells during persistent hepatitis C virus infection. *J Virol* 2005;79:7852–9.

256. Smyk-Pearson S, Golden-Mason L, Klarquist J, et al. Functional suppression by FoxP3+CD4+CD25(high) regulatory T cells during acute hepatitis C virus infection. *J Infect Dis* 2008;197:46–57.

257. Feld JJ, Hoofnagle JH. Mechanism of action of interferon and ribavirin in treatment of hepatitis C. *Nature* 2005;436:967–72.

258. Thomas E, Feld JJ, Li Q, Hu Z, Fried MW, Liang TJ. Ribavirin potentiates interferon action by augmenting interferon-stimulated gene induction in hepatitis C virus cell culture models. *Hepatology* 2011;53:32–41.

259. Crotty S, Cameron CE, Andino R. RNA virus error catastrophe: direct molecular test by using ribavirin. *Proc Natl Acad Sci USA* 2001;98:6895–900.

260. Tilg H. New insights into the mechanisms of interferon alfa: an immunoregulatory and anti-inflammatory cytokine. *Gastroenterology* 1997;112:1017–21.

261. Cramp ME, Rossol S, Chokshi S, Carucci P, Williams R, Naoumov NV. Hepatitis C virus-specific T-cell reactivity during interferon and ribavirin treatment in chronic hepatitis C. *Gastroenterology* 2000;118:346–55.

262. Lohr HF, Schmitz D, Arenz M, Weyer S, Gerken G, Meyer zum Buschenfelde KH. The viral clearance in interferon-treated chronic hepatitis C is associated with increased cytotoxic T cell frequencies. *J Hepatol* 1999;31:407–15.

263. Lauer GM, Lucas M, Timm J, et al. Full-breadth analysis of CD8+ T-cell responses in acute hepatitis C virus infection and early therapy. *J Virol* 2005;79:12979–88.

264. Rahman F, Heller T, Sobao Y, et al. Effects of antiviral therapy on the cellular immune response in acute hepatitis C. *Hepatology* 2004;40:87–97.

265. Schirren CA, Jung MC, Worzfeld T, et al. Hepatitis C virus-specific CD4+ T cell response after liver transplantation occurs early, is multispecific, compartmentalizes to the liver, and does not correlate with recurrent disease. *J Infect Dis* 2001;183:1187–94.

266. Schirren CA, Zachoval R, Gerlach JT, et al. Antiviral treatment of recurrent hepatitis C virus (HCV) infection after liver transplantation: association of a strong, multispecific, and long-lasting CD4+ T cell response with HCV-elimination. *J Hepatol* 2003;39:397–404.

267. Badr G, Bedard N, Abdel-Hakeem MS, et al. Early interferon therapy for hepatitis C virus infection rescues polyfunctional, long-lived CD8+ memory T cells. *J Virol* 2008;82:10017–31.

268. Gaudieri S, Rauch A, Pfafferott K, et al. Hepatitis C virus drug resistance and immune-driven adaptations: relevance to new antiviral therapy. *Hepatology* 2009;49:1069–82.

269. Der SD, Zhou A, Williams BR, Silverman RH. Identification of genes differentially regulated by interferon alpha, beta, or gamma using oligonucleotide arrays. *Proc Natl Acad Sci USA* 1998;95:15623–8.

270. Diago M, Castellano G, Garcia-Samaniego J, et al. Association of pretreatment serum interferon gamma inducible protein 10 levels with sustained virological response to peginterferon plus ribavirin therapy in genotype 1 infected patients with chronic hepatitis C. *Gut* 2006;55:374–9.

271. Golden-Mason L, Klarquist J, Wahed AS, Rosen HR. Cutting edge: programmed death-1 expression is increased on immunocytes in chronic hepatitis C virus and predicts failure of response to antiviral therapy: race-dependent differences. *J Immunol* 2008;180:3637–41.

272. Nascimbeni M, Mizukoshi E, Bosmann M, et al. Kinetics of CD4+ and CD8+ memory T-cell responses during hepatitis C virus rechallenge of previously recovered chimpanzees. *J Virol* 2003;77:4781–93.

273. Lanford RE, Guerra B, Chavez D, et al. Cross-genotype immunity to hepatitis C virus. *J Virol* 2004;78:1575–81.

274. Major ME, Mihalik K, Puig M, et al. Previously infected and recovered chimpanzees exhibit rapid responses that control hepatitis C virus replication upon rechallenge. *J Virol* 2002;76:6586–95.

275. Bassett SE, Guerra B, Brasky K, et al. Protective immune response to hepatitis C virus in chimpanzees rechallenged following clearance of primary infection. *Hepatology* 2001;33:1479–87.

276. Bukh J, Thimme R, Meunier JC, et al. Previously infected chimpanzees are not consistently protected against reinfection or persistent infection after reexposure to the identical hepatitis C virus strain. *J Virol* 2008;82:8183–95.

277. Lai ME, Mazzoleni AP, Argiolu F, et al. Hepatitis C virus in multiple episodes of acute hepatitis in polytransfused thalassaemic children. *Lancet* 1994;343:388–90.

278. Mehta SH, Cox A, Hoover DR, et al. Protection against persistence of hepatitis C. *Lancet* 2002;359:1478–83.

279. Zhang P, Zhong L, Struble EB, et al. Depletion of interfering antibodies in chronic hepatitis C patients and vaccinated chimpanzees reveals broad cross-genotype neutralizing activity. *Proc Natl Acad Sci USA* 2009;106:7537–41.

280. Yu MY, Bartosch B, Zhang P, et al. Neutralizing antibodies to hepatitis C virus (HCV) in immune globulins derived from anti-HCV-positive plasma. *Proc Natl Acad Sci USA* 2004;101:7705–10.

281. Krawczynski K, Alter M, Tankersley DL, et al. Effect of immune globulin on the prevention of experimental hepatitis C virus infection. *J Infect Dis* 1996;173:822–8.

282. Farci P, Alter HJ, Wong DC, et al. Prevention of hepatitis C virus infection in chimpanzees after antibody-mediated in vitro neutralization. *Proc Natl Acad Sci USA* 1994;91:7792–6.

283. Choo Q-L, Kuo G, Ralston R, et al. Vaccination of chimpanzees against infection by the hepatitis C virus. *Proc Natl Acad Sci USA* 1994;91:1294–8.

284. Houghton M, Abrignani S. Prospects for a vaccine against the hepatitis C virus. *Nature* 2005;436:961–6.

285. Forns X, Payette PJ, Ma X, et al. Vaccination of chimpanzees with plasmid DNA encoding the hepatitis C virus (HCV) envelope E2 protein modified the infection after challenge with homologous monoclonal HCV. *Hepatology* 2000;32:618–25.

286. Rollier C, Depla E, Drexhage JA, et al. Control of heterologous hepatitis C virus infection in chimpanzees is associated with the quality of vaccine-induced peripheral T-helper immune response. *J Virol* 2004;78:187–96.

287. Folgori A, Capone S, Ruggeri L, et al. A T-cell HCV vaccine eliciting effective immunity against heterologous virus challenge in chimpanzees. *Nat Med* 2006;12:190–7.

288. Major M. Prophylactic and therapeutic vaccination against hepatitis C virus (HCV): developments and future perspectives. *Viruses* 2009;1:144–65.

289. Te HS, Jensen DM. Epidemiology of hepatitis B and C viruses: a global overview. *Clin Liver Dis* 2010;14:1–21, vii.

290. Alter MJ. Epidemiology of hepatitis C virus infection. *World J Gastroenterol* 2007;13:2436–41.

291. Alter MJ, Kruszon-Moran D, Nainan OV, et al. The prevalence of hepatitis C virus infection in the United States, 1988 through 1994. *N Engl J Med* 1999;341:556–62.

292. Rustgi VK. The epidemiology of hepatitis C infection in the United States. *J Gastroenterol* 2007;42:513–21.

293. Cohen J. The scientific challenge of hepatitis C. *Science* 1999;285:26–30.

294. Wasley A, Alter MJ. Epidemiology of hepatitis C: geographic differences and temporal trends. *Semin Liver Dis* 2000;20:1–16.

295. Shepard CW, Finelli L, Alter MJ. Global epidemiology of hepatitis C virus infection. *Lancet Infect Dis* 2005;5:558–67.

296. Ghany MG, Strader DB, Thomas DL, Seeff LB. Diagnosis, management, and treatment of hepatitis C: an update. *Hepatology* 2009;49:1335–74.

297. Davis GL, Alter MJ, El-Serag H, Poynard T, Jennings LW. Aging of hepatitis C virus (HCV)-infected persons in the United States: a multiple cohort model of HCV prevalence and disease progression. *Gastroenterology* 2010;138:513–21.

298. Mitchell AE, Colvin HM, Palmer Beasley R. Institute of Medicine recommendations for the prevention and control of hepatitis B and C. *Hepatology* 2010;51:729–33.

299. Armstrong GL, Simard EP, Wasley A, McQuillan GM, Kuhnert WL, Alter MJ. The prevalence of hepatitis C virus infection in the United States, 1999–2002 [Abstract]. *Hepatology* 2004;40:176A.

300. Armstrong GL, Alter MJ, McQuillan GM, Margolis HS. The past incidence of hepatitis C virus infection: implications for the future burden of chronic liver disease in the United States. *Hepatology* 2000;31:777–82.

301. Armstrong GL, Wasley A, Simard EP, McQuillan GM, Kuhnert WL, Alter MJ. The prevalence of hepatitis C virus infection in the United States, 1999 through 2002. *Ann Intern Med* 2006;144:705–14.

302. Alter MJ. Epidemiology of hepatitis C. *Hepatology* 1997;26:S62–5.

303. Centers for Disease Control and Prevention. Statistics and surveillance. In: *Hepatitis C Information for Healthcare Professionals*. Atlanta, GA: Centers for Disease Control and Prevention, 2010. http://www.cdc.gov/hepatitis/HCV/StatisticsHCV.htm.

304. Omland LH, Krarup H, Jepsen P, et al. Mortality in patients with chronic and cleared hepatitis C viral infection: a nationwide cohort study. *J Hepatol* 2010;53:36–42.

305. Gidding HF, Topp L, Middleton M, et al. The epidemiology of hepatitis C in Australia: notifications, treatment uptake and liver transplantations, 1997–2006. *J Gastroenterol Hepatol* 2009;24:1648–54.

306. Garfein RS, Vlahov D, Galai N, Doherty MC, Nelson KE. Viral infections in short-term injection drug users: the prevalence of the hepatitis C, hepatitis B, human immunodeficiency, and human T-lymphotropic viruses. *Am J Public Health* 1996;86:655–61.

307. Hagan H, Pouget ER, Williams IT, et al. Attribution of hepatitis C virus seroconversion risk in young injection drug users in 5 US cities. *J Infect Dis* 2010;201:378–85.

308. Karmochkine M, Carrat F, Dos Santos O, Cacoub P, Raguin G. A case–control study of risk factors for hepatitis C infection in patients with unexplained routes of infection. *J Viral Hepat* 2006;13:775–82.

309. Koblin BA, Factor SH, Wu Y, Vlahov D. Hepatitis C virus infection among noninjecting drug users in New York City. *J Med Virol* 2003;70:387–90.

310. Galperim B, Cheinquer H, Stein A, Fonseca A, Lunge V, Ikuta N. Intranasal cocaine use does not appear to be an independent risk factor for HCV infection. *Addiction* 2004;99:973–7.

311. Conry-Cantilena C, Melpolder JC, Alter HJ, Gorlin JB, Mascotti K. Intranasal drug use among volunteer whole-blood donors: results of survey C. *Transfusion* 1998;38:512–13.

312. Scheinmann R, Hagan H, Lelutiu-Weinberger C, et al. Non-injection drug use and hepatitis C virus: a systematic review. *Drug Alcohol Depend* 2007;89:1–12.

313. Perz JF, Thompson ND, Schaefer MK, Patel PR. US outbreak investigations highlight the need for safe injection practices and basic infection control. *Clin Liver Dis* 2010;14:137–51, x.

314. Strickland GT. Liver disease in Egypt: hepatitis C superseded schistosomiasis as a result of iatrogenic and biological factors. *Hepatology* 2006;43:915–22.

315. Frank C, Mohamed MK, Strickland GT, et al. The role of parenteral antischistosomal therapy in the spread of hepatitis C virus in Egypt. *Lancet* 2000;355:887–91.

316. Pepin J, Lavoie M, Pybus OG, et al. Risk factors for hepatitis C virus transmission in colonial Cameroon. *Clin Infect Dis* 2010;51:768–76.

317. Kiyosawa K, Tanaka E, Sodeyama T, et al. Transmission of hepatitis C in an isolated area in Japan: community-acquired infection. The South Kiso Hepatitis Study Group. *Gastroenterology* 1994;106:1596–602.

318. Fischer GE, Schaefer MK, Labus BJ, et al. Hepatitis C virus infections from unsafe injection practices at an endoscopy clinic in Las Vegas, Nevada, 2007–2008. *Clin Infect Dis* 2010;51:267–73.

319. Krause G, Trepka MJ, Whisenhunt RS, et al. Nosocomial transmission of hepatitis C virus associated with the use of multidose saline vials. *Infect Control Hosp Epidemiol* 2003;24:122–7.

320. Schreiber GB, Busch MP, Kleinman SH, Korelitz JJ. The risk of transfusion-transmitted viral infections. The Retrovirus Epidemiology Donor Study. *N Engl J Med* 1996;334:1685–90.

321. Cunningham MJ, Macklin EA, Neufeld EJ, Cohen AR. Complications of beta-thalassemia major in North America. *Blood* 2004;104:34–9.

322. Hassan M, Hasan S, Castro O, Giday S, Banks A, Smoot D. HCV in sickle cell disease. *J Natl Med Assoc* 2003;95:864–7, 872–64.

323. DeVault KR, Friedman LS, Westerberg S, Martin P, Hosein B, Ballas SK. Hepatitis C in sickle cell anemia. *J Clin Gastroenterol* 1994;18:206–9.

324. Key NS, Negrier C. Coagulation factor concentrates: past, present, and future. *Lancet* 2007;370:439–48.

325. Goedert JJ, Eyster ME, Lederman MM, et al. End-stage liver disease in persons with hemophilia and transfusion–associated infections. *Blood* 2002;100:1584–9.

326. Eyster ME, Diamondstone LS, Lien JM, Ehmann WC, Quan S, Goedert JJ. Natural history of hepatitis C virus infection in multitrans-fused hemophiliacs: effect of coinfection with human immunodeficiency virus. The Multicenter Hemophilia Cohort Study. *J Acquir Immune Defic Syndr* 1993;6:602–10.

327. Fried MW, Kroner BL, Preiss LR, Wilhelmsen K, Goedert JJ. Hemophilic siblings with chronic hepatitis C: familial aggregation of spontaneous and treatment-related viral clearance. *Gastroenterology* 2006;131:757–64.

328. Tagliaferri A, Rivolta GF, Iorio A, et al. Mortality and causes of death in Italian persons with haemophilia, 1990–2007. *Haemophilia* 2010;16:437–46.

329. Fried MW, Peter J, Hoots K, et al. Hepatitis C in adults and adolescents with hemophilia: a randomized, controlled trial of interferon alfa-2b and ribavirin. *Hepatology* 2002;36:967–72.

330. Maor Y, Schapiro JM, Bashari D, et al. Treatment of hepatitis C in patients with haemophilia – the Israeli National Hemophilia Center experience. *Haemophilia* 2008;14:336–42.

331. Alavian SM, Tabatabaei SV, Keshvari M, et al. Peginterferon alpha-2a and ribavirin treatment of patients with haemophilia and hepatitis C virus infection: a single-centre study of 367 cases. *Liver Int* 2010;30:1173–80.

332. Fried MW, Shindo M, Fong TL, Fox PC, Hoofnagle JH, Di Bisceglie AM. Absence of hepatitis C viral RNA from saliva and semen of patients with chronic hepatitis C. *Gastroenterology* 1992;102:1306–8.

333. Leruez-Ville M, Kunstmann JM, De Almeida M, Rouzioux C, Chaix ML. Detection of hepatitis C virus in the semen of infected men. *Lancet* 2000;356:42–3.

334. Nguyen O, Sheppeard V, Douglas MW, Tu E, Rawlinson W. Acute hepatitis C infection with evidence of heterosexual transmission. *J Clin Virol* 2010;49:65–8.

335. Thomas DL, Zenilman JM, Alter HJ, et al. Sexual transmission of hepatitis C virus among patients attending sexually transmitted diseases clinics in Baltimore – an analysis of 309 sex partnerships. *J Infect Dis* 1995;171:768–75.

336. Tohme RA, Holmberg SD. Is sexual contact a major mode of hepatitis C virus transmission? *Hepatology*; 52:1497–505.

337. Bottieau E, Apers L, Van Esbroeck M, Vandenbruaene M, Florence E. Hepatitis C virus infection in HIV-infected men who have sex with men: sustained rising incidence in Antwerp, Belgium, 2001–2009. *Euro Surveill* 2010;15:19673.

338. Urbanus AT, van de Laar TJ, Stolte IG, et al. Hepatitis C virus infections among HIV-infected men who have sex with men: an expanding epidemic. *AIDS* 2009;23:F1–7.

339. Indolfi G, Resti M. Perinatal transmission of hepatitis C virus infection. *J Med Virol* 2009;81:836–43.

340. Mast EE, Hwang LY, Seto DS, et al. Risk factors for perinatal transmission of hepatitis C virus (HCV) and the natural history of HCV infection acquired in infancy. *J Infect Dis* 2005;192:1880–9.

341. Mofenson LM, Brady MT, Danner SP, et al. Guidelines for the prevention and treatment of opportunistic infections among HIV-exposed and HIV-infected children: recommendations from CDC, the National Institutes of Health, the HIV Medicine Association of the Infectious Diseases Society of America, the Pediatric Infectious Diseases Society, and the American Academy of Pediatrics. *MMWR Recomm Rep* 2009;58:1–166.

342. McIntyre PG, Tosh K, McGuire W. Caesarean section versus vaginal delivery for preventing mother to infant hepatitis C virus transmission. *Cochrane Database Syst Rev* 2006;1:CD005546.

343. Pembrey L, Newell ML, Tovo PA. The management of HCV infected pregnant women and their children European paediatric HCV network. *J Hepatol* 2005;43:515–25.

344. Network EPHCV. Effects of mode of delivery and infant feeding on the risk of mother-to-child transmission of hepatitis C virus. European Paediatric Hepatitis C Virus Network. *Br J Obstet Gynaecol* 2001;108:371–7.

345. Michelin A, Henderson DK. Infection control guidelines for prevention of health care-associated transmission of hepatitis B and C viruses. *Clin Liver Dis* 2010;14:119–36, ix–x.

346. MacCannell T, Laramie AK, Gomaa A, Perz JF. Occupational exposure of health care personnel to hepatitis B and hepatitis C: prevention and surveillance strategies. *Clin Liver Dis* 2010;14:23–36, vii.

347. Corey KE, Servoss JC, Casson DR, et al. Pilot study of postexposure prophylaxis for hepatitis C virus in healthcare workers. *Infect Control Hosp Epidemiol* 2009;30:1000–5.

348. Puro V, De Carli G, Cicalini S, et al. European recommendations for the management of healthcare workers occupationally exposed to hepatitis B virus and hepatitis C virus. *Euro Surveill* 2005;10:260–4.

349. Anon. Updated US Public Health Service guidelines for the management of occupational exposures to HBV, HCV, and HIV and recommendations for postexposure prophylaxis. *MMWR Recomm Rep* 2001;50:1–52.

350. National Institutes of Health Consensus Development Conference Statement. Management of hepatitis C 2002 (June 10–12, 2002). *Gastroenterology* 2002;123:2082–99.

351. Alter HJ, Purcell RH, Shih JW, et al. Detection of antibody to hepatitis C virus in prospectively followed transfusion recipients with acute and chronic non-A, non-B hepatitis. *N Engl J Med* 1989;321:1494–500.

352. Alter MJ, Margolis HS, Krawczynski K, et al. The natural history of community-acquired hepatitis C in the United States. The Sentinel Counties Chronic non-A, non-B Hepatitis Study Team. *N Engl J Med* 1992;327:1899–905.

353. Choo QL, Weiner AJ, Overby LR, Kuo G, Houghton M, Bradley DW. Hepatitis C virus: the major causative agent of viral non-A, non-B hepatitis. *Br Med Bull* 1990;46:423–41.

354. Alter MJ, Kuhnert WL, Finelli L. Guidelines for laboratory testing and result reporting of antibody to hepatitis C virus. Centers for Disease Control and Prevention. *MMWR Recomm Rep* 2003;52:1–13.

355. Gretch DR. Diagnostic tests for hepatitis C. *Hepatology* 1997;26:S43–7.

356. Chevaliez S, Pawlotsky JM. Diagnosis and management of chronic viral hepatitis: antigens, antibodies and viral genomes. *Best Pract Res Clin Gastroenterol* 2008;22:1031–48.

357. Zaaijer HL, Cuypers HT, Reesink HW, Winkel IN, Gerken G, Lelie PN. Reliability of polymerase chain reaction for detection of hepatitis C virus. *Lancet* 1993;341:722–4.

358. Le Guillou-Guillemette H, Lunel-Fabiani F. Detection and quantification of serum or plasma HCV RNA: mini review of commercially available assays. *Methods Mol Biol* 2009;510:3–14.

359. Zoulim F. New nucleic acid diagnostic tests in viral hepatitis. *Semin Liver Dis* 2006;26:309–17.

360. Chevaliez S, Bouvier-Alias M, Brillet R, Pawlotsky JM. Overestimation and underestimation of hepatitis C virus RNA levels in a widely used real-time polymerase chain reaction-based method. *Hepatology* 2007;46:22–31.

361. Vermehren J, Kau A, Gartner BC, Gobel R, Zeuzem S, Sarrazin C. Differences between two real-time PCR-based hepatitis C virus (HCV) assays (RealTime HCV and Cobas AmpliPrep/Cobas TaqMan) and one signal amplification assay (Versant HCV RNA 3.0) for RNA detection and quantification. *J Clin Microbiol* 2008;46:3880–91.

362. Sarrazin C, Shiffman ML, Hadziyannis SJ, et al. Definition of rapid virologic response with a highly sensitive real-time PCR-based HCV RNA assay in peginterferon alfa-2a plus ribavirin response-guided therapy. *J Hepatol* 2010;52:832–8.

363. Simmonds P, Bukh J, Combet C, et al. Consensus proposals for a unified system of nomenclature of hepatitis C virus genotypes. *Hepatology* 2005;42:962–73.

364. Blatt LM, Mutchnick MG, Tong MJ, et al. Assessment of hepatitis C virus RNA and genotype from 6807 patients with chronic hepatitis C in the United States. *J Viral Hepat* 2000;7:196–202.

365. Weck K. Molecular methods of hepatitis C genotyping. *Expert Rev Mol Diagn* 2005;5:507–20.

366. Alter MJ, Seeff LB, Bacon BR, Thomas DL, Rigsby MO, Di Bisceglie AM. Testing for hepatitis C virus infection should be routine for persons at increased risk for infection. *Ann Intern Med* 2004;141:715–17.

367. Farci P, Alter HJ, Wong D, et al. A long-term study of hepatitis C virus replication in non-A, non-B hepatitis. *N Engl J Med* 1991;325:98–104.

368. Mosley JW, Operskalski EA, Tobler LH, et al. Viral and host factors in early hepatitis C virus infection. *Hepatology* 2005;42:86–92.

369. Alter M, Margolis H, Krawczynski K, et al. The natural history of community-acquired hepatitis C in United States. The Sentinel Counties Chronic non-A,non-B Hepatitis Study team. *N Engl J Med* 1992;327:1899–905.

370. Barrera JM, Francis B, Ercilla G, et al. Improved detection of anti-HCV in post-transfusion hepatitis by a third-generation ELISA. *Vox Sang* 1995;68:15–18.

371. Villano SA, Vlahov D, Nelson KE, Cohn S, Thomas DL. Persistence of viremia and the importance of long-term follow-up after acute hepatitis C infection. *Hepatology* 1999;29:908–14.

372. Marcellin P. Hepatitis C: the clinical spectrum of the disease. *J Hepatol* 1999;31(Suppl 1):9–16.

373. Wiegand J, Jackel E, Cornberg M, et al. Long-term follow-up after successful interferon therapy of acute hepatitis C. *Hepatology* 2004;40:98–107.

374. Alter HJ, Conry-Cantilena C, Melpolder J, et al. Hepatitis C in asymptomatic blood donors. *Hepatology* 1997;26:S29–33.

375. Seeff LB, Hollinger FB, Alter HJ, et al. Long-term mortality and morbidity of transfusion-associated non-A, non-B, and type C hepatitis: a National Heart, Lung, and Blood Institute collaborative study. *Hepatology* 2001;33:455–63.

376. Thomas DL, Astemborski J, Rai RM, et al. The natural history of hepatitis C virus infection. *JAMA* 2000;284:450–6.

377. Vogt M, Lang T, Frosner G, et al. Prevalence and clinical outcome of hepatitis C infection in children who underwent cardiac surgery before the implementation of blood-donor screening. *N Engl J Med* 1999;341:866–70.

378. Locasciulli A, Testa M, Pontisso P, et al. Prevalence and natural history of hepatitis C infection in patients cured of childhood leukemia. *Blood* 1997;90:4628–33.

379. Wiese M, Berr F, Lafrenz M, Porst H, Oesen U. Low frequency of cirrhosis in a hepatitis C (genotype 1b) single-source outbreak in germany: a 20-year multicenter study. *Hepatology* 2000;32:91–6.

380. Kenny-Walsh E. Clinical outcomes after hepatitis C infection from contaminated anti-D immune globulin. *N Engl J Med* 1999;340:1228–33.

381. Page K, Hahn JA, Evans J, et al. Acute hepatitis C virus infection in young adult injection drug users: a prospective study of incident infection, resolution, and reinfection. *J Infect Dis* 2009;200:1216–26.

382. Rauch A, Kutalik Z, Descombes P, et al. Genetic variation in IL28B is associated with chronic hepatitis C and treatment failure: a genome-wide association study. *Gastroenterology* 2010;138:1338–45, e1331–7.

383. Thio CL, Thomas DL, Carrington M. Chronic viral hepatitis and the human genome. *Hepatology* 2000;31:819–27.

384. Tillmann HL, Thompson AJ, Patel K, et al. A polymorphism near IL28B is associated with spontaneous clearance of acute hepatitis C virus and jaundice. *Gastroenterology* 2010;139:1586–92, e1581.

385. Kim AY, Kuntzen T, Timm J, et al. Spontaneous control of HCV is associated with expression of HLA–B*57 and preservation of targeted epitopes. *Gastroenterology* 2011;140:686–96.

386. Alric L, Fort M, Izopet J, et al. Genes of the major histocompatibility complex class II influence the outcome of hepatitis C virus infection. *Gastroenterology* 1997;113:1675–81.

387. Thursz M, Yallop R, Goldin R, Trepo C, Thomas HC. Influence of MHC class II genotype on outcome of infection with hepatitis C virus. The HENCORE group. Hepatitis C European Network for Cooperative Research. *Lancet* 1999;354:2119–24.

388. Piasecki BA, Lewis JD, Reddy KR, et al. Influence of alcohol use, race, and viral coinfections on spontaneous HCV clearance in a US veteran population. *Hepatology* 2004;40:892–9.

389. Lehmann M, Meyer MF, Monazahian M, Tillmann HL, Manns MP, Wedemeyer H. High rate of spontaneous clearance of acute hepatitis C virus genotype 3 infection. *J Med Virol* 2004;73:387–91.

390. Merican I, Sherlock S, McIntyre N, Dusheiko GM. Clinical, biochemical and histological features in 102 patients with chronic hepatitis C virus infection. *Q J Med* 1993;86:119–25.

391. Barkhuizen A, Rosen HR, Wolf S, Flora K, Benner K, Bennett RM. Musculoskeletal pain and fatigue are associated with chronic hepatitis C: a report of 239 hepatology clinic patients. *Am J Gastroenterol* 1999;94:1355–60.

392. Cacoub P, Ratziu V, Myers RP, et al. Impact of treatment on extrahepatic manifestations in patients with chronic hepatitis C. *J Hepatol* 2002;36:812–18.

393. Forton DM, Thomas HC, Murphy CA, et al. Hepatitis C and cognitive impairment in a cohort of patients with mild liver disease. *Hepatology* 2002;35:433–9.

394. Foster GR, Goldin RD, Thomas HC. Chronic hepatitis C virus infection causes a significant reduction in quality of life in the absence of cirrhosis. *Hepatology* 1998;27:209–12.

395. Spiegel BM, Younossi ZM, Hays RD, Revicki D, Robbins S, Kanwal F. Impact of hepatitis C on health related quality of life: a systematic review and quantitative assessment. *Hepatology* 2005;41:790–800.

396. Rodger AJ, Jolley D, Thompson SC, Lanigan A, Crofts N. The impact of diagnosis of hepatitis C virus on quality of life. *Hepatology* 1999;30:1299–301.

397. Ware JE Jr, Bayliss MS, Mannocchia M, Davis GL. Health-related quality of life in chronic hepatitis C: impact of disease and treatment response. The Interventional Therapy Group. *Hepatology* 1999;30:550–5.

398. Bruce MG, Bruden D, McMahon BJ, et al. Hepatitis C infection in Alaska Natives with persistently normal, persistently elevated

or fluctuating alanine aminotransferase levels. *Liver Int* 2006;26:
643–9.

399. Haber MM, West AB, Haber AD, Reuben A. Relationship of aminotransferases to liver histological status in chronic hepatitis C. *Am J
Gastroenterol* 1995;90:1250–7.

400. Healey CJ, Chapman RW, Fleming KA. Liver histology in hepatitis
C infection: a comparison between patients with persistently normal
or abnormal transaminases. *Gut* 1995;37:274–8.

401. McCormick SE, Goodman ZD, Maydonovitch CL, Sjogren MH.
Evaluation of liver histology, ALT elevation, and HCV RNA titer in
patients with chronic hepatitis C. *Am J Gastroenterol* 1996;91:1516–22.

402. Giannini E, Risso D, Botta F, et al. Validity and clinical utility of
the aspartate aminotransferase–alanine aminotransferase ratio in
assessing disease severity and prognosis in patients with hepatitis C virus-related chronic liver disease. *Arch Intern Med* 2003;163:
218–24.

403. Sheth SG, Flamm SL, Gordon FD, Chopra S. AST/ALT ratio predicts
cirrhosis in patients with chronic hepatitis C virus infection. *Am J
Gastroenterol* 1998;93:44–8.

404. Seeff LB. Natural history of chronic hepatitis C. *Hepatology*
2002;36:S35–46.

405. Freeman AJ, Dore GJ, Law MG, et al. Estimating progression
to cirrhosis in chronic hepatitis C virus infection. *Hepatology*
2001;34:809–16.

406. Thein HH, Yi Q, Dore GJ, Krahn MD. Estimation of stage-specific
fibrosis progression rates in chronic hepatitis C virus infection: a
meta-analysis and meta-regression. *Hepatology* 2008;48:418–31.

407. Collier JD, Woodall T, Wight DG, Shore S, Gimson AE, Alexander GJ. Predicting progressive hepatic fibrosis stage on subsequent
liver biopsy in chronic hepatitis C virus infection. *J Viral Hepat*
2005;12:74–80.

408. Colletta C, Smirne C, Fabris C, et al. Value of two noninvasive methods to detect progression of fibrosis among HCV carriers with normal aminotransferases. *Hepatology* 2005;42:838–45.

409. Ryder SD, Irving WL, Jones DA, Neal KR, Underwood JC. Progression of hepatic fibrosis in patients with hepatitis C: a prospective
repeat liver biopsy study. *Gut* 2004;53:451–5.

410. Wilson LE, Torbenson M, Astemborski J, et al. Progression of liver
fibrosis among injection drug users with chronic hepatitis C. *Hepatology* 2006;43:788–95.

411. Wali M, Lewis S, Hubscher S, et al. Histological progression during short-term follow-up of patients with chronic hepatitis C virus
infection. *J Viral Hepat* 1999;6:445–52.

412. Tong MJ, el-Farra NS, Reikes AR, Co RL. Clinical outcomes after
transfusion-associated hepatitis C. *N Engl J Med* 1995;332:1463–6.

413. Adinolfi LE, Giordano MG, Andreana A, et al. Hepatic fibrosis plays
a central role in the pathogenesis of thrombocytopenia in patients
with chronic viral hepatitis. *Br J Haematol* 2001;113:590–5.

414. Degos F, Christidis C, Ganne-Carrie N, et al. Hepatitis C virus
related cirrhosis: time to occurrence of hepatocellular carcinoma and
death. *Gut* 2000;47:131–6.

415. Davila JA, Morgan RO, Shaib Y, McGlynn KA, El-Serag HB. Hepatitis C infection and the increasing incidence of hepatocellular carcinoma: a population-based study. *Gastroenterology* 2004;127:1372–80.

416. Chiba T, Matsuzaki Y, Abei M, et al. Multivariate analysis of risk factors for hepatocellular carcinoma in patients with hepatitis C virus-
related liver cirrhosis. *J Gastroenterol* 1996;31:552–8.

417. El-Serag HB, Rudolph KL. Hepatocellular carcinoma: epidemiology
and molecular carcinogenesis. *Gastroenterology* 2007;132:2557–76.

418. Ohki T, Tateishi R, Sato T, et al. Obesity is an independent risk factor for hepatocellular carcinoma development in chronic hepatitis C
patients. *Clin Gastroenterol Hepatol* 2008;6:459–64.

419. El-Serag HB, Mason AC. Rising incidence of hepatocellular carcinoma in the United States. *N Engl J Med* 1999;340:745–50.

420. Konishi I, Hiasa Y, Shigematsu S, et al. Diabetes pattern on the 75
g oral glucose tolerance test is a risk factor for hepatocellular carcinoma in patients with hepatitis C virus. *Liver Int* 2009;29:1194–201.

421. Ohata K, Hamasaki K, Toriyama K, et al. Hepatic steatosis is a risk
factor for hepatocellular carcinoma in patients with chronic hepatitis C virus infection. *Cancer* 2003;97:3036–43.

422. Davila JA, Morgan RO, Shaib Y, McGlynn KA, El-Serag HB. Diabetes increases the risk of hepatocellular carcinoma in the United
States: a population based case control study. *Gut* 2005;54:533–9.

423. Bruix J, Sherman M. Management of hepatocellular carcinoma. *Hepatology* 2005;42:1208–36.

424. Di Bisceglie AM, Sterling RK, Chung RT, et al. Serum alpha-
fetoprotein levels in patients with advanced hepatitis C: results from
the HALT-C trial. *J Hepatol* 2005;43:434–41.

425. Fattovich G, Giustina G, Degos F, et al. Morbidity and mortality in
compensated cirrhosis type C: a retrospective follow-up study of
384 patients. *Gastroenterology* 1997;112:463–72.

426. Planas R, Balleste B, Alvarez MA, et al. Natural history of decompensated hepatitis C virus-related cirrhosis. A study of 200 patients.
J Hepatol 2004;40:823–30.

427. Murray KF, Carithers RL Jr. AASLD practice guidelines: evaluation
of the patient for liver transplantation. *Hepatology* 2005;41:1407–32.

428. Thuluvath PJ, Guidinger MK, Fung JJ, Johnson LB, Rayhill SC, Pelletier SJ. Liver transplantation in the United States, 1999–2008. *Am J
Transplant* 2010;10:1003–19.

429. Berenguer M. What determines the natural history of recurrent hepatitis C after liver transplantation? *J Hepatol* 2005;42:448–56.

430. Wise M, Bialek S, Finelli L, Bell BP, Sorvillo F. Changing trends in
hepatitis C-related mortality in the United States, 1995–2004. *Hepatology* 2008;47:1128–35.

431. Poynard T, Bedossa P, Opolon P. Natural history of liver fibrosis progression in patients with chronic hepatitis C. The OBSVIRC,
METAVIR, CLINIVIR, and DOSVIRC groups. *Lancet* 1997;349:
825–32.

432. Poynard T, Ratziu V, Charlotte F, Goodman Z, McHutchison J,
Albrecht J. Rates and risk factors of liver fibrosis progression in
patients with chronic hepatitis c. *J Hepatol* 2001;34:730–9.

433. Poynard T, Mathurin P, Lai CL, et al. A comparison of fibrosis progression in chronic liver diseases. *J Hepatol* 2003;38:257–65.

434. Di Martino V, Lebray P, Myers RP, et al. Progression of liver fibrosis
in women infected with hepatitis C: long-term benefit of estrogen
exposure. *Hepatology* 2004;40:1426–33.

435. Yu MW, Chang HC, Chang SC, et al. Role of reproductive factors in
hepatocellular carcinoma: impact on hepatitis B- and C-related risk.
Hepatology 2003;38:1393–400.

436. El-Serag HB, Davila JA, Petersen NJ, McGlynn KA. The continuing
increase in the incidence of hepatocellular carcinoma in the United
States: an update. *Ann Intern Med* 2003;139:817–23.

437. Wiley TE, Brown J, Chan J. Hepatitis C infection in African Americans: its natural history and histological progression. *Am J Gastroenterol* 2002;97:700–6.

438. Sterling RK, Stravitz RT, Luketic VA, et al. A comparison of the spectrum of chronic hepatitis C virus between Caucasians and African
Americans. *Clin Gastroenterol Hepatol* 2004;2:469–73.

439. Ghany MG, Kleiner DE, Alter H, et al. Progression of fibrosis in
chronic hepatitis C. *Gastroenterology* 2003;124:97–104.

440. Fontaine H, Nalpas B, Poulet B, et al. Hepatitis activity index is a
key factor in determining the natural history of chronic hepatitis C.
Hum Pathol 2001;32:904–9.

441. Kleiner DE. The liver biopsy in chronic hepatitis C: a view from the
other side of the microscope. *Semin Liver Dis* 2005;25:52–64.

442. Thorburn D, Curry G, Spooner R, et al. The role of iron and
haemochromatosis gene mutations in the progression of liver disease in chronic hepatitis C. *Gut* 2002;50:248–52.

443. Bonkovsky HL, Troy N, McNeal K, et al. Iron and HFE or TfR1 mutations as comorbid factors for development and progression of chronic hepatitis C. *J Hepatol* 2002;37:848–54.

444. Erhardt A, Maschner-Olberg A, Mellenthin C, et al. HFE mutations and chronic hepatitis C: H63D and C282Y heterozygosity are independent risk factors for liver fibrosis and cirrhosis. *J Hepatol* 2003;38:335–42.

445. Tung BY, Emond MJ, Bronner MP, Raaka SD, Cotler SJ, Kowdley KV. Hepatitis C, iron status, and disease severity: relationship with HFE mutations. *Gastroenterology* 2003;124:318–26.

446. Giannini E, Mastracci L, Botta F, et al. Liver iron accumulation in chronic hepatitis C patients without HFE mutations: relationships with histological damage, viral load and genotype and alpha-glutathione S-transferase levels. *Eur J Gastroenterol Hepatol* 2001;13:1355–61.

447. Hezode C, Cazeneuve C, Coue O, et al. Liver iron accumulation in patients with chronic active hepatitis C: prevalence and role of hemochromatosis gene mutations and relationship with hepatic histological lesions. *J Hepatol* 1999;31:979–84.

448. Larson AM, Taylor SL, Bauermeister D, Rosoff L Jr, Kowdley KV. Pilot study of the relationship between histologic progression and hepatic iron concentration in chronic hepatitis C. *J Clin Gastroenterol* 2003;37:406–11.

449. Di Bisceglie AM, Bonkovsky HL, Chopra S, et al. Iron reduction as an adjuvant to interferon therapy in patients with chronic hepatitis C who have previously not responded to interferon: a multicenter, prospective, randomized, controlled trial. *Hepatology* 2000;32:135–8.

450. Sartori M, Andorno S, Rossini A, et al. Phlebotomy improves histology in chronic hepatitis C males with mild iron overload. *World J Gastroenterol* 2010;16:596–602.

451. Fontana RJ, Israel J, LeClair P, et al. Iron reduction before and during interferon therapy of chronic hepatitis C: results of a multicenter, randomized, controlled trial. *Hepatology* 2000;31:730–6.

452. Fargion S, Fracanzani AL, Rossini A, et al. Iron reduction and sustained response to interferonalpha therapy in patients with chronic hepatitis C: results of an Italian multicenter randomized study. *Am J Gastroenterol* 2002;97:1204–10.

453. Goodman ZD, Ishak KG. Histopathology of hepatitis C virus infection. *Semin Liver Dis* 1995;15:70–81.

454. Kumar D, Farrell GC, Fung C, George J. Hepatitis C virus genotype 3 is cytopathic to hepatocytes: reversal of hepatic steatosis after sustained therapeutic response. *Hepatology* 2002;36:1266–72.

455. Conjeevaram HS, Kleiner DE, Everhart JE, et al. Race, insulin resistance and hepatic steatosis in chronic hepatitis C. *Hepatology* 2007;45:80–7.

456. Ong JP, Younossi ZM, Speer C, Olano A, Gramlich T, Boparai N. Chronic hepatitis C and superimposed nonalcoholic fatty liver disease. *Liver* 2001;21:266–71.

457. Adinolfi LE, Gambardella M, Andreana A, Tripodi MF, Utili R, Ruggiero G. Steatosis accelerates the progression of liver damage of chronic hepatitis C patients and correlates with specific HCV genotype and visceral obesity. *Hepatology* 2001;33:1358–64.

458. Hourigan LF, Macdonald GA, Purdie D, et al. Fibrosis in chronic hepatitis C correlates significantly with body mass index and steatosis. *Hepatology* 1999;29:1215–19.

459. Hu KQ, Kyulo NL, Esrailian E, et al. Overweight and obesity, hepatic steatosis, and progression of chronic hepatitis C: a retrospective study on a large cohort of patients in the United States. *J Hepatol* 2004;40:147–54.

460. Poynard T, Ratziu V, McHutchison J, et al. Effect of treatment with peginterferon or interferon alfa-2b and ribavirin on steatosis in patients infected with hepatitis C. *Hepatology* 2003;38:75–85.

461. Camma C, Bruno S, Di Marco V, et al. Insulin resistance is associated with steatosis in nondiabetic patients with genotype 1 chronic hepatitis C. *Hepatology* 2006;43:64–71.

462. Petta S, Camma C, Di Marco V, et al. Insulin resistance and diabetes increase fibrosis in the liver of patients with genotype 1 HCV infection. *Am J Gastroenterol* 2008;103:1136–44.

463. Roudot-Thoraval F, Bastie A, Pawlotsky JM, Dhumeaux D. Epidemiological factors affecting the severity of hepatitis C virus-related liver disease: a French survey of 6,664 patients. The Study Group for the Prevalence and the Epidemiology of Hepatitis C Virus. *Hepatology* 1997;26:485–90.

464. Cacciola I, Pollicino T, Squadrito G, Cerenzia G, Orlando ME, Raimondo G. Occult hepatitis B virus infection in patients with chronic hepatitis C liver disease. *N Engl J Med* 1999;341:22–6.

465. Kamal SM, Turner B, He Q, et al. Progression of fibrosis in hepatitis C with and without schistosomiasis: correlation with serum markers of fibrosis. *Hepatology* 2006;43:771–9.

466. Weber R, Sabin CA, Friis-Moller N, et al. Liver-related deaths in persons infected with the human immunodeficiency virus: the D:A:D study. *Arch Intern Med* 2006;166:1632–41.

467. Benhamou Y, Bochet M, Di Martino V, et al. Liver fibrosis progression in human immunodeficiency virus and hepatitis C virus coinfected patients. The Multivirc Group. *Hepatology* 1999;30:1054–8.

468. Allory Y, Charlotte F, Benhamou Y, Opolon P, Le Charpentier Y, Poynard T. Impact of human immunodeficiency virus infection on the histological features of chronic hepatitis C: a case–control study. The MULTIVIRC group. *Hum Pathol* 2000;31:69–74.

469. Graham CS, Baden LR, Yu E, et al. Influence of human immunodeficiency virus infection on the course of hepatitis C virus infection: a meta-analysis. *Clin Infect Dis* 2001;33:562–9.

470. Benhamou Y, Di Martino V, Bochet M, et al. Factors affecting liver fibrosis in human immunodeficiency virus- and hepatitis C virus-coinfected patients: impact of protease inhibitor therapy. *Hepatology* 2001;34:283–7.

471. Marine-Barjoan E, Saint-Paul MC, Pradier C, et al. Impact of antiretroviral treatment on progression of hepatic fibrosis in HIV/hepatitis C virus co-infected patients. *Aids* 2004;18:2163–70.

472. Martin-Carbonero L, Benhamou Y, Puoti M, et al. Incidence and predictors of severe liver fibrosis in human immunodeficiency virus-infected patients with chronic hepatitis C: a European collaborative study. *Clin Infect Dis* 2004;38:128–33.

473. Brau N, Salvatore M, Rios-Bedoya CF, et al. Slower fibrosis progression in HIV/HCV-coinfected patients with successful HIV suppression using antiretroviral therapy. *J Hepatol* 2006;44:47–55.

474. Mehta SH, Thomas DL, Torbenson M, et al. The effect of antiretroviral therapy on liver disease among adults with HIV and hepatitis C coinfection. *Hepatology* 2005;41:123–31.

475. Qurishi N, Kreuzberg C, Luchters G, et al. Effect of antiretroviral therapy on liver-related mortality in patients with HIV and hepatitis C virus coinfection. *Lancet* 2003;362:1708–13.

476. Hutchinson SJ, Bird SM, Goldberg DJ. Influence of alcohol on the progression of hepatitis C virus infection: a meta-analysis. *Clin Gastroenterol Hepatol* 2005;3:1150–9.

477. Corrao G, Arico S. Independent and combined action of hepatitis C virus infection and alcohol consumption on the risk of symptomatic liver cirrhosis. *Hepatology* 1998;27:914–19.

478. Monto A, Patel K, Bostrom A, et al. Risks of a range of alcohol intake on hepatitis C-related fibrosis. *Hepatology* 2004;39:826–34.

479. National Institutes of Health. NIH Consensus Statement on Management of Hepatitis C: 2002. *NIH Consens State Sci Statements* 2002;19:1–46.

480. Hezode C, Roudot-Thoraval F, Nguyen S, et al. Daily cannabis smoking as a risk factor for progression of fibrosis in chronic hepatitis C. *Hepatology* 2005;42:63–71.

481. Ishida JH, Peters MG, Jin C, et al. Influence of cannabis use on severity of hepatitis C disease. *Clin Gastroenterol Hepatol* 2008;6:69–75.

482. Modi AA, Feld JJ, Park Y, et al. Increased caffeine consumption is associated with reduced hepatic fibrosis. *Hepatology*; 51:201–9.

483. Freedman ND, Everhart JE, Lindsay KL, et al. Coffee intake is associated with lower rates of liver disease progression in chronic hepatitis C. *Hepatology* 2009;50:1360–9.

484. Cacoub P, Poynard T, Ghillani P, et al. Extrahepatic manifestations of chronic hepatitis C. MULTIVIRC Group. Multidepartment Virus C. *Arthritis Rheum* 1999;42:2204–12.

485. Sansonno D, De Vita S, Iacobelli AR, Cornacchiulo V, Boiocchi M, Dammacco F. Clonal analysis of intrahepatic B cells from HCV-infected patients with and without mixed cryoglobulinemia. *J Immunol* 1998;160:3594–601.

486. Lunel F, Musset L, Cacoub P, et al. Cryoglobulinemia in chronic liver diseases: role of hepatitis C virus and liver damage. *Gastroenterology* 1994;106:1291–300.

487. Sene D, Ghillani-Dalbin P, Thibault V, et al. Longterm course of mixed cryoglobulinemia in patients infected with hepatitis C virus. *J Rheumatol* 2004;31:2199–206.

488. Sansonno D, Lauletta G, De Re V, et al. Intrahepatic B cell clonal expansions and extrahepatic manifestations of chronic HCV infection. *Eur J Immunol* 2004;34:126–36.

489. Ferri C, Monti M, La Civita L, et al. Hepatitis C virus infection in non-Hodgkin's Bcell lymphoma complicating mixed cryoglobulinaemia. *Eur J Clin Invest* 1994;24:781–4.

490. Giannelli F, Moscarella S, Giannini C, et al. Effect of antiviral treatment in patients with chronic HCV infection and t(14;18) translocation. *Blood* 2003;102:1196–201.

491. Gisbert JP, Garcia-Buey L, Pajares JM, Moreno-Otero R. Prevalence of hepatitis C virus infection in B-cell non-Hodgkin's lymphoma: systematic review and meta-analysis. *Gastroenterology* 2003;125:1723–32.

492. Giordano TP, Henderson L, Landgren O, et al. Risk of non-Hodgkin lymphoma and lymphoproliferative precursor diseases in US veterans with hepatitis C virus. *JAMA* 2007;297:2010–17.

493. de Sanjose S, Benavente Y, Vajdic CM, et al. Hepatitis C and non-Hodgkin lymphoma among 4784 cases and 6269 controls from the International Lymphoma Epidemiology Consortium. *Clin Gastroenterol Hepatol* 2008;6:451–8.

494. Bronowicki JP, Bineau C, Feugier P, et al. Primary lymphoma of the liver: clinical-pathological features and relationship with HCV infection in French patients. *Hepatology* 2003;37:781–7.

495. Perrone A, Deramo MT, Spaccavento F, Santarcangelo P, Favoino B, Antonaci S. Hepatitis C virus (HCV) genotypes, human leucocyte antigen expression and monoclonal gammopathy prevalence during chronic HCV infection. *Cytobios* 2001;106(Suppl 1):125–34.

496. Andreone P, Zignego AL, Cursaro C, et al. Prevalence of monoclonal gammopathies in patients with hepatitis C virus infection. *Ann Intern Med* 1998;129:294–8.

497. Gisbert JP, Garcia-Buey L, Pajares JM, Moreno-Otero R. Prevalence of hepatitis C virus infection in porphyria cutanea tarda: systematic review and meta-analysis. *J Hepatol* 2003;39:620–7.

498. Azim J, McCurdy H, Moseley RH. Porphyria cutanea tarda as a complication of therapy for chronic hepatitis C. *World J Gastroenterol* 2008;14:5913–15.

499. Carrozzo M, Gandolfo S, Carbone M, et al. Hepatitis C virus infection in Italian patients with oral lichen planus: a prospective case–control study. *J Oral Pathol Med* 1996;25:527–33.

500. Arrieta JJ, Rodriguez-Inigo E, Casqueiro M, et al. Detection of hepatitis C virus replication by in situ hybridization in epithelial cells of anti-hepatitis C virus-positive patients with and without oral lichen planus. *Hepatology* 2000;32:97–103.

501. Abdallah MA, Ghozzi MY, Monib HA, et al. Necrolytic acral erythema: a cutaneous sign of hepatitis C virus infection. *J Am Acad Dermatol* 2005;53:247–51.

502. Tabibian JH, Gerstenblith MR, Tedford RJ, Junkins-Hopkins JM, Abuav R. Necrolytic acral erythema as a cutaneous marker of hepatitis C: report of two cases and review. *Dig Dis Sci* 2010;55:2735–43.

503. White DL, Ratziu V, El-Serag HB. Hepatitis C infection and risk of diabetes: a systematic review and meta-analysis. *J Hepatol* 2008;49:831–44.

504. Petit JM, Bour JB, Galland-Jos C, et al. Risk factors for diabetes mellitus and early insulin resistance in chronic hepatitis C. *J Hepatol* 2001;35:279–83.

505. Moucari R, Asselah T, Cazals-Hatem D, et al. Insulin resistance in chronic hepatitis C: association with genotypes 1 and 4, serum HCV RNA level, and liver fibrosis. *Gastroenterology* 2008;134:416–23.

506. Milner KL, van der Poorten D, Trenell M, et al. Chronic hepatitis C is associated with peripheral rather than hepatic insulin resistance. *Gastroenterology* 2010;138:932–41, e931–3.

507. Romero-Gomez M, Fernandez-Rodriguez CM, Andrade RJ, et al. Effect of sustained virological response to treatment on the incidence of abnormal glucose values in chronic hepatitis C. *J Hepatol* 2008;48:721–7.

508. Arase Y, Suzuki F, Suzuki Y, et al. Sustained virological response reduces incidence of onset of type 2 diabetes in chronic hepatitis C. *Hepatology* 2009;49:739–44.

509. Mosnier JF, Degott C, Marcellin P, Henin D, Erlinger S, Benhamou JP. The intraportal lymphoid nodule and its environment in chronic active hepatitis C: an immunohistochemical study. *Hepatology* 1993;17:366–71.

510. Murakami J, Shimizu Y, Kashii Y, et al. Functional B-cell response in intrahepatic lymphoid follicles in chronic hepatitis C. *Hepatology* 1999;30:143–50.

511. Racanelli V, Sansonno D, Piccoli C, D'Amore FP, Tucci FA, Dammacco F. Molecular characterization of B cell clonal expansions in the liver of chronically hepatitis C virus-infected patients. *J Immunol* 2001;167:21–9.

512. Monto A, Alonzo J, Watson JJ, Grunfeld C, Wright TL. Steatosis in chronic hepatitis C: relative contributions of obesity, diabetes mellitus, and alcohol. *Hepatology* 2002;36:729–36.

513. Rubbia-Brandt L, Fabris P, Paganin S, et al. Steatosis affects chronic hepatitis C progression in a genotype specific way. *Gut* 2004;53:406–12.

514. Perlemuter G, Sabile A, Letteron P, et al. Hepatitis C virus core protein inhibits microsomal triglyceride transfer protein activity and very low density lipoprotein secretion: a model of viral-related steatosis. *FASEB J* 2002;16:185–94.

515. Peters MG, Terrault NA. Alcohol use and hepatitis C. *Hepatology* 2002;36:S220–5.

516. Bruno S, Shiffman ML, Roberts SK, et al. Efficacy and safety of peginterferon alfa-2a (40KD) plus ribavirin in hepatitis C patients with advanced fibrosis and cirrhosis. *Hepatology*; 51:388–97.

517. The French METAVIR Cooperative Study Group. Intraobserver and interobserver variations in liver biopsy interpretation in patients with chronic hepatitis C. *Hepatology* 1994;20:15–20.

518. Bedossa P, Dargere D, Paradis V. Sampling variability of liver fibrosis in chronic hepatitis C. *Hepatology* 2003;38:1449–57.

519. Colloredo G, Guido M, Sonzogni A, Leandro G. Impact of liver biopsy size on histological evaluation of chronic viral hepatitis: the smaller the sample, the milder the disease. *J Hepatol* 2003;39:239–44.

520. Guido M, Rugge M. Liver biopsy sampling in chronic viral hepatitis. *Semin Liver Dis* 2004;24:89–97.

521. Ishak K, Baptista A, Bianchi L, et al. Histological grading and staging of chronic hepatitis. *J Hepatol* 1995;22:696–9.

522. Knodell RG, Ishak KG, Black WC, et al. Formulation and application of a numerical scoring system for assessing histological activity in asymptomatic chronic active hepatitis. *Hepatology* 1981;1:431–5.

523. Maylin S, Martinot-Peignoux M, Moucari R, et al. Eradication of hepatitis C virus in patients successfully treated for chronic hepatitis C. *Gastroenterology* 2008;135:821–9.

524. Barton AL, Banner BF, Cable EE, Bonkovsky HL. Distribution of iron in the liver predicts the response of chronic hepatitis C infection to interferon therapy. *Am J Clin Pathol* 1995;103:419–24.

525. Iezzoni JC, Gaffey MJ, Stacy EK, Normansell DE. Hepatocytic globules in end-stage hepatic disease: relationship to alpha1-antitrypsin phenotype. *Am J Clin Pathol* 1997;107:692–7.

526. Eigenbrodt ML, McCashland TM, Dy RM, Clark J, Galati J. Heterozygous alpha 1-antitrypsin phenotypes in patients with end stage liver disease. *Am J Gastroenterol* 1997;92:602–7.

527. Propst T, Propst A, Dietze O, Judmaier G, Braunsteiner H, Vogel W. High prevalence of viral infection in adults with homozygous and heterozygous alpha 1-antitrypsin deficiency and chronic liver disease. *Ann Intern Med* 1992;117:641–5.

528. Wiesner RH, Sorrell M, Villamil F. Report of the first International Liver Transplantation Society expert panel consensus conference on liver transplantation and hepatitis C. *Liver Transpl* 2003;9:S1–9.

529. Dixon LR, Crawford JM. Early histologic changes in fibrosing cholestatic hepatitis C. *Liver Transpl* 2007;13:219–26.

530. Liang Y, Shilagard T, Xiao SY, et al. Visualizing hepatitis C virus infections in human liver by two-photon microscopy. *Gastroenterology* 2009;137:1448–58.

531. Swain MG, Lai MY, Shiffman ML, et al. A sustained virologic response is durable in patients with chronic hepatitis C treated with peginterferon alfa-2a and ribavirin. *Gastroenterology* 2011;139:1593–601.

532. McGreal N, Jensen DM. Sustained viral response after interferon-based therapy in chronic hepatitis C: more evidence to support a life-long cure. *Liver Int* 2009;29:481–2.

533. Nelson DR, Davis GL, Jacobson I, et al. Hepatitis C virus: a critical appraisal of approaches to therapy. *Clin Gastroenterol Hepatol* 2009;7:397–414; quiz 366.

534. Radkowski M, Gallegos-Orozco JF, Jablonska J, et al. Persistence of hepatitis C virus in patients successfully treated for chronic hepatitis C. *Hepatology* 2005;41:106–14.

535. Radkowski M, Horban A, Gallegos-Orozco JF, et al. Evidence for viral persistence in patients who test positive for anti-hepatitis C virus antibodies and have normal alanine aminotransferase levels. *J Infect Dis* 2005;191:1730–3.

536. George SL, Bacon BR, Brunt EM, Mihindukulasuriya KL, Hoffmann J, Di Bisceglie AM. Clinical, virologic, histologic, and biochemical outcomes after successful HCV therapy: a 5-year follow-up of 150 patients. *Hepatology* 2009;49:729–38.

537. Marcellin P, Boyer N, Gervais A, et al. Long-term histologic improvement and loss of detectable intrahepatic HCV RNA in patients with chronic hepatitis C and sustained response to interferon-alpha therapy. *Ann Intern Med* 1997;127:875–81.

538. Bruno S, Stroffolini T, Colombo M, et al. Sustained virological response to interferon-alpha is associated with improved outcome in HCV-related cirrhosis: a retrospective study. *Hepatology* 2007;45:579–87.

539. Alberti A. Impact of a sustained virological response on the long-term outcome of hepatitis C. *Liver Int* 2011;31(Suppl 1):18–22.

540. Veldt BJ, Heathcote EJ, Wedemeyer H, et al. Sustained virologic response and clinical outcomes in patients with chronic hepatitis C and advanced fibrosis. *Ann Intern Med* 2007;147:677–84.

541. Backus L, Boothroyd DB, Phillips BR, Mole LA. Impact of sustained virological response to pegylated interferon/ribavirin on all-cause mortality by HCV genotype in a large real-world cohort: the US Department of Veterans Affairs' experience [Abstract]. *Hepatology* 2010;52:428A.

542. Darling JM, Fried MW. Optimizing treatment regimens in hepatitis C. *Clin Liver Dis* 2006;10:835–50.

543. Fried MW. The role of triple therapy in HCV genotype 1-experienced patients. *Liver Int* 2011;31(Suppl 1):58–61.

544. Hoofnagle JH, Mullen KD, Jones DB, et al. Treatment of chronic non-A,non-B hepatitis with recombinant human alpha interferon. A preliminary report. *N Engl J Med* 1986;315:1575–8.

545. Davis GL, Balart LA, Schiff ER, et al. Treatment of chronic hepatitis C with recombinant interferon alfa. A multicenter randomized, controlled trial. Hepatitis Interventional Therapy Group. *N Engl J Med* 1989;321:1501–6.

546. Di Bisceglie AM, Martin P, Kassianides C, et al. Recombinant interferon alfa therapy for chronic hepatitis C. A randomized, double-blind, placebo-controlled trial. *N Engl J Med* 1989;321:1506–10.

547. Poynard T, Bedossa P, Chevallier M, et al. A comparison of three interferon alfa-2b regimens for the long-term treatment of chronic non-A, non-B hepatitis. Multicenter Study Group. *N Engl J Med* 1995;332:1457–62.

548. Carithers RL Jr, Emerson SS. Therapy of hepatitis C: meta-analysis of interferon alfa-2b trials. *Hepatology* 1997;26:S83–8.

549. Lindsay KL, Davis GL, Schiff ER, et al. Response to higher doses of interferon alfa-2b in patients with chronic hepatitis C: a randomized multicenter trial. Hepatitis Interventional Therapy Group. *Hepatology* 1996;24:1034–40.

550. Thevenot T, Regimbeau C, Ratziu V, Leroy V, Opolon P, Poynard T. Meta-analysis of interferon randomized trials in the treatment of viral hepatitis C in naive patients: 1999 update. *J Viral Hepat* 2001;8:48–62.

551. Brillanti S, Garson J, Foli M, et al. A pilot study of combination therapy with ribavirin plus interferon alfa for interferon alfa-resistant chronic hepatitis C. *Gastroenterology* 1994;107:812–17.

552. Gilbert BE, Knight V. Biochemistry and clinical applications of ribavirin. *Antimicrob Agents Chemother* 1986;30:201–5.

553. Chung RT, Gale M Jr, Polyak SJ, Lemon SM, Liang TJ, Hoofnagle JH. Mechanisms of action of interferon and ribavirin in chronic hepatitis C: summary of a workshop. *Hepatology* 2008;47:306–20.

554. Maag D, Castro C, Hong Z, Cameron CE. Hepatitis C virus RNA-dependent RNA polymerase (NS5B) as a mediator of the antiviral activity of ribavirin. *J Biol Chem* 2001;276:46094–8.

555. Cornberg M, Hinrichsen H, Teuber G, et al. Mycophenolate mofetil in combination with recombinant interferon alfa-2a in interferon-nonresponder patients with chronic hepatitis C. *J Hepatol* 2002;37:843–7.

556. Feld JJ, Nanda S, Huang Y, et al. Hepatic gene expression during treatment with peginterferon and ribavirin: identifying molecular pathways for treatment response. *Hepatology* 2007;46:1548–63.

557. Feld JJ, Lutchman GA, Heller T, et al. Ribavirin improves early responses to peginterferon through improved interferon signaling. *Gastroenterology* 2010;139:154–62, e154.

558. Di Bisceglie AM, Conjeevaram HS, Fried MW, et al. Ribavirin as therapy for chronic hepatitis C. A randomized, double-blind, placebo-controlled trial. *Ann Intern Med* 1995;123:897–903.

559. Bodenheimer HC Jr, Lindsay KL, Davis GL, Lewis JH, Thung SN, Seeff LB. Tolerance and efficacy of oral ribavirin treatment of chronic hepatitis C: a multicenter trial. *Hepatology* 1997;26:473–7.

560. Hoofnagle JH, Lau D, Conjeevaram H, Kleiner D, Di Bisceglie AM. Prolonged therapy of chronic hepatitis C with ribavirin. *J Viral Hepat* 1996;3:247–52.

561. McHutchison JG, Gordon SC, Schiff ER, et al. Interferon alfa-2b alone or in combination with ribavirin as initial treatment for chronic hepatitis C. Hepatitis Interventional Therapy Group. *N Engl J Med* 1998;339:1485–92.

562. Poynard T, Marcellin P, Lee SS, et al. Randomised trial of interferon alpha2b plus ribavirin for 48 weeks or for 24 weeks versus interferon alpha2b plus placebo for 48 weeks for treatment of chronic infection with hepatitis C virus. International Hepatitis Interventional Therapy Group (IHIT). *Lancet* 1998;352:1426–32.

563. Pedder SC. Pegylation of interferon alfa: structural and pharmacokinetic properties. *Semin Liver Dis* 2003;23(Suppl 1):19–22.

564. Zeuzem S, Welsch C, Herrmann E. Pharmacokinetics of peginterferons. *Semin Liver Dis* 2003;23(Suppl 1):23–8.

565. Jain A, Jain SK. PEGylation: an approach for drug delivery. A review. *Crit Rev Ther Drug Carrier Syst* 2008;25:403–47.

566. Glue P, Fang JW, Rouzier-Panis R, et al. Pegylated interferon-alpha2b: pharmacokinetics, pharmacodynamics, safety, and preliminary efficacy data. Hepatitis C Intervention Therapy Group. *Clin Pharmacol Ther* 2000;68:556–67.

567. McHutchison JG, Lawitz EJ, Shiffman ML, et al. Peginterferon alfa-2b or alfa-2a with ribavirin for treatment of hepatitis C infection. *N Engl J Med* 2009;361:580–93.

568. Fried MW, Shiffman ML, Reddy KR, et al. Combination of peginterferon alfa-2a plus ribavirin in patients with chronic hepatitis C virus infection. *N Engl J Med* 2002;347:975–82.

569. Manns MP, McHutchison JG, Gordon SC, et al. Peginterferon alfa-2b plus ribavirin compared with interferon alfa-2b plus ribavirin for initial treatment of chronic hepatitis C: a randomised trial. *Lancet* 2001;358:958–65.

570. Hadziyannis SJ, Sette H Jr, Morgan TR, et al. Peginterferon-alpha2a and ribavirin combination therapy in chronic hepatitis C: a randomized study of treatment duration and ribavirin dose. *Ann Intern Med* 2004;140:346–55.

571. Davis GL. Monitoring of viral levels during therapy of hepatitis C. *Hepatology* 2002;36:145–51.

572. Fried MW, Hadziyannis SJ, Shiffman ML, Messinger D, Zeuzem S. Rapid virological response is the most important predictor of sustained virological response across genotypes in patients with chronic hepatitis C virus infection. *J Hepatol* 2011;55:69–75.

573. Ferenci P, Fried MW, Shiffman ML, et al. Predicting sustained virological responses in chronic hepatitis C patients treated with peginterferon alfa-2a (40 KD)/ribavirin. *J Hepatol* 2005;43:425–433.

574. Ferenci P. Predicting the therapeutic response in patients with chronic hepatitis C: the role of viral kinetic studies. *J Antimicrob Chemother* 2004;53:15–18.

575. Jensen DM, Morgan TR, Marcellin P, et al. Early identification of HCV genotype 1 patients responding to 24 weeks peginterferon alpha-2a (40 kd)/ribavirin therapy. *Hepatology* 2006;43:954–60.

576. Zeuzem S, Poordad F. Pegylated-interferon plus ribavirin therapy in the treatment of CHC: individualization of treatment duration according to on-treatment virologic response. *Curr Med Res Opin* 2010;26:1733–43.

577. Zeuzem S, Buti M, Ferenci P, et al. Efficacy of 24 weeks treatment with peginterferon alfa-2b plus ribavirin in patients with chronic hepatitis C infected with genotype 1 and low pretreatment viremia. *J Hepatol* 2006;44:97–103.

578. Craxi A, Zuckerman E, Koutsounas S, et al. PREDICT study final results: efficacy and safety of a 24-wk regimen of peginterferon alfa-2b plus weight-based ribavirin in patients with chronic hepatitis C virus (HCV) genotype 1 (G1) with low viral load who achieve rapid viral response. *Hepatology* 2009;50:693A (Abstract).

579. Ferenci P, Laferl H, Scherzer TM, et al. Peginterferon alfa-2a and ribavirin for 24 weeks in hepatitis C type 1 and 4 patients with rapid virological response. *Gastroenterology* 2008;135:451–8.

580. Mangia A, Minerva N, Bacca D, et al. Individualized treatment duration for hepatitis C genotype 1 patients: a randomized controlled trial. *Hepatology* 2008;47:43–50.

581. Berg T, Weich V, Teuber G, et al. Individualized treatment strategy according to early viral kinetics in hepatitis C virus type 1-infected patients. *Hepatology* 2009;50:369–77.

582. Mangia A, Santoro R, Minerva N, et al. Peginterferon alfa-2b and ribavirin for 12 vs. 24 weeks in HCV genotype 2 or 3. *N Engl J Med* 2005;352:2609–17.

583. Shiffman ML, Suter F, Bacon BR, et al. Peginterferon alfa-2a and ribavirin for 16 or 24 weeks in HCV genotype 2 or 3. *N Engl J Med* 2007;357:124–34.

584. Singal AK, Freeman DH Jr, Anand BS. Meta-analysis: interferon improves outcomes following ablation or resection of hepatocellular carcinoma. *Aliment Pharmacol Ther* 2010;32:851–8.

585. Drusano GL, Preston SL. A 48-week duration of therapy with pegylated interferon alpha 2b plus ribavirin may be too short to maximize long-term response among patients infected with genotype-1 hepatitis C virus. *J Infect Dis* 2004;189:964–70.

586. Berg T, von Wagner M, Nasser S, et al. Extended treatment duration for hepatitis C virus type 1: comparing 48 versus 72 weeks of peginterferon-alfa-2a plus ribavirin. *Gastroenterology* 2006;130:1086–97.

587. Pearlman BL, Ehleben C, Saifee S. Treatment extension to 72 weeks of peginterferon and ribavirin in hepatitis C genotype 1–infected slow responders. *Hepatology* 2007;46:1688–94.

588. Buti M, Lurie Y, Zakharova NG, et al. Randomized trial of peginterferon alfa-2b and ribavirin for 48 or 72 weeks in patients with hepatitis C virus genotype 1 and slow virologic response. *Hepatology* 2010;52:1201–7.

589. Farnik H, Lange CM, Sarrazin C, Kronenberger B, Zeuzem S, Herrmann E. Meta-analysis shows extended therapy improves response of patients with chronic hepatitis C virus genotype 1 infection. *Clin Gastroenterol Hepatol* 2010;8:884–90.

590. Snoeck E, Wade JR, Duff F, Lamb M, Jorga K. Predicting sustained virological response and anaemia in chronic hepatitis C patients treated with peginterferon alfa-2a (40KD) plus ribavirin. *Br J Clin Pharmacol* 2006;62:699–709.

591. Wade JR, Snoeck E, Duff F, Lamb M, Jorga K. Pharmacokinetics of ribavirin in patients with hepatitis C virus. *Br J Clin Pharmacol* 2006;62:710–14.

592. Lindahl K, Stahle L, Bruchfeld A, Schvarcz R. High-dose ribavirin in combination with standard dose peginterferon for treatment of patients with chronic hepatitis C. *Hepatology* 2005;41:275–9.

593. McHutchison JG, Manns M, Patel K, et al. Adherence to combination therapy enhances sustained response in genotype-1-infected patients with chronic hepatitis C. *Gastroenterology* 2002;123:1061–9.

594. Reddy KR, Shiffman ML, Morgan TR, et al. Impact of ribavirin dose reductions in hepatitis C virus genotype 1 patients completing peginterferon alfa-2a/ribavirin treatment. *Clin Gastroenterol Hepatol* 2007;5:124–9.

595. Bronowicki JP, Ouzan D, Asselah T, et al. Effect of ribavirin in genotype 1 patients with hepatitis C responding to pegylated interferon alfa-2a plus ribavirin. *Gastroenterology* 2006;131:1040–8.

596. Jarvis SM, Thorn JA, Glue P. Ribavirin uptake by human erythrocytes and the involvement of nitrobenzylthioinosine-sensitive (es)-nucleoside transporters. *Br J Pharmacol* 1998;123:1587–92.

597. De Franceschi L, Fattovich G, Turrini F, et al. Hemolytic anemia induced by ribavirin therapy in patients with chronic hepatitis C virus infection: role of membrane oxidative damage. *Hepatology* 2000;31:997–1004.

598. Fried MW. Side effects of therapy for hepatitis C and their management. *Hepatology* 2002;36:237–44.

599. Sulkowski MS, Shiffman ML, Afdhal NH, et al. Hepatitis C virus treatment-related anemia is associated with higher sustained virologic response rate. *Gastroenterology* 2010;139:1602–11, e1601.

600. Reau N, Hadziyannis SJ, Messinger D, Fried MW, Jensen DM. Early predictors of anemia in patients with hepatitis C genotype 1 treated with peginterferon alfa-2a (40KD) plus ribavirin. *Am J Gastroenterol* 2008;103:1981–8.

601. Afdhal NH, Dieterich DT, Pockros PJ, et al. Epoetin alfa maintains ribavirin dose in HCV-infected patients: a prospective, double-blind, randomized controlled study. *Gastroenterology* 2004;126:1302–11.

602. Shiffman ML, Salvatore J, Hubbard S, et al. Treatment of chronic hepatitis C virus genotype 1 with peginterferon, ribavirin, and epoetin alpha. *Hepatology* 2007;46:371–9.

603. Bertino G, Ardiri A, Boemi PM, et al. Epoetin alpha improves the response to antiviral treatment in HCV-related chronic hepatitis. *Eur J Clin Pharmacol* 2010;66:1055–63.

604. Tanaka N, Ishida F, Tanaka E. Ribavirin-induced pure red-cell aplasia during treatment of chronic hepatitis C. *N Engl J Med* 2004;350:1264–5.

605. Fellay J, Thompson AJ, Ge D, et al. ITPA gene variants protect against anaemia in patients treated for chronic hepatitis C. *Nature* 2010;464:405–8.

606. Thompson AJ, Fellay J, Patel K, et al. Variants in the ITPA gene protect against ribavirin-induced hemolytic anemia and decrease the need for ribavirin dose reduction. *Gastroenterology* 2010;139:1181–9.

607. Poordad F, Lawitz E, Shiffman ML, et al. Virologic response rates of weight-based taribavirin versus ribavirin in treatment-naive patients with genotype 1 chronic hepatitis C. *Hepatology* 2010;52:1208–15.

608. Benhamou Y, Afdhal NH, Nelson DR, et al. A phase III study of the safety and efficacy of viramidine versus ribavirin in treatment-naive patients with chronic hepatitis C: ViSER1 results. *Hepatology* 2009;50:717–26.

609. Marcellin P, Gish RG, Gitlin N, et al. Safety and efficacy of viramidine versus ribavirin in ViSER2: randomized, double-blind study in therapy naive hepatitis C patients. *J Hepatol* 2010;52:32–8.

610. Afdhal NH, McHutchison JG, Zeuzem S, et al. Hepatitis C pharmacogenetics: state of the art in 2010. *Hepatology* 2010;53:336–45.

611. Balagopal A, Thomas DL, Thio CL. IL28B and the control of hepatitis C virus infection. *Gastroenterology* 2010;139:1865–76.

612. Suppiah V, Moldovan M, Ahlenstiel G, et al. IL28B is associated with response to chronic hepatitis C interferon-alpha and ribavirin therapy. *Nat Genet* 2009;41:1100–4.

613. Thompson AJ, Muir AJ, Sulkowski MS, et al. Interleukin-28B polymorphism improves viral kinetics and is the strongest pretreatment predictor of sustained virologic response in genotype 1 hepatitis C virus. *Gastroenterology* 2010;139:120–9, e118.

614. Mangia A, Thompson AJ, Santoro R, et al. An IL28B polymorphism determines treatment response of hepatitis C virus genotype 2 or 3 patients who do not achieve a rapid virologic response. *Gastroenterology* 2010;139:821–7, e821.

615. Honda M, Sakai A, Yamashita T, et al. Hepatic ISG expression is associated with genetic variation in interleukin 28B and the outcome of IFN therapy for chronic hepatitis C. *Gastroenterology* 2010;139:499–509.

616. Urban TJ, Thompson AJ, Bradrick SS, et al. IL28B genotype is associated with differential expression of intrahepatic interferon-stimulated genes in patients with chronic hepatitis C. *Hepatology* 2010;52:1888–96.

617. Dill MT, Duong FH, Vogt JE, et al. Interferon-induced gene expression is a stronger predictor of treatment response than IL28B genotype in patients with hepatitis C. *Gastroenterology* 2011;140:1021–31.

618. Darling JM, Aerssens J, Fanning G, et al. Quantitation of pretreatment serum interferon-gamma-inducible protein-10 improves the predictive value of an IL28B gene polymorphism for hepatitis C treatment response. *Hepatology* 2011;53:14–22.

619. Snow KK, Bonkovsky HL, Fontana RJ, et al. Changes in quality of life and sexual health are associated with low-dose peginterferon therapy and disease progression in patients with chronic hepatitis C. *Aliment Pharmacol Ther* 2010;31:719–34.

620. Bernstein D, Kleinman L, Barker CM, Revicki DA, Green J. Relationship of health-related quality of life to treatment adherence and sustained response in chronic hepatitis C patients. *Hepatology* 2002;35:704–8.

621. Russo MW, Fried MW. Side effects of therapy for chronic hepatitis C. *Gastroenterology* 2003;124:1711–19.

622. Conjeevaram HS, Fried MW, Jeffers LJ, et al. Peginterferon and ribavirin treatment in African American and Caucasian American patients with hepatitis C genotype 1. *Gastroenterology* 2006;131:470–7.

623. Raison CL, Borisov AS, Broadwell SD, et al. Depression during pegylated interferon-alpha plus ribavirin therapy: prevalence and prediction. *J Clin Psychiatry* 2005;66:41–8.

624. Evon DM, Verma A, Dougherty KA, et al. High deferral rates and poorer treatment outcomes for HCV patients with psychiatric and substance use comorbidities. *Dig Dis Sci* 2007;52:3251–8.

625. Evon DM, Verma A, Simpson K, Galanko JA, Dougherty KA, Fried MW. Psychiatric symptoms during interferon treatment for hepatitis C: experiences from a tertiary care hepatology centre. *Aliment Pharmacol Ther* 2008;27:1071–80.

626. Raison CL, Demetrashvili M, Capuron L, Miller AH. Neuropsychiatric adverse effects of interferon-alpha: recognition and management. *CNS Drugs* 2005;19:105–23.

627. Evon DM, Ramcharran D, Belle SH, Terrault NA, Fontana RJ, Fried MW. Prospective analysis of depression during peginterferon and ribavirin therapy of chronic hepatitis C: results of the Virahep-C study. *Am J Gastroenterol* 2009;104:2949–58.

628. Raison CL, Woolwine BJ, Demetrashvili MF, et al. Paroxetine for prevention of depressive symptoms induced by interferon-alpha and ribavirin for hepatitis C. *Aliment Pharmacol Ther* 2007;25:1163–74.

629. Kraus MR, Schafer A, Al-Taie O, Scheurlen M. Prophylactic SSRI during interferon alpha re-therapy in patients with chronic hepatitis C and a history of interferon-induced depression. *J Viral Hepat* 2005;12:96–100.

630. Kraus MR, Schafer A, Schottker K, et al. Therapy of interferon-induced depression in chronic hepatitis C with citalopram: a randomised, double-blind, placebo-controlled study. *Gut* 2008;57:531–6.

631. Carella C, Mazziotti G, Morisco F, et al. Long-term outcome of interferon-alpha-induced thyroid autoimmunity and prognostic influence of thyroid autoantibody pattern at the end of treatment. *J Clin Endocrinol Metab* 2001;86:1925–9.

632. Kim ET, Kim LH, Lee JI, Chin HS. Retinopathy in hepatitis C patients due to combination therapy with pegylated interferon and ribavirin. *Jpn J Ophthalmol* 2009;53:598–602.

633. Panetta JD, Gilani N. Interferon-induced retinopathy and its risk in patients with diabetes and hypertension undergoing treatment for chronic hepatitis C virus infection. *Aliment Pharmacol Ther* 2009;30:597–602.

634. Slavenburg S, Heijdra YF, Drenth JP. Pneumonitis as a consequence of (peg)interferon–ribavirin combination therapy for hepatitis C: a review of the literature. *Dig Dis Sci* 2010;55:579–85.

635. Everson GT, Trotter J, Forman L, et al. Treatment of advanced hepatitis C with a low accelerating dosage regimen of antiviral therapy. *Hepatology* 2005;42:255–62.

636. Everson GT. Treatment of hepatitis C in the patient with decompensated cirrhosis. *Clin Gastroenterol Hepatol* 2005;3:S106–12.

637. Morgan TR, Ghany MG, Kim HY, et al. Outcome of sustained virological responders with histologically advanced chronic hepatitis C. *Hepatology* 2010;52:833–44.

638. Singal AG, Volk ML, Jensen D, Di Bisceglie AM, Schoenfeld PS. A sustained viral response is associated with reduced liver-related morbidity and mortality in patients with hepatitis C virus. *Clin Gastroenterol Hepatol* 2010;8:280–8, e281.

639. Muir AJ, Bornstein JD, Killenberg PG. Peginterferon alfa-2b and ribavirin for the treatment of chronic hepatitis C in blacks and non-Hispanic whites. *N Engl J Med* 2004;350:2265–71.

640. Jeffers LJ, Cassidy W, Howell CD, Hu S, Reddy KR. Peginterferon alfa-2a (40 kd) and ribavirin for black American patients with chronic HCV genotype 1. *Hepatology* 2004;39:1702–8.

641. Rodriguez-Torres M, Jeffers LJ, Sheikh MY, et al. Peginterferon alfa-2a and ribavirin in Latino and non-Latino whites with hepatitis C. *N Engl J Med* 2009;360:257–67.

642. Simard EP, Engels EA. Cancer as a cause of death among people with AIDS in the United States. *Clin Infect Dis* 2010;51:957–62.

643. Loko MA, Salmon D, Carrieri P, et al. The French national prospective cohort of patients co-infected with HIV and HCV (ANRS CO13 HEPAVIH): early findings, 2006–2010. *BMC Infect Dis* 2010;10:303.

644. Sulkowski MS, Thomas DL. Hepatitis C in the HIV-infected person. *Ann Intern Med* 2003;138:197–207.

645. Sulkowski MS, Thomas DL, Chaisson RE, Moore RD. Hepatotoxicity associated with antiretroviral therapy in adults infected with human immunodeficiency virus and the role of hepatitis C or B virus infection. *JAMA* 2000;283:74–80.

646. Vispo E, Barreiro P, Pineda JA, et al. Low response to pegylated interferon plus ribavirin in HIV-infected patients with chronic hepatitis C treated with abacavir. *Antivir Ther* 2008;13:429–37.

647. Amorosa VK, Slim J, Mounzer K, et al. The influence of abacavir and other antiretroviral agents on virological response to HCV therapy among antiretroviral-treated HIV-infected patients. *Antivir Ther* 2010;15:91–9.

648. Reiberger T, Kosi L, Maresch J, et al. Mitochondrial toxicity is associated with virological response in patients with HIV and hepatitis C virus coinfection treated with ribavirin and highly active antiretroviral therapy. *J Infect Dis* 2010;202:156–60.

649. Gluud LL, Marchesini E, Iorio A. Peginterferon plus ribavirin for chronic hepatitis C in patients with human immunodeficiency virus. *Am J Gastroenterol* 2009;104:2335–41; quiz 2342.

650. Pineda JA, Caruz A, Rivero A, et al. Prediction of response to pegylated interferon plus ribavirin by IL28B gene variation in patients coinfected with HIV and hepatitis C virus. *Clin Infect Dis* 2010;51:788–95.

651. Aparicio E, Parera M, Franco S, et al. IL28B SNP rs8099917 is strongly associated with pegylated interferon-alpha and ribavirin therapy treatment failure in HCV/HIV-1 coinfected patients. *PLoS One* 2010;5:e13771.

652. Chung RT, Andersen J, Volberding P, et al. Peginterferon alfa-2a plus ribavirin versus interferon alfa-2a plus ribavirin for chronic hepatitis C in HIV-coinfected persons. *N Engl J Med* 2004;351:451–9.

653. Torriani FJ, Rodriguez-Torres M, Rockstroh JK, et al. Peginterferon alfa-2a plus ribavirin for chronic hepatitis C virus infection in HIV-infected patients. *N Engl J Med* 2004;351:438–50.

654. Crespo M, Sauleda S, Esteban JI, et al. Peginterferon alpha-2b plus ribavirin vs interferon alpha-2b plus ribavirin for chronic hepatitis C in HIV-coinfected patients. *J Viral Hepat* 2007;14:228–38.

655. Rodriguez-Torres M, Slim J, Bhatti L, et al. Standard- versus high-dose ribavirin in combination with peginterferon alfa-2a (40KD) in genotype 1 HCV patients co-infected with HIV: final results of the PARADIGM study [Abstract]. *Hepatology* 2009;50:1022A (Abstract).

656. Meyers CM, Seeff LB, Stehman-Breen CO, Hoofnagle JH. Hepatitis C and renal disease: an update. *Am J Kidney Dis* 2003;42:631–57.

657. Martin P, Fabrizi F. Hepatitis C virus and kidney disease. *J Hepatol* 2008;49:613–24.

658. Aroldi A, Lampertico P, Montagnino G, et al. Natural history of hepatitis B and C in renal allograft recipients. *Transplantation* 2005;79:1132–6.

659. Rahnavardi M, Hosseini Moghaddam SM, Alavian SM. Hepatitis C in hemodialysis patients: current global magnitude, natural history, diagnostic difficulties, and preventive measures. *Am J Nephrol* 2008;28:628–40.

660. Fabrizi F, Dixit V, Messa P, Martin P. Pegylated interferon monotherapy of chronic hepatitis C in dialysis patients: meta-analysis of clinical trials. *J Med Virol* 2010;82:768–75.

661. Berenguer M. Treatment of chronic hepatitis C in hemodialysis patients. *Hepatology* 2008;48:1690–9.

662. Fabrizi F, Lunghi G, Dixit V, Martin P. Meta-analysis: anti-viral therapy of hepatitis C virus-related liver disease in renal transplant patients. *Aliment Pharmacol Ther* 2006;24:1413–22.

663. Zylberberg H, Carnot F, Mamzer MF, Blancho G, Legendre C, Pol S. Hepatitis C virus-related fibrosing cholestatic hepatitis after renal transplantation. *Transplantation* 1997;63:158–60.

664. Toth CM, Pascual M, Chung RT, et al. Hepatitis C virus-associated fibrosing cholestatic hepatitis after renal transplantation: response to interferon-alpha therapy. *Transplantation* 1998;66:1254–8.

665. Saadoun D, Landau DA, Calabrese LH, Cacoub PP. Hepatitis C-associated mixed cryoglobulinaemia: a crossroad between autoimmunity and lymphoproliferation. *Rheumatology (Oxford)* 2007;46:1234–42.

666. Iannuzzella F, Vaglio A, Garini G. Management of hepatitis C virus-related mixed cryoglobulinemia. *Am J Med* 2010;123:400–8.

667. Vigano M, Lampertico P, Rumi MG, et al. Natural history and clinical impact of cryoglobulins in chronic hepatitis C: 10-year prospective study of 343 patients. *Gastroenterology* 2007;133:835–42.

668. Maheshwari A, Ray S, Thuluvath PJ. Acute hepatitis C. *Lancet* 2008;372:321–32.

669. Gerlach JT, Diepolder HM, Zachoval R, et al. Acute hepatitis C: high rate of both spontaneous and treatment-induced viral clearance. *Gastroenterology* 2003;125:80–8.

670. Kamal SM. Acute hepatitis C: a systematic review. *Am J Gastroenterol* 2008;103:1283–97; quiz 1298.

671. Wiegand J, Buggisch P, Boecher W, et al. Early monotherapy with pegylated interferon alpha-2b for acute hepatitis C infection: the HEP-NET acute-HCV-II study. *Hepatology* 2006;43:250–6.

672. Jaeckel E, Cornberg M, Wedemeyer H, et al. Treatment of acute hepatitis C with interferon alfa-2b. *N Engl J Med* 2001;345:1452–7.

673. Kamal SM, Moustafa KN, Chen J, et al. Duration of peginterferon therapy in acute hepatitis C: a randomized trial. *Hepatology* 2006;43:923–31.

674. Loomba R, Rivera MM, McBurney R, et al. The natural history of acute hepatitis C: clinical presentation, laboratory findings and treatment outcomes. *Aliment Pharmacol Ther* 2011;33:559–65.

675. Fried MW. Genotype 1: managing the non-responders and relapsers. In: Foster GR, Reddy KR, eds. *Clinical Dilemmas in Viral Liver Disease*. Oxford: Wiley-Blackwell, 2009:38–42.

676. Singal AG, Waljee AK, Shiffman M, Bacon BR, Schoenfeld PS. Meta-analysis: re-treatment of genotype I hepatitis C nonresponders and relapsers after failing interferon and ribavirin combination therapy. *Aliment Pharmacol Ther* 2010;32:969–83.

677. Bacon BR, Shiffman ML, Mendes F, et al. Retreating chronic hepatitis C with daily interferon alfacon-1/ribavirin after nonresponse to pegylated interferon/ribavirin: DIRECT results. *Hepatology* 2009;49:1838–46.

678. Poynard T, Colombo M, Bruix J, et al. Peginterferon alfa-2b and ribavirin: effective in patients with hepatitis C who failed interferon alfa/ribavirin therapy. *Gastroenterology* 2009;136:1618–28, e1612.

679. Jensen DM, Marcellin P, Freilich B, et al. Re-treatment of patients with chronic hepatitis C who do not respond to peginterferon-alpha2b: a randomized trial. *Ann Intern Med* 2009;150:528–40.

680. Di Bisceglie AM, Shiffman ML, Everson GT, et al. Prolonged therapy of advanced chronic hepatitis C with low-dose peginterferon. *N Engl J Med* 2008;359:2429–41.

681. Lok AS, Everhart JE, Wright EC, Morgan TR, Di Bisceglie AM, Kim HY. Maintenance peginterferon therapy to prevent hepatocellular carcinoma in patients with advanced chronic hepatitis C: extended follow-up results from the HALT-C trial [Abstract]. *Hepatology* 2010;52:428A.

682. Afdhal N, Freilich B, Levine R, et al. Colchicine vs peginterferon alfa-2b long-term therapy: results of the 4-year COPILOT trial [Abstract]. *J Hepatol* 2008;48:54.

683. Shimakami T, Lanford RE, Lemon SM. Hepatitis C: recent successes and continuing challenges in the development of improved treatment modalities. *Curr Opin Pharmacol* 2009;9:537–44.

684. Steinkuhler C, Biasiol G, Brunetti M, et al. Product inhibition of the hepatitis C virus NS3 protease. *Biochemistry* 1998;37:8899–905.

685. Susser S, Welsch C, Wang Y, et al. Characterization of resistance to the protease inhibitor boceprevir in hepatitis C virus-infected patients. *Hepatology* 2009;50:1709–18.

686. Kieffer TL, Sarrazin C, Miller JS, et al. Telaprevir and pegylated interferon-alpha-2a inhibit wild-type and resistant genotype 1 hepatitis C virus replication in patients. *Hepatology* 2007;46:631–9.

687. Olsen DB, Eldrup AB, Bartholomew L, et al. A 7-deaza-adenosine analog is a potent and selective inhibitor of hepatitis C virus replication with excellent pharmacokinetic properties. *Antimicrob Agents Chemother* 2004;48:3944–53.

688. Tomei L, Altamura S, Bartholomew L, et al. Characterization of the inhibition of hepatitis C virus RNA replication by nonnucleosides. *J Virol* 2004;78:938–46.

689. Le PS, Kang H, Harris JF, et al. Selection and characterization of replicon variants dually resistant to thumb- and palm-binding nonnucleoside polymerase inhibitors of the hepatitis C virus. *J Virol* 2006;80:6146–54.

690. Najera I, Le Pogam S, Seshaadri A, et al. A high barrier to resistance may contribute to the robust antiviral effect demonstrated by R1626 in HCV genotype 1-infected treatment-naive patients. *Hepatology* 2007;46:813A [Abstract].

691. Biswal BK, Cherney MM, Wang M, et al. Crystal structures of the RNA-dependent RNA polymerase genotype 2a of hepatitis C virus reveal two conformations and suggest mechanisms of inhibition by non-nucleoside inhibitors. *J Biol Chem* 2005;280:18202–10.

692. Gao M, Nettles RE, Belema M, et al. Chemical genetics strategy identifies an HCV NS5A inhibitor with a potent clinical effect. *Nature* 2010;465:96–100.

693. Lanford RE, Hildebrandt-Eriksen ES, Petri A, et al. Therapeutic silencing of microRNA-122 in primates with chronic hepatitis C virus infection. *Science* 2010;327:198–201.

694. Einav S, Gerber D, Bryson PD, et al. Discovery of a hepatitis C target and its pharmacological inhibitors by microfluidic affinity analysis. *Nat Biotechnol* 2008;26:1019–27.

695. Lamarre D, Anderson PC, Bailey M, et al. An NS3 protease inhibitor with antiviral effects in humans infected with hepatitis C virus. *Nature* 2003;426:186–9.

696. Hinrichsen H, Benhamou Y, Wedemeyer H, et al. Short-term antiviral efficacy of BILN 2061, a hepatitis C virus serine protease inhibitor, in hepatitis C genotype 1 patients. *Gastroenterology* 2004;127:1347–55.

697. Perni RB, Almquist SJ, Byrn RA, et al. Preclinical profile of VX-950, a potent, selective, and orally bioavailable inhibitor of hepatitis C virus NS3-4A serine protease. *Antimicrob Agents Chemother* 2006;50:899–909.

698. Lin K, Perni RB, Kwong AD, Lin C. VX-950, a novel hepatitis C virus (HCV) NS3-4A protease inhibitor, exhibits potent antiviral activities in HCv replicon cells. *Antimicrob Agents Chemother* 2006;50:1813–22.

699. Reesink HW, Zeuzem S, Weegink CJ, et al. Rapid decline of viral RNA in hepatitis C patients treated with VX-950: a phase Ib, placebo-controlled, randomized study. *Gastroenterology* 2006;131:997–1002.

700. Sarrazin C, Kieffer TL, Bartels D, et al. Dynamic hepatitis C virus genotypic and phenotypic changes in patients treated with the protease inhibitor telaprevir. *Gastroenterology* 2007;132:1767–77.

701. Zhou Y, Muh U, Hanzelka BL, et al. Phenotypic and structural analyses of hepatitis C virus NS3 protease Arg155 variants: sensitivity to telaprevir (VX-950) and interferon alpha. *J Biol Chem* 2007;282:22619–28.

702. Kieffer TL, Sarrazin C, Miller JS, et al. Telaprevir and pegylated interferon-alpha-2a inhibit wild-type and resistant genotype 1 hepatitis C virus replication in patients. *Hepatology* 2007;46:631–9.

703. Forestier N, Reesink HW, Weegink CJ, et al. Antiviral activity of telaprevir (VX-950) and peginterferon alfa-2a in patients with hepatitis C. *Hepatology* 2007;46:640–8.

704. McHutchison JG, Everson GT, Gordon SC, et al. Telaprevir with peginterferon and ribavirin for chronic HCV genotype 1 infection. *N Engl J Med* 2009;360:1827–38.

705. Hezode C, Forestier N, Dusheiko G, et al. Telaprevir and peginterferon with or without ribavirin for chronic HCV infection. *N Engl J Med* 2009;360:1839–50.

706. Jacobson IM, McHutchison JG, Dusheiko G, et al.; ADVANCE Study Team. Telaprevir for previously untreated chronic hepatitis C virus infection. *N Engl J Med* 2011;364(25):2405–16.

707. Sherman KE, Flamm SL, Afdhal NH, et al. Tealprevir in combination with peginterferon alfa-2a and ribavirin for 24 or 48 weeks in treatment-naive genotype 1 HCV patients who achieved and extended rapid virological response: final results of the phase 3 ILLUMINATE study [Abstract]. *Hepatology* 2010;52:late breaker abstract 2.

708. Sarrazin C, Rouzier R, Wagner F, et al. SCH 503034, a novel hepatitis C virus protease inhibitor, plus pegylated interferon alpha-2b for genotype 1 nonresponders. *Gastroenterology* 2007;132:1270–8.

709. Schiff E, Poordad F, Jacobson I, et al. Boceprevir combination therapy in null responders: response dependent on interferon responsiveness. *J Hepatol* 2008;48:S46.

710. Kwo PY, Lawitz EJ, McCone J, et al. Efficacy of boceprevir, an NS3 protease inhibitor, in combination with peginterferon alfa-2b and ribavirin in treatment-naive patients with genotype 1 hepatitis C infection (SPRINT-1): an open-label, randomised, multicentre phase 2 trial. *Lancet* 2010;376:705–16.

711. Poordad F, McCone J Jr, Bacon BR, et al.; SPRINT-2 Investigators. Boceprevir for untreated chronic HCV genotype 1 infection. *N Engl J Med* 2011;364(13):1195–206.

712. McHutchison JG, Manns MP, Muir AJ, et al. Telaprevir for previously treated chronic HCV infection. *N Engl J Med* 2010;362:1292–303.

713. Zeuzem S, Andreone P, Pol S, et al.; REALIZE Study Team. Telaprevir for retreatment of HCV infection. *N Engl J Med* 2011;364(25):2417–28.

714. Bacon BR, Gordon SC, Lawitz E, et al.; HCV RESPOND-2 Investigators. Boceprevir for previously treated chronic HCV genotype 1 infection. *N Engl J Med* 2011;364(13):1207–17.

715. Neumann AU, Lam NP, Dahari H, et al. Hepatitis C viral dynamics in vivo and the antiviral efficacy of interferon-alpha therapy. *Science* 1998;282:103–7.

716. Rong L, Dahari H, Ribeiro RM, Perelson AS. Rapid emergence of protease inhibitor resistance in hepatitis C virus. *Sci Transl Med* 2010;2:30–2.

717. McHutchison J, Everson G, Gordon S, et al. Telaprevir with peginterferon and ribavirin for chronic HCV genotype 1 infection. *N Engl J Med* 2009;360:1827–38.

718. Sarrazin C, Rouzier R, Wagner F, et al. SCH 503034, a novel hepatitis C virus protease inhibitor, plus pegylated interferon alpha-2b for genotype 1 nonresponders. *Gastroenterology* 2007;132:1270–8.

719. Reesink H, Fanning G, Abou Farha K, et al. Rapid HCV-RNA decline with once-daily TMC435: a Phase I study in healthy volunteers and hepatitis C patients. *Gastroenterology* 2010;138:913–21.

720. Seiwert S, Andrews S, Jiang Y, et al. Preclinical characteristics of the hepatitis C virus NS3/4A protease inhibitor ITMN-191 (R7227). *Antimicrob Agents Chemother* 2008;52:4432–41.

721. Liverton N, Carroll S, Dimuzio J, et al. MK-7009: a potent and selective inhibitor of hepatitis C virus NS3/4A protease. *Antimicrob Agents Chemother* 2010;54:305–11.

722. Lin C, Gates C, Rao B, et al. In vitro studies of cross-resistance mutations against two hepatitis C virus serine protease inhibitors, VX-950 and BILN 2061. *J Biol Chem* 2005;280:36784–91.

723. Yi M, Tong X, Skelton A, et al. Mutations conferring resistance to SCH6, a novel hepatitis C virus NS3/4A protease inhibitor. Reduced RNA replication fitness and partial rescue by second-site mutations. *J Biol Chem* 2006;281:8205–15.

724. Tong X, Bogen S, Chase R, et al. Characterization of resistance mutations against HCV ketoamide protease inhibitors. *Antiviral Res* 2008;77:177–85.

725. Susser S, Welsch C, Wang Y, et al. Characterization of resistance to the protease inhibitor boceprevir in hepatitis C virus-infected patients. *Hepatology* 2009;50:1709–18.

726. He Y, King M, Kempf D, et al. Relative replication capacity and selective advantage profiles of protease inhibitor-resistant hepatitis C virus (HCV) NS3 protease mutants in the HCV genotype 1b replicon system. *Antimicrob Agents Chemother* 2008;52:1101–10.

727. Zhou Y, Bartels D, Hanzelka B, et al. Phenotypic characterization of resistant Val36 variants of hepatitis C virus NS3-4A serine protease. *Antimicrob Agents Chemother* 2008;52:110–20.

728. Tong X, Chase R, Skelton A, Chen T, Wright-Minogue J, Malcolm B. Identification and analysis of fitness of resistance mutations against the HCV protease inhibitor SCH 503034. *Antiviral Res* 2006;70: 28–38.

729. Shimakami T, Welsch C, Yamane D, et al. Protease inhibitor-resistant hepatitis C virus mutants with reduced fitness from impaired production of infectious virus. *Gastroenterology* 2011;140:667–75.

730. Gane EJ, Roberts SK, Stedman CA, et al. Oral combination therapy with a nucleoside polymerase inhibitor (RG7128) and danoprevir for chronic hepatitis C genotype 1 infection (INFORM-1): a randomised, double-blind, placebo-controlled, dose-escalation trial. *Lancet* 2010;376:1467–75.

731. Zeuzem S, Buggisch P, Agarway K, et al. Dual, triple, and quadruple combination treatment with a protease inhibitor (GS9256) and a polymerase inhibitor (GS9190) alone and in combination with ribavirin or PEGIFN/RBV for up to 28 days in treatment naive genotype 1 HCV subjects [Abstract]. *Hepatology* 2010;52:late breaker abstract 1.

732. Lok A, Gardiner D, Lawitz E, et al. Quadruple therapy with BMS-790052, BMS-650032 and PEG-IFN/RBV for 24 weeks results in 100% SVR12 in HCV genotype 1 null responders [Late breaker abstract O1356]. Association for the Study of the Liver conference (EASL) March 30 – April 3, 2011; Berlin, Germany.

733. Racanelli V, Rehermann B. Hepatitis C virus infection: when silence is deception. *Trends Immunol* 2003;24:456–64.

734. Bowen DG, Walker CM. Adaptive immune responses in acute and chronic hepatitis C virus infection. *Nature* 2005;463:946–952.

PART VI

Alcohol and Drug-induced Liver Disease

Overview

Willis C. Maddrey

Fortunately, significant progress is being made in identifying the mechanisms through which drugs harm the liver. Based on new observations, researchers are developing innovative ways to identify groups of patients who are at heightened risk. The potential for causing hepatotoxicity is a factor to be reckoned with in the development of any new drug. Attention must be paid to hepatic effects during the design process with continued attention throughout drug testing. The process of obtaining regulatory approval is often influenced by what happens to the liver. It is necessary to develop provisional plans for ongoing assessment to detect any hepatic issues that may arise once a new agent is on the market.

With the identification of new disease-related targets, there are remarkable arrays of novel drug candidates and biologic agents filling the developmental pipelines of pharmaceutical companies throughout the world. Furthermore, there is a parallel universe of agents, often poorly defined, used as herbal remedies. With each new drug evaluated, attention is given to an assessment of its risk profile with special consideration directed towards recognition of hepatic abnormalities that are or may be related to the drug.

Many promising agents have failed because of recognition of adverse hepatic events. In an individual patient, when abnormal liver test results are noted or, in rare situations in which clinically apparent liver injury appears, the focus of clinical attention may shift from concerns over treatment of the primary problem to a salvage operation to minimize serious liver injury. Regulatory agencies are keenly aware of the importance of hepatic risk which, if identified, may delay or prevent approval. The evaluation process for a new agent does not end with approval and release.

How the hepatic risks are presented and explained to clinicians have important consequences. The confidence a clinician has in prescribing a new agent is affected if there are special warnings regarding the potential risk

of hepatic injury. A black box warning can significantly limit the use of a drug. It is widely appreciated that once a drug is marketed, liver changes that were not apparent during structured clinical trials may be detected. It only takes a case or two of serious hepatic injury to cause a promising agent in the late stages of development to be abandoned or lead to the recall of a drug already on the market.

Loss of an effective drug because of hepatotoxicity is a manifestation of a therapeutic promise gone awry. The approaches by which a hepatic signal caused by a drug is identified and ways to estimate the extent of risk are becoming more refined. Factors that influence the risk of developing a hepatic reaction to an individual agent include the age and sex of the patient, the state of nutrition (obesity or malnutrition), interactions with other drugs, the hepatic effects of the underlying disease for which the drug is being used, and the ever-present concerns regarding the use of alcohol.

We now know there is much more to the story of drug-induced hepatotoxicity than attributing liver abnormalities to exposure to a damaging reactive intermediate. Extensive evaluations of drug metabolism have been broadened and encompass consideration of the roles of cytochrome P450s, nuclear receptors, transporters, and many other pathways.

Considerable attention is being given to the role of immune responses, both innate and delayed, that develop as the result of exposure to drug metabolites. These may determine the initiation and progression of drug-induced liver injury.

The stories of the evolution of knowledge regarding the hepatic risks of drugs, including acetaminophen, isoniazid, phenytoin, halothane, diclofenac, statins, and amoxicillin-clavulanic acid, are only a few of those fully described in the chapter on "Drug-induced liver injury." The list of drugs that affect the liver in some way goes on and on, and it is important for the clinician to know the risk profile of the agents that he or she uses. Drug-induced hepatic injury can mimic almost all liver diseases – from hepatitis, to fat accumulation, cholestasis, granulomas, and even the development of benign and malignant hepatic tumors. In some patients, such as those receiving treatment for cancer, human immunodeficiency virus (HIV), and fungal disorders, the number of drugs the patient is receiving may be overwhelming. In that setting, if liver abnormalities are detected, the issue is which suspect caused the injury. A clinician may have to diligently search for the culprit causing liver changes. The important first step is to consider the possibility that the observed liver abnormalities may have been caused by a drug. Once the possibility is considered, the search for the causative agent begins. An important confirmation that a drug was the cause of injury is if resolution occurs following its withdrawal.

Now new windows of understanding are opening. The concept of idiosyncrasy is being better understood. When only one in many thousands of individuals receiving a drug develops an adverse reaction, there must be a reason that this person was singled out. The genetic underpinnings controlling drug metabolism, disposition, and the immune responses occurring at many stages are increasingly being defined. There are evolving new concepts regarding the influences of the interplay between the genetic profile of the patient and the conditioning effects of risk factors. A few of the new observations appear to be relevant to increasing our understanding. The extent of metabolism of a given agent is important – drugs that are highly metabolized are riskier. Furthermore, the dose required to obtain the desired therapeutic effect has a role – the lower the needed dose of a drug, the smaller the risk.

The liver is faced with new challenges whenever a novel chemical is presented. Most of the time, the liver rapidly adapts. The concept of hepatic adaptation to the newly administered drug is of considerable interest. It is well known that many agents cause some elevations in aminotransferase levels soon after their initial introduction with a subsequent return to normal despite continued administration. Adaptation (tolerance) may occur in a variety of ways. One is through the development of enhanced pathways to dispose of reactive intermediates, thereby reducing or abolishing the hepatic effects, or in others, adjustment in the intensity of innate immune responses. The inability of a few individuals to adapt may well be a major contributor to the development of clinically apparent disease.

Among the guidelines to judge the risk of drug-induced hepatocellular injury is the observation by Dr Hyman Zimmermann that patients who have elevated aminotransferase levels associated with clinical jaundice are at increased risk of proceeding to an unfavorable outcome. If a drug, during development, causes even a few patients to have considerable elevations of aminotransferases and bilirubin, that drug receives special attention. Large-scale studies from around the world have confirmed the validity of the Zimmermann observation that there is an approximate 10% risk of mortality (or need for liver transplantation) in patients who have elevated aminotransferase levels (greater than three times the upper limit of normal) and elevated serum bilirubin levels (greater than two times the upper limit of normal). Furthermore, increased attention is paid to those drugs that cause slight increases in aminotransferase levels in many patients – the "where there is smoke, there is fire" concept.

Pre-drug genetic profiling is receiving increasing attention. There is much to be gained from determining if an individual has genetically influenced risk factors and under what circumstances that patient is at increased risk. It may be that a genetically susceptible individual will only develop serious hepatic disease if any of several environmental factors (e.g., obesity or alcohol use) are present. Important information has come from the genomic profiling of a few patients who have an unquestioned adverse hepatic reaction to an agent and comparing these patients with a control group who did not have a reaction. However, there are several problems with a widespread application of this approach. One of these is the difficulty in obtaining index cases of clearly related liver injury from a particular drug. There may be very few affected individuals even in a large trial. A second issue is making sure that the comparator individuals have similar characteristics, including ancestry. It is abundantly clear that the adverse reactions from some therapeutic agents vary remarkably in different racial groups. Of course, these observations apply to considerations of likely benefit as well as risks.

It is well established that only a few patients with an allele that predisposes to hepatic injury from a specific drug will develop a clinically apparent liver problem when exposed. Identifying the multiple hits required to cause significant injury is a challenge. How to effectively use genetic profiling during drug development to identify patients who are likely to have a problem is an area of intense research. As a result of identifying genetically susceptible individuals, some useful agents – which in the past would have been (or have been) discarded during development or even withdrawn from the market – may be reintroduced to patients who are shown on screening not to be genetically predisposed to develop an adverse hepatic event.

The future of understanding ways to make drugs safer is bright and in the two chapters devoted to drug-induced liver injury our colleagues have provided a sturdy platform.

Whereas severe drug-induced liver injuries caused by approved drugs are quite rare, alcohol-induced liver diseases are quite common. Clinicians of many disciplines are fully versed in caring for patients who are chronic alcoholics. Alcohol has been known to have adverse health consequences throughout recorded history. In many western countries, alcohol remains the most important cause of cirrhosis and its consequences. From epidemiologic studies, there is no question that there are dose and duration of exposure relationships between the use of alcohol and the development of liver disorders. However, individual responses to alcohol use and abuse vary widely.

Liver injury caused by alcohol is an established precursor to the development of cirrhosis and hepatocellular carcinoma. The medical status of patients with chronic alcoholism and liver disease is complex with the often coexistent presence of cardiomyopathy, pancreatitis, predisposition to infection, propensity to accidents, vitamin deficiencies, and a wide variety of neurologic problems. The interactions between alcohol abuse, obesity, nonalcoholic steatohepatitis, and chronic hepatitis C and B are well recognized. In many patients, there may be several causes that contribute to the progression of hepatic fibrosis. Often the excessive use of alcohol appears to be the most important. There is considerable evidence that there are interactions between alcohol-induced hepatic injury and injury related to chronic hepatitis C and hepatitis B. It is established that patients with chronic hepatitis C respond less readily to presently available therapy if alcohol intake is continued during treatment.

Fatty liver occurs regularly in patients who use alcohol in excess. Once considered benign, alcohol-induced fatty liver has been shown to be a contributor in the progression of liver disease and the role of metabolically active fat is being given attention at many research centers around the world.

The search for genetic factors that predispose some patients who use alcohol in excess to progress to cirrhosis and, conversely, others, even those who consume prodigious amounts of alcohol, not to develop serious injury, goes on. In the chapter on "Alcoholic liver disease" the current state of knowledge of the role of genetic influences on the responses to alcohol and the progression of some patients to cirrhosis is fully presented.

The important role of the stellate cell as a production center for collagen has received considerable attention. Many influences, including acetaldehyde, a variety of cytokines, and reactive oxidative products lead to stellate cell transformation. It would be a great stride forward if methods could be developed to modulate the formation of collagen and to stimulate the degradation of already established fibrosis. A way to preferentially induce stellate cell apoptosis would be a welcome advance.

There are hopes (not yet realized) that new pharmacologic approaches that decrease the craving for alcohol will augment current efforts directed to the treatment of alcoholism. For patients with severe alcohol-induced necrosis (alcoholic hepatitis), the judicious use of pentoxyphylline and corticosteroids are helpful, at least in the short run. The use of agents to inhibit proinflammatory cytokines has fallen from favor because of risks of infection, but careful patient selection and attention to dose may resurrect interest in this approach. The role of liver transplantation in patients who have alcohol-induced cirrhosis has been an area fraught with discussion and emotion. However, the favorable follow-up results of liver transplantation in these patients cannot be denied. Hopefully, the day will soon come when advances in stem-cell biology will find a role in the patient with advanced cirrhosis caused by alcohol.

CHAPTER 26

Alcoholic Liver Disease

Srinivasan Dasarathy & Arthur J. McCullough

Department of Pathobiology, Cleveland Clinic Foundation, Cleveland, OH, USA

Key concepts

- About 90% of heavy drinkers (more than 60 g alcohol per day) show evidence of fatty livers, while only 10–35% develop alcoholic hepatitis and 5–15% develop cirrhosis.

- The daily intake of alcohol that results in liver injury varies and depends on a number of risk factors. Alcoholic liver disease develops at lower doses in females, Hispanics, obese subjects, and patients with hepatitis C infection.

- Insights into the pathogenesis of alcohol-induced liver injury have improved significantly but the translation into clinical benefit has been slow. Interactions amongst the products of alcohol metabolism, hepatic parenchymal and nonparenchymal cells, and cytokine release all contribute to the injury and progression of disease.

- The importance of continued abstinence and correction of nutritional deficiencies are major components in the long-term management of alcoholic liver disease.

- Alcoholic hepatitis has a variable mortality and the prognosis is determined most commonly by the modified discriminant function. The model of end-stage liver disease is being increasingly used to predict outcome in alcoholic hepatitis even though standard cutoff values are not available.

- Anti-inflammatory therapy with corticosteroids and anticytokine therapy with pentoxifylline are effective and evidence-based therapies for patients with severe alcoholic hepatitis. Response to corticosteroids after 1 week of therapy is being used increasingly to predict outcome of therapy.

- Patients with end-stage alcoholic liver disease should be considered for liver transplantation. Six months of abstinence is still considered to be a requirement prior to transplant, but this length of time may be adjusted on an individual basis.

- Liver transplantation is now considered standard of care in patients with decompensated alcoholic cirrhosis and the results are similar to nonalcoholic patients. Recidivism remains a concern and a number of models are being identified to predict post-transplant alcohol abuse. Liver transplantation for acute alcoholic hepatitis continues to be a matter of debate.

Alcohol is the most frequently used and socially acceptable hepatotoxin worldwide [1]. Geographic patterns of alcohol intake and the prevalence of alcoholic liver disease are changing constantly and recent reports question the stabilization of its use in western European countries, Canada, and Australia [2,3]. Approximately two thirds of adult Americans drink some alcohol [4]. The majority drink light or moderate amounts and do so without problems [5–8]; however, a subgroup of drinkers become dependent on alcohol and have the disease of alcoholism or alcohol use disorders [9–11]. Another group of drinkers are alcohol abusers (and problem drinkers) who experience negative consequences of drinking (e.g., unemployment, loss of family, or accidental injury or death). These patients are not considered to be alcohol dependent [8,12]. Failure to recognize alcoholism remains a significant problem and impairs both the prevention and management of alcoholic liver disease (ALD) [12,13]. The clinical features of *t*olerance, *p*hysical dependence, *i*mpaired control, and *c*raving which define *al*coholism (Table 26.1), as well as their acronym TyPICal, are suggested as aids to the clinician for making the diagnosis. For more complete and formal diagnostic criteria of alcohol use disorders, publications by various organizations including the American Psychiatric Association and the World Health Organization are recommended [14,15].

Disease spectrum

Alcohol affects the liver depending on the dose and the duration of use or abuse [16–18]. The spectrum of

Schiff's Diseases of the Liver, Eleventh Edition. Edited by Eugene R. Schiff, Willis C. Maddrey and Michael F. Sorrell.
© 2012 John Wiley & Sons, Ltd. Published 2012 by John Wiley & Sons, Ltd.

Table 26.1 Characteristics of alcoholism, based on the acronym TyPICal, which is used as an aid in the diagnosis of alcoholism.

Characteristic	Clinical feature
Tolerance	A state of adaptation in which increasing amounts of alcohol are needed to produce the desired effects
Physical dependence	A typical withdrawal syndrome appears upon interruption of drinking, which is relieved by alcohol itself or other drugs in the alcohol/sedative group
Impaired control	Total alcohol intake cannot invariably be regulated once drinking has begun at any drinking occasion
Craving	A dysphoria of abstinence that leads to relapse

alcohol-related liver injury varies from asymptomatic hepatomegaly to profound hepatocellular failure and portal hypertension [19–21]. Pathologically this is translated into fatty infiltration of the hepatocytes at the stage of asymptomatic hepatomegaly to frank cirrhosis with decompensation in the end stage [19,22,23]. There are at least five histologic manifestations of ALD and these include: fatty liver or steatosis, acute alcoholic hepatitis, chronic hepatitis, hepatic fibrosis, and cirrhosis

[24]. Of these, chronic hepatitis is a stage that has been reported in ALD but its diagnosis has been questioned [25,26].

Figure 26.1 displays the different stages and evolution of ALD and Table 26.2 lists the histologic characteristics and describes their prevalence in the different stages of ALD [24]. Even though these are considered to be distinct stages, multiple stages can exist simultaneously in a given patient [19]. Fatty liver develops in about 90% of those who drink more than 60 g/day of alcohol but may also occur with lower levels of alcohol use [27–29]. Fat localizes initially to the perivenular or centrilobular region of the liver [27,30,31]. Decreased energy stores due to hypoxia and a shift in lipid metabolism, along with a shift in the redox reactions caused by the preferential oxidation of alcohol in zone 3 of the hepatic lobule, are the reasons for this localization (Fig. 26.2) [27,32]. Simple, uncomplicated fatty liver is usually asymptomatic and considered reversible [33]. Once fatty infiltration is severe, particularly with a mixed (macro-/microvesicular) pattern and associated with giant mitochondria or perivenular fibrosis[31,34], progression to fibrosis and cirrhosis occur in up to 8–20% of patients [35].

Progression of ALD culminates in scarring and development of cirrhosis [36]. Although it is usually micronodular, it is occasionally mixed micro- and macronodular

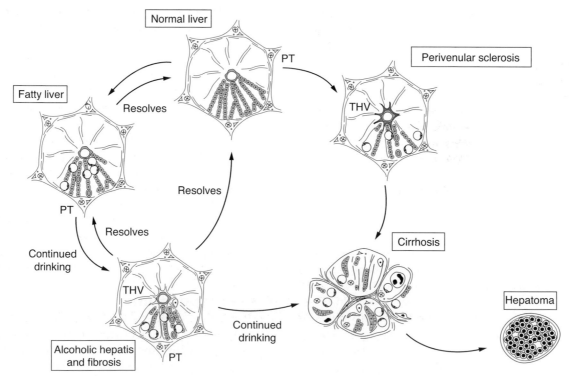

Figure 26.1 Progression and potential regression amongst the various histologic stages of alcoholic liver disease. PT, portal tract; THV, terminal hepatic venule.

Table 26.2 Histologic characteristics of alcoholic liver disease.

	Fatty liver	Alcoholic hepatitis	Cirrhosis	Cirrhosis–alcoholic hepatitis
Ballooning degeneration with PMNs	73%	97%	76%	35%
Mallory bodies	0%	76%	19%	95%
Mega mitochondria	100%	32%	8%	13%
Sclerosing hyaline necrosis	4%	68%	3%	44%
Fibrosis	31%	54%	100%	100%
Fat (moderate to severe)	69%	82%	27%	43%
Perivenular fibrosis	4.9	19%	–	–

PMNs, polymorphonuclear cells.
Data from reference [24].

[21,37]. Fibrogenesis is believed to start in the perivenular area and is influenced by the amount of alcohol ingested [31,38]. Perivenular fibrosis and deposition of fibronectin occurs in 40–60% of patients who ingest more than 40–80 g/day for an average of 25 years. However, the thickness of the perivenular fibrosis does not correlate with the amount of alcohol ingested. It should also be noted that the occurrence of the fibrotic features was more than twice that of the frequency of cirrhosis. Although this may be partly related to sampling error, the disparity between the frequency of fibrosis and the development of cirrhosis suggests that factors other than fibrogenesis are involved in the progression to cirrhosis in patients with ALD [35,39,40].

Figure 26.3 shows the estimated prevalence of the different histologic forms of alcohol-mediated liver injury amongst heavy drinkers [24]. This emphasizes the heterogeneity of the patient populations with regard to disease severity and individual susceptibility to alcohol. Amongst patients who are heavy drinkers, 90–100% will show histologic evidence of fatty liver but only 10–35% will develop alcoholic hepatitis and 8–20% will develop cirrhosis [35,41,42].

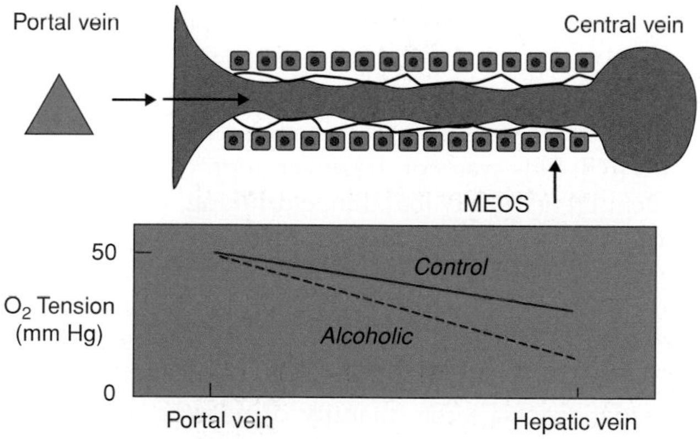

Risk factors

Only a subset of individuals who ingest significant amounts of alcohol progress beyond fatty liver and develop alcoholic hepatitis or cirrhosis. Therefore, other factors must play a role in placing these individuals at risk for developing these more severe forms of ALD [43,44]. A number of risk factors have been proposed (Fig. 26.4), but none of them can either singly or in combination completely explain the reason why only a subset of those ingesting large amounts of alcohol develop ALD [45,46].

Figure 26.2 Oxygen gradient between the portal area (zone 1) and the pericentral area (zone 3) of the hepatic lobule. The metabolism of alcohol increases oxygen consumption and causes the largest gradient in zone 3. MEOS, microsomal ethanol oxidizing system.

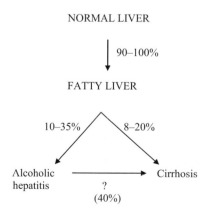

Figure 26.3 Percentage of heavy drinkers who develop the different stages of alcoholic liver disease.

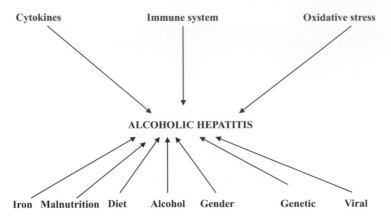

Figure 26.4 Risk factors that may be cofactors required for the development of advanced alcoholic liver disease.

Ethnicity

Ethnic differences in the prevalence of alcohol-related liver disease and associated mortality have changed with time [47]. In the first half of the twentieth century, when reporting of mortality was done for Caucasians and non-Caucasians (comprised predominantly of African-Americans), the mortality was significantly higher for the former. By the mid-1950s, this reversed and the mortality for non-Caucasians exceeded that of Caucasians. Later, when data were published for different ethnic groups, a two-fold increase in transaminases occurred more frequently in Hispanics and blacks than in Caucasians [48, 49]. South Asian (Indian) non-Muslim men have also been observed to have a higher rate of alcoholic cirrhosis at a younger age and after a shorter duration of alcohol abuse [50]. It is not clear if the ethnic differences are the result of genetic polymorphisms, the quantity or type of alcoholic beverages consumed, or co-morbidities [47].

Alcohol

The quantity of alcohol ingested (independent from the form in which it is consumed) is the an important risk factor for the development of ALD [51–53]. A significant correlation exists between per capita consumption and the prevalence of cirrhosis but this relation is not linear [54, 55]. Epidemiologic evidence exists for a marked reduction in the prevalence of ALD with diminished alcohol ingestion during war rationing, prohibition, and increased cost [56,57].

Available evidence indicates that there is an increased risk of developing cirrhosis with the ingestion of >60–$80\,g/day$ of alcohol in men and $>20\,g/day$ in women consumed for 10 years or longer [18,47,58]. Even in these groups, only 6–41% of those drinking at these levels develop cirrhosis [18,47,59]. In the Dionysos study, even in patients with very high daily alco-

hol intake ($>120\,g/day$) only 13.5% developed alcohol-induced liver damage [58,60]. The risk of cirrhosis or non-cirrhotic chronic liver disease also increased with a total lifetime alcohol intake of more than 100 kg or daily intake of $>30\,g/day$ [58]. The odds of developing cirrhosis or noncirrhotic liver disease with a daily alcohol intake of $>30\,g/day$ was 13.7 and 23.6, respectively, when compared with nondrinkers.

The type of alcohol consumed may also determine the risk of development of liver disease [61]. In a large survey of over 30,000 persons in Denmark, beer or spirits were found to be more likely to be associated with liver disease. It was also observed that in people who drank heavily, consumption of wine lowered the all-cause mortality [62,63]. It is, however, unclear if wine drinking was itself protective or was a surrogate for other healthy behavior such as the consumption of fruit and vegetables [63]. Alcoholic beverages that contain a higher content of short chain aliphatic alcohols have been associated with a high prevalence of liver cirrhosis [64].

Another factor that has been identified is the contribution of the pattern of drinking to the development of liver injury. Drinking outside meal times has been reported to increase the risk of alcoholic liver disease by 2.7-fold compared with those who consumed alcohol only at meal times [65]. This was not, however, reproduced in a subsequent French study [66]. Binge drinking, which may be considered to be a form of outside meal drinking, and has been defined by some workers as five drinks for men and four drinks for women, has also been shown to increase the risk of ALD and all-cause mortality [67,68]. Binge drinking has also been shown to be associated with the degradation of a large quantity of mitochondrial DNA that contributes to steatohepatitis as well as reperfusion injury, both of which result in significant damage to the hepatocytes and potentially to the nonparenchymal hepatic cells [69]. Increasing evidence is accumulating that

Table 26.3 Relative risk of alcoholic liver disease (ALD) at different levels of alcohol intake.

Weekly units of alcohol	Alcoholic cirrhosis		Alcoholic liver disease	
	Men	Women	Men	Women
<1	3.7	1.09	1.8	1.0
1–6	1.0	1.0	1.0	1.0
7–13	0.9	4.1[a]	1.1	2.9[a]
14–27	1.6	3.1[a]	1.4	2.9[a]
28–41	7.0[a]	16.8[a]	3.8[a]	7.3[a]
42–69	13.0[a]	NR	5.9[a]	NR
≥70	18.1[a]	NR	9.1	NR

[a]Represents a statistically significant increased relative risk of having ALD.
NR, not reported.
Data from Figure 1 in reference [55].

the pattern of binge drinking is common in early adulthood, predicts alcohol abuse behavior in later adulthood, and increases the risk of ALD [2,70].

Gender

Women have been found to be twice as sensitive to alcohol and to develop more severe ALD at lower doses and with a shorter duration of alcohol consumption than men [27,71–75]. As compared with men, in whom 80 g of daily alcohol was considered to be a hazardous amount, early data suggested the hazardous level to be 60 g/day in women [76]. Since the majority of those individuals developing ALD ingested more than 35 units per week, a "safe" limit of alcohol intake had been suggested to be 21 units/week in men and 14 units/week in women [76,77]. However, data from the Copenhagen City study suggest that a lower quantity, more than 7 units/week, may be toxic in women [55,78]. The data in Table 26.3 and Fig. 26.5 confirm the association between increased alcohol intake and ALD, the lower threshold toxic dose, and the increased female susceptibility for ALD. On a practical level 1 unit of alcohol (1 ounce of "spirits" (40% alcohol), one 12-ounce beer (5% alcohol), or one 4-ounce glass of wine (12.5% alcohol) contains approximately 10 g of alcohol for wine and spirits, and 14.4 g of alcohol for beer. This is based on a specific gravity of 0.8 for alcohol and the average alcohol content of beer. These amounts may vary depending on the actual alcohol content of the beer, which varies significantly amongst commercial brands (Table 26.4), as well as the size of the pour for wine and spirits.

This increased female susceptibility has been related to gender-dependent differences in the hepatic metabolism of alcohol [27,79]. An alteration in gastric metabolism

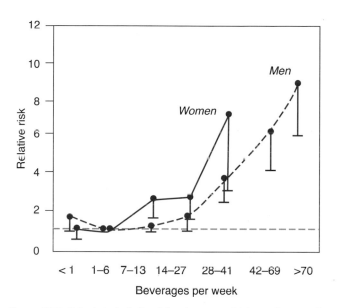

Figure 26.5 Risk of alcoholic liver injury increases with increasing quantity of alcohol intake. This risk is higher in females at all doses of alcohol ingestion.

Table 26.4 Alcohol content of commercial beer.

Brand	Alcohol content (%)	
	Light	Regular
Molson	2.41	3.88
Budweiser	3.88	4.82
Busch	4.12	5.19
Miller	4.40	4.80
Stroh's	4.45	4.68
Michelob	4.52	4.99

of alcohol is another explanation to explain female susceptibility to developing ALD [71,79–81]. First-pass gastric metabolism of alcohol does indeed exist in humans [79], but gastric metabolism of alcohol may not be large (10–30% at most), decreases with gastric injury, may not occur during most standard meals or realistic life conditions, and may vary among races since it has not been observed in Orientals [82,83]. Furthermore, the lack of increased risk of ALD in postgastrectomy patients has also refuted this hypothesis [84]. Experimental evidence exists for estrogen-induced endotoxemia and exaggerated hepatic inflammatory response to alcohol [85,86].

Malnutrition and diet

Dietary habits and nutritional status may also be important risk factors for the development of ALD [18,20, 87–89]. Early studies conducted in hospitalized chronic alcoholic patients with liver disease led to the misconception that protein-calorie malnutrition was a necessary risk factor for ALD [89,90]. However, alcohol is directly hepatotoxic and does not require preexisting malnutrition to result in liver injury [91,92]. In addition, even though alcohol adversely affects energy and protein metabolism, the prevalence and extent of protein-calorie malnutrition are similar in alcoholic and nonalcoholic cirrhosis [93].

Micronutrient abnormalities also potentially aggravate liver disease. Hepatic vitamin A depletion activates the stellate cells and results in hepatic fibrosis with alcohol abuse. Vitamin E levels are depressed in alcoholic cirrhosis and may contribute to enhanced membrane lipid peroxidation and hepatocyte damage [94].

Other nutritional disorders, including obesity, and dietary habits may be important risk factors [18,95,96]. Data from France suggest that obesity may be an independent risk factor for developing ALD (Fig. 26.6) [96]. In alcoholic patients from China, excess body weight

was associated with a 5.6-fold increase in risk of ALD [65]. Increased tumor necrosis factor activity and hepatic insulin resistance, which are associated with obesity, seem to contribute to the aggravation of ALD [97]. Obesity also makes the liver susceptible to alcohol-mediated injury by metabolic activation of CYP2E1, oxidant stress, and immune hyperreactivity in the liver [98]. It is currently unclear whether the hepatotoxic consequences of obesity and ethanol ingestion are additive or synergistic. High-fat diets are also necessary to promote alcohol-induced liver disease in animals (Fig. 26.7) [99,100]. Polyunsaturated fats in the diet have been shown to aggravate the hepatotoxic effects of alcohol in animal studies but no corroborating human data exist as yet [101]. The incidence of cirrhosis also appears lower than expected in countries with high intakes of saturated fat – an epidemiologic finding that is independent from other risk factors and supported by animal data [102,103]. The clinical significance of these observations is not yet known.

Recently, there is increasing interest in identifying the abnormal signaling pathways involved in the muscle loss in cirrhosis due to both the direct effects of alcohol as well as portosystemic shunting. Myostatin is a transforming growth factor β (TGF-β) superfamily member that has been shown to inhibit both skeletal muscle growth and protein synthesis following portosystemic shunting [104]. Furthermore, rats fed alcohol have an increased skeletal muscle expression of myostatin [105]. Recently, plasma concentrations of myostatin have been reported to be elevated in patients with cirrhosis [106]. These observations are of great clinical interest because of the potential to inhibit myostatin and thereby increase muscle mass without altering the underlying disorder.

Genetic factors

Environmental factors alone cannot explain the variable susceptibility to alcohol, and genetic factors appear to provide a predisposition to both alcoholism and ALD [107–110]. There has been growing interest in defining genetic factors, which include functional polymorphisms in genes that may contribute to the pathophysiology of ALD [111–113].

Alcohol metabolism

Much of the initial work focused on genes involved in the metabolism of alcohol: alcohol dehydrogenase (ADH), acetaldehyde dehydrogenase (ALDH), and the cytochrome P450 system (CYP4502E1) [114–117]. The most common reported abnormality is an increased frequency of *ADH321* (the gene that encodes for the γ-1ADH isoenzyme that is capable of faster alcohol metabolism to acetaldehyde), which when combined with abnormalities in the ALDH2-2 allele (slow acetaldehyde metabolism) results in high acetaldehyde concentration [114,118,119].

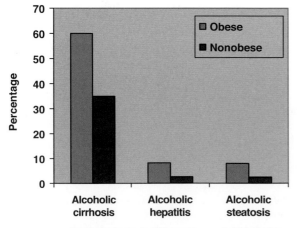

Figure 26.6 Prevalence of obesity in different forms of alcoholic liver disease in obese and nonobese patients. (Adapted from Naveau et al. [96].)

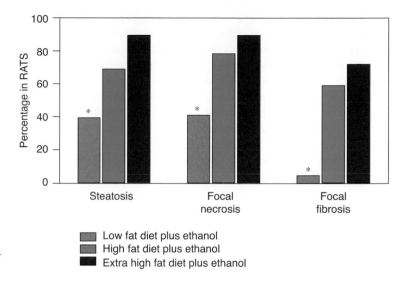

Figure 26.7 The effect of a high-fat diet on the severity of liver disease with alcohol feeding in experimental rats. *, $P < 0.05$.

Such an abnormality may be responsible for some of the hepatotoxicity of alcohol and mediates the flushing and enhanced alcohol sensitivity commonly observed in Asians [120–122]. Patients in Japan have a higher frequency of ADH2-1, and an increased frequency of ALDH2-1 has been reported in patients who were alcoholics (with or without liver disease) than in controls [123]. However, the data regarding a specific ADH/ALDH pattern in patients with ALD are conflicting.

The genetic pattern of P4502E1 (the microsomal enzyme primarily involved in alcohol metabolism) has been studied because it generates reactive oxygen species (ROS) when metabolizing alcohol [122,124]. A specific polymorphism identified as the c2 allele has been shown to result in an increased expression of hepatic CYP2E1 activity. An increased prevalence of the c2 allele has been reported in Japanese but not Chinese alcoholic subjects with ALD [123,125,126]. A higher prevalence of the c2 allele in Mexican-Americans than Caucasians has also been reported [127]. However, a meta-analysis of nine independent studies has shown that there was no relation between the c2 allele and the development of ALD among Caucasians [116,128].

Mitochondrial dysfunction

Mitochondrial dysfunction has been identified in the liver of patients with ALD, and a reduced activity of the mitochondrial form of superoxide dismutase 2 (SOD2) was expected to have a reduced activity. In French patients with ALD, a polymorphism in the gene with a valine to alanine mutation at position 1183 of the *SOD2* gene was observed but this resulted unexpectedly in an increase in SOD2 activity [129]. In a subsequent study from England, no association was observed between SOD2 polymorphism and ALD [130]. Polymorphisms in glutathione-*S*-transferase type $\mu 1$ and $\theta 1$ have also been reported to

occur more frequently in patients with advanced forms of ALD [112].

Cytokines and the immune system

Data supporting a role for the endotoxin-mediated release of cytokines in the pathogenesis of ALD have suggested a different set of candidate genes with a potential role in disease susceptibility [131–133]. Small studies that have reported an association between advanced ALD and promoter polymorphisms in the genes encoding the endotoxin receptor CD14 and interleukin 10 (IL10) need further confirmation [134–137].

These abnormalities suggested an upregulation of immune response in these patients [138,139]. Reported targets of this immune response are autoantigens, which include alcohol dehydrogenase, cytochrome P450 isoforms CYP2E1/CYP3AH, and endogenous protein adducts to ethanol metabolites or products of lipid peroxidation [140,141]. Polymorphisms in tumor necrosis factor α (TNF-α) (associated with alcoholic hepatitis), type I collagen (associated with cirrhosis) genes, and the gene encoding cytotoxic T-lymphocyte-associated antigen 4 (CTLA-4) (which functions as a suppressor of T-cell mediated immune response in patients with ALD) have been reported [139,142–147]. Studies from England and Spain have reported polymorphisms in the gene encoding for IL10, a cytokine that downregulates inflammatory response, that results in lower levels of IL10 in patients with ALD [143,148].

An integrated view of genetic polymorphisms and the consequent immune mediated liver injury has been suggested by the observations that CTLA-4 gene polymorphism and lower activity was associated with an increase in antibodies to the hydroxyethyl CYP2E1 adducts and development of liver disease [147,149]. Despite interesting and valuable new information in this area, there is variability in the reported association between genetic and phenotypic abnormalities in different studies and racial populations. Specific genetic abnormalities for a susceptibility to alcohol abuse and the development of ALD have not yet been firmly established [128].

Based on extensive published data on the role of gene polymorphisms in ALD, early reports of association have not been confirmed across populations or in subsequent, more rigorous studies [150]. Hence the role of gene polymorphisms, even though interesting, needs validation by large-scale cross-ethnic and cross-national studies.

Viral infection

There is a strong association between hepatitis C and ALD [151,152]. Unlike hepatitis B, hepatitis C infection appears to be strongly involved in the development of advanced ALD [153]. An increased prevalence of hepatitis C virus (HCV) has been reported in patients with ALD (Fig. 26.8) [154,155]. Hepatic injury by alcohol is synergistic with that of HCV because HCV plus alcohol predisposes to more advanced liver injury than alcohol alone [152,156, 157]. Compared to ALD patients without HCV infection, ALD patients with HCV infection have more severe histologic features, develop their disease at a younger age, have decreased survival, and have a higher incidence of hepatocellular carcinoma (HCC) [151,152,158]. The progression of fibrosis is most rapid in male patients who continue to abuse alcohol [153,159]. Although a daily dose of >50 g of alcohol has been shown to be a risk factor for fibrosis in patients with HCV infection, even a moderate consumption of alcohol (<50 g/day) has been shown to result in a dose-dependent increase in liver disease [157,160]. Despite these observations, the precise toxic threshold is not known and maybe lower and nonuniform amongst patients at risk. The estimated rate of progression is shown in Fig. 26.9 [41,153,160–163]. The prevalence of HCV also increases proportionally as the liver injury

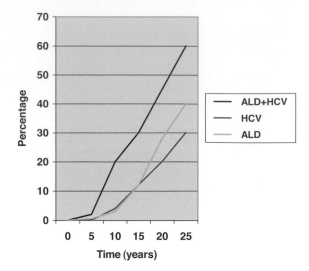

Figure 26.9 Progression of fibrosis with alcoholic liver disease (ALD) and hepatitis C virus (HCV). (Data from references [41,153,160–163].)

becomes more severe, with the relative risk for developing cirrhosis estimated at 8.7 in ALD patients with anti-HCV [164–166]. A French study showed that both mortality and the length of hospital stay was longer in patients with alcohol abuse and hepatitis C [163]. In addition, the presence of HCV is reported to be the major risk factor for the development of HCC [167]. In patients with alcoholic cirrhosis, the 10-year absolute cumulative occurrence risk of HCC has been reported to be as high as 81% in anti-HCV-positive patients as compared with 19% in anti-HCV-negative patients [157,168–170]. Although one study has questioned this association between progression of HCV and alcohol consumption [171], the consensus of data is highly suggestive of an unfavorable interaction between them [151]. Patients with hepatitis C should therefore be strongly urged to abstain from alcohol.

Iron overload

There is increasing recognition that iron accumulation with chronic alcohol consumption contributes to progressive hepatocellular injury. Both iron-rich beverages like wine and stimulation of exogenous iron absorption from food contribute to this [35,172]. An inadequate upregulation of the iron hormone hepcidin and an increase in transferrin receptor Trf1 have been suggested to contribute to the iron accumulation in both parenchymal and Kupffer cells [173,174]. Both alcohol and the reactive oxygen species generated during ethanol metabolism have been suggested to result in the alteration in iron-metabolizing genes [35,152]. Increased iron accumulation with alcohol not only contributes to hepatocellular injury, but also is believed to be a significant factor in the development of HCC in these patients [152].

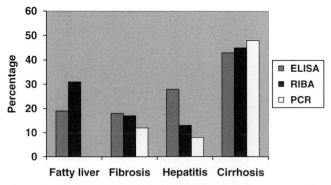

Figure 26.8 Prevalence of various markers of hepatitis C in patients with different forms of alcoholic liver disease. ELISA, enzyme-linked immunosorbent assay; PCR, polymerase chain reaction; RIBA, recombinant immunoblot assay.

Diagnosis

The diagnosis of ALD is often made in the context of a history of significant alcohol intake, physical signs of liver disease, and supporting laboratory data [20,175,176]. However, denial of alcohol abuse is significant [177,178]. Physicians usually identify less than 50% of their patients with drinking problems and institute specific recommendations even less frequently [179,180]. Both the physical findings and laboratory evidence for ALD may be absent or nonspecific, especially in patients with mild ALD or early cirrhosis [21,181–183]. Therefore, the clinician has to rely on indirect evidence of alcohol abuse, such as questionnaires, information from family members, or nonhepatic laboratory tests to suggest or strengthen a clinical suspicion of ALD [184–186].

General screening

Screening for alcohol abuse and failure to treat the same is common in clinical practice [187]. Alcohol abuse or alcohol dependence is diagnosed based on the amount of alcohol ingested, the social and psychologic consequences of alcohol abuse, the presence of other alcohol-related diseases, and past incidents of trauma (such as frequent falls, lacerations, burns, fractures, or emergency department visits) [188,189]. The diagnosis of ALD consists of both the documentation of alcohol abuse and evidence of liver disease [21,138]. Both clinical and supporting laboratory data for liver disease and alcohol abuse are required for this. Furthermore, alcohol may be one of a number of factors causing the liver disease and the specific contributory role of alcohol alone may be difficult to assess in a patient with multifactorial liver disease. Biochemical tests have been considered to be less sensitive than verbal tests in screening for alcohol abuse [190,191]. Biochemical tests have, however, been considered useful in identifying relapse after abstinence [190,192,193].

A combination of patient self-reports with corroboration from the family or close friends is considered essential in the diagnosis of alcohol abuse. Various questionnaires that have been used in the past for the detection of alcohol dependence and abuse include the CAGE and MAST (Michigan alcoholism screening test) tests [190,194,195]. The alcohol use disorders identification test (AUDIT) is a ten-item questionnaire that has been discussed in detail in previous editions of this textbook (Box 26.1) [196]. The major perceived limitation of the full AUDIT questionnaire is the length of time required to administer it. A number of brief screening instruments have been developed that include CRAFT, brief AUDIT, and RAPS4 [197,198]. The details of these instruments are beyond the scope of this review and have been discussed elsewhere [199]. The brief screening questionnaire,

Box 26.1 Alcohol use disorders identification test (AUDIT) questionnaire. This consists of ten questions with scores assigned to the answers.

1 How often do you have a drink containing alcohol?
0 Never
1 Monthly or less
2 Two to 4 times a month
3 Two to 3 times a week
4 Four or more times a week

2 How many drinks containing alcohol do you have on a typical day when you are drinking?
0 One or 2
1 Three or 4
2 Five or 6
3 Seven to 9
4 Ten or more

3 How often do you have six or more drinks on one occasion?
0 Never
1 Less than monthly
2 Monthly
3 Weekly
4 Daily or almost daily

4 How often during the last year have you found that you were not able to stop drinking once you had started?
0 Never
1 Less than monthly
2 Monthly
3 Weekly
4 Daily or almost daily

5 How often during the last year have you failed to do what was normally expected from you because of drinking?
0 Never
1 Less than monthly
2 Monthly
3 Weekly
4 Daily or almost daily

6 How often during the last year have you needed a first drink in the morning to get yourself going after a heavy drinking session?
0 Never
1 Less than monthly
2 Monthly
3 Weekly
4 Daily or almost daily

7 How often during the last year have you had a feeling of guilt or remorse after drinking?
0 Never
1 Less than monthly
2 Monthly
3 Weekly
4 Daily or almost daily

8 How often during the last year have you been unable to remember what happened the night before because you had been drinking?
0 Never
1 Less than monthly

2 Monthly

3 Weekly

4 Daily or almost daily

9 Have you or someone else been injured as a result of your drinking?

0 No

2 Yes, but not in the last year

4 Yes, during the last year

10 Has a relative, friend, doctor, or other health worker been concerned about your drinking or suggested that you should cut down?

0 No

2 Yes, but not in the last year

4 Yes, during the last year

RAPS4 (rapid alcohol problems screen 4), has been compared to CAGE in patients from the National Alcohol Survey [200]. The RAPS4 had a higher sensitivity (0.86) compared with CAGE (0.67). Both had similar specificity (0.95 versus 0.98) across gender and ethnicity. Comparing brief versions of the AUDIT to the full AUDIT in the primary care setting showed variable sensitivity and specificity of the brief versions [198]. A quantity frequency (QF) score that includes questions on drinking frequency can be added to RAPS and the combined instrument, RAPS-QF, outperformed CAGE. It appears that quantity frequency will be a major component of brief questionnaires that are being developed to replace the full AUDIT.

Clinical differentiation of the different stages of ALD is difficult at times and there is no single marker that definitively establishes the etiology of liver disease to be alcohol and laboratory tests are often needed to confirm the diagnosis. Recent studies have suggested that the brief versions may be adequate to diagnose alcohol abuse [201,202]. Recently published American Association for the Study of Liver Diseases (AASLD) guidelines suggest that regardless of the screening instrument selected, it is important for clinicians to incorporate screening into their clinical practice because this may improve the ability of clinicians to predict long-term clinical outcomes [195].

Physical examination

On physical examination, patients with ALD may show a constellation of abnormalities that are related to portal hypertension (ascites, splenomegaly, abdominal wall collaterals, and a venous hum), alcohol abuse and hepatic injury (cutaneous telangiectasia, palmar erythema, finger clubbing, Dupuytren contractions, and peripheral neuropathy), and feminization (gynecomastia and hypogonadism). Detailed discussions of the physical signs have been published recently and will not be discussed here [21,191,203].

Although some of the physical findings are more commonly observed in ALD (parotid enlargement, Dupuytren contracture, and especially those associated with alcohol abuse and feminization) than in non-ALD, no single physical finding or constellation of findings is 100% specific or sensitive for ALD [204]. Furthermore, there is significant interobserver variability for most of these physical findings, which is dependent on the experience of the examiner and the physical finding being sought [203,204]. When present, certain findings on physical examination such as ascites, poor nutritional status, and cutaneous telangiectasia indicate significant liver injury and poor prognosis [205–207]. However, even in the absence of significant liver injury, physical findings associated with alcohol abuse may be present and then subsequently improve with abstinence [208]. Physical examination of the liver, which may be normal in the presence of ALD, does not provide accurate information regarding liver volume [209]. Its major role is to define the characteristics of the consistency of the liver's lower edge rather than to delineate disease etiology or liver volume.

Other organ dysfunction in ALD includes cardiomyopathy, skeletal muscle wasting, pancreatic dysfunction, and alcoholic neurotoxicity that may coexist with ALD. Evidence of these must be sought during the clinical examination so that appropriate treatment may be provided [210–212]. Prognosis in these patients is determined by evidence of clinical decompensation, including encephalopathy, ascites, edema, and gastrointestinal bleeding [195]. Recently, in a large study from Sweden, the prognosis of patients with ALD was reported to be worse and the clinical course to be more aggressive than in nonalcoholic liver disease [213]. The authors recognized that this may, however, be due to continued alcohol use or abuse, poor follow-up, and noncompliance with therapy in these patients.

In summary, physical examination alone is unable to either establish the diagnosis of ALD or delineate ALD from non-ALD and must be considered in the context of the patient's history and laboratory findings.

Laboratory abnormalities

The various laboratory tests used to diagnose ALD are shown in Box 26.2. Low sensitivity and specificity limit the usefulness of γ-glutamyltransferase (GGT) to diagnose alcohol abuse [214–216]. Serum transaminases have been used in the diagnosis of ALD [217]; serum aspartate aminotransferase (AST) is raised only 2–6 times in severe acute alcoholic hepatitis. Levels of AST >500 IU/L or ALT >200 IU/L should suggest an etiology other than alcoholic hepatitis. In about 70% of patients the AST : ALT ratio is higher than 2, but this is of greater value in noncirrhotic patients; ratios greater than 3 are essentially

Box 26.2 Typical laboratory abnormalities in alcoholic liver disease.

Serum enzymes

- AST>>>ALT
- AST usually <500 IU and ALT <200 IU
- Alkaline phosphatase and γ-glutamyl transpeptidase: both usually elevated to a variable degree

Immunoglobulins

- Both IgG and IgA are elevated

Metabolic alterations

- Hyperglycemia
- Hypertriglyceridemia
- Hyperuricemia
- Electrolyte abnormalities
- Low potassium, magnesium, and phosphorus

Tests of liver function

- Serum albumin, prothrombin time, and serum bilirubin: usually normal until significant liver injury is present

Hematologic abnormalities

- Mild anemia is common (usually macrocytic)
- Platelets (normal to markedly decreased)
- Elevated white blood cell count
- Leukemoid reactions associated with alcoholic hepatitis

diagnostic for ALD, with the specificity increasing as the ratio increases. Macrocytosis is seen in individuals abusing alcohol but lacks sensitivity. A combination of raised GGT and mean corpuscular volume (MCV) has a sensitivity of 30–40% for diagnosing alcohol abuse. Serum carbohydrate-deficient transferrin (CDT) is a specific and sensitive test for alcohol use independent of liver disease but is more accurate in men ingesting over 60 g daily alcohol [218]. Frequent determination of serum ethanol levels during the patient's visits to the physician's office is another simple but often ignored method of assessing alcohol use. Other sensitive indices include fucosylated haptoglobin and serum secretory immunoglobulin A (IgA), but both need prospective testing at multiple centers before their validity can be confirmed [219–221]. A direct comparison of four markers of alcohol consumption showed that the overall accuracies of GGT and CDT were the highest to detect alcohol drinking, while sialic acid and P3NP (amino terminal of pro-collagen III) were of value in differentiating liver disease from alcohol abuse [222]. Serum hyaluronic acid has been used alone [223] and in combination with other tests [224] to detect the stage of liver disease in ALD. These and other promising biomarkers require additional studies in this area [34].

In symptomatic patients, nonspecific findings include elevated uric acid, lactate, and triglycerides and a decrease in magnesium, glucose phosphate, and potassium. Polyclonal hyperglobulinemia and an increase in circulating IgA also occur with ALD [225]. It must be reiterated that no specific laboratory test exists that is specific for ALD.

Nonalcoholic steatohepatitis (NASH) is a distinct clinical entity with histologic features suggestive of alcohol abuse with little or no alcohol ingestion [226]. This is seen in association with other features of the metabolic syndrome [227]. There are many similarities in the pathogenesis of NASH and alcoholic steatohepatitis, but the critical component of the injury in ALD is the consumption of significant amounts of alcohol. There are no reliable laboratory tests or histologic patterns that reliably differentiate NASH from alcoholic steatohepatitis.

Liver biopsy

A liver biopsy is useful but not essential in the management of ALD [228]. The role of liver biopsy in ALD is shown in Box 26.3. A liver biopsy is helpful in establishing the diagnosis, because as many as 20% of patients with alcohol abuse have non-ALD or other coexisting forms of liver disease [229]. Clinical and biochemical indicators are poor markers of the severity of liver disease and a biopsy is needed to establish the stage and severity of the liver disease [228,230]. A biopsy assumes greater importance in patients who continue to have abnormal liver tests after a period of abstinence of approximately 3–4 months. Liver biopsy is usually safe with a low morbidity and mortality, but precautions should be taken as for any other patient undergoing a liver biopsy. In patients with a diagnosis of acute alcoholic hepatitis with a coagulation profile precluding a percutaneous liver biopsy, consideration should be given to performing a transjugular biopsy.

Box 26.3 Role of liver biopsy in alcoholic liver disease.

Diagnosis

- Confirm diagnosis
- Exclude other causes of liver disease (primary or concomitant)
- Assess extent of liver damage

Prognosis (adverse)

- Neutrophilic infiltration
- Stenosis of central veins
- Number of hepatic stellate cells, giant stellate cells, and lipid vesicles in stellate cells
- Number of Kupffer cells
- Degree of liver cell necrosis
- Perivenous fibrosis

Therapeutic decision

- Prior to steroid therapy

The histologic features of alcohol-induced hepatic injury include steatosis (fatty change), lobular hepatitis, periportal fibrosis, Mallory bodies, nuclear vacuolation, bile duct proliferation, and fibrosis or cirrhosis [19]. The development of large droplet (macrovesicular) steatosis (fatty liver) is the earliest and most common manifestation of ALD. It is often clinically asymptomatic and completely reversible on abstinence [231]. It is most prominent in the centrilobular regions but in severe cases may involve the entire lobule [232]. It is most commonly diagnosed on ultrasound, demonstrating fatty change with increased echogenicity of the liver parenchyma [233].

Alcoholic hepatitis is characterized by liver cell damage, neutrophilic infiltration of the lobules, and fibrosis [24,207]. Steatosis and hepatitis may exist independent of each other and do not imply a continuum of changes. The liver cell damage in alcoholic hepatitis includes hepatocyte necrosis, ballooning degeneration, and lobular inflammation that affect the perivenular regions in the earliest stages [38]. Ballooning is secondary to the accumulation of protein and water. Mallory bodies are irregular, refractile, eosinophilic, cytoplasmic structures with a beaded form that stain positive for ubiquitin [234]. They have been shown to be aggregated cytokeratin intermediate filaments as well as other proteins. Mallory bodies, giant mitochondria, neutrophilic infiltration, and fibrosis may be seen in other conditions besides ALD [235]. In contrast to their presence in simple fatty liver, megamitochondria in alcoholic hepatitis have been reported to be associated with a milder form of alcoholic hepatitis, a lower incidence of cirrhosis, and fewer complications with a good long-term survival [236]. Alcoholic hepatitis is associated with perivenular and pericellular fibrosis as a consequence of hepatic stellate cell (HSC) activation. Compared with patients who consume alcohol and have normal hepatic histology, inactive cirrhosis, or active alcoholic cirrhosis, patients with acute alcoholic hepatitis without cirrhosis had a 2–5-fold increase in the number of HSCs and a 7–15-fold increase in the number of giant HSCs. There was also a marked increase (15–20-fold) in the number of lipid vesicles in the giant HSCs [237]. These changes are associated with an increase in the extent of perisinusoidal collagenization. Perivenular fibrosis is considered to be a harbinger to future cirrhosis, especially in patients who continue to abuse alcohol or those who are coinfected with HCV [31,166]. Sclerosing hyaline necrosis is a more extensive degree of alcoholic hepatitis and is associated with extensive fibrosis [238]. The number of Kupffer cells and serum levels of TNF-α, IL6, and IL12 were significantly higher in patients with ALD than in controls [239]. In patients with severe steatohepatitis, there is stenosis of the central veins and the degree of stenosis correlates with the amount of ascites and

hyperbilirubinemia and the peripheral leukocyte counts [240]. Histologically, the appearance of Mallory bodies increases significantly as venoocclusive lesions become more severe, but these lesions do not correlate with the degree of sinusoidal neutrophilic infiltration.

There are a number of nonalcoholic hepatic disorders (NASH, total parenteral nutrition, and certain drugs – corticosteroids, amiodarone, and synthetic estrogens) that may mimic ALD histologically and have been reviewed extensively elsewhere [241,242]. In particular, it may be necessary to perform a liver biopsy in order to identify other diseases that may mimic ALD clinically. Histologic differentiation between these diseases may be difficult. Perivenular fibrosis, which is similar but not identical to that often described in ALD, has been described in hepatitis C infection [164,243,244]. This emphasizes the need for a detailed evaluation of the histology and appropriate clinical correlation in these diseases. Excessive iron accumulation with siderosis of both hepatocytes and Kupffer cells occurs in up to two thirds of patients with ALD [245]. This is secondary to increased intestinal absorption, prior transfusion, or, rarely, spur cell anemia [246]. A liver biopsy should be performed in those patients who have biochemical findings suggestive of iron overload (total iron-binding capacity (TIBC) saturation >45%) in order to rule out hereditary hemochromatosis (HHC), by calculating the hepatic iron index. This is because both HCV infection and ALD can each individually cause biochemical abnormalities suggestive of HHC [247,248]. In the alcoholic patient without cirrhosis, the presence of moderate periportal hemosiderosis should warrant testing for *HFE* (the abnormal gene in the majority of patients with hemochromatosis), in addition to biochemical tests of iron overload (serum iron, TIBC, ferritin) [248]. The diagnosis of *HFE*-HHC in patients with clinical features consistent with *HFE*-HHC and/or biochemical evidence of iron overload is based on the results of the screening tests, transferring iron saturation, and serum ferritin concentration, and of confirmatory tests such as molecular genetic testing for the p.C282Y and p.H63D mutations in the *HFE* gene and/or histologic assessment of hepatic iron stores on liver biopsy [172].The current guidelines published by the AASLD recommend that for patients with a diagnosis of severe alcoholic hepatitis, liver biopsy should be done only if medical treatment is contemplated and if there is reasonable uncertainty about the underlying diagnosis [195].

Imaging studies
Imaging studies have been used to diagnose the presence of liver disease but may not have a specific role in establishing alcohol as the etiology of liver disease. The diagnosis of fatty change, established cirrhosis, and HCC are suggested by ultrasound or computed tomography (CT)

scan and confirmed by other laboratory investigations [228,249]. Altered echogenicity of the liver has been considered to be moderately sensitive but not specific to diagnose fatty change that is associated with alcoholic liver injury. Established cirrhosis can be suspected on CT or magnetic resonance imaging (MRI) based on the findings of a lobular surface of the liver with altered density, but the etiology cannot be established with certainty. Enlargement of the caudate lobe and right posterior notch has been suggested to identify alcohol as the etiology of liver disease [250]. Evidence of portal collaterals and a dilated portal–splenic axis suggest the presence of associated portal hypertension [251]. The major value of imaging studies is to exclude other causes of abnormal liver function tests in a patient who abuses alcohol, such as obstructive biliary pathology or infiltrative and neoplastic diseases of the liver [252]. Another tool for the diagnosis of ALD is hepatic ^{31}P magnetic resonance spectroscopy [253]. This is used to calculate hepatic energy metabolism and phospholipid membrane metabolism. Lower phosphodiesterase to adenosine triphosphate (ATP) ratios have been reported in patients with alcoholic cirrhosis.

Endoscopy

Upper gastrointestinal endoscopy in patients with ALD is used electively to establish the presence of esophagogastric varices and emergently to identify the source of gastrointestinal bleeding. In the clinical situation of alcohol abuse, upper gastrointestinal bleeding may be secondary to a variety of causes that include: Mallory–Weiss tear, peptic ulcer disease, direct alcohol-induced gastric mucosal erosions and injury, portal hypertensive bleeding from varices, or congestive gastropathy secondary to cirrhosis [254,255]. Endoscopy has both diagnostic and therapeutic value in an alcoholic patient with active upper gastrointestinal bleeding.

Pathogenesis

An in-depth discussion of the pathophysiology of alcohol-induced liver disease is beyond the scope of this chapter and several recent major reviews exist [35,256–259]. However, a general understanding of the mechanisms of alcohol-mediated liver damage is essential because it forms the basis of current therapeutic strategies.

In the past, it has been considered that whole-liver tissue analysis would provide an understanding of the pathogenesis of ALD. However, the liver consists of both hepatic parenchymal cells (65%) and nonparenchymal cells (endothelial cells, Kupffer cells/hepatic macrophages, hepatic stellate cells, bile duct epithe-

lial cells, and pit cells/liver natural killer cells) [260–263]. All these cellular components are involved in the pathogenesis of ALD (Table 26.5). Even though the nonparenchymal cells constitute less than a third of the liver volume, they have distinct functions and are involved in cellular homeostasis, hepatocyte support, chemokine release, hepatocyte injury, fibrosis, and cell death [237,239,261,264,265].

Alcohol-induced liver injury is the result of a complex interaction between alcohol metabolism and inflammatory and immune responses that result in cellular injury [35,256]. These include oxidative stress and the consequent inflammatory cellular responses that cause direct injury to hepatocytes in addition to the activation of hepatic nonparenchymatous cells (Fig. 26.10). Additionally, indirect damage to the liver occurs because of endotoxin/cytokine activation, immune-mediated mechanisms, and induction of fibrogenesis [266]. Superimposed on these hepatotoxic mechanisms is the impairment of hepatic regeneration by alcohol, though rat studies have questioned this [267,268].

Direct hepatocyte injury

Hepatocytes are the primary site of alcohol oxidation and there are two major oxidative pathways involved: the alcohol and aldehyde dehydrogenase pathway and the microsomal ethanol oxidizing system (MEOS), the major component of which is CYP2E1 (Fig. 26.10) [270,271]. Thus, ethanol oxidation generates reactive free radicals leading to oxidative stress that is reinforced by depletion of glutathione and vitamin E (antioxidants) [272, 273]. Oxidative stress induces the transcription of several cytokines and the release of growth factors from different cells in the liver that interact with the immune cells mediating hepatocyte injury [262,266,274].

Alcohol dehydrogenase pathway

Alcohol dehydrogenase is an enzyme that produces acetaldehyde, which causes direct hepatocyte damage and immune-mediated damage by the formation of acetaldehyde adducts that are potent immunogens [141, 275]. In addition to acetaldehyde, other aldehydes produced as a result of free radical generation include malondialdehyde (MDA), which has been shown to combine with the cytochrome c oxidase subunits IV and V of mitochondria [141]. Antiacetaldehyde adduct IgA and IgG as well as anti-MDA adduct antibodies were found in a significantly higher number of patients with severe alcoholic hepatitis and cirrhosis [225]. Additionally, acetaldehyde and MDA can form hybrid adducts with proteins (MAA adducts), which are also highly immunogenic [276]. These suggest that the ADH pathway provides a strong immunologic mechanism in the pathogenesis of ALD.

Table 26.5 Role of cellular and subcellular organelles in the pathophysiology of alcoholic liver disease.

Target	Mediator	Consequence
Hepatocytes		
Cytochrome P450IIE1	Reactive oxygen species	Lipid peroxidation

Abnormal methionine metabolism
  SAMe
  S-adenosyl homocysteine
	Transmethylation reaction	Nucleic acid, protein, phospholipids

Mitochondria	GSH depletion Membrane fluid abnormality Electron transport chain Mitochondrial DNA breaks	Reactive oxygen species Megamitochondria Defective ATP depletion Apoptosis induction
Hepatocyte growth	Impaired protein synthesis Inhibits calcium mobilization Reduced DNA synthesis	Impaired regeneration
Increased expression of protooncogenes	Increased regenerative proliferation	Hepatoma
Matrix remodeling and deposition	Hepatocyte communication	Impaired apoptosis, regeneration
Kupffer cell/macrophages		
Alcohol-induced damage	Cytokine release Defective IL10 release Defective regulation of local inflammation	Increased TNF-α expression Increased apoptosis Hepatocyte inflammatory cell infiltration
Iron overload (increased absorption)	Impaired function	Endotoxemia
Sinusoidal endothelial cells		
Inflammatory cell Migration	ICAM expression increased	Hepatocyte injury
Hypoxemia	Microvascular circulation abnormalities	
Hepatic T lymphocytes		
Increased activation	TNF-α release	Hepatocyte apoptosis
Hepatic stellate cells		
Oxidative stress Endotoxemia Differential MAT expression	Activation	Lobular fibrosis

ATP, adenosine triphosphate; ICAM, intracellular adhesion molecule; IL10, interleukin 10; MAT, methionine adenosyl transferase; SAMe, *S*-adenosyl methionine; TNF-α, turmor necrosis factor α.

Acetaldehyde also significantly enhances the DNA binding of two major transcription factors: nuclear factor κB (NF-κB) and activator protein 1 (AP-1), and increases their transactivating activities [277]. These observations suggest that acetaldehyde plays a major role in regulating the expression of proinflammatory cytokines by activating NF-κB and AP-1 [278]. Other transcriptional regulators that may be involved are the early growth response 1 (Egr 1), which is regulated by the mitogen-activated protein kinase (MAPK) signaling cascade, and the Janus kinase-associated signal transducer and activator transcription factor (JAK-STAT) [256,257]. Many of these data, however, are from in vitro cell culture and animal models and human application and relevance is not yet clear.

Cytochrome P4502E1 pathway

Cytochrome P4502E1 (CYP2E1) is a component of the MEOS enzyme pathway that plays a major role in inducing oxidative stress and alcohol-induced hepatocellular damage [279]. After chronic ethanol ingestion, a 5–10-fold induction of CYP2E1 occurs that not only metabolizes ethanol but is also responsible for the activation of xenobiotics to toxic metabolites [122,124,279]. This increases the vulnerability of patients who abuse alcohol to solvents, xenobiotic compounds used in industry and therapy, as well as vitamin A precursors (β-carotene and retinol) [280–282]. In contrast to the ADH pathway, which is not inducible in humans, CYP2E1 is induced in humans by ethanol ingestion, and increases the production of ROS and consequent membrane peroxidation that results in

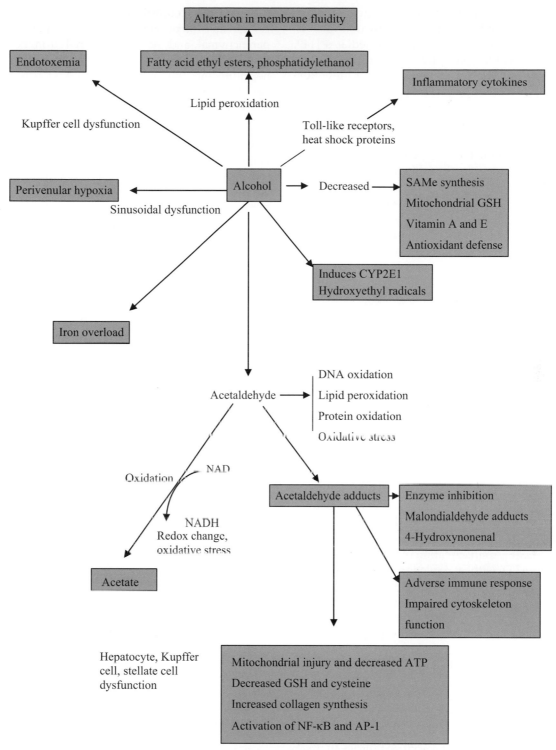

Figure 26.10 Pathogenesis of the role of the hepatocyte and alcohol oxidative pathways in the pathogenesis of alcoholic liver disease. AP-1, activator protein 1; ATP, adenosine triphosphate; CYP2E1, cytochrome P450 system; GSH, glutathione; NAD/NADH, nicotinamide adenine dinucleotide (reduced); NF-κB, nuclear factor κB; SAMe, S-adenosyl methionine.

cell damage [270,283]. There is increased generation of superoxide radical and free radical production, including the 1-hydroxyethyl free radical intermediates [149, 284]. Normally, cellular protective mechanisms against oxidative stress prevent the adverse effects of these ROS [285]. In the presence of liver disease and malnutrition, with maximal activation of the system, the detrimental responses predominate and result in tissue injury [286]. Other cytochromes like P4501A2 and -3A4 are also induced and may contribute to the cell injury and ROS generation associated with ethanol ingestion [122].

The CYP2E1 system may not be as essential in the pathogenesis of ALD [287]. CYP2E1 knock-out mice have been shown to be as susceptible to the hepato-injurious effects of ethanol [288]. The induction of other cytochrome enzymes (CYP1A, CYP2A, CYP2B, and CYP3A) also occurs with ethanol and may contribute to the oxidative damage associated with ethanol ingestion. The dissociation of CYP2E1 and ALD is also suggested by the prevention of experimental ALD with gadolinium chloride despite induction of CYP2E1 [289]. Nonetheless, the majority of data suggest that CYP2E1 is involved in the pathogenesis of ALD [260]. Furthermore, studies that have attempted to question the role of CYP2E1 have examined the early stages of ALD, while CYP2E1 plays a role later in the progression of ALD. Finally, levels of CYP2E1 are much lower in mice than rats or humans and caution must be exercised before extrapolating the findings in mice to humans [260].

Abnormal methionine metabolism

The liver plays a central role in methionine metabolism, with the formation of *S*-adenosyl methionine (SAMe) in the presence of the enzyme methionine adenosyl transferase (MAT) [290]. An inactivation of hepatic MAT activity occurs in ALD with a depletion of hepatic SAMe and glutathione (GSH) and decreased transmethylation reactions. These result in impaired antioxidant defense, altered phospholipid composition, and membrane fluidity and possibly altered DNA stability [59]. Finally, the homocysteine that is released as a consequence of altered MAT activity may stimulate hepatic stellate cells and promote hepatic fibrosis [291,292].

Role of hepatic mitochondria

Mitochondrial dysfunction has been observed in alcohol-fed animal models [293]. Increased synthesis of ROS, decreases in mitochondrial membrane potentials, increased oxidative modification, as well as single strand breaks in mitochondrial DNA have been reported [293,294]. These may be inducers of apoptosis and result in hepatocyte death in ALD. Dysregulated apoptosis has been suggested as a key pathogenic event in ALD with activation of effector caspases [262,295–297].

Role of iron accumulation

As already mentioned earlier, the role of increased parenchymal and nonparenchymal iron accumulation results from oxidative stress-mediated suppression of hepcidin and the induction of transferrin receptor 1. Additionally, iron accumulation also contributes to hepatocarcinogenesis [35,173,174].

Other molecular signaling abnormalities

A number of abnormalities are being recognized, including alcohol-mediated inhibition of critical intracellular energy sensor adenosine monophosphate (AMP) kinase, peroxisome proliferator activator receptor γ, coactivator protein α, and sirtuin 1 in the development and progression of ALD [35,298]. Plasminogen activator inhibitor 1 levels were reported to be elevated after alcohol exposure in mice [299]. A detailed review of these is beyond the scope of this current review especially since these mechanistic studies have been conducted in cultured hepatocytes/hepatoma cells or animal models and it is currently unknown if these can be directly translated to human disease pathogenesis.

Indirect hepatocyte injury

Hepatic macrophages (Kupffer cells) generate cytokines (such as TNF-α and TGF-β) that may accentuate or promote liver cell injury [35,262,274]. The role of TNF-α in alcoholic hepatitis is not clear [300]. Elevated serum levels of TNF-α in alcoholic hepatitis have been correlated with disease severity and mortality [142]. The TNF-α receptor 1 knock-out mice are resistant to alcohol-induced liver damage, as shown in Fig. 26.11 [301]. These studies suggest that TNF-α aggravates liver injury in ALD [256,302]. The contribution of Kupffer cells is supported by an attenuated alcohol-mediated hepatic injury by blocking Kupffer cell function [303]. Furthermore, MAT is expressed in

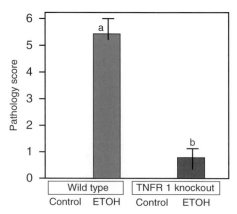

Figure 26.11 Tumor necrosis factor receptor (TNFR) 1 knock-out mice are less prone to alcohol-mediated hepatic injury compared to wild-type control mice. ETOH, alcohol; a, *P* <0.01 versus control; b, *P* = NS versus control.

both Kupffer cells as well as sinusoidal endothelial cells, and an alteration in expression of this enzyme system in the three groups of cells (hepatocytes, macrophages, endothelial cells) could contribute to the pathogenesis of injury in ALD [260]. Liver-associated T lymphocytes mediate injury and these may be responsible for both immune-mediated and nonimmune-mediated (via the release of cytokines) hepatic injury [304]. Hepatic stellate cells may be responsible for both matrix remodeling and regulation of local inflammation [237]. An alteration in stellate cell activation may result in fibrosis as well as cell death in ALD [305,306]. Products of lipid peroxidation have the ability to activate the HSC and stimulate fibrogenesis [307]. Increasing evidence is accumulating that in addition to direct oxidative stress-induced injury to hepatocytes, innate immune responses in Kupffer cells, fibrotic events in the stellate cells, and activation of hepatic sinusoidal cells all contribute to the spectrum of alcohol-mediated liver injury. Emerging data show the role of toll-like receptor-mediated signaling in Kupffer cells, and their regulation by heat shock proteins accompanies the activation of a number of transcription factors resulting in hepatocellular injury and fibrosis [256]. The contribution of nonhepatic cellular components to hepatic injury is not entirely understood and warrants further studies to examine the role of these cell types.

Prognostic factors

Alcoholic cirrhosis has a worse prognosis than other forms of cirrhosis (Table 26.6) [308]. A number of adverse prognostic factors for the long-term outcome in ALD have been suggested. They include the development of cirrhosis, ascites, portal hypertension (especially with evidence of encephalopathy), spontaneous bacterial peritonitis, hepatic encephalopathy, hepatorenal syndrome,

Table 26.6 Survival of patients with different types of cirrhosis.

Etiology	N	5-year survival	10-year survival
Alcohol	82	23%[a]	7%[a]
Cryptogenic	13	33%	20%
HCV	62	38%	24%
HBV	42	48%	20%
Hemochromatosis	20	41%	22%
Autoimmune	16	46%	23%
PBC	36	56%	39%

[a]P <0.05 versus other forms of cirrhosis.
HBV, hepatitis B virus; HCV, hepatitis C virus; PBC, primary biliary cirrhosis.
Adapted from Pessione et al. [308].

coagulopathy, severe hyperbilirubinemia, hypoalbuminemia, severe malnutrition, decreased galactose elimination capacity, α-fetoprotein, increasing age, histologic evidence of hepatic inflammation, continued alcohol abuse, and coinfection with other hepatotropic virus infection [20,309–312]. Iron overload and bacterial infections also predict poor outcome in ALD [313,314].

Scoring system for disease severity

Clinical progress in the therapy of ALD has been limited in part by the lack of accurate predictors of prognosis. This has also resulted in difficulty in comparing outcomes and the results of different treatments due to the nonhomogeneity in the predictors used. Accurate prediction of the prognosis of the most severe form of alcoholic liver disease, alcoholic hepatitis, is necessary to develop reliable treatment strategies for this disease. The modified Maddrey discriminant function (DF), which includes prothrombin time and bilirubin levels, is the most widely used predictor of severity of alcoholic hepatitis [315]. Values of ≥32 are associated with a mortality of 35–40% and are used to identify patients who will benefit from corticosteroid therapy. A patient with a DF of <32 has a survival of 83–90% and these patients do not benefit from corticosteroids [316]. The major limitation of the Maddrey DF is that even though it is a continuous scale, it is effectively used as a dichotomous test at the cutoff of 32. Once patients have a value of ≥32, they are at risk of dying, but this risk is not specified. The presence of encephalopathy has been included by some workers to predict outcome and the decision to start corticosteroids [317]. The model for end-stage liver disease (MELD) and the Glasgow alcoholic hepatitis scale (GAHS) have been used more recently to predict outcome in patients with acute alcoholic hepatitis [317–319]. A MELD score of 21 or higher had the best sensitivity and specificity in predicting 90-day mortality [320]. Other authors have also used the MELD, and a score of 11 has been used as a cutoff to predict outcome [321]. These studies have compared MELD with the Maddrey DF and found MELD to be either equally sensitive and specific or superior to the DF in predicting the outcome in acute alcoholic hepatitis [317].

The limitations of MELD include the difficulty in calculating the score at the bedside, the variable predictive value amongst studies, and the inclusion of serum creatinine, which limits its usefulness in the presence of hyperbilirubinemia as this reduces the accuracy of creatinine measurement [322]. The GAHS has been validated in a large population of patients studied up to day 84, allowing assessment of not only the short-term outcome at days 28–30 but also the intermediate clinical course of the disease [319]. The key components of GAHS include age, white blood cell count, blood urea, prothrombin time, and

Table 26.7 Five-year survival in alcoholic liver disease showing the effect of abstinence.

Time period of study (years)	N	Survival (%)		Reference
		Stopped drinking	Continued drinking	
5	122	57[a]	27	Pessione et al. [308]
4	45	87	55	Merkel et al. [310]
3	54	45[a]	20	Borowsky et al. [327][b]
7	258	77[a]	48	Brunt et al. [328]
8	168	70[a]	44	Juhl & Tygstrup [330]
12	278	63[a]	40	Powell & Klatskin [331]
7	100	72[a]	44	Verrill et al. [332]

[a]$P < 0.05$ versus continued drinking, as stated in the text or estimated from life table analysis.
[b]Data in Borowsky et al.'s study were for 2-year survival for heavy drinking versus total abstinence.

serum bilirubin [318,319]. It is still unclear if GAHS can be universally applied, and both MELD and GAHS need to be extensively studied by different groups before they are accepted as a predictor of outcome and replace the widely used Maddrey DF. Dynamic models that incorporate changes in laboratory values have been used that include changes in MELD or DF at 1 week, a change of ≥ 2 in MELD in the first week, and the bilirubin response at 1 week [317,323]. Despite these reports, the DF remains the most commonly and widely accepted prognostic measure in acute alcoholic hepatitis. It has also been used in patients with acute on chronic alcoholic liver disease even though it has been validated only in patients with acute alcoholic hepatitis.

Abstinence

Abstinence is a major goal of therapy and remains a fundamental factor in the management of ALD [308,324]. It is perhaps the most important but difficult therapeutic

intervention for ALD [271,325]. A recent review of 118 studies on survival in cirrhosis found only 12 of these examined the effect of alcohol intake on outcome [326]. Abstinence has been shown to improve the outcome and histologic features of hepatic injury, to reduce portal pressure, and to decrease progression to cirrhosis (Table 26.7), but this effect may be lower in female patients [71,240,310, 327–332]. Furthermore, a survival analysis of abstinent alcoholic cirrhotics infected with HCV when compared with patients with HCV cirrhosis who had never consumed alcohol showed no difference [333].This improvement can be relatively rapid, and in 66% of patients abstaining from alcohol a significant improvement was observed in 3 months [208,334]. Continued alcohol ingestion results in increased portal hypertensive bleeding especially in patients who have bled in the past and worsens both short- and long-term survival [255]. The deleterious effect of continued alcohol ingestion on the outcome compared with the abstinent population is shown in Fig. 26.12.

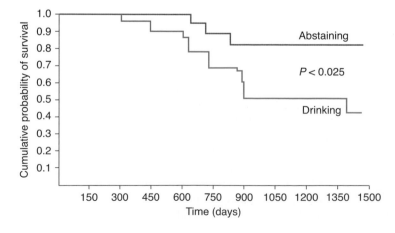

Figure 26.12 Effect of abstinence on long-term survival (Kaplan–Meier survival curve). (From Merkel et al. [310].)

Recidivism is the major risk in all patients at any time following abstinence [335,336]. Estimates of recidivism vary depending on the time course of follow-up, the definition chosen and the population studied. Over the course of 1 year, relapse rates range from 67% to 81% [337]. No controlled trials exist on the benefits of alcohol abstinence and the effects of recurrent drinking on ALD. Cohort studies, however, have consistently demonstrated that abstinence does improve survival at all stages of the disease [308,327]. Several drugs have been tried to help sustain abstinence. Naltrexone, a pure opioid antagonist controls the craving for alcohol. A Cochrane systematic review of the use of naltrexone and nalmefene in 29 randomized controlled trials concluded that short-term treatment with naltrexone lowered the risk of relapse of alcohol abuse [338]. Naltrexone, however, has the potential to cause hepatocellular injury that is of importance especially in patients who continue to drink. Acamprosate (acetylhomotaurine) is a novel drug with structural similarities to excitatory amino acids and γ-aminobutyric acid (GABA) and is associated with a reduction in withdrawal symptoms [339]. In 15 controlled trials, the efficacy of acamprosate has been demonstrated in reducing withdrawal symptoms but the effects on survival are not yet available [340]. The primary benefit of acamprosate is for patients who have become abstinent but it is not effective in inducing remission [195]. Recently, newer agents are being considered but their short- and long-term efficacy and safety in alcoholic liver disease are currently unknown [341]. Few studies have examined the benefit of interventions to induce abstinence and maintain it in patients with alcoholic cirrhosis. One study using baclofen, a GABA-B receptor antagonist, has shown benefit in maintaining abstinence [342]. The AASLD practice guidelines recommend strict abstinence in patients with ALD and have graded abstinence to class 1b on the evidence base [195].

Exercise has been shown to ameliorate the alcohol-induced hepatic injury in rats [343]. It is possible that a healthy behavior pattern in humans would reinforce abstinence in addition to its beneficial effect on ALD [63]. Human studies should be encouraged given the multiple beneficial effects of exercise. Before recommending exercise in patients with ALD, the possible underlying cardiomyopathy and hepatopulmonary syndrome of cirrhosis need to be excluded.

Hepatic inflammation

The presence of hepatic inflammation appears to be the single most important prognostic histologic factor in patients with ALD [20,344,345]. In a study of 217 patients (140 cirrhotics and 77 noncirrhotics) with biopsy-proven ALD, the presence of hepatitis indicated a poor prognosis [345]. Patients with cirrhosis and hepatitis had increased 1- and 5-year mortality rates of 27% and 47%, respectively. This contrasts with cirrhotic patients without hepatitis who had a survival rate similar to patients with no cirrhosis or hepatitis. These data have been indirectly confirmed as the presence of polymorphonuclear cells on liver biopsy was found to be a prognostic factor for early and late survival [311].

Hepatitis C

As discussed previously, the presence of HCV is another factor that causes inflammation in these patients [152, 346]. The decision to use antiviral therapy in those ALD patients with HCV infection should be determined on an individual basis. Since the data available indicate that active drinking will reduce the efficacy of interferon therapy for HCV infection, the potential use of interferon or other antiviral agents must be decided on an individual basis [347–349]. However, the potential efficacy of antiviral therapy may be improved by abstinence and therefore the potential for HCV therapy may be a motivational factor [348]. A recent Dutch study, however, suggested that response to therapy is maintained even in patients with alcohol use but this needs to be validated given previous data to the contrary [350].

Interaction with other drugs

The activation of the microsomal oxidative enzyme pathways also enhances the hepatotoxicity of other drugs, especially acetaminophen. A combination of an enhanced cytochrome P450 system and decreased hepatic glutathione results in severe toxicity. A significant proportion (64%) of patients who developed acetaminophen toxicity are reported to be alcohol abusers [351,352]. Furthermore, the majority of patients reported taking doses that were well below the accepted toxic range [353]. Awareness and suspicion of the diagnosis are the most important factors in the management of these patients. Diagnostic clues include very high aspartate transaminase (above 1,000 U/L) and a prolonged prothrombin time. Early and accurate diagnosis is essential due to the high mortality and need for early therapy [354].

Therapy

Therapy is based on the stage of the disease at which it is started and the pathogenetic event being targeted (Table 26.8) [271,355]. The primary treatment modalities that have been evaluated in the acute phase of alcoholic hepatitis include agents to suppress inflammation (corticosteroids) and anticytokine therapy (pentoxifylline, infliximab, etanercept), nutritional improvement (enteral and parenteral supplements including amino acids, anabolic steroids), modifiers of metabolism

Table 26.8 Pathophysiology of alcoholic liver disease and potential therapies.

Direct injury		Indirect injury	
Proposed treatment[a]	**Mechanism**	**Proposed treatment**[a]	**Mechanism**
PUL[3]	Membrane damage	Antibiotics, nutrition	'Gut' function
S-adenosylmethionine	Oxidative stress	Anti-TNF-α[2]	Cytokines
N-acetylcysteine[3]	Oxidative stress	Pentoxifylline[1], steroids	Cytokines
PTU[2]	Hypermetabolism	γ-Interferon	Cytokines
		Steroids[1]	**Immunologic mechanism**
		Colchicine[2], PUL[3]	Fibrogenesis

Regenerative capacity:
nutrition[3], oxandrolone[3], hepatotropic agents

[a] Some therapies were investigated in randomized, placebo-controlled trials and were found to be either: (1) effective, (2) ineffective, or (3) possibly effective.
PUL, polyunsaturated lecithin; PTU, propylthiouracil.

(propylthiouracil), and inhibitors of hepatic fibrosis (colchicine) [59]. Once cirrhosis is established, complications of cirrhosis – which include evidence of chronic hepatic failure (encephalopathy, ascites) as well as portal hypertension (variceal bleeding) – are treated along similar lines as in patients with non-ALD with additional attention given to other organ dysfunction associated specifically with alcohol [355,356].

Treatment of alcoholic hepatitis

Therapy for acute alcoholic hepatitis is determined partly on factors that estimate mortality. These indices are calculated based on laboratory tests, and the most commonly used index is the Maddrey discriminant function: ((prothrombin time prolongation over controls in seconds) × 4.6) + serum bilirubin in mg/dL [316]. A number of previously used predictors such as the Child–Turcotte–Pugh score and the combined clinical and laboratory index have fallen out of favor due to low diagnostic accuracy [345,357]. The MELD and GAHS have been gaining interest as accurate predictors of outcome [319]. The Lille scoring system of the response to therapy at 1 week is considered to be a robust measure of outcome as well as of response to therapy [358,359].

A number of biomarkers have been suggested to diagnose the severity of alcoholic hepatitis but are not yet in routine clinical practice [360,361].

Corticosteroids
Rationale
Corticosteroids have been used to suppress the inflammatory and immune response directed against neoanti-

gens that is induced by acetaldehyde adducts, which include liver-specific lipoprotein, liver membrane antigen, Mallory bodies, and epitopes of protein–aldehyde adducts in the liver [362]. Specific immune targets that have been considered targets of corticosteroids include malondialdehyde and acetaldehyde adducts, autoantibodies to P4502E1 and P4503A4, and antibodies to liver membrane antigen [363]. There is enhanced cytotoxicity of lymphocytes towards hepatocytes in patients with alcoholic hepatitis [262,364]. Steroids also exert a direct antifibrotic effect by suppressing the expression of extracellular matrix proteins in the liver [133]. Finally, inhibition of cytokine synthesis in response to gut-derived endotoxins by glucocorticoids also contributes to their beneficial effects in ALD.

Clinical trials
Corticosteroids have been the most extensively used treatment of alcoholic hepatitis but their efficacy still remains controversial. Of a total of 13 randomized controlled trials, five showed that corticosteroids reduce mortality compared with placebo, while eight others found no difference in outcomes (Table 26.9) [365–377]. Although the results are not consistent, differences in study design may explain the different outcomes. These include variability in dose and duration of therapy, selection of patients (e.g., varying time intervals before randomization or inconsistent use of disease severity scoring), possible misclassification (a consequence of inclusion without liver biopsy), and severity of illness, concomitant medical problems, or medications, as well as undiagnosed chronic viral hepatitis infections. Despite these variations,

Table 26.9 Results of randomized controlled trials of corticosteroid use in patients with alcoholic hepatitis showing the different death rates.

N	Deaths with placebo (95% CI; range)	Deaths with steroid (95% CI; range)	RR	Reference	Date
37	6/17 (0.35; 0.14–0.62)	1/20 (0.05; 0.0013–0.25)	0.143	Helman et al. [365]	1971
20	7/9 (0.77; 0.44–0.93)	6/11 (0.55; 0.28–0.79)	1	Porter et al. [368]	1971
45	9/25 (0.36; 0.2–0.56)	7/29 (0.35; 0.18–0.57)	1	Campra et al. [498]	1973
33	5/16 (0.31; 0.14–0.56)	6/12 (0.5; 0.25–0.75)	1	Blitzer et al. [366]	1977
14	7/7 (1.0; 0.63–1.0)	2/7 (0.29; 0.09–0.65)	0.29	Lesesne et al. [375]	1978
27	6/31 (0.194; 0.09–0.36)	1/24 (0.042) (0.009–0.20)	0.22	Maddrey et al. [367]	1978
27	7/15 (0.47; 0.25–0.75)	6/12 (0.5; 0.25–0.75)	1	Shumaker et al. [376]	1978
28	7/13 (0.54; 0.29–0.77)	8/15 (0.53; 0.3–0.75)	1	Depew et al. [372]	1980
55	16/28 (0.57; 0.39–0.74)	17/27 (0.63; 0.44–0.79)	1	Theodossi et al. [371]	1982
178	50/88 (0.57; 0.46–0.67)	55/90 (0.61; 0.51–0.71)	1	Mendenhall et al. [370]	1984
45	2/21 (0.095; 0.029–0.29)	1/24 (0.042; 0.0098–0.20)	1	Bories et al. [373]	1987
66	11/31 (0.36; 0.21–0.53)	2/35 (0.057; 0.108–0.19)	0.16	Carithers et al. [374]	1989
61	16/29 (0.55; 0.37–0.72)	4/32 (0.125; 0.05–0.28)	0.23	Ramond et al. [369]	1992

CI, confidence interval; RR, relative risk.
Summarized from O'Shea and McCullough [377].

two separate meta-analyses [378,379] found a benefit to the use of steroids. One meta-aggression using a different statistical weighting of the different trials [380] suggested no benefit of corticosteroid therapy after attempting to control for potential confounders. In one meta-analysis, steroid treatment provided a protective efficacy of 27% of patients with hepatic encephalopathy, which increased to 40% among higher quality trials and in 51% of patients without gastrointestinal bleeding (Table 26.10) [378]. In the most recent meta-analysis, no statistical effect of steroids on mortality in alcoholic hepatitis was reported but it did demonstrate an improvement in outcome in patients with encephalopathy and/or a DF of ≥ 32 [381].

Table 26.10 A meta-analysis of the efficacy of corticosteroid use in patients with alcoholic hepatitis with or without hepatic encephalopathy.

Trial characteristic	N	RR (95% CI)[a]	Protective efficacy (1 – RR)
With hepatic encephalopathy			
All trials	11	0.73 (0.58–0.92)	27%
GI bleeding excluded	7	0.49 (0.33–0.72)	51%
GI bleeding not excluded	4	1.06 (0.76–1.48)	NS
Quality score ≥4	7	0.56 (0.38–0.83)	44%
Quality score <4	3	1.05 (0.75–1.47)	NS
"Best estimate"[b]	5	0.64 (0.42–0.97)	36%
Without hepatic encephalopathy			
All trials	9	1.07 (0.68–1.71)	NS
GI bleeding excluded	5	1.01 (0.36–2.81)	NS
GI bleeding not excluded	4	1.21 (0.72–2.04)	NS
Quality score ≥4	6	1.02 (0.47–2.26)	NS
Quality score <4	3	1.18 (0.65–2.13)	NS
"Best estimate"[b]	4	1.01 (0.35–2.91)	NS

[a]If the 95% CI includes unity (1) then there is no significant therapeutic benefit (or protective efficacy) of corticosteroids for that subgroup.
[b]Best estimate is based on those trials with: (i) a quality score of 4; (ii) a baseline equivalence between groups; and (iii) an exclusion of active GI bleeding.
CI, confidence interval; GI, gastrointestinal; N, number of trials; NS, not significant; RR, relative risk.

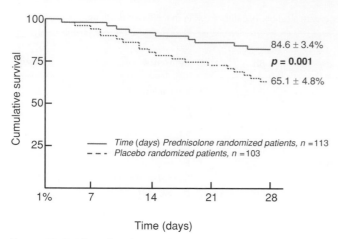

Figure 26.13 Effect of corticosteroids on the mortality of patients with alcoholic hepatitis (discriminant function score ≥32) undergoing the 28-day treatment. Data are from three randomized controlled trials [369,370,374].

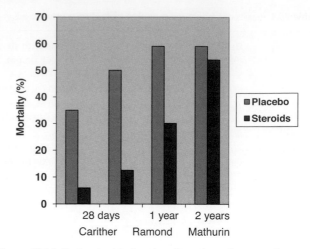

Figure 26.14 Corticosteroids show benefit on 1-year but not at 2-year mortality figures in alcoholic hepatitis [31,369,374].

The major limitation of these meta-analyses was that they were not designed to analyze individual patient data. A reanalysis of the pooled raw data from the three recent placebo-controlled randomized trials, restricted to patients with a DF ≥32, concluded that patients treated with corticosteroids had a significantly higher survival at 28 days than those given placebo: 84.6% versus 65% (Fig. 26.13) [315,316]. Therapy with corticosteroids, age, and serum creatinine were the independent predictors of outcome in these patients. Based on these data, the number needed to treat was calculated to be 5 (i.e., five patients treated to prevent one death). A recent analysis of individual data from five randomized controlled trials showed that corticosteroids significantly improved 28-day survival in patients with severe alcoholic hepatitis. The survival benefit was mainly observed in patients classified as responders by the Lille model [382].

In addition to these observations on the short-term benefits of corticosteroids in acute alcoholic hepatitis, a follow-up study showed that steroids improved the survival at 1 year but not 2 years in these patients (Fig. 26.14) [312]. The long-term benefit of corticosteroids in acute alcoholic hepatitis is uncertain. A number of factors may contribute to these results and include recidivism, co-morbidities, and progression of disease.

These observations provide a number of suggestions for the management of alcoholic hepatitis [377]. Approximately five to seven patients need to be treated to avoid one death. This necessitates careful selection of patients to avoid the side effects of corticosteroids in the other four to six patients who will derive no clinical benefits or may suffer the adverse effects of corticosteroids. This means excluding patients with active infection and being certain of the diagnosis (liver biopsy may be nec-

essary) because histologically confirmed alcoholic hepatitis correlates poorly with the clinical impression of alcoholic hepatitis [311]. As many as 28% of patients with a clinical picture of alcoholic hepatitis do not have histologic features of alcoholic hepatitis on liver biopsy. Only patients with severe disease (as defined by the presence of hepatic encephalopathy, the DF, the MELD score, or the GAHS) should be treated with corticosteroids. Another recently identified marker is the early change in bilirubin (ECB) at 7 days, which has been shown to accurately identify those patients not likely to respond to corticosteroids [323]. Finally, based on pharmacologic considerations (prednisone is converted to its active form, prednisolone, in the liver), published data indicate that prednisolone (40 mg daily for 4 weeks followed by a taper) should be used rather than prednisone. One may conclude from these observations that corticosteroids reduce mortality by up to 25% in alcoholic hepatitis, but the mortality still remains high (44%) in patients treated with corticosteroids. Therefore, other therapies or combination of therapies need to be considered [315].

Anticytokine therapy

Rationale

Cytokines are essential to the processes of hepatocyte inflammation, cell death, and regeneration. Serum levels of TNF, as well as, IL1, IL6, and IL8 are elevated in alcoholic hepatitis [266,383,384]. Human studies have shown that levels of soluble TNF receptors correlate linearly with an increased risk of mortality and that serum levels of TNF are high on admission and correlate with mortality [385]. In addition, monocytes from patients with alcoholic hepatitis produce TNF-α at higher levels than controls in response to endotoxin. Based on these observations, clinical trials have been performed using therapy targeted towards blocking TNF-α.

Pentoxifylline
Rationale
Pentoxifylline is a phosphodiesterase inhibitor used in the treatment of peripheral vascular disease based on its ability to increase erythrocyte flexibility, reduce blood viscosity, and inhibit platelet aggregation [386]. Pentoxifylline also reduces the production of TNF-α, IL5, IL10, and IL12 [387]. It also has been shown to decrease the transcription of IL2 and TNF-α promoters in transiently transfected normal T cells, to inhibit the activation of NF-κB and nuclear factor of activated T cells, and to stimulate the activation of protein-1 and cAMP response element-binding proteins. In an animal model of cirrhosis it reduced portal pressure [388].

Clinical trials
A 4-week double-blind prospective randomized trial in 101 hospitalized patients with severe alcoholic hepatitis (Maddrey score ≥32) treated with either pentoxifylline (400 mg three times a day) or placebo showed a significantly decreased mortality with pentoxifylline therapy (23% with pentoxifylline and 42% with placebo) (Fig. 26.15) [386]. Hepatorenal syndrome was the major cause of death in both groups, but significantly more frequent in the placebo group. The difference in mortality between the two groups suggests a number needed to treat of 4.7, which is almost identical to the number arrived at by Mathurin et al. when comparing the use of steroids and placebo [311]. In another study, 29 patients who did not respond to corticosteroids (absence of early decline of bilirubin) were switched to pentoxifylline for 28 days and compared with 58 matched patients who continued corticosteroids. No survival benefit was observed

with pentoxifylline at 2 months [389]. The mechanism whereby pentoxifylline decreased the development of hepatorenal syndrome is unclear, but could be related to either direct effects on the liver (through any of the above possible mechanisms) or, alternatively, by a direct renal effect. Plasma concentration of TNF-α did not decrease with pentoxifylline during the study [386] and suggests a TNF-α-independent mechanism for this therapy.

Infliximab
Clinical trials
Two small uncontrolled pilot studies using infliximab (IgG1 monoclonal antibody to TNF) suggested a benefit in alcoholic hepatitis [390,391]. A subsequent randomized controlled trial using infliximab (10 mg/kg) in combination with prednisolone (40 mg/day) versus prednisolone alone was begun in a total of 36 patients [392]. The trial was terminated prematurely because of the significantly higher mortality related to infection in the infliximab group compared with the controls (39% versus 11%) (Fig. 26.16). This study has been criticized based on the specifics of the study design (especially in the relatively high dose of infliximab) as well as the premise for the use of such therapy [393].

Etanercept
Etanercept, a P75-soluble TNF receptor–Fc fusion protein neutralizes soluble TNF and excludes an effect on membrane bound TNF. A single study in 13 patients with moderate or severe alcoholic hepatitis for a 2-week duration showed that the 30-day survival rate for patients receiving etanercept was 92% [394]. Adverse events (including an infection, hepatorenal decompensation, and gastrointestinal bleeding) necessitated premature discontinuation of etanercept in 23% of patients. In a multicenter, randomized, double-blind, placebo-controlled study of

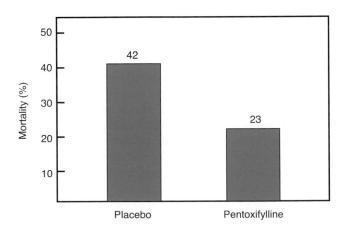

Figure 26.15 Pentoxifylline lowers mortality in acute alcoholic hepatitis compared with placebo.

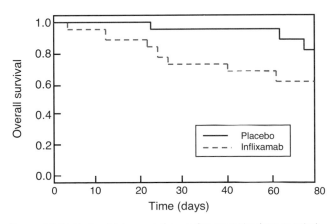

Figure 26.16 Kaplan–Meier survival curve demonstrating lower survival with infliximab compared with placebo when administered to patients with acute alcoholic hepatitis. (Adapted from Naveau et al. [392].)

etanercept in 48 patients with severe alcoholic hepatitis (MELD score ≥15) no difference in 1-month mortality rates was found between the two groups. However, 6-month mortality was significantly higher in the patients treated with etanercept (57.7% versus 22.7%). Serious adverse events were also significantly higher in those patients treated with etanercept [395].

In summary, the results of measures directed against TNF-α appear controversial. Based on the data from the studies using infliximab and etanercept in alcoholic hepatitis, the extent to which complete TNF inhibition (via antibody or receptor blockade) is beneficial is unknown and there may be concerns about serious adverse events, including higher mortality, in the treated patients. In addition, questions have been raised regarding the extent to which TNF inhibition is of benefit in this disease as TNF has been shown to be important in hepatic regeneration [267].

Antioxidants
Rationale
A major mechanism of alcohol-related liver injury is mediated by the generation of superoxides, the induction of cytochrome P4502E1 activity, and the product of inducible nitric oxide synthetase-related oxidative stress (Fig. 26.17) [396,397].

In vitro studies indicate that oxidative stress sensitizes lymphocytes to TNF-α-mediated cytotoxicity that is mediated through the cellular death domain pathways [398]. In addition, blood vitamin E levels and mitochondrial glutathione are decreased by ethanol [399,400].

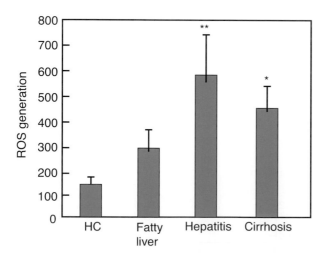

Figure 26.17 Nonstimulated neutrophils release greater quantities of reactive oxygen species (ROS) in patients with alcohol-induced liver injury compared with placebo. The release of ROS is greater with increasing severity of liver injury. HC, healthy controls; *, $P < 0.05$ versus HC; **, $P < 0.01$ versus HC.

These lead to an imbalance between alcohol-induced oxidative stress and the endogenous components of cellular defense against oxidative stress. Antioxidants also attenuate NF-κB activation and TNF-α production in monocytes of patients with alcoholic hepatitis and rat Kupffer cells in vitro [383].

Clinical trials
Vitamin E when used alone was not shown to be significantly beneficial in either alcoholic hepatitis or alcoholic cirrhosis [401,402]. However, neither of these studies were optimally designed and there are data suggesting that vitamin E when combined with other antioxidants may improve outcome in alcoholic hepatitis [403].

N-acetylcysteine (NAC) has been used either alone or in combination with other antioxidants. A combination (NAC, β-carotene, vitamins C and E, selenium, methionine, allopurinol, and desferrioxamine) had lower 30-day survival when compared with corticosteroids in patients with alcoholic hepatitis but this survival difference was lost at 1 year of follow-up [404]. In another study in patients with severe alcoholic hepatitis, stratified by gender and corticosteroid therapy, the response to a loading dose of NAC (150 mg/kg) followed by 100 mg/kg/day for 1 week and daily doses of vitamins A–E, biotin, selenium, zinc, manganese, copper, magnesium, folic acid, and coenzyme Q for 6 months was examined. Antioxidant therapy was found to have no benefit either alone or in combination with corticosteroids at 6 months [405]. In another study published only as an abstract, 87 patients with alcoholic hepatitis (Maddrey DF ≥32) were randomized to corticosteroids with or without NAC. Patients in the NAC arm had a better 1-month survival but this did not persist at 3 and 6 months. A more recent study of intravenous NAC failed to demonstrate any survival benefit at 6 months [406]. These data suggest that despite initial promise, NAC does not seem to confer major survival benefits and any further use of this agent should be as part of clinical studies.

Nutritional supplementation
Rationale
Nutritional therapy for ALD is based on the observations of a high prevalence of protein-calorie malnutrition in ALD, which consists of skeletal muscle loss or sarcopenia, loss of fat mass, and cachexia that includes both muscle and fat loss [91,94,407]. A combination of liver disease, as well as direct toxicity of alcohol on skeletal muscle protein metabolism, contribute to this high prevalence of sarcopenia and cachexia in these patients. The metabolic abnormalities in ALD that contribute to nutritional deficiencies are shown in Box 26.4. Aggressive nutritional therapy should supply optimal nutritional replacement to correct preexisting malnutrition and to provide sufficient amino

Box 26.4 Nutritional deficiency, poor intake, and consequent metabolic derangements in alcoholic liver disease.

Related to hepatic dysfunction

- Poor intake: anorexia, change in mental status, and abdominal distension (ascites)
- Malabsorption: portal hypertensive enteropathy and bile salt deficiency
- Metabolic derangement: decreased respiratory quotient and protein synthesis. Increased amino acid oxidation and resting energy expenditure

Related to alcohol

- Energy metabolism: anorexia and inhibition of ATP production
- Protein synthesis: increased protein breakdown and decreased synthesis.
- Cytokine mediated: TNF-induced apoptosis and decreased DNA synthesis. Increased energy expenditure

Micronutrient imbalances

- Thiamine, folic acid, pyridoxine, vitamin A, vitamin C, vitamin K, hypocalcemia, hypomagnesemia, low selenium, and zinc. Choline and lecithin low

ATP, adenosine triphosphate; TNF, tumor necrosis factor.

acids to encourage hepatic regeneration and reverse sarcopenia. Adequate protein intake is to be encouraged because the previously considered risks of encephalopathy have been found to be overstated. The nutritional requirements in ALD are shown in Table 26.11.

Clinical trials

In a large trial of over 200 patients with ALD, 100% prevalence of nutritional deficiency was reported [408]. Furthermore, protein-calorie malnutrition correlated with short- and long-term mortality and the degree of liver dysfunction in patients with ALD, and improved nutritional status correlated with increased survival [408]. Based on these observations, amino acid infusions have been used in the therapy of alcoholic hepatitis [409]. A total of eight randomized controlled trials and six open labeled trials have been published in patients with alcoholic hepatitis, six studies showing beneficial results and two negative results [195,410,411]. The beneficial results were related to improved histology and/or liver function tests. Improved survival was only reported in a single study [412]. Overall mortality in all studies combined was 17% in the treated group and 9.6% in the control group ($P > 0.05$). In the two studies reporting a negative result, there was a large proportion of patients with inactive cirrhosis rather than active hepatitis [413,414]. As is true with all artificial feedings, the enteral route is preferred over the parenteral route if possible. Based on these results, one may conclude that routine protein restriction is not needed in patients with alcoholic hepatitis with or without cirrhosis even if encephalopathy is present provided oral feeds can be tolerated. However, if encephalopathy worsens with protein-based diets, special amino acid formulations enriched in branched chain amino acids should be considered [415].

A number of trials have examined various nutritional therapies for patients with cirrhosis (Table 26.12). These trials demonstrate that both short-term [416–419] and long-term nutritional intervention provides therapeutic benefit for a number of important clinical outcomes [420–422]. Nutritional therapies have also been used successfully in cirrhotic patients undergoing liver transplant and cirrhotic patients with hepatocellular cancer [423]. Practical guidelines for daily dietary feeding in ALD are shown in Box 26.5.

Myostatin antagonists are currently being tried in human disease with early promising results and, if found

Table 26.11 Nutritional requirements in patients with alcoholic liver disease.

	Protein (g/kg/day)	Energy (kcal/kg/day)	Energy substrate	
			% CHO	% Fat
Alcoholic hepatitis	1.0–1.5	30–40	67–80%	20–33%
Cirrhosis (uncomplicated)	1.0–1.5	30–40	67–80%	20–33%
Cirrhosis (complicated):				
Malnutrition	1.0–1.8	40–50	72%	28%
Cholestasis	1.0–1.5	30–40	73–80%	20–27%
Encephalopathy:				
grade 1 or 2	0.5–1.2	25–40	75%	25%
grade 3 or 4	0.5	25–40	75%	25%
Liver transplant				
Peritransplant	1.2–1.75	30–50	70–80%	20–30%
Post-transplant	1.0	30–35	70%	≤30%

Table 26.12 Nutritional therapy in patients with alcoholic liver disease.

N	Patient profile	Therapy	Benefit	Reference
Short-term studies				
31	Decompensated alcoholic liver disease	Hospitalized enteral feeding (Isocal® 1.5 g protein/kg)	Encephalopathy, serum bilirubin, antipyrine clearance	Kearns et al. [417]
26	Malnourished cirrhosis	Standard oral diet (30–35 kcal/kg daily)	Improved nutritional status and nitrogen balance	Campillo et al. [418]
35	Severely malnourished cirrhotics	Hospitalized enteral feeding (2,115 kcal)	Child score Improved survival (P = 0.065)	Cabré et al. [437]
Long-term studies				
71	Alcoholic cirrhosis and hepatitis	Enteral tube feeding (2,000 kcal/day) or steroids	Higher mortality due to steroids related to infection	Cabré et al. [416]
174	Advanced cirrhosis	BCAA versus lactalbumin/ maltrodextrin 14.4 g/day	Improved Child score Trend to improved survival	Marchesini et al. [419]
64	Chronic encephalopathy	BCAA versus casein supplements (0.24 g/kg)	Encephalopathy Nitrogen balance Bilirubin	Marchesini et al. [420]
32	Symptomatic cirrhosis BCAA/AAA <1.0	BCAA supplements (16 g) Enteral supplements (1,000 kcal)	Delayed death Less frequent hospitalization for sepsis	Yoshida et al. [421]
51	Decompensated alcoholic cirrhosis	Oral supplements (1,000 kcal + 34 g protein)	Less frequent hospitalizations for infections	Hirsch et al. [422]
31	Child B and C	Nutritional supplement (Ensure®) 1,000 kcal + 35 g protein	Improved nutrition and cell-mediated immunity	

AAA, anti-F actin antibody; BCAA, branched chain amino acid.

effective, will form a novel method of reversing the sarcopenia of alcoholic cirrhosis [424].

Other evaluated agents
A number of other agents have been evaluated and these include propylthiouracil, colchicines, and anabolic steroids.

Propylthiouracil
Rationale
Alcoholic hepatitis is associated with a hypermetabolic state with increased energy expenditure and oxygen consumption by the hepatocytes [425]. This could be blocked by propylthiouracil.

Clinical trials
There have been two controlled trials of short-term propylthiouracil in alcoholic hepatitis [426,427]. No difference in mortality was reported in these studies. A Cochrane meta-analysis of six randomized controlled clinical trials of propylthiouracil in patients with alcoholic liver disease (includes steatosis, fibrosis, hepatitis, and/or cirrhosis) found no significant difference between placebo and propylthiouracil in the all-cause or liver-related mortality, complications of liver disease, or liver histology [428].

Colchicine
Rationale
Colchicine inhibits collagen production, increases hepatic collagenase activity, mobilizes ferritin deposits, and inhibits cytokine production.

Clinical trials
There have been two studies reported on the use of colchicine in the therapy of alcoholic hepatitis with no therapeutic benefit [429,430]. A Cochrane review of 15 randomized trials including 1,714 patients concluded that colchicine has no role in alcoholic hepatitis outside controlled clinical trials [431].

Anabolic steroids
Rationale
The anabolic steroids testosterone and oxandrolone have been shown to improve hepatic histology in fatty liver and improve the synthetic functions [377]. In contrast to testosterone, oxandrolone has higher nitrogen-retaining and myotrophic properties. Co-treatment with nutritional supplementation may result in further improved results.

Box 26.5 Guidelines for daily dietary feeding in alcoholic liver disease.

- Protein = 1.0–1.5 g/kg BW
- Total calories = 1.2–1.4 × REE with a minimum of 30 kcal/kg BW:
  50–55% as carbohydrate (preferably as complex carbohydrates)
  30–35% as fat (preferably high in unsaturated fat and with
  adequate essential fatty acids)
- Nutrition should be given enterally by voluntary oral intake and/or
  by small-bore feeding tube; PPN is second choice; TPN is last choice
- Salt and water intake should be adjusted for patient's fluid volume
  and electrolyte status
- Liberal multivitamins and minerals
- Specialized BCAA-enriched supplements are not usually necessary:
  Most patients tolerate standard AA supplements
  Reserve BCAA formulations for patients who cannot tolerate the
  necessary amount of standard AAs (which maintain nitrogen
  balance) without precipitating encephalopathy
  Avoid supplements providing only BCAAs; they do not maintain
  nitrogen balance
  Conditionally essential AAs as well as all essential AAs are
  needed
  Conditionally essential AAs are those that normally can be
  synthesized from other precursors, but cannot be synthesized
  in cirrhotic patients. These include choline, cystine, taurine
  and tyrosine
- Night time snack consisting of 500–700 cal should be given

AA, amino acid; BCAA, branched chain amino acid; BW, body
weight; PPN, peripheral parenteral nutrition; REE, resting energy
expenditure; TPN, total parenteral nutrition.

Adapted from reference [1998].

Clinical trials

A multicenter trial of oxandralone in alcoholic hepatitis showed no difference in 30-day hospital mortality compared with placebo [370]. However, patients with moderate but not severe disease had improved 6-month survival. The Cochrane systematic meta-analysis of anabolic steroids in alcoholic hepatitis did not show a benefit in mortality, complications, or other outcome measures [432].

We conclude that all these other evaluated agents have a secondary role, if any, as an experimental option in alcoholic hepatitis.

Liver transplantation

Even though liver transplantation has been traditionally considered to be the definitive therapy for ALD once cirrhosis has developed and patients have been abstinent, there is increasing interest in offering this option for patients with severe alcoholic hepatitis [315,322]. However, spontaneous improvement may occur with absti-

nence making transplantation unnecessary and, without adequate abstinence, it is believed that the risk of recidivism is high [208,433–435].

Long-term management of alcoholic liver disease

Although less acute than alcoholic hepatitis, continuous long-term management is an important component of the treatment of patients with ALD.

Nutritional therapy

Protein-calorie malnutrition is widely prevalent in ALD [408] and is associated with many of the major complications observed in cirrhosis (infection, encephalopathy, ascites) and indicates a poor prognosis. Consequently the importance for the clinician to recognize and understand the significance of malnutrition in these patients has been emphasized. Current literature on nutritional management of alcoholic cirrhosis has been reviewed recently [436].

Enteral feeding for 3–4 weeks in hospitalized, severely malnourished, or decompensated cirrhotic patients improved survival ($P < 0.065$), hepatic encephalopathy, liver function, and Child–Pugh score, as compared with controls receiving a standard oral diet [437]. In longer term studies, Marchesini and co-workers compared equinitrogenous amounts of dietary branched chain amino acids (BCAAs) versus casein supplements in patients with chronic hepatic encephalopathy for 3–6 months [420]. BCAAs significantly improved encephalopathy, nitrogen balance, and serum bilirubin compared with casein. Hirsch supplemented 34 g of protein and 1,000 kcal to a regular diet in decompensated alcoholic cirrhotics and reduced hospitalizations for infections over a 1-year period [422]. These studies are important because they emphasize the concept that patient selection and long-term therapy may be important factors for employing and demonstrating the benefits of nutritional therapy. Because standard nutritional supplements are effective and the cost of BCAAs is high, the use of BCAA-enriched formulations should be restricted to patients who cannot tolerate nutritionally required amounts of standard formulations.

Changes in dietary feeding patterns may also be beneficial. After an overnight fast, cirrhotic patients obtain more than 70% of nonprotein-calories from fat as compared with 40% in normal volunteers [438]. Therefore, patients with alcoholic cirrhosis have early recruitment of alternative fuels and have metabolic profiles similar to those observed with prolonged fasting. Consequently it has been demonstrated that patients with cirrhosis should not be allowed to starve for extended periods of time and require frequent interval feedings, in particular a night time snack and morning feeding that improve nitrogen balance [195,439–441].

It now seems clear that long-term aggressive nutritional therapy is necessary and reasonable for these patients. General goals and practical points for nutritional therapy in chronic liver disease (see Table 26.11 and Box 26.5) have been suggested, but three additional points need to be emphasized [411,442]. First, nutritional assessment should be an ongoing process. Second, multiple feedings, emphasizing breakfast and a night time snack, with a regular oral diet at higher than usual dietary intakes (1.2–1.5 g/kg for protein and 35–40 kcal/kg for energy) seem indicated [439–441]. Third, during intermittent acute illness or exacerbations of the underlying chronic liver disease, above normal protein (1.5–2.0 g/kg and 40–45 kcal/kg for energy) feeds improve protein-calorie malnutrition [411,438,442].

Propylthiouracil

The hypermetabolic state induced by alcohol ingestion can be ameliorated by propylthiouracil [425]. Direct vasodilator effects of propylthiouracil and well as its antioxidant potential have been suggested to be of value in alcoholic cirrhosis.

Clinical trials

In a large prospective study, involving 310 patients, therapy with propylthiouracil for up to 2 years showed improved survival in the treated group compared to placebo [443]. However, a Cochrane review of propylthiouracil in alcoholic liver disease reviewed six randomized controlled trials with a total of 710 patients administered propylthiouracil or placebo. There was no significant benefit of propylthiouracil compared to placebo on mortality (both total and liver related), complications of liver disease, or liver histology. There was an increase in nonserious adverse effects that was not significant [428].

S-adenosyl methionine

Rationale

S-adenosyl methionine is produced from methionine and ATP in the presence of the enzyme SAMe synthetase, also known as methionine adenosyl transferase (MAT) [444]. SAMe is the principal biologic methyl donor involved in transmethylation, transulfuration, and aminopropylation. The transulfuration pathway is responsible for GSH synthesis – the main cellular antioxidant. Impaired MAT activity occurs in cirrhosis resulting in impaired methionine metabolism with increased levels of methionine and homocysteine [291]. Deficient MAT results in low SAMe levels and hence low GSH. Exogenous GSH is not useful therapeutically because it does not penetrate the hepatocytes. Cysteine is a precursor of GSH, and methionine is the precursor of cysteine. Cysteine and methionine

administration have been unsuccessful in correcting the deficiency of GSH. Oral administration of SAMe bypasses the deficit in SAMe synthesis from methionine.

Clinical trials

Oral SAMe administration has been shown to be effective in humans studies in ALD after a few initial disappointing results [444,445]. SAMe supplementation improved survival in patients with alcoholic cirrhosis who were Child class A and B [445]. In contrast, the Cochrane data base, based on eight randomized controlled trials with 330 patients in different stages of ALD, did not demonstrate any significant effect of SAMe on mortality, liver-related mortality, complications, or liver transplantation in patients with ALD [446]. It concluded that SAMe should not be used for ALD outside randomized clinical trials.

Colchicine

Colchicine has been used in alcoholic cirrhosis with beneficial results reported but few hepatologists prescribe this agent. This may be related to doubts cast on the results of the largest study that reported on the use of colchicine in cirrhosis [447], its potential toxicity, and need for long-term use before any potential benefits can be observed. A systematic meta-analysis by the Cochrane group showed that a total of 14 randomized trials with 1,150 patients have been studied (patients with alcoholic fibrosis, alcoholic hepatitis, and/or alcoholic cirrhosis as well as patients with viral-induced or cryptogenic fibrosis and/or cirrhosis) [431]. The results showed that there was no benefit on overall mortality, liver-related mortality, liver function tests, or histology, with an increased risk of adverse effects related to colchicine therapy. Based on the evidence currently available, colchicine cannot be recommended in the therapy of established alcoholic cirrhosis.

Antiviral therapy

Alcohol use even in moderate quantities has been suggested to worsen the course of hepatitis C [157,448]. Additionally, it has been shown that the response rates to interferon-based treatment protocols are less effective in the presence of active alcohol use [449]. It is therefore recommended that therapy for hepatitis C be started only in patients who become abstinent. If hepatitis C can be eradicated, the long-term prognosis of ALD should improve.

Liver transplantation for ALD

Alcoholic liver disease is the second most common indication for orthotopic liver transplantation (OLT) for chronic liver disease in the western world [450,451]. In the United States, even though specific candidate selection criteria vary from center to center, patients with ALD are transplanted in virtually all programs [452]. The reasons for the resistance to transplant patients with ALD include the pretransplant socioethical issues of donating organs to patients who have perceived self-inflicted liver disease while others who did not pursue such an active self-injurious course wait and potentially die [453,454]. Other concerns include questions regarding the patient's ability to comply with the complex clinical protocols and immunosuppressive regimens after the transplantation, the rate of recidivism to a behavior of alcohol abuse, and recurrence of injury to the transplanted liver [335]. As the number of OLTs in ALD increases, it is becoming more acceptable to transplant these patients as their outcome after OLT is similar to that in nonalcoholic patients [454,455].

Six months of abstinence has been recommended as a minimal listing criterion allowing chemical dependency issues to be resolved during this period. Adherence to the 6-month abstinence could result in a resolution of the anti-inflammatory effects of recent alcohol consumption and thus may make OLT unnecessary in a subset of these patients [434]. The requirement for a fixed abstinence period, the so-called 6-month rule, as a predictor of future abstinence is arbitrary but used most often [456]. However, many abstinence experts are skeptical about this rule because it ignores the complex nature of addictive behavior and it does not accurately predict future drinking by alcoholic candidates for liver transplantation [455–457]. Others, however, have demonstrated that duration of abstinence predicts post-transplant recidivism and recommend at least 6 months of abstinence [433, 435]. A recent study that predicted trajectories of alcohol consumption after liver transplantation also suggested that a period of abstinence is an independent predictor of post-transplant recidivism [458]. These studies, along with recent data indicating that a period of abstinence will permit the recovery of liver function [208], suggest that a minimum of 6 months abstinence is a reasonable recommendation despite many opinions to the contrary.

An evaluation of the peritransplant period in ALD showed that patients were more ill at the time of OLT and likely to have prolonged intensive care unit stays and increased blood product requirements [459]. Decreased acute and chronic rejection after OLT have been reported in patients with ALD compared with nonalcoholic subjects and is probably related to the depression in cellular immunity from the alcohol abuse prior to the OLT [460–462]. There have been a total of 22 published reports on the outcome of liver transplantation in alcoholic patients in over 11,500 patients followed over 11 years, with the largest number being from the European Transplant Registry (Table 26.13) [335,451,459,463–485]. Short-term (1-year) graft survival and patient survival are similar in patients with alcoholic and nonalcoholic cirrhosis.

One third to one half of alcoholic liver recipients will report some use of alcohol in the first 5 years after transplantation [454]. A recent report has reviewed the published data on recidivism after liver transplantation [450]. Rates of recidivism at 3–5 years after OLT have been reported at between 11% and 49% [325,335,468,469, 475,481,486]. It should be emphasized that the rate of recidivism depends on the method used to assess alcohol use and abuse. Higher rates have been reported with objective criteria like urine and blood alcohol levels, carbohydrate-deficient transferring, or a detailed structured interview rather than unstructured questioning of the patient [487,488]. However, recipients who relapse into alcohol use after OLT have similar or potentially lower graft failure rates compared to non-ALD patients. Poor follow-up attendance and noncompliance with therapy is observed in only a minority of patients, and graft rejection rates are similar for patients with ALD (acute rejection 41%, chronic rejection 5.6%) compared with the non-ALD patients (acute rejection 43.7%, chronic rejection 6.2%) [451,454,489]. Since length of sobriety seems to be the most powerful predictor of recidivism, OLT should be offered to appropriately selected patients with ALD [458].

One of the issues that is still unresolved is the role of OLT in acute alcoholic hepatitis. In studies using retrospective histologic analysis of the explanted liver, superimposed alcoholic hepatitis did not worsen the outcome after OLT [490,491]. However, patients in these studies had been abstinent for 3–12 months, had a Maddrey DF <32, and had variable clinical and biologic features of alcoholic hepatitis at the time of OLT. Therefore, the role of OLT in acute alcoholic hepatitis is unresolved at this time [322]. With the availability of living donor transplantation and extended criteria donor, this is likely to further the debate on this issue.

Potential new treatment options

Various nonconventional treatment options have been considered promising in the therapy of ALD. Recently, advances in the understanding of the pathogenesis of ALD have suggested new targets for more successful intervention. Some of the nontraditional treatment options include the following:

1 *Silymarin.* Silymarin (milk thistle) is a mixture of flavinolignans (silibinin, silidianin, silichristin, silybin), of which silybin is the most active [492]. The exact mechanism of action of silymarin is not yet clear but is most likely related to its antioxidant properties. There have been six published trials of silymarin in patients with ALD in doses ranging from 80 to 420 mg/day for time periods of 4 weeks to 6 years with a total of 302 patients treated with silymarin and 305 patients with placebo [492]. Normalization of liver function tests, improvement in liver histology, and possibly longer survival were observed in a significantly higher proportion of patients treated with silymarin compared with

Table 26.13 Results of liver transplantation for patients with alcoholic liver disease.

N	1-year survival	5-year survival	10-year survival	Recidivism	Reference
64	49 (2 years)	–	–	45%	Mackie et al. [335]
51	–	64	–	33	Burra & Lucey [451]
123	84	72	–	19.7	Bellamy et al. [459]
27	93	–	–	21	Gish et al. [463]
18	73 (6 months)	–	–	27.2	Stefanini et al. [464]
42	74	71 (3 years)	–	7	Zibari et al. [465]
40	79	–	–	95	Howard & Fahy [466]
59	80	77	–	34	Lucey et al. [467]
43	100	–	–	19	Osorio et al. [468]
53	–	–	–	32	Pageaux et al. [469]
56	36	–	–	9%	Goldar-Najafi et al. [470]
185	–	72	–	20	Jain et al. [471]
56	–	–	–	8.4	Pereira & Williams [472]
35	74 (2 years)	–	–	–	Dhar et al. [473]
56	–	–	–	50	Tang et al. [474]
44	–	–	–	18	Fabrega et al. [475]
83	74	–	–	12	Kumar et al. [476]
24	66	–	–	17	Bird et al. [477]
41	83	71	–	13	Knechtle et al. [478]
167	–	96.8	–	17.1	Platz et al. [479]
41	–	–	–	8.2	Gerhardt et al. [480]
80	67	49	–	12.8	Berlakovich et al. [481]
305	95	87	82 (abstinent) 68 (recidivism)	27	Schmeding et al. [484]
9,880	84	73	58	–	Burra et al. [482]
300	96	88	76	19	Pfitzmann et al. [483]
110	79	68	64	12	Immordino et al. [490]
49	–	–	78 (9 years)	28	Biselli et al. [485]

placebo. No adverse effects were reported. A Cochrane systematic review and meta-analysis of the 13 published studies of silymarin in ALD and hepatitis B- or C-related liver diseases showed that the overall methodologic quality of the studies was low. Based on high-quality trials, milk thistle does not significantly influence the course of patients with alcoholic and/or hepatitis B or C liver diseases [493].

2 *Other agents.* Thalidomide, misoprostol, adiponectin, and probiotics have been shown in preliminary reports to have anticytokine properties [393,494–496]. However, it must be emphasized that in the past many promising treatments have not passed the test of time as treatment for ALD and alcoholic hepatitis. Emerging data suggest a role for TNF-α-mediated apoptosis in alcoholic hepatitis, and therapy targeting this cytokine to inhibit apoptosis may be effective [497]. However, current poor results with TNF-α antagonists (infliximab, etanercept) are concerning and need to be considered before planning future trials.

3 *Complementary and alternative medications.* A number of alternative treatment options in addition to those dis-

cussed above have been reviewed [377,492]. There are not adequate clinical data available to make any recommendations since most of these studies were in animal models or in vitro systems.

Future directions

In light of a still incomplete understanding of the involved pathophysiologic mechanisms and conflicting data regarding the efficacy of specific interventional therapies of ALD, a conservative approach seems justified. These include general supportive care, aggressive nutritional interventions, and the judicious use of corticosteroids and pentoxifylline in selected patients with severe alcoholic hepatitis. In addition, abstinence from alcohol, treating the co-morbidities of obesity and hepatitis C, and continuous nutritional monitoring are prudent on a long-term basis, with liver transplantation offered for select patients with progressive disease. Algorithms have been proposed for both alcoholic hepatitis and long-term management of ALD (Figs 26.18 and 26.19). Although these

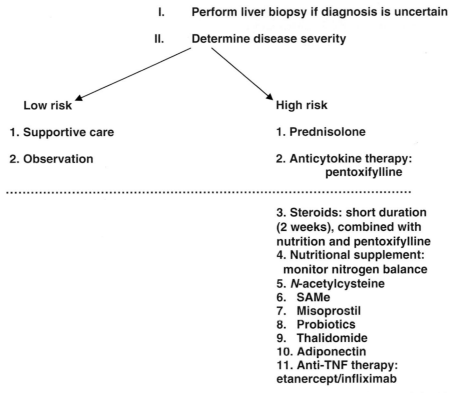

I.   **Perform liver biopsy if diagnosis is uncertain**

II.   **Determine disease severity**

Low risk

1. **Supportive care**

2. **Observation**

High risk

1. **Prednisolone**

2. **Anticytokine therapy:**
   pentoxifylline

3. **Steroids: short duration**
(2 weeks), combined with
nutrition and pentoxifylline
4. **Nutritional supplement:**
   monitor nitrogen balance
5. ***N*-acetylcysteine**
6. **SAMe**
7. **Misoprostil**
8. **Probiotics**
9. **Thalidomide**
10. **Adiponectin**
11. **Anti-TNF therapy:**
etanercept/infliximab

Figure 26.18 Proposed therapeutic algorithm for alcoholic hepatitis. High-risk patients are those with severe disease as defined by a modified discriminant function ≥ 32, the presence of encephalopathy, or a MELD score ≥ 18–21. Therapies under the broken line remain experimental but merit further study. SAMe, S-adenosyl methionine; TNF, tumor necrosis factor.

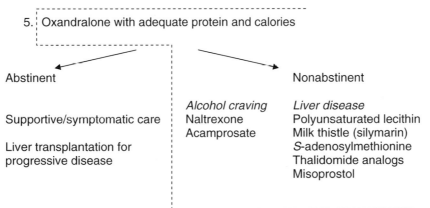

1. Emphasize abstinence

2. Determine histology

3. Nutritional manipulation
      i.   Frequent feeding with night time snack
      ii. Be vigilant for increasing protein requirements
      iii. Micronutrient replacement, care regarding vitamin A and iron toxicity
4. Treat co-morbidities

5. Oxandralone with adequate protein and calories

Abstinent

Supportive/symptomatic care

Liver transplantation for
progressive disease

Alcohol craving
Naltrexone
Acamprosate

Nonabstinent

Liver disease
Polyunsaturated lecithin
Milk thistle (silymarin)
S-adenosylmethionine
Thalidomide analogs
Misoprostol

Figure 26.19 Proposed therapeutic algorithm for the long-term management of alcoholic liver disease. Liver biopsy is indicated if diagnosis is uncertain, especially if there is serologic evidence of iron overload or viral infection. Both hepatitis C and obesity (if patient is abstinent) should be treated if present. Therapies within the broken line remain experimental but merit further study.

algorithms are by necessity incomplete, they are provided to stimulate different approaches to this disease and to emphasize several of the following important issues:

1 Abstinence and dietary manipulation should be emphasized in the long-term management of these patients. The issue of abstinence from alcohol will play an important role in determining medical treatment as well as candidacy for liver transplantation.

2 The high prevalence of hepatitis C must be considered regarding its potential influence upon prognosis and therapeutic strategies.

3 Future therapeutic directions should aim at specific pathophysiologic mechanisms of alcohol-induced hepatocellular damage as well as the regulation of hepatic regeneration in this disease. Combination therapy targeting both direct and indirect mechanisms of alcohol-induced hepatocellular damage as well as the regenerative capacity of the injured liver may prove to be necessary after assessment of disease severity and prognosis. Clinical trials of combined therapy are needed and include:

- A mechanism to reduce hypermetabolism and centrilobular hypoxia/ischemia.
- A means to maintain or enhance gut integrity. The role of nutrition needs to be investigated. Furthermore, more objective and systemic ways to assess the function and integrity of the intestinal mucosa are required.
- The role of bowel sterilization with antibiotics to decrease bacterial translocation and endotoxin- and cytokine-mediated liver damage.
- Modification of immunologic mechanisms.
- Altering cytokine-mediated inflammation and fibrosis. Potential therapeutic interventions include antibodies or antagonists to specific cytokines of pathogenetic importance and drugs that modulate the actions of these cytokines. Despite the available, somewhat compelling animal and in vitro data, therapies directed against anti-TNF may be particularly helpful but the poor outcome of published trials must be considered before new studies are undertaken.
- The inhibition of fibrogenesis by blocking factors, which promote fibrogenesis, and by stimulating collagen degradation or suppressing collagen gene expression.
- The regulation of iron metabolism, altering iron accumulation to reduce the progression of fibrosis and development of hepatocellular carcinoma.
- Hepatotropic agents to maximize the capacity of cell repair.
- Exploring new strategies to decrease lipid peroxidation and its sequelae. SAMe, N-acetylcysteine, and vitamin E may be particularly relevant in this area.

- Orthotopic and living donor liver transplantation are a realistic option for alcoholic cirrhosis and increasing evidence supports a period of abstinence before listing. Their roles in alcoholic hepatitis continue to remain a matter of debate.

Conclusions

Alcoholic liver disease is a common illness, which develops in only a subgroup of people who chronically use or abuse alcohol. The hepatotoxic dose of alcohol is nonuniform and dependent on incompletely understood risk factors, which include gender, ethnicity, hepatitis C, nutritional status (particularly obesity), iron accumulation, and possibly genetic factors. These factors, in addition to a variable natural history and changing epidemiology, especially with regard to binge drinking and pathophysiology, can make ALD difficult to diagnose and frustrating to manage.

The management of the complications of chronic liver disease (ascites, portal hypertension-associated bleeding, encephalopathy, and hepatocellular) is similar in alcoholic and nonalcoholic liver disease. However, abstinence remains the cornerstone of therapy for ALD. There is also consensus for the use of corticosteroids and pentoxifylline in severe alcoholic hepatitis, for maintaining good nutritional status, for treating co-morbidities in all forms of ALD, and for liver transplantation in carefully selected patients with end-stage ALD. No other therapies can be recommended at the present time, although nascent data suggest that a number of newer therapies may be effective, as discussed above. The recently published practice guidelines for the management of ALD provide evidence-based therapy.

Building on our increased knowledge of the molecular basis of ALD, a greater understanding of the pathophysiology of ALD, the interactive role of other cofactors in causing hepatotoxicity, and translation to human disease need to remain a major focus of alcohol research.

Annotated references

Breitkopf K, Nagy LE, Beier JI, Mueller S, Weng H, Dooley S. Current experimental perspectives on the clinical progression of alcoholic liver disease. *Alcohol Clin Exp Res* 2009;33(10):1647–55.

Mandrekar P, Szabo G. Signalling pathways in alcohol-induced liver inflammation. *J Hepatol* 2009;50(6):1258–66.

Purohit V, Gao B, Song BJ. Molecular mechanisms of alcoholic fatty liver. *Alcohol Clin Exp Res* 2009;33(2):191–205.
These are detailed reviews of the current concepts in alcoholic liver disease. They discuss the epidemiology, pathogenetic mechanisms, role of different cell types, and molecular mechanisms in the pathogenesis of ALD.

Burra P, Senzolo M, Adam R, et al., ELITA and ELTR Liver Transplant Centers. Liver transplantation for alcoholic liver disease in Europe: a study from the ELTR (European Liver Transplant Registry). *Am J Transplant* 2010;10(1):138–48.

Karim Z, Intaraprasong P, Scudamore CH, et al. Predictors of relapse to significant alcohol drinking after liver transplantation. *Can J Gastroenterol* 2010;24(4):245–50.

Tan HH, Virmani S, Martin P. Controversies in the management of alcoholic liver disease. *Mt Sinai J Med* 2009;76(5):484–98.
These may be considered to be the most comprehensive studies on liver transplantation in ALD and recidivism. The current beliefs, myths, and facts are discussed. The evolution of the current status of transplantation for ALD is discussed emphasizing as a conclusion that abstinent alcoholic cirrhosis is considered an appropriate indication for liver transplantation.

Cabré E, Gassull MA. Nutrition in liver disease. *Curr Opin Clin Nutr Metab Care* 2005;8(5):545–51.

Leevy CM, Moroianu SA. Nutritional aspects of alcoholic liver disease. *Clin Liver Dis* 2005;9(1):67–81.

Stickel F, Hoehn B, Schuppan D, Seitz HK. Review article: nutritional therapy in alcoholic liver disease. *Aliment Pharmacol Ther* 2003;18(4):357–73.
These studies emphasize the role of nutritional evaluation, supplementation, and maintenance in the short- and long-term treatment of alcoholic liver disease.

Dunn W, Jamil LH, Brown LS, et al. MELD accurately predicts mortality in patients with alcoholic hepatitis. *Hepatology* 2005;41(2):353–8.

Mathurin P, O'Grady J, Carithers RL, et al. Corticosteroids improve short-term survival in patients with severe alcoholic hepatitis: meta-analysis of individual patient data. *Gut* 2010;60:255–60.

O'Shea RS, Dasarathy S, McCullough AJ. Alcoholic liver disease. *Hepatology* 2010;51(1):307–328.

Tilg H, Day CP. Management strategies in alcoholic liver disease. *Nat Clin Pract Gastroenterol Hepatol* 2007;4(1):24–34.
These are the most recent studies on the prognostic criteria and current treatment options in severe alcoholic hepatitis. Both acute and long term effects of prednisolone and the acute effects of pentoxifylline suggest beneficial effects in severe alcoholic hepatitis.

Mullen KD, Dasarathy S. Potential new therapies for alcoholic liver disease. *Clin Liver Dis* 1998;2:851–81.
This article reviews many of the potential new therapies, specifically nontraditional treatment, for alcoholic liver disease that could not be discussed in detail in this chapter.

References

1. Windle M, Windle RC. Adolescent tobacco, alcohol, and drug use: current findings. *Adolesc Med* 1999;10(1):153–63, vii.
2. Brandish E, Sheron N. Drinking patterns and the risk of serious liver disease. *Expert Rev Gastroenterol Hepatol* 2010;4(3):249–52.
3. Chikritzhs TN, Allsop SJ, Moodie AR, Hall WD. Per capita alcohol consumption in Australia: will the real trend please step forward? *Med J Aust* 2010;193(10):594–7.
4. Welte J, Barnes G, Wieczorek W, Tidwell MC, Parker J. Alcohol and gambling pathology among US adults: prevalence, demographic patterns and comorbidity. *J Stud Alcohol* 2001;62(5):706–12.
5. Caetano R, Tam T, Greenfield T, Cherpitel C, Midanik L. DSM-IV alcohol dependence and drinking in the US population: a risk analysis. *Ann Epidemiol* 1997;7(8):542–9.
6. Tam TW, Midanik LT. The effect of screening on prevalence estimates of alcohol dependence and social consequences. *J Stud Alcohol* 2000;61(4):617–21.
7. Greenfield TK, Midanik LT, Rogers JD. A 10-year national trend study of alcohol consumption, 1984–1995: is the period of declining drinking over? *Am J Public Health* 2000;90(1):47–52.
8. Gordis E. Advances in research on alcoholism and what they promise for future treatment and prevention. *Med Health R I* 1999;82(4):121.
9. Li TK, Hewitt BG, Grant BF. The alcohol dependence syndrome, 30 years later: a commentary. The 2006 H. David Archibald lecture. *Addiction* 2007;102(10):1522–30.
10. Hasin D, Paykin A, Meydan J, Grant B. Withdrawal and tolerance: prognostic significance in DSM-IV alcohol dependence. *J Stud Alcohol* 2000;61(3):431–8.
11. Corrao G, Bagnardi V, Vittadini G, Favilli S. Capture–recapture methods to size alcohol related problems in a population. *J Epidemiol Community Health* 2000;54(8):603–10.
12. Chick J, Erickson CK. Conference summary: consensus conference on alcohol dependence and the role of pharmacotherapy in its treatment. *Alcohol Clin Exp Res* 1996;20(2):391–402.
13. Kitchens JM. Does this patient have an alcohol problem? *JAMA* 1994;272(22):1782–7.
14. American Psychiatric Association. *Diagnostic and Statistical Manual of Mental Disorders* 4th edn. Washington, DC: APA, 1994.
15. World Health Organization. *World Health Organization. The ICD/10 classification of mental and behavioural disorders: clinical descriptions and diagnostic guidelines*, 10th revision. Geneva: WHO, 1992.
16. Lieber CS. Alcoholic liver disease: new insights in pathogenesis lead to new treatments. *J Hepatol* 2000;32(1 Suppl):113–28.
17. Day PC. [Genetic background of alcoholic liver disease.] *Orv Hetil* 2000;141(4):163–7.
18. Day CP. Who gets alcoholic liver disease: nature or nurture? (Extended abstract). *Acta Gastroenterol Belg* 2003;66(4):290–1.
19. Lefkowitch JH. Morphology of alcoholic liver disease. *Clin Liver Dis* 2005;9(1):37–53.
20. Mendez-Sanchez N, Meda-Valdes P, Uribe M. Alcoholic liver disease. An update. *Ann Hepatol* 2005;4(1):32–42.
21. Menon KV, Gores GJ, Shah VH. Pathogenesis, diagnosis, and treatment of alcoholic liver disease. *Mayo Clin Proc* 2001;76(10):1021–9
22. Liew CT. The clinicopathological spectrum of alcoholic liver disease – an autopsy survey of 441 cases. *Changgeng Yi Xue Za Zhi* 1990;13(2):72–85.
23. Cameron RG, Neuman MG. Novel morphologic findings in alcoholic liver disease. *Clin Biochem* 1999;32(7):579–84.
24. MacSween RN, Burt AD. Histologic spectrum of alcoholic liver disease. *Semin Liver Dis* 1986 Aug;6(3):221–232.
25. Crapper RM, Bhathaland PS, Mackay IR. Chronic active hepatitis in alcoholic patients. *Liver* 1983;3(5):327–37.
26. Anderson S, Nevins CL, Green LK, El Zimaity H, Anand BS. Assessment of liver histology in chronic alcoholics with and without hepatitis C virus infection. *Dig Dis Sci* 2001;46(7):1393–8.
27. Crabb DW. Pathogenesis of alcoholic liver disease: newer mechanisms of injury. *Keio J Med* 1999;48(4):184–8.
28. Lieber CS, Spritz N. Effects of prolonged ethanol intake in man: role of dietary adipose, and endogenously synthesized fatty acids in the pathogenesis of the alcoholic fatty liver. *J Clin Invest* 1966;45(9):1400–11.
29. Lieber CS, Jones DP, DeCarli LM. Effects of prolonged ethanol intake: production of fatty liver despite adequate diets. *J Clin Invest* 1965;44: 1009–21.
30. Hegedus G. [Pathology of alcoholic liver disease]. *Orv Hetil* 2000;141(7):331–6.
31. Worner TM, Lieber CS. Perivenular fibrosis as precursor lesion of cirrhosis. *JAMA* 1985;254(5):627–30.
32. Poli G. Pathogenesis of liver fibrosis: role of oxidative stress. *Mol Aspects Med* 2000;21(3):49–98.
33. Mach T. Fatty liver – current look at the old disease. *Med Sci Monit* 2000;6(1):209–16.
34. Naveau S, Raynard B, Ratziu V, et al. Biomarkers for the prediction of liver fibrosis in patients with chronic alcoholic liver disease. *Clin Gastroenterol Hepatol* 2005;3(2):167–74.

35. Breitkopf K, Nagy LE, Beier JI, Mueller S, Weng H, Dooley S. Current experimental perspectives on the clinical progression of alcoholic liver disease. *Alcohol Clin Exp Res* 2009;33(10): 1647–55.

36. Lieber CS. Pathogenesis and treatment of liver fibrosis in alcoholics: 1996 update. *Dig Dis* 1997;15(1–2):42–66.

37. Christensen E, Schlichting P, Andersen PK, et al. Updating prognosis and therapeutic effect evaluation in cirrhosis with Cox's multiple regression model for time-dependent variables. *Scand J Gastroenterol* 1986;21(2):163–74.

38. Savolainen V, Perola M, Lalu K, Penttila A, Virtanen I, Karhunen PJ. Early perivenular fibrogenesis – precirrhotic lesions among moderate alcohol consumers and chronic alcoholics. *J Hepatol* 1995; 23(5):524–31.

39. Diehl AM. Alcoholic liver disease: natural history. *Liver Transpl Surg* 1997;3(3):206–11.

40. Beier JI, McClain CJ. Mechanisms and cell signaling in alcoholic liver disease. *Biol Chem* 2010;391(11):1249–64.

41. Teli MR, Day CP, Burt AD, Bennett MK, James OF. Determinants of progression to cirrhosis or fibrosis in pure alcoholic fatty liver. *Lancet* 1995;346(8981):987–90.

42. Orholm M, Sorensen TI, Bentsen K, Hoybye G, Eghoje K, Christoffersen P. Mortality of alcohol abusing men prospectively assessed in relation to history of abuse and degree of liver injury. *Liver* 1985;5(5):253–60.

43. Day CP, Yeaman SJ. The biochemistry of alcohol-induced fatty liver. *Biochim Biophys Acta* 1994;1215(1–2):33–48.

44. Stewart S, Jones D, Day CP. Alcoholic liver disease: new insights into mechanisms and preventative strategies. *Trends Mol Med* 2001;7(9):408–13.

45. Bird GL, Williams R. Factors determining cirrhosis in alcoholic liver disease. *Mol Aspects Med* 1988;10(2):97–105.

46. Lindros KO. Alcoholic liver disease: pathobiological aspects. *J Hepatol* 1995;23(Suppl 1):7–15.

47. Mandayam S, Jamal MM, Morgan TR. Epidemiology of alcoholic liver disease. *Semin Liver Dis* 2004;24(3):217–32.

48. Stinson FS, Grant BF, Dufour MC. The critical dimension of ethnicity in liver cirrhosis mortality statistics. *Alcohol Clin Exp Res* 2001;25(8):1181–7.

49. Stewart SH, Connors GJ. Ethnicity, alcohol drinking and changes in transaminase activity among heavy drinkers. *J Natl Med Assoc* 2007;99(5):564–9.

50. Wickramasinghe SN, Corridan B, Izaguirre J, Hasan R, Marjot DH. Ethnic differences in the biological consequences of alcohol abuse: a comparison between south Asian and European males. *Alcohol Alcohol* 1995;30(5):675–80.

51. Savolainen VT, Liesto K, Mannikko A, Penttila A, Karhunen PJ. Alcohol consumption and alcoholic liver disease: evidence of a threshold level of effects of ethanol. *Alcohol Clin Exp Res* 1993;17(5): 1112–17.

52. Rehm J, Taylor B, Mohapatra S, et al. Alcohol as a risk factor for liver cirrhosis: a systematic review and meta-analysis. *Drug Alcohol Rev* 2010;29(4):437–45.

53. Patra J, Taylor B, Irving H, et al. Alcohol consumption and the risk of morbidity and mortality for different stroke types – a systematic review and meta-analysis. *BMC Public Health* 2010;10: 258.

54. Kamper-Jorgensen M, Gronbaek M, Tolstrup J, Becker U. Alcohol and cirrhosis: dose–response or threshold effect? *J Hepatol* 2004;41(1):25–30.

55. Becker U, Deis A, Sorensen TI, et al. Prediction of risk of liver disease by alcohol intake, sex, and age: a prospective population study. *Hepatology* 1996;23(5):1025–9.

56. Batey RG. Wine, the tax man and alcohol-related disease. *Med J Aust* 1995;162(11):565.

57. Seitz HK, Salaspuro M, Savolainen M, et al. From alcohol toxicity to treatment. *Alcohol Clin Exp Res* 2005;29(7):1341–50.

58. Bellentani S, Saccoccio G, Costa G, et al. Drinking habits as cofactors of risk for alcohol induced liver damage. The Dionysos Study Group. *Gut* 1997;41(6):845–50.

59. Seitz HK, Lieber CS, Stickel F, Salaspuro M, Schlemmer HP, Horie Y. Alcoholic liver disease: from pathophysiology to therapy. *Alcohol Clin Exp Res* 2005;29(7):1276–81.

60. Bellentani S, Pozzato G, Saccoccio G, et al. Clinical course and risk factors of hepatitis C virus related liver disease in the general population: report from the Dionysos study. *Gut* 1999;44(6):874–80.

61. Bode C, Bode JC, Erhardt JG, French BA, French SW. Effect of the type of beverage and meat consumed by alcoholics with alcoholic liver disease. *Alcohol Clin Exp Res* 1998;22(8):1803–5.

62. Becker U, Gronbaek M, Johansen D, Sorensen TI. Lower risk for alcohol-induced cirrhosis in wine drinkers. *Hepatology* 2002;35(4): 868–75.

63. Everhart JE. In vino veritas? *J Hepatol* 2003;38(2):245–6.

64. Szucs S, Sarvary A, McKee M, Adany R. Could the high level of cirrhosis in central and eastern Europe be due partly to the quality of alcohol consumed? An exploratory investigation. *Addiction* 2005;100(4):536–42.

65. Lu XL, Luo JY, Tao M, et al. Risk factors for alcoholic liver disease in China. *World J Gastroenterol* 2004;10(16):2423–6.

66. Pelletier S, Vaucher E, Aider R, et al. Wine consumption is not associated with a decreased risk of alcoholic cirrhosis in heavy drinkers. *Alcohol Alcohol* 2002;37(6):618–21.

67. Wechsler H, Austin SB. Binge drinking: the five/four measure. *J Stud Alcohol* 1998;59(1):122–4.

68. Barrio E, Tome S, Rodriguez I, et al. Liver disease in heavy drinkers with and without alcohol withdrawal syndrome. *Alcohol Clin Exp Res* 2004;28(1):131–6.

69. Mansouri A, Gaou I, De KC, et al. An alcoholic binge causes massive degradation of hepatic mitochondrial DNA in mice. *Gastroenterology* 1999;117(1):181–90.

70. Mathurin P, Deltenre P. Effect of binge drinking on the liver: an alarming public health issue? *Gut* 2009;58(5):613–17.

71. Pares A, Caballeria J, Bruguera M, Torres M, Rodes J. Histological course of alcoholic hepatitis. Influence of abstinence, sex and extent of hepatic damage. *J Hepatol* 1986;2(1):33–42.

72. Loft S, Olesen KL, Dossing M. Increased susceptibility to liver disease in relation to alcohol consumption in women. *Scand J Gastroenterol* 1987;22(10):1251–6.

73. Norton R, Batey R, Dwyer T, MacMahon S. Alcohol consumption and the risk of alcohol related cirrhosis in women. *Br Med J (Clin Res Ed)* 1987;295(6590):80–2.

74. Sato N, Lindros KO, Baraona E, et al. Sex difference in alcohol-related organ injury. *Alcohol Clin Exp Res* 2001;25(5 Suppl ISBRA): S40–5.

75. Eagon PK. Alcoholic liver injury: influence of gender and hormones. *World J Gastroenterol* 2010;16(11):1377–84.

76. Lelbach WK. Quantitative aspects of drinking in alcoholic liver cirrhosis. In: Khanna HM: Israel Y, eds. *Alcoholic Liver Pathology*. Toronto: Addiction Research Foundation, 1975: 118.

77. Lelbach WK. Epidemiology of alcoholic liver disease. *Prog Liver Dis* 1976;5: 494–515.

78. Becker PU, Deis A, Sorensen TI, et al. [Alcohol intake and risk of liver disease – significance of gender. A population study.] *Ugeskr Laeger* 1997;159(24):3782–6.

79. Frezza M, di Padova C, Pozzato G, Terpin M, Baraona E, Lieber CS. High blood alcohol levels in women. The role of decreased gastric alcohol dehydrogenase activity and first-pass metabolism. *N Engl J Med* 1990;322(2):95–9.

80. Nanji AA, French SW. Female to male mortality ratios for alcohol-related disorders: possible indicator of susceptibility in different sexes. *Adv Alcohol Subst Abuse* 1987;6(3):89–95.

81. Van Thiel DH. Gender differences in the susceptibility and severity of alcohol- induced liver disease. *Alcohol Alcohol Suppl* 1991;1:9–18.

82. Yin SJ, Liao CS, Wu CW, et al. Human stomach alcohol and aldehyde dehydrogenases: comparison of expression pattern and activities in alimentary tract. *Gastroenterology* 1997;112(3):766–75.

83. Yin SJ, Han CL, Liao CS, Wu CW. Expression, activities, and kinetic mechanism of human stomach alcohol dehydrogenase. Inference for first-pass metabolism of ethanol in mammals. *Adv Exp Med Biol* 1997;414: 347–55.

84. Frezza M, Buda A, Terpin MM, et al. Gastrectomy, lack of gastric first pass metabolism of ethanol and alcoholic liver disease. Results of a multicentre study. *Ital J Gastroenterol Hepatol* 1997;29(3):243–8.

85. Nanji AA, Jokelainen K, Fotouhinia M, et al. Increased severity of alcoholic liver injury in female rats: role of oxidative stress, endotoxin, and chemokines. *Am J Physiol Gastrointest Liver Physiol* 2001;281(6):G1348–56.

86. Yin M, Ikejima K, Wheeler MD, et al. Estrogen is involved in early alcohol-induced liver injury in a rat enteral feeding model. *Hepatology* 2000;31(1):117–23.

87. Aleynik MK, Lieber CS. Dilinoleoylphosphatidylcholine decreases ethanol-induced cytochrome P4502E1. *Biochem Biophys Res Commun* 2001;288(4):1047–51.

88. Sarin SK, Dhingra N, Bansal A, Malhotra S, Guptan RC. Dietary and nutritional abnormalities in alcoholic liver disease: a comparison with chronic alcoholics without liver disease. *Am J Gastroenterol* 1997,92(5).777–83.

89. French SW. Nutrition in the pathogenesis of alcoholic liver disease. *Alcohol Alcohol* 1993;28(1):97–109.

90. Jacobs RM, Sorrell MF. The role of nutrition in the pathogenesis of alcoholic liver disease. *Semin Liver Dis* 1981;1(3):244–53.

91. Mendenhall CL, Moritz TE, Roselle GA, et al. Protein energy malnutrition in severe alcoholic hepatitis: diagnosis and response to treatment. The VA Cooperative Study Group #275. *JPEN J Parenter Enteral Nutr* 1995;19(4):258–65.

92. Mendenhall C, Roselle GA, Gartside P, Moritz T. Relationship of protein calorie malnutrition to alcoholic liver disease: a reexamination of data from two Veterans Administration Cooperative Studies. *Alcohol Clin Exp Res* 1995;19(3):635–41.

93. McCullough AJ, O'Connor JF. Alcoholic liver disease: proposed recommendations for the American College of Gastroenterology. *Am J Gastroenterol* 1998;93(11):2022–36.

94. Leevy CM, Moroianu SA. Nutritional aspects of alcoholic liver disease. *Clin Liver Dis* 2005;9(1):67–81.

95. Iturriaga H, Bunout D, Hirsch S, Ugarte G. Overweight as a risk factor or a predictive sign of histological liver damage in alcoholics. *Am J Clin Nutr* 1988;47(2):235–8.

96. Naveau S, Giraud V, Borotto E, Aubert A, Capron F, Chaput JC. Excess weight risk factor for alcoholic liver disease. *Hepatology* 1997;25(1):108–11.

97. Diehl AM. Obesity and alcoholic liver disease. *Alcohol* 2004;34(1):81–7.

98. Clouston AD, Powell EE. Interaction of non-alcoholic fatty liver disease with other liver diseases. *Best Pract Res Clin Gastroenterol* 2002;16(5):767–81.

99. Nanji AA, French SW. Dietary factors and alcoholic cirrhosis. *Alcohol Clin Exp Res* 1986;10(3):271–3.

100. Mezey E. Dietary fat and alcoholic liver disease. *Hepatology* 1998;28(4):901–5.

101. Tipoe GL, Liong EC, Leung TM, Nanji AA. A voluntary oral-feeding rat model for pathological alcoholic liver injury. *Methods Mol Biol* 2008;447: 11–31.

102. Nanji AA. Role of different dietary fatty acids in the pathogenesis of experimental alcoholic liver disease. *Alcohol* 2004;34(1):21–5.

103. Nanji AA, Zakim D, Rahemtulla A, et al. Dietary saturated fatty acids down-regulate cyclooxygenase-2 and tumor necrosis factor alfa and reverse fibrosis in alcohol-induced liver disease in the rat. *Hepatology* 1997;26(6):1538–45.

104. Dasarathy S, McCullough AJ, Muc S, et al. Sarcopenia associated with portostemic shunting is reversed by follistatin. *J Hepatol* 2011;54: 915–21.

105. Lang CH, Frost RA, Svanberg E, Vary TC. IGF-I/IGFBP-3 ameliorates alterations in protein synthesis, eIF4E availability, and myostatin in alcohol-fed rats. *Am J Physiol Endocrinol Metab* 2004;286(6):E916–26.

106. Garcia PS, Cabbabe A, Kambadur R, Nicholas G, Csete M. Brief-reports: elevated myostatin levels in patients with liver disease: a potential contributor to skeletal muscle wasting. *Anesth Analg* 2010;111(3):707–9.

107. Uhl GR, Liu QR, Walther D, Hess J, Naiman D. Polysubstance abuse-vulnerability genes: genome scans for association, using 1,004 subjects and 1,494 single-nucleotide polymorphisms. *Am J Hum Genet* 2001;69(6):1290–300.

108. Brown K. Alcohol hepatotoxicity: a genotypic predisposition? *Am J Gastroenterol* 1992;87(5):677–8.

109. Enoch MA, Goldman D. Genetics of alcoholism and substance abuse. *Psychiatr Clin North Am* 1999;22(2):289–99, viii.

110. Goldman D, Bergen A. General and specific inheritance of substance abuse and alcoholism. *Arch Gen Psychiatry* 1998;55(11):964–5

111. Harada S, Okubo T, Tsutsumi M, Takase S, Muramatsu T. Investigation of genetic risk factors associated with alcoholism. *Alcohol Clin Exp Res* 1996;20(9 Suppl):293A–296A.

112. Ladero JM, Martinez C, Garcia-Martin E, et al. Polymorphisms of the glutathione S-transferases mu-1 (GSTM1) and theta-1 (GSTT1) and the risk of advanced alcoholic liver disease. *Scand J Gastroenterol* 2005;40(3):348–53.

113. Roberts-Thomson IC, Butler WJ. Polymorphism, alcohol and alcoholic liver disease. *J Gastroenterol Hepatol* 2004;19(12):1421–2.

114. Borras E, Coutelle C, Rosell A, et al. Genetic polymorphism of alcohol dehydrogenase in europeans: the ADH2*2 allele decreases the risk for alcoholism and is associated with ADH3*1. *Hepatology* 2000;31(4):984–9.

115. Wong NA, Rae F, Bathgate A, Smith CA, Harrison DJ. Polymorphisms of the gene for microsomal epoxide hydrolase and susceptibility to alcoholic liver disease and hepatocellular carcinoma in a Caucasian population. *Toxicol Lett* 2000;115(1):17–22.

116. Wong NA, Rae F, Simpson KJ, Murray GD, Harrison DJ. Genetic polymorphisms of cytochrome p4502E1 and susceptibility to alcoholic liver disease and hepatocellular carcinoma in a white population: a study and literature review, including meta-analysis. *Mol Pathol* 2000;53(2):88–93.

117. Monzoni A, Masutti F, Saccoccio G, Bellentani S, Tiribelli C, Giacca M. Genetic determinants of ethanol-induced liver damage. *Mol Med* 2001;7(4):255–62.

118. Enomoto N, Takada A, Date T. Genotyping of the aldehyde dehydrogenase 2 (ALDH2) gene using the polymerase chain reaction: evidence for single point mutation in the ALDH2 gene of ALDH2-deficiency. *Gastroenterol Jpn* 1991;26(4):440–7.

119. Wan YJ, Poland RE, Lin KM. Genetic polymorphism of CYP2E1, ADH2, and ALDH2 in Mexican-Americans. *Genet Test* 1998;2(1):79–83.

120. Wall TL, Shea SH, Chan KK, Carr LG. A genetic association with the development of alcohol and other substance use behavior in Asian Americans. *J Abnorm Psychol* 2001;110(1):173–8.

121. McCarthy DM, Wall TL, Brown SA, Carr LG. Integrating biological and behavioral factors in alcohol use risk: the role of ALDH2 status and alcohol expectancies in a sample of Asian Americans. *Exp Clin Psychopharmacol* 2000;8(2):168–75.

122. Sun AY, Ingelman-Sundberg M, Neve E, et al. Ethanol and oxidative stress. *Alcohol Clin Exp Res* 2001;25(5 Suppl ISBRA):S237–43.

123. Tanaka F, Shiratori Y, Yokosuka O, Imazeki F, Tsukada Y, Omata M. Polymorphism of alcohol-metabolizing genes affects drinking behavior and alcoholic liver disease in Japanese men. *Alcohol Clin Exp Res* 1997;21(4):596–601.

124. Gonzalez FJ. Role of cytochromes P450 in chemical toxicity and oxidative stress: studies with CYP2E1. *Mutat Res* 2005;569(1–2):101–10.

125. Tsutsumi M, Takada A, Wang JS. Genetic polymorphisms of cytochrome P4502E1 related to the development of alcoholic liver disease. *Gastroenterology* 1994;107(5):1430–5.

126. Chao YC, Young TH, Tang HS, Hsu CT. Alcoholism and alcoholic organ damage and genetic polymorphisms of alcohol metabolizing enzymes in Chinese patients. *Hepatology* 1997;25(1):112–17.

127. Gordillo-Bastidas E, Panduro A, Gordillo-Bastidas D, et al. Polymorphisms of alcohol metabolizing enzymes in indigenous Mexican population: unusual high frequency of CYP2E1*c2 allele. *Alcohol Clin Exp Res* 2010;34(1):142–9.

128. Stickel F, Osterreicher CH. The role of genetic polymorphisms in alcoholic liver disease. *Alcohol Alcohol* 2006;41(3):209–24.

129. Degoul F, Sutton A, Mansouri A, et al. Homozygosity for alanine in the mitochondrial targeting sequence of superoxide dismutase and risk for severe alcoholic liver disease. *Gastroenterology* 2001;120(6):1468–74.

130. Stewart SF, Leathart JB, Chen Y, et al. Valine-alanine manganese superoxide dismutase polymorphism is not associated with alcohol-induced oxidative stress or liver fibrosis. *Hepatology* 2002;36(6):1355–60.

131. Fujimoto J. Gene therapy for liver cirrhosis. *J Gastroenterol Hepatol* 2000;15(Suppl):D33–6.

132. Horie Y, Kato S, Ohki E, Tamai H, Ishii H. Role of endothelin in endotoxin-induced hepatic microvascular dysfunction in rats fed chronically with ethanol. *J Gastroenterol Hepatol* 2001;16(8):916–22.

133. McClain CJ, Song Z, Barve SS, Hill DB, Deaciuc I. Recent advances in alcoholic liver disease. IV. Dysregulated cytokine metabolism in alcoholic liver disease. *Am J Physiol Gastrointest Liver Physiol* 2004;287(3):G497–502.

134. Meiler C, Muhlbauer M, Johann M, et al. Different effects of a CD14 gene polymorphism on disease outcome in patients with alcoholic liver disease and chronic hepatitis C infection. *World J Gastroenterol* 2005;11(38):6031–7.

135. Martins A, Cortez-Pinto H, Machado M, et al. Are genetic polymorphisms of tumour necrosis factor alpha, interleukin-10, CD14 endotoxin receptor or manganese superoxide dismutase associated with alcoholic liver disease? *Eur J Gastroenterol Hepatol* 2005;17(10):1099–104.

136. Jarvelainen HA, Orpana A, Perola M, Savolainen VT, Karhunen PJ, Lindros KO. Promoter polymorphism of the CD14 endotoxin receptor gene as a risk factor for alcoholic liver disease. *Hepatology* 2001;33(5):1148–53.

137. Grove J, Daly AK, Bassendine MF, Gilvarry E, Day CP. Interleukin 10 promoter region polymorphisms and susceptibility to advanced alcoholic liver disease. *Gut* 2000;46(4):540–5.

138. Walsh K, Alexander G. Alcoholic liver disease. *Postgrad Med J* 2000;76(895):280–6.

139. Neuman MG, Brenner DA, Rehermann B, et al. Mechanisms of alcoholic liver disease: cytokines. *Alcohol Clin Exp Res* 2001;25(5 Suppl ISBRA):S251–3.

140. Niemela O, Parkkila S, Juvonen RO, Viitala K, Gelboin HV, Pasanen M. Cytochromes P450 2A6, 2E1, and 3A and production of protein–aldehyde adducts in the liver of patients with alcoholic and non-alcoholic liver diseases. *J Hepatol* 2000;33(6):893–901.

141. Thiele GM, Worrall S, Tuma DJ, Klassen LW, Wyatt TA, Nagata N. The chemistry and biological effects of malondialdehyde–acetaldehyde adducts. *Alcohol Clin Exp Res* 2001;25(5 Suppl ISBRA):S218–24.

142. Shangareeva ZA, Viktorova TV, Sagidullin AF. [The TNF family genes polymorphisms (−308G/A TNF and +252A/G LTA) and alcoholic liver disease.] *Mol Biol (Mosk)* 2004;38(6):1014–16.

143. Ladero JM, Fernandez-Arquero M, Tudela JI, et al. Single nucleotide polymorphisms and microsatellite alleles of tumor necrosis factor alpha and interleukin-10 genes and the risk of advanced chronic alcoholic liver disease. *Liver* 2002;22(3):245–51.

144. Ingelman-Sundberg M, Johansson I, Yin H, et al. Ethanol-inducible cytochrome P4502E1: genetic polymorphism, regulation, and possible role in the etiology of alcohol-induced liver disease. *Alcohol* 1993;10(6):447–52.

145. Bathgate AJ, Pravica V, Perrey C, Hayes PC, Hutchinson IV. Polymorphisms in tumour necrosis factor alpha, interleukin-10 and transforming growth factor beta1 genes and end-stage liver disease. *Eur J Gastroenterol Hepatol* 2000;12(12):1329–33.

146. Valenti L, De Feo T, Fracanzani AL, et al. Cytotoxic T-lymphocyte antigen-4 A49G polymorphism is associated with susceptibility to and severity of alcoholic liver disease in Italian patients. *Alcohol Alcohol* 2004;39(4):276–80.

147. Vidali M, Stewart SF, Rolla R, et al. Genetic and epigenetic factors in autoimmune reactions toward cytochrome P4502E1 in alcoholic liver disease. *Hepatology* 2003;37(2):410–19.

148. Lim S, Crawley E, Woo P, Barnes PJ. Haplotype associated with low interleukin-10 production in patients with severe asthma. *Lancet* 1998;352(9122):113.

149. Dupont I, Lucas D, Clot P, Menez C, Albano E. Cytochrome P4502E1 inducibility and hydroxyethyl radical formation among alcoholics. *J Hepatol* 1998;28(4):564–71.

150. Machado M, Cortez-Pinto H. Are genes really important in alcoholic liver disease? *Eur J Gastroenterol Hepatol* 2008;20(12):1244–8.

151. Szabo G, Wands JR, Eken A, et al. Alcohol and hepatitis C virus—interactions in immune dysfunctions and liver damage. *Alcohol Clin Exp Res* 2010;34(10):1675–86.

152. Mueller S, Millonig G, Seitz HK. Alcoholic liver disease and hepatitis C: a frequently underestimated combination. *World J Gastroenterol* 2009;15(28):3462–71.

153. Poynard T, Ratziu V, Charlotte F, Goodman Z, McHutchison J, Albrecht J. Rates and risk factors of liver fibrosis progression in patients with chronic hepatitis c. *J Hepatol* 2001;34(5):730–9.

154. Yamanaka T, Shiraki K, Nakazaawa S, et al. Impact of hepatitis B and C virus infection on the clinical prognosis of alcoholic liver cirrhosis. *Anticancer Res* 2001;21(4B):2937–40.

155. Maddrey WC. Alcohol-induced liver disease. *Clin Liver Dis* 2000;4(1):115–31, vii.

156. Degos F. Hepatitis C and alcohol. *J Hepatol* 1999;31(Suppl 1):113–18.

157. Monto A, Patel K, Bostrom A, et al. Risks of a range of alcohol intake on hepatitis C-related fibrosis. *Hepatology* 2004;39(3):826–34.

158. Bhattacharya R, Shuhart MC. Hepatitis C and alcohol: interactions, outcomes, and implications. *J Clin Gastroenterol* 2003;36(3):242–52.

159. Harris DR, Gonin R, Alter HJ, et al. The relationship of acute transfusion-associated hepatitis to the development of cirrhosis in the presence of alcohol abuse. *Ann Intern Med* 2001;134(2):120–4.

160. Hezode C, Lonjon I, Roudot-Thoraval F, Pawlotsky JM, Zafrani ES, Dhumeaux D. Impact of moderate alcohol consumption on histological activity and fibrosis in patients with chronic hepatitis C, and specific influence of steatosis: a prospective study. *Aliment Pharmacol Ther* 2003;17(8):1031–7.

161. Freeman AJ, Dore GJ, Law MG, et al. Estimating progression to cirrhosis in chronic hepatitis C virus infection. *Hepatology* 2001;34(4 Pt 1):809–16.

162. Hutchinson SJ, Bird SM, Goldberg DJ. Influence of alcohol on the progression of hepatitis C virus infection: a meta-analysis. *Clin Gastroenterol Hepatol* 2005;3(11):1150–9.

163. Tsui JI, Pletcher MJ, Vittinghoff E, Seal K, Gonzales R. Hepatitis C and hospital outcomes in patients admitted with alcohol-related problems. *J Hepatol* 2006;44: 262–6.

164. Brillanti S, Masci C, Siringo S, Di Febo G, Miglioli M, Barbara L. Serological and histological aspects of hepatitis C virus infection in alcoholic patients. *J Hepatol* 1991;13(3):347–50.

165. Yokoyama H, Ishii H, Moriya S, et al. Relationship between hepatitis C virus subtypes and clinical features of liver disease seen in alcoholics. *J Hepatol* 1995;22(2):130–4.

166. Tanaka T, Yabusako T, Yamashita T, et al. Contribution of hepatitis C virus to the progression of alcoholic liver disease. *Alcohol Clin Exp Res* 2000;24(4 Suppl):S112–16.

167. Horie Y, Ishii H, Hibi T. [National survey of alcoholic liver disease in Japan.] *Nihon Arukoru Yakubutsu Igakkai Zasshi* 2004;39(6):505–10.

168. Fasani P, Sangiovanni A, De Fazio C, et al. High prevalence of multinodular hepatocellular carcinoma in patients with cirrhosis attributable to multiple risk factors. *Hepatology* 1999;29(6).1704–7.

169. Marsano LS, Pena LR. The interaction of alcoholic liver disease and hepatitis C. *Hepatogastroenterology* 1998;45(20):331–9.

170. Monto A, Wright TL. The epidemiology and prevention of hepatocellular carcinoma. *Semin Oncol* 2001;28(5):441–9.

171. Anand BS, Thornby J. Alcohol has no effect on hepatitis C virus replication: a meta-analysis. *Gut* 2005;54(10):1468–72.

172. Purohit V, Russo D, Salin M. Role of iron in alcoholic liver disease: introduction and summary of the symposium. *Alcohol* 2003;30(2):93–7.

173. Iqbal T, Diab A, Ward DG, et al. Is iron overload in alcohol-related cirrhosis mediated by hepcidin? *World J Gastroenterol* 2009;15(46):5864–6.

174. Kohgo Y, Ohtake T, Ikuta K, Suzuki Y, Torimoto Y, Kato J. Dysregulation of systemic iron metabolism in alcoholic liver diseases. *J Gastroenterol Hepatol* 2008;23(Suppl 1):S78–81.

175. Levitsky J, Mailliard ME. Diagnosis and therapy of alcoholic liver disease. *Semin Liver Dis* 2004;24(3):233–47.

176. Alcohol and disease. Proceedings of the first Acta Medica Scandinavica International Symposium. Stockholm, Sweden, November 22–23, 1984. *Acta Med Scand Suppl* 1985;703: 1–290.

177. Grant BF. Barriers to alcoholism treatment: reasons for not seeking treatment in a general population sample. *J Stud Alcohol* 1997;58(4):365–71.

178. Eckardt MJ, Rawlings RR, Martin PR. Biological correlates and detection of alcohol abuse and alcoholism. *Prog Neuropsychopharmacol Biol Psychiatry* 1986;10(2):135–44.

179. McQuade WH, Levy SM, Yanek LR, Davis SW, Liepman MR. Detecting symptoms of alcohol abuse in primary care settings. *Arch Fam Med* 2000;9(9):814–21.

180. D'Amico EJ, Paddock SM, Burnam A, Kung FY. Identification of and guidance for problem drinking by general medical providers: results from a national survey. *Med Care* 2005;43(3):229–36.

181. Sharpe PC, McBride R, Archbold GP. Biochemical markers of alcohol abuse. *Q J Med* 1996;89(2):137–44.

182. Goldberg DM, Kapur BM. Enzymes and circulating proteins as markers of alcohol abuse. *Clin Chim Acta* 1994;226(2):191–209.

183. Rosman AS, Lieber CS. Diagnostic utility of laboratory tests in alcoholic liver disease. *Clin Chem* 1994;40(8):1641–51.

184. Umbricht-Schneiter A, Santora P, Moore RD. Alcohol abuse: comparison of two methods for assessing its prevalence and associated morbidity in hospitalized patients. *Am J Med* 1991;91(2):110–18.

185. Pulford J, McCormick R, Wheeler A, Firkin P, Scott I, Robinson G. Alcohol assessment: the practice, knowledge, and attitudes of staff working in the general medical wards of a large metropolitan hospital. *N Z Med J* 2007;120(1257):U2608.

186. Chang G, Goetz MA, Wilkins-Haug L, Berman S. Identifying prenatal alcohol use: screening instruments versus clinical predictors. *Am J Addict* 1999;8(2):87–93.

187. Lucey MR, Weinrieb RM. Alcohol and substance abuse. *Semin Liver Dis* 2009;29(1):66–73.

188. Prytz H, Melin T. Identification of alcoholic liver disease or hidden alcohol abuse in patients with elevated liver enzymes. *J Intern Med* 1993;233(1):21–6.

189. Aertgeerts B, Buntinx F. Screening for alcohol abuse. *Br J Gen Pract* 2001;51(467):492–3.

190. Girela E, Villanueva E, Hernandez-Cueto C, Luna JD. Comparison of the CAGE questionnaire versus some biochemical markers in the diagnosis of alcoholism. *Alcohol Alcohol* 1994;29(3):337–43.

191. Levine J. The relative value of consultation, questionnaires and laboratory investigation in the identification of excessive alcohol consumption. *Alcohol Alcohol* 1990;25(5):539–53.

192. Helander A, Eriksson CJ. Laboratory tests for acute alcohol consumption: results of the WHO/ISBRA Study on State and Trait Markers of Alcohol Use and Dependence. *Alcohol Clin Exp Res* 2002;26(7).1070–7.

193. Aalto M, Seppa K. Use of laboratory markers and the audit questionnaire by primary care physicians to detect alcohol abuse by patients. *Alcohol Alcohol* 2005;40(6):520–3.

194. Soderstrom CA, Smith GS, Kufera JA, et al. The accuracy of the CAGE, the Brief Michigan Alcoholism Screening Test, and the Alcohol Use Disorders Identification Test in screening trauma center patients for alcoholism. *J Trauma* 1997;43(6):962–9.

195. O'Shea RS, Dasarathy S, McCullough AJ. Alcoholic liver disease. *Hepatology* 2010;51(1):307–28.

196. McCullough AJ. Alcoholic liver disease. In: Schiff ER, Sorrell MF, Maddrey WC, eds. *Diseases of the Liver*, 8th edn. 1999. Philadelphia, PA: Lippincott Raven Press: 941–71.

197. Fiellin DA, Reid MC, O'Connor PG. Screening for alcohol problems in primary care: a systematic review. *Arch Intern Med* 2000;160(13):1977–89.

198. Gomez A, Conde A, Santana JM, Jorrin A. Diagnostic usefulness of brief versions of Alcohol Use Disorders Identification Test (AUDIT) for detecting hazardous drinkers in primary care settings. *J Stud Alcohol* 2005;66(2):305–8.

199. Kelly TM, Donovan JE, Chung T, Cook RL, Delbridge TR. Alcohol use disorders among emergency department-treated older adolescents: a new brief screen (RUFT-Cut) using the AUDIT, CAGE, CRAFFT, and RAPS-QF. *Alcohol Clin Exp Res* 2004;28(5):746–53.

200. Cherpitel CJ. Screening for alcohol problems in the US general population: comparison of the CAGE, RAPS4, and RAPS4-QF by gender, ethnicity, and service utilization. Rapid Alcohol Problems Screen. *Alcohol Clin Exp Res* 2002;26(11):1686–91.

201. Meneses-Gaya C, Zuardi AW, Loureiro SR, et al. Is the full version of the AUDIT really necessary? Study of the validity and internal construct of its abbreviated versions. *Alcohol Clin Exp Res* 2010;34(8):1417–24.

202. Aertgeerts B, Buntinx F, Kester A. The value of the CAGE in screening for alcohol abuse and alcohol dependence in general clinical populations: a diagnostic meta-analysis. *J Clin Epidemiol* 2004;57(1):30–9.

203. Espinoza P, Ducot B, Pelletier G, et al. Interobserver agreement in the physical diagnosis of alcoholic liver disease. *Dig Dis Sci* 1987;32(3):244–7.

204. Cozzolino G, Francica G, Lonardo A, Cerini R, Cacciatore L. [Variability of the clinical and laboratory aspects in the presentation of chronic liver diseases in relation to their etiology. Analysis of a case study and review of the literature.] *Minerva Med* 1985;76(16): 753–60.

205. Chedid A, Mendenhall CL, Gartside P, French SW, Chen T, Rabin L. Prognostic factors in alcoholic liver disease. VA Cooperative Study Group. *Am J Gastroenterol* 1991;86(2):210–16.

206. Colic-Cvrlje V, Naumovski-Mihalic S, Prskalo M, Colic A, Cvjeticanin B, Sabaric B. Prognosis for the patients with alcoholic and nonalcoholic liver disease. *Coll Antropol* 2000;24(1):249–52.

207. Bode JC, Kruse G, Mexas P, Martini GA. [Alcoholic fatty liver, alcoholic hepatitis and alcoholic cirrhosis. Drinking behavior and incidence of clinical, clinico-chemical and histological findings in 282 patients.] *Dtsch Med Wochenschr* 1984;109(40):1516–21.

208. Vanlemmens C, Di M, V, Milan C, et al. Immediate listing for liver transplantation versus standard care for Child–Pugh stage B alcoholic cirrhosis: a randomized trial. *Ann Intern Med* 2009; 150(3):153–61.

209. Leung NW, Farrant P, Peters TJ. Liver volume measurement by ultrasonography in normal subjects and alcoholic patients. *J Hepatol* 1986;2(2):157–64.

210. Neundorfer B, Claus D. [Differential diagnosis, pathogenesis and therapy of alcoholic polyneuropathy.] *Fortschr Neurol Psychiatr* 1986;54(8):241–7.

211. Anderson P, Cremona A, Paton A, Turner C, Wallace P. The risk of alcohol. *Addiction* 1993;88(11):1493–508.

212. Preedy VR, Adachi J, Ueno Y, et al. Alcoholic skeletal muscle myopathy: definitions, features, contribution of neuropathy, impact and diagnosis. *Eur J Neurol* 2001;8(6):677–87.

213. Stokkeland K, Ebrahim F, Ekbom A. Increased risk of esophageal varices, liver cancer, and death in patients with alcoholic liver disease. *Alcohol Clin Exp Res* 2010;34(11):1993–9.

214. Krastev Z, Mateva L, Danev S, Nikolov R. Clinical meaning of GGT activity in follow-up of patients with alcohol- related liver injury and cholestasis. *Ital J Gastroenterol* 1992;24(4):185–7.

215. Sillanaukee P, Massot N, Jousilahti P, et al. Dose response of laboratory markers to alcohol consumption in a general population. *Am J Epidemiol* 2000;152(8):747–51.

216. Nystrom M, Perasalo J, Pikkarainen J, Salaspuro M. Conventional laboratory tests as indicators of heavy drinking in young university students. *Scand J Prim Health Care* 1993;11(1):44–9.

217. Nalpas B, Vassault A, Charpin S, Lacour B, Berthelot P. Serum mitochondrial aspartate aminotransferase as a marker of chronic alcoholism: diagnostic value and interpretation in a liver unit. *Hepatology* 1986;6(4):608–14.

218. Caldwell SH, Halliday JW, Fletcher LM, et al. Carbohydrate-deficient transferrin in alcoholics with liver disease. *J Gastroenterol Hepatol* 1995;10(2):174–8.

219. Mathurin P, Vidaud D, Vidaud M, et al. Quantification of apolipoprotein A-I and B messenger RNA in heavy drinkers according to liver disease. *Hepatology* 1996;23(1):44–51.

220. Chambers W, Thompson S, Skillen AW, Record CO, Turner GA. Abnormally fucosylated haptoglobin as a marker for alcoholic liver disease but not excessive alcohol consumption or non-alcoholic liver disease. *Clin Chim Acta* 1993;219(1–2):177–82.

221. Seilles E, Rossel M, Vuitton DA, et al. Serum secretory IgA and secretory component in patients with non-cirrhotic alcoholic liver diseases. *J Hepatol* 1995;22(3):278–85.

222. Anttila P, Jarvi K, Latvala J, Romppanen J, Punnonen K, Niemela O. Biomarkers of alcohol consumption in patients classified according to the degree of liver disease severity. *Scand J Clin Lab Invest* 2005;65(2):141–51.

223. Pares A, Deulofeu R, Gimenez A, et al. Serum hyaluronate reflects hepatic fibrogenesis in alcoholic liver disease and is useful as a marker of fibrosis. *Hepatology* 1996;24(6):1399–403.

224. Rosenberg WM, Voelker M, Thiel R, et al. Serum markers detect the presence of liver fibrosis: a cohort study. *Gastroenterology* 2004;127(6):1704–13.

225. Viitala K, Israel Y, Blake JE, Niemela O. Serum IgA, IgG, and IgM antibodies directed against acetaldehyde-derived epitopes: relationship to liver disease severity and alcohol consumption. *Hepatology* 1997;25(6):1418–24.

226. Brunt EM. Nonalcoholic steatohepatitis: definition and pathology. *Semin Liver Dis* 2001;21(1):3–16.

227. Reid AE. Nonalcoholic steatohepatitis. *Gastroenterology* 2001;121(3): 710–23.

228. Bird GL. Investigation of alcoholic liver disease. *Baillieres Clin Gastroenterol* 1993;7(3):663–82.

229. Levin DM, Baker AL, Riddell RH, Rochman H, Boyer JL. Nonalcoholic liver disease. Overlooked causes of liver injury in patients with heavy alcohol consumption. *Am J Med* 1979;66(3):429–34.

230. Poynard T, Ratziu V, Bedossa P. Appropriateness of liver biopsy. *Can J Gastroenterol* 2000;14(6):543–8.

231. Hill DB, Kugelmas M. Alcoholic liver disease. Treatment strategies for the potentially reversible stages. *Postgrad Med* 1998;103(4):261–8, 273.

232. Lieber CS. Alcoholic liver injury: pathogenesis and therapy in 2001. *Pathol Biol (Paris)* 2001;49(9):738–52.

233. Saverymuttu SH, Joseph AE, Maxwell JD. Ultrasound scanning in the detection of hepatic fibrosis and steatosis. *Br Med J (Clin Res Ed)* 1986;292(6512):13–15.

234. Jensen K, Gluud C. The Mallory body: theories on development and pathological significance (Part 2 of a literature survey). *Hepatology* 1994;20(5):1330–42.

235. Diehl AM, Goodman Z, Ishak KG. Alcohollike liver disease in nonalcoholics. A clinical and histologic comparison with alcohol-induced liver injury. *Gastroenterology* 1988;95(4):1056–62.

236. Chedid A, Mendenhall CL, Tosch T, et al. Significance of megamitochondria in alcoholic liver disease. *Gastroenterology* 1986;90(6):1858–64.

237. Reeves HL, Burt AD, Wood S, Day CP. Hepatic stellate cell activation occurs in the absence of hepatitis in alcoholic liver disease and correlates with the severity of steatosis. *J Hepatol* 1996;25(5): 677–83.

238. Xu GF, Wang XY, Ge GL, et al. Dynamic changes of capillarization and peri-sinusoid fibrosis in alcoholic liver diseases. *World J Gastroenterol* 2004;10(2):238–43.

239. Duryee MJ, Klassen LW, Freeman TL, Willis MS, Tuma DJ, Thiele GM. Lipopolysaccharide is a cofactor for malondialdehyde–acetaldehyde adduct-mediated cytokine/chemokine release by rat sinusoidal liver endothelial and Kupffer cells. *Alcohol Clin Exp Res* 2004;28(12):1931–8.

240. Marbet UA, Bianchi L, Meury U, Stalder GA. Long-term histological evaluation of the natural history and prognostic factors of alcoholic liver disease. *J Hepatol* 1987;4(3):364–72.

241. Kanel GC. Hepatic lesions resembling alcoholic liver disease. *Pathology (Phila)* 1994;3(1):77–104.

242. Pounder DJ. Problems in the necropsy diagnosis of alcoholic liver disease. *Am J Forensic Med Pathol* 1984;5(2):103–9.

243. Coelho-Little ME, Jeffers LJ, Bernstein DE, et al. Hepatitis C virus in alcoholic patients with and without clinically apparent liver disease. *Alcohol Clin Exp Res* 1995;19(5):1173–6.

244. Regev A, Jeffers LJ. Hepatitis C and alcohol. *Alcohol Clin Exp Res* 1999;23(9):1543–51.

245. Adams PC. Iron overload in viral and alcoholic liver disease. *J Hepatol* 1998;28(Suppl 1):19–20.

246. Pascoe A, Kerlin P, Steadman C, et al. Spur cell anaemia and hepatic iron stores in patients with alcoholic liver disease undergoing orthotopic liver transplantation. *Gut* 1999;45(2):301–5.

247. Bell H, Skinningsrud A, Raknerud N, Try K. Serum ferritin and transferrin saturation in patients with chronic alcoholic and nonalcoholic liver diseases. *J Intern Med* 1994;236(3):315–22.

248. Fletcher LM, Halliday JW, Powell LW. Interrelationships of alcohol and iron in liver disease with particular reference to the iron-binding proteins, ferritin and transferrin. *J Gastroenterol Hepatol* 1999;14(3):202–14.

249. Schiano TD, Bodian C, Schwartz ME, Glajchen N, Min AD. Accuracy and significance of computed tomographic scan assessment of hepatic volume in patients undergoing liver transplantation. *Transplantation* 2000;69(4):545–50.

250. Okazaki H, Ito K, Fujita T, Koike S, Takano K, Matsunaga N. Discrimination of alcoholic from virus-induced cirrhosis on MR imaging. *AJR Am J Roentgenol* 2000;175(6):1677–81.

251. Sharma MP, Dasarathy S, Misra SC, Saksena S, Sundaram KR. Sonographic signs in portal hypertension: a multivariate analysis. *Trop Gastroenterol* 1996;17(2):23–9.

252. Vilgrain V. Ultrasound of diffuse liver disease and portal hypertension. *Eur Radiol* 2001;11(9):1563–77.

253. Schlemmer HP, Sawatzki T, Sammet S, et al. Hepatic phospholipids in alcoholic liver disease assessed by proton-decoupled 31P magnetic resonance spectroscopy. *J Hepatol* 2005;42(5):752–9.

254. Kaufman DW, Kelly JP, Wiholm BE, et al. The risk of acute major upper gastrointestinal bleeding among users of aspirin and ibuprofen at various levels of alcohol consumption. *Am J Gastroenterol* 1999;94(11):3189–96.

255. Kelly JP, Kaufman DW, Koff RS, Laszlo A, Wiholm BE, Shapiro S. Alcohol consumption and the risk of major upper gastrointestinal bleeding. *Am J Gastroenterol* 1995;90(7):1058–64.

256. Mandrekar P, Szabo G. Signalling pathways in alcohol-induced liver inflammation. *J Hepatol* 2009;50(6):1258–66.

257. Szabo G, Bala S. Alcoholic liver disease and the gut–liver axis. *World J Gastroenterol* 2010;16(11):1321–9.

258. Beier JI, Arteel GE, McClain CJ. Advances in alcoholic liver disease. *Curr Gastroenterol Rep* 2011;13: 56–64.

259. Miranda-Mendez A, Lugo-Baruqui A, Armendariz-Borunda J. Molecular basis and current treatment for alcoholic liver disease. *Int J Environ Res Public Health* 2010;7(5):1872–88.

260. Tsukamoto H, Lu SC. Current concepts in the pathogenesis of alcoholic liver injury. *FASEB J* 2001;15(8):1335–49.

261. Wang BY, Ju XH, Fu BY, Zhang J, Cao YX. Effects of ethanol on liver sinusoidal endothelial cells-fenestrae of rats. *Hepatobiliary Pancreat Dis Int* 2005;4(3):422–6.

262. Leevy CB, Elbeshbeshy HA. Immunology of alcoholic liver disease. *Clin Liver Dis* 2005;9(1):55–66.

263. Chedid A, Arain S, Snyder A, Mathurin P, Capron F, Naveau S. The immunology of fibrogenesis in alcoholic liver disease. *Arch Pathol Lab Med* 2004;128(11):1230–8.

264. Vapaatalo H, Mervaala E. Clinically important factors influencing endothelial function. *Med Sci Monit* 2001;7(5):1075–85.

265. Hines IN, Wheeler MD. Recent advances in alcoholic liver disease III. Role of the innate immune response in alcoholic hepatitis. *Am J Physiol Gastrointest Liver Physiol* 2004;287(2):G310–14.

266. Latvala J, Hietala J, Koivisto H, Jarvi K, Anttila P, Niemela O. Immune responses to ethanol metabolites and cytokine profiles differentiate alcoholics with or without liver disease. *Am J Gastroenterol* 2005;100(6):1303–10.

267. Akerman PA, Cote PM, Yang SQ, et al. Long-term ethanol consumption alters the hepatic response to the regenerative effects of tumor necrosis factor-alpha. *Hepatology* 1993;17(6):1066–73.

268. Zhang M, Gong Y, Corbin I, et al. Light ethanol consumption enhances liver regeneration after partial hepatectomy in rats. *Gastroenterology* 2000;119(5):1333–9.

269. Diehl AM. Recent events in alcoholic liver disease. V. Effects of ethanol on liver regeneration. *Am J Physiol Gastrointest Liver Physiol* 2005;288(1):G1–6.

270. Masalkar PD, Abhang SA. Oxidative stress and antioxidant status in patients with alcoholic liver disease. *Clin Chim Acta* 2005;355(1–2):61–5.

271. Sougioultzis S, Dalakas E, Hayes PC, Plevris JN. Alcoholic hepatitis: from pathogenesis to treatment. *Curr Med Res Opin* 2005;21(9):1337–46.

272. Medina J, Moreno-Otero R. Pathophysiological basis for antioxidant therapy in chronic liver disease. *Drugs* 2005;65(17):2445–61.

273. Pemberton PW, Smith A, Warnes TW. Non-invasive monitoring of oxidant stress in alcoholic liver disease. *Scand J Gastroenterol* 2005;40(9):1102–8.

274. Cohen JI, Nagy LE. Pathogenesis of alcoholic liver disease: interactions between parenchymal and non-parenchymal cells. *J Dig Dis* 2011;12: 3–9.

275. Holstege A, Bedossa P, Poynard T, et al. Acetaldehyde-modified epitopes in liver biopsy specimens of alcoholic and nonalcoholic patients: localization and association with progression of liver fibrosis. *Hepatology* 1994;19(2):367–74.

276. Patel VB, Worrall S, Emery PW, Preedy VR. Protein adduct species in muscle and liver of rats following acute ethanol administration. *Alcohol Alcohol* 2005;40(6):485–93.

277. Roman J, Gimenez A, Lluis JM, et al. Enhanced DNA binding and activation of transcription factors NF-kappa B and AP-1 by acetaldehyde in HEPG2 cells. *J Biol Chem* 2000;275(19):14684–90.

278. Jokelainen K, Reinke LA, Nanji AA. Nf-kappab activation is associated with free radical generation and endotoxemia and precedes pathological liver injury in experimental alcoholic liver disease. *Cytokine* 2001;16(1):36–9.

279. Lieber CS. Microsomal ethanol oxidizing system (MEOS): the first 30 years (1968–1998) – a review. *Alcohol Clin Exp Res* 1999;23(6):991–1007.

280. Meskar A, Plee-Gautier E, Amet Y, Berthou F, Lucas D. [Alcohol-xenobiotic interactions. Role of cytochrome P450 2E1.] *Pathol Biol (Paris)* 2001;49(9):696–702.

281. Ni R, Leo MA, Zhao J, Lieber CS. Toxicity of beta-carotene and its exacerbation by acetaldehyde in HepG2 cells. *Alcohol Alcohol* 2001;36(4):281–5.

282. Leo MA, Aleynik SI, Aleynik MK, Lieber CS. Beta-carotene beadlets potentiate hepatotoxicity of alcohol. *Am J Clin Nutr* 1997;66(6):1461–9.

283. Zima T, Fialova L, Mestek O, et al. Oxidative stress, metabolism of ethanol and alcohol-related diseases. *J Biomed Sci* 2001;8(1):59–70.

284. Clot P, Parola M, Bellomo G, et al. Plasma membrane hydroxyethyl radical adducts cause antibody-dependent cytotoxicity in rat hepatocytes exposed to alcohol. *Gastroenterology* 1997;113(1):265–76.

285. Dryden GW Jr, Deaciuc I, Arteel G, McClain CJ. Clinical implications of oxidative stress and antioxidant therapy. *Curr Gastroenterol Rep* 2005;7(4):308–16.

286. Oh SI, Kim CI, Chun HJ, Park SC. Chronic ethanol consumption affects glutathione status in rat liver. *J Nutr* 1998;128(4):758–63.

287. Kono H, Bradford BU, Yin M, et al. CYP2E1 is not involved in early alcohol-induced liver injury. *Am J Physiol* 1999;277(6 Pt 1): G1259–67.

288. Kono H, Bradford BU, Rusyn I, et al. Development of an intragastric enteral model in the mouse: studies of alcohol-induced liver disease using knockout technology. *J Hepatobiliary Pancreat Surg* 2000;7(4):395–400.

289. Koop DR, Klopfenstein B, Iimuro Y, Thurman RG. Gadolinium chloride blocks alcohol-dependent liver toxicity in rats treated chronically with intragastric alcohol despite the induction of CYP2E1. *Mol Pharmacol* 1997;51(6):944–50.

290. Lu SC, Mato JM. Role of methionine adenosyltransferase and S-adenosylmethionine in alcohol-associated liver cancer. *Alcohol* 2005;35(3):227–34.

291. Lu SC, Huang ZZ, Yang H, Mato JM, Avila MA, Tsukamoto H. Changes in methionine adenosyltransferase and S-adenosylmethionine homeostasis in alcoholic rat liver. *Am J Physiol Gastrointest Liver Physiol* 2000;279(1):G178–85.

292. Aleynik S, Lieber CS. Role of S-adenosylmethionine in hyperhomocysteinemia and in the treatment of alcoholic liver disease. *Nutrition* 2000;16(11–12):1104–8.

293. Cunningham CC, Bailey SM. Ethanol consumption and liver mitochondria function. *Biol Signals Recept* 2001;10(3–4):271–82.

294. Garcia-Ruiz C, Morales A, Colell A, et al. Feeding S-adenosyl-L-methionine attenuates both ethanol-induced depletion of mitochondrial glutathione and mitochondrial dysfunction in periportal and perivenous rat hepatocytes. *Hepatology* 1995;21(1): 207–14.

295. Neuman MG. Apoptosis in diseases of the liver. *Crit Rev Clin Lab Sci* 2001;38(2):109–66.

296. Ji C, Mehrian-Shai R, Chan C, Hsu YH, Kaplowitz N. Role of CHOP in hepatic apoptosis in the murine model of intragastric ethanol feeding. *Alcohol Clin Exp Res* 2005;29(8):1496–503.

297. Feldstein AE, Gores GJ. Apoptosis in alcoholic and nonalcoholic steatohepatitis. *Front Biosci* 2005;10: 3093–9.

298. Purohit V, Gao B, Song BJ. Molecular mechanisms of alcoholic fatty liver. *Alcohol Clin Exp Res* 2009;33(2):191–205.

299. Arteel GE. New role of plasminogen activator inhibitor-1 in alcohol-induced liver injury. *J Gastroenterol Hepatol* 2008;23(Suppl 1): S54–9.

300. Ramaiah S, Rivera C, Arteel G. Early-phase alcoholic liver disease: an update on animal models, pathology, and pathogenesis. *Int J Toxicol* 2004;23(4):217–31.

301. Yin M, Wheeler MD, Kono H, et al. Essential role of tumor necrosis factor alpha in alcohol-induced liver injury in mice. *Gastroenterology* 1999;117(4):942–52.

302. Ronis MJ, Korourian S, Blackburn ML, Badeaux J, Badger TM. The role of ethanol metabolism in development of alcoholic steatohepatitis in the rat. *Alcohol* 2010;44(2):157–69.

303. Adachi Y, Bradford BU, Gao W, Bojes HK, Thurman RG. Inactivation of Kupffer cells prevents early alcohol-induced liver injury. *Hepatology* 1994;20(2):453–60.

304. Cao Q, Batey R, Pang G, Clancy R. Ethanol-altered liver-associated T cells mediate liver injury in rats administered concanavalin A (Con A) or lipopolysaccharide (LPS). *Alcohol Clin Exp Res* 1999;23(10):1660–7.

305. Elsharkawy AM, Oakley F, Mann DA. The role and regulation of hepatic stellate cell apoptosis in reversal of liver fibrosis. *Apoptosis* 2005;10(5):927–39.

306. Greenwel P. Acetaldehyde-mediated collagen regulation in hepatic stellate cells. *Alcohol Clin Exp Res* 1999;23(5):930–3.

307. Nieto N, Greenwel P, Friedman SL, Zhang F, Dannenberg AJ, Cederbaum AI. Ethanol and arachidonic acid increase alpha 2(I) collagen expression in rat hepatic stellate cells overexpressing cytochrome P450 2E1. Role of H2O2 and cyclooxygenase-2. *J Biol Chem* 2000;275(26):20136–45.

308. Pessione F, Ramond MJ, Peters L, et al. Five-year survival predictive factors in patients with excessive alcohol intake and cirrhosis. Effect of alcoholic hepatitis, smoking and abstinence. *Liver Int* 2003;23(1):45–53.

309. Mendenhall CL, Chedid A, French SW, et al. Alpha-fetoprotein alterations in alcoholics with liver disease. V.A. Cooperative Study Groups. *Alcohol Alcohol* 1991;26(5–6):527–34.

310. Merkel C, Marchesini G, Fabbri A, et al. The course of galactose elimination capacity in patients with alcoholic cirrhosis: possible use as a surrogate marker for death. *Hepatology* 1996;24(4): 820–3.

311. Mathurin P, Duchatelle V, Ramond MJ, et al. Survival and prognostic factors in patients with severe alcoholic hepatitis treated with prednisolone. *Gastroenterology* 1996;110(6):1847–53.

312. Gluud C, Henriksen JH, Nielsen G. Prognostic indicators in alcoholic cirrhotic men. *Hepatology* 1988;8(2):222–7.

313. Rosa H, Silverio AO, Perini RF, Arruda CB. Bacterial infection in cirrhotic patients and its relationship with alcohol. *Am J Gastroenterol* 2000;95(5):1290–3.

314. Ganne-Carrie N, Christidis C, Chastang C, et al. Liver iron is predictive of death in alcoholic cirrhosis: a multivariate study of 229 consecutive patients with alcoholic and/or hepatitis C virus cirrhosis: a prospective follow up study. *Gut* 2000;46(2):277–82.

315. Mathurin P. Corticosteroids for alcoholic hepatitis – what's next? *J Hepatol* 2005;43(3):526–33.

316. Mathurin P, Mendenhall CL, Carithers RL Jr, et al. Corticosteroids improve short-term survival in patients with severe alcoholic hepatitis (AH): individual data analysis of the last three randomized placebo controlled double blind trials of corticosteroids in severe AH. *J Hepatol* 2002;36(4):480–7.

317. Srikureja W, Kyulo NL, Runyon BA, Hu KQ. MELD score is a better prognostic model than Child–Turcotte–Pugh score or discriminant function score in patients with alcoholic hepatitis. *J Hepatol* 2005;42(5):700–6.

318. Forrest EH, Evans CD, Stewart S, et al. Analysis of factors predictive of mortality in alcoholic hepatitis and derivation and validation of the Glasgow alcoholic hepatitis score. *Gut* 2005;54(8):1174–9.

319. Tilg H, Kaser A. Predicting mortality by the Glasgow alcoholic hepatitis score: the long awaited progress? *Gut* 2005;54(8):1057–9.

320. Dunn W, Jamil LH, Brown LS, et al. MELD accurately predicts mortality in patients with alcoholic hepatitis. *Hepatology* 2005; 41(2):353–8.

321. Sheth M, Riggs M, Patel T. Utility of the Mayo End-Stage Liver Disease (MELD) score in assessing prognosis of patients with alcoholic hepatitis. *BMC Gastroenterol* 2002;2: 2.

322. Mathurin P. Is alcoholic hepatitis an indication for transplantation? Current management and outcomes. *Liver Transpl* 2005;11(11 Suppl 2):S21–4.

323. Mathurin P, Abdelnour M, Ramond MJ, et al. Early change in bilirubin levels is an important prognostic factor in severe alcoholic hepatitis treated with prednisolone. *Hepatology* 2003;38(6):1363–9.

324. Tonnesen H, Rosenberg J, Nielsen HJ, et al. Effect of preoperative abstinence on poor postoperative outcome in alcohol misusers: randomised controlled trial. *Br Med J* 1999;318(7194):1311–16.

325. Newton SE. Recidivism and return to work posttransplant. *Recipients with substance abuse histories.* J Subst Abuse Treat 1999; 17(1–2):103–8.

326. D'Amico G, Garcia-Tsao G, Pagliaro L. Natural history and prognostic indicators of survival in cirrhosis: a systematic review of 118 studies. *J Hepatol* 2006;44(1):217–31.

327. Borowsky SA, Strome S, Lott E. Continued heavy drinking and survival in alcoholic cirrhotics. *Gastroenterology* 1981;80(6):1405–9.

328. Brunt PW, Kew MC, Scheuer PJ, Sherlock S. Studies in alcoholic liver disease in Britain. I. Clinical and pathological patterns related to natural history. *Gut* 1974;15(1):52–8.

329. Luca A, Garcia-Pagan JC, Bosch J, et al. Effects of ethanol consumption on hepatic hemodynamics in patients with alcoholic cirrhosis. *Gastroenterology* 1997;112(4):1284–9.

330. Juhl E, Tygstrup N. [Alcoholic liver cirrhosis – the influence of interrupted alcohol consumption and prednisone.] *Nord Med* 1971;86(45):1312.

331. Powell WJ Jr., Klatskin G. Duration of survival in patients with Laennec's cirrhosis. Influence of alcohol withdrawal, and possible effects of recent changes in general management of the disease. *Am J Med* 1968;44(3):406–20.

332. Verrill C, Markham H, Templeton A, Carr NJ, Sheron N. Alcohol-related cirrhosis – early abstinence is a key factor in prognosis, even in the most severe cases. *Addiction* 2009;104(5):768–74.

333. Serra MA, Escudero A, Rodriguez F, del Olmo JA, Rodrigo JM. Effect of hepatitis C virus infection and abstinence from alcohol on survival in patients with alcoholic cirrhosis. *J Clin Gastroenterol* 2003;36(2):170–4.

334. Veldt BJ, Laine F, Guillygomarc'h A, et al. Indication of liver transplantation in severe alcoholic liver cirrhosis: quantitative evaluation and optimal timing. *J Hepatol* 2002;36(1):93–8.

335. Mackie J, Groves K, Hoyle A, et al. Orthotopic liver transplantation for alcoholic liver disease: a retrospective analysis of survival, recidivism, and risk factors predisposing to recidivism. *Liver Transpl* 2001;7(5):418–27.

336. Miguet M, Monnet E, Vanlemmens C, et al. Predictive factors of alcohol relapse after orthotopic liver transplantation for alcoholic liver disease. *Gastroenterol Clin Biol* 2004;28(10 Pt 1):845–51.

337. Miller WR, Walters ST, Bennett ME. How effective is alcoholism treatment in the United States? *J Stud Alcohol* 2001;62(2):211–20.

338. Srisurapanont M, Jarusuraisin N. Opioid antagonists for alcohol dependence. *Cochrane Database Syst Rev* 2005;1: CD001867.

339. Palmer AJ, Neeser K, Weiss C, Brandt A, Comte S, Fox M. The long-term cost-effectiveness of improving alcohol abstinence with adjuvant acamprosate. *Alcohol Alcohol* 2000;35(5):478–92.

340. Mason BJ. Acamprosate in the treatment of alcohol dependence. *Expert Opin Pharmacother* 2005;6(12):2103–15.

341. Olive MF. Pharmacotherapies for alcoholism: the old and the new. *CNS Neurol Disord Drug Targets* 2010;9(1):2–4.

342. Addolorato G, Leggio L, Ferrulli A, et al. Effectiveness and safety of baclofen for maintenance of alcohol abstinence in alcohol-dependent patients with liver cirrhosis: randomised, double-blind controlled study. *Lancet* 2007;370(9603):1915–22.

343. Trudell JR, Lin WQ, Chrystof DA, Kirshenbaum G, Ardies CM. Induction of HSP72 in rat liver by chronic ethanol consumption combined with exercise: association with the prevention of ethanol-induced fatty liver by exercise. *Alcohol Clin Exp Res* 1995;19(3):753–8.

344. Bouchier IA, Hislop WS, Prescott RJ. A prospective study of alcoholic liver disease and mortality. *J Hepatol* 1992;16(3):290–7.

345. Orrego H, Blake JE, Blendis LM, Medline A. Prognosis of alcoholic cirrhosis in the presence and absence of alcoholic hepatitis. *Gastroenterology* 1987;92(1):208–14.

346. Gitto S, Micco L, Conti F, Andreone P, Bernardi M. Alcohol and viral hepatitis: a mini-review. *Dig Liver Dis* 2009;41(1):67–70.

347. Okazaki T, Yoshihara H, Suzuki K, et al. Efficacy of interferon therapy in patients with chronic hepatitis C. Comparison between non-drinkers and drinkers. *Scand J Gastroenterol* 1994;29(11):1039–43.

348. Ohnishi K, Matsuo S, Matsutani K, et al. Interferon therapy for chronic hepatitis C in habitual drinkers: comparison with chronic hepatitis C in infrequent drinkers. *Am J Gastroenterol* 1996;91(7):1374–9.

349. Oshita M, Hayashi N, Kasahara A, et al. Increased serum hepatitis C virus RNA levels among alcoholic patients with chronic hepatitis C. *Hepatology* 1994;20(5):1115–20.

350. Lindenburg CE, Lambers FA, Urbanus AT, et al. Hepatitis C testing and treatment among active drug users in Amsterdam: results from the DUTCH-C project. *Eur J Gastroenterol Hepatol* 2011;23: 23–31.

351. Johnston SC, Pelletier LL Jr. Enhanced hepatotoxicity of acetaminophen in the alcoholic patient. Two case reports and a review of the literature. *Medicine (Baltimore)* 1997;76(3):185–91.

352. Kuffner EK, Dart RC. Acetaminophen use in patients who drink alcohol: current study evidence. *Am J Manag Care* 2001;7(19 Suppl): S592–6.

353. Tanaka E, Yamazaki K, Misawa S. Update: the clinical importance of acetaminophen hepatotoxicity in non-alcoholic and alcoholic subjects. *J Clin Pharm Ther* 2000;25(5):325–32.

354. Kozer E, Koren G. Management of paracetamol overdose: current controversies. *Drug Saf* 2001;24(7):503–12.

355. Lieber CS. New concepts of the pathogenesis of alcoholic liver disease lead to novel treatments. *Curr Gastroenterol Rep* 2004;6(1): 60–5.

356. Zhang FK, Zhang JY, Jia JD. Treatment of patients with alcoholic liver disease. *Hepatobiliary Pancreat Dis Int* 2005;4(1):12–17.

357. Orrego H, Israel Y, Blake JE, Medline A. Assessment of prognostic factors in alcoholic liver disease: toward a global quantitative expression of severity. *Hepatology* 1983;3(6):896–905.

358. Mathurin P. The use of corticosteroids in severe alcohol hepatitis: we need to look beyond this controversy. *J Hepatol* 2010;53(2): 392–3.

359. Louvet A, Naveau S, Abdelnour M, et al. The Lille model: a new tool for therapeutic strategy in patients with severe alcoholic hepatitis treated with steroids. *Hepatology* 2007;45(6):1348–54.

360. Castera L, Hartmann DJ, Chapel F, et al. Serum laminin and type IV collagen are accurate markers of histologically severe alcoholic hepatitis in patients with cirrhosis. *J Hepatol* 2000;32(3):412–18.

361. Thabut D, Naveau S, Charlotte F, et al. The diagnostic value of biomarkers (AshTest) for the prediction of alcoholic steato-hepatitis in patients with chronic alcoholic liver disease. *J Hepatol* 2006;44(6):1175–85.

362. Thiele GM, Freeman TL, Klassen LW. Immunologic mechanisms of alcoholic liver injury. *Semin Liver Dis* 2004;24(3):273–87.

363. Israel Y. Antibodies against ethanol-derived protein adducts: pathogenic implications. *Gastroenterology* 1997;113(1):353–5.

364. Lieber CS. Hepatic, metabolic, and nutritional disorders of alcoholism: from pathogenesis to therapy. *Crit Rev Clin Lab Sci* 2000; 37(6):551–84.

365. Helman RA, Temko MH, Nye SW, Fallon HJ. Alcoholic hepatitis. Natural history and evaluation of prednisolone therapy. *Ann Intern Med* 1971;74(3):311–21.

366. Blitzer BL, Mutchnick MG, Joshi PH, Phillips MM, Fessel JM, Conn HO. Adrenocorticosteroid therapy in alcoholic hepatitis. A prospective, double-blind randomized study. *Am J Dig Dis* 1977; 22(6):477–84.

367. Maddrey WC, Boitnott JK, Bedine MS, Weber FL Jr, Mezey E, White RI Jr. Corticosteroid therapy of alcoholic hepatitis. *Gastroenterology* 1978;75(2):193–9.

368. Porter HP, Simon FR, Pope CE, Volwiler W, Fenster LF. Corticosteroid therapy in severe alcoholic hepatitis. A double-blind drug trial. *N Engl J Med* 1971;284(24):1350–5.

369. Ramond MJ, Poynard T, Rueff B, et al. A randomized trial of prednisolone in patients with severe alcoholic hepatitis. *N Engl J Med* 1992;326(8):507–12.

370. Mendenhall CL, Anderson S, Garcia-Pont P, et al. Short-term and long-term survival in patients with alcoholic hepatitis treated with oxandrolone and prednisolone. *N Engl J Med* 1984;311(23):1464–70.

371. Theodossi A, Eddleston AL, Williams R. Controlled trial of methyl-prednisolone therapy in severe acute alcoholic hepatitis. *Gut* 1982;23(1):75–9.

372. Depew W, Boyer T, Omata M, Redeker A, Reynolds T. Double-blind controlled trial of prednisolone therapy in patients with severe acute alcoholic hepatitis and spontaneous encephalopathy. *Gastroenterology* 1980;78(3):524–9.

373. Bories P, Guedj JY, Mirouze D, Yousfi A, Michel H. [Treatment of acute alcoholic hepatitis with prednisolone. 45 patients.] *Presse Med* 1987;16(16):769–72.

374. Carithers RL Jr, Herlong HF, Diehl AM, et al. Methylprednisolone therapy in patients with severe alcoholic hepatitis. A randomized multicenter trial. *Ann Intern Med* 1989;110(9):685–90.

375. Lesesne HR, Bozymski EM, Fallon HJ. Treatment of alcoholic hepatitis with encephalopathy. Comparison of prednisolone with caloric supplements. *Gastroenterology* 1978;74: 169–73.

376. Shumaker JB, Resnick RH, Galambos JT, Makopour H, Iber FL. A controlled trial of 6-methylprednisolone in acute alcoholic hepatitis. With a note on published results in encephalopathic patients. *Am J Gastroenterol* 1978;69(4):443–9.

377. O'Shea RS, McCullough AJ. Treatment of alcoholic hepatitis. *Clin Liver Dis* 2005;9(1):103–34.

378. Imperiale TF, O'Connor JB, McCullough AJ. Corticosteroids are effective in patients with severe alcoholic hepatitis. *Am J Gastroenterol* 1999;94(10):3066–8.

379. Daures JP, Peray P, Bories P, et al. [Corticoid therapy in the treatment of acute alcoholic hepatitis. Results of a meta-analysis.] *Gastroenterol Clin Biol* 1991;15(3):223–8.

380. Christensen E, Gluud C. Glucocorticoids are ineffective in alcoholic hepatitis: a meta-analysis adjusting for confounding variables. *Gut* 1995;37(1):113–18.

381. Rambaldi A, Saconato HH, Christensen E, Thorlund K, Wetterslev J, Gluud C. Systematic review: glucocorticosteroids for alcoholic hepatitis – a Cochrane Hepato-Biliary Group systematic review with meta-analyses and trial sequential analyses of randomized clinical trials. *Aliment Pharmacol Ther* 2008;27(12):1167–78.

382. Mathurin P, O'Grady J, Carithers RL, et al. Corticosteroids improve short-term survival in patients with severe alcoholic hepatitis: meta-analysis of individual patient data. *Gut* 2011;60: 255–60.

383. Hill DB, Barve S, Joshi-Barve S, McClain C. Increased monocyte nuclear factor-kappaB activation and tumor necrosis factor production in alcoholic hepatitis. *J Lab Clin Med* 2000;135(5):387–95.

384. Neuman MG. Cytokines – central factors in alcoholic liver disease. *Alcohol Res Health* 2003;27(4):307–16.

385. Spahr L, Giostra E, Frossard JL, Bresson-Hadni S, Rubbia-Brandt L, Hadengue A. Soluble TNF-R1, but not tumor necrosis factor alpha, predicts the 3-month mortality in patients with alcoholic hepatitis. *J Hepatol* 2004;41(2):229–34.

386. Akriviadis E, Botla R, Briggs W, Han S, Reynolds T, Shakil O. Pentoxifylline improves short-term survival in severe acute alcoholic hepatitis: a double-blind, placebo-controlled trial. *Gastroenterology* 2000;119(6):1637–48.

387. Jimenez JL, Punzon C, Navarro J, Munoz-Fernandez MA, Fresno M. Phosphodiesterase 4 inhibitors prevent cytokine secretion by T lymphocytes by inhibiting nuclear factor-kappaB and nuclear factor of activated T cells activation. *J Pharmacol Exp Ther* 2001;299(2): 753–9.

388. Sanchez S, Albornoz L, Bandi JC, Gerona S, Mastai R. Pentoxifylline, a drug with rheological effects, decreases portal pressure in an experimental model of cirrhosis. *Eur J Gastroenterol Hepatol* 1997;9(1):27–31.

389. Louvet A, Diaz E, Dharancy S, et al. Early switch to pentoxifylline in patients with severe alcoholic hepatitis is inefficient in non-responders to corticosteroids. *J Hepatol* 2008;48(3):465–70.

390. Spahr L, Rubbia-Brandt L, Frossard JL, et al. Combination of steroids with infliximab or placebo in severe alcoholic hepatitis: a randomized controlled pilot study. *J Hepatol* 2002;37(4):448–55.

391. Tilg H, Jalan R, Kaser A, et al. Anti-tumor necrosis factor-alpha monoclonal antibody therapy in severe alcoholic hepatitis. *J Hepatol* 2003;38(4):419–25.

392. Naveau S, Chollet-Martin S, Dharancy S, et al. A double-blind randomized controlled trial of infliximab associated with prednisolone in acute alcoholic hepatitis. *Hepatology* 2004;39(5):1390–7.

393. McClain CJ, Hill DB, Barve SS. Infliximab and prednisolone: too much of a good thing? *Hepatology* 2004;39(6):1488–90.

394. Menon KV, Stadheim L, Kamath PS, et al. A pilot study of the safety and tolerability of etanercept in patients with alcoholic hepatitis. *Am J Gastroenterol* 2004;99(2):255–60.

395. Boetticher NC, Peine CJ, Kwo P, et al. A randomized, double-blinded, placebo-controlled multicenter trial of etanercept in the treatment of alcoholic hepatitis. *Gastroenterology* 2008;135(6): 1953–60.

396. Parlesak A, Schafer C, Paulus SB, Hammes S, Diedrich JP, Bode C. Phagocytosis and production of reactive oxygen species by peripheral blood phagocytes in patients with different stages of alcohol-induced liver disease: effect of acute exposure to low ethanol concentrations. *Alcohol Clin Exp Res* 2003;27(3):503–8.

397. Arteel GE. Oxidants and antioxidants in alcohol-induced liver disease. *Gastroenterology* 2003;124(3):778–90.

398. Liu H, Jones BE, Bradham C, Czaja MJ. Increased cytochrome P-450 2E1 expression sensitizes hepatocytes to c-Jun-mediated cell death from TNF-alpha. *Am J Physiol Gastrointest Liver Physiol* 2002;282(2): G257–66.

399. Bjorneboe GE, Johnsen J, Bjorneboe A, et al. Some aspects of antioxidant status in blood from alcoholics. *Alcohol Clin Exp Res* 1988; 12(6):806–10.

400. Kurose I, Higuchi H, Kato S, et al. Oxidative stress on mitochondria and cell membrane of cultured rat hepatocytes and perfused liver exposed to ethanol. *Gastroenterology* 1997;112(4): 1331–43.

401. Mezey E, Potter JJ, Rennie-Tankersley L, Caballeria J, Pares A. A randomized placebo controlled trial of vitamin E for alcoholic hepatitis. *J Hepatol* 2004;40(1):40–6.

402. de la Maza MP, Petermann M, Bunout D, Hirsch S. Effects of long-term vitamin E supplementation in alcoholic cirrhotics. *J Am Coll Nutr* 1995;14(2):192–6.

403. Wenzel G, Kuklinski B, Ruhlmann C, Ehrhardt D. [Alcohol-induced toxic hepatitis – a "free radical" associated disease. Lowering fatality by adjuvant antioxidant therapy.] *Z Gesamte Inn Med* 1993; 48(10):490–6.

404. Phillips M, Curtis H, Portmann B, Donaldson N, Bomford A, O'Grady J. Antioxidants versus corticosteroids in the treatment of severe alcoholic hepatitis – a randomised clinical trial. *J Hepatol* 2006;44(4):784–90.

405. Stewart S, Prince M, Bassendine M, et al. A randomized trial of antioxidant therapy alone or with corticosteroids in acute alcoholic hepatitis. *J Hepatol* 2007;47(2):277–83.

406. Moreno C, Langlet P, Hittelet A, et al. Enteral nutrition with or without *N*-acetylcysteine in the treatment of severe acute alcoholic hepatitis: a randomized multicenter controlled trial. *J Hepatol* 2010;53(6):1117–22.

407. Bunout D. Nutritional and metabolic effects of alcoholism: their relationship with alcoholic liver disease. *Nutrition* 1999;15(7–8): 583–9.

408. Mendenhall CL, Anderson S, Weesner RE, Goldberg SJ, Crolic KA. Protein-calorie malnutrition associated with alcoholic hepatitis. Veterans Administration Cooperative Study Group on Alcoholic Hepatitis. *Am J Med* 1984;76(2):211–22.

409. O'Keefe SJ, Ogden J, Dicker J. Enteral and parenteral branched chain amino acid-supplemented nutritional support in patients with encephalopathy due to alcoholic liver disease. *JPEN J Parenter Enteral Nutr* 1987;11(5):447–53.

410. Fulton S, McCullough AJ. Treatment of alcoholic hepatitis. *Clin Liver Dis* 1998;2: 799–819.

411. Nompleggi DJ, Bonkovsky HL. Nutritional supplementation in chronic liver disease: an analytical review. *Hepatology* 1994;19(2):518–33.

412. Nasrallah SM, Galambos JT. Aminoacid therapy of alcoholic hepatitis. *Lancet* 1980;2(8207):1276–7.

413. Naveau S, Pelletier G, Poynard T, et al. A randomized clinical trial of supplementary parenteral nutrition in jaundiced alcoholic cirrhotic patients. *Hepatology* 1986;6(2):270–4.

414. Calvey H, Davis M, Williams R. Controlled trial of nutritional supplementation, with and without branched chain amino acid enrichment, in treatment of acute alcoholic hepatitis. *J Hepatol* 1985;1(2):141–51.

415. DerSimonian R. Parenteral nutrition with branched-chain amino acids in hepatic encephalopathy: meta analysis. *Hepatology* 1990;11(6):1083–4.

416. Cabré E, Gonzalez-Huix F, bad-Lacruz A, et al. Effect of total enteral nutrition on the short-term outcome of severely malnourished cirrhotics. A randomized controlled trial. *Gastroenterology* 1990;98(3):715–20.

417. Kearns PJ, Young H, Garcia G, et al. Accelerated improvement of alcoholic liver disease with enteral nutrition. *Gastroenterology* 1992;102(1):200–5.

418. Campillo B, Bories PN, Leluan M, Pornin B, Devanlay M, Fouet P. Short-term changes in energy metabolism after 1 month of a regular oral diet in severely malnourished cirrhotic patients. *Metabolism* 1995;44(6):765–70.

419. Marchesini G, Bianchi G, Merli M, et al. Nutritional supplementation with branched-chain amino acids in advanced cirrhosis: a double-blind, randomized trial. *Gastroenterology* 2003;124(7):1792–801.

420. Marchesini G, Dioguardi FS, Bianchi GP, et al. Long-term oral branched-chain amino acid treatment in chronic hepatic encephalopathy. A randomized double-blind casein-controlled trial. The Italian Multicenter Study Group. *J Hepatol* 1990;11(1):92–101.

421. Yoshida T, Muto Y, Moriwaki H, Yamato M. Effect of long-term oral supplementation with branched-chain amino acid granules on the prognosis of liver cirrhosis. *Gastroenterol Jpn* 1989;24(6):692–8.

422. Hirsch S, Bunout D, de la Maza P, et al. Controlled trial on nutrition supplementation in outpatients with symptomatic alcoholic cirrhosis. *JPEN J Parenter Enteral Nutr* 1993;17(2):119–24.

423. Cabré E, Gassull MA. Nutrition in liver disease. *Curr Opin Clin Nutr Metab Care* 2005;8(5):545–51.

424. Kung T, Springer J, Doehner W, Anker SD, von Haehling S. Novel treatment approaches to cachexia and sarcopenia: highlights from the 5th Cachexia Conference. *Expert Opin Investig Drugs* 2010;19(4):579–85.

425. Mezey E. Commentary on the hypermetabolic state and the role of oxygen in alcohol-induced liver injury. *Recent Dev Alcohol* 1984;2:135–41.

426. Orrego H, Kalant H, Israel Y, et al. Effect of short-term therapy with propylthiouracil in patients with alcoholic liver disease. *Gastroenterology* 1979;76(1):105–15.

427. Halle P, Pare P, Kaptein E, Kanel G, Redeker AG, Reynolds TB. Double-blind, controlled trial of propylthiouracil in patients with severe acute alcoholic hepatitis. *Gastroenterology* 1982;82(5 Pt 1):925–31.

428. Rambaldi A, Gluud C, Rambaldi A. Propylthiouracil for alcoholic liver disease. *Cochrane Database Syst Rev* 2005;4: CD002800.

429. Akriviadis EA, Steindel H, Pinto PC, et al. Failure of colchicine to improve short-term survival in patients with alcoholic hepatitis. *Gastroenterology* 1990;99(3):811–18.

430. Trinchet JC, Beaugrand M, Callard P, et al. Treatment of alcoholic hepatitis with colchicine. Results of a randomized double blind trial. *Gastroenterol Clin Biol* 1989;13(6–7):551–5.

431. Rambaldi A, Gluud C. Colchicine for alcoholic and non-alcoholic liver fibrosis and cirrhosis. *Cochrane Database Syst Rev* 2005;2: CD002148.

432. Rambaldi A, Iaquinto G, Gluud C. Anabolic-androgenic steroids for alcoholic liver disease. *Cochrane Database Syst Rev* 2003;1: CD003045.

433. Karim Z, Intaraprasong P, Scudamore CH, et al. Predictors of relapse to significant alcohol drinking after liver transplantation. *Can J Gastroenterol* 2010;24(4):245–50.

434. Mukherjee S, Sorrell MF. Immediate listing for liver transplantation for alcoholic cirrhosis: curbing our enthusiasm. *Ann Intern Med* 2009;150(3):216–17.

435. Tandon P, Goodman KJ, Ma MM, et al. A shorter duration of pre-transplant abstinence predicts problem drinking after liver transplantation. *Am J Gastroenterol* 2009;104(7):1700–6.

436. Stickel F, Hoehn B, Schuppan D, Seitz HK. Review article. Nutritional therapy in alcoholic liver disease. *Aliment Pharmacol Ther* 2003;18(4):357–73.

437. Cabré E, Rodriguez-Iglesias, Caballere J, et al. Short- and long-term outcome of severe alcohol-induced hepatitis treated with steroids or enteral nutrition: a multicenter randomized trial. *Hepatology* 2000 Jul;32(1):36–42.

438. McCullough AJ, Bugianesi E. Protein-calorie malnutrition and the etiology of cirrhosis. *Am J Gastroenterol* 1997;92(5):734–8.

439. Swart GR, Zillikens MC, van Vuure JK, van den Berg JW. Effect of a late evening meal on nitrogen balance in patients with cirrhosis of the liver. *Br Med J* 1989;299(6709):1202–3.

440. Zillikens MC, van den Berg JW, Wattimena JL, Rietveld T, Swart GR. Nocturnal oral glucose supplementation. The effects on protein metabolism in cirrhotic patients and in healthy controls. *J Hepatol* 1993;17(3):377–83.

441. Verboeket-van de Venne WP, Westerterp KR, van Hoek B, Swart GR. Energy expenditure and substrate metabolism in patients with cirrhosis of the liver: effects of the pattern of food intake. *Gut* 1995;36(1):110–16.

442. Lochs H, Plauth M. Liver cirrhosis: rationale and modalities for nutritional support – the European Society of Parenteral and Enteral Nutrition consensus and beyond. *Curr Opin Clin Nutr Metab Care* 1999;2(4):345–9.

443. Orrego H, Blake JE, Blendis LM, Compton KV, Israel Y. Long-term treatment of alcoholic liver disease with propylthiouracil. *N Engl J Med* 1987;317(23):1421–7.

444. Lieber CS. S-adenosyl-L-methionine: its role in the treatment of liver disorders. *Am J Clin Nutr* 2002;76(5):S1183–7.

445. Martinez-Chantar ML, Garcia-Trevijano ER, Latasa MU, et al. Importance of a deficiency in S-adenosyl-L-methionine synthesis in the pathogenesis of liver injury. *Am J Clin Nutr* 2002;76(5):S1177–82.

446. Rambaldi A, Gluud C. S-adenosyl-L-methionine for alcoholic liver diseases (Cochrane review). *Cochrane Database Syst Rev* 2001;4: CD002235.

447. Kershenobich D, Uribe M, Suarez GI, Mata JM, Perez-Tamayo R, Rojkind M. Treatment of cirrhosis with colchicine. A double-blind randomized trial. *Gastroenterology* 1979;77(3):532–6.

448. Szabo G, Weinman SA, Gao B, Polyak SJ, Mandrekar P, Thiele GM. RSA 2004: Combined Basic Research Satellite Symposium – session four: hepatitis virus and alcohol interactions in immunity and liver disease. *Alcohol Clin Exp Res* 2005;29(9):1753–7.

449. Safdar K, Schiff ER. Alcohol and hepatitis C. *Semin Liver Dis* 2004;24(3):305–15.

450. Tan HH, Virmani S, Martin P. Controversies in the management of alcoholic liver disease. *Mt Sinai J Med* 2009;76(5):484–98.

451. Burra P, Lucey MR. Liver transplantation in alcoholic patients. *Transpl Int* 2005;18(5):491–8.

452. Hoofnagle JH, Kresina T, Fuller RK, et al. Liver transplantation for alcoholic liver disease: executive statement and recommendations. Summary of a National Institutes of Health workshop held December 6–7, 1996, Bethesda, Maryland. *Liver Transpl Surg* 1997;3(3):347–50.

453. McMaster P. Transplantation for alcoholic liver disease in an era of organ shortage. *Lancet* 2000;355(9202):424–5.

454. Zetterman RK. Liver transplantation for alcoholic liver disease. *Clin Liver Dis* 2005;9(1):171–81.

455. Perney P, Bismuth M, Sigaud H, et al. Are preoperative patterns of alcohol consumption predictive of relapse after liver transplantation for alcoholic liver disease? *Transpl Int* 2005;18(11):1292–7.

456. Shawcross DL, O'Grady JG. The 6-month abstinence rule in liver transplantation. *Lancet* 2010;376(9737):216–17.

457. Vargas HE, Krahn L. The transplantation candidate with alcohol misuse: the selection minefield. *Liver Transpl* 2008;14(11):1559–60.

458. DiMartini A, Dew MA, Day N, et al. Trajectories of alcohol consumption following liver transplantation. *Am J Transplant* 2010;10(10):2305–12.

459. Bellamy CO, DiMartini AM, Ruppert K, et al. Liver transplantation for alcoholic cirrhosis: long term follow-up and impact of disease recurrence. *Transplantation* 2001;72(4):619–26.

460. Wiesner RH, Lombardero M, Lake JR, Everhart J, Detre KM. Liver transplantation for end-stage alcoholic liver disease: an assessment of outcomes. *Liver Transpl Surg* 1997;3(3):231–9.

461. Bathgate AJ, Hynd P, Sommerville D, Hayes PC. The prediction of acute cellular rejection in orthotopic liver transplantation. *Liver Transpl Surg* 1999;5(6):475–9.

462. Farges O, Saliba F, Farhamant H, et al. Incidence of rejection and infection after liver transplantation as a function of the primary disease: possible influence of alcohol and polyclonal immunoglobulins. *Hepatology* 1996;23(2):240–8.

463. Gish RG, Lee A, Brooks L, Leung J, Lau JY, Moore DH. Long-term follow-up of patients diagnosed with alcohol dependence or alcohol abuse who were evaluated for liver transplantation. *Liver Transpl* 2001;7(7):581–7.

464. Stefanini GF, Biselli M, Grazi GL, et al. Orthotopic liver transplantation for alcoholic liver disease: rates of survival, complications and relapse. *Hepatogastroenterology* 1997;44(17):1356–9.

465. Zibari GB, Edwin D, Wall L, et al. Liver transplantation for alcoholic liver disease. *Clin Transplant* 1996;10(6 Pt 2):676–9.

466. Howard L, Fahy T. Liver transplantation for alcoholic liver disease. *Br J Psychiatry* 1997;171: 497–500.

467. Lucey MR, Brown KA, Everson GT, et al. Minimal criteria for placement of adults on the liver transplant waiting list: a report of a national conference organized by the American Society of Transplant Physicians and the American Association for the Study of Liver Diseases. *Liver Transpl Surg* 1997;3(6):628–37.

468. Osorio RW, Ascher NL, Avery M, Bacchetti P, Roberts JP, Lake JR. Predicting recidivism after orthotopic liver transplantation for alcoholic liver disease. *Hepatology* 1994;20(1 Pt 1): 105–10.

469. Pageaux GP, Michel J, Coste V, et al. Alcoholic cirrhosis is a good indication for liver transplantation, even for cases of recidivism. *Gut* 1999;45(3):421–6.

470. Goldar-Najafi A, Gordon FD, Lewis WD, et al. Liver transplantation for alcoholic liver disease with or without hepatitis C. *Int J Surg Pathol* 2002;10(2):115–22.

471. Jain A, DiMartini A, Kashyap R, Youk A, Rohal S, Fung J. Long-term follow-up after liver transplantation for alcoholic liver disease under tacrolimus. *Transplantation* 2000;70(9):1335–42.

472. Pereira SP, Williams R. Alcohol relapse and functional outcome after liver transplantation for alcoholic liver disease. *Liver Transpl* 2001;7(3):204–5.

473. Dhar S, Omran L, Bacon BR, Solomon H, Di Bisceglie AM. Liver transplantation in patients with chronic hepatitis C and alcoholism. *Dig Dis Sci* 1999;44(10):2003–7.

474. Tang H, Boulton R, Gunson B, Hubscher S, Neuberger J. Patterns of alcohol consumption after liver transplantation. *Gut* 1998;43(1):140–5.

475. Fabrega E, Crespo J, Casafont F, De las Heras G, de la Pena J, Pons-Romero F. Alcoholic recidivism after liver transplantation for alcoholic cirrhosis. *J Clin Gastroenterol* 1998;26(3):204–6.

476. Kumar S, Stauber RE, Gavaler JS, et al. Orthotopic liver transplantation for alcoholic liver disease. *Hepatology* 1990;11(2):159–64.

477. Bird GL, O'Grady JG, Harvey FA, Calne RY, Williams R. Liver transplantation in patients with alcoholic cirrhosis: selection criteria and rates of survival and relapse. *Br Med J* 1990;301(6742): 15–17.

478. Knechtle SJ, Fleming MF, Barry KL, et al. Liver transplantation for alcoholic liver disease. *Surgery* 1992;112(4):694–701.

479. Platz KP, Mueller AR, Spree E, et al. Liver transplantation for alcoholic cirrhosis. *Transpl Int* 2000;13(Suppl 1):S127–30.

480. Gerhardt TC, Goldstein RM, Urschel HC, et al. Alcohol use following liver transplantation for alcoholic cirrhosis. *Transplantation* 1996;62(8):1060–3.

481. Berlakovich GA, Steininger R, Herbst F, Barlan M, Mittlbock M, Muhlbacher F. Efficacy of liver transplantation for alcoholic cirrhosis with respect to recidivism and compliance. *Transplantation* 1994;58(5):560–5.

482. Burra P, Senzolo M, Adam R, et al. Liver transplantation for alcoholic liver disease in Europe: a study from the ELTR (European Liver Transplant Registry). *Am J Transplant* 2010;10(1): 138–48.

483. Pfitzmann R, Schwenzer J, Rayes N, Seehofer D, Neuhaus R, Nussler NC. Long-term survival and predictors of relapse after orthotopic liver transplantation for alcoholic liver disease. *Liver Transpl* 2007;13(2):197–205.

484. Schmeding M, Heidenhain C, Neuhaus R, Neuhaus P, Neumann UP. Liver Transplantation for alcohol-related cirrhosis: a single centre long-term clinical and histological follow-up. *Dig Dis Sci* 2011;56: 236–43.

485. Biselli M, Gramenzi A, Del GM, et al. Long term follow-up and outcome of liver transplantation for alcoholic liver disease: a single center case–control study. *J Clin Gastroenterol* 2010;44(1):52–7.

486. Cuadrado A, Fabrega E, Casafont F, Pons-Romero F. Alcohol recidivism impairs long-term patient survival after orthotopic liver transplantation for alcoholic liver disease. *Liver Transpl* 2005;11(4): 420–6.

487. DiMartini A, Day N, Dew MA, et al. Alcohol use following liver transplantation: a comparison of follow-up methods. *Psychosomatics* 2001;42(1):55–62.

488. DiMartini A, Day N, Lane T, Beisler AT, Amanda DM, Anton R. Carbohydrate deficient transferrin in abstaining patients with end-stage liver disease. *Alcohol Clin Exp Res* 2001;25(12):1729–33.

489. Burra P, Mioni D, Cillo U, et al. Long-term medical and psychosocial evaluation of patients undergoing orthotopic liver transplantation for alcoholic liver disease. *Transpl Int* 2000;13(Suppl 1): S174–8.

490. Immordino G, Gelli M, Ferrante R, et al. Alcohol abstinence and orthotopic liver transplantation in alcoholic liver cirrhosis. *Transplant Proc* 2009;41(4):1253–5.

491. Wells JT, Said A, Agni R, et al. The impact of acute alcoholic hepatitis in the explanted recipient liver on outcome after liver transplantation. *Liver Transpl* 2007;13(12):1728–35.

492. Mullen KD, Dasarathy S. Potential new therapies for alcoholic liver disease. *Clin Liver Dis* 1988;2: 851–81.

493. Rambaldi A, Jacobs BP, Iaquinto G, Gluud C. Milk thistle for alcoholic and/or hepatitis B or C liver diseases – a systematic Cochrane Hepato-Biliary Group review with meta-analyses of randomized clinical trials. *Am J Gastroenterol* 2005;100(11):2583–91.

494. Austin AS, Mahida YR, Clarke D, Ryder SD, Freeman JG. A pilot study to investigate the use of oxpentifylline (pentoxifylline) and thalidomide in portal hypertension secondary to alcoholic cirrhosis. *Aliment Pharmacol Ther* 2004;19(1):79–88.

495. Yokota T, Oritani K, Takahashi I, et al. Adiponectin, a new member of the family of soluble defense collagens, negatively regulates the growth of myelomonocytic progenitors and the functions of macrophages. *Blood* 2000;96(5):1723–32.

496. Li Z, Yang S, Lin H, et al. Probiotics and antibodies to TNF inhibit inflammatory activity and improve nonalcoholic fatty liver disease. *Hepatology* 2003;37(2):343–50.

497. Day CP. Apoptosis in alcoholic hepatitis: a novel therapeutic target? *J Hepatol* 2001;34(2):330–3.

498. Campra JL, Hamlin EM Jr, Kirshbaum RJ, et al. Prednisone therapy of acute alcoholic hepatitis. Report of a controlled trial. *Ann Intern Med* 1973;79(5):625–31.

Multiple choice questions

26.1 The most effective therapy for acute alcoholic hepatitis with hepatic encephalopathy is which of the following?

  a Infliximab.
  b Corticosteroids.
  c Etanercept.
  d Lactulose.

26.2 Liver transplantation is considered a standard therapeutic option in patients with decompenstated alcoholic cirrhosis because of which of the following?

  a The graft and patient survival are similar to that in nonalcoholic cirrhosis.
  b Recidivism rates are low even without abstinence.
  c Mortality is higher than with cirrhosis of other etiologies.
  d There is a lower risk of post-transplant complications in alcoholic cirrhosis than in post-hepatitis cirrhosis.

Answers to the multiple choice questions can be found in the Appendix at the end of the book.

These multiple choice questions are also available for you to complete online.
Visit http://www.schiffsdiseasesoftheliver.com/

CHAPTER 27
Drug-induced Liver Disease

Shivakumar Chitturi & Geoffrey C. Farrell

Department of Hepatic Medicine, Australian National University Medical School and Gastroenterology and Hepatology Unit, Canberra Hospital, Garran, Australia

Key concepts

- Over 300 agents in current use have been implicated in causing drug-induced liver injury (DILI), but there is strong evidence for causality with fewer than 30.
- Most implicated drugs cause liver disease in fewer than one in 10,000 persons exposed; the frequency of hepatotoxicity is variously influenced by genetic factors, age, gender, intake of other drugs or alcohol, nutritional status and preexisting liver disease.
- Interactions between drugs, liver, and other diseases can increase risk and worsen DILI; examples include highly active antiretroviral treatment and hepatitis C virus infection; tamoxifen and nonalcoholic fatty liver disease; methotrexate, diabetes, and hepatic fibrosis; and antituberculosis drugs with chronic hepatitis B and hepatitis C.
- The clinicopathologic spectrum of DILI ranges from nonspecific injury to acute and chronic hepatitis, granulomatous hepatitis, cholestatic reactions, vascular lesions and hepatic tumors.
- Although characteristic "signature" patterns are observed with some drugs, others are associated with diverse clinical syndromes.
- While the liver biochemistry profile may aid initial evaluation, liver biopsy remains the gold standard for defining the type and extent of drug-induced liver disease.
- Pathogenic mechanisms underlying DILI include dose-dependent injury, metabolic idiosyncrasy, and immunoallergic reactions. The

latter may be part of the reactive metabolite syndrome, a multisystem disorder with hallmarks of hypersensitivity.
- Supportive measures remain the cornerstone in management. Early recognition of drug toxicity and immediate withdrawal of the offending drug are critical. *N*-acetylcysteine remains pivotal in managing acetaminophen overdoses. It has also shown to be of value in acute liver failure (grades I and II encephalopathy) resulting from drugs other than acetaminophen. Corticosteroids are not routinely recommended, but may be valuable in selected cases showing pronounced hypersensitivity characteristics (e.g., allopurinol). Anecdotal evidence favors the use of ursodeoxycholic acid in the setting of protracted cholestasis. Early consultation with a liver transplant centre is mandatory for individuals developing progressive impairment of liver function.
- Serial liver test profiles are often recommended to facilitate early detection of liver injury. However, with few exceptions, the sensitivity and cost-effectiveness of this approach remains untested.
- Clinical evaluation of symptoms that could be drug related is critical in facilitating early detection of DILI.
- Herbal hepatotoxicity and use of recreational drugs (of abuse) should now be considered in the differential diagnosis of all liver disorders.

Introduction

Terminology and definitions

Hepatotoxicity is liver injury caused by foreign compounds (*xenobiotics*). These include prescribed and nonprescribed therapeutic agents (*drugs*), including "over-the-counter" pharmacologic agents, herbal and other complementary and alternative medicines (CAM), and a vast array of other organic and inorganic substances that may be ingested deliberately or accidentally. The latter compounds may contaminate the environment, workplace, or home. Thus, xenobiotics include pesticides, herbicides, and plant, fungal, and microbial products, each of which may have toxic and/or carcinogenic

properties. The present chapter will concentrate on drug-induced liver injury (DILI), in which hepatotoxicity is caused by medicinal drugs or those used by individuals for therapeutic, nutritional, or recreational purposes; the latter including drugs of abuse. While passing reference is made to other hepatotoxins, the interested reader is referred to specialized texts for a comprehensive coverage of environmental and industrial hepatotoxicity [1,2].

Injury to the liver is largely defined by increased blood levels of proteins that are liberated from damaged hepatocytes; a typical example is alanine aminotransferase (ALT). In order to implicate a drug as the cause of ALT elevation we need to know: (i) that there is no other

Schiff's Diseases of the Liver, Eleventh Edition. Edited by Eugene R. Schiff, Willis C. Maddrey and Michael F. Sorrell.
© 2012 John Wiley & Sons, Ltd. Published 2012 by John Wiley & Sons, Ltd.

hepatic process that could account for the test abnormality (e.g., steatosis); (ii) that the logistics (particularly the temporal relationships) relating the drug intake and liver test abnormality are consistent and compelling, and (3) that ALT elevation really means that the liver is injured. There is often a considerable amount of uncertainty in each of these three areas. Some practical implications will be dealt with in later sections on hepatic adaptation (physiologic responses by the liver when exposed to drugs) and diagnosis.

We have avoided the term "hepatic dysfunction" in this text because of the confusion between injury, adaptation, and indices that truly reflect functions of the liver. Likewise, the pathologically meaningless term "transaminitis" (an ALT elevation without histologic evidence of liver injury) will not be used; DILI is now preferable and in widespread use. When the presence of a major (five-fold or greater) elevation of ALT clearly indicates liver injury, or when one or more of the *functions of the liver* are abnormal (e.g., low levels of plasma proteins like albumin and clotting factors synthesized by the liver, or clinicopathologic evidence of impaired bile flow (*cholestasis*)), it is *highly probable* that a drug to which the person has been exposed is the cause of liver disease. Ideally, however, the definition of *drug-induced liver disease* requires histopathologic characterization rather than syndromic recognition of liver test abnormalities. Although the distinction between injury and disease is sometimes artificial, because they clearly overlap, it will be maintained wherever possible in this chapter so as to provide insights into the clinical significance of hepatic adverse drug reactions.

As new drugs emerge, the evidence that they induce liver injury is often weak and circumstantial. It is sometimes hotly debated because of the implications for further use and marketing of valuable therapeutic agents, or for medicolegal implications [3]. In order to partly meet the challenge of possible newer types of DILI that are not yet well defined, we have included a section on "emerging therapies." Another definitional challenge is that drugs may sometimes alter physiologic parameters that impact on hepatic viability. In particular, some drugs can profoundly reduce hepatic blood flow and oxygen delivery, induce hyperthermia, or modify arterial supply to major bile ducts, each of which can result in liver injury that may be minor or profound. Cocaine, general anesthetic agents, alcohol, intra-arterial floxuridine, and "ecstasy" are agents that most likely produce liver injury by such indirect mechanisms rather than by direct hepatotoxicity or adverse drug reactions.

Another challenge for defining drug-induced liver disease is the increasing number of circumstances in which drug ingestion appears to contribute to chronic liver disease or hepatic tumours. The lead time ("*latent period*") to onset or diagnosis of such associations is many months or years. As a result, repeated observations and case–control studies are essential to ensure they are not chance associations, while experimental evidence from laboratory or animal studies is desirable in order to invoke biologically plausible mechanistic explanations for this type of effect of the drug on the liver.

Thus, there is no "gold standard" by which drugs can be proved to have a unique etiologic role in liver disease, particularly as some of the disorders with which they are associated appear very similar or identical to syndromes associated with other causes. Further, it is increasingly apparent that drugs may interact with each other or with other hepatotoxins (particularly alcohol) as part of *interactive hepatotoxicity*, as well as with viruses (human immunodeficiency virus (HIV), hepatitis B virus (HBV, and hepatitis C virus (HCV)), immune mechanisms (HIV/acquired immune deficiency syndrome (AIDS) and bone marrow transplantation), and metabolic factors (nonalcoholic steatohepatitis (NASH)) to accentuate or cause liver injury. Such interactions may be exceedingly difficult to recognize or to prove, and near impossible to quantify as "relative risk" by conventional epidemiologic techniques. The evidence implicating the involvement of drugs in liver injury associated with more complex medical settings will be discussed in a later section.

Dose-dependent hepatotoxicity and hepatic drug reactions

Some agents possess a high degree of *intrinsic hepatotoxic potential*; they cause *dose-dependent liver injury* in humans and usually many other species. The history of industrial hepatotoxicity is replete with such examples, including dimethylnitrosamine, carbon tetrachloride, tetrachloroethane, trinitrotoluene, phosphorus, tannic acid, and vinyl chloride. Some early therapeutic drugs and anesthetic agents (arsenicals, chloroform) have also been assigned to this category, although older studies are inadequate in ascertaining causal mechanisms because viral hepatitis, hepatic perfusion, and tissue oxygenation could not be assessed by contemporary criteria. Among today's drugs, very few are dose-dependent hepatotoxins (Box 27.1). For those that are, as illustrated by acetaminophen, it is not the chemical structure of the parent drug that is responsible for the liver injury, but rather the production of chemically reactive metabolites that interfere with the integrity of the liver. It follows that for most dose-dependent hepatotoxins, a range of host factors predicate the amount of reactive (toxic) metabolites that accumulate, thereby determining the risk of liver injury for a given dose of the toxicant.

The vast majority (more than 95%) of drugs implicated as causing DILI are clearly *not* dose-dependent human hepatotoxins, although some of them (usually

Box 27.1 Examples of dose-dependent hepatotoxins.

- Acetaminophen (paracetamol)
- Drugs used in cancer chemotherapy (especially used with radiotherapy); cyclophosphamide, busulphan, bis-chlorethyl-nitrosourea.
- Amodiaquine
- Hycanthone
- Carbon tetrachloride, dimethylnitrosamine, methylenedianiline
- Plant and fungal toxins: pyrrolizidine alkaloids, aflatoxin
- Ethanol
- Metals: copper, iron, mercury
- Bile salts

at high, nonpharmacologic doses) produce experimental liver injury. This relative "intrinsic hepatotoxic potential" tends to be roughly proportional to the risk of liver injury in humans [2]. There is also evidence for a few agents that liver injury is partially dose dependent (e.g., perhexiline maleate, tacrine, dantrolene, cyclophosphamide, sex steroids, and cyclosporine). However, the frequency with which such agents cause liver injury among those exposed is either low or extremely small, ranging from 0.5–2% with chlorpromazine and isoniazid, through more typical rates of 1–10 cases per 100,000 persons exposed, to even lower rates (e.g., one case per 1,000,000 persons exposed) with minocycline, and some of the oxypenicillins and nonsteroidal anti-inflammatory drugs (NSAIDs) (Table 27.1).

It is clear that for these rare, dose-independent, unpredictable or *idiosyncratic drug reactions* to occur, it is the host response to the drug that often determines liver injury, not the dose or chemical structures of the agent and its metabolites. Idiosyncratic hepatotoxicity is difficult to reproduce in other species, and it is therefore hard

Table 27.1 Frequencies of some types of idiosyncratic drug-induced liver diseases.

Frequency[a]	Drugs
5 to 20/1,000 exposed	Isoniazid, chlorpromazine, dantrolene
1 to 2.5/10,000 exposed	Estrogen-induced cholestasis
0.5 to 20/10,000 exposed	Ketoconazole
1 to 10/100,000 exposed	Diclofenac, sulindac, phenytoin, flucloxacillin
0.5 to 3/100,000 exposed	Amoxicillin-clavulanate, nitrofurantoin, terbinafine, dicloxacillin
≤1 to 10/1,000,000 exposed	Minocycline

[a]Based on published data referred to in the text.

to ascertain the pathogenetic mechanisms involved. Clinical recognition will always remain a challenge because most doctors will never encounter individual reactions, or will observe them no more often than once or twice in a professional lifetime.

Two broad types of pathogenic mechanism could account for idiosyncratic hepatic drug reactions. The first is *metabolic idiosyncrasy*, in which pathways of drug metabolism or disposition favor drug accumulation or formation of toxic metabolites. The underlying determinants include pharmacogenetic variability of drug metabolism, and expression of "antistress" and antioxidant cell defense pathways. The metabolic idiosyncrasy concept now needs to be extended to consider ways in which the liver, a highly adaptable organ, normally counters the "stress" of potentially damaging chemicals. Thus, using experimental toxicants, it has become evident that foreign compounds, drug metabolites, and resultant oxidative stress can stimulate or interrupt intracellular signaling pathways that converge on target genes involved in stress responses, cell death, or cell cycle regulation. Alternatively, they may directly activate transcriptional regulators to the same effect, or more indirectly interfere with cell integrity and cell death pathways by their interactions with mitochondrial function and integrity. The latter includes mitochondrial DNA (mtDNA) and the unique "guardian role" of mitochondria for cell survival as well as in energy generation. Drugs can alter the regulation of adenosine triphosphate (ATP)-dependent transporters that actively pump drug metabolites out of hepatocytes, particularly via canalicular pathways that are physiologically engaged in the generation of bile flow. Drugs, reactive metabolites and oxidative stress can interact with the cytoskeletal determinants of cellular transport, receptor signaling, and cell–cell communication (see Chapter 28). Recently, the concept of partial dose dependency has been raised again in cases of idiosyncratic liver injury (it was originally noted by Hyman Zimmerman among others in the 1980s); drugs with daily doses greater than 50 mg have been overrepresented in cases of significant hepatotoxicity. Whether this is related to overrepresentation of drug classes with higher doses (NSAIDs, antimicrobials) or true dose dependency needs to be verified [4]. Likewise, it has been "rediscovered" [2] that drugs undergoing significant hepatic metabolism are more often implicated in causing hepatic injury when compared with drugs that do not [5].

The alternative pathogenic mechanism underlying idiosyncratic hepatic drug reactions is an *immunoallergic* response. This refers to classic "hypersensitivity" in the sense that repeated exposure results in an exaggerated and unhelpful tissue-based or systemic injurious inflammatory response. Immunoallergic reactions are even less well understood than metabolic idiosyncrasy for their role in DILI. The possible immunologic mechanisms have been reviewed elsewhere [6,7]. Some are examples of drug-induced autoimmunity in which the liver is the principal organ involved, implying that the drug (or its metabolites) has induced immune dysregulation [6]. Syndromes of chronic hepatitis with hyperglobulinemia and autoantibodies (e.g., with nitrofurantoin, minocycline, or diclofenac) are examples of such an immune-based mechanism. There is increasing evidence that, for a subset of reactions, reactive metabolites are involved with recruiting inflammatory mechanisms, as haptens with molecular mimicry [8,9]. Regulation of hepatic cytokines may also be important as shown by studies of drug hepatotoxicity in mice with targeted disruptions of interleukin 4 (IL4), IL10, or cyclooxygenase 2 mediators that help prevent allergic hepatitis [7]. Recruitment of eosinophils to the liver in the later stages of idiosyncratic drug reactions may depend on expression of the chemokine eotaxin [10].

It is often not possible to clearly distinguish between what seem like diametrically different causative mechanisms. They may overlap, particularly because hepatic inflammatory reactions appear to evoke the liver's own innate immunity, as seen by the presence of liver lymphocytes and activated Kupffer cells (resident macrophages) as well as by the activation of toll-like receptors (TLRs) [11]. Ultimately, it is most likely that the principal factors predicating idiosyncratic drug reactions are *genetically determined* [12,13]. This provides a challenge for future studies directed at prevention, and for timely interventions to avoid the adverse clinical outcomes that are unacceptably common for some agents and reactions (see "Improving outcomes" below).

Importance of drug-induced liver disease

The importance of drug-induced liver disease is summarized in Box 27.2. The pertinent factors are the disproportionate frequency, severity, and potential for preventing serious hepatic adverse drug reactions in older people. Some newer aspects include the potential of drugs to produce synergistic hepatotoxicity in persons with, for example, viral hepatitis, HIV/AIDS, HBV/HCV, and NASH, as discussed later (in the section on the role of drugs in multifactorial disease). The low frequency of reactions for many commonly used drugs can delay the recognition of DILI; continued ingestion of the causative agent is the single most important determinant of adverse outcome. In addition to the key responsibility of physicians for early diagnosis and stopping exposure to potentially implicated agents, they have moral, ethical, and medicolegal responsibilities to prevent, mitigate, and report iatrogenic disease.

The increasing number of pharmacologic agents associated with DILI is a major challenge for clinicians [2,12,

Box 27.2 Factors that contribute to the importance of drug-induced liver disease (DILI).

- About 6% of all adverse drug reactions result in DILI
- DILI occurs with a higher frequency among severe adverse drug reactions
- DILI is the most frequent cause for post-marketing withdrawal of medications
- DILI is a preventable or correctable cause of acute and chronic liver disease
- About 5% of cases of jaundice or acute hepatitis in the community result from DILI
- A higher proportion (10–40% depending on age) of cases of hepatitis admitted to hospital are due to DILI
- DILI is an important cause of acute liver failure (more than 50% of cases in United States: 36% from acetaminophen, 16% idiosyncratic hepatic drug reactions)
- DILI is a common cause of undiagnosed liver injury, particularly among persons aged more than 50 years
- More than 300 currently used drugs are cited in the literature as potential causes of DILI
- A low frequency of liver injury leads to cases often being overlooked, and difficulty in attributing causality to drugs
- One agent may cause more than one pattern of DILI
- Early diagnosis and stopping drug exposure are critically important in avoiding progression and poor outcomes
- A poor understanding of pathogenic mechanisms in DILI makes reactions difficult to predict and prevent
- The role of drugs is important in synergistic hepatotoxicity with viral hepatitis, NASH, HIV/AIDS, bone marrow, and organ transplantation
- There is a moral/ethical responsibility to prevent or minimize iatrogenic disease
- There are medicolegal implications of this responsibility (informed consent, practice standards, due diligence, etc.)

AIDS, acquired immune deficiency syndrome; HIV, human immunodeficiency virus; NASH, nonalcoholic steatohepatitis.

14–20]. In addition to case recognition, this invokes consideration of what level of patient information should be regarded as appropriate at the time of prescribing drugs, and how that information should be imparted to the consumer.

Diversity of clinical expression

Drugs have become the greater mimickers of "natural" liver diseases. Thus hepatic drug reactions range from nonspecific abnormalities of liver tests (which may represent minor degrees of liver injury or hepatic adaptation), through clinicopathologic features of cholestasis, acute hepatitis, and acute liver failure, to more exotic syndromes like hepatic sinusoidal or venous outflow obstruction syndromes, nodular regenerative hyperplasia

(NRH), chronic hepatitis resembling autoimmune hepatitis, hepatic fibrosis, NASH, cirrhosis, and benign or malignant liver tumors. It therefore remains crucial that physicians should always consider a possible drug or toxic etiology, irrespective of the pattern of liver injury. A common pitfall is to impute causality to known causes of liver disease that happen to be present (HCV, alcohol, and gallstones are common "confounders") in what are actually cases of DILI. Another challenge is the propensity of some drugs to cause more than one clinicopathologic syndrome, as discussed later for oral contraceptive steroids (OCSs), diclofenac, and nitrofurantoin.

Epidemiology and risk factors

Epidemiology

In discussing how commonly a drug causes liver injury, it is important to note that the term "incidence" (the number of new cases in a period of time) is not particularly helpful because the onset of adverse drug reactions is nonlinear with time; they tend to occur within the first few weeks or months of treatment. A better descriptor is the proportion of persons exposed to the agent who develop the reaction. This proportion is best described by the *frequency of the reaction* within the affected group; the latter is expressed ideally as the number of persons exposed, but surrogate estimates are often used, such as the number of prescriptions written or the number of person-years of drug ingestion. Other estimates of the frequency of adverse drug reactions or risk of hepatotoxicity come from prescription event monitoring or record linkage conducted prospectively by health maintenance groups, and from case–control studies. More commonly used methods include voluntary (or mandated) reporting of reactions to agencies that monitor adverse drug reactions or drug manufacturers. However, this approach is weakened by the inherent inaccuracies of case definition and the vagaries of case documentation, factors that depend on the skill and motivation of observers.

Drugs that carry a high frequency of liver injury are usually recognized as hepatotoxic during phase III trials, which typically involve hundreds or a few thousand persons, or during the first 2 years of post-marketing surveillance (which may involve hundreds of thousands or millions of subjects) [3]. Nefazodone, bromfenac, lumiracoxib, and troglitazone are examples of agents withdrawn because of a high frequency of severe liver injury. More often, recognition of DILI comes several years after the release of a new agent, often with a flurry of case reports, small series, and analyses of larger repositories of information held by drug-monitoring authorities or pharmaceutical companies. More recent examples include amoxicillin-clavulanate, oxypenicillins, diclofenac, sulin-

dac, and troglitazone [21–24]. Such "mini-epidemics" serve principally to highlight how often early reactions to the implicated agents may have been overlooked, or become evident during massive prescribing of vigorously marketed new drugs. The latter phenomenon is illustrated by hepatic reactions to flucloxacillin in Australia, where the number of prescriptions written per million people greatly exceeded that of any other country [25].

Reliable information about the risk of liver injury is available for less than 30 of the 300 or so currently used drugs that have been implicated as possible or likely causes of drug-induced liver disease (Table 27.1). The most significant issue confounding the epidemiology of DILI is the lack of diagnostic accuracy in case definition. As discussed next, this depends entirely on probabilistic evidence surrounding the onset of the reaction and its resolution or recurrence in relation to drug exposure, on the exclusion of other hepatobiliary diseases, and occasionally on ancillary evidence of an adverse drug reaction.

When drugs contribute to but are not the unique cause of liver disease, it may be possible to assign a relative risk. This has been attempted in the case of OCSs and liver tumours [26,27], OCSs and hepatic venous outflow obstruction [28], aspirin and Reye syndrome [29], and methotrexate and hepatic fibrosis among those who drink appreciable quantities of alcohol [30].

Risk factors for incidence and severity

The factors that increase the risk of DILI may include dose, duration of treatment, blood levels, the site of metabolism, age, gender, coincidental metabolic disorders or genetic predisposition to hypersensitivity reactions, concomitant exposure to other drugs or environmental agents, and underlying liver disease (Table 27.2).

Genetic factors

It seems likely that host predisposition to idiosyncratic hepatic drug reactions may simply reflect the dual requirements for altered expression of relevant genes and for exposure to particular drugs under particular circumstance; halothane, OCS cholestasis, valproic acid, and phenytoin reactions are those for which more than one case has occurred in the same family [11]. Phenytoin is an example of the reactive metabolite syndrome (RMS) pattern of severe skin reactions often associated with systemic involvement, amongst which DILI is common [31]. Known causative agents for RMS, its risk factors, and clinical features are summarized in Table 27.3. Individuals have a 25% likelihood of developing adverse drug toxicity if a first-degree relative has experienced a similar reaction; the chances are even higher with other risk factors such as HIV/AIDS, systemic lupus erythematosus (SLE),

Table 27.2 Risk factors for the incidence and severity of drug-induced liver diseases.

Risk factor	Representative agents	Importance
Age	Isoniazid, nitrofurantoin, halothane, troglitazone	Age >60 years increases frequency and severity
	Valproic acid, salicylates	More common in children
Gender	Halothane, minocycline, nitrofurantoin, dextropropoxyphene	More common in women, especially chronic hepatitis
	Amoxicillin-clavulanate, azathioprine	More common in men
Dose	Acetaminophen, some herbal medicines	Risk of hepatotoxicity depends on blood levels
	Anticancer drugs; perhexiline, tacrine, oxypenicillins, dantrolene	Partial relationship to dose
	Methotrexate, vitamin A	Total dose, dose frequency, and duration of exposure influence risk of hepatic fibrosis
Genetic factors	Halothane, phenytoin, sulfonamides	Multiple cases in families, in vitro test results
	Amoxicillin-clavulanate	Strong HLA association
	Diclofenac	Association with specific gene polymorphisms (see text)
	Valproic acid	Familial cases, association with mitochondrial enzyme deficiencies
Other drug reactions	Isoflurane, halothane, enflurane	Cross-sensitivity reported between these classes of drugs
	Erythromycins, other macrolide antibiotics	
	Diclofenac, ibuprofen	
	Sulfonamides, COX-2 inhibitors	
Concomitant drugs	Acetaminophen	Isoniazid, zidovudine, and phenytoin lower hepatotoxic dose threshold and increase severity
	Valproic acid	Other anticonvulsants increase risk
Excessive alcohol use	Acetaminophen hepatotoxicity	Lowers dose threshold and worsens outcome
	Isoniazid, methotrexate	Increases risk of liver injury and hepatic fibrosis
Nutritional status:		
Obesity	Halothane, tamoxifen, methotrexate	Increases risk of liver injury, NASH, or hepatic fibrosis
fasting	Acetaminophen	Increases risk of hepatotoxicity
Liver disease	Hycanthone, pemoline	Increases risk of liver injury
	Antituberculosis chemotherapy, ibuprofen	Increases risk of liver injury with chronic hepatitis B and C
Other diseases:		
Diabetes mellitus	Methotrexate	Increases risk of hepatic fibrosis
Psoriasis	Methotrexate	Increases risk of hepatic fibrosis
HIV/AIDS	Sulfonamides (cotrimoxazole)	Increases risk of hypersensitivity
Renal failure	Tetracycline, methotrexate	Increases risk of liver injury and hepatic fibrosis
Organ transplantation	Azathioprine, thioguanine, busulfan	Increases risk of vascular toxicity

AIDS, acquired immune deficiency syndrome; COX-2, cyclooxygenase 2; HIV, human immunodeficiency virus; HLA, human leukocyte antigen; NASH, nonalcoholic steatohepatitis.

and antecedent intake of valproic acid or corticosteroids (Table 27.3).

As well as determining the expression and inducibility of cytochrome P450 (CYP) pathways of drug oxidation, conjugation reactions, and antioxidant enzymes (Chapter 28), genetic factors encode ATP-dependent pathways of drug elimination from hepatocytes, through the canalicular membrane into bile or via the basolateral membrane into sinusoidal blood [32]. Regulation of the immune response, including hepatic innate immunity, is also genetically determined. Other genes encode the structure of the cytoskeleton, heat shock proteins, and

cellular resistance against activated cell death pathways, all potential variables in the pathogenesis of DILI. The characterization of which genes are involved in hepatic reactions to clinically relevant agents provides an outstanding challenge in the field of drug-induced liver disease, as reviewed elsewhere [33]. The likelihood that more than one "abnormality" (genetic polymorphisms, extreme variation) is required before tissue destructive responses occur would explain the rarity of most reactions. Already it is known that inherited defects of mitochondrial metabolism and mtDNA repair clearly predispose to valproate hepatotoxicity [33,34] (see later section

Table 27.3 The reactive metabolite syndrome and hepatic drug reactions

Drugs implicated	Risk factors	Clinical and laboratory features
Sulfonamides	First-degree relative with serious rash to same drug (1 in 4 risk), or metabolically cross-reacting drug	Onset: 1–6 weeks (up to 12 weeks)
Clozapine		Sentinel symptoms: fever, pharyngitis, malaise, headache, periorbital edema, otalgia/headache, mouth ulcers, rhinorrhea
Anticonvulsants (phenytoin, lamotrigine, phenobarbital, carbamazepine)	HIV/AIDS (100-fold increased risk)	Serious rash: erythematous, Stevens–Johnson syndrome, toxic epidermal necrolysis, erythema multiforme
	Systemic lupus erythematosus (10-fold increased risk)	
Some NSAIDs		Lymphadenopathy (16%), splenomegaly
Aminopenicillins	Corticosteroids at time of starting drug (4.4-fold increased risk)	Hepatic reactions: cholestasis, hepatitis, granulomas (13%)
Chinese herbal medicines		Nephritis (9%)
Quinolones	Valproic acid at time of starting new anticonvulsant (4–10-fold increased risk)	Pneumonitis (6%)
Protease inhibitors (nevirapine, abacavir)		Hematologic (neutropenia, thrombocytopenia) (5%)
		Encephalitis/meningitis (5%)
Allopurinol		Myositis (4%)
Minocycline		Colitis (2%)
		Arthritis, transient hypothyroidism
		Blood tests: neutrophilia (shift to left); atypical lymphocytes, acute phase reactants (early); eosinophilia (often late)

AIDS, acquired immune deficiency syndrome; HIV, human immunodeficiency virus; NSAIDs, nonsteroidal anti-inflammatory drugs.

below), and there are strong associations between human leukocyte antigens (HLA) and cholestatic drug reactions to amoxicillin-clavulanate, flucloxacillin, and tiopronin [35–39]. Weaker associations between HLA molecules and particular types of drug hepatitis have been also reported [40].

Age and sex

The frequency and severity of hepatic drug reactions both increase with age (Table 27.2). The explanations are likely to be multifactorial and include: increased exposure, higher probability of multiple drug therapy, and biologic effects of aging on drug disposition, especially altered hepatic uptake as the result of decreases in blood flow and/or diffusion of drugs across the hepatic microvasculature into hepatocytes [41]. Conversely, a small number of DILIs are more common in children, particularly those that involve mitochondrial injury, such as valproic acid hepatotoxicity and Reye syndrome.

Women are more likely than men to develop drug-induced hepatitis after exposure to nitrofurantoin, sulfonamides, diclofenac, minocycline, troglitazone, and halothane. Chronic hepatitis caused by the first four of these agents (and historically with methyldopa and oxyphenisatin) has an even higher (80–90%) female gender predominance. Some cholestatic reactions are more common in men (Table 27.2); these include amoxicillin-clavulanate- and azathioprine-induced vascular injury in transplant recipients, as well as anabolic steroids for reason of their greater use by men. The biologic explanation for sex differences in some types of hepatic drug reactions remains unclear.

Exposure to other drugs and toxins

Patients taking more than one agent have an increased risk of adverse drug reactions, including DILI [42–45]. Particularly relevant examples include acetaminophen, isoniazid, valproic acid, and anticancer drugs [43–46]. A possible relationship between agents that alter canalicular bile pathways has also been intimated, including interactive hepatotoxicity between OCSs and other drugs to produce prolonged cholestatic reactions [42].

Chronic excessive intake of ethanol is a risk factor for hepatotoxicity with acetaminophen, isoniazid, nicotinamide, and methotrexate.

Nutritional status

Fasting predisposes to acetaminophen hepatotoxicity because of its effects on drug conjugation and oxidation pathways, as well as on hepatic glutathione (GSH) levels. It has also been proposed that malnutrition increases the risk and severity of hepatotoxicity from drugs used to treat tuberculosis [47], but controlled studies are lacking. Overnutrition (obesity) increases the risk of halothane hepatitis. The increased risk of NASH and hepatic fibrosis amongst those taking methotrexate, estrogens, tamoxifen, or corticosteroids (Table 27.2) will be discussed later.

Past history, and other medical disorders

Instances of cross-reactivity to similar agents have been reported with haloalkane anesthetics (halothane, enflurane, isoflurane), isoniazid and pyrazinamide, sulfonamides and some cyclooxygenase 2 (COX-2) inhibitors, some NSAIDs, and macrolide antibiotics. Such cross-reactivity is surprisingly uncommon, but a history of any previous adverse drug reaction increases the risk of DILI to other agents. It is again emphasized that *a previous reaction to the same drug* is the single most important factor predisposing to acute liver failure or chronic liver disease from DILI.

Renal failure predisposes to methotrexate-induced hepatic fibrosis and tetracycline-induced fatty liver, while renal and other solid organ transplantation is a risk factor for hepatic vascular injury with azathioprine. Likewise, disorders associated with hepatic venous outflow obstruction, such as venoocclusive disease (VOD) (now termed the sinusoidal obstruction syndrome, SOS; the terms VOD and SOS will be used interchangeably in this chapter), are attributed to cancer chemotherapeutic agents prescribed during bone marrow transplantation (as well as with radiotherapy) [48]. Rheumatoid arthritis, and possibly SLE, appears to increase the risk of salicylate hepatotoxicity and sulfasalazine-induced hepatitis. The risk of drug reactions (including hepatitis) to both sulfonamides and sulfones is greatly increased among persons with HIV/AIDS and also in SLE (Table 27.3), while diabetes (as well as obesity, alcohol, renal failure, and preexisting liver disease – see below) predisposes individuals to hepatic fibrosis during methotrexate therapy.

Preexisting liver disease

Early studies of chlorpromazine, halothane, and methyldopa reactions clearly demonstrated that other liver disorders, including alcoholic cirrhosis and cholestatic liver diseases, did not predispose to these archetypical examples of idiosyncratic drug hepatitis. On the other hand, for a few agents where partial dose dependency or metabolic mechanisms appear likely, preexisting liver disease may be a risk factor for incidence and severity (Table 27.2). These drugs include nicotinamide (niacin), hycanthone, pemoline, and some anticancer drugs [49–52]. The risk of methotrexate-induced hepatic fibrosis is also increased in the presence of other forms of liver disease [53]. More recently, interactions between chronic viral hepatitis and accentuation of liver injury have been described, including an apparently heightened risk of reactions to anti-

tuberculosis chemotherapy, ibuprofen, flutamide, cyproterone acetate, and highly active antiretroviral therapy (HAART) [54–60].

Improving outcomes

Prevention

Given the central role of the liver in drug metabolism and disposition, and the rarity of most types of liver injury with what are otherwise valuable therapeutic agents, it is impossible to completely prevent all cases of DILI. General approaches to primary prevention include appropriate use of drugs (nonpharmacological approaches whenever possible, optimal choice of agents based on efficacy and safety, case selection, avoiding polypharmacy where possible, avoiding excessive dosage), restricted availability and blister-packaging of over-the-counter medication (see section on acetaminophen below) [61], physician and public education about possible drug side effects, how to recognize and what to do about them, and monitoring for adverse drug reactions. Conveying appropriate recommendations about dose limitations for agents like acetaminophen, nicotinamide, and complementary and alternative medicine (CAM) would prevent many instances of DILI.

Careful adherence to dosage guidelines (or use of blood levels) has virtually abolished severe cases of methotrexate-induced hepatic fibrosis (see later section), tetracycline-induced mitochondrial injury, and aspirin hepatitis. Avoiding repeated halothane administration within a 28-day period, or in people with suspected previous halothane sensitivity, would prevent many cases of this serious form of drug-induced hepatitis.

For selected agents with known hepatotoxicity, and particularly when treatment is likely to extend for longer than 2–4 weeks, it may be appropriate to first establish that liver function tests (LFTs) are normal before starting treatment, and then estimate LFTs or conduct other safety monitoring during therapy. However, although such "LFT monitoring" is often suggested as one approach to prevent serious outcomes of DILI (particularly by authors of single case reports, and by manufacturers who share liability in litigation cases), there is little evidence to support this as a general policy [62,63]. Thus, the high costs and inconvenience of such screening, the need to determine appropriate testing intervals (4 weeks is usually too long for agents that can cause acute liver failure), the weak specificity of abnormal results for identifying serious hepatotoxic potential, and the difficulty of defining a threshold at which the drug should be discontinued, all thwart the logistics of monitoring drug treatment with liver tests. It particularly needs to be appreciated that 7.5% of subjects receiving placebo in clinical trials have persistently raised ALT levels [64]. In the absence of symptoms, it is difficult to specify a level of ALT abnormality at which treatment should be discontinued. Generally, it is recommended that the drug be stopped if ALT exceeds five times the upper limit of normal (ULN) (approximately 250 U/L). More importantly, *any* abnormality of serum bilirubin or albumin concentration or prothrombin time and the presence of any symptoms are clear indications to stop therapy.

In practice, there are few agents for which liver test monitoring is strongly endorsed, as discussed in later sections – these include methotrexate, isoniazid, etretinate and other synthetic retinoids, ketoconazole, anticancer drugs, and prolonged therapy with minocycline. Conversely, the "statins" (3-hydroxy-3-methylglutaryl coenzyme A (HMG-CoA) reductase inhibitors) are a group of commonly used drugs that rarely cause significant liver injury [65], and for which the recommendation (by the manufacturers) for LFT monitoring is now considered inappropriate.

Management

The most important aspect is early recognition and discontinuation of a putative causative agent. At each visit, patients should be warned to report any untoward new symptoms, and particularly fever, systemic symptoms (e.g., malaise: "I don't feel these tablets agree with me, doctor;" see also the sentinel symptoms listed in Table 27.3), anorexia, nausea, and vomiting. Presentation after jaundice has developed is often too late to avoid a severe reaction, with its potential for developing liver failure or prolonged cholestasis. When patients report symptoms of a possible drug reaction, physicians should immediately check liver tests to establish whether or not there has been a change from baseline; in cases of doubt, the agent should be discontinued.

Following drug discontinuation, most adverse drug reactions will resolve spontaneously, rapidly, and completely, but this is not always the case. Drugs with a prolonged half-life are particularly associated with protracted hepatic drug reactions. Amiodarone, etretinate, ketoconazole, and hypervitaminosis A are examples, but a delayed resolution of liver injury with several other drugs can occur on some occasions. In severe reactions, hospitalization is advisable, and further evaluation is carried out if the diagnosis is unclear. Otherwise, relief of symptoms is all that is required. As for any type of hepatic injury, older age carries an increased risk of severe liver injury. Repeated vomiting, deepening jaundice, and development of even subtle laboratory or clinical features of liver failure are indications for admission. Transfer to a liver failure unit should be considered

and/or discussions with a liver transplant team should be initiated before the decline into hepatic coma, bleeding from coagulation disorder, sepsis, and hepatorenal failure.

In cases of dose-dependent hepatotoxicity, approaches to management include testing for drug levels and monitoring the clinical condition of the poisoned person. Attempts to remove unabsorbed drug by aspiration of the stomach contents should be considered for agents like acetaminophen, metals, and toxic mushrooms; other approaches (administration of charcoal or other resins or osmotic cathartics) are generally unlikely to be effective, although they have been advocated for poisoning with toxic mushrooms [66]. Likewise, approaches to remove residual drug from the body, such as with chelating resins for drugs with an enterohepatic circulation [67], or by hemodialysis, passage of blood through charcoal columns, or forced diuresis are not effective for most hepatotoxins.

Acetaminophen hepatotoxicity is the only drug-induced liver disorder for which a specific antidote (*N*-acetylcysteine) is available [42]. However, *N*-acetylcysteine has been shown to improve liver transplant-free survival in patients with acute liver failure arising from drugs other than acetaminophen. However, the benefit of this agent is confined to patients with early (grade I to II) but not late (grades III to IV) stages of hepatic encephalopathy [68]. Two agents that have been proposed to control protracted hepatic drug reactions are corticosteroids and ursodeoxycholic acid. There are few clear guidelines for their use, and the evidence of efficacy is confined to uncontrolled reports among individual cases or in small series. Older studies with corticosteroids found limited or no efficacy among cases of severe drug hepatitis for methyldopa, iproniazid, isoniazid, chlorpromazine, halothane, phenytoin, and oxyphenisatin [42]. More recent observations indicate occasional responses, particularly when DILI is associated with vasculitis (allopurinol, sulfonamides), and in some (but not all) cases of chronic hepatitis [42]. A reasonable approach is to observe the course for 3–6 weeks after stopping the drug (unless there is evidence of further deterioration), reserving corticosteroids for cases that fail to show clinical or biochemical improvement, or where the distinction between autoimmune and drug-induced chronic hepatitis remains in doubt.

Some experienced clinicians still favor a short course of corticosteroids ("steroid whitewash") to hasten recovery in persons with prolonged drug-induced cholestasis. If the mechanistic basis for such efficacy can be established (upregulating bile acid-metabolizing enzymes (CYP3A4) and canalicular transporters responsible for bile flow via pregnane-X receptors are examples), more appropriate pharmacologic agents to stimulate clinical resolution could eventually be identified. Meanwhile, corticosteroids have a range of unpleasant or severe side effects; our preference would be to use ursodeoxycholic acid (15 mg/kg body weight) in such cases. A reasonable body of uncontrolled data indicates that about two thirds of such cases will experience a reduction of pruritus and other symptoms, and acceleration of biochemical improvement. Ursodeoxycholic acid is safe, well tolerated, and has been used with frequent success in patients presenting with cholestatic liver injury attributed to amoxicillin-clavulanate, flucloxacillin, and flutamide [69–71], as well as cyclosporine (which is not a form of cholestasis) [72]. Other approaches to treating pruritus are discussed in Chapter 21 and elsewhere [73]. During prolonged cholestatic reactions, fat-soluble vitamin deficiency should be corrected.

Diagnosis

Diagnosis of DILI is always presumptive as it is based on a logistic approach, rather than on absolute criteria and specific diagnostic tests. As a result, there will be varying degrees of certainty about the diagnosis flowing from the strength of supporting evidence. In estimating the likelihood of diagnosis ("*causality assessment*") [74,75], evidence is sought by first considering whether the link between drug ingestion and liver injury is plausible, then excluding other disorders, seeking the presence of any positive features of adverse drug reactions, and finally by assessing indicative features of the liver histology. Attempts have been made to compile these lines of evidence into diagnostic "scales" that give weight to various features [76,77]. Regrettably, these fall down in relation to less common or atypical types of drug-induced liver disease, which are those most difficult to diagnose. They have particular limitations for cases with a long delay between the start of drug ingestion and recognition of liver injury [74,77]. Further, there is uncertainty about the weight that should be given to the need for rechallenge (rarely done in practice), alcohol consumption, and interobserver reliability [78]. Using a structured expert review of suspected cases gave better results than the widely used RUCAM score but the interobserver variation in reporting remains an issue [79].

Clinical suspicion

Some situations in which DILI may be particularly likely are summarized in Box 27.3. Meticulous attention should be paid to the drug history, returning to it as a special investigation with consideration of nonprescribed medications, CAM, and environmental toxins. It may be per-

---

Box 27.3 Some situations in which drugs are a particularly likely cause of liver disease.

- The person has started new treatment (including CAM) in the last 3–6 months
- The presence of extrahepatic manifestations, especially rash, lymphadenopathy, and eosinophilia (see also Table 27.3)
- The acute hepatitis is not readily accounted for by hepatitis viruses, other infections, or metabolic or immunologic disorders
- There are atypical features of liver disease – mixed "hepatocellular and cholestatic" reactions, or hepatitis with microvesicular steatosis
- Cholestasis with normal bile duct calibre on hepatobiliary imaging
- Cholestasis after common causes have been excluded, particularly in the elderly
- Histologic features suggest DILD (see text) in cases of cholestasis or acute hepatitis, and hepatitis with hepatic granulomas
- Chronic hepatitis without autoantibodies or hyperglobulinemia
- Abnormal liver tests in complex medical situations
- Obscure or poorly explained liver disease among those taking sex steroids, immunosuppressive agents, or other drugs (including CAM) for years

CAM, complementary and alternative medicine; DILD, drug-induced liver disease.

---

tinent to direct inquiry to other household members and primary care providers, and to examine all medications being taken or the contents of drug cupboards, bedside tables and lockers, etc.

Time of onset in relation to drug ingestion

Dose-dependent hepatotoxins usually produce overt evidence of liver injury within hours or a few days (see section on acetaminophen). For adverse hepatic drug reactions, there is a *latent period* between commencing the drug and the development of symptoms and/or abnormal liver tests. With immunoallergic types of drug hepatitis, granulomatous hepatitis and drug-induced cholestasis, this is within 4 months (typically 2–10 weeks) in more than three quarters of cases. Occasionally liver injury becomes evident only after the drug is stopped; for amoxicillin-clavulanate this period may be up to 6 weeks. With other types of drug hepatitis presumed to be instances of metabolic idiosyncrasy, the latent period to onset tends to be longer, often 6–26 weeks. For drug-induced chronic liver disease (chronic hepatitis, steatohepatitis, syndromes related to vascular injury), exposure may have been 6 months or longer than 1 year before clinical onset is apparent. Exploring the *chronological relationships* between drug ingestion and the onset and resolution of liver injury is the most important consideration in the diagnosis of DILI [80].

Repeated drug ingestion

Some drugs almost never cause liver injury after the first exposure, but the risk of hepatotoxicity increases with each subsequent treatment course. Halothane, dacarbazine, and nitrofurantoin are recognized examples. For a much broader range of compounds, a personal history of previous reaction to the drug (*inadvertent rechallenge*) is common with severe or prolonged liver injury; isoniazid, NSAIDs, Chinese herbal medicines, germander and chaparral are examples.

In order to provide stronger evidence of causality, *deliberate rechallenge* has been used in the past, employing a single and smaller than usual dose of the suspected hepatotoxin. It has proven particularly valuable to incriminate agents not previous known to be associated with liver injury, and to identify which agent was responsible when the person was taking more than one potentially hepatotoxic drug. A positive response is connoted by a recurrence of fever or other symptoms, and/or a two-fold increase of ALT or serum alkaline phosphatase (SAP) [78]; this strongly implicates the drug as the cause of liver injury. However, the application of rechallenge in practice is greatly limited by safety considerations, it should never be conducted without the fullest consideration by both the person involved and their family, and with reference to an Institutional Human Ethics Review Board. Particularly note that deliberate rechallenge is potentially dangerous and should never be attempted for the types of reactions listed in Table 27.3.

Response to discontinuation of the drug

Dechallenge should be followed by improvement in liver tests within days or weeks of stopping the drug; some guidelines have been provided [80]. There are clear exceptions. In DILI caused by ketoconazole, troglitazone, coumarol, etretinate, amiodarone, and minocycline, severe reactions may resolve slowly (months), or incompletely, sometimes with further decline of hepatic function after drug discontinuation. Some instances of drug-induced cholestasis can also be prolonged but failure of jaundice to resolve in suspected hepatic drug reactions more often indicates an alternative diagnosis (e.g., malignant biliary obstruction) is likely and should be reinvestigated.

Clinical features

While the clinicopathologic syndrome associated with exposure to a particular drug may be a useful aid to diagnosis, the diversity of reactions to individual drugs is such that absence of the "drug signature" (or "syndromic recognition") test should *not* be used to exonerate a given drug as the cause of liver injury. In most respects, the clinical features of drug hepatitis or drug-induced cholestasis are not dissimilar from those found with other causes of these disorders. However, identifying specific risk factors for hepatotoxicity (e.g., prolonged fasting, or chronic excessive alcohol intake in a person regularly taking acetaminophen) or the presence of extrahepatic features of drug hypersensitivity (Table 27.3) may suggest the correct diagnosis.

Exclusion of other disorders

It is critical to exclude other liver diseases before attributing liver injury to drugs (Box 27.4). In earlier work, [81] nearly two thirds of reactions reported as drug-induced chronic hepatitis were subsequently ascribed to chronic hepatitis C. Contemporary serologic, viral, immunologic, and imaging tests have facilitated the early diagnosis of most acute viral, vascular, and metabolic liver disorders. Likewise, the cause of cholestasis, and particularly mechanical obstruction of the biliary tract, is usually easy to identify with modern imaging. Approaches to making the correct diagnosis of a drug reaction when the clinical and laboratory features resemble autoimmune hepatitis include the course after discontinuation of the drug, and the response to a short course (4–6 weeks) of corticosteroids if there is not rapid improvement after stopping the drug. If there is an impressive response to

---

Box 27.4 Drug-induced liver disease is a diagnosis of exclusion. The following factors should be considered.

- Hepatitis viruses: serology and molecular virology (especially HCV RNA)
- Other infectious agents: EBV, CMV, HIV, HSV, and *Coxiella burnettii*
- Autoimmune hepatitis: ANAs, SMAs, LKMs, and immunoglobulin G levels
- Acute biliary obstruction: exclude cholangitis
- Metabolic disorders: Wilson disease, α_1-antitrypsin deficiency, and risk factors for NAFLD/NASH (serum lipids, fasting blood glucose or abnormal glucose tolerance test, insulin, family history of diabetes, features of the metabolic syndrome)
- Vascular disorders of liver: risk factors and imaging with vascular phase (Chapter 33)
- Alcohol
- Bacterial infection
- Hepatic metastases
- Systemic malignancy or lymphoma

ANAs, antinuclear antibodies; CMV, cytomegalovirus; EBV, Epstein–Barr virus; HCV, hepatitis C virus; HIV, human immunodeficiency virus; HSV, herpes simplex virus; LKMs, liver–kidney microsomal antibodies; NAFLD, nonalcoholic fatty liver disease; NASH, nonalcoholic steatohepatitis; SMAs, smooth muscle antibodies.

corticosteroids followed by relapse after reducing the dose, it allows the physician to assume that the case is actually one of autoimmune hepatitis.

Liver biopsy

The liver biopsy plays a special role in excluding other hepatobiliary disorders, but it may also provide positive evidence to corroborate DILI. Biopsy is most strongly indicated when the cause of liver disease remains in doubt; for example, there may be ambiguous evidence of autoimmunity, or the pattern of reaction may be very unusual or not previously reported for the drug in question. Details such as whether continued treatment with this medication is highly desirable, and whether or not there is rapid improvement after stopping the drug, may influence the decision on whether or not to perform liver biopsy. As for any indication, the justification for liver biopsy must satisfy the question as to "whether the likelihood that this will make a difference to management of the person justifies the inconvenience, discomfort and risks of the procedure". Informed consent is clearly mandatory, and it may be valuable to record in the medical record (or on a signed consent form) why the biopsy is considered valuable in this particular case.

There are no histologic features that are pathognomonic for drug-induced liver disease, and indeed some, such as the presence of occasional eosinophils, are often overinterpreted. Nonetheless, some patterns of hepatic lesions may suggest to an experienced liver pathologist that a drug or toxin could be implicated (Box 27.5). The reader is referred to Chapter 7 for examples of hepatic histopathology in drug-induced liver disease, and to the excellent detailed illustrations found in texts such as Hall [82] and Zimmerman [2], as well as earlier editions of this book.

Box 27.5 Histologic changes that may indicate the operation of drug-induced liver disease.

- Zonal lesions, including necrosis and/or steatosis
- Microvesicular steatosis (often results from mitochondrial injury)
- Necrotic lesions of disproportionate severity for the clinical picture
- Mixed hepatitis and cholestasis
- Destructive bile duct lesions
- Prominent neutrophils, and (in later stages) eosinophils (more than 25%)
- Granulomas
- Vascularity of hepatic tumors: sinusoidal dilatation and peliosis
- Vascular lesions
- Florid steatohepatitis: resembles alcohol-related steatohepatitis more than typical "primary" nonalcoholic steatohepatitis

---

Specific diagnostic tests

As reviewed elsewhere [7,12], there are no completely validated specific tests for any type of drug-induced liver disease. Interesting data have been presented about the relative specificity of some drug-induced autoantibodies, including anti-M6 (antimitochondrial antibodies) with iproniazid, anti-LKM-2 (against CYP2C9) with tienilic acid, anti-CYP1A2 with dihydralazine, and anti-CYP2E1 with halothane. A test that detects antibodies against trifluoroacetylated (TFA) proteins has been advocated for halothane and other haloalkane-related hepatotoxicity (see later section). However, all such tests have minimal applicability in clinical practice because of their unavailability and lack of standardization, including agreement on what comprises a significant titer of antibodies.

Identifying one causative agent among many

Having established with near certainty that one or more drugs are responsible for an individual case of liver disease, an additional challenge may be to identify which among several is the guilty party. In general, the agent started most recently before the onset of liver injury is the one most likely to be responsible; new and nonproprietary medicines should also heighten suspicion. Otherwise, the drug with the most hepatotoxic track record becomes the prime contender. Whenever possible, all potential hepatotoxins, including therapeutic agents, should be discontinued. If the patient's condition and laboratory tests improve, the drug(s) that seem unlikely to be responsible can be carefully reintroduced.

Clinicopathologic syndromes

The initial "labeling" of cases with apparent DILI relied heavily on the profile of liver test abnormalities (Table 27.4) and not histopathology, which provides a more definitive classification. It should be noted that clinical and laboratory features are not always congruent with liver pathology, and there is much overlap between categories. Thus, although the histologic changes usually mirror the biochemical abnormalities, certain caveats should be borne in mind. First, the alteration of liver enzymes is not synonymous with liver injury and can represent hepatocyte adaptation (below). Second, liver tests may underestimate the severity of liver disease, as with the fairly modest changes in aminotransferase (AT) that may accompany acute liver failure from drug-induced microvesicular steatosis. Conversely, drugs such as estrogens may be associated with a major increase in AT despite bland cholestasis on biopsy, while others (methotrexate, vinyl chloride, arsenic) can cause cirrhosis

Table 27.4 Definition of patterns of liver injury.

| | Liver injury | | |
	Hepatocellular	Cholestatic	Mixed
ALT >2–3 × ULN	ALT >2–3 × ULN *and* normal SAP	SAP >2 × ULN	ALT >2–3 × ULN *and* SAP >2 × ULN
or	*or*	*or*	*or*
>2 × ULN conjugated bilirubin *or* elevated AST, SAP, and total bilirubin (one of these must be >2 × ULN)	ALT : SAP ratio ≥5*	ALT : SAP ratio ≤2*	ALT : SAP ratio between 2 and 5*

*The ALT and SAP values are expressed as multiples of the upper limit of normal. Note that these patterns are a relatively poor guide to the histologic nature of liver disease (see text).
ALT, alanine aminotransferase; AST, aspartate aminotransferase; SAP, serum alkaline phosphatase; ULN, upper limit of normal.

with minimal or no change in biochemical tests. Third, the pattern of liver tests is most often mixed or relatively nonspecific; this occurs with granulomatous hepatitis, steatohepatitis, cholestatic hepatitis, chronic hepatitis, and minor nonspecific patterns of liver injury.

A relatively simple approach to clinicopathologic classification of drug-induced liver disease is outlined in Table 27.5.

Hepatic adaptation

Many drugs induce abnormal liver tests without causing symptoms or biochemical evidence of *significant* liver disease. Minor elevations of ALT may be transient. In reality, these may indicate minor degrees of nonprogressive injury to key organelles such as mitochondria or cell membranes, without causing cell death and without recruiting an inflammatory response. The nonprogression (often resolution) of these changes may result from the induction of protective processes, such as antioxidant and antiapoptotic pathways; in this sense, minor forms of chemical liver injury are often followed by adaptation of the liver to withstand continuing or more substantial insults. Experimental work has demonstrated the hepatoprotective effects of a small dose of CCl₄ against subsequent massive poisoning, and the phenomenon of ischemic preconditioning substantially abrogates subsequent ischemic or reperfusion injury. The mechanisms of these adaptive processes are of potential importance to the understanding of DILI.

Other forms of "hepatic adaptation" include drug-induced hyperbilirubinemia, as observed with such agents as rifampicin, flavaspidic acid, and cyclosporine, and "induction of hepatic enzymes." Hyperbilirubinemia is best understood as a direct interference with pathways of bilirubin uptake, conjugation, and canalicular excretion into bile. Sustained elevation of enzymes such as γ-glutamyl transpeptidase (GGTP) and serum alkaline phosphatase is seen with phenytoin and other anticonvulsants, rifampicin, alcohol, and warfarin. Because such agents induce hepatic CYP enzymes, this phenomenon is often referred to as "microsomal enzyme induction;" the actual relationship between the activity of drug oxidases and the increased plasma levels of these non-microsomal enzymes is less clear. Potential explanations are that the indirect effects of increased CYP enzyme activity on bile acid metabolism produce more "detergent" metabolites that liberate these enzymes from the hepatocyte plasma membranes, or that stimulate increased synthesis of alkaline phosphatase and GGTP—both these mechanisms may apply. It is important clinically to recognize the difference between these biochemical changes and cholestasis; for example, serum bile acid levels increase with cholestasis or liver injury not with hepatic adaptation.

A morphologic or ultrastructural consequence of microsomal enzyme induction by drugs is the presence of ground glass cytoplasm in hepatocytes, as seen by light microscopy. This results from hypertrophy of the endoplasmic reticulum, which can be confirmed by electron microscopy.

Drug-induced acute hepatitis

Many drugs are associated with acute hepatocellular injury (Box 27.6). There is a latent period between starting treatment and the onset of symptoms or liver test abnormalities. This tends to be shorter (2–6 weeks) for agents clearly associated with immunoallergic mechanisms (see Table 27.3), and more variable and longer for those presumed to be due to metabolic idiosyncrasy. There are often prodromal features of fever, malaise, and other

Table 27.5 Clinicopathologic classification of drug-induced liver disease.

Category	Description	Examples
Hepatic adaptation	No symptoms; raised GGTP and SAP (occasionally ALT) Hyperbilirubinemia	Phenytoin, warfarin, rifampin Rifampin
Dose-dependent hepatotoxicity	Very short interval to onset; symptoms of hepatitis; zonal, bridging, and massive necrosis; ALT >5 × ULN, often >2,000 U/L	Acetaminophen, nicotinic acid, amodiaquine
Other cytopathic changes		
Acute steatosis	Microvesicular steatosis, diffuse or zonal; partially dose-dependent, severe liver injury, features of mitochondrial toxicity (lactic acidosis, pancreatitis)	Valproic acid, didanosine, HAART, fialuridine, L-asparaginase, some herbal medicines, ecstasy
Acute hepatitis	Onset within 1–20 weeks; sentinel symptoms of hepatitis; focal, bridging, and massive necrosis; ALT >5 × ULN; extrahepatic features of drug allergy in some cases (Table 27.3)	Isoniazid, dantrolene, nitrofurantoin, halothane, sulfonamides, phenytoin, disulfiram, etretinate, ketoconazole, terbinafine, troglitazone
Chronic hepatitis	Duration >3 months; interface hepatitis, bridging necrosis, fibrosis, cirrhosis; clinical/laboratory features of chronic liver disease; autoantibodies in some cases	Nitrofurantoin, etretinate, diclofenac, minocycline, mesalamine
Granulomatous hepatitis	Hepatic granulomas with varying hepatitis and cholestasis; raised ALT, SAP, GGTP	Allopurinol, carbamazepine, hydralazine, quinidine, quinine, phenylbutazone
Steatohepatitis	Onset delayed (6–18 months); steatosis, focal necrosis, Mallory hyaline, pericellular fibrosis, cirrhosis; chronic liver disease, portal hypertension	Perhexiline, amiodarone, tamoxifen, toremifene; rarely nifedipine, diltiazem
Cholestasis without hepatitis	Cholestasis, no inflammation; SAP >2 × ULN	Oral contraceptives, androgens, cyclosporin A
Cholestatic hepatitis	Cholestasis with inflammation; symptoms of hepatitis; raised ALT and SAP	Chlorpromazine, tricyclic antidepressants, erythromycins, amoxicillin-clavulanate, angiotensinogen-converting enzyme inhibitors
Cholestasis with bile duct injury	Bile duct lesions and cholestatic hepatitis; clinical features of cholangitis	Chlorpromazine, flucloxacillin, dextropropoxyphene, carmustine, paraquat
Chronic cholestasis	Cholestasis present >3 months	Chlorpromazine, flucloxacillin, trimethoprim-sulfamethoxazole (Table 27.6)
Vanishing bile duct syndrome	Ductopenia; resembles primary biliary cirrhosis but antimitochondrial antibodies absent	
Sclerosing cholangitis	Strictures of large bile ducts	Intra-arterial floxuridine, intralesional scolicidals
Vascular disorders	Sinusoidal dilatation, peliosis, noncirrhotic portal hypertension, NRH, SOS (VOD)	Anabolic steroids, oral contraceptives, vinyl chloride, Thorotrast® (Table 27.6)
Liver tumors	Focal nodular hyperplasia, hepatic adenoma, hepatocellular carcinoma, angiosarcoma	Anabolic steroids, oral contraceptives, vinyl chloride, Thorotrast (Table 27.6)

ALT, alanine aminotransferase; GGTP, γ-glutamyl transpeptidase; HAART, highly active antiretroviral therapy; NRH, nodular regenerative hyperplasia; SAP, serum alkaline phosphatase; SOS, sinusoidal obstruction syndrome; ULN, upper limit of normal; VOD, venoocclusive disease.

"sentinel symptoms" (Table 27.3), followed by rash, lymphadenopathy, or other systemic features of drug hypersensitivity. Clinical features that resemble acute viral hepatitis soon follow, or may be the presenting symptoms; anorexia, nausea, vomiting, and lassitude are prominent among these. Jaundice is present in severe cases. AT levels are raised (see Table 27.4) proportionately more than

serum alkaline phosphatase. Serum bilirubin and indices of hepatic synthetic function such as prothrombin time and serum albumin concentration are variably altered depending on the severity and duration of liver injury.

The histologic lesions consist mainly of focal hepatic necrosis, with apoptotic (acidophil) bodies and a mixed inflammatory infiltrate. Bridging necrosis is present in

Box 27.6 Drugs associated with acute liver failure.

Analgesics/NSAIDs
- Acetaminophen[a]
- Bromfenac[b]
- Diclofenac
- Etodolac
- Ibuprofen
- Leflunomide
- Nimesulide
- Oxaprozin
- Piroxicam
- Tienilic acid

Cardiovascular drugs
- Amiodarone
- Captopril
- Ecarazine
- Enalapril
- Lisinopril
- Labetalol

Endocrine drugs
- Carbimazole
- Propylthiouracil
- Troglitazone[b]

Neuropsychiatric drugs
- Carbamazepine
- Chlormethiazole
- Felbamate
- Lamotrigine
- Nefazodone
- Pemoline
- Phenytoin
- Tacrine
- Tetrabamate
- Tolcapone
- Topiramate
- Valproic acid

Antimicrobial drugs
- Amoxicillin-clavulanic acid
- Ciprofloxacin, ofloxacin, trovofloxacin
- Co-trimoxazole
- Dapsone
- Fialuridine[b]

- Flucloxacillin
- Highly active antiretroviral treatment
- Isoniazid, rifampin, pyrazinamide
- Ketoconazole, itraconazole
- Lamotrigine
- Minocycline
- Sulfonamides (many)
- Terbinafine
- Tetracycline (intravenous)

Gastrointestinal drugs
- Ebrotidine
- Omeprazole
- Ranitidine

General anesthetics
- Enflurane
- Halothane
- Isoflurane

Oncotherapeutic drugs
- Carboplatin
- Chlorambucil
- Cyproterone acetate
- Flutamide
- Gemcitabine
- Imatinib mesylate

Miscellaneous drugs, including herbal medicines and self-administered agents
- Allopurinol
- Chaparral[a]
- Cocaine[a]
- Disulfiram
- Germander
- Herbal slimming aids
- Hydrazine sulfate
- Interferon-α,[a] interferon-β
- Kava
- 3,4-Methylenedioxymethamphetamine ("ecstasy")
- Nicotinic acid[a]
- Zafirlukast

Environmental agents
- Carbon tetrachloride[a]
- Mushroom poisoning[a]

[a]Dose-dependent hepatotoxicity.
[b]Withdrawn.

severe cases and may lead to chronic hepatitis if the causative agent is not withdrawn.

Zonal necrosis is a typical feature of severe liver injury caused by drugs and with chemical or plant toxins. *Zone 3 lesions* (centrilobular or perivenular) are seen with acetaminophen and carbon tetrachloride toxicity but can also occur in acute SOS (or VOD). The overrepresentation of zone 3 lesions in cases of DILI is related to the high metabolic activity of this zone, which generates reactive metabolites. By comparison, isolated *zone 1* (phosphorus or iron poisoning) and *zone 2 lesions* (cocaine toxicity) are extremely rare.

Severe acute hepatitis may culminate in *acute liver failure*. Massive or submassive hepatic necrosis is often present. Acetaminophen (see later section) is the leading cause of drug-induced acute liver failure worldwide, but regional differences exist. Other drugs that have been associated with acute liver failure are listed in Box 27.6.

Mitochondrial injury

Fatty liver (steatosis) can be seen in the vicinity of zonal necrotic lesions or may be the predominant manifestation. Microvesicular steatosis results from mitochondrial injury; decreased numbers of mitochondria are often found. There is often evidence of other organ involvement, particularly pancreatitis, nephrotoxicity, encephalopathy, and metabolic acidosis. The clinical syndrome resembles acute fatty liver of pregnancy. Patients present with nausea, vomiting, abdominal pain, and rapidly evolving encephalopathy. Liver biopsies show accumulation of small fat droplets (microvesicular steatosis) in hepatocytes in a zonal or diffuse distribution. Biochemical features include profound hepatocellular dysfunction with hypoglycemia, coagulopathy, hyperammonemia, and lactic acidemia. There may be a rise in serum bilirubin and AT levels, but these are less pronounced than in other forms of acute hepatotoxicity or hepatitis. Historically, this syndrome was associated with the use of tetracycline in pregnant women, Reye syndrome caused by use of aspirin in febrile young children with influenza B and some other viral infections, and with sodium valproate in very young children with predisposing factors (see later section). Currently, the most important cause is HAART, particularly the nucleos(t)ide inhibitors, but amphetamine analogs used recreationally, especially ecstasy, and buprenorphine misuse can produce similar lesions [83]. The drugs associated with microvesicular steatosis are listed in Box 27.7.

Unlike acute microvesicular steatosis, drug-induced *steatohepatitis* is a type of hepatocellular injury associated with chronic liver disease. Hepatic decompensation can occur. Some drugs associated with steatohepatitis have also been implicated as causing acute liver failure but progression to cirrhosis or liver complications is generally

Box 27.7 Drugs associated with microvesicular steatosis.

- Amiodarone
- Aspirin (Reye syndrome in febrile children)[a]
- Fialuridine[b]
- Highly active antiretroviral treatment (HAART)
- Industrial toxins: dimethylformamide, selenium
- NSAIDs: ibuprofen, piroxicam, pirprofen[b], tolmetin
- Riluzole
- Tetrabamate (Atrium™)
- Tetracycline (historical)
- Ticlopidine
- Valproic acid
- Vitamin A

[a]Declining incidence since health warnings have been issued about the use of aspirin in young children.
[b]Withdrawn.
NSAIDs, nonsteroidal anti-inflammatory drugs.

slower. Implicated drugs are listed in Box 27.8. The histologic features are indistinguishable from alcoholic steatohepatitis, with varying degrees of steatosis, focal lobular inflammation with polymorphonuclear cells, hepatocellular necrosis, and Mallory bodies. Excluding ethanol abuse is critical. The changes also resemble those found in NASH (Chapter 32). Thus, some associations between drugs used for complications of the metabolic syndrome (diabetes, hypertension, cardiac failure) and steatohepatitis may be fortuitous, while other agents (corticosteroids, estrogens, tamoxifen) may exacerbate NASH due to effects on insulin resistance and lipid turnover. Drug-induced steatohepatitis often causes hepatic fibrosis

Box 27.8 Drugs associated with steatohepatitis.

- Amiodarone
- Coralgil (4,4-diethylaminoethoxyhexestrol)[a]
- Estrogens[b]
- Glucocorticosteroids[b]
- Oxaliplatin
- Perhexiline maleate
- Methotrexate
- Methyldopa[b]
- Nifedipine[b]
- Tamoxifen
- Toremifene, ?raloxifene
- Verapamil[b]

[a]Withdrawn.
[b]More likely to be a fortuitous association resulting from association with risk factors for nonalcoholic steatohepatitis (see text).

in the pericentral (perivenular, or acinar zone 3) and pericellular distribution, a pattern typical for other causes of steatohepatitis. Cirrhosis can develop, leading to hepatic decompensation.

Cholestasis

There are several different syndromes of drug-induced cholestasis (Table 27.6) [84,85]. *Bland cholestasis* occurs without symptoms of hepatitis. Liver biopsies show intrahepatic cholestasis without significant hepatic inflammation. This syndrome is associated with OCS use and occurs more often in women with a family or personal history of cholestasis of pregnancy (Chapter 11). Pruritus is often troublesome, but jaundice is less common. Recovery is the rule but complete resolution can be protracted in some cases.

In *cholestatic hepatitis*, liver histology shows lobular and portal tract inflammation as well as cholestasis. As with other forms of drug hepatitis, clinical onset is with flu-like symptoms but this is soon followed by features of hepatitis, such as anorexia, vomiting, jaundice, and right hypochondrial pain. The latter can be severe and can be misinterpreted as acute cholecystitis. Drugs that cause cholestatic hepatitis can also cause *bile duct injury*; dextropropoxyphene [86] and methylenedianiline (an epoxyresin hardener associated with cases of liver injury or jaundice following industrial exposure or food contamination, most infamously as "the Epping jaundice") cause a striking syndrome of cholangitis [87]. Cholangiolytic (interlobular bile duct) injury is prominent in many cases of drug-induced cholestatic hepatitis. When lesions are severe enough, this can lead to ductopenia or the *vanishing bile duct syndrome* (VBDS).

VBDS is characterized by progressive destruction of segments of the biliary tree [88,89]. Over 30 drugs have been implicated [90–94] but those causing the highest risk of this outcome after drug-induced cholestatic hepatitis are chlorpromazine (7% of cases), the oxypenicillins (particularly flucloxacillin (10–30% of cases)), and the erythromycins (5% of cases) (Box 27.9). The main predictor of VBDS after cholestatic hepatitis may be the initial severity of the bile duct damage [89]. The clinical features resemble primary biliary cirrhosis (PBC) with jaundice, and liver tests indicating cholestasis, hypercholesterolemia, xanthomas, and other manifestations of chronic cholestasis. However, unlike PBC, antimitochondrial antibodies are absent. Hepatic fibrosis is not usually prominent, but biliary cirrhosis can sometimes develop. Resolution may take up to 2 years and is sometimes incomplete.

Large duct bile duct lesions ("sclerosing cholangitis") are an uncommon type of drug-induced injury. Well-characterized historical examples include intra-arterial

Table 27.6 Clinicopathologic syndromes of drug-induced cholestasis.

Type	Clinical and laboratory features	Examples
Acute forms		
Cholestasis without hepatitis ("bland" cholestasis)	Prodromal symptoms, then intense pruritus; SAP >3 × ULN; AT rise is often transient (rarely >3–5 × ULN); bilirubin <12 mg/dL	Estrogens, anabolic steroids, tamoxifen, azathioprine
Cholestasis with hepatitis[a]	Right upper quadrant or generalized abdominal pain; jaundice often present; can simulate acute cholangitis; pruritus less impressive; SAP >3 × ULN in 70%, AT >2–5 × ULN	Chlorpromazine, other phenothiazines, macrolide antibiotics, oxypenicillins, tricyclic antidepressants, amoxicillin-clavulanate, ketoconazole, NSAIDs (sulindac, piroxicam), captopril, enalapril, azathioprine
Cholestasis with bile duct injury[a] (cholangiolytic)	Resembles acute cholangitis (often with cholestatic hepatitis)	Dextropropoxyphene, flucloxacillin, paraquat, methylenedianiline
Chronic forms		
Vanishing bile duct syndrome (see Box 27.9)	Chronic cholestasis; resembles PBC but antimitochondrial antibodies are absent	Chlorpromazine, flucloxacillin, and other oxypenicillins
Large bile duct strictures (similar to sclerosing cholangitis)	Chronic cholestasis; resembles sclerosing cholangitis (but strictures at junction of right and left hepatic ducts)	Floxuridine, intralesional scolicides (2% formaldehyde, hypertonic saline, iodine solution, absolute alcohol, silver nitrate)

[a]Several drugs implicated in causing cholestatic hepatitis may also produce bile duct injury.
AT, aminotransferase; NSAIDs, nonsteroidal anti-inflammatory drugs; PBC, primary biliary cirrhosis; SAP, serum alkaline phosphatase; ULN, upper limit of normal.

floxuridine infusions (which cause an ischemic cholangiopathy) and intracavitary instillation of scolicidal agents [95]. Current practices of targeted chemotherapy for hepatic malignancy, and ultrasound-guided scolicidal therapy have a low risk of drug-induced biliary injury.

Box 27.9 Drugs associated with the vanishing bile duct syndrome.

- Amitriptyline, imipramine
- Amoxicillin-clavulanic acid*
- Ampicillin
- Azathioprine
- Barbiturates
- Carbamazepine*
- Chlorpromazine*
- Chlorthiazide
- Cimetidine
- Clindamycin
- Co-trimoxazole*
- Cyproheptadine
- Erythromycin esters*
- Estradiol, norandrostenolone, methyltestosterone*
- Flucloxacillin*, dicloxacillin
- Glycyrrhizin (a component of Chinese herbal medicines)
- Gold
- Haloperidol
- Ibuprofen
- Itraconazole
- D-Penicillamine
- Phenytoin*
- Prochloperazine*
- Terbinafine
- Tetracycline[a]
- Thiabendazole
- Tiopronin
- Tolbutamide

[a]More than one reported case.
Original references can be obtained from those cited in references [1999,1994,2003].

Granulomatous hepatitis

Hepatic granulomas are associated with numerous infective, inflammatory, vasculitic, and neoplastic disorders (Chapter 40) [96]. Older studies found that nearly one third of cases of hepatic granulomas were attributable to drugs [97], and it seems likely that drugs remain an important cause of "granulomatous hepatitis." In drug reactions, granulomatous hepatitis may be the sole manifestation of liver injury, but more commonly granulomas accompany other histologic features and represent one of several patterns of hepatic response to injury. Thus, granulomas have been described with many drugs that are better known for other types of pathology, especially acute hepatitis (nitrofurantoin, methyldopa, halothane), but also cholestatic hepatitis (chlorpromazine, phenylbutazone, carbamazepine) and steatohepatitis (amiodarone, calcium channel blockers) (Box 27.10).

The clinical presentation is indistinguishable from other causes or idiopathic granulomatous hepatitis (Chapter 40). Thus, profound lethargy, fever, night sweats, rigors, myalgia, and weight loss are prominent. There is tender hepatomegaly and the spleen is enlarged in 25% of cases. Other extrahepatic manifestations include rashes, particularly a form typifying small vessel vasculitis, lymphadenopathy, and bone marrow granulomas [14]. Serum ALT is often raised, but typically less than serum alkaline phosphatase and GGTP. Jaundice is much less common than with other types of drug-induced acute

Box 27.10 Drugs associated with hepatic granulomas.

Analgesics/NSAIDs
- Acetaminophen
- Aspirin
- Clometacin
- Phenylbutazone[a]

Antiepileptics
- Carbamazepine*
- Chlorpromazine
- Phenytoin*

Antimicrobials
- Amoxicillin-clavulanate
- Cephalexin
- Dapsone
- Dicloxacillin, oxacillin
- Isoniazid
- Mebendazole
- Nitrofurantoin
- Norfloxacin
- Penicillin G, penicillin V
- Pyrazinamide
- Quinine[a]
- Sulfonamides (many)[a]

Cardiovascular drugs
- Amiodarone
- Diltiazem

- Disopyramide
- Hydralazine[a]
- Methyldopa
- Procainamide[a]
- Quinidine[a]

Endocrine drugs
- Chlorpropamide
- Glibenclamide
- Methimazole
- Tolbutamide

Miscellaneous, including herbal medicines
- Allopurinol[a]
- Chaparral
- Etanercept
- Glibenclamide
- Gold
- Halothane
- Interferon-α
- Mesalamine
- Methotrexate
- Rosiglitazone
- Tacrine
- Tetrabamate
- Ticlopidine

[a]Well-characterized examples with causality proven. Note that the high frequency with which hepatic granulomas are found in liver biopsies is such that other associations may be fortuitous. NSAIDs, nonsteroidal anti-inflammatory drugs.

hepatitis, but has been observed when cases overlap with cholestatic hepatitis; carbamazepine and hydralazine are examples. Withdrawal of the offending drug leads to rapid resolution in most cases. A short course of corticosteroids may hasten recovery in special circumstances, particularly cases associated with vasculitis or other extrahepatic complications such as interstitial nephritis; allopurinol and sulfonamides are examples.

Drug-induced chronic hepatitis

Chronic hepatitis is defined by the persistence of symptoms and biochemical or histologic abnormalities for longer than 3 months [14]. All drugs implicated as causing chronic hepatitis have also been associated with acute reactions. Continued ingestion of the drug beyond the phase of acute hepatitis is one of the key factors that leads to the development of chronic hepatitis, cirrhosis, and liver failure. Early recognition and timely withdrawal of the offending drug are therefore crucial.

A distinctive type of drug-induced chronic hepatitis resembling autoimmune hepatitis (AIH) is described. This probably comes about through the process of drug-induced immune dysregulation. The relatively few agents that cause this type of liver disease include nitrofurantoin, diclofenac, methyldopa, and minocycline. More than 80% of reported cases are in women. Characteristic features include fever and arthralgia in addition to signs of chronic liver disease, hypergammaglobulinemia, and antinuclear and/or smooth muscle antibodies.

A second pattern of drug-induced chronic hepatitis is characterized by autoantibodies directed against specific hepatic microsomal proteins (e.g., tienilic acid, halothane). Yet other agents (e.g., etretinate, germander) can be associated with chronic hepatic inflammation and liver cell injury (hepatitis) in the absence of autoantibodies or autoimmune manifestations. Finally, a picture of classic AIH may emerge after an episode of drug-induced acute hepatitis. It is unclear whether the emergence of AIH is related to the unmasking of latent AIH or whether the drug directly induces AIH in susceptible persons.

Hepatic fibrosis

Hepatic fibrosis may be the end result of chronic hepatitis, chronic hepatototoxicity, steatohepatitis, or chronic cholestasis with bile duct injury. However, some drugs and chemicals such as methotrexate, vitamin A, and arsenic can provoke an intense fibrotic reaction *without* a prominent inflammatory response. With these agents, other profibrogenic risk factors, especially ethanol but possibly also obesity, diabetes, insulin resistance, and iron overload, can accelerate fibrogenesis (discussed later for vitamin A and methotrexate).

Vascular lesions

Drugs and chemicals are the most important cause of vascular lesions of the liver. These include histologic curiosities, such as sinusoidal dilatation, through to clinically important disorders such as peliosis hepatis, SOS (VOD), Budd–Chiari syndrome, nodular regenerative hyperplasia, and other causes of noncirrhotic portal hypertension (Table 27.7).

Causative drugs include sex steroids, alkylating chemotherapeutic agents (cyclophosphamide, busulfan, melphalan, dactinomycin), and immunosuppressive agents (azathioprine). In current practice, SOS (or VOD) most often occurs in the setting of bone marrow transplantation, but in the past it was synonymous with pyrrolizidine alkaloid hepatotoxicity resulting from the ingestion of brewed herbal tea mixtures (e.g., "Jamaican morning sickness") [98] or from plant alkaloid contamination of herbal medicines such as comfrey [99]. Epidemics of VOD have also reported in areas where pyrrolizidine alkaloid-contaminated wheat flour has been consumed,

Table 27.7 Drug-induced vascular disorders and tumors.

Vascular lesions	Examples
Vascular disorders	
Peliosis hepatis	Anabolic steroids, azathioprine, oral contraceptives, 6-thioguanine, Thorotrast®
Hepatic sinusoidal obstruction syndrome (venous outflow obstruction, including venoocclusive disease)	Oral contraceptives, pyrrolizidine alkaloids, 6-thioguanine, dacarbazine, gemcitabine
Noncirrhotic portal hypertension	Vitamin A, methotrexate, arsenic, vinyl chloride, azathioprine
Nodular regenerative hyperplasia	Azathioprine, 6-thioguanine, busulfan
Tumors	
Hemangioma	Oral contraceptives (trophic effect on preexisting lesions only)
Focal nodular hyperplasia	?Oral contraceptives (see text)
Hepatic adenoma	Oral contraceptives, anabolic steroids
Hepatocellular carcinoma	Anabolic steroids, danazol, oral contraceptives, Thorotrast, vinyl chloride
Angiosarcoma	Vinyl chloride, thorium dioxide, arsenic

particularly in South Asia and the Middle East. Hepatic vein and portal vein thrombosis can occur in OCS users, although latent or overt myeloproliferative disorders or inherited procoagulant states (such as factor V Leiden) [100] are usually also found in cases of venous thrombosis at these sites (Chapter 33).

Hepatic neoplasms

Drugs and toxins are a rare cause of liver tumors (Chapters 35 and 36), but some associations exist, as exemplified by OCSs and *hepatic adenomas*. OCS use is recorded in over 80% of patients with hepatic adenomas, and there is a strong relationship with dose and duration of estrogen therapy [101,102]. Further, evidence of estrogen dependence of these tumors is evident; regression occurs in a significant proportion of patients after discontinuing OCSs [103]. As discussed later, surgery is still required in most cases.

The relationship between estrogens and *focal nodular hyperplasia* is less clearly etiologic (see later section). As for cavernous hemangiomas, sex steroids, and particularly estrogens, may have trophic effects on these two benign hepatic neoplasms, especially on their vascularity, although this remains controversial [104]; estrogens are therefore not the primary causative factor.

Malignant tumors such as *hepatocellular carcinoma* (HCC) are caused by chronic viral hepatitis in more than 80% of cases (Chapter 36), but in parts of Africa and Asia the ingestion of aflatoxin- or other fungal toxin-contaminated food may play a synergistic role in carcinogenesis. Estrogens increase the risk of HCC in long-term OCS users, but this effect is weak and is overwhelmed in importance by chronic HBV and HCV infection in regions endemic for these viruses [27].

Angiosarcoma is an uncommon liver tumor that was classically associated with the radiocontrast agent Thorotrast® (see also Chapter 36), vinyl chloride monomer, arsenic, and, rarely, androgen use.

Role of drugs in multifactorial liver disease

Viral hepatitis

Patients with chronic hepatitis B or C may be at increased risk of liver injury during chemotherapy for tuberculosis and cancer, during HAART, and after the intake of ibuprofen and possibly other NSAIDs [57–59]. Successful antiviral treatment for chronic hepatitis C reduces the risk of antiretroviral drug hepatotoxicity [105].

A common problem is the person who regularly attends the liver clinic with mild-to-moderate ALT elevation associated with chronic viral hepatitis, who then presents with an ALT >300 U/L. Particularly for chronic hepatitis C, changes due to hepatotoxic drugs are more likely than spontaneous fluctuations of disease severity; drugs are almost always the cause with ALT values that greatly exceed 1,000 U/L. A common culprit is acetaminophen taken in moderate daily dosage when there are factors such as concomitant medication, prolonged fasting, or chronic alcohol excess (see later section). Another frequent scenario is that the person has tried Chinese herbal medicines or some other form of CAM.

Highly active antiretroviral therapy

Abnormal liver tests and clinical evidence of liver disease are common in persons with HIV/AIDS. Contributory factors include chronic hepatitis B or C, hepatobiliary infections and infestations, lymphoma and other tumors, and possibly direct effects of HIV infection (Chapter 41). However, drugs remain the commonest cause of liver injury in this setting. When monotherapy was used against HIV, individual nucleos(t)ide analogs (e.g., didanosine, zidovudine) were associated with uncommon episodes of severe cytopathic liver injury. As discussed later, it seems likely that drug combinations that include protease inhibitors as well as nucleos(t)ide analogs are more toxic than individual agents.

Bone marrow transplantation

As discussed in Chapter 10, hepatobiliary complications of hematopoietic cell transplantation are common, often serious and may be multifactorial in origin. Bone marrow transplantation particularly increases the risk of vascular complications, such as VOD and nodular regenerative hyperplasia. Thus while SOS (or VOD) complicates at least 1% of cases during the use of anticancer drugs, its risk can be as high as 54% after bone marrow transplantation, depending on the regimen used [42]. Of 103 patients undergoing bone marrow transplantation in one series, NRH was present in 23% and SOS (VOD) in 9% [106].

The clinical features are those of portal hypertension, often complicated by bleeding esophageal varices and ascites. Hepatic encephalopathy can occur after an episode of severe upper gastrointestinal hemorrhage. Liver tests may be normal or show minor nonspecific changes. The diagnosis is made histologically; a wedge biopsy may be necessary. In general, the prognosis for NRH is good; complete reversibility may occur in some drug-induced cases [106].

Metabolic syndrome and non-alcoholic steatohepatitis

Steatohepatitis is a form of chronic liver disease in which fatty change is associated with focal liver cell injury, Mallory hyaline, inflammation with mixed cellularity, including polymorphonuclear cells, and progressive hepatic fibrosis in a pericentral (zone 3) and pericellular distribution (Chapter 32). While alcohol is a common etiology, steatohepatitis can be associated with diabetes, obesity, and several drugs (e.g., perhexiline maleate [107] and amiodarone [108]); the term "drug-induced steatohepatitis" is now preferred to "secondary NASH".

Among drugs associated with steatohepatitis during the last 20 years, causality is harder to prove because NASH is so common among patients with insulin resistance, diabetes, and metabolic syndrome (Chapter 32). Thus, calcium channel blockers used for arterial hypertension have been associated with steatohepatitis [109, 110] and methyldopa has been reported to cause cirrhosis in obese middle-aged women [111,112]; these associations may be fortuitous. Other drugs, including estrogens [113], tamoxifen, and glucocorticosteroids may precipitate NASH because of their effects on metabolic risk factors: insulin resistance, type 2 diabetes, obesity, and hypertriglyceridemia. A recent addition to this list is oxaliplatin-based chemotherapy for metastatic colorectal cancer; hepatic steatosis (20–25%) and less commonly NASH (up to 5%) are described. The presence of steatohepatitis confers increased morbidity and poor outcome after liver resection [114].

Postoperative jaundice

Drug-induced liver injury is a common cause of postoperative liver disease. It is usually easy to distinguish underlying hepatobiliary disorders and bilirubin transport abnormalities resulting from tissue hypoxia or systemic infection ("benign postoperative cholestasis" or "jaundice in sick patients") from drug reactions. Halothane-induced liver injury is one of the classic types of hepatic drug reactions but has become much less common now that halothane has been almost completely replaced (in some countries) with equally acceptable and less hepatotoxic agents. Other than halothane, which causes a typical "signature syndrome," few other anesthetics cause significant liver injury. Some cases have been attributed to isoflurane; the evidence and practical implications are discussed later. Postoperative liver injury is also observed with antibiotics (especially amoxicillin-clavulanate, and less commonly with synthetic penicillins or cephalosporins), analgesics (particularly acetaminophen given alone or in drug combinations), dextropropoxyphene, tranquilizers, antidepressants, and (undisclosed) use of herbal medicines.

Liver disease associated with particular classes of drugs

Antimicrobial agents

Penicillins

Hepatic injury associated with natural penicillins (penicillin G, penicillin V) is poorly documented [14]. It has been usually recorded in the setting of anaphylaxis, suggesting a possible ischemic basis for the liver injury rather than direct toxicity [115]. In contrast, the semisynthetic penicillins have been implicated in many hepatic drug reactions, including hepatocellular injury, bland cholestasis, and cholestatic hepatitis that may lead to VBDS (Table 27.8) [116–118].

Oxacillin

There are many reports of abnormal liver tests, mainly raised AT [119,120], with oxacillin. Isolated instances of cholestatic hepatitis or acute hepatitis have also been reported. Most reported cases have occurred in the setting of high-dose, prolonged (>2 weeks), intravenous treatment. Children may be particularly susceptible to this adverse reaction [121]. Onset is within 2 to 43 days. Although eosinophilia has been described, features of hypersensitivity are not conspicuous. The liver test abnormalities usually normalize when the drug is withdrawn.

Table 27.8 Hepatic injury associated with antimicrobial agents.

Drug	Pattern of liver injury	Comments
Amoxicillin, carbenicillin	Minor, nonspecific increase in aminotransferases	
Amoxicillin-clavulanate	Cholestatic hepatitis with bile duct injury; acute hepatitis (15% of cases)	Associated with vanishing bile duct syndrome, granuloma and cirrhosis (single case)
Ampicillin	Acute hepatitis, mixed hepatocellular–cholestatic injury, with granulomatous hepatitis	Rarely vanishing bile duct syndrome; cross-hepatotoxicity with cefuroxime
Ampicillin-sulbactam	Cholestatic hepatitis	Single case
Cephalosporins	Minor liver injury, acute hepatitis, cholestatic hepatitis	Rare, mild, and reversible; granulomas (cephalexin); biliary sludge (ceftriaxone)
Chloramphenicol	Hepatocellular, cholestasis	Hepatic injury rare; also reported with chloramphenicol eye drops
Co-trimoxazole	Acute hepatitis, cholestatic hepatitis, granulomatous hepatitis, vanishing bile duct syndrome	Cholestasis recorded with trimethoprim alone; increased risk with HIV/AIDS
Erythromycin	Cholestatic hepatitis	Also with azithromycin, clarithromycin, roxithromycin, and telithromycin (acute liver failure, acute hepatitis)
Flucloxacillin	Cholestasis with bile duct injury; vanishing bile duct syndrome	Similar toxicity with oxacillin, cloxacillin, and dicloxacillin, but possibly less frequent and less severe
Minocycline	Acute and chronic hepatitis	Autoimmune hepatitis-type features (see text)
Nitrofurantoin	Acute and chronic hepatitis, granulomatous hepatitis, cirrhosis	Declining incidence; was common in long-term users (>6 months)
Penicillin G, penicillin V	Acute hepatitis, granulomatous hepatitis	Very rare; hypersensitivity features often present
Quinolones	Mainly cholestasis; rarely hepatitis and fulminant hepatic failure	Overall low incidence; granulomas (norfloxacin)
Sulfonamides	Acute hepatitis, cholestatic hepatitis, granulomatous hepatitis, vanishing bile duct syndrome	Similar toxicity with sulfones, sulfasalazine, and pyrimethamine-sulfadoxine
Tetracycline	Microvesicular steatosis	Rarely vanishing bile duct syndrome
Trovafloxacin	Fulminant hepatic failure	Now withdrawn

AIDS, acquired immune deficiency syndrome; HIV, human immunodeficiency virus.

Flucloxacillin

Over 600 cases of cholestatic hepatitis have been reported, mainly from Europe, Scandinavia, and Australia [122–126]. The frequency of liver injury is between 1 and 10 cases per 100,000 persons exposed [123,125]. Risk factors for flucloxacillin-induced liver injury are high daily doses, prolonged courses (>2 weeks), and age over 55 years [123]. Symptoms usually begin after 1–9 weeks, but can be delayed for up to 6 weeks after the antibiotic course is completed. Nausea, anorexia, and vomiting herald the onset of hepatitis, and are followed by jaundice and pruritus. Constitutional symptoms and weight loss are often striking. Blood tests reflect severe hepatitis with high AT, serum alkaline phosphatase, and GGTP values. Bilirubin levels can be markedly raised [125]. Liver histology shows cholestatic hepatitis with bile duct injury and ductopenia [124]. This is a very severe form of drug-induced liver disease with reported mortality up to 5%. Although most patients recover after drug withdrawal, prolonged cholestasis is observed in 10–30%, and in some cases this can lead to cirrhosis. Management is supportive in the acute phases, but with continued cholestasis ursodeoxycholic acid appears to benefit approximately two thirds of cases [70]. The postulation of an idiosyncratic basis for flucloxacillin liver toxicity is supported by the identification of reactive metabolites capable of inducing cytotoxicity in biliary epithelial cells [127]. However, more recent data showing an association between this hepatic adverse reaction and the presence of a specific HLA allele (HLA-B*5701) invoke the role of inappropriate T-cell responses as a basis for the hepatotoxicity [38]. On the other hand, patients with flucloxacillin-related DILI have certain polymorphisms within pregnane-X receptors, an important nuclear receptor relevant to bile metabolism and canalicular secretion. Accumulation of the drug is a likely consequence [128]. If, as suggested, drug metabolites could induce adduct formation by covalent binding to cellular proteins and in turn, generating a robust immune response, then both these processes could contribute to DILI [129].

Cloxacillin and dicloxacillin

Some data indicate that cholestatic hepatitis may be less common and possibly less severe with cloxacillin and dicloxacillin, compared with flucloxacillin [126], but this remains unproven and controversial. In other respects, the liver injury and clinical course resemble the flucloxacillin reaction described earlier.

Amoxicillin-clavulanate (Augmentin®)

At least 150 cases of cholestatic liver injury have been attributed to amoxicillin-clavulanate [130,131]. The clavulanate component has been implicated because such toxicity is rare with amoxicillin, whereas other clavulanate–penicillin compounds such as Timentin® (ticarcillin-clavulanate) can cause cholestasis [132]. The frequency of liver injury has been estimated at 1.1–2.7 cases per 100,000 persons exposed [23]. Male gender, age over 60 years, and prolonged courses of treatment are risk factors for hepatic injury. A prospective study from Spain, where Augmentin accounts for 13% of cases of idiosyncratic DILI, noted that acute hepatitis was significantly more common in patients under 55 years (64%) and in those receiving short courses of treatment (mean of 8.8 days) as compared with cholestatic/mixed hepatocellular–cholestatic reactions, which were seen in patients over 55 years (40%) and with longer treatment regimes (mean of 12.7 days) [133]. Although there is a strong association with DRB1*1501-DRB5*0101-DQB1*062 [36,37], this haplotype does not appear to influence the clinical expression and outcomes of amoxicillin-clavulanate hepatitis. Persons with glutathione-S-transferase null genotypes (GSTM1, GSTT1), who are unable to detoxify electrophilic compounds, are also susceptible to amoxicillin-clavulanate hepatotoxicity (odds ratio (OR), 2.8) [134]. These genotypes also did not correlate with clinical expression or outcome.

Onset is within 6 weeks (mean, 18 days) of beginning therapy, and rarely up to 8 weeks after its completion. Hypersensitivity features such as fever, rash, and eosinophilia are seen in 30–60% of patients [130]. Bland cholestasis or cholestatic hepatitis is observed in biopsied cases [130]. Bile duct injury and perivenular bilirubinostasis with ceroid pigment deposits are often present. Other histologic features include hepatic granulomas, biliary ductopenia [135] and, rarely, cirrhosis [136]. The major-

ity of patients recover but this can take up to 4 months. Fatalities are rare [136].

Quinolones

Transient AT increases are recorded in 2–3% of recipients but serious liver injury is infrequent, with the exception of trovafloxacin, which was withdrawn due to severe hepatotoxicity [137]. Among the reported cases, cholestatic liver injury predominates, usually occurring within 2–21 days [138,139]. Ciprofloxacin [139], norfloxacin [140], ofloxacin [141], gatifloxacin [142], and moxifloxacin [143] have all been implicated. Instances of hepatocellular injury have also been recorded, including acute liver failure with ciprofloxacin [139] and ofloxacin [141]. Acute cholestatic hepatitis followed by prolonged cholestasis and biliary ductopenia were observed with gatifloxacin [142]. Two elderly subjects with renal impairment developed acute hepatocellular injury with levofloxacin, presumably a consequence of altered pharmacokinetics because levofloxacin undergoes renal elimination [144].

Tetracycline

Tetracycline hepatotoxicity was characterized by microvesicular steatosis resulting in acute liver failure. Risk factors included the administration of high intravenous doses (usually >2 g/day) of tetracycline in pregnancy [42], or to men taking estrogens. The other important risk factor was renal failure, which reduces tetracycline clearance. The clinical features resembled those now seen in some cases of severe liver injury associated with HAART (see later section). Tetracycline hepatotoxicity is attributed to impaired hepatic lipid transport and inhibition of mitochondrial β-oxidation of fatty acids [2]. It is no longer observed now that tetracycline is contraindicated in pregnancy.

Oral tetracycline has been associated with two cases of prolonged cholestasis with bile duct injury; bilirubin levels remained elevated for nearly 3 years in one of these patients [92]. A recent population-based study found that current or past users of oral tetracycline were 2.7–3.7 times more likely to develop liver injury than controls, whereas persons on doxycycline were not at additional risk [145].

Minocycline

Minocycline, a semisynthetic tetracycline used in treating acne, is an important cause of drug-induced liver disease [146–148]. A systematic review identified 65 published cases, while 493 (6%) of over 8,000 adverse drug reactions attributed to minocycline reported to an international pharmacovigilance center were liver related [147]. Two modes of presentation are described. Those presenting with "early-onset" hepatitis (within 5 weeks) exhibit prominent hypersensitivity features such as exfoliative dermatitis, lymphadenopathy, and eosinophilia; this is typical of the reactive metabolite syndrome (see Table 27.3). Among such cases, six of 16 were in persons of African-Carribean ethnicity, suggesting possible racial susceptibility. By contrast, long-term minocycline recipients (>12 months) present with a clinical and histologic picture simulating autoimmune hepatitis, with fever, arthralgia (>70%), antinuclear and/or smooth muscle antibodies (>90%), and raised globulins [149]. Other features of drug-induced SLE may be present, including arthritis and nephritis [148]. The absence of tissue eosinophilia in some cases may divert attention from a drug etiology. Nearly half (48%) of those affected have been women, most (94%) aged less than 40 years, and many of them in their adolescent years [150]. This reflects, in part, the age of those exposed to prolonged minocycline for the treatment of acne. Autoimmune hepatitis evolving to cirrhosis has been described in a 15-year-old male who continued using minocycline after the onset of symptoms [151].

Most patients recover completely after minocycline is discontinued. However, both acute and chronic hepatitis can be severe, with a few patients needing liver transplantation or dying from liver failure [148]. Occasional patients seemed to benefit from a short course of immunosuppressive therapy, but it is unclear whether spontaneous resolution would have occurred. Among fatal cases, additional factors such as myocarditis or concurrent viral infections may have contributed to the mortality [147].

It is unclear how minocycline induces AIH. The sera of one affected patient contained antibodies that reacted with 50 and 90 kD proteins expressed by human hepatoma cell lines, and with rat CYP proteins [152]. This raises the possibility of molecular mimicry between drug-induced autoantibodies and host proteins. The suggestion that minocycline could have triggered latent AIH seems less plausible because most affected patients recover without immunosuppression, and hepatitis occurs in those who do not exhibit the usual HLA haplotypes (HLA-DR3 and -DR4) associated with AIH [153].

Sulfonamides

Sulfonamides have long been implicated as causing acute and chronic hepatitis, cholestatic, granulomatous, or mixed reactions, and rarely fulminant hepatic failure [154, 155]. Persons with HIV/AIDS [156] are particularly susceptible, implicating immune dysregulation in the pathogenesis of the hepatic injury. On the other hand, 90% of patients with sulfonamide hypersensitivity in one series were identified as slow acetylators [157]; reduced activity of the acetylation pathway may contribute to defec-

tive detoxification of a sulfonamide metabolite, or facilitate the CYP-mediated production of a nitroso metabolite [158]. How this triggers an apparent immune-mediated liver injury is unclear.

Sulfonamide-induced liver injury occurs usually in the setting of systemic drug hypersensitivity (see Table 27.3). Symptoms begin early (within 2 weeks) of starting therapy. Associated features include a rash (occasionally with the Stevens–Johnson syndrome), vasculitis, lymphadenopathy, pancreatitis, neuropathy, pancytopenia, and renal failure [42,115].

Sulfonamide combinations: co-trimoxazole, sulfasalazine, fansidar

In addition to other types of sulfonamide-induced liver injury, prolonged cholestasis with biliary ductopenia has been attributed to co-trimoxazole [159]. Significant liver injury has occurred in recipients of sulfasalazine (see below) and pyrimethamine-sulfadoxine (Fansidar®) [160].

Sulfasalazine and mesalamine

Sulfasalazine has been associated with several reports of acute hepatitis [161]. Sulfasalzine-associated hepatic injury was observed more often in patients with rheumatoid arthritis than in inflammatory bowel disease [42, 162]. Reactions are often severe, and at least ten deaths have been recorded. Fever, rash, and arthralgia usually develop within 1–4 weeks. The liver injury was originally ascribed to the sulfonamide component (sulfapyridine). However, other 5-aminosalicylic acid (5-ASA) compounds, including mesalamine (mesalazine) and olsalazine, can also cause acute hepatitis, implicating the 5 ASA moiety in at least some cases [163, 164]. Sulfasalazine- and mesalamine-related hepatic drug reactions occur with similar frequency (6 and 3.2 per million prescriptions, respectively) [162]. A more recent British surveillance study estimated the frequency of sulfasalazine-related DILI at 0.4% of patients treated [165]. Five of the ten reported cases in this series of patients with rheumatoid arthritis were of Afro-Caribbean ancestry (who only constituted ~12% of the cohort), highlighting possible ethnic differences in the risk of DILI. Mesalazine has also been associated with cholestasis [166] and rarely chronic hepatitis (one report) with hypergammaglobulinemia and antinuclear and smooth muscle antibodies [163].

Dapsone (4,4-diaminodiphenylsulfone)

Liver involvement occurs as part of a severe hypersensitivity syndrome ("sulfone syndrome"). This reaction, another example of the RMS (see above) is reported in up to 1.3% of dapsone recipients [167]. Most cases occurred within 6 weeks. Liver histology shows acute hepatitis or cholestatic hepatitis. Hepatic granulomas or acute cholangitis are also described [168]. Resolution occurs within 4 weeks of stopping dapsone. Acute liver failure and death are uncommon but have been reported in severe cases. Corticosteroids have been used with success in some cases. However, untreated patients have also recovered whilst fatalities are recorded despite corticosteroid use [167].

Nitrofurantoin

Cases of significant hepatotoxicity still occur with this commonly prescribed urinary tract antiseptic. In a recent survey from Michigan, nitrofurantoin accounted for three of 32 (10%) cases of drug-induced hepatitis [169]. Acute and chronic hepatitis are the most characteristic hepatic syndromes, but varying degrees of cholestasis can occur, as do granulomas.

Nitrofurantoin-induced chronic hepatitis simulates AIH. It is seen only in individuals using nitrofurantoin for more than 6 months; in some cases, exposure has been intermittent and to very small doses of nitrofurantoin, such as those found in cow's milk [170]. Positive rechallenge is well documented, and may occur even after 17 years [171]. The clinical features are those of chronic hepatitis with fatigue, malaise, and nausea, with raised ALT, hypoalbuminaemia, and hyperglobulinemia. Antinuclear antibodies (80%) and smooth muscle antibodies (70%) are often present. Cirrhosis is present in up to 20% of patients with nitrofurantoin-induced chronic hepatitis. Nitrofurantoin is also an important cause of pulmonary fibrosis, and concurrent liver and lung injury are observed in about 20% of persons developing nitrofurantoin hepatitis [172].

Clinical recovery follows nitrofurantoin withdrawal, but the course may be prolonged and sometimes recovery is incomplete [2]. Corticosteroids are not routinely used, but seem to have accelerated recovery in occasional cases [173]. Monitoring liver tests is not likely to be clinically useful or cost-effective.

Erythromycins and other macrolide antibiotics

Erythromycin estolate was recognized as a paradigm of cholestatic hepatitis in the early 1970s, but similar toxicity, albeit far less commonly, has been reported with all the erythromycin esters (rarely with erythromycin base), and with other macrolides, such as clarithromycin [14]. The presence of fever and serum and tissue eosinophilia, along with an accelerated response to rechallenge, is consistent with immunoallergic idiosyncrasy, although intrinsic toxicity may also contribute [174].

Symptoms begin 2–25 days after commencing treatment [114]. Nausea, anorexia, vomiting, and abdominal pain are common. Abdominal pain may be quite severe and mimics acute cholecystitis. Before this syndrome was appreciated, inappropriate cholecystectomy was often performed. Dark urine (bilirubinuria), jaundice, and itch may also occur. The biochemical profile shows raised AT and alkaline phosphatase, with hyperbilirubinemia in severe cases. Peripheral eosinophilia can occur. Liver biopsies show intrahepatic cholestasis and portal inflammation, often accompanied by numerous eosinophils. Rare cases have been associated with chronic cholestasis, with biliary ductopenia on histologic sections.

Most recover after the drug is withdrawn, although liver test abnormalities may take up to 4 months to subside. Cross-sensitivity between erythromycin preparations has been reported [115]. Intravenous erythromycin lactobionate [175] has been implicated in a case of fulminant hepatitis.

Clarithromycin [176], azithromycin [177], and roxithromycin [178] have also been associated with cholestasis or mixed hepatocellular–cholestatic injury. Two reports of fulminant hepatic failure have accrued for clarithromycin; one of these patients was also receiving disulfiram (see also below) [179]. Forty-two cases of acute hepatocellular injury involving telithromycin, a ketolide antibiotic, were reported to the US Food and Drug Administration (FDA) [180]. There were four deaths and one patient required a liver transplant. The frequency of severe liver injury was estimated at one per 370,000 prescriptions. Most cases occurred early (2–43 days; median, 10 days) and presented with fever, abdominal pain, and jaundice. Ascites was present in 17%, and interestingly occurred even in resolving cases suggesting either severe liver injury or a possible serositis. Eosinophilia was present in 19%, raising a possibility of a hypersensitivity reaction [180].

Antituberculous drugs

Of the current antituberculous drugs, hepatotoxicity is an important complication of isoniazid, rifampin, and pyrazinamide, particularly when used in combination. Risk factors for liver injury are shown in Box 27.11. Except for a single report of cholestasis [181], ethambutol appears to be devoid of hepatic adverse effects. Among drugs used in former times, severe hepatocellular injury and cholestasis were recorded with p-aminosalicyclic acid, often as part of a multisystem syndrome with hypersensitivity features [2], and acute hepatocellular injury with prothionamide and ethionamide [2]. Ethionamide is still used rarely as a second-line antituberculous drug. Rifabutin causes liver enzyme changes, but these are usually part of hepatic adaptation; hepatitis has not been a problem.

Box 27.11 Risk factors for antituberculosis treatment-related hepatotoxicity.

- Age over 60 years
- Serum albumin <35 g/L
- Female gender
- Increased serum bilirubin, preexisting chronic liver disease
- Hepatitis B surface antigen positivity
- Genetic factors: HLA haplotype associations, glutathione-S-transferase mutations
- Multidrug regimens, particularly containing pyrazinamide; ?dosing regimen (daily use more toxic than thrice-weekly regimen)
- Excess alcohol consumption
- CYP2E1 status

CYP2E1, cytochrome P450 2E1; HLA, human leucocyte antigen.

Isoniazid

Frequency and risk factors

The hepatotoxic potential of isoniazid (INH) was established by landmark studies in the late 1960s and early 1970s [182–185]. Minor elevations (less than three-fold) of serum AT occur in 10–20% of subjects during the first 3 months of treatment. These abnormalities often settle with continued treatment and a progressive rise is uncommon. Jaundice occurs in approximately 1% of recipients of INH, but in more than 2% of those aged 50 years or older. In general, liver injury is rare in persons under the age of 20 but severe hepatitis can occur even in children; over a 10-year period (1987–97), eight children required liver transplantation in the United States (0.2% of pediatric liver transplants) [186].

Persons with a history of excessive alcohol use and women, especially of African-American and Hispanic ethnicity, are also at increased risk of toxicity [187]. The presence of hepatitis B, hepatitis C, HIV, or extrapulmonary tuberculosis (OR, 2.3) has been suggested as a risk factor [188]. The relative risk of developing hepatotoxicity if the person was hepatitis C- or HIV-positive was five-fold and four-fold, respectively, and 14-fold with HIV/HCV coinfection. Antituberculous therapy could be reinstituted after successful antiviral therapy against HCV. In another study, persons who were hepatitis B surface antigen (HBsAg) positive were more likely to sustain liver injury than HBsAg-negative individuals [187]. Further, those with positive replication status (i.e., HBeAg-positive) had a higher likelihood of developing hepatotoxicity with INH than those with "inactive" hepatitis B (7.7-fold increased risk). Discontinuation rates were also higher in the former group. Opposing views were expressed in a case–control study [189], in which malnutrition was the only determinant of hepatotoxicity.

Evidence on the influence of the acetylator phenotype has been conflicting. Initial studies conveyed the impression that fast acetylators were at increased risk, but other reports have suggested that the acetylator status is either not a predictor of toxicity [190] or that slow acetylators are more susceptible [191].

Metabolic idiosyncrasy is postulated as the basis for INH toxicity through the generation of a toxic metabolite, most likely hydrazine. This could explain why the risk of severe liver injury is enhanced by concomitant intake of rifampicin [192], and why pyrazinamide (which is structurally similar to both INH and nicotinamide (a dose-dependent hepatotoxin discussed later)) is also associated with an increased risk of more severe hepatotoxicity. Persons carrying certain genetic polymorphisms [193] in key enzymes (e.g., CYP2E1) that enhance reactive metabolite formation, or in those involved in detoxification processes (e.g., glutathione-S-transferase) [194], may be predisposed to INH-induced liver injury. An association with certain HLA haplotypes (absence of HLA-DQA1*0102 antigen, and the presence of HLA-DQB1*0201 antigen) was observed in North Indian patients (Box 27.11) [195].

Clinical features, outcome, and management

Prodromal features are those of nonspecific drug reactions or resemble viral hepatitis. Because of the often vague nature of these symptoms, patients taking INH should be warned (repeatedly) about the potential significance of malaise, fatigue, anorexia, nausea, vomiting, and dark urine. Jaundice is the presenting symptom in 10% of patients. Fever, rash, eosinophilia, or other manifestations of drug hypersensitivity are rare. Presentation is within 4 weeks of starting INH in 15% of cases; half the cases present within 2 months, but onset may be delayed from 3 to 12 months in the remainder. A marked rise of AT levels is common, with peak values as high as 4,000 IU/L. Liver biopsy shows lobular hepatitis, often with marked hydropic changes of hepatocytes, and bridging (submassive) or massive (panlobular) hepatic necrosis in fatal cases. Cases associated with apparent chronic hepatitis (without autoimmune features) and cirrhosis have been described rarely, mostly before HCV testing was introduced. These seemed to have been cases of chronic hepatotoxicity not chronic hepatitis, and patients generally recovered after discontinuation of the drug.

Rapid resolution of symptoms and liver test abnormalities occurs when INH is stopped before the onset of liver failure. The almost universal feature of cases leading to liver transplantation or fatal liver failure, from the early 1970s until the present time [184], is continued ingestion of INH after the commencement of symptoms. The case fatality of jaundiced patients exceeds 10%. Management of liver failure is supportive; corticosteroids are of no benefit. Liver transplantation has been performed successfully [196]. In less severe cases, combination anti-tuberculous treatment can be reintroduced. Guidelines vary as to the method of reintroduction; some advocate introducing one drug at a time (often at lower doses) whereas others have found no difference in the incidence of hepatotoxicity between patients with sequentially introduced drug regimens and those prescribed the full drug combination [197].

Prevention

In the United States, a 9-month course of INH is recommended for tuberculin-positive family members of patients with tuberculosis. Monitoring of ALT, aspartate aminotransferase (AST), and bilirubin is recommended at baseline in high-risk groups (HIV- or HCV-positive individuals, history of alcoholism, previous liver disease, pregnant women, and those presenting in the postpartum period) and during treatment (if baseline values are abnormal and in high-risk groups) [198]. It is now generally agreed that patients taking INH (or other forms of antituberculosis chemotherapy) should be advised to seek medical attention as soon as new symptoms develop, even if these seem nonspecific and relatively minor. Biochemical monitoring does not effectively substitute for clinical monitoring [198]. Thus, one study found that no more than 0.15% of over 11,000 clinically monitored patients receiving INH developed significant hepatotoxicity [198]. In contrast, the most noteworthy aspect of US case reports of liver failure attributable to antituberculosis chemotherapy that resulted in death or liver transplantation has been the failure of patients to report early symptoms, and/or the failure of health care workers to recognize the significance of those symptoms, thereby allowing continued intake of INH [199].

Rifampin

A meta-analysis showed that regimens combining INH and rifampin were associated with a higher incidence of hepatotoxicity (2.5%) than regimens without this combination (1.1%) [200]. Rifampin probably increases both the risk and severity of INH-associated liver disease [192]. The potent CYP-inducing properties of rifampin (exerted via pregnane-X receptors) could facilitate the production of reactive isoniazid metabolites.

On some occasions, rifampin may itself be hepatotoxic, as shown by cases with positive rechallenge and in situations where it is used alone (for example, to relieve pruritus) [201]. In the latter setting (typically in persons with PBC), the frequency of rifampin hepatitis (7.3–12.5%) may be higher than generally recognized [201]. Liver test abnormalities usually occur within 2 months, rarely as late as 14 months, and they mostly conform to a mild hepatocellular pattern [202]. The clinical features resemble viral hepatitis. Histologic features include focal hep-

atocellular necrosis and apoptosis (acidophilic bodies), especially in zone 3, portal inflammation, and cholestasis. Patients recover when rifampin is stopped. However, continued use of rifampin has been associated with jaundice and impaired hepatic synthetic function; histology showed severe interface and intra-acinar hepatitis together with bridging and confluent necrosis. Therefore, rifampin monotherapy should be initiated at a low dose (150 mg/day) and the dose should be titrated to the clinical response. Rifampin can also be associated with hyperbilirubinemia, possibly due to impairment of canalicular drug transporters [203]. This transport defect is unrelated to hepatocellular injury or cholestasis, and resembles reactions to cyclosporine.

Interstitial nephritis, described with an intermittent use of rifampin, can accompany the liver injury. Conversely, in one series of 60 patients with rifampin nephrotoxicity, concurrent hepatotoxicity was present in 25% [204].

Increased liver enzymes were reported in 12% of recipients treated with high-dose rifabutin, a rifamycin antibiotic. Serious liver injury has not been reported.

Pyrazinamide

Pyrazinamide causes dose-dependent liver injury. High-dose pyrazinamide (40–50 mg/kg) was associated with a greater frequency of hepatotoxicity than the doses used in current regimens (25–35 mg/kg). The concurrent administration of pyrazinamide with isoniazid-rifampin increases the risk of hepatotoxicity compared to dual therapy (OR, 2.8) [205,206].

Significant liver injury has been also documented with a recently approved 2-month rifampin and pyrazinamide regimen for treating latent tuberculosis infection (LTBI). Twenty-three cases of acute hepatitis were reported [207], all developing in the second month of treatment. There were seven deaths and the case fatality rate was estimated to be 0.9 per 1,000 treatment initiations. In some cases, patients continued taking their medications after the onset of symptoms. On the other hand, one patient developed symptoms 6 weeks after the drugs were stopped and eventually needed a liver transplant 1 month later. Many restrictions have been placed in using this drug combination for LTBI. Recommendations include frequent liver test monitoring, the absence of alcohol abuse or history of INH toxicity, and the need for monitoring by experienced physicians [207]. An alternative combination of pyrazinamide with levofloxacin has also fallen out of favor due to the increased frequency of side effects, including DILI [208]. The least toxic prophylactic regimen being explored is using rifampin monotherapy for 4 months; this also has better adherence rates than the 9-month INH-based schedule [208].

Perceptions of the excellent safety of antitubercular drugs in children have been challenged by a report of

Table 27.9 Liver injury associated with antifungal drugs.

Drug	Pattern of liver injury	Comments
Amphotericin	Hepatocellular	Rare
Fluconazole	Raised alanine aminotransferase in 25% of recipients, rarely hepatitis, and fatal hepatic necrosis	Patients with HIV/AIDS may be particularly susceptible
Flucytosine	Transient rise in aminotransferases (10%); hepatic necrosis	Dose-dependent liver injury
Griseofulvin	Cholestasis	Mallory bodies in mice; liver toxicity in humans is rare
Itraconazole	Acute hepatitis, prolonged cholestasis (two cases) with bilary ductopenia (vanishing bile duct syndrome); acute liver failure	Pulse therapy appears safer than continuous dose regimens
Ketoconazole	Hepatitis, cholestasis, fulminant liver failure, and cirrhosis (single case)	Frequency of liver injury approximately 20 per 10,000 persons exposed
Terbinafine	Cholestasis, vanishing bile duct syndrome, and acute liver failure	Frequency of liver injury approximately 1 per million persons exposed

AIDS, acquired immune deficiency syndrome; HIV, human immunodeficiency virus.

hepatotoxicity in Japanese children less than 5 years of age [209]. Ohkawa et al. studied 117 pediatric recipients of antituberculosis treatment. Of these, 8% developed hepatotoxicity; all eight were below 5 years of age and four were receiving pyrazinamide [209].

Antifungal drugs

Liver injury with the oral "azole" antifungal agents is best documented for ketoconazole (Table 27.9), but itraconazole, voriconazole, and fluconazole have been implicated in a few reports [210–213]. Itraconazole is largely perceived as being nonhepatotoxic. However, among more than 69,000 patients who received an oral antifungal agent, ketoconazole and itraconazole were most often associated with DILI; the respective relative risks were 228 and 17.7 compared to nonusers [214]. Further, an FDA public health advisory has been issued after receiving 40 reports of acute liver failure in association with itraconazole; there were 22 deaths and two patients needed liver transplantation. In view of the serious nature of possible (albeit rare) liver injury, a diagnosis of onychomycosis should be clearly established before starting antifungal treatment. Liver test abnormalities are frequent in patients receiving voriconazole but hepatocellular injury is usually mild and reversible [210].

Ketoconazole

Between 5% and 17% of recipients of ketoconazole develop abnormal liver tests. Previous estimates of symptomatic hepatitis varied between 0.7 and 5 per 10,000 persons exposed [210,215] but recent estimates are higher (~20 per 10,000 persons exposed) [214,216]. Biochemical tests most often reflect a hepatocellular pattern, but cholestatic or mixed hepatocellular–cholestatic reactions are also common. Women (female : male ratio 2 : 1) and persons over 40 years of age are particularly susceptible [210,216].

Symptoms develop within 6 weeks in 60% of patients, but can be delayed up to 6 months [210,217]. Jaundice occurs in 50% of those developing acute hepatitis, but up to one third may present with nonspecific symptoms such as nausea, anorexia, and vomiting. Fever, rash, eosinophilia, and other immunoallergic characteristics are uncommon. Liver injury is therefore hypothesized to be a sequel of metabolic idiosyncrasy [218]. Rarely, acute hepatitis and even anaphylaxis can occur rapidly within 1–3 days of rechallenge in persons who have previously received repeated courses [219]. Unintentional positive rechallenge can occur as late as 30 months after the first reaction [220]. Fulminant hepatic failure requiring liver transplantation has been reported [221].

The common histologic changes are diffuse hepatocellular necrosis, particularly evident in zone 3, but cholestasis can be prominent [210]. Recovery is usual after drug discontinuation but progressive liver disease can occur if the drug is continued beyond the onset of symptoms. Several instances of protracted jaundice have been described. Evolution to cirrhosis has been described after an initial episode of acute hepatitis [222].

Table 27.10 Liver injury associated with antiparasitic agents.

Drug	Pattern of liver injury	Reference
Albendazole	Raised aminotransferases (20%), acute hepatitis	Choi et al. 2008 [231]
Amodiaquine	Severe hepatitis (one in 15,000 exposed); dose dependent	El-Mufti et al. 1993 [232]
Antimonials	Steatosis	Zimmerman 1999 [2]
Artemisinin	Raised aminotransferases (0.9%), acute hepatocellular injury	CDC 2009 [233]
Atovaquone-proguanil	Transient alterations in aminotransferases	Looareesuwan et al. 1999 [234]
Chlorguanide	Acute hepatitis (single case)	Oostweegel et al. 1998 [235]
Mebendazole	Acute hepatitis, granulomatous hepatitis	Colle et al. 1999 [236]
Mefloquine	Transient rise in aminotransferases, fatty liver (one case)	Gotsman et al. 2000 [237], Grieco et al. 1999 [238]
Metronidazole	Hepatocellular, cholestasis (few cases)	Lam & Bank 1995 [239], Hestin et al. 1994 [240]
Ornidazole	Acute hepatitis, acute cholestatic hepatitis, chronic hepatitis	Tabak et al. 2003 [241]
Quinacrine	Acute hepatitis, cholangitis	Scoazec et al. 2003 [242]
Quinine	Granulomatous hepatitis (usual presentation), mixed hepatocellular–cholestatic reactions	Farver & Lavin 1999 [243], Katz et al. 1983 [244]
Thiabendazole	Cholestasis, vanishing bile duct syndrome, cirrhosis, sicca syndrome	Rex et al. 1983 [245], Roy et al. 1989 [246]

Terbinafine

An elevation of AT ($>2 \times$ ULN) is observed in 3.3% of those treated with terbinafine, but the frequency of symptomatic hepatitis is substantially lower (approximately two per 10,000 persons exposed) [223]. Hepatocellular mixed or bland cholestatic reactions have been reported. Most patients are aged over 50 years. No clear gender differences have been observed [224]. Onset is within 3–8 weeks but the symptoms can appear as long as 2 months after stopping the drug. Liver biopsies show hepatocyte degeneration and canalicular cholestasis with variable portal tract inflammation [84]. Prolonged cholestasis with progressive biliary ductopenia and portal fibrosis [225] can occur. Terbinafine hepatotoxicity has mimicked acute rejection in a liver transplant recipient [226]. Although a rare association, the FDA has received at least 16 reports of fulminant liver failure possibly linked to terbinafine [227]. Such an outcome has been estimated at one per 1 million persons exposed [223]. Recovery is usual with drug discontinuation. There have been anecdotal reports of ursodeoxycholic acid hastening recovery in a few protracted cases [228]. Terbinafine-associated liver injury is probably idiosyncratic because hypersensitivity features are unusual. The recent identification of a hepatotoxic metabolite of terbinafine is consistent with this hypothesis [229]. Liver injury associated with other antifungal drugs is summarized in Table 27.9.

Agents used to treat parasitic infestations

Pyrimethamine-sulfadoxine (Fansidar) has been linked with severe hepatotoxicity with a frequency of approximately one per 100,000 prescriptions. Deaths from hepatic necrosis have been recorded. Because liver injury has been attributed to pyrimethamine as well as sulfonamides (see earlier), it is not clear which component is responsible, or whether interaction between the two components is important [230]. The hepatotoxicity of other antiparasitic agents is summarized in Table 27.10.

Antiretroviral therapy

The frequency of hepatic injury with HAART, which now typically includes three to four agents, is at least 10%. The agents used can be broadly categorized as nucleoside (or nucleotide) reverse transcriptase inhibitors (NRTIs), non-nucleoside reverse transcriptase inhibitors, protease inhibitors, and the more recent additions, integrase inhibitors and fusion (entry inhibitors) [247].

Nucleos(t)ide reverse transcriptase inhibitors

Mitochondrial toxicity is a group-specific feature [248]. The first-generation NRTIs, zidovudine, didanosine, and stavudine, have most often been implicated in causing DILI [249]. These agents inhibit mitochondrial DNA polymerase-γ, a key enzyme involved in mitochondrial DNA replication. An additional mechanism of hepatotoxicity may involve oxidative stress, the consequences of impaired oxidative phosphorylation and fatty acyl β-oxidation, and insulin resistance. Reported risk factors for mitochondrial drug toxicity among people with HIV infection include obesity, female gender, and absence of AIDS-defining illness [248]; one study was unable to confirm the gender predisposition or influence of HIV status [248]. Mitochondrial toxicity is unusual with second-generation NRTIs such as lamivudine, tenofovir, and abacavir.

The hallmarks of mitochondrial hepatotoxicity are extensive microvesicular and/or macrovesicular steatosis, lactic acidosis (sometimes with a shock-like state), and liver test abnormalities progressing to acute liver failure. Asymptomatic hyperlactatemia is common, especially with stavudine [250], but life-threatening lactic acidosis/hepatic steatosis is rare; the estimated risk is 1–15 per 1,000 person-years of antiretroviral use [249]. Onset is usually within 6 months (range, 3–17 months) of starting treatment. The presenting symptoms are nonspecific: nausea, vomiting, diarrhea, dyspnoea, lethargy, and abdominal pain. In many cases there are extrahepatic manifestations, such as myopathy or peripheral neuropathy, and in severe cases pancreatitis and renal failure may follow the onset of the lactic acidosis and liver injury. The discontinuation of drugs is mandatory, but despite this deaths still occur [251].

Non-nucleoside reverse transcriptase inhibitors

Persons receiving nevirapine or abacavir (non-NRTIs) can develop severe hypersensitivity within 6 weeks, manifested by fever, rash, and eosinophilia. In such individuals, further use of these agents is contraindicated (see Table 27.3). Nevirapine has also been implicated in causing severe hepatotoxicity [252], highlighted by cases involving health care workers who developed liver injury after receiving nevirapine as part of postexposure prophylaxis [253]. The FDA received 12 reports of such hepatotoxic reactions during 1997 through 2000; seven recipients developed acute hepatitis, four had asymptomatic increases in serum AT, and one person developed acute liver failure. It is noteworthy that in some cases there was not adherence to the recommended 2-week dose escalation regimen [253].

Nevirapine is no longer recommended for postexposure prophylaxis and should be used with caution in individuals with liver disease and in pregnancy [253]. Sequential toxicity with nevirapine followed by efavirenz has been reported in an HIV/HCV coinfected person [254]. While one study reported a lower frequency of liver toxicity with efavirenz (8%) as compared with nevirapine (15%), there are other reports that did not show significant differences in hepatotoxicity [255]. A combination of genetic, immune, and host factors (low body mass index, pregnancy) have been identified that could help predict nevirapine reactions. In one predominantly Caucasian cohort, HIV-positive individuals with a CD4 percentage over 25% and who also carried the HLA-DRB1*0101 haplotype were at risk of developing liver toxicity with rash/and or fever. Screening for this HLA hap-

lotype could prevent one in 14 potentially fatal reactions [256] among Caucasians with a CD4 percentage over 25%, but these findings have not been replicated [257]. Abacavir hypersensitivity is also associated with certain HLA haplotypes; the presence of HLA-B*5701, HLA-DR7, and HLA-DQ3 had a positive predictive value of 100% in predicting such a reaction [258].

Protease inhibitors

Elevated liver enzymes are common with this class of drugs, but clinical hepatitis is infrequent with the exception of ritonavir (see below) [259]. The agents most often implicated are ritonavir and indinavir. Indinavir and atazanavir may also be associated with unconjugated hyperbilirubinemia in 6–40% of treated persons resulting from inhibition of uridine diphosphate (UDP)-glucuronosyl transferase, a finding that is of no clinical consequence [260]. Severe acute hepatitis can rarely occur with indinavir and atazanavir [261,262]. The association with peripheral and/or tissue eosinophilia in some biopsied cases involving indinavir suggests an immunoallergic form of liver injury [262].

Acute hepatitis has also been reported in 3–30% of those prescribed ritonavir [263]. The illness runs a mild course, and the liver injury responds favorably to drug withdrawal. Rarely, acute liver failure may develop. In these cases, liver histology has shown severe microvesicular steatosis, cholestasis, and extensive fibrosis [263]. By contrast, the combination of low-dose ritonavir (200 mg/day) with other protease inhibitors is not associated with an increased frequency of severe liver injury when compared with protease inhibitors such as nelfinavir or efavirenz [263].

Two studies have addressed the potential impact of underlying chronic viral hepatitis on the toxicity of protease inhibitors. Although hepatotoxicity was more frequent, the liver injury was rapidly reversible in most cases; this suggests that there is no overall detrimental effect of protease inhibitors used in HIV/HCV or HIV/HBV coinfected persons [264]. However, the FDA has raised concerns about the hepatotoxic potential of a regimen involving low-dose ritonavir and tipranavir, a nonpeptidic protease inhibitor, especially in patients coinfected with HBV or HCV infections [265].

Newer anti-HIV drugs

Of these, raltegravir (an integrase inhibitor) and maraviroc and enfuvirtide (fusion inhibitors) have not been associated with significant hepatotoxicity. An earlier member of the latter group (aplaviroc) was associated with hepatotoxicity and has been withdrawn [266]. Raltegravir has been used successfully in patients who have experienced liver injury with other anti-HIV drugs [267].

Monitoring for HAART hepatotoxicity

A few general rules have emerged (Chapter 41). Baseline and serial monitoring of liver tests should be routine. Grade 4 hepatotoxicity (AT × 10 ULN or bilirubin 5 × ULN) warrants immediate discontinuation and use of an alternative drug combination. For lesser changes, frequent monitoring (1–2 weeks) is suggested, with treatment being continued only if there are no signs and symptoms of hyperlactatemia, hepatitis, or hypersensitivity [255].

Cardiovascular drugs

Angiotensin-converting enzyme inhibitors

Drug-induced liver disease is a rare but important complication of this widely prescribed class of drugs. Onset of liver injury has varied from 2 weeks to 4 years after starting treatment [268]. Cholestatic liver toxicity predominates. Recovery is usual but may be protracted (up to 6 months). Fatalities or advanced liver injury (ductopenia, cirrhosis) are infrequent [268].

Captopril is the oldest and possibly most hepatotoxic representative. Reactions to it and to enalapril usually manifest as cholestatic hepatitis, but hepatocellular or mixed hepatocellular reactions can occur both in adults and rarely in children [268]. Enalapril-related cholestatic hepatitis can culminate in biliary ductopenia. However, the short-term outcome seems favorable after drug withdrawal [269]. Hypersensitivity features such as fever, skin rashes, and eosinophilia can accompany captopril hepatotoxicity [268]. Fulminant hepatic failure has been attributed to lisinopril [270], while fosinopril has been associated with bland cholestasis [271]. Three instances of cholestatic liver injury have been recorded with ramipril; liver histology showed cholestasis, bile duct necrosis, bile extravasation, and ductular proliferation. Prolonged cholestasis was observed in one case (14 months); liver biopsy showed biliary cirrhosis [268].

Methyldopa

Methyldopa is much less prescribed now, but it retains a place in managing obstetric hypertension. The history of methyldopa-induced liver injury remains relevant because of the range of hepatic disorders it can produce. These encompass a spectrum of toxicity that includes: asymptomatic elevation of AT, acute hepatitis, chronic hepatitis, cirrhosis, bland cholestasis, cholestatic hepatitis, steatosis, and hepatic granulomas [15,272]. Ten percent to 30% have abnormal liver tests without overt liver disease, and these changes often resolve despite continuation of the drug [2]. Acute hepatitis occurs in less than 0.1% of recipients, usually within 3 months of starting methyldopa; up to 50% present within 2–4 weeks.

The clinical presentation resembles acute viral hepatitis, with anorexia, nausea, and vomiting, followed by jaundice. Serum AT levels are elevated (5–30 × ULN), with moderately raised serum alkaline phosphatase. Liver biopsies show focal or confluent hepatocellular necrosis, acidophilic bodies, and mixed portal/periportal inflammatory infiltrates. Bridging hepatic necrosis and massive hepatic necrosis can occur. Tissue or peripheral eosinophilia is rare. Most patients recover after withdrawal of the drug. However, mortality among patients presenting with jaundice is 10% or higher [272].

Chronic hepatitis or cirrhosis have been reported as the first clinical manifestations of liver injury [272]. In such cases, liver histology shows confluent areas of lobular collapse, periportal necrosis, and inflammation; the latter includes plasma cells and occasional eosinophils [272]. Fibrous septa and established cirrhosis may also be present. Older reports of middle-aged women with steatosis and cirrhosis attributed to long-term methyldopa therapy may have confused drug reactions with NASH [109].

The pathogenesis of methyldopa-induced liver injury has been attributed to either immunologic or metabolic idiosyncrasy; this dramatically illustrates the uncertainty of indirect criteria used to assign etiopathogenic mechanisms of drug-induced liver disease. Female preponderance, positive rechallenge, presence of autoantibodies (antinuclear antibody (ANA), less commonly smooth muscle antibody (SMA)), hypergammaglobulinemia, and a positive Coombs' test have been cited in favor of an immune basis, but many of these characteristics are also observed in patients receiving methyldopa but showing no signs of liver injury. Conversely, there is some evidence that methyldopa can be metabolized to a reactive intermediate (semiquinone or quinone) [2], and this could cause membrane injury or generate a neoantigen target for an immune-mediated hepatodestructive response.

Beta-blockers

The hepatotoxic potential of β-blockers is very low, but reactions to acebutalol, propranolol [2], metoprolol [273] (both hepatocellular), atenolol (hepatitis and cholestasis) [274,275], carvedilol (mixed hepatocellular–cholestatic) [276], and labetalol [277] have been described. Labetalol has been implicated in over 11 reports of acute hepatitis, including three fatal cases [277]; histology showed massive or submassive hepatic necrosis or chronic hepatitis.

Calcium channel blockers

Liver injury associated with the calcium channel antagonists (verapamil, nifedipine, diltiazem) is infrequent. Most reported cases were hepatocellular in nature [278], but other presentations include cholestasis, granulomatous hepatitis (diltiazem) [279], and steatohepatitis (nifedipine and diltiazem) [280]. As discussed earlier, the association of calcium channel blockers with steatohepatitis may be fortuitous because hypertension is a component of the metabolic syndrome, which predisposes to NASH.

Diuretics

Of the currently used thiazides, chlorthiazide, [14], chlorthalidone, and hydrochlorthiazide [2] have been linked with rare instances of cholestasis. Ticrynafen (tienilic acid), a uricosuric diuretic, now withdrawn, was associated with acute and chronic hepatocellular injury. The case fatality rate was 10% [281]. Experimental studies of tienilic acid toxicity have been of interest because they provide an illustration of drug-induced autoimmune hepatitis. Circulating antibodies directed against hepatic CYP2C9 (which catalyzes oxidation of tienilic acid) were often present in the sera of affected patients [282]. There are a few anecdotal reports of acute hepatitis with spironolactone [14,283].

Hydralazine

Acute hepatitis with bridging necrosis is an occasional complication of hydralazine treatment. Granulomas [284] and cholestasis have also been described [285].

Other antihypertensive agents

Although their overall hepatotoxic potential appears low, cases of liver injury have accrued with all drugs within the angiotensin II receptor antagonist group. Most cases have occurred within 5 months of commencement. Tasosartan was withdrawn at the preregistration stage because of hepatotoxicity [286]. Losartan, valsartan, and candesartan have been implicated in causing acute hepatitis or cholestatic hepatitis [287,288]. Early resolution has been the rule after stopping these agents. Exceptions include two reports of prolonged cholestasis (for 1 year) following irbesartan-associated cholestatic hepatitis and biliary ductopenia accompanied by portal–portal fibrosis with candesartan [287]. Irbesartan has also been implicated in triggering an acute hepatitis with histologic features of AIH. Although autoantibodies were absent, the subsequent course, including steroid responsiveness and relapse with steroid withdrawal, was indistinguishable from AIH [288].

Antiarrhythmic drugs

Amiodarone

Raised ATs (1–5-fold) are observed in up to 25% of amiodarone recipients, but clinically significant liver disease occurs only in 0.6% [289]. The typical histologic lesion is a form of steatohepatitis indistinguishable from NASH and alcoholic liver disease [289,290], with microvesicular and

macrovesicular steatosis, hydropic change, Mallory bodies, neutrophilic infiltrates, and pericellular and perivenular fibrosis. Micronodular cirrhosis is present in 15–50% [291] of cases. Other manifestations include granulomas, cholangitis [292], and acute liver failure. The latter may result from severe acute hepatitis or a Reye syndrome-like illness [293], which has been reported within a few days of starting treatment. Amiodarone can also cause acute hepatic injury [294], within hours to days after an intravenous loading dose. Rapid resolution follows drug withdrawal, although a single loading dose can be fatal. In a few cases, positive rechallenge has been observed. The vehicle (polysorbate 80) may be responsible for the hepatotoxicity associated with parenteral amiodarone preparations; the successful reintroduction of oral amiodarone in such cases supports this hypothesis [294].

The onset of amiodarone-induced chronic liver disease is delayed and insidious; most patients have received treatment for at least a year (median, 21 months) [14]. Symptoms include fatigue, weight loss, nausea, vomiting, and abdominal swelling due to ascites. Hepatomegaly, jaundice, and other features of chronic liver disease are evident. Liver test abnormalities are often seemingly minor, even in cases with hepatic decompensation. AT values are increased at least five-fold above normal, with the AST : ALT ratio close to unity; this differs from alcoholic hepatitis. There is a minor increase in serum alkaline phosphatase. In more severe cases there may be jaundice, hypoalbuminemia, and prolongation of prothrombin time. Chronic liver injury from amiodarone is associated with prolonged storage of the drug in the liver, which therefore appears radioopaque on computed tomography (CT) examination because of the iodine content of this iodinated benzofuran derivative [295]. Electron microscopy shows lysosomal inclusions, (representing phospholipidosis) in hepatocytes and other liver cells [296]. The presence of hepatocytes with granular cytoplasm has been suggested as an early marker of amiodarone toxicity [297].

In less severe cases, biochemical resolution occurs between 2 weeks and 4 months after stopping amiodarone. However, in advanced cases the mortality is high, with a progressive decline in liver function despite discontinuing treatment. A likely explanation is that tissue levels of the drug remain high for some time due to the prolonged retention of amiodarone and its principal metabolite N-desethylamiodarone in hepatic lysosomes.

Prevention of amiodarone toxicity by baseline and serial monitoring of liver tests has been suggested [298]. In many cases, this is impractical because of the high frequency of abnormal liver tests in people treated with amiodarone due to such factors as cardiac failure, other drugs, or NASH. Further, the presence of right heart failure or prior liver test abnormalities has not been shown to engender a greater risk of hepatotoxicity [299,300]. Moreover, in one uncontrolled study the cardiac mortality after stopping amiodarone exceeded the total mortality among those who continued the drug despite suspected adverse reactions [291]. Another recommendation is measurement of serum amiodarone levels in long-term amiodarone recipients; ALT elevations were minimal in those with a serum amiodarone concentration of less than 1.5 mg/L [298].

The pathogenesis of phospholipidosis acquired from amiodarone is unclear, but may be related to inhibition of the lysosomal phospholipases, A1 and A2 [301]. Phospholipidosis is a constant association with steatohepatitis, but in animal studies appeared not to be related to it pathogenetically. A series of elegant studies from Hôpital Beaujon in Paris has shown that amiodarone, an amphiphilic cationic compound, accumulates in the anionic milieu of the mitochondrial matrix, and this leads to disruption of mitochondrial electron transport and impairment of fatty acid β-oxidation resulting in microvesicular steatosis, generation of oxidative stress, and lipid peroxidation [109,302].

Other antiarrhythmic drugs

Quinidine is an infrequent cause of hepatocellular injury. Fever and elevated AT levels occur 1–24 weeks after commencing therapy [303]. Liver histology shows hepatic necrosis and granulomas [304]. Recovery is usual after stopping the drug. Procainamide has been associated with hepatic granulomas, hepatocellular injury, and intrahepatic cholestasis [14,305]. Propafenone has been implicated in at least nine cases of predominantly cholestatic jaundice [306]. Most reported cases occurred within 2–6 weeks (range, 2–28 weeks). Liver biopsies showed portal tract inflammation with prominent cholangiolitis. No fatalities were recorded. Resolution occurred several months after drug cessation [306].

Anticoagulants

Unfractionated heparin and low molecular weight heparins can both cause elevation of serum ATs [307]. At least four cases of cholestasis have accrued with unfractionated heparin [307]. Of the currently used oral anticoagulants, the coumarin derivatives (warfarin, phenprocoumon, dicoumarol, acenocoumarol) have been associated with transient increases in liver enzymes, which usually settle without changing therapy. Occasionally, they may cause hepatocellular or mixed hepatocellular–cholestatic injury and bland cholestasis [307]. Several instances of acute hepatitis, including subacute liver failure requiring liver transplantation, have been reported from Germany, where phenprocoumon is used extensively [308]. An alternative coumarin or reintroduction of phenprocoumon can be considered in mild cases. However,

reintroduction may be unsuccessful and further cross-reactivity with other coumarins can also occur. In such cases, long-term anticoagulation has been achieved with low molecular weight heparin. Phenindione is now withdrawn; it was associated with severe hypersensitivity reactions and liver injury in up to 10% of recipients [14].

Lipid lowering drugs

Hydroxymethylglutaryl-coenzyme A reductase inhibitors ("statins")

Overall, this class of drugs is not strongly associated with significant hepatic injury, although there appears to be discordance between literature reports and data contributed to drug safety surveillance authorities. The frequency of hepatotoxicity is estimated at approximately one per 100,000 patient-years of exposure; comparative figures for NSAID liver injury are between 2.2 and 50 per 100,000 patient-years of exposure [309]. One to three percent of statin recipients develop a dose-related rise in ATs [309]. These abnormalities settle rapidly with discontinuation of treatment and often also if therapy is not interrupted. Baseline liver test abnormalities do not connote a greater risk of liver injury with the statins. In one study the frequency of severe hepatoxicity (serum bilirubin >3 mg/dL or AT 10 × ULN or baseline values) between a cohort with and without baseline elevation of liver tests was 0.6% and 0.2%, respectively (*P* not significant) [310]. Further, the safety of statins in patients with compensated chronic liver disease has been reiterated [311,312].

Lovastatin [314], pravastatin [315], atorvastatin [316], and simvastatin [317] have been implicated in a few cases of cholestatic hepatitis. Interlobular bile duct injury and prolonged cholestasis have been noted with atorvastatin [316]. Acute liver failure has also been attributed to lovastatin. This is an extremely rare event (less than one per 1 million patient treatment years) and its frequency is similar to the background rates for idiosyncratic acute liver failure in the community. In one Italian study, fluvastatin was associated with the highest rate of hepatic reactions among the statins [318]. Autoimmune hepatitis has been associated with atorvastatin, but the drug appears to have unmasked preexisting AIH rather than induced immune liver injury by itself [319].

Although monitoring liver enzymes is often recommended, this is neither likely to predict toxicity [320] nor to be cost-effective. In the AFCAPS/TEXCAPS study, only 18 of 100,000 AT estimations performed were raised more than three times the upper limit of normal; in none of these instances, did the affected person develop hepatitis [320]. Like amiodarone, the benefits of continued treatment may outweigh the potential (but low) risks of liver injury.

Other lipid lowering drugs

Rare cases of acute hepatitis and cholestatic hepatitis have been attributed to the fibrates [321]. A few cases of chronic hepatitis with portal or bridging fibrosis have been described in persons also receiving statins [322]. Serologic and histologic features resembling AIH were observed but these resolved after the drugs were discontinued. Other than one report of hepatocellular injury with colestipol, bile acid sequestrants have not been implicated in causing liver injury [323]. Reports of AIH and cholestatic hepatitis have been attributed to ezetimibe [324]. Profound conjugated hyperbilirubinemia (bilirubin 648 μmol/L) has been described in a patient with probable nonalcoholic fatty liver disease (NAFLD) related cirrhosis and mild preexisting hyperbilirubinemia [325]. Ezetimibe, in combination with simvastatin, has been also implicated in a case of acute liver failure necessitating liver transplantation [326].

Nicotinic acid (niacin)

The hepatotoxic potential of nicotinic acid has been recognized for more than 60 years. This is a dose-dependent hepatotoxin with liver injury occurring at doses exceeding 2 g/day, but there are rare instances of low-dose (500 mg/day) sustained release (SR) niacin also causing fulminant hepatic failure [327]. Patients taking sulfonylurea drugs and those with preexisting liver disease, particularly alcoholic hepatitis, are at increased risk of nicotinamide hepatotoxicity [328,329].

Both the crystalline unmodified immediate release (IR) and SR preparations have been associated with liver injury [42,330]. SR preparations have improved bioavailability and are therefore more potent (about twice) than equivalent IR preparations; a dose reduction of 50–70% has been recommended [330]. Hepatotoxicity often occurred when the formulation of nicotinamide was changed without appropriate dose modification.

The symptoms of nicotinamide hepatotoxicity begin as early as 1 week to as long as 4 years after initiating therapy. Fatigue, malaise, anorexia, and jaundice are typical features, usually resolving completely when the drug is stopped. Liver biopsies show hepatic necrosis and centrilobular cholestasis. Well-documented cases of fulminant hepatitis have also been attributed to nicotinamide, some necessitating liver transplantation [42,330].

Niaspan is an extended release preparation of nicotinamide with IR characteristics. Its hepatotoxic potential appears to be minimal. Less than 3% of recipients developed elevated AT greater than two times above ULN; most were also receiving statins. Liver tests normalized with dose reduction [331].

Drugs used in the treatment of endocrine disorders

Oral contraceptive and anabolic steroids

Both oral contraceptive steroids and the 17-alkylated anabolic steroids are associated with cholestasis, vascular lesions, and hepatic neoplasms. However, the strength of associations varies with each condition. OCSs are clearly associated with benign hepatic neoplasms, whereas their association with HCC is controversial. By contrast, HCC is well documented in users of anabolic steroids. Likewise, hepatic and portal vein thrombosis is an established adverse effect of OCSs, but not with anabolic steroids. Other vascular lesions, such as peliosis hepatis, are more often observed with anabolic steroids than with OCSs.

Oral contraceptive steroids
Cholestasis
The frequency of cholestasis with OCSs is 2.5 per 10,000 women exposed. Genetic factors influence the frequency of this complication, with a particularly high incidence among women in Chile and Scandinavia. Individuals with a previous history of cholestasis of pregnancy are at high risk (50%). Mild prodromal symptoms, such as anorexia and nausea, followed by pruritus, develop 2–3 months after starting OCSs (rarely as late as 9 months). Serum alkaline phosphatase is moderately elevated, and this is accompanied by a transient increase in ATs, occasionally exceeding 10 × ULN; GGTP levels are often normal. The development of chronic cholestasis is extremely rare [84]. In general, recovery occurs within days to weeks after drug cessation. Hormonal replacement therapy (HRT) is safe in patients with liver disease, but jaundiced patients may experience an increase in bilirubin levels; they should be monitored with liver tests [84]

Benign neoplasms
Oral contraceptive steroids can induce enlargement of preexisting hemangiomas through their trophic effects on the vascular endothelium [332]. Recurrences of hemangiomas have also been described in patients with a history of previously resected lesions [333]. A role for estrogens in the pathogenesis of *focal nodular hyperplasia* (FNH) is plausible because these lesions occur principally in young women (up to 86%) [334]. However, unlike liver adenomas, an increased incidence of FNH has not been observed historically commensurate with the increasing use of OCSs after 1960. Further, FNH can occur in men and other persons not using OCSs [334]. A study of over 200 patients with FNH failed to show a relationship between OCSs or with size or number of FNH lesions [334]. Discontinuation of OCSs did not generally influence the size of FNH, and estrogen-dependent tumors were rare. The authors suggested that hepatic adenomas,

misclassified as FNH, could account for the apparent growth of FNH reported previously with OCSs.

The association between OCSs and *hepatic adenomas* was described nearly 40 years ago. The increasing frequency of this neoplasm paralleled the rising use of OCSs. In the 1970s and 1980s, the annual risk was approximately 3–4 per 100,000 exposed persons [26,102], but this risk is probably now lower with the lower dose estrogen preparations currently used. There is also a relationship with duration of OCS use, so that the risk (compared with nonusers) for long-term OCS users (>10 years) is increased 100-fold. Patients with liver adenomas usually present with a painless or tender right upper quadrant mass, or occasionally with hemoperitoneum secondary to hepatic rupture. Adenomas usually regress after OCSs are withdrawn [103]. However, surgery is recommended for larger lesions to avert possible rupture [335] and because of the small but definite risk of malignant transformation. To prevent hepatic adenomas, an OCS with lower estrogenic potency is preferred. Long uninterrupted periods of OCS use should also be avoided.

Hepatocellular carcinoma

The relative risk for HCC is increased two-fold among women who have ever taken OCSs, and it is increased seven-fold in long-term users (>8 years) compared with age-matched controls [27,336,337]. However, it must be emphasized that estrogen-related HCC is rare, accounting for less than 1% of primary liver cancer in western countries. In countries with a high prevalence of HCC, OCS use is not an independent risk factor owing to the far greater importance of chronic viral hepatitis and aflatoxin [27]. Median age at presentation is 30 years (versus 55 years with other cancers), and HCC occurs at least 5 years after starting intake of combination OCS. The tumors are well differentiated, including fibrolamellar HCC, and have a better short-term outcome than HCC due to other causes [14], but most are eventually lethal.

Anabolic steroids
Cholestasis

At high doses, anabolic steroids often produce reversible bland cholestasis, usually within 1–6 months of beginning treatment. Prolonged jaundice with ductopenia is a very rare complication [338]. Acute hepatitis is also an unusual sequel following self-ingestion of high-dose anabolic steroids [339].

Benign neoplasms

The association with hepatic adenomas is less robust. Many reports were from patients with Fanconi anemia [340], a disorder caused by genomic instability and a resultant high background incidence of neoplasms. However, reports of adenomas among female body builders and in persons taking anabolic steroids for other indications [341] show a probable etiologic association. Oral and parenteral androgens are both implicated [337]. Spontaneous hepatic rupture of a presumed hepatic adenoma has been reported; this patient was also receiving warfarin [342].

Hepatic adenomas were identified in three of 11 long-term users of danazol [343], all patients with hereditary angioneurotic edema. Similar lesions have been also described in patients with SLE and endometriosis. For this reason, surveillance ultrasonography is suggested in long-term recipients of danazol [343] and also for former anabolic steroid users; liver tumors have been described up to 24 years after steroid discontinuation [337]. These tumors can regress with androgen withdrawal [344], but this is not always the case and surgical resection may be required. Danazol has also been implicated in one case of acute hepatic failure in a patient with aplastic anaemia; the liver at autopsy showed diffuse necrosis [345].

Hepatocellular carcinoma

Several cases of HCC have been documented [346], but confounding factors such as viral hepatitis were not clearly excluded in earlier cases. Because some of these tumors metastasize very late and sometimes regress [347], doubts have been expressed about their true nature. It is sometimes difficult to distinguish well-differentiated HCC from adenomas [348]. Further, hepatic adenoma and HCC can coexist. Four reports of HCC have been attributed to long-term danazol use [349]; the underlying diseases were hereditary angioneurotic edema, SLE, and chronic idiopathic thrombocytopenic purpura. These liver tumors were large, well-differentiated carcinomas that did not show regression with drug withdrawal. Serum α-fetoprotein levels were normal in three of the four cases.

Estrogen receptor antagonists

The range of tamoxifen hepatotoxicity includes hepatic steatosis, NASH, and rare instances of submassive hepatic necrosis and even cirrhosis. Of these, the association with hepatic steatosis and NASH is most striking. In one series of 66 women with breast cancer who had received tamoxifen for 3–5 years, 24 showed radiologic evidence of hepatic steatosis [350]. In another study, liver biopsies were obtained from 15 women with moderate-to-severe hepatic steatosis (as designated by a liver:spleen CT ratio of <0.5); 14 showed NASH [351]. The median time to development of NAFLD is around 2 years [352,353]. Beyond 2 years, the incidence of NAFLD was not significantly different from subjects receiving placebo [352]. The metabolic profile of these women resembled that of most patients with NASH; half were obese, and hepatic steatosis correlated with increases in body mass index (BMI) [354]. In one multivariate analysis, independent factors associated with NAFLD included tamoxifen use (OR, 8.2) and BMI (OR, 1.13) [353]. Tamoxifen can also induce hypertriglyceridemia, a risk factor for NASH. It therefore seems possible that tamoxifen may play a synergistic role with other factors like hyperlipidemia, obesity, and insulin resistance to cause NASH. A more direct role for tamoxifen has been postulated recently based on the results of a study showing inhibition of intrahepatic fatty acid synthesis, which contributes to steatosis [355].

Physicians should be aware of the high frequency of hepatic steatosis (approximately 30%), as determined by hepatic imaging, or NASH in women treated with tamoxifen. Monitoring patients for this adverse effect should include physical examination for hepatomegaly and liver tests. Some authors have also recommended that hepatic imaging (ultrasonography or CT) be performed annually [356]. Liver biopsy is required to establish the severity of the disorder, particularly if liver test abnormalities fail to resolve after stopping tamoxifen, and also to exclude metastatic breast cancer in difficult cases. Many cases improve after stopping tamoxifen [353]; the median time to normalization was 23 months [range, 5–56 months]. Tamoxifen remains a valuable agent for the treatment of breast cancer, and it is not yet clear whether treatment should always be withdrawn permanently. Preliminary experience with bezafibrate appears promising, with improvement in liver imaging characteristics and AT being demonstrated in a small series [351]. An alternate strategy is to attempt optimization of the metabolic milieu, especially in persons with preexisting hepatic steatosis because they have a threefold risk of developing abnormal glucose tolerance with follow-up [354].

Toremifene, a tamoxifen analog, is associated with a lower frequency (<10%) of steatosis or steatohepatitis [356]. Raloxifene, a selective estrogen receptor modulator, has been implicated in two cases of liver injury, one case with acute hepatocellular injury accompanied by eosinophilia, and NASH in the other. Causality could not be clearly established in the second case because this patient could have had preexisting NAFLD as there were features of the metabolic syndrome [357,358].

Antithyroid drugs

The estimated frequency of hepatotoxicity from antithyroid drugs is less than 0.5% [359]. Methimazole and carbimazole have rarely been incriminated in reports of cholestasis or cholestatic hepatitis [360]. By contrast, propylthiouracil reactions usually result in acute hepatitis [361,362], which can be severe. Hypersensitivity features are frequently present. Histologic appearances range from portal inflammation, hepatic granulomas, and cholestasis in milder forms of hepatitis, to submassive or massive hepatic necrosis in severe cases [362]. Chronic

hepatitis is a rare complication. Ten acute liver failure-related deaths, including one in pregnancy, have been identified from a review of 36 published cases and an additional case report [361,362]. There is a higher than expected frequency of liver injury among children receiving propylthiouracil as compared with methimazole [363]. Most patients recover, but continued ingestion of the drug after symptoms develop can lead to a poor outcome.

Anesthetic agents

Halothane

In the first years after the introduction of halothane in the mid-1950s, most cases of postoperative massive liver necrosis were readily attributable to nonanesthetic causes, such as shock and hypoxia. However, cases of *unexplained massive hepatic necrosis after anesthesia* appeared to be more common after halothane than after the use of other agents [364]. The clinical syndrome was characteristic, and the temporal relationships between exposure to halothane and the development of liver injury were convincing. This evidence, together with the observations of recurrence after deliberate or inadvertent rechallenge eventually led to the acceptance of *halothane hepatitis* as a real entity. Rare cases of halothane-induced liver injury have also occurred after workplace exposure among anesthetists, surgeons, nurses, and laboratory staff, and after halothane sniffing for "recreational" use. Despite its rarity, the severity of cases of halothane hepatitis and the greater availability of equally acceptable agents have contributed to the virtual abandonment of halothane in industrialized nations, but halothane use remains relevant in many parts of Asia and Africa where cases of liver injury still accrue [365].

Two types of postoperative liver injury have followed the use of halothane. Minor elevations of ALT occur between the first and tenth postoperative day in 10–20% of patients, all of whom remain asymptomatic. The risk of hepatic enzyme abnormalities is higher after a second halothane anesthetic than for agents like enflurane, isoflurane, and desflurane [14,366]. This change in liver tests is rapidly reversible. Its relationship to the more severe lesions of halothane hepatitis is unclear. Potentially the changes could be explained by minor nonspecific toxic injury or by ischemia–reperfusion consequent to the profound reduction of hepatic blood flow that can be ascribed to halothane anesthesia. Halothane hepatitis is a rare, dose-independent hepatic drug reaction. After one halothane anesthetic, the frequency is very low (about one per 10,000 persons), but after two or more halothane exposures within a 28-day period, this increases to 15 per 10,000 exposed persons [14].

The reaction is unrelated to the type of surgery, duration of anesthesia, or to the presence of underlying liver disease. Halothane hepatitis is extremely rare in children, and more severe in those over 40 years of age. Two thirds of cases are in women. A key feature is repeated exposure to halothane within a relatively short period of time; this is observed in 80% of cases. Further, many patients give a history of previous unexplained, delayed-onset fever, nausea, or jaundice in the postoperative period. Onset of liver injury is earlier after a repeat administration of halothane, and typically increases in severity with each exposure. Obesity is another risk factor, possibly related to increased halothane storage in adipose tissue or the induction of hepatic CYP2E1, an enzyme involved in halothane metabolism. The induction of CYP enzymes has been implicated experimentally in the pathogenesis of halothane-induced liver injury, and one study indicated that co-administration of antiepileptic drugs predisposed patients to halothane hepatitis [367]. A genetic predisposition to halothane-induced liver injury is evident in guinea pigs, and there are human data to invoke familial predisposition, such as instances of several closely related family members experiencing halothane hepatitis [368,369]. Likewise, with the use of an in vitro test that detected injury to peripheral blood mononuclear cells after exposure to phenytoin epoxide, increased susceptibility was noted among patients with halothane hepatitis and their relatives [370].

Fever is common in the first 48 hours after any major surgery, but fever associated with an adverse reaction to halothane is typically delayed until 3–14 days; occasionally a rash is noted. Jaundice occurs within 21 days of halothane exposure, with the median time to onset 9 days after a single anesthetic and 5 days after multiple exposures. Jaundice is usually preceded or accompanied by symptoms of hepatitis. The liver may be swollen and tender, but in severe cases it decreases in size as a result of extensive hepatic necrosis. Liver failure ensues, with bruising, bleeding, clouding of consciousness, and onset of hepatic coma or hepatorenal failure. Renal failure may develop as part of the hepatorenal syndrome, but acute tubular necrosis could result from a nephrotoxic effect of halothane, as has been better documented for methoxyflurane. Liver histology may show zonal, bridging, or panlobular necrosis.

In milder cases, symptoms may not be attributed to a halothane reaction. It is therefore crucial to elicit a full history of earlier anesthetic exposures to prevent fatal cases of halothane-induced liver injury. In more severe cases, hepatic failure may follow a fulminant course. Apart from acetaminophen hepatotoxicity, halothane was the leading cause of drug-induced liver failure until the mid-1980s. The reported mortality is 10–80%, but the higher rates reflect referral to specialized centers [371,372]. In most cases, though, symptoms resolve within 5–14 days and recovery is complete. Rare cases have been reported in which repeated exposure with halothane was implicated as the cause of chronic liver disease [373].

Although an immunologic mechanism has been invoked as part of the causative mechanism [6], immunosuppressive agents do not alter the clinical outcome. Management centers on intensive medical support. Liver transplantation must be considered in cases with a poor prognosis, as presaged by previous episodes, early onset, a serum bilirubin level of more than 200 μmol/L (10 mg/dL), and a prolongation of prothrombin time. In adults, halothane-induced liver disease could have been prevented in 90% of reported cases by attention to the previous history and adherence to safety guidelines. As many as two thirds of cases occur in individuals with a history of previous reactions to halothane, and the majority of cases are associated with repeated use of halothane within 28 days, especially in obese, middle-aged women.

Because halothane may leach out of the tubing of anesthetic devices, prevention of recurrence in sensitized patients requires that the equipment used for anesthesia should never have been exposed to halothane. Cross-sensitivity between halothane and other haloalkane anesthetics is best documented for methoxyflurane, an agent that is no longer used because of nephrotoxicity. Cross-sensitivity with enflurane is likely and for isoflurane is possible, as described later, but it has not been reported for desflurane and sevoflurane.

There is no readily available diagnostic test for halothane hepatitis. Some interest has surrounded use of an antibody test claimed to be 80% sensitive [8], but independent validation is lacking and the test is not widely available. Diagnosis therefore requires careful consideration of the present and past relationships of liver injury to halothane exposure, and excluding other causes of postoperative jaundice.

Other anesthetic agents

Other than halothane, general anesthetic agents in current use have rarely been associated with postoperative liver failure and massive hepatic necrosis. However, the evidence that such agents cause idiosyncratic hepatic drug reactions is strong only for enflurane [14,374,375]. The likelihood that individual haloalkane anesthetics can cause liver injury is related to the extent to which they are metabolized by hepatic CYP enzymes: 20% for halothane, 2% for enflurane, 1% for sevoflurane, and 0.2% or less for isoflurane and desflurane. Accordingly, the estimated frequency of enflurane-related hepatitis is much less than for halothane. The clinical syndrome is similar, with onset of fever within 3 days and jaundice in 3–19 days. At least one case was proved by positive rechallenge [374]. Two thirds of patients had previously been exposed to either enflurane or halothane.

The possibility that isoflurane could be responsible for DILI is more contentious. More than 50 suspected cases were reported to the FDA by 1986, but in two thirds of these another potential cause of liver injury seemed more likely [375]. In the remainder, isoflurane was only one of several possible factors that could cause hepatic damage. There have been a few case reports in which isoflurane seemed to be the likely cause of fatal hepatotoxicity, either because of repeated exposure to isoflurane in the absence of other potential causes of liver injury [376] or because isoflurane had been administered after possible previous sensitization to halothane [377] or enflurane [378]. Isoflurane should be regarded as a possible but very rare cause of hepatotoxicity; the pathogenic mechanism remains unclear.

The newer haloalkane anesthetics, sevoflurane and desflurane appear mostly free from adverse hepatic events, although rare reports have noted an association of liver injury after desflurane and also with sevoflurane [379], including three fatal cases with submassive hepatic necrosis [380]. Two of three cases involved reexposure to sevoflurane, raising the possibility of an immune-mediated hepatic reaction. The lack of trifluoroacetylated protein formation with sevoflurane no longer exonerates it from causing liver damage – another potential reactive metabolite (compound A) produced by the reaction of sevoflurane with carbon dioxide absorbents in the anesthetic circuit could be responsible [379]. Further, immunoglobulin G4 (IgG4) subclass antibodies to CYP2E1 and a 58 kD endoplasmic protein (ERp58) have been documented in cases of desflurane hepatitis [381]. Unlike patients with liver injury, a different subclass of antibodies (IgG1) has been demonstrated in asymptomatic anesthesiologists exposed to volatile anesthetics [382].

Drugs used in the management of diabetes mellitus

Thiazolidinediones

Troglitazone
Elevated AT levels were noted in 0.5–1.9% of clinical trial recipients [383] but reports of acute liver failure only emerged in the postmarketing phase [384]. Troglitazone was implicated in over 75 instances of fatal hepatotoxicity or liver failure requiring hepatic transplantation [384] before it was withdrawn in 1999. The frequency of acute liver failure was estimated at 240 per 1 million person-years of troglitazone exposure [384].

Troglitazone is metabolized by CYP3A4 and CYP2C8. Unlike the newer thiazolidinediones, it has a unique α-tocopherol side chain that is metabolized to a quinone. This raises the possibility of quinone-related liver injury, similar to acetaminophen or methyldopa hepatotoxicity.

However, the quinone metabolite is less toxic than the parent compound and an alternative hypothesis implicating mitochondrial injury leading to cell death (via necrosis or apoptosis) is currently favored [386,387]. A potentially aggravating factor is bile salt-induced apoptosis resulting from inhibition of the bile salt export pump (Bsep) by troglitazone or by co-administration of cholestasis-inducing drugs such as glibenclamide [388]. Abrogation of inherent cytoprotective mechanisms (e.g., reduction in heat shock protein 70 levels) may also contribute [389]. Finally, features of drug allergy are unusual [383]. Taken together, the existing data are consistent with an idiosyncratic metabolic form of liver injury. However, the evidence for any of these pathways is weak and/or indirect and speculative, as reviewed elsewhere [385,386].

Risk factors for troglitazone hepatotoxicity have not been clearly defined. Reported cases were generally in older women and obese persons, but this represents the common phenotype of those with type 2 diabetes; detailed epidemiologic studies have not been performed [390]. In Japan, persons carrying mutations of CYP2C19 were overrepresented (50%) in a small series of eight patients with troglitazone-induced hepatocellular injury as compared to those without liver injury (13%) [391]. Likewise, Japanese subjects carrying the combined glutathione S transferase GSTT1 GSTM1 null phenotype were three times more likely to develop liver injury. However, this phenotype was present in only about 21–59% of those developing liver toxicity, suggesting that other factors may be important [391]. There is no evidence that preexisting liver disease or other drugs predispose to troglitazone hepatotoxicity, although a progressive course reported in one patient was attributed to concurrent simvastatin and troglitazone [392]. Interaction with NASH, which occurs in at least 20% of obese individuals with type 2 diabetes, has not been explored thoroughly [392]. However, many patients affected by troglitazone-induced liver injury had normal liver tests before starting troglitazone treatment.

The onset of troglitazone hepatotoxicity was often as long as 9 months, and sometimes more than 12 months, after starting treatment [393]; rare cases have had a much earlier onset (3 days) [394]. Patients presented with nausea, fatigue, jaundice, vomiting, and symptoms of liver failure. Progression from jaundice to encephalopathy, liver failure, or death was often rapid (average 24 days) [394], even after detection of biochemical abnormalities before the development of symptoms, and in some cases deterioration continued despite cessation of troglitazone intake. Only 13% survived without receiving a liver transplant [394]. Histology from biopsies, explants, or autopsies showed submassive or massive hepatic necrosis, with postcollapse scarring, bile duct proliferation, and some eosinophils [395]. Severe cholestasis has also been reported [396], but this is sometimes observed in other cases of fulminant hepatic failure (e.g., valproate) and does not necessarily imply any different pathogenic mechanism. The progressive nature of liver injury has been highlighted by patients developing micronodular cirrhosis and portal hypertension after surviving the initial episode of liver injury [397].

Rosiglitazone and pioglitazone

By comparison with troglitazone, serious liver injury is infrequent with these second-generation thiazolidinediones [398]. In clinical trials, a raised ALT ($>3 \times$ ULN) was reported in 0.25% and 0.26% of patients treated with rosiglitazone and pioglitazone, respectively [398]. However, analysis of data derived from the FDA's Adverse Event Reporting System revealed 21 cases of significant hepatotoxicity involving both drugs. The onset of liver injury was within 3 months (median, 9 weeks). Rarely, liver injury can occur beyond 1 year of use [399]. Liver histology appearances have varied from cholestatic hepatitis [400], bile duct injury, or granulomatous hepatitis [401] through to submassive hepatic necrosis in fatal cases. Although earlier case reports noted resolution within 3 months in most cases, the recent FDA series highlighted a more ominous course with a case fatality rate of 81% [402]. Assuming that only 10% of adverse drug reactions are reported, the number needed to harm was calculated as 44,000 patient-years of exposure for rosiglitazone and 52,000 patient-years for pioglitazone. However, the validity of these data have been questioned by the manufacturers [403,404] who point to the lack of liver toxicity in clinical trials, the presence of confounding factors, and the known background risk of acute liver failure in patients with type 2 diabetes receiving oral hypoglycemic drugs (1/10,000 person-years) [405]. On balance, it does appear that the risk of liver injury is lower than that for troglitazone but occasional cases of hepatotoxicity can occur with these two drugs, as well as with any treatment for diabetes [405]. Rosiglitazone has been withdrawn due to its cardiac toxicity, and pioglitazone is being actively studied in trials involving patients with NAFLD.

The FDA recommends baseline liver tests when considering treatment with pioglitazone or rosiglitazone, as well as periodic monitoring. If ALT levels remain persistently elevated ($>3 \times$ ULN), the drug should be discontinued. As with isoniazid, symptoms suggestive of hepatitis should be assessed immediately. Individuals who have developed jaundice with troglitazone should not receive these thiazolidinediones, although cross-toxicity was not a problem in one reported case [400]. However, biochemical screening is not infallible; it cannot identify cases when there is rapid transition from normal AT to liver failure within 1 or 2 weeks [417]. Further, the trogli-

tazone episode has highlighted the low compliance ($<5\%$) with monitoring recommendations. Finally, the positive predictive value of abnormal liver tests is likely to be suboptimal in patients with type 2 diabetes [406] because of confounding factors such as NAFLD/NASH, chronic hepatitis C, or concomitant drug therapy.

Oral hypoglycemic drugs

Liver injury (typically hepatocellular) was common with older sulfonylureas, such as carbutamide, metahexamide, and chlorpropamide [2,14]. Of the currently used agents, tolbutamide, tolazamide, glibenclamide, and glimepiride have rarely been associated with cholestasis or cholestatic hepatitis [2,407–410]. Considering the structural relationship of sulfonylureas to sulfonamides, it is perhaps not surprising that hypersensitivity phenomena (fever, skin rash, eosinophilia) were present in some cases [410]. Most cases resolved after drug withdrawal, but chronic cholestasis progressing to VBDS has been described with tolbutamide and tolazamide [14]. Death from liver failure has been reported in two patients, one of whom had cirrhosis [410]. There are three reports of acute hepatitis induced by gliclazide, with hypersensitivity features present in one case [411]. Glibenclamide has also been associated with hepatocellular liver injury, and with hepatic granulomas [407].

Other antidiabetic agents that have been rarely associated with liver injury include metformin, repaglinide, acarbose, and human insulin (Table 27.11) [411–415].

Analgesics and drugs used to treat rheumatologic diseases

Acetaminophen

Acetaminophen (paracetamol) hepatotoxicity is an important cause of drug-induced liver injury in most countries [416,417]; currently it accounts for approximately 50% of cases of acute liver failure in the United States [417]. When used in recommended doses (1–4 g/day) acetaminophen is extremely safe [418], but single doses exceeding 15–25 g may cause severe liver injury that is fatal in up to a quarter of cases. Acetaminophen hepatotoxicity usually follows deliberate self-poisoning in an attempted suicidal or parasuicidal gesture. However, up to 30% of cases of acetaminophen hepatotoxicity admitted to hospital now result from "therapeutic misadventure" in which the daily dose has not greatly exceeded recommended safe limits but in which specific risk factors were present (see below) [419,420]. Daily doses of 2–6 g have been associated with fatal hepatotoxicity. Cases associated with actual therapeutic doses are rare and may represent inadequate/unreliable disclosure and documentation as well as other risk factors (see below) and late presentation.

Table 27.11 Liver injury associated with drugs used in diabetes mellitus.

Drug	Pattern of liver injury	Comments
Acarbose (glucosidase inhibitor)	Acute hepatitis; most reported cases from Spain (to date). Cholestasis with voglibose (another glucosidase inhibitor)	Positive rechallenge
Human insulin	Mixed liver injury; all reports from Japan. Resolved when changed to porcine insulin	Positive rechallenge
Metformin (biguanide)	Cholestatic hepatitis, cholestasis, acute hepatitis	Very rare
Repaglinide	Acute hepatocellular injury	Single report
Sulfonylureas	Acute hepatitis, cholestasis, cholestatic hepatitis, vanishing bile duct syndrome, granulomatous hepatitis	Usually reversible but fatalities reported
Thiazolidinediones:		
Troglitazone	Submassive or massive hepatic necrosis, cholestasis	Many fatal cases
Rosiglitazone	Acute cholestatic hepatitis, granulomatous hepatitis	Withdrawn from use
Pioglitazone	Acute hepatocellular injury, cholestatic hepatitis, fulminant hepatic failure	Few reports, fatalities rare

Risk factors

Acetaminophen causes dose-dependent liver injury but individual susceptibility is also important. Thus death has followed the ingestion of single doses of 7.5 g in adults or 150 mg/kg in children, whereas survival has been recorded with massive overdoses (50 g or more) [421]. Age alters individual susceptibility: liver injury has been described even in neonates, but children are considered to be relatively resistant to acetaminophen poisoning [423]. This has been attributed to differences in disposition and metabolism of the drug, but relatively larger liver and kidney sizes (as a proportion of total body weight) is an alternative explanation [423]. However, there is increasing recognition that both intentional and unintentional acetaminophen toxicity can occur in children. Prescribing errors have often been involved in these cases, including the use of adult doses, wrong dosing intervals, concomitant use of other acetaminophen-containing or hepatotoxic products, and host factors – particularly fasting, undernutrition, and drug–drug interactions. Rectal preparations of acetaminophen were implicated in a few cases. The bioavailability of acetaminophen in this formulation can vary up to nine-fold. Furthermore, the slower onset of action encourages repetitive use and consequent cumulative toxicity [424]. Although acetaminophen self-poisoning is more common in women, fatal acetaminophen hepatotoxicity occurs more frequently in men; this is largely due to alcoholism and late presentation [21].

The risk of liver injury is also influenced by concomitant medication use; in one study, NSAIDs and fibrates were associated with a decreased risk of fatal liver injury in women while statins were protective in both sexes. In addition, sympathetic stimulants (in men) and ethanol (in both sexes) increased the likelihood of such toxicity [425]. Conversely, concurrent use of angiotensin-converting enzyme inhibitors or angiotensin receptor II antagonists in younger subjects was associated with a reduced likelihood of death. Finally, Gilbert syndrome, – hereditary unconjugated hyperbilirubinemia due to a polymorphism in the promoter sequence of the conjugating enzyme, bilirubin UDP-glucuronyl transferase – lowers the threshold for acetaminophen hepatotoxicity due to lower activity of the glucuronidation pathway of acetaminophen metabolism.

Clinical features

The clinical evolution of liver injury follows three phases. In the first, anorexia, nausea, and vomiting are prominent. This may last from 12 to 24 hours before symptoms often subside, so that the person often feels well during the second phase, which lasts another 24 hours. Signs of hepatic failure, often with renal insufficiency, appear 48–72 hours after ingestion of acetaminophen (phase 3). Pain over the liver may be pronounced. It is accompanied by jaundice, hypoglycemia, coagulopathy, renal failure, lactic acidosis, and encephalopathy. Myocardial injury has also been described [421]. Renal failure can occur, with or without significant liver injury. In untreated subjects, death occurs between 4 and 18 days after drug ingestion, usually from cerebral edema and/or sepsis from multiorgan failure.

ALT levels are markedly elevated (2,000–10,000 IU/L); indeed, when the cause of acute liver injury is unclear (for example, in an unconscious individual or in a person with chronic hepatitis C), such high AT levels should arouse suspicion of acetaminophen toxicity. These high ALT values are unusual in viral hepatitis but may occur with ischemic hepatitis, and with other forms of DILI, including herbal toxicity (see later section). The following clinical and laboratory indices predicate a poor outcome of acetaminophen hepatotoxicity: prothrombin time >100 seconds, serum creatinine >300 μmol/L, a single finding of a pH of <7.3 after adequate fluid replacement, or grade 3 or 4 encephalopathy in patients with a normal pH [426]. Other prognostic indices proposed include the APACHE II score and blood lactate, phosphate, and α-fetoprotein levels [427]. None of these indices has been widely adopted, and they await independent validation.

Histology

This includes zone 3 necrosis, with submassive (bridging) or panacinar (massive) necrosis in severe cases [14]. Inflammatory activity is inconspicuous and resolution occurs without fibrosis. Chronic liver injury has been described in patients consuming moderate doses of acetaminophen (2–6 g each day) for many months. Preexisting liver disease or concurrent alcohol intake were not always excluded in such individuals [14], and the rapid resolution after discontinuing acetaminophen abuse implies a form of chronic hepatotoxicity rather than a syndrome of drug-induced chronic hepatitis.

Acetaminophen toxicity with therapeutic doses ("therapeutic misadventure")

Enhanced susceptibility to acetaminophen toxicity is now well recognized both in alcoholic and nonalcoholic individuals. At least 200 instances of inadvertent hepatotoxicity have been recorded in heavy drinkers, which have followed acetaminophen intake for between 1 day and several weeks. In one series, 40% of individuals had taken acetaminophen in excess of 6 g/day [419], but 35% had taken doses below 4 g/day. In other reports, hepatotoxicity has occurred after as little as 1.5–2 g of acetaminophen a day. Data from the US Acute Liver Failure Group revealed that 60% of persons who had taken an unintentional overdose were using an acetaminophen–narcotic combination. It has been suggested that addiction (and, later, tolerance) to the narcotic component induces repetitive use that may not always be recalled or disclosed by the patient [417]. Alcohol enhances CYP2E1 activity, and accompanying malnutrition may contribute to GSH depletion. As in acute self-poisoning cases, AST and ALT are often 40–1,000-fold elevated above the upper limit of normal. This allows ready distinction of cases of acetaminophen hepatotoxicity from alcoholic hepatitis.

The importance of chronic excessive alcohol intake as a potentiator for susceptibility to acetaminophen hepatotoxicity has recently been challenged because in many case reports invoking such an interaction the person had clearly taken a hepatotoxic dose of acetaminophen [418]. Nonetheless, the authors' experience is that therapeutic misadventures with acetaminophen are a common and clinically important type of DILI [428]. A recent study of alcohol–acetaminophen interaction was conducted in an alcohol detoxification unit, with all trial participants receiving 1 g acetaminophen q.i.d. for 2 days

or placebo [429]. No differences in hepatotoxicity were observed between the two groups. However, the investigators' assertion that acetaminophen can be safely used in patients with chronic alcohol abuse has been criticized on several grounds, including the selection of persons with serum AT levels of less than 120 U/L, which could have excluded a subset with significant underlying liver disease. The FDA recommends that persons taking more than three drinks of alcohol daily should not receive acetaminophen.

In nonalcoholic patients, fasting has emerged as one of the most important risk factors [430], particularly after near complete deprivation of carbohydrate intake for at least 48 hours. This is a particularly important risk factor for acetaminophen hepatotoxicity in young children. Fasting decreases the activity of hepatic conjugation pathways (both glucuronidation and sulfation) for acetaminophen elimination, increases CYP2E1 activity, and depletes hepatic GSH levels. However, others have contended that fasting has been overstated as a risk factor for acetaminophen hepatotoxicity [431]. They maintain that earlier studies were flawed because CYP2E1 and GSH measurements had not been carried out simultaneously; depletion of GSH is also accompanied by a decrease in CYP2E1 activity [432].

Concurrent medications (isoniazid, zidovudine, phenytoin, and other anticonvulsants) are also important. These agents compete for the "safe" conjugation pathways, and may also induce CYP3A4 (phenytoin) or CYP2E1 (isoniazid), the net effect of which is to promote CYP-mediated oxidation of acetaminophen to its reactive intermediate, *N*-acetyl-*p*-benzoquinone imine (NAPQI). However, human studies do not appear to support a phenytoin–acetaminophen adverse interaction. It is contended that phenytoin induces CYP3A4 only, a relatively minor metabolic pathway; further, it enhances glucuronidation, a key detoxification step [431]. Severe cardiopulmonary disease and renal failure have also been described as settings for acetaminophen hepatotoxicity [432], although the importance of metabolic factors or impaired (fluctuating) hepatic blood flow was not clarified in these studies.

Mechanism of liver injury and the basis for antidote therapy

Acetaminophen undergoes metabolism to glucuronide and sulfate conjugates, which are excreted in the urine. Normally, only a small proportion (~5%) of acetaminophen is oxidized to NAPQI. This reaction is catalyzed by CYP2E1 (which increases with fasting, INH, and chronic alcohol intake) and, to a lesser extent, by CYP3A4 (induced by anticonvulsants, several other drugs, and possibly alcohol). The small amounts of NAPQI formed with pharmacologic doses of acetaminophen are readily detoxified by hepatic GSH; hepatorenal injury only occurs when GSH reserves are depleted. This provides a rationale for administering *N*-acetylcysteine and methionine, known thiol donors that can replenish intracellular GSH stores [421]. NAPQI binds cellular proteins, including oxidation of thiol groups in mitochondria leading to mitochondrial permeability transition [433]. The ensuing mitochondrial dysfunction generates profound oxidative stress and also facilitates peroxynitrite formation; the latter can also undergo covalent binding with key proteins and further aggravate mitochondrial dysfunction. These events culminate in nuclear and cytoplasmic swelling, cytoplasmic vacuolization, and mitochondrial swelling (oncotic necrosis or oncosis) of hepatocytes and sinusoidal endothelial cells. While apoptosis also occurs, oncosis is considered the principal mode of cell death [434].

Immune mechanisms (in particular, the hepatic innate system) have been increasingly implicated in acetaminophen hepatotoxicity. Acetaminophen-induced hepatocyte death leads to the release of free DNA and the subsequent activation of Toll-like receptor 9 (TLR-9). This activates nuclear factor κB (NF-κB) to increase production of interleukin 1 (IL1) and other cytokines and chemokines leading to neutrophil recruitment. The end result is the amplification of the initial toxic insult [435]. Depletion of natural killer cells (NK cells) and natural killer cell with T-cell receptors (NKT cells) also protects against acetaminophen liver toxicity in mice [436]. As expected, such reduction in liver injury was accompanied by decreased expression of proinflammatory cytokines and chemokines, and reduced neutrophil recruitment.

Prevention of liver injury

Adherence to the recommended therapeutic dose should be stressed as a public health measure. However, both prescribers and consumers should be made aware of the increased risk of acetaminophen toxicity in those who consume excess alcohol and in the setting of prolonged fasting, cardiorespiratory disease, and where other drugs are also being used. Recently, doubts have been expressed about the safety of acetaminophen in patients with underlying liver disease. Although acetaminophen is not contraindicated in such persons, the finding of detectable serum levels of acetaminophen in 20% of persons with acute viral hepatitis-related acute liver failure has raised questions about the safety of acetaminophen in both acute and chronic liver disease [437]. There is a public health need to revise downwards and promulgate altered dosage guidelines for acetaminophen when used in regular daily doses under any of the above high-risk circumstances.

To reduce the impact of impulsive self-poisoning, attempts have been made to restrict pack sizes and change the packing (to bubble packs) of acetaminophen by legislation in the United Kingdom. This has been associated with a 66% reduction in the number of liver transplants for acetaminophen overdose, as well as a reduction in mortality (by 21%) [438]. However, the impact has not been uniform, with only a transient decline in Scotland, and it remains unclear whether the decline in adverse outcomes is attributable to this measure alone [438].

Management of acetaminophen overdose

Gastric lavage with a wide-bore tube is performed in all patients presenting within 4 hours of acetaminophen overdose. Activated charcoal and osmotic cathartics are of no benefit. Serum levels of acetaminophen are often determined at baseline, but a 4-hour postingestion level is a more reliable predictor of the risk of liver injury [439]. The need for antidote treatment is assessed from blood acetaminophen levels by reference to well-established nomograms [440,441]. The 4-hour serum acetaminophen concentration may be misleading in overdoses with extended release preparations [442]; blood acetaminophen levels should be estimated after a further 4–6 hours [442]. In persons presenting with nonaccidental or staggered ingestion of acetaminophen, the total dose ingested and time from ingestion to presentation are important determinants of liver injury. In these cases, hepatotoxicity is likely if the time interval exceeds 24 hours or if the total acetaminophen dose exceeds 150 mg/kg (75 mg/kg in high-risk individuals); *N*-acetylcysteine (NAC) therapy is initiated beyond these thresholds [443].

NAC is the principal antidote. By functioning as a thiol donor, NAC replenishes hepatocellular cytosolic and mitochondrial glutathione stores, and also provides mitochondrial energy substrates [444]. Significant hepatotoxicity is rare when NAC is administered within 16 hours of drug ingestion. Beyond 16 hours, oxidation of acetaminophen to NAPQI is complete and thiol donation is unlikely to prevent hepatocyte or renal tubular cell death. Nevertheless, the benefits of NAC have been shown to extend to patients presenting up to 24 hours after the ingestion, even in patients with acute liver failure [445]. The beneficial effects of NAC in acute liver failure were attributed to improved tissue oxygen delivery [445], although this has been disputed [446].

NAC is administered intravenously in Europe and Australia, and by mouth in the United States [441,447]. The intravenous regimen is now approved by the FDA for persons who cannot or will not tolerate oral NAC.

Treatment protocol

An oral loading dose of 140 mg/kg is followed by 4-hour administration of half this dose for up to 72 hours. Oral

NAC can be discontinued after 48 hours in persons meeting specific criteria at that time (normal liver tests and undetectable acetaminophen levels) [448]. Intravenous administration involves a loading dose (150 mg/kg) of NAC given slowly over 15 minutes, followed by a 4-hour infusion (50 mg/kg) and a 100 mg/kg infusion over 16 hours. A third intravenous (48 hour) protocol has also been evaluated [449]. It has been suggested that, for high-risk patients, the incidence of hepatotoxicity is lower with the oral and 48-hour intravenous regimens when compared to 20-hour intravenous infusion, but direct comparisons have not been performed. A retrospective study using historical controls favoured the use of 20-hour IV NAC for patients presenting within 12 hours of ingestion, and a 72-hour oral NAC regimen for late presentations (>18 hours postingestion) [450]. Only the 20-hour intravenous protocol has been approved by the FDA.

Anaphylactoid reactions to IV NAC are relatively common (6–15%) [451]. They are generally mild and rarely lead to treatment discontinuation, but severe reactions can occur. Male gender and a family history of allergy (OR, 2.89) were identified as risk factors for the development of an anaphylactoid reaction [452]; paradoxically, high plasma acetaminophen concentrations [453] were found to be protective. Guidelines to deal with such reactions [451] include observation during drug administration (with appropriate antidotes readily available), discontinuing the infusion with the onset of angioedema or respiratory symptoms, the administration of antihistaminics, and resumption of the infusion after 1 hour if there are no persistent symptoms. For minor reactions, such as flushing, the infusion can be slowed or continued uninterrupted [451].

Other thiol donors such as methionine may be effective but must be administered within 10 hours. Methionine solutions need to be freshly prepared and often cause troublesome vomiting; their use is restricted to patients with hypersensitivity to NAC. Managing acetaminophen overdoses in pregnant women and in children is along usual lines; in one small study, NAC did not have any major adverse effects to the fetus [454].

Treatment of acute liver failure is described in Chapter 19. Assessment for liver transplantation requires consideration of the psychosocial factors underlying self-poisoning, and the likelihood of survival without transplantation. When liver transplantation has been performed, survival rates exceed 70% [455,456] and long-term outcomes appear reasonable. Still, there are real concerns with regards to noncompliance with medications and the prospect of repeated self-harm in survivors, stressing the need for detailed psychiatric evaluation and support before and after transplantation [455,456].

Dextropropoxyphene

Adverse drug reactions are rare with this opioid analgesic but important, particularly as liver injury may occur in the postoperative period or in other medically complex situations. At least 25 cases of cholestasis with bile duct injury have been reported [86], some proved by inadvertent rechallenge. The majority of those affected are women. Abdominal pain is the most impressive symptom. It is often severe and resembles pain from other causes of cholangitis with which it is often confused, particularly as jaundice is usually present. However, the large bile ducts appear normal at cholangiography. Liver histology shows portal tract edema, irregularity and necrosis of the biliary epithelium, bile ductular proliferation, and a peribiliary infiltrate of neutrophils and eosinophils. Cholestasis is usually evident. Recovery occurs within 1–3 months of stopping dextropropoxyphene.

Nonsteroidal anti-inflammatory drugs

NSAIDs are among the most commonly used prescription and nonprescription drugs, with up to 15% of the population using them in any one year. AT abnormalities are observed in up to 15% of patients taking NSAIDs, but overt hepatotoxicity is much less common with currently used agents. There are distinct differences in the frequency of hepatic injury associated with individual NSAIDs [457], with some agents being virtually free from reported hepatotoxicity and others such as bromfenac, benoxaprofen, and ibufenac having been withdrawn because of fatal liver injury (Table 27.12) [458]. Several pharmacoepidemiologic studies have attempted to categorize risk factors associated with NSAID-associated liver injury, and also to ascertain the hepatotoxic potential of individual NSAIDs. The results of these studies have been conflicting, which could be attributed to methodologic differences, including study settings (hospital versus ambulatory care) and study definitions. Focusing on studies with significant clinical events (i.e., hospitalization and death), Rubenstein and colleagues conducted a systematic review and found a slight (but not significant) increase in the risk of liver injury for current as compared with former NSAID users (OR, 1.2–1.7; P = NS) [458]. Contrary to general belief, women and the elderly were not found to be at greater risk. However, in another study carried out in an ambulatory care setting in France, gender differences were striking; after adjustment for confounding factors, there was a significant association between liver injury and NSAID use in women (OR, 6.49 (1.67–25.2)) [459]. Other risk factors identified in the Rubenstein review were rheumatoid arthritis (as compared with osteoarthritis) and use of nimesulide or sulindac.

Table 27.12 Liver injury associated with salicylates and nonsteroidal anti-inflammatory drugs.

Drug	Pattern of liver injury	Comments
Aspirin and other salicylates	Dose-dependent hepatocellular injury, Reye syndrome (febrile children)	Similar toxicity with sodium salicylate, mesalamine; diflunisal causes cholestasis
Bromfenac	Acute hepatitis, fulminant hepatic failure	Withdrawn from clinical use
Clometacin	Acute or chronic hepatitis, cholestatic hepatitis, cirrhosis, granulomatous hepatitis	Fatalities recorded. Female predominance (chronic hepatitis); some reported cases were later found to have hepatitis C virus infection
COX-2 inhibitors	Cholestatic hepatitis (few reports) with celecoxib or rofecoxib	Overall incidence low
Diclofenac	Acute hepatitis, chronic hepatitis	Women, older patients with osteoarthritis
Ibuprofen	Acute hepatitis, vanishing bile duct syndrome (rare); hepatotoxic potential is low	Hepatocellular injury with pirprofen, fenoprofen, flurbiprofen, and ketoprofen; cholestasis (tiaprofenic acid)
Indomethacin	Acute hepatitis, cholestasis, massive hepatic necrosis (rare)	Low incidence of toxicity
Naproxen	Mixed liver injury	Low incidence of toxicity
Nimesulide	Acute hepatitis, acute liver failure, cholestasis	Female predominance (with acute hepatitis)
Phenylbutazone	Acute hepatitis, cholestasis, granulomatous hepatitis	Similar toxicity as oxyphenbutazone
Piroxicam	Hepatocellular, cholestasis, massive/submassive hepatic necrosis (at least six reports)	Low incidence. Isoxicam and droxicam cause acute cholestatic hepatitis
Oxaprozin	Hepatocellular, fulminant hepatitis	
Sulindac	Cholestatic hepatitis (predominant), acute hepatitis	Hypersensitivity features common

COX-2, cyclooxygenase 2

NSAID-associated hepatic disease encompasses a clinicopathologic spectrum from acute self-limited hepatitis, cholestasis, cholestatic hepatitis, and hepatic granulomas to fulminant hepatic failure, chronic hepatitis, and chronic cholestasis with ductopenia (Table 27.12) [458]. Consistent with the diverse chemical structures of NSAIDs, both immunologic and metabolic idiosyncratic mechanisms have been invoked.

Sulindac

Sulindac is structurally related to indomethacin but has been implicated more often in DILI. Cholestatic reactions predominate, although appreciable hepatic inflammation was noted in 25% of cases [460]. Sulindac has also been associated with acute pancreatitis, and this may cause extrahepatic biliary obstruction. Women appear more susceptible to liver injury (female:male ratio 3.5:1). Nearly 70% of affected individuals are over 50 years old [460]. Hypersensitivity features characteristic of the RMS are common; these include fever, eosinophilia, and cutaneous reactions, including Stevens–Johnson syndrome. Other proposed mechanisms of liver injury include inhibition of multiple hepatic transport proteins by the drug or its metabolites [461] and a synergistic interaction with

tumour necrosis factor α (TNF-α); the latter is particularly relevant to the use of sulindac in inflammatory states [462]. Resolution often follows drug cessation but protracted cholestasis can occur. The overall case fatality rate is approximately 5%, attributable both to sequelae of systemic hypersensitivity reactions (Stevens–Johnson syndrome, nephrotoxicity) as well as the liver injury.

Ibuprofen

Ibuprofen rarely causes significant hepatic injury. In the few reported cases, the reactions have been hepatocellular or mixed hepatocellular–cholestatic [14]. There are three case reports of VBDS, including two pediatric cases with associated Stevens–Johnson syndrome; two of these were referred for liver transplantation and the other had prolonged cholestasis [463,464]. The presence of rash, fever, and eosinophilia is suggestive of an immunoallergic reaction. Rare cases of subacute liver failure have followed therapeutic doses as well as ibuprofen overdose. Explant histology showed submassive necrosis [463] or microvesicular steatosis [465]. Recent reports of acute hepatitis induced by ibuprofen ingestion among HCV-positive patients are of interest, but need to be confirmed [57].

Other propionic acid derivatives

Bromfenac has been implicated in several cases of acute liver failure resulting in death or necessitating liver transplantation (Table 27.12) [466]. In most cases, treatment had been instituted for more than 90 days before patients developed malaise and fatigue, followed by symptoms of severe hepatitis that progressed to liver failure over 5 to 37 days. There were no extrahepatic features of drug allergy. The liver pathology showed confluent or zonal necrosis and a predominantly lymphocyte infiltrate. Other propionic acid derivatives associated with liver injury include fenoprofen, ketoprofen, pirprofen, and tiaprofenic acid [15,42].

Diclofenac

Diclofenac has been implicated in more than 200 published cases of hepatic injury [467], some severe and with occasional fatalities. In several cases, causality has been proved by inadvertent rechallenge. Significant hepatotoxicity occurs in about 1–5 per 100,000 persons exposed [24]. Acute hepatitis or mixed hepatocellular–cholestatic injury is characteristic, but chronic hepatitis resembling autoimmune hepatitis has been reported [468]. Women, the elderly, and patients with osteoarthritis appear to be susceptible to diclofenac-induced liver injury. A comparative study of diclofenac with nabumetone found a better safety profile for the latter in elderly patients, with no patient developing an ALT elevation >2 × ULN as compared to 4% in the diclofenac group [469]. However, the relevance of ALT elevation to cases of overt liver disease is unclear.

A prodromal illness or symptoms of hepatitis herald the onset of liver injury, most often within 3 months (range, 1–11 months) of starting diclofenac treatment. This is followed by jaundice and liver failure in severe cases. Fever and rash occur in 25%. Liver tests usually reflect acute hepatitis, but some features of cholestasis may be present; jaundice occurred in 50% of reported cases [467]. In some cases, the clinicopathologic features of ascites, hypoalbuminemia, and hyperglobulinemia indicate chronic liver disease. Liver biopsies usually show acute lobular hepatitis, but confluent necrosis may be seen in severe cases. In chronic cases, periportal inflammation (interface hepatitis) and fibrous expansion of portal tracts are noteworthy.

Resolution usually follows cessation of diclofenac, although fatalities have been recorded, particularly in elderly subjects. Corticosteroids were used successfully in a few cases of chronic diclofenac-induced hepatitis when no clinical improvement had been evident at 3 months after drug discontinuation [469]. Cross-sensitivity between NSAIDs is rare, but has been reported with ibuprofen in a person with a history of diclofenac

hepatitis; another had an adverse reaction to tiaprofenic acid [468].

Pathogenic mechanisms involved in diclofenac toxicity include oxidative stress alone or in combination with mitochondrial injury [470]. In certain cases, immune mechanisms may be relevant, especially in those presenting with chronic hepatitis. The presence of diclofenac metabolite–protein adducts in liver tissue raises the possibility of liver injury resulting from direct disruption of critical cellular functions or by elicitation of an immune response to these neoantigens [471]. Supporting this hypothesis is the finding that certain polymorphisms favoring a T helper cell 2 (Th2) mediated antibody response were found more often among patients with diclofenac hepatotoxicity than in healthy controls and persons receiving diclofenac without hepatotoxicity [471]. Genetic susceptibility to diclofenac toxicity is supported by an increased frequency of polymorphisms within genes (*UGT2B7*, *CYP2C8*) encoding metabolic pathways involved in the formation and biliary excretion of bile (*ABCC2*) [472].

Piroxicam

The frequency of hepatic injury with this oxicam derivative is low [14]. Acute hepatitis and cholestasis have been described, and there have been at least six cases of massive or submassive hepatic necrosis [14]. The reaction appears to be dose independent, and immunoallergic features have not been conspicuous. Other oxicam derivatives implicated occasionally in cases of acute cholestatic hepatitis include isoxicam and droxicam [42].

Salicylates

Aspirin causes dose-dependent hepatic injury, usually with increased AT levels. Overt jaundice is uncommon, occurring in less than 5% of those affected [14]. Patients with hypoalbuminemia, juvenile rheumatoid arthritis, and SLE are especially susceptible to salicylate-induced liver injury [14]. Hepatitis resolves rapidly after drug withdrawal and usually does not recur after reintroduction of salicylates at a lower dose. Blood levels of salicylate should not exceed 24 mg/L [14]. Only one death has been recorded [473]. Focal necrosis and lobular inflammation are usual. Other salicylates can cause similar injury [474]. Epidemiologic studies have linked the use of aspirin in febrile children with Reye syndrome but concerted public health campaigns have lead to a major decline (near abolition) in incidence in this disorder.

Ticlopidine is not an NSAID but is discussed here with aspirin because it also inhibits platelet aggregation and is often used for similar indications. Unlike aspirin, ticlopidine-induced hepatotoxicity is dose independent and associated predominantly with cholestasis. More than 30 cases have been reported [475]. The majority of cases have been in individuals over 55 years old. The onset of symptoms is between 2 and 12 weeks. Rarely, symptoms may commence 1 month after the drug is withdrawn [476]. Histology shows bland cholestasis but cholestatic hepatitis with bile duct injury has been described. Recovery is usual within 3–6 months, but occasionally may take longer than a year [477]. Eosinophilia in some cases and a positive in vitro T-cell stimulation study to ticlopidine have been cited as favoring an immune basis for the liver injury [477]. An association with several HLA subtypes has been reported in Japanese patients; of these, HLA-A*3303 has been linked to cholestatic pattern of liver toxicity (OR, 36.5) [478]. This allele is more common in Asians (11.7%) than in Caucasians (0.53%) and its role in non-Japanese cases awaits clarification.

Although corticosteroids appear to have aided recovery in some cases, their routine use cannot be justified in this older group of patients (mean age, 67 years). One report of cytomegalovirus-associated acute hepatitis following corticosteroid therapy in this setting is a timely reminder of the risks associated with steroid use in this group [479].

Clopidogrel has been successfully substituted for ticlopidine in patients with cholestasis but it is also associated with hepatocellular or hepatocellular–cholestatic injury [480]. Of the 13 reported cases, the onset was between 3 days and 6 months. Positive rechallenge has been documented. All recovered within 1–6 months [480].

Cyclooxygenase 2 inhibitors

In clinical trials, the frequency of hepatic dysfunction (0.8%) with celecoxib was not significantly different from placebo-treated (0.9%) subjects [481]. A recent pooled analysis of 41 studies reiterated these findings and highlighted the lower frequency of hepatic adverse events (1.1%) as compared with diclofenac (4.2%) [482]. However, celecoxib has been now incriminated in a few reports of severe acute cholestatic hepatitis [483]; two patients developed acute liver failure and needed liver transplantation [483]. Another had alcoholic cirrhosis, which raises questions of celecoxib safety in persons with reduced hepatic reserve [484].

Symptoms suggestive of liver injury develop between 4 days to up to 3 weeks after commencing celecoxib. Pruritus, jaundice, and malaise are accompanied by a mixed hepatocellular–cholestatic biochemical profile. Peripheral eosinophilia has been observed in some cases. Resolution occurs within 4 months of discontinuing celecoxib.

Rofecoxib, now withdrawn due to cardiovascular toxicity, was associated with a few reports of cholestatic hepatitis, some prolonged [485].

Nimesulide, another NSAID with preferential COX-2 selectivity has also been associated with several instances of hepatocellular injury, cholestasis, and occasional cases of fulminant hepatic failure [486–488]. Six of 32 patients

with acute liver failure of unknown cause presenting to an Irish liver transplant unit between 1994 and 2007 had received nimesulide in the past 6 months; causality assessment implicated this drug in all six cases [487]. Five were middle-aged women, but equal gender distribution was noted in a report from an Italian registry. The latter report emphasized the high frequency (78%) of patients presenting with jaundice (34% for other drugs) among the nimesulide group. Three of their 14 cases developed signs of liver failure. Interestingly, many of the 14 cases had received a single dose of the medication [488].

Allopurinol

Granulomatous hepatitis is a typical feature of liver injury with allopurinol [489]. Other manifestations include increased ATs in asymptomatic persons, cholestasis, and hepatocellular injury, which can be occasionally severe enough to progress to fulminant hepatic failure. Severe centrilobular hemorrhagic necrosis resembling Budd–Chiari syndrome has also been described [490]. Exfoliative dermatitis, fever, eosinophilia, interstitial nephritis, and microangiopathic vasculitis may be present in these cases. In a few severe cases, corticosteroids have been used with apparent benefit [491].

Benzbromarone, a uricosuric agent, now withdrawn, has been implicated in causing chronic hepatitis, cirrhosis, and fulminant hepatic failure [42]. However, this has been disputed by a review of published data by Lee et al., where only one of four published cases had incontrovertible evidence of DILI [492].

Gold

Hepatic toxicity of gold (gold sodium thiomalate) is usually characterized by mild cholestatic hepatitis. Onset is within 1–4 weeks. Fever, rash, and eosinophilia are often present. Liver biopsies show canalicular cholestasis with minimal hepatocellular degeneration or portal tract inflammation. Resolution is the rule; fatalities are extremely rare [42]. Rarely, prolonged cholestasis with ductopenia and other accompanying features of VBDS (sialadenitis, sicca syndrome) can occur [493]. Hypersensitivity features such as skin rash and peripheral and tissue eosinophilia were present in this case.

Hepatocellular injury is less common, but can be severe, resulting in death [494]. This severe reaction to gold appears to be dose dependent and is more likely the consequence of metabolic toxicity than for cases presenting with cholestatic hepatitis. Submassive or massive hepatic necrosis with a mixed inflammatory infiltrate is observed on liver biopsies. Resolution can be slow [495]. Gold accumulates in the lysosomes ("aurosomes") in persons undergoing long-term crysotherapy. It has been proposed that liver injury occurs when the lysosomal storage capacity for gold is exceeded [495]. Other gold compounds containing the same aurothio side group as gold sodium thiomalate (gold thiosulfate, aurothioglucose) are also associated with similar liver injury. Recently, acute cholestatic hepatitis has been reported following an overdose of gold potassium cyanide, a nonaurothiogold compound used in electroplating [496].

Penicillamine

Used in the treatment of Wilson disease and as a disease-modifying agent in rheumatoid arthritis, D-penicillamine has been associated with a range of side effects from nephrotoxicity to provoking autoimmune phenomena. Liver injury is less frequent. Most reports are of cholestatic hepatitis in association with hypersensitivity features [42]. These occur within 2 weeks of commencing treatment. The prognosis is good with resolution occurring within a few weeks after cessation of penicillamine; fatalities are rare [497].

Leflunomide

Leflunomide is a disease-modifying antirheumatic drug. Its principal metabolite, A771726, is highly metabolized and eliminated via the liver. CYP2C9 is probably involved in its metabolism. In clinical trials, 5% of recipients showed mild, reversible changes in AT levels. Concerns about significant liver toxicity were first highlighted by the European Medicines Evaluation agency, which had received 296 reports of hepatic adverse effects, including 15 cases of liver failure with nine of these cases having a fatal outcome. However, assigning a cause–effect relationship has proved problematic because many (78%) were receiving other potentially hepatotoxic drugs, including NSAIDs and methotrexate. Further, other confounding factors were present: alcohol use, abnormal baseline liver tests, heart failure, and failure to comply with recommended doses. The low hepatotoxic potential of leflunomide compared with methotrexate was confirmed in two large cohorts involving over 40,000 patients [498]. A special committee of the FDA concluded that the risk of hepatotoxicity was small with leflunomide, thereby permitting its continued usage [499].

Special caution is advised when leflunomide is used with methotrexate. AT increases are seen more often in persons receiving this combination (22%) as compared with recipients of methotrexate plus placebo (5%). However, normalization of AT was achieved without dose change (59%) or a single dose decrease (29%) [500]. Nevertheless, continued vigilance is necessary because early changes of cirrhosis were observed in a patient taking both these drugs [500]. It has been also suggested that persons carrying a low metabolizing activity polymorphism (e.g., CYP2C9*3) may be at an increased risk of liver injury [501].

The manufacturer recommends baseline and monthly monitoring of liver tests for the first 6 months and thereafter every 2 months. Minor ALT changes ($<2 \times$ ULN) should prompt retesting in 2–4 weeks. Dose reduction (from 20 to 10 mg) is suggested if ALT increases above $2 \times$ ULN. Increases of ALT greater than $3 \times$ ULN or persistent ALT abnormalities should prompt drug withdrawal, together with the use of cholestyramine to facilitate the elimination of leflunomide.

Oncotherapeutic and immunosuppressive drugs

Systemic malignancy is commonly associated with abnormal liver tests [14]. In addition to the direct and indirect effects of neoplastic cells, radiotherapy, sepsis, concurrent medication, viral hepatitis, parenteral nutrition, and hypoxemia may contribute to hepatic liver test abnormalities. This makes it difficult to interpret changes or assign liver toxicity to individual drugs. Interactive toxicity between individual oncotherapeutic drugs also merits special consideration. This is exemplified by the development of hepatic SOS (VOD) with combination chemotherapy, and the potentiation of doxorubicin hepatotoxicity by 6-mercaptopurine.

Antimetabolites and antibiotics are more often linked to significant liver injury than are alkylating agents. Hepatocellular injury is characteristic, but a wide range of histologic lesions may be encountered [15,502]. Steatosis is often present, especially with dactinomycin, L-asparaginase, and methotrexate. Cholestasis is typically associated with the hormonal agents, but can be a feature of liver injury with azathioprine and IL2. A range of vascular lesions, including peliosis hepatis, SOS (VOD), and NRH have been observed, usually in the setting of bone marrow or renal transplantation. Chronic hepatitis can rarely occur with doxorubicin and azathioprine, but cirrhosis is distinctly uncommon, except with methotrexate (discussed below). The hepatotoxicity of commonly used oncotherapeutic agents is summarized in Table 27.13. More in-depth discussions of the subject can be obtained from recent reviews and texts [2,15, 502,503].

Methotrexate

The hepatotoxic potential of methotrexate was recognized soon after it was introduced in the 1950s for the treatment of acute childhood leukemia; significant hepatic fibrosis and cirrhosis were reported in up to 25% of patients [14]. Methotrexate is now used more often in a low-dose weekly regimen for treating rheumatoid arthritis, psoriasis, and other immunologic conditions, including inflammatory bowel disease. The hepatoxicity of low-dose regimens is much lower, but is still debated [504,505]. Although ultrastructural changes can occur,

Table 27.13 Liver injury associated with oncotherapeutic drugs.

Drug	Pattern of liver injury
Antimetabolites	
Azathioprine	Cholestasis, vascular injury, peliosis hepatis, SOS (VOD)
Capecitabine	Hyperbilirubinemia (likely related to hemolysis)
Cytosine arabinoside	Raised AT (with low doses), cholestasis, or hepatocellular injury (with high doses)
5-Fluorouracil	Rare liver injury with intravenous and intra-arterial route (particularly when associated with levamisole); hepatic steatosis; floxuridine causes PSC-like lesions
Gemcitabine	Transient AT changes, cholestatic hepatitis leading to acute liver failure, SOS (VOD)
6-Mercaptopurine	Bland cholestasis, hepatocellular or mixed injury, fatal hepatic necrosis (rare)
Methotrexate	Steatosis, hepatic fibrosis, cirrhosis
6-Thioguanine	SOS (VOD) (in combination treatment), peliosis, hepatocellular injury, or cholestasis (rare)
Antibiotics	
Bleomycin	Low incidence of liver toxicity
Cyclosporin	Mild cholestasis (more accurately – impaired bilirubin transport), usually reversible with dose modification
Dactinomycin	Hepatopathy–thrombocytopenia syndrome (with vincristine), clinically resembles SOS (VOD)
Daunorubicin	SOS (VOD) (in combination treatment)
Doxorubicin	Rarely acute or chronic hepatitis; hepatotoxicity enhanced by 6-mercaptopurine
Mithramycin (plicamycin)	Raised AT (in up to 100%); occasionally centrilobular necrosis, steatosis
Mitomycin C	SOS (VOD), steatosis
Mitoxantrone	Minor increase in AT
Spindle inhibitors	
Paclitaxel, docetaxel	Minor increase in AT
Vincristine	Transient liver enzyme changes; synergistic with irradiation in producing liver injury
Platinum	Liver injury rare
Carboplatin	Acute liver failure (one case), SOS (VOD) (with etoposide)
Cisplatin	Raised AT (high doses), steatosis, cholestasis, minor hepatic necrosis
Oxaliplatin	SOS (VOD)
Topoisomerase inhibitors	
Etoposide	Frequent liver test abnormalities (high dose); occasionally severe hepatitis (standard dose)
Irinotecan, topotecan	Abnormal liver tests; hepatic steatosis and nonalcoholic steatohepatitis (irinotecan)
Alkylating agents	Low incidence of liver injury with this group
Busulfan	Cholestasis, porphyria cutanea tarda, NRH, SOS (VOD) (in combination treatment)
Capecitabine	Hepatocellular
Chlorambucil	Hepatocellular, cholestatic hepatitis, acute liver failure
Cyclophosphamide	Hepatocellular, SOS (VOD) (in combination treatment), steatosis
Ifosfamide	Liver injury rare, cholestasis (two cases)
Melphalan	Minor increase in AT
Thiotepa	Severe hepatotoxicity resembling phosphorus poisoning (rare)
Nitrosoureas	
BCNU, CCNU, streptozotocin	Minor increase in AT; rare fatalities from liver injury (BCNU, CCNU)
Hormonal agents	
Aminoglutethamide	Cholestasis
Flutamide	Cholestatic hepatitis, fulminant hepatic failure; megesterol acetate associated with cholestasis
Tamoxifen	Steatosis, NASH, rarely submassive hepatic necrosis and cirrhosis
Miscellaneous drugs	
Amsacrine	Hepatocellular injury, cholestasis, rarely fatal hepatic necrosis
L-Asparaginase	Microvesicular steatosis, hepatic necrosis, coagulopathy (also with pegasparaginase)
Dacarbazine (DTIC)	SOS (VOD)
Procarbazine, hydroxyurea	Hepatocellular injury

AT, aminotransferases; NASH, nonalcoholic steatohepatitis; NRH, nodular regenerative hyperplasia; PSC, primary sclerosing cholangitis; SOS, sinusoidal obstruction syndrome; VOD, venoocclusive disease.

Original references can be obtained from those cited in references [2,14,532].

Table 27.14 Risk factors for methotrexate liver toxicity.

Risk factor	Importance	Implications for prevention
Age >60 years	Increased risk (? reduced renal clearance)	Greater care in use of methotrexate for older people
Dose	Incremental dose	5–15 mg/week very safe
	Dose frequency	Weekly bolus (pulse) safer than daily schedules
	Duration of therapy	Consider review of hepatic status every 2–3 years
	Cumulative (total) dose	Review hepatic status after each 2 g methotrexate given
Alcohol consumption	Increased risk with daily levels of >15 g (1–2 standard drinks)	Avoid methotrexate use if intake not curbed Consider pretreatment liver biopsy
Obesity, diabetes, metabolic syndrome	Increased risk	Consider pretreatment and progress liver biopsies
Preexisting liver disease	Greatly increased risk Particularly related to alcohol, obesity, and diabetes (NASH)	Pretreatment liver biopsy mandatory Avoid methotrexate, or schedule progress biopsies according to severity of hepatic fibrosis, total dose, and duration of methotrexate therapy. Monitor liver tests during therapy (see text)
Folate supplements	Increased risk of liver injury in persons not receiving folic acid	Concurrent folate therapy recommended
Systemic disease	Risk greater with psoriasis than rheumatoid arthritis	None
Impaired renal function	Reduced systemic clearance of methotrexate	Reduce dose; greater caution with use

NASH, nonalcoholic steatohepatitis.

clinically significant liver disease is now rarely if ever encountered.

The development of hepatic fibrosis during methotrexate therapy is greatly influenced by the factors listed in Table 27.14. Pretreatment variables, such as older age, renal failure, preexisting liver disease, and risk factors for NASH (diabetes, obesity) should be carefully considered before commencing treatment with methotrexate [504]. Alcohol intake, preexisting liver disease, and the total and incremental dose are the most important of these risk factors. In earlier studies, a cumulative methotrexate dose of 3 g was associated with histologic progression in 20% of cases, but only 3% had advanced fibrotic changes [505]. In a meta-analysis of 15 studies, moderate or heavy drinkers (>100 g/week) were more likely to have advanced histologic changes (18%) and to show histologic progression (73%) [505]. Compared to those with rheumatoid arthritis, individuals with psoriasis were also more likely to have advanced changes (7.7% versus 2.7%) and histologic progression (33% versus 24%). Finally, it is noteworthy that preexisting liver test abnormalities are observed in 25–50% of individuals with psoriasis and rheumatoid arthritis.

Clinical features and laboratory data

Minor increases in ALT are seen 1–2 days after starting methotrexate treatment. These changes bear little rele-

vance to the development of hepatic fibrosis, which can only be assessed by liver biopsy. Clinical features are absent or nonspecific for liver disease until complications of portal hypertension and liver failure develop. In these now rare advanced cases, hepatosplenomegaly, ascites, muscle wasting, thrombocytopenia, and hypoalbuminemia can be noted, but jaundice, hyperbilirubinemia, and coagulation disturbances are distinctly uncommon.

Histology

A specific scoring system, devised by Roenigk, is widely used for grading liver histology in methotrexate users [506]. In this system, grades 1 and 2 indicate a variable amount of steatosis, nuclear pleomorphism, and necroinflammatory activity but fibrosis is absent. Higher grades reflect increasing degrees of fibrosis, as follows: grade 3A (few septa), grade 3B (bridging fibrosis), and grade 4 (cirrhosis). The pattern of hepatic fibrosis includes striking pericellular fibrosis, a feature of both alcoholic steatohepatitis and NASH; the possibility that methotrexate itself causes steatohepatitis or accentuates fibrogenesis among persons with underlying "metabolic NASH" has been suggested [53]. However, cases have been reported in which hepatic fibrosis appeared in livers with a relative paucity (or complete absence) of portal and lobular inflammation. Because the extent of hepatic fibrosis is the

Table 27.15 Guidelines for monitoring hepatotoxicity in patients with rheumatoid arthritis and psoriasis during methotrexate treatment.

Approach	Psoriasis (Said et al. 1997 [510], Roenigk et al. 1998 [512])	Rheumatoid arthritis (Kremer et al. 1994 [511])
Pretreatment (laboratory tests)	Routine liver tests, full blood count, urinalysis, blood urea, creatinine, creatinine clearance, hepatitis B/C serology Not mandatory	Same as psoriasis
Pretreatment (liver biopsy)	*Early treatment biopsy* (2–4 months) in patients with risk factors for liver disease (past/current ethanol intake of >1–2 drinks/day, abnormal liver tests, familial liver disease, diabetes, obesity, exposure to hepatotoxic drugs)	Recommended in patients with history of excessive ethanol intake, abnormal baseline AST values, and chronic hepatitis B/C virus infection[a]
During treatment (laboratory tests)	Liver tests at 4–8 weeks (1 week after last dose) Frequent monitoring during initial treatment, during dose escalation, and during episodes where blood methotrexate levels could be elevated (dehydration, impaired renal function, NSAID use) With significant and persistent abnormalities, withhold methotrexate for 1–2 weeks and repeat tests If abnormalities persist, consider liver biopsy	Recommended in patients with history of excessive ethanol intake, abnormal baseline AST, and chronic hepatitis B/C virus infection
During treatment (liver biopsy)	This is with no risk factors for liver disease and normal physical exam and liver tests Liver biopsy is recommended after a cumulative methotrexate dose of 1.5 g[b] If biopsy is normal, repeat at subsequent 1–1.5 g cumulative doses[c]	Liver biopsy recommended if five of nine AST determinations within 12 months (six of 12 if tests are performed monthly) are above the upper limit of normal or serum albumin falls (to less than normal) in controlled rheumatoid arthritis

[a]Current understanding would add "risk factors for NAFLD/NASH, especially the metabolic syndrome."
[b]The authors agree that this should now be 2–4 g.
[c]The authors agree that this should now be for additional 2 g cumulative doses (modified by earlier biopsy findings).
AST, aspartate aminotransferase; NAFLD, nonalcoholic fatty liver disease; NASH, nonalcoholic steatohepatitis; NSAID, nonsteroidal anti-inflammatory drug.

only important abnormality in those taking methotrexate. Richards and colleagues have proposed a new semi-quantitative method for the evaluation of liver biopsies in patients with rheumatoid arthritis [507]. The objective is to provide greater sensitivity for detecting early hepatic fibrosis than the Roenigk system, and further validation will be of interest.

Prevention of methotrexate fibrosis

Co-prescription of folic acid is associated with a lower risk of liver injury (OR (CI), 0.10 (0.04–0.21)) [508] without sacrificing efficacy. However, its impact on preventing hepatic fibrosis is unknown [509]. Guidelines have been published for monitoring methotrexate therapy [504,510–512] in patients with rheumatoid arthritis and psoriasis (summarized in Table 27.15). A recent development has been a set of guidelines drawn up by an international panel of rheumatologists [513]. Their recommendations endorse gradual dose escalation of methotrexate, co-prescription of folic acid, and checking ALT/AST alone with blood counts and creatinine every 1–1.5 months until a stable dose is reached and 1–3 monthly thereafter. If the ALT/AST levels rise to 3 × ULN, the panel recommends stopping methotrexate, but the drug can be reintroduced at a lower dose following liver test normalization. Persistently elevated ALT/AST levels greater than 3 × ULN should prompt further diagnostic studies.

A revised threshold for liver biopsy has also been proposed [514]. In this British retrospective study, advanced liver fibrosis was found in 2.6% and 8.2% of patients with psoriasis who had received a cumulative dose of 4 and 5 g, respectively. On this basis, liver biopsy was recommended after a cumulative methotrexate dose of 5 g [514]. The value of liver biopsies to assess methotrexate hepatotoxicity in diseases other than psoriasis and rheumatoid arthritis has not been established. In a study of 32 patients with inflammatory bowel disease receiving long-term methotrexate (mean dose 2.6 g; follow-up 131 weeks), histologic changes were common but minor, and significant fibrosis was rare [514]. Similar considerations apply to methotrexate use in sarcoidosis: hepatic reactions were common, but it proved difficult to separate drug toxicity from sarcoidosis-related liver features [515].

Noninvasive methods for assessing hepatic fibrosis such as assessment of serum biomarkers of hepatic fibrosis and dynamic hepatic scintigraphy, have been proposed as alternatives to liver biopsy but are yet to be validated [42].

Thiopurines

The thiopurines, azathioprine, 6-mercaptopurine, and to a lesser extent 6-thioguanine (6-TG) are extensively used in the management of autoimmune disorders and inflammatory bowel disease [516]. Other than early hypersensitivity reactions, the risk of liver toxicity is relatively high (mean, 1.4% per patient per year). However, underreporting is common. In a prospective series, up to 10% showed DILI [517]. Further, liver test monitoring for thiopurine DILI has not been as well emphasized as the need for full blood counts (to identify myelotoxicity). Monitoring serum thiopurine metabolite levels is not routine but may be helpful if the clinical response is suboptimal or if there are concerns about drug toxicity. Generally, only 6-TG metabolites are measured and the dose of thiopurine increased if there is suboptimal response. However, liver injury can still occur in some individuals who preferentially metabolize the thiopurine to 6-methylmercaptopurine metabolites; the latter have been previously associated with hepatotoxicity. Thus, if monitoring is to be undertaken, it is suggested that both 6-methylmercaptopurine and 6-thioguanine metabolites should be measured [518].

Azathioprine

Azathioprine, the prodrug of 6-mercaptopurine, is an immunosuppressive "steroid-sparing" agent often used in inflammatory bowel and autoimmune diseases (Chapter 22). Hepatic complications are rare. When these complications develop, they may be severe and diverse, and often occur very late after starting the drug. All these factors provide a challenge for appropriate diagnosis and management. DILI associated with azathioprine includes bland cholestasis, cholestatic hepatitis with bile duct injury [519], zonal necrosis, and vascular toxicity [520,521]. The latter encompasses diverse syndromes of SOS (VOD), peliosis hepatis, NRH, and noncirrhotic portal hypertension [521]. HCC has also been recorded in a long-term recipient [522]. Indirect hepatic effects of azathioprine, such as opportunistic infections (e.g., cytomegalovirus) or, rarely, liver infiltration from lymphoma should always be considered. DILI resolves in mild cases but the course may be progressive in severe cases. 6-Mercaptopurine has been successfully used in cases of azathioprine hepatotoxicity [523]. However, 6-mercaptopurine causes dose-dependent hepatocellular necrosis, possibly by favouring 6-methylmercaptopurine

production, which can be fatal. Rarely, it is associated with cholestasis [14].

6-Thioguanine

Vascular toxicity, particularly hepatic SOS (VOD), is a characteristic feature of 6-TG hepatotoxicity (see Table 27.13) in the context of hematologic malignancies. Less well recognized is the development of NRH in persons with inflammatory bowel disease. In one study conducted in Los Angeles, 111 patients with inflammatory bowel disease receiving 6-TG were examined for potential hepatotoxic effects. An increase in liver enzymes and reduced platelet counts were found in 26% [524]. These were seen more often in men, and in those with preferential 6-methylmercaptopurine production during treatment with 6-mercaptopurine or azathioprine. Liver histology was available in 38 cases. Reticulin-stained sections showed NRH in 20 cases (53%); conventional hematoxylin and eosin (H&E) sections identified NRH in only four of these cases. Ultrastructural studies demonstrated sinusoidal collagen deposition in 60% (14 of 23), a figure significantly higher than that observed with conventional trichrome stains (34%). SOS (VOD) was observed in one case [525]. NRH was present more often (76%) in patients with abnormal laboratory tests than among those without such abnormalities (33%). NRH may be a consequence of dose-dependent toxicity; no cases of NRH were identified in a Dutch series of 28 cases treated with lower doses of 6-TG than in the American report cited above [526].

Cyclosporine A

Between 6% and 86% of organ transplant recipients receiving cyclosporine develop abnormal liver tests [15, 527]. However, these changes are mild and self-limiting. They consist of a transient increase in serum alkaline phosphatase, accompanied by a slight elevation in bilirubin and AT. Most patients do not develop symptoms of cholestasis or hepatitis. The biochemical changes are most evident in the first month after transplantation. However, up to 32% of cases may be associated with prolonged liver test abnormalities [527]. Long-term recipients of cyclosporine are also at risk of developing biliary calculi [528], the consequence of altered bile flow and biliary lipid composition. Cyclosporine-induced liver test abnormalities usually settle with dose reduction or discontinuation of treatment. There is anecdotal evidence that ursodeoxycholic acid may be beneficial in this setting [72].

In experimental models, cyclosporine induces cholestasis by inhibiting Bsep-mediated taurocholate transport, culminating in decreased bile flow [529]. It also disturbs bile salt kinetics by inhibiting bile salt synthesis, reducing the size of the bile salt pool, and increases cholesterol saturation in bile by reducing phospholipid secretion.

Sirolimus

Increases in AT have been observed in liver and renal transplant recipients of sirolimus [530]. Such cases were initially misdiagnosed as representing allograft rejection and were managed (unsuccessfully) with dose escalation. Resolution occurred only when sirolimus was withdrawn. Liver biopsies have shown sinusoidal congestion or mild hepatitis.

Anticonvulsants

Phenytoin

Raised GGTP and serum alkaline phosphatase levels are very often observed in the absence of hepatic injury among people taking phenytoin. This usually reflects enhanced hepatic enzyme synthesis (a form of hepatic adaptation), but in those without adequate sunlight exposure, it is important to exclude vitamin D deficiency arising from enhanced hepatic metabolism of this vitamin. Acute hepatitis, including severe cholestatic hepatitis leading to VBDS, is a very rare but important side effect of phenytoin [2,531], usually as part of the reactive metabolite syndrome (see Table 27.3). There may be an increased rate of hepatic reactions among Afro-Americans compared with whites [42]. Onset is usually within 6 weeks. Biochemical features reflect hepatocellular necrosis with high AT levels, but mixed patterns may occur. In phenytoin hepatitis, liver biopsies show diffuse hepatocellular degeneration and multiple acidophilic (apoptotic) bodies, bridging necrosis, and a prominent lymphocytic or mixed cell inflammatory infiltrate containing neutrophils and eosinophils. Hepatic granulomas may also be present. The combined appearances of lymphocyte beading, mitotic hepatocytes, and granulomas mimic infectious mononucleosis [2].

Phenytoin was one of the first drugs associated with hypersensitivity features now regarded as characteristic of the RMS (also known as the anticonvulsant hypersensitivity syndrome or "pseudomononucleosis" syndrome) [42]. Fever, severe forms of rash, lymphadenopathy, leukocytosis, and Stevens–Johnson syndrome are frequent, and the key link is with visceral involvement including the liver, kidney, bone marrow, and lung (see Table 27.3). Resolution occurs with phenytoin withdrawal, but the case fatality rate of patients developing liver injury is up to 20%. Continued ingestion of phenytoin after the onset of symptoms is associated with a poor outcome. Treatment consists of supportive measures. Corticosteroids have not proved beneficial.

Although the presence of hypersensitivity features suggests immunologic idiosyncrasy, it now seems likely that the primary abnormality is related to the generation of a highly reactive arene oxide metabolite. If detoxification of this metabolite by epoxide hydrolase is inadequate, it binds to cellular macromolecules or initiates oxidative stress, causing cell injury with apoptosis or necrosis. The way in which this reactive metabolite incites profound drug hypersensitivity is less clear, but neoantigenic determinants of immune reactivity, cytokine mobilization, and defects in cell defenses against oxidative stress and proinflammatory stressors are potential candidates. A genetic deficiency of this enzyme has been identified in patients and their family members [532]. Another key enzyme in phenytoin metabolism is CYP2C9; phenytoin-associated VBDS has been described in a patient heterozygous for CYP2C9*3 (an allele conferring low enzyme activity) [532].

Carbamazepine

Liver disorders comprise approximately 10% of adverse drug reactions with carbamazepine [14]. The frequency of liver injury is estimated at 16 cases per 100,000 treatment-years [14]. Granulomatous hepatitis with varying degrees of hepatocellular injury and cholestasis have been reported [42,533,534]. Children may also be affected, including neonates of women receiving carbamazepine in pregnancy [535]. Onset is within 6–8 weeks. The hallmarks of hypersensitivity (fever, rash, angioedema, eosinophilia, and raised IgE levels) are often observed, linking this reaction as part of the RMS observed with other aromatic anticonvulsants (phenytoin, phenobarbitone) metabolized via arene oxides.

Submassive or massive hepatic necrosis has been noted in a few patients. Multiple hepatocellular adenomas were described in a man receiving carbamazepine for 17 years [536], but there is no evident biologic basis for an etiopathogenic role of the drug in this syndrome. The case fatality rate of carbamazepine hepatitis is 10% among those with hepatocellular reactions. Some reported cases of fulminant liver failure were also associated with concurrent acetaminophen intake or antituberculous therapy [537]; the role of interactive hepatotoxicity needs to be considered in such severe cases. Patients presenting with granulomatous and/or cholestatic reactions usually survive, although bile duct injury and VBDS may rarely occur.

Lamotrigine

Indications for lamotrigine include partial and generalized seizures, and as adjunctive therapy in children with refractory epilepsy. Early reports of liver test abnormalities were wrongly attributed to status epilepticus. Subsequently, a small but definite risk of hepatotoxicity was documented [538]. However, attributing causality can be difficult because other potentially hepatotoxic antiepileptic drugs are often co-prescribed.

Acute hepatitis has been reported in ten persons, including two instances of fulminant hepatic failure.

Symptoms developed within 2–3 weeks (range, 6–39 days). Extrahepatic features such as rash, disseminated intravascular coagulopathy, and rhabdomyolysis were sometimes present. Liver biopsies showed acute hepatic necrosis or focal hepatitis with mild portal inflammation [538]. Progressive hepatic necrosis culminating in fatal acute liver failure has been documented. In most other reported reactions, liver injury settled within a few weeks of stopping lamotrigine. Lamotrigine is structurally different from the aromatic anticonvulsants (phenytoin, phenobarbital, carbamazepine). Although in vitro cross-reactivity has been reported in patients with a history of reactions to the older antiepileptic drugs [539], there is no documented clinical cross-reactivity between lamotrigine and these agents.

Valproic acid (sodium valproate)

Risk factors

Up to 40% of recipients of valproic acid (VPA) develop reversible increases in ATs. These changes are frequently observed within the first 2 months of treatment and are unrelated to the rare severe form of liver injury. VPA-associated hepatic injury is independent of dose and duration of treatment. It occurs predominantly in children, particularly those aged less than 3 years. Among 37 fatal cases noted in a retrospective analysis of 400,000 persons taking VPA between 1978 and 1984, children younger than 10 years represented 73% (27 of 37 affected) [540]. Risk factors include a family history of mitochondrial enzyme deficiencies (including urea cycle, long chain fatty acid metabolism defects), Friedreich ataxia, Reye syndrome, having a sibling affected by VPA hepatotoxicity, and multiple drug therapy. There are 26 published cases of VPA liver toxicity in adults [541]. The overall risk of liver injury among persons taking VPA is between one per 500 persons exposed among high-risk groups to less than one in 37,000 in low-risk groups [542]. An association between use of VPA for complex partial seizures and hepatotoxicity has been recently noted [543]. The explanation lies in a genetic polymorphism in the mtDNA repair enzyme, DNA polymerase-γ (POLG). Thus, all four children aged between 3 and 18 years who developed severe VPA-induced liver injury at the Seattle Children's hospital while being treated for complex partial seizures, were genotyped to have POLG mutations. The authors are aware of unpublished data indicating a high frequency of the genetic predisposition factor among a large cohort of VPA hepatotoxicity cases in North America, and it is a strong candidate for the predisposition to this disorder.

Onset, clinical features, and laboratory findings

Symptoms begin 4–12 weeks after starting VPA and are often nonspecific; lethargy, malaise, poor feeding, somno-

lence, worsening seizures, muscle weakness, and facial swelling are important new symptoms among children prescribed VPA. They may be followed by features more readily attributable to hepatotoxicity, including anorexia, nausea, vomiting, weight loss, right upper quadrant discomfort, or abdominal pain. Jaundice, hypoglycemia, ascites, coagulation disorders, and encephalopathy indicate liver failure with imminent coma and death. Another presentation is with fever and tender hepatomegaly suggestive of Reye syndrome. The prognosis is better in such cases. Yet others exhibit prominent neurologic features, such as ataxia and confusion, with little evidence of hepatic involvement. Additional extrahepatic features observed among patients with VPA hepatotoxicity include thrombocytopenia, pancreatitis, and alopecia. The biochemical features resemble those described earlier for other mitochondrial hepatotoxins: a modest rise in bilirubin and ALT is accompanied by hypoalbuminemia, hyperammonemia, and profound impairment in serum levels of clotting factors synthesized by the liver.

Pathology

Histologic appearances include submassive or massive hepatic necrosis in two thirds of cases [544], and zonal or diffuse microvesicular steatosis in the others; steatosis may also accompany hepatic necrosis. Bile duct injury has been observed in a few cases, but as part of massive or submassive necrosis in which any additional significance is questionable.

Management, outcome, and prevention

This includes supportive measures for underlying metabolic defects and managing acute liver failure. In one retrospective study, L-carnitine supplementation reduced mortality [545]; 20 (48%) of 42 patients treated with L-carnitine survived, as against only five (10%) of 50 patients managed by aggressive supportive care alone. The place of liver transplantation is unclear; it has been performed successfully in some cases, but in others led to worsening of neurologic disease [546].

At least 60 deaths from VPA hepatotoxicity are recorded and the mortality remains high. Prevention is possible by adherence to prescribing guidelines; these include avoiding VPA in combination with other drugs in the first 3 years of life and in children with mitochondrial enzyme defects. Monitoring liver tests is unhelpful because of the high frequency of nonspecific liver test abnormalities. Children and their parents should be urged to report any new symptoms developing within the first 6 months of VPA therapy. In the future, genetic screening for POLG polymorphisms may become appropriate.

Mechanism of liver injury

Unlike the aromatic anticonvulsants, VPA hepatotoxicity is rarely accompanied by manifestations of the RMS [547].

Metabolic idiosyncrasy is probably the principal mechanism of VPA toxicity. Glucuronidation and β-oxidation are the principal pathways of VPA metabolism, but VPA may be metabolized by CYP enzymes to 4-en-VPA, a pathway that is accentuated in persons taking concurrent medications (particularly other anticonvulsants), which induces CYPs. Some VPA oxy-metabolites, and notably 4-en-VPA, inhibit mitochondrial fatty acid β-oxidation. Other metabolic effects of VPA therapy include secondary carnitine deficiency, therapeutic correction of which may be valuable (see above).

Topiramate

A woman receiving topiramate and carbamazepine developed acute liver failure. The explanted liver showed centrilobular necrosis [548]. Another person prescribed topiramate for a bipolar affective disorder developed raised ALT (>700 U/L), hypoalbuminemia, and mild hyperammonemia. Resolution occurred after topiramate was discontinued and other medications including VPA could be resumed without ill effects [549]. By contrast, topiramate used as an add-on anticonvulsant induced acute liver failure [550], which resolved only after VPA was withdrawn.

Felbamate

Cases of acute hepatitis and fatal fulminant hepatic failure have been attributed to felbamate [551]. The majority of affected individuals were women. The overall frequency of liver injury and liver-related death was estimated, respectively, at one per 7,000 and one per 125,000 persons exposed. Half the reported cases occurred between 3 and 6 months (range, 2 weeks to 8 months). The generation of atropaldehyde, a reactive metabolite, could be critical to felbamate toxicity [552]. Felbamate should be reserved for treating refractory epilepsy, especially the Lennox–Gastaut syndrome.

Gabapentin

This drug has been implicated in causing cholestatic hepatitis [553]. Another report of liver injury attributed to gabapentin has been disputed because other potentially hepatotoxic medicines had been co-prescribed [554]. The Committee on Safety of Medicines UK has received reports of four other unpublished cases of jaundice, including one other cholestatic drug reaction. Overall, this drug has low hepatotoxic potential.

Antipsychotic agents, sedative–hypnotics, and antidepressant drugs

Chlorpromazine

Chlorpromazine is historically one of the most important causes of drug-induced liver disease, both because of the relatively high frequency of idiosyncratic reac-

Table 27.16 Liver injury associated with antipsychotic, sedative–hypnotic and antidepressant drugs.

Drug	Nature of liver injury
Antipsychotic drugs	
Chlorpromazine	Cholestasis, vanishing bile duct syndrome
Clozapine	Hepatocellular injury, acute liver failure
Haloperidol	Cholestasis, vanishing bile duct syndrome
Quetiapine	Acute liver failure (single case)
Risperidone	Raised aminotransferases, cholestatic hepatitis
Sedative–hypnotics	
Barbiturates	Cholestatic or hepatocellular injury
Benzodiazepine	Hepatocellular injury, chronic hepatitis (bentazepam)
Chlormezanone	Cholestasis, hepatocellular injury, acute liver failure
Antidepressants	
Monoamine oxidase inhibitors	Acute hepatitis
Tetracyclic antidepressants	Cholestasis with mianserin, maprotiline
Tricyclic antidepressants	Hepatocellular or cholestatic injury, vanishing bile duct syndrome (amitriptyline, imipramine)
Selective serotonin reuptake inhibitors:	
Fluoxetine	Acute hepatitis, chronic hepatitis
Paroxetine	Raised aminotransferases, chronic hepatitis (one case)
Sertraline	Acute hepatitis (when used alone and also in combination with other drugs), cholestatic hepatitis
Citalopram	Cholestasis
Other antidepressants:	
Bupropion	Raised aminotransferases in trials; acute hepatitis (one case), cholestatic hepatitis
Fluvoxamine	Acute hepatitis
Nefazodone	Raised aminotransferases, occasionally subacute liver failure
Trazodone	Acute and chronic hepatitis, cholestasis, fatal hepatic necrosis
Venlafaxine	Acute hepatitis with zone 3 necrosis, mixed liver injury. Low-dose venlafaxine is associated with hepatocellular injury in a patient with chronic hepatitis B

tions, but also because it is the archetypical example of a drug causing cholestatic hepatitis (Table 27.16). VBDS and other complications, such as massive hepatic necrosis, also occur occasionally. Full descriptions of chlorpromazine hepatitis may be found elsewhere [2,14,555]. The essential features are recapitulated here because of what chlorpromazine has taught us about hepatic drug reactions, and because the agent is still used.

Chlorpromazine is associated with cholestatic hepatitis in 0.2–2% of recipients; the risk increases with age and is higher in women. The onset of prodromal symptoms occurs within 1–6 weeks [555]. Fever and nonspecific systemic complaints are present in over half the patients, but rash is uncommon. Jaundice, pruritus, and generalized or right upper quadrant pain occur later. Serum alkaline phosphatase is elevated more than threefold, along with a moderate rise in the AT and a variable increase in serum bilirubin, depending on severity. Peripheral blood eosinophilia is present in 10–40%. Liver histology is characterized by centrilobular cholestasis, portal inflammation, mild parenchymal injury, and occasionally bile duct damage [555]. Resolution occurs within 12 weeks in the majority of cases, but about 7% develop VBDS.

The brisk response to rechallenge suggests immunoallergic idiosyncrasy but there is evidence of a toxic component to the liver injury. Chlorpromazine, and particularly its hydroxylated metabolites, inhibit plasma membrane Na^+/K^+-ATPase, alter membrane fluidity, and actin polymerization. Genetically determined defects in sulfoxidation of chlorpromazine (the sulfoxide metabolite is inert) have been postulated but are unproven [556].

A similar pattern of cholestatic liver injury has been described less frequently with prochlorperazine [557] and other neuroleptics such as haloperidol [558], pimozide, and sulpiride, including rare cases of VBDS [42].

Sedative–hypnotics

Liver injury is extremely rare with the benzodiazepines and other minor tranquilizers, anxiolytics, or hypnotics. Both hepatocellular and cholestatic reactions are described, but often from times preceding accurate diagnosis of all forms of viral hepatitis [14].

Antidepressants

Monoamine oxidase inhibitors

Iproniazid was one of the first drugs associated with acute hepatitis [2]. These reactions occurred in 1% of recipients and were often severe, including instances of fatal fulminant liver failure. The hydrazine substituent (which iproniazid partly shares with isoniazid, ethionamide, pyrazinamide, and nicotinamide) was probably the hepatotoxic moiety [559]. Hydrazine sulfate can cause severe hepatorenal toxicity [559]. Phenelzine and isocarboxazid have also been associated with occasional instances of hepatocellular injury, but monoamine oxidase inhibitors are now rarely prescribed.

Tricyclic antidepressants

These agents bear structural resemblance to the phenothiazines and are an occasional cause of cholestatic or less commonly hepatocellular injury. Recovery following drug cessation is usual, but prolonged cholestasis has been observed with amitriptyline and imipramine [42].

Selective serotonin reuptake inhibitors and other modern antidepressants

Liver enzyme alterations in asymptomatic persons have been observed with fluoxetine and paroxetine [560]. A few reports of acute and chronic hepatitis have been attributed to the use of selective serotonin reuptake inhibitors (SSRIs) (Table 27.16) [560]. In all reported cases, the liver injury subsided with drug discontinuation.

Nefazodone has been withdrawn after being implicated in inducing acute and subacute liver failure [561]. A Spanish pharmacovigilance study examining antidepressant hepatotoxicity found that nefazodone had the highest frequency of liver injury among these drugs (28.96 per 100,000 patient-years); the comparative figures for fluoxetine, paroxetine, sertraline, and citalopram were less than two per 100,000 patient-years [562]. Of 32 cases of liver injury analyzed by the Canadian adverse drug monitoring programme, 26 (81%) were classified as severe. About half the patients recovered after drug withdrawal but three patients progressed to acute liver failure [563] necessitating liver transplantation. Centrilobular, massive, or submassive hepatic necrosis was observed on histology. Two thirds of affected persons were women aged between 30 and 70 years. While most had been taking the drug for between 3 and 6 months, early liver injury (within 4 weeks) has also been reported [564]. Bioactivation of nefazodone to a reactive quinone-imine metabolite may underlie its hepatotoxicity [565].

Trazodone has been implicated in cases of acute and chronic hepatocellular injury [566]. The onset is usually within 6 months (range, 4 days to 18 months). Positive rechallenge within 2 days of reinstituting the drug has been described [566]. Recovery is complete within 2 months of discontinuing trazodone. Occasional reports note the occurrence of severe hepatotoxicity with combinations of antidepressants or antidepressants with other neuroleptics [42].

The liver toxicity associated with other antidepressants is summarized in Table 27.16 [560].

Cognition modifiers

Tacrine

This reversible cholinesterase inhibitor was formerly used in treating Alzheimer disease. Following initial concerns about possible hepatotoxicity, a seminal observational study was conducted [567]. ALT values greater than the ULN, 3 × ULN, and 20 × ULN were recorded in 49%, 25%, and 2%, respectively. Among individuals in whom treatment was discontinued due to abnormal liver enzyme changes, biochemical resolution invariably occurred, and 88% were able to resume long-term therapy (usually at a lower dose); there were no fatalities [567]. Only few cases of overt hepatic disease have been reported. Histologic appearances range from mild lobular hepatitis to centrilobular hepatic necrosis, steatosis, and granulomatous hepatitis [568].

The mechanism of tacrine-induced liver injury remains unclear. Hypersensitivity features were observed only infrequently and rechallenge did not produce an exaggerated rise in ALT. Genetic predisposition to tacrine hepatotoxicity may contribute; polymorphisms associated with glutathione-S-transferase and IL6 genes have been described [569].

Donepezil

This acetylcholinesterase inhibitor has been implicated in two cases of acute hepatitis [570]. One of these patients who developed fulminant hepatic failure had also been taking sertraline.

Methylphenidate

This sympathomimetic amine is prescribed for pediatric attention deficit disorder (ADD) and narcolepsy and is also self-administered by intravenous injection in "recreational" use. Hepatocellular injury is documented with therapeutic (oral) and intravenous use [571,572]. The latter reactions are more severe and have been associated with multiorgan failure involving the liver, kidney, pancreas, lung, and central nervous system [572]. A single report has implicated this drug in an autoimmune hepatitis-type presentation. This patient had undergone a liver transplant for chronic hepatitis C and presented with deranged liver tests and had serologic and histologic characteristics consistent with AIH. Partial improvement in liver tests was noted after drug withdrawal but a short course of prednisolone was also used later [573].

Pemoline

This psychostimulant, now withdrawn, was used in children with ADD. Clinical trials revealed mild, reversible liver injury in around 2% of recipients. However, instances of serious liver toxicity were subsequently reported to the FDA; of 13 cases presenting with fulminant hepatic failure, 11 died or required liver transplantation [574]. Onset was usually within 4 weeks but could be delayed for up to 1 year. Liver histology showed focal necrosis, mild steatosis, or portal inflammation.

Rash, fever, or eosinophilia were infrequent [575]. Moreover, the observation of a similar rise in serum AT in twins with ADD supports a hypothesis of genetically determined individual susceptibility [576]. On the other hand, the existence of distinctive cases of steroid-responsive chronic liver disease resembling AIH indicates that immunoallergic mechanisms could also be involved [577]. Zimmerman suggested that persons prescribed pemoline should be monitored for serum AT changes, but it is noted that the onset of acute liver failure can be extremely rapid [575].

Other drugs used in the treatment of neurologic diseases

Riluzole

This glutamate antagonist is approved for the treatment of amyotrophic lateral sclerosis. Increased ALT was observed in 1.3–10% of clinical trial recipients. Two cases of acute hepatitis with microvesicular steatosis have since been reported, with onset respectively at 4 and 8 weeks after starting treatment [578]. Rarely, hepatocellular injury may be delayed for as long as 6 months [579]. Liver test abnormalities settle shortly after riluzole is stopped.

Dantrolene

Dantrolene is a skeletal muscle relaxant used against spasticity. The frequency of liver injury is about 1%. A feature has been the severity (the case fatality is approximately 28%) of the liver injury [580], which in some cases progressed even after stopping dantrolene. Most were over 30 years of age. Up to one third of affected persons were asymptomatic, while others had developed symptoms of hepatitis. Hepatocellular necrosis, often submassive or massive, was the usual histologic characteristic [580]. Chronic hepatitis and cirrhosis have also been observed [581]. Liver tests should be performed every 2 weeks for the first 6 weeks of dantrolene therapy. The drug should be stopped if there is no clinical benefit.

Other drugs with muscle relaxant properties that have been rarely associated with liver injury include phenyramidol (hepatocellular injury), chlormezanone (cholestasis, hepatocellular injury, acute liver failure), and baclofen (serum AT changes) [42].

Tolcapone

This catechol-O-methyltransferase (COMT) inhibitor is approved for Parkinson disease. In preclinical trials, significant ALT elevations (>3 × ULN) were present in 1–3% of recipients. Tolcapone has now been implicated in at least four cases of acute liver failure [582], all in women older than 70 years. They presented with jaundice and high ALT levels. Centrilobular necrosis was observed at autopsy in one case. Ultrastructural changes included mitochondrial swelling with disruption of cristae and reduced matrix density. Patients developing severe hepatotoxicity had not been monitored as recommended [582]. With strict monitoring, hepatocellular injury is infrequent (0.04%); most have only elevated AT without clinically significant liver disease [583].

The mechanism of tolcapone hepatotoxicity could be related to the uncoupling of mitochondrial oxidative phosphorylation, and also through interactions with fatty acid β-oxidation and bile acid synthesis [584]. It is relevant that entacapone, another COMT inhibitor, does not exhibit similar toxicity at comparable concentrations [585]. As compared with tolcapone, entacapone has a greater binding affinity with glucuronidation enzymes, but a lower capacity for penetrating the mitochondrial outer membrane [585]. Of three recent cases of hepatic injury attributed to entacapone, there were confounding factors in two [586]. Overall, the experience with entacapone (over 300,000 patient-years) has confirmed its generally safe track record [586].

Drugs of abuse

3,4-Methylenedioxymetamphetamine ("ecstasy")

This widely used recreational agent has been associated with more than 30 cases of acute liver injury, including several deaths from acute liver failure [587]. In Spain, up to 25% of cases of unexplained acute liver failure in young adults were attributable to 3,4-methylenedioxymetamphetamine (MDMA) [588]. Liver injury was initially described as part of a hyperthermic syndrome with rhabdomyolysis, acute renal failure, and coagulopathy. This was precipitated by vigorous muscle exercise, dehydration, and increased ambient temperatures, particularly during all-night "rave" dancing [588]. However, acute hepatitis can be the sole manifestation of MDMA toxicity; it can occur following ingestion of even a single tablet, although many of the reported cases have involved consumption of MDMA for longer periods.

MDMA is demethylated in the liver by CYP2D6. It was suggested that persons with low-level expression of CYP2D6 (the debrisoquine slow metabolizer phenotype) could be susceptible to MDMA-induced hepatitis, but this has been challenged [42]. Liver biopsies may show acute lobular hepatitis or zone 3 or massive hepatic necrosis, but others have observed chronic cases with hepatic fibrosis [589].

MDA (methylene dianiline) may be confused with MDMA [590] if used in similar settings. This is illustrated by a report of cholestasis in participants of a "technoparty" who had their alcoholic beverage spiked with MDA. Unlike MDMA, which primarily causes hepatocellular injury, MDA toxicity manifests as cholestasis, as exemplified by the 1965 outbreak of jaundice in Epping, England, where bread flour had been contaminated with MDA [86]. Acute right upper quadrant abdominal

pain (similar to erythromycin hepatitis) is a prominent symptom.

Phencyclidine

Severe phencyclidine ("angel dust") overdose can lead to submassive hepatic necrosis (accompanied by hyperthermia, rhabdomyolysis, and respiratory and renal failure) [42].

Cocaine

Cocaine is a dose-dependent hepatotoxin in mice [14]. Massive doses self-administered to humans cause liver injury in association with shock and other toxic phenomena [591]. Rarely, cocaine can cause acute hepatitis without altered systemic hemodynamics and following intranasal (as opposed to parenteral) use [592]. In rodents, the histologic lesions include extensive centrilobular, midzonal, or panlobular necrosis, together with microvesicular steatosis [14]. Gender and genetic differences, as well as the activity of CYP enzymes, determine this varied histologic spectrum.

Clinical presentation of cocaine hepatotoxicity is with raised serum AT (over ten-fold in 40% of cases), nearly always accompanied by hypotension, hyperpyrexia, renal failure, myoglobulinuria, and disseminated intravascular coagulation [593]. The high mortality is illustrated by one series of 39 patients, among whom more than 40% died [593]. Thrombotic microangiopathy is a rare complication; early recognition and institution of plasma exchange can be life-saving for this hematologic disorder [594]. The mechanism of liver injury may vary between species – in rodents it involves drug metabolism to toxic, oxy- or nitro-metabolites and factors pertaining to host defenses [2]. In humans, systemic hypotension and hypoxia (and possibly hyperthermia) are more likely to contribute to the liver injury [593] than the direct effects of cocaine on the liver. Induction of hepatic CYP2E1 by alcohol can potentiate the hepatotoxic effects of cocaine experimentally [42].

Drugs used in aversion therapy and treatment of alcohol withdrawal

Tetrabamate (Atrium®)

This drug combination (febarbamate, difebarbamate, and phenobarbital) has been used in France and Spain to treat alcohol withdrawal, tremor, and depression. Phenobarbital is an extremely rare cause of liver injury (cases are similar to phenytoin hepatitis) [14], whereas difebarbamate and febarbamate have not been previously implicated in hepatotoxicity. However, use of the combined preparation (tetrabamate) has been implicated in causing acute hepatitis [595]. Onset of symptoms was between 15 days to 2 years after commencing tetrabamate

[595]. Most recovered after stopping tetrabamate, but two deaths from liver failure were recorded; both occurred in patients who continued taking tetrabamate after the onset of symptoms. Histology shows acute hepatocellular necrosis. Other lesions also described include cholestasis, microvesicular steatosis, and granulomatous hepatitis.

Hypersensitivity features were prominent in some individuals, including the presence of antinuclear and/or smooth muscle antibodies. Therefore, immunologic idiosyncrasy may contribute to the liver injury, but genetic differences in drug metabolism could have also been responsible [42]. Phenobarbital, a potent CYP enzyme inducer, could have also potentially enhanced the production of toxic metabolites from the other co-constituents (cf. VPA and the RMS).

Disulfiram

Disulfiram has been incriminated in over 100 instances of acute hepatocellular injury [596]. Recovery is usual within 2 weeks, but liver tests can take up to 3 months to normalize. The high AT readings distinguish these reactions from alcoholic hepatitis. Rarely, acute liver failure may develop [597] and liver transplantation becomes necessary; the youngest patient undergoing this procedure was only 16 years old [597]. The overall mortality in jaundiced patients was 16% in one series [596]. The frequency of fatal liver injury is estimated at one per 30,000 treated persons per year. Although abnormal AT in the absence of advanced liver disease at baseline does not necessarily predict an increased risk of liver toxicity, patients with underlying cirrhosis may be susceptible to severe liver injury (five of seven reported cases) [596]. The presence of eosinophils (as opposed to hepatocyte dropout) on liver biopsies has been associated with a more favorable outcome.

Cyanamide produces a characteristic ground glass appearance of hepatocytes, which resembles LaFora bodies [598]. This is a form of hepatic adaptation rather than liver injury. The intense immunohistochemical staining of these cytoplasmic inclusions with a polyglucosan-reactive monoclonal antibody suggests that they are derived from altered glucose metabolism [598]. However, cyanamide can rarely cause acute hepatitis, and serial liver biopsies from alcohol-abstinent recipients of cyanamide showed portal–portal and portal–central fibrosis [42].

Chlormethiazole

Previously implicated in only one case of acute cholestatic hepatitis, chlormethiazole has greater hepatotoxic potential than previously appreciated [42]. DILI may be underreported in the context of alcohol withdrawal because of difficulties in separating drug toxicity from the underlying alcoholic liver disease. Hepatocellular or mixed liver injury was described in three recent cases wehre patients were receiving disulfiram for indications other than alcohol withdrawal (insomnia, depression); all were over 70 years of age and treated for less than 2 months. One developed fatal acute liver failure and histology showed submassive necrosis. The other two patients recovered within 2 months.

Antihistamines: H1 receptor antagonists

Transient AT changes are observed in less than 2% of recipients of cetirizine but four reports of liver toxicity have accrued; three were hepatocellular reactions and one patient developed cholestasis [599]. The appearance of a rash, eosinophilia, and the presence of antiliver–kidney microsomal antibodies in two cases is suggestive of drug hypersensitivity. Positive rechallenge (inadvertent) has been reported [42].

Cholestatic drug reactions are also described with terfenadine, cinnarizine, chlorpheniramine, and pizotyline [42]. Loratadine has been linked to two reports of hepatocellular injury, including one patient who developed subfulminant hepatic failure and was transplanted; the liver explant showed massive hepatic necrosis [600].

Gastric acid-lowering agents

H2 receptor antagonists

Although these agents have a good safety profile, serious hepatotoxicity led to the withdrawal of oxmetadine, ebrotidine, and niperotidine, and rare episodes of liver injury have been reported with other members of this group [42]. Cross-reactivity between famotidine and cimetidine has been described [42], but there is no overall evidence of a class effect on hepatotoxicity among these structurally variable drugs.

Compared to nonusers, the relative risk for liver injury was 5.5 for cimetidine and 1.7 for ranitidine (and 2.1 for omeprazole) [601]. The frequency of hepatotoxicity with cimetidine and ranitidine has been estimated at 3–6 per 100,000 and one per 100,000 prescriptions, respectively [601]. The risk of liver injury with cimetidine is highest with doses exceeding 800 mg/day and at the onset of treatment. Cimetidine, ranitidine, and famotidine usually cause acute hepatitis or cholestatic hepatitis [602]. Of 170 cases of H2 receptor antagonist toxicity reported to the Australian Adverse Drug Reaction Advisory Committee, hepatotoxicity constituted 4–8% of reactions. The majority of affected individuals were over 50 years of age [602] and, in this report, hepatic reactions were more frequently reported with ranitidine than with cimetidine or famotidine. Supportive evidence of hypersensitivity features were recorded in a few patients. Others have reported Stevens–Johnson syndrome in association with ranitidine use in two patients with preexisting severe liver disease;

it was suggested that altered hepatic metabolism may have contributed, but no data were presented to support this [42]. However, others point out that markers of hypersensitivity and positive rechallenge have not been consistently demonstrated, leading them to propose an alternative hypothesis for liver injury [42]. In a rat model, significant hepatocellular injury could be elicited in the presence of lipopolysaccharide-induced liver inflammation. On this basis, they suggest that similar mechanisms may underlie human ranitidine hepatotoxicity because these cases were characterized by a preceding cluster of symptoms that could be attributed to endotoxemia (fever, diarrhea, abdominal pain). In turn, the ensuing endotoxemia-related hepatic inflammation could render the hepatocytes susceptible to ranitidine-related liver injury. Interestingly, in the same rat model, co-administration of LPS with famotidine, a less frequent cause of hepatotoxicity, did not elicit significant liver injury

Proton pump inhibitors

A few reports of acute hepatitis or mixed hepatocellular–cholestatic liver injury [42] have been ascribed to the proton pump inhibitors. Although omeprazole was implicated in one case of fulminant hepatic failure, concurrent acetaminophen use was not clearly excluded (see earlier) [42]. Fulminant hepatic failure has also been attributed to rabeprazole [42]. However, the role of rabeprazole in causing fulminant hepatitis appears equally less conclusive because terbinafine had also been prescribed. The authors' assertion that terbinafine hepatotoxicity is usually mild is not consistent with other data presented to the FDA (see earlier section).

Antispasmodic drugs

Two cases of acute hepatocellular injury have been reported with alverine, a smooth muscle relaxant. In the first report, the accompanying peripheral and tissue eosinophilia along with antinuclear antibodies directed against a component of the nuclear envelope (lamin A and C) suggested immune-mediated liver injury. These features were absent in the second case. Both patients recovered after alverine was discontinued [603].

Emerging drugs

A clinical challenge with drug-induced liver disease is provided by instances of hepatotoxicity attributable to recently introduced drugs (Table 27.17). The frequency of liver injury with these drugs will not be known until larger studies are conducted.

Alfuzosin

Three reports of liver injury (hepatocellular and mixed hepatocellular–cholestatic) have been recorded with this

Table 27.17 Liver injury associated with emerging drugs.

Drug	Nature of liver injury
Alfuzosin	Hepatocellular or mixed hepatocellular–cholestatic injury
Beta-interferon	Raised AT common; clinically significant liver injury rare; can trigger autoimmune hepatitis
Bosentan, sitaxsentan	Raised AT in 8–32%; acute hepatitis
Imatinib mesylate and other tyrosine kinase inhibitors	Raised AT in 35%; acute hepatitis, massive or submassive hepatic necrosis (rare); acute liver failure also with sunitinib; raised AT and/or bilirubin with lapatinib
Infliximab and other tumor necrosis factor antagonists	Bland cholestasis, cholestatic hepatitis with bile duct injury, hepatic granulomas (etanercept), autoimmune hepatitis-like features, reactivation of chronic hepatitis B, acute liver failure (rare)
Leukotriene antagonists (zafirlukast, montelukast)	Submassive or massive hepatic necrosis (zafirlukast), acute hepatitis, cholestatic hepatitis (montelukast)
Orlistat	Cholestatic hepatitis, subacute liver failure (single cases only)
Ximelagatran	Raised AT in 6%; acute liver failure (relationship with drug not definitely established)

AT, aminotransferase.

α$_1$-adrenoceptor antagonist used to treat benign prostatic hyperplasia [41,604]. Features of cholestasis with spotty hepatocyte necrosis and pericellular fibrosis with giant cell formation were noted at liver histology [604]. One of these patients had underlying chronic liver disease [604]. Because alfuzosin is extensively metabolized in the liver, it is possible that the ensuing hepatotoxicity in this case was a consequence of increased drug levels. Normalization of liver tests was complete within 6 months of stopping the drug [42].

Bosentan

This endothelin antagonist is prescribed for primary pulmonary hypertension, chronic heart failure, and hypertension. Dose-dependent reversible AT (up to 3 × ULN) increases were observed in 10% of clinical trial recipients, and in 7.6% in a recent postmarketing surveillance report [605]. In a pivotal trial of patients with primary pulmonary hypertension, AT increases of eight times ULN were observed in 3% and 7% of those assigned to the 125 mg b.i.d. group and 250 mg b.i.d. arms, respectively [605]. The pharmacokinetics of bosentan is unaltered by mild hepatic function impairment (Child–Pugh class A) but the drug is contraindicated if more severe liver disease is present. Reversible acute hepatocellular injury has been described after commencing methotrexate in a patient with scleroderma-related pulmonary arterial hypertension who had been on bosentan for 15 months [606]. Other drug interactions with consequent acute hepatocellular injury have been documented with co-prescription of bosentan/clarithromycin and bosentan/glibenclamide (glyburide) (29% show AT changes) [42]. The latter reaction is probably related to the synergistic effects of the two agents – in a rat model, bosentan inhibited the canalicular bile acid transporter, Bsep [607]. Patients with chronic heart failure also appear to be at an increased risk of liver injury, with up to 18% showing AT elevations in one study.

Dose-dependent AT increases have been reported with sitaxsentan, a selective endothelin receptor antagonist. The cumulative risk of developing raised AT (up to 3 × ULN) after 9 months with the 100 and 300 mg daily doses has been estimated at 8% and 32%, respectively [608]. In addition, six cases of acute hepatocellular injury have accrued with this drug [608]. Onset was within 4 months. Most patients recovered but the liver injury can be severe. One died from pneumonia with evidence of persistent jaundice (bilirubin >200 µmol/L) and another required a liver transplant. Liver histology appearances were consistent with acute hepatitis. Apparent response to corticosteroids in one case and evidence of eosinophil infiltration within the portal tracts in another raises the possibility of an immune reaction. Liver toxicity could be a class effect of this group of drugs because cross-toxicity between bosentan and sitaxentan has been reported [608]. However, to date, ambrisentan has not been associated with such toxicity.

Interferons

Interferon-α has been associated with acute "flares" in patients with hepatitis C, sometimes resulting in viral clearance. It may also rarely activate latent AIH [42]. This may occur if the autoimmune etiology of chronic hepatitis has not been correctly appreciated at diagnosis, or it may represent a direct immune-mediated complication of interferon.

Beta-interferon is used in relapsing–remitting multiple sclerosis. The analysis of pooled data from six randomized controlled trials involving over 2,800 subjects has shown that AT increases are frequent (67% of subjects by 24 months) [609]; most (75%) of these increases occur within 6 months. AT changes settled spontaneously or after dose reduction (in 5%), and only a minority (0.4%) had their medication withdrawn. A retrospective chart review of 844 patients in British Columbia com-

pared three different preparations of interferon-β-1b with respect to their hepatotoxic potential [610]. AT increases of up to 2.5 × ULN, 5 × ULN, and >5 × ULN were found in 23–39%, 1.9–7.8%, and 0–1.9%, respectively; the lowest figures were recorded with the intramuscular preparation of interferon-β-1b. Despite the high frequency of AT changes observed with the β-interferons, clinically significant toxicity is restricted to a few case reports of acute hepatitis [611]. Of the two reported patients developing fulminant hepatic failure [611], one was also receiving nefazodone. Unmasking of AIH has also been observed with interferon-β [42].

Pegylated interferon-α has a higher rate of AT abnormalities than conventional recombinant interferon-α but clinically significant hepatotoxicity has not been reported.

Imatinib mesylate and other tyrosine kinase inhibitors

Imatinib mesylate is approved for chronic myeloid leukemia and gastrointestinal stromal tumors (GISTs). Adverse effects include fluid overload from salt retention and abnormal liver tests; up to 3.5% of treated cases showed AT and/or serum bilirubin changes (median time to onset, 100 days) [42]. These abnormalities usually settled with dose reduction and the drug was withdrawn in only 0.5% of cases on account of hepatotoxicity. A few reports of acute hepatitis have since accrued, including five cases of acute liver failure [612]. Concurrent acetaminophen intake was recorded in two of these cases. Most were patients with myeloproliferative disease but some had advanced GISTs [613]. Positive rechallenge has been documented. Histologic appearances showed acute hepatitis with extensive lobular and portal inflammation or focal hepatic necrosis in less severe cases, and submassive hepatic necrosis in those presenting with acute liver failure [614]. Corticosteroids have been used successfully to achieve resolution in some cases [613] while liver transplantation was needed to rescue patients developing acute liver failure. Interestingly, another structurally similar tyrosine kinase inhibitor, nilotinib, has been used without evidence of cross-hepatotoxicity. On the other hand, there have been reports of acute hepatocellular injury and fatal hepatic failure with sunitinib [615]. Concurrent acetaminophen use was recorded in the latter case; severe hepatic centrilobular necrosis with steatosis was noted at autopsy [615]. Lapatinib, used in treating advanced breast cancer, has also been implicated in hepatotoxicity. Elevations in AT (>3 × ULN) and total bilirubin (>1.5 × ULN) is seen in 6.4% and 8.1%, respectively. The presence of four specific HLA alleles have been correlated with ALT rises; the strongest link is with HLA-DQA1*0201 with an odds ratio of 2.6 (increasing to 18 in cases with ALT >8 × ULN) [616].

Leukotriene antagonists

This group of drugs is used to treat asthma, and includes zileuton, zafirlukast, and montelukast. As a group, reversible increases in AT ($>2 \times$ ULN) were recorded in up to 3% of leukotriene antagonist recipients in preclinical trials. Zileuton, the first member of this drug class, was implicated in a single case of acute hepatocellular injury. It has been superceded by zafirlukast and montelukast [617].

Zafirlukast

Over 100 cases of disturbed liver function with zafirlukast have been collated and published online by the manufacturers. These include 46 reports of hepatitis and 14 cases of acute liver failure. The risk of developing acute liver failure was estimated at less than one per 100,000 patient-years. Assigning causality is difficult because details of concomitant drug intake or preexisting liver disease were not provided. Nevertheless, detailed descriptions of clinically significant hepatic injury have been published elsewhere [617]. In these two case series, jaundice was observed in seven of nine cases. Two patients progressed to acute liver failure and needed liver transplantation. Symptoms were delayed until 6 months (range, 1.5–13 months) after starting zafirlukast. Inadvertent rechallenge reproduced the liver injury in one case. Liver explants showed submassive or massive hepatic necrosis. It is important to note that, in persons developing acute liver failure, prodromal features of hepatitis were not always present. The apparent response to corticosteroids in four cases, three of whom had hypersensitivity features such as skin rash and peripheral and tissue eosinophilia, is suggestive of immune-mediated liver injury. However, in another report the absence of hypersensitivity features and the long latent period (13 months) are more consistent with idiosyncratic liver injury [42]. Cross-reactivity with montelukast has not been described [42]. Periodic monitoring of liver tests is suggested [617]. However, the long latent period, lack of prodromal symptoms, and also the relentless progression of liver injury even after drug withdrawal cast doubts on the validity of routine surveillance [617].

Montelukast

Three reports of acute hepatitis have been documented with montelukast. Time to onset of liver injury has been variable (1 month to 2 years) [41,618]. Recovery was complete in all cases. Biochemical resolution can be slow and AT ($>2 \times$ ULN) remained elevated for more than 1 year after drug withdrawal. Liver histology showed acute hepatitis or cholestatic hepatitis [617]. A lymphocyte transformation test was reported as positive in one case, supporting a cause–effect relationship [618].

Infliximab and tumour necrosis factor antagonists

Transient AT elevations were recorded with infliximab in combination with methotrexate but no major hepatic adverse effects were noted in clinical trials. However, several reports of hepatotoxicity have since accrued for infliximab and other TNF antagonists including adalimumab, etanercept, and natalizumab [619]. The frequency of liver injury has been estimated at six and 28 per 100,000 patient-years of exposure with infliximab and natalizumab, respectively [619,620]. As expected with the profile of patients with rheumatologic disorders, most have occurred in women (12 of 17 cases; mean age, 43 years) who have also been receiving other hepatotoxic drugs (methotrexate, azathioprine). The onset of symptoms was usually after 4 weeks; occasionally they were delayed beyond 1 year or developed as early as after the first infusion (four of six cases with natalizumab). The clinical presentation is that of an acute hepatitis or with bland cholestasis. AT elevations range from 2 to $50 \times$ ULN, but jaundice or impaired liver synthetic function is uncommon. Antinuclear, smooth muscle, and other autoantibodies are often present (64%). Liver histology appearances have varied from typical acute hepatitic features and autoimmune hepatitis-like patterns through to bland cholestasis, bile duct injury, bridging fibrosis, and granulomatous hepatitis [619]. One patient with severe liver injury required liver transplantation. Otherwise, recovery within 6 weeks is the rule. Corticosteroids have been used with apparent success in the majority of cases with autoimmune features. A successful switch to another TNF-α blocker, etanercept, has been described in patients with infliximab hepatotoxicity [621]. Whether the TNF antagonists are directly hepatotoxic or whether they trigger autoimmune hepatocellular and bile duct damage is not clear. In addition, there are now well-documented cases of chronic hepatitis B reactivation (both HBsAg-positive and HBsAg-negative cases) following infliximab and adalimumab treatment in patients with inflammatory bowel disease and other rheumatologic disorders; antiviral prophylaxis is recommended in rheumatoid arthritis (Chapter 24).

Ximelagatran

This thrombin inhibitor, now withdrawn, was associated with increased AT ($>3 \times$ ULN) in 7.9% of long-term recipients. Most (96%) of these biochemical changes decreased to less than two-fold above ULN irrespective of whether the drug was continued or withdrawn. Symptomatic cases have been rare [622]. AT increases were correlated with the presence of certain HLA alleles (DRB1*0701, DQA1*0201) [623]. Three cases of acute liver failure were attributed to this drug but a definitive relationship was not clearly established. Risk factors for liver injury included prolonged treatment of over 3 months (OR, 6.7), deep vein thrombosis (OR, 5.2), and when used for stroke prophylaxis in patients with atrial fibrillation (OR, 8.3) [622].

Hepatotoxicity of herbal medicines

Whether herbal medicines have any therapeutic benefits in liver disease has yet to be defined, as reviewed elsewhere [624]. However, the growing popularity of complementary and alternative medicine in industrialized societies has brought about an increasing number of cases of herbal hepatotoxicity [625]. Many herbal products have been used for centuries, in part because of their excellent safety record, so that recognition of DILI has seemed surprising. Explanations include nonadherence to recommended doses and concurrent intake of other agents, including conventional medicines (like acetaminophen). Toxicity may also result from the use of newer, more biologically active formulations. For instance, a 78-year-old woman developed acute hepatitis soon after using a ready-made powder formulation of a fungal extract, linghzi (*Ganoderma lucidum*), despite having used this herbal compound previously for a year without toxicity [42]. The only difference was that earlier treatment had been home prepared and presumably was not as concentrated as the marketed product that caused the adverse reaction. Individual susceptibility may also be an important determinant of herbal toxicity. Kava, a reasonably safe and widely used anxiolytic agent with rare hepatotoxicity, appears more likely to cause acute hepatitis [626] in Caucasians with the slow debrisoquine phenotype (low expression of CYP2D6) (also see below under "Kava"). The same phenotype has also been implicated in facilitating senna-associated hepatocellular injury where altered pharmacokinetics with a prolongation of serum half-life and high metabolite levels were demonstrated [42]. In comparison with these agents, others such as the pyrrolizidine alkaloids have substantial hepatotoxic potential.

Some herbal preparations (for example, jin bu huan) could incite an immunoallergic mechanism of liver injury. Others could aggravate preexisting liver disease, as noted with ma huang, which can exacerbate AIH [627]. Rarely, herbal medicines may trigger latent AIH (e.g., dai-saiko-to, black cohosh) [628,629]. Such interactions between herbal medicines and preexisting liver disease are poorly understood. This is an important aspect because many patients with viral hepatitis use herbal remedies, and disclosure is not always forthcoming.

Recurring themes among reports of herbal hepatotoxicity are delayed diagnosis, product contamination, or botanical misidentification [625]. The latter two issues can be rectified by exclusive use of agents prepared according to codes of good manufacturing practice. Relevant legislation governing the sale of herbal products is in place in some countries, but the international availability of herbal medicines by mail and internet ordering partly abrogates such improvements. Greater awareness of possible herbal hepatotoxicity is required on the part of physicians and the public so as to avoid the problem of delayed diagnosis. The implications of continued intake of hepatotoxic chemicals after the onset of liver injury are identical whether it is a conventional medicinal agent or a herbal product. Natural products, often equated with "safety," may be easily overlooked by the patient and doctor. Items not readily identified include skin creams, "natural" sedatives, herbal tea infusions, health tonics, and so-called energy vitalizers.

Some herbal products can complicate the management of patients with chronic liver disease by exacerbating a bleeding tendency (gingko) or by antagonizing the antimineralocorticoid action of spironolactone (glycyrrhizin, licorice) [625]. Agents with immunostimulant actions, such as *Echinacea* and *St John's wort*, can interfere with immunosuppressive therapy and provoke allograft rejection [625].

Herbal hepatoxicity encompasses a range of hepatic pathology from acute hepatitis, steatosis, and fibrosis, through to SOS and submassive or massive hepatic necrosis. Table 27.18 provides an updated account of contemporary agents implicated in significant liver injury, and some well-characterized and illustrative examples are briefly outlined below. More detailed accounts are available in recent reviews [629,630].

Chaparral

Chaparral (*Larrea tridentate*) is marketed as tablets, capsules, or herbal tea infusions. It is used as a dietary "energy" supplement and as a cure for numerous ailments ranging from chicken pox to cancer. Cholestatic hepatitis is the predominant mode of presentation, but chaparral has been associated with acute hepatitis, subacute hepatic necrosis, and acute liver failure [631]. Hepatotoxicity is at least partly dose dependent; dosage recommendations were exceeded in some severe cases [631]. At least three patients have developed end-stage liver disease requiring hepatic transplantation.

Germander

Used as a traditional remedy for many centuries, germander became popular as a slimming aid in the 1980s, particularly in France and Italy. More than 30 cases of liver injury were recorded, mostly in middle-aged women. Acute hepatitis developed 8 weeks after the ingestion of germander capsules or herbal teas [632]. Presence of ANAs, SMAs, and, transiently, antimitochondrial M2 antibodies have been recorded occasionally [633]. Although most patients recovered, several fatalities from

Table 27.18 Herbal remedies and dietary supplements implicated as causing toxic liver injury.

Herbal remedy	Indications	Toxic constituent	Pattern of liver injury
Atractylis gummifera	Purgative, emetic, diuretic	Potassium atractylate and gummiferin	Acute liver failure
Black cohosh	Menopausal symptoms	Not known; contains diterpenoids	Acute liver failure; can trigger autoimmune hepatitis
Boh-gol-zhee	Herbal tea	*Psoralea corylifolea*	Zone 3 hepatic necrosis, acute cholestatic hepatitis
Camphor	Rubefacient	Cyclic terpenes	Abnormal liver tests, encephalopathy
Carp capsules (raw carp gallbladder)	Rheumatism, visual acuity	Cyprinol	Liver enzyme changes (no biopsy) with acute renal failure, hepatic necrosis (rats)
Cascara sagrada	Laxative	Many; ?anthraquinones	Cholestatic hepatitis, portal hypertension
Centella asiatica	Obesity, leprosy, wound care	Pentacyclic triterpenic saponosides	Acute hepatitis, granulomatous hepatitis, cirrhosis
Chaparral leaf	Multiple uses	*Larrea tridentate*	Zone 3 necrosis, massive hepatic necrosis, chronic hepatitis, cholestasis
Chaso, onshido; sennomotokounou	Slimming aid	*N*-nitrosofenfluramine	Submassive or massive hepatic necrosis, acute hepatitis
Chinese herbal medicines (see text)	Multiple uses; skin diseases, health tonic, viral hepatitis	Many; *Dictamnus dasycarpus* present in six cases (in combination)	Liver injury (no histology), acute hepatitis, SOS (VOD), VBDS
Comfrey; gordolobo yerba tea; maté tea; Chinese herbal tea	Health tonic	Pyrrolizidine alkaloids, Compositae	SOS (VOD)
Dai-saiko-to (TJ-9)[a]	Liver disease, especially chronic viral hepatitis	Scutellaria, glycyrrhizin	Acute and chronic hepatitis
Fu fang qing dai wan	Psoriasis	Unknown (multiple herbs)	Acute hepatitis
Germander (tea, capsules) and related *Teucrium* species	Weight reduction, health tonic	Neoclerodane diterpenes (*Teucrium chamaedrys* L.)	Acute and chronic hepatitis, zone 3 necrosis, fibrosis, cirrhosis, acute liver failure (*T. capitatum, T. polium*); zone 3 hepatic necrosis, hepatic fibrosis (*T. polium*)
Greater celandine	Gallstones	*Chelidonium majus*	Acute hepatitis, cholestatic hepatitis, fibrosis
"Green juice"	Dietary supplement	Contains vegetable extracts and micronutrients	Granulomatous hepatitis
Green tea extracts (Exolise®, Hydroxycut®, The Right Approach®)	Herbal tea	?Epigallocatechin-3-gallate	Acute hepatocellular injury, cholestatic hepatitis, submassive or massive hepatic necrosis
Herbalife®	Health supplement	Not known	Acute hepatitis, cholestasis, bile duct injury, giant cell hepatitis, SOS (VOD) (?due to contaminant)
Isabgol	Laxative	Not identified	Giant cell hepatitis (one report)
Jin bu huan anodyne tablets	Sedation, analgesic	*Lycopodium serratum*	Acute and chronic hepatitis, steatosis, fibrosis
Kava	Anxiety disorders	Kavalactone	Diffuse hepatocellular necrosis, cholestatic hepatitis; isolated GGTP increase
Kombucha "mushroom"	Health tonic	Yeast–bacteria aggregate; contains usnic acid	Acute hepatitis
Linghzi	Multiple uses	*Ganoderma lucidum*	Acute cholestatic hepatitis
LipoKinetix®	Slimming aid	?Ephedra, ?usnic acid	Acute hepatitis, acute liver failure

Table 27.18 (Continued)

Herbal remedy	Indications	Toxic constituent	Pattern of liver injury
Lycopodium similiaplex	Insomnia	*Lycopodium serratum* and *Chelidonium majus*	Acute hepatitis
Ma-huang	Slimming aid	Ephedrine	Acute hepatitis; exacerbates autoimmune hepatitis
Margosa oil	Health tonic	*Azadirachza indica*	Reye syndrome
Mediterranean remedy	Anti-inflammatory agent	*Teucrium polium*	Zone 3 necrosis, acute liver failure, fibrosis
Mixed preparations: mistletoe, skullcap, valerian	Herbal tonics	Not identified; ?scutellaria. Skullcap has diterpenoids (cf. germander)	Liver injury (no histologic studies)
"Natural laxatives"	Cathartic	Senna, podophyllin, aloin	Senna (acute hepatitis, cholestatic hepatitis)
			Cascara (acute cholestatic hepatitis, bridging hepatic fibrosis)
Noni juice	Food supplement	*Morinda citrafolia*	Hepatocellular injury including cases of acute or subacute liver failure
Oil of cloves	Dental pain	Eugenol	Dose-dependent hepatotoxin, zonal necrosis
Pennyroyal oil (squawmint)	Abortifacient, herbal drug	Pulegone metabolites	Confluent hepatocellular necrosis
Prostata	Prostatism	Saw palmetto	Hepatitis, fibrosis
Red yeast rice	Hypercholesterolemia	HMG CoA reductase inhibitors including lovastatin	Acute hepatitis
Shark cartilage	Food supplement	Not identified	Abnormal liver tests (no histology)
Sho-saiko-to (TJ-9)[a]	Health tonic, viral hepatitis	Scutellaria, glycyrrhizin, others	Zonal/bridging necrosis, fibrosis, microvesicular steatosis
Shou-wu-pian	Dizziness, premature graying of hair, liver disease	*Polygonum multiflorum* (?anthraquinones); ?stilbene glycosides	Acute hepatitis, acute cholestatic hepatitis
Usnic acid	Slimming aid	Usnic acid	Acute liver failure
Zulu remedy	Health tonic	*Callilepsis laureola*	Hepatic necrosis

[a]TJ-9 is used in Japan and China; there are several alternative spellings, including sho-saiko-to and dai-saiko-to.
GGTP, γ-glutamyl transpeptidase; HMG-CoA, 3-hydroxy-3-methylglutaryl coenzyme A; SOS, sinusoidal obstruction syndrome; VBDS, vanishing bile duct syndrome; VOD, venoocclusive disease.

liver failure have been recorded. In some individuals, chronic hepatitis or cirrhosis was evident at presentation. Other case studies suggest that unfavorable outcomes are related more often to continued or repeated drug ingestion after the onset of liver injury. Early recrudescence of liver test abnormalities following rechallenge is suggestive of immunologic idiosyncrasy. The identification of a microsomal target for germander-induced autoantibodies is consistent with this proposal [634]. On the other hand, the demonstration that the constitutive neoclordane diterpenoids in germander are metabolized by CYP3A enzymes to epoxides that can deplete GSH and incite oxidative stress-dependent apoptosis favors a reactive metabolite mechanism of liver injury [635].

Herbal products derived from closely allied medicinal plants *Teucrium polium* L. and *Teucrium capitatum* L. have also been associated with acute liver failure and acute hepatitis with bridging necrosis, respectively [636].

Jin bu huan

Jin bu huan has been implicated in several cases of acute hepatitis [637]. The onset of symptoms occurred after a mean of 20 weeks (range, 7–52 weeks). Focal hepatic necrosis with numerous eosinophils, minor lobular hepatitis with microvesicular steatosis, and bridging fibrosis have been described. Resolution occurred within 8 weeks of discontinuation, but chronic hepatitis has been reported with long-term use [638].

Levo-tetrohydropalmatine, the active ingredient, is structurally similar to the hepatotoxic pyrrolizidine alkaloids (see next). Despite being banned in the United States and Canada since 1994, new cases of jin bu huan toxicity continue to accrue, stressing the need for continued vigilance.

Kava

Extracts of *Piper methysticum* have been used as a traditional ceremonial beverage ("Kava," "Kava Kava") in South Pacific countries. Elsewhere, they are dispensed by alternative medical practitioners as anxiolytics or sedatives. Over 60 cases of hepatotoxicity have been reported worldwide [639]. Most reported cases have occurred in users of alcohol or acetone extracts of the herb, but traditional preparations of kava, which are aqua based, have also been rarely implicated in causing liver injury [640]. The frequency of kava-associated liver injury has been estimated at 0.24–0.26 per million daily doses. Many of the affected individuals have been women (female : male ratio 3 : 1). These included 11 patients with acute liver failure who required liver transplantation [641]; the explants showed pan-acinar necrosis. In less severe cases, cholestatic or lobular hepatitis was noted. Symptoms of liver injury were reported to begin 3–16 weeks after starting ingestion (range, 2 weeks to 2 years; median, 4.5 months). Reversible increase in GGTP has also been recorded in kava users [42], but this appears unrelated to the marked rise in AT seen in patients developing liver injury and could instead reflect adaptation (microsomal enzyme induction).

The hepatotoxic potential of kava has been disputed by phytomedicine practitioners, who cite its safe track record and the presence of alcohol or concurrent hepatotoxic medications in some reports. However, there are well-documented cases occurring in the absence of such confounding factors. Moreover, positive rechallenge has been documented in at least two cases [639].

The active ingredients in kava are collectively termed kavapyrones (or kavalactones). The mechanism of liver injury is unclear but the following have been suggested: inhibition of CYP enzymes, inhibition of cyclooxygenases COX-1 and COX-2, or depletion of hepatic glutathione. An immunoallergic basis has been postulated due to the lack of dose dependency; it is further supported by the presence of autoantibodies, eosinophilia, positive lymphocyte transformation tests, and also the successful use of corticosteroids in some cases. However, metabolic idiosyncrasy appears more plausible as the above "immune" phenomena are lacking in the majority of cases [639,642]. As noted above, the debrisoquine slow metabolizer phenotype may predispose to kava hepatitis in Caucasians. However, studies involving affected Pacific islanders have not confirmed such a relationship [640], which is not surprising given the low prevalence (~1%) of CYP2D6 deficiency in these ethnic groups [626].

Pyrrolizidine alkaloids

Ingestion of these plant alkaloids is endemic in Africa and Jamaica, usually as herbal tea mixtures or extracts derived from mashing and boiling herbal or plant material (decoctions) or even as an enema [629]. Such preparations have been associated with hepatic VOD (SOS), fibrosis, and cirrhosis. Pyrrolizidine alkaloid contamination has also been found in cases of SOS associated with the consumption of Chinese herbal teas and comfrey [630]. In India and Afghanistan, epidemics of SOS have occurred following the contamination of wheat flour with pyrrolizidine alkaloids [643]. In the acute form of SOS, the typical manifestations are abdominal pain, ascites, hepatomegaly, and raised ATs. Liver failure can occur, even during the acute phase, but recovery is also possible. On the other hand, the prognosis is poor for individuals presenting with the chronic form of this disease. Death occurs from liver failure.

Herbal slimming aids

Several cases of acute liver injury have been reported in association with herbal weight reduction remedies [644]. In Japan, 12 women presented with jaundice, fatigue, diarrhea, and a biochemical picture of hepatocellular injury, 5–45 days after commencing Chaso® or Onshido® [645]. Of these, two developed acute liver failure; one survived after a liver transplant and the other died 6 weeks after admission. Pathologic findings were of massive or submassive hepatic necrosis or acute hepatitis. Over 400 cases of hepatotoxicity associated with herbal weight loss aids were reported to the Japanese Health Ministry in 2002; Chaso and Onshido use were recorded in 21 and 135 cases, respectively. *N*-nitrosofenfluramine has been identified as a potential hepatotoxin with these two products, and is a recognized hepatocarcinogen. Other *N*-nitrosofenfluramine-containing compounds associated with liver toxicity include Sennomotokounou® and LipoKinetix® (see below). Over 100 cases, including two deaths from Sennomotokounou liver toxicity were reported to the Japanese Ministry of Health, Labour, and Welfare [644]. Individual susceptibility may be important because the frequency of liver injury appears to be low; the CYP2C19 poor metabolizer phenotype was present in one of two patients with acute hepatitis. An immunoallergic basis was postulated for the other patient, who lacked this phenotype, but developed peripheral and tissue (liver) eosinophilia.

LipoKinetix, a dietary supplement, has been implicated in seven cases of acute hepatocellular injury in Los Angeles, USA [646]. Five of these were Japanese nationals. The onset of liver injury was within 3 months of ingestion (many within 1 month). Three patients developed acute liver failure but eventually recovered. Recovery was complete within 3 months. Liver histology was not available. The toxic ingredient was not identified among this multicomponent herbal product; potential candidates include ephedra alkaloids or usnic acid. The latter, marketed as a "fat burner," works by uncoupling oxidative phosphorylation. It has been implicated in causing acute liver failure in a 35-year-old woman [647]. The disruption in mitochondrial bioenergetics and generation of oxidative stress could be central to usnic acid hepatotoxicity. Interestingly, usnic acid is also present in kombucha "mushroom", a multipurpose tonic previously implicated in cases of hepatocellular injury [644]. It has also been suggested that usnic acid could be the primary hepatotoxin in LipoKinetix-related liver toxicity. However, the absence of lactic acidosis argues against the involvement of usnic acid, a primary mitochondrial toxin [644]. Another herbal slimming aid, now withdrawn, Hydroxycut® was implicated in several instances of acute hepatitis, including a few reports of acute liver failure necessitating liver transplantation [648].

Natural and synthetic retinoids

Hypervitaminosis A

Risk factors

Vitamin A is a dose-dependent hepatotoxin. Historically, cases of acute hypervitaminosis A with liver injury occurred among arctic travelers who were forced to consume large quantities of polar bear liver. Today, liver injury more often follows self-medication with vitamin A preparations, although rare instances of hypervitaminosis A have followed consumption of large amounts of raw liver alone or in combination with β-carotene-rich vitamins [649,650].

Hepatic injury occurs both with acute ingestion of massive doses (>600,000 IU) and with prolonged ingestion of smaller doses [651]. The mean daily dose of vitamin A in reported cases has been 96,000 IU, and the average duration of ingestion has been 7.2 years (range, 11 days to 30 years) representing a mean cumulative dose of 229 million units [652]. Cirrhosis has occurred in persons with a daily intake of 25,000 IU for 6 years or longer [652]. It is therefore noteworthy that up to 3% of vitamin supplements in the United States recommended for daily use contain 25,000 IU or more of vitamin A. In patients with renal failure, vitamin A doses as low as 4,000 IU/day can lead to hepatotoxicity [653].

Diagnosis: presentation, clinical features, and laboratory findings

In a Belgian series, only about a third of 41 cases were identified correctly at presentation; the average delay in diagnosis was 18 months [652]. Hypervitaminosis A is associated with hepatotoxicity in about 50% of cases. Other features of hypervitaminosis are usually present, such as fatigue, myalgia, bone pain, dry skin, alopecia, gingivitis, xanthosis, headache, neuropsychiatric disturbances, hypercalcemia, and growth retardation [654]. The liver is often enlarged. Splenomegaly, ascites, and signs of portal hypertension are present in severe cases, but jaundice is not usually found.

The clinicopathologic spectrum of hypervitaminosis A-related liver disease includes minor alteration of liver enzymes, peliosis hepatis [655], noncirrhotic portal hypertension with perisinusoidal fibrosis, sclerosis of central veins, and cirrhosis. Decompensated chronic liver disease can occur in the absence of cirrhosis and may be irreversible. Liver enzyme changes are nonspecific. Hypoalbuminemia, prolongation of prothrombin time, and hyperglobulinemia (with predominant IgM) are seen in advanced cases [652]. An increased plasma level of retinyl esters (>10%) as a proportion of total serum vitamin A (normal <8%) has been suggested as a marker of hypervitaminosis A [656], but this is not supported by the NHANES III survey, which showed no correlation between retinyl esters and liver test abnormalities [657]. Further, plasma vitamin A levels may also be normal in patients with hepatic fibrosis [652]. A demonstration of increased hepatic vitamin A stores and the characteristic histologic appearances are a more reliable guide to diagnosis.

Liver pathology

Stellate cells store vitamin A in the liver. As expected, liver biopsies of people with hypervitaminosis A show stellate cell hypertrophy and hyperplasia. This can give rise to sinusoidal compression and a typical honeycombed ("Swiss cheese") appearance. Perisinusoidal fibrosis is often striking, whereas hepatocellular injury is usually minimal. Microvesicular steatosis and focal degeneration have also been reported [658]. Vitamin A deposition is readily detected on fresh liver sections by the characteristic greenish autofluorescence after irradiation with ultraviolet light.

Course and management

Gradual improvement usually occurs after vitamin A is discontinued, but progression from noncirrhotic portal hypertension to cirrhosis may continue [659]. Features of liver failure with established cirrhosis at diagnosis indicate a poor prognosis; most patients die or require hepatic transplantation [660]. This is because turnover of vitamin A stores is very slow [half-life, 58–286 days]. Abstinence from alcohol is advised because ethanol can potentiate vitamin A hepatotoxicity [661].

Synthetic retinoids

Etretinate is an aromatic synthetic retinoid (structurally unrelated to vitamin A) used in the management of psoriasis and other dyskeratotic skin disorders. Abnormal liver tests are found in up to 20% of recipients of etretinate but overt liver injury is less common (<1%). Acute and chronic hepatitis, mild cholestasis and cirrhosis have all been reported [662]. Features of drug allergy are usually not present, although eosinophilia was reported in one case [663]. Recovery can be delayed because of the long tissue half-life of etretinate (120 days). Corticosteroids appeared to induce a clinical response in one report of etretinate-induced chronic hepatitis [662]. It is recommended that patients taking etretinate be monitored with regular liver tests. If the liver enzymes are raised (>3 × ULN), the options are to either perform a liver biopsy to assess the significance of liver injury or discontinue etretinate [14].

Acitretin, the major metabolite of etretinate, has a shorter half-life (50 hours). A large study evaluating sequential liver biopsies on recipients of acitretin did not show significant histologic progression [664]. However, acitretin has also been associated with a few reports of acute hepatitis, including one instance of acute cholestatic hepatitis with bile-duct injury accompanied by marked hyperbilirubinemia (70 mg/dL) [665]. Progressive fibrosis and cirrhosis can occur, despite stopping acitretin [666]. Periodic monitoring of liver function tests is recommended.

References

1. Farrell GC. Liver disease due to environmental toxins. In: Farrell GC, ed. *Drug-induced Liver Disease*. Edinburgh: Churchill Livingstone, 1994:511–49.
2. Zimmerman HJ. *Hepatotoxicity: the adverse effects of drugs and other chemicals on the liver*, 2nd edn. Philadelphia: Lippincott Williams and Wilkins, 1999.
3. Chalasani N, Björnsson E. Risk factors for idiosyncratic drug-induced liver injury. *Gastroenterology* 2010;138:2246–59.
4. Lammert C, Bjornsson E, Niklasson A, et al. Oral medications with significant hepatic metabolism at higher risk for hepatic adverse events. *Hepatology* 2010;51:615–20.
5. Mackay IR. The immunological mediation of drug reactions affecting the liver. In: Farrell GC, ed. *Drug-induced Liver Disease*. Edinburgh: Churchill Livingstone, 1994;61–81.
6. Bissell DM, Gores GJ, Laskin DL, et al. Drug-induced liver injury: mechanisms and test systems. *Hepatology* 2001;33:1009–13.
7. Smith GCM, Kenna JG, Harrison DJ, et al. Autoantibodies to hepatic microsomal carboxylesterase in halothane hepatitis. *Lancet* 1993;342:963–4.
8. Gut J, Christen U, Huwyler J, et al. Molecular mimicry of trifluoroacetylated human liver protein adducts by constitutive proteins and immunochemical evidence for its impairment in halothane hepatitis. *Eur J Biochem* 1992;210:569–76.
9. Pham B-N, Bernuau J, Durand F, et al. Eotaxin expression and eosinophil infiltrate in the liver of patients with drug-induced liver disease. *J Hepatol* 2001;34:537–47.
10. Imaeda AB, Watanabe A, Sohail MA, et al. Acetaminophen-induced hepatotoxicity in mice is dependent on Tlr9 and the Nalp3 inflammasome. *J Clin Invest* 2009;119:305–14.
11. Teoh N, Chitturi S, Farrell GC. Liver disease caused by drugs, anesthetics, and toxins. In: Feldman M, Friedman LS, Brandt LJ, eds. *Sleisenger and Fordtran's Gastrointestinal and Liver Disease*, 9th edn. Philadelphia: WB Saunders, 2010:1413–46.
12. Larrey D, Pageaux GP. Genetic predisposition to drug-induced hepatotoxicity. *J Hepatol* 1997;26(Suppl 2):12–21.
13. Henderson CJ, Wolf CR, Kitteringham N, et al. Increased resistance to acetaminophen hepatotoxicity in mice lacking glutathione S-transferase Pi. *Proc Natl Acad Sci USA* 2000;97:12741–5.
14. Farrell GC. *Drug-induced Liver Disease*. Edinburgh: Churchill Livingstone, 1994.
15. Lee WM. Drug-induced hepatotoxicity. *N Engl J Med* 1995;333:1118–27.
16. Lewis JH. Drug-induced liver disease. *Med Clin North Am* 2000;84:1275–311.
17. Biour M, Poupon R, Grange JD, et al. Drug-induced hepatotoxicity. The 13th updated edition of the bibliographic database of drug-related liver injuries and responsible drugs. *Gastroenterol Clin Biol* 2000;24:1052–91.
18. Stricker BHCh. Drug-induced hepatic injury. In: Dukes MNG, ed. *Drug-induced Disorders*, vol 5, 2nd edn. Amsterdam: Elsevier, 1992.
19. Larrey D. Drug-induced liver diseases. *J Hepatol* 2000;32(Suppl. 1):77–88.
20. Farrell GC. Drug-induced hepatic injury. *J Gastroenterol Hepatol* 1997;12:S242–50.
21. Larrey D, Vial T, Micaleff A, et al. Hepatitis associated with amoxicillin-clavulanic acid combination. Report of 15 cases. *Gut* 1992;33:368–71.
22. Garcia Rodriguez LA, Stricker BH, Zimmerman HJ. Risk of acute liver injury associated with the combination of amoxicillin and clavulanic acid. *Arch Intern Med* 1996;156:1327–32.
23. Kromann-Andersen H, Pedersen A. Reported adverse reactions to and consumption of nonsteroidal anti-inflammatory drugs in Denmark over a 17-year period. *Dan Med Bull* 1988;35:187–92.
24. Neuschwander-Tetri BA, Isley WL, Oki JC, et al. Troglitazone-induced hepatic failure leading to liver transplantation. *Ann Intern Med* 1998;129:38–41.
25. McNeil JJ, Grabsch EA, McDonald MM. Postmarketing surveillance: strengths and limitations. The flucloxacillin-dicloxacillin story. *Med J Aust* 1999;170:270–3.
26. Rooks JB, Ory HW, Ishak KG, et al. Epidemiology of hepatocellular adenoma. The role of oral contraceptive use. *JAMA* 1979;242:644–8.
27. Prentice RL. Epidemiologic data on exogenous hormones and hepatocellular carcinoma and selected other cancers. *Prevent Med* 1991;20:38–46.
28. Valla D, Benhamou J-P. Drug-induced vascular and sinusoidal lesions of the liver. *Bailliere's Clin Gastroenterol* 1988;2:481–500.
29. Hurwitz ES, Barrett MJ, Bregman D, et al. Public health service study of Reye's syndrome and medications. *JAMA* 1987;257:1905–11.
30. Whiting-O'Keefe QE, Fye KH, Sack KD. Methotrexate and histologic hepatic abnormalities: a meta-analysis. *Am J Med* 1991;90:711–16.
31. Knowles SR, Uetrecht J, Shear NH. Idiosyncratic drug reactions: the reactive metabolite syndromes. *Lancet* 2000;356:1587–91.
32. Stieger B, Fattinger K, Madon J, et al. Drug- and estrogen-induced cholestasis through inhibition of the hepatocellular bile export pump (Bsep) of rat liver. *Gastroenterology* 2000;118:422–30.
33. Daly AK. Drug-induced liver injury: past, present and future. *Pharmacogenomics* 2010;11:607–11.

34. Uusimaa J, Hinttala R, Rantala H, et al. Homozygous W748S mutation in the POLG1 gene in patients with juvenile-onset Alpers syndrome and status epilepticus. *Epilepsia* 2008;49:1038–45.

35. Krahenbuhl S, Brandner S, Kleinle S, et al. Mitochondrial diseases represent a risk factor for valproate-induced fulminant liver failure. *Liver* 2000;20:346–8.

36. O'Donohue J, Oien KA, Donaldson P, et al. Co-amoxiclav jaundice: clinical and histological features and HLA class II association. *Gut* 2000;47:717–20.

37. Hautekeete ML, Horsmans Y, Van Waeyenberge C, et al. HLA association of amoxicillin-clavulanate-induced hepatitis. *Gastroenterology* 1999;117:1181–6.

38. Daly AK, Donaldson PT, Bhatnagar P, et al. HLA-B*5701 genotype is a major determinant of drug-induced liver injury due to flucloxacillin. *Nat Genet* 2009;41:816–19.

39. Kurosaki M, Takagi H, Mori M. HLA-A33/B44/DR6 is highly related to intrahepatic cholestasis induced by tiopronin. *Dig Dis Sci* 2000;45:1103–8.

40. Berson A, Fréneaux E, Larrey D, et al. Possible role of HLA in hepatotoxicity. An exploratory study in 71 patients with drug-induced idiosyncratic hepatitis. *J Hepatol* 1994;20:336–42.

41. Le Couteur DG, Cogger VC, Markus AM, et al. Pseudocapillarization and associated energy limitation in the aged rat liver. *Hepatology* 2001;33:537–43.

42. Chitturi S, Farrell GC. In: Schiff ER, Sorrell MF, Maddrey WC, eds. *Schiff's Diseases of the Liver*, 9th edn. Philadelphia: Lippincott Williams and Wilkins, 2003:1059–128.

43. Hokkanen OT, Sotaniemi EA. Liver injury and multiple drug therapy. *Arch Toxicol Suppl* 1978;1:173–6.

44. Smith DW, Cullity GJ, Silberstein EP. Fatal hepatic necrosis associated with multiple anticonvulsant therapy. *Aust NZ J Med* 1988;18:575–81.

45. Perez Gutthann S, Garcia Rodriguez LA. The increased risk of hospitalizations for acute liver injury in a population with exposure to multiple drugs. *Epidemiology* 1993;4:496–501.

46. Moertel CG, Fleming TR, Macdonald JS, et al. Hepatic toxicity associated with fluorouracil plus levamisole adjuvant therapy. *J Clin Oncol* 1993;11:2386–90.

47. Singh J, Garg PK, Tandon RK. Hepatotoxicity due to antituberculosis therapy. Clinical profile and reintroduction of therapy. *J Clin Gastroenterol* 1996;22:211–14.

48. McDonald GB, Sharma P, Matthews DE, et al. Venoocclusive disease of the liver after bone marrow transplantation: diagnosis, incidence, and predisposing factors. *Hepatology* 1984;4:116–22.

49. Seaman WE, Ishak KG, Plotz PH. Aspirin-induced hepatotoxicity in patients with systemic lupus erythematosus. *Ann Intern Med* 1974;80:1–8.

50. Gray DR, Morgan T, Chretien SD, et al. Efficacy and safety of controlled-release niacin in dyslipoproteinemic veterans. *Ann Intern Med* 1994;121:252–8.

51. Nehra A, Mullick F, Ishak KG, et al. Pemoline-associated hepatic injury. *Gastroenterology* 1990;99:1517–19.

52. Marotta PJ, Roberts EA. Pemoline hepatotoxicity in children. *J Pediatr* 1998;132:894–7.

53. Langman G, Hall PM, Todd G. Role of non-alcoholic steatohepatitis in methotrexate-induced liver injury. *J Gastroenterol Hepatol* 2001;16:1395–401.

54. Dennis EW. Fatal hepatic necrosis in association with the use of hycanthone. *S Afr Med J* 1978;54:137–8.

55. Wong WM, Wu PC, Yuen MF, et al. Antituberculosis drug-related liver dysfunction in chronic hepatitis B infection. *Hepatology* 2000;31:201–6.

56. Sulkowski MS, Thomas DL, Chaisson RE, et al. Hepatotoxicity associated with antiretroviral therapy in adults infected with human immunodeficiency virus and the role of hepatitis C or B virus. *JAMA* 2000;283:74–80.

57. Riley TR 3rd, Smith JP. Ibuprofen-induced hepatotoxicity in patients with chronic hepatitis C: a case series. *Am J Gastroenterol* 1998;93:1563–5.

58. Pu YS, Liu CM, Kao JH, et al. Antiandrogen hepatotoxicity in patients with chronic viral hepatitis. *Eur Urol* 1999;36:293–7.

59. Benson GB. Hepatotoxicity following the therapeutic use of antipyretic analgesics. *Am J Med* 1983;75(Suppl):85–93.

60. Gordin FM, Simon GL, Wofsy CB, et al. Adverse reactions to trimethoprim-sulfamethoxazole in patients with acquired immunodeficiency syndrome. *Ann Intern Med* 1984;100:495–9.

61. Poulin C. Prevention of paracetamol poisoning. *Lancet* 2000;355:2009–10.

62. Peters TS. Do preclinical testing strategies help predict human hepatotoxic potentials? *Toxicol Pathol* 2005;33:146–54.

63. Smith CC, Bernstein LI, Davis RB, et al. Screening for statin-related toxicity: the yield of transaminase and creatine kinase measurements in a primary care setting. *Arch Intern Med* 2003;163:657–9.

64. Rosenzweig P, Miget N, Brohier S. Transaminase elevation on placebo during phase I trials. *Br J Clin Pharmacol* 1999;48:19–23.

65. Chalasani N. Statins and hepatotoxicity: focus on patients with fatty liver. *Hepatology* 2005;41:690–5.

66. Pond SM, Olson KR, Woo OF, et al. Amatoxin poisoning in northern California, 1982–1983. *West J Med* 1984;145:204–9.

67. Cohn WJ, Boylan JJ, Blanke RV, et al. Treatment of chlordecone (Kepone) toxicity with cholestyramine. Results of a controlled clinical trial. *N Engl J Med* 1978;298:243–8.

68. Lee WM, Hynan LS, Rossaro L, et al. Intravenous N-acetylcysteine improves transplant-free survival in early stage non-acetaminophen acute liver failure. *Gastroenterology* 2009;137:856–64.

69. Katsinelos P, Vasiliadis T, Xiarchos P, et al. Ursodeoxycholic acid (UDCA) for the treatment of amoxicillin-clavulanate potassium (Augmentin)-induced intra-hepatic cholestasis: report of two cases. *Eur J Gastroenterol Hepatol* 2000;12:365–8.

70. Piotrowicz A, Polkey M, Wilkinson M. Ursodeoxycholic acid for the treatment of flucloxacillin-associated cholestasis. *J Hepatol* 1995;22:119–20.

71. Cicognani C, Malavolti M, Morselli-Labate AM, et al. Flutamide-induced toxic hepatitis. Potential utility of ursodeoxycholic acid administration in toxic hepatitis. *Dig Dis Sci* 1996;41:2219–21.

72. Kallinowski B, Theilmann L, Zimmermann R, et al. Effective treatment of cyclosporine-induced cholestasis in heart-transplanted patients treated with ursodeoxycholic acid. *Transplantation* 1991;51:1128–9.

73. Franco J. Pruritus. *Curr Treatment Options Gastroenterol* 1999;2:451–6.

74. Kaplowitz N. Causality assessment versus guilt-by-association in drug hepatotoxicity. *Hepatology* 2001;33:308–10.

75. Danan G, Benichou C. Causality assessment of adverse reactions to drugs – I. A novel method based on the conclusions of international consensus meetings: application to drug-induced liver injuries. *J Clin Epidemiol* 1993;46:1323–30.

76. Maria VA, Victorino RM. Development and validation of a clinical scale for the diagnosis of drug induced hepatitis. *Hepatology* 1997;26:664–9.

77. Lucena MI, Camargo R, Andrade RJ, et al. Comparison of two clinical scales for causality assessment in hepatotoxicity. *Hepatology* 2001;33:123–30.

78. Lewis JH, Larrey D, Olsson R, et al. Utility of the Roussel Uclaf Causality Assessment Method (RUCAM) to analyze the hepatic findings in a clinical trial program: evaluation of the direct thrombin inhibitor ximelagatran. *Int J Clin Pharmacol Ther* 2008;46:327–39.

79. Rockey DC, Seeff LB, Rochon J, et al.; US Drug-induced Liver Injury Network. Causality assessment in drug-induced liver injury using a

structured expert opinion process: comparison to the Roussel–Uclaf causality assessment method. *Hepatology* 2010;51:2117–26.

80. Benichou C. Criteria for drug-induced liver disorders. Report of an International Consensus Meeting. *J Hepatol* 1990;11:272–6.

81. Laurent-Puig P, Dussaix E, de Paillette L, et al. Prevalence of hepatitis C RNA in suspected drug-induced liver diseases [Letter]. *J Hepatol* 1993;19:487–9.

82. Hall P de la M. Histological diagnosis of drug-induced liver disease. In: Farrell GC, ed. *Drug-induced Liver Disease*. Edinburgh: Churchill Livingstone, 1994:115–51.

83. Berson A, Gervais A, Cazals D, et al. Hepatitis after intravenous buprenorphine misuse in heroin addicts. *J Hepatol* 2001;34:346–50.

84. Chitturi S, Farrell GC. Drug-induced cholestasis. *Semin Gastrointest Dis* 2001;12:113–24.

85. Geubel AP, Sempoux SL. Drug and toxin-induced bile duct disorders. *J Gastroenterol Hepatol* 2000;15:1232–8.

86. Rosenberg WMC, Ryley NG, Trowell JM, et al. Dextropropoxyphene induced hepatotoxicity: a report of nine cases. *J Hepatol* 1993; 19:470–4.

87. Kopelman H, Robertson MH, Sanders PG, et al. The Epping jaundice. *Br Med J* 1966;5486:514–16.

88. Desmet VJ. Vanishing bile duct syndrome in drug-induced liver disease. *J Hepatol* 1997;26(Suppl 1):31–5.

89. Degott C, Feldmann G, Larrey D, et al. Drug-induced prolonged cholestasis in adults: a histological semiquantitative study demonstrating progressive ductopenia. *Hepatology* 1992;15:244–51.

90. Forbes GM, Jeffrey GP, Shilkin KB, et al. Carbamazepine hepatotoxicity: another cause of the vanishing bile duct syndrome. *Gastroenterology* 1992;102:1385–8.

91. Hunt CM, Washington K. Tetracycline-induced bile duct paucity and prolonged cholestasis. *Gastroenterology* 1994;107:1844–7.

92. Srivastava M, Perez-Atayde A, Jonas MM. Drug-associated acute-onset vanishing bile duct and Stevens–Johnson syndromes in a child. *Gastroenterology* 1998;115:743–6.

93. Chawla A, Kahn E, Yunis EJ, et al. Rapidly progressive cholestasis: an unusual reaction to amoxicillin/clavulanic acid therapy in a child. *J Pediatr* 2000;136:121–3.

94. Lazarczyk DA, Duffy M. Erythromycin-induced primary biliary cirrhosis. *Dig Dis Sci* 2000;45:1115–18.

95. Suleyman M, Hekimoglu B, Yücesoy C, et al. Percutaneous treatment of hepatic hydatid cysts: an alternative to surgery. *Am J Roentgenol* 1999;172:83–9.

96. Lefkowitch JH. Hepatic granulomas. *J Hepatol* 1999;30(Suppl):40–5.

97. McMaster KR, Hennigar GR. Drug-induced granulomatous hepatitis. *Lab Invest* 1981;44:61–73.

98. McDermott WV, Ridker PM. The Budd–Chiari syndrome and hepatic veno-occlusive disease. Recognition and treatment. *Arch Surg* 1990;125:525–7.

99. Ridker PM, Ohkuma S, McDermott WV, et al. Hepatic venocclusive disease associated with the consumption of pyrrolizidine-containing dietary supplements. *Gastroenterology* 1985;88:1050–4.

100. Deltenre P, Denninger MH, Hillaire S, et al. Factor V Leiden related Budd–Chiari syndrome. *Gut* 2001;48:264–8.

101. Edmondson HA, Henderson B, Benton B. Liver-cell adenomas associated with use of oral contraceptives. *N Engl J Med* 1976;294:470–2.

102. Ishak KG. Hepatic lesions caused by anabolic and contraceptive steroids. *Semin Liver Dis* 1981;1:116–28.

103. Aseni P, Sansalone CV, Sammartino C, et al. Rapid disappearance of hepatic adenoma after contraceptive withdrawal. *J Clin Gastroenterol* 2001;33:234–6.

104. Mathieu D, Zafrani ES, Anglade MC, et al. Association of focal nodular hyperplasia and hepatic hemangioma. *Gastroenterology* 1989;97:154–7.

105. Labarga P, Soriano V, Vispo ME, et al. Hepatotoxicity of antiretroviral drugs is reduced after successful treatment of chronic hepatitis C in HIV-infected patients. *J Infect Dis* 2007;196:670–6.

106. McDonald GB, Hinds MS, Fisher LD, et al. Veno-occlusive disease of the liver and multiorgan failure after bone marrow transplantation: a cohort study of 355 patients. *Ann Intern Med* 1993;118:255–67.

107. Snover DC, Weisdorf S, Bloomer J, et al. Nodular regenerative hyperplasia of the liver following bone marrow transplantation. *Hepatology* 1989;9:443–8.

108. Morgan MY, Reshef R, Shah RR, et al. Impaired oxidation of debrisoquine in patients with perhexiline liver injury. *Gut* 1984; 25:1057–64.

109. Farrell GC. Drugs and steatohepatitis. *Semin Liver Dis* 2002; 22:185–94.

110. Babany G, Uzzan F, Larrey D, et al. Alcoholic-like liver lesions induced by nifedipine. *J Hepatol* 1989;9:252–5.

111. Beaugrand M, Denis J, Callard P. Tous les inhibiteurs calciques peuvent-ils entrainer des lesions d'hepatite alcoolique? *Gastroenterol Clin Biol* 1987;1:76.

112. Sotaniemi EA, Hokkanen OT, Ahokas JT, et al. Hepatic injury and drug metabolism in patients with alpha-methyldopa-induced liver damage. *Eur J Clin Pharmacol* 1977;12:429–35.

113. Seki K, Minami Y, Nishikawa M, et al. Nonalcoholic steatohepatitis induced by massive doses of synthetic estrogen. *Gastroent Jpn* 1983;18:197–203.

114. Choti MA. Chemotherapy-associated hepatotoxicity: do we need to be concerned? *Ann Surg Oncol* 2009;16:2391–4.

115. Reddy KR, Schiff ER. Hepatotoxicity of antimicrobial, antifungal, and antiparasitic agents. *Gastroenterol Clin North Am* 1995;24:923–36.

116. Chitturi S, George J. Hepatotoxicity of commonly used drugs: nonsteroidal anti-inflammatory drugs, antihypertensives, antidiabetic agents, anticonvulsants, lipid-lowering agents, psychotropic drugs. *Semin Liver Dis* 2002;22:169–83.

117. Koklu S, Yuksel O, Yolcu OF, et al. Cholestatic attack due to ampicillin and cross-reactivity to cefuroxime. *Ann Pharmacother* 2004;38:1539–40.

118. Koklu S, Yuksel O, Filik L, et al. Recurrent cholestasis due to ampicillin. *Ann Pharmacother* 2003;37:395.

119. Taylor C, Corrigan K, Steen S, et al. Oxacillin and hepatitis. *Ann Intern Med* 1979;90:857–8.

120. Bruckstein AH, Attia AA. Oxacillin hepatitis. Two patients with liver biopsy, and review of the literature. *Am J Med* 1978;64:519–22.

121. Lee CY, Chen PY, Huang FL, Chi CS. Reversible oxacillin-associated hepatitis in a 9-month-old boy. *J Paediatr Child Health* 2008;44:146–8.

122. Koek GH, Sticker BHCh, Blok APR, et al. Flucloxacillin-associated hepatic injury. *Liver* 1994;14:225–9.

123. Fairley CK, McNeil JJ, Desmond P. Risk factors for development of flucloxacillin-associated jaundice. *Br Med J* 1993;306:233–5.

124. Eckstein RP, Dowsett JF, Lunzer MR. Flucloxacillin induced liver disease: histopathological findings at biopsy and autopsy. *Pathology* 1993;25:223–8.

125. Olsson R, Wiholm BE, Sand C, et al. Liver damage from flucloxacillin, cloxacillin and dicloxacillin. *J Hepatol* 1992;15:154–61.

126. Gosbell IB, Turnidge JD, Tapsall JW, et al. Toxicities of flucloxacillin and dicloxacillin – is there really a diference. *Med J Aust* 2000;173:500–1.

127. Lakehal F, Dansette PM, Becquemont L, et al. Indirect cytotoxicity of flucloxacillin toward human biliary epithelium via metabolite formation in hepatocytes. *Chem Res Toxicol* 2001;14:694–701.

128. Andrews E, Armstrong M, Tugwood J, et al. A role for the pregnane X receptor in flucloxacillin-induced liver injury. *Hepatology* 2010;51:1656–64.

129. Jenkins RE, Meng X, Elliott VL, et al. Characterisation of flucloxacillin and 5-hydroxymethyl flucloxacillin haptenated HSA in vitro and in vivo. *Proteomics Clin Appl* 2009;3:720–9.

130. Reddy KR, Brillant P, Schiff ER. Amoxicillin-clavulanate potassium-associated cholestasis. *Gastroenterology* 1989;96:1135–41.

131. Hautekeete ML, Brenard R, Horsmans Y, et al. Liver injury related to amoxicillin-clavulanic acid: interlobular bile-duct lesions and extrahepatic manifestations. *J Hepatol* 1995;22:71–7.

132. Ryan J, Dudley FJ. Cholestasis with ticarcillin-potassium clavulanate (Timentin). *Med J Aust* 1992;156:291.

133. Lucena MI, Andrade RJ, Fernández MC, et al. Determinants of the clinical expression of amoxicillin-clavulanate hepatotoxicity: a prospective series from Spain. *Hepatology* 2006;44:850–6.

134. Lucena MI, Andrade RJ, Martínez C, et al. Glutathione S-transferase m1 and t1 null genotypes increase susceptibility to idiosyncratic drug-induced liver injury. *Hepatology* 2008;48:588–96.

135. Richardet JP, Mallat A, Zafrani ES, et al. Prolonged cholestasis with ductopenia after administration of amoxicillin/clavulanic acid. *Dig Dis Sci* 1999;44:1997–2000.

136. Jordan T, Gonzalez M, Casado M, et al. Amoxicillin-clavulanic acid induced hepatotoxicity with progression to cirrhosis. *Gastroenterol Hepatol* 2002;25:240–3.

137. Lazarczyk DA, Goldstein NS, Gordon SC. Trovafloxacin hepatotoxicity. *Dig Dis Sci* 2001;46:925–6.

138. Lucena MI, Andrade RJ, Sanchez-Martinez H, et al. Norfloxacin-induced cholestatic jaundice. *Am J Gastroenterol* 1998;93:2309–11.

139. Zimpfer A, Propst A, Mikuz G, et al. Ciprofloxacin-induced acute liver injury: case report and review of literature. *Virchows Arch* 2004;444:87–9.

140. Romero-Gomez M, Suarez Garcia E, Fernandez MC, et al. Norfloxacin-induced acute cholestatic hepatitis in a patient with alcoholic liver cirrhosis. *Am J Gastroenterol* 1999;94:2324–5.

141. Gonzalez Carro P, Huidobro ML, Zabala AP, et al. Fatal subfulminant hepatic failure with ofloxacin. *Am J Gastroenterol* 2000;95:1606.

142. Cheung O, Chopra K, Yu T, et al. Gatifloxacin-induced hepatotoxicity and acute pancreatitis. *Ann Intern Med* 2004;140:73–4.

143. Soto S, Lopez-Roses L, Avila S, et al. Moxifloxacin-induced acute liver injury. *Am J Gastroenterol* 2002;97:1853–4.

144. Schwalm JD, Lee CH. Acute hepatitis associated with oral levofloxacin therapy in a hemodialysis patient. *Can Med Assoc J* 2003;168:847–8.

145. Heaton PC, Fenwick SR, Brewer DE. Association between tetracycline or doxycycline and hepatotoxicity: a population based case–control study. *J Clin Pharm Ther* 2007;32:483–7.

146. Gough A, Chapman S, Wagstaff K, et al. Minocycline induced autoimmune hepatitis and systemic lupus erythematosus-like syndrome. *Br Med J* 1996;312:169–72.

147. Lawrenson RA, Seaman HE, Sundstrom, et al. Liver damage associated with minocycline use in acne: a systematic review of the published literature and pharmacovigilance data. *Drug Safety* 2000;23:333–49.

148. Ford TJ, Dillon JF. Minocycline hepatitis. *Eur J Gastroenterol Hepatol* 2008;20:796–9.

149. Goldstein NS, Bayati N, Silverman AL, et al. Minocycline as a cause of drug-induced autoimmune hepatitis. Report of four cases and comparison with autoimmune hepatitis. *Am J Clin Pathol* 2000;114:591–8.

150. Ramakrishna J, Johnson AR, Banner BF. Long-term minocycline use for acne in healthy adolescents can cause severe autoimmune hepatitis. *J Clin Gastroenterol* 2009;43:787–90.

151. Chamberlain MC, Schwarzenberg SJ, Akin EU, Kurth MH. Minocycline induced autoimmune hepatitis with subsequent cirrhosis. *J Pediatr Gastroenterol Nutr* 2006;42:232–5.

152. Herzog D, Hajoui O, Russo P, et al. Study of immune reactivity of minocycline-induced chronic active hepatitis. *Dig Dis Sci* 1997;42:110–13.

153. Nietsch HH, Libman BS, Pansze TW, et al. Minocycline-induced hepatitis [Letter]. *Am J Gastroenterol* 2000;95:2994.

154. Carson JL, Strom BL, Duff A, et al. Acute liver disease associated with erythromycins, sulfonamides, and tetracyclines. *Ann Intern Med* 1993;119:576–83.

155. Ilario MJM, Ruiz JE, Axiotis CA. Acute fulminant hepatic failure in a woman treated with phenytoin and trimethoprim-sulfamethoxazole. *Arch Path Lab Med* 2000;124:1800–3.

156. Gordon FM, Simon GL, Wofsy CB, et al. Adverse reactions to trimethoprim-sulfamethoxazole in patients with the acquired immunodeficiency syndrome. *Ann Intern Med* 1984;100:495–9.

157. Rieder MJ, Shear NH, Kanee A, et al. Prominence of slow acetylator phenotype among patients with sulfonamide hypersensitivity reactions. *Clin Pharmacol Ther* 1991;49:13–17.

158. Cribb AE, Spielberg SP. Sulfamethoxazole is metabolized to the hydroxylamine in humans. *Clin Pharmacol Ther* 1992;51:522–6.

159. Yao F, Behling CA, Saab S, et al. Trimethoprim-sulfamethoxazole-induced vanishing bile duct syndrome. *Am J Gastroenterol* 1997;92:167–9.

160. Olsen VV, Loft S, Christensen KD, et al. Serious reactions during malaria prophylaxis with pyrimethamine-sulfadoxine. *Lancet* 1994;2:994.

161. Gulley RM, Mirza A, Kelley C. Hepatotoxicity of salicylazolpyridine. A case report and review of the literature. *Am J Gastroenterol* 1979;72:561–4.

162. Ransford RA, Langman MJ. Sulphasalazine and mesalazine: serious adverse reactions re-evaluated on the basis of suspected adverse reaction reports to the Committee on Safety of Medicines. *Gut* 2002;51:536–9.

163. Deltenre P, Berson A, Marcellin P, et al. Mesalamine (5 aminosalicylic acid) induced chronic hepatitis. *Gut* 1999;44:886–8.

164. Mulder H, Gratama S. Azodisalicylate (Dipentum)-induced hepatitis? *J Clin Gastroenterol* 1989;11:708–11.

165. Jobanputra P, Amarasena R, Maggs F, et al. Hepatotoxicity associated with sulfasalazine in inflammatory arthritis: a case series from a local surveillance of serious adverse events. *BMC Musculoskelet Disord* 2008;9:48.

166. Stoschus B, Meybehm M, Spengler U, et al. Cholestasis associated with mesalazine therapy in a patient with Crohn's disease. *J Hepatol* 1997;26:425–8.

167. Lee KB, Nashed TB. Dapsone-induced sulfone syndrome. *Ann Pharmacother* 2003;37:1044–6.

168. Itha S, Kumar A, Dhingra S, et al. Dapsone induced cholangitis as a part of dapsone syndrome: a case report. *BMC Gastroenterol* 2003;3:21.

169. Galan MV, Potts JA, Silverman AL et al. Hepatitis in a United States tertiary referral center. *J Clin Gastroenterol* 2005;39:64–7.

170. Berry WR, Warren GH, Reichen J. Nitrofurantoin-induced cholestatic hepatitis from cow's milk in a teenaged boy. *West J Med* 1984;140:278–80.

171. Paiva LA, Wright PJ, Koff RS. Long-term hepatic memory for hypersensitivity to nitrofurantoin. *Am J Gastroenterol* 1992;87:891–3.

172. Schattner A, Von der Walde J, Kozak N, et al. Nitrofurantoin-induced immune-mediated lung and liver disease. *Am J Med Sci* 1999;317:336–40.

173. Amit G, Cohen P, Ackerman Z. Nitrofurantoin-induced chronic active hepatitis. *Isr Med Assoc J* 2002;4:184–6.

174. Viluksela M, Vainio PJ, Tuominen RK. Cytotoxicity of macrolide antibiotics in cultured human liver cell line. *Antimicrob Chemother* 1996;38:465–73.

175. Gholson CF, Warren GH. Fulminant hepatic failure associated with intravenous erythromycin lactobionate. *Arch Intern Med* 1990;150:215–16.
176. Fox JC, Szyjkowski RS, Sanderson SO, et al. Progressive cholestatic liver disease associated with clarithromycin treatment. *J Clin Pharmacol* 2002;42:676–80.
177. Suriawinata A, Min AD. A 33-year-old woman with jaundice after azithromycin use. *Semin Liver Dis* 2002;22:207–10.
178. Pedersen FM, Bathum L, Fenger C. Acute hepatitis and roxithromycin. *Lancet* 1993;341:251–2.
179. Masia M, Gutierrez F, Jimeno A, et al. Fulminant hepatitis and fatal toxic epidermal necrolysis (Lyell disease) coincident with clarithromycin administration in an alcoholic patient receiving disulfiram therapy. *Arch Intern Med* 2002;162:474–6.
180. Brinker AD, Wassel RT, Lyndly J, et al. Telithromycin-associated hepatotoxicity: clinical spectrum and causality assessment of 42 cases. *Hepatology* 2009;49:250–7.
181. Gulliford M, Mackey AD, Prowse K. Cholestatic jaundice induced by ethambutol. *Br Med J* 1986;292:866.
182. Garibaldi RA, Drusin RE, Ferebee SH, et al. Isoniazid-associated hepatitis: report of an outbreak. *Am Rev Resp Dis* 1972;106:357–65.
183. Maddrey WC, Boitnott JK. Isoniazid hepatitis. *Ann Intern Med* 1973;79:1–12.
184. Black M, Mitchell JR, Zimmerman HJ, et al. Isoniazid-associated hepatitis in 114 patients. *Gastroenterology* 1975;69:289–302.
185. Mitchell JR, Zimmerman HJ, Ishak KG, et al. Isoniazid liver injury: clinical spectrum, pathology and probable pathogenesis. *Ann Intern Med* 1976;84:181–92.
186. Wu SS, Chao CS, Vargas JH, et al. Isoniazid-related hepatic failure in children: a survey of liver transplantation centers. *Transplantation* 2007;84:173–9.
187. Tostmann A, Boeree MJ, Aarnoutse RE, et al. Antituberculosis drug-induced hepatotoxicity: concise up-to-date review. *J Gastroenterol Hepatol* 2008;23:192–202.
188. Marzuki OA, Fauzi AR, Ayoub S, Kamarul Imran M. Prevalence and risk factors of anti-tuberculosis drug-induced hepatitis in Malaysia. *Singapore Med J* 2008;49:688–93.
189. Singh J, Arora A, Garg PK, et al. Antituberculosis treatment-induced hepatotoxicity: role of predictive factors. *Postgrad Med J* 1995;71:359–62.
190. Gurumurthy P, Krishnamurthy MS, Nazareth O, et al. Lack of relationship between hepatic toxicity and acetylator phenotype in three thousand South Indian patients during treatment with isoniazid for tuberculosis. *Am Rev Respir Dis* 1984;129:58–61.
191. Ohno M, Yamaguchi I, Yamamoto I, et al. Slow N-acetyltransferase 2 genotype affects the incidence of isoniazid and rifampicin-induced hepatotoxicity. *Int J Tuberc Lung Dis* 2000;4:256–61.
192. Pessayre D, Bentata M, Degott C, et al. Isoniazid rifampicin fulminant hepatitis: a possible consequence of enhancement of isoniazid hepatotoxicity by enzyme induction. *Gastroenterology* 1977;72:284–9.
193. Sun F, Chen Y, Xiang Y, Zhan S. Drug-metabolising enzyme polymorphisms and predisposition to anti-tuberculosis drug-induced liver injury: a meta-analysis. *Int J Tuberc Lung Dis* 2008;12:994–1002.
194. Leiro V, Fernández-Villar A, Valverde D, et al. Influence of glutathione S-transferase M1 and T1 homozygous null mutations on the risk of antituberculosis drug-induced hepatotoxicity in a Caucasian population. *Liver Int* 2008;28:835–9.
195. Sharma SK, Balamurugan A, Saha PK, et al. Evaluation of clinical and immunogenetic risk factors for the development of hepatotoxicity during antituberculosis treatment. *Am J Respir Crit Care Med* 2002;166:916–19.
196. Farrell FJ, Keeffe EB, Man KM, et al. Treatment of hepatic failure secondary to isoniazid hepatitis with liver transplantation. *Dig Dis Sci* 1994;39:2255–9.
197. Sharma SK, Singla R, Sarda P, et al. Safety of 3 different reintroduction regimens of antituberculosis drugs after development of antituberculosis treatment-induced hepatotoxicity. *Clin Infect Dis* 2010;50:833–9.
198. Nolan CM, Goldberg SV, Buskin SE. Hepatotoxicity associated with isoniazid preventive therapy: a 7-year survey from a public health tuberculosis clinic. *JAMA* 1999;281:1014–18.
199. Centers for Disease Control and Prevention (CDC). Severe isoniazid-associated liver injuries among persons being treated for latent tuberculosis infection – United States, 2004–2008. *MMWR Morb Mortal Wkly Rep* 2010;59:224–9.
200. Steele MA, Burk RF, DesPrez M. Toxic hepatitis with isoniazid and rifampin: a meta-analysis. *Chest* 1991;99:465–71.
201. Prince MI, Burt AD, Jones DE. Hepatitis and liver dysfunction with rifampicin therapy for pruritus in primary biliary cirrhosis. *Gut* 2002;50:436–9.
202. Scheuer PJ, Summerfield JA, Lal S, et al. Rifampicin hepatitis. A clinical and histological study. *Lancet* 1974;1:421–5.
203. Capelle P, Dhumeaux D, Mora M, et al. Effect of rifampicin on liver function in man. *Gut* 1972;13:366–71.
204. Covic A, Goldsmith DJ, Segall L, et al. Rifampicin-induced acute renal failure: a series of 60 patients. *Nephrol Dial Transplant* 1998;13:924–9.
205. Chang KC, Leung CC, Yew WW, et al. Hepatotoxicity of pyrazinamide:cohort and case–control analyses. *Am J Respir Crit Care Med* 2008;177:1391–6.
206. Durand F, Bernuau J, Pessayre D, et al. Deleterious influence of pyrazinamide on the outcome of patients with fulminant or subfulminant liver failure during antituberculous treatment including isoniazid. *Hepatology* 1995;21:929–32.
207. Centers for Disease Control and Prevention (CDC); American Thoracic Society. Update: adverse event data and revised American Thoracic Society/CDC recommendations against the use of rifampin and pyrazinamide for treatment of latent tuberculosis infection – United States, 2003. *MMWR Morb Mortal Wkly Rep* 2003;52:735–9.
208. Menzies D, Long R, Trajman A, et al. Adverse events with 4 months of rifampin therapy or 9 months of isoniazid therapy for latent tuberculosis infection: a randomized trial. *Ann Intern Med* 2008;149:689–97.
209. Ohkawa K, Masayuki H, Ohno K. Risk factors for antituberculous chemotherapy-induced hepatotoxicity in Japanese pediatric patients. *Clin Pharmacol Ther* 2002;72:220–6.
210. Stricker BH, Blok AP, Bronkhorst FB, et al. Ketoconazole-associated hepatic injury. A clinicopathological study of 55 cases. *J Hepatol* 1986;3:399–406.
211. Amigues I, Cohen N, Chung D, et al. Hepatic safety of voriconazole after allogeneic hematopoietic stem cell transplantation. *Biol Blood Marrow Transplant* 2010;16:46–52.
212. Talwalkar JA, Soetikno RE, Carr-Locke DL, et al. Severe cholestasis related to itraconazole for the treatment of onychomycosis. *Am J Gastroenterol* 1999;94:3632–3.
213. Jacobson MA, Hanks DK, Ferrel LD. Fatal acute hepatic necrosis due to fluconazole. *Am J Med* 1994;96:188–90.
214. Garcia Rodriguez LA, Duque A, Castellsague J, et al. A cohort study on the risk of acute liver injury among users of ketoconazole and other antifungal drugs. *Br J Clin Pharmacol* 1999;48:847–52.
215. Lewis JH, Zimmerman HJ, Benson GD, et al. Hepatic injury associated with ketoconazole therapy. Analysis of 33 cases. *Gastroenterology* 1984;86:503–13.
216. Chien RN, Yang LJ, Lin PY, et al. Hepatic injury during ketoconazole therapy in patients with onychomycosis: a controlled cohort study. *Hepatology* 1997;25:103–7.

217. Lake-Bakaar G, Scheuer PJ, Sherlock S. Hepatic reactions associated with ketoconazole in the United Kingdom. *Br Med J* 1987;294:419–22.

218. Rodriguez RJ, Buckholz CJ. Hepatotoxicity of ketoconazole in Sprague–Dawley rats: glutathione depletion, flavin-containing monooxygenases-mediated bioactivation and hepatic covalent binding. *Xenobiotica* 2003;33:429–41.

219. Lin CL, Hu JT, Yang SS, Shin CY, Huang SH. Unexpected emergence of acute hepatic injury in patients treated repeatedly with ketoconazole. *J Clin Gastroenterol* 2008;42:432–3.

220. Chien RN, Sheen IS, Liaw YF. Unintentional rechallenge resulting in a causative relationship between ketoconazole and acute liver injury. *Int J Clin Pract* 2003;57:829–30.

221. Knight TE, Shikuma CY, Knight J. Ketoconazole-induced fulminant hepatitis necessitating liver transplantation. *J Am Acad Dermatol* 1991;25:398–400.

222. Kim TH, Kim BH, Kim YW, et al. Liver cirrhosis developed after ketoconazole-induced acute hepatic injury. *J Gastroenterol Hepatol* 2003;18:1426–9.

223. Gupta AK, Del Rosso JQ, Lynde CW, et al. Hepatitis associated with terbinafine therapy: three case reports and a review of the literature. *Clin Exp Dermatol* 1998;23:64–7.

224. Ajit C, Suvannasankha A, Zaeri N, et al. Terbinafine-associated hepatotoxicity. *Am J Med Sci* 2003;325:292–5.

225. Anania FA, Rabin L. Terbinafine hepatotoxicity resulting in chronic biliary ductopenia and portal fibrosis. *Am J Med* 2002;112:741–2.

226. Lovell MO, Speeg KV, Havranek RD, et al. Histologic changes resembling acute rejection in a liver transplant patient treated with terbinafine. *Hum Pathol* 2003;34:187–9.

227. Anon. Itraconazole, terbinafine possibly linked to liver failure. *Am J Health Syst Pharm* 2001;58:1076.

228. Agca E, Akcay A, Simsek H. Ursodeoxycholic acid for terbinafine induced toxic hepatitis. *Ann Pharmacother* 2004;38:1088–9.

229. Iverson SL, Uetrecht JP. Identification of a reactive metabolite of terbinafine: insights into terbinafine-induced hepatotoxicity. *Chem Res Toxicol* 2001;14:175–81.

230. Phillips-Howard PA, West LJ. Serious adverse drug reactions to pyrimethamine-sulphadoxine, pyrimethamine-dapsone and to amodiaquine in Britain. *J R Soc Med* 1990;83:82–5.

231. Choi GY, Yang HW, Cho SH, et al. Acute drug-induced hepatitis caused by albendazole. *J Korean Med Sci* 2008;23:903–5.

232. El-Mufti M, Kamag A, Ibrahim H, et al. Albendazole therapy of hydatid disease: 2-year follow-up of 40 cases. *Ann Trop Med Parasitol* 1993;87:241–6.

233. Centers for Disease Control and Prevention (CDC). Hepatitis temporally associated with an herbal supplement containing artemisinin – Washington, 2008. *MMWR Morb Mortal Wkly Rep* 2009;58:854–6.

234. Looareesuwan S, Wilairatana P, Chalermrut K, et al. Efficacy and safety of atovaquone/proguanil compared with mefloquine for treatment of acute *Plasmodium falciparum* malaria in Thailand. *Am J Trop Med Hyg* 1999;60:526–32.

235. Oostweegel LM, Beijnen JH, Mulder JW. Hepatitis during chloroguanide prophylaxis. *Ann Pharmacother* 1998;32:1023–5.

236. Colle I, Naegels S, Hoorens A, et al. Granulomatous hepatitis due to mebendazole. *J Clin Gastroenterol* 1999;28:44–5.

237. Gotsman I, Azaz-Livshits T, Fridlender Z, et al. Mefloquine-induced acute hepatitis. *Pharmacotherapy* 2000;20:1517–19.

238. Grieco A, Vecchio FM, Natale L, et al. Acute fatty liver after malaria prophylaxis with mefloquine. *Lancet* 1999;353:295–6.

239. Lam S, Bank S. Hepatotoxicity caused by metronidazole overdose. *Ann Intern Med* 1995;122:803.

240. Hestin D, Hanesse B, Frimat L, et al. Metronidazole-associated hepatotoxicity in a hemodialyzed patient. *Nephron* 1994;68:286.

241. Tabak F, Ozaras R, Erzin Y, et al. Ornidazole-induced liver damage: report of three cases and review of the literature. *Liver Int* 2003;23:351–4.

242. Scoazec JY, Krolak-Salmon P, Casez O, et al. Quinacrine-induced cytolytic hepatitis in sporadic Creutzfeldt–Jakob disease. *Ann Neurol* 2003;53:546–7.

243. Farver DK, Lavin MN. Quinine-induced hepatotoxicity. *Ann Pharmacother* 1999;33:32–4.

244. Katz B, Weetch M, Chopra S. Quinine-induced granulomatous hepatitis. *Br Med J* 1983;286:264–5.

245. Rex D, Lumeng L, Eble J, et al. Intrahepatic cholestasis and sicca complex after thiabendazole. Report of a case and review of the literature. *Gastroenterology* 1983;85:718–21.

246. Roy MA, Nugent FW, Aretz HT. Micronodular cirrhosis after thiabendazole. *Dig Dis Sci* 1989;34:938–4.

247. Soriano V, Puoti M, Garcia-Gascó P, et al. Antiretroviral drugs and liver injury. *AIDS* 2008;22:1–13.

248. Brinkman K, ter Hofstede HJM, Burger DM, et al. Adverse effects of reverse transcriptase inhibitors: mitochondrial toxicity as common pathway. *AIDS* 1998;12:1735–44.

249. Ogedegbe AO, Sulkowski MS. Antiretroviral-associated liver injury. *Clin Liver Dis* 2003;7:475–99.

250. John M, Moore CB, James IR, et al. Chronic hyperlactatemia in HIV-infected patients taking antiretroviral therapy. *AIDS* 2001;15:717–23.

251. Sundar K, Suarez M, Banogon PE, et al. Zidovudine-induced fatal lactic acidosis and hepatic failure in patients with acquired immunodeficiency syndrome: report of two patients and review of the literature. *Crit Care Med* 1997;25:1425–30.

252. Verdon R, Six M, Rousselot, et al. Efavirenz-induced acute eosinophilic hepatitis. *J Hepatol* 2001;31:783–5.

253. Anon. Serious adverse events attributed to nevirapine regimens for postexposure prophylaxis after HIV exposures worldwide, 1997–2000. *JAMA* 2001;285:402–3.

254. Piroth L, Grappin M, Sgro C, et al. Recurrent NNRTI-induced hepatotoxicity in an HIV–HCV-coinfected patient. *Ann Pharmacother* 2000;34:534–5.

255. Ogedegbe AO, Sulkowski MS. Antiretroviral-associated liver injury. *Clin Liver Dis* 2003;7:475–99.

256. Martin AM, Nolan D, James I, et al. Predisposition to nevirapine hypersensitivity associated with HLA-DRB1*0101 and abrogated by low CD4 T-cell counts. *AIDS* 2005;19:97–9.

257. Manfredi R, Calza L. Nevirapine versus efavirenz in 742 patients: no link of liver toxicity with female sex, and a baseline CD4 cell count greater than 250 cells/microl. *AIDS* 2006;20:2233–6.

258. Mallal S, Nolan D, Witt C, et al. Association between presence of HLA-B*5701, HLA-DR7, and HLA-DQ3 and hypersensitivity to HIV-1 reverse-transcriptase inhibitor abacavir. *Lancet* 2002;359:727–32.

259. Flexner C. HIV-protease inhibitors. *N Eng J Med* 1998;338:1281–92.

260. Sulkowski MS. Drug-induced liver injury associated with antiretroviral therapy that includes HIV-1 protease inhibitors. *Clin Infect Dis* 2004;38(Suppl 2):S90–7.

261. Eholie SP, Lacombe K, Serfaty L, et al. Acute hepatic cytolysis in an HIV-infected patient taking atazanavir. *AIDS* 2004;18:1610–11.

262. Bräu N, Leaf HL, Wieczorek RL, et al. Severe hepatitis in three AIDS patients treated with indinavir [Letter]. *Lancet* 1997;349:924.

263. Sulkowski MS, Mehta SH, Chaisson RE, et al. Hepatotoxicity associated with protease inhibitor-based antiretroviral regimens with or without concurrent ritonavir. *AIDS* 2004;18:2277–84.

264. den Brinker M, Wit FW, Wertheim-van Dillen PM, et al. Hepatitis B and C virus co-infection and the risk for hepatotoxicity of highly active antiretroviral therapy in HIV-1 infection. *AIDS* 2000;14:2895–902.

265. Chan-Tack KM, Struble KA, Birnkrant DB. Intracranial hemorrhage and liver-associated deaths associated with tipranavir/ritonavir: review of cases from the FDA's Adverse Event Reporting System. *AIDS Patient Care STDS* 2008;22:843–50.

266. Ortu F, Weimer LE, Floridia M, et al. Raltegravir, tenofovir and emtricitabine in an HIV-infected patient with HCV chronic hepatitis, NNRTI intolerance and protease inhibitors-induced severe liver toxicity. *Eur J Med Res* 2010;15:81–3.

267. Nichols WG, Steel HM, Bonny T, et al. Hepatotoxicity observed in clinical trials of aplaviroc GW873140. *Antimicrob Agents Chemother* 2008;52:858–65.

268. Yeung E, Wong FS, Wanless IR, et al. Ramipril-associated hepatotoxicity. *Arch Pathol Lab Med* 2003;127:1493–7.

269. Macias FM, Campos FR, Salguero TP, et al. Ductopenic hepatitis related to Enalapril. *J Hepatol* 2003;39:1091–2.

270. Larrey D, Babany G, Bernuau J, et al. Fulminant hepatitis after lisinopril administration. *Gastroenterology* 1990;99:1832–3.

271. Chou JW, Yu CJ, Chuang PH, et al. Successful treatment of fosinopril-induced severe cholestatic jaundice with plasma exchange. *Ann Pharmacother* 2008;42:1887–92.

272. Maddrey WC, Boitnott JK. Severe hepatitis from methyldopa. *Gastroenterology* 1975;68:351–60.

273. Larrey D, Henrion J, Heller F, et al. Metoprolol-induced hepatitis: rechallenge and drug oxidation phenotyping. *Ann Intern Med* 1988;108:67–8.

274. Schwartz MS. Atenolol-associated cholestasis. *Am J Gastroenterol* 1989;184:1084–6.

275. Yusuf SW, Mishra RM. Hepatic dysfunction associated with atenolol. *Lancet* 1995;346:192.

276. Hagmeyer KO, Stein J. Hepatotoxicity associated with carvedilol. *Ann Pharmacother* 2001;35:1364–6.

277. Clark J, Zimmerman HJ, Tanner L. Labetalol hepatotoxicity. *Ann Intern Med* 1990;113:210–13.

278. Kumar KL, Colley CA. Verapamil-induced hepatotoxicity. *West J Med* 1994;160:485–6.

279. Toft E, Vyberg M, Therkelsen K. Diltiazem-induced granulomatous hepatitis. *Histopathology* 1991;18:474–5.

280. Babany G, Uzzan F, Larrey D, et al. Alcoholic-like liver lesions induced by nifedipine. *Hepatology* 1989;9:252–5.

281. Zimmerman HJ, Lewis JH, Ishak KG, et al. Ticrynafen-associated hepatic injury: analysis of 340 cases. *Hepatology* 1984;4:315–23.

282. Beaune P, Dansette PM, Mansuy D, et al. Human antiendoplasmic reticulum autoantibodies appearing in a drug-induced hepatitis are directed against a human liver cytochrome P-450 that hydroxylates the drug. *Proc Natl Acad Sci USA* 1987;84:551–7.

283. Thai KE, Sinclair RD. Spironolactone-induced hepatitis. *Australas J Dermatol* 2001;42:180–2.

284. Jori GP, Peschle C. Hydralazine disease associated with transient granulomas in the liver: a case report. *Gastroenterology* 1973;64:1163–7.

285. Stewart GW, Peart WS, Boylston AW. Obstructive jaundice, pancytopenia and hydralazine [Letter]. *Lancet* 1981;1:207.

286. Andrade RJ, Lucena MI, Fernandez MC, et al. Cholestatic hepatitis related to use of irbesartan: a case report and a literature review of angiotensin II antagonist-associated hepatotoxicity. *Eur J Gastroenterol Hepatol* 2002;14:887–90.

287. Basile G, Villari D, Gangemi S, et al. Candesartan cilexetil-induced severe hepatotoxicity. *J Clin Gastroenterol* 2003;36:273–5.

288. Annicchiarico BE, Siciliano M. Could irbesartan trigger autoimmune cholestatic hepatitis? *Eur J Gastroenterol Hepatol* 2005;17:247–8.

289. Lewis JH, Mullick F, Ishak KG, et al. Histopathologic analysis of suspected amiodarone hepatotoxicity. *Hum Pathol* 1990;21:59–67.

290. Simon JB, Manley PN, Brien JF, et al. Amiodarone hepatotoxicity simulating alcoholic liver disease. *N Engl J Med* 1984;311:167–72.

291. Lewis JH, Ranard RC, Caruso A, et al. Amiodarone hepatotoxicity: prevalence and clinicopathologic correlations among 104 patients. *Hepatology* 1989;9:679–85.

292. Chang CC, Petrelli M, Tomashefski JF, et al. Severe intrahepatic cholestasis caused by amiodarone toxicity after withdrawal of the drug: a case report and review of the literature. *Arch Pathol Lab Med* 1999;123:251–6.

293. Richer M, Roberts S. Fatal hepatotoxicity following oral administration of amiodarone. *Ann Pharmacother* 1995;29:582.

294. Bravo AE, Drewe J, Schlienger RG, et al. Hepatotoxicity during rapid intravenous loading with amiodarone: description of three cases and review of the literature. *Crit Care Med* 2005;33:128–34.

295. Beuers U, Heuck A. Images in hepatology. Iodine accumulation in the liver during long-term treatment with amiodarone. *J Hepatol* 1997;26:439.

296. Poucell S, Ireton J, Valencia-Mayoral P, et al. Amiodarone-associated phospholipidosis and fibrosis of the liver. Light, immunohistochemical, and electron microscopic studies. *Gastroenterology* 1984;86:926–36.

297. Jain D, Bowlus CL, Anderson JM, et al. Granular cells as a marker of early amiodarone hepatotoxicity. *J Clin Gastroenterol* 2000;31:241–3.

298. Pollak PT, Shafer SL. Use of population modeling to define rational monitoring of amiodarone hepatic effects. *Clin Pharmacol Ther* 2004;75:342–51.

299. Mattar W, Juliar B, Gradus-Pizlo I, Kwo PY. Amiodarone hepatotoxicity in the context of the metabolic syndrome and right-sided heart failure. *J Gastrointest Liver Dis* 2009;18:419–23.

300. Kum LC, Chan WW, Hui HH, et al. Prevalence of amiodarone-related hepatotoxicity in 720 Chinese patients with or without baseline liver dysfunction. *Clin Cardiol* 2006;29:295–9.

301. Heath MF, Costa-Jussa FR, Jacobs JM, et al. The induction of pulmonary phospholipidosis and the inhibition of lysosomal phospholipases by amiodarone. *Br J Exp Pathol* 1985;66:391–7.

302. Berson A, De Beco V, Letteron P, et al. Steatohepatitis-inducing drugs cause mitochondrial dysfunction and lipid peroxidation in rat hepatocytes. *Gastroenterology* 1998;114:764–74.

303. Knobler H, Levij IS, Gavish D, et al. Quinidine-induced hepatitis. A common and reversible hypersensitivity reaction. *Arch Intern Med* 1986;146:526–8.

304. Bramlet DA, Posalaky Z, Olson R. Granulomatous hepatitis as a manifestation of quinidine hypersensitivity. *Arch Intern Med* 1980;140:395–7.

305. Chuang L, Tunier A, Akhtar N, et al. Possible case of procainamide-induced intrahepatic cholestatic jaundice. *Ann Pharmacother* 1993;27:434–7.

306. Cocozzella D, Curciarello J, Corallini O, et al. Propafenone hepatotoxicity: report of two new cases. *Dig Dis Sci* 2003;48:354–7.

307. Carlson MK, Gleason PP, Sen S. Elevation of hepatic transaminases after enoxaparin use: case report and review of unfractionated and low-molecular-weight heparin-induced hepatotoxicity. *Pharmacotherapy* 2001;21:108–13.

308. Schimanski CC, Burg J, Mohler M, et al. Phenprocoumon-induced liver disease ranges from mild acute hepatitis to subacute liver failure. *J Hepatol* 2004;41:67–74.

309. Tolman KG. Defining patient risks from expanded preventive therapies. *Am J Cardiol* 2000;85:E15–19.

310. Farmer JA, Torre-Amione G. Comparative tolerability of the HMG-CoA reductase inhibitors. *Drug Saf* 2000;23:197–213.

311. Lewis JH, Mortensen ME, Zweig S, et al. Efficacy and safety of high-dose pravastatin in hypercholesterolemic patients with well-compensated chronic liver disease: results of a prospective, randomized, double-blind, placebo-controlled, multicenter trial. *Hepatology* 2007;46:1453–63.

312. Ravins AL, Manos MM, Ackerson L, et al. Hepatic effects of lovastatin exposure in patients with liver disease: a retrospective cohort study. *Drug Saf* 2008;31:325–34.

313. Chalasani N, Aljadhey H, Kesterson J, et al. Patients with elevated liver enzymes are not at higher risk for statin hepatotoxicity. *Gastroenterology* 2004;126:1287–92.

314. Grimbert S, Pessayre D, Degott C, Benhamou JP. Acute hepatitis induced by HMG-CoA reductase inhibitor, lovastatin. *Dig Dis Sci* 1994;39:2032–3.

315. Hartleb M, Rymarczyk G, Januszewski K. Acute cholestatic hepatitis associated with pravastatin. *Am J Gastroenterol* 1999;94:1388–90.

316. Rahier JF, Rahier J, Leclercq I, Geubel AP. Severe acute cholestatic hepatitis with prolonged cholestasis and bile-duct injury following atorvastatin therapy: a case report. *Acta Gastroenterol Belg* 2008;71:318–20.

317. Ballare M, Campanini M, Catania E, et al. Acute cholestatic hepatitis during simvastatin administration. *Recenti Prog Med* 1991;82:233–5.

318. Conforti A, Magro L, Moretti U, et al. Fluvastatin and hepatic reactions: a signal from spontaneous reporting in Italy. *Drug Saf* 2006;29:1163–72.

319. Pelli N, Setti M, Ceppa P, et al. Autoimmune hepatitis revealed by atorvastatin. *Eur J Gastroenterol Hepatol* 2003;15:921–4.

320. Downs JR, Clearfield M, Tyroler IIA, et al. Air Force/Texas Coronary Atherosclerosis Prevention Study (AFCAPS/TEXCAPS): additional perspectives on tolerability of long-term treatment with lovastatin. *Am J Cardiol* 2001;87:1074–9.

321. Hajdu D, Aiglová K, Vinklerová I, et al. Acute cholestatic hepatitis induced by fenofibrate. *J Clin Pharm Ther* 2009;34:599–602.

322. Punthakee Z, Scully LJ, Guindi MM, et al. Liver fibrosis attributed to lipid lowering medications: two cases. *J Intern Med* 2001;250:249–54.

323. Sirmans SM, Beck JK, Banh HL, et al. Colestipol-induced hepatotoxicity. *Pharmacotherapy* 2001;21:513–16.

324. Stolk MF, Becx MC, Kuypers KC, et al. Severe hepatic side effects of ezetimibe. *Clin Gastroenterol Hepatol* 2006;4:908–11.

325. Ritchie SR, Orr DW, Black PN. Severe jaundice following treatment with ezetimibe. *Eur J Gastroenterol Hepatol* 2008;20:572–3.

326. Tuteja S, Pyrsopoulos NT, Wolowich WR, et al. Simvastatin-ezetimibe-induced hepatic failure necessitating liver transplantation. *Pharmacotherapy* 2008;28:1188–93.

327. Hodis HN. Acute hepatic failure associated with the use of low-dose sustained-release niacin. *JAMA* 1990;264:181.

328. Gray DR, Morgan T, Chretien SD, et al. Efficacy and safety of controlled-release niacin in dyslipoproteinemic veterans. *Ann Intern Med* 1994;121:252–8.

329. Rader JI, Calvert RJ, Hathcock JN. Hepatic toxicity of unmodified and time-release preparations of niacin. *Am J Med* 1992;92:77–81.

330. Mullin GE, Greenson JK, Mitchel MC. Fulminant hepatic failure after ingestion of sustained-release nicotinic acid. *Ann Intern Med* 1989;111:253–5.

331. Goldberg A, Alagona P, Capuzzi DM, et al. Multiple-dose efficacy and safety of an extended-release form of niacin in the management of hyperlipidemia. *Am J Cardiol* 2000;85:1100–5.

332. Xiao X, Hong L, Sheng M. Promoting effect of estrogen on the proliferation of hemangioma vascular endothelial cells in vitro. *J Pediatr Surg* 1999;34:1603–5.

333. Conter RL, Longmire WP Jr. Recurrent hepatic hemangiomas: possible association with estrogen therapy. *Ann Surg* 1988;207:115–19.

334. Mathieu D, Kobeiter H, Maison P, et al. Oral contraceptive use and focal nodular hyperplasia of the liver. *Gastroenterology* 2000;118:560–84.

335. Reddy KR, Kligerman S, Levi J, et al. Benign and solid tumors of the liver: relationship to sex, age, size of tumors, and outcome. *Am Surg* 2001;67:173–8.

336. La Vecchia C, Negri E, Parazzini F. Oral contraceptives and primary liver cancer. *Br J Cancer* 1989;59:460–1.

337. La Vecchia C, Altieri A, Franceschi S, et al. Oral contraceptives and cancer: an update. *Drug Saf* 2001;24:741–54.

338. Glober GA, Wilkerson JA. Biliary cirrhosis following the administration of methyltestosterone. *JAMA* 1968;204:170–3.

339. Stimac D, Milic S, Dintinjana RD, et al. Androgenic/anabolic steroid-induced toxic hepatitis. *J Clin Gastroenterol* 2002;35:350–2.

340. Touraine RL, Bertrand Y, Foray P, et al. Hepatic tumours during androgen therapy in Fanconi anaemia. *Eur J Pediatr* 1993;152:691–3.

341. Westaby D, Portmann B, Williams R. Androgen related primary hepatic tumors in non-Fanconi patients. *Cancer* 1983;51:1947–52.

342. Patil JJ, O'Donohoe B, Loyden CF, Shanahan D. Near-fatal spontaneous hepatic rupture associated with anabolic androgenic steroid use: a case report. *Br J Sports Med* 2007;41:462–3.

343. Bork K, Pitton M, Harten P, et al. Hepatocellular adenomas in patients taking danazol for hereditary angio-oedema. *Lancet* 1999;353:1066–7.

344. Middleton C, McCaughan GW, Painter DM, et al. Danazol and hepatic neoplasia: a case report. *Aust NZ J Med* 1989;19:733–5.

345. Hayashi T, Takahashi T, Minami T, et al. Fatal acute hepatic failure induced by danazol in a patient with endometriosis and aplastic anemia. *J Gastroenterol* 2001;36:783–6.

346. Farrell GC, Joshua DE, Uren RF, et al. Androgen-induced hepatoma. *Lancet* 1975;1:430–2.

347. McCaughan GW, Bilous MJ, Gallagher ND. Long-term survival with tumor regression in androgen-induced liver tumors. *Cancer* 1985;56:2622–6.

348. Anthony PP. Hepatoma associated with androgenic steroids? *Lancet* 1975;1:685–6.

349. Confavreux C, Seve P, Broussolle C, et al. Danazol-induced hepatocellular carcinoma. *Q J Med* 2003;96:317–18.

350. Ogawa Y, Murata Y, Nishioka A, et al. Tamoxifen-induced fatty liver in patients with breast cancer [Letter]. *Lancet* 1998;351:725.

351. Ogawa Y, Murata Y, Saibara T, et al. Follow-up CT findings of tamoxifen-induced non-alcoholic steatohepatitis (NASH) of breast cancer patients treated with bezafibrate. *Oncol Rep* 2003;10:1473–8.

352. Bruno S, Maisonneuve P, Castellana P, et al. Incidence and risk factors for non-alcoholic steatohepatitis: prospective study of 5408 women enrolled in Italian tamoxifen chemoprevention trial. *Br Med J* 2005;330:932.

353. Saphner T, Triest-Robertson S, Li H, Holzman P. The association of nonalcoholic steatohepatitis and tamoxifen in patients with breast cancer. *Cancer* 2009;115:3189–95.

354. Elefsiniotis IS, Pantazis KD, Ilias A, et al. Tamoxifen induced hepatotoxicity in breast cancer patients with pre-existing liver steatosis: the role of glucose intolerance. *Eur J Gastroenterol Hepatol* 2004;16:593–8.

355. Lelliott CJ, Lopez M, Curtis RK, et al. Transcript and metabolite analysis of the effects of tamoxifen in rat liver reveals inhibition of fatty acid synthesis in the presence of hepatic steatosis. *FASEB J* 2005;19:1108–19.

356. Hamada N, Ogawa Y, Saibara T, et al. Toremifene-induced fatty liver and NASH in breast cancer patients with breast-conservation treatment. *Int J Oncol* 2000;17:1119–23.

357. Vilches AR, Perez V, Suchecki DE. Raloxifene-associated hepatitis. *Lancet* 1998;352:1524–5.

358. Takamura T, Shimizu A, Komura T, et al. Selective estrogen receptor modulator raloxifene-associated aggravation of nonalcoholic steatohepatitis. *Intern Med* 2007;46:579–81.

359. Williams KV, Nayak S, Becker D, et al. Fifty years of experience with propylthiouracil-associated hepatotoxicity: what have we learned? *J Clin Endocrinol Metab* 1997;82:1727–33.

360. Schwab GP, Wetscher GJ, Vogl W, et al. Methimazole-induced cholestatic liver injury, mimicking sclerosing cholangitis. *Langenbecks Arch Chir* 1996;381;225–7.

361. Kim HJ, Kim BH, Yan YS, et al. The incidence and clinical characteristics of symptomatic propylthiouracil-induced hepatic injury in patients with hyperthyroidism: a single-center retrospective study. *Am J Gastroenterol* 2001;96:165–9.

362. Ruiz JK, Rossi GV, Vallejos HA, et al. Fulminant hepatic failure associated with propylthiouracil. *Ann Pharmacother* 2003;37:224–8.

363. Rivkees SA, Szarfman A. Dissimilar hepatotoxicity profiles of propylthiouracil and methimazole in children. *J Clin Endocrinol Metab* 2010 (Epub).

364. National Halothane Study. Summary of the national halothane study: possible association between halothane anesthesia and post-operative hepatic necrosis. *JAMA* 1966;197:123–34.

365. Eghtesadi-Araghi P, Sohrabpour A, Vahedi H, Saberi-Firoozi M. Halothane hepatitis in Iran: a review of 59 cases. *World J Gastroenterol* 2008;14:5322–6.

366. Wright R, Eade OE, Chisholm M, et al. Controlled prospective study of the effect on liver function of multiple exposures to halothane. *Lancet* 1975;1:817–20.

367. Schmidt CC, Suttner SW, Piper SN, et al. Comparison of the effects of desflurane and isoflurane anaesthesia on hepatocellular function assessed by alpha glutathione *S*-transferase. *Anaesthesia* 1999;4:1207–11.

368. Hoft RH, Bunker JP, Goodman HI, et al. Halothane hepatitis in three pairs of closely related women. *N Engl J Med* 1981;304:1023–4.

369. Nomura F, Hatano H, Ohnishi K, et al. Effects of anticonvulsant agents on halothane-induced liver injury in human subjects and experimental animals. *Hepatology* 1986;6:952–6.

370. Farrell GC, Prendergast D, Murray M. Halothane hepatitis. Detection of a constitutional susceptibility factor. *N Engl J Med* 1985;313:1300–14.

371. Böttiger LE, Dalén E, Hallén B. Halothane-induced liver damage: an analysis of the material reported to the Swedish Adverse Drug Reaction Committee, 1966–1973. *Acta Anesth Scand* 1976;20:40–6.

372. Inman HW, Mushkin WW. Jaundice after repeated exposure to halothane: an analysis of reports to the Committee on Safety of Medicines. *Br Med J* 1974;1:5–10.

373. Klatskin G, Kimberg DV. Recurrent hepatitis attributable to halothane sensitization in an anesthetist. *N Engl J Med* 1969;280:515–22.

374. Lewis JH, Zimmerman HJ, Ishak KG, et al. Enflurane hepatotoxicity. A clinicopathologic study of 234 cases. *Ann Intern Med* 1983;98:984–92.

375. Eger EI II, Smuckler EA, Ferrell LD, et al. Is enflurane hepatotoxic? *Anesth Analg* 1986;65:21–30.

376. Turner GB, O'Rourke D, Scott GO, et al. Fatal hepatotoxicity after re-exposure to isoflurane: a case report and review of the literature. *Eur J Gastroenterol Hepatol* 2000;12:955–9.

377. Hasan F. Isoflurane hepatotoxicity in a patient with a previous history of halothane-induced hepatitis. *Hepatogastroenterology* 1998;45:518–22.

378. Weitz J, Kienle P, Bohrer H, et al. Fatal hepatic necrosis after isoflurane anaesthesia. *Anaesthesia* 1997;52:892–5.

379. Lehmann A, Neher M, Kiessling AH, et al. Case report: fatal hepatic failure after aortic valve replacement and sevoflurane exposure. *Can J Anaesth* 2007;54:917.

380. Turillazzi E, D'Errico S, Neri M, et al. A fatal case of fulminant hepatic necrosis following sevoflurane anesthesia. *Toxicol Pathol* 2007;35:840–5.

381. Anderson JS, Rose NR, Martin JL, et al. Desflurane hepatitis associated with hapten and autoantigen-specific IgG4 antibodies. *Anesth Analg* 2007;104:1452–3.

382. Njoku DB, Mellerson JL, Talor MV, et al. Role of CYP2E1 immunoglobulin G4 subclass antibodies and complement in pathogenesis of idiosyncratic drug-induced hepatitis. *Clin Vaccine Immunol* 2006;13:258–65.

383. Watkins PB, Whitcomb RW. Hepatic dysfunction associated with troglitazone [Letter]. *N Engl J Med* 1998;338:916–17.

384. Graham DJ, Drinkard CR, Shatin D. Incidence of idiopathic acute liver failure and hospitalized liver injury in patients with troglitazone. *Am J Gastroenterol* 2003;98;175–9.

385. Chojkier M. Troglitazone and liver injury: in search of answers. *Hepatology* 2005;41:229–30.

386. Smith MT. Mechanisms of troglitazone hepatotoxicity. *Chem Res Toxicol* 2003;16:679–87.

387. Bova MP, Tam D, McMahon G, et al. Troglitazone induces a rapid drop of mitochondrial membrane potential in liver HepG2 cells. *Toxicol Lett* 2005;155:41–50.

388. Funk C, Ponelle C, Scheuermann G, et al. Cholestatic potential of troglitazone as a possible factor contributing to troglitazone-induced hepatotoxicity: in vivo and in vitro interaction at the canalicular bile salt export pump (Bsep) in the rat. *Mol Pharmacol* 2001;59:627–35.

389. Malik AH, Prasad P, Saboorian MH, et al. Hepatic injury due to troglitazone. *Dig Dis Sci* 2000;45:210–14.

390. Kumashiro R, Kubota T, Koga Y, et al. Association of troglitazone-induced liver injury with mutation of the cytochrome P450 2C19 gene. *Hepatol Res* 2003;26:337–42.

391. Watanabe I, Tomita A, Shimizu M, et al. A study to survey susceptible genetic factors responsible for troglitazone-associated hepatotoxicity in Japanese patients with type 2 diabetes mellitus. *Clin Pharmacol Ther* 2003;73:435–55.

392. Caldwell SH, Hespenheide EE, von Borstel RW. Myositis, microvesicular hepatitis, and progression to cirrhosis from troglitazone added to simvastatin. *Dig Dis Sci* 2001;46:376–8.

393. Iwase M, Yamaguchi M, Yoshinari M, et al. A Japanese case of liver dysfunction after 19 months of troglitazone treatment. *Diabetes Care* 1999;22:1382–4.

394. Graham DJ, Green L, Senior JR, et al. Troglitazone-induced liver failure: a case study. *Am J Med* 2003;114:299–306.

395. Shibuya A, Watanabe M, Yoshikuni F, et al. An autopsy case of troglitazone-induced fulminant hepatitis. *Diabetes Care* 1998;21:2140–3.

396. Menon KVN, Angulo P, Lindor KD. Severe cholestatic hepatitis from troglitazone in a patient with nonalcoholic steatohepatitis and diabetes mellitus. *Am J Gastroenterol* 2001;96:1631–4.

397. Julie NL, Julie IM, Kende AI, Wilson GL. Mitochondrial dysfunction and delayed hepatotoxicity: another lesson from troglitazone. *Diabetologia* 2008;51:2108–16.

398. Marcy TR, Britton ML, Blevins SM. Second-generation thiazolidinediones and hepatotoxicity. *Ann Pharmacother* 2004;38:1419–23.

399. Gouda HE, Khan A, Schwartz J, et al. Liver failure in a patient treated with long-term rosiglitazone therapy. *Am J Med* 2001;111:584–5.

400. Bonkovsky HL, Azar R, Bird S, et al. Severe cholestatic hepatitis caused by thiazolidinediones: risks associated with substituting rosiglitazone for troglitazone. *Dig Dis Sci* 2002;47:1632–7.

401. Dhawan M, Agrawal R, Ravi J, et al. Rosiglitazone-induced granulomatous hepatitis. *J Clin Gastroenterol* 2002;34:582–4.

402. Floyd JS, Barbehenn E, Lurie P, Wolfe SM. Case series of liver failure associated with rosiglitazone and pioglitazone. *Pharmacoepidemiol Drug Saf* 2009;18:1238–43.

403. Osei SY, Koro CE, Cobitz AR, Kolatkar NS, Stender M. Commentary on 'Case series of liver failure associated with rosiglitazone and pioglitazone' by Floyd et al. *Pharmacoepidemiol Drug Saf* 2009;18:1244–6.

404. Beiderbeck AB, Sakaguchi M. Commentary on 'Case series of liver failure associated with rosiglitazone and pioglitazone' by James Floyd et al. *Pharmacoepidemiol Drug Saf* 2009;18:1247–9.

405. Chan KA, Truman A, Gurwitz JH, et al. A cohort study of the incidence of serious acute liver injury in diabetic patients treated with hypoglycemic agents. *Arch Intern Med* 2003;163:728–34.

406. Jick SS, Stender M, Myers MW. Frequency of liver disease in type 2 diabetic patients treated with oral antidiabetic agents. *Diabetes Care* 2000;22:2067–71.

407. Saw D, Pitman E, Maung M, et al. Granulomatous hepatitis associated with glyburide. *Dig Dis Sci* 1996;41:322–5.

408. Gregory DH, Zaki GF, Sarosi GA, et al. Chronic cholestasis following prolonged tolbutamide administration. *Arch Pathol* 1967;84:194.

409. Heurgue A, Bernard-Chabert B, Higuero T, et al. Glimepiride-induced acute cholestatic hepatitis. *Ann Endocrinol (Paris)* 2004;65:174–5.

410. Clarke BF, Campbell JW, Ewing DJ, et al. Generalized hypersensitivity reaction and visceral arteritis with fatal outcome during glibenclamide therapy. *Diabetes* 1974;23:739–42.

411. Chitturi S, Le V, Kench J, et al. Gliclazide-induced acute hepatitis with hypersensitivity features. *Dig Dis Sci* 2002;47:1107–10.

412. Desilets DJ, Shorr AF, Moran KA, et al. Cholestatic jaundice associated with the use of metformin. *Am J Gastroenterol* 2001;96:2257–8.

413. Nan DN, Hernandez JL, Fernandez-Ayala M, et al. Acute hepatotoxicity caused by repaglinide. *Ann Intern Med* 2004;141:823.

414. Andrade RJ, Lucena M, Vega JL, et al. Acarbose-associated hepatotoxicity [Letter]. *Diabetes Care* 1998;21:2029–30.

415. Tawata M, Ikeda M, Kodama Y, et al. A type 2 diabetic patient with liver dysfunction due to human insulin. *Diabetes Res Clin Pract* 2000;49:17–21.

416. Makin AJ, Wendon J, Williams R. A 7-year experience of severe acetaminophen-induced hepatotoxicity (1987–1993). *Gastroenterology* 1995;109:1907–16.

417. Lee WM. Acetaminophen and the US Acute Liver Failure Study Group: lowering the risks of hepatic failure. *Hepatology* 2004;40:6–9.

418. Prescott LF. Paracetamol, alcohol and the liver. *Br J Clin Pharmacol* 2000;49:291–301.

419. Zimmerman HJ, Maddrey WC. Acetaminophen (paracetamol) hepatotoxicity with regular intake of alcohol: analysis of instance of therapeutic misadventure. *Hepatology* 1995;22:767–73.

420. Johnston SC, Pelletier LL Jr. Enhanced hepatotoxicity of acetaminophen in the alcoholic patient: two cases reports and a review of the literature. *Medicine (Baltimore)* 1997;76:185–91.

421. Prescott LF, Critchley JAJH. The treatment of acetaminophen poisoning. *Ann Rev Pharmacol Toxicol* 1983;23:87–101.

422. Isbister GK, Bucens IK, Whyte IM. Paracetamol overdose in a preterm neonate. *Arch Dis Child Fetal Neonatal Ed* 2001;85:F70–2.

423. Tenenbein M. Why young children are resistant to acetaminophen poisoning. *J Pediatrics* 2000;137:891–2.

424. American Academy of Pediatrics, Committee on Drugs. Acetaminophen toxicity in children. *Pediatrics* 2001;108:1020–4.

425. Suzuki A, Yuen N, Walsh J, et al. Co-medications that modulate liver injury and repair influence clinical outcome of acetaminophen-associated liver injury. *Clin Gastroenterol Hepatol* 2009;7:882–8.

426. O'Grady JG, Alexander GJ, Hayllar KM, et al. Early indicators of prognosis in fulminant hepatic failure. *Gastroenterology* 1989;97:439–45.

427. Farrell GC, Chitturi S. Drug-induced hepatic injury (prevention). In: Wolfe MM, Davis GL, Farraye FA, Giannella RA, Malagelada J-R, Steer ML, eds. *Therapy of Digestive Disorders*. Philadelphia: WB Saunders, 2005:565–78.

428. Brotodihardjo A, Batey RG, Farrell GC, et al. Hepatotoxicity from paracetamol self-poisoning in western Sydney: a continuing challenge. *Med J Aust* 1992;157:382–5.

429. Kuffner EK, Dart RC, Bogdan GM, et al. Effect of maximal daily doses of acetaminophen on the liver of alcoholic patients: a randomized, double-blind, placebo-controlled trial. *Arch Intern Med* 2001;161:2247–52.

430. Whitcomb DC, Block GD. Association of acetaminophen hepatotoxicity with fasting and ethanol use. *JAMA* 1994;272:1845–50.

431. Rumack BH. Acetaminophen misconceptions. *Hepatology* 2004;40:10–15.

432. Bonkovsky HL, Kane RE, Jones DP, et al. Acute hepatic and renal toxicity from low doses of acetaminophen in the absence of alcohol abuse or malnutrition: evidence for increased susceptibility to drug toxicity due to cardiopulmonary and renal insufficiency. *Hepatology* 1994;19:1141–8.

433. Hinson JA, Reid AB, McCullough SS, et al. Acetaminophen-induced hepatotoxicity: role of metabolic activation, reactive oxygen/nitrogen species, and mitochondrial permeability transition. *Drug Metab Rev* 2004;36:805–22.

434. Jaeschke H, Knight TR, Bajt ML. The role of oxidant stress and reactive nitrogen species in acetaminophen hepatotoxicity. *Toxicol Lett* 2003;144:279–88.

435. Imaeda AB, Watanabe A, Sohail MA, et al. Acetaminophen-induced hepatotoxicity in mice is dependent on Tlr9 and the Nalp3 inflammasome. *J Clin Invest* 2009;119:305–14.

436. Liu ZX, Govindarajan S, Kaplowitz N. Innate immune system plays a critical role in determining the progression and severity of acetaminophen hepatotoxicity. *Gastroenterology* 2004;127:1760–74.

437. Rezende G, Roque-Afonso AM, Samuel D, et al. Viral and clinical factors associated with the fulminant course of hepatitis A infection. *Hepatology* 2003;38:613–18.

438. Morgan O, Griffiths C, Majeed A. Impact of paracetamol pack size restrictions on poisoning from paracetamol in England and Wales: an observational study. *J Public Health* 2005;27:19–24.

439. Vale JA, Proudfoot AT. Paracetamol (acetaminophen) poisoning. *Lancet* 1995;346:547–52.

440. Rumack BH, Matthew H. Acetaminophen poisoning and toxicity. *Pediatrics* 1975;55:871–6.

441. Prescott LF, Illingworth RN, Critchley JAJH et al. Intravenous N-acetylcysteine: the treatment of choice for paracetamol poisoning. *Br Med J* 1979;2:1097–100.

442. Zed PJ, Krenzelok EP. Treatment of acetaminophen overdose. *Am J Health Syst Pharm* 1999;56:1081–93.

443. Dargan PI, Jones AL. Acetaminophen poisoning: an update for the intensivist. *Crit Care* 2002;6:108–10.

444. Saito C, Zwingmann C, Jaeschke H. Novel mechanisms of protection against acetaminophen hepatotoxicity in mice by glutathione and N-acetylcysteine. *Hepatology* 2010;51:246–54.

445. Keays R, Harrison PM, Wendon JA, et al. Intravenous acetylcysteine in paracetamol induced fulminant hepatic failure: a prospective controlled trial. *Br Med J* 1991;303:1026–9.

446. Walsh TS, Hopton P, Philips BJ. The effect of n-acetylcysteine on oxygen transport and uptake in patients with fulminant hepatic failure. *Hepatology* 1998;27:1332–40.

447. Smilkstein MJ, Knapp GL, Kulig KW, et al. Efficacy of oral N-acetylcysteine in the treatment of acetaminophen overdose: analysis of the national multicenter study (1976 to 1985). *N Eng J Med* 1988;319:1557–62.

448. Betten DP, Cantrell FL, Thomas SC, et al. A prospective evaluation of shortened course oral N-acetylcysteine for the treatment of acute acetaminophen poisoning. *Ann Emerg Med* 2007;50:272–9.

449. Smilkstein MJ, Bronstein AC, Linden C, et al. Acetaminophen overdose: a 48 hour intravenous N-acetylcysteine treatment protocol. *Ann Emerg Med* 1991;20:1058–63.

450. Yarema MC, Johnson DW, Berlin RJ, et al. Comparison of the 20-hour intravenous and 72-hour oral acetylcysteine protocols for

the treatment of acute acetaminophen poisoning. *Ann Emerg Med* 2009;54:606–14.

451. Bailey B, McGuigan MA. Management of anaphylactoid reactions to intravenous *N*-acetylcysteine. *Ann Emerg Med* 1998;31:710–15.
452. Pakravan N, Waring WS, Sharma S, et al. Risk factors and mechanisms of anaphylactoid reactions to acetylcysteine in acetaminophen overdose. *Clin Toxicol (Phila)* 2008;46:697–702.
453. Waring WS, Stephen AF, Robinson OD, et al. Lower incidence of anaphylactoid reactions to *N*-acetylcysteine in patients with high acetaminophen concentrations after overdose. *Clin Toxicol* 2008;46:496–500.
454. Horowitz RS, Dart RC, Jarvie DR, et al. Placental transfer of *N*-acetylcysteine following human maternal acetaminophen poisoning. *J Toxicol Clin Toxicol* 1997;35:447–51.
455. Bernal W, Wendon J, Rela M, et al. Use and outcome of liver transplantation in acetaminophen-induced acute liver failure. *Hepatology* 1998;27:1050–5.
456. Cooper SC, Aldridge RC, Shah T, et al. Outcomes of liver transplantation for paracetamol (acetaminophen)-induced hepatic failure. *Liver Transpl* 2009;15:1351–7.
457. Rodriguez LAG, Gutthann SP, Walker AM, et al. The role of non-steroidal anti-inflammatory drugs in acute liver injury. *Br Med J* 1992;305:865–8.
458. Rubenstein JH, Laine L. Systematic review: the hepatotoxicity of non-steroidal anti-inflammatory drugs. *Aliment Pharmacol Ther* 2004;20:373–80.
459. Lacroix I, Lapeyre-Mestre M, Bagheri H, et al. Nonsteroidal anti-inflammatory drug-induced liver injury: a case–control study in primary care. *Fundam Clin Pharmacol* 2004;18:201–6.
460. Tarazi EM, Harter JG, Zimmermann HJ, et al. Sulindac-associated hepatic injury: analysis of 91 cases reported to the Food and Drug Administration. *Gastroenterology* 1993;104:569–74.
461. Lee JK, Paine M, Brouwer K. Sulindac and its metabolites inhibit multiple transport proteins in rat and human hepatocytes. *J Pharmacol Exp Ther* 2010;334:410–18.
462. Zou W, Beggs KM, Sparkenbaugh EM, et al. Sulindac metabolism and synergy with tumor necrosis factor-alpha in a drug–inflammation interaction model of idiosyncratic liver injury. *J Pharmacol Exp Ther* 2009;331:114–21.
463. Javier Rodríguez-Gonzalez F, Montero JL, Puente J, et al. Orthotopic liver transplantation after subacute liver failure induced by therapeutic doses of ibuprofen. *Am J Gastroenterol* 2002;97:2476–7.
464. Taghian M, Tran TA, Bresson-Hadni S, et al. Acute vanishing bile duct syndrome after ibuprofen therapy in a child. *J Pediatr* 2004;145:273–6.
465. Alam I, Ferrell LD, Bass NM. Vanishing bile duct syndrome temporally associated with ibuprofen use. *Am J Gastroenterol* 1996;91:1626–30.
466. Fontana RJ, McCashland TM, Benner KG, et al. Acute liver failure associated with prolonged use of bromfenac leading to liver transplantation. The Acute Liver Failure Study Group. *Liver Transpl Surg* 1999;5:480–4.
467. Banks AT, Zimmerman HJ, Ishak KG, et al. Diclofenac-associated hepatotoxicity: analysis of 180 cases reported to the Food and Drug Administration as adverse reactions. *Hepatology* 1995;22:820–7.
468. Scully LJ, Clarke D, Bar J. Diclofenac induced hepatitis. 3 cases with features of autoimmune chronic active hepatitis. *Dig Dis Sci* 1993;38:744–51.
469. Iveson TJ, Ryley NG, Kelly PMA, et al. Diclofenac associated hepatitis. *J Hepatol* 1990;10:85–9.
470. Boelsterli UA. Diclofenac-induced liver injury: a paradigm of idiosyncratic drug toxicity. *Toxicol Appl Pharmacol* 2003;192:307–22.

471. Aithal GP, Ramsay L, Daly AK, et al. Hepatic adducts, circulating antibodies, and cytokine polymorphisms in patients with diclofenac hepatotoxicity. *Hepatology* 2004;39:1430–40.
472. Daly AK, Aithal GP, Leathart JB, et al. Genetic susceptibility to diclofenac-induced hepatoxicity: contribution of UGT2B7, CYP2C8, and ABCC2 genotypes. *Gastroenterology* 2007;132:272–281.
473. Scully RE, Galdabini JJ, Mcneely BU. Case records of the Massachusetts General Hospital. Weekly clinicopathological exercises. Case 22 – 1977. *N Engl J Med* 1977;296:1337–46.
474. Zimmerman HJ. Effects of aspirin and acetaminophen on the liver. *Arch Intern Med* 1981;141:333–42.
475. Iqbal M, Goenka P, Young MF, et al. Ticlopidine-induced cholestatic hepatitis: report of three cases and review of the literature. *Dig Dis Sci* 1998;43:2223–6.
476. Kubin CJ, Sherman O, Hussain KB, et al. Delayed-onset ticlopidine-induced cholestatic jaundice. *Pharmacotherapy* 1999;19:1006–10.
477. Amaro P, Nunes A, Macoas F, et al. Ticlopidine-induced prolonged cholestasis: a case report. *Eur J Gastroenterol Hepatol* 1999;11;673–6.
478. Hirata K, Takagi H, Yamamoto M, et al. Ticlopidine-induced hepatotoxicity is associated with specific human leukocyte antigen genomic subtypes in Japanese patients: a preliminary case–control study. *Pharmacogenomics J* 2008;8:29–33.
479. Leone N, Giordanino C, Baronio M, et al. Ticlopidine-induced cholestatic hepatitis successfully treated with corticosteroids: a case report. *Hepatology Research* 2004;28:109–12.
480. Goyal RK, Srivastava D, Lessnau KD. Clopidogrel-induced hepatocellular injury and cholestatic jaundice in an elderly patient: case report and review of the literature. *Pharmacotherapy* 2009;29:608–12.
481. Maddrey WC, Maurath CJ, Verburg KM, et al. The hepatic safety and tolerability of the novel cyclooxygenase-2 inhibitor celecoxib. *Am J Ther* 2000;284:1247–55.
482. Soni P, Shell B, Cawkwell G, Li C, Ma H. The hepatic safety and tolerability of the cyclooxygenase-2 selective NSAID celecoxib: pooled analysis of 41 randomized controlled trials. *Curr Med Res Opin* 2009;25:1841–51.
483. El Hajj II, Malik SM, Alwakeel HR, Shaikh OS, Sasatomi E, Kandil HM. Celecoxib-induced cholestatic liver failure requiring orthotopic liver transplantation. *World J Gastroenterol* 2009;15:3937–9.
484. Alegria P, Lebre L, Chagas C. Celecoxib-induced cholestatic hepatotoxicity in a patient with cirrhosis. *Ann Intern Med* 2002;137:75.
485. Linares P, Vivas S, Jorquera F, et al. Severe cholestasis and acute renal failure related to rofecoxib. *Am J Gastroenterol* 2004;99:1622–3.
486. Van Steenbergen W, Peeters P, De Bondt J, et al. Nimesulide-induced acute hepatitis: evidence from six cases. *J Hepatol* 1998;29:135–41.
487. Walker SL, Kennedy F, Niamh N, McCormick PA. Nimesulide associated fulminant hepatic failure. *Pharmacoepidemiol Drug Saf* 2008;17:1108–12.
488. Licata A, Calvaruso V, Cappello M, et al. Clinical course and outcomes of drug-induced liver injury: nimesulide as the first implicated medication. *Dig Liver Dis* 2010;42:143–8.
489. Vanderstigel M, Zafrani ES, Lejonc JL, et al. Allopurinol hypersensitivity syndrome as a cause of hepatic fibrin-ring granulomas. *Gastroenterology* 1986;90:188–90.
490. Mete N, Yilmaz F, Gulbahar O, et al. Allopurinol hypersensitivity syndrome as a cause of hepatic centrilobular hemorrhagic necrosis. *J Investig Allergol Clin Immunol* 2003;13:281–3.
491. Al-Kawas FH, Seeff LB, Berendson RA, et al. Allopurinol hepatotoxicity. Report of two cases and review of the literature. *Ann Intern Med* 1981;95:588–90.
492. Lee MH, Graham GG, Williams KM, et al. A benefit–risk assessment of benzbromarone in the treatment of gout. Was its withdrawal from the market in the best interest of patients? *Drug Saf* 2008;31:643–65.

493. Basset C, Vadrot J, Denis J, et al. Prolonged cholestasis and ductopenia following gold salt therapy. *Liver Int* 2003;23:89–93.

494. Watkins PB, Schade R, Mills AS, et al. Fatal hepatic necrosis associated with parenteral gold therapy. *Dig Dis Sci* 1988;33:1025–9.

495. Fleischner GM, Morecki R, Hanaichi T, et al. Light- and electron-microscopical study of a case of gold salt-induced hepatotoxicity. *Hepatology* 1991;14:422–5.

496. Wu ML, Tsai WJ, Ger J, et al. Cholestatic hepatitis caused by acute gold potassium cyanide poisoning. *J Toxicol Clin Toxicol* 2001;39:739–43.

497. Jacobs JW, Van der Weide FR, Kruijsen MW. Fatal cholestatic hepatitis caused by D-penicillamine. *Br J Rheumatol* 1994;33:770–3.

498. Suissa S, Ernst P, Hudson M, et al. Newer disease-modifying antirheumatic drugs and the risk of serious hepatic adverse events in patients with rheumatoid arthritis. *Am J Med* 2004;117:87–92.

499. Goldkind L, Simon LS. FDA Meeting March 2003: update on the safety of new drugs for rheumatoid arthritis. Part III: Safety and efficacy update on leflunomide (Arava). Available at http://www.rheumatology.org/publications/hotline/0503leffda.asp?aud_mem. (accessed March 25, 2005).

500. Kremer JM, Genovese MC, Cannon GW, et al. Concomitant leflunomide therapy in patients with active rheumatoid arthritis despite stable doses of methotrexate. A randomized, double-blind, placebo-controlled trial. *Ann Intern Med* 2002;137:726–33.

501. Sevilla-Mantilla C, Ortega L, Agundez JA, et al. Leflunomide-induced acute hepatitis. *Dig Liver Dis* 2004;36:82–4.

502. King PD, Perry MC. Hepatotoxicity of chemotherapy. *Oncologist* 2001;6:172–6.

503. Field KM, Michael M. Part II: Liver function in oncology: towards safer chemotherapy use. *Lancet Oncol* 2008;9:1181–90.

504. Lewis JH, Schiff E. Methotrexate induced chronic liver injury: guidelines for detection and prevention. *Am J Gastroenterol* 1988;88:1337–45.

505. Whiting-O'Keefe QE, Fye KH, Sack KD. Methotrexate and histologic hepatic abnormalities: a meta-analysis. *Am J Med* 1991;90:711–16.

506. Roenigk HH, Auerbach R, Maibach HI, et al. Methotrexate in psoriasis: revised guidelines. *J Am Acad Dermatol* 1988;19:145–56.

507. Richard S, Guerret S, Gerard F, et al. Hepatic fibrosis in rheumatoid arthritis patients treated with methotrexate: application of a new semi quantitative scoring system. *Rheumatology (Oxford)* 2000;39:50–4.

508. Hoekstra M, van Ede AE, Haagsma CJ, et al. Factors associated with toxicity, final dose, and efficacy of methotrexate in patients with rheumatoid arthritis. *Ann Rheum Dis* 2003;62:423–6.

509. Whittle SL, Hughes RA. Folate supplementation and methotrexate treatment in rheumatoid arthritis: a review. *Rheumatology (Oxford)* 2004;43:267–71.

510. Said S, Jeffes EW, Weinstein GD. *Methotrexate.* Clin Dermatol 1997;15:781–97.

511. Kremer JM, Alarcon GS, Lightfoot RW Jr, et al. Methotrexate for rheumatoid arthritis: suggested guidelines for monitoring liver toxicity. *Arth Rheum* 1994;7:316–28.

512. Roenigk HH Jr, Auerbach R, Maibach H, et al. Methotrexate in psoriasis: consensus conference. *J Am Acad Dermatol* 1998;38:478–85.

513. Visser K, Katchamart W, Loza E, et al. Multinational evidence-based recommendations for the use of methotrexate in rheumatic disorders with a focus on rheumatoid arthritis: integrating systematic literature research and expert opinion of a broad international panel of rheumatologists in the 3E Initiative. *Ann Rheum Dis* 2009;68:1086–93.

514. Aithal GP, Haugk B, Das S, et al. Monitoring methotrexate-induced hepatic fibrosis in patients with psoriasis: are serial liver biopsies justified? *Aliment Pharmacol Ther* 2004;19:391–9.

515. Te HS, Schiano TD, Kuan SF, et al. Hepatic effects of long-term methotrexate use in the treatment of inflammatory bowel disease. *Am J Gastroenterol* 2000;95:3150–6.

516. Gisbert JP, González-Lama Y, Maté J. Thiopurine-induced liver injury in patients with inflammatory bowel disease: a systematic review. *Am J Gastroenterol* 2007;102(7):1518–27.

517. Bastida G, Nos P, Aguas M, et al. Incidence, risk factors and clinical course of thiopurine-induced liver injury in patients with inflammatory bowel disease. *Aliment Pharmacol Ther* 2005;22:775–82.

518. Gardiner SJ, Gearry RB, Burt MJ, et al. Severe hepatotoxicity with high 6-methylmercaptopurine nucleotide concentrations after thiopurine dose escalation due to low 6-thioguanine nucleotides. *Eur J Gastroenterol Hepatol* 2008;20:1238–42.

519. Sobesky R, Dusoleil A, Condat B, et al. Azathioprine-induced destructive cholangitis. *Am J Gastroenterol* 2001;96:616–17.

520. Sterneck M, Weisner R, Ascher N, et al. Azathioprine hepatotoxicity after liver transplantation. *Hepatology* 1991;14:806–10.

521. Mion F, Napoleon B, Berger F, et al. Azathioprine induced liver disease: nodular regenerative hyperplasia of the liver and perivenous fibrosis in a patient treated for multiple sclerosis. *Gut* 1991;32:715–17.

522. Russmann S, Zimmermann A, Krahenbuhl S, et al. Veno-occlusive disease, nodular regenerative hyperplasia and hepatocellular carcinoma after azathioprine treatment in a patient with ulcerative colitis. *Eur J Gastroenterol Hepatol* 2001;13:287–90.

523. Bermejo F, López-Sanromán A, Algaba A, et al. Mercaptopurine rescue after azathioprine-induced liver injury in inflammatory bowel disease. *Aliment Pharmacol Ther* 2010;31:120–4.

524. Dubinsky MC, Vasiliauskas EA, Singh H, et al. 6-Thioguanine can cause serious liver injury in inflammatory bowel disease patients. *Gastroenterology* 2003;125:298–303.

525. Geller SA, Dubinsky MC, Poordad FF, et al. Early hepatic nodular hyperplasia and submicroscopic fibrosis associated with 6-thioguanine therapy in inflammatory bowel disease. *Am J Surg Pathol* 2004;28:1204–11.

526. de Boer NK, Zondervan PE, Gilissen LP, et al. Absence of nodular regenerative hyperplasia after low-dose 6-thioguanine maintenance therapy in inflammatory bowel disease patients. *Dig Liver Dis* 2008;40:108–13.

527. Kassianides C, Nussenblatt R, Palestine AG, et al. Liver injury from cyclosporine A. *Dig Dis Sci* 1990;35:693–7.

528. Spes CH, Angermann CE, Beyer RW, et al. Increased incidence of cholelithiasis in heart transplant recipients receiving cyclosporine therapy. *J Heart Transplant* 1990;9:404–7.

529. Kullak-Ublick GA, Stieger B, Meier PJ. Enterohepatic bile salt transporters in normal physiology and liver disease. *Gastroenterology* 2004;126:322–42.

530. Neff GW, Ruiz P, Madariaga JR, et al. Sirolimus-associated hepatotoxicity in liver transplantation. *Ann Pharmacother* 2004;38:1593–6.

531. Mullick F, Ishak KG. Hepatic injury associated with diphenylhydantoin therapy. A clinicopathologic study of 20 cases. *Am J Clin Pathol* 1980;74:442–52.

532. Citerio G, Nobili A, Airoldi L, et al. Severe intoxication after phenytoin infusion: a preventable pharmacogenetics adverse reaction. *Neurology* 2003;60:1395–6.

533. Williams SJ, Ruppin DC, Grierson JM, et al. Carbamazepine hepatitis: the clinicopathological spectrum. *J Gastroenterol Hepatol* 1986;1:159–68.

534. Horowitz S, Patwardhan R, Marcus E. Hepatotoxic reactions associated with carbamazepine therapy. *Epilepsia* 1988;29:149–54.

535. Frey B, Braegger CP, Ghelfi D. Neonatal cholestatic hepatitis from carbamazepine exposure during pregnancy and breast feeding. *Ann Pharmacother* 2002;36:644–7.

536. Tazawa K, Yasuda M, Ohtani Y, et al. Multiple hepatocellular adenomas associated with long-term carbamazepine. *Histopathology* 1999;35:92–4.

537. Berkowitz FE, Henderson SL, Fajman N, et al. Acute liver failure caused by isoniazid in a child receiving carbamazepine. *Int J Tuberc Lung Dis* 1998;2:603–6.

538. Overstreet K, Costanza C, Behling C, et al. Fatal progressive hepatic necrosis associated with lamotrigine treatment: a case report and literature review. *Dig Dis Sci* 2002;47:1921–5.

539. Bavdekar SB, Muranjan MN, Gogtay NJ, et al. Anticonvulsant hypersensitivity syndrome: lymphocyte toxicity assay for the confirmation of diagnosis and risk assessment. *Ann Pharmacother* 2004;38:1648–50.

540. Dreifuss FE, Santilli N, Langer DH, et al. Valproic acid hepatic fatalities: a retrospective review. *Neurology* 1987;37:379–85.

541. Konig SA, Schenk M, Sick C, et al. Fatal liver failure associated with valproate therapy in a patient with Friedreich's disease: review of valproate hepatotoxicity in adults. *Epilepsia* 1999;40:1036–40.

542. Bryant AE III, Dreifuss FE. Valproic acid hepatic fatalities. III. US experience since 1986. *Neurology* 1996;46:465–9.

543. Saneto RP, Lee IC, Koenig MK, et al. POLG DNA testing as an emerging standard of care before instituting valproic acid therapy for pediatric seizure disorders. *Seizure* 2010;19:140–6.

544. Zimmerman HJ, Ishak KG. Valproate-induced hepatic injury: analyses of 23 fatal cases. *Hepatology* 1982;2:591–7.

545. Bohan TP, Helton E, McDonald I, et al. Effect of L-carnitine treatment for valproate-induced hepatotoxicity. *Neurology* 2001;56:1405–9.

546. Thomson MA, Lynch S, Strong R, et al. Orthotopic liver transplantation with poor neurologic outcome in valproate-associated liver failure: a need for critical risk–benefit appraisal in the use of valproate. *Transplant Proc* 2000;32:200–3.

547. Huang YL, Hong HS, Wang ZW, et al. Fatal sodium valproate-induced hypersensitivity syndrome with lichenoid dermatitis and fulminant hepatitis. *J Am Acad Dermatol* 2003;49:316–19.

548. Bjoro K, Gjerstad L, Bentdal O, et al. Topiramate and fulminant liver failure. *Lancet* 1998;352:1119.

549. Doan RJ, Clendenning M. Topiramate and hepatotoxicity. *Can J Psychiatry* 2000;45:937–8.

550. Bumb A, Diederich N, Beyenburg S. Adding topiramate to valproate therapy may cause reversible hepatic failure. *Epileptic Disord* 2003;5:157–9.

551. O'Neil MG, Perdun CS, Wilson MB, et al. Felbamate-associated fatal acute hepatic necrosis. *Neurology* 1996;46:1457–9.

552. Dieckhaus CM, Thompson CD, Roller SG, et al. Mechanisms of idiosyncratic drug reactions: the case of felbamate. *Chem Biol Interact* 2002;142:99–117.

553. Richardson CE, Williams DW, Kingham JG. Gabapentin induced cholestasis. *Br Med J* 2002;325:635.

554. Hauben M. Re: Lasso-de-la-Vega et al. gabapentin as a probable cause of hepatotoxicity and eosinophilia. *Am J Gastroenterol* 2002;97:2156–7.

555. Ishak KG, Irey NS. Hepatic injury associated with the phenothiazines. Clinicopathologic and follow-up study of 36 patients. *Arch Pathol* 1972;93:283–304.

556. Watson RG, Olomu A, Clements D, et al. A proposed mechanism for chlorpromazine jaundice – defective hepatic sulphoxidation combined with rapid hydroxylation. *J Hepatol* 1988;7:72–8.

557. Lok AS, Ng IO. Prochlorperazine-induced chronic cholestasis. *J Hepatol* 1988;6:369–73.

558. Dincsoy HP, Saelinger DA. Haloperidol-induced chronic cholestatic liver disease. *Gastroenterology* 1982;83:694–700.

559. Hainer MI, Tsai N, Komura ST, et al. Fatal hepatorenal failure associated with hydrazine sulfate. *Ann Intern Med* 2000;133:877–80.

560. Selim K, Kaplowitz N. Hepatotoxicity of psychotropic drugs. *Hepatology* 1999;29:1347–51.

561. Aranda-Michel J, Koehler A, Bejarano PA, et al. Nefazodone-induced liver failure:report of three cases. *Ann Intern Med* 1999;130:285–8.

562. Carvajal Garcia-Pando A, Garcia del Pozo J, Sanchez AS, et al. Hepatotoxicity associated with the new antidepressants. *J Clin Psychiatry* 2002;63:135–7.

563. Stewart DE. Hepatic adverse reactions associated with nefazodone. *Can J Psychiatry* 2002;47:375–7.

564. Tzimas GN, Dion B, Deschenes M. Early onset, nefazodone-induced fulminant hepatic failure. *Am J Gastroenterol* 2003;98:1663–4.

565. Kalgutkar AS, Vaz AD, Lame ME, et al. Bioactivation of the nontricyclic antidepressant nefazodone to a reactive quinine-imine species in human liver microsomes and recombinant cytochrome P450 3A4. *Drug Metab Dispos* 2005;33:243–53.

566. Fernandes NF, Martin RR, Schenker S. Trazodone-induced hepatotoxicity: a case report with comments on drug-induced hepatotoxicity. *Am J Gastroenterol* 2000;95:532–5.

567. Watkins PB, Zimmerman HJ, Knapp MJ, et al. Hepatotoxic effects of tacrine administration in patients with Alzheimer's disease. *JAMA* 1994;271:992–8.

568. Ames DJ, Bhathal PS, Davies BM, et al. Heterogeneity of adverse hepatic reactions to tetrahydroaminoacridine. *Aust NZ J Med* 1990;20:193–5.

569. Carr DF, Alfirevic A, Tugwood JD, et al. Molecular and genetic association of interleukin-6 in tacrine-induced hepatotoxicity. *Pharmacogenet Genomics* 2007;17:961–72.

570. Dierckx RI, Vandewoude MF. Donepezil-related toxic hepatitis. *Acta Clin Belg* 2008;63:339–42.

571. Goodman CR. Hepatotoxicity due to methylphenidate hydrochloride. *NY State J Med* 1972;72:2339–40.

572. Stecyk O, Loludice TA, Demeter S, et al. Multiple organ failure resulting from intravenous abuse of methylphenidate hydrochloride. *Ann Emerg Med* 1985;14:597–9.

573. Lewis JJ, Iezzoni JC, Berg CL. Methylphenidate-induced autoimmune hepatitis. *Dig Dis Sci* 2007;52:594–7.

574. Rosh JR, Dellert SF, Narkewicz M, et al. Four cases of severe hepatotoxicity associated with pemoline: possible autoimmune pathogenesis. *Pediatrics* 1998;101:921–3.

575. Nehra A, Mullick F, Ishak KG, et al. Pemoline-associated hepatic injury. *Gastroenterology* 1990;99:1517–19.

576. Marotta PJ, Roberts EA. Pemoline hepatotoxicity in children. *J Pediatr* 1998;132:894–7.

577. Sterling MJ, Kane M, Grace ND. Pemoline-induced autoimmune hepatitis. *Am J Gastroenterol* 1996;91:2233–4.

578. Remy A-J, Camu W, Ramos J, et al. Acute hepatitis after riluzole administration. *J Hepatol* 1999;30:527–30.

579. Castells LI, Gamez J, Cervera C, et al. Icteric toxic hepatitis associated with riluzole. *Lancet* 1998;351:648.

580. Wilkinson SP, Portmann B, Williams R. Hepatitis from dantrolene sodium. *Gut* 1979;20:33–6.

581. Chan CH. Dantrolene sodium and hepatic injury. *Neurology* 1990;40:1427–32.

582. Borges N. Tolcapone in Parkinson's disease: liver toxicity and clinical efficacy. *Expert Opin Drug Saf* 2005;4:69–73.

583. Truong DD. Tolcapone: review of its pharmacology and use as adjunctive therapy in patients with Parkinson's disease. *Clin Interv Aging* 2009;4:109–13.

584. Fischer JJ, Michaelis S, Schrey AK, et al. Capture compound mass spectrometry sheds light on the molecular mechanisms of liver toxicity of two Parkinson drugs. *Toxicol Sci* 2010 (Epub).

585. Korlipara LV, Cooper JM, Schapira AH. Differences in toxicity of the catechol-O-methyl transferase inhibitors, tolcapone and

entacapone to cultured human neuroblastoma cells. *Neuropharmacology* 2004;46:562–9.

586. Brooks DJ. Safety and tolerability of COMT inhibitors. *Neurology* 2004;62:S39–46.

587. Henry JA, Jeffreys KJ, Dawling S. Toxicity and deaths from 3,4-methylenedioxymethamphetamine ("ecstasy"). *Lancet* 1992;340:384.

588. Andreu V, Mas A, Bruguera M, et al. Ecstasy: a common cause of severe acute hepatotoxicity. *J Hepatol* 1998;29:394–7.

589. Case records of the Massachusetts General Hospital. Weekly clinico-pathological exercises. Case 6 – 2001. A 17-year-old girl with marked jaundice and weight loss. *N Engl J Med* 2001;344:591–9.

590. Tillmann HL, van Pelt FN, Martz W, et al. Accidental intoxication with methylene dianiline p,p'-diaminodiphenylmethane: acute liver damage after presumed ecstasy consumption. *J Toxicol Clin Toxicol* 1997;35:35–40.

591. Perino LE, Warren GHH, Levine JS. Cocaine-induced hepatotoxicity in humans. *Gastroenterology* 1987;93:176–80.

592. Peyriere H, Mauboussin JM. Cocaine-induced acute cytologic hepatitis in HIV-infected patients with nonactive viral hepatitis. *Ann Intern Med* 2000;132:1010–11.

593. Silva MO, Roth D, Reddy KR, et al. Hepatic dysfunction accompanying acute cocaine intoxication. *J Hepatol* 1991;12:312–15.

594. Balaguer F, Fernandez J, Lozano M, et al. Cocaine-induced acute hepatitis and thrombotic microangiopathy. *JAMA* 2005;293:797–8.

595. Lopez-Torres E, Lucena MI, Andrade RJ, et al. Tetrabamate-induced hepatotoxicity. Report of seven cases and literature review. *Gastroenterol Hepatol* 2002;25:589–93.

596. Djörnsson E, Nordlinder H, Olsson R. Clinical characteristics and prognostic markers in disulfiram-induced liver injury. *J Hepatol* 2006;44:001–7.

597. Mohanty SR, LaBrecque DR, Mitros FA, et al. Liver transplantation for disulfiram-induced fulminant hepatic failure. *J Clin Gastroenterol* 2004;38:292–5.

598. Hashimoto K, Hoshii Y, Takahashi M, et al. Use of a monoclonal antibody against Lafora bodies for the immunocytochemical study of ground-glass inclusions in hepatocytes due to cyanamide. *Histopathology* 2001;39:60–5.

599. Pompili M, Basso M, Grieco A, et al. Recurrent acute hepatitis associated with use of cetirizine. *Ann Pharmacother* 2004;38:1844–7.

600. Schiano TD, Bellary SV, Cassidy MJ, et al. Subfulminant liver failure and severe hepatotoxicity caused by loratadine use. *Ann Intern Med* 1996;125:738–40.

601. Black M. Hepatotoxic and hepatoprotective potential of histamine (H2)-receptor antagonists. *Am J Med* 1987;83:68–75.

602. Fisher AA, Le Couteur DG. Nephrotoxicity and hepatotoxicity of histamine H2 receptor antagonists. *Drug Saf* 2001;24:39–57.

603. Malka D, Pham BN, Courvalin JC, et al. Acute hepatitis caused by alverine associated with anti-lamin A and C autoantibodies. *J Hepatol* 1997;27:399–403.

604. Kim SY, Kim BH, Dong SH, et al. Alfuzosin-induced acute liver injury. *Korean J Hepatol* 2007;13:414–18.

605. Humbert M, Segal ES, Kiely DG, Carlsen J, Schwierin B, Hoeper MM. Results of European post-marketing surveillance of bosentan in pulmonary hypertension. *Eur Respir J* 2007;30:338–44.

606. Dwyer N, Jones G, Kilpatrick D. Severe hepatotoxicity in a patient on bosentan upon addition of methotrexate: reversible with resumption of methotrexate without bosentan. *J Clin Rheumatol* 2009;15:88–9.

607. Fattinger K, Funk C, Pantze M, et al. The endothelin antagonist bosentan inhibits the canalicular bile salt export pump: a potential mechanism for hepatic adverse reactions. *Clin Pharmacol Ther* 2001;69:223–31.

608. Lavelle A, Sugrue R, Lawler G, et al. Sitaxentan-induced hepatic failure in two patients with pulmonary arterial hypertension. *Eur Respir J* 2009;34:770–1.

609. Francis GS, Grumser Y, Alteri E, et al. Hepatic reactions during treatment of multiple sclerosis with interferon-beta-1a: incidence and clinical significance. *Drug Saf* 2003;26:815–27.

610. Tremlett HL, Yoshida EM, Oger J. Liver injury associated with the beta-interferons for MS: a comparison between the three products. *Neurology* 2004;62:628–31.

611. Wallack EM, Callon R. Liver injury associated with the beta-interferons for MS. *Neurology* 2004;63:1142–3.

612. Ridruejo E, Cacchione R, Villamil AG, et al. Imatinib-induced fatal acute liver failure. *World J Gastroenterol* 2007;13:6608–111.

613. Tonyali O, Coskun U, Yildiz R, et al. Imatinib mesylate-induced acute liver failure in a patient with gastrointestinal stromal tumors. *Med Oncol* 2009 (Epub).

614. Lin NU, Sarantopoulos S, Stone JR, et al. Fatal hepatic necrosis following imatinib mesylate therapy. *Blood* 2003;102:3455–6.

615. Weise AM, Liu CY, Shields AF. Fatal liver failure in a patient on acetaminophen treated with sunitinib malate and levothyroxine. *Ann Pharmacother* 2009;43:761–6.

616. http://www.aasld.org/conferences/Documents/Presentation Library/2010Hepatoxicity_SessionII_Spraggs.pdf.

617. Davern TJ, Bass NM. Leukotriene antagonists. *Clin Liver Dis* 2003;7:501–12.

618. Russmann S, Iselin HU, Meier D, et al. Acute hepatitis associated with montelukast. *J Hepatol* 2003;38:694–5.

619. Mancini S, Amorotti E, Vecchio S, Ponz de Leon M, Roncucci L. Infliximab-related hepatitis: discussion of a case and review of the literature. *Intern Emerg Med.* 2010 (Epub).

620. Bezabeh S, Flowers CM, Kortepeter C, Avigan M. Clinically significant liver injury in patients treated with natalizumab. *Aliment Pharmacol Ther* 2010;31:1028–35.

621. Carlsen KM, Riis L, Madsen OR. Toxic hepatitis induced by infliximab in a patient with rheumatoid arthritis with no relapse after switching to etanercept. *Clin Rheumatol* 2009;28:1001–3.

622. Testa L, Andreotti F, Biondi Zoccai GG, et al. Ximelagatran/melagatran against conventional anticoagulation: a meta-analysis based on 22,639 patients. *Int J Cardiol* 2007;122:117–24.

623. Kindmark A, Jawaid A, Harbron CG, et al. Genome-wide pharmacogenetic investigation of a hepatic adverse event without clinical signs of immunopathology suggests an underlying immune pathogenesis. *Pharmacogenomics J* 2008;8:186–95.

624. Seeff LB, Lindsay KL, Bacon BR, et al. Complementary and alternative medicine in chronic liver disease. *Hepatology* 2001;34:595–603.

625. Chitturi S, Farrell GC. Herbal hepatotoxicity: an expanding but poorly defined problem. *J Gastroenterol Hepatol* 2000;15:1093–9.

626. Russmann S, Lauterburg BH, Helbling A. Kava hepatotoxicity. *Ann Intern Med* 2001;135:68–9.

627. Borum ML. Fulminant exacerbation of autoimmune hepatitis after the use of ma huang. *Am J Gastroenterol* 2001;96:1654–5.

628. Cohen SM, O'Connor AM, Hart J, et al. Autoimmune hepatitis associated with the use of black cohosh: a case study. *Menopause* 2004;11:575–7.

629. Larrey D, Pageaux GP. Hepatotoxicity of herbal remedies and mushrooms. *Semin Liver Dis* 1995;15:183–8.

630. Stedman C. Herbal hepatotoxicity. *Semin Liver Dis* 2002;22:195–206.

631. Sheikh NM, Philen RM, Love LA. Chaparral-associated hepatotoxicity. *Arch Intern Med* 1997;157:913–19.

632. Larrey D, Vial T, Pauwels A, et al. Hepatitis after germander (*Teucrium chamaedrys*): another instance of herbal medicine hepatotoxicity. *Ann Intern Med* 1992;117:129–32.

633. Polymeros D, Kamberoglou D, Tzias V. Acute cholestatic hepatitis caused by *Teucrium polium* (golden germander) with transient

appearance of antimitochondrial antibody. *J Clin Gastroenterol* 2002;34:100–1.

634. De Berardinis V, Moulis C, Maurice M, et al. Human microsomal epoxide hydrolase is the target of germander-induced autoantibodies on the surface of human hepatocytes. *Mol Pharmacol* 2000;58:542–51.

635. Fau D, Lekehal M, Farrell G, et al. Diterpenoids from germander, an herbal medicine, induce apoptosis in isolated rat hepatocytes. *Gastroenterology* 1997;113:1334–46.

636. Mattei, Dourakis SP, Papanikolaou IS, et al. Acute hepatitis associated with herb (*Teucrium capitatum* L.) administration. *Eur J Gastroenterol Hepatol* 2002;14:693–5.

637. Woolf GM, Petrovic LM, Rojter SE, et al. Acute hepatitis associated with the Chinese herbal product Jin Bu Huan. *Ann Intern Med* 1994;121:729–35.

638. Picciotti A, Campo N, Brizzolara R, et al. Chronic hepatitis induced by Jin Bu Huan. *J Hepatol* 1998;28:165–7.

639. Stickel F, Baumuller HM, Seitz K, et al. Hepatitis induced by kava (Piper methysticum rhizoma). *J Hepatol* 2003;39:62–7.

640. Russmann S, Barguil Y, Cabalion P, et al. Hepatic injury due to traditional aqueous extracts of kava root in New Caledonia. *Eur J Gastroenterol Hepatol* 2003;15:1033–6.

641. Hepatic toxicity possibly associated with kava-containing products – United States, Germany, and Switzerland, 1999–2002. *MMWR Morb Mortal Wkly Rep* 2002;51:1065–7.

642. Teschke R, Schwarzenboeck A, Hennermann KH. Kava hepatotoxicity: a clinical survey and critical analysis of 26 suspected cases. *Eur J Gastroenterol Hepatol* 2008;20:1182–93.

643. Tandon BN, Tandon HD, Tandon RK, et al. An epidemic of veno-occlusive disease of liver in central India. *Lancet* 1976;2:271–2.

644. Chitturi S, Farrell GC. Hepatotoxic slimming aids and other herbal hepatotoxins. *J Gastroenterol Hepatol* 2008;23:366–73.

645. Adachi M, Saito H, Kobayashi H, et al. Hepatic injury in 12 patients taking the herbal weight loss AIDS Chaso or Onshido. *Ann Intern Med* 2003;139:488–92.

646. Favreau JT, Ryu ML, Braunstein G, et al. Severe hepatotoxicity associated with the dietary supplement LipoKinetix. *Ann Intern Med* 2002;136:590–5.

647. Neff GW, Reddy KR, Durazo FA, et al. Severe hepatotoxicity associated with the use of weight loss diet supplements containing ma huang or usnic acid. *J Hepatol* 2004;41:1062–4.

648. Fong TL, Klontz KC, Canas-Coto A, et al. Hepatotoxicity due to hydroxycut: a case series. *Am J Gastroenterol* 2010 (Epub).

649. Leo MA, Lieber CS. Hypervitaminosis A: a liver lover's lament. *Hepatology* 1988;8:412–17.

650. Nagai K, Hosaka H, Kubo S, et al. Vitamin A toxicity secondary to excessive intake of yellow–green vegetables, liver and laver. *J Hepatol* 1999;31:142–8.

651. Kowalski TE, Falestiny M, Furth E, et al. Vitamin A hepatotoxicity: a cautionary note regarding 25,000 IU supplements. *Am J Med* 1994;97:523–8.

652. Geubel AP, De Galocsy C, Alves N, et al. Liver damage caused by therapeutic vitamin A administration: estimation of dose-related toxicity in 41 cases. *Gastroenterology* 1991;100:1701–9.

653. Doyle S, Conlon P, Royston D. Vitamin A induced stellate cell hyperplasia and fibrosis in renal failure. *Histopathology* 2000;36:90–1.

654. Inkeles SB, Conner WE, Illingworth DR. Hepatic and dermatologic manifestations of chronic hypervitaminosis A in adults. Report of two cases. *Am J Med* 1986;80:491–6.

655. Zafrani ES, Bernuau D, Feldmann G. Peliosis-like ultrastructural changes of the hepatic sinusoids in human chronic hypervitaminosis A: report of three cases. *Hum Pathol* 1984;15:1166–70.

656. Olson JA. Serum levels of vitamin A and carotenoids as reflectors of nutritional status. *J Nat Cancer Inst* 1984;73:1439–44.

657. Ballew C, Bowman BA, Russell RM, et al. Serum retinyl esters are not associated with biochemical markers of liver dysfunction in adult participants in the third National Health and Nutrition Examination Survey (NHANES III), 1988–1994. *Am J Clin Nutr* 2001;73:934–40.

658. Farrell GC, Bhathal PS, Powell LW. Abnormal liver function in chronic hypervitaminosis A. *Am J Dig Dis* 1977;22:724–8.

659. Jorens PG, Michielsen PP, Pelckmans PA, et al. Vitamin A abuse: development of cirrhosis despite cessation of vitamin A. A six-year clinical and histopathologic follow-up. *Liver* 1992;12:381–6.

660. Russell RM, Boyer JL, Bagheri SA, et al. Hepatic injury from chronic hypervitaminosis a resulting in portal hypertension and ascites. *N Engl J Med* 1974;291:435–40.

661. Weber FL Jr, Mitchell GE Jr, Powell DE, et al. Reversible hepatotoxicity associated with hepatic vitamin A accumulation in a protein-deficient patient. *Gastroenterology* 1982;82:118–23.

662. Kamm MA, Davies DJ, Breen KJ. Acute hepatitis due to etretinate. *J Gastroenterol Hepatol* 1988;3:663–6.

663. Weiss VC, West DP, Ackerman R et al. Hepatotoxic reactions in a patient treated with etretinate. *Arch Dermatol* 1984;120:104–6.

664. Roenigk HH Jr, Callen JP, Guzzo CA, et al. Effects of acitretin on the liver. *J Am Acad Dermatol* 1999;41:584–8.

665. Kreiss C, Amin S, Nalesnik MA, et al. Severe cholestatic hepatitis in a patient taking acitretin. *Am J Gastroenterol* 2002;97:775–7.

666. van Ditzhuijsen TJ, van Haelst UJ, et al. Severe hepatotoxic reaction with progression to cirrhosis after use of a novel retinoid (acitretin). *J Hepatol* 1990;11:185–8.

Multiple choice questions

27.1 With respect to acetaminophen hepatotoxicity, all of the following statements are true except which one?

a Acetaminophen is the leading cause of acute liver failure in the United States.
b Concomitant use of statins increases the risk of acetaminophen hepatotoxicity.
c Intravenous *N*-acetylcysteine is an alternative to oral *N*-acetylcysteine in treating patients at risk of significant liver injury.
d *N*-acetylcysteine replenishes cytosolic and mitochondrial glutathione and also provides mitochondrial energy substrates.
e *N*-acetylcysteine can be beneficial even in patients presenting with acute liver failure.

27.2 A strong genetic predisposition to developing drug-induced liver injury has been reported for all the following drugs except which one?

a Nevirapine.
b Abacavir.
c Flucloxacillin.
d Atorvastatin.
e Sodium valproate.

Answers to the multiple choice questions can be found in the Appendix at the end of the book.

These multiple choice questions are also available for you to complete online.
Visit http://www.schiffsdiseasesofthecliver.com/

CHAPTER 28

Mechanisms of Drug-induced Liver Injury

Paul B. Watkins

Institute for Drug Safety Sciences, University of North Carolina at Chapel Hill, NC, USA

Key concepts

- An initial event in drug-induced liver injury (DILI) is often accumulation of a reactive metabolite over a "threshold." This occurs when the rate at which the reactive metabolite is produced exceeds the rate at which it can be safely eliminated.
- Reactive metabolites can injury cells in many ways, including creating oxidative stress and covalent binding. The mitochondria appear to be a particularly important target for these effects.
- Liver injury can stimulate an innate immune response, which can amplify the death of hepatocytes. The extent of this "collateral damage" appears to be largely based on a balance of pro- and anti-inflammatory cytokines.
- Drug-induced liver injury can resolve spontaneously despite continuation of drug therapy due to adaptation. This can involve

- altered regulation of hepatocyte enzymes and transporters and probably downregulation of the innate immune response.
- There is increasing evidence that rare or idiosyncratic DILI may result from an adaptive immune attack on the liver. This may occur in response to drug–protein adducts acting as antigens and mild drug-mediated liver injury acting as a "danger signal."
- Genomic approaches currently being undertaken should improve our understanding of the mechanisms that underlie DILI. This should lead to improved methods of preclinical safety testing of new drugs and to personalized medicine tests to improve the safety of existing drugs.

Drug-induced liver injury (DILI) has been traditionally divided into two categories: predictable and unpredictable (or "idiosyncratic"). In reality, these classifications are two ends of a spectrum, with some drugs sharing features of both. Predictable liver toxins produce dose-dependent injury that typically occurs within days of dosing; essentially all patients will develop liver injury if they receive a sufficiently high dose. Drugs that are predictable toxins are generally identified in preclinical (animal) studies, or during the early clinical trials specifically designed to look for dose-related toxicity. If liver toxicity occurs at doses likely to be near those required for significant therapeutic benefit, the drug is generally abandoned from further development. As a result, there are few predictable hepatotoxins in therapeutic use today. One example of a drug that is a predictable hepatotoxin is acetaminophen. As with all predictable toxins, subtoxic exposures can generally be safely tolerated as "the dose makes the poison."

In contrast to predictable toxicity, idiosyncratic toxicity is not clearly dose related and is typically delayed weeks to months after starting dosing. With a true idiosyncratic toxin, only a very small fraction of the total treated

patients are susceptible to liver injury even when receiving high doses (i.e., it is the *host* that makes the poison). Animal models, while having value in identifying predictable liver toxins in man, generally are of little help in identifying drugs capable of causing idiosyncratic toxicity. If the toxicity occurs in less than one in 1,000 patients receiving the drug, the toxicity might not be recognized during preapproval clinical trials, and only become evident after regulatory approval for marketing and widespread usage. Recognition that an otherwise good drug can cause idiosyncratic hepatotoxicity often leads to regulatory actions that limit access of patients to that drug, even when most patients are at no risk for toxicity. Idiosyncratic hepatotoxicity has been the major reason for regulatory actions concerning drugs, including failure to approve, marketing restrictions, and withdrawal from the market place [1]. Idiosyncratic hepatotoxicity therefore poses a great problem for physicians, patients, and the pharmaceutical industry. Until the mechanisms underlying idiosyncratic hepatotoxicity are further identified, it is unlikely that industry will be able to design this liability out of new drugs. The vast majority of research on the mechanisms underlying DILI has involved predictable hepatotoxins, particularly acetaminophen. Furthermore, it is generally assumed that the mechanisms underlying predictable toxicity are relevant to idiosyncratic toxicity, but that the latter occurs because of genetic or nongenetic factors that are present only in susceptible patients.

Mechanisms of predictable hepatotoxicity

Most predictable hepatotoxins, including environmental compounds like aflatoxin B1, bromobenzene, and carbon tetrachloride, are relatively harmless to the liver. These, and most other predictable hepatotoxins, are converted in the liver to reactive, or toxic, metabolites generated from the parent (or "protoxin") [2,3]. A general scheme for hepatotoxicity mechanisms involving reactive metabolites is shown in Fig. 28.1. The liver is particularly susceptible to generating reactive metabolites because it is the major organ responsible for drug metabolism and elimination. Furthermore, many of the same enzymes involved in the safe elimination of drugs (nontoxic pathways) have also been implicated in creating reactive and potentially toxic metabolites.

When a reactive metabolite is involved in toxicity, it usually represents only a small fraction of the total metabolism of the drug. Hepatocytes are generally capa-

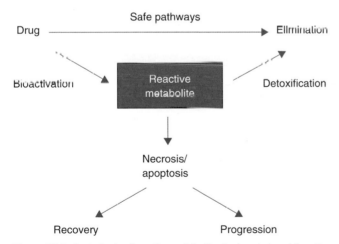

Figure 28.1 Central role of reactive metabolites in drug-induced liver. For most drugs, the major routes of elimination involve the production of metabolites that are safely excreted and therefore represent no threat to the liver cells. Drugs that produce liver injury generally appear to do so through "bioactivation" to reactive or toxic metabolites, which often result from relatively minor metabolic pathways. Fortunately, the liver generally has adequate ability to detoxify these metabolites, allowing their safe elimination. However, under certain circumstances, the reactive metabolite can accumulate in the hepatocyte above a threshold for toxicity, resulting in hepatocyte damage through a variety of mechanisms discussed in the text. For a given level of hepatocyte injury, the outcome may be complete recovery or progression to death, depending on the response of the innate immune system.

ble of efficiently detoxifying and eliminating reactive metabolites once formed, preventing toxicity. A generally held concept is that the initiating event in predictable hepatotoxicity is the accumulation of the reactive metabolite above some threshold. Accumulation occurs when the relative rates of production of the reactive metabolite exceed its rate of safe removal.

The rate of production of a reactive metabolite in the hepatocyte reflects the intrinsic activity of the enzyme responsible for this conversion (termed "bioactivation" in Fig. 28.1) and the concentration of the parent molecule surrounding the enzyme within the hepatocyte. The concentration of the parent molecule chiefly reflects: (i) the competing rates of uptake into, and efflux out of, the hepatocyte; and (ii) the rate of conversion of the parent molecule to safe and readily excreted metabolites (the competing "safe pathways" shown in Fig. 28.1).

Safe pathways of drug metabolism and transport

The rates of uptake and efflux of drugs (and metabolites) in most cases does not reflect passive diffusion, but rather the activities of specific transport proteins [4,5]. There has been great progress in the identification and characterization of these transporters (Fig. 28.2). Uptake transporters are present on the basolateral membrane of the hepatocyte and efflux transporters are present on both the basolateral and canalicular membranes. Once inside the hepatocyte, the rate of conversion of the parent molecule to nontoxic metabolites reflects the activities of a variety of enzymes traditionally divided into two categories: phase 1 and phase 2. Phase 1 reactions result in a direct modification of the primary structure of the drug, usually resulting in the insertion of an oxygen atom in the form of a hydroxyl (-OH) group. Phase 2 reactions involve covalent binding (conjugation) of the drug to polar ligands, usually glucuronic acid or sulfate, often to the hydroxyl group resulting from phase 1 metabolism. The terms phase 1 and phase 2 refer to the fact that often, but not always, drugs must first be subjected to phase 1 metabolism before they can be conjugated. Metabolites generated by phase 1 and phase 2 enzymes are generally actively secreted into bile or back into the systemic circulation for elimination by the kidneys into urine. In most instances, this process appears to reflect active transport by many of the same proteins involved in the efflux of parent drugs (Fig. 28.2). Active efflux of metabolites from the hepatocyte is sometimes termed phase 3.

It is now appreciated that most (but not all) of what was described as phase 1 drug metabolism is the result of the activity of a large family of enzymes termed cytochromes P450, now termed simply P450s or CYPs (pronounced "sips"). Liver P450s metabolize most drugs in use today; in many and perhaps most instances, metabolism by a

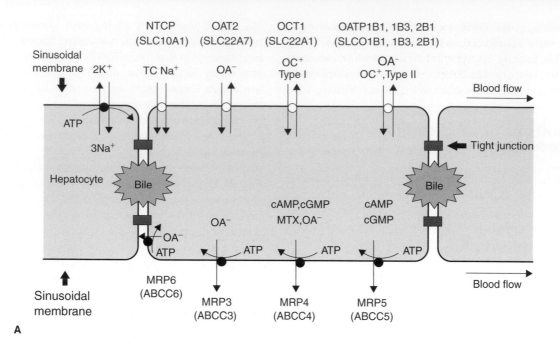

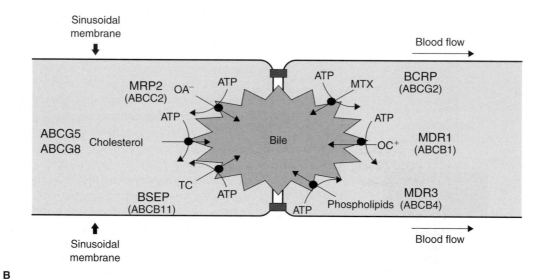

Figure 28.2 Uptake and efflux transporters in the hepatocyte. (A) Basolateral transporters: the uptake of serum bile acids results from the action of neutral taurocholate protein (NTCP) and to a lesser extent organic anion transport polypepetides (OATPs), which are also involved in the uptake of many drugs. Multidrug resistance-associated proteins (MRPs) are chiefly involved with the efflux of drug and their metabolites, particularly glucuronide and sulfate conjugates. During the recovery phase of hepatotoxicity due to acetaminophen or carbon tetrachloride, there is downregulation of NTCP and several OATPs, and upregulation of several MRPs, including MRP3 and MRP4. The aggregate effects of these changes, which reduce the hepatocyte content of potentially injurious bile acids and xenobiotics, likely account in part for adaptation to hepatotoxicity with recurrent dosing. (B) Canalicular transporters: bile salt excretory protein (BSEP) is the major bile acid efflux pump. Multidrug resistance transporter 1 (MDR1) and MRP2 are responsible for biliary excretion of most xenobiotics and their metabolites. During the recovery phase of hepatotoxicity due to acetaminophen or carbon tetrachloride, there is upregulation of MRP2 and probably MDR1 and BSEP. These changes compliment the altered regulation in basolateral transporters and should further reduce the hepatocyte content of potentially injurious bile acids and xenobiotics and thereby contribute to adaptation with recurrent dosing. ATP, adenosine triphosphate; cAMP, cyclic adenosine monophosphate; cGMP, cyclic guanosine monophosphate; MTX, methotrexate; OA, organic anionx; OAT, organic anion transporter; OC, organic cation; OCT, organic cation transporter. (Adapted from Chandra and Brouwer [4].)

P450 is rate limiting in the elimination of the parent drug. Most P450s important for drug metabolism derive from three gene families, now termed CYP1, CYP2, and CYP3 [6]. Within each P450 family, there are subfamilies designated by capital letters. Each subfamily generally contains multiple members, designated by Arabic numbers usually reflecting the order in which they were discovered.

A list of the major P450s involved in human drug metabolism is shown in Table 28.1. In many instances, a single P450 represents the major pathway of metabolism of a drug but a single P450 can generally metabolize many different drugs. To identify the P450s that metabolize drugs in development, many pharmaceutical companies use high throughput technology [7] and some are utilizing computer-based (in silico) modeling [8].

The best studied phase 2 enzymes involved in the elimination of nontoxic metabolites are the uridine 5'-diphosphate (UDP) glucuronyltransferases, and the sulfotransferases, which catalyze conjugation to glucuronic acid and sulfate, respectively. Conjugation generally results in enhanced water solubility and elimination in urine and stool. As with the P450s, the UDP glucuronyltransferases and sulfotransferases arise from multigene families [9,10]. High throughput means of assessing which phase 2 enzymes metabolize drugs have been developed [11].

Enzymes involved in generating reactive metabolites

It appears that the initiating step in drug-induced liver injury often involves creation in the liver of a reactive metabolite from the parent molecule (see Fig. 28.1). Reactive metabolites are generally minor products of drug metabolism, and their reactivity can make them very short lived and difficult to detect in biologic systems. For this reason, identifying the precise structure of a reactive metabolite can be challenging.

P450s are the major enzymes capable of generating reactive and potentially toxic metabolites. The identical enzymes involved in the safe metabolism of drugs are those that have been most implicated in the production of hepatotoxic metabolites (see Table 28.1 for examples). In general, P450s are expressed in the highest concentration in zone 3 hepatocytes, and this in part accounts for the predominance of pericentral necrosis in some forms of DILI (such as that due to acetaminophen) [12]. Interspecies differences in P450 catalytic activities and regulation probably contribute to the imperfect ability of preclinical animal studies to identify human hepatotoxins [13].

Not all reactive metabolites are produced by P450s. Some reactive metabolites, such as acylglucuronides [14], are products of phase 2 metabolism. For example, glucuronide metabolites of diclofenac and valproic acid has been shown to covalently bind multiple proteins in the hepatocyte, and this covalent binding may contribute to hepatoxicity rarely associated with these drugs [15–17].

Enzymes involved in the safe elimination of reactive metabolites

Minor reactive metabolites are probably commonly produced during the metabolism of drugs. Fortunately, the liver usually has the ability to dispose of these metabolites before they can cause injury. The major safe elimination pathway for reactive metabolites involves conjugation to glutathione (GSH). Although GSH is synthesized in every cell in the body, the liver is the major site of its synthesis. Under usual conditions, the hepatocyte cytosolic concentration of GSH is quite high (~ 10 mm). GSH may conjugate to reactive metabolites spontaneously, but this reaction is usually catalyzed by the glutathione-S-transferases [18]. The resultant conjugates are generally nonreactive and readily excreted into bile or urine. GSH conjugates are pumped from the liver cell into bile by transporters, principally multidrug resistance-associated protein 2 (MRP2) (Fig. 28.2).

There are three families of glutathione transferases (GSTs): cytosolic, mitochondrial, and microsomal. The cytosolic GSTs are those most involved in drug metabolism and are divided into seven classes, designated alpha, mu, pi, sigma, theta, omega, and theta [19, 20]. Each class has several members designated by arabic numbers. For example, GSTM1 is the first of five members of the mu gene family.

The important role of GSH conjugation has led to the development of sophisticated methods to detect GSH conjugates in liver microsomes and whole animals [21]. The production of GSH conjugates from a drug generally means that reactive metabolites have been formed. However, in whole-animal studies, GSH conjugates may be undetectable if they enter bile and are eliminated in stool, or broken down by intestinal bacteria. In addition, not all reactive metabolites depend on GSH for safe elimination. One important class of reactive metabolites is the epoxides, which can be safely eliminated through the action of microsomal epoxide hydrolase [22]. In addition to functioning in the catalysis of detoxification reactions, it has recently been appreciated that GSTs and epoxide hydrolases play a role in intracellular signaling that may be linked to cell death pathways [23,24].

How reactive metabolites cause hepatotoxicity

There appear to be many potential ways in which toxic metabolites can injure hepatocytes, but the most common mechanisms appear to involve oxidative stress and covalent binding.

Table 28.1 Some characteristics of the main human liver P450s.

P450	Substrates	Inhibitors	Inducers
CYP1A2	Tacrine Theophylline Tolcapone[a] [135] Dihydralazine[a] [136] Flutamide[a] [137]	Fluvoxamine	Cigarette smoke Charcoal broiled foods Omeprazole
CYP2A6	Halothane[a] [138] Nicotine	8-Methoxy psoralen	None known
CYP2B6	Bupropion Carbamazepine[a] [139] Ticlopidine	None known	rif, phen, carb, pheno, SJW
CYP2C8	Paclitaxel Rosiglitazone	None known	rif, phen, carb, pheno, SJW
CYP2C9	Diclofenac[a] [140] Warfarin Tienilic acid[a] [141] Phenytoin Valproate	Fluvoxamine	rif, phen, carb, pheno, SJW
CYP2C19	Omeprazole Mephenytoin Diazepam Phenytoin[a] [142] Flutamide[a] [143]	Sulfinpyrazone Ticlopidine Fluvoxamine	rif, phen, carb, pheno, SJW
CYP2D6	Debrisoquine Metoprolol and other ß-blockers Amitriptyline and other neuroleptics Codeine Chlorpromazine[a] [144] Thioridazine[a] [144]	Fluoxetine and other SSRIs Quinidine	None identified
CYP2E1	Acetaminophen[a] [145] Ethanol Tolcapone[a] [135] Isoniazid[a] [146] Halothane [138]	Disulfram Ethanol	Ethanol Isoniazid
CYP3A4	Erythromycin Cyclosporine A Carbamazepine[a] [139] Midazolam/triazolam Lovastatin and other statins Saquinavir and other protease inhibitors Trazodone[a] [147] Nefazodone[a] [148] Troglitazone[a] [149] Nevirapine[a] [150]	Ketoconazole and other azoles Troleandomycin Rotinavir	rif, phen, carb, pheno, SJW

[a]Drugs metabolized to reactive metabolites that are implicated in hepatotoxicity.
carb, carbamazepine; rif, rifampin; phen, phenytoin, phenol, phenobarbital; SJW, Saint John's wort; SSRI, selective serotonin reuptake inhibitor.

Oxidative stress

The liver is the largest solid organ in the body, and its numerous metabolic functions require substantial energy. Energy is largely provided by adenosine triphosphate (ATP), which is derived from the reduction of molecular oxygen to water in mitochondria through a process termed oxidative phosphorylation. In the process of generating ATP and water, up to 5% of oxygen is converted to superoxide anion (O_2^-) and its metabolites, which are collectively termed reactive oxygen species (ROS).

ROS can also be produced outside of the mitochondria as a by-product of metabolism by cytochromes P450, particularly CYP2E1 [25] and CYP3A4 [26]. ROS can alter normal physiologic functions in the hepatocyte by reacting with proteins, DNA, or lipids [27–29]. For example, ROS can initiate lipid peroxidation. This is a self-propagating chain reaction whereby unsaturated fatty acids of membranes are broken down to volatile small molecules (such as F2-isoprostanes) that can be measured in breath [30,31].

ROS usually do not accumulate in hepatocytes because there exist multiple mechanisms for their deactivation to less harmful species, including reactions catalyzed by glutathione peroxidase, superoxide dismutase (SOD), and catalase. Moreover, as ROS deplete protective mechanisms, the cell mounts a coordinated "antioxidant response." This involves activation of NF E2 related factor (NFR2), which mediates transcriptional activation of a cassette of genes that include those coding for GSH synthesis, GSTs, and certain uridine diphosphate glucuronosyltransferases (UGTs) [31].

The term "oxidative stress" has traditionally been used for the situation where the production of ROS exceeds the capabilities of antioxidant defenses, resulting in an accumulation of ROS [27]. However, it has recently become clear that in addition to the direct damaging effects of ROS through oxidation of proteins, lipids, and DNA, ROS can alter cell signaling pathways leading to cell death through either apoptosis or necrosis. For example, depletion of GSH, which occurs as a result of ROS, has been shown to sensitize hepatocytes to the injurious effects of certain cytokines, probably by inhibiting the transcription nuclear factor κB (NF-κB) [32]. ROS have also been shown to activate the transcription factor c-jun N-terminal kinase (JNK), which can result in activation of cell death pathways. It has therefore been proposed that the term "oxidative stress" be defined by these and related alterations in cell signaling typically but not exclusively observed in states of ROS accumulation [33].

Covalent binding

A variety of experimental evidence supports the view that covalent binding of reactive metabolites to proteins can alter their function, contributing to or causing hep-

atotoxicity [3,34–36]. For example, the location of covalently bound protein adducts within the acinus correlates well with the location of hepatocyte damage due to acetaminophen [37] and cocaine [38]. In addition, experimental manipulations that increase or decrease the rate of covalent binding (such as treatment with inducers or inhibitors of specific P450s) proportionately increase or decrease the sensitivity of the liver to toxicity [38–40]. However, the simple magnitude of covalent binding produced by a drug does not accurately predict hepatotoxicity [15,34]. For example, there exist structural analogs of acetaminophen that have relatively little hepatotoxic potential, but nonetheless covalently bind to hepatic proteins at rates comparable to, or actually higher than, observed with acetaminophen [41]. In addition, under certain experimental conditions, hepatocyte injury produced by cocaine can be prevented without influencing the extent of covalent binding to hepatocyte proteins [42]. It has therefore become clear that covalent binding to protein does not always result in toxicity. Indeed, covalent binding may in some instances represent an adaptive mechanism for the hepatocyte. For example, it has been speculated that certain cytosolic proteins identified as targets for acetaminophen covalent binding may function to protect the cell by inactivating reactive metabolites [43].

In view of the discrepancies between total covalent binding and toxicity, the idea has emerged that toxicity is caused by covalent binding to specific proteins critical to cell viability [44]. During acetaminophen hepatotoxicity, multiple enzymes important to the hepatocyte undergo covalent modification that results in the loss of catalytic activity [36]. The identity of specific proteins targeted by a given metabolite probably reflects several factors. First, if the metabolite is extremely reactive, it is likely to be very short lived; hence, binding can only occur to proteins that are located in close proximity to the enzyme that produced the metabolite. The closest protein to the metabolite when it is created is the enzyme that produced it. Hence, when a specific P450 is identified as the target for covalent binding, it is likely that this is the enzyme responsible for the generation of the reactive metabolite [45]. If the implicated metabolite is less reactive and longer lived, it may diffuse from the site where it was formed to bind to more distant proteins. Which specific proteins are affected also reflects the chemical nature of the metabolite and target protein. Acetaminophen, and the structurally similar but not hepatotoxic compound 3'-hydroxyacetanilide, produce comparable amounts of total covalent binding in the liver [41]. However, covalent binding with acetaminophen occurs largely in mitochondria, whereas AMAP forms adducts predominantly in other cellular compartments [46]. Specific binding to critical mitochondrial proteins may therefore account for the differences in hepatotoxic potential of acetaminophen and AMAP. On the other hand, the selective binding to mitochondrial proteins may simply indicate that the reactive metabolite reached the mitochondria where it might initiate other processes responsible for toxicity.

Role of mitochondria as a target for drug-induced liver injury

The mitochondria are the cell's major source of energy by creating ATP. With complete loss of functioning mitochondria, the ATP-dependent sodium and potassium ion pumps at the plasma membrane cease to function, and the hepatocyte swells and ruptures in the process known as necrosis. Programmed cell death, or apoptosis, requires energy and therefore some functioning mitochondria are required. There is increasing evidence that mitochondria are critical targets during DILI and other types of adverse reactions to drugs [33,47,48].

As discussed above, loss of mitochondrial function could result from covalent binding of a reactive metabolite to key proteins involved in several critical processes. In addition, reactive metabolites could cause toxicity by damaging mitochondrial DNA [49]. Most mitochondrial proteins are encoded by genes present in the cell nucleus, however some vital mitochondrial proteins involved in oxidative phosphorylation are the products of genes contained within the mitochondria. Mitochondria are relatively deficient in DNA repair enzymes, and hence DNA mutations caused by reactive metabolites (or resulting from oxidative stress) can accumulate over time. For example, some antiviral drugs (fialuridine (FIAU) and azidothymidine (AZT) for example) are believed to have caused liver failure due to gradually accumulating mutations in mitochondrial genes [50,51].

Mitochondrial dysfunction can also occur as a consequence of depletion of mitochondrial glutathione [33,52]. Mitochondria are particularly susceptible to GSH depletion because they do not synthesize GSH and must import it from the cytosol. Mitochondria also lack catalase, and therefore place greater reliance on glutathione peroxidase to handle ROS. The activity of glutatione peroxidase activity is critically dependent on the concentration of GSH within the mitochondria, with a rapid fall in activity as GSH concentrations (usually 10–15 mM) fall below 2–3 mM. Greater than 90% depletion of mitochondrial GSH therefore significantly impairs the mitochondria's ability to safely dispose of ROS. Because ROS are constantly produced in mitochondria, even in totally healthy hepatocytes, depletion of mitochondrial GSH by reactive metabolites may be sufficient to cause hepatocyte injury and death through oxidative stress.

Mitochondria also play a central role in the initiation of apoptosis. It has been theorized that mitochondria evolved from a primitive bacterium that, when the earth's oxygen atmosphere began to emerge, entered and became part of early eukaryotic cells [53]. A bacterial origin would also account for why mitochondria have their own set of genes. According to the theory, the relationship between the bacterium and the eukaryotic cell was symbiotic. The bacterium's rudimentary machinery for oxidative phosphorylation provided the eukaryote with a means for survival in what would have otherwise been a toxic environment. The bacterium also benefited in most instances from the controlled environment afforded by the host cell. It has been further theorized that, in case the relationship ceased to be symbiotic, the bacterium retained or developed the ability to kill the cell and thereby "go it alone" [54]. According to this theory, as the bacteria evolved to become permanent residents in cells (i.e., mitochondria), these death mechanisms remained.

The mechanisms whereby mitochondria initiate apoptosis have been largely clarified. The critical event appears to be depolarization of the inner membrane of the mitochondria, termed mitochondrial permeability transition (MTP), that results from opening of pores in the inner membrane [55,56]. MTP results in a loss of the proton gradient required for the generation of ATP. If MTP occurs in all or most mitochondria there will be insufficient ATP generation to sustain vital physiologic functions. However, a further effect of MTP pore opening is swelling of the mitochondria and eventual rupture of the outer mitochondrial membrane. When the mitochondria ruptures, cytochrome c is released into the cytosol, causing activation of certain caspases that initiate apoptosis. Evidence suggests that MTP may be a common pathway for hepatocyte apoptosis resulting from diverse signals that may be involved in some forms of hepatotoxicity, including ligand binding to plasma membrane death receptors (FAS and tumor necrosis factor receptor (TNFr)), release of calcium from the endoplasmic reticulum, and release of lysosomal enzymes [56,57]. Apoptosis requires ATP, so the energy status of the hepatotocyte (i.e., how many mitochondria remain functional) appears to determine whether death will be by apoptosis or necrosis. Features of both necrosis and apoptosis can be present in a dying hepatocyte, termed "necrapoptosis" [58,59].

Progression versus recovery

Once liver injury has begun, it can either progress to liver failure or can subside with recovery (see Fig. 28.1). It was originally assumed that the critical variable here was how much damage was done by the reactive metabolite, such as the extent of critical covalent binding or extent of oxidative stress. Although this is clearly an important variable, it has recently become clear that there are many factors that can influence the outcome that are "down stream" of the events discussed so far. These factors can both reverse toxicity or accelerate the death of injured or dying hepatocytes or even cause the death of healthy hepatocytes.

One factor that limits the progression of liver injury is increased tolerance to the hepatotoxin. For example, it has been shown that mice recurrently exposed to certain halogenated hydrocarbons develop hepatic necrosis after 1 week of treatment, but the liver injury can largely resolve despite continued exposure (Fig. 28.3) [60]. This indicates that the liver has the ability to reverse even severe hepatotoxicity through a process termed adaptation. Adaptation may account for why therapeutic dosing of acetaminophen is generally safe despite the fact that it

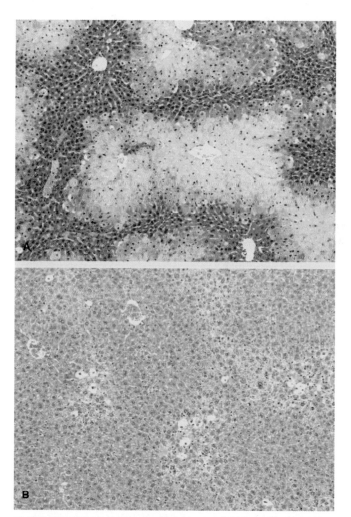

Figure 28.3 Adaptation to direct hepatotoxicity. Mice were exposed to recurrent doses of bromodichloromethane. (A) At 1 week, pericentral necrosis was observed in the mice. (B) Those that survived this initial injury had substantial recovery with absence of liver necrosis at 3 weeks, despite continued exposure to the toxicant. This is a dramatic example of the ability of the liver to adapt to hepatotoxins, which may reflect alterations in the expression of drug-metabolizing enzymes, transporters, or components of the innate immune response. (Reproduced from Torti et al. [60] with permission from Oxford University Press.)

causes alanine aminotransferase (ALT) elevations exceeding three times the upper limits of normal in one third of healthy adults [61]. It has also been shown that rats given gradually increasing doses of acetaminophen can develop complete tolerance to doses that would cause severe toxicity to treatment naïve rats [62]. This progressive tolerance also appears to occur in man; there has been one report of a narcotic/acetaminophen abuser who claimed to consume up to 65 g of acetaminophen daily yet had no clinical evidence of significant liver injury [62].

Adaptation to hepatotoxicity can involve an altered regulation of genes involved in determining reactive metabolite accumulation. For example, when rodents are exposed to increasing doses of acetaminophen there is downregulation of the P450s involved in producing the reactive metabolite (N-acetyl-p-benzoquinone imine (NAPQI)) and an increase in hepatocyte GSH content [62]. In addition, it has been shown that during the recovery phase of acute exposure to acetaminophen or carbon tetrachloride, there is downregulation of certain basolateral uptake transporters (Na(+)-taurocholate cotransporting polypeptide (NTCP) and several organic anionic transporting polypeptides (OATPs)) and upregulation of basolateral and canalicular efflux transporters (including MRP3, MRP4, and MRP2) [63–66]. This appears to protect the cell by *preventing uptake* and *accelerating removal* of xenobiotics and potentially toxic bile acids. These effects could result from a combination of the antioxidant response and the acute phase reaction chiefly mediated by Nrf-2 activation and interleukin 6 (IL6), respectively [67,68]. In addition, regenerating (young) hepatocytes have reduced P450 activity and increased GSH levels and should therefore be less prone to toxic injury [69]. These mechanisms for adapatation are likely to be operative in patients. One human study demonstrated that after subfulminant liver injury, the regenerative hepatocytes contained increased levels of several transporters, including the major multidrug resistence transporter 1 (MDR1) [70].

Other factors that can determine progression or regression of injury involve mediators of inflammation controlled by the innate immune system [71]. The innate immune response, unlike the adaptive immune response, is not antigen-specific, has no memory, and can be immediately activated by pathogens. It is the coordinated and rapid release of certain cytokines and other biologic mediators that neutralize pathogens and, together with natural killer T cells and tissue macrophages, kill infected cells. Mechanisms involved in activation of the innate immune system in response to bacteria have been extensively studied. Various components of bacteria and viruses, termed pathogen-associated molecular patterns or PAMPs, activate toll-like receptors (TLRs) on mammalian cells that upregulate expression of pro-IL1β [72]. Pro-IL1β is not active until cleaved by caspase 1, which is expressed when mammalian cells are injured or dying. Products of dying cells, termed damage-associated molecular patterns or DAMPs, activate receptor complexes termed inflammasomes, resulting in transcription of caspase 1 [73]. This two-step process makes sense since it permits the detection of pathogen infection anywhere the blood circulation may take the PAMPs but then focuses the inflammatory response where tissue damage is occurring. A recent finding is that DNA fragments resulting from hepatocyte necrosis can both activate TLRs and a certain inflammasome, resulting in the production of both IL-1β and caspase 1 [74]. Hence toxicity resulting in hepatocyte necrosis appears to be sufficient to activate a full innate immune attack on the liver.

The innate immune response is beneficial if it limits the spread of infection by killing and disposing of infected cells and pathogens. However, promotion of hepatocyte death by an innate immune response is not beneficial in the setting of toxic injury. Hence, it is not surprising that the elimination of various components of an innate immune response can reduce the degree of liver necrosis in response to acetaminophen [75,76]. Examples of components of the innate immune response that increase susceptibility to acetaminophen hepatotoxicity include interferon γ [77], macrophage inhibitory factor (MIF) [78], and tumor necrosis factor (TNF) [79]. However, the situation is complex since the loss of CD44, a lymphocyte surface protein involved in trafficking into tissues, appears to increase susceptibility to acetaminophen hepatotoxicity in both rodents and humans [80]. In addition, some cytokines reduce susceptibility to acetaminophen hepatotoxicity [81,82]. Whether an injury progresses or resolves may therefore depend on the balance of pro- and anti-inflammatory cytokines released in the liver; the factors that determine this balance during an episode of hepatotoxicity remain unclear.

The ability to downregulate the innate immune response may be particularly important in the liver [74, 75,83,84]. During evolution, some degree of hepatotoxicity probably occurred as a result of dietary consumption of naturally occurring hepatotoxic substances, such as natural insecticides made by plants, or fungal and bacterial products resulting from food spoilage. A reasonable hypothesis is that factors counteracting the innate immune response evolved in the liver to limit needless liver inflammation and hepatocyte injury as a result of recurrent encounters with these hepatotoxins.

It should be noted that most cytokines are produced in the liver by Kupffer cells and, during an innate immune response, other types of macrophages that are recruited to the liver. One study has suggested that the activation of inflammasones by DAMPs occurs in the sinusoidal endothelial cells [74]. This points out the potential limitations of studying hepatotoxicity mechanisms in isolated hepatocytes and emphasizes the need for more complex culture systems.

Other issues that may determine whether liver injury progresses or regresses have been identified. Soluble factors released from dying hepatocytes (such as calpain [85, 86]) may kill adjacent healthy hepatotcytes. In addition, it has been shown that liver injury caused by one predictable toxin can be "amplified" by pretreatments that hinder the liver's ability to regenerate [87].

Variation in susceptibility to predictable hepatotoxicity

Increased susceptibility to predictable hepatotoxicity could occur from any of the conditions outlined in Box 28.1. For example, some drugs either inhibit or increase (induce) the activity of certain drug-metabolizing enymes (see Table 28.1) and transporters. If safe pathways are induced or bioactivation pathways are inhibited, there should be less toxicity at a given dose of hepatotoxin. Alternatively, if safe pathways are inhibited and bioactivation pathways are induced, susceptiblity to toxicity should increase. However, the induction of metabolic pathways usually involves the activation of transcription factors that result in the transcription of multiple genes [88]. The deleterious effects of induction of the bioactivation pathway may therefore be offset by the simultaneous induction of safe elimination. An example where variation in susceptibility to toxicity can result from nongenetic factors is acetaminophen hepatotoxicity.

Increased susceptibility to acetaminophen hepatotoxicity

Chronic consumption of ethanol appears to increase susceptibility to acetaminophen hepatotoxicity [89]. Chronic ethanol consumption can increase CYP2E1 activity (see Table 28.1), and this provides an attractive explanation for incremental risks in ethanol consumers. However, early animal [90,91] and human [92] studies did not show increases in NAPQI formation when acetaminophen was given during or immediately after ingestion of ethanol. Indeed, these studies suggested that ethanol consumption actually reduces the rate of production of NAPQI, protecting the liver from toxicity. This is explained by the observation that the induction of CYP2E1 that occurs involves stabilization of the enzyme (reduced degradation), and that this occurs when ethanol is bound to the enzyme as substrate [93,94]. Prolonged intoxication therefore results in an accumulation of CYP2E1, but the enzyme activity is reduced because the induced CYP2E1 is inhibited by ethanol (Fig. 28.4). When ingestion is stopped, and ethanol is cleared from the liver, the accumulated CYP2E1

Box 28.1 Some potential reasons for increased susceptibility to predictable hepatotoxicity.

Decreased activity of safe elimination pathways
- Genetic: polymorphisms in phase 1 and 2 enzymes or transporters
- Nongenetic: drug interactions involving enzyme/transporter inhibition, nutrition, and inflammation

Increased activity of enzymes making reactive metabolites
- Genetic: gene duplication (CYP2D6)
- Nongenetic: induction of P450s

Reduced elimination of reactive metabolites
- Genetic: polymorphisms in elimination enzymes (e.g., glutathione transferases, epoxid hydrolase) or transporters (e.g., MRP2)
- Nongenetic: drug interactions involving enzyme/transporter inhibition, inflammation nutrition, and cofactor depletion (e.g., glutathione)

Variation in proteins and pathways targeted by reactive pathways
- Genetic: polymorphisms in proteins involved in target pathways (e.g., inherited defects in oxidative phosphorylation proteins)
- Nongenetic: drug effects (e.g., aspirin inhibition of oxidative phosphorylation), nutrition, and concomitant disease

Variation in the innate immune response
- Genetic: polymorphisms in cytokines and proteins involved in Kuppfer cells and lymphocyte function
- Nongenetic: inflammation and nutrition

Variation in ability to regenerate hepatocytes
- Genetic: polymorphisms in genes important in regeneration
- Nongenetic: effects of other drugs/xenobiotics, age, nutrition, and inflammation

Variation in ability to adapt to toxicity
- Genetic: polymorphisms in enzymes and transporters and proteins involved in their regulation or in innate immune response elements
- Nongenetic: effects of other drugs/xenobiotics, age, nutrition, and inflammation

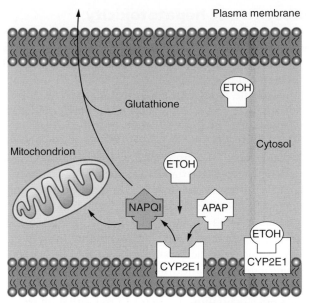

Figure 28.4 Effect of ethanol on acetaminophen toxicity. Acetaminophen is converted by cytochrome P450 2E1 (CYP2E1) to the reactive metabolite N-acetyl-p-benzoquinone imine (NAPQI), which then conjugates to glutathione and are safely excreted. If the production of NAPQI is rapid enough to deplete available cytosolic glutathione stores, NAPQI travels to mitochondria where it covalently binds to critical proteins and depletes mitchondrial glutathione, resulting in oxidative stress. Ethanol binds tightly to the substrate-binding site of CYP2E1, preventing acetaminophen from being metabolized to NAPQI. This accounts for the observation that acutely intoxicated rodents produce less NAPQI and are resistant to acetaminophen toxicity. However, the intracellular half-life of CYP2E1 is prolonged when bound to ethanol, so the enzyme accumulates in an inactive form during intoxication. When ethanol consumption ceases and ethanol is removed from the liver, the accumulated CYP2E1 becomes fully active and the rate of NAPQI formation increases until the CYP2E1 levels return to baseline (probably not more than 24 hours). This effect is very modest in social drinkers but can become significant when very large amounts of ethanol are consumed for prolonged periods. APAP, acetaminophen; ETOH, ethyl alcohol. (Reproduced from Thummel et al. [94] with permission from Nature.)

is no longer inhibited, and the aggregate CYP2E1 activity is increased above baseline levels [94]. However, stabilization against degradation is also reversed, resulting in a relatively rapid fall of enzyme activity to the preethanol exposure level. This results in a narrow window of susceptibility that probably lasts less than 24 hours [94]. This effect of inhibition followed by transient induction is also mimicked by some other substrates of CYP2E1, including isoniazid [95]. This may account for reports of enhanced susceptiblity to acetaminophen toxicity in patients treated with isoniazid [95,96].

Chronic alcoholics are also likely to have reduced hepatocyte concentrations of GSH, particularly mitochondrial GSH [97], limiting their ability to safely eliminate NAPQI once formed.

Another clinical situation that appears to increase susceptibility to acetaminophen toxicity is fasting [98]. This should result in reduced GSH levels, but should also cause depletion of the glucose available to make the UGT cofactor glucuronic acid, reducing the ability for safe elimination of acetaminophen by glucuronidation. It has also been proposed that liver hypoxia due to cardiopulmonary insufficiency can increase susceptibility to acetaminophen toxicity due to reduced glucuronidation capacity [99]. Patients with Gilbert syndrome have a reduced activity of the form of UGT that conjugates bilirubin (UGT1A1) and it has been reported that these patients may have increased susceptibility to acetaminophen toxicity. However, this seems unlikely since the major UGT involved in conjugation of acetaminophen is not UGT1A1.

Idiosyncratic hepatotoxicity

Understanding of the processes involved in the production of liver toxicity from reactive metabolites has greatly improved our understanding of variation in susceptibility to predictable liver toxins, particularly acetaminophen. Evidence that the mechanisms underlying predictable hepatotoxicity are also important in idiosyncratic hepatotoxicity has come from genetic studies. Susceptibility to idiosyncratic DILI from various drugs has been associated with genetic variation that leads to a reduced or increased function of transport proteins or in enzymes involved in bioactivation and detoxification [100]. This suggests that the mechanisms shown in Fig. 28.1 are relevant to understanding idiosyncratic toxicity. The rarity of idiosyncratic hepatotoxicity could be explained by interpatient variation in the multiple metabolic and transport functions as well as multiple mechanisms that may underlie a failure to adapt to the initial injury. The rarity of susceptible individuals could be explained if multiple susceptibility factors were required to manifest the toxicity.

One feature of idiosyncratic hepatotoxicity that is difficult to explain based on the mechanisms shown in Fig. 28.1 is the prolonged latency characteristic for this type of injury. Two theories have been proposed that directly link mechanisms of predictable toxicity to this latency. The first proposes that toxicity is initiated by a coincident episode of inflammation and the second proposes a cumulative, clinically occult injury.

Inflammatory stress hypothesis

It has been shown that rats or mice treated with a nonhepatotoxic dose of an inflammagen such as lipopolysaccharide (LPS) become susceptible to liver injury when treated with several drugs capable of causing idiosyncratic hepatotoxicity, including diclofenac and sulindac [101,102]. These observations support the idea that idiosyncratic hepatotoxicity might result from the same mechanisms as predictable hepatotoxicity (see Fig. 28.1), but that the threshold for hepatocyte injury is lowered by a concurrent mild infection, or occasional leak of bacterial products from the intestine [103]. The mechanisms whereby mild inflammation could initiate DILI are not clear, but this phenomenon has been reproduced in cultured human hepatocytes [104]. Certain cytokines released during inflammation alter the intracellular signaling pathways, and this can have many consequences, including a substantial alteration in expression of various liver enzymes and transporters [105]. Such sudden alterations could result in the increased production of a toxic metabolite initiating injury or could reduce the liver's ability to adapt to the injury. Also, partial activation of the innate immune system could result in an exaggerated injury where adaptation might otherwise have occurred.

Clinical support for the inflammation hypothesis is sparce, however. Although chronic hepatitis B may predispose patients to idiosyncratic hepatotoxicity from antituberculosis drugs [106], there are no data to suggest that the injuries occur with shorter latency in these patients. In addition, many drugs causing idiosyncratic hepatotoxicity display a characteristic latency interval that would be difficult to ascribe to random inflammatory events.

Progressive injury hypothesis

According to this hypothesis, injury to the hepatocyte begins soon after the start of drug dosing in susceptible individuals, but does not become clinically manifest until weeks or months later. This is easiest to understand with mitochondrial injuries, such as the depletion of mitochondrial DNA, which could gradually reduce the number of functioning mitochondria. There may be no clinical consequences apparent until mitochondrial function falls below a critical level. As hepatocytes begin to die, this would place more metabolic demand on the remaining but already compromised hepatocytes. This could result in what appears to be a sudden onset of severe liver injury after a prolonged latency. Support for the progressive injury hypothesis has come from a mouse model deficient in superoxide dismutase, an enzyme important in reducing oxidative stress in mitochondria. These mice are phenotypically normal but develop a delayed hepatotoxicity when treated with some drugs capable of idiosyncratic hepatotoxicity in man [107]. In addition, recent evidence supports the idea that genetic deficiency in SOD may increase susceptibility to idiosyncratic hepatotoxicity from multiple different drugs in patients [108].

Adaptive immune response

It is generally accepted that adaptive (as opposed to innate) immune mechanisms underlie the liver injury produced by some drugs. For example, liver injury due to halothane, phenytoin, and sulfonamides characteristically present with fever, rash, and eosinophilia – the classic clinical hallmarks of hypersensitivity [109]. This type of liver injury characteristically occurs within the first month of starting therapy with the drug, similar to the time required to become fully immunized to a vaccine. Reexposure after an episode of toxicity generally results in more rapid onset of the toxicity and greater severity of the injury, as would be expected with a hypersensitivity reaction.

There is also increasing evidence that adaptive immune mechanisms may be involved in idiosyncratic hepatotoxicity, even in the absence of clinical signs of hypersensitivity. For example, methyldopa-induced liver injury is not usually associated with peripheral eosinophilia, fever, or rash, but recurs promptly and may be more severe upon rechallenge, consistent with an immune mechanism [110]. Tacrine-induced liver disease also has no hypersensitivity features [111] yet recurs promptly upon rechallenge, consistent with an immunologic mechanism. The idea that the adaptive immune system is involved in many forms of hepatotoxicity is also supported by lymphocyte proliferation studies. These studies are performed by isolating peripheral blood lymphocytes from patients who have experienced hepatotoxicity, and determining whether a subpopulation of the T lymphocytes proliferate upon exposure to the implicated drugs. A proliferative response implies that the drug has stimulated an adaptive, cell-mediated immunity. The test is often positive in adverse drug reactions resulting from hypersensitivity, but in one study [112], 56% of 95 patients with liver injury to diverse drugs demonstrated lymphocyte proliferation in response to exposure to the implicated drug. In contrast, proliferation was not observed in any of 35 control individuals who had been exposed to the same drugs without evidence of liver toxicity. In 70% of the patients with a positive test, there were no clinical signs suggestive of hypersensitivity. Although observations with lymphocyte transformation support a role for an adaptive immune response in DILI, these studies alone would also be consistent with an adaptive immune response as a result of, not the cause of, the liver injury.

The most convincing data to support a role for the acquired immune system in idiosyncratic DILI has come from genetic studies in patients who have experienced idiosyncratic DILI. Table 28.2 lists some identified associations between DILI susceptibility and human leukocyte antigens (HLAs), also called the major histocompatibility complex (MHC) antigens. These are proteins on the surface of certain cells (antigen-presenting cells) that hold and present antigens to the helper T cells. In the case of drugs, it has been assumed that the antigen is the reactive metabolite covalently bound to a liver protein. It should be noted that the HLA risk alleles listed in Table 28.2 are quite common in the population so only a small subpopulation of individuals with these risk alleles will develop DILI when treated with the listed drug. Some

of the associations observed are very strong. For example, a person with the HLA-B*5701 allele is 80-fold more likely to develop DILI after treatment with the antibiotic flucloxacillin. This has suggested that HLA genotyping might be useful in screening patients for susceptibility prior to treatment with certain drugs, or using HLA genotyping to aid in the diagnosis of DILI due to certain drugs.

The immune system will not generally attack healthy cells just because they contain new antigens on their surface. As with the innate immune response, a second signal is necessary to mount an adaptive immune response. This "danger signal" was first proposed by Matzinger [113] and is consistent with the observation that vaccines only work when given with adjuvants that cause tissue injury at the site of injection. It appears that the DAMPs resulting from tissue injury (that mediate the second signal required for an innate immune response) also are capable of mediating the second signal required for the acquire immune response [114].

The involvement of an acquired immune response could account for the characteristic latency of idiosyncratic DILI and also provides another important locus for interpatient variation to account for the rarity of these events. A unified theory would be that an individual who develops idiosyncratic DILI would have to have the appropriate factors (see Box 28.1) to create sufficient amounts of a reactive metabolite to cause hepatocyte injury, to trigger an innate immune response, and to release DAMPs to provide the "danger signal." In addition, the individual must have a susceptibility HLA allele or adapation and resolution of injury will occur. Consistent with this hypothesis, susceptibility to DILI from ticlopidine has been recently associated with a polymorphism in CYP2B6 as well as with HLA-A*3303 [115]. In addition, susceptibility to flucloxacillin-induced liver injury has been associated with a polymorphism in the region of the pregnene X nuclear receptor (PXR) that activates transcription of a variety of drug-metabolizing enzymes and drug transporters [116]. This hypothesis would also explain why drugs that cause serious idiosyncratic DILI usually also cause much more frequent elevations in serum aminotransferases in clinical trials, and why the

Table 28.2 Some HLA associations with susceptibility to drug-induced liver injury.

Drug	Prevalence	Risk allele	Frequency	Relative risk	Reference
Augmentin	<0.001	HLA-DRB1*1501	0.15	4	Holden 2010 [154]
Flucloxacillin	<0.001	HLA-B*5701	0.04	81	Daly et al. 2009 [156]
Lapatinib	0.09	HLA-DRB1*0701	0.08	9	Spraggs 2010 [152]
Lumiracoxib	0.013	HLA-DRB1*1501	0.15	13	Singer et al. 2010 [153]
Ticlopidine	<0.001	HLA-A*3303	0.07	36	Hirata et al. 2008 [155]
Ximelagatran	0.08	HLA-DRB1*0701	0.08	4	Kindmark et al. 2008 [151]

episodes of severe DILI tend to occur with a latency characteristic of the transient ALT elevations [117]. For example, the anticoagulant ximelagatran was withdrawn from worldwide markets because of severe DILI, including liver failure. In clinical trials, about 10% of patients treated with ximelagatran developed ALT elevations that characteristically occurred between 1 and 6 months of treatment [118]. In most cases, the ALT elevations were transient, but rare cases of severe and fatal liver injury have been reported. In most instances, these severe events occurred within the latency period for ALT elevations, consistent with the idea that patients with severe injury arise out of the group with milder and transient liver injuries.

It should be noted that although an adaptive immune response to predictable liver injury is an attractive hypothesis to explain idiosyncratic hepatotoxicity, two observations do not support it. If the above hypothesis was correct, we would expect the initial liver injury to occur soon after starting treatment, but ALT elevations are characteristically delayed in clinical trials with drugs capable of causing idiosyncratic DILI. In addition, HLA allele associations should only be found with severe liver injuries and not with milder reversible ALT elevations. However, in the cases examined to date, the HLA associations exist with the minor ALT elevations as well as with the more severe liver injuries.

Hepatotoxicity not related to reactive metabolites

Although it is generally believed that reactive metabolites are the initiating events in most forms of DILI, this is not always the case. For example, ximelagatran has never been demonstrated to have reactive metabolites [114]. In some cases, the parent drug may directly interfere with crucial hepatocyte functions, resulting in toxicity. One example of this is interference with the homeostasis of bile acids, some of which can be toxic to cells, particularly to mitochondria [119]. The concentration of bile acids within the hepatocyte is governed by the rates of synthesis, uptake, and efflux of bile acids, which are usually tightly regulated. If a drug interferes with this homeostasis, toxicity could result. For example, it has been demonstrated that troglitazone and bosentan inhibit bile salt excretory protein (BSEP) (see Fig. 28.2) and this may contribute to the hepatoxicity observed with these drugs [120–123]. Glyburide has also been shown to inhibit BSEP, and this may explain why patients taking this drug appear to be at higher risk of developing liver toxicity from bosentan [123]. An interesting observation is that bosentan does not cause liver toxicity in the rat [120]. This may relate to the observation that whereas bosentan is a potent inhibitor of BSEP in both mouse and man, it is

also a potent inhibitor of NTCP in just the rat [124]. Since NTCP transports bile acids into the hepatocyte, inhibition of both uptake and efflux in the rat may result in little change in hepatocyte concentrations of bile acids.

Pharmaceutical industry and preclinical drug testing

Idiosyncratic hepatotoxicity is the major single organ toxicity that results in abandonment of drug development programs and regulatory actions concerning drugs. Pharmaceutical companies are currently spending many millions of dollars to improve the ways drug candidates are screened for hepatotoxic potential. No consensus has yet been reached and practices vary.

One approach has been to try to "humanize" preclinical testing by using cultured human hepatocytes [125], mice that express human genes relevant to toxicity (such as human P450s and certain nuclear receptors) [126,127], or, recently, mice with stem cell-derived human livers [128]. There are potential problems with each of these approaches. Many important genes stop being expressed in cultured hepatocytes [129] and, as discussed above, cell types other than hepatocytes, such as Kuppfer cells and sinusoidal endothelial cells, may be important missing elements in current cell culture systems. A problem with humanized mice is that we do not yet know which are the relevant human genes to put into the mice. Putting a human liver into a mouse may also not represent a great advance since it is unlikely that the stem cells would be obtained from an individual susceptible to such a rare event as DILI.

Another approach taken is to screen compounds for the ability to form reactive metabolites. The rationale is that if the formation of a reactive metabolite is an essential step in idiosyncratic hepatotoxicity (see Fig. 28.1), understanding the many potential processes that culminate in liver injury are irrelevant if no reactive metabolite is made [21,130,131]. Although the concept of reactive metabolite screening is attractive, it is largely being abandoned in candidate drug selection. One problem is that most drugs generate reactive metabolites to some degree, and some safe drugs would be discarded unnecessarily [132]. For example, acetaminophen causes substantial covalent binding in the liver, as discussed previously. However, acetaminophen is quite safe when taken as directed.

Finally, there has been the broad application of current genomic technology to traditional preclinical toxicity testing [133]. This technology allows simultaneous quantitation of thousands of mRNAs (the "transcriptome"), proteins (the "proteome"), and endogenous metabolites (the "metabolome"). Some companies have treated rats or human hepatocytes with known hepatotoxic and non-toxic drugs and examined time-dependent changes in the liver transcriptome, liver and serum proteome, and liver, serum, and urine metabolome. The goal is to find specific patterns that predict hepatotoxicity potential. Proteome and metabolome analyses have yet to become a standard part of preclinical testing. However, at least several companies have selected a set of mRNA transcripts that appear to correlate with certain forms of hepatotoxicity and are routinely measuring them, along with traditional serologic markers (like ALT) and pathologic evaluation, in the lead candidate selection process. In another recent study [134], florescent probes and automated confocal microscopy was used to assess the effects of a panel of drugs, both safe and those known to cause idiosyncratic DILI, on a variety of physiologic processes in cultured human hepatocytes.

It remains to be determined whether the application of genomic technology to new animal and culture models will reduce the risk of idiosyncratic hepatotoxicity for new drugs currently in the development pipeline.

Conclusions and future directions

The understanding of mechanisms underlying predictable liver toxicity, particularly acetaminophen-induced liver injury, has improved substantially in recent years. There has been identification of mechanisms that determine the extent of initial liver injury, and those involved in the balance between recovery and progression. It seems logical that variation in the activities of the proteins that underlie those mechanisms, which may reflect both genetic and nongenetic factors, will in part account for susceptibility to idiosyncratic hepatotoxicity. The recent finding of HLA allele associations with susceptibility to DILI from certain drugs has provided further support of an acquired immune component to at least some forms of DILI, and have provided plausible explanations for the characteristic latency. The data to date suggest that there are multiple mechanisms that can underlie idiosyncratic hepatotoxicity, and some may be relatively drug or drug class specific. However, it also seems likely that key components of susceptibility that lie in the "downstream" events, such as failure to adapt or progression of injury, may not be molecule specific. Fully elucidating these mechanisms will require studying many people who have actually experienced idiosyncratic hepatotoxicity. The Drug Induced Liver Injury Network, supported by the National Institute for Diabetes, Digestive and Kidney Diseases, and the Severe Adverse Events Consortium supported by the pharmaceutical industry, are creating a registry of such individuals, collecting genomic DNA, and have begun genetic studies. This will undoubtedly remain an exciting area of research.

Annoted references

Jones DP, Lemasters JJ, Han D, Boelsterli UA, Kaplowitz N. Mechanisms of pathogenesis in drug hepatotoxicity putting the stress on mitochondria. *Mol Interv* 2010;10:98–111.
A comprehensive review of the multiple roles that mitochondria are likely to play in drug-induced liver injury.

Roth RA, Ganey PE. Intrinsic versus idiosyncratic drug-induced hepatotoxicity – two villains or one? *J Pharmacol Exp Ther* 2010;332:692–7.
A concise review about the potential role of inflammation and predictable toxicity mechanisms that may underlie idiosyncratic hepatotoxicity.

Stieger B. Role of the bile salt export pump, BSEP, in acquired forms of cholestasis. *Drug Metab Rev* 2010;42:437–45.
A comprehensive review of the role that the major bile salt transport protein, BSEP, plays in drug-induced liver injury.

Uetrecht J. Idiosyncratic drug reactions: past, present, and future. *Chem Res Toxicol* 2008;21:84–92.
An excellent concise review of mechanisms underlying idiosyncratic drug-induced liver injury with an emphasis on the role of the acquired immune system.

Watkins PB, Seeff LB. Drug-induced liver injury: summary of a single topic clinical research conference. *Hepatology* 2006;43:618–31.
This is a series of brief summaries of talks presented at a 2-day symposium on drug-induced liver injury.

References

1. Watkins PB. Idiosyncratic liver injury: challenges and approaches. *Toxicol Pathol* 2005;33(1):1–5.
2. Gillette JR. Keynote address. man, mice, microsomes, metabolites, and mathematics 40 years after the revolution *Drug Metab Rev* 1995;27(1–2):1–44.
3. Srivastava A, Maggs JL, et al. Role of reactive metabolites in drug-induced hepatotoxicity. *Handbook Exp Pharmacol* 2010;196.165–94.
4. Chandra P, Brouwer KL. The complexities of hepatic drug transport: current knowledge and emerging concepts. *Pharm Res* 2004;21(5):719–35.
5. Klaassen CD, Aleksunes LM Xenobiotic, bile acid, and cholesterol transporters: function and regulation. *Pharmacol Rev* 2010;62(1):1–96.
6. Lewis DF, Ito Y. Human CYPs involved in drug metabolism: structures, substrates and binding affinities. *Expert Opin Drug Metab Toxicol* 2010;6(6):661–74.
7. Harper TW, Brassil PJ. Reaction phenotyping: current industry efforts to identify enzymes responsible for metabolizing drug candidates. *AAPS J* 2008;10(1):200–7.
8. Vaz RJ, Zamora I, et al. The challenges of in silico contributions to drug metabolism in lead optimization. *Expert Opin Drug Metab Toxicol* 2010;6(7):851–61.
9. Mackenzie PI, Bock KW, et al. Nomenclature update for the mammalian UDP glycosyltransferase (UGT) gene superfamily. *Pharmacogenet Genomics* 2005;15(10):677–85.
10. Lindsay J, Wang LL, et al. Structure, function and polymorphism of human cytosolic sulfotransferases. *Curr Drug Metab* 2008;9(2):99–105.
11. Trubetskoy O, Finel M, et al. High-throughput screening technologies for drug glucuronidation profiling. *J Pharm Pharmacol* 2008;60(8):1061–7.
12. Gumucio JJ. Hepatocyte heterogeneity: the coming of age from the description of a biological curiosity to a partial understanding of its physiological meaning and regulation. *Hepatology* 1989;9(1):154–60.
13. Watkins P. Role of cytochromes P450 in drug induced liver disease. In: Kaplowitz N, DeLeve LD, eds. *Drug-induced Liver Disease*. New York: Marcel Dekker, 2002.

14. Skonberg C, Olsen J, et al. Metabolic activation of carboxylic acids. *Expert Opin Drug Metab Toxicol* 2008;4(4):425–38.

15. Boelsterli UA. Mechanisms of NSAID-induced hepatotoxicity: focus on nimesulide. *Drug Saf* 2002;25(9):633–48.

16. Cannell GR, Bailey MJ, et al. Inhibition of tubulin assembly and covalent binding to microtubular protein by valproic acid glucuronide in vitro. *Life Sci* 2002;71(22):2633–43.

17. Madsen KG, Skonberg C, et al. Bioactivation of diclofenac in vitro and in vivo: correlation to electrochemical studies. *Chem Res Toxicol* 2008;21(5):1107–19.

18. Rinaldi R, Eliasson E, et al. Reactive intermediates and the dynamics of glutathione transferases. *Drug Metab Dispos* 2002;30(10):1053–8.

19. Hayes JD, Flanagan JU, et al. Glutathione transferases. *Annu Rev Pharmacol Toxicol* 2005;45:51–88.

20. Dourado DF, Fernandes PA, et al. Mammalian cytosolic glutathione transferases. *Curr Protein Pept Sci* 2008;9(4):325–37.

21. Liebler DC, Guengerich FP. Elucidating mechanisms of drug-induced toxicity. *Nat Rev Drug Discov* 2005;4(5):410–20.

22. Morisseau C, Hammock BD. Epoxide hydrolases: mechanisms, inhibitor designs, and biological roles. *Annu Rev Pharmacol Toxicol* 2005;45:311–33.

23. Decker M, Arand M, et al. Mammalian epoxide hydrolases in xenobiotic metabolism and signalling. *Arch Toxicol* 2009;83(4):297–318.

24. Ruzza P, Rosato A, et al. Glutathione transferases as targets for cancer therapy. *Anticancer Agents Med Chem* 2009;9(7):763–77.

25. Sakurai K, Cederbaum AI. Oxidative stress and cytotoxicity induced by ferric-nitrilotriacetate in HepG2 cells that express cytochrome P450 2E1. *Mol Pharmacol* 1998;54(6):1024–35.

26. Puntarulo S, Cederbaum AI. Production of reactive oxygen species by microsomes enriched in specific human cytochrome P450 enzymes. *Free Radical Biol Med* 1998;24(7–8):1324–30.

27. Sies H. Oxidative stress: from basic research to clinical application. *Am J Med* 1991;91(3C):S31–8.

28. Ray SD, Lam TS, et al. Oxidative stress is the master operator of drug and chemically-induced programmed and unprogrammed cell death: implications of natural antioxidants in vivo. *Biofactors* 2004;21(1–4):223–32.

29. Ganeva MG, Getova DP, et al. Adverse drug reactions and reactive oxygen species. *Folia Med (Plovdiv)* 2008;50(1):5–11.

30. Basu S. F2-isoprostanes in human health and diseases: from molecular mechanisms to clinical implications. *Antioxid Redox Signal* 2008;10(8):1405–34.

31. Li W, Kong AN. Molecular mechanisms of Nrf2-mediated antioxidant response. *Mol Carcinog* 2009;48(2):91–104.

32. Lou H, Kaplowitz N. Glutathione depletion down-regulates tumor necrosis factor alpha-induced NF-kappaB activity via IkappaB kinase-dependent and -independent mechanisms. *J Biol Chem* 2007;282(40):29470–81.

33. Jones DP, Lemasters JJ, et al. Mechanisms of pathogenesis in drug hepatotoxicity putting the stress on mitochondria. *Mol Interv* 2010;10(2):98–111.

34. Cohen SD, Pumford NR, et al. Selective protein covalent binding and target organ toxicity. *Toxicol Appl Pharmacol* 1997;143(1):1–12.

35. Pumford NR, Halmes NC, et al. Covalent binding of xenobiotics to specific proteins in the liver. *Drug Metab Rev* 1997;29(1–2):39–57.

36. Park BK, Kitteringham NR, et al. The role of metabolic activation in drug-induced hepatotoxicity. *Annu Rev Pharmacol Toxicol* 2005;45:177–202.

37. Bartolone JB, Cohen SD, et al. Immunohistochemical localization of acetaminophen-bound liver proteins. *Fundam Appl Toxicol* 1989;13(4):859–62.

38. Roth L, Harbison RD, et al. Cocaine hepatotoxicity: influence of hepatic enzyme inducing and inhibiting agents on the site of necrosis. *Hepatology* 1992;15(5):934–40.

39. Mitchell JR, Jollows DJ. Progress in hepatology. Metabolic activation of drugs to toxic substances. *Gastroenterology* 1975;68(2):392–410.

40. Peterson FJ, Knodell RG, et al. Prevention of acetaminophen and cocaine hepatotoxicity in mice by cimetidine treatment. *Gastroenterology* 1983;85(1):122–9.

41. Roberts SA, Price VF, et al. Acetaminophen structure-toxicity studies: in vivo covalent binding of a nonhepatotoxic analog, 3-hydroxyacetanilide. *Toxicol Appl Pharmacol* 1990;105(2):195–208.

42. Goldlin c, Boelsterli UA. Dissociation of covalent protein adduct formation from oxidative injury in cultured hepatocytes exposed to cocaine. *Xenobiotica* 1994;24(3):251–64.

43. Birge RB, Bartolone JB, et al. Acetaminophen hepatotoxicity: correspondence of selective protein arylation in human and mouse liver in vitro, in culture, and in vivo. *Toxicol Appl Pharmacol* 1990;105(3):472–82.

44. Park KB, Dalton-Brown E, et al. Selection of new chemical entities with decreased potential for adverse drug reactions. *Eur J Pharmacol* 2006;549(1–3):1–8.

45. Lopez Garcia MP, Dansette PM, et al. Human–liver cytochromes P-450 expressed in yeast as tools for reactive-metabolite formation studies. Oxidative activation of tienilic acid by cytochromes P-450 2C9 and 2C10. *Eur J Biochem* 1993;213(1):223–32.

46. Tirmenstein MA, Nelson SD. Subcellular binding and effects on calcium homeostasis produced by acetaminophen and a nonhepatotoxic regioisomer, 3'-hydroxyacetanilide, in mouse liver. *J Biol Chem* 1989;264(17):9814–19.

47. Dykens JA, Will Y. The significance of mitochondrial toxicity testing in drug development. *Drug Discov Today* 2007;12(17–18):777–85.

48. Pessayre D, Mansouri A, et al. Mitochondrial involvement in drug-induced liver injury. *Handbook Exp Pharmacol* 2010; (196):311–65.

49. Pessayre D, Mansouri A, et al. Hepatotoxicity due to mitochondrial dysfunction. *Cell Biol Toxicol* 1999;15(6):367–73.

50. Lewis W, Dalakas MC. Mitochondrial toxicity of antiviral drugs. *Nature Med* 1995;1(5):417–22.

51. Nunez M, Soriano V. Hepatotoxicity of antiretrovirals: incidence, mechanisms and management. *Drug Saf* 2005;28(1):53–66.

52. Fernandez-Checa JC, Kaplowitz N. Hepatic mitochondrial glutathione: transport and role in disease and toxicity. *Toxicol Appl Pharmacol* 2005;204(3):263–73.

53. Margulis L. Archaeal–eubacterial mergers in the origin of Eukarya: phylogenetic classification of life. *Proc Natl Acad Sci USA* 1996;93(3):1071–6.

54. Frade JM, Michaelidis TM. Origin of eukaryotic programmed cell death: a consequence of aerobic metabolism? *Bioessays* 1997;19(9):827–32.

55. Kim JS, He L, et al. Role of the mitochondrial permeability transition in apoptotic and necrotic death after ischemia/reperfusion injury to hepatocytes. *Curr Mol Med* 2003;3(6):527–35.

56. Lemasters JJ, Theruvath TP, et al. Mitochondrial calcium and the permeability transition in cell death. *Biochim Biophys Acta* 2009;1787(11):1395–401.

57. Lemasters JJ. Dying a thousand deaths: redundant pathways from different organelles to apoptosis and necrosis. *Gastroenterology* 2005;129(1):351–60.

58. Lemasters JJ. V. Necrapoptosis and the mitochondrial permeability transition: shared pathways to necrosis and apoptosis. *Am J Physiol* 1999;276(1 Pt 1):G1–6.

59. Malhi H, Gores GJ, et al. Apoptosis and necrosis in the liver: a tale of two deaths? *Hepatology* 2006;43(2 Suppl 1):S31–44.

60. Torti VR, Cobb AJ, et al. Nephrotoxicity and hepatotoxicity induced by inhaled bromodichloromethane in wild-type and p53-heterozygous mice. *Toxicol Sci* 2001;64(2):269–80.

61. Watkins PB, Kaplowitz N, et al. Aminotransferase elevations in healthy adults receiving 4 grams of acetaminophen daily: a randomized controlled trial. *JAMA* 2006;296(1):87–93.

62. Shayiq RM, Roberts DW, et al. Repeat exposure to incremental doses of acetaminophen provides protection against acetaminophen-induced lethality in mice: an explanation for high acetaminophen dosage in humans without hepatic injury. *Hepatology* 1999;29(2):451–63.

63. Nakatsukasa H, Silverman JA, et al. Expression of multidrug resistance genes in rat liver during regeneration and after carbon tetrachloride intoxication. *Hepatology* 1993;18(5):1202–7.

64. Geier A, Kim SK, et al. Hepatobiliary organic anion transporters are differentially regulated in acute toxic liver injury induced by carbon tetrachloride. *J Hepatol* 2002;37(2):198–205.

65. Aleksunes LM, Slitt AM, et al. Differential expression of mouse hepatic transporter genes in response to acetaminophen and carbon tetrachloride. *Toxicol Sci* 2005;83(1):44–52.

66. Aleksunes LM, Slitt AL, et al. Induction of Mrp3 and Mrp4 transporters during acetaminophen hepatotoxicity is dependent on Nrf2. *Toxicol Appl Pharmacol* 2008;226(1):74–83.

67. Salminen WF Jr, Voellmy R, et al. Differential heat shock protein induction by acetaminophen and a nonhepatotoxic regioisomer, 3'-hydroxyacetanilide, in mouse liver. *J Pharmacol Exp Ther* 1997;282(3):1533–40.

68. Siewert E, Dietrich CG, et al. Interleukin-6 regulates hepatic transporters during acute-phase response. *Biochem Biophys Res Commun* 2004;322(1):232–8.

69. Roberts E, Ahluwalia MB, et al. Resistance to hepatotoxins acquired by hepatocytes during liver regeneration. *Cancer Res* 1983;43(1):28–34.

70. Ros JE, Libbrecht L, et al. High expression of MDR1, MRP1, and MRP3 in the hepatic progenitor cell compartment and hepatocytes in severe human liver disease. *J Pathol* 2003;200(5):553–60.

71. Tosi MF. Innate immune responses to infection. *J Allergy Clin Immunol* 2005;116(2):241–9, quiz 250.

72. Mogensen TH. Pathogen recognition and inflammatory signaling in innate immune defenses. *Clin Microbiol Rev* 2009;22(2):240–73.

73. Bianchi ME. DAMPs, PAMPs and alarmins: all we need to know about danger. *J Leukoc Biol* 2007;81(1):1–5.

74. Imaeda AB, Watanabe A, et al. Acetaminophen-induced hepatotoxicity in mice is dependent on Tlr9 and the Nalp3 inflammasome. *J Clin Invest* 2009;119(2):305–14.

75. Kaplowitz N. Idiosyncratic drug hepatotoxicity. *Nat Rev Drug Discov* 2005;4(6):489–99.

76. Masson MJ, Collins LA, et al. The role of cytokines in the mechanism of adverse drug reactions. *Handbook Exp Pharmacol* 2010;196:195–231.

77. Liu ZX, Govindarajan S, et al. Innate immune system plays a critical role in determining the progression and severity of acetaminophen hepatotoxicity. *Gastroenterology* 2004;127(6):1760–74.

78. Bourdi M, Reilly TP, et al. Macrophage migration inhibitory factor in drug-induced liver injury: a role in susceptibility and stress responsiveness. *Biochem Biophys Res Commun* 2002;294(2):225–30.

79. Chiu H, Gardner CR, et al. Role of tumor necrosis factor receptor 1 (p55) in hepatocyte proliferation during acetaminophen-induced toxicity in mice. *Toxicol Appl Pharmacol* 2003;193(2):218–27.

80. Harrill AH, Watkins PB, et al. Mouse population-guided resequencing reveals that variants in CD44 contribute to acetaminophen-induced liver injury in humans. *Genome Res* 2009;19(9):1507–15.

81. Bourdi M, Masubuchi Y, et al. Protection against acetaminophen-induced liver injury and lethality by interleukin 10: role of inducible nitric oxide synthase. *Hepatology* 2002;35(2):289–98.

82. Masubuchi Y, Bourdi M, et al. Role of interleukin-6 in hepatic heat shock protein expression and protection against acetaminophen-induced liver disease. *Biochem Biophys Res Commun* 2003;304(1):207–12.

83. Ju C, Pohl LR. Tolerogenic role of Kupffer cells in immune-mediated adverse drug reactions. *Toxicology* 2005;209(2):109–12.

84. Adams DH, Ju C, et al. Mechanisms of immune-mediated liver injury. *Toxicol Sci* 2010;115(2):307–21.

85. Mehendale HM, Limaye PB. Calpain: a death protein that mediates progression of liver injury. *Trends Pharmacol Sci* 2005;26(5):232–6.

86. Limaye PB, Bhave VS, et al. Upregulation of calpastatin in regenerating and developing rat liver: role in resistance against hepatotoxicity. *Hepatology* 2006;44(2):379–88.

87. Mehendale HM. Tissue repair: an important determinant of final outcome of toxicant-induced injury. *Toxicol Pathol* 2005;33(1):41–51.

88. Kohle C, Bock KW. Coordinate regulation of human drug-metabolizing enzymes, and conjugate transporters by the Ah receptor, pregnane X receptor and constitutive androstane receptor. *Biochem Pharmacol* 2009;77(4):689–99.

89. Zimmerman HJ, Maddrey WC. Acetaminophen (paracetamol) hepatotoxicity with regular intake of alcohol: analysis of instances of therapeutic misadventure. *Hepatology* 1995;22(3):767–73 (erratum in *Hepatology* 1995;22(6):1898).

90. Sato C, Nakano M, et al. Prevention of acetaminophen-induced hepatotoxicity by acute ethanol administration in the rat: comparison with carbon tetrachloride-induced hepatoxicity. *J Pharmacol Exp Ther* 1981;218(3):805–10.

91. Altomare E, Leo MA, et al. Interaction of acute ethanol administration with acetaminophen metabolism and toxicity in rats fed alcohol chronically. *Alcohol Clin Exp Res* 2984;8(4):405–8.

92. Banda PW, Quart BD. The effect of mild alcohol consumption on the metabolism of acetaminophen in man. *Res Commun Chem Pathol Pharmacol* 1982;38(1):57–70.

93. Roberts BJ, Song BJ, et al. Ethanol induces CYP2E1 by protein stabilization. Role of ubiquitin conjugation in the rapid degradation of CYP2E1. *J Biol Chem* 1995;270(50):29632–5.

94. Thummel KE, Slattery JT, et al. Ethanol and production of the hepatotoxic metabolite of acetaminophen in healthy adults. *Clin Pharmacol Ther* 2000;67(6):591–9.

95. Chien JY, Thummel KE, et al. Pharmacokinetic consequences of induction of CYP2E1 by ligand stabilization. *Drug Metab Dispos* 1997;25(10):1165–75.

96. Murphy R, Swartz R, et al. Severe acetaminophen toxicity in a patient receiving isoniazid. *Ann Intern Med* 1990;113(10):799–800 (erratum in *Ann Intern Med* 1991;114(3):253, see comments).

97. Reed DJ. Mitochondrial glutathione and chemically induced stress including ethanol. *Drug Metab Rev* 2004;36(3–4):569–82.

98. Whitcomb DC, Block GD. Association of acetaminophen hepatotoxicity with fasting and ethanol use. *JAMA* 1994;272(23):1845–50.

99. Bonkovsky HL, Kane RE, et al. Acute hepatic and renal toxicity from low doses of acetaminophen in the absence of alcohol abuse or malnutrition: evidence for increased susceptibility to drug toxicity due to cardiopulmonary and renal insufficiency. *Hepatology* 1994;19(5):1141–8.

100. Andrade RJ, Robles M, et al. Drug-induced liver injury: insights from genetic studies. *Pharmacogenomics* 2009;10(9):1467–87.

101. Zou W, Beggs KM, et al. Sulindac metabolism and synergy with tumor necrosis factor-alpha in a drug-inflammation interaction model of idiosyncratic liver injury. *J Pharmacol Exp Ther* 2009;331(1):114–21.

102. Deng X, Stachlewitz RF, et al. Modest inflammation enhances diclofenac hepatotoxicity in rats: role of neutrophils and bacterial translocation. *J Pharmacol Exp Ther* 2006;319(3):1191–9.

103. Deng X, Luyendyk JP, et al. Inflammatory stress and idiosyncratic hepatotoxicity: hints from animal models. *Pharmacol Rev* 2009;61(3):262–82.

104. Cosgrove BD, Alexopoulos LG, et al. Cytokine-associated drug toxicity in human hepatocytes is associated with signaling network dysregulation. *Mol Biosyst* 2010;6(7):1195–206.

105. Morgan ET, Goralski KB, et al. Regulation of drug-metabolizing enzymes and transporters in infection, inflammation, and cancer. *Drug Metab Dispos* 2008;36(2):205–16.

106. Bliven EE, Podewils LJ. The role of chronic hepatitis in isoniazid hepatotoxicity during treatment for latent tuberculosis infection. *Int J Tuberc Lung Dis* 2009;13(9):1054–60.

107. Boelsterli UA, Hsiao CJ. The heterozygous Sod2(+/−) mouse: modeling the mitochondrial role in drug toxicity. *Drug Discov Today* 2008;13(21–22):982–8.

108. Lucena MI, Garcia-Martin E, et al. Mitochondrial superoxide dismutase and glutathione peroxidase in idiosyncratic drug-induced liver injury. *Hepatology* 2010;52(1):303–12.

109. Park BK, Pirmohamed M, et al. Idiosyncratic drug reactions: a mechanistic evaluation of risk factors. *Br J Clin Pharmacol* 1992;34(5): 377–95.

110. Rehman OU, Keith TA, et al. Methyldopa-induced submassive hepatic necrosis. *JAMA* 1973;224(10):1390–2.

111. Watkins PB, Zimmerman HJ, et al. Hepatotoxic effects of tacrine administration in patients with Alzheimer's disease. *JAMA* 1994; 271(13):992–8.

112. Maria VA, Victorino RM. Diagnostic value of specific T cell reactivity to drugs in 95 cases of drug induced liver injury. *Gut* 1997;41(4): 534–40.

113. Matzinger P. Tolerance, danger, and the extended family. *Annu Rev Immunol* 1994;12:991–1045.

114. Uetrecht J. Idiosyncratic drug reactions: past, present, and future. *Chem Res Toxicol* 2008;21(1):84–92.

115. Ariyoshi N, Iga Y, et al. Enhanced susceptibility of HLA-mediated ticlopidine-induced idiosyncratic hepatotoxicity by CYP2B6 polymorphism in Japanese. *Drug Metab Pharmacokinet* 2010;25(3): 298–306.

116. Andrews E, Armstrong M, et al. A role for the pregnane X receptor in flucloxacillin-induced liver injury. *Hepatology* 2010;51(5):1656–64.

117. Watkins PB, Seligman PJ, et al. Using controlled clinical trials to learn more about acute drug-induced liver injury. *Hepatology* 2008;48(5):1680–9.

118. Lewis JH, Larrey D, et al. Utility of the Roussel Uclaf Causality Assessment Method (RUCAM) to analyze the hepatic findings in a clinical trial program: evaluation of the direct thrombin inhibitor ximelagatran. *Int J Clin Pharmacol Ther* 2008;46(7):327–39.

119. Palmeira CM, Rolo AP. Mitochondrially-mediated toxicity of bile acids. *Toxicology* 2004;203(1–3):1–15.

120. Fattinger K, Funk C, et al. The endothelin antagonist bosentan inhibits the canalicular bile salt export pump: a potential mechanism for hepatic adverse reactions. *Clin Pharmacol Ther* 2001;69(4):223–31.

121. Funk C, Ponelle C, et al. Cholestatic potential of troglitazone as a possible factor contributing to troglitazone-induced hepatotoxicity: in vivo and in vitro interaction at the canalicular bile salt export pump (Bsep) in the rat. *Mol Pharmacol* 2001;59(3):627–35.

122. Kemp DC, Zamek-Gliszczynski MJ, et al. Xenobiotics inhibit hepatic uptake and biliary excretion of taurocholate in rat hepatocytes. *Toxicol Sci* 2005;83(2):207–14.

123. Stieger B. Role of the bile salt export pump, BSEP, in acquired forms of cholestasis. *Drug Metab Rev* 2010;42(3):437–45.

124. Leslie EM, Watkins PB, et al. Differential inhibition of rat and human Na+-dependent taurocholate cotransporting polypeptide (NTCP/SLC10A1) by bosentan: a mechanism for species differences in hepatotoxicity. *J Pharmacol Exp Ther* 2007;321(3):1170–8.

125. Dambach DM, Andrews BA, et al. New technologies and screening strategies for hepatotoxicity: use of in vitro models. *Toxicol Pathol* 2005;33(1):17–26.

126. Gonzalez FJ, Yu AM. Cytochrome P450 and xenobiotic receptor humanized mice. *Annu Rev Pharmacol Toxicol* 2006;46:41–64.

127. Cheng J, Ma X, et al. Rifampicin-activated human pregnane X receptor and CYP3A4 induction enhance acetaminophen-induced toxicity. *Drug Metab Dispos* 2009;37(8):1611–21.

128. Strom SC, Davila J, et al. Chimeric mice with humanized liver: tools for the study of drug metabolism, excretion, and toxicity. *Methods Mol Biol* 2010;640:491–509.

129. Jaeschke H. Are cultured liver cells the right tool to investigate mechanisms of liver disease or hepatotoxicity? *Hepatology* 2003;38(4):1053–5.

130. Uetrecht J. Screening for the potential of a drug candidate to cause idiosyncratic drug reactions. *Drug Discov Today* 2003;8(18):832–7.

131. Evans DC, Watt AP, et al. Drug–protein adducts: an industry perspective on minimizing the potential for drug bioactivation in drug discovery and development. *Chem Res Toxicol* 2004;17(1):3–16.

132. Tang W, Lu AY. Metabolic bioactivation and drug-related adverse effects: current status and future directions from a pharmaceutical research perspective. *Drug Metab Rev* 2010;42(2):225–49.

133. Wills Q, Mitchell C. Toxicogenomics in drug discovery and development – making an impact. *Altern Lab Anim* 2009;37(Suppl 1): 33–7.

134. Xu JJ, Henstock PV, et al. Cellular imaging predictions of clinical drug-induced liver injury. *Toxicol Sci* 2008;105(1):97–105.

135. Smith KS, Smith PL, et al. In vitro metabolism of tolcapone to reactive intermediates: relevance to tolcapone liver toxicity. *Chem Res Toxicol* 2003;16(2):123–8.

136. Belloc C, Gauffre A, et al. Epitope mapping of human CYP1A2 in dihydralazine-induced autoimmune hepatitis. *Pharmacogenetics* 1997;7(3):181–6.

137. Kang P, Dalvie D, et al. Bioactivation of flutamide metabolites by human liver microsomes. *Drug Metab Dispos* 2008;36(7):1425–37.

138. Kharasch ED, Hankins DC, et al. Human halothane metabolism, lipid peroxidation, and cytochromes P(450)2A6 and P(450)3A4. *Eur J Clin Pharmacol* 2000;55(11–12):853–9.

139. Pearce RE, Uetrecht J, et al. Pathways of carbamazepine bioactivation in vitro. II. The role of human cytochrome P450 enzymes in the formation of 2-hydroxyiminostilbene. *Drug Metab Dispos* 2005;33(12):1819–26.

140. Yan Z, Li J, et al. Detection of a novel reactive metabolite of diclofenac: evidence for CYP2C9-mediated bioactivation via arene oxides. *Drug Metab Dispos* 2005;33(6):706–13.

141. Lecoeur S, Andre C, et al. Tienilic acid-induced autoimmune hepatitis: anti-liver and-kidney microsomal type 2 autoantibodies recognize a three-site conformational epitope on cytochrome P4502C9. *Mol Pharmacol* 1996;50(2):326–33.

142. Cuttle L, Munns AJ, et al. Phenytoin metabolism by human cytochrome P450: involvement of P450 3A and 2C forms in secondary metabolism and drug–protein adduct formation. *Drug Metab Dispos* 2000;28(8):945–50.

143. Kang P, Dalvie D, et al. Identification of a novel glutathione conjugate of flutamide in incubations with human liver microsomes. *Drug Metab Dispos* 2007;35(7):1081–8.

144. Wen B, Zhou M. Metabolic activation of the phenothiazine antipsychotics chlorpromazine and thioridazine to electrophilic iminoquinone species in human liver microsomes and recombinant P450s. *Chem Biol Interact* 2009;181(2):220–6.

145. Laine JE, Auriola S, et al. Acetaminophen bioactivation by human cytochrome P450 enzymes and animal microsomes. *Xenobiotica* 2009;39(1):11–21.

146. Yue J, Peng RX, et al. CYP2E1 mediated isoniazid-induced hepatotoxicity in rats. *Acta Pharmacol Sin* 2004;25(5):699–704.

147. Kalgutkar AS, Henne KR, et al. Metabolic activation of the nontricyclic antidepressant trazodone to electrophilic quinone-imine and epoxide intermediates in human liver microsomes and recombinant P4503A4. *Chem Biol Interact* 2005;155(1–2):10–20.

148. Kalgutkar AS, Vaz AD, et al. Bioactivation of the nontricyclic antidepressant nefazodone to a reactive quinone-imine species in human liver microsomes and recombinant cytochrome P450 3A4. *Drug Metab Dispos* 2005;33(2):243–53.

149. He K, Talaat RE, et al. Metabolic activation of troglitazone: identification of a reactive metabolite and mechanisms involved. *Drug Metab Dispos* 2004;32(6):639–46.

150. Wen B, Chen Y, et al. Metabolic activation of nevirapine in human liver microsomes: dehydrogenation and inactivation of cytochrome P450 3A4. *Drug Metab Dispos* 2009;37(7):1557–62.

151. Kindmark A, Jawaid A, et al. Genome-wide pharmacogenetic investigation of a hepatic adverse event without clinical signs of immunopathology suggests an underlying immune pathogenesis. *Pharmacogenomics J* 2008;8(3):186–95.

152. Spraggs C. (2010). HLA-DQA1*0201is a major determinant of lapatinib-induced hepatotoxicityrisk in women with advanced breast cancer. w.aasld.org/conferences/Documents/Presentation Library/2010Hepatoxicity_SessionII_Spraggs.pdf, 2010.

153. Singer JB, Lewitzky S, et al. A genome-wide study identifies HLA alleles associated with lumiracoxib-related liver injury. *Nat Genet* 2010;42(8):711–14.

154. Holden A. Introduction to session II: Genetics and Genomics Associated with DILI24. http://www.aasld.org/conferences/Documents/PresentationLibrary/2010Hepatoxicity_SessionII_Holden.pdf, 2010.

155. Hirata K, Takagi H, et al. Ticlopidine-induced hepatotoxicity is associated with specific human leukocyte antigen genomic subtypes in Japanese patients: a preliminary case–control study. *Pharmacogenomics J* 2008;8(1):29–33.

156. Daly AK, Donaldson PT, et al. HLA-B*5701 genotype is a major determinant of drug-induced liver injury due to flucloxacillin. *Nat Genet* 2009;41(7):816–19.

Genetic and Metabolic Disease

PART VII

Genetic and Metabolic Disease

CHAPTER 29
Wilson Disease

Michael L. Schilsky[1] & *Anthony S. Tavill*[2]

[1] Yale New Haven Transplant Center, Yale University Medical Center, New Haven, CT, USA
[2] Case Western Reserve University, Cleveland Clinic, Cleveland, OH, USA

Key concepts

- Wilson disease is a genetic disorder in which copper accumulates in the liver and brain in excess of normal metabolic needs. The accumulation is based on an inherited defect in the hepatic biliary excretion of copper.
- The inheritance pattern is autosomal recessive. Homozygotes for this disorder, numbering about 1 in 30,000 of the population, inherit disease-specific mutations of both alleles of the gene for Wilson disease, *ATP7B*, on chromosome 13. The disease does not develop in heterozygotes with a mutation of a single *ATP7B* allele, and they do not require treatment.
- The diagnosis of Wilson disease is established by a combination of clinical and biochemical findings or by molecular genetic studies. Biochemical findings include most notably a decrease in levels of circulating ceruloplasmin, and a hepatic copper concentration above 250 mg/g dry weight of liver in most affected individuals. Clinical findings include the presence of corneal Kayser–Fleischer rings, stigmata of chronic liver disease, and neurologic findings.

- Molecular genetic studies demonstrating two disease-specific mutations of *ATP7B* may be used to establish a diagnosis of Wilson disease. Most patients are compound heterozygotes with two different mutations, but clinical and biochemical evaluation are needed to demonstrate phenotypic expression and to stage the disease.
- In most symptomatic patients, treatment with metal chelating agents is effective in stabilizing or reversing the disease. Asymptomatic patients may be treated with metal chelating agents or zinc salts. In all circumstances, lifelong pharmacologic treatment is required and results in excellent patient survival.
- Acute liver failure in Wilson disease or hepatic insufficiency unresponsive to medical therapy is best treated with orthotopic liver transplantation, which, by providing the liver with a normal physiologic capacity for copper excretion, is curative.

History

In 1912, while serving as a senior resident at the National Hospital for Nervous Diseases in London, Kinnier Wilson published his work "Progressive lenticular degeneration: a familial nervous disease associated with cirrhosis of the liver" as part of his dissertation for the Edinburgh MD degree [1]. Correctly, he speculated that the brain disease, characterized by extrapyramidal features, was caused by the liver disease. However, his concept of a "morbid toxin" produced by the cirrhotic liver, although strictly correct, could not have anticipated the much later insights into the role of the liver in copper metabolism and the vulnerability of certain areas of the brain to the toxic effects of excessive copper deposition. It was not until 33 years later that Glazebrook [2] detected a marked excess of copper in the basal ganglia of a patient dying of Wilson disease and surmised from the recognized accumulation of copper in the liver that the inability of the liver to excrete copper was the dysfunction responsible for the lenticular degeneration, a pathogenetic association later confirmed by other workers [3,4].

In 1902 and 1903 the first descriptions of corneal pigmented rings, now recognized eponymously as Kayser–Fleischer (K-F) rings, were based on observations in patients with neurologic disease [5,6]. Fleischer [7] was the first to associate three seminal features of Wilson diseases – namely, corneal pigmentation, neuropsychiatric disease, and hepatic cirrhosis – and another 10 years passed before the first hypothesis was proposed that the corneal pigmentation is caused by the pathologic deposition of copper [8,9]. Recognition of the value of a low serum ceruloplasmin concentration in the diagnosis of Wilson disease came from the observations of Scheinberg and Gitlin [10], who first reported this phenomenon in 96% of Wilson disease homozygotes. However, Sternlieb and Scheinberg [11] subsequently recognized that up to 20% of heterozygotes also have low

Schiff's Diseases of the Liver, Eleventh Edition. Edited by Eugene R. Schiff, Willis C. Maddrey and Michael F. Sorrell.
© 2012 John Wiley & Sons, Ltd. Published 2012 by John Wiley & Sons, Ltd.

ceruloplasmin concentrations without any other clinical manifestations of Wilson disease. This observation and the presence of a normal ceruloplasmin in a small minority of Wilson disease homozygotes, and the lack of copper accumulation in patients with a defect in ceruloplasmin biosynthesis (aceruloplasminemia), argued against a direct pathogenetic role for ceruloplasmin in the accumulation of copper in tissues in cases of Wilson disease. With the understanding that the clinical features of Wilson disease are the result of copper toxicity in the various affected tissues of the body, the rationale for chelation therapy became apparent. The first chelation agent used for the treatment of Wilson disease in 1951 was British anti-lewisite (BAL), or dimercaptopropanol [12, 13]. This drug, which is lipophilic and therefore administered intramuscularly, provided the first effective therapy for a previously untreatable disorder. BAL was developed as a war time expedient as an antidote to arsenic gas. The principle on which its action was based depended on its two sulfydryl groups for the binding and inactivation of arsenic. Unfortunately BAL has a high incidence of toxic reactions, is painful for the recipient, and while also effective in the chelation of copper it has many toxic, adverse effects. As Walshe pointed out in his review of the pharmacologic treatment of Wilson disease [14], BAL, while offering significant progress, was limited in its application to copper toxicity by both toxicity and tachyphylaxis, thereby prompting the search for an oral copper chelator excreted through the kidneys.

John Walshe of Cambridge University, while working at the Boston City Hospital, introduced the first effective oral chelation therapy in the form of penicillamine and demonstrated its cupriuretic action and role in the symptomatic improvement of patients with life-threatening features of Wilson disease [15]. It was the incidental finding of the excretion of dimethylcysteine in the urine following the administration of penicillin that led Walshe to postulate that this breakdown amino acid product of the antibiotic (also known as D-penicillamine) might have copper chelating properties. That hypothesis was borne out in clinical practice, and with pharmaceutical industry collaboration the D-isomer of dimethylcysteine became the favored treatment for the copper overload of Wilson disease, with very promising benefits for both the hepatic and neurologic components of the disease. Sternlieb and Scheinberg [11] subsequently expanded the use of this drug to include the treatment of asymptomatic (or presymptomatic) patients with Wilson disease by showing its effectiveness in preventing disease progression.

Walshe [16] proceeded to develop another, safer chelating agent, triethylene tetramine dihydrochloride (trientine), which proved a valuable alternative agent in the treatment of those patients intolerant of the toxic effects of penicillamine. The development of trientine took place initially in Walshe's own laboratory before being taken up by industry and marketed as an orphan drug. It had powerful copper chelating ability with clinical benefits comparable to that of penicillamine but without the adverse effects of precipitating a lupus-like syndrome.

Walshe [17] was also instrumental in the initial human use of tetrathiomolybdate, currently an investigational drug in the United States and United Kingdom. Its mode of action is probably through tight binding of copper both in the intestine and the tissues, with the potential for reducing both its absorption from the intestine and its toxicity in the tissues.

The possibility of preventing the toxic accumulation of copper in Wilson disease by blocking the intestinal absorption of copper with oral zinc therapy was first considered by Schouwink [18]. Oral zinc therapy would not be regarded as appropriate for the management of newly diagnosed, symptomatic Wilson disease because it is ineffective in the removal of accumulated copper from the tissues and therefore it has not been licensed by the US Food and Drug Administration (FDA) for this purpose. Studies have shown, however, that it is a valuable alternative to chelation agents for long-term maintenance therapy based on its effectiveness in preventing copper reaccumulation [19,20].

A development that revolutionized the treatment of a subset of patients with Wilson disease presenting with acute liver failure was orthotopic liver transplantation [OLT), which effectively cures the disease [21]. The phenotypic reversion from a diseased to a normal state in transplant recipients demonstrates the central role of the liver in Wilson disease and copper metabolism.

The recognition of Wilson disease as an inherited disorder, defined by a complex of signs and symptoms, has evolved in less than a century to the point at which we are now able to define the molecular basis for the pathophysiology of this disorder. Milestones in this process, which culminated in the identification of the gene for Wilson disease, designated *ATP7B*, and the recognition of disease-specific mutations, are reviewed in subsequent text and outlined in Table 29.1.

Genetics

Although Wilson correctly recorded the familial nature of the disease, it was Hall in 1921 [22] who demonstrated its inheritance, later shown to be autosomal recessive [23]. Subsequently, the linkage of Wilson disease to the locus of the red cell *esterase-D* gene placed the gene for Wilson disease on the long arm of chromosome 13 [24], and additional studies further delineated its chromosomal localization [25,26].

A breakthrough in the understanding of the molecular basis of the defect of copper metabolism in Wilson disease was the discovery of the gene for Menkes disease,

Table 29.1 Milestones in the genetics of Wilson disease.

Year	Milestone	Reference
1912	Recognition of Wilson disease as an inherited disorder	Wilson 1912 [1]; Groth et al. 1973 [21]
1953	Pattern of inheritance described as autosomal recessive	Hall 1921 [22]; Bearn and Kunkel 1953 [23]
1985	Localization of disease locus to chromosome 13 by linkage with esterase D	Frydman et al. 1985 [24]
1986–1993	Localization of the responsible gene to a specific region in chromosome 13	Houwen et al. 1990 [25]; Bowcock et al. 1988 [26]
1992–1993	Identification of the gene for Menkes disease as a putative copper-transporting P-type ATPase	Vulpe et al. 1993 [27]; Chelly et al. 1993 [28]
1993	Identification of the gene for Wilson disease, *ATP7B*, and disease-specific mutations	Bull et al. 1993 [32]; Mercer et al. 1993 [29]; Petrukhin et al. 1993 [31]; Tanzi et al. 1993 [30]
1994 to present	Continued studies on disease-specific mutations and polymorphisms of *ATP7B*	Yamaguchi et al. 1993 [33]; Petrukhin et al. 1994 [34]

ATPase, adenosine triphosphatase.

another rare inherited disease of copper metabolism, and the identification of its gene product, ATP7A, a cation-transporting P-type adenosine triphosphatase (ATPase) involved in copper transport in many tissues [27–29]. The extrapolation of the copper-transporting P-type ATPase to the Wilson disease model led to the hypothesis that a mutation in the gene for a liver-specific copper transporter might be responsible for the association between the defective incorporation of copper into ceruloplasmin, failure of biliary secretion of copper, and accumulation of copper in the liver.

The isolation and identification of the gene for Wilson disease, designated *ATP7B*, followed closely the discovery of the gene for Menkes disease. The identification of the specific gene was accomplished almost simultaneously by three independent laboratories [30–33]. The detection of specific mutations unique to individuals with clinical and biochemically proven disease confirmed the identity of the responsible gene [30,31].

The *ATP7B* gene is contained within an approximately 80 kb region of DNA containing 22 exons (exon 22 being contained in a rare transcript); these encode an approximately 7.8 kb messenger RNA that is highly expressed in the liver [34]. Analysis of the gene sequence indicates that ATP7B belongs to a family of ATP-dependent metal transporters that are highly conserved through evolution [35]. A schema of the *ATP7B* gene showing specific regions of known homology to ATPases and metal transporters is shown in Fig. 29.1.

Screening for mutations of *ATP7B* has led to the identification of a large number (>300) of disease-specific mutations and polymorphisms of the gene [31,32,35–37].

Most of the mutations thus far identified are point mutations that result in amino acid substitutions. However, deletions, insertions, missense, and splice site mutations have also been reported. A summary of the mutations and polymorphisms of the gene can be found in the following website: http://www.wilsondisease .med.ualberta.ca/database.asp. When particular mutations are found frequently among members of a specific population or ethnic group, direct mutational analysis

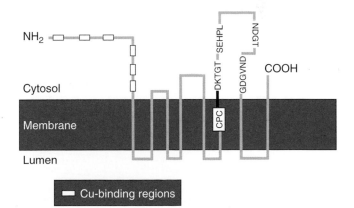

Cu-binding regions

Figure 29.1 Predicted major structural features of the Wilson disease gene product (ATP7B). ATP7B, as a member of a class of heavy metal-transporting adenosine triphosphatases (ATPases), is predicted to contain the following structural features: cysteine-rich metal-binding regions near the amino terminus, a transduction and phosphatase domain, multiple transmembrane regions with one containing the amino acids cysteine-proline-cysteine (CPC), a phosphorylation domain (DKTGT), an ATP-binding region (NDGT), a hinge region (GDGVND), and a conserved domain for metal-transforming ATPase, critical for copper (Cu) transfer (SEHPL). (Adapted from Petrukhin et al. [34] and Cox [36].)

for these mutations is particularly useful and may expedite diagnosis. Haplotype analysis (polymorphism analysis of the region surrounding *ATP7B*) has proved useful for genetic screening of siblings of probands, though advances in DNA sequencing technology and its wider availability makes direct mutational analysis the testing of choice (see subsequent text). The most frequently observed point mutation, which results in a change from histidine to glutamine (H1069Q), is present in nearly 30% of patients of European descent [31,37]. In only a single population in Austria has the frequency of this mutation been reported to be higher (up to 65%) [38]. Most mutations are clustered about several transmembrane regions of the protein and in another region predicted to be involved in ATP binding. Some evidence indicates that mutations that result in a loss of the expression of the ATP7B protein may cause more severe phenotypic expression; however, not all studies support this conclusion. Another study suggests that expression of another gene, *APOE*, may modify the phenotype of Wilson disease. Polymorphisms in other genes involved in copper metabolism may also modify the disease phenotype, as suggested by studies of *MURR1* or *COMMD1* [39], a member of the commander family of proteins, the gene responsible for copper toxicosis in Bedlington terriers but whose function in copper export is not yet certain. XIAP (X-linked inhibitor of apoptosis) is another protein

that is influenced by copper concentration that modifies the threshold for apoptosis [40]. Further investigations are ongoing that aim to correlate specific phenotypic presentations or manifestations of Wilson disease with *ATP7B* genotype and the expression of other potential modifying genes.

Pathophysiology

Copper is an essential cofactor for many enzymes and proteins and is important for the mobilization of tissue iron stores. The normal pathways for copper metabolism are outlined in Fig. 29.2. Ingested copper is extracted from the portal circulation by hepatocytes by the cell surface human copper transporter (hCTR1) [41]. Intracellular copper then interacts with low molecular weight ligands such as glutathione [42], metallothionein [43], and HAH1 [44], which serve as transfer or storage agents. It is subsequently used for cellular metabolic needs, incorporated into the secretory glycoprotein ceruloplasmin, or excreted into bile.

The passage of copper from hepatocytes to bile is critical for homeostasis of this metal because copper excreted into bile undergoes minimal enterohepatic recirculation [45]. The transport of hepatocellular copper to bile is thought to involve a vesicular pathway that is dependent

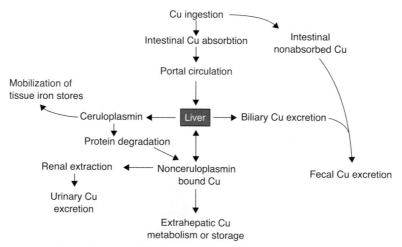

Figure 29.2 Copper (Cu) metabolism and pathophysiology of Wilson disease. Dietary copper is absorbed in the proximal small intestine, whereas nonabsorbed copper or copper bound within shed enterocytes passes into the feces. Absorbed copper is bound mainly to albumin in the portal circulation, from which it is avidly extracted by hepatocytes. Hepatocellular copper is bound to ligands and used for metabolic needs, transferred to endogenous chelators, incorporated into ceruloplasmin, or excreted into bile. Biliary copper does not undergo enterohepatic recycling and is therefore excreted in the feces. In Wilson disease, biliary copper excretion is reduced, and copper accumulates within hepatocytes. The incorporation of copper into ceruloplasmin is also impaired in Wilson disease; as a result,

circulating levels of this protein are decreased in most patients. When cellular stores are overloaded or after a hepatocellular injury, the amount of copper released into the circulation is increased. Extraction of the excess of nonceruloplasmin-bound copper by the kidneys leads to an increase in urinary copper excretion and extrahepatic deposition of this metal. The dietary intake of copper is approximately 5 mg/24 h, with intestinal absorption varying between 25% and 60% of intake. Fecal excretion is approximately 4.9 mg/24 h, and urinary copper excretion and renal excretion do not usually exceed 50 μg/24 h (maximum 100 μg/24 h). In Wilson disease, nonceruloplasmin-bound copper is the precursor of the excessive copper deposited in the tissues.

results in a decrease in biliary copper excretion, which is responsible for the hepatic accumulation of this metal in Wilson disease [4,49–51].

Ceruloplasmin is a serum glycoprotein that contains six copper atoms per molecule. It is synthesized predominantly in the liver. Copper is thought to be incorporated into apoprotein ceruloplasmin in the Golgi apparatus [52] and the copper-containing holoprotein secreted from the hepatocyte. Newly transported copper, which is used for ceruloplasmin biosynthesis, must also cross organelle membranes to enter into the protein biosynthetic pathway, a process that is dependent on ATP7B and is absent or diminished in most patients with Wilson disease. A reduction of the incorporation of copper into ceruloplasmin is believed to lead to a reduced circulating level of this protein in most patients with Wilson disease because the noncopper-containing apoprotein is less stable and undergoes more rapid degradation in vivo.

When copper accumulates beyond the cellular capacity for its safe storage, hepatocellular injury may result. Toxic effects of excess copper include the generation of free radicals, lipid peroxidation of membranes and DNA, inhibition of protein synthesis, and alterations in the levels of cellular antioxidants [53]. Recent data suggest that both hepatocellular necrosis and apoptosis may be triggered by copper-induced cell damage [54,55]. When copper-induced injury occurs, the functional status of the liver is determined by the delicate balance between injury, cell death, and the regenerative capacity of liver cells.

When the capacity of the liver to store copper is exceeded, or when hepatocellular damage results in the release of cellular copper into the circulation, levels of noceruloplasmin-bound copper in the circulation become elevated. It is from this pool that the extrahepatic deposition of copper is thought to occur. The brain is the most critical extrahepatic site of copper accumulation, and copper-induced neuronal injury is responsible for the neurologic and psychiatric manifestations of Wilson disease and the characteristic changes on radiologic imaging studies of the brain.

Pathology

The evolution of pathologic changes in the tissues of patients with Wilson disease (see [53] for a review) follows the relative rates of accumulation of copper in the various body organs. Because the primary genetic defect resides in the liver and because the liver is the predominant storage organ for copper, it is not surprising that the earliest pathologic manifestations are hepatic in nature. As copper "spills" over to other organs from the liver, pathologic manifestations become evident in the brain, kidneys, eyes, red blood cells, and joints.

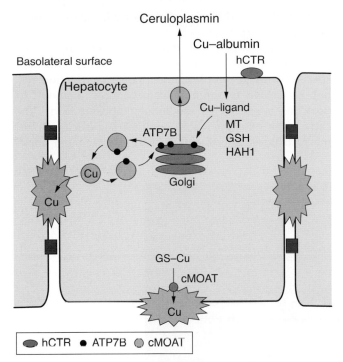

Figure 29.3 Cellular pathways of copper (Cu) metabolism. Newly absorbed copper, loosely bound to albumin, is transported across the plasma membrane of the hepatocyte, where it is transported by a variety of ligands to the Golgi apparatus. There, the ATP7B protein serves to transport it across the Golgi into ceruloplasmin for secretion into the circulation. Excretion into bile may occur by vesicular secretion, by transcanalicular association with glutathione (GSH) through the canalicular multispecific organic anion transporter (cMOAT), or by copper-transporting adenosine triphosphatase in the canalicular membrane. GS-Cu, copper glutathione; HAH1, human homolog of Atx1p, a copper chaperone; hCTR, human copper transporter; MT, metallothionein.

on the function of ATP7B. This protein appears to be present mainly in the *trans*-Golgi network of liver cells under basal conditions (Fig. 29.3) [46]. Interestingly, in recent studies of the homologous Menkes disease protein, ATP7A, this protein was observed to alter its intracellular localization in response to increases in the level of copper [47]. Although studies of ATP7B protein suggest that it also redistributes to a vesicular compartment in response to copper loading [46], how the redistribution affects the function of the protein remains to be determined. It is presumed that the vesicular pathway is critical for biliary copper excretion. However, other investigators suggest that ATP7B protein resides in a pericanalicular region and relocates directly to the canalicular membrane in response to increased cellular copper [48]. If the ATP7B protein is present at this site, it would be involved in the direct transfer of copper to bile. Whether the ATP7B protein resides in the canalicular membrane or whether copper is delivered through this site by vesicular transport, the absence or diminished function of ATP7B

Hepatic pathology

Macroscopically, the liver may be only mildly enlarged in the early stages of life. Later, without treatment, the liver pathology progresses in most patients to fibrosis and cirrhosis. The nodular transformation of cirrhosis is a mixed macronodular–micronodular pattern, in which the nodules may vary in color depending on the degree of copper accumulation (Fig. 29.4A). The rate of pathologic change varies greatly between patients, and in some cases steatosis and fibrosis without cirrhosis may persist for decades [56].

At a microscopic level, the evidence of copper accumulation in early infancy may be subtle and non-specific. Diffuse cytoplasmic copper accumulation may not be visible by immunohistochemical methods for detecting copper (e.g., rhodanine, rubeanic acid). This early stage of copper accumulation is associated with macrosteatosis, microsteatosis, and glycogenated nuclei,

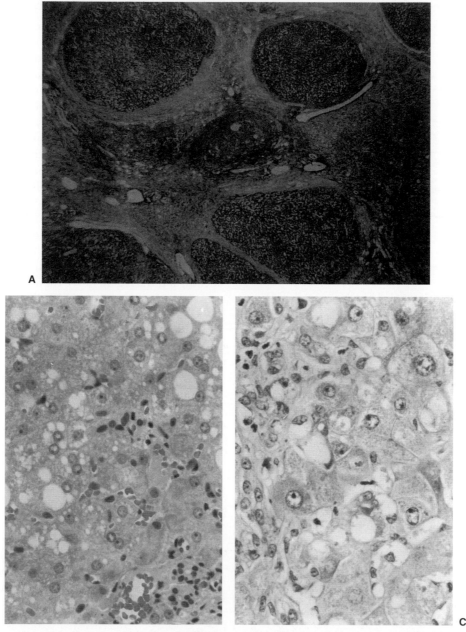

Figure 29.4 Light microscopic findings in liver in Wilson disease. (A) Masson trichrome stain of liver from a patient with established cirrhosis reveals broad bands of fibrosis intersecting variably sized nodules with varied staining characteristics. Original ×80. (B) Prominent microvesicular and macrovesicular steatosis and some inflammatory cells in a specimen from an asymptomatic patient with Wilson disease. Original ×250. (C) Hepatocellular ballooning and degeneration in a biopsy specimen from a patient with acute Wilsonian hepatitis. Original ×250.

features that may be seen in a variety of other conditions (Fig. 29.4B) [57]. Sternlieb [58] emphasized the almost ubiquitous presence of distinctive mitochondrial changes at this early stage of the disease. The ultrastructural abnormalities range from enlargement and separation of the inner and outer mitochondrial membranes, with widening of the intercristal spaces, to increases in the density and granularity of the matrix or replacement by large vacuoles. Pleomorphic changes may also be seen in distorted peroxisomes and endoplasmic reticulum, with nuclei showing glycogen inclusions. With progression of the disease, copper-associated protein is sequestered in lysosomes, appearing as electron-dense pericanalicular structures visible on light microscopy as granules detectable by copper immunohistochemistry (Fig. 29.5).

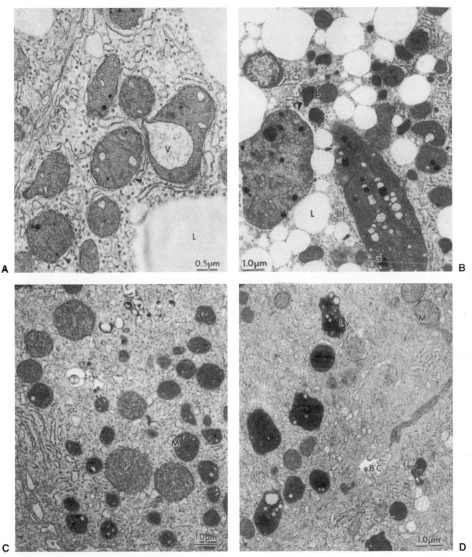

Figure 29.5 Electron micrographs of fine sections of liver biopsy specimens obtained from untreated patients with Wilson disease, showing portions of hepatocytes. (A) Ten-year-old asymptomatic girl with normal physical findings: aspartate aminotransferase, 76 IU/L; alanine aminotransferase, 55 IU/L; serum ceruloplasmin, 21.4 mg/dL; hepatic copper, 1,258 μg/g of dry tissue. Some of the mitochondria display vacuoles (V) with granular material. Note the separation of the inner from outer membrane (arrowheads), with the creation of an enlarged intermembranous space. L, lipid droplet. (B) Nineteen-year-old woman with a history of progressive fatigue, found to have Kayser–Fleischer rings 2 months after an episode of hemolytic anemia with jaundice: serum ceruloplasmin, 12.7 mg/dL; hepatic copper, 591 μg/g of dry tissue. The mitochondria are markedly pleomorphic, some displaying multiple, pathognomonic abnormalities: gigantism, increased matrical density, separation of inner from outer membrane (arrowhead), vacuoles, dilated cristae, crystals, and enlarged dense granules (G). P, peroxisomes. (C) Ten-year-old asymptomatic girl with a serum ceruloplasmin level below 1 mg/dL and a hepatic copper concentration of 1,029 μg/g of dry tissue. Mitochondria (M) display dilated cristae; the markedly enlarged peroxisomes (P) with grainy matrices are strikingly abnormal. (D) In a 20-year-old woman with severe neurologic Wilson disease, the hepatocellular cytoplasm appears virtually normal except for the abundance of electron-dense, peribiliary, lysosomal granules (Ly). BC, bile canaliculus; M, mitochondria.

If the condition is untreated or unrecognized, the initial stages of Wilson disease progress to an intermediate hepatic stage. This is characterized by periportal inflammation with mononuclear cellular infiltrates, erosion of the limiting lobular plates, lobular necrosis, and bridging fibrosis, features indistinguishable from those of chronic active hepatitis of many other causes [57]. Cirrhosis is virtually invariable at this stage of disease, with either a micronodular or a mixed macronodular–micronodular histologic pattern. Mallory bodies may be visible in up to 50% of biopsy specimens.

In patients presenting with acute liver failure, parenchymal necrosis with hepatocellular ballooning, apoptotic bodies, cholestasis, and collapse of the liver may predominate (Fig. 29.4C). In some of these individuals with acute liver failure, the liver has significant collapse and bridging fibrosis, but cirrhosis may not be present (M. Schilsky and J. Lefkowitch, personal observations, 2005).

A histochemical confirmation of copper deposition may be helpful; however, a negative result does not exclude copper overload. Rhodanine and rubeanic acid may show dense granular lysosomal copper deposition in hepatocytes at the stage of cirrhotic nodular regeneration. Staining at this stage often shows marked variability from nodule to nodule (Fig. 29.6). Paradoxically, the results of immunohistochemical staining for copper are usually negative in the earlier stages of the disease when the hepatocyte copper is diffusely distributed in the cytoplasm [59]. A more sensitive stain, Timms sulfide, is more effective in detecting cytoplasmic copper-binding proteins, although it is not routinely utilized. Overall, the opinion of most hepatopathologists is that histochemical copper stains should not be routinely used for the diagnosis of Wilson disease (see below) because of their lack of sensitivity [60].

Neuropathology

Macroscopically, most of the overt neuropathologic changes in advanced Wilson disease are concentrated in the lenticular nuclei. These show atrophy and discoloration, with cystic degeneration, pitting, and fissuring of the cut surfaces. Similar changes have been described in the thalamus, subthalamic region, and even the cerebral white matter [61].

Microscopically, the major pathologic changes occur in those parts of the central nervous system with the highest copper levels. Scheinberg and Sternlieb [61] calculated that the concentrations are highest in the thalamus, followed by the putamen and cerebral cortex. Neuroglial changes are the most distinctive in Wilson disease, with an increase in the number of astrocytes in the gray matter of the lenticular nuclei. Swollen glia may undergo cavitation and liquefaction, which create small cavities with an overall appearance of spongiform degeneration. Neuronal loss is accompanied by gliosis and astrocytosis and the production of glial fibrillary protein. The characteristic astrocytes seen within areas of lenticular degeneration are Alzheimer type I and II cells and, distinctively for Wilson disease, Opalski cells [62]. Opalski cells are large cells, up to 35 μm in diameter, with fine granular cytoplasm and slightly eccentric nuclei (single or multiple) that Scheinberg and Sternlieb [61] suggested originate from degenerating astrocytes. It is unclear at the present time whether the glial changes are secondary to the stimulation of metallothionein protein synthesis by copper in selective areas of the brain populated by protoplasmic astrocytes or whether the selective targeting of glial cells is related to other, as yet unidentified, factors.

Miscellaneous pathologic changes

Functional changes in the kidneys are often disproportionate to any observable changes on light microscopy.

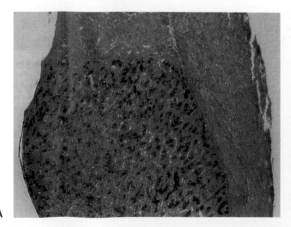
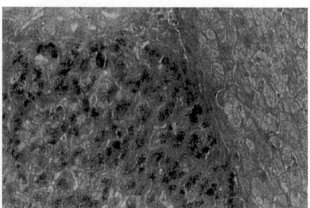

Figure 29.6 Liver section stained with rhodanine to show a lobule with heavy lysosomal copper deposition and the adjoining liver tissue with minimal copper staining. (A) Low power original ×110; (B) high power original ×200.

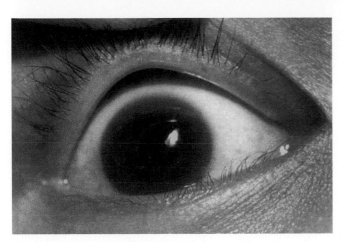

Figure 29.7 Kayser–Fleischer ring in a 17-year-old patient with neurologic symptoms of Wilson disease.

Proximal or distal tubular dysfunction leading to tubular proteinuria, bicarbonate loss, aminoaciduria, glycosuria, hyperphosphaturia, uricosuria, and hypercalciuria is common. Glomerular abnormalities, in the form of hypercellularity, basement membrane thickening, hyalinization, and fibrosis, have been described [61]. Penicillamine-induced immune complex nephropathy has been described. Bone pathology and periarticular abnormalities have been observed, accounting for osteoporosis, osteomalacia, spontaneous fractures, adult rickets, osteoarthritis, osteochondritis dissecans, chondrocalcinosis, and subchondral cyst formation [61]. Involvement of the spine and knee joints is the most common distribution of skeletal and articular abnormalities.

Ophthalmologic findings include K-F rings and sunflower cataracts. The K-F rings, most marked at the upper and lower poles of the cornea, are caused by the granular deposition of elemental copper on the inner surface of the cornea in the Descemet membrane (Fig. 29.7). The rings have a golden brown or green appearance on slit-lamp examination. The sunflower cataracts, with radiating centrifugal extensions, are associated with the granular deposition of copper in the anterior and posterior lens capsule.

Both the K-F rings and sunflower cataracts are reversible with effective treatment.

Diagnosis

The diagnosis of Wilson disease should be considered in any person aged between 3 and 40 years with unexplained hepatic, neurologic, or psychiatric disease, although rare cases have been diagnosed in persons in the sixth, seventh, and even eighth decades of life [56]. In particular, this diagnosis must be excluded unequivocally in children or young adults who present with unusual extrapyramidal or cerebellar motor disorders, atypical psychiatric disease, unexplained hemolysis, or elevated liver enzyme levels or other manifestations of liver disease, with or without a family history of liver or neurologic disease. Failure to do so will lead to unnecessary and preventable demise. In most cases, the diagnosis can be made by a combination of clinical and biochemical testing. In practice, three levels of tests may be undertaken to confirm the diagnosis of Wilson disease (Table 29.2). The presence of K-F rings and a reduced serum concentration of ceruloplasmin are sufficient to establish the diagnosis. However, in the absence of K-F rings, it may be necessary to proceed to a liver biopsy for a quantitative copper determination to confirm the diagnosis.

Molecular testing is currently available for Wilson disease. There are two types of testing that may be employed. Haplotype analysis that looks for familial inheritance of polymorphisms around the *ATP7B* gene can be considered for use in screening the siblings of affected persons, however direct mutational analysis is now available and is the preferred testing technique. Newer methodology has made the molecular screening of the entire coding region of *ATP7B* less cumbersome and time consuming, although some targeting of specific exons with higher frequencies of mutations makes sense, particularly in individual populations in which specific mutations are present at higher frequency. There is a need to identify disease-specific mutations of the gene to firmly

Table 29.2 Diagnostic tests in Wilson disease.

Level 1[a]	Level 2[a]	Level 3
Low serum ceruloplasmin[1]	Liver copper concentration[2]	
Slit-lamp examination for K-F rings		Ultrastructural studies of hepatocytes
Raised serum-free copper level[3]	24-hour urine copper[4]	Molecular genetic studies for Wilson disease

[a]Normal values: (1) 20–50 mg/dL; (2) <250 μg/g dry weight; (3) <10 μg/dL; (4) <50 μg/24 hours. Values in Wilson disease: (1) <20 mg/dL; (2) >250 μg/g dry weight; (3) >25 μg/dL; (4) >100 μg/24 hours.
K-F, Kayser–Fleischer.

establish the diagnosis in the absence of pathognomonic biochemical abnormalities. Although molecular studies may detect the disease, it may still be useful to fully characterize all patients with standard clinical and biochemical testing to better understand the degree of disease involvement, as well as to provide confirmation of the diagnosis. Given the current relatively high cost and complexity of this testing, molecular testing is not useful as a screening test for Wilson disease in the population at large. However, for patients in whom there is difficulty in determining the diagnosis by clinical and biochemical testing, and for family screening, molecular testing should prove extremely useful.

Concentration of ceruloplasmin

A test to determine the serum concentration of ceruloplasmin is routinely available in all clinical laboratories. It is most useful, when measured by means of enzymatic methods, to determine oxidase activity, because this best reflects the copper content of the protein, although immunologic assays are frequently utilized. The normal range is 20–50 mg/dL. About 95% of homozygotes with Wilson disease have values of less than 20 mg/dL. Up to 5% of all homozygotes and up to 15–50% of persons with liver disease may have normal levels, which is defined as concentrations above 20 mg/dL [61,63]. In some cases, normal levels are present in patients with active liver disease, probably as a consequence of acute-phase responses in the liver or estrogen supplementation. Homozygotes rarely have serum concentrations exceeding 30 mg/dL. Low serum concentrations of ceruloplasmin may also be observed in hypoproteinemic states, such as protein-calorie malnutrition, nephrotic syndrome, protein-losing enteropathy, and other forms of severe decompensated liver disease, and in up to 20% of asymptomatic heterozygous carriers of the gene for Wilson disease. Rarer causes of serum ceruloplasmin deficiency include hereditary aceruloplasminemia and Menkes disease.

Concentration of circulating copper not bound to ceruloplasmin

The total concentration of copper in plasma or serum represents ceruloplasmin-bound copper plus nonceruloplasmin-bound ("free") copper, which is bound mainly to albumin, peptides, or amino acids. Because the former is reduced in proportion to the degree of hypoceruloplasminemia, the total copper may be low in the face of a typically raised free copper concentration. To calculate the latter, the plasma ceruloplasmin copper concentration (approximately the ceruloplasmin level in mg/dL multiplied by 3) is subtracted from the total copper concentration (in µg/dL). The value for total plasma copper ranges from 80 to 120 µg/dL and the value for nonceruloplasmin-bound copper is usually 10% of the total value (8–12 µg/dL). In Wilson disease, levels of nonceruloplasmin-bound copper are typically above 25 µg/dL in symptomatic patients before treatment. Recently a direct assay for nonceruloplasmin copper in serum was introduced, but it is not yet widely available [64].

Slit-lamp detection of Kayser–Fleischer rings

It is essential that all patients in whom Wilson disease is suspected undergo a slit-lamp examination, performed by an experienced ophthalmologist, for the detection of K-F rings. These rings are present in patients with neurologic disease, with only rare exceptions, but they may be absent, particularly in younger patients with hepatic manifestations only (see Fig. 29.7). Another finding that may suggest Wilson disease is the presence of sunflower cataracts, also best observed by slit-lamp examination.

Urinary excretion of copper

The copper excreted in urine is derived from the free copper circulating in plasma, which represents filterable, nonceruloplasmin-bound copper. The rate of excretion may exceed 100 µg/24 h in symptomatic patients. In patients presenting with chronic liver disease, the urinary copper level is elevated above normal levels but may not reach diagnostic levels of more than 100 µg/24 h. False-positive increases in urinary copper level may be seen in the face of significant proteinuria and urinary loss of ceruloplasmin, and rarely in other liver diseases where copper storage is increased or in acute liver failure. A provocative test for urinary copper excretion with the use of the chelating agent penicillamine has been studied in children [65] but may be no better than changing the threshold of urinary copper excretion to 40 µg of copper in 24 hours [66]. When urinary excretion of copper is tested, it is crucial that a metal-free container be used and that the adequacy of the collection be monitored by correlation with volume excreted or with creatinine excretion.

Concentration of copper in the liver

Normal concentrations of copper in the liver rarely exceed 50 µg/g dry weight of liver. Most patients homozygous for Wilson disease have levels above 250 µg/g, whereas the concentration of copper in the liver of heterozygotes, although commonly elevated above normal, typically does not exceed 250 µg/g [61]. The hepatic copper concentrations may also be elevated in other liver diseases, particularly chronic cholestatic diseases such as primary biliary cirrhosis and primary sclerosing cholangitis. However, these disorders are usually readily distinguishable from Wilson disease on the basis of serologic and histologic criteria.

A recent study by Ferenci et al. [67] suggested that in some individuals confirmed to have Wilson disease by molecular studies, hepatic copper content does not reach 250 µg/g dry weight of liver. On the basis of these results, these investigators proposed a lower threshold for considering Wilson disease: 70 µg copper/g dry weight liver. However, no data are presented in this study on heterozygotes in whom hepatic copper may easily exceed this threshold. Therefore, the previous cutoff of 250 µg copper/g dry weight liver may better differentiate heterozygotes and homozygotes with Wilson disease, but this should not be the sole criterion for excluding the diagnosis if there is appropriate histology or clinical signs of disease. In patients for whom the diagnosis remains uncertain despite extensive clinical and biochemical evaluation, molecular studies will help in confirming or refuting the diagnosis of Wilson disease.

Liver biopsy specimens for a quantitative copper determination should be obtained with a (Tru-Cut or Jamshidi) needle and placed dry in a copper-free vessel. About 1 cm of a 1.6 mm diameter core of liver should be dried overnight at 56°C in a vacuum oven or, alternatively, frozen immediately before being shipped to a laboratory specializing in microchemical analysis for copper. The remainder of the specimen can be fixed in the usual manner for histopathologic examination. In asymptomatic patients, the hepatic copper level is higher than that in patients with established cirrhosis. Specimens with extensive fibrosis and fewer parenchymal cells may yield copper concentrations that are nondiagnostic, and therefore the result of hepatic copper quantification should be correlated with the histologic, clinical, and biochemical data. If the diagnosis of Wilson disease is considered after specimens are processed, liver tissue can be removed from paraffin and copper quantitation performed after extraction of the paraffin and drying of the specimen. These specimens are often smaller, and larger errors in the estimation of tissue copper may occur if too little of the specimen remains for analysis.

Molecular genetic studies
The identification of the gene for Wilson disease has enabled the molecular genetic diagnosis of this disorder. There are now numerous disease-specific mutations of the gene described; however, the most common mutation is present in only 15–30% of most populations [37,38]. This makes most patients compound heterozygotes, possessing different mutations on each allele of *ATP7B*. Direct de novo analysis for the presence of disease-specific mutations is now possible, given the advances in DNA sequencing and screening technology. The ability to establish the diagnosis by this methodology depends on distinguishing disease-specific mutations from polymorphisms of the gene and is further limited by the fact that some

of the noncoding regions of the gene, which may also affect gene expression, are not analyzed. It is also possible to screen family members of an affected person by haplotype analysis. This process involves inspecting the patterns of polymorphisms of the DNA in the region surrounding the Wilson disease gene to determine whether mutant regions present in the affected person have been inherited by family members [31]. Future developments in DNA analysis should make it possible to screen for disease-specific mutations in an even more cost-effective manner, so that de novo population screening will one day prove practical. At present, genetic testing should be used for screening families and used in concert with standard clinical and biochemical testing as discussed above.

Ultrastructural studies
In cases in which indeterminate hepatic copper concentrations make it difficult to distinguish between heterozygotes and homozygotes, ultrastructural analysis for the pathognomonic mitochondrial abnormalities described by Sternlieb [58] may be helpful. The performance of these studies requires proper specimen handling and the assistance of pathologists skilled in electron microscopy, obviously with forethought to process the specimen appropriately for such analysis.

Clinical manifestations

Patients with symptomatic Wilson disease most frequently present with liver disease or neurologic/psychiatric symptoms. Affected persons detected by family screening are often asymptomatic (also termed *presymptomatic*). The failure to initiate specific treatment for Wilson disease or the disruption of ongoing treatment results in progression to hepatic insufficiency, neuropsychiatric disease, and ultimately hepatic failure and death.

The clinical spectrum of liver diseases associated with Wilson disease is broad (Box 29.1). Younger patients identified by family screening or serial evaluations of isolated biochemical abnormalities are most often asymptomatic. Some patients present with chronic liver disease indistinguishable from other forms of chronic active hepatitis, with or without specific symptoms. In patients with cirrhosis and hepatic insufficiency, jaundice, ascites, edema, or other stigmata of chronic liver disease, including hepatic encephalopathy, may be observed. When untreated, the liver disease progresses to cirrhosis with hepatic insufficiency, liver failure, and death. Some patients, most often in their second decade of life, present with acute hepatitis and an associated nonimmunopathic hemolytic anemia, which without the life-saving intervention of OLT is frequently fatal (see below). Among patients

Box 29.1 Clinical presentations of Wilson disease.

- Asymptomatic (presymptomatic)
- Hepatic disease
- Asymptomatic with only biochemical abnormalities
- Chronic active hepatitis
- Cirrhosis with hepatic insufficiency and associated signs and symptoms
- Acute hepatitis with or without hemolytic anemia
- Neurologic signs and symptoms
- Dystonia with rigidity and contractures
- Tremors
- Dysarthria and dysphonia
- Gait disturbance
- Choreiform movements
- Psychiatric symptoms
- Range from neuroses to psychoses
- Renal disease
- Aminoaciduria
- Nephrocalcinosis
- Hematologic disease
- Hemolysis

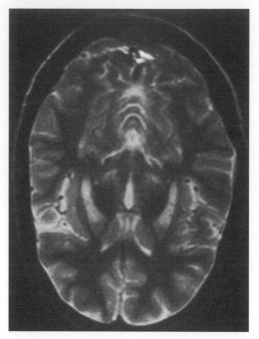

Figure 29.8 Magnetic resonance image of the brain of a 21-year-old woman with dysarthria, dysphagia, slurred speech, and tremors caused by Wilson disease. Note the hyperintensity in the region of the basal ganglia.

presenting with Wilsonian acute hepatitis, the female to male ratio is almost 2:1 [68].

Patients in whom the first presenting symptoms of Wilson disease are either neurologic or psychiatric are frequently older than those who present with hepatic symptoms. Most patients with central nervous system involvement are believed to have significant liver disease at the time of presentation. However, hepatic histology is not generally available for these patients because the diagnosis is often established on the basis of a decreased ceruloplasmin level and the presence of K-F rings. Neurologic disease may be manifested as motor abnormalities with parkinsonian characteristics of dystonia, hypertonia and rigidity, chorea or athetosis, tremors, and dysarthria [69]. Disabling muscle spasms can lead to contractures, dysarthria, dysphonia, and dysphagia. At this stage of disease, magnetic resonance imaging or computed tomography of the brain may be useful in delineating changes in the basal ganglia (Fig. 29.8).

Wilson disease infrequently presents with abnormalities of other organ systems. Changes induced by copper toxicity in the kidneys include nephrocalcinosis, hematuria, and aminoaciduria [61] and those in the skeletal system include arthritis, arthralgias, and premature osteoarthrosis [61]. Myocardial copper accumulation can cause cardiomyopathy and arrhythmias [70,71], although these are rarely manifested clinically. A more indolent form of hemolytic anemia unassociated with acute hepatitis may occasionally be seen [72].

The diagnosis of Wilson disease in the setting of acute hepatitis deserves special mention because of several unique features. In this setting, acute hepatitis is associated with a nonimmunopathic hemolytic anemia with unconjugated hyperbilirubinemia and markedly elevated serum and urinary levels of copper. Most of these patients are in the second decade of life, and K-F rings may not yet be apparent. Paradoxically, levels of serum alkaline phosphatase are frequently depressed [73–75], and this feature led to the observation that a ratio of alkaline phosphatase to bilirubin of less than 2 might be diagnostic of Wilsonian acute hepatitis [75,76]. We and others have observed some patients with Wilsonian acute hepatitis in whom this ratio was above 2 [68]. However, when an alkaline phosphatase:bilirubin ratio of <4 and aspartate aminotransferase (AST) to alanine aminotransferase (ALT) ratio of >2.2 are used in combination, a nearly 100% identification of Wilson disease can be made in patients with acute liver failure [77].

Treatment

The therapeutic options in Wilson disease include pharmacologic treatment and OLT. The aim of medical therapy is to abolish symptoms, if present, and prevent the worsening or progression of disease. Successful therapy may be gauged by clinical improvement or stabilization and by the normalization of biochemical parameters

Table 29.3 (a) Treatment and (b) follow-up management in Wilson disease (WD) patients.

(a)

Medical therapy for WD treatment	Chemical form	Route of administration
British antilewisite (BAL)	Dimercaptopropanol	Intramuscular
Penicillamine	Dimethylcysteine	Oral
Trientine	Trientine dihydrochloride	Oral
Zinc salts	Zinc sulfate, zinc gluconate, zinc acetate	Oral
Tetrathiomolybdate (experimental)	–	Oral

(b)

Maintenance therapy for WD	Oral maintenance dose (adult)	Comments	Monitoring of efficacy and compliance
Penicillamine	750–1,000 mg in three to four divided doses	Monitor for lupus-like reactions and marrow suppression; requires supplemental pyridoxine, and dose reduction for surgery and pregnancy	Nonceruloplasmin Cu <10 μg/dL Urine Cu >250 μg/24 h
Trientine	750–1,000 mg in three to four divided doses	Monitor for sideroblastic anemia; requires dose reduction for surgery and pregnancy	Nonceruloplasmin Cu <10 μg/dL Urine Cu >250 μg/24 h
Zinc salts	150 mg in three divided doses	Occasional gastric intolerance	Nonceruloplasmin Cu <10 μg/dL Urine zinc >1,000 μg/24 h Urine Cu <150 μg/24 h

Cu, copper.

of liver function and copper metabolism. Serial liver biopsies have no role in the management of Wilson disease. Repeated liver biopsies should be performed only to exclude concurrent illness or as part of an experimental treatment protocol. Liver transplantation should be reserved for patients with severe hepatic insufficiency or liver failure occurring in the context of acute hepatitis or end-stage liver disease. Transplant recipients subsequently have a normal donor phenotype with respect to copper metabolism, and with rare exception, they do not require further therapy specific to Wilson disease.

Pharmacologic treatments for Wilson disease include chelating agents and zinc salts (Table 29.3). Chelating agents (e.g., penicillamine, trientine, BAL, and tetrathiomolybdate) remove copper from potentially toxic sites within cells and detoxify and/or excrete the remaining copper. Zinc salts act mainly by blocking the intestinal absorption of dietary copper, but also stimulate the biosynthesis of endogenous chelators in the liver, such as metallothioneins, that help detoxify the remaining metal [43].

The treatment of asymptomatic patients and maintenance therapy for previously symptomatic patients are identical (Table 29.3). Patients with hepatic insufficiency or chronic active hepatitis evident only on biochemical testing or histologic examination of the liver should be considered symptomatic, and treated with chelation therapy for adequate copper removal before their medications are changed or the doses of chelator reduced for maintenance therapy (see subsequent text). The largest experience for long-term treatment is still with penicillamine, whereas trientine and zinc salts are alternative agents with fewer potential side effects. Both these alternative agents, previously used only for penicillamine-intolerant patients, should now be considered for the initial therapy of asymptomatic patients and for long-term use as maintenance therapy. Regardless of the specific agent chosen, monitoring for efficacy and patient compliance is crucial.

Chelation therapy is indicated as the primary therapy for symptomatic patients with hepatic or neurologic/psychiatric disease. As mentioned in the preceding text, the greatest experience thus far is with penicillamine.

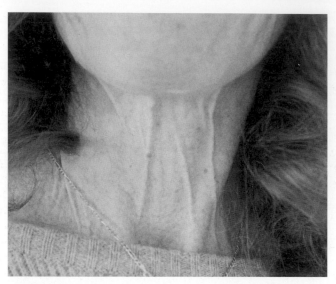

Figure 29.9 Progeric change (appearance of premature aging) in the skin of the neck, characteristic of patients on long-term penicillamine treatment.

The reported incidence of penicillamine-induced side effects varies greatly [61,78], although worsening of neurologic symptoms has been observed in about 10% of symptomatic patients during the early phase of penicillamine therapy. Whether this worsening would have occurred with the use of alternative agents is uncertain and awaits the systematic evaluation of alternative agents as the primary treatment for neurologically affected patients. Late, dermatologic effects of penicillamine include progeric changes in the skin, often visible around the neck (Fig. 29.9), and the cheloid-like lesions of elastosis perforans serpiginosa, which may appear anywhere on the body (Fig. 29.10). Trientine has proved

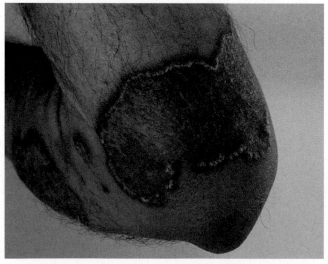

Figure 29.10 The cheloid-like lesions of elastosis perforans serpiginosa on the elbow of this penicillamine-treated patient may appear on different areas of the body.

to be an effective treatment for penicillamine-intolerant patients [79], and experience is growing in the utilization of this agent as a first-line therapy for hepatic and neurologic disease [79–82]. Zinc salts may be used as an alternative initial therapy for patients who cannot tolerate penicillamine or trientine. Although it has been reported that zinc is an effective treatment for symptomatic patients, it may be delayed in its effective onset of action and therefore chelation agents are preferable in this setting.

Once clinical and biochemical stabilization has been achieved, typically within 2 to 6 months of the initiation of treatment for most patients, but somewhat longer for more severely affected persons, maintenance therapy should be considered. Tetrathiomolybdate, first used to treat animals with copper toxicosis, is currently an experimental agent undergoing evaluation as an initial treatment for patients with neurologic symptoms. Initial reports on the use of tetrathiomolybdate in this setting suggest no worsening of neurologic symptoms and a rapid reduction in circulating nonceruloplasmin-bound copper during the first 8 weeks of therapy [83]. However, studies directly comparing the efficacy of this agent with trientine did not show statistically significant differences in neurologic and speech scores over a 4-year observation period [84].

BAL, the first available treatment for Wilson disease, is now rarely used, and only as adjunctive therapy for patients with neurologic/psychiatric symptoms refractory to chelation therapy with penicillamine or trientine alone [85]. This drug, used in conjunction with oral therapy with penicillamine or trientine, is administered intramuscularly in an oil base. As a lipophilic compound, BAL has the theoretical advantage of possibly crossing the blood–brain barrier more easily. The main drawback of BAL therapy is the difficulty and discomfort involved in administering it and the lack of objective parameters outside clinical evaluation to determine its efficacy.

The dietary consumption of foods with a high copper content should be avoided during the initial phases of treatment. These include organ meats such as liver, in addition to nuts, shellfish, and chocolate. During the maintenance phase of therapy, liberalization of the diet is permitted.

OLT should be considered for patients with Wilsonian acute liver failure and for those with severe hepatic insufficiency unresponsive to medical therapy [68]. Two different series that retrospectively reviewed the data on OLT for patients with Wilson disease found 1-year survival rates after transplantation to be about 80% [68,86], and, more recently, 1-year patient survival was found to be about 87% [87]. In this last report, acute renal insufficiency was observed more often in patients who underwent transplantation for acute liver failure secondary to Wilson disease than in those who underwent transplantation for acute liver failure of other causes. The acute renal insufficiency resolved without long-term renal damage. During the acute phase of acute liver failure, when toxic copper complexes are being released into the circulation, plasmapheresis, exchange transfusion, and albumin dialysis have been utilized in an effort to further reduce copper-induced toxicity. These interventions may be helpful in reducing comorbidity and stabilizing the patient, but they have not precluded the need for OLT. Neurologic symptoms may improve after transplantation [68,88]. However, it is our opinion that transplantation should not be used for patients with neurologic symptoms in the absence of hepatic failure, especially given the current shortage of donor organs. After the perioperative period of OLT, with rare exceptions, no further specific therapy for Wilson disease is necessary.

Living donor transplantation has been performed for acute liver failure secondary to Wilson disease in a few children and in some adults as well. Partial grafts from heterozygous parents have been successful, with good organ function in both donor and recipient [89].

The treatment of pregnant women with Wilson disease and persons with Wilson disease who must undergo surgical interventions deserves special mention. The goal of treatment in pregnant patients is to maintain adequate disease control in the mother, reduce her risk for bleeding, and prevent interference with wound healing and the possibility of teratogenicity. Pregnancies have been successful in patients taking penicillamine, trientine, or zinc [90–94]. For patients being maintained on chelation therapy, the dosage of penicillamine or trientine should be lowered whenever possible early in the course of the pregnancy. The suggested dosage is 500 mg/day, and monitoring during each trimester is advised. Zinc therapy can be maintained uninterrupted at full dosage during pregnancy and postpartum [94]. Dose reduction during pregnancy is recommended as the medications D-penicillamine and trientine have known teratogenicity. Furthermore, the reduction in dosage helps prevent impaired collagen cross-linking due to copper depletion in lysyl oxidase.

When patients with Wilson disease maintained on chelating agents must undergo surgery, the dose of their medication should be reduced preoperatively and perioperatively to avoid interference with wound healing. The dosage of penicillamine or trientine can be reduced to 250–500 mg daily during this time and rapidly advanced to a maintenance dosage once wound healing has taken place. No adjustment of the dosage is required for patients on zinc therapy, either perioperatively or postoperatively.

We cannot overemphasize that the key to the long-term success of pharmacotherapy for Wilson disease is patient adherence to the use of medications. This can

be monitored by history and clinical examinations to detect any changes in the symptoms or signs of liver or neurologic disease, pill counts, screening for biochemical evidence of hepatic dysfunction, measurement of urinary copper or zinc excretion, periodic slit-lamp examinations, and, importantly, biochemical testing for nonceruloplasmin-bound copper. This last test is the standard by which pharmacotherapeutic doses should be determined and is the single best parameter for gauging the adequacy of treatment. Nonceruloplasmin-bound copper is a derived number, estimated from the difference between the total serum copper content and the copper content of ceruloplasmin, determined by its oxidase activity (approximately three times the value for ceruloplasmin in mg/dL). In healthy persons and appropriately treated patients, the value for nonceruloplasmin-bound copper should be 8–12 μg/dL or less. In untreated, inadequately treated, and noncompliant patients, this value is frequently elevated above 25 μg/dL (Fig. 29.11).

The interpretation of the results of urinary copper excretion must take into account the mode of treatment, ability to collect a complete sample, avoidance of contamination, and appropriate analysis of copper content. During the early phase of treatment with chelating agents, values for urinary copper excretion are frequently greater than 1,000 μg/24 h. These decline to about

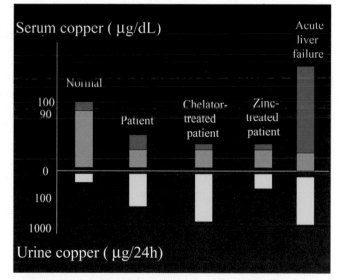

Figure 29.11 Copper parameters in normal, untreated, and treated Wilson disease. In normal patients ceruloplasmin accounts for ~90% of serum copper. In untreated Wilson disease, the percent of copper not bound to ceruloplasmin in the circulation is increased, as is the urine copper. In patients treated with copper chelators, the nonceruloplasmin-bound copper is reduced and the urine copper is increased. In zinc-treated patients, the nonceruloplasmin-bound copper is reduced and the urine copper typically is less than 100 μg/24 h. In acute liver failure, nonceruloplasmin-bound copper and urine copper are markedly increased. Ceruloplasmin-bound copper: blue; nonceruloplasmin-bound copper: green.

250–500 µg/24 h over time, and despite the continuous use of chelation agents, the values for urinary copper excretion tend to remain at about this level (Fig. 29.11). Values below 250 µg/24 h suggest noncompliance with therapy, overtreatment, or an incorrect diagnosis from the outset.

The values for 24-hour urinary copper excretion in patients on zinc therapy are not significantly elevated because zinc acts to prevent copper absorption [95]. However, a rise in urinary copper excretion to above 125 µg/24 h may indicate noncompliance or inadequate therapy, and, if so, they are likely to be accompanied by an increase in the nonceruloplasmin-bound copper level. Urinary and plasma levels of zinc may also be used to monitor compliance with zinc therapy.

The prognosis for patients who comply with pharmacotherapy for Wilson disease is excellent, even if cirrhosis or chronic hepatitis is present at the time of diagnosis [96]. Patients with neurologic or psychiatric symptoms of Wilson disease may continue to recover for months to years after the initiation of treatment. In some patients with neurologic disease or hepatic insufficiency, symptoms or biochemical abnormalities persist but stabilize with treatment. At present, the best way to determine whether and to what extent a patient's disease is reversible is to await a response to treatment.

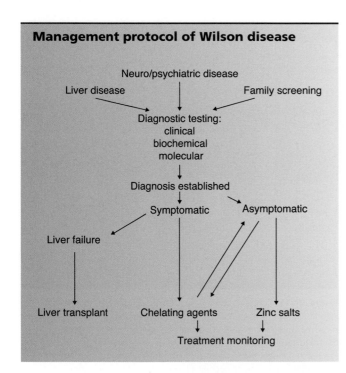

Management protocol of Wilson disease

Neuro/psychiatric disease
Liver disease
Family screening
→
Diagnostic testing:
clinical
biochemical
molecular
↓
Diagnosis established
Symptomatic   Asymptomatic
Liver failure
↓
Liver transplant   Chelating agents   Zinc salts
↓
Treatment monitoring

Annotated references

Brewer GJ, Johnson VD, Dick RD, et al. Treatment of Wilson's disease with zinc. XVII: Treatment during pregnancy. *Hepatology* 2000;31: 364–70.
Successful outcomes were achieved for pregnancy in Wilson disease patients on zinc but rare birth defects were still present. Highlights the importance of maintaining treatment for Wilson disease during pregnancy.

Frommer DJ. Defective biliary excretion of copper in Wilson's disease. *Gut* 1974;15:125–9.
Describes the lower copper content in biliary secretions in patients with Wilson disease.

Gollan JL, Deller DT. Studies on the nature and excretion of biliary copper in man. *Clin Sci* 1973;44:9–15.
Studies on the complexes of copper excreted by the liver that were then analyzed in biliary secretions in man.

O'Reilly S, Weber PM, Oswald M, et al. Abnormalities of the physiology of copper. *Arch Neurol* 1971;25:28–32.
Describes the lower copper content of biliary secretions in man and in the stool of patients with Wilson disease.

Petrukhin K, Fischer SG, Pirastu M, et al. Mapping, cloning and genetic characterization of the region containing the Wilson disease gene. *Nat Genet* 1993;5:338–43.
Critical steps in identifying the gene for Wilson disease were localization of the gene to chromosome 13, further sublocalization on this chromosome, and identification of the Menkes disease gene as a copper-transporting adenosine triphosphatase.

Roberts EA, Schilsky ML. AASLD Practice Guidelines. Diagnosis and treatment of Wilson disease: an update. *Hepatology* 2008;47:2089–111.
A review of the evidence-based literature on diagnosing and treating Wilson disease formulated into practical guidelines for the American Association for the Study of Liver Diseases.

Scheinberg IH, Gitlin D. Deficiency of ceruloplasmin in patients with hepatolenticular degeneration (Wilson's disease). *Science* 1952;116: 484–5.
This article describes for the first time the reduction of ceruloplasmin in the circulation of patients with Wilson disease, after which ceruloplasmin determination became part of the diagnostic evaluation for Wilson disease.

Schilsky ML, Scheinberg IH, Sternlieb I. Liver transplantation for Wilson's disease: indications and outcome. *Hepatology* 1994;19:583–7.
This study of patients with Wilson disease who were treated with OLT at multiple transplantation centers confirmed and extended prior observations that OLT is curative for Wilson disease and established that it should be considered for patients with acute Wilsonian hepatitis and those with severe hepatic insufficiency unresponsive to medical therapy.

Sternlieb I. Wilson's disease and pregnancy. *Hepatology* 2000;31:531–2.
This article and accompanying editorial highlight the dilemmas encountered in the management of female patients with Wilson disease during pregnancy. Brewer et al. who favor zinc as an alternative to chelating agents for primary and maintenance therapy, reported 26 pregnancies in 19 patients that were successful for both mother and fetus, except for two developmental defects (one major) in a fetus. Sternlieb in his accompanying editorial offers combined data from three groups representing major international referral centers that attest to the safety and efficacy of penicillamine and trientine when the dose is appropriately adjusted.

Sternlieb I, Scheinberg IH. Prevention of Wilson's disease in asymptomatic patients. *N Engl J Med* 1968;278:352–9.
The treatment of asymptomatic (presymptomatic) patients, now the standard of practice, was not accepted before this important clinical study.

Sternlieb I, van den Hamer CJA, Morell AG, et al. Lysosomal defect of hepatic copper excretion in Wilson's disease (hepatolenticular degeneration). *Gastroenterology* 1973;64:99–105.
An important step in understanding the pathophysiology of Wilson disease and normal human copper metabolism was the recognition that biliary copper excretion is critical in copper homeostasis and that a reduction of biliary copper excretion leads to an accumulation of copper in the liver and toxicity.

Walshe JM. Copper chelation in patients with Wilson's disease: a comparison of penicillamine and triethylene tetramine dihydrochloride. *Q J Med* 1973;42:441–52.

The introduction of the first two oral copper-chelating agents effective in reversing or stabilizing symptoms of Wilson disease by this distinguished physician revolutionized treatment, which had previously relied on the intramuscular administration of BAL.

Walshe JM. The conquest of Wilson's disease. *Brain* 2009;132:2289–95.

A succinct account of the development of chelating and other pharmacologic agents for the management of Wilson disease from a pioneer in the field.

Wilson SAK. Progressive lenticular degeneration: a familial nervous disease associated with cirrhosis of the liver. *Brain* 1912;34:295–509.

Original description of Wilson disease as a progressive lenticular degeneration with associated cirrhosis of the liver.

References

1. Wilson SAK. Progressive lenticular degeneration: a familial nervous disease associated with cirrhosis of the liver. *Brain* 1912;34:295–509.

2. Glazebrook AJ. Wilson's disease. *Edinburgh Med J* 1945;52:83–7.

3. Gibbs K, Walshe JM. Biliary excretion of copper in Wilson's disease. *Lancet* 1980;2:538.

4. Frommer DJ. Defective biliary excretion of copper in Wilson's disease. *Gut* 1974;15:125–9.

5. Kayser B. Ueber ein Fall von angeborenen grunlicher. Verfarbung der cornea. *Klin Monatsbl Augenheilkd* 1902;40:22–5.

6. Fleischer B. Zwei weitere Falle von grunlicher Verfarbung der Kornea. *Klin Monatsbl Augenheilkd* 1903;41:489–91.

7. Fleischer B. Ueber eine der "Pseudosclerose" nahestehende bisher unbekante Krankheit (gekennzeignet durch Tremor, psychische Storungen, braunliche Pigmentierung bestimmter Gewebe, insbezondere Hornhautperipherie, Lebercirrhose). *Dtsch Z Nervenheilkd* 1912;44:179–201.

8. Jess A. Hornhautverkupferung in Form des Fleischerschen Pigmentringes bei der Pseudosclerose. *Klin Monatsbl Augenheilkd* 1922;69:218.

9. Siermerling E, Oloff H. Pseudosclerose mit Cornealring und doppelseitiger Scheinkatarakt, die nur bei seitlicher Beleuchtung sichtbar und die nach der Verletzung durch Kupfersplitter entstehenden Katarakten ahnlich ist. *Klin Wochenschr* 1922;1:1087–9.

10. Scheinberg IH, Gitlin D. Deficiency of ceruloplasmin in patients with hepatolenticular degeneration (Wilson's disease). *Science* 1952;116:484–5.

11. Sternlieb I, Scheinberg IH. Prevention of Wilson's disease in asymptomatic patients. *N Engl J Med* 1968;278:352–9.

12. Cumings JN. The effect of BAL in hepatolenticular degeneration. *Brain* 1951;74:10–22.

13. Denny Brown D, Porter H. The effect of BAL (2,3 dimercaptopropanol) on hepatolenticular degeneration (Wilson's disease). *N Engl J Med* 1951;245:917–25.

14. Walshe JM. The conquest of Wilson's disease. *Brain* 2009;132:2289–2295.

15. Walshe JM. Disturbances of amino acid metabolism following liver injury. *Q J Med* 1953;22:483–507.

16. Walshe JM. Copper chelation in patients with Wilson's disease: a comparison of penicillamine and triethylene tetramine dihydrochloride. *Q J Med* 1973;42:441–52.

17. Walshe JM. Tetramolybdate (MoS4) as an anti-copper agent in man. In: Scheinberg IH, Walshe JM, eds. *Orphan Diseases and Orphan Drugs.* Manchester: University Press, 1986:76–86.

18. Schouwink G. De hepatoberebrale degeneratie, met een onderzoek naar de zinkstofwisseling. Thesis, University of Amsterdam, 1961.

19. Hoogenraad TU, van Hattum J, Van den Hamer CJ. Management of Wilson's disease with zinc sulphate. Experience in a series of 27 patients. *J Neurol Sci* 1987;77:137–46.

20. Brewer GJ, Dick RD, Yuzbasiyan-Gurkan V, et al. Treatment of Wilson's disease with zinc. XIII. Therapy with zinc in presymptomatic patients from the time of diagnosis. *J Lab Clin Med* 1994;123:849–58.

21. Groth CG, Dubois RS, Corman J, et al. Metabolic effects of hepatic transplantation in Wilson's disease. *Transplant Proc* 1973;1:829–33.

22. Hall HC. *La Dègènèrescence Hèpato-lenticulaire: maladie de Wilson-pseudosclèrose.* Paris: Masson, 1921.

23. Bearn AG, Kunkel HG. Genetic and biochemical aspects of Wilson's disease. *Am J Med* 1953;15:442–6.

24. Frydman M, Bonne-Tammir B, Farrer LA, et al. Assignment of the gene for Wilson disease to chromosome 13: linkage to the esterase D locus. *Proc Natl Acad Sci USA* 1985;82:1819–21.

25. Houwen RH, Scheffer H, Te-Meerman GJ, et al. Close linkage of the Wilson's disease locus to D13S12 in the chromosomal region 13q21 and not to EDD in 13q14. *Hum Genet* 1990;85:560–2.

26. Bowcock AM, Farrer LA, Hebert JM, et al. Eight closely linked loci place the Wilson disease locus within 13q14-q21. *Am J Hum Genet* 1988;43:664–74.

27. Vulpe C, Levinson B, Whitney S, et al. Isolation of a candidate gene for Menkes disease and evidence that it encodes a copper-transporting ATPase. *Nat Genet* 1993;3:7–13.

28. Chelly J, Tumer Z, Tonnesen T, et al. Isolation of a candidate gene for Menkes' disease that encodes a potential heavy metal-binding protein. *Nat Genet* 1993;3:14–19.

29. Mercer JFB, Livingston J, Hall B, et al. Isolation of a partial candidate gene for Menkes' disease by positional cloning. *Nat Genet* 1993;3:20–5.

30. Tanzi RE, Petrukhin K, Chernov I, et al. The Wilson's disease gene is a copper-transporting ATPase with homology to the Menkes' disease gene. *Nat Genet* 1993;5:344–50.

31. Petrukhin K, Fischer SG, Pirastu M, et al. Mapping, cloning and genetic characterization of the region containing the Wilson disease gene. *Nat Genet* 1993;5:338–43.

32. Bull PC, Thomas GR, Rommens JM, et al. The Wilson disease gene is a putative copper transporting P-type ATPase similar to the Menkes gene. *Nat Genet* 1993;5:327–37.

33. Yamaguchi Y, Heiny ME, Gitlin JD. Isolation and characterization of a human liver cDNA as a candidate gene for Wilson's disease. *Biochem Biophys Res Commun* 1993;197:271–7.

34. Petrukhin K, Lutsenko S, Chernov I, et al. Characterization of the Wilson's disease gene encoding a P-type copper transporting ATPase: genomic organization, alternative splicing, and structure/function predictions. *Hum Mol Genet* 1994;3:1647–56.

35. Solioz M, Vulpe C. CPx-type ATPases: a class of P-type ATPases that pump heavy metals. *Trends Biochem Sci* 1996;21:237–41.

36. Cox DW. Molecular advances in Wilson disease. In: Boyer JL, Ockner RK, eds. *Progress in Liver Disease.* Philadelphia: WB Saunders, 1996:245–64.

37. Shah AB, Chernov I, Zhang HT, et al. Identification and analysis of mutations in the Wilson disease gene (ATP7B): population frequencies, genotype-phenotype correlation, and functional analyses. *Am J Hum Genet* 1997;61:317–28.

38. Maier-Dobersberger T, Ferenci P, Polli C, et al. Detection of the His 1069 Glu mutation in Wilson disease by rapid polymerase chain reaction. *Ann Intern Med* 1997;127:21–6.

39. Stuehler B, Reichert J, Stremmel W. et al. Analysis of the human homologue of the canine copper toxicosis gene MURR1 in Wilson disease patients. *J Mol Med* 2004;82(9):629–34.

40. Mufti AR, Burstein E, Csomos RA, et al. XIAP Is a copper binding protein deregulated in Wilson's disease and other copper toxicosis disorders. *Mol Cell* 2006;21(6):775–85.

41. Zhou B, Gitscher J. hCTR1: a human gene for copper uptake identified by complementation in yeast. *Proc Natl Acad Sci USA* 1997;94:7481–6.

42. Freedman JH, Ciriolo MR, Peisach J. The role of glutathione in copper metabolism and toxicity. *J Biol Chem* 1989;264:5598–605.

43. Schilsky ML, Blank RR, Czaja MJ, et al. Hepatocellular copper toxicity and its attenuation by zinc. *J Clin Invest* 1989;84:1562–8.

44. Klomp LW, Liu SJ, Yuan DS, et al. Identification and functional expression of HAH1, a novel human gene involved in copper homeostasis. *J Biol Chem* 1997;272:9221–6.

45. Lewis KO. The nature of the copper complexes in bile and their relationship to the absorption and excretion of copper in normal subjects and in Wilson's disease. *Gut* 1973;14:221–32.

46. Hung IH, Suzuki M, Yamaguchi Y, et al. Biochemical characterization of the Wilson disease protein and functional expression in the yeast Saccharomyces cerevisiae. *J Biol Chem* 1997;272:21461–6.

47. Petris MJ, Mercer JFB, Culvenor JG, et al. Ligand-regulated transport of the Menkes' copper P-type ATPase efflux pump from the Golgi apparatus to the plasma membrane: a novel mechanism of regulated trafficking. *EMBO J* 1996;15:6084–95.

48. Roelofsen H, Wolters H, Van Luyn MJ, et al. Copper-induced apical trafficking of ATP7B in polarized hepatoma cells provides a mechanism for biliary copper excretion. *Gastroenterology* 2000;119:782–93.

49. O'Reilly S, Weber PM, Oswald M, et al. Abnormalities of the physiology of copper. *Arch Neurol* 1971;25:28–32.

50. Sternlieb I, van den Hamer CJA, Morell AG, et al. Lysosomal defect of hepatic copper excretion in Wilson's disease (hepatolenticular degeneration). *Gastroenterology* 1973;64:99–105.

51. Gollan JL, Deller DT. Studies on the nature and excretion of biliary copper in man. *Clin Sci* 1973;44:9–15.

52. Terada K, Kawarda Y, Muira N, et al. Copper incorporation into ceruloplasmin in rat livers. *Biochim Biophys Acta* 1995;1270:58–62.

53. Sternlieb I. Copper and zinc. In: Arias IM, Boyer JL, Fausto N, et al., eds. *The Liver: biology and pathobiology*, Vol. 3. New York: Raven Press, 1994:585–96.

54. Ferenci P, Gilliam TC, Gitlin JD, et al. An international symposium on Wilson's and Menkes' diseases. *Hepatology* 1996;24:952–8.

55. Strand S, Hofmann WJ, Grambihler A, et al. Hepatic failure and liver cell damage in acute Wilson's disease involve CD95 (APO-1/Fas)-mediated apoptosis. *Nat Med* 1998;4:588–93.

56. Ala A, Borjigin J, Rochwarger A, et al. Wilson disease in septuagenarian siblings: raising the bar for diagnosis. *Hepatology* 2005;41:668–70.

57. Alt E, Sternlieb I, Goldfischer S. The cytopathology of metal overload [Review]. *Int Rev Exp Pathol* 1990;31:165–88.

58. Sternlieb I. Mitochondrial and fatty changes in hepatocytes of patients with Wilson's disease. *Gastroenterology* 1968;55:354–67.

59. Goldfischer S, Sternlieb I. Changes in the distribution of hepatic copper in relation to the progression of Wilson's disease (hepatolenticular degeneration). *Am J Pathol* 1968;53:883–901.

60. Pilloni L, Lecca S, Van Eycken P, et al. Value of histochemical stains for copper in the diagnosis of Wilson's disease. *Histopathology* 1998;33:28–33.

61. Scheinberg IH, Sternlieb I. *Wilson's Disease*. Philadelphia, PA: WB Saunders, 1984.

62. Opalski A. Type spècial de cellules neurologiqes dans la dègènèrescence lenticulaire progressive. *Z Gesamte Neurol Psychiatrie* 1930;124:420.

63. Steindl P, Ferenci P, Dienes HP, et al. Wilson's disease in patients presenting with liver disease: a diagnostic challenge. *Gastroenterology* 1997;113:212–18.

64. McMillin GA, Travis JJ, Hunt JW. Direct measurement of free copper in serum or plasma ultrafiltrate. *Am J Clin Pathol* 2009;131:160–5.

65. Martins da Costa C, Baldwin D, Portmann B, et al. Value of urinary copper excretion after penicillamine challenge in the diagnosis of Wilson's disease. *Hepatology* 1992;15:609–15.

66. Schilsky ML. Non-invasive testing for Wilson disease: revisiting the d-penicillamine challenge test. *J Hepatol* 2007;47:172–3.

67. Ferenci P, Steindl-Munda P, Vogel W, et al. Diagnostic value of quantitative hepatic copper determination in patients with Wilson's disease. *Clin Gastroenterol Hepatol* 2005;3(8):811–18.

68. Schilsky ML, Scheinberg IH, Sternlieb I. Liver transplantation for Wilson's disease: indications and outcome. *Hepatology* 1994;19:583–7.

69. Walshe JM, Yealland M. Chelational treatment of neurological Wilson's disease. *Q J Med* 1993;86:197–204.

70. Factor SM, Cho S, Sternlieb I, et al. The cardiomyopathy of Wilson's disease: myocardial alterations in nine cases. *Virchows Arch* 1982;397:301–11.

71. Kuan P. Fatal cardiac complications of Wilson's disease. *Am Heart J* 1982;104:314–16.

72. Roberts EA, Schilsky ML. AASLD Practice Guidelines. Diagnosis and treatment of Wilson disease: an update. *Hepatology* 2008;47:2089–111.

73. Wilson RA, Clayson KJ, Leon S. Unmeasurable serum alkaline phosphatase activity in Wilson's disease associated with fulminant hepatic failure and hemolysis. *Hepatology* 1987;7:613–15.

74. Shaver WA, Bhatt H, Combes B. Low serum alkaline phosphatase activity in Wilson's disease. *Hepatology* 1986;6:859–63.

75. Berman DH, Leventhal RI, Gavaler JS, et al. Clinical differentiation of fulminant wilsonian hepatitis for other causes of hepatic failure. *Gastroenterology* 1991;100:1129–34.

76. McCullough AJ, Fleming CR, Thistle JL, et al. Diagnosis of Wilson's disease presenting as fulminant hepatic failure. *Gastroenterology* 1983;84:161–7.

77. Korman JD, Volenberg I, Balko J, et al.; Pediatric and Adult Acute Liver Failure Study Groups. Screening for Wilson disease in acute liver failure: a comparison of currently available diagnostic tests. *Hepatology* 2008;48:1167–74.

78. Brewer GJ, Terry CA, Aisen AM, et al. Worsening of neurologic syndrome in patients with Wilson's disease with metal penicillamine therapy. *Arch Neurol* 1987;44:490–3.

79. Scheinberg IH, Jaffe ME, Sternlieb I. The use of trientine in preventing the effects of interrupting penicillamine therapy in Wilson's disease. *N Engl J Med* 1987;317:209–13.

80. Santos-Silva EE, Sarles J, Buts JP, et al. Successful medical treatment of severely decompensated Wilson disease. *J Pediatr* 1996;128:285–7.

81. Saito H, Watanabe K, Sahera M, et al. Triethylene-tetramine (trien) therapy for Wilson's disease. *Tohoku J Exp Med* 1991;164:29–35.

82. Askari FK, Greenson J, Dick RD, et al. Treatment of Wilson's disease with zinc. XVIII. Initial treatment of the hepatic decompensation presentation with trientine and zinc. *J Lab Clin Med* 2003;142:385–90.

83. Brewer GJ, Johnson V, Dick RD, et al. Treatment of Wilson disease with ammonium tetrathiomolybdate. *Arch Neurol* 1996;53:1017–25.

84. Brewer GJ, Askari F, Lorincz MT, et al. Treatment of Wilson disease with ammonium tetrathiomolybdate: IV. Comparison of tetrathiomolybdate and trientine in a double-blind study of treatment of the neurologic presentation of Wilson disease. *Arch Neurol* 2006;63:521–7.

85. Scheinberg IH, Sternlieb I. Treatment of the neurologic manifestations of Wilson's disease. *Arch Neurol* 1995;52:339.

86. Bellary S, Hassanein T, Van Thiel D. Liver transplantation for Wilson's disease. *J Hepatol* 1995;23:373–81.

87. Emre S, Atillasoy EO, Ozdemir S, et al. Orthotopic liver transplantation for Wilson's disease: a single center experience. *Liver Transpl* 2001;72:1232–6.

88. Chen CL, Chen YS, Lui CC, et al. Neurologic improvement of Wilson's disease after liver transplantation. *Transplant Proc* 1997;29:497–8.

89. Asonuma K, Inomata Y, Kashara M, et al. Living related liver transplantation from heterozygote genetic carriers to children with Wilson's disease. *Pediatr Transplant* 1999;3:201–5.

90. Scheinberg IH, Sternlieb I. Pregnancy in penicillamine-treated patients with Wilson's disease. *N Engl J Med* 1975;293:1300–2.

91. Walshe JM. Pregnancy in Wilson's disease. *Q J Med* 1977;181:73–83.

92. Walshe JM. The management of pregnancy in Wilson's disease treated with trientine. *Q J Med* 1986;58:81–7.

93. Brewer GJ, Johnson VD, Dick RD, et al. Treatment of Wilson's disease with zinc. XVII: Treatment during pregnancy. *Hepatology* 2000;31:364–70.

94. Sternlieb I. Wilson's disease and pregnancy. *Hepatology* 2000;31:531–2.

95. Brewer GJ, Yuzbasiyan-Gurkan V. Wilson's disease. *Medicine* 1992;71:139–64.

96. Schilsky ML, Scheinberg IH, Sternlieb I. Prognosis of wilsonian chronic active hepatitis. *Gastroenterology* 1991;100:762–7.

Multiple choice questions

29.1 **What clinical and biochemical tests help diagnose Wilson disease?**

   a Ceruloplasmin.
   b Slit-lamp examination for Kayser–Fleischer rings.
   c 24-hour urine copper.
   d Liver copper content.
   e Molecular testing for ATP7B mutations.
   f All of the above.

29.2 **Which of the following is not true for patients with acute liver failure due to Wilson disease?**

   a Serum and urine copper are extremely elevated.
   b Hemolytic anemia is caused by nonimmune-mediated mechanisms.
   c Transplantation is indicated for these patients.
   d Advanced fibrosis or cirrhosis is always present in the liver of the patient.
   e Exchange transfusion, albumin dialysis, plasmapheresis, or other methods aimed at copper removal from the circulation may help stabilize a patient awaiting transplantation.
   f Living donor transplant using a parent as a donor is never possible for these patients.

29.3 **Which of the following treatments are not useful as a treatment for Wilson disease?**

   a D-penicillamine.
   b Trientine.
   c Zinc.
   d Desferrioxamine.
   e Liver transplant.

Answers to the multiple choice questions can be found in the Appendix at the end of the book.

These multiple choice questions are also available for you to complete online.
Visit http://www.schiffsdiseasesoftheliver.com/

CHAPTER 30

Hemochromatosis and Iron Storage Disorders

Bruce R. Bacon & Robert S. Britton

School of Medicine, Division of Gastroenterology and Hepatology, Saint Louis University, St Louis, MO, USA

Key concepts

- An increase in systemic iron levels is the consequence of: (i) inherited excessive intestinal absorption of dietary iron (hereditary hemochromatosis); (ii) ineffective erythropoiesis or chronic liver disease; or (iii) parenteral iron administration. Excessive intracellular deposition of iron ultimately results in tissue and organ damage.
- Hereditary hemochromatosis (HH) constitutes several inherited disorders characterized by an increased intestinal absorption of iron with its subsequent accumulation in tissues. Most (approximately 90%) patients with HH have mutations in the *HFE* gene, and *HFE*-related HH is one of the most common inherited disorders among whites, with a frequency of about one in 250.
- Two independent mutations of the *HFE* gene are principally responsible for *HFE*-related HH. These mutations result in a change of cysteine to tyrosine at amino acid 282 (C282Y) and of histidine to aspartic acid at amino acid 63 (H63D) of the HFE protein. Approximately 95% of persons with *HFE*-related HH are homozygous for the C282Y mutation. Population studies indicate that the penetrance of the C282Y mutation is incomplete, and genetic modifiers may be involved. Some compound heterozygotes with copies of both the C282Y and H63D mutations have a clinically significant degree of iron overload.
- Mutations in the iron-related genes encoding for hemojuvelin, hepcidin, ferroportin, transferrin receptor 2 (TFR2), divalent metal transporter 1, and ferritin result in non-*HFE*-related HH.
- The pathogenesis of nearly all forms of HH involves an inappropriately low expression of the iron-regulatory hormone hepcidin, which acts to decrease the export of iron from absorptive enterocytes and reticuloendothelial cells. Hepcidin is highly expressed in hepatocytes, and it is proposed that HFE protein, TFR2, and hemojuvelin all play a role in the hepatic iron-signaling pathway that regulates hepcidin expression. The C282Y mutation causes functional inactivation of the HFE protein, leading to low hepcidin expression with a resultant increase in duodenal iron absorption.
- In *HFE*-related HH, the excess iron is preferentially deposited in the cytoplasm of parenchymal cells of various organs and tissues, including the liver, pancreas, heart, endocrine glands, skin, and joints. Damage can result in micronodular cirrhosis of the liver and atrophy of the pancreas (primarily islets). Hepatocellular carcinoma, usually in the presence of cirrhosis, is another consequence of excess iron deposition in the liver. Symptoms are related to damage of the involved organs and include liver failure (from cirrhosis), diabetes mellitus, arthritis, cardiac dysfunction (arrhythmias and failure), and hypogonadotropic hypogonadism.
- The diagnosis of iron overload includes serum iron studies (elevated transferrin saturation, elevated serum ferritin levels), genetic testing, and sometimes liver biopsy to assess the hepatic iron concentration and degree of liver injury. In cases of *HFE*-related HH, liver biopsy is usually not indicated if the patient has normal liver enzyme levels and a serum ferritin level below 1,000 ng/mL. Because regular phlebotomy therapy prevents or reverses the accumulation of excess iron and prevents the complications of HH, it is important to identify persons with this inherited disorder early in the disease process.

History

The first medical description of a patient with hemochromatosis was by Trousseau [1] in the French pathology literature in 1865 (Table 30.1). Twenty-four years later, the German pathologist von Recklinghausen [2] was the first to use the term *hemochromatosis*; he thought that the pigmentation ("chrom") in the tissues of patients with the disorder was caused by something circulating in their blood ("hemo"). In 1935, Joseph Sheldon [3], a British geriatrician, published a monograph describing the 311 cases of hemochromatosis that existed in the world literature up to that time. Sheldon concluded that hemochromatosis is an inherited disorder in which tissue injury and damage result from excess iron deposition. He drew accurate conclusions without the techniques of modern molecular medicine available today. The situation was somewhat confused by MacDonald [4], a pathologist at the Boston City Hospital, who believed that hemochromatosis was a nutritional disorder, possibly because he

---

Schiff's Diseases of the Liver, Eleventh Edition. Edited by Eugene R. Schiff, Willis C. Maddrey and Michael F. Sorrell.
© 2012 John Wiley & Sons, Ltd. Published 2012 by John Wiley & Sons, Ltd.

Table 30.1 Milestones in *HFE*-related hereditary hemochromatosis.

Year	Event	Reference
~1–300 AD	C282Y mutation of *HFE* in Celtic population	
1865	First case described	Trousseau [1]
1889	Coined the term hemochromatosis	von Recklinghausen [2]
1935	Postulated HH is an inherited defect of iron metabolism	Sheldon [3]
1950	First liver biopsy in HH, and first phlebotomy therapy	Davis & Arrowsmith [189]
1976	Benefit of phlebotomy therapy described	Bomford & Williams [190]
1976	Linkage to HLA-A	Simon et al. [6]
1985	Benefit of early diagnosis and therapy	Niederau et al. [102]
1996	*HFE* gene cloned, and C282Y and H63D mutations described	Feder et al. [7]
1998	*Hfe* knock-out mouse has iron overload	Zhou et al. [45]
2001	Hepcidin as iron-regulatory hormone	Nicolas et al. [73]
2003	Low hepcidin expression in *HFE*-related HH	Bridle et al. [79]
1997 to present	Cell biology of iron-related proteins	Many

HH, hereditary hemochromatosis; HLA, human leukocyte antigen.

saw many alcoholic patients who happened to be of Irish descent. It is now known that the prevalence of homozygosity for *HFE*-related hereditary hemochromatosis (HH) is high in the Irish population, approaching 1 in 70 persons [5]. In 1976, Marcel Simon et al. [6] definitively showed that classic hemochromatosis is inherited as an autosomal recessive disorder, with linkage to the human leukocyte antigen (HLA) region of the human genome; the gene for hemochromatosis is located on the short arm of chromosome 6. It took another 20 years until the research group at Mercator Genetics successfully identified and cloned the hemochromatosis gene by means of a positional cloning approach using DNA samples from well-documented patients with hemochromatosis in the United States [7]. In 1996, Feder et al. [7] identified *HFE*, a novel major histocompatibility complex (MHC) class I-like gene; homozygosity for a single missense mutation (C282Y) of *HFE* was found in 83% of the patients who were studied. Quickly, several other groups reported their findings in series of patients with hemochromatosis, and homozygosity for the C282Y mutation was found in about 85–90% of typical patients [8]. This discovery has yielded significant benefits in clinical medicine and hepatology, including more accurate diagnosis of *HFE*-related HH, improved family screening, and evaluation of the role of *HFE* mutations in other liver diseases. Additionally, there has been a wealth of new information about the cellular and molecular mechanisms of iron homeostasis, including the discovery of the iron-regulatory hormone hepcidin. In this chapter, we highlight the new advances in the area of HH and other iron storage disorders, interdigitating these discoveries with the classic pathologic and clinical features seen in these patients.

Classification of iron overload syndromes

Many terms have been used in the past to describe HH, such as idiopathic, primary, and familial. The term *hereditary hemochromatosis* should be reserved to describe inherited disorders of iron metabolism that lead to tissue iron loading (Box 30.1). The most common form of this disease, *HFE*-related HH, is caused primarily by homozygosity for the C282Y mutation in the *HFE* gene. However, other heritable forms of iron overload have also been recognized (non-*HFE*-related HH). These include: (i) autosomal recessive forms of HH characterized by rapid iron accumulation and caused by mutations in the genes for hemojuvelin and hepcidin (also called juvenile hemochromatosis) [9,10]; (ii) an autosomal dominant form of HH caused by mutations in the ferroportin gene [11,12]; (iii) an autosomal recessive form of HH resulting from mutations in the gene for transferrin receptor 2 (*TFR2*) [13]; and (iv) rare forms of HH resulting from mutations in the *divalent metal transporter 1 (DMT1)* gene [14] or in the regulatory region of ferritin messenger RNA [15]. Some other types of iron overload may have a heritable component but the genes involved have not yet been identified. For example, African iron overload is a familial disorder of iron loading prevalent in sub-Saharan Africa that is exacerbated by the ingestion of iron-rich home-brewed beer [16]. The degree of iron loading can be similar to that in *HFE*-related HH, but the cellular and lobular distribution of iron is different. In addition, a rare disorder termed congenital alloimmune (neonatal) iron overload is characterized by severe neonatal liver injury in association with parenchymal iron accumulation and extrahepatic siderosis [17,18].

Box 30.1 Classification of iron overload syndromes.

Hereditary hemochromatosis

- *HFE*-related:
    C282Y/C282Y
    C282Y/H63D
    Other *HFE* mutations
- Non-*HFE*-related:
    Hemojuvelin (*HJV*) mutations (autosomal recessive)
    Hepcidin (*HAMP*) mutations (autosomal recessive)
    Ferroportin (*SLC40A1*) mutations (autosomal dominant)
    Transferrin receptor 2 (*TFR2*) mutations (autosomal recessive)
    Divalent metal transporter 1 (*SLC11A2*) mutations (rare)
    Ferritin regulatory mutations (rare)
- Miscellaneous:
    African iron overload
    Congenital alloimmune (neonatal) iron overload (rare)

Secondary iron overload

- Anemia caused by ineffective erythropoiesis:
    Thalassemia major
    Sideroblastic anemias
- Congenital dyserythropoietic anemias
- Congenital atransferrinemia:
    Aceruloplasminemia
- Liver disease:
    Alcoholic liver disease
    Chronic viral hepatitis B and C
    Porphyria cutanea tarda
    Nonalcoholic steatohepatitis
    After portacaval shunt
- Miscellaneous:
    Excessive iron ingestion

Parenteral iron overload

- Red blood cell transfusions
- Iron–dextran injections
- Associated with long-term dialysis

Several noninherited syndromes of iron overload are known. In secondary iron overload, an underlying disorder causes an increase in iron absorption; examples are disorders of ineffective erythropoiesis and liver disease [19]. Parenteral iron overload is an iatrogenic disorder in which blood transfusions or iron–dextran injections are given to patients who are anemic [20].

In *HFE*-related HH, it has become clear from population studies that not all individuals who have the C282Y/C282Y genotype become iron loaded. This observation indicates that there are many nonexpressing C282Y homozygotes in the population [21–23] and has led to a four-category description of *HFE*-related HH: (i) genetic predisposition with no other abnormality; (ii) iron overload (approximately 2–5 g) but without symptoms or tissue damage; (iii) iron overload with early symptoms (i.e.,

lethargy, arthralgias); and (iv) iron overload with organ damage, particularly cirrhosis.

HFE-related hereditary hemochromatosis

Since the work of Simon et al. in the mid-1970s [6], it has been known that the major gene for HH is located on the short arm of chromosome 6 in the HLA region of the genome. In 1996, investigators at Mercator Genetics used a positional cloning approach to identify *HFE* as the responsible gene [7]. *HFE* codes for a novel MHC class I-like protein that requires interaction with β_2-microglobulin (β_2M) for normal presentation on the cell surface [7]. Structural homology with other MHC class I proteins and X-ray crystallographic studies indicate that HFE protein has a large extracellular domain with three α-loops, a single transmembrane region, and a short cytoplasmic tail [7,24]. In the original work by Feder et al. [7], two missense mutations were identified in *HFE*, one resulting in a change of cysteine to tyrosine at amino acid 282 (C282Y) and the second causing a change of histidine to aspartate at amino acid 63 (H63D). Other *HFE* mutations have been identified, but their frequency is low and their clinical impact is limited. Feder et al. [7] reported that 148 (83%) of 178 patients with typical phenotypic HH were homozygous for the C282Y mutation while eight (4%) patients were compound heterozygotes, with one allele containing the C282Y mutation and the other allele containing the H63D mutation. These findings were confirmed by subsequent studies that showed that 60–100% (mean value, 84%) of patients with typical phenotypic HH were homozygous for C282Y [8]. Of interest, approximately 6% of these patients had a clinical syndrome phenotypically similar to that of patients with typical HH but were negative for either *HFE* mutation [8]. Some of these patients may have had mutations in known iron-related genes or in as yet unidentified genes involved in iron metabolism.

HFE gene and protein

The *HFE* gene is expressed at relatively low levels in most human tissues [7]. However, unlike other classic MHC class I genes, *HFE* is rarely expressed in lymphopoietic and hematopoietic cells [7]. Little is known of the regulation of *HFE* gene expression. In contrast to the expression of genes for other MHC molecules, *HFE* expression is not induced in cultured cells by various cytokines. Sequences known to confer transcriptional regulation by cellular metal ion content have not been identified in the *HFE* gene. Furthermore, sequences homologous to iron-responsive elements (IREs) have not been identified in either the 3'- or 5'-untranslated region of *HFE* mRNA. However, several splice variants of human *HFE* mRNA have been identified. An HFE transcript lacking exons 6 and 7 has been detected (by means of reverse transcription followed by polymerase chain reaction) in human duodenum, spleen, breast, skin, and testicle [25]. Because this transcript does not include the sequences encoding the transmembrane and cytoplasmic domains, it is predicted to encode a secretory form of HFE protein. HFE splice variant transcripts lacking exon 2 and/or a portion of exon 4 have been identified in a human liver cell line, a colon carcinoma cell line, and an ovarian cell line [26]. Deletion of exon 2 is predicted to eliminate the α_1-loop of HFE protein, whereas deletion of a portion of exon 4 is predicted to affect the α_3-loop. The levels of protein expression and physiologic roles of the splice variant HFE transcripts are not yet known.

The *HFE* gene encodes a 343-amino acid protein consisting of a 22-amino acid signal peptide, a large extracellular domain, a single transmembrane domain, and a short cytoplasmic tail [7]. HFE protein is widely expressed in several organs including the liver, placenta, and gastrointestinal tract (i.e., epithelium of esophagus, stomach, duodenum, small intestine, and colon) [27]. The extracellular domain of HFE protein consists of three loops (α_1, α_2, and α_3), with intramolecular disulfide bonds within the second and third loops. The structure of HFE protein is therefore similar to that of other MHC class I proteins. The two common *HFE* mutations, C282Y and H63D, are in the extracellular domain. Crystallographic studies demonstrate that the α_1- and α_2-loops of HFE protein form a superdomain consisting of antiparallel β-strands topped by two antiparallel α-helices [24]. The groove between the antiparallel α-helices is analogous to the peptide-binding groove in antigen-presenting MHC class I proteins. Several lines of evidence, however, suggest that HFE protein does not participate in antigen presentation. The groove between the α-helices in HFE protein is physically narrower than that in antigen-presenting MHC class I molecules, so that the ability to bind peptides is precluded. Indeed, N-terminal sequencing performed on acid eluates from HFE protein found no evidence of peptide binding [24]. HFE protein, like other MHC class I molecules, is physically associated with β_2M. This association has been demonstrated in the human duodenum and placenta [27], and in cultured cells [28–30].

C282Y mutation of *HFE*

The C282Y mutation results in the substitution of tyrosine for cysteine at amino acid 282 in the α_3-loop and abolishes the disulfide bond in this domain [7]. Loss of the disulfide bond was predicted to interfere with the interaction of β_2M with HFE protein [7]. Indeed, C282Y mutant protein expressed in cell culture systems demonstrates diminished binding with β_2M and decreased presentation at the cell surface in comparison with wild-type HFE protein [28,29]. The C282Y mutant protein is retained in the endo-

plasmic reticulum and middle Golgi compartments, fails to undergo late Golgi processing, and is subject to accelerated degradation [29]. However, some C282Y mutant protein in patients with HH reaches the cell surface, as detected by immunohistochemistry, although at reduced levels [31]. Definitive proof that this mutation can cause HH was provided when knock-in of the C282Y mutation in mice resulted in iron overload [32].

The C282Y mutation is present in most, but not all, patients with a clinical diagnosis of HH. The proportion of patients with HH who are homozygous for C282Y varies in different populations. In the United States, Britain, Australia, Canada, and France, approximately 85–90% of patients with a clinical diagnosis of HH are homozygous for C282Y [8], but a lower frequency (60%) has been reported in Italy [33]. Conversely, population studies have revealed that the clinical features of HH do not develop in many C282Y homozygotes [21–23]. This observation suggests incomplete penetrance of the C282Y mutation and raises the possibility that other genes involved in iron homeostasis may act as modifiers of the HH phenotype [34,35].

The prevalence of the C282Y mutation is greatest in whites of European ancestry. In this population, the carrier frequency ranges from 10% to 15% [5,8,17,18]. In other ethnic populations, the C282Y mutation is less common and is always associated with the ancestral white haplotype [36,37]. Such studies suggest that the C282Y mutation occurred once on an ancestral (possibly Celtic) haplotype that spread from northern Europe to other regions of the world [38,39]. The observation that the haplotype containing the C282Y mutation extends for approximately 7 megabases suggests that the mutation arose during the last 2,000 years [40]. It has been proposed that the C282Y mutation, associated with increased iron absorption and the accumulation of body iron stores, provided a selective advantage to a population in which the availability of dietary iron was limited or in which intestinal parasitic infections caused a loss of iron.

H63D mutation of *HFE*

The most common *HFE* mutation in the general population is a missense mutation that results in the substitution of aspartate for histidine at amino acid 63 (H63D) of the HFE protein [7]. The H63D mutation is found at a frequency of 15–40% in white populations [8], but homozygosity for H63D appears to increase the risk for iron loading only slightly [41]. However, the frequency of compound heterozygosity for the H63D and C282Y mutations is greater in patients with iron overload than that predicted for the general population [7,8]. It is estimated that the risk for iron loading of the C282Y/H63D compound heterozygote is nearly 200-fold lower than that for the C282Y homozygote [42]. The population distribution of the H63D mutation differs somewhat from that of C282Y. The highest frequencies of H63D are found in European countries bordering the Mediterranean, the Middle East, and the Indian subcontinent [39]. The H63D mutation has been found on many haplotypes, which suggests that this less consequential mutation may have arisen historically multiple times and in different populations. Because the haplotype comprising the H63D mutation is shorter (approximately 700 kb) than that of the C282Y mutation, it is thought to be evolutionarily older [40].

Other mutations of *HFE*

HFE mutations other than C282Y and H63D have been identified in isolated patients with iron overload [43,44]. These include missense mutations (e.g., S65C, G93R, I105T, Q127H), splice site mutations (e.g., IVS3+1 G/T, IVS5+1 G/A), frameshift mutations (e.g., V68ΔT, P160ΔC), and nonsense mutations (e.g., R74X, E168X, W169X). Each symptomatic patient carrying one of the missense mutations has carried the C282Y or H63D mutation on the other allele. The two identified splice site mutations cause altered mRNA splicing and exon skipping, resulting in abnormal variants of HFE protein. The frameshift and nonsense mutations result in the production of truncated forms of HFE protein. The relative contribution of *HFE* mutations other than C282Y or H63D to the overall incidence of *HFE*-related HH is small.

Experimental disruption of the *Hfe* gene in mice

Transgenic methodology has provided important information about the functional consequences of *Hfe* gene disruption in the whole animal. Four different murine models have been generated: an exon 4 knock-out [45], an exon 3 disruption/exon 4 knock-out [32], an exon 2–3 knock-out [46], and a C282Y knock-in (32)[32]. These mice manifest increases in hepatic iron levels [32,45,46], transferrin saturation (TS) [45], and intestinal iron absorption [46]. No immunologic consequences of *Hfe* disruption have been observed in mice [46]. Like patients with *HFE*-related HH, these mice demonstrate relative sparing of iron loading in reticuloendothelial (RE) cells [32,45]. Interestingly, iron loading in mice that are homozygous for the C282Y mutation is less severe than that in *Hfe* knock-out mice, which indicates that the C282Y mutation is not a null allele [32]. Strain differences determine the severity of iron accumulation in *Hfe* knock-out mice, supporting the concept that there are genetic modifiers of the HH phenotype [35,47].

Determinants of duodenal iron absorption

An increase in intestinal iron absorption is a key characteristic of HH [48–50], and, therefore, understanding the pathogenesis of HH requires a review of the determinants of duodenal iron absorption. Because there are no significant physiologic mechanisms to regulate iron loss, iron homeostasis is dependent on tightly linking body iron requirements (approximately 1 mg/day) with intestinal iron absorption. Nearly all absorption of dietary iron occurs in the duodenum, where iron may be taken up either as ionic iron or as heme [50]. The absorption of both forms of iron is increased in patients with HH. Uptake of heme occurs by an as yet unidentified transporter. Absorption of ionic iron across the enterocytes occurs in two stages: uptake across the apical membrane and transfer across the basolateral membrane (Fig. 30.1). Before uptake, ionic iron requires reduction from the ferric to the ferrous state. This is accomplished by the ferric reductases (such as Dcytb), which are expressed on the luminal surface of duodenal enterocytes [51]. The ferrous iron crosses the apical membrane using the transporter DMT1 [52,53]. Iron taken up by the enterocyte may be stored as ferritin (and excreted in the feces when the senescent enterocyte is sloughed) or transferred across the basolateral membrane to the plasma. This latter process occurs through the transporter ferroportin [54–56]. The basolateral transfer of iron requires oxidation of iron to the ferric state by the ferroxidase, hephaestin [57]. In addition to increased uptake of iron from the diet, patients with *HFE*-related HH demonstrate increased basolateral transfer of iron from the enterocytes to the plasma, and this may be a driving force behind the increased intestinal iron absorption observed in *HFE*-related HH [49]. Some studies on patients with *HFE*-related HH [58–60] and *Hfe* knock out mice [61,62] have demonstrated increased expression of mRNAs encoding DMT1 and ferroportin. However, not all investigators have observed upregulation of DMT1 and ferroportin expression in patients with HH [63,64] or in *Hfe* knock-out mice [65,66]. In *Hfe* knock-out mice, these discrepancies may be due to differences in mouse strain [47] or age [67].

Several biologic factors influence the rate of dietary iron absorption. Reduction in body iron stores, increased erythropoietic activity, decreased blood hemoglobin content, and decreased blood oxygen saturation increase the absorption of iron from the diet [50]. In contrast, the presence of systemic inflammation decreases dietary iron absorption. All these factors are thought to act by influencing the levels of hepcidin, an iron-regulatory hormone.

Dysregulation of hepcidin in hereditary hemochromatosis

Hepcidin is a 25-amino acid peptide, first identified in urine and plasma as an antimicrobial peptide [68–70]. However, its role in influencing systemic iron status has become paramount, and it is now considered to be the principal iron-regulatory hormone [71,72]. The first

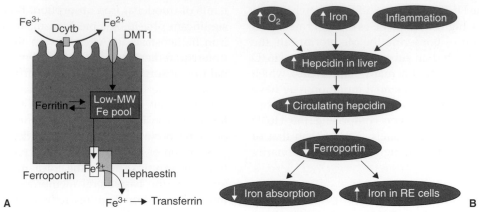

Figure 30.1 Iron absorption and the role of hepcidin. (A) Absorption of dietary ionic iron across the duodenal villus enterocyte occurs in two stages: uptake across the apical membrane and transfer across the basolateral membrane. Ferric reductases (such as Dcytb) are expressed on the luminal surface of duodenal enterocyte and are required for the reduction of ferric to ferrous iron, which then crosses the apical membrane via divalent metal transporter (DMT1). Iron taken up by the enterocyte is thought to enter a low molecular weight (MW) iron pool and is then stored as ferritin or transferred across the basolateral membrane to the plasma. On the basolateral surface of the enterocyte iron is oxidized to the ferric state by hephaestin, a ferroxidase and transported via ferroportin. Ferric iron is then bound to transferrin in the circulation. (B) Hepcidin expression by the liver is upregulated by increased iron, inflammation, or increased oxygen availability. The functional activity of ferroportin is decreased by hepcidin by binding to it and causing its internalization and degradation. In reticuloendothelial (RE) cells, this results in iron sequestration while in duodenal enterocytes it leads to decreased basolateral iron transfer and, therefore, decreased dietary iron absorption. Patients with hereditary hemochromatosis have low hepcidin expression with a consequent increase in iron absorption.

evidence that hepcidin is involved in iron homeostasis came from the observation that liver hepcidin mRNA expression is increased in mice with dietary iron loading [70]. The fortuitous discovery that knock-out of the hepcidin gene in the mouse led to a HH-like phenotype established the critical role of hepcidin as a negative regulator of intestinal iron absorption [73,74]. It was later discovered that hepcidin mutations are responsible for one form of juvenile hemochromatosis [10]. Factors regulating intestinal iron absorption (i.e., iron status, erythropoietic activity, hemoglobin levels, oxygen content, and inflammation) also regulate liver hepcidin expression (see Fig. 30.1). In each of these situations, intestinal iron absorption varies inversely with liver hepcidin expression. For example, animals with dietary iron overload [70] or systemic inflammation [75] have higher hepatic hepcidin mRNA levels, whereas animals subjected to hypoxia or hemolytic anemia have lower mRNA levels [76]. Hepcidin is an acute-phase reactant and plays a central role in the hypoferremia of inflammation (i.e., anemia of chronic diseases) [75,77]. Hepcidin acts to decrease the functional activity of the iron exporter ferroportin by binding to it and causing its internalization and degradation [78]. In the duodenal enterocyte, this leads to decreased basolateral iron transfer and, therefore, decreased dietary iron absorption.

Dysregulation of hepcidin expression is thought to play a key role in the pathogenesis of HH. Bridle et al. [79] demonstrated that patients with *HFE*-related HH have low hepatic expression of hepcidin, as do *Hfe* knock-out mice, despite excess hepatic iron stores [79–81]. In addition, urinary hepcidin levels are low in patients with HH caused by mutations in *HFE*, *TFR2*, and *HJV* [75,82–85]. Therefore, it is proposed that low circulating levels of hepcidin in these forms of HH cause increased ferroportin-mediated efflux of iron from both RE cells (resulting in iron sparing) and duodenal enterocytes (resulting in increased iron absorption).

Iron-dependent regulation of hepcidin in hepatocytes is mediated by bone morphogenetic protein 6 (BMP6) [86,87]. BMP6 binds to specific receptors on hepatocytes, and this triggers SMAD-dependent activation of hepcidin expression. Selective inhibition of BMP signaling abrogates iron-induced upregulation of hepcidin [87]. Interestingly, hemojuvelin is a BMP co-receptor, facilitating the binding of BMP6 to its receptor [86].

The molecular mechanisms by which HFE and TFR2 influence iron-dependent regulation of hepcidin remain unclear [13,86–88]. Mutations of *TFR2* cause a rare form of HH in humans [13] and *Tfr2* mutant mice have a HH phenotype [89]. Despite hepatic iron loading, hepcidin expression is low in patients with *TFR2*-related HH [85] and in *Tfr2* mutant mice [90]. This suggests that TFR2 protein is necessary for the appropriate transduction of the signal between body iron status and hepcidin expression [13,88]. Likewise, HFE protein may also modulate the BMP6 signaling pathway within hepatocytes because inactivating mutations of HFE result in low hepcidin expression and iron overload [96]. HFE protein binds avidly to the classic TFR1 [91], but it is not yet clear whether this interaction plays a part in the signaling pathway to hepcidin.

Non-*HFE*-related hereditary hemochromatosis

Although *HFE* mutations account for the vast majority of HH, other forms of HH have been recognized and are generally grouped together as non-*HFE*-related HH (see Box 30.1) [92]. Mutations in two different genes, *HJV* and *HAMP*, cause forms of juvenile HH. The *HJV* gene encodes hemojuvelin, a glycosylphosphatidylinositol-anchored protein that has substantial expression in hepatocytes. More than 25 disease-causing mutations have been described in *HJV* [9]. As a co-receptor of BMP6, hemojuvelin is involved in regulating the hepcidin pathway, and patients with *HJV*-associated HH [84] and *Hjv* knock-out mice [93,94] have a low hepcidin expression that is responsible for increased iron absorption. Inactivating mutations of the *HAMP* gene (that encodes hepcidin) also produce a form of juvenile HH [10].

Two distinct types of ferroportin mutations cause autosomal dominant HH [95,96]. The first type of mutation results in ferroportin inactivation, while the second type interferes with the interaction between ferroportin and hepcidin (but ferroportin retains its iron export capability). Inactivating ferroportin mutations cause a cellular distribution of iron loading that differs from that of *HFE*-related HH because iron is retained primarily in RE cells rather than hepatocytes [97]. Moreover, TS values tend to be lower than those in *HFE*-related HH. Individuals with the second type of ferroportin mutation fail to respond to hepcidin and therefore demonstrate a more classic HH phenotype. In both forms of ferroportin-related HH (unlike other types of HH), hepcidin expression is elevated rather than decreased [97].

Mutations in the *TFR2* gene produce an autosomal recessive type of HH that is clinically similar to *HFE*-related HH [13]. It is not yet known how these uncommon mutations of *TFR2* result in iron overload, but it is possible that they cause abnormal iron signaling to hepcidin within hepatocytes, the predominant site of *TFR2* expression [88].

DMT1 mediates iron uptake at the intestinal brush border and across the membrane of acidified endosomes in cells such as erythyroid precursors [98,99]. A single patient with severe hypochromic microcytic anemia and iron overload has been reported to carry a homozygous mutation (E399D) of DMT1 [14]. Cell biology studies suggest that E399D DMT1 protein has a partial loss of function that may limit iron availability to erythyroid precursor cells. The resulting anemia may subsequently stimulate dietary iron absorption, mediated by the partially functional DMT1 in enterocytes [100]. This may explain the distinguishing iron overload seen in this patient, along with microcytic anemia.

Ferritin, which is composed of H and L subunits, plays an important role in iron storage and intracellular iron distribution. Synthesis of both ferritin subunits is controlled by an iron-regulatory protein, which binds to the IRE in the 5'-untranslated region of the H- and L-ferritin mRNAs [101]. Kato et al. [15] identified a single point mutation (A49U) in the IRE motif of H-ferritin mRNA in four members of a Japanese family affected by dominantly inherited iron overload. When the mutated H-ferritin mRNA is expressed in cultured cells, there is an increase in iron uptake, suggesting that the A49U mutation may be responsible for tissue iron deposition.

Hereditary hemochromatosis

Clinical features

In older series of patients with typical phenotypic HH, a number of symptoms and physical findings generally associated with the disorder have been delineated (Boxes 30.2 and 30.3). Symptoms include fatigue, malaise, abdominal pain, arthralgias, and impotence. Physical findings include hepatomegaly, skin pigmentation, diabetes, and cardiac abnormalities [102–104]. All physicians should be aware of this constellation of symptoms and findings, but most patients who now come to medical attention have few of these signs or symptoms.

Box 30.2 Symptoms in patients with hereditary hemochromatosis.

Asymptomatic
- Abnormal serum iron study results on routine screening chemistry panel
- Evaluation of abnormal liver test results
- Identified by family screening
- Identified by population screening

Nonspecific, systemic symptoms
- Weakness
- Fatigue
- Lethargy
- Apathy
- Weight loss

Specific, organ-related symptoms
- Abdominal pain (hepatomegaly)
- Arthralgias (arthritis)
- Diabetes (pancreas)
- Amenorrhea (cirrhosis)
- Loss of libido and impotence (pituitary, cirrhosis)
- Congestive heart failure (heart)
- Arrhythmias (heart)

Box 30.3 Physical findings in patients with hereditary hemochromatosis.

Asymptomatic
- No physical findings
- Hepatomegaly

Symptomatic

Liver
- Hepatomegaly
- Cutaneous stigmata of chronic liver disease
- Splenomegaly
- Liver failure: ascites, encephalopathy

Joints
- Arthritis
- Joint swelling

Heart
- Dilated cardiomyopathy
- Congestive heart failure

Skin
- Increased pigmentation

Endocrine
- Diabetes
- Testicular atrophy
- Hypogonadism
- Hypothyroidism

More recent series in which patients were identified by family studies, abnormal iron study results on routine screening chemistry panels, or population surveys indicate that most patients are asymptomatic, even on spe-

cific questioning about the symptoms of HH [105,106]. When symptoms are present, they are the same as those described above, with fatigue and arthralgias being the most common. Therefore, in the face of abnormal iron study results, clinicians should not expect to see the usual symptoms or findings of "classic" HH but should recognize that many C282Y homozygotes are asymptomatic. Alcohol and chronic hepatitis C are potentiating factors in the development of hepatic fibrosis in patients with *HFE*-related HH [107–109].

Diagnosis

Once the diagnosis of HH is being considered for a patient after either an evaluation of the symptoms and findings listed in Boxes 30.2 and 30.3, or a workup for abnormal results of screening iron studies or a family study, then a definitive diagnosis is relatively straightforward [107–109]. The fasting TS ((serum iron level divided by transferrin level or total iron-binding capacity) × 100) and the serum levels of ferritin and liver enzymes should be determined (Table 30.2). It is important that the TS be obtained in the fasting state because the serum iron level varies diurnally, and many breakfast cereals that are highly fortified with iron can raise the serum iron level shortly after ingestion. An elevated TS ($\geq$45%) is recognized as the most common early phenotypic marker of HH; some patients who are homozygous for the C282Y mutation have elevated TS with a normal ferritin level. The sensitivity and specificity of these tests are difficult to determine when young persons are being evaluated (in whom increased iron stores may not have developed) or when patients have co-morbidities, such as chronic

Table 30.2 Diagnostic criteria for *HFE*-related hereditary hemochromatosis.

Measurements	Normal subjects	Patients with *HFE*-related HH
Blood (fasting)		
Serum iron (μg/dL)	60–180	180–300
Serum transferrin (mg/dL)	220–410	200–300
Transferrin saturation (%)	20–50	45–100
Serum ferritin (ng/mL):		
Men	20–200	150–6,000
Women	15–150	120–6,000
***HFE* mutation analysis**	wt/wt	C282Y/C282Y (homozygote)
		C282Y/H63D (compound heterozygote)
Liver		
Hepatic iron concentration:		
μg/g dry weight	300–1,500	1,500–30,000
μmol/g dry weight	5–27	27–550
Liver histology (Perls' Prussian blue stain)	0, 1+	2+ to 4+

wt, wild type.

liver disease (in which values may be falsely elevated). For example, serum ferritin levels are elevated in more than 50% of patients with alcoholic liver disease [110,111], nonalcoholic steatohepatitis (NASH) [107], or chronic viral hepatitis [112–114] in the absence of HH. Furthermore, other inflammatory disorders (e.g., inflammatory arthropathies) and various neoplastic disorders (e.g., lymphoproliferative disorders) may cause ferritin levels to rise without any increase in iron stores. Therefore, many results of serum iron studies can be false-positive or false-negative, and reliance on these laboratory values alone may cause significant problems in the diagnosis. The use of HFE mutation analysis significantly improves diagnostic accuracy in these challenging patients.

When evaluating the results of HFE genotyping obtained from screening family members or from population studies, it is valuable to remember that the C282Y mutation has incomplete penetrance. This is highlighted by the results of two large North American population studies comprising approximately 100,000 and 41,000 primary care patients [22,23]. In these two populations, a substantial proportion (27% and 60%, respectively) of female C282Y homozygotes had a TS of less than 45% or 50%, respectively, while the values were smaller (16% and 25%) for male C282Y homozygotes with a TS of less than 50%. Similarly, more than 40% of female C282Y homozygotes (43% and 46%) in these populations had serum ferritin levels in the normal range (<200 ng/mL), while the corresponding values in male C282Y homozygotes were 12% and 24% (serum ferritin levels of <300 or 250 ng/mL, respectively). Therefore, for C282Y homozygotes without increases in TS or ferritin level (termed nonexpressing C282Y homozygotes), it seems likely that many will not develop a clinically significant degree of iron overload in their lifetimes. Periodic follow-up measurements of serum ferritin levels at about 5-year intervals may be warranted in such individuals, with initiation of phlebotomy therapy if the values rise above normal.

In the past, if either a fasting TS or a ferritin level was elevated in an otherwise uncomplicated patient, a liver biopsy was performed to establish or disprove the diagnosis of HH. Perls' Prussian blue staining was used for histochemical iron analysis, and the hepatic iron concentration was also measured, with subsequent calculation of the hepatic iron index (HII). In current practice, if a patient has an abnormal result on iron studies, HFE mutation analysis is performed; if the patient is found to be a C282Y homozygote or a compound heterozygote (C282Y/H63D), and has normal liver enzymes and a serum ferritin level below 1,000 ng/mL, then a liver biopsy is not required before commencing phlebotomy treatment. Accordingly, as genetic testing has become more widely available and better understood, fewer liver biopsies are being performed. Four reports

from France, United States, and Australia have shown that if the parameters mentioned earlier are used, no patient with significant fibrosis will be missed even if a liver biopsy is not performed [109,115–119]. An algorithm for the evaluation of possible HFE-related HH is shown in Fig. 30.2.

On the other hand, if a patient has elevated liver enzymes or a ferritin level above 1,000 ng/mL, a liver biopsy may be performed, and the typical findings of HFE-related HH should be recognized. Iron deposition occurs preferentially within the hepatocytes in the periportal region (acinar zone 1) of the hepatic lobule; the gradient of iron deposition decreases toward the pericentral region (acinar zone 3) (Fig. 30.3). With high levels of iron loading, Kupffer cell aggregates (siderotic nodules), iron deposition in bile duct epithelial cells, and increased fibrosis are found in the portal tracts. In other liver diseases associated with increased iron deposition (e.g., alcoholic liver disease, NASH, chronic viral hepatitis), the distribution of iron is usually panlobular, with increased amounts of iron found in sinusoidal lining cells (Kupffer cells) and hepatocytes. The histologic evaluation of iron staining – with a recognition of the pattern seen in HFE-related HH as opposed to that associated with secondary iron overload – provides important complementary information to the clinician caring for a patient with liver disease and abnormal iron study results. It has been reported that a non-HH pattern of iron distribution reliably predicts the absence of homozygosity for C282Y or the compound heterozygous state [118]. Conversely, the HH pattern of iron deposition can be seen in other forms of liver disease in the absence of C282Y homozygosity [118].

The HII was introduced in a classic paper by the Brisbane group in 1986 [119]. It is based on the concept that in patients with HH the hepatic iron concentration increases progressively with age, whereas in HH heterozygotes or in patients with various forms of liver disease with secondary iron overload, it does not. The HII was originally introduced as a means of differentiating HH homozygotes from both HH heterozygotes and patients with alcoholic liver disease and secondary iron overload, but it quickly came to be used as a surrogate test for HH homozygosity. The HII is calculated by dividing the hepatic iron concentration (in µmol/g dry weight of liver) by the patient's age (in years). In several studies, patients with homozygous HH had an HII above 1.9. Now that investigations have been performed with HFE mutation analysis used as the "gold standard" for the diagnosis of HFE-related HH, it is clear that many patients who are C282Y homozygotes have an HII below 1.9 [116]. Therefore, with the availability of genetic testing, the determination of the hepatic iron concentration and HII has little diagnostic value for HFE-related HH.

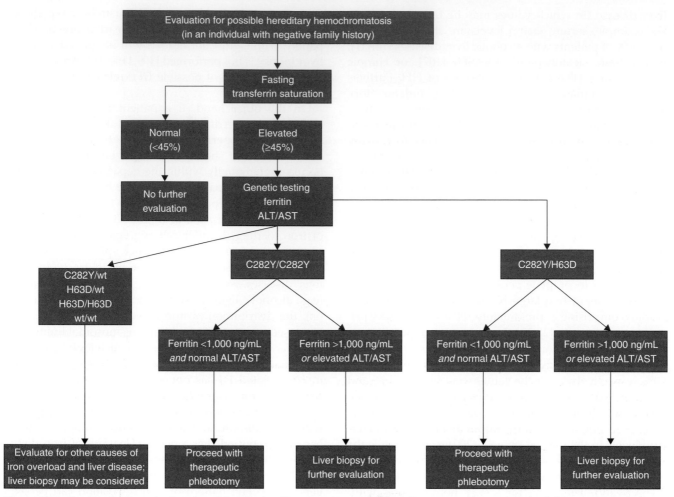

Figure 30.2 Algorithm for the evaluation of possible *HFE*-related hereditary hemochromatosis in a person with a negative family history. ALT, alanine aminotransferase; AST, aspartate aminotransferase; wt, wild type.

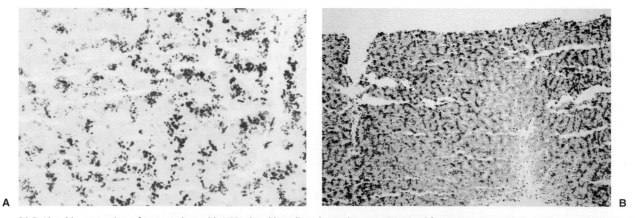

Figure 30.3 Liver biopsy specimen from a patient with *HFE*-related hereditary hemochromatosis stained for storage iron with Perls' Prussian blue stain. The hepatic iron concentration was elevated to 9,840 μg/g dry weight. Iron deposition is found preferentially in hepatocytes (A; original ×400) in the periportal region (acinar zone 1) of the hepatic lobule, with a decrease in the gradient toward the pericentral region (acinar zone 3) (B; original ×200). (Courtesy of Dr Elizabeth M. Brunt.)

Treatment

The treatment of HH remains relatively straightforward [107–109]. Once the diagnosis has been established by standard iron studies, genetic testing, or liver biopsy, treatment should be initiated with routine therapeutic phlebotomy. Patients should be encouraged to undergo weekly therapeutic phlebotomy with removal of 500 mL (1 U) of whole blood, which represents approximately 200–250 mg of iron, depending on the hemoglobin level. Some patients can tolerate the removal of 2 or even 3 U of blood per week, but 1 U per week is comfortable for most patients. Occasionally, older patients may only be able to tolerate the removal of 0.5 U every other week. Therapeutic phlebotomy should be performed until iron-limited erythropoiesis develops, which is identified by the failure of the hemoglobin level and hematocrit to recover before the next phlebotomy. It is reasonable to monitor the TS and ferritin levels periodically (every 3 months) to predict the return to normal iron stores and encourage patients who are undergoing phlebotomy. Phlebotomy should be continued until the serum ferritin level is less than 50 ng/mL and the TS is less than 50%. It is not necessary for patients to become iron deficient, just depleted of their excess iron stores. Usually, in otherwise uncomplicated patients, each unit of blood removed reduces the serum ferritin level by about 30 ng/mL. This can be a useful way of predicting the depletion of iron stores. Once standard therapeutic phlebotomy has been completed, patients require maintenance phlebotomy. Because in most patients approximately 2–3 mg of iron is absorbed per day in excess of their needs, they can be maintained in normal iron balance if 1 U of blood (200–250 mg of iron) is removed from them every 3 months.

With treatment, patients generally have an improved sense of well-being, and pain/fullness in the right upper quadrant is reduced (Box 30.4). If liver enzyme abnormalities are present, they will normalize with treatment.

Box 30.4 Response to phlebotomy therapy in hereditary hemochromatosis.

- Reduction of tissue iron stores to normal levels
- Improved survival if condition is diagnosed and treated before the development of cirrhosis and diabetes
- Improved sense of well-being and energy levels
- Improved cardiac function
- Improved control of diabetes
- Reduction in abdominal pain
- Decrease in skin pigmentation
- Normalization of elevated liver enzymes
- Reversal of hepatic fibrosis (approximately 30% of cases)
- No reversal of established cirrhosis
- No (or only minimal) improvement in arthropathy
- No reversal of testicular atrophy

Also, if patients require management of diabetes, the need for insulin or oral agents may decrease with successful phlebotomy therapy. On the other hand, testicular atrophy, arthropathy, and established cirrhosis generally are not reversible. Patients with established cirrhosis are still at risk for the development of hepatocellular carcinoma [102,120–122], and they should be screened periodically (every 6 months) with abdominal imaging and measurement of α-fetoprotein levels.

Family and population screening

Once a proband with *HFE*-related HH has been identified, family screening is necessary [107–109,123]. It is recommended that all first-degree relatives undergo *HFE* mutation analysis. In the past, HLA haplotyping was recommended as a surrogate genetic test, but with the availability of *HFE* mutation analysis, HLA typing is no longer recommended. Both the C282Y and H63D mutations should be analyzed. If a family member is found to be a C282Y homozygote or a compound heterozygote (C282Y/H63D), then therapeutic phlebotomy may be initiated if serum parameters indicate iron overload, such as an elevated ferritin level or TS. Individuals who are C282Y heterozygotes (C282Y/wt), H63D homozygotes (H63D/H63D), or H63D heterozygotes (H63D/wt) are not at risk for progressive iron overload. The issue of screening children by genetic testing raises questions of possible genetic discrimination and stigmatization [123]. These issues are not yet resolved at a societal level, but it may be useful to have the spouse of a proband undergo genetic testing to predict the genotype in a child [124]. Because C282Y and H63D are such common mutations, occurring in approximately 35% of persons singly or in combination, the chance that the spouse will have a mutation of *HFE* is approximately 1 in 3. If the spouse is homozygous for wild-type *HFE*, then the children do not require genetic testing because they are obligate heterozygotes and are not at increased risk for excess iron storage. In children who are C282Y homozygotes or compound heterozygotes, ferritin levels should be measured yearly and phlebotomy instituted when ferritin levels become elevated.

After the original discovery of *HFE*, it was thought that population screening using genetic testing might be ideal for *HFE*-related HH. Some of the reasons favoring screening are that C282Y homozygosity is common in white populations, there is a long latent phase before the development of disease manifestations, and treatment is simple and effective [21–23,125,126]. More than 15 studies have used *HFE* genotyping in population studies, and it has become evident that the C282Y mutation has incomplete penetrance, both in terms of serum iron parameters (i.e., TS and ferritin) and clinical impact (i.e., signs, symptoms, and morbidity) [22,23,125]. Incomplete penetrance of the C282Y mutation raises serious concerns about the cost-effectiveness of large-scale population screening, as does the issue of genetic discrimination about health and life insurance [127,128]. Alternative screening approaches such as targeted screening of high-risk groups (e.g., patients with diabetes) and workplace screening may prove efficacious [129,130]. At the present time, general population screening is not recommended and the most cost-effective methods of early detection of *HFE*-related HH appear to be family screening and evaluation of potential cases by primary care physicians with a high index of clinical suspicion [128,131].

Analysis of *HFE* mutations in patients with liver disease

Clinicians must frequently determine whether a patient has liver disease with abnormal parameters of iron metabolism or *HFE*-related HH with elevated liver enzymes. Abnormal results of blood iron studies are common in patients with a variety of liver diseases. These are generally associated with hepatocellular types of liver disease rather than the cholestatic syndromes. Approximately 50% of patients with alcoholic liver disease [110, 111], NASH [132,133], or chronic viral hepatitis (B and C) [112–114] have abnormalities in serum iron parameters. Typically, these abnormalities are limited to an elevated serum ferritin level, but some patients may also have an elevated TS. The hepatic iron concentration is typically normal or slightly elevated, and if the HII is calculated, it is usually normal. *HFE* mutation analysis has been applied to groups of patients with alcoholic liver disease, chronic hepatitis C virus (HCV), NASH, and porphyria cutanea tarda (PCT).

It has been known for more than 20 years that results of iron studies are frequently abnormal in patients with alcoholic liver disease [110,111]. Patients with acute alcoholic hepatitis can present with ferritin levels above 1,000 ng/mL and a TS above 100%. These values return to normal with abstinence and recovery from alcoholic hepatitis. Parameters of iron metabolism can also be abnormal in patients with chronic alcoholic liver disease. When *HFE* mutations are examined in patients with chronic alcoholic liver disease, the prevalence of C282Y or H63D is not greater than that in the control population [134, 135]. Additionally, the absence of a relationship between *HFE* mutations and hepatic iron levels in patients with alcoholic liver disease suggests that the abnormal iron parameters (whether blood studies or hepatic iron concentration) are caused by factors other than *HFE* mutations [134].

A relationship between the hepatic iron concentration and the response to treatment with interferon monotherapy of patients with chronic HCV has been reported [136,137]. Studies in the 1990s demonstrated a higher hepatic iron concentration in patients with chronic HCV who did not respond to treatment with interferon monotherapy than in those who did [136–139]. This concept led to the use of therapeutic phlebotomy to deplete iron stores before initial interferon therapy or retreatment with interferon. Iron depletion results in reduced levels of serum alanine aminotransferase (ALT) but does not significantly improve the rate of sustained virologic response (HCV RNA levels undetectable after 6 months without therapy) [140–143]. In addition, hepatic iron concentration is not an independent predictor of response to combined therapy with interferon and ribavirin [144]. In a long-term study in patients with HCV who failed to respond to interferon, phlebotomy combined with a low iron diet decreased ALT activity, histologic inflammation and fibrosis, and the hepatic levels of 8-hydroxy-deoxyguanosine (a marker of DNA damage) [145]. These results suggest that iron depletion can slow the progression of liver damage in HCV and may reduce the risk for developing hepatocellular carcinoma.

Other studies have suggested that the effect of an increased hepatic iron concentration may be synergistic with that of HCV in causing hepatic fibrosis [146–149]. Studies in which *HFE* mutation analysis was performed in patients with HCV, like those carried out in patients with alcoholic liver disease, showed no difference in the prevalence of C282Y or H63D mutations in comparison with a control population [141,147,148,150–152]. Some studies have reported that the presence of *HFE* mutations (especially C282Y) in patients with HCV is associated with an increase in fibrosis and cirrhosis [141,147,153], but other studies have not confirmed this association [149,151,152,154]. Further investigation is needed to determine the potential role of *HFE* mutations and iron in HCV-induced liver injury and to confirm that long-term iron removal by phlebotomy decreases the progression of hepatic fibrosis and the incidence of hepatocellular carcinoma in patients with HCV.

Results of serum iron studies are often abnormal in patients with NASH [132,133,155–158] and stainable hepatic iron may also be present. A number of investigations have assessed the prevalence of *HFE* mutations in NASH and the potential role of hepatic iron in disease severity. In several studies, it has been observed that patients with NASH have a higher prevalence of the C282Y mutation (usually heterozygotes) [157–160], but this is not always the case [161]. Not all patients with NASH with elevated hepatic iron levels have the C282Y mutation, indicating that other factors are involved. Some studies also observed an increase in hepatic fibrosis in patients with NASH who carry the C282Y mutation [157,158]. While two reports found an association of increased hepatic iron with the development of fibrosis in NASH [157,158], other investigations have not found this

Table 30.3 Prevalence of *HFE* mutations and hepatitis C virus in patients with porphyria cutanea tarda.

Country	No. of patients	Percentage with C282Y/C282Y	Percentage with at least one C282Y mutation	Percentage with at least one H63D mutation	Percentage HCV antibody-positive	Reference
United States	70	19	42	31	56	Bonkovsky et al. 1998 [169]
United States	108	19	41	29	59	Bulaj et al. 2000 [170]
Britain	41	17	44	32	NR	Roberts et al. 1997 [171]
Sweden	117	17	40	31	NR	Harper et al. 2004 [172]
Germany	190	12	49	54	15	Tannapfel et al. 2001 [173]
Australia	27	11	44	44	26	Stuart et al. 1998 [174]
Hungary	50	6	16	36	44	Nagy et al. 2004 [175]
Italy	68	0	3	50	78	Sampietro 1998 [176]

HCV, hepatitis C virus; NR, not reported.

association [159,161,162]. Regardless of iron levels and *HFE* mutations, several small trials indicate that phlebotomy therapy decreases ALT levels in patients with NASH [163–166], but the potential beneficial effects on hepatic histopathology have not been systematically evaluated.

In PCT, the role of abnormal iron stores in disease progression has been known for many years [167,168]. In addition, some patients with PCT also have chronic HCV, and alcohol consumption is known to be another risk factor. Studies from the United States, Europe, and Australia have shown that 16–49% of patients with PCT have at least one C282Y mutation in *HFE* and 6–19% are C282Y homozygotes (Table 30.3) [169–175]. The situation is different for Italian patients with PCT, in whom the prevalence of the C282Y mutation is not increased; rather, the prevalence of the H63D mutation is elevated [176]. Therapeutic phlebotomy is beneficial in PCT, inducing a reduction in liver enzyme abnormalities and regression of the skin lesions [167,168]. Patients should also be counseled about abstaining from alcohol, and if they have HCV they should be offered a course of antiviral therapy once their excess iron stores have been depleted.

In summary, all patients with PCT should undergo *HFE* mutation analysis and HCV testing, and phlebotomy therapy is definitely beneficial. For patients with alcoholic liver disease, the role of *HFE* mutation analysis seems to be limited because *HFE* mutations do not appear to contribute to the iron abnormalities seen in these patients. For patients with chronic HCV and NASH, it is reasonable to request *HFE* mutation analysis if the parameters of iron metabolism are abnormal (elevated ferritin level or TS), but the relationships between *HFE* mutations and abnormal iron parameters are not as clear as those in PCT. In patients with HCV or NASH, phlebotomy may be beneficial in decreasing ALT activity and ameliorating liver damage, but additional long-term studies of iron depletion are needed to further assess the possible beneficial effects on the development of cirrhosis and hepatocellular carcinoma.

Other iron storage disorders

Secondary and parenteral iron overload

Disorders of erythropoiesis and some forms of chronic liver disease can cause increased iron absorption and deposition in tissues (see Box 30.1). In these disorders, the iron overload is said to be secondary because the increased absorption of dietary iron is a consequence of an underlying condition [19,177,178]. A common factor in the iron-loading anemias is refractory anemia, characterized by hypercellular bone marrow and ineffective erythropoiesis. These conditions, which include β-thalassemia and the sideroblastic anemias, can be associated with clinical and pathologic consequences similar to those seen in *HFE*-related HH. In patients with disorders of erythropoiesis who undergo blood transfusions, the iron burden can be increased rapidly by the combined effects of increased iron absorption and the transfusion of iron (in hemoglobin). Therefore, iron toxicity to the liver, heart, and pancreas may develop many years earlier than in patients with *HFE*-related HH [179]. To minimize iron-induced toxicity in patients with iron-loading anemias, intensive chelation therapy with desferrioxamine or other chelators is required; this is started at the time when a commitment to long-term transfusion is made [19].

Parenteral iron overload is iatrogenic and results from transfusions of red blood cells, injections of iron–dextran, or long-term dialysis [19,20]. Parenteral iron deposition is initially confined to cells of the RE system, including the Kupffer cells of the liver. When transfusions are required in disorders of erythropoiesis, parenchymal and RE iron overload can coexist. With long-term parenteral iron overload, iron also accumulates in the parenchyma, presumably through the uptake of iron released from RE cells. The degree of structural and functional damage to the liver and endocrine organs generally parallels the degree of parenchymal iron overload. Sensitive magnetic resonance imaging (MRI) techniques are now available that accurately measure hepatic iron concentration noninvasively [180–182], and these may be particularly useful for ongoing assessment of chelation efficacy in patients with disorders of erythropoiesis.

African iron overload and congenital alloimmune iron overload

The iron overload that occurs in people living in sub-Saharan Africa is now considered to be the result of a non-*HFE*-related genetic trait that can be exacerbated by dietary iron loading [16]. Some persons with African iron overload consume an iron-rich beverage made from fermented maize, but iron overload also occurs in persons who do not drink it. The distribution of accumulated iron in African iron overload is different from that in *HFE*-related HH in that the ratio of the splenic iron concentration to hepatic iron concentration is higher in African iron overload. In addition, iron-loaded Kupffer cells are prominent in African iron overload, whereas the Kupffer cells are relatively spared in *HFE*-related HH. Nevertheless, both African iron overload and *HFE*-related HH can result in portal fibrosis and cirrhosis, and the risk for hepatocellular carcinoma is increased [183]. Associations of African iron overload with diabetes mellitus, peritonitis, scurvy, and osteoporosis have been described [16]. It has been reported that non-*HFE*-related iron overload may occur in African-Americans [184–186], but further investigations are needed to determine the genetic basis, prevalence, and clinical consequences of this condition.

Congenital alloimmune iron overload (also known as neonatal iron overload) is a rare disorder (fewer than 250 cases are reported in the literature) in which severe liver disease is associated with parenchymal iron loading, relative sparing of Kupffer cells, and extrahepatic siderosis [17,18,187]. Most cases have a fatal outcome, and treatment with desferrioxamine or an antioxidant cocktail has not been effective [188]. Some successful orthotopic liver transplantations have been performed in infants with neonatal iron overload, but long-term survival after this procedure has been disappointing [188]. Some cases show evidence of autosomal recessive inheritance, but without mutations in the genes for *HFE*, $\beta_2 M$, heme oxygenase, TFR1, or ferritin [17]. Neonatal iron overload recurs within sibships at a rate higher than that predicted for simple Mendelian autosomal recessive inheritance, suggesting the role of a maternal factor [17]. Immunomodula-

tion with intravenous high-dose immunoglobulin during pregnancy lessens the severity of disease, strongly suggesting that recurrent neonatal iron overload is an alloimmune condition causing liver injury [18,187].

Conclusions

With the discovery of *HFE* and other genes involved in iron homeostasis, our understanding of the normal physiology of iron absorption and the pathophysiology associated with mutations of these genes has been dramatically enhanced. *HFE* mutation analysis has greatly improved the ability to diagnose *HFE*-related HH accurately, to perform careful family screening, and to evaluate patients with liver disease and abnormal results of iron studies. Interestingly, population studies have revealed that many C282Y homozygotes do not have clinically significant iron overload, suggesting the influence of modifier genes. With a better understanding of the genes that modulate iron homeostasis, the reasons for the phenotypic variability of C282Y homozygotes may be discovered. Mutations in the iron-related genes encoding for hemojuvelin, hepcidin, ferroportin, TFR2, DMT1, and ferritin result in non-*HFE*-related HH. The pathogenesis of nearly all forms of HH involves an inappropriately low expression of hepcidin, an iron-regulatory hormone that acts to decrease the export of iron from duodenal enterocytes and RE cells. As a consequence of this low hepcidin expression, patients with HH having phenotypic expression have increased absorption of dietary iron and an elevated TS. Timely phlebotomy treatment of patients with *HFE*-related HH prevents cirrhosis and other iron-induced toxicity.

Acknowledgments

The research work of the authors was supported in part by a grant from the US Department of Health and Human Services (NIH DK-41816). The authors thank Rosemary O'Neill and Mary Ann Barrale for excellent assistance.

Annotated references

Bacon BR. Hemochromatosis: diagnosis and management. *Gastroenterology* 2001;120:718–25.
   This article provides recommendations about the diagnosis and management of HH.

Bottomley SS. Secondary iron overload disorders. *Semin Hematol* 1998;35:77–86.
   A comprehensive review of the causes and consequences of secondary iron overload.

Camaschella C. BMP6 orchestrates iron metabolism. *Nat Genet* 2009;41:386–8.
   This article reviews the important role of bone morphogenetic protein 6 in regulating iron metabolism.

Feder JN, Gnirke A, Thomas W, et al. A novel MHC class 1-like gene is mutated in patients with hereditary haemochromatosis. *Nat Genet* 1996;13:399–408.

This landmark article describes the cloning of the HFE gene and reports the two major mutations responsible for HFE-related HH (C282Y and H63D).

Nelson JE, Kowdley KV. Non-*HFE* hemochromatosis: genetics, pathogenesis, and clinical management. *Curr Gastroenterol Rep* 2005;7: 71–80.

This review article delineates the causes, consequences, and treatment of non-HFE-related HH.

Nemeth E, Ganz T. The role of hepcidin in iron metabolism. *Acta Haematol* 2009;122:78–86.

A review that summarizes the actions of hepcidin as a key regulator of iron homeostasis.

Pietrangelo A. Hereditary hemochromatosis: pathogenesis, diagnosis, and treatment. *Gastroenterology* 2010;139:393–408.

The molecular basis, diagnosis, and treatment of HH are described in this review article.

Zhou XY, Tomatsu S, Fleming RE, et al. *HFE* gene knockout produces mouse model of hereditary hemochromatosis. *Proc Natl Acad Sci USA* 1998;95:2492–7.

This report shows definitively that the functional loss of HFE protein results in iron overload, and it establishes a mouse model for HFE-related HH.

References

1. Trousseau A. *Glycosurie, diabète sucré. Clinique médicale de l'Hôtel-Dieu de Paris*, Vol. 2, 2nd edn. Paris: Balliere, 1865:663.
2. von Recklinghausen FD. Über Hämochromatose. *Tagebl Versamml Natur Ärzte Heidelberg* 1889;62:324.
3. Sheldon JH. *Haemochromatosis*. London: Oxford University Press, 1935.
4. MacDonald RA. *Hemochromatosis and Hemosiderosis*. Springfield, IL: Charles C Thomas, 1964.
5. Byrnes V, Ryan E, Barrett S, Kenny P, Mayne P, Crowe J. Genetic hemochromatosis, a Celtic disease: is it now time for population screening? *Genet Test* 2001;5(2):127–30.
6. Simon M, Bourel M, Fauchet R, Genetet B. Association of HLA-A3 and HLA-B14 antigens with idiopathic haemochromatosis. *Gut* 1976;17(5):332–4.
7. Feder JN, Gnirke A, Thomas W, et al. A novel MHC class I-like gene is mutated in patients with hereditary haemochromatosis. *Nat Genet* 1996;13(4):399–408.
8. Bacon BR, Powell LW, Adams PC, Kresina TF, Hoofnagle JH. Molecular medicine and hemochromatosis: at the crossroads. *Gastroenterology* 1999;116(1):193–207.
9. Papanikolaou G, Samuels ME, Ludwig EH, et al. Mutations in HFE2 cause iron overload in chromosome 1q-linked juvenile hemochromatosis. *Nat Genet* 2004;36(1):77–82.
10. Roetto A, Papanikolaou G, Politou M, et al. Mutant antimicrobial peptide hepcidin is associated with severe juvenile hemochromatosis. *Nat Genet* 2003;33(1):21–2.
11. Njajou OT, Vaessen N, Joosse M, et al. A mutation in SLC11A3 is associated with autosomal dominant hemochromatosis. *Nat Genet* 2001;28(3):213–14.
12. Montosi G, Donovan A, Totaro A, et al. Autosomal-dominant hemochromatosis is associated with a mutation in the ferroportin (SLC11A3) gene. *J Clin Invest* 2001;108(4):619–23.
13. Camaschella C, Roetto A, Cali A, et al. The gene TFR2 is mutated in a new type of haemochromatosis mapping to 7q22. *Nat Genet* 2000;25(1):14–15.
14. Mims MP, Guan Y, Pospisilova D, et al. Identification of a human mutation of DMT1 in a patient with microcytic anemia and iron overload. *Blood* 2005;105(3):1337–42.
15. Kato J, Fujikawa K, Kanda M, et al. A mutation, in the iron-responsive element of H ferritin mRNA, causing autosomal dominant iron overload. *Am J Hum Genet* 2001;69(1):191–7.
16. Gordeuk VR. African iron overload. *Semin Hematol* 2002;39(4):263–9.
17. Knisely AS, Mieli-Vergani G, Whitington PF. Neonatal hemochromatosis. *Gastroenterol Clin North Am* 2003;32(3):877–89, vi–vii.
18. Whitington PF, Hibbard JU. High-dose immunoglobulin during pregnancy for recurrent neonatal haemochromatosis. *Lancet* 2004; 364(9446):1690–8.
19. Bottomley SS. Secondary iron overload disorders. *Semin Hematol* 1998;35(1):77–86.
20. Burns DL, Pomposelli JJ. Toxicity of parenteral iron dextran therapy. *Kidney Int Suppl* 1999;69:S119–24.
21. Olynyk JK, Cullen DJ, Aquilia S, Rossi E, Summerville L, Powell LW. A population-based study of the clinical expression of the hemochromatosis gene. *N Engl J Med* 1999;341(10):718–24.
22. Adams PC, Reboussin DM, Barton JC, et al. Hemochromatosis and iron-overload screening in a racially diverse population. *N Engl J Med* 2005;352(17):1769–78.
23. Beutler E, Felitti VJ, Koziol JA, Ho NJ, Gelbart T. Penetrance of 845G → A (C282Y) HFE hereditary haemochromatosis mutation in the USA. *Lancet* 2002;359(9302):211–18.
24. Lebron JA, Bennett MJ, Vaughn DE, et al. Crystal structure of the hemochromatosis protein HFE and characterization of its interaction with transferrin receptor. *Cell* 1998;93(1):111–23.
25. Jeffrey GP, Basclain K, Hajek J, Chakrabarti S, Adams PC. Alternate splicing produces a soluble form of the hereditary hemochromatosis protein HFE. *Blood Cells Mol Dis* 1999;25(1):61–7.
26. Rhodes DA, Trowsdale J. Alternate splice variants of the hemochromatosis gene Hfe. *Immunogenetics* 1999;49(4):357–9.
27. Parkkila S, Waheed A, Britton RS, et al. Association of the transferrin receptor in human placenta with HFE, the protein defective in hereditary hemochromatosis. *Proc Natl Acad Sci USA* 1997;94(24):13198–202.
28. Feder JN, Tsuchihashi Z, Irrinki A, et al. The hemochromatosis founder mutation in HLA-H disrupts beta2-microglobulin interaction and cell surface expression. *J Biol Chem* 1997;272(22): 14025–8.
29. Waheed A, Parkkila S, Zhou XY, et al. Hereditary hemochromatosis: effects of C282Y and H63D mutations on association with beta2-microglobulin, intracellular processing, and cell surface expression of the HFE protein in COS-7 cells. *Proc Natl Acad Sci USA* 1997;94(23):12384–9.
30. Gross CN, Irrinki A, Feder JN, Enns CA. Co-trafficking of HFE, a nonclassical major histocompatibility complex class I protein, with the transferrin receptor implies a role in intracellular iron regulation. *J Biol Chem* 1998;273(34):22068–74.
31. Parkkila S, Niemela O, Britton RS, et al. Molecular aspects of iron absorption and HFE expression. *Gastroenterology* 2001;121(6): 1489–96.
32. Levy JE, Montross LK, Cohen DE, Fleming MD, Andrews NC. The C282Y mutation causing hereditary hemochromatosis does not produce a null allele. *Blood* 1999;94(1):9–11.
33. Carella M, D'Ambrosio L, Totaro A, et al. Mutation analysis of the HLA-H gene in Italian hemochromatosis patients. *Am J Hum Genet* 1997;60(4):828–32.
34. Whitfield JB, Cullen LM, Jazwinska EC, et al. Effects of HFE C282Y and H63D polymorphisms and polygenic background on iron stores in a large community sample of twins. *Am J Hum Genet* 2000;66(4): 1246–58.
35. Fleming RE, Holden CC, Tomatsu S, et al. Mouse strain differences determine severity of iron accumulation in Hfe knockout model of hereditary hemochromatosis. *Proc Natl Acad Sci USA* 2001;98(5): 2707–11.

36. Chang JG, Liu TC, Lin SF. Rapid diagnosis of the HLA-H gene Cys 282 Tyr mutation in hemochromatosis by polymerase chain reaction – a very rare mutation in the Chinese population. *Blood* 1997; 89(9):3492–3.

37. Cullen LM, Gao X, Easteal S, Jazwinska EC. The hemochromatosis 845 G→A and 187 C→G mutations: prevalence in non-Caucasian populations. *Am J Hum Genet* 1998;62(6):1403–7.

38. Jazwinska EC, Pyper WR, Burt MJ, et al. Haplotype analysis in Australian hemochromatosis patients: evidence for a predominant ancestral haplotype exclusively associated with hemochromatosis. *Am J Hum Genet* 1995;56(2):428–33.

39. Merryweather-Clarke AT, Pointon JJ, Jouanolle AM, Rochette J, Robson KJ. Geography of HFE C282Y and H63D mutations. *Genet Test* 2000;4(2):183–98.

40. Rochette J, Pointon JJ, Fisher CA, et al. Multicentric origin of hemochromatosis gene (HFE) mutations. *Am J Hum Genet* 1999; 64(4):1056–62.

41. Gochee PA, Powell LW, Cullen DJ, Du Sart D, Rossi E, Olynyk JK. A population-based study of the biochemical and clinical expression of the H63D hemochromatosis mutation. *Gastroenterology* 2002;122(3):646–51.

42. Risch N. Haemochromatosis, HFE and genetic complexity. *Nat Genet* 1997;17(4):375–6.

43. Barton JC, Sawada-Hirai R, Rothenberg BE, Acton RT. Two novel missense mutations of the HFE gene (I105T and G93R) and identification of the S65C mutation in Alabama hemochromatosis probands. *Blood Cells Mol Dis* 1999;25(3–4):147–55.

44. Pointon JJ, Wallace D, Merryweather-Clarke AT, Robson KJ. Uncommon mutations and polymorphisms in the hemochromatosis gene. *Genet Test* 2000;4(2):151–61.

45. Zhou XY, Tomatsu S, Fleming RE, et al. HFE gene knockout produces mouse model of hereditary hemochromatosis. *Proc Natl Acad Sci USA* 1998;95(5):2492–7.

46. Bahram S, Gilfillan S, Kuhn LC, et al. Experimental hemochromatosis due to MHC class I HFE deficiency: immune status and iron metabolism. *Proc Natl Acad Sci USA* 1999;96(23):13312–17.

47. Dupic F, Fruchon S, Bensaid M, et al. Inactivation of the hemochromatosis gene differentially regulates duodenal expression of iron-related mRNAs between mouse strains. *Gastroenterology* 2002;122(3):745–51.

48. Powell LW, Campbell CB, Wilson E. Intestinal mucosal uptake of iron and iron retention in idiopathic haemochromatosis as evidence for a mucosal abnormality. *Gut* 1970;11(9):727–31.

49. McLaren GD, Nathanson MH, Jacobs A, Trevett D, Thomson W. Regulation of intestinal iron absorption and mucosal iron kinetics in hereditary hemochromatosis. *J Lab Clin Med* 1991;117(5): 390–401.

50. Anderson GJ, Frazer DM, McLaren GD. Iron absorption and metabolism. *Curr Opin Gastroenterol* 2009;25(2):129–35.

51. McKie AT, Barrow D, Latunde-Dada GO, et al. An iron-regulated ferric reductase associated with the absorption of dietary iron. *Science* 2001;291(5509):1755–9.

52. Gunshin H, Mackenzie B, Berger UV, et al. Cloning and characterization of a mammalian proton-coupled metal-ion transporter. *Nature* 1997;388(6641):482–8.

53. Fleming MD, Trenor CC 3rd, Su MA, et al. Microcytic anaemia mice have a mutation in Nramp2, a candidate iron transporter gene. *Nat Genet* 1997;16(4):383–6.

54. Donovan A, Brownlie A, Zhou Y, et al. Positional cloning of zebrafish ferroportin1 identifies a conserved vertebrate iron exporter. *Nature* 2000;403(6771):776–81.

55. McKie AT, Marciani P, Rolfs A, et al. A novel duodenal iron-regulated transporter, IREG1, implicated in the basolateral transfer of iron to the circulation. *Mol Cell* 2000;5(2):299–309.

56. Abboud S. A novel mammalian iron-regulated protein involved in intracellular iron metabolism. *J Biol Chem* 2000;2000(275):19906–12.

57. Vulpe CD, Kuo YM, Murphy TL, et al. Hephaestin, a ceruloplasmin homologue implicated in intestinal iron transport, is defective in the sla mouse. *Nat Genet* 1999;21(2):195–9.

58. Zoller H, Pietrangelo A, Vogel W, Weiss G. Duodenal metal-transporter (DMT-1, NRAMP-2) expression in patients with hereditary haemochromatosis. *Lancet* 1999;353(9170):2120–3.

59. Zoller H, Koch RO, Theurl I, et al. Expression of the duodenal iron transporters divalent-metal transporter 1 and ferroportin 1 in iron deficiency and iron overload. *Gastroenterology* 2001;120(6): 1412–19.

60. Rolfs A, Bonkovsky HL, Kohlroser JG, et al. Intestinal expression of genes involved in iron absorption in humans. *Am J Physiol Gastrointest Liver Physiol* 2002;282(4):G598–607.

61. Fleming RE, Migas MC, Zhou X, et al. Mechanism of increased iron absorption in murine model of hereditary hemochromatosis: increased duodenal expression of the iron transporter DMT1. *Proc Natl Acad Sci USA* 1999;96(6):3143–8.

62. Griffiths WJ, Sly WS, Cox TM. Intestinal iron uptake determined by divalent metal transporter is enhanced in HFE-deficient mice with hemochromatosis. *Gastroenterology* 2001;120(6):1420–9.

63. Stuart KA, Anderson GJ, Frazer DM, et al. Duodenal expression of iron transport molecules in untreated haemochromatosis subjects. *Gut* 2003;52(7):953–9.

64. Kelleher T, Ryan E, Barrett S, et al. Increased DMT1 but not IREG1 or HFE mRNA following iron depletion therapy in hereditary haemochromatosis. *Gut* 2004;53(8):1174–9.

65. Canonne-Hergaux F, Levy JE, Fleming MD, Montross LK, Andrews NC, Gros P. Expression of the DMT1 (NRAMP2/DCT1) iron transporter in mice with genetic iron overload disorders. *Blood* 2001;97(4): 1138–40.

66. Herrmann T, Muckenthaler M, van der Hoeven F, et al. Iron overload in adult Hfe-deficient mice independent of changes in the steady-state expression of the duodenal iron transporters DMT1 and Ireg1/ferroportin. *J Mol Med* 2004;82(1):39–48.

67. Ajioka RS, Levy JE, Andrews NC, Kushner JP. Regulation of iron absorption in Hfe mutant mice. *Blood* 2002;100(4):1465–9.

68. Krause A, Neitz S, Magert HJ, et al. LEAP-1, a novel highly disulfide-bonded human peptide, exhibits antimicrobial activity. *FEBS Lett* 2000;480(2-3):147–50.

69. Park CH, Valore EV, Waring AJ, Ganz T. Hepcidin, a urinary antimicrobial peptide synthesized in the liver. *J Biol Chem* 2001;276(11): 7806–10.

70. Pigeon C, Ilyin G, Courselaud B, et al. A new mouse liver-specific gene, encoding a protein homologous to human antimicrobial peptide hepcidin, is overexpressed during iron overload. *J Biol Chem* 2001;276(11):7811–19.

71. Nicolas G, Viatte L, Bennoun M, Beaumont C, Kahn A, Vaulont S. Hepcidin, a new iron regulatory peptide. *Blood Cells Mol Dis* 2002; 29(3):327–35.

72. Nemeth E, Ganz T. The role of hepcidin in iron metabolism. *Acta Haematol* 2009;122:78–86.

73. Nicolas G, Bennoun M, Devaux I, et al. Lack of hepcidin gene expression and severe tissue iron overload in upstream stimulatory factor 2 (USF2) knockout mice. *Proc Natl Acad Sci USA* 2001;98(15):8780–5.

74. Fleming RE, Sly WS. Hepcidin: a putative iron-regulatory hormone relevant to hereditary hemochromatosis and the anemia of chronic disease. *Proc Natl Acad Sci USA* 2001;98(15):8160–2.

75. Nemeth E, Valore EV, Territo M, Schiller G, Lichtenstein A, Ganz T. Hepcidin, a putative mediator of anemia of inflammation, is a type II acute-phase protein. *Blood* 2003;101(7):2461–3.

76. Nicolas G, Chauvet C, Viatte L, et al. The gene encoding the iron regulatory peptide hepcidin is regulated by anemia, hypoxia, and inflammation. *J Clin Invest* 2002;110(7):1037–44.

77. Weinstein DA, Roy CN, Fleming MD, Loda MF, Wolfsdorf JI, Andrews NC. Inappropriate expression of hepcidin is associated with iron refractory anemia: implications for the anemia of chronic disease. *Blood* 2002;100(10):3776–81.

78. Nemeth E, Tuttle MS, Powelson J, et al. Hepcidin regulates cellular iron efflux by binding to ferroportin and inducing its internalization. *Science* 2004;306(5704):2090–3.

79. Bridle KR, Frazer DM, Wilkins SJ, et al. Disrupted hepcidin regulation in HFE-associated haemochromatosis and the liver as a regulator of body iron homoeostasis. *Lancet* 2003;361(9358):669–73.

80. Ahmad KA, Ahmann JR, Migas MC, et al. Decreased liver hepcidin expression in the Hfe knockout mouse. *Blood Cells Mol Dis* 2002;29(3):361–6.

81. Muckenthaler M, Roy CN, Custodio AO, et al. Regulatory defects in liver and intestine implicate abnormal hepcidin and Cybrd1 expression in mouse hemochromatosis. *Nat Genet* 2003;34(1):102–7.

82. Nemeth E, Roetto A, Garozzo G, Ganz T, Camaschella C. Hepcidin is decreased in TFR2 hemochromatosis. *Blood* 2005;105(4):1803–6.

83. Detivaud L, Nemeth E, Boudjema K, et al. Hepcidin levels in humans are correlated with hepatic iron stores, hemoglobin levels, and hepatic function. *Blood* 2005;106(2):746–8.

84. Papanikolaou G, Tzilianos M, Christakis JI, et al. Hepcidin in iron overload disorders. *Blood* 2005;105(10):4103–5.

85. Kemna E, Tjalsma H, Laarakkers C, Nemeth E, Willems H, Swinkels D. Novel urine hepcidin assay by mass spectrometry. *Blood* 2005;106(9):3268–70.

86. Andriopoulos B Jr, Corradini E, Xia Y, et al. BMP6 is a key endogenous regulator of hepcidin expression and iron metabolism. *Nat Genet* 2009;41(4):482–7.

87. Camaschella C. BMP6 orchestrates iron metabolism. *Nat Genet* 2009;41:386–8.

88. Fleming RE. Advances in understanding the molecular basis for the regulation of dietary iron absorption. *Curr Opin Gastroenterol* 2005;21(2):201–6.

89. Fleming RE, Ahmann JR, Migas MC, et al. Targeted mutagenesis of the murine transferrin receptor-2 gene produces hemochromatosis. *Proc Natl Acad Sci USA* 2002;99(16):10653–8.

90. Kawabata H, Fleming RE, Gui D, et al. Expression of hepcidin is down-regulated in TfR2 mutant mice manifesting a phenotype of hereditary hemochromatosis. *Blood* 2005;105(1):376–81.

91. Giannetti AM, Snow PM, Zak O, Bjorkman PJ. Mechanism for multiple ligand recognition by the human transferrin receptor. *PLoS Biol* 2003;1(3):E51.

92. Pietrangelo A. Non-HFE hemochromatosis. *Hepatology* 2004;39(1):21–9.

93. Huang FW, Pinkus JL, Pinkus GS, Fleming MD, Andrews NC. A mouse model of juvenile hemochromatosis. *J Clin Invest* 2005;115(8):2187–91.

94. Niederkofler V, Salie R, Arber S. Hemojuvelin is essential for dietary iron sensing, and its mutation leads to severe iron overload. *J Clin Invest* 2005;115(8):2180–6.

95. De Domenico I, Ward DM, Nemeth E, et al. The molecular basis of ferroportin-linked hemochromatosis. *Proc Natl Acad Sci USA* 2005;102(25):8955–60.

96. Drakesmith H, Schimanski LM, Ormerod E, et al. Resistance to hepcidin is conferred by hemochromatosis-associated mutations of ferroportin. *Blood* 2005;106(3):1092–7.

97. Camaschella C. Understanding iron homeostasis through genetic analysis of hemochromatosis and related disorders. *Blood* 2005;106(12):3710–17.

98. Mims MP, Prchal JT. Divalent metal transporter 1. *Hematology* 2005;10(4):339–45.

99. Gunshin H, Fujiwara Y, Custodio AO, Direnzo C, Robine S, Andrews NC. Slc11a2 is required for intestinal iron absorption and erythropoiesis but dispensable in placenta and liver. *J Clin Invest* 2005;115(5):1258–66.

100. Lam-Yuk-Tseung S, Mathieu M, Gros P. Functional characterization of the E399D DMT1/NRAMP2/SLC11A2 protein produced by an exon 12 mutation in a patient with microcytic anemia and iron overload. *Blood Cells Mol Dis* 2005;35(2):212–16.

101. Pantopoulos K. Iron metabolism and the IRE/IRP regulatory system: an update. *Ann NY Acad Sci* 2004;1012:1–13.

102. Niederau C, Fischer R, Sonnenberg A, Stremmel W, Trampisch HJ, Strohmeyer G. Survival and causes of death in cirrhotic and in noncirrhotic patients with primary hemochromatosis. *N Engl J Med* 1985;313(20):1256–62.

103. Edwards CQ, Cartwright GE, Skolnick MH, Amos DB. Homozygosity for hemochromatosis: clinical manifestations. *Ann Intern Med* 1980;93(4):519–25.

104. Milder MS, Cook JD, Stray S, Finch CA. Idiopathic hemochromatosis, an interim report. *Medicine (Baltimore)* 1980;59(1):34–49.

105. Adams PC, Kertesz AE, Valberg LS. Clinical presentation of hemochromatosis: a changing scene. *Am J Med* 1991;90(4):445–9.

106. Bacon BR, Sadiq SA. Hereditary hemochromatosis: presentation and diagnosis in the 1990s. *Am J Gastroenterol* 1997;92(5):784–9.

107. Bacon BR. Hemochromatosis: diagnosis and management. *Gastroenterology* 2001;120(3):718–25.

108. Tavill AS. Diagnosis and management of hemochromatosis. *Hepatology* 2001;33(5):1321–8.

109. Powell LW. Broadsheet number 54. Hereditary hemochromatosis. *Pathology* 2000;32(1):24–36.

110. Chapman RW, Morgan MY, Laulicht M, Hoffbrand AV, Sherlock S. Hepatic iron stores and markers of iron overload in alcoholics and patients with idiopathic hemochromatosis. *Dig Dis Sci* 1982;27(10):909–16.

111. Fletcher LM, Halliday JW, Powell LW. Interrelationships of alcohol and iron in liver disease with particular reference to the iron-binding proteins, ferritin and transferrin. *J Gastroenterol Hepatol* 1999;14(3):202–14.

112. Di Bisceglie AM, Axiotis CA, Hoofnagle JH, Bacon BR. Measurements of iron status in patients with chronic hepatitis. *Gastroenterology* 1992;102(6):2108–13.

113. Bonkovsky HL, Banner BF, Rothman AL. Iron and chronic viral hepatitis. *Hepatology* 1997;25(3):759–68.

114. Tung BY. Iron and viral hepatitis. *Viral Hepatitis* 1999;5:63–76.

115. Guyader D, Jacquelinet C, Moirand R, et al. Noninvasive prediction of fibrosis in C282Y homozygous hemochromatosis. *Gastroenterology* 1998;115(4):929–36.

116. Bacon BR, Olynyk JK, Brunt EM, Britton RS, Wolff RK. HFE genotype in patients with hemochromatosis and other liver diseases. *Ann Intern Med* 1999;130(12):953–62.

117. Morrison ED, Brandhagen DJ, Phatak PD, et al. Serum ferritin level predicts advanced hepatic fibrosis among US patients with phenotypic hemochromatosis. *Ann Intern Med* 2003;138(8):627–33.

118. Brunt EM, Olynyk JK, Britton RS, et. al. Histological evaluation of iron oerload in liver biopsies: relationship to HFE mutations. *Am J Gastroenterol* 2000;2000:1788–93.

119. Bassett ML, Halliday JW, Powell LW. Value of hepatic iron measurements in early hemochromatosis and determination of the critical iron level associated with fibrosis. *Hepatology* 1986;6(1):24–9.

120. Deugnier YM, Guyader D, Crantock L, et al. Primary liver cancer in genetic hemochromatosis: a clinical, pathological, and pathogenetic study of 54 cases. *Gastroenterology* 1993;104(1):228–34.

121. Kowdley KV. Iron, hemochromatosis, and hepatocellular carcinoma. *Gastroenterology* 2004;127(5 Suppl 1):S79–86.

122. Harrison SA, Bacon BR. Relation of hemochromatosis with hepatocellular carcinoma: epidemiology, natural history, pathophysiology, screening, treatment, and prevention. *Med Clin North Am* 2005;89(2):391–409.

123. Adams PC, Brissot P, Powell LW. EASL international consensus conference on haemochromatosis. *J Hepatol* 2000;33:485–504.

124. Adams PC. Implications of genotyping of spouses to limit investigation of children in genetic hemochromatosis. *Clin Genet* 1998;53(3):176–8.

125. Asberg A, Hveem K, Thorstensen K, et al. Screening for hemochromatosis: high prevalence and low morbidity in an unselected population of 65,238 persons. *Scand J Gastroenterol* 2001;36(10):1108–15.

126. Wilson JM. The principles and practice of screening for disease. *Public Health Pap WHO* 1968;34:26–39.

127. Adams PC, Arthur MJ, Boyer TD, et al. Screening in liver disease: report of an AASLD clinical workshop. *Hepatology* 2004;39(5):1204–12.

128. Galhenage SP, Viiala CH, Olynyk JK. Screening for hemochromatosis: patients with liver disease, families, and populations. *Curr Gastroenterol Rep* 2004;6(1):44–51.

129. DuBois S, Kowdley KV. Review article: targeted screening for hereditary haemochromatosis in high-risk groups. *Aliment Pharmacol Ther* 2004;20(1):1–14.

130. Delatycki MB, Allen KJ, Nisselle AE, et al. Use of community genetic screening to prevent HFE-associated hereditary haemochromatosis. *Lancet* 2005;366(9482):314–16.

131. Powell LW, Dixon JL, Hewett DG. Role of early case detection by screening relatives of patients with HFE-associated hereditary haemochromatosis. *Best Pract Res Clin Haematol* 2005;18(2):221–34.

132. Bacon BR, Farahvash MJ, Janney CG, Neuschwander-Tetri BA. Nonalcoholic steatohepatitis: an expanded clinical entity. *Gastroenterology* 1994;107(4):1103–9.

133. Marchesini G, Brizi M, Bianchi G, et al. Nonalcoholic fatty liver disease: a feature of the metabolic syndrome. *Diabetes* 2001;50(8):1844–50.

134. Grove J, Daly AK, Burt AD, et al. Heterozygotes for HFE mutations have no increased risk of advanced alcoholic liver disease. *Gut* 1998;43(2):262–6.

135. Lauret E, Rodriguez M, Gonzalez S, et al. HFE gene mutations in alcoholic and virus-related cirrhotic patients with hepatocellular carcinoma. *Am J Gastroenterol* 2002;97(4):1016–21.

136. Van Thiel DH, Friedlander L, Fagiuoli S, Wright HI, Irish W, Gavaler JS. Response to interferon alpha therapy is influenced by the iron content of the liver. *J Hepatol* 1994;20(3):410–15.

137. Olynyk JK, Reddy KR, Di Bisceglie AM, et al. Hepatic iron concentration as a predictor of response to interferon alfa therapy in chronic hepatitis C. *Gastroenterology* 1995;108(4):1104–9.

138. Piperno A, Sampietro M, D'Alba R, et al. Iron stores, response to alpha-interferon therapy, and effects of iron depletion in chronic hepatitis C. *Liver* 1996;16(4):248–54.

139. Fargion S, Fracanzani AL, Sampietro M, et al. Liver iron influences the response to interferon alpha therapy in chronic hepatitis C. *Eur J Gastroenterol Hepatol* 1997;9(5):497–503.

140. Fong TL, Han SH, Tsai NC, et al. A pilot randomized, controlled trial of the effect of iron depletion on long-term response to alpha-interferon in patients with chronic hepatitis C. *J Hepatol* 1998;28(3):369–74.

141. Fontana RJ, Israel J, LeClair P, et al. Iron reduction before and during interferon therapy of chronic hepatitis C: results of a multicenter, randomized, controlled trial. *Hepatology* 2000;31(3):730–6.

142. Di Bisceglie AM, Bonkovsky HL, Chopra S, et al. Iron reduction as an adjuvant to interferon therapy in patients with chronic hepatitis C who have previously not responded to interferon: a multicenter, prospective, randomized, controlled trial. *Hepatology* 2000;32(1):135–8.

143. Yano M, Hayashi H, Wakusawa S, et al. Long term effects of phlebotomy on biochemical and histological parameters of chronic hepatitis C. *Am J Gastroenterol* 2002;97(1):133–7.

144. Rulyak SJ, Eng SC, Patel K, McHutchison JG, Gordon SC, Kowdley KV. Relationships between hepatic iron content and virologic response in chronic hepatitis C patients treated with interferon and ribavirin. *Am J Gastroenterol* 2005;100(2):332–7.

145. Kato J, Kobune M, Nakamura T, et al. Normalization of elevated hepatic 8-hydroxy-2'-deoxyguanosine levels in chronic hepatitis C patients by phlebotomy and low iron diet. *Cancer Res* 2001;61(24):8697–702.

146. Beinker NK, Voigt MD, Arendse M, Smit J, Stander IA, Kirsch RE. Threshold effect of liver iron content on hepatic inflammation and fibrosis in hepatitis B and C. *J Hepatol* 1996;25(5):633–8.

147. Smith BC, Gorve J, Guzail MA, et al. Heterozygosity for hereditary hemochromatosis is associated with more fibrosis in chronic hepatitis C. *Hepatology* 1998;27(6):1695–9.

148. Martinelli AL, Franco RF, Villanova MG, et al. Are haemochromatosis mutations related to the severity of liver disease in hepatitis C virus infection? *Acta Haematol* 2000;102(3):152–6.

149. Negro F, Samii K, Rubbia-Brandt L, et al. Hemochromatosis gene mutations in chronic hepatitis C patients with and without liver siderosis. *J Med Virol* 2000;60(1):21–7.

150. Piperno A, Vergani A, Malosio I, et al. Hepatic iron overload in patients with chronic viral hepatitis: role of HFE gene mutations. *Hepatology* 1998;28(4):1105–9.

151. Hezode C, Cazeneuve C, Coue O, et al. Liver iron accumulation in patients with chronic active hepatitis C: prevalence and role of hemochromatosis gene mutations and relationship with hepatic histological lesions. *J Hepatol* 1999;31(6):979–84.

152. Kazemi-Shirazi L, Datz C, Maier-Dobersberger T, et al. The relation of iron status and hemochromatosis gene mutations in patients with chronic hepatitis C. *Gastroenterology* 1999;116(1):127–34.

153. Tung BY, Emond MJ, Bronner MP, Raaka SD, Cotler SJ, Kowdley KV. Hepatitis C, iron status, and disease severity: relationship with HFE mutations. *Gastroenterology* 2003;124(2):318–26.

154. Lal P, Fernandes H, Koneru B, Albanese E, Hameed M. C282Y mutation and hepatic iron status in hepatitis C and cryptogenic cirrhosis. *Arch Pathol Lab Med* 2000;124(11):1632–5.

155. Angulo P, Keach JC, Batts KP, Lindor KD. Independent predictors of liver fibrosis in patients with nonalcoholic steatohepatitis. *Hepatology* 1999;30(6):1356–62.

156. Youssef W, McCullough AJ. Diabetes mellitus, obesity, and hepatic steatosis. *Semin Gastrointest Dis* 2002;13(1):17–30.

157. George DK, Goldwurm S, MacDonald GA, et al. Increased hepatic iron concentration in nonalcoholic steatohepatitis is associated with increased fibrosis. *Gastroenterology* 1998;114(2):311–18.

158. Bonkovsky HL, Jawaid Q, Tortorelli K, et al. Non-alcoholic steatohepatitis and iron: increased prevalence of mutations of the HFE gene in non-alcoholic steatohepatitis. *J Hepatol* 1999;31(3):421–9.

159. Chitturi S, Weltman M, Farrell GC, et al. HFE mutations, hepatic iron, and fibrosis: ethnic-specific association of NASH with C282Y but not with fibrotic severity. *Hepatology* 2002;36(1):142–9.

160. Valenti L, Dongiovanni P, Fracanzani AL, et al. Increased susceptibility to nonalcoholic fatty liver disease in heterozygotes for the mutation responsible for hereditary hemochromatosis. *Dig Liver Dis* 2003;35(3):172–8.

161. Bugianesi E, Manzini P, D'Antico S, et al. Relative contribution of iron burden, HFE mutations, and insulin resistance to fibrosis in nonalcoholic fatty liver. *Hepatology* 2004;39(1):179–87.

162. Younossi ZM, Gramlich T, Bacon BR, et al. Hepatic iron and nonalcoholic fatty liver disease. *Hepatology* 1999;30(4):847–50.

163. Agrawal S, Bonkovsky HL. Management of nonalcoholic steatohepatitis: an analytic review. *J Clin Gastroenterol* 2002;35(3):253–61.

164. Facchini FS, Hua NW, Stoohs RA. Effect of iron depletion in carbohydrate-intolerant patients with clinical evidence of nonalcoholic fatty liver disease. *Gastroenterology* 2002;122(4):931–9.

165. Valenti L, Fracanzani AL, Fargion S. Effect of iron depletion in patients with nonalcoholic fatty liver disease without carbohydrate intolerance. *Gastroenterology* 2003;124(3):866; author reply, 7.

166. Piperno A, Vergani A, Salvioni A, et al. Effects of venesections and restricted diet in patients with the insulin-resistance hepatic iron overload syndrome. *Liver Int* 2004;24(5):471–6.

167. Elder GH. Porphyria cutanea tarda. *Semin Liver Dis* 1998; 18(1):67–75.

168. Bonkovsky HL, Obando JV. Role of HFE gene mutations in liver diseases other than hereditary hemochromatosis. *Curr Gastroenterol Rep* 1999;1(1):30–7.

169. Bonkovsky HL, Poh-Fitzpatrick M, Pimstone N, et al. Porphyria cutanea tarda, hepatitis C, and HFE gene mutations in North America. *Hepatology* 1998;27(6):1661–9.

170. Bulaj ZJ, Phillips JD, Ajioka RS, et al. Hemochromatosis genes and other factors contributing to the pathogenesis of porphyria cutanea tarda. *Blood* 2000;95(5):1565–71.

171. Roberts AG, Whatley SD, Morgan RR, Worwood M, Elder GH. Increased frequency of the haemochromatosis Cys282Tyr mutation in sporadic porphyria cutanea tarda. *Lancet* 1997;349(9048):321–3.

172. Harper P, Floderus Y, Holmstrom P, Eggertsen G, Gafvels M. Enrichment of HFE mutations in Swedish patients with familial and sporadic form of porphyria cutanea tarda. *J Intern Med* 2004;255(6):684–8.

173. Tannapfel A, Stolzel U, Kostler E, et al. C282Y and H63D mutation of the hemochromatosis gene in German porphyria cutanea tarda patients. *Virchows Arch* 2001;439(1):1–5.

174. Stuart KA, Busfield F, Jazwinska EC, et al. The C282Y mutation in the haemochromatosis gene (HFE) and hepatitis C virus infection are independent cofactors for porphyria cutanea tarda in Australian patients. *J Hepatol* 1998;28(3):404–9.

175. Nagy Z, Koszo F, Par A, et al. Hemochromatosis (HFE) gene mutations and hepatitis C virus infection as risk factors for porphyria cutanea tarda in Hungarian patients. *Liver Int* 2004;24(1):16–20.

176. Sampietro M, Piperno A, Lupica L, et al. High prevalence of the His63Asp HFE mutation in Italian patients with porphyria cutanea tarda. *Hepatology* 1998;27(1):181–4.

177. Wickramasinghe SN. Congenital dyserythropoietic anemias. *Curr Opin Hematol* 2000;7(2):71–8.

178. Harris ZL, Klomp LW, Gitlin JD. Aceruloplasminemia: an inherited neurodegenerative disease with impairment of iron homeostasis. *Am J Clin Nutr* 1998;67(5 Suppl):S972–7.

179. Modell CB, Beck J. Long-term desferrioxamine therapy in thalassemia. *Ann NY Acad Sci* 1974;232:201–10.

180. Gandon Y, Olivie D, Guyader D, et al. Non-invasive assessment of hepatic iron stores by MRI. *Lancet* 2004;363(9406):357–62.

181. St Pierre TG, Clark PR, Chua-anusorn W, et al. Noninvasive measurement and imaging of liver iron concentrations using proton magnetic resonance. *Blood* 2005;105(2):855–61.

182. Wood JC, Enriquez C, Ghugre N, et al. MRI R2 and R2* mapping accurately estimates hepatic iron concentration in transfusion-dependent thalassemia and sickle cell disease patients. *Blood* 2005;106(4):1460–5.

183. Mandishona E, MacPhail AP, Gordeuk VR, et al. Dietary iron overload as a risk factor for hepatocellular carcinoma in Black Africans. *Hepatology* 1998;27(6):1563–6.

184. Wurapa RK, Gordeuk VR, Brittenham GM, Khiyami A, Schechter GP, Edwards CQ. Primary iron overload in African Americans. *Am J Med* 1996;101(1):9–18.

185. Barton JC, Acton RT, Rivers CA, et al. Genotypic and phenotypic heterogeneity of African Americans with primary iron overload. *Blood Cells Mol Dis* 2003;31(3):310–19.

186. Gordeuk VR, McLaren CE, Looker AC, Hasselblad V, Brittenham GM. Distribution of transferrin saturations in the African-American population. *Blood* 1998;91(6):2175–9.

187. Whitington PF. Neonatal hemochromatosis: a congenital alloimmune hepatitis. *Semin Liver Dis* 2007;27(3):243–50.

188. Sigurdsson L, Reyes J, Kocoshis SA, Hansen TW, Rosh J, Knisely AS. Neonatal hemochromatosis: outcomes of pharmacologic and surgical therapies. *J Pediatr Gastroenterol Nutr* 1998;26(1): 85–9.

189. Davis WD Jr, Arrowsmith WR. The effect of repeated bleeding in hemochromatosis. *J Lab Clin Med* 1950;36(5):814–15.

190. Bomford A, Williams R. Long term results of venesection therapy in idiopathic haemochromatosis. *Q J Med* 1976;45(180):611–23.

Multiple choice questions

30.1 Which of the following molecules interacts with ferroportin to regulate iron absorption by enterocytes?

- **a** Hemojuvelin.
- **b** Hepcidin.
- **c** Hephaestin.
- **d** Transferrin receptor 2.
- **e** Hemopexin.

30.2 In which of the following clinical scenarios would a liver biopsy be recommended?

HFE genotype	Ferritin (ng/mL)	ALT (IU/mL)
a. C282Y/H63D	800	25
b. C282Y/C282Y	608	12
c. C282Y/wt	645	35
d. C282Y/C282Y	1,586	68
e. H63D/wt	253	38

Answers to the multiple choice questions can be found in the Appendix at the end of the book.

These multiple choice questions are also available for you to complete online.
Visit http://www.schiffsdiseasesoftheliver.com/

CHAPTER 31
Alpha-1 Antitrypsin Deficiency

David H. Perlmutter

Department of Cell Biology and Physiology, University of Pittsburgh School of Medicine and Children's Hospital of Pittsburgh of UPMC, Pittsburgh, PA, USA

Key concepts

- Homozygous protease inhibitor phenotype ZZ (PIZZ) α_1-antitrypsin (α_1-AT) deficiency, which has an incidence of one in 2,000 to one in 3,000 live births, is the most common genetic cause of liver disease in children. It is also causes more chronic liver disease and hepatocellular carcinoma in adults than previously appreciated. It is the most frequent genetic cause of chronic obstructive pulmonary disease (COPD)/emphysema.
- α_1-AT is an approximately 55 kDa secretory glycoprotein that inhibits destructive neutrophil proteases, elastase, cathepsin G, and proteinase 3. Plasma α_1-AT is predominantly derived from the liver, and its level increases 3–5-fold during the host response to tissue injury and inflammation. It is the archetype of a family of structurally related circulating serine protease inhibitors termed serpins.
- Although COPD is predominantly caused by a loss-of-function mechanism in which uninhibited proteolytic activity destroys the connective tissue backbone of the lung, liver disease is caused by a gain-of-toxic function mechanism attributable to the toxic effects of polymerized/aggregated mutant α_1-AT molecules retained within the endoplasmic reticulum (ER) of liver cells.
- Screening studies by Sveger in Sweden have shown that only 8% of the PIZZ population have clinically significant liver disease in the first

30 years of life. These results provide the basis for the concept that genetic and/or environmental modifiers determine whether a homozygote develops clinically significant liver disease. One series of studies has suggested that a subgroup of PIZZ individuals are predisposed to liver injury because of an inefficient degradation of mutant α_1-ATZ within the ER.
- Altered migration of the abnormal α_1-AT molecule in isoelectric focusing gels is the basis of the diagnosis of α_1-AT deficiency.
- Management of α_1-AT deficiency-associated liver disease is mostly supportive. Liver replacement therapy has been used successfully for severe liver injury.
- Although clinical efficacy has not been demonstrated, many patients with emphysema due to α_1-AT deficiency are being treated by means of intravenous and intratracheal aerosol administration of purified plasma α_1-AT. An increasing number of patients with severe emphysema are undergoing lung transplantation.
- Advances in understanding how cells degrade mutant α_1-ATZ and how cells activate protective signaling responses when mutant α_1-AT accumulates in the ER have led to novel concepts for pharmacologic strategies.

Incidence

The incidence of homozygous protease inhibitor phenotype ZZ (PIZZ) α_1-antitrypsin (α_1-AT) deficiency is highest among people of Scandinavian and northern European descent at one in 1,600 to one in 2,000 live births [1]. Although the incidence of the homozygous deficiency state in North American white populations was originally reported to be one in 6,700 live births [2], more recent studies have demonstrated an incidence of one in 2,000 to one in 3,000 [3].

Clinical manifestations

Liver disease

Liver involvement is often first noticed at the age of 1–2 months because of persistent jaundice. Conjugated bilirubin levels in the blood and serum transaminase levels are mildly to moderately elevated. The liver may be enlarged. Such infants are usually admitted to the hospital with a diagnosis of neonatal hepatitis syndrome and undergo a detailed diagnostic evaluation [4]. Infants may also be initially evaluated for α_1-AT deficiency because

Schiff's Diseases of the Liver, Eleventh Edition. Edited by Eugene R. Schiff, Willis C. Maddrey and Michael F. Sorrell.
© 2012 John Wiley & Sons, Ltd. Published 2012 by John Wiley & Sons, Ltd.

of an episode of gastrointestinal bleeding, bleeding from the umbilical stump, or bruising [5]. A small number of affected infants have hepatosplenomegaly, ascites, and liver synthetic dysfunction in early infancy. An even smaller number have severe fulminant hepatic failure in infancy [6]. A few cases are recognized initially because of a cholestatic clinical syndrome characterized by pruritus and hypercholesterolemia. The clinical features among these infants resemble those of extrahepatic biliary atresia, but histologic examination shows a paucity of intrahepatic bile ducts.

Liver disease associated with α_1-AT deficiency may be discovered in late childhood or early adolescence, when the patient is seen with abdominal distension due to hepatosplenomegaly or ascites or with upper intestinal bleeding caused by esophageal variceal hemorrhage. In some of these cases, there is a history of unexplained prolonged obstructive jaundice during the neonatal period. In others, there is no evidence of any previous liver injury, even when the neonatal history is carefully reviewed.

α_1-AT deficiency should be considered in the differential diagnosis for any adult who has chronic hepatitis, cirrhosis, portal hypertension, or hepatocellular carcinoma of unknown origin. An autopsy study in Sweden showed a higher risk of cirrhosis among adults with α_1-AT deficiency than was previously suspected, and indicated that α_1-AT deficiency has a strong association with primary liver cancer [7]. This study raised the possibility that the risk of clinical liver disease is as high as 25% among men in the fifth and sixth decades of life (Box 31.1).

The only prospective data on the course of α_1-AT deficiency-associated liver injury are from the Swedish nationwide screening study conducted by Sveger [1]. In this study, 200,000 newborn infants were screened and 127 PIZZ individuals were identified. Fourteen of the 127 had prolonged obstructive jaundice and nine of the 14

had severe liver disease, as indicated by clinical and laboratory criteria. Another eight of the 127 PIZZ infants had mildly abnormal serum bilirubin or serum transaminase levels or hepatomegaly. Approximately 50% of the rest of the 127 only had abnormal transaminase levels [8]. Published results of follow-up studies of the original cohort of 127 PIZZ children at 26 years of age [9] showed marginal elevations in serum transaminase levels in 4–9% with no evidence of liver dysfunction. Issues not addressed by the Sveger study are whether 26-year-olds with α_1-AT deficiency have persistent subclinical histologic abnormalities, despite a lack of clinical or biochemical evidence of liver injury, and whether liver disease will eventually become clinically evident during adulthood.

It is still not clear what clinical manifestations or abnormal laboratory test results can be used to predict a poor prognosis for patients with α_1-AT deficiency-associated liver disease. Results of one study suggested that persistence of hyperbilirubinemia, hard hepatomegaly, early development of splenomegaly, and progressive prolongation of prothrombin time were indicators of poor prognosis [10]. In another study, elevated transaminase levels, prolonged prothrombin time, and a lower trypsin inhibitor capacity correlated with a worse prognosis [11]. However, this author and his colleagues have found that some children with α_1-AT deficiency-associated liver disease can lead relatively normal lives for years after the development of hepatosplenomegaly and mild prolongation of prothrombin time. In a review of 44 patients with α_1-AT deficiency seen in the specialty practice at St Louis Children's Hospital, 17 patients had cirrhosis, portal hypertension, or both [12]. Nine of the 17 patients with cirrhosis or portal hypertension had a prolonged, relatively uneventful course for at least 4 years after the diagnosis of cirrhosis or portal hypertension. Two of these patients eventually underwent liver transplantation, but seven were leading relatively healthy lives for as long as 23 years after being diagnosed as having severe α_1-AT deficiency-associated liver disease. Patients with a prolonged stable course could be differentiated from those with a rapidly progressive course on the basis of overall life functioning but not on the basis of other more conventional clinical or biochemical criteria. Therefore, prediction of poor prognosis for α_1-AT deficiency-associated liver disease and for the timing of liver transplantation depends more on the overall functioning of the child than on histologic findings or laboratory data.

It is not clear whether heterozygotes for the Z allele of α_1-AT are predisposed to liver disease. Early studies of liver biopsy collections suggested that there was a relation between heterozygosity and the development of liver disease [13]. A retrospective study at the Mayo Clinic showed a higher prevalence of heterozygosity for α_1-ATZ in liver transplant recipients than in the general

---

Box 31.1 Liver disease associated with α_1-antitrypsin deficiency.

Clinical features
- Prolonged jaundice in an infant
- Neonatal hepatitis syndrome
- Mild elevation of transaminase levels in a toddler
- Portal hypertension in a child or adolescent
- Severe liver dysfunction in a child or adolescent
- Chronic hepatitis in an adult
- Cryptogenic cirrhosis in an adult
- Hepatocellular carcinoma in an adult

Diagnostic features
- Diminished serum levels of α_1-antitrypsin
- Abnormal mobility of α_1-antitrypsin in isoelectric focusing (PIZ)
- Periodic acid–Schiff-positive, diastase-resistant globules in liver cells

population, including a group of patients without another explanation for liver disease [14]. However, both these studies were biased in ascertainment and did not include concurrent prospective controls. Results of a cross-sectional study of patients with α_1-AT deficiency in a referral-based Austrian university hospital, who were reexamined with the most sophisticated and sensitive assays available, suggested that liver disease in heterozygotes can be accounted for, to a great extent, by infections with hepatitis B or C virus or by autoimmune disease [15]. Although this author suspects that liver disease can be caused by genetic and/or environmental modifiers in some heterozygotes, because of lack of clarity on this issue it is always wise to search for other causes of clinical liver disease in heterozygotes for the α_1-ATZ allele.

Liver disease has been described for several other allelic variants of α_1-AT. Children with compound heterozygosity type PISZ are affected by liver injury in a manner similar to that of PIZZ children [1,8,9]. There are several reports of liver disease in α_1-AT deficiency-type PIMMalton [16,17]. This is a particularly interesting association because the abnormal PIMMalton α_1-AT molecule has been shown to undergo polymerization and retention within the endoplasmic reticulum (ER) [17]. Liver disease has been detected in single patients with several other α_1-AT allelic variants, such as PIMDuarte [18], PIW [19], and PIFZ [20], but it is not clear whether other causes of liver injury for which there are more sophisticated diagnostic assays, such as infection with hepatitis C and autoimmune hepatitis, have been completely excluded in these cases.

Lung disease

The association between α_1-AT deficiency and the premature development of chronic obstructive pulmonary disease (COPD) is well documented [21]. Cigarette smoking markedly accelerates this destructive lung disease, reduces the quality of life, and markedly shortens the longevity of these persons [22]. There is still, however, wide variability in the incidence and severity of destructive lung disease within the α_1-AT-deficient population [3]. There are even PIZZ individuals who smoke but do not have any symptoms of lung disease or pulmonary function abnormalities or do not experience them until the seventh or eighth decade of life. Although results of one study have suggested the possibility that a subtle degree of hyperinflation can be detected with pulmonary function testing in infants with α_1-AT deficiency [23], results of other studies did not show any significant difference between the pulmonary function of PIZZ individuals aged 13–30 years and that of age-matched controls [24,25]. Clinical symptoms of COPD in α_1-AT-deficient individuals do not begin until the third decade of life. The usual initial symptoms are shortness of breath,

wheezing, cough, sputum production, and frequent chest infections [21].

There is still limited information about the incidence of liver disease among persons with α_1-AT deficiency and emphysema. In one recent study of 22 PIZZ patients with emphysema, there was an elevated transaminase level in ten patients, and cholestasis was present in one patient [26]. Liver biopsies were not performed in this study and may be necessary for the accurate determination of the extent of liver injury in these patients.

Alpha-1 antitrypsin structure, function, and physiology

Alpha-1 antitrypsin gene structure

Alpha-1 antitrypsin is encoded by a 12.2 kb gene on chromosome 14q31-32.3 [27]. There is a sequence-related gene approximately 12 kb downstream. Because there is no evidence that it is expressed, the downstream gene is considered a pseudogene. The gene is composed of five exons and four introns (Fig. 31.1) [28]. Exon I_C, the 5' portion of exon II, and the 3' portion of exon V are noncoding regions. The first intron is 5.3 kb long, contains a short open reading frame, an Alu family sequence, and a pseudotranscription initiation codon. Apparently, the short open reading frame does not code for protein. The α_1-AT messenger RNA expressed in the liver is 1.4 kb long [29]. In macrophages, the α_1-AT mRNA is slightly longer [29]. There are three forms of α_1-AT mRNA in macrophages, depending on transcription initiation sites in two upstream exonic structures (exons I_A and I_B) [29,30].

Alpha-1 antitrypsin protein structure

Alpha-1 antitrypsin is a single-chain, approximately 55 kDa polypeptide with 394 amino acids and three asparagine-linked complex carbohydrate side chains [31]. There are two major serum isoforms depending on the presence of a biantennary or triantennary configuration of the carbohydrate side chains. α_1-AT is the archetype of a family of structurally related proteins called serpins (serine protease inhibitors), which includes antithrombin III, α_1-antichymotrypsin, C1 inhibitor, α_2-antiplasmin, protein C inhibitor, heparin cofactor II, plasminogen activator inhibitors I and II, and protease nexin I [31]. A serpin-like structure is also found in several cellular proteins, trophic factors, and circulating carrier proteins, such as corticosteroid- and thyroid hormone-binding globulin.

Many studies of the structural characteristics of α_1-AT have shown that it is essentially composed of two central β-sheets surrounded by a small β-sheet and nine α-helices. The dominant structure is the five-stranded, β-pleated sheet called the A sheet (Fig. 31.2). A mobile

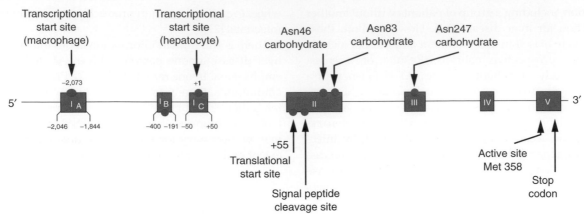

Figure 31.1 Structure of the α_1-antitrypsin gene (not to scale).

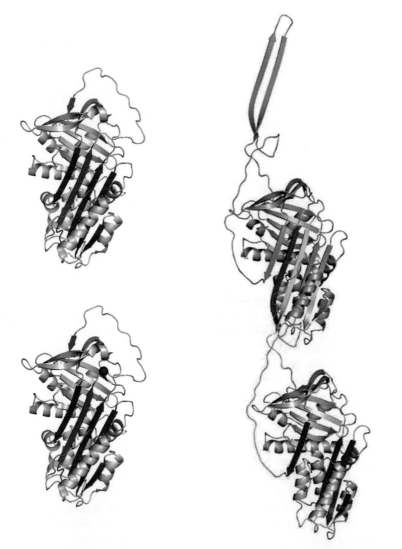

Figure 31.2 Ribbon diagrams of the normal α_1-antitrypsin molecule (A), mutant α_1-ATZ molecule (B), and polymerized α_1-ATZ molecule (C) according to the new domain swapping model. The position of the lysine substitution for glutamate 342 that characterizes the α_1-ATZ molecule is shown as a dark blue ball. That position lies within strand s5A, which is shown in pink. The reactive site loop, which becomes strand s4a, is shown in yellow. This color scheme makes it possible to see the swap of strand s4a and s5a together from the bottom α_1-ATZ molecule into the top molecule of the polymer structure. Strands s4a and s5a of the top molecule are shown in green, presumably being swapped into another α_1-ATZ molecule. The hydrophobic linker region is shown in teal blue. (Adapted from Yamasaki et al. [100] with permission from Nature.)

reactive center loop rises above a gap in the center of the A sheet [31,32].

Protease inhibitor system for classification of structural variants of α_1-antitrypsin

Variants of α_1-AT in humans are classified according to the PI phenotype system, as defined by agarose electrophoresis or isoelectric focusing of plasma in polyacrylamide at acid pH [33]. The PI classification system assigns a letter to variants according to migration of the major isoform. For example, the most common normal variant migrates to an intermediate isoelectric point, designated M. Persons with the most common severe deficiency have an α_1-AT allelic variant that migrates to a high isoelectric point, designated Z (Fig. 31.3). Even greater polymorphic variation of α_1-AT has been detected by means of restriction fragment length and direct DNA sequence analysis. With these techniques, in addition to isoelectric focusing, investigators have identified more than 100 allelic variants [34].

Normal allelic variants

The most common normal variant of α_1-AT is termed M1 and is found in 65–70% of whites in the United States [2].

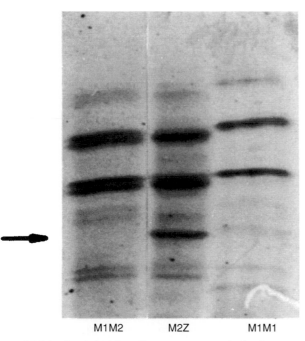

M1M2   M2Z   M1M1

Figure 31.3 Isoelectric focusing of human serum samples for the diagnosis of α_1-antitrypsin deficiency. Serum samples from a person with the normal M1M2 variant, from an M2Z heterozygote, and from a person with the normal M1M1 variant were subjected to isoelectric focusing with the anode at top and cathode at bottom. Migration of the Z allele is indicated by the arrow. (Courtesy of J. A. Pierce, St Louis, MO. Reproduced from Perlmutter [164] with permission from Elsevier.)

There are many rare normal allelic variants with allelic frequencies of less than 0.1%. For each of these variants, serum concentration and functional activity of α_1-AT are within the normal range.

Null allelic variants

Alpha-1 antitrypsin variants in which α_1-AT is not detectable in serum are called null allelic variants (Table 31.1). The inheritance of a null allelic variant with another null variant or a deficiency variant is associated with premature development of emphysema. There is no evidence for liver injury in persons with null variants who were examined in detail [34]. Potential molecular mechanisms for the null phenotype have been identified by DNA sequence analysis of a number of null variants [34–37]. They include deletion of all α_1-AT coding exons, substitutions that result in stop codons, frameshift mutations, and single base substitutions. In at least three cases, the frameshift mutation resulted in an abnormal truncated protein that is retained in the ER (null$_{HongKong}$, null$_{Clayton}$, null$_{Saarbrucken}$) [35–38].

Dysfunctional variants

α_1-AT$_{Pittsburgh}$ is the most well-characterized dysfunctional variant [39], which was identified in a 14-year-old boy who died of an episodic bleeding disorder. A single amino acid substitution, Met to Arg at residue 358, converted α_1-AT from an elastase inhibitor to a thrombin inhibitor. The episodic nature of the illness was attributed to changes in the synthesis of the mutant protein during the host response to acute inflammation and tissue injury, the acute phase response. The α_1-AT M$_{Mineral Springs}$ and null$_{Ludwigshafen}$ probably are other examples of dysfunctional variants [37,40].

Deficiency variants

Several variants of α_1-AT that are associated with a reduction in serum concentrations have been described and are called deficiency variants (Table 31.2). Some of these variants are not associated with clinical disease, such as the S variant [18,41]. Other deficiency variants are associated only with emphysema, such as M$_{Heerlen}$, M$_{Procida}$, and P$_{Lowell}$ [34]. In two persons with M$_{Malton}$ and one with M$_{Duarte}$, hepatocyte α_1-AT inclusions and liver disease have been found with emphysema [16–18]. In one person with the α_1-AT S$_{Iiyama}$ variant, emphysema and hepatocyte inclusions were reported, but this patient did not have liver disease [42]. The most common deficiency variant, the Z variant, is associated with emphysema and liver disease, as discussed later.

Alpha-1 antitrypsin function

Alpha-1 antitrypsin is an inhibitor of serine proteases in general, but its most important targets are neutrophil

Table 31.1 Null variants of α_1-antitrypsin.

Variant	Clinical disease				
	Defect	Site	Liver	Lung	Cellular defect
Null$_{GraniteFalls}$	Single base deletion	Tyr160	−	+	No detectable RNA
Null$_{Bellingham}$	Single base deletion	Lys217	−	+	No detectable RNA
Null$_{Mattawa}$	Single base insertion	Phe353	−	+	?IC degradation
Null$_{HongKong}$	Dinucleotide deletion	Leu318	−	+	IC accumulation
Null$_{Ludwigshafen}$	Single base substitution	Isoleu92–Asp	−		?Accelerated catabolism
Null$_{Clayton}$	Single base insertion	Glu363	−	+	IC accumulation
Null$_{Bolton}$	Single base deletion	Glu363	−	+	?IC degradation
Null$_{IsoladiProcida}$	Deletion	Exons II–V	−	+	Unknown
Null$_{Riedenburg}$	Deletion	Exons II–V	−	+	Unknown
Null$_{Newport}$	Single base substitution	Gly115–Ser	−	+	Unknown
Null$_{BonnyBlue}$	Intron deletion		−	+	Unknown
Null$_{NewHope}$	Two base substitutions	Gly320–Glu Glu342–Lys	−	+	Unknown
Null$_{Trastavere}$	Single base substitution	Trp194–stop	−	+	Unknown
Null$_{Kowloon}$	Single base substitution	Tyr38–stop	−	+	Unknown
Null$_{Saarbruecken}$	Single base insertion	Pro362–stop	−	+	IC accumulation
Null$_{Lisbon}$	Single base substitution	Thr68–Ile	−	+	Unknown
Null$_{West}$	Intron deletion	−	−	+	Unknown

IC, intracellular; ?, not proven.

Table 31.2 Deficiency variants of α_1-antitrypsin.

Variant	Clinical disease				
	Defect	Site	Liver	Lung	Cellular defect
Z	Single base substitution M1 (Ala213)	Glu342–Lys	+	+	IC accumulation
S	Single base substitution	Glu264–Val	−	−	IC accumulation
M$_{Heerlen}$	Single base substitution	Pro369–Leu	−	+	IC accumulation
M$_{Procida}$	Single base substitution	Leu41–Pro	−	+	IC accumulation
M$_{Malton}$	Single base deletion	Phe52	?	+	IC accumulation
M$_{Duarte}$	Unknown	Unknown	?	+	Unknown
S$_{Iiyama}$	Single base substitution	Ser53–Phe	−	+	?IC degradation
P$_{Duarte}$	Two base substitutions	Arg101–His Asp256–Val	?	+	Unknown
P$_{Lowell}$	Single base substitution	Asp256–Val	−	+	?IC degradation
W$_{Bethesda}$	Single base substitution	Ala336–Thre	−	+	?Accelerated catabolism
Z$_{Wrexham}$	Single base substitution	Ser19–Leu	?	?	Unknown
F	Single base substitution	Arg223–Cys	−	−	Unknown
T	Single base substitution	Glu264–Val	−	−	Unknown
I	Single base substitution	Arg39–Cys	−	−	IC degradation
M$_{Palermo}$	Single base deletion	Phe51	−	−	Unknown
M$_{Nichinan}$	Single base deletion and single base substitution	Phe52 Gly148–Arg	−	−	Unknown
Z$_{Ausburg}$	Single base substitution	Glu342–Lys	−	−	Unknown

IC, intracellular; ?, not proven.

elastase, cathepsin G, and proteinase 3, proteases released by activated neutrophils. Several lines of evidence suggest that inhibition of neutrophil elastase is the major physiologic role of α_1-AT. First, persons with α_1-AT deficiency are susceptible to premature development of emphysema, a lesion that can be induced in experimental animals by means of the instillation of excessive amounts of neutrophil elastase [43]. These observations have led to the concept that destructive lung disease may result from perturbations of the net balance of elastase and α_1-AT within the local environment of the lung [44]. Second, the kinetics of association for α_1-AT and neutrophil elastase are more favorable, by several orders of magnitude, than those for α_1-AT and any other serine protease [45]. Third, α_1-AT constitutes more than 90% of the neutrophil elastase inhibitory activity in the one body fluid that has been examined – pulmonary alveolar lavage fluid [44].

α_1-AT acts competitively by allowing its target enzymes to bind directly to a substrate-like region within its reactive center loop. The reaction between enzyme and inhibitor is essentially of second order, and the resulting complex contains one molecule of each of the reactants. A reactive site peptide bond within the inhibitor is hydrolyzed during the formation of the enzyme–inhibitor complex. The complex of α_1-AT and serine protease is a covalently stabilized structure resistant to dissociation by denaturing compounds, including sodium dodecyl sulfate and urea. The interaction between α_1-AT and serine protease is suicidal in that the modified inhibitor is no longer able to bind with or inactivate the enzyme. There is also a profound alteration in the structure of the enzyme, including disruption of the catalytic site, such that the enzyme becomes inactive and subject to proteolytic destruction [46]. Studies have shown that the irreversible trapping of target enzyme is mediated by a profound conformational change in α_1-AT, such that the cleaved reactive-loop binding-enzyme inserts into the gap in the A sheet. Carrell and Lomas [47] likened the inhibitory mechanism to a mousetrap: The active inhibitor circulates in the metastable, stressed form and then springs into the stable, relaxed form to lock the complex with its target protease.

The net functional activity of α_1-AT in complex biologic fluids may be modified by several factors. First, the reactive site methionine may be oxidized and thereby rendered inactive as an elastase inhibitor [48]. In vitro, α_1-AT is oxidatively inactivated by oxidants released by activated neutrophils and alveolar macrophages of cigarette smokers [49,50]. Second, the functional activity of α_1-AT may be modified by proteolytic inactivation. Several members of the metalloproteinase family, including collagenase and *Pseudomonas* elastase, and the thiol protease family can cleave and inactivate α_1-AT [51]. Studies

have shown that the pathogenesis of bullous pemphigoid may involve uninhibited neutrophil elastase activity at the dermal–epidermal junction because α_1-AT is cleaved and inactivated by matrix metalloproteinase 9 (MMP-9)–gelatinase B in the skin [52,53]. Third, DNA, which is often released from neutrophils at sites of inflammatory activation and phagocytosis, can impair the cathepsin G inhibitory activity of α_1-AT [54].

Although α_1-AT from the plasma or liver of persons with PIZZ α_1-AT deficiency is functionally active [55], there may be a decrease in its specific elastase inhibitory capacity. Ogushi et al. [56] showed that the kinetics of association with neutrophil elastase and the stability of complexes with neutrophil elastase were significantly decreased for α_1-AT isolated from PIZZ plasma. There was no decrease in the functional activity of α_1-AT in individuals homozygous for the S variant.

Results of several studies have indicated that α_1-AT protects experimental animals from the lethal effects of tumor necrosis factor [57]. Most of the evidence from these studies indicates that this protective effect is due to inhibition of the synthesis and release of platelet-activating factor from neutrophils [58], presumably through the inhibition of neutrophil-derived proteases. The antiapoptotic effect of α_1-AT on vascular smooth muscle cells [59] also probably involves the inhibition of extracellular matrix degradation by neutrophil-derived proteases.

Results of several studies indicate that α_1-AT has functional activities other than the inhibition of serine protease. The carboxyl-terminal fragment of α_1-AT, which can be generated during the formation of a complex with serine protease or during proteolytic inactivation by oxidants, thiolproteinases, or metalloproteinases, is a potent neutrophil chemoattractant [60]. The chemotactic response is equivalent to that elicited by formyl-methionyl-leucyl-phenylalanine. The carboxyl-terminal fragment of α_1-AT is also responsible for an increase in synthesis of α_1-AT in human monocytes and macrophages when these cells are incubated with exogenous neutrophil elastase [61]. In each case, the biologic effect is mediated by the interaction of a pentapeptide neodomain within the carboxyl-terminal fragment of α_1-AT and a novel cell surface receptor, the serpin–enzyme complex (SEC) receptor [62–64]. This mechanism may also be responsible for the neutrophil chemotactic effect of α_1-AT polymers [65], an effect that could explain the excessive neutrophil infiltration that characterizes the lungs of patients homozygous for the polymerization-prone α_1-ATZ.

Several studies have suggested that α_1-AT inhibits human immunodeficiency virus 1 (HIV-1) [66,67]. This effect appears to involve inhibition of viral entry and does not require protease inhibitory activity. A synthetic peptide from the region around the reactive site of α_1-AT has more potent anti-HIV activity but it was not proven that this peptide region mediates the effect of the intact protein [68].

There have been several reports that α_1-AT alters immune and inflammatory activities through effects on white blood cells that are distinct from its protease inhibitory activites, but investigation of the responsible mechanisms has produced confusing results [2,68,69].

Biosynthesis of α_1-antitrypsin

The predominant site of synthesis of plasma α_1-AT is the liver. This is most clearly shown by conversion of plasma α_1-AT to the donor phenotype after orthotopic liver transplantation [70]. α_1-AT is synthesized in human hepatocellular carcinoma cells as a 52 kDa precursor, undergoes post-translational, dolichol phosphate-linked glycosylation at three asparagine residues [71], and undergoes tyrosine sulfation [72]. It is secreted as a 55 kDa native single-chain glycoprotein with a half-time for secretion of 35–40 minutes.

Tissue-specific expression of α_1-AT in human hepatocellular carcinoma cells is directed by structural elements within a 750-nucleotide region upstream of the hepatocyte transcriptional start site in exon I_C. Within these regions are structural elements that are recognized by nuclear transcription factors, including hepatocyte nuclear factor 1α (HNF-1α), HNF-1β, hepatocyte nuclear factor 1α (HNF-1α), HNF-4, and HNF-3 [73]. HNF-1α and HNF-4 appear to be particularly important for the expression of the human α_1-AT gene in liver cells and intestinal epithelial cells [74]. Two distinct regions within the proximal element bind these two transcription factors. Substitution of five nucleotides at positions 77 to 72 disrupts binding of HNF-1α and dramatically reduces expression of the human α_1-AT gene in the liver of transgenic mice [75]. Substitution of four nucleotides at positions 118 to 115 disrupts the binding of HNF-4 but does not alter expression of the human α_1-AT gene in the liver of adult transgenic mice. The latter mutation does reduce expression of human α_1-AT in the liver during embryonic development.

Plasma concentrations of α_1-AT increase three- to five-fold during the host response to inflammation or tissue injury [76]. The source of this additional α_1-AT has always been considered the liver; therefore, α_1-AT is known as a *positive hepatic acute-phase reactant*. Synthesis of α_1-AT in human hepatocellular carcinoma cells (e.g., HepG2, Hep3B) is upregulated by interleukin 6 (IL6) but not by IL1 or tumor necrosis factor [77]. Plasma concentrations of α_1-AT also increase during pregnancy and during treatment with estrogens or androgens [78].

α_1-AT is also synthesized and secreted in primary cultures of human blood monocytes and bronchoalveolar and breast milk macrophages [79]. Expression of α_1-AT in monocytes and macrophages is influenced by products generated during inflammation, such as bacterial lipopolysaccharide [80] and IL6 [77]. Expression of α_1-AT in monocytes and tissue macrophages is also regulated by a feed-forward mechanism that is triggered by its functional activity. This regulatory mechanism was elucidated when it was discovered that synthesis of α_1-AT by monocytes increased when neutrophil elastase was added to the incubation medium [61]. This effect was later attributed to the formation of elastase–α_1-AT complexes that could interact with a specific cell surface receptor [62]. The effect on α_1-AT synthesis could be elicited by synthetic peptides corresponding to a domain in the carboxyl-terminal fragment of the α_1-AT molecule that is exposed only after the structural rearrangement that accompanies complex formation or proteolytic modification. This class of receptor molecules was called SEC receptors because the receptors recognize the highly conserved domains of other SECs, such as antithrombin III–thrombin, α_1-antichymotrypsin–cathepsin G, and, to a lesser extent, C1 inhibitor–C1s and tissue plasminogen activator–plasminogen activator inhibitor I complexes, as well as that of α_1-AT–elastase complexes [62,81]. Substance P, several other tachykinins, and bombesin bind to the SEC receptor through a similar pentapeptide sequence [82], indicating that expression of α_1-AT can be upregulated at sites of tissue inflammation by neuropeptides and peptide hormones as well as by cytokines. Although the pharmacologic and physiologic characteristics of the SEC receptor still appear to be distinct the receptor has not been purified and its primary structure has not been determined.

α_1-AT mRNA has been isolated from several tissues in transgenic mice [83], but in many cases it has not been possible to determine whether this mRNA is in ubiquitous tissue macrophages or other cell types. α_1-AT is synthesized in enterocytes and Paneth cells, as indicated by the results of studies with intestinal epithelial cell lines, ribonuclease protection assays of human intestinal RNA, and in situ hybridization analysis in cryostat sections of human intestinal mucosa [84]. Expression of α_1-AT in enterocytes increases markedly during differentiation from crypt to villus, in response to IL6, and during inflammation in vivo. α_1-AT is also synthesized by pulmonary epithelial cells [85,86]. Synthesis of α_1-AT in pulmonary epithelial cells is less responsive to regulation by IL6 than by a related cytokine, oncostatin M [86]. Moreover, there is evidence that HNF-1β, and not HNF-1α, HNF-4, or HNF-3, plays a predominant cell-specific role in transcription of the α_1-AT gene in pulmonary epithelial cells [87].

Clearance and distribution of α_1-antitrypsin

The half-life of α_1-AT in plasma is approximately 5 days [2,34]. It is estimated that the daily production rate of α_1-AT is 34 mg/kg body weight, 33% of the intravascular pool of α_1-AT being degraded daily. There is a slight increase in the rate of clearance of radiolabeled α_1-ATZ compared with that of PIM α_1-AT when infused into PIMM individuals, but this difference does not account for the decrease in serum levels of α_1-AT in persons with the deficiency [2,34]. The low-density lipoprotein receptor-related protein (LRP) family probably plays a major role in the clearance and catabolism of α_1-AT when it is in complex with neutrophil elastase [88]. The SEC receptor may be involved in the clearance and catabolism of both complex and modified forms of α_1-AT [81,89], but this has not yet been tested in vivo. The mechanism of clearance of native α_1-AT is not yet known [90].

α_1-AT diffuses into most tissues and is found in most body fluids [44]. Its concentration in lavage fluid from the lower respiratory tract is approximately equivalent to that in serum. α_1-AT is also found in feces, and increased fecal concentrations of α_1-AT correlate with the presence of inflammatory lesions of the bowel [91]. In each case, it is assumed that α_1-AT is derived from serum. However, local sites of synthesis, such as macrophages and epithelial cells, may make important contributions to the α_1-AT pool in these tissues and body fluids.

Mechanism for deficiency of α_1-antitrypsin in PIZZ individuals

The mutant α_1-ATZ molecule is characterized by a single nucleotide substitution that results in a single amino acid substitution, Lys for Glu342 [92,93]. There is a selective decrease in the secretion of α_1-AT, the abnormal protein accumulating in the ER [94,95]. The defect is not specific to liver cells because it also affects extrahepatic sites of α_1-AT synthesis, such as macrophages [94] and transfected cell lines [96,97]. Site-directed mutagenesis studies have shown that this single amino acid substitution is sufficient to produce the cellular defect [98]. Once translocated into the lumen of the ER, the mutant α_1-AT protein is relatively inefficient in traversing the remainder of the secretory pathway because it is abnormally folded. Only 10–15% of newly synthesized α_1-ATZ reach the extracellular fluid in cell line models or the blood and body fluids in vivo.

Several studies have provided evidence that the substitution of glutamate 342 by lysine in the α_1-ATZ variant decreases the stability of the molecule in its monomeric form and increases the likelihood that it will form polymers [99]. Studies by Lomas and Carrell showed for the first time polymers of α_1-ATZ in the ER of liver cells in biopsy specimens from patients with α_1-AT deficiency [99]. A recent study by Yamasaki et al., which elucidated the crystal structure of a stable serpin dimmer, has provided the basis for an interesting new model in which a domain swapping mechanism explains the formation of polymers and insoluble aggregates of α_1-ATZ [100]. The model predicts that the final step in the folding of the serpin molecule is the incorporation of strand s5a into the central β-sheet A. The substitution of lysine for glutamate 342 that characterizes the ATZ molecule lies within strand s5a and this substitution further disrupts the usual intramolecular interactions with Lys290 on strand s6a and Thr203. Because of these effects, the region, which is destined to form strand s5a in the α_1-ATZ protein, becomes flexible and unstructured in a way that favors domain swapping of strand s5a together with the reactive center loop/strand s4a between adjacent α_1-ATZ molecules. Presumably domain swapping between adjacent α_1-ATZ molecules leads to progressive linear polymerization. Finally, the unfolding event that leads to domain swapping is predicted to expose a 30-residue helical linker region. Because this linker is hydrophobic it is possible to envision lateral association between linear polymers that would produce the tangled aggregates seen by Lomas and Carrell in the ER of liver cells in AT deficiency [99]. This model provides explanations for several phenomena that have been somewhat mysterious in the past: (i) how the α_1-ATZ molecule transitions from a relatively normally folded but still polymerogenic intermediate into polymers and insoluble aggregates; (ii) how a small number (10–15%) of α_1-ATZ molecules are kinetically capable of folding into a conformation that can traverse the secretory pathway; and (iii) how the accumulation of polymeric α_1-ATZ in the ER does not activate the unfolded protein response (see below) because the structure of the polymer closely resembles the relaxed conformation of the normally folded monomer.

Polymers have also been found in the plasma of patients with the PIS$_{\text{Iiyama}}$ α_1-AT variant and the PIM$_{\text{Malton}}$ α_1-AT variant [101,102]. The mutations in α_1-AT PIS$_{\text{Iiyama}}$ (Ser53 to Phe) [42] and α_1-AT PIM$_{\text{Malton}}$ (Phe52 deletion) [17] affect residues that provide a ridge for the sliding movement opening the A sheet. According to the domain swapping model of Yamasaki et al., these mutations would be expected to slow the final folding step from a polymerogenic intermediate with an exposed strand 5A to the native state with the strand incorporated in β-sheet A. It is interesting that the hepatocytic α_1-AT globules have been found in a few patients with these two variants. Recent observations suggest that the α_1-ATS variant also undergoes polymerization [103] and that this may account for its retention in the ER, although to a milder extent than that for α_1-ATZ [41].

Polymerization also appears to occur for other serpins in clinical deficiency states, including antithrombin deficiency [104] and C1 inhibitor deficiency [105]. A striking example of this phenomenon is the familial dementia associated with Collins bodies. Studies by Davis et al. [106] have shown that these neuronal inclusion bodies contain a polymerized mutant neuroserpin.

Several studies have suggested that polymerization is the cause of retention of α_1-ATZ in the ER of liver cells. The most powerful of these are studies showing partial correction of the secretory defect by the insertion of a second mutation into the α_1-ATZ protein that suppresses polymerization [107–109]. However, these studies do not exclude the possibility that there is an abnormality in folding that is distinct from the tendency to polymerize and is also partially corrected by the second, experimentally introduced mutation. More recent studies cast some doubt on the concept that polymerization is the cause of ER retention. First, naturally occurring variants of α_1-AT, in which the carboxyl terminal tail is truncated – including a double mutant with the substitution that characterizes the Z allele together with the substitution that results in carboxyl terminal truncation – are retained in the ER of liver cells although they do not form polymers [38]. Second, only a minor proportion (approximately 18%) of the intracellular pool of α_1-ATZ at steady state in model cell lines is in the form of polymers [38,110]. Moreover, because the remainder of α_1-ATZ in the ER in vivo is in the form of heterogeneous soluble complexes with multiple ER chaperones [110], the principles by which purified α_1-ATZ polymerizes in vitro are probably not applicable to what happens in live cells in vivo. Taken together, the extant data suggest that polymerization is not the cause by which α_1-ATZ is retained in the ER of liver cells but rather is the result of its retention. Nonetheless, the polymerogenic properties of the Z mutant are still likely to be critical determinants in the pathobiology of liver disease.

To understand how alteration in the folding of α_1-AT might result in retention within the ER, we must consider what is known about the biology of protein secretion. Most newly synthesized secretory proteins are translocated into the lumen of the ER together with membrane proteins. Before being transported to their final destination, these nascent secretory and membrane polypeptide chains undergo a series of post-translational modifications, including glycosylation, formation of disulfide bonds, oligomerization, and folding. Folding is facilitated by interaction with resident ER proteins, termed molecular chaperoness. One family has been referred to as the polypeptide chain-binding protein family and includes several heat-shock proteins, GRP78/BiP and GRP94, protein disulfide isomerase, ERp57, and Erp72 [111]. Lectins including the calcium-binding phosphoproteins calnexin and calreticulin as well as OS9, also have molecular chaperone activity within the ER [112].

It is still not clear, however, whether the mechanism by which the secretory proteins are transported out of the ER involves one of three possible alternatives: (i) the protein encodes a transport signal by which it is recognized for selective removal from the ER and is concentrated as cargo in a departing vesicle; (ii) the protein encodes a signal for retention in the ER and restricts it from entering a departing vesicle; or (iii) the protein lacks both transport and retention signals and enters, by means of bulk flow, the budding vesicles at its prevailing concentration in the ER. Several cargo receptors, which direct transport out of the ER, have been identified, but so far we know of only a select group of secretory protein ligands governed by this mechanism. Nyfeler et al. recently provided evidence that the lectin ER Golgi intermediate compartment 53 kD protein (ERGIC-53) is an export receptor for α_1-AT [113]. Most importantly, ERGIC-53 failed to recognize mutant α_1-ATZ [113]. This could mean that polymerization/aggregation prevents α_1-ATZ from being presented to ERGIC-53 or that the altered folding pathway of α_1-ATZ prevents an essential ligand domain from being available to bind to ERGIC-53. The implications of these observations, together with those of the domain swapping model for polymerization/aggregation of α_1-ATZ from Yamasaki et al. [100], will be critical in conceptualizing novel therapeutic strategies in the future.

Pathogenesis of liver injury in PIZZ individuals

Liver damage in the classic form of α_1-AT deficiency is caused by accumulation of mutant α_1-AT molecules in the ER of liver cells, constituting a gain-of-toxic-function mechanism. Experimental results with transgenic mice provide the most compelling evidence for the gain-of-toxic-function mechanism and completely exclude the possibility that liver damage is caused a loss-of-function mechanism that might involve "proteolytic attack" as a consequence of diminished serum α_1-AT concentrations. Transgenic mice carrying the mutant Z allele of the human α_1-AT gene develop periodic acid–Schiff (PAS)-positive, diastase-resistant intrahepatic globules and liver injury early in life [114,115]. Because there are normal levels of α_1-AT and presumably other antielastases in these animals, as directed by endogenous murine genes, the liver injury cannot be attributed to proteolytic attack.

It has been difficult to reconcile the accumulation theory with the observations of Sveger [8,9], who showed that only a subset of α_1-AT-deficient persons sustain clinically significant liver damage. These observations have therefore led to the concept that modifiers, either genetic or environmental, predispose a subgroup of homozygotes to liver disease and/or protect the remainder of the population from liver disease. Furthermore, we have theorized that these putative modifiers affect the pathways responsible for the disposal of mutant ATZ and/or the protective signaling pathways that are activated by accumulation of ATZ in the ER [116]. This theory envisions "secondary" alterations that are subtle, in the sense that they are clinically silent when inherited or acquired by a host who has not inherited the mutation of ATZ. Furthermore, the modifiers are likely to be heterogeneous among patients and their families because this would explain the rather remarkable diversity in natural history of liver disease that has been observed. One study [117] has provided substantiation for this theory by showing a delay in intracellular disposal of ATZ after gene transfer into cell lines from homozygotes with known liver disease (susceptible hosts) compared with cell lines from homozygotes who had no evidence of liver disease (protected hosts) (Figs 31.4 and 31.5).

Because the pathways for degradation of the α_1-ATZ that is retained in the ER are obvious candidates for putative modifiers of liver disease by the gain-of-toxic function mechanism, we and others have sought to characterize the pathways. Early studies in both yeast and mammalian cell lines showed that the proteasome participates in the degradation of mutant α_1-ATZ [118–121]. In fact, degradation of mutant α_1-ATZ by the proteasome

was one of the original observations that led to the recognition of the ER-associated degradation (ERAD) pathway. ERAD is a pathway by which proteins in the lumen or membrane of the ER are targeted for degradation by retrograde translocation into cytoplasm where ubiquitination and proteasomal degradation take place (reviewed in [111]). We know now that there are different types of ERAD for luminal and membrane proteins and there may even be further subspecialization for different types of luminal proteins, but the exact chaperones and proteins that recognize α_1-ATZ and mediate its transport into the cytoplasm are not yet elucidated. It is even possible that transport of α_1-ATZ from the ER to cytoplasm involves proteasome-mediated "extraction" or "dislocation" [122]. Studies using a cell-free microsomal translocation system suggest that α_1-ATZ degradation by the proteasome occurs by both ubiquitin-dependent and -independent mechanisms [119].

Nevertheless, there was evidence from these studies of the proteasomal pathway in mammalian cell lines, of cell-free microsomal translocation systems, and of yeast that this pathway could not completely account for the disposal of ATZ. Autophagy was first implicated in AT deficiency when a marked increased in autophagosomes were observed in fibroblast cell lines engineered for the expression of ATZ [123]. Increased autophagosomes were observed in the liver of PiZ mice and in liver biopsy specimens from patients [123].

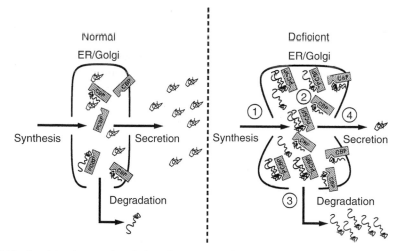

Figure 31.4 Conceptual model for liver injury in α_1-antitrypsin (α_1-AT) deficiency. Polypeptide chain-binding proteins (PCBP) and membrane-associated calcium-binding proteins (CBP) are shown as hatched bars. The α_1-AT molecules that are unfolded or misfolded are shown as long wavy lines, and those that are maturely folded are shown as condensed masses. (A) In the normal state, α_1-AT enters the secretory pathway (endoplasmic reticulum, ER) unfolded. Interaction with PCBP or CBP facilitates folding into a mature state and allows dissociation from the PCBP or CBP in a form competent for secretion. A relatively minor proportion of the α_1-AT molecules that do not fold into the mature state are directed into a pathway for degradation in, or through, the ER. (B) In a person with α_1-AT deficiency, only a minor proportion of the mutant α_1-AT molecules achieve the mature, folded state that allows secretion. There is a net accumulation of α_1-AT molecules in the ER and an increase in α_1-AT molecules directed into the pathway for degradation. Further intracellular accumulation of α_1-AT, which is potentially hepatotoxic, could result from increased synthesis of α_1-AT (1), abnormalities in interaction with PCBP or CBP (2), abnormalities in degradative enzymes (3), or abnormalities in bulk flow that allow secretion (4) of 10–15% of the newly synthesized mutant α_1-ATZ molecules.

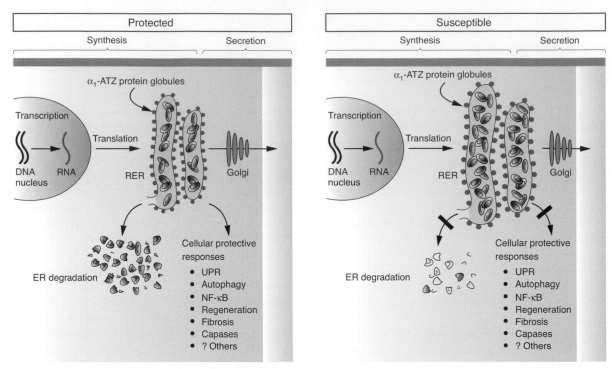

Figure 31.5 Difference in endoplasmic reticulum (ER) degradation of α_1-ATZ protein in protected and susceptible hosts. The blocks in ER degradation and cellular response pathways in susceptible hosts are represented by small dark bars. DNA, deoxyribonucleic acid; NF-κB, nuclear factor κB; RER, rough endoplasmic reticulum; RNA, ribonucleic acid; UPR, unfolded protein response; ?, not proven.

Autophagy is a catabolic process by which the cell digests its internal constituents to generate amino acids in response to nutrient starvation and other stress states. It also appears to play a role in homeostasis, cell growth, and cell differentiation. It begins with the formation of a membranous platform around a targeted region of the cell. This platform becomes a double-membrane vesicle as it envelopes cytoplasm together with parts of or entire subcellular organelles. Eventually this autophagosome fuses with the lysosome for degradation of its contents.

Thus, the presence of abundant autophagosomes in the liver in AT deficiency and its models raised the possibility that autophagy could be involved in degrading the mutant ATZ that is retained in the ER. Indeed the initial study went on to show that the disposal of ATZ was partially abrogated by chemical inhibitors of autophagy, including 3-methyladenine, wortmannin, and LY-294002 [123]. However, because these drugs have other cellular effects and therefore cannot be considered specific for autophagy, we sought to provide genetic evidence that autophagy participated in the disposal of ATZ. For this we engineered an embryonic fibroblast cell line (MEF) from an ATG5-null mouse for expression of ATZ [124]. The results showed a marked delay in degradation of ATZ in the ATG5-null compared to the wild-type MEFs. Furthermore in the ATG5-null cell line it became possible to observe massive accumulation of ATZ with very large inclusions throughout the cytoplasm. Therefore, in addition to providing definitive evidence that it contributes to the disposal of ATZ, these studies suggested that autophagy plays a "homeostatic" role in the AT-deficient state by preventing toxic cytoplasmic accumulation of ATZ through piecemeal digestion of insoluble aggregates.

A study by Kruse et al. [125] using a completely different strategy also demonstrated the importance of autophagy in the disposal of ATZ. This group expressed human ATZ in a library of yeast mutants and screened for mutants that were impaired for degradation of ATZ. One of the mutants corresponded to the yeast homolog of mammalian ATG6. In the absence of this ATG6 homolog or the homolog of ATG16 there was a marked delay in the disposal of human ATZ. These studies were particularly revealing because a delay in the degradation of ATZ was most apparent in the autophagy-deficient yeast strains when ATZ was expressed at high levels. At lower levels of expression, ATZ was degraded at a rate not signicantly different from that in wild-type yeast. These results are consistent with the notion that at lower levels of expression ATZ in the ER is predominantly soluble and can be degraded by the proteasome, whereas at higher levels of expression it is more likely to undergo transition to insoluble polymers/aggregates that require autophagy for disposal.

Kruse et al. also discovered that a mutant subunit of fibrinogen that forms insoluble aggregates in the ER of liver cells in an inherited form of fibrinogen deficiency depends on autophagy for disposal [126]. This type of fibrinogen deficiency has been associated with a chronic liver disease characterized by distinct fibrillar aggregates in the ER of liver cells. These results substantiate the concept that chronic liver disease can be caused by accumulation of an aggregation-prone protein in the ER and that autophagy is specialized for the disposal of aggregation-prone proteins that accumulate in the ER.

The presence of increased hepatic autophagosomes in AT deficiency could potentially indicate that there is some defect in the clearance of autophagosomes rather than an increase in the formation of autophagosomes. We have recently investigated this issue by monitoring LC3 isoform conversion in a cell line model with inducible expression of ATZ. The results indicate that ATZ expression is sufficient to elicit LC3 conversion and that conversion is further accentuated by the presence of lysosomal inhibitors (N. Maurice and D. H. Perlmutter, unpublished results). Thus, at least within the context of a cell line model, accumulation of ATZ in the ER results in increased formation of autophagosomes and increased autophagic flux without a defect in clearance.

Several lines of evidence suggest that there are one or more other pathways that contribute to disposal of ATZ. A pathway that depends on a tyrosine phosphatase activity has been described [127]. The studies of Kruse et al. indicated that ATZ could be transported to the trans-Golgi and then targeted to the lysosome of yeast [125] but a comparable pathway has not be described in mammalian cells.

Modifiers that affect the function of any of these pathways could increase susceptibility to liver disease according to our theory. Indeed, a single nucleotide polymorphism (SNP) in the downstream flanking region of ER mannosidase I has been implicated in early-onset liver disease among AT-deficient individuals [128]. Because ER mannosidase I plays a role in ERAD, a polymorphism that affects its function would be a prime candidate for a modifier of liver disease in AT deficiency. However, further epidemiologic studies are needed to determine if this SNP is truly affecting liver disease susceptibility and further cellular studies are needed to identify how it alters ATZ accumulation. A SNP in the upstream flanking region of the AT gene itself has also been implicated in liver disease susceptibility [129]. There is no reason to believe that this SNP would affect the disposal of ATZ. The logical explanation for the effect of this polymorphism would be to increase expression of ATZ, but the published results did not substantiate that notion. Furthermore, the study could have led to an entirely different conclusion with a

legitimate alternate way of classifying one of the patient groups.

According to our theory for the pathogenesis of liver disease in AT deficiency, modifiers would also be predicted to alter the functioning of cellular signaling pathways that might be activated to protect the cell from aggregated proteins. To address this we began a series of studies designed to determine what signaling pathways were activated when ATZ accumulated in the ER. We reasoned that this would require cell line and mouse model systems with inducible rather than constitutive expression of ATZ because the latter would potentially permit adaptations that could obscure the primary signaling effects. A series of studies using these kinds of systems have shown that the autophagic response and the nuclear factor κB (NF-κB) signaling pathway, but not the unfolded protein response, are activated when ATZ accumulates in the ER [124,130]. Activation of the autophagic response was shown by investigating the liver of a novel mouse model with hepatocyte-specific inducible expression of ATZ, the Z mouse, bred onto the GFP-LC3 mouse background. LC3 is an autophagosomal membrane-specific protein, so the GFP-LC3 mouse makes green fluorescent autophagosomes. Green fluorescent autophagosomes appear in the liver of the GFP-LC3 mouse only after 24 hours of starvation. In the Z × GFP-LC3 mouse green fluorescent autophagosomes are seen merely by allowing hepatocyte expression of the ATZ gene to be induced [130]. GFP+ autophagosomes are not seen in the liver of the Saar × GFP-LC3 mouse, which has hepatocyte-specific inducible expression of the AT Saar variant that accumulates in the ER but does not polymerize. Thus, autophagy is activated when ATZ accumulates in the ER and the autophagic pathway then plays a critical role in disposal of ATZ and in preventing massive intracellular aggregates.

Activation of NF-κB is another hallmark of the cellular response to ATZ accumulation [130]. One of the most interesting aspects of the NF-κB signaling pathway under these circumstances is that it is associated with a rather limited set of downstream transcriptional targets [131]. Indeed the most significant change in expression that could be attributable to NF-κB is downregulation of Egr-1, a transcription factor that is essential for hepatocyte proliferation and the hepatic regenerative response [132]. Our most recent studies have indicated that the downregulation of Egr-1 in the liver of the Z mouse when ATZ expression is induced is directly attributable to the action of NF-κB (A. Mukherjee and D. H. Perlmutter, unpublished results). Furthermore, the complex of proteins that assembles to form NF-κB when ATZ accumulates in the ER has a profile that is entirely distinct from that which forms when cells are treated with tumor necrosis factor (TNF) or tunicamycin

(A. Mukherjee and D. H. Perlmutter, unpublished results). Finally, mating of the PiZ mouse to a mouse model with conditional hepatocyte-specific deficiency of NF-κB activity shows more severe inflammation, fibrosis, steatosis, dysplasia, and more hepatocytes with globules (A. Mukherjee, T. Hidvegi and D. H. Perlmutter, unpublished results), indicating that NF-κB signaling is intended to protect the liver from the effects of ATZ accumulation. Together, the data on NF-κB suggest that it plays a particularly important role in the effects of ATZ on cell proliferation, survival, and ultimately the predisposition to hepatic carcinogenesis in AT deficiency.

The absence of the unfolded protein response (UPR) is also noteworthy [130]. For one, it means that activation of autophagy and NF-κB in cells that accumulate mutant ATZ is independent of the UPR, another distinct characteristic of the cellular response in the AT deficiency state. With what is known about the mechanism by which the UPR is initiated it has always been relatively easy to understand how polymerized and aggregated would not elicit the UPR. Results of recent structural studies by Huntington and colleagues provide an explanation for why soluble monomeric ATZ does not get recognized by the UPR apparatus. Those results suggest that the monomeric ATZ intermediate adopts a conformation that resembles the wild-type molecule [100] and therefore would not be recognized as unfolded.

Genomic analysis of liver from the Z mouse has identified other changes in gene expression that are attributable to the cellular response to ATZ [131]. One of these changes, upregulation of the regulator of G signaling 16 (RGS16), may represent a mechanism by which autophagy is activated in the liver in AT deficiency. We have found that the RGS16 response is characteristic and specific for ATZ. Because RGS16 anatagonizes Gαi3, and Gαi3 plays a role in inhibiting hepatic autophagy [133], we have hypothesized that increased RGS16 when ATZ accumulates in the ER leads to reversal of the inhibition of autophagy that would otherwise pertain in resting hepatocytes. There is still relatively limited information about how RGS16 is upregulated and where in the cell it acts to antagonize Gαi3.

Together the results of the foregoing studies indicate that degradation of α$_1$-ATZ is a complex process that may involve more than one pathway and at least several sequential steps in each pathway. Furthermore, signaling pathways that are presumably designed to protect the cell from the toxic effects of aggregated proteins are activated by accumulation of α$_1$-ATZ in the ER. Theoretically, each of these pathways or its individual steps may be affected in an α$_1$-AT-deficient patient who is "susceptible" to liver disease; that is, there may be heterogeneity among susceptible hosts in the mechanism by which ER degradation is delayed.

Mechanism of liver injury

There is still relatively little information about the mechanism by which ER retention of α$_1$-ATZ leads to liver cell injury. In transgenic mice that express the human α$_1$-ATZ gene, there are focal areas of liver cell necrosis, microabcesses with an accumulation of neutrophils, regenerative activity in the form of multicellular liver plates, and focal nodule formation during the neonatal period [134]. Nodular clusters of altered hepatocytes that lack α$_1$-AT immunoreactivity are also found during the neonatal period. With aging, there is a decrease in the number of hepatocytes containing α$_1$-ATZ globules; there is also an increase in the number of nodular aggregates of α$_1$-AT-negative hepatocytes and the development of perisinusoidal fibrosis [134]. Within 6 weeks, there are dysplastic changes in these aggregates. Adenoma occurs within 1 year, and invasive hepatocellular carcinoma occurs between 1 and 2 years of age [135]. The histopathology of α$_1$-ATZ transgenic mice is remarkably similar to that of hepatitis B virus surface antigen in transgenic mice and is particularly interesting because hepatitis B virus is retained in the ER or the ER–Golgi intermediate compartment of hepatocytes, often called *ground-glass hepatocytes* [136]. It is still unclear why liver injury in the transgenic mouse model of α$_1$-AT deficiency is somewhat milder and less fibrogenic than that in children with α$_1$-AT deficiency-associated liver disease. It is possible that strain-specific factors condition the response to injury, just as there are apparently host-specific factors that affect the response to injury in α$_1$-AT-deficient infants [117].

A series of studies showing the presence of hepatic mitochondrial injury in α$_1$-AT deficiency [137] have raised the possibility that liver damage is mediated by oxidative mechanisms. Mitochondrial damage was evident in both cell line and transgenic mouse models of α$_1$-AT deficiency including mitochondrial depolarization and activation of caspase 3. Treatment of the PIZ mouse model with cyclosporin A, an inhibitor of mitochondrial depolarization, resulted in less histologic damage and complete reversal of mortality associated with the experimental stress of starvation [137].

Rudnick et al. examined the proliferation of hepatocytes in the PIZ mouse model [138], and the results have led to a new theory for the mechanism by which α$_1$-AT deficiency is predisposed to hepatocellular carcinoma. This study showed that there was increased hepatocellular proliferation in the liver at baseline. The increase was 5–10-fold above that in controls and highly significant statistically; it represented a relatively low number of BrdU-positive hepatocytes (2–3% detected over 72 hours of continuous labeling). These data indicate that liver injury in the mouse model is relatively mild and appropriately corresponds to the smoldering and slowly progressing liver disease seen in most α_1-AT-deficient patients. Four other important observations were made. First, the increase in proliferation was proportional to the number of hepatocytes with globules containing the retained α_1-ATZ. This suggested that the globule-containing hepatocytes were producing a regenerative signal or signals. Second, the proliferating hepatocytes were almost entirely the ones devoid of globules. This suggested that retention of α_1-ATZ inhibits cell proliferation and that cells with a lesser accumulation of α_1-ATZ have a selective proliferative advantage in the damaged liver. Third, both globule-containing and globule-devoid hepatocytes proliferated when the PIZ mice were subjected to partial hepatectomy. This suggested that the block in proliferation of globule-containing hepatocytes is relative; that is, that they would proliferate if the stimulus were as powerful as the one generated after partial hepatectomy. Fourth, although globule-containing hepatocytes were more likely than globule-devoid hepatocytes to be undergoing cell death [139] there were still many globule-containing hepatocytes in the liver of α_1-AT-deficient patients that had not undergone death. This suggested that the globule-containing hepatocytes were "sick but not dead."

These observations constitute the basis for a new paradigm for the pathogenesis of hepatic cancer in α_1-AT deficiency and, perhaps, other chronic liver diseases. Globule-devoid hepatocytes, which are probably progenitors or at least young cells with less time to accumulate the mutant protein, have a selective proliferative advantage in the liver of the deficient individual. They are chronically stimulated in "trans" by signals that are generated by globule-containing hepatocytes that are "sick but not dead." The cancer-prone state is then engendered by having cells that are unable to die at the appropriate time and cells that are chronically dividing in the inflamed milieu. This paradigm is consistent with what has been found in the liver of the Z#2 mouse model of α_1-AT deficiency [135]. Most of the liver (>90%) becomes α_1-AT-negative as the mouse ages. This probably represents the selective proliferation of the globule-devoid hepatocytes, the progenitor cells. Adenomas and then carcinomas arise in these regions in more than 80% of the mice. This paradigm also appears to apply to the predilection for hepatic cancer in several other forms of chronic liver disease [140]. The origin of the globule-devoid hepatocytes has not been determined but these cells are known to have a lesser proportion of polymerized/aggregated α_1-ATZ than the globule-containing hepatocytes [141]. Therefore we have speculated that these cells are younger and engendered with a selective proliferative advantage when in the presence of the globule-containing hepatocytes.

Diagnosis

The diagnosis of α_1-AT deficiency is established by means of serum α_1-AT phenotype determination in isoelectric focusing or by means of agarose electrophoresis at acid pH. Serum concentrations can be used for screening, with follow-up PI typing of any values below normal (85–215 mg/dL). A retrospective study of all pediatric patients who had both serum concentrations and PI typing done at one center indicated that the serum concentration determination had a positive predictive value of 94% and a negative predictive value of 100% for homozygous α_1-AT deficiency [142]. However, because of the inherent limitations of retrospectively defining a patient population for the analysis, the results of the study are not necessarily applicable to each diagnostic situation that might be encountered. It is wise to get a phenotype together with the serum level in most cases of neonatal hepatitis or unexplained chronic liver disease in older children, adolescents, and adults. Serum concentrations of α_1-AT may be helpful, when used with the phenotype, to differentiate persons homozygous for the Z allele from SZ compound heterozygotes, both of whom may develop liver disease. In some cases, phenotype determinations of parents and other relatives are necessary to insure the distinction between ZZ and SZ allotypes, a distinction important for genetic counseling. Serum concentrations of α_1-AT are occasionally misleading. For example, serum α_1-AT concentrations may increase during the host response to inflammation, even in homozygous PIZZ individuals, and give a falsely reassuring impression.

The distinctive histologic feature of homozygous PIZZ α_1-AT deficiency, PAS-positive, diastase-resistant globules in the ER of hepatocytes, substantiates the diagnosis (Fig. 31.6). The presence of these inclusions should not

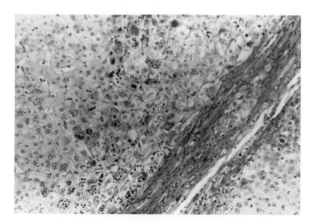

Figure 31.6 Histologic appearance of liver biopsy specimen of a patient with homozygous PIZZ α_1-antitrypsin deficiency. Micrograph shows periodic acid–Schiff (PAS)-positive, diastase-resistant globules in hepatocytes, especially periportal ones, adjacent to a broad band of fibrous tissue. PAS, diastase, original ×40. (Courtesy of Dr C. Coffin, St Louis, MO.)

be interpreted as confirming the diagnosis of α_1-AT deficiency. Similar structures are occasionally found in PIMM individuals with other liver diseases [143]. The inclusions are eosinophilic, round to oval, and 1–40 μm in diameter. They are most prominent in periportal hepatocytes but may also be present in Kupffer cells and cells of biliary ductular lineage [144]. There may be evidence of variable degrees of hepatocellular necrosis, inflammatory cell infiltration, periportal fibrosis, or cirrhosis. There may also be evidence of bile duct epithelial cell destruction, and occasionally there is a paucity of intrahepatic bile ducts.

Treatment

The most important principle in the treatment of patients with α_1-AT deficiency is avoidance of cigarette smoking, which markedly accelerates the destructive lung disease associated with α_1-AT deficiency, reduces the quality of life, and significantly shortens the longevity of these patients [2].

There is no specific therapy for α_1-AT deficiency-associated liver disease. Therefore, clinical care largely involves supportive management of symptoms caused by liver dysfunction and the prevention of complications. Progressive liver dysfunction and failure in children have been managed with orthotopic liver transplantation, with survival rates approaching 90% at 1 year and 80% at 5 years [145]. Approximately 70–80 patients with this deficiency undergo liver transplantation in the United States annually. Nevertheless, a number of PIZZ individuals with severe liver disease, even cirrhosis or portal hypertension, may have a relatively low rate of disease progression and lead a relatively normal life for extended periods. With the availability of living related donor transplantation techniques, it may be possible to treat these patients expectantly for some time. Children with α_1-AT deficiency, mild liver dysfunction (elevated transaminase levels or hepatomegaly), and without functional impairment may never need liver transplantation.

Numerous studies have shown that a class of compounds called chemical chaperones can reverse the cellular mislocalization or misfolding of mutant plasma membrane, and lysosomal, nuclear, and cytoplasmic proteins [146]. These compounds include glycerol, trimethylamine oxide, deuterated water, and 4-phenylbutyric acid (PBA). This author and his colleagues have found that glycerol and PBA mediate a marked increase in the secretion of α_1-ATZ in a model cell culture system [147]. Oral administration of PBA was also well tolerated by PIZ mice (transgenic for the human α_1-ATZ gene) and consistently mediated an increase in blood levels of human α_1-AT, reaching 20–50% of the levels present in PIM mice and healthy humans. However, in a pilot study

in patients with α_1-AT deficiency, PBA did not mediate an increase in serum levels of α_1-AT [148]. However it was not clear whether this was because the patients could not tolerate the doses necessary to have chemical chaperone activity. It is important to note that the mechanism of action of chemical chaperones has not been elucidated, but in some cases it may involve histone deacetylase inhibitory activity that mimics the changes in the transcriptional program of the cell during stress states [146].

Recently the emergence of drugs that enhance the function of endogenous degradation pathways [149–152] has raised the possibility that these drugs might be considered in patients with AT deficiency. Drugs that enhance proteasomal activity [149] or the ERAD pathway [150] should certainly be further investigated. By enhancing the degradation of soluble forms of mutant α_1-ATZ this strategy may reduce the load of α_1-ATZ in the ER in such a way that it prevents the high levels of accumulation that drive the formation of insoluble polymers and aggregates. Drugs that enhance autophagy would also be very appealing in that they would target the insoluble forms of α_1-ATZ that appear to be integral to hepatic fibrosis and carcinogenesis. Several US Food and Drug Administration (FDA)-approved drugs that have recently been shown to enhance the autophagic disposal of aggregation-prone proteins that cause neurodegenerative diseases [151,152] are currently being investigated in cell line and mouse models of α_1-AT deficiency. Ultimately it would be ideal to investigate these drugs together with small molecules that alter the conformation of the mutant α_1-ATZ in such a way that insoluble α_1-ATZ is destroyed in the liver and soluble α_1-ATZ is secreted, thereby preventing both liver and lung disease in α_1-AT deficiency. The recently described domain swapping mechanism for the polymerization of α_1-ATZ [100] provides a basis for believing that only relatively minor changes in the kinetics of folding and degradation would be needed to facilitate secretion of the soluble forms of α_1-ATZ.

Patients with COPD associated with α_1-AT deficiency have undergone replacement therapy with α_1-AT purified from recombinant plasma and administered intravenously or by means of intratracheal aerosol [34]. This therapy is associated with improvement in α_1-AT serum concentrations and in α_1-AT and neutrophil elastase inhibitory capacity in bronchoalveolar lavage fluid without significant side effects. Although results of initial studies have suggested that there is a slower decline in forced expiratory volume in patients undergoing replacement therapy, this occurred only in a subgroup of patients, and the study was not randomized [153]. It is not clear why there has not been a more impressive clinical response to date. This could mean that therapy is instituted only for patients with established and progressive COPD, too late in the course for clinical efficacy. It is also possible that replacement therapy is unable to reverse unregulated longstanding pericellular proteolysis [154] or even that the loss-of-function mechanism does not completely account for the lung damage. Protein replacement therapy is not used for patients with liver disease because there is no information to support the notion that deficient serum levels of α_1-AT are mechanistically related to liver injury.

A number of patients with severe emphysema from α_1-AT deficiency have undergone lung transplantation in the last 10 years. The latest data from the St Louis International Lung Transplantation Registry show that 91 patients with emphysema and α_1-AT deficiency had undergone single or bilateral lung transplantation by 1993. The actuarial survival rate among patients in this category who underwent transplantation between 1987 and 1994 was approximately 50% for 5 years. Lung function and exercise tolerance were significantly improved [155].

Replacement of α_1-AT by means of somatic gene therapy has been discussed in the literature [34]. This strategy is potentially less expensive than replacement therapy with purified protein and can alleviate the need for intravenous or inhalation therapy. Again, this form of therapy will be useful only in ameliorating COPD because liver disease associated with α_1-AT deficiency is not caused by deficient levels of α_1-AT in the serum or tissue. Of course, it would be helpful to know whether replacement therapy with purified α_1-AT, as it is currently applied, is effective in ameliorating COPD in this deficiency before embarking on clinical trials involving gene therapy. There are still major issues that must be addressed before gene therapy becomes a realistic alternative [156]. Several novel types of gene therapy – such as repair of mRNA by means of trans-splicing ribozymes and chimeric RNA/DNA oligonucleotides, triplex-forming oligonucleotides, small fragment homologous replacement, or RNA silencing [157] – are theoretically attractive alternative strategies for the management of liver disease in α_1-AT deficiency because they would prevent the synthesis of mutant α_1-ATZ protein and ER retention.

Studies have shown that transplanted hepatocytes can repopulate the diseased liver in several mouse models, including a mouse model of a childhood metabolic liver disease called hereditary tyrosinemia [158,159]. Replication of the transplanted cells occurs only when there is injury or regeneration in the liver because the transplanted hepatocytes have a selective proliferative advantage in the presence of the hepatocyte that are damaged by the metabolic abnormality [159]. These results provide evidence that it may be possible to use hepatocyte transplantation techniques to manage hereditary tyrosinemia and, perhaps, other metabolic liver diseases in which the defect is cell autonomous. For example, α_1-AT deficiency involves a cell-autonomous defect and we already know that the globule-devoid hepatocytes have a selective proliferative advantage [138] and thus it would be an excellent candidate for this strategy.

A recent study described a novel approach that depends on the latest advances in viral-mediated gene transfer and gene repair technology together with the selective proliferative advantage of relatively healthy hepatocytes on a background of damaged hepatocytes to correct a mouse metabolic defect [160]. Adeno-associated virus 8 was used to carry a wild-type sequence for repairing the mutant gene in a mouse model of hereditary tryrosinemia. With correction of the metabolic defect the transduced hepatocytes had a selective proliferative advantage. This approach would also be applicable for α_1-AT deficiency.

Genetic counseling

Restriction fragment length polymorphisms detected with synthetic oligonucleotide probes [161] and family studies [162] allow prenatal diagnosis of α_1-AT deficiency. Nevertheless, it is not clear how prenatal diagnosis of this deficiency should be used and how families should be counseled about the diagnosis. The data reviewed earlier indicate that 85–90% of individuals with α_1-AT deficiency do not have evidence of liver disease at 18 years of age and that nonsmoking PIZZ individuals may not develop emphysema or even pulmonary function abnormalities until 60–70 years of age. These data could support a counseling strategy in which amniocentesis and abortion are discouraged. The only other data on this subject come from two studies with conflicting results. Results of one study suggested that the incidence of significant liver disease among siblings at risk is 78% [162]. The results of the other suggested that the incidence is 21% [11]. These studies, however, were retrospective and heavily influenced by bias in ascertainment of patients. The issue will not be resolved until it is studied prospectively, as, for example, in the Swedish population [1].

Population screening

Results of several studies have suggested that population screening for α_1-AT deficiency would be efficacious. First, there is evidence that knowledge of and counseling about the consequences of α_1-AT deficiency are associated with a reduced rate of smoking among affected adolescents [163]. Second, although there was initially some evidence for adverse psychologic effects, more recent results have indicated that there are no significant negative psychosocial consequences in adults who were informed about their deficiency in a follow-up study after neonatal screening in Sweden [163]. These data should give new momentum to reconsider screening programs for α_1-AT deficiency.

Annotated references

Eriksson S, Carlson J, Velez R. Risk of cirrhosis and primary liver cancer in α1-antitrypsin deficiency. *N Engl J Med* 1986;314:736–9.
Demonstration of predisposition to cirrhosis and hepatocellular carcinoma in α_1-AT deficiency.

Hidvegi T, Schmidt BZ, Hale P, Perlmutter DH. Accumulation of mutant α1-antitrypsin Z in the ER activates caspases-4 and -12, NFκB and BAP31 but not the unfolded protein response. *J Biol Chem* 2005;280:39002–15.
This study used powerful new inducible systems to characterize the adaptive signaling pathways that are activated in cells which accumulate the mutant α_1-AT Z molecule.

Huntington JA, Read RJ, Carrell RW. Structure of a serpin–protease complex shows inhibition by deformation. *Nature* 2000;407:923–6.
Description of the crystal structure of the α_1-AT–trypsin complex provides a structural basis for the mechanism of enzyme inhibition by α_1-AT.

Kamimoto T, Shoji S, Mizushima N, et al. The intracellular inclusions containing mutant α-1-antitrypsin Z are propagated in the absence of autophagic activity. *J Biol Chem* 2006;281:4467–76.
This study provides genetic evidence for the participation of the autophagic response in disposal of α_1-ATZ and for specific activation of the hepatic autophagic response in a mouse model of α_1-AT deficiency.

Kruse KB, Brodsky JL, McCracken AA. Characterization of an ERAD gene as VPS30/ATG6 reveals two alternative and functionally distinct protein quality control pathways: One for soluble A1PiZ and another for aggregates of A1PiZ. *Mol Biol Cell* 2006;17:203–12.
This study discovered the essential role for autophagy in the disposal of α_1-ATZ in yeast, particularly when high levels of insoluble mutant protein accumulate in the ER.

Lomas DA, Evans DL, Finch JJ, et al. The mechanism of Z α1-antitrypsin accumulation in the liver. *Nature* 1992;357:605–7.
This is the original description of the tendency for α_1-ATZ to undergo polymerization.

Piitulainen E, Carlson J, Ohlsson K, Sveger T. Alpha1-antitrypsin deficiency in 26-year-old subjects: lung, liver and protease/protease inhibitor studies. *Chest* 2005;128: 2076–81.
These are the most recent results for liver disease from the nationwide screening study of α_1-AT deficiency initiated in Sweden in the 1970s. It is the only unbiased study of the disease.

Qu D, Teckman TH, Omura S, et al. Degradation of mutant secretory protein, α1-antitrypsin Z, in the endoplasmic reticulum requires proteasome activity. *J Biol Chem* 1996;271:22791–5.
This paper provides evidence that degradation of α_1-ATZ in the ER requires interaction with the molecular chaperone calnexin, ubiquitin system, and proteasome.

Rudnick DA, Liao Y, An J-K, et al. Analyses of hepatocellular proliferation in a mouse model of α1-antitrypsin deficiency. *Hepatology* 2004;39:1048–53.
Evidence for increased hepatocellular proliferation and basis for carcinogenesis in α_1-AT deficiency.

Teckman JH, An J-K, Blomenkamp K, et al. Mitochondrial autophagy and injury in the liver α1-antitrypsin deficiency. *Am J Physiol* 2004;286:G851–62.
Evidence for mitochondrial autophagy and injury cell line, transgenic mouse models of α_1-AT deficiency, and demonstration that cyclosporin A prevents liver injury and mortality.

Wu Y, Whitman I, Molmenti E, et al. A lag in intracellular degradation of mutant α1-antitrypsin correlates with the liver disease phenotype in homozygous PIZZ α1-antitrypsin deficiency. *Proc Natl Acad Sci USA* 1994;91:9014–18.
This is the original description of a defect in the degradation of α_1-ATZ in the ER that predisposes a subgroup of persons with α_1-AT deficiency to liver disease.

Yamasaki M, Li W, Johnson DJD, Huntington JA. Crystal structure of a stable dimer reveals the molecular basis of serpin polymerization. *Nature* 2008;455:1255–8.
This study describes the structure of a stable serpin dimer and provides evidence that polymerization of serpins involves a domain swapping mechanism. The mutation that characterizes the disease-associated Z allele lies within the domain that is swapped. This new model for polymerization of α_1-ATZ has enormous implications for the pathobiology of liver disease.

References

1. Sveger T. Liver disease in α1-antitrypsin deficiency detected by screening of 200,000 infants. *N Engl J Med* 1976;294:1316–21.
2. Wilson-Cox D. Alpha-1-antitrypsin deficiency. In: Scriver CB, Beaudet AL, Sly WS, et al., eds. *The Metabolic Basis of Inherited Disease*. New York: McGraw-Hill, 1989: 2409–37.
3. Silverman EK, Sandhaus RA. Clinical practice. Alpha1-antitrypsin deficiency. *N Engl J Med* 2009;360:2749–57.
4. Sharp HL, Bridges RA, Krivit W. Cirrhosis associated with alpha-1-antitrypsin deficiency: a previously unrecognized inherited disorder. *J Lab Clin Med* 1969;73:934–9.
5. Hope PL, Hall MA, Millward-Sadler GH, et al. Alpha-1-antitrypsin deficiency presenting as a bleeding diathesis in the newborn. *Arch Dis Child* 1982;57:68–70.
6. Ghishan FR, Gray GF, Greene HL. α1-Antitrypsin deficiency presenting with ascites and cirrhosis in the neonatal period. *Gastroenterology* 1983;85:435–8.
7. Eriksson S, Carlson J, Velez R. Risk of cirrhosis and primary liver cancer in α1-antitrypsin deficiency. *N Engl J Med* 1986;314:736–9.
8. Sveger T. α1-Antitrypsin deficiency in early childhood. *Pediatrics* 1978;62:22–35.
9. Piitulainen E, Carlson J, Ohlsson K, Sveger T. Alpha1-antitrypsin deficiency in 26-year-old subjects: lung, liver and protease/protease inhibitor studies. *Chest* 2005;128:2076–81.
10. Nebbia G, Hadchouel M, Odievre M, et al. Early assessment of evolution of liver disease associated with α1-antitrypsin deficiency in childhood. *J Pediatr* 1983;102:661–5.
11. Ibarguen E, Gross CR, Savik SK, et al. Liver disease in α1-antitrypsin deficiency: prognostic indicators. *J Pediatr* 1990;117:864–70.
12. Volpert D, Molleston JP, Perlmutter DH. α1-Antitrypsin deficiency-associated liver disease progresses slowly in some children. *J Pediatr Gastroenterol Nutr* 2000;31:258–63.
13. Hodges JR, Millward-Sadler GH, Barbatis C, et al. α1-Anti-trypsin deficiency in adults with chronic active hepatitis and cryptogenic cirrhosis. *N Engl J Med* 1981;304:357–60.
14. Graziadel IW, Joseph JJ, Wiesner RH, et al. Increased risk of chronic liver failure in adults with heterozygous α1-antitrypsin deficiency. *Hepatology* 1998;28:1058–63.
15. Propst T, Propst A, Dietze O, et al. High prevalence of viral infections in adults with homozygous and heterozygous α1-antitrypsin deficiency and chronic liver disease. *Ann Intern Med* 1992;117:641–5.
16. Reid CL, Wiener GJ, Cox DW, et al. Diffuse hepatocellular dysplasia and carcinoma associated with the Mmalton variant of α1-antitrypsin. *Gastroenterology* 1987;93:181–7.
17. Curiel DT, Holmes MD, Okayama H, et al. Molecular basis of the liver and lung disease associated with α1-antitrypsin deficiency allele Mmalton. *J Biol Chem* 1989;264:13938–45.

18. Crowley JJ, Sharp HL, Freier E, et al. Fatal liver disease associated with α1-antitrypsin deficiency PIM1/PIMduarte. *Gastroenterology* 1987;93:242–4.

19. Clark P, Chong AYH. Rare alpha-1-antitrypsin allele PIW and a history of infant liver disease. *Am J Med Genet* 1993;45:674–6.

20. Kelly CP, Tyrrell DNM, McDonald GSA, et al. Heterozygous FZ α1-antitrypsin deficiency associated with severe emphysema and hepatic disease: case report and family study. *Thorax* 1989;44:758–9.

21. Brantly ML, Paul LD, Miller BH, et al. Clinical features and history of the destructive lung disease associated with alpha-1-antitrypsin deficiency of adults with pulmonary symptoms. *Am Rev Respir Dis* 1988;128:327–36.

22. Janus ED, Philips NT, Carrell RW. Smoking, lung function and α1-antitrypsin deficiency. *Lancet* 1985;1:152–4.

23. Hird MF, Greenough A, Mieli-Vergani G, et al. Hyperinflation in children with liver disease due to α1-antitrypsin deficiency. *Pediatr Pulmonol* 1991;11:212–16.

24. Wiebicke W, Niggermann B, Fischer A. Pulmonary function in children with homozygous alpha-1-protease inhibitor deficiency. *Eur J Pediatr* 1996;155:603–7.

25. Bernspang B, Wollmer P, Sveger T, Piitulainen E. Lung function in 30-year-old alpha-1-antitrypsin-deficient individuals. *Respir Med* 2009;103:861–5.

26. Schonfeld JV, Brewer N, Zotz R, et al. Liver function in patients with pulmonary emphysema due to severe alpha-1-antitrypsin deficiency (PIZZ). *Digestion* 1996;57:165–9.

27. Rabin M, Watson M, Kidd V, et al. Regional location of α1-antichymotrypsin and α1-antitrypsin genes on human chromosome 14. *Somat Cell Mol Genet* 1986;12:209–14.

28. Long GL, Chandra T, Woo SLC, et al. Complete nucleotide sequence of the cDNA for human α1-antitrypsin and the gene for the S variant. *Biochemistry* 1984;23:4828–37.

29. Perlino E, Cortese R, Ciliberto G. The human α1-antitrypsin gene is transcribed from two different promoters in macrophages and hepatocytes. *EMBO J* 1987;6:2767–71.

30. Hafeez W, Ciliberto G, Perlmutter DH. Constitutive and modulated expression of the human α1-antitrypsin gene: different transcriptional initiation sites used in three different cell types. *J Clin Invest* 1992;89:1214–22.

31. Silverman GA, Bird PI, Carrell RW, et al. The serpins are an expanding superfamily of structurally similar but functionally diverse proteins. Evolution, mechanism of inhibition, novel functions, and a revised nomenclature. *J Biol Chem* 2001;276:33293–6.

32. Elliott PR, Abrahams JP, Lomas DA. Wild type α1-antitrypsin is in the canonical inhibitory conformation. *J Mol Biol* 1998;275:419–25.

33. Pierce JA, Eradio BG. Improved identification of antitrypsin phenotypes through isoelectric focusing with dithioerythritol. *J Lab Clin Med* 1979;94:826–31.

34. Crystal RG. Alpha-1-antitrypsin deficiency, emphysema and liver disease: genetic basis and strategies for therapy. *J Clin Invest* 1990;95:1343–52.

35. Brantly M, Lee JH, Hildeshiem J, et al. α1-Antitrypsin gene mutation hot spot associated with the formation of a retained and degraded null variant. *Am J Respir Cell Mol Biol* 1997;16:225–31.

36. Sifers RN, Brashears-Macatee S, Kidd VJ, et al. A frameshift mutation results in a truncated α1-antitrypsin that is retained within the rough endoplasmic reticulum. *J Biol Chem* 1988;263:7330–5.

37. Frazier GC, Siewersen MA, Hofker MH, et al. A null deficiency allele of α1-antitrypsin, QO Ludwigshafen, with altered tertiary structure. *J Clin Invest* 1990;86:1878–84.

38. Lin L, Schmidt B, Teckman J, et al. A naturally occurring nonpolymerogenic mutant of α1-antitrypsin characterized by prolonged retention in the endoplasmic reticulum. *J Biol Chem* 2001;276:33893–8.

39. Owen MC, Brennan SO, Lewis JH, et al. Mutation of antitrypsin to antithrombin: α1-antitrypsin Pittsburgh (358 Met-Arg) – a fatal bleeding disorder. *N Engl J Med* 1983;309:694–8.

40. Curiel DT, Vogelmeier C, Hubbard RC, et al. Molecular basis of α1-antitrypsin deficiency and emphysema associated with α1-antitrypsin M mineral springs allele. *Mol Cell Biol* 1990;10:47–56.

41. Teckman JH, Perlmutter DH. The endoplasmic reticulum degradation pathway for mutant secretory proteins α1-antitrypsin Z and S is distinct from that for an unassembled membrane protein. *J Biol Chem* 1996;271:J13215–20.

42. Seyama K, Nukiwa T, Takabe K, et al. Siiyma serine 53 (TCC) of phenylalanine 53 (TCC): a new α1-antitrypsin deficient variant with mutation on a predicted conserved residue of the serpin backbone. *J Biol Chem* 1991;266:12627–32.

43. Senior RM, Tegner H, Kuhn C, et al. The induction of pulmonary emphysema with human leukocyte elastase. *Am Rev Respir Dis* 1977;116:469–75.

44. Gadek JE, Fells GA, Zimmerman RL, et al. Antielastase of the human alveolar structures: implication for the protease-antiprotease theory of emphysema. *J Clin Invest* 1981;68:889–98.

45. Travis J, Salvesen GS. Human plasma proteinase inhibitors. *Annu Rev Biochem* 1983;52:655–709.

46. Huntington JA, Read RJ, Carrell RW. Structure of a serpin-protease complex shows inhibition of deformation. *Nature* 2000;407:923–6.

47. Carrell RW, Lomas DA. Conformational disease. *Lancet* 1997;350:134–6.

48. Carp H, Janoff A. Possible mechanisms of emphysema in smokers: in vitro suppression of serum elastase inhibitory capacity by fresh cigarette smoke and its prevention by antioxidants. *Am Rev Respir Dis* 1978;118:617–21.

49. Ossanna PJ, Test ST, Matheson NR, et al. Oxidative regulation and neutrophil elastase-alpha-1-proteinase inhibitor interactions. *J Clin Invest* 1986;72:1939–51.

50. Hubbard RC, Ogushi F, Fells GA, et al. Oxidants spontaneously released by alveolar macrophages of cigarette smokers can inactivate the active site of α1-antitrypsin, rendering it ineffective as an inhibitor of neutrophil elastase. *J Clin Invest* 1987;80:1289–95.

51. Mast AE, Enghild J, Nagase H, et al. Kinetics and physiologic relevance of the inactivation of α1-proteinase inhibitor, α1-antichymotrypsin, and antithrombin III by matrix metalloproteinases-1 (tissue collagenase), -2 (72-kDa gelatinase/type IV collagenase), and -3 (stromelysin). *J Biol Chem* 1991;266:15810–16.

52. Liu Z, Zhou X, Shapiro SD, et al. The serpin α1-proteinase inhibitor is a critical substrate for gelatinase B/MMP-9 in vivo. *Cell* 2000;102:647–55.

53. Liu Z, Shapiro SD, Zhou X, et al. A critical role for neutrophil elastase in experimental bullous pemphigoid. *J Clin Invest* 2000;105:113–23.

54. Duranton J, Boudier C, Belorgey D, et al. DNA strongly impairs the inhibition of cathepsin G by α1-antichymotrypsin and α1-proteinase inhibitor. *J Biol Chem* 2000;275(6):3787–92.

55. Bathurst IC, Travis J, George PM, et al. Structural and functional characterization of the abnormal Z α1-antitrypsin isolated from human liver. *FEBS Lett* 1984;177:179–83.

56. Ogushi F, Fells GA, Hubbard RC, et al. Z-type α1-antitrypsin is less competent than M1-type α1-antitrypsin as an inhibitor of neutrophil elastase. *J Clin Invest* 1987;89:1366–74.

57. Libert C, Van Molle W, Brouckaert P, et al. α1-Antitrypsin inhibits the lethal response to TNF in mice. *J Immunol* 1996;157:5126–9.

58. Camussi G, Tetta C, Bussolino F, et al. Synthesis and release of platelet-activating factor is inhibited by plasma α1-proteinase inhibitor or α1-antichymotrypsin and is stimulated by proteinases. *J Exp Med* 1988;168:1293–306.

59. Ikari Y, Mulvihill E, Schwartz SM. α1-Proteinase inhibitor, α1-antichymotrypsin, and α2-macroglobulin are the antiapoptotic factors of vascular smooth muscle cells. *J Biol Chem* 2001;276:11798–803.

60. Banda MJ, Rice AG, Griffin GL, et al. The inhibitory complex of human α1-proteinase inhibitor and human leukocyte elastase is a neutrophil chemoattractant. *J Exp Med* 1988;167:1608–15.

61. Perlmutter DH, Travis J, Punsal PI. Elastase regulates the synthesis of its inhibitors, α1-proteinase inhibitor, and exaggerates the defect in homozygous PIZZ α1-proteinase inhibitor deficiency. *J Clin Invest* 1988;81:1774–80.

62. Perlmutter DH, Glover GI, Rivetna M, et al. Identification of a serpin–enzyme complex (SEC) receptor on human hepatoma cells and human monocytes. *Proc Natl Acad Sci USA* 1990;87:3753–7.

63. Joslin G, Fallon RJ, Bullock J, et al. The SEC receptor recognizes a pentapeptide neo-domain of α1-antitrypsin–protease complexes. *J Biol Chem* 1991;266:11281–8.

64. Joslin G, Griffin GLI, August AM, et al. The serpin–enzyme complex (SEC) receptor mediate the neutrophil chemotactic effect of α1-antitrypsin–elastase complexes and amyloid–β-peptide. *J Clin Invest* 1992;90:1150–4.

65. Parmar JS, Mahadeva R, Reed BJ, et al. Polymers of alpha(1)-antitrypsin are chemotactic for human neutrophils: a new paradigm for the pathogenesis of emphysema. *Am J Respir Cell Mol Biol* 2002;26:723–30.

66. Shapiro L, Pott GB, Ralston AH. Alpha-1-antitrypsin inhibits human immunodeficiency virus type 1. *FASEB J* 2001;15:115–22.

67. Munch J, Standker L, Adermann K, et al. Discovery and optimization of a natural HIV-1 entry inhibitor targeting the gp41 fusion peptide. *Cell* 2007;129:263–75.

68. Lewis EC, Mizrahi M, Toledano M, et al. α1-Antitrypsin monotherapy induces immune tolerance during islet allograft transplantation in mice. *Proc Natl Acad Sci USA* 2008;105:16236–41.

69. Pott GB, Chan ED, Dinarello CA, Shapiro L. α-1-Antitrypsin is an endogenous inhibitor of proinflammatory cytokine production in whole blood. *J Leukoc Biol* 2009;85:886–95.

70. Hood JM, Koep LJ, Peters RL, et al. Liver transplantation for advanced liver disease with α1-antitrypsin deficiency. *N Engl J Med* 1980;302:272–6.

71. Lodish HF, Kong N. Glucose removal from N-linked oligosaccharides is required for efficient maturation of certain secretory glycoproteins from the rough endoplasmic reticulum to the Golgi complex. *J Cell Biol* 1987;104:221–30.

72. Liu MC, Yu S, Sy J, et al. Tyrosine sulfation of proteins from human hepatoma cell line HepG2. *Proc Natl Acad Sci USA* 1985;82:7160–4.

73. DeSimone V, Cortese R. Transcription factors and liver-specific genes. *J Biol Biophys Acta* 1992;1132:119–26.

74. Hu C, Perlmutter DH. Regulation of α1-antitrypsin gene expression in human intestinal epithelial cell line Caco2 by HNF1α and HNF4. *Am J Physiol* 1999;276:G1181–94.

75. Triposi M, Abbott C, Vivian M, et al. Disruption of the LF-A1 and LF-B1, binding sites in the human alpha-1-antitrypsin gene, has a differential effect during development in transgenic mice. *EMBO J* 1991;10:3177–82.

76. Dickson I, Alper CA. Changes in serum proteinase inhibitor levels following bone surgery. *Clin Chim Acta* 1974;54:381–5.

77. Perlmutter DH, May LT, Sehgal PB. Interferon β2/interleukin-6 modulates synthesis of α1-antitrypsin in human mononuclear phagocytes and in human hepatoma cells. *J Clin Invest* 1989;264:9485–90.

78. Laurell CB, Rannevik G. A comparison of plasma protein changes induced by danazol, pregnancy and estrogens. *J Clin Endocrinol Metab* 1979;49:719–25.

79. Perlmutter DH, Cole FS, Kilbridge P, et al. Expression of the α1-proteinase inhibitor gene in human monocytes and macrophages. *Proc Natl Acad Sci USA* 1985;82:795–9.

80. Barbey-Morel C, Pierce JA, Campbell EJ, et al. Lipopolysaccharide modulates the expression of α1-proteinase inhibitor and other serine proteinase inhibitors in human monocytes and macrophages. *J Exp Med* 1987;166:1041–54.

81. Joslin G, Wittwer A, Adams S, et al. Cross-competition for binding of α1-antitrypsin (α-1-AT)–elastase complexes to the serpin–enzyme complex receptor by other serpin–enzyme complexes and by proteolytically modified α-1-AT. *J Biol Chem* 1993;268:1886–93.

82. Joslin G, Krause JE, Hershey AD, et al. Amyloid-β peptide, substance P and bombesin bind to the serpin–enzyme complex receptor. *J Biol Chem* 1991;266:21897–902.

83. Kelsey GD, Povey S, Bygrave AE, et al. Species- and tissue-specific expression of human alpha-1-antitrypsin in transgenic mice. *Genes Dev* 1987;1:161–70.

84. Molmenti EP, Perlmutter DH, Rubin DC. Cell-specific expression of α1-antitrypsin in human intestinal epithelium. *J Clin Invest* 1993;92:2022–34.

85. Venembre P, Boutten A, Seta N, et al. Secretion of α1-antitrypsin by alveolar epithelial cells. *FEBS Lett* 1994;346:171–4.

86. Cichy J, Potempa J, Travis J. Biosynthesis of α1-proteinase inhibitor by human lung-derived epithelial cells. *J Biol Chem* 1997;272(13):8250–5.

87. Hu C, Perlmutter DH. Cell-specific involvement of HNF1-β in alpha-1-antitrypsin gene expression in human respiratory epithelial cells. *Am J Physiol Lung Cell Mol Physiol* 2002;282:L757–65.

88. Kounnas MZ, Church FC, Argraves WS, et al. Cellular internalization and degradation of antithrombin-III–thrombin, heparin cofactor II–thrombin, and α1-antitrypsin–trypsin complexes is mediated by the low density lipoprotein receptor-related protein. *J Biol Chem* 1996;271:6523–9.

89. Perlmutter DH, Joslin G, Nelson P, et al. Endocytosis and degradation of α1-antitrypsin–proteinase complexes is mediated by the SEC receptor. *J Biol Chem* 1990;265:16713–16.

90. Mast AE, Enghild JJ, Pizzo SV, et al. Analysis of plasma elimination kinetics and conformation stabilities of native, proteinase-complexed and reactive site cleaved serpins: comparison of α1-proteinase inhibitor, α1-antichymotrypsin, antithrombin III, α2-antiplasmin, angiotensinogen, and ovalbumin. *Biochemistry* 1991;30:1723–30.

91. Thomas DW, Sinatra FR, Merritt RJ. Random fecal alpha-1-antitrypsin concentration in children with gastrointestinal disease. *Gastroenterology* 1981;80:776–82.

92. Kidd VJ, Walker RB, Itakura K, et al. α1-Antitrypsin deficiency detection by direct analysis of the mutation of the gene. *Nature* 1983;304:230–4.

93. Jeppsson JO. Amino acid substitution Glu-Lys in α1-antitrypsin PIZ. *FEBS Lett* 1976;65:195–7.

94. Perlmutter DH, Kay RM, Cole FS, et al. The cellular defect in α1-proteinase inhibitor deficiency is expressed in human monocytes and xenopus oocytes injected with human liver mRNA. *Proc Natl Acad Sci USA* 1985;82:6918–21.

95. Foreman RC, Judah JD, Colman A. Xenopus oocytes can synthesize but do not secrete the Z variant of human α1-antitrypsin. *FEBS Lett* 1984;169:84–8.

96. McCracken AA, Kruse KB, Brown JL. Molecular basis for defective secretion of variants having altered potential for salt bridge formation between amino acids 240 and 242. *Mol Cell Biol* 1989;9:1408–14.

97. Sifers RN, Hardick CP, Woo SLC. Disruption of the 240–342 salt bridge is not responsible for the defect of the PIZ α1-antitrypsin variant. *J Biol Chem* 1989;264:2997–3001.

98. Wu Y, Foreman RC. The effect of amino acid substitutions at position 342 on the secretion of human α1-antitrypsin from *Xenopus* oocytes. *FEBS Lett* 1990;268:21–3.

99. Lomas DA, Evans DL, Finch JJ, et al. The mechanism of Z α1-antitrypsin accumulation in the liver. *Nature* 1992;357:605–7.

100. Yamasaki M, Li W, Johnson DJD, Huntington JA. Crystal structure of a stable dimer reveals the molecular basis of serpin polymerization. *Nature* 2008;455:1255–8.

101. Lomas DA, Finch JT, Seyama K, et al. α1-Antitrypsin Siiyama (Ser53 Phe): further evidence for intracellular loop-sheet polymerization. *J Biol Chem* 1993;268:15333–5.

102. Lomas DA, Elliott PR, Sidhar SK, et al. α1-Antitrypsin MMalton (Phe52 deleted) forms loop-sheet polymers in vivo: evidence for the C-sheet mechanism of polymerization. *J Biol Chem* 1995;270:16864–74.

103. Elliott PR, Stein PE, Bilton D, et al. Structural explanation for the deficiency of S α1-antitrypsin. *Nat Struct Biol* 1996;3:910–11.

104. Beauchamp NJ, Pike RN, Daly M, et al. Antithrombins wibble and wobble (T85M/K): archetypal conformational disease with in vivo latent-transition, thrombosis and heparin activation. *Blood* 1998;92:2696–706.

105. Eldering E, Verpy E, Roem D, et al. Carboxyl-terminal substitutions in the serpin C1 inhibitor that cause loop over insertion and subsequent multimerization. *J Biol Chem* 1995;270:2579–87.

106. Davis RL, Shrimpton AE, Holohan PD, et al. Familial dementia caused by polymerization of mutant neuroserpin. *Nature* 1999;401:376–9.

107. Kim J, Lee KN, Yi GS, et al. A thermostable mutation located at the hydrophobic core of α1-antitrypsin suppresses the folding defect of the Z-type variant. *J Biol Chem* 1995;270:8597–601.

108. Sidhar SK, Lomas DA, Carrell RW, et al. Mutations which impede loop-sheet polymerization enhance the secretion of human α1-antitrypsin deficiency variants. *J Biol Chem* 1995;270:8393–6.

109. Kang HA, Lee KN, Yu MH. Folding and stability of the Z and Siiyama genetic variants of human α1-antitrypsin. *J Biol Chem* 1997;272:510–16.

110. Schmidt B, Perlmutter DH. GRP78, GRP94 and GRP170 interact with α1 AT mutants that are retained in the endoplasmic reticulum. *Am J Physiol Gastrointest Liver Physiol* 2005;289:G444–55.

111. Brodsky JL, Wojcikiewicz RJ. Substrate-specific mediators of ER-associated degradation. *Curr Opin Cell Biol* 2009;21:516–21.

112. Maattanen P, Gehring K, Bergeron JJM, Thomas DY. Protein quality control in the ER: the recognition of misfolded proteins. *Semin Cell Develop Biol* 2010;21:500–11.

113. Nyfeler B, Reiterer V, Wendeler MW, et al. Identification of ERGIC-53 as an intracellular transport receptor of α1-antitrypsin. *J Cell Biol* 2008;180:705–12.

114. Dycaico JM, Grant SGN, Felts K, et al. Neonatal hepatitis induced by α1-antitrypsin: a transgenic mouse model. *Science* 1988;242:1404–12.

115. Carlson JA, Rogers BB, Sifers RN, et al. Accumulation of PIZ antitrypsin causes liver damage in transgenic mice. *J Clin Invest* 1988;83:1183–90.

116. Perlmutter DH. Liver injury in α1 AT deficiency: an aggregated protein induces mitochondrial injury. *J Clin Invest* 2002;110:233–8.

117. Wu Y, Whitman I, Molmenti E, et al. A lag in intracellular degradation of mutant α1-antitrypsin correlates with the liver disease phenotype in homozygous PIZZ α1-antitrypsin deficiency. *Proc Natl Acad Sci USA* 1994;91:9014–18.

118. Werner ED, Brodsky JL, McCracken AA. Proteasome-dependent endoplasmic reticulum-associated protein degradation: an unconventional route to a familiar fate. *Proc Natl Acad Sci USA* 1996;93:13797–801.

119. Qu D, Teckman TH, Omura S, et al. Degradation of mutant secretory protein, α1-antitrypsin Z, in the endoplasmic reticulum requires proteasome activity. *J Biol Chem* 1996;271:22791–5.

120. Teckman JH, Gilmore R, Perlmutter DH. The role of ubiquitin in proteasomal degradation of mutant α1-antitrypsin Z in the endoplasmic reticulum. *Am J Physiol* 2000;278:G38–48.

121. Teckman JH, Burrows J, Hidvegi T, et al. The proteasome participants in degradation of mutant α1-antitrypsin Z in the endoplasmic reticulum of hepatoma-derived hepatocytes. *J Biol Chem* 2001;276:44865–72.

122. Mayer T, Braun T, Jentsch S. Role of the proteasome in membrane extraction of a short-lived ER-transmembrane protein. *EMBO J* 1998;17:3251–7.

123. Teckman JH, Perlmutter DH. Retention of the mutant secretory protein α-1-antitrypsin Z in the endoplasmic reticulum induces autophagy. *Am J Physiol* 2000;279:G961–74.

124. Kamimoto T, Shoji S, Mizushima N, et al. The intracellular inclusions containing mutant α-1-antitrypsin Z are propagated in the absence of autophagic activity. *J Biol Chem* 2006;281:4467–76.

125. Kruse KB, Brodsky JL, McCracken AA. Characterization of an ERAD gene as VPS30/ATG6 reveals two alternative and functionally distinct protein quality control pathways: one for soluble A1PiZ and another for aggregates of A1PiZ. *Mol Biol Cell* 2006;17:203–12.

126. Kruse K, Dear A, Kaltenbrun ER, et al. Mutant fibrinogen cleared from the endoplasmic reticulum via endoplasmic reticulum-associated protein degradation and autophagy: an explanation for liver disease. *Am J Pathol* 2006;168:1300–8.

127. Cabral CM, Liu Y, Moremen KW, Sifers RN. Organizational diversity among distinct glycoprotein endoplasmic reticulum-associated degradation programs. *Mol Cell Biol* 2002;13:2639–50.

128. Pan S, Huang L, McPherson J, et al. Single nucleotide polymorphism-mediated translational suppression of endoplasmic reticulum mannosidase I modifies the onset of end-stage liver disease in alpha-1-antitrypsin deficiency. *Hepatology* 2009;50:275–81.

129. Chappell S, Hadzic N, Stockley R, Guetta-Baranes T, Morgan K, Kalsheker N. A polymorphism of the alpha-1-antitrypsin gene represents a risk factor for liver disease. *Hepatology* 2008;47.127–32.

130. Hidvegi T, Schmidt BZ, Hale P, Perlmutter DH. Accumulation of mutant α1-antitrypsin Z in the ER activates caspases-4 and -12, NFκB and BAP31 but not the unfolded protein response. *J Biol Chem* 2005;280:39002–15.

131. Hidvegi T, Mirnics K, Hale P, Ewing M, Beckett C, Perlmutter DH. Regulator of G signaling 16 is a marker for the distinct endoplasmic reticulum stress state associated with aggregated mutant α1-antitrypsin Z in the classical form of α1-antitrypsin deficiency. *J Biol Chem* 2007;282:27769–80.

132. Liao Y, Shikapwashya ON, Shteyer E, Dieckgraefe BK, Hruz PW, Rudnick DA. Delayed hepatocellular mitotic progression and impaired liver regeneration in early growth response-1-deficient mice. *J Biol Chem* 2004;279:43107–16.

133. Gohla A, Klement K, Piekorz RP, et al. An obligatory requirement for the heterotrimeric G protein Gαi3 in the antiautophagic action of insulin in the liver. *Proc Natl Acad Sci USA* 2007;104:3003–8.

134. Geller SA, Nichols WS, Dycaico MJ, et al. Histopathology of α1-antitrypsin liver disease in a transgenic mouse model. *Hepatology* 1990;12:40–7.

135. Geller SA, Nichols WS, Kim SS, et al. Hepatocarcinogenesis is the sequel to hepatitis in Z#2 α1-antitrypsin transgenic mice: histopathological and DNA ploidy studies. *Hepatology* 1994;19:389–97.

136. Chisari FV. Hepatitis B virus transgenic mice: insights into the virus and the disease. *Hepatology* 1995;22:1317–25.

137. Teckman JH, An JK, Blomenkamp K, et al. Mitochondrial autophagy and injury in the liver in α1-antitrypsin deficiency. *Am J Physiol* 2004;286:G851–62.

138. Rudnick DA, Liao Y, An JK, et al. Analyses of hepatocellular proliferation in a mouse model of α1-antitrypsin deficiency. *Hepatology* 2004;39:1048–55.

139. Linblad D, Blomenkamp K, Teckman J. Alpha-1-antitrypsin mutant Z protein content in individual hepatocytes correlates with cell death in a mouse model. *Hepatology* 2007;46:1228–35.

140. Rudnick DA, Perlmutter DH. Alpha-1-Antitrypsin deficiency: a new paradigm for hepatocellular carcinoma in genetic liver disease. *Hepatology* 2005;42:514–21.

141. An JK, Blomenkamp K, Lindblad D, Teckman JH. Quantitative isolation of alpha1AT mutant Z polymers from human and mouse livers and the effect of heat. *Hepatology* 2005;41:160–7.

142. Steiner SJ, Gupta SK, Croffie JM, et al. Serum levels of α1-antitrypsin predict phenotypic expression of the α1-antitrypsin gene. *Dig Dis Sci* 2003;48:1793–6.

143. Qizibash A, Yong-Pong O. Alpha-1-antitrypsin liver disease: differential diagnosis of PAS-positive diastase-resistant globules in liver cells. *Am J Clin Pathol* 1983;79:697–702.

144. Yunis EJ, Agostini RM, Glew RH. Fine structural observations of the liver in α1-antitrypsin deficiency. *Am J Clin Pathol* 1976;82:265–86.

145. Kemmer N, Kaiser T, Zacharias V, Neff GW. Alpha-1-antitrypsin deficiency: outcomes after liver transplantation. *Transplant Proc* 2008;40:1492–4.

146. Powers ET, Morimoto RI, Dillin A, Kelly JW, Balch WE. Biological and chemical approaches to diseases of proteostasis deficiency. *Annu Rev Biochem* 2009;78:959–91.

147. Burrows JAJ, Willis LK, Perlmutter DH. Chemical chaperones mediate increased secretion of mutant α1-antitrypsin (α1-AT) Z: a potential pharmacological strategy for prevention of liver injury and emphysema in α1-AT deficiency. *Proc Natl Acad Sci USA* 2000;97:1796–801.

148. Teckman JH. Lack of effect of oral 4-phenylbutyrate on serum alpha-1-antitrypsin in patients with alpha-1-antitrypsin deficiency: a preliminary study. *J Ped Gastroenterol Nutr* 2004;39:34–7.

149. Boelens J, Lust S, Offner F, Bracke ME, Vanhoecke BW. The endoplasmic reticulum: a taget for new anticancer drugs [Review]. *In Vivo* 2007;21:215–26.

150. Hotamisligil GS. Endoplasmic reticulum stress and the inflammatory basis of metabolic disease. *Cell* 2007;140:900–17.

151. Renna M, Jimenez-Sanchez M, Sarkar S, Rubinsztein DC. Chemical inducers of autophagy that enhance the clearance of mutant proteins in neurodegenerative diseases. *J Biol Chem* 2010;285:11061–7.

152. Zhang L, Yu J, Pan H, et al. Small molecule regulators of autophagy identified by image-based high-throughput screen. *Proc Natl Acad Sci USA* 2007;104:19023–8.

153. The Alpha-1-Antitrypsin Deficiency Registry Study Group. Survival and FEV1 decline in individuals with severe deficiency of α1-antitrypsin. *Am J Respir Crit Care Med* 1998;158:49–59.

154. Campbell EF, Campbell MA, Boukedes SS, et al. Quantum proteolysis by neutrophils: implications for pulmonary emphysema in α1-antitrypsin deficiency. *J Clin Invest* 1999;104:337–44.

155. Cassivi SD, Meyers BF, Battafarano RJ, et al.. Thirteeen-year experience in lung transplantation for emphysema. *Ann Thorac Surg* 2002;74:1663–9.

156. Wang L, Wang H, Bell P, et al. Systematic evaluation of AAV vectors for liver directed gene transfer in murine models. *Mol Ther* 2010;18:118–25.

157. Grimm D, Kay MA. Therapeutic application of RNAi: is mRNA targeting finally ready for prime time? *J Clin Invest* 2007;117:3633–41.

158. Rhim JA, Sandgen EP, Degen JL, et al. Replacement of disease mouse liver by hepatic cell transplantation. *Science* 1994;263:1149–52.

159. Overturf K, Al-Dhalimy M, Tanguay R, et al. Hepatocytes corrected by gene therapy are selected in vivo in a murine model of hereditary tyrosinaemia type I. *Nat Genet* 1996;12:266–73.

160. Paulk NK, Wursthorn K, Wand Z, Finegold MJ, Kay MA, Grompe M. Adeno-associated virus gene repair corrects a mouse model of hereditary tyrosinemia in vivo. *Hepatology* 2010;51:1200–8.

161. Kidd VJ, Golbus MS, Wallace RB, et al. Prenatal diagnosis of α1-antitrypsin deficiency by direct analysis of the mutation site in the genes. *N Engl J Med* 1984;310:639–42.

162. Psacharopoulos HT, Mowat AP, Cook PJL, et al. Outcome of liver disease associated with α1-antitrypsin deficiency (PIMZ): implications for genetic counselling and antenatal diagnosis. *Arch Dis Child* 1983;58:882–7.

163. Sveger T, Thelin T, McNeil TF. Young adults with α1-antitrypsin deficiency identified neonatally: their health, knowledge about and adaptation to the high-risk condition. *Acta Paediatr* 1997;86:37–40.

164. Perlmutter DH. Alpha-1-antitrypsin deficiency. In: Snape WJ, ed. *Consultations in Gastroenterology*. Philadelphia: WB Saunders; 1996:793.

Multiple choice questions

31.1 The histologic hallmark of the liver disease associated with α_1-AT deficiency is which of the following?

    a Steatosis.
    b Congo red-positive amyloid fibrils in hepatic macrophages.
    c PAS-positive, diastase-resistant globules in hepatocytes.
    d Peroxisomal proliferation.

31.2 Alternative strategies for treatment of severe liver disease due to α_1-AT deficiency include which of the following?

    a Liver transplantation.
    b Monthly infusions of purified α_1-AT.
    c Sodium benzoate to scavenge ammonia.
    d *N*-acetylcysteine.

Answers to the multiple choice questions can be found in the Appendix at the end of the book.

These multiple choice questions are also available for you to complete online.
Visit http://www.schiffsdiseasesoftheliver.com/

CHAPTER 32

Nonalcoholic Fatty Liver Disease

Stephen H. Caldwell, Curtis K. Argo & Abdullah M. S. Al-Osaimi

Division of Gastroenterology and Hepatology, Department of Internal Medicine, University of Virginia Health System, Charlottesville, VA, USA

Key concepts

- Nonalcoholic fatty liver disease (NAFLD) is one of the most common liver disorders worldwide. It is defined as liver fat exceeding 5–10% by weight and exists as a spectrum from steatosis (which is usually stable) to steatohepatitis or nonalcoholic steatohepatitis (NASH) (cellular ballooning, necroapoptosis, inflammation, and fibrosis) which progresses to cirrhosis in 15–20%. Progression is often associated with lower (even normal) aminotransferases and loss of steatosis – advanced cases may present as "cryptogenic cirrhosis." Cirrhotic complications and hepatocellular cancer occur at a slightly slower rate of progression compared to hepatitis C cirrhosis but NASH-related cirrhosis is an increasing indication for liver transplantation.

- Obesity with insulin resistance, type 2 diabetes, hyperlipidemia, and metabolic syndrome are major risk factors. Nonobese patients with fatty liver often have central obesity, insulin resistance, and physical deconditioning on exercise testing ("metabolic obesity") although some may have primary lipoprotein disorders or possibly toxin exposure (toxin-associated steatohepatitis). Ethnic variation in NAFLD is due to the *PNPLA3* (patatin-like phospholipase 3) gene, which influences the relation of steatosis to obesity and insulin resistance.

- Hepatic fat accumulation results from de novo lipogenesis from carbohydrate substrate, uptake of circulating fatty acids from lipolysis in adipose tissue, and uptake of very low-density lipoprotein-derived low-density lipoprotein remnants or circulating dietary chylomicron remnants. Lipid peroxidation, a branching chain reaction attack mediated by free radicals, is the most consistent mechanistic finding in NASH. Malondialdehyde and lipofuschin are common end products. Excessive free fatty acids alter permeability of mitochondria (cytochrome c) and lipophagic lysosomes (cathepsin), both of which result in the activation of apoptotic cell death pathways. Disturbed cytoskeleton metabolism (keratin 18 degradation) probably contributes to cellular ballooning and necrotic cell death. Oxidative injury to the phospholipid monolayer of small fat droplets (and associated PAT proteins) contributes to endoplasmic reticulum injury and likely impairs the disposal of fatty acids which might otherwise proceed through incorporation into fat droplet triglyceride.

- The diagnosis of steatosis can be made noninvasively by conventional imaging such as ultrasound, computed tomography or magnetic resonance (MR) imaging, although quantification and accuracy at levels less than 20% triglyceride require MR spectroscopy (or

modifications of conventional MR). The diagnosis of NASH requires an adequate biopsy sample, which also allows determination of fibrosis stage. Noninvasive markers of NASH are emerging and may soon provide alternatives, especially as means of following progression or response to therapy. These include measures of elasticity and blood markers of collagen metabolism and keratin fragments as indices of cell death.

- Survival in NAFLD is influenced by its association with the metabolic syndrome. The risk of liver-related death is increased, as is the risk of cardiovascular disease and non-liver cancers. The dominant course in a given patient is difficult to predict. This constellation of abnormalities presents the clinician with significant challenges. For example, conventional therapies for type 2 diabetes (angiotensin-converting enzyme inhibitors or aspirin) may be problematic in patients with portal hypertension due to fluid retention. Anticoagulant therapy in patients with coronary disease (stents), metabolic syndrome, and underlying cirrhosis is another challenging area.

- Exercise and dietary changes are key elements of treatment and may result in histologic improvement. Conditioning exercise with (or without) weight loss can reduce liver fat. Alterations in dietary composition (type of sweeteners and polyunsaturated fats) also influence disease expression. Voluntary adoption of such lifestyle changes can improve histology and introduces confounding variables in pharmacologic studies. This requires consideration of other end-points in treatment trials, including anthropometric indices and measures of insulin signaling, hepatic fat, physical conditioning, and systemic markers of fibrosis and cell death.

- A number of randomized and controlled pharmacologic trials are now available. From these, the thiazolidinediones can reduce steatosis, inflammation, and ballooning but cause weight gain, carry possible vascular risk with some agents, and have less effect on fibrosis. Higher dose vitamin E, possibly in combination with cytoprotective agents, appears promising but requires further study and carries concerns of long-term safety. Statins and fibrates appear ineffective but further study of these agents is needed. As an alternative in some patients, bariatric surgery improves liver histology along with parameters of the metabolic syndrome but carries significant risk if cirrhosis is already present. Long-term follow-up suggests a slight increase in fibrosis can also be seen.

Schiff's Diseases of the Liver, Eleventh Edition. Edited by Eugene R. Schiff, Willis C. Maddrey and Michael F. Sorrell.
© 2012 John Wiley & Sons, Ltd. Published 2012 by John Wiley & Sons, Ltd.

Nonalcoholic fatty liver disease (NAFLD) is an umbrella term that includes a range of conditions including nonalcoholic steatohepatitis (NASH); both of these terms were coined two or more decades ago [1,2]. This disease is now recognized worldwide as a potentially serious condition, which can progress to cirrhosis, liver failure, and hepatocellular cancer [3]. The spectrum of severity from very mild to very severe reflects the normal role of the liver in systemic lipid metabolism – capable of lipid synthesis from carbohydrate substrates, fat storage, and importantly lipoprotein secretion, but also subject to significant lipid-induced injury.

Terminology and diagnostic criteria

Although criteria and the name itself continue to be debated, the term NASH is widely accepted as the more severe form of NAFLD (Box 32.1) [4]. NAFLD or liver

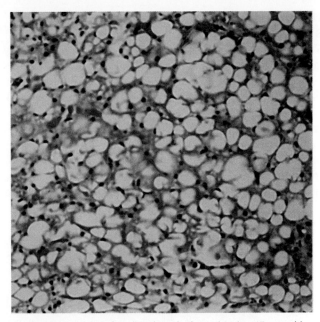

Figure 32.1 Non-NASH fatty liver (NNFL). The patient is a 47-year-old female with mild obesity, hepatomegaly, minimal past ethanol exposure, and an idiopathic, neurodegenerative disease. The biopsy showed only minimal inflammation and no fibrosis. No inciting agents were identified to explain the liver condition. NNFL is variably referred to as simple steatosis, pure steatosis, and NAFL in publications. Hematoxylin and eosin (H&E), original ×200.

> **Box 32.1 Definitions and terms.**
>
> - *Nonalcoholic fatty liver disease (NAFLD):* indicates the presence of fatty infiltration of the liver, defined as fat exceeding 5–10% of weight and frequently taken as >5–10% macrosteatotic hepatocytes in biopsy specimens. Microsteatosis is an underappreciated aspect because of limitations of routine staining techniques. The term NAFLD includes the term NASH
> - *Nonalcoholic steatohepatitis (NASH):* a type of NAFLD with inflammation, ballooned hepatocytes, necroapoptosis (cell death), and fibrosis, usually beginning around the central vein, which may progress to cirrhosis
> - *Non-NASH fatty liver (NNFL):* nonalcoholic fatty infiltration with no or minimal inflammation, and no fibrosis. We use this term to include what others have referred to as simple steatosis, nonalcoholic fatty liver (NAFL), pure steatosis, and bland steatosis. This form of fatty liver is more stable over time
> - *"Primary" NAFLD or NASH:* a term occasionally encountered in the literature. It usually indicates typical NAFLD or NASH associated with central obesity and often type 2 diabetes mellitus but without a specific, additional etiology. The likelihood that many cases of "secondary" NAFLD or NASH represent unrecognized or exacerbated "primary" NAFLD or NASH makes the term less useful
> - *"Secondary" NAFLD or NASH:* NAFLD or NASH associated with a specific, nonalcohol-related problem such as a drug- or toxin-induced cause
> - *Toxin-associated steatohepatitis (TASH):* NAFLD or NASH associated with a specific toxin or medication. Toxins implicated to date include petrochemical exposure in the oil industry and severe vinyl chloride exposure. Medications that have been associated with fatty liver include methotrexate and tamoxifen
> - *"Presumed" NASH or NAFLD:* a number of epidemiologic studies have utilized a presumptive diagnosis of NAFLD or NASH based on abnormal liver enzymes, negative viral studies, and echogenic or 'bright' liver on ultrasonography consistent with fatty infiltration

steatosis is technically defined as fat exceeding 5–10% of the liver *by weight* although it is usually estimated as fat identifiable in more than 5–10% of hepatocytes by light microscopy [5]. While NASH has become a well-known term, fatty liver without evidence of progressive injury or significant ethanol exposure (see below) is less clear and it is variably referred to as simple steatosis, pure fatty liver, or nonalcoholic fatty liver (NAFL) (Fig. 32.1). In this chapter, we have elected to use the term non-NASH fatty liver (NNFL) for this condition, which carries a better prognosis than NASH [6]. The diagnosis of either NASH or NNFL is a clear example of a "clinicopathologic" diagnosis (dependent on both clinical and histologic parameters).

Clinical criteria of nonalcoholic steatohepatitis

By definition, the criteria for NASH require the presence of steatosis and cell injury and the exclusion of alcohol as an etiology. The acceptable level of alcohol consumption is variable but can be conservatively taken as daily alcohol intake not exceeding 20 g/day in males and 10 g/day in females – levels below the risk level (30 g/day in males and 20 g/day in females) [7–9]. These cutoffs leave an unresolved gray area where a patient prone to NASH may consume alcohol close to the threshold or have significant past exposure. These issues are further discussed below.

Histologic criteria of nonalcoholic steatohepatitis

The term NASH indicates more severe cellular injury compared with NNFL. Important histologic features of NASH include lobular and/or portal inflammation, ballooned hepatocytes often containing Mallory–Denk bodies, and fibrosis (usually sinusoidal in a pericentral vein or zone 3 distribution) (Figs 32.2 and 32.3) [10,11]. Fat droplets are typically mixed macro-, medio-, and microvesicular (Fig. 32.4). Other characteristic findings include foci of necrosis, occasional apoptotic bodies, lipogranulomas, and glycogenated nuclei. Age-related patterns of injury are reported: a portal-dominant pattern is characteristic of pediatric NASH [12]. Substantial concordance between observers is evident for the extent of steatosis, and the distribution and severity of fibrosis [13]. Balloon degeneration has been more controversial but recent characterization of these cells as keratin deficient and containing small fat droplets associated with dilated endoplasmic reticulum (ER) may lead to refined clinical characterization [14,15]. The degree of fibrosis has been organized into a staging system [16]. Other refinements in histology include the NASH activity index (NAI) and NAFLD activity score (NAS) by Kleiner et al. (see below).

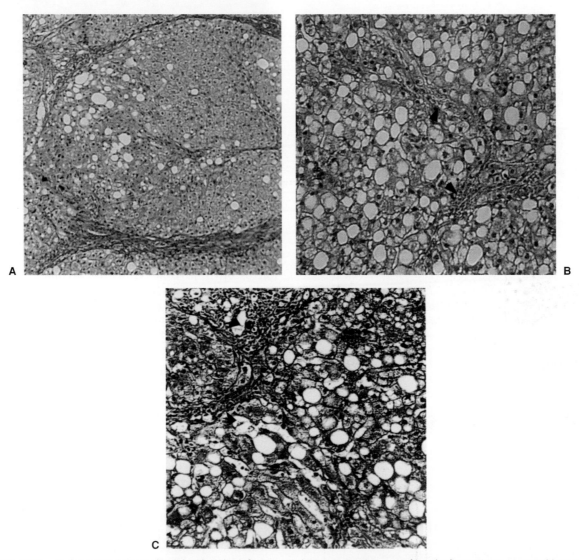

Figure 32.2 (A) Nonalcoholic steatohepatitis (NASH) with cirrhosis from a 65-year-old female with moderate obesity and type 2 diabetes. She did not have complications of portal hypertension. The presence of macrovesicular steatosis, inflammation, and cirrhosis allowed the diagnosis of NASH with cirrhosis (stage 4). H&E, original ×100. (B) Early stage 3 (bridging fibrosis) with H&E stain (original ×200). (C) The same biopsy accentuating the presence of bridging with a Masson trichrome stain (original ×200). The latter two specimens are from the first patient's 40-year-old son who had mild liver enzyme abnormalities and mild (mostly truncal) obesity (BMI = 30 kg/m²) without diabetes. NASH with fibrosis, mildly apparent on the H&E stain (B), is accentuated with trichrome staining (C) which demonstrated bridging consistent with stage 3. These slides also illustrate a familial pattern seen in about 20% of patients.

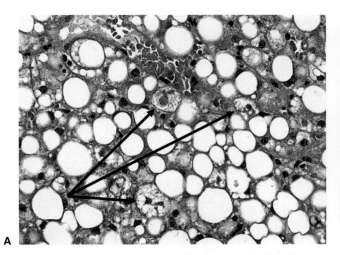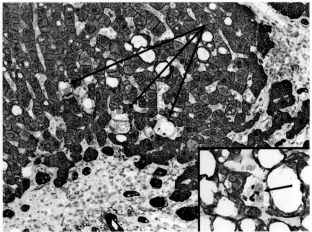

Figure 32.3 Hepatocellular ballooning and Mallory–Denk bodies. (A) The arrows indicate ballooned hepatocytes with Mallory–Denk bodies evident as perinuclear material in two of the cells by H&E staining. (B) With antikeratin8/18 immunohistochemistry, ballooned hepatocytes are "empty" of keratin (arrows) but the Mallory–Denk bodies are accentuated as dark brown-staining masses. (Courtesy of Dr Carolyn Lackner.)

Presumed nonalcoholic fatty liver disease

In epidemiologic studies, the diagnosis of "presumed NAFLD" may be made on the basis of noninvasive testing. In general, such studies have utilized abnormal transaminases in the absence of other known liver disease and/or liver ultrasound to make the diagnosis of fatty liver. The relationship between the diagnosis of presumed NAFLD and the histologic activity, stage, and prognosis is unreliable. Indeed, this constitutes one of the major limitations of these studies.

Cryptogenic cirrhosis

While diverse causes are recognized, NASH can progress to a late stage with loss of steatosis which is sometimes called "cryptogenic cirrhosis" (Fig. 32.5) [17–19]. Typical patients are 60 years old with only mild liver enzyme elevation and more often are or were obese and diabetic compared with control groups (Fig. 32.6) [20–29]. A *history* of obesity must be specifically sought due to nutritional changes characteristic of advancing cirrhosis – especially loss of body fat [30]. Histologically, residual cellular ballooning and glycogenated nuclei serve as clues to prior NASH from studies in patients undergoing serial biopsy [31]. Loss of steatosis may be due to altered blood flow, decreased sinusoidal permeability, and impaired lipoprotein delivery as the liver becomes fibrotic or to more fundamental changes in hepatocyte metabolism related to the proliferation of progenitor cells [32–34]. In a series of patients undergoing transplantation for cryptogenic cirrhosis, definitive features of NASH were evident in 17 of 30 patients and minor features were seen in an additional ten patients [35]. The incidence of steatosis and steatohepatitis after transplantation for cryptogenic cirrhosis further supports this relationship [36–38]. A proposed classification is shown in Box 32.2.

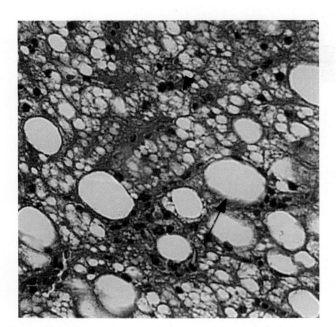

Figure 32.4 Micro- and macrovesicular steatosis in nonalcoholic steatohepatitis. The arrowhead indicates a cell with small droplets of fat in addition to the more apparent and typical large droplet, macrovesicular, steatosis (arrow). Special stains or fixation techniques, such as osmium tetroxide fixation (not shown), can be used to accentuate the often overlooked microvesicular component. H&E, original ×400.

Focal steatosis and focal fat sparing

In a series of patients with fatty liver detected radiographically, focal steatosis was evident in approximately 15% and focal sparing (usually of the caudate lobe) was seen in 9% [39]. Variation in blood flow is thought to explain both and altered insulin exposure is a suspected factor [40,41].

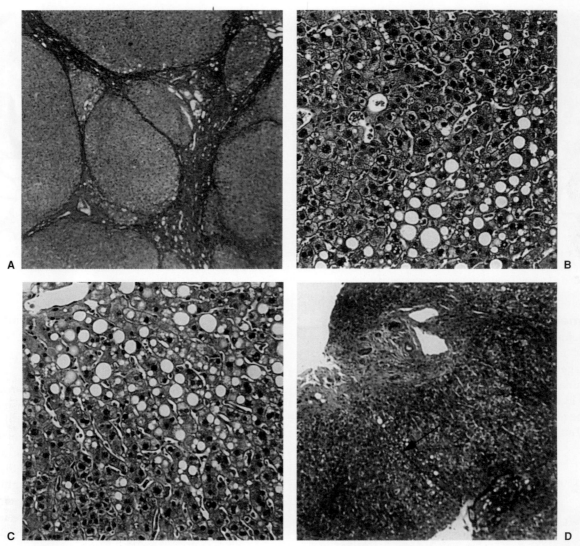

Figure 32.5 Development of nonalcoholic steatohepatitis following transplantation for cryptogenic cirrhosis. (A) Explanted liver from an obese, diabetic male showing "bland" cirrhosis. H&E, original ×40. (B) Two years later a repeat biopsy for abnormal liver enzymes revealed steatosis. H&E, original ×200. (C) The steatosis was persistent and associated with mild inflammation at 3 years. H&E, original ×200. (D) Four years after transplantation the patient developed ascites and a repeat biopsy showed early cirrhosis with bridging and diminished fatty infiltration. The arrow indicates a fibrous band. H&E, original ×100.

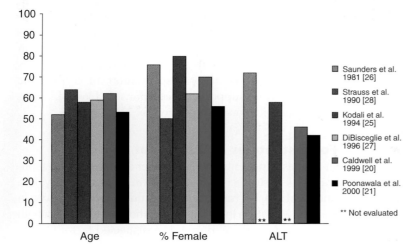

Saunders et al. 1981 [26]
Strauss et al. 1990 [28]
Kodali et al. 1994 [25]
DiBisceglie et al. 1996 [27]
Caldwell et al. 1999 [20]
Poonawala et al. 2000 [21]

** Not evaluated

Figure 32.6 Past series of cryptogenic cirrhosis patients. Previous case series have shown a predominance of females, onset in sixth or seventh decade, and mildly abnormal alanine aminotransferase (ALT) levels. The y axis represents age in years, percent females, or mean serum ALT. Series are included in the references cited in the text.

Box 32.2 Proposed classification of cryptogenic cirrhosis.

- Class 1: Cirrhosis with features of steatohepatitis
  - 1a: NASH with cirrhosis
  - 1b: Cirrhosis with features of NASH
  - 1c: Bland cirrhosis with NASH risk factors (obesity, hyperlipidemia, diabetes)
- Class 2: Cirrhosis with features of autoimmune disease
- Class 3: Cirrhosis with features of viral hepatitis
- Class 4: Cirrhosis with features of alcoholic liver disease (i.e., history of lifelong significant alcohol consumption)
- Class 5: Cirrhosis with features of biliary disease
- Class 6: Bland cirrhosis with no specific histologic or historical diagnostic features

Adapted from Argo and Caldwell [64] and Caldwell [473].

Histologically, the lesions vary from simple steatosis to frank steatohepatitis.

Historical perspective

Early observations

A long recognized association between the liver and fat storage is revealed in the origin of the Latin word for liver *ficatum* and the corresponding modern Greek term *sycoti*, both of which derived from the common name for fattened animal livers, *iecur ficatum* and *hepar sykoton* (D. Tiniakou, personal communication). A scientific appreciation of fatty liver emerged in the nineteenth century when Virchow classified various types of fatty infiltration of the liver [42]. The color, shape, and firmness of fatty liver were described and fat globules were proven to be within hepatocytes [43]. Morgan, in the 1870s, described an association of fatty liver with obesity and overeating [44]. This was extended many years later by Zelman who reported liver fibrosis and cirrhosis in obese patients without significant alcohol consumption [45]. The concept resurfaced in the 1970s in patients who had undergone intestinal bypass for morbid obesity [46].

The ethanol conundrum

Cutoffs for classification as "*non*-alcoholic" versus "alcoholic" steatohepatitis (NASH versus ASH) remain unresolved. Clearly, there are patients with NASH and related cirrhosis without a history of ethanol exposure (teetotalers). Prior to this recognition, a common experience was nicely summarized by Ludwig in his original description of NASH [2]:

> ...we have encountered patients who did not drink, who had not been subject to bypass surgery, and who had not taken

drugs that may produce steatohepatitis, yet had in their liver biopsy specimens changes that were thought to be characteristic of alcoholic liver disease In these instances, the biopsy evidence sometimes caused clinicians to persevere unduly in their attempts to wrench from the patient an admission of excessive alcohol or to obtain a confirmation of such habits from relatives of the patients. Thus, the misinterpretation of the biopsy in this poorly understood and hitherto unnamed condition caused embarrassment to the patient and physician.

Nonetheless, about 10% of patients classified as having NASH actually have had significant lifetime exposure to ethanol when a more structured history is obtained [47]. Intuitively, synergy between ASH and NASH seems likely because obesity is a risk for more severe alcohol-related liver disease [48]. However, studies suggest *moderate* consumption either reduces or does not worsen histology in NASH – an effect possibly mediated by changes in insulin signaling [49–51]. Conventional histologic features do not reliably distinguish ASH from NASH, with the exception of glycogenated nucleii (increased in NASH) [52]. Immunohistochemical stains may help but are not established [53]. Proposed laboratory tests have largely fallen short [54] although aminotransferase ratios may provide guidance: the aspartate aminotransferase (AST) to alanine aminotransferase (ALT) ratio is typically <1 in early or mild NASH, >1 and <2 in more severe NASH, and >2 in more severe ASH (see section below on laboratory findings). For these reasons, a gray area is likely to persist and a careful history remains the common means of assessing alcohol consumption.

Hepatogenous diabetes

Complicating the relationships between insulin resistance and NAFLD is the relationship between cirrhosis and diabetes referred to as "hepatogenous diabetes" [55]. A number of papers have established an increased prevalence of diabetes in cirrhosis of various etiologies [56]. Impaired insulin sensitivity is postulated to explain this [57]. The role of abnormal cirrhosis-related skeletal muscle metabolism has yet to be fully investigated [58].

Epidemiology and prevalence

Nonalcoholic fatty liver disease is one of the most common liver disorders [3,59–63]. The prevalence of NAFLD (including both NNFL and NASH) is as high as 38% depending on criteria and region studied [64,65]. In 150 consecutive patients with abnormal liver enzymes for at least 6 months, 42% had fatty liver while 15% had hepatitis C [66]. In 81 patients with abnormal liver enzymes and a negative serologic workup, 50% of the patients had steatosis and 32% had steatohepatitis [67].

Box 32.3 Conditions associated with nonalcoholic fatty liver.

Metabolic factors
- Metabolic syndrome:
    Obesity (especially truncal or central obesity)
    Type 2 diabetes mellitus or hyperinsulinemia
    Hypertension
    Hyperlipidemia (especially hypertriglyceridemia)
- Polycystic ovary disease

Genetic/metabolic conditions associated with fatty infiltration of the liver
- Lipodystrophies
- Mitochondrial diseases
- Weber–Christian disease
- Wilson disease

Toxin-associated steatohepatitis
- Medications:
    Methotrexate
    Amiodarone
    Tamoxifen
    Nucleoside analogs
- Work-related toxins:
    Carbon tetrachloride
    Percholorethylene
    Ethyl bromide
    Petrochemicals
    Vinyl chloride

Parenteral nutrition and malnutrition
- Total parenteral nutrition
- Kwashiorkor
- Celiac disease

NAFLD accounts for about one third of cases of chronic liver disease in primary care [68]. Obesity, type 2 diabetes, and hyperlipidemia are the most constant conditions associated with steatosis and are predictors of more severe histologic disease [69,70]. An overview of conditions associated with NAFLD is shown in Box 32.3.

Obesity

There is a 4.6-fold increased risk of fatty liver in obese patients compared with nonobese patients by ultrasound imaging [8]. In an autopsy study, steatosis was found in approximately 70% of obese versus 35% of lean patients, and steatohepatitis was found in 18.5% of obese versus 2.7% of lean patients [71]. In a compilation of 12 studies of 1,620 patients undergoing bariatric surgery (body mass index (BMI) usually $>35 \, kg/m^2$), histology revealed steatosis (NNFL) in 85–90%, NASH in 25–30%, and unexpected cirrhosis in 1–2% (Fig. 32.7) [72]. In a series of consecutive obese patients with abnormal liver enzymes approximately 30% had at least septal fibrosis and 10% had cirrhosis [73]. However, the relationship between obesity and fatty liver is significantly influenced by both ethnicity and the degree of physical conditioning (see below).

Insulin resistance and type 2 diabetes mellitus

Insulin resistance is very common in NAFLD [74–76]. It can be demonstrated in major insulin targets including adipose tissue (persistent lipolysis), muscle (diminished glucose disposal), and liver (failure to suppress glucose release). The progression to overt diabetes depends on pancreatic islet cell vitality but it is thought that steatosis usually precedes this development in susceptible populations [77]. However, as with obesity, ethnicity significantly influences these relationships (see below). In general, it is estimated that up to 75% of type 2 diabetic patients have fatty infiltration [78,79]. Liver injury worsens with the degree of abnormal glucose metabolism, and the existence of diabetes in patients with NAFLD more than doubles the prevalence of cirrhosis from 10% to 25% [80,81].

Hyperlipidemia

The prevalence of NAFLD in different forms of hyperlipidemia remains uncertain. One study using noninvasive imaging showed that two thirds of patients with

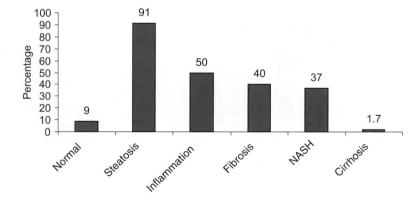

Figure 32.7 Liver histology in a series of severely obese patients (BMI >35 kg/m²). Only 9% had normal histology while 1–2% had previously unidentified cirrhosis. Approximately 90% had steatosis and one third of these met criteria for nonalcoholic steatohepatitis (NASH) with varying degrees of fibrosis in 40%. (Data from Machado et al. [72].)

hypertriglyceridemia and one third with hypercholesterolemia had fatty liver [82]. This is probably an underestimation as hyperlipidemia is reported in up to 92% of
NASH patients, although a wide range has been noted
[83]. Postprandial lipid profiles as opposed to fasting
profiles may be especially relevant [84]. The complexity of these relationships is reflected in the mechanistic
role of lipoproteins in NASH, ethnic variation in lipid
metabolism, overlapping risks of NASH and atherosclerotic vascular disease, and suspected heterogeneity in
lipid phenotypes in NAFLD.

Metabolic syndrome

Steatosis and central adiposity are independent risk
factors for the metabolic syndrome, united by underlying insulin resistance and lipotoxicity [85,86]. An
unexplained elevation of liver enzymes, attributable to
NAFLD, is seen in 7% of individuals with metabolic
syndrome defined by the Adult Treatment Panel III
criteria (Box 32.4) [87,88]. However, the prevalence of
NAFLD in the general population, the prevalence of
metabolic syndrome among patients with NAFLD, and
the frequency of normal liver enzymes even with histologic disease suggest that the prevalence of NAFLD in
metabolic syndrome is much higher although influenced
by genetic/ethnic factors (discussed below) [89,90]. While
closely related, it is evident that fatty liver in itself does
not cause metabolic syndrome but constitutes a feature of
this syndrome [91].

Normal body mass index

Nonalcoholic fatty liver disease has been well documented in patients with normal BMI [5]. Such individuals
are characterized by visceral adiposity, hyperinsulinemia,
and physical deconditioning [92]. These findings are consistent with the concept of "metabolic obesity" in patients
with a lower BMI and NAFLD and the role of body fat

distribution and physical deconditioning in the development of this disorder [93–95].

Pediatric patients

Nonalcoholic fatty liver disease is a potentially serious
problem in children, where it is also associated with obesity and the metabolic syndrome [96,97]. Severity varies
but fibrosis and cirrhosis were described in 18 of 24
patients in one series [98]. Recently acquired rather than
longstanding obesity increases the risk of fatty infiltration. Male preponderance and prominent portal tract
injury are characterisitic [99]. Ethnic influences are similar to adult disease, with a greater risk among children of
Hispanic or northern European compared with those of
African-American descent [100].

Nonalcoholic steatohepatitis in other liver diseases

Nonalcoholic fatty liver disease coexists with and influences other liver diseases [101]. Steatosis mediated by
core protein metabolism and microsomal triglyceride
transfer protein (MTTP) is associated with hepatitis C
(especially genotype 3) and probably accelerates progression [102,103]. Many hepatitis C virus (HCV) patients
have coexisting risk factors for NASH, suggesting a synergistic effect in some [104]. Obesity, insulin resistance,
and steatosis negatively influence response to antiviral
therapy [105]. Occult hemochromatosis and iron loading
has also been suggested as a factor in the progression
of NASH [106]. However, hyperferritinemia in NAFLD
correlates more closely with insulin resistance than with
iron overload or *HFE* gene mutations and can be reversed
with weight loss [107]. Steatosis has also been recognized
as a potential factor in the progression of primary biliary cirrhosis (PBC) [108]. Histologic features of autoimmune hepatitis are sometimes seen with NASH. It is
likely that this represents two separate diseases although
weight gain with steroid therapy may explain an
association.

Genetic factors

Ethnic variation

The prevalence of NAFLD varies among high-risk groups
depending on ethnicity (Fig. 32.8) [109–111]. People of
Hispanic descent in the United States have a higher
prevalence, while people of primarily African-American
descent have a lower than expected prevalence relative
to rates of obesity and diabetes compared with people
of Asian or northern European descent. The findings
reflect ethnic differences in the distribution of body fat
and lipoprotein metabolism [112–114]. Importantly, ethnic variation reveals a dissociation between fatty liver,

---

Box 32.4 Adult Treatment Panel III clinical features of the metabolic syndrome.[a]

- Abdominal obesity:
    Men: waist circumference >102 cm (>40 inches)
    Women: waist circumference >88 cm (>35 inches)
- Triglycerides: ≥ 150 mg/dL
- High-density lipoprotein cholesterol:
    Men: <40 mg/dL
    Women: <50 mg/dL
- Blood pressure: ≥130/≥85 mmHg
- Fasting glucose: ≥110 mg/dL

[a] Although specific criteria are noted, this syndrome can also be
viewed as a continuum.

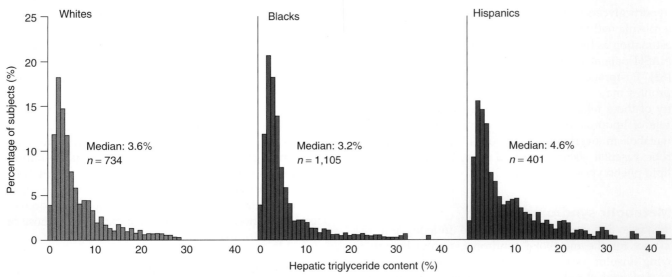

Figure 32.8 Distribution of hepatic triglycerides content by ethnicity as assessed by ^{1}H-magnetic resonance spectroscopy. The distribution of hepatic triglycerides content was skewed toward lower levels in blacks and slightly higher levels in Hispanics. (Reproduced from Browning et al. [111] with permission from Wiley.)

hyperlipidemia, and insulin resistance. Although liver fat generally correlates to intraperitoneal fat, African-Americans have lower intraperitoneal fat, lower liver fat, and lower blood triglycerides despite similar levels of insulin resistance as Hispanic-Americans [115]. Similar ethnic variation has been described in cryptogenic cirrhosis [116].

Familial factors

A high prevalence of afflicted first-degree relatives is seen in NASH [117–119]. There is an association with obesity, diabetes, and cryptogenic cirrhosis within kindreds. The findings likely represent a combination of both genetic risk and common health habits. The demonstration of insulin resistance among relatives of type 2 diabetics and impaired skeletal muscle mitochondrial metabolism in their offspring supports a strong genetic component [120, 121]. Moreover, a prospective study using spectroscopy among siblings and parents of overweight probands with and without fatty liver detected fatty liver in 17% of siblings and 37% of parents in the group without fatty liver compared to 59% and 78%, respectively, in the group with fatty liver [122].

Genetic variation

Given the complexity of organ injury in NASH, it is not surprising that a number of associations have been identified in genes regulating fat and glucose metabolism, oxidative stress, the mitochondrial antioxidant system, keratins, and cytokine activity [123,124]. A gene coding

for a phospholipase-like protein called PNPLA3 (patatin-like phospholipase 3) or adiponutrin has been identified as a major predictor of steatosis within different ethnic groups [125]. PNPLA3 may function primarily in the transfer of fatty acids between lipids. The gene is highly conserved and appears to be regulated in part by dietary fat [126]. Apolipoprotein C3 variants may also influence the risk of steatosis, together with fasting and postprandial triglyceride clearance possibly mediated by altered chylomicron metabolism [127]. Polymorphisms in transcription factor 7-like 2 (TCF7L2) and MTTP influence NASH risks through postprandial lipidemia, adipokine secretion, and metabolism of oxidized low-density lipoprotein (LDL) [128,129]. A synergistic association between angiotensinogen and transforming growth factor β1 (TGF-β1) genotypes has also been described in patients with more severe NASH [130].

Clinical and laboratory findings

Symptoms and signs

Typical signs and symptoms and laboratory findings are summarized in Box 32.5. Fatigue and right upper quadrant discomfort (often positional) are common but an absence of more specific symptoms was noted in 48–100% of patients in a compilation of studies [131]. Discomfort may be mistaken for gallstone disease. Hepatomegaly is usually due to steatosis but may be due to glycogenosis in diabetic patients [132]. Clinical findings of obesity

Box 32.5 Symptoms, signs, and laboratory features of nonalcoholic fatty liver disease.

Symptoms
- Asymptomatic (48–100%)
- Fatigue (~70%)
- Right upper quadrant pain (up to 50%)
- Occasional neurologic deficits (possibly part of systemic lipotoxicity)
- Obstructive sleep apnea
- Polycystic ovarian syndrome-related complaints

Signs
- Hepatomegaly
- Acanthosis nigricans
- Palmer erythema and spider angiomata (with development of cirrhosis)

Laboratory features
- Elevated aspartate aminotransferase (AST) and alanine aminotransferase (ALT) levels (usually <2 times upper limit of normal)
- Elevated γ-glutamyltransferase (GGT) level
- Mildly elevated alkaline phosphatase level
- Antinuclear antibody (ANA) positive (~30%)
- Increased serum immunoglobulin A (IgA) level in about 20%
- Elevated iron indices in 20–60% (usually without actual hemochromatosis)
- Hyperuricemia

and metabolic syndrome include diabetes, hyperlipidemia, hypertension, vascular disease, polycystic ovary syndrome, and sleep apnea [133–135]. Changes in body composition due to aging and cirrhosis may mask a history of prior obesity [30]. A relationship between hypercoagulability in metabolic syndrome and steatohepatitis is increasingly recognized [136–138]. Acanthosis nigricans may be present especially in children, but also in adults. The presence of a "buffalo hump" may indicate more severe histologic disease. Palmer erythema or spider angiomata suggest the presence of cirrhosis. A subacute form of NASH with unexplained sudden decompensation has also been recognized [139].

Common laboratory findings

Many patients present with abnormal ALT and/or AST, detected on screening or in treatment for weight loss, hypertension, diabetes, or hyperlipidemia. AST and ALT levels average 55 and 74 IU/L, respectively [140]. AST is partly mitochondrial in origin (mAST) [141]. An AST:ALT ratio of <1 suggests mild disease, while values >1 often indicate fibrosis [142]. However, patients with advanced disease, including cirrhosis, may have normal aminotransferases [143]. This results in part from dimin-

ished inflammation as fibrosis progresses (see below). In addition, obesity in the general population has resulted in a spuriously rising "normal" reference range – an issue that has yet to be uniformly resolved [144,145]. Antidiabetic and antilipidemic medications also influence this relationship in both directions.

Other laboratory abnormalities

Autoantibodies such as antinuclear antibody are seen in about one third of NASH patients [146]. Abnormal iron indices are seen in 20–60% of patients but usually are not associated with genetic hemochromatosis, although ferritin elevation may be a marker for more severe disease [147,148]. Hyperuricemia may be present as in metabolic syndrome. Low platelets warrant an additional search for hypersplenism and cirrhosis [149]. Similar to alcoholic steatohepatitis, elevation of serum immunoglobulin A (IgA) may be seen [150]. Thyroid dysfunction has been suggested as an association in some patients.

Tests of insulin resistance, dyslipidemia, and physical conditioning

The HOMA (homeostatic model assessment) and QUICKI (quantitative insulin sensitivity check index) are used to estimate insulin resistance although these tests have limitations [151]. Both utilize mathematical manipulation (derived from euglycemic clamp testing) of fasting insulin and glucose levels. The addition of free fatty acid levels to the QUICKI improves its accuracy [152]. Lipoprotein profiles in NAFLD are incompletely defined. The VAP (vertical analytic profile) panel and nuclear magnetic resonance-based techniques may be useful to define lipid particle size. Although not widely available, measures of exercise capacity by bicycle ergometry to determine oxygen utilization (VO_{2peak}) may also be useful to discern "metabolic obesity" and correlate to the degree of insulin resistance [153].

Noninvasive markers of liver injury and fibrosis

See the section on the role of liver biopsies below.

Findings of lipodystrophy

Fatty liver is common in the lipodystrophies [154]. These disorders, congenital or acquired, are possibly more prevalent than commonly thought. A familial form of partial lipodystrophy with NAFLD and cirrhosis is reported among females with the acquired variety [155]. Typical features include diabetes, elevated triglycerides, and focal or diffuse loss of subcutaneous fat. Histologic NASH was observed in eight of ten patients who had improvement with leptin replacement [156].

Lipodystrophy related to antiretroviral therapy is discussed further below.

Findings suggestive of mitochondrial disease

Mitochondrial abnormalities in the liver suggest that systemic mitochondrial disease may be present and influenced by genetic mitochondrial heteroplasmy [157, 158]. Cryptogenic cirrhosis is seen in mitochondrial disease and insulin resistance is a feature of the MIDD syndrome (maternally inherited diabetes and deafness) and Madelung disease (both associated with mitochondrial DNA mutations) [159–161]. Similar hepatic mitochondrial DNA mutations have been identified in NASH [162]. Symptoms suggestive of systemic mitochondrial disease include depression, ophthalmoplegia, neurodegenerative diseases, deafness, lipomatosis, and gut dysmotility [163].

Weber–Christian disease

Nodular panniculitis with fat necrosis, especially over the lower extremeties, is the most distinguishing features of Weber–Christian disease. Steatohepatitis suggests a systemic disorder of fat metabolism [164]. Immunosuppression has been reported to be effective therapy indicating an autoimmune component [165].

Liver imaging

Liver imaging plays an important role in the clinical evaluation of NAFLD (Fig. 32.9) and in epidemiologic studies of the disease [166]. However, conventional techniques are unable to grade or stage NASH and are insensitive to hepatic fat that is less than 20% by weight [167,168]. Cross-sectional imaging is also used to assess fat distri-

bution (visceral versus peripheral fat) by determining the fat area at specific levels such as L4–5 [169,170]. Ultrasonography detects steatosis by echogenicity and sound attenuation with defined criteria [171]. Ultrasonic elastography measures liver stiffness as a marker of fibrosis. Sensitivity and specificity for stage 3–4 fibrosis is 91% and 75%, respectively ($>7.9\,kPa$) but failure to acquire a signal increases with a BMI of $>30\,kg/m^2$ [172].

Unenhanced computed tomography (CT) relies on attenuation differences between the liver and spleen [173]. A "liver : spleen ratio" (in Hounsfield units) of <1 is consistent with steatosis. Sensitivity and specificity for fatty liver were 84% and 99%, respectively, for a spleen minus liver value of ≥ 10 Hounsfield units in one study [174]. Conventional spin-echo magnetic resonance imaging (MRI) is insensitive in detecting steatosis. However, refinements including "in–out of phase imaging" improve fat detection [175]. Improved signal processing (using the Dixon technique) provides quantitative estimates expressed as percentage triglyceride content. Magnetic resonance proton spectroscopy is the most accurate means of quantifying steatosis (Fig. 32.10) [176]. In one study, the correlation between fat measured in liver biopsies and proton spectroscopy was 0.9 ($P < 0.001$) [177]. ^{31}P spectroscopy is capable of measuring adenosine triphosphate (ATP), lipid peroxidation, and the phospholipid content of the liver [178,179].

Role of liver biopsy

Liver biopsy remains the standard for confirming the diagnosis, staging fibrosis, grading activity, and judging response to treatment. Clinically, biopsy is often deferred until failure of a conservative course of exercise and diet unless the evaluation indicates more advanced disease

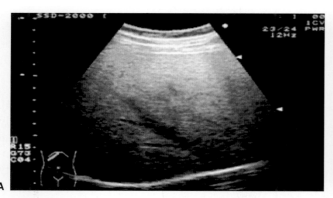
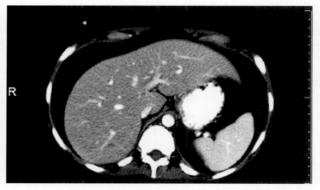

Figure 32.9 Radiologic imaging of NAFLD. (A) Sonographic appearance of NAFLD demonstrating a heterogeneous appearing echotexture with findings of "bright liver" in the parenchyma. (B) Computed tomography (CT) appearance of NAFLD showing a relatively hypodense liver compared to the spleen (liver:spleen ratio <1).

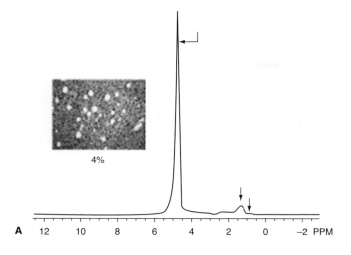

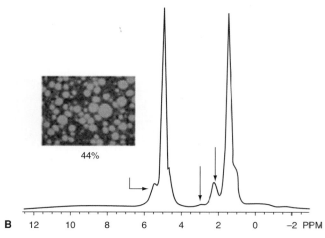

Figure 32.10 Magnetic resonance proton spectroscopy to measure hepatic fat content. (A) A patient with lower triglyceride content (4%) with a strong water signal and relatively weak methyl and methylene signal from triglyceride. (B) A patient with high triglyceride content (44%) evident by the sharp peak from the methyl and methylene groups. Small peaks can provide an estimation of the amount of unsaturated fatty acids. (Reproduced from Browning [176] with permission from Elsevier.)

or when there is a question of medication-induced injury. Limitations and risks inherent to biopsy have led to study of noninvasive "surrogate" markers.

Noninvasive surrogates

Clinical predictors of histology (Box 32.6) should be regarded cautiously due to the high number of exceptions; they most consistently include age (>40–50 years), the degree of obesity, the degree of diabetes or insulin resistance, features of the metabolic syndrome, family history of liver disease, aminotransferase elevation, and an AST : ALT ratio >1 [180–182]. Of note, the use of statins and some antidiabetic agents may spuriously change the AST : ALT ratio, thus limiting the use of this sim-

> **Box 32.6 Predictors of more severe histology in nonalcoholic steatohepatitis (NASH).**
>
> - Age >40–50 years
> - Degree of obesity
> - Hypertension
> - Overt diabetes mellitus
> - Hypertriglyceridemia
> - Elevated ALT
> - Elevated AST
> - AST : ALT ratio >1
> - Elevated serum IgA level
> - Family history of NASH or cryptogenic cirrhosis
>
> ALT, alanine aminotransferase; AST, aspartate aminotransferase; IgA, immunoglobulin A.

ple test. Other blood markers include indices of collagen metabolism (fibrosis), markers of cell death (M30 keratin 18 fragments), adipocytokine indices of insulin resistance (adiponectin and resistin), and markers of oxidative injury [183–185]. Clinical and laboratory variables have been combined into composite scores but none have gained uniform acceptance [186].

Limitations of liver biopsy

The limitations of biopsy include risk, patient inconvenience, performance in obese patients, and sampling error. Although always warranting careful caution, complications with liver biopsy are low and available techniques offer improved safety [187]. Sampling error is well recognized with all types of liver biopsy and may represent regional variation within the liver [188]. Fibrosis staging error is reduced by obtaining a specimen >2 cm in length (1.5 mm diameter) with a minimal length of 1.5 cm core using a 15–16 gauge needle [189].

Biopsy scoring

Composite scores provide a useful means of globally evaluating the biopsy (Table 32.1). Key parameters were combined into the NASH activity index (NAI) and the more commonly used NAFLD activity score (NAS) [190–191]. The NAI ranges from 0 to 12 and accounts for steatosis, necroinflammatory activity, and hepatocyte injury, each of which is scored from 0 to 4. The NAS uses a scale of 0 to 8 to score steatosis (0–3), lobular and/or portal inflammation (0–3), and cellular ballooning (0–2). Fibrosis stage is staged separately between 1 and 4, where 3 is bridging fibrosis and 4 is cirrhosis. Limitations of these systems include the imprecise and narrow ballooned cell scores and the stages of fibrosis intermediate between bridging fibrosis and cirrhosis ("incomplete" cirrhosis).

Table 32.1 Histology scoring systems in nonalcoholic fatty liver disease (NAFLD).

	Steatosis	Inflammation (lobular)	Hepatocyte injury (ballooning)	Maximum score	Fibrosis
NASH grade and stage (Brunt)	0–3	0–3	0–2	8	0–4
	0 = none	0 = no foci	0 = absent		0 = none
	1 = <33%	1 = 1–2 foci/mpf	1 = present in z3		1 = sinusoidal
	2 = 33–66%	2 = 3–4 foci/mpf	2 = marked in z3		2 = sinusoidal and periportal
	3 = >66%	3 = >4 foci/mpf			3 = bridging fibrosis
					4 = cirrhosis
NAI (NASH activity index) (Promrat)	0–4	0–4	0–4	12	0–4
	0 = <5%	0 = no foci	0 = absent		0 = none
	1 = 5–25%	1 = <1 foci/2 mpf	1 = only z3, <50% of CVs		1 = perisinusoidal
	2 = 25–50%	2 = 1 foci/1–2 mpf	2 = only z3, >50% of CVs		2 = perisinusoidal and periportal
	3 = 50–75%	3 = 1–2 foci/mpf	3 = Both z2 and z3 (1/3 to 2/3)		3 = bridging fibrosis
	4 = >75%	4 = >2 foci/mpf	4 = All zones (>2/3)		4 = cirrhosis/regeneration
NAS (NAFLD activity score CRN revision) (Kleiner)	0–3	0–3	0–2	8	0–4
	0 = <5%	0 = no foci	0 = absent		0 = none
	1 = 5–33%	1 = <2 foci/mpf	1 = few ballooned cells		1 = perisinusoidal or periportal
	2 = 33–66%	2 = 2–4 foci/mpf	2 = many/prominent ballooning		1A = mild, z3, perisinusoidal
	3 = >66%	3 = >4 foci/mpf			1B = moderate, z3, perisinusoidal
					1C = portal/periportal
					2 = perisinusoidal and portal/periportal
					3 = bridging fibrosis
					4 = cirrhosis

CRN, xxx; CVs, central veins; mpf, medium power field (defined as ×20 ocular); NASH, nonalcoholic steatohepatitis; z2, zone 2; z3, zone 3.

Better understanding of pathophysiology will likely lead to refinements of composite scoring.

Natural history and prognosis

Mortality in NAFLD is influenced by underlying histology and co-morbidities associated with the metabolic syndrome [192,193]. Although cardiovasacular disease is a leading cause of death (see below), obesity is a risk for cirrhosis-related death [194,195]. In type 2 diabetes, although cardiac deaths exceed liver-related deaths (19.5% versus 6.4%), the O/E ratio (observed/expected deaths) is higher for cirrhosis than for heart disease (2.67 versus 1.81) [196]. Nonhepatic cancer is another prominent cause of death in this group. Although it remains unclear which of these (vascular, cancer, or cirrhosis) is dominant in a given patient, serial biopsy studies and longer follow-up in cohort studies over the past 20 years have improved our understanding [197].

Clinical course based on the initial biopsy

In a retrospective study of adults, the overall and cirrhosis-related mortality was increased compared to crude death rates when steatosis was accompanied by inflammation, fibrosis, or ballooned cells (i.e., NASH) [198]. In contrast, NNFL appears to be relatively stable over time [6,199]. Older age (>40–50 years), higher BMI (>30 kg/m^2), diabetes, and abnormal aminotransferases are consistent predictors of more severe histology on the initial biopsy [70,74,200–202]. The diverging course between NASH and NNFL indicates that NASH usually begins as such rather than progressing from an initial stage of NNFL [203].

Histologic progression over time

Although serial biopsy studies have limitations due to variable technique, criteria, and incomplete data, existing studies offer essential observations [204–207]. Over 5–6

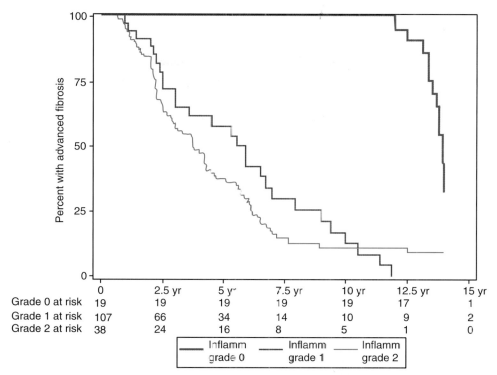

Figure 32.11 Histologic progression in nonalcoholic steatohepatitis. Kaplan–Meier curves showing the differences in progression to stage 3 or 4 fibrosis between patients with inflammation on the initial biopsy versus those without inflammation. (Reproduced from Argo et al. [208] with permission from Elsevier.)

years, histologic improvement can be seen but worsening fibrosis occurs more frequently than improvement (38% versus 21%) [208]. The risk of progression is associated with older age and the presence of inflammation on the initial biopsy (Fig. 32.11). One third of patients develop bridging fibrosis or cirrhosis.

Long-term mortality in nonalcoholic fatty liver disease

Based on four long-term cohort studies, the overall mortality from the initial diagnosis over 10–15 years is 10–12%, being significantly higher in NASH versus NNFL (Table 32.2) [209–212]. Over the same period, the

Table 32.2 Long-term natural history studies of nonalcoholic fatty liver disease (NAFLD) and nonalcoholic steatohepatitis (NASH): past cohorts followed over time.

	Adams et al. 2005 [207]	Ekstedt et al. 2006 [210]		Ong et al. 2008 [211]	Rafiq et al. 2009 [212]	
	NAFLD	**NNFL**	**NASH**	**NAFLD**	**NNFL**	**NASH**
Approximate baseline period[a]	1980–2000	1988–1993		1988–1994	1979–1987	
N	435	58	71	817	74	57
Male/female	213/222	—	—	—	45/29	24/33
Age at diagnosis	49 ± 15	47 ± 12	55 ± 12	—	53 ± 25	54 ± 12
Follow-up (years)	7.6 ± 4	13.7 ± 1.3		8.4	19.5	15
Portal HTN complication	13 (3.1%)	0 (0%)	7 (9.8%)	—	—	—
Death due to CAD	13 (2.9%)	5 (8.6%)	11 (15.5%)	20 (2.4%)	15 (20.3%)	7 (12.3%)
Death due to non-liver malignancy	15 (3.4%)	1 (1.7%)	4 (5.6%)	19 (2.3%)	9 (12.2%)	5 (8.8%)
Death due to liver-related complication	7 (1.6%)	0 (0%)	2 (2.8%)	5 (0.6%)	2 (2.7%)	10 (17.5%)

[a]This indicates the approximate period during which patients were initially encountered
CAD, coronary artery disease; HTN, hypertension; NNFL, non-NASH fatty liver.

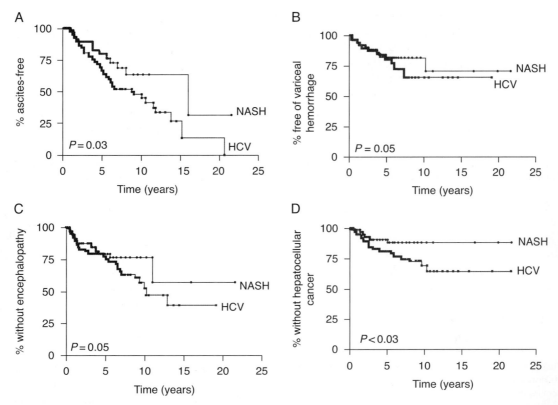

Figure 32.12 Comparison of complications in nonalcoholic steatohepatitis (NASH) cirrhosis versus cirrhosis due to hepatitis C (HCV). The course is similar in the two diseases but slightly slower in NASH cirrhosis. The figure depicts the hazard of developing (A) ascites, (B) variceal hemorrhage, (C) encephalopathy, and (D) hepatocellular cancer, and are shown as "time to failure" via the Kaplan–Meier method. (Reproduced from Sanyal et al. [214] with permission from Wiley-Blackwell.)

risk of decompensated cirrhosis was 5–10% and for hepatocellular cancer it was 1–2%. The leading causes of death overall were coronary artery disease (10%), extrahepatic malignancy (5%), and cirrhosis-related death (2%) – expressed as a percentage of the original cohort. Cirrhosis deaths exceeded cardiac deaths among NASH patients in one study [213]. These circumstances present clinical challenges as it is increasingly likely that patients with metabolic syndrome suffer from both coronary disease and cirrhosis – two conditions with often conflicting management strategies.

Prognosis of nonalcoholic steatohepatitis-related cirrhosis

Once cirrhosis develops, the risk of developing a major complication of portal hypertension is reported to be 17%, 23%, and 52% at 1, 3, and 10 years, respectively, indicating a progressive condition [213]. In a study comparing 152 NASH–cirrhosis patients with 150 patients with cirrhosis from hepatitis C, the number of patients free of a given complication (bleeding, ascites, encephalopathy, hepatocellular cancer) over 10–20 years revealed that patients with NASH–cirrhosis were similar to those with hepati-

tis C-related cirrhosis but progressed at a slightly slower rate (Fig. 32.12) [214].

Cryptogenic cirrhosis

A close association between NASH and cryptogenic cirrhosis is evident in different populations, in post-transplantation studies, and in "look-back" histologic studies (see above as well) [17–37]. About one half present with a major complication of portal hypertension. Although there is confusion in nomenclature between NASH–cirrhosis and cryptogenic cirrhosis, these conditions constitute an increasingly common indication for liver transplantation, estimated at 5–10% of liver transplants [215].

Hepatocellular cancer

Epidemilogic studies show an increased risk of hepatocellular cancer (HCC) in both obese and diabetic patients [216,217] and case series confirm progression of NASH to cirrhosis to HCC [17,218,219]. HCC is especially common in NASH–cirrhosis and it tends to be diagnosed at a later stage possibly due to inadequate surveillance [220,221]. While NASH–cirrhosis or obesity-related cryptogenic cirrhosis constitute the primary associations, HCC is reported in NNFL, suggesting that steatosis alone is a risk [222–224]. HCC screening is recommended in NASH–cirrhosis or cryptogenic cirrhosis although optimal schedules are uncertain. Tumorogenesis in this setting may represent unique cancer biology. Molecular events include proliferation of progenitor cells observed in human and experimental NAFLD [225].

Experimental and animal models

Small animal models
Experimental models, usually in rodents, have been reviewed extensively [226]. Classic models include the ob/ob mouse, which has a congenital deficiency of leptin, the FA/FA rat, which has an impaired leptin receptor, and the methionine-choline deficient (MCD) diet rodent. While often helpful, the models often have limitations such as absence of insulin resistance in the MCD models [227]. Recent studies have focused on dietary manipulations such as trans fat or fructose content or high fat with toxin exposure and others have utilized the zebra fish as a model of fat metabolism [228–230].

Large animal steatosis
Fatty liver is seen in cows, hens, cats, and some pigs [231,232]. It is a common disorder in cats [233]. Seasonal variation in steatosis is seen in wild deer [234]. Palmipedes (migratory geese) develop fatty liver before migration and utilize fat as a preferred source of energy for muscle metabolism [235]. This has been exploited in the production of foie gras wherein geese are fed a corn-based diet resulting in an increase in liver size in as little as 2 weeks from 100 to 800 g. Mixed micro- and macrosteatosis is evident with increased susceptibility to accidental mycotoxin exposure [236]. Steatosis involves increased synthesis and altered very low-density lipoprotein (VLDL) secretion [237,238]. These relationships illustrate the role of the liver in the evolution of adipose and energy metabolism and thermoregulation [239].

Pathogenesis

Nonalcoholic fatty liver disease and especially NASH can be viewed as conditions within the spectrum of the metabolic syndrome and systemic lipotoxicity [240]. Steatosis and oxidative injury known as the "two hit" hypothesis encapsulates the consistent role played by oxidative injury [241]. A cascade of events leads eventually to cellular ballooning, cell death, organ fibrosis, and cirrhosis. Although fat necrosis may occur from the direct release of fat from swollen hepatocytes in NAFLD [242],

cell injury results predominantly from the indirect effects of intracellular lipid peroxidation and the toxicity of fatty acids on organelles (Fig. 32.13).

Local cellular factors

Steatosis
Steatosis exists when fat stores exceed 5–10% of the organ by weight [5,243]. Fat is derived from the uptake of plasma fatty acids (nonesterified fatty acids (NEFAs)) released by lipolysis of adipose tissue, the uptake of VLDL-derived LDL remnants or circulating dietary chylomicron remnants, and from de novo lipogenesis (DNL) from carbohydrate precursors [244]. Both triglycerides (mostly as unsaturated fatty acids) and free fatty acids (mostly as saturated fatty acids) are increased in steatosis [245]. The disposal of fatty acids proceeds by several routes: incorporation into triglyceride in cytoplasmic lipid droplets, export as lipoproteins such as VLDL, oxidation especially via mitochondrial β-oxidation, or formation of phospholipids as membrane components. Recycling through autophagy is another key aspect (see below). The regulation of these pathways depends on energy homeostasis influenced by peroxisome proliferators-activated receptor (PPAR) activity and the adrenergic nervous system [246–248]. The transcription factors sterol regulatory element binding protein (SREBP), governed by insulin and dietary fatty acids, and carbohydrate response element binding protein (CREBP), governed by glucose levels, regulate lipid metabolism [249–251]. SREBP and CREBP stimulate nuclear transcription of the enzymes responsible for fatty acid synthesis and their incorporation into triglyceride in lipid droplets or exported as VLDLs.

De novo lipogenesis from carbohydrates
Adenosine triphosphate-dependent synthesis of the 16-carbon palmitic acid begins with translocation of carbohydrate-derived acetyl-coenzyme A (acetyl-CoA) subunits which pass through the mitochondrial membrane to the cytosol as citrate. Acetyl-CoA carboxylase (ACC) then activates the formation of malonyl-CoA from acetyl-CoA. Importantly, ACC is activated by insulin and inactivated by epinephrine, glucagons, and long chain fatty acids (the end-product). Through a series of repetitive cytosolic condensations catalyzed by fatty acid synthase (FAS), molecules of malonyl-CoA are assembled into palmitic acid. As a control, malonyl-CoA inhibits fatty acid β-oxidation by blocking carnitine, which shuttles fatty acids into the mitochondrion. Once formed, palmitic acid undergoes elongation in the ER to longer chain fatty acids or desaturation and esterification to glycerol to form mono-, di-, and triglycerides. The latter is incorporated in the ER via MTTP into VLDLs for export in

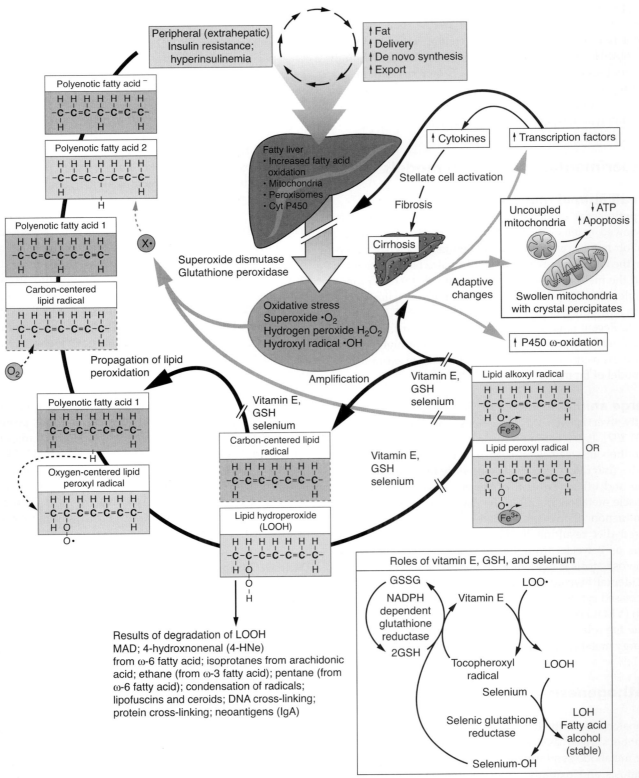

Figure 32.13 Lipid peroxidation and cell injury. (A) Lipid peroxidation is a branching chain reaction stimulated by free radical attack (super oxide, hydroxyl radical) on lipid constituents. Unsaturated fatty acids are especially susceptible and lose an electron to the radical. This produces a *carbon-centered lipid radical* which reacts with oxygen to form an *oxygen-centered lipid peroxyl radical*. This reacts with a second fatty acid to form another lipid free radical (propagation) and a *lipid hydroperoxide*. The latter is unstable and, in the presence of iron and another fatty acid, reacts to form yet another lipid radical (amplification). Lipid hydroperoxide degrades to malondialdehyde (MDA), ethane, or pentane or reacts with other radicals to form a stable pigment (lipofuscins). It may also cross-link with DNA or cellular proteins impairing their function. Lipid radicals are neutralized through combination with tocopherols (vitamin E). (*Continued*)

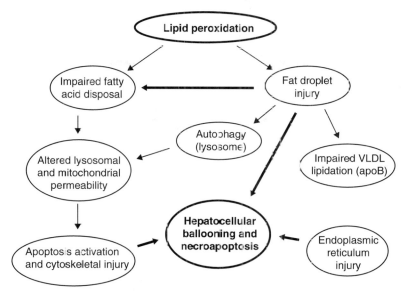

Figure 32.13 (*Continued*) The latter is then restored by shuffling the radical groups to glutathione (GSH) via selenium. ATP, adenosine triphosphate; GSSG, oxidized gluatathione, IgA, immunoglobulin A; _OH, fatty acid alcohol; NADPH, nicotinamide adenine dinucleotide phosphate (reduced form). (B) Cell injury appears to result from a cascade of events initiated by lipid peroxidation, which triggers lipid droplet dysfunction, endoplasmic reticulum "stress," autophagosome formation, and mitochondrial cysfunction. Fatty acids cause activation of apoptosis through changes in lysosome and mitochondrial permeability. Caspases (apoptosis pathway) contribute to cytoskeletal injury and ballooning and Mallory–Denk body formation. Necroapoptotic cell death stimulates fibrotic pathways amplified by systemic factors such as cytokines. VLDL, very low-density lipoprotein.

association with apolipoprotein B100 [252]. Triglyceride synthesis in human NAFLD results from the uptake of adipose-derived NEFAs (59%), DNL (26%), and dietary fat (15%) based on nutrition studies with radiolabeled precursors [253].

Lipid composition (lipidomics)

Variation in fat droplet size and density reflects different types of component fatty acids [254,255]. Incorporation of NEFA into droplet triglyceride depends on the activity of diacylglycerol acyltransferase 1 (Dgat1) [256]. Lipidomic analysis shows a stepwise increase from normal to NASH in the triacylglycerol to diacylglycerol ratio, indicating a relative increase in triacylglycerol in more advanced disease [257]. The ratio of n6 : n3 polyunsaturated fatty acid is higher in NASH possibly due to the diminished triacylglycerol content of eicosapentanoic acid and docosahexanoic acid. Free fatty acids were not different but phosphatidylcholine was decreased in NNFL and NASH, while the free cholesterol to phosphotidylcholine ratio was increased. Ceramide, a toxic lipid intermediary, has been detected more in obese patients with fatty liver versus those without although its role is uncertain [258].

Lipoproteins

Although lipid trafficking and lipoprotein metabolism are important factors [259], no dominant pattern of fasting lipoproteins is established in NAFLD. In some cases, primary lipoprotein disorders might constitute a separate and/or overlapping entity. VLDL secretion is increased in human NAFLD but plateaus at a hepatic triglyceride content of 10%, indicating limited compensation for increased uptake of NEFAs. The secretion of apolipoprotein B100, a component of VLDL, is insufficient and may promote the secretion of a larger VLDL particle with greater triglyceride content [260,261]. Differences in ApoA1 (a component of high-density lipoprotein) are also described [262]. The role of *postprandial* lipid metabolism and intestinal chylomicrons is an emerging area [263].

Lipid peroxidation

The most enduring finding that distinguishes NASH from NNFL is lipid peroxidation (see Fig. 32.13) [264–267]. This process is evident as the accumulation of oxidative by-products such as 4-HNE (4-hydroxynonenal), MDA (malondialdehyde), nitrotyrosine, and 8-hydroxydeoxyguanine, and systemically as adducts of oxidized phospholipids and 11-HETE (hydroxyeicosatetraenoic acid), a by-product of arachidonic acid oxidative injury [185,268]. Lipid peroxidation is a branching, chain reaction attack on unsaturated fatty acids that produces another free radical and a lipid hydroperoxide [269–271]. It is sparked by superoxide radicals derived especially from mitochondrial oxidative-phosphorylation in the electron transport chain. The superoxide radical is metabolized via superoxide dismutase to hydrogen peroxide, which in the presence of Fe^{2+}

(Fenton or Haber–Weiss reaction) decays to hydroxyl radicals. Hydroxyl radicals catalyze peroxidation of fatty acids damaging membranes, cellular proteins, and DNA [272]. Oxidation of the phospholipid monolayer of fat droplets (including PAT proteins (perilipin-adipose differentiation protein-tail interacting protein)) and constituents of the ER may be particularly relevant to cellular ballooning, impaired disposal of fatty acids, and hepatic insulin resistance [265,273–275]. The speed of these pathologic reactions in vivo, whether in seconds, minutes, hours, days or longer, is uncertain.

Lipid droplets, VLDL lipidation, and lipophagy

Lipid droplets are composed of a hydrophobic core of triglycerides and lesser amounts of cholesterol esters surrounded by a phospholipid monolayer [276]. They form at the site of fatty acid acyl transferases in the ER in association with the cytoskeleton [277]. Droplets are associated with lipoprotein-like proteins known as PAT proteins which govern lipase activity and are themselves regulated by PPAR-γ agonists [278–282]. Their growth appears to occur predominantly by fusion [283]. Through the activity of the MTTP enzyme at the ER, droplets normally serve as a source for triglycerides in VLDL synthesis. Because oxidative injury to the droplet surface alters PAT protein expression, it is likely that secretion and fusion is disturbed in NASH [284]. Consistent with this, the smallest droplets in alcoholic steatohepatitis resemble precursors of VLDLs [285,286]. Autophagy of fat droplets ('lipophagy'), which forms an autophagosome (lysosome), appears to be a key compensatory and regulatory pathway [287]. Altered permeability of the lysosome mediated by free fatty acids is a trigger of cell death pathways (see below).

Endoplasmic reticulum dysfunction

Experimentally, small droplet accumulation is associated with the formation of cholesterol-rich "Apo-B crescents" at sites in the ER [288]. We speculate that this is directly related to dysfunction of the ER. The latter is evident in human NASH as the unfolded protein response ("ER stress"), which activates proinflammatory pathways such as interleukin 8, nuclear factor κB (NF-κB), and c-jun N-terminal kinase (JNK) [289,290]. Thus, impaired Apo-B100 interaction with lipid droplets at the ER provides a link between oxidative stress, droplet accumulation, altered VLDL secretion, the ER stress reaction, and activation of proinflammatory pathways [291–293].

Mitochondrial dysfunction and adenosine triphosphate homeostasis

An association between steatosis and diminished ATP was observed over 50 years ago and later confirmed using ^{31}P magnetic resonance spectroscopy in vivo [294,295]. The evolutionary history of the mitochondrion places it centrally in critical pathways including fatty acid synthesis and oxidation, oxidative-phosphorylation, and apoptosis signaling [296,297]. Morphologic abnormalities in NASH include enlargement and formation of crystalline arrays, which may represent phospholipid phase transitions (Fig. 32.14) [298]. It likely results from an impaired electron transport chain (in part due to uncoupling protein) [299,300] and accounts for the poor function of steatotic livers in transplantation due to ischemia [301, 302]. Whether or not fatty acid oxidation is decreased in NAFLD is unclear as a net increase in mitochondrial β-oxidation has been reported in NASH and in obesity [303,304]. Changes in permeability cause the release of cytochrome c and apoptosis signaling (see below). Mitochondrial cholesterol content may contribute to changes in permeability [305].

Cell death, fibrosis, and the ductal reaction

Cell death results from a combination of apoptosis signaling and focal necrosis resulting in a process best described as "necroapoptosis" or "apoptonecrosis" [306]. Excessive free fatty acids due to diminished fatty acid-binding protein [307] (and possibly to impaired fat droplet function) alter autophagosome permeability, leading to the release of cathepsins (lysosomal proteases), which then alter mitochondrial permeability, leading to the release of cytochrome c and activation of proapoptotic caspases [308–310]. Caspase 3 in particular causes fragmentation of keratin 18, possibly contributing to the formation of Mallory–Denk bodies and to the release of keratin 18 fragments detectable in serum [311,312]. Although apoptotic pathways are diffusely activated, necrosis appears to dominate histologically, possibly as a result of an ATP deficit, fat droplet accumulation, and cytoskeletal injury – all of which appear to contribute to cellular ballooning. Cell death stimulates inflammation and activation of hepatic stellate cells to produce collagen [313]. This process is mediated at least in part by activation of toll-like receptors [314]. Compensatory repair is characterized by increased activity of progenitor cells recognized as the "ductular reaction" in the portal tracts [315].

Cytochrome P450 and peroxisomal metabolism

Induction of cytochrome P450 2E1 (CYP2E1) has been described as a possible source of oxidative stress through microsomal ω-oxidation of fatty acids [316]. Expression of CYP2E1 is influenced by dietary fat and colocalizes to markers of lipid peroxidation [317]. Its role is uncertain as experimental overexpression of CYP2E1 is protective against oxidative injury and decreases apoptosis but increases the risk of necrosis induced by fatty acid

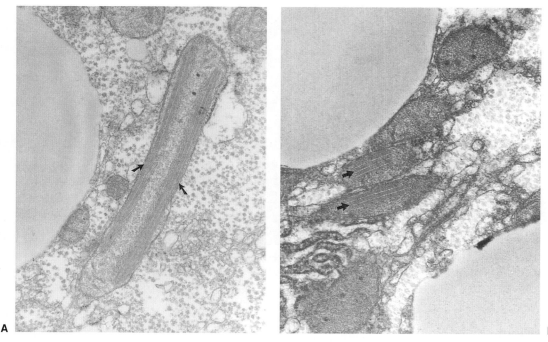

Figure 32.14 Deformed mitochondria with crystalline inclusions in nonalcoholic steatohepatitis. (A) An elongated mitochondrion with two bundles of parallel, crystalline structures (arrows) near a large fat droplet. (B) Two mitochondria cut tangentially showing crystalline inclusions (arrows) in an area of cytoplasm between two large fat droplets. Note the paucity of normal cristae.

exposure [318]. Peroxisomes are involved in numerous potentially relevant lipid-related metabolic pathways and morphologic abnormalities have been described in human fatty liver [319,320]. Although not well defined, it is possible that genetic abnormalities, nutritional abnormalities, or adaptive changes in the peroxisome may contribute in some patients.

Ballooned cells

Hepatocyte ballooning is a major histologic feature of NASH evident in all scoring systems, but a consensus definition has remained elusive [321–323]. Ballooning is conventionally defined at the light level based on hematoxylin and eosin (H&E) staining as cellular enlargement 1.5–2 times the normal diameter (normal up to $30\,\mu m$) with rarefied cytoplasm [324,325]. Recent advances have shown that ballooning is associated with injury to the cytoskeleton evident as diminished cytokeratin 8 and 18, the presence of Mallory–Denk bodies, and the detection of cytokeratin 18 fragments (M30), suggesting impairment of cell size regulation [326–328]. Further work has revealed an association between the accumulation of small and medium fat droplets and morphologic changes in the ER (Fig. 32.15) [15]. These studies show cytoskeletal injury also in smaller cells, suggesting that this pattern exists as a spectrum. Experimentally, abnormal keratin metabolism may also play a role in mitochondrial dys-

morphology [329]. Correlation of injury to the cytoskeleton and serum keratin 18 (M30) fragment levels is emerging.

Systemic factors

Insulin resistance and systemic inflammatory changes

Although insulin resistance is neither sufficient nor essential for NAFLD (see above), it is present in the majority of NAFLD patients and is intertwined with disease pathogenesis. Insulin resistance (evident in adipose tissue, skeletal muscle, and liver) is mediated by lipid accumulation, free fatty acids, and altered mitochondrial metabolism [330–332]. Manifestations include decreased muscle utilization of glucose, mobilization of fatty acids from adipose tissue (lipolysis), and unrestrained hepatic glucose output. Biochemically, insulin resistance is characterized by a shift from tyrosine phosphorylation in the insulin receptor substrate to serine phosphorylation resulting in diminished insulin-stimulated activity in *metabolic pathways* (mediated by phosphatidylinositol 3-kinase (PI3-kinase), Akt, and mTOR) and *mitogenic pathways* (mediated by Ras, Raf, and mitogen-activated protein or MAP-kinase). Inflammatory changes in adipose tissue are characterized by ER stress and JNK activation, which stimulates the production of systemically active cytokines, which contribute to the shift from tyrosine to

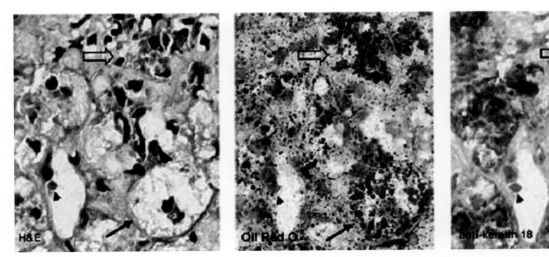

Figure 32.15 Relationship between cellular ballooning, small droplet fat accumulation, and cytoskeletal injury. Serial imaging of a frozen section using oil red O to accentuate the small lipid droplets in ballooned cells, in comparison to H&E and antikeratin 18 stains. The long arrow indicates a ballooned hepatocyte. The arrowhead indicates a landmark red blood cell in a central vein. The open arrow indicates a focus of necrosis with densely staining fat droplet remnants. (Reproduced from Caldwell et al. [15] with permission from Elsevier.)

serine phosphorylation [333,334]. Tumor necrosis factor α (TNF-α) and interleukins 6 and 8 act through their effects on a modulator of cytokine activity known as SOCS (suppressor of cytokine signaling) [335].

Adipocytokines and lipokines

Adipose-derived "adipokines" (adiponectin, leptin, resistin, visfatin) modulate insulin signaling. Adiponectin is the most abundant protein in the adipocyte and participates in glucose homeostasis via receptors in muscle (adipoR1) and liver (adipoR2) where it activates adenosine monophosphate (AMP) kinase and promotes fatty acid oxidation [336–338]. Depressed production of adiponectin has a prominent role in NAFLD and successful therapy is often associated with the recovery of normal levels. Recently, adipose-derived "lipokines," including C16:1n7-palmitoleate, have been proposed as additional systemic modulators of hepatic fat and insulin activity in skeletal muscle [339].

Other systemic changes

Alterations in small bowel permeability and associated bacterial overgrowth in NAFLD patients have been implicated in the activation of inflammatory mediators through exposure to substances such as endotoxin in portal blood [340,341]. The latter may partly explain the previously reported association between celiac disease and NAFLD due to increased gut permeability in celiac disease [342]. Whether or not systemic exposure to environmental pollutants such as bisphenol A significantly alters insulin resistance and manifestations of the metabolic syndrome remains controversial [343].

Energy homeostasis

Steatosis can be viewed as a component of integrated systems involved with energy (and thermoregulatory) homeostasis including the adrenergic system, the adipose organ, the thyroid axis, and insulin/glucagon signaling. While the insulin axis is the best characterized with regard to fatty liver, a broader understanding is helpful in understanding the disease. This is evident by the recently described presence of cold-activated brown adipose tissue in healthy men and its inverse relationship to obesity [344]. Factors governing these relations are unclear. Adrenergic modulation of hepatic inflammation has been demonstrated in animal models and may play a role in human fatty liver [345]. Liver fat metabolism in migratory Palmipedes may also be instructive (see above).

Other conditions associated with NAFLD/NASH ("secondary" NASH)

The foregoing has focused on what may be referred to as "primary" NAFLD associated with insulin resistance. Other conditions are sometimes referred to as "secondary" NAFLD (see Boxes 32.1 and 32.3) although overlapping risks often make the distinction less clear.
- *Jejunoileal bypass.* Historically, older forms of bariatric surgery played a role in the recognition of NAFLD/ NASH due to a severe form of NASH following jejunoileal bypass [346]. Stimulation of TNF by bacterial overgrowth and endotoxin production, micronutrient deficiency, and rapid weight loss were conditions etiologically implicated. Modern forms of bariatric surgery

are much less likely to exacerbate NASH and may indeed ameliorate the condition (see below).

- *Medication-induced.* A number of medications have been implicated as causes of steatohepatitis. For some, including nifedipine, methotrexate, and tamoxifen, the association may be one of medication use in patients at risk for NASH and possible exacerbation of underlying disease [347–349]. Steatosis has been associated with exposure to anabolic steroids among body builders in the absence of obesity [350] and amiodarone has long been associated with phospholipidosis and steatohepatitis, although this seems less common now possibly due to lower dosing [351]. Acquired lipodystrophy, insulin resistance, and steatosis has been well described with therapy for human immunodeficiency virus (HIV) infection [352]. Obesity also appears to increase the risk of chemotherapy-associated steatohepatitis in colorectal cancer liver metastatic disease [353].

- *Parenteral nutrition, malnutrition, and celiac disease.* Liver disease, often with macro- and microvesicular steatosis, is a potentially severe side effect of total parenteral nutrition (TPN) [354,355]. Both the amount and composition of infused lipid appear to affect the expression of liver disease [356]. Choline deficiency may play a role in some patients. At the opposite end of the spectrum, steatosis in kwashiorkor results from impaired hepatic lipid export due to protein malnutrition (diminished apolipoprotein B) [357]. Celiac disease can be seen in up to 3–4% of NASH patients even in the absence of significant weight loss [358]. In this situation, celiac disease is postulated to exacerbate intrahepatic inflammation.

- *Solvents and industrial agents.* A variety of toxins have been implicated in the development of fatty liver diseases [359]. Better described agents include carbon tetrachloride (now rarely used), dimethylformamide, perchloro-ethylene, and more recently petrochemical derivatives [360]. These forms of steatohepatitis have been termed TASH (toxicant-associated steatohepatitis) and can also be seen with high exposures to vinyl chloride [361]. Although these conditions may be dissociated from insulin resistance, vinyl chloride exposure was associated with insulin resistance in the absence of obesity.

- *Wilson disease and other inherited metabolic diseases.* Macro- and microvesicular steatosis are well known features of Wilson disease [362]. It should be considered particularly with steatohepatitis in a younger individual. It is not known how often the carrier state for mutations in the copper-transporting ATPase gene could influence NASH [363]. Macrovesicular steatosis is seen in other inherited metabolic diseases, most of which present in childhood. These include glycogen storage diseases, galactosemia, tyrosinemia, heterozygous hypobetalipoproteinemia, and abetalipoproteine-

mia. The latter disorders involve impaired formation of VLDL due to decreased synthesis of apolipoprotein B [364,365]. Lipid storage diseases (cholesterol ester, Niemann–Pick, Tay–Sachs, and Gaucher disease) can have fatty infiltration of the liver with cholesterol esters, sphingolipids, phospholipids, sphingomyelin, gangliosides, or glucocerebrosides. Presentation in infancy (although not exclusively) and distribution in the reticuloendothelial cells distinguish the lipid storage disorders [366].

Obese, diabetic patients with newly discovered cirrhosis

The silent progression of NASH to cirrhosis has led increasingly to the incidental discovery of cirrhosis in patients with obesity and type 2 diabetes [367]. While therapy aimed at diabetes may ameliorate steatohepatitis in an early stage (see below), there is little knowledge on the effects of commonly employed medications such as aspirin and angiotensin-converting enzyme (ACE) inhibitors in the setting of NASH-related cirrhosis. However, it should be noted that portosystemic shunting results in the "hyperdynamic state" of cirrhosis, a hallmark of which is systemic vasodilatation and changes in renal hemodynamics. In this setting, ACE inhibitors and nonsteroidal anti-inflammatory drugs (NSAIDs) including aspirin may exacerbate fluid retention and ascites. Thus, treatment in these patients needs to include a reconsideration of conventional tenets of diabetes management. Another emerging area is that of overlapping atherosclerotic vascular disease and NASH cirrhosis (see section on natural history above). This situation increasingly results in the need for balancing anticoagulation strategies with portal hypertension-related bleeding risks.

Treatment

Overview of therapy: who should be treated

Patient selection and the relative risk–benefit of intervention remain some of the most challenging aspects of treating NAFLD. NASH carries the major risk for cirrhosis (relative to NNFL) and thus warrants stronger consideration for pharmacologic treatment (Table 32.3). However, there is consensus that dietary changes and exercise are cornerstones of initial intervention although variable compliance complicates the interpretation of pharmaceutical trials [368]. Most such studies account for weight loss and some for dietary changes but few account for physical conditioning, which can also influence the outcome. These variables likely explain the placebo effect

Table 32.3 Selected randomized, controlled trials of therapy for nonalcoholic steatohepatitis (NASH) with histologic end-points: key differences between active and control groups are shown in comments. Improvement in control groups (placebo effect) is seen consistently in pharmacologic studies and probably reflects voluntary lifestyle changes.

	N	Agent	Daily dose	Duration	Comments	Reference
Lifestyle modifications	25	Diet, exercise	Diet 25 kcal/kg IBW, jogging b.i.d.	3 months	Decreased steatosis compared to control group; mild improvement in inflammation, fibrosis; BMI decreased by 3 over study period in intervention group	Ueno et al. 1997 [388]
	53	Diet, exercise	25–30 kcal/kg, 45 min/day	24 months	Improvement in ALT, steatosis, inflammation, NAS. No additional benefit of adding vitamin E 600 IU/day or vitamin C	Nobil et al. 2008 [389]
	23	Exercise	Graded by effort	4 weeks	Significant reduction in visceral and especially liver fat even without weight loss	Johnson et al. 2009 [383]
	31	Diet, exercise	<1500 kcal, 200 min/week	48 weeks	Significant improvements in NAS, steatosis, inflammation, ballooning (weight loss 9.3% in lifestyle intervention group)	Promrat et al. 2010 [390]
Weight loss agents	50	Orlistat	360 mg	36 weeks	Vitamin E 800 IU/day in all patients. Improvement seen in multiple histologic parameters dependent on weight loss but independent of orlistat use	Harrison et al. 2009 [401]
Thiazolidinediones	20	Pioglitazone	30 mg	6 months	Improvement in steatosis and inflammation, no improvement in fibrosis	Sanyal 2004
	55	Pioglitazone	45 mg	6 months	Improvement in ALT, steatosis, inflammation; no significant improvement in fibrosis	Belfort et al. 2006 [431]
	74	Pioglitazone	45 mg	12 months	Improvement in ALT, ballooning, fibrosis; no improvement in steatosis	Aithal et al. 2008 [432]
	53	Rosiglitazone	8 mg	3 years	Improvement in ALT, steatosis; no significant improvement in inflammation, fibrosis	Ratziu et al. 2010 [435]
	163	Pioglitazone	30 mg	96 weeks	Improvement in ALT, steatosis, ballooning, inflammation, NAS, fibrosis	Sanyal et al. 2010 [419]
Cytoprotective agents	166	UDCA	13–15 mg/kg	24 months	Improvement in multiple parameters but no different than placebo	Lindor et al. 2004 [410]
	48	UDCA + vitamin E	12–15 mg/kg 800 IU/day	2 years	Improvement in AST, steatosis; no significant improvement in inflammation, fibrosis	Dufour et al. 2006 [412]
	185	UDCA	23–28 mg/kd	18 months	No improvement in steatosis, NAS, fibrosis	Leuschner et al. 2010 [411]
	74	Carnitine	2 g	24 weeks	Improvement in ALT, steatosis, ballooning, inflammation, NAS, fibrosis; placebo effect also observed	Malaguamera 2010
Antioxidants	45	Vitamins E and C	1000 IU 1000 mg	6 months	Slight improved fibrosis; no improvement in steatosis, inflammation	Harrison et al. 2003 [418]
	167	Vitamin E	800 IU	2 years	Improved ALT, steatosis, ballooning, inflammation, NAS	Sanyal et al. 2010 [419]
	55	Betaine	20 g	12 months	No improvement in ALT, steatosis, ballooning, inflammation, NAS, fibrosis	Abdelmalek et al. 2009 [424]
HMG-CoA reductase inhibitors	16	Simvastatin	40 mg	12 months	No improvement in ALT; no improvement in steatosis, ballooning, inflammation, NAS, or fibrosis	Nelson et al. 2009 [459]

ALT, alanine aminotransferase; BMI, body mass index; HMG-CoA, 3-hydroxy-3-methylglutaryl coenzyme A; IBW, xxx; NAS, nonalcoholic fatty liver disease activity score; UDCA, ursodeoxycholic acid.

and sometimes the failure of agents in randomized controlled trials (RCTs) that appeared promising in pilot studies [369,370].

End-points of therapy

Because progression to cirrhosis carries a severe prognosis, the primary end-point of therapy remains improvement in histology, although sampling error is a potential problem which requires that studies report biopsy details (length and/or portal tracts). Surrogate markers for liver injury include serum aminotransferases, hepatic fat content by imaging techniques, and serologic markers of fibrosis such as collagen metabolites or cell injury such as keratin fragments (see above). Other measures include anthropometrics (weight, BMI, waist circumference), physical conditioning (VO_{2max} by ergometry), measures of insulin signaling, and adipocytokine/cytokine levels such as adiponectin, TNF-α, and TGF-β. Novel markers of histologic injury, especially in the research setting, include immunohistochemistry for oxidative cell injury, fat stains (oil red O), digital quantitative imaging for fibrosis, hepatocyte ultrastructure, and markers of stellate cell activation [371]. These parameters are used as surrogates for cell injury and thus for progression to cirrhosis. Although cirrhosis is an established prognositic indicator, ultimately any intervention will require translation into outcomes of liver-related morbidity and mortality; such studies will, however, require many years to accrue.

Initial intervention

Optimistically, diet modification and exercise can be accomplished in obese patients with success as high as 80% of patients achieving dietary goals and 36% achieving exercise goals [372]. Pessimistically, even intensive counseling to reduce fat intake (<30% of daily calories) and to engage in regular physical activity produces only a modest 5% sustained weight loss [373,374]. However, successful intervention can significantly reduce liver fat even with modest changes. In the Tuebingen Lifestyle Intervention Program (TULIP) study, the degree of physical deconditioning correlated both to baseline liver fat content and inversely to response to lifestyle intervention [375].

Exercise alone

The relative benefit of exercise *without* weight loss (i.e., the "fit fat") versus dietary weight loss has been explored in experimental and clinical NAFLD [376,377]. Exercise affects insulin signaling and calorie disposal through interactions with skeletal muscle substrate utilization, PPAR signaling, and mitochondrial metabolism [378–380]. Although the optimal "dose" remains to be determined, the most effective "conditioning" exercise

is that which just passes beyond the lactate threshold – a level usually associated with some degree of discomfort [381,382]. Compared to a control group who received only stretching advice, a treated group who underwent 4 weeks of graded exercise (three 30–45-minute sessions per week at 50% baseline VO_{2peak} for 1 week, 60% for 1 week, and 70% for 2 weeks) had a 12% reduction in visceral fat and a 21% reduction in liver fat without overall weight loss [383]. It seems likely that the efficacy of this approach will depend on earlier intervention.

Dietary weight loss and exercise in adults and children

Diet *and* exercise-induced weight loss is effective in NAFLD although very rapid loss should be viewed cautiously [384,385]. Weight reduction through nutritional counseling is associated with improved aminotransferases and histology, usually in parallel to improved insulin signaling [386,387]. Significant improvement in aminotransferases and histology was seen in adults treated with diet (25 kcal/kg ideal body weight/day) and exercise (walking and jogging) for 3 months compared to a control group [388]. Similarly, improvement was seen in metabolic and histologic parameters (steatosis, inflammation, ballooning) after 2 years intervention in pediatric cases [389]. In another 2-year controlled trial in adults, lifestyle intervention resulted in 9% weight loss versus 0.2% in controls [390]. Seventy-two percent of the lifestyle intervention group versus 30% of controls had a reduction in the histologic score (NAS) by 3 or more or to ≤ 2 points post-treatment. Specific diet plans such as low carbohydrate diets [391] or reduced calorie diet may be less important than finding one that is sustainable.

Dietary composition (omega 3 fatty acids, fructose, and fast food)

Changes in dietary composition appear to be particularly important. Fast food hyperalimentation with two such meals per day for 4 weeks caused significant increases in aminotransferases and hepatic fat in a study of young healthy volunteers [392]. Elimination of this source of food could reasonably be expected to lead to improvement in these parameters. Dietary fats effect the composition of cell and organelle membranes, insulin sensitivity, gene regulation (PPARs), adipocyte differentiation, and prostaglandin metabolism (altered especially by the relative content of n6 versus n3 polyunsaturated fatty acids (PUFAs)) [393–395]. Although there has been concern regarding PUFAs in alcoholic steatohepatitis [396], animal and limited human studies of omega 3 (n3) supplements as EPA (eicosapentaenoic acid) and DHA (docosahexanoic acid) have been encouraging but are yet to be substantiated [397]. Cohort studies using food frequency questionnaires have indicated that concentrated fructose sweeteners, especially in beverages such as soft drinks, are associated with increased fatty liver independent of metabolic syndrome and greater fibrosis in patients with NASH [398,399]. This may in part be attributable to the metabolism of concentrated fructose, which is particularly steatogenic [400].

Weight loss agents

Orlistat (tetrahydrolipostatin) decreases fat absorption by inhibiting lipase. In spite of several promising pilot studies, an RCT showed similar weight loss in both groups and improved insulin signaling and histology in subjects losing ≥9% body weight regardless of treatment with orlistat or not [401]. Less clear is the role of other weight loss agents such as sibutramine (a serotonin and norepinephrin reuptake inhibitor) and potential appetite modulators such as leptin, amylin, or the incretins (glucagon-like peptide 1, glucose-dependent insulinotropic polypeptide). Endocannabinoids such as rimonabant as weight loss agents are no longer under study to our knowledge due to concerns over side effects.

Weight reduction surgery

Gastric bypass, biliointestinal bypass, and gastric banding are effective in reducing weight, improving insulin resistance, and improving liver histology in NASH in selected patients [402–404]. Accepted indications include a BMI of >40 kg/m^2 (after failure of conventional weight loss measures) or a BMI of ≥35 kg/m^2 with a co-morbidity such as heart disease, diabetes mellitus, hyperlipidemia, or sleep apnea. NASH per se is not typically included as one of these co-morbidities although given the morbidity and mortality associated with steatohepatitis, this is likely to change. On the other hand, limitations of bariatric surgery include resource utilization, long-term effects, and application in patients with incidentally discovered cirrhosis. In the latter, mortality is increased at 4% and progressive liver dysfunction is seen in 12% [405]. In contrast, structured 5-year follow-up biopsies reveal only mild increased fibrosis in the majority of patients with initially early-stage fibrosis [406].

Ursodeoxcholic acid, L-carnitine, and other cytoprotective agents

The possible benefits of ursodeoxcholic acid (UCDA) include effects on mitochondrial membrane stability, blood flow, and immunomodulation [407]. Histologic and biochemical improvement were noted in pilot studies but the results from larger controlled trials have been variable [408,409]. In a 2-year RCT of 166 patients, both groups had similar improvement in aminotransferases and follow-up biopsy (available in only two thirds), consistent with a strong placebo [410]. Similar results were noted in an 18-month controlled trial of high-dose UDCA

(23–28 mg/kg/day) in 185 patients where no significant differences were noted in multiple histologic parameters although improved inflammation approached significance [411]. On the other hand, combination therapy has been more promising: UDCA (12–15 mg/kg/day) and vitamin E (800 IU/day) for 2 years versus single or double placebo controls showed significant improvement in the NAS only in the group treated with combination therapy [412]. L-Carnitine at a dose of 1 g twice daily has been compared with placebo in a 24-week trial. Metabolic and histologic parameters improved in both groups but significantly more so in the carnitine-treated subjects [413]. Other potential cytoprotective agents include taurine, triacetyl uridine, pentoxifylline, and possibly probiotics through indirect mechanisms.

Antioxidants (vitamin E, betaine, and others)

Vitamin E refers to a family of tocopherols and tocotrienols that exhibit antioxidant activity. Available forms usually contain only α-tocopherol – whether other forms are more or less effective is uncertain [414]. Small and short-term human studies (mostly with α-tocopherol) have shown improvement in serologic markers of inflammation but variable histologic results and unclear differentiation from control groups [415–417]. However, a 6-month, placebo-controlled combination study (vitamin E 1,000 IU plus vitamin C 1,000 mg daily) showed improvement in fibrosis although no improvement in inflammation or necrosis was seen [418]. These results were supported in a recent 2-year controlled trial of 247 nondiabetic adults, comparing α-tocopherol (800 IU/day) with placebo and pioglitazone (see below) [419]. Although there were methodologic criticisms (histologic criteria and tocopherol metabolism), significantly greater improvement was seen in key parameters, including steatosis, inflammation, and ballooning, compared with placebo [420]. Toxicity has not been reported in these studies although there remains some theoretical concern regarding higher doses [421,422]. Betaine (trimethylglycine), a methyl donor, promotes conversion of phosphotidyl-ethanolamine to phosphotidylcholine and the export of fat as VLDL [423]. Steatosis was blunted in a 1-year, randomized, placebo-controlled trial but other metabolic and histologic parameters were unchanged compared with placebo [424]. Other potential agents, which to our knowledge have not been adequately studied, include silymarin (milk thistle extract), N-acetylcysteine (converted to glutathione in the liver), glycyrrhizin, and lazaroids (21-aminosteroids).

Antidiabetic agents

Insulin-sensitizing agents have emerged as the most studied form of pharmacologic therapy [425]. Most adequately controlled studies have focused on the thiazolidinediones and metformin, while less is known about the effects of sulfonylureas, insulin, incretins, or agents such as acipimox (inhibits peripheral lipolysis), although the latter does not appear to lower hepatic fat with short-term exposure [426].

Thiazolidinediones

Thiazolidinediones (TZDs: rosiglitazone and pioglitazone) are ligands of PPAR-γ, a nuclear receptor normally activated by fatty acids that regulates gene expression of enzymes involved in lipid and glucose metabolism and which is usually expressed in adipose tissue, intestines, macrophages, and muscle. The receptor, the ligand, and a coactivator form a heterodimer with retinoid X receptor which binds to the response element of specific genes [427]. The most profound effect of TZDs is in adipocyte differentiation [428]. As a result, TZDs cause increased peripheral but decreased central adiposity [429]. A number of potentially relevant nonhypoglycemic effects are also reported [430].

The most consistent effects in human NASH studies have been improved aminotransferases, reduced hepatic steatosis and histologic inflammation, improved insulin signaling, a mild or zero impact on fibrosis even with extended therapy (up to 3 years in the FLIRT 2 study with rosiglitazone), and overall weight gain of several kilograms in most but not all patients (Fig. 32.16) [431–435]. Similar results have been seen with both pioglitazone and rosiglitazone although pioglitazone appears to be slightly more effective. A relapse of necroinflammation occurs after the discontinuation of therapy but can be ameliorated with sustained adherence to dietary changes and increased exercise [436,437]. Because PPAR-γ receptors are not highly expressed in human liver, the effects in NASH are likely to primarily involve indirect mechanisms [438]. In the largest study to date, although troubled by methodologic issues (see above), 47% of

pioglitazone-treated patients versus 36% of vitamin E-treated patients and 21% of placebo-treated patients had resolution of steatohepatitis after 2 years of therapy [420].

Uncommon idiosyncratic hepatotoxicity led to the withdrawal of troglitazone (the first widely available TZD) [439]. Very rare hepatotoxicity has been reported with rosiglitazone and pioglitazone [440,441]. The effect of shifting fat stores on myocyte function, exercise tolerance, and endurance in these patients has not been adequately addressed. Other side effects of concern include possible precipitation of edema and congestive heart failure and osteoporosis [436,442]. However, of greatest concern is the risk of cardiovascular events in rosiglitazone-treated patients that appears to be related to changes in lipoprotein metabolism (much less evident or nonexistent with pioglitazone) [443,444].

Metformin

Metformin is an insulin-sensitizing, oral biguanide approved for use in type 2 diabetes in the United States since 1995 [445]. The biguanides exert changes in cellular bioenergetics, reduce hepatic glucose production, and increase peripheral glucose utilization [446]. A major site of action is the mitochondria and signaling is via AMP-activated protein kinase [447] – this pathway is similarly activated with exercise, suggesting that in some ways metformin simulates the effects of exercise on glucose transport. Lactic acidosis appears to be uncommon but caution is warranted in renal insufficiency [448]. Favorable studies in early rodent models, its mild side effect profile (especially the absence of weight gain), and early pilot data in humans sustained an interest in its use in NASH. However, conflicting data have led to the general impression that the agent is usually well tolerated in adult NASH but is not particularly effective in resolving histologic injury [449–452]. A large controlled pediatric study remains in progress.

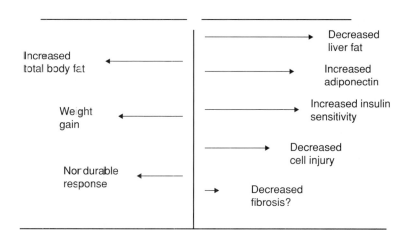

Figure 32.16 The relative effects of thiazolidinediones in nonalcoholic steatohepatitis. Limitations are shown to the left and potential benefits to the right. The length of the arrow indicates relative benefit.

Antihyperlipidemic agents (fibrates and statins)

Fibrates act on PPAR-α receptors located in the liver, heart, muscle, and kidney (normally activated by fatty acids) that stimulate fatty acid oxidation. Promising results with gemfibrozil were not recognized in a histology-based controlled trial of fenofibrate [453–454]. Whether there are differences between the agents is not known. Based on the natural history of NASH (an increased risk of cardiovascular death; see above), the lack of overt evidence of increased hepatic toxicity, and their efficacy in atherosclerosis, HMG-CoA reductase inhibitors or statins are widely prescribed in NASH patients and appear relatively safe [455]. However, the interaction of these agents and NAFLD/NASH is complex and presently not well explored [456]. Whether fibrosis is decreased or possibly increased is unclear from a long-term cohort study where mean fibrosis scores improved but the percentage of patients with advanced stage fibrosis appeared to increase [457]. Favorable therapeutic results in early pilot studies were not confirmed in a subsequent histology-based RCT [458,459].

Other agents (caspase inhibitors, adrenergics, and angiotensin receptor blockers)

Because of the role of apoptosis pathway activation (see above), a great deal of interest has centered on caspase inhibition as a possible therapeutic avenue in experimental models [460,461]. However, the effects on necrosis pathways, the relative risk–benefit with chronic therapy, and the costs of this approach are uncertain. The effects of the adrenergic system on NAFLD have also been explored and may offer an avenue of pharmacologic therapy [462,463]. Angiotensin receptor blockers may modulate fibrosis pathways and are also reported in an uncontrolled study in human NASH [464,465]. As evident from the foregoing discussion, controlled trials are needed to determine its efficacy.

Liver transplantation, disease recurrence, and donor organs

Although there is confusion in nomenclature between NASH-cirrhosis and many cases of cryptogenic cirrhosis, NASH as a designated indication for transplantation appears to be increasing in the Unted States. Whether this represents a true increase, or a greater acceptance of NASH as a cause of advanced cirrhosis, is unclear. Transplant eligibility is complicated by co-morbidities related to the metabolic syndrome [466,467]. Thus, many centers restrict candidacy by BMI (usually $<40 \, \text{kg/m}^2$). Recurrent (and de novo) NAFLD and NASH after transplantation is reported and may be progressive (see Fig. 32.5) [216,468]. The relative risks of different immunosuppression regimens is not clearly established although weight gain is predictive. Compared with other causes, overall long-term post-transplant survival for NASH-cirrhosis is similar, although early survival is diminished in those with an age over 60 years, BMI $\geq 30 \, \text{kg/m}^2$, and diabetes [469–471]. Steatosis in donor livers is associated with poor graft function likely due to disturbed ATP homeostasis [472]. This problem is magnified in living-related donation where accurate diagnosis of steatosis in a partial donor is essential.

Annotated references

Aithal GP, Thomas JA, Kaye PV, et al. Randomized, placebo-controlled trial of pioglitazone in nondiabetic subjects with nonalcoholic steatohepatitis. *Gastroenterology* 2008;135:1176–84.

Belfort R, Harrison SA, Brown K, et al. A placebo-controlled trial of pioglitazone in subjects with nonalcoholic steatohepatitis. *N Engl J Med* 2006;355:2297–307.

Ratziu V, Giral P, Jacqueminet S, et al. Rosiglitazone for nonalcoholic steatohepatitis: one-year results of the randomized placebo-controlled Fatty Liver Improvement with Rosiglitazone Therapy (FLIRT) Trial. *Gastroenterology* 2008;135:100–10.

Sanyal AJ, Chalasani N, Kowdley KV, et al. Pioglitazone, vitamin E, or placebo for nonalcoholic steatohepatitis. *N Engl J Med* 2010;362:1675–85.

A number of randomized controlled pharmacologic trials have been reported. The thiazolidinediones (TZDs) are the best studied group of agents. The most consistent effects of the TZDs are reduction of steatosis, inflammation, and ballooning, but they have a limited effect on fibrosis and increased body weight due to peripheral adipose accumulation in many but not all patients. Weight gain and vascular risk with some agents limits the application of the TZDs. Higher dose vitamin E, possibly in combination with cytoprotective agents, appears promising but requires further study and carries concerns of long-term safety.

Argo CK, Northup PG, Al-Osaimi AM, et al. Systematic review of risk factors for fibrosis progression in non-alcoholic steatohepatitis. *J Hepatol* 2009;51:371–9.

Ekstedt M, Franzen LE, Mathiesen UL, et al. Long-term follow-up of patients with NAFLD and elevated liver enzymes. *Hepatology* 2006;44:865–73.

Rafiq N, Bai C, Fang Y, et al. Long-term follow-up of patients with non-alcoholic fatty liver. *Clin Gastroenterol Hepatol* 2009;7:234–8.

The natural history of NAFLD and NASH has come into much sharper focus. From histologic studies using paired biopsies over time, inflammation appears to be a key predictor of progression to advanced fibrosis seen in about 15% of cases over about 5–10 years. Patients with histologic NASH compared with those with non-NASH fatty liver have significantly diminished survival. Leading causes of death are cardiovascular disease, nonhepatic cancers, and cirrhosis-related disease. The dominant pattern in a given patient is difficult to predict and it is increasingly apparent that many patients develop coronary disease in the setting of cirrhosis, presenting the clinician with complex challenges.

Browning JD, Szczepaniak LS, Dobbins R, et al. Prevalence of hepatic steatosis in an urban population in the United States: impact of ethnicity. *Hepatology* 2004;40:1387–95.

Romeo S, Kozlitina J, Xing C, et al. Genetic variation in PNPLA3 confers susceptibility to nonalcoholic fatty liver disease. *Nat Genet* 2008;40:1461–5.

Schwimmer JB, Celedon MA, Lavine JE, et al. Heritability of nonalcoholic fatty liver disease. *Gastroenterology* 2009;136:1585–92.

These studies have established significant ethnic variation and familial risk in the prevalence of NAFLD and elucidated the complex relationships between obesity, insulin resistance, and fatty liver within these groups. Much of the variation is conferred by a gene product called PNPLA3 (adiponutrin) which is a lipase that appears to be especially active in the endoplasmic reticulum.

Caldwell S, Ikura Y, Dias D, et al. Hepatocellular ballooning in NASH. *J Hepatol* 2010;53:719–23.

Kleiner DE, Brunt EM, Van Natta ML, et al. Nonalcoholic Steatohepatitis Clinical Research Network. Design and validation of a histologic scoring system for NAFLD. *Hepatology* 2005;41:1313–21.

Lackner C, Gogg-Kamerer M, Zatloukal K, et al. Ballooned hepatocytes in steatohepatitis: The value of keratin immunohistochemistry for diagnosis. *J Hepatol* 2008;48:821–8.

Key histologic parameters have been combined into a widely utilized composite score (the NASH activity score or NAS) which facilitates assessment of therapeutic interventions and comparison between different studies. Interobserver variation in the criteria of ballooning has been problematic. It now appears that these cells are depleted of keratin 8 and 18 and contain small fat droplets as well as dilated endoplasmic reticulum – features that may lend themselves to more refined scoring.

Caldwell SH, Oelsner DH, Iezzoni JC, et al. Cryptogenic cirrhosis: clinical characterization and risk factors for underlying disease. *Hepatology* 1999;29:664–9.

Maheshwari A, Thuluvath PJ. Cryptogenic cirrhosis and NAFLD: are they related? *Am J Gastroenterol* 2006;101:664–8.

Cryptogenic cirrhosis remains a common diagnostic problem. The potential for NASH to progress to a late stage of characterized by cirrhosis with loss of steatosis was first noted 20 years ago. Subsequently, a number of studies compiled and compared in this work confirmed that in most regions of the world, NASH is the most common cause of cryptogenic cirrhosis usually in association with prior obesity and diabetes although other causes are recognized such as silent autoimmune hepatitis.

Donnelly KL, Smith CI, Schwarzenberg SJ, et al. Sources of fatty acids in liver and secreted via lipoproteins in patients with nonalcoholic fatty liver disease. *J Clin Invest* 2005;115:1343–51.

Feldstein AE, Wieckowska A, Lopez AR, et al. Cytokeratin-18 fragment levels as noninvasive biomarkers for nonalcoholic steatohepatitis: A multicenter validation study. *Hepatology* 2009;50:1072–8.

Fujita K, Nozaki Y, Wada K, et al. Dysfunctional very-low-density lipoprotein synthesis and release is a key factor in nonalcoholic steatohepatitis pathogenesis. *Hepatology* 2009;50:772–80.

Puri P, Baillie RA, Wiest MM, et al. A lipidomic analysis of nonalcoholic fatty liver disease. *Hepatology* 2007;46:1081–90.

Singh R, Kaushik S, Wang Y, et al. Autophagy regulates lipid metabolism. *Nature* 2009;458:1131–5.

These studies have demonstrated key pathologic mechanisms of cell injury in NAFLD/NASH. Lipid accumulation results from both increased de novo synthesis from carbohydrate substrate and uptake of nonesterified fatty acids from peripheral fat lipolysis. Impaired apo-B function contributes to lipid accumulation by insufficient VLDL secretion relative to the total fat content of the liver. Lysosomal recycling of accumulated small fat droplets is regulated through a process called lipophagy. Caspase activation results from the effects of fatty acids on lysosomal and mitochondrial permeability and results in fragmentation of the elements of the cytoskeleton including keratin 18 fragments.

Johnson NA, Sachinwalla T, Walton DW, et al. Aerobic exercise training reduces hepatic and visceral lipids in obese individuals without weight loss. *Hepatology* 2009;50:1105–12.

Nobili V, Manco M, Devito R, et al. Lifestyle intervention and antioxidant therapy in children with nonalcoholic fatty liver disease: a randomized, controlled trial. *Hepatology* 2008;48:119–28.

Promrat K, Kleiner DE, Niemeier HM, et al. Randomized controlled trial testing the effects of weight loss on nonalcoholic steatohepatitis. *Hepatology* 2010;51:121–9.

Ueno T, Sugawara H, Sujaku K, et al. Therapeutic effects of restricted diet and exercise in obese patients with fatty liver. *J Hepatol* 1997;27:103–7.

These studies have clearly demonstrated histologic improvement of NASH with conservative measures of exercise and dietary changes. Exercise alone (without net weight loss) also diminishes liver fat. Such voluntary lifestyle changes constitute the most important intervention but are successful in only about 20–30%. Outcomes are enhanced with more structured programs. Voluntary adoption introduces a confounding variable into pharmacologic studies which is challenging but essential to account for.

References

1. Schaffner F, Thaler H. Nonalcoholic fatty liver disease. *Prog Liver Dis* 1986;8:283–98.
2. Ludwig J, Viggiano TR, McGill DB, Ott BJ. Nonalcoholic steatohepatitis: Mayo Clinic experiences with a hitherto unnamed disease. *Mayo Clin Proc* 1980;55:434–8.
3. Lazo M, Clark JM. The epidemiology of nonalcoholic fatty liver disease: a global perspective. *Semin Liver Dis* 2008;28:339–50.
4. Brunt EM. What's in a NAme? *Hepatology* 2009;50:663–7.
5. Cairns SR, Peters TJ. Biochemical analysis of hepatic lipid in alcoholic and diabetic and control subjects. *Clin Sci* 1983;65:645–52.
6. Teli MR, James OFW, Burt AD, Bennett MK, Day CP. The natural history of nonalcoholic fatty liver: a followup study. *Hepatology* 1995;22:1714–19.
7. Becker U, Deis A, Sorensen TIA, et al. Prediction of liver disease by alcohol intake, sex and age: a prospective population study. *Hepatology* 1996;23:1025–9.
8. Bellentani S, Saccoccio G, Masutti F, et al. Prevalence of and risk factors for hepatic steatosis in northern Italy. *Ann Intern Med* 2000;132:112–17.
9. Ferrell GC, George J, Hall P, McCullough AJ. Overview: an Introduction to NASH and related fatty liver disorders. In: Farrell GC, George J, Hall P, McCullough AJ, eds. *Fatty Liver Disease; NASH and Related Disorders.* Malden, MA: Blackwell Publishing, 2005:1-12.
10. Yeh MM, Brunt EM. Pathology of nonalcoholic fatty liver disease. *Am J Clin Pathol* 2007;128 837–47.
11. Burt AD, Mutton A, Day CP. Diagnosis and interpretation of steatosis and steatohepatitis. *Semin Diagn Pathol* 1998;15:246–58.
12. Brunt EM. Histopathology of non-alcoholic fatty liver disease. *Clin Liv Dis* 2009;13:533–44.
13. Younossi ZM, Gramlich T, Liu YC, et al. Nonalcoholic fatty liver disease: an assessment of variability in pathological interpretation. *Mod Pathol* 1998;11:560–5.
14. Lackner C, Gogg-Kamerer M, Zatloukal K, Stumptner C, Brunt EM, Denk H. Ballooned hepatocytes in steatohepatitis: the value of keratin immunohistochemistry for diagnosis. *J Hepatol* 2008;48:821–8.
15. Caldwell S, Ikura Y, Dias D, et al. Hepatocellular ballooning in NASH. *J Hepatol* 2010;53:719–23.
16. Brunt EM, Janney CG, Di Bisceglie AM, Neuschwander-Tetri BA, Bacon BR. Nonalcoholic steatohepatitis: a proposal for grading and staging the histologic lesions. *Am J Gastroenterol* 1999;94:2467–74.
17. Powell EE, Cooksley WG, Hanson R, Searll J, Halliday JW, Powell LW. The natural history of nonalcoholic steatohepatitis: A followup study of forty-two patients for up to 21 years. *Hepatology* 1990;11:74–80.
18. Abdelmmalek M, Ludwig J, Lindor KD. Two cases from the spectrum of nonalcoholic steatohepatitis. *J Clin Gastroenterol* 1995;20:127–30.
19. Berg T, Neuhaus R, Klein R, et al. Distinct enzyme profiles in patients with cryptogenic cirrhosis reflect heterogeneous causes with different outcomes after liver transplantation (OLT): A long-term documentation before and after OLT. *Transplantation* 2002;74:792–8.

20. Caldwell SH, Oelsner DH, Iezzoni JC, Hespenheide EE, Battle EH, Driscoll CJ. Cryptogenic cirrhosis: clinical characterization and risk factors for underlying disease. *Hepatology* 1999;29:664–9.

21. Poonawala A, Nair SP, Thuluvath PJ. Prevalence of obesity and diabetes in patients with cryptogenic cirrhosis: a case–control study. *Hepatology* 2000;32:689–92.

22. Mendiola AE, Gish RG. Risk factors for NASH in patients with cryptogenic cirrhosis. *Gastroenterology* 2001;120:A545

23. Clark JM, Diehl AM. Nonalcoholic fatty liver disease: an under-recognized cause of cryptogenic cirrhosis. *JAMA* 2003;289:3000–4.

24. Caldwell SH, Crespo DM. The spectrum expanded: cryptogenic cirrhosis and the natural history of nonalcoholic fatty liver disease. *J Hepatol* 2004;40:578–84.

25. Kodali VP, Gordon SC, Silverman AL, McGray DG. Cryptogenic liver disease in the United States: further evidence for non-A, non-B, non-C hepatitis. *Am J Gastroenterol* 1994;89:1836–9.

26. Saunders JB, Walters JR, Davies AP, Paton A. A twenty year prospective study of cirrhosis. *Br Med J* 1981;282:263–6.

27. DiBisceglie AM, Bacon BR, Neuschwander-Tetri BA, Yun A, Kim JP. Role of hepatitis G virus in cryptogenic liver disease. *Gastroenterology* 1996;110:A1181.

28. Strauss E, Lacet CMC, Caly WR, Fukushima JT, Gayotta LCC. Cryptogenic cirrhosis: clinical-biochemical comparison with alcoholic and viral etiologies. *Arch Gastroenterol* 1990;27:46–52.

29. Maheshwari A. Thuluvath PJ. Cryptogenic cirrhosis and NAFLD: are they related? *Am J Gastroenterol* 2006;101:664–8.

30. Crawford DHG, Shepherd RW, Halliday JW, et al. Body composition in nonalcoholic cirrhosis: the effect of disease etiology and severity on nutritional compartments. *Gastroenterology* 1994;106:1611–17.

31. Caldwell SH, Lee VD, Kleiner DE, et al. NASH and cryptogenic cirrhosis: a histological analysis. *Ann Hepatol* 2009;8:346–52.

32. Schaffner F, Popper H. Capillarization of hepatic sinusoids. *Gastroenterology* 1963;44:239–42.

33. Nosadini R, Avogaro A, Mollo F, et al. Carbohydrate and lipid metabolism in cirrhosis. Evidence that hepatic uptake of gluconeogenic precursors and of free fatty acids depends on effective hepatic flow. *J Clin Endocr Metab* 1984;58:1125–32.

34. Matsui O, Kadoya M, Takahashi S, et al. Focal sparing of segment IV in fatty livers shown by sonography and CT: correlation with aberrant gastric venous drainage. *Am J Roentgenol* 1995;164:1137–40.

35. Contos MJ, Cales W, Sterling RK, et al. Development of nonalcoholic fatty liver disease after orthotopic liver transplantation for cryptogenic cirrhosis. *Liver Transpl* 2001;7:363–73.

36. Ong J, Younossi ZM, Reddy V, et al. Cryptogenic cirrhosis and post-transplantation non-alcoholic fatty liver disease. *Liver Transpl* 2001;7:797–801.

37. Ayata G, Gordon FD, Lewis WD, et al. Cryptogenic cirrhosis: clinicopathologic findings at and after liver transplantation. *Hum Pathol* 2002;33:1098–104.

38. Yalamanchili K, Saadeh S, Klintmalm GB, Jennings LW, Davis GL. Nonalcoholic fatty liver disease after liver transplantation for cryptogenic cirrhosis or nonalcoholic fatty liver disease. *Liver Transpl* 2010;16:431–9.

39. El-Hassan AY, Ibrahim EM, Al-Mulhim FA, Nabhan AA, Chammas MY. Fatty infiltration of the liver: analysis of prevalence, radiological and clinical features and influence on patient management. *Br J Radiol* 1992;65:774–8.

40. Gale ME, Gerzof SG, Robbins AH. Portal architecture: a differential guide to fatty infiltration of the liver on computerized tomography. *Gastrointest Radiol* 1983;8:231–6.

41. Burrows CJ, Jones AW. Hepatic subcapsular steatosis in patients with insulin dependent diabetes receiving dialysis. *J Clin Pathol* 1994;47:274–5.

42. Bockus HL. In: *Gastro-Enterology*, Vol. III. Philadelphia, PA: WB Saunders, 1946:385–92.

43. Budd G. *On Diseases of the Liver*. Philadelphia, PA: Lea and Blanchard, 1846:227. University of Virginia Historical Collection.

44. Morgan W. The Liver and its Diseases, both Functional and Organic. Their history, anatomy, chemistry, pathology, physiology, and treatment. London: Homoeopathic Pub. Co., 1877:144. University of Virginia Historical Collection.

45. Zelman S. The liver in obesity. *Arch Intern Med* 1958;90:141–56.

46. McGill DB, Humphreys SR, Baggenstoss AH, Dickson ER. Cirrhosis and death after jejunoileal shunt. *Gastroenterology* 1972;63:872–7.

47. Hayashi PH, Harrison SA, Torgerson S, Perez TA, Nochajski T, Russell M. Cognitive lifetime drinking history in nonalcoholic fatty liver disease: some cases may be alcohol related. *Am J Gastroenterol* 2004;99:76–81.

48. Naveau S, Giraud V, Borotto E, Aubert A, Capron F, Chaput J-C. Excess weight risk factor for alcoholic liver disease. *Hepatology* 1997;25:108–11.

49. Dixon JB, Bathal PS, O'Brien PE. Nonalcoholic fatty liver disease: predictors of nonalcoholic steatohepatitis and liver fibrosis in the severely obese. *Gastroenterology* 2001;121:91–100.

50. Davies MJ, Baer DJ, Judd JT, Brown ED, Campbell WS, Taylor PR. Effects of moderate alcohol intake on fasting insulin and glucose concentrations and insulin sensitivity in postmenopausal women. *JAMA* 2003;287:2559–62.

51. Cotrim HP, Freitas LA, Alves E, Almeida A, May DS, Caldwell S. Effects of light-to-moderate alcohol consumption on steatosis and steatohepatitis in severely obese patients. *Eur J Gastroenterol Hepatol* 2009;21:969–72.

52. Pinto HC, Baptista A, Camilo ME, Valenta A, Saragoca A, de Moura MC. Nonalcoholic steatohepatitis. Clinicopathological comparison with alcoholic hepatitis in ambulatory and hospitalized patients. *Dig Dis Sci* 1996;41:172–9.

53. Sanderson SO, Smyrk TC. The use of protein tyrosine phosphatase 1B and insulin receptor immunostains to differentiate nonalcoholic from alcoholic steatohepatitis in liver biopsy specimens. *Am J Clin Pathol* 2005;123:503–9.

54. Mihas AA, Tavassoli M. Laboratory markers of ethanol intake and abuse: a critical appraisal. *Am J Med Sci* 1992;303:415–28.

55. Perseghin G, Mazzaferro V, Sereni LP, et al. Contribution of reduced insulin sensitivity and secretion to the pathogenesis of hepatogenous diabetes: effect of liver transplantation. *Hepatology* 2000;31:694–703.

56. Petrides AS. Liver disease and diabetes mellitus. *Diabetes Rev* 1994;2:2–18.

57. Petrides AS, Stanley T, Matthews DE, Vogt C, Bush AJ, Lambeth H. Insulin resistance in cirrhosis: prolonged reduction of hyperinsulinemia normalizes insulin sensitivity. *Hepatology* 1998;28:141–9.

58. Jacobsen EB, Hamberg O, Quistorff B, Ott P. Reduced mitochondrial adenosine triphosphate synthesis in skeletal muscle in patients with Child–Pugh class B and C cirrhosis. *Hepatology* 2001;34:7–12.

59. Byron D, Minuk GY. Profile of an urban hospital-based practice. *Hepatology* 1996;24:813–15.

60. Sorbi D, McGill DB, Thistle JL, Therneau TM, Henry J, Lindor KD. An assessment of the role of liver biopsies in asymptomatic patients with chronic liver test abnormalities. *Am J Gastroenterol* 2000;95:3206–10.

61. Kim WR, Brown RS, Terrault NA, El-Serag H. Burden of liver disease in the Unites States: summary of a workshop. *Hepatology* 2002;36:227–42.

62. Clark JM, Brancati FL, Diehl AM. The prevalence and etiology of elevated aminotransferase levels in the United States. *Am J Gastroenterol* 2003;98:960–7.

63. Bedogni G, Miglioli L, Masutti F, Tiribelli C, Marchesini G, Bellentani S. Prevalence of and risk factors for nonalcoholic fatty liver disease: the Dionysos nutrition and liver study. *Hepatology* 2005;42: 44–52.

64. Argo CK, Caldwell SH. Epidemiology and natural history of nonalcoholic steatohepatitis. *Clin Liver Dis* 2009;13:511–31.

65. Flegal KM, Carroll MD, Ogden CL, Curtin LR. Prevalence and trends in obesity among US adults, 1999–2008. *JAMA* 2010;303: 235–41.

66. Mathieson UL, Franzen LE, Fryden A, Foberg U, Bodemar G. The clinical significance of slightly too moderately elevated liver transaminase values in asymptomatic patients. *Scan J Gastroenterol* 1999;34:85–91.

67. Daniel S, Ben-Menachem T, Vasudevan G, Ma CK, Blumenkehl M. Prospective evaluation of unexplained chronic liver transaminase abnormalities in asymptomatic and symptomatic patients. *Am J Gastroenterol* 1999;94:3010–14.

68. Navarro VJ, St Louis T, Bell BZ, Sofair AN. Chronic liver disease in the primary care practices of Waterby, Connecticut. *Hepatology* 2003;38:1062.

69. Angulo P, Keach JC, Batts KP, Lindor KD. Independent predictors of liver fibrosis in patients with nonalcoholic steatohepatitis. *Hepatology* 1999;30:1356–62.

70. Ong JP, Elariny H, Collantes R, et al. Predictors of nonalcoholic steatohepatitis and advanced fibrosis in morbidly obese patients. *Obes Surg* 2005;15:310–15.

71. Wanless IR, Lentz JS. Fatty liver hepatitis (steatohepatitis) and obesity: an autopsy study with anlysis of risk factors. *Hepatology* 1990;12:1106–10.

72. Machado M, Marques-Vidal P, Cortez-Pinto H. Hepatic histology in obese patients undergoing bariatric surgery. *J Hepatol* 2006;45: 600–6.

73. Ratziu V, Giral P, Charlotte F, et al. Liver fibrosis in overweight patients. *Gastroenterology* 2000;118:1117–23.

74. Marchesini G, Brizi M, Morselli-Labate AM, et al. Association of nonalcoholic fatty liver diseae with insulin resistance. *Am J Med* 1999;107:450–5.

75. Guidorizzi de Siqueira AC, Cotrim HP, Rocha R, et al. Non-alcoholic fatty liver disease and insulin resistance: importance of risk factors and histological spectrum. *Eur J Gastroenterol Hepatol* 2005;17: 837–41.

76. Chitturi S, Abeygunasekera S, Farrell GC, et al. NASH and insulin resistance: insulin hypersecretion and specific association with the insulin resistance syndrome. *Hepatology* 2002;35:373–9.

77. Batman PA, Scheuer PJ. Diabetic hepatitis preceeding the onset of glucose intolerance. *Histopathology* 1985;9:237–43.

78. Silverman JF, Pories WJ, Caro JF. Liver pathology in diabetes mellitus and morbid obesity. *Pathol Annu* 1989;24:275–302.

79. Guerrero R, Vega GL, Grundy SM, Browning JD. Ethnic differences in hepatic steatosis: an insulin resistance paradox? *Hepatology* 2009;49:791–801.

80. Silverman JF, O'Brien KF, Long S, et al. Liver pathology in morbidly obese patients with and without diabetes. *Am J Gastroenterol* 1990;85:1349–55.

81. Younossi ZM, Gramlich T, Matteoni CA, Boparai N, McCullough AJ. Nonalcoholic fatty liver disease in patients with type 2 diabetes. *Clin Gastroenterol Hepatol* 2004;2:262–5.

82. Assy N, Kaita K, Mymin D, Levy C, Rosser B, Minuk G. Fatty infiltration of liver in hyperlipidemic patients. *Dig Dis Sci* 2000;45:1929–34.

83. McCullough AJ. The clinical features, diagnosis, and natural history of nonalcoholic fatty liver disease. *Clin Liver Dis* 2004;8:521–33.

84. Gambino R, Cassader M, Pagano G, Durazzo M, Musso G. Polymorphism in microsomal triglyceride transfer protein: a lik between liver disease and atherogenic postprandial lipid profile in NASH? *Hepatology* 2007;45:1097–107.

85. Reaven GM. Role of insulin resistance in human diabetes. *Diabetes* 1988;37:1595–607.

86. Nguyen-Duy T-B, Nichaman MZ, Church TS, Blair SN, Ross R. Visceral and liver fat are independent predictors of metabolic risk factors in men. *Am J Physiol Endocrinol Metab* 2003;284:E1065–71.

87. Park Y-W, Zhu S, Palaniappan L, Heshka S, Carnethon MR, Heymsfield SB. The metabolic syndrome. *Arch Intern Med* 2003;163: 427–36.

88. Liangpunsakul S, Chalasani N. Unexplained elevations in alanine aminotransferase in individuals with the metabolic syndrome: results from the third National Health and Nutrition Survey (NHANES III). *Am J Med Sci* 2005;329:111–16.

89. Pagano G, Pacini G, Musso G, et al. Nonalcoholic steatohepatitis, insulin resistance and metabolic syndrome: further evidence for an etiologic association. *Hepatology* 2002;35:367–72.

90. Hamaguchi M, Kojima T, Takeda N, et al. The metabolic syndrome as a predictor of nonalcoholic fatty liver disease. *Ann Intern Med* 2005;143:722–8.

91. Amarro A, Fabbrini E, Kars M, et al. Dissociation between intrahepatic triglyceride content and insulin resistance in familial hypobetalipoproteinemia. *Gastroenterology* 2010;139:149–53.

92. Banerji MA, Faridi N, Atluri R, Chaiken RL, Lebovitz HE. Body composition, visceral fat, leptin, and insulin resistance in Asian Indian men. *J Clin Endocrinol Metab* 1999;84:137–44.

93. Kral JG, Schaffner F, Pierson RN, Wang J. Body fat topography as an independent predictor of fatty liver. *Metabolism* 1993;42:548–51.

94. Ruderman N, Chisolm D, Pi-Sunyer X, Schneider S. The metabolically obese, normal-weight individual revisited. *Diabetes* 1998;47: 699–713.

95. Wildman RP, Munter P, Reynolds K, et al. The obese without cardiometabolic risk factor clustering and the normal weight with cardiometabolic risk factor clustering. *Arch Intern Med* 2008;168: 1617–24.

96. Schwimmer JB, Behling C, Newbury R, et al. Histopathology of pediatric nonalcoholic fatty liver disease. *Hepatology* 2005;42:641–9.

97. Fatton HM, Yates K, Unalp-Arida A, et al. Association between metabolic syndrome and liver histology among children with nonalcoholic fatty liver disease. *Am J Gastroenterol* 2010;105:2093–102.

98. Rashid M, Roberts EA. Nonalcoholic steatohepatitis in children. *J Pediatr Gastroenterol Nutr* 2000;30:48–53.

99. Schwimmer JB, Deutsch R, Rauch JB, Behling C, Newbury R, Lavine JE. Obesity, insulin resistance, and other clinicaopathological correlates of pediatric nonalcoholic fatty liver disease. *J Pediatr* 2003;143:500–5.

100. Schwimmer JB, McGreal N, Deutsch R, Finegold MJ, Lavine JE. Influence of gender, race, and ethnicity on suspected fatty liver in obese adolescents. *Pediatrics* 2005;115:561–5.

101. Brunt EM, Ramrakhiani S, Cordes BG, et al. Concurrence of histological features of steatohepatitis with other forms of chronic liver disease. *Mod Pathol* 2003;16:49–56.

102. Mirandola S, Realdon S, Iqbal J, et al. Liver microsomal triglyceride transfer protein is involved in hepatitis C liver steatosis. *Gastroenterology* 2006;130:1661–9.

103. Leandro G, Mangia A, Hui J, et al. HCV Meta-Analysis (on) Individual Patients' Data Study Group. Relationship between steatosis, inflammation, and fibrosis in chronic hepatitis C: a meta-analysis of individual patient data. *Gastroenterology* 2006;130:1636–42.

104. Solis-Herruzo JA, Perez-Carreras M, Rivas E, et al. Factors associated with the presence of nonalcoholic steatohepatitis in patients with chronic hepatitis C. *Am J Gastroenterol* 2005;100:1091–8.

105. Charlton MR, Pockros PJ, Harrison SA. Impact of obesity on treatment of chronic hepatitis C. *Hepatology* 2006;43:1177–86.

106. Bonkovsky H, Jawaid Q, Tortorelli K, et al. Non-alcoholic steatohepatitis and iron: increased prevalence of mutations of the HFE gene in non-alcoholic steatohepatitis. *J Hepatol* 1999;31:421–9.

107. Powell EE, Jonsson JR, Clouston AD. Steatosis: co-factor in other liver diseases. *Hepatology* 2005;42:5–13.

108. Sorrentino P, Terracciano L, D'Angelo S, et al. Oxidative stress and steatosis are cofactors of liver injury in primary biliary cirrhosis. *J Gastroenterol* 2010;45:1053–62.

109. Caldwell SH, Harris DM, Hespenheide EE. Is NASH under diagnosed among African Americans? *Am J Gastroenterol* 2002;97:1496–500.

110. Weston SR, Leyden W, Murphy R, et al. Racial and ethnic distribution of nonalcoholic fatty liver in persons with newly diagnosed chronic liver disease. *Hepatology* 2005;41:372–9.

111. Browning JD, Szczepaniak LS, Dobbins R, et al. Prevalence of hepatic steatosis in an urban population in the United States: impact of ethnicity. *Hepatology* 2004;40:1387–95.

112. Perry AC, Applegate EB, Jackson ML, et al. Racial differences in visceral adipose tissue but not anthropometric markers of health-related variables. *J Appl Physiol* 2000;89:636–43.

113. Yanoyski JA, Yanovski SZ, Filmer KM, et al. Differences in body composition of black and white girls. *Am J Clin Nutr* 1996;64:833–9.

114. Sumner AE, Finley KB, Genovese DJ, Criqui MH, Boston RC. Fasting triglyceride and the triglyceride-HDL cholesterol ratio are not markers of insulin resistance in African Americans. *Arch Intern Med* 2005;165:1395–400.

115. Guerrero R, Vega GL, Grundy SM, Browning JD. Ethnic differences in hepatic steatosis: an insulin resistance paradox? *Hepatology* 2009;49:791–801.

116. Browning JD, Kumar KS, Saboorian MH, Thiele DL. Ethnic differences in the prevalence of cryptogenic cirrhosis. *Am J Gastroenterol* 2004;99:292–8.

117. Struben VMD, Hespenheide EE, Caldwell SH. Nonalcoholic steatohepatitis and cryptogenic cirrhosis within kindreds. *Am J Med* 2000;108:9–13.

118. Willner IR, Waters B, Patil SR, Reuben A, Morelli J, Riely CA. Ninety patients with nonalcoholic steatohepatitis: insulin resistance, familial tendency, and severity of disease. *Am J Gastroenterol* 2001;96:2957–61.

119. Abdelmalek MF, Liu C, Shuster J, Nelson DR, Asal NR. Familial aggregation of insulin resistance in first-degree relatives of patients with nonalcoholic fatty liver disease. *Clin Gastroenterol Hepatol* 2006;4:1162–9.

120. Laws A, Stefanick ML, Reaven GM. Insulin resistance and hypertriglyceridemia in nondiabetic relatives of patients with noninsulin-dependent diabetes mellitus. *J Clin Endocr Metab* 1989;69:343–7.

121. Petersen KF, Dufour S, Befroy D, Garcia R, Shulman GI. Impaired mitochondrial activity in the insulin-resistant offspring of diabetes with type 2 diabetes. *N Engl J Med* 2004;350:664–71.

122. Schwimmer JB, Celedon MA, Lavine JE, et al. Heritability of nonalcoholic fatty liver disease. *Gastroenterology* 2009;136:1585–92.

123. Day CP. Genetic and environmental susceptibility to non-alcoholic fatty liver disease. *Dig Dis* 2010;28:255–60.

124. Diehl AM. Genetic susceptibility to hepatic statosis. *N Engl J Med* 2010;362:1082–9.

125. Romeo S, Kozlitina J, Xing C, et al. Genetic variation in PNPLA3 confers susceptibility to nonalcoholic fatty liver disease. *Nat Genet* 2008;40:1461–5.

126. Hoekstra M, Li Z, Kruijt JK, Van Eck M, Van Berkel TJ, Kuiper J. The expression level of non-alcoholic fatty liver disease-related gene PNPLA3 in hepatocytes is highly influenced by hepatic lipid status. *J Hepatol* 2010;52:244–51.

127. Petersen KF, Dufour S, Hariri A, et al. Apolipoprotein C3 gene variants in nonalcoholic fatty liver disease. *N Engl J Med* 2010;362:1082–9.

128. Gambino R, Cassader M, Pagano G, Durazzo M, Musso G. Polymorphism in microsomal triglyceride transfer protein: a link between liver disease and atherogenic postprandial lipid profile in NASH? *Hepatology* 2007;45:1097–107.

129. Musso G, Gambino R, Pacini G, Pagano G, Durazzo M, Cassader M. Transcription factor 7-like 2 polymorphism modulates glucose and lipid homeostasis, adipokine profile, and hepatocyte apoptosis in NASH. *Hepatology* 2009;49:426–35.

130. Dixon JB, Bhathal PS, Jonsson JR, Dixon AF, Powell EE, O'Brien PE. Pro-fibrotic polymorphisms predictive of advanced liver fibrosis in the severely obese. *J Hepatol* 2003;39:967–71.

131. Reid AE. Nonalcoholic steatohepatitis. *Gastroenterology* 2001;121:710–23.

132. Chatila R, West AB. Hepatomegaly and abnormal liver tests due to glycogenosis in adults with diabetes. *Medicine* 1996;75:327–33.

133. Cortez-Pinto H, Camilo ME, Baptista A, de Oliveira AG, De Moura MC. Non-alcoholic fatty liver: another feature of the metabolic syndrome. *Clin Nutr* 1999;18:353–8.

134. Marchesini G, Brizi M, Bianchi G, et al. Nonalcoholic fatty liver disease: a feature of the metabolic syndrome. *Diabetes* 2001;50:1844–50.

135. Diehl AK. Cholelithiasis and the insulin resistance syndrome. *Hepatology* 2000;31:528–30.

136. Mertens I, Van Gaal LF. Visceral fat as a determinant of fibrinolysis and hemostasis. *Semin Vasc Med* 2005;5:48–55.

137. Villanova N, Moscatiello S, Ramilli S, et al. Endothelial dysfunction and cardiovascular risk profil in nonalcoholic fatty liver disease. *Hepatology* 2005;42:473–80.

138. Hickman IJ, Sullivan CM, Flight S, et al. Altered clot kinetics in patients with non-alcoholic fatty liver disease. *Ann Hepatol* 2009;8:331–8.

139. Caldwell SH, Hespenheide EE. Subacute liver failure in obese females. *Am J Gastroenterol* 2002;97:2058–62.

140. Neuschwander-Tetri BA, Clark JM, Bass NM, et al. NASH Clinical Research Network. Clinical, laboratory and histological associations in adults with nonalcoholic fatty liver disease. *Hepatology* 2010;52:913–24.

141. Fletcher LM, Kwoh-Gain I, Powell EE, Powell LW, Halliday JW. Markers of chronic alcohol ingestion in patients with nonalcoholic steatohepatitis: an aid to diagnosis. *Hepatology* 1991;13:455–9.

142. Nanji AA, French SW, Freeman JB. Serum alanine aminotransferase to aspartate aminotransferase ratio and degree of fatty liver in morbidly obese patients. *Enzyme* 1986;36:266–9.

143. Mofrad P, Contos MJ, Haque M, et al. Clinical and histological spectrum of nonalcoholic fatty liver disease associated with normal ALT values. *Hepatology* 2003;37:1286–92.

144. Suzuki A, Angulo P, Lymp J, et al. Chronological development of elevated aminotransferases in a nonalcoholic population. *Hepatology* 2005;41:64–71.

145. Neuschwander-Tetri BA, Unalp A, Creer MH; Nonalcoholic Steatohepatitis Clinical Research Network. Influence of local reference populations on upper limits of normal for serum alanine aminotransferase levels. *Arch Intern Med* 2008;168:663–6.

146. Cotler SJ, Kanji K, Keshavarzian A, Jensen DM, Jakate S. Prevalence and significance of autoantibodies in patients with non-alcoholic steatohepatitis. *J Clin Gastroenterol* 2004;38:801–4.

147. Younossi ZM, Gramlich T, Bacon B, et al. Hepatic iron and nonalcoholic fatty liver disease. *Hepatology* 1999;30:847–50.

148. Fracanzani AL, Valenti L, Bugianesi E, et al. Risk of severe liver disease in nonalcoholic fatty liver disease with normal aminotransferase levels: a role for insulin resistance and diabetes. *Hepatology* 2008;48:792–8.

149. Caldwell SH, Han K, Hess CE. Thrombocytopenia and unrecognized cirrhosis. *Ann Intern Med* 1997;127:572–3.

150. Nagore N, Scheuer PJ. Does a linear pattern of sinusoidal IgA deposition distinguish between alcoholic and diabetic liver disease? *Liver* 1988;8:281–6.

151. Wallace TM, Levy JC, Matthews DR. Use and abuse of HOMA modeling. *Diabetes Care* 2004;27:1487–95.

152. Perseghin G, Caumo A, Caloni M, Testolin G, Luzi L. Incorporation of the fasting plasma FFA concentration into QUICKI improves its association with insulin sensitivity in nonobese individuals. *J Clin Endocrinol Metab* 2001;86:4776–81.

153. Neuschwander-Tetri BA. Lifestyle modification as the primary treatment of NASH. *Clin Liver Dis* 2009;13:649–65.

154. Garg A. Acquired and inherited lipodystrophies. *N Engl J Med* 2004;350:1220–34.

155. Powell EE, Searle J, Mortimer R. Steatohepatitis associated with limb lipodystrophy. *Gastroenterology* 1989;97:1022–4.

156. Javor ED, Ghany MG, Cochran EK, et al. Leptin reverses nonalcoholic steatohepatitis in patients with severe lipodystrophy. *Hepatology* 2005;41:753–60.

157. Caldwell SH, Swerdlow RH, Khan EM, et al. Mitochondrial abnormalities in non-alcoholic steatohepatitis. *J Hepatol* 1999;31:430–4.

158. Sanyal AJ, Campbell-Sargent C, Mirshahi F, et al. Nonalcoholic steatohepatitis: association of insulin resistance and mitochondrial abnormalities. *Gastroenterology* 2001;120:1183–92.

159. Carrozzo R, Hirano M, Fromenty B, Casali C, Santorelli FM, Bonilla E. Multiple mtDNA deletions features in autosomal dominant and recessive diseases suggest distinct pathogeneses. *Neurology* 1998;50:99–106.

160. Feliciani C, Amerio P. Madelung's disease: inherited from an ancient Mediterranean population? *N Engl J Med* 1999;340:1481.

161. Guillausseau P-J, Massin P, Dubois-LaForgue D, et al. Maternally inherited diabetes and deafness: a multicenter study. *Ann Intern Med* 2001;134:721–8.

162. Bohan A, Droogan O, Nolan N, et al. Mitochondrial DNA abnormalities without significant deficiency of intramitochondrial fatty acid β-oxidation enzymes in a well-defined subgroup of patients with nonalcoholic steatohepatitis (NASH). *Hepatology* 2000;32 A387.

163. Al-Osaimi AM, Berg CL, Caldwell SH. Intermittent disconjugate gaze: a novel finding in nonalcoholic steatohepatitis and cryptogenic cirrhosis. *Hepatology* 2005;41:943.

164. Wasserman JM, Thung SN, Berman R, Bodenheimer HC, Sigal SH. Hepatic Weber–Christian disease. *Semin Liver Dis* 2001;21:115–18.

165. Amarapurkar DN, Patel ND, Amarapurkar AD. Panniculitis and liver disease (hepatic Weber Christian disease). *J Hepatol* 2005;42:146–52.

166. Siegelman ES, Rosen MA. Imaging of steatosis. *Semin Liver Dis* 2001;21:71–80.

167. Colli A, Fraquelli M, Andreoletti M, Marino B, Zuccoli E, Conte D. Severe liver fibrosis or cirrhosis: accuracy of US for detection – analysis of 300 cases. *Radiology* 2003;227:89–94.

168. Saadeh S, Younossi ZM, Remer EM, et al. The utility of radiological imaging in nonalcoholic fatty liver disease. *Gastroenterology* 2002;123:745–50.

169. Abate N, Burns D, Peshock RM, Garg A, Grandy SM. Estimation of adipose tissue mass by magnetic resonance imaging: validation against dissection in human cadavers. *J Lipid Res* 1994;35:1490–6.

170. Tornaghi G, Raiteri R, Pozzato C, et al. Anthropometric or ultrasonic measurements in assessment of visceral fat? A comparative study. *Int J Obesity* 1994;18:771–5.

171. Joesh AE, Saverymuttu SH, al-Sam S, Cook MG, Maxwell JD. Comparison of liver histology with ultrasonography in assessing diffuse parenchymal liver disease. *Clin Radiol* 1991;43:26–31.

172. Wong VW-C, Vergniol J, Wong GL-H, et al. Diagnosis of fibrosis and cirrhosis using liver stiffness measurement in non-alcoholic fatty liver disease. *Hepatology* 2010;51:454–62.

173. Jacobs JE, Birnbaum BA, Shapiro MA, et al. Diagnostic criteria for fatty infiltration of the liver on contrast-enhanced helical CT. *AJR Am J Roentgenol* 1998;171:659–64.

174. Alpern MB, Lawson TL, Foley DW, et al. Focal hepatic masses and fatty infiltration detected by enhanced dynamic CT. *Radiology* 1986;158:45–9.

175. Fishbein MH, Gardner KG, Potter CJ, Schmalbrock P, Smith MA. Introduction of fast MR imaging in the assessment of hepatic steatosis. *Magn Reson Imaging* 1997;15:287–93.

176. Browning JD. New imaging techniques for non-alcoholic steatohepatitis. *Clin Liver Dis* 2009;13:607–19.

177. Thomsen C, Becker U, Winkler K, Christoffersen P, Jensen M, Henriksen C. Quantification of liver fat using magnetic resonance spectroscopy. *Magn Reson Imaging* 1994;12:487–95.

178. Schlemmer H-P, Sawatzki T, Sammet S, et al. Hepatic phospholipids in alcoholic liver disease assessed by proton-decoupled 31P magnetic resonance spectroscopy. *J Hepatol* 2005;42:752–9.

179. Solga SF, Horska A, Clark JM, Diehl AM. Hepatic 31P magnetic resonance spectroscopy: a hepatologist's user guide. *Liver Int* 2005;25:490–500.

180. Yu AS, Keefe EB. Elevated AST or ALT in nonalcoholic fatty liver disease: accurate predictor of disease? *Am J Gastroenterol* 2003;98: 955–6.

181. Ryan MC, Best JD, Wilson AM, Jenkins AJ, Slavin J, Desmond PV. Associations between liver histology and severity of the metabolic syndrome in subjects with nonalcoholic fatty liver disease. *Diabetes Care* 2005;28:1222–4.

182. Shah AG, Lydecker A, Murray K, Tetri BN, Contos MJ, Sanyal AJ; Nash Clinical Research Network. Comparison of noninvasive markers of fibrosis in patients with nonalcoholic fatty liver disease. *Clin Gastroenterol Hepatol* 2009;7:1104–12.

183. Feldstein AE, Wieckowska A, Lopez AR, Liu YC, Zein NN, McCullough AJ. Cytokeratin-18 fragment levels as noninvasive biomarkers for nonalcoholic steatohepatitis: a multicenter validation study. *Hepatology* 2009;50:1072–8.

184. Younossi ZM, Page S, Rafiq N, et al. A biomarker panel for nonalcoholic steatohepatitis (NASH) and NASH-related fibrosis. *Obes Surg* 2011;21:431–9.

185. Albano E, Mottaran E, Vidali M, et al. Immune response towards lipid peroxidation products as a predictor of progression of non-alcoholic fatty liver disease to advanced fibrosis. *Gut* 2005;54: 987–93.

186. Pagadala M, Zein CO, McCullough AJ. Predictors of steatohepatitis and advanced fibrosis in non-alcoholic fatty liver disease. *Clin Liver Dis* 2009;13 591–606.

187. Rockey DC, Caldwell SH, Goodman ZD, Nelson RC, Smith AD; American Association for the Study of Liver Diseases. Liver biopsy. *Hepatology* 2009;49:1017–44.

188. Merrimar RB, Ferrell LD, Patti MG, et al. Correlation of paired liver biopsies in morbidly obese patients with suspected nonalcoholic fatty liver disease. *Hepatology* 2006;44:874–80.

189. Ratziu V, Charlotte F, Heurtier A, et al. LIDO Study Group. Sampling variability of liver biopsy in nonalcoholic fatty liver disease. *Gastroenterology* 2005;125:1898–906.

190. Promrat K, Lutchman G, Uwaifo GI, et al. A pilot study of pioglitazone treatment for NASH. *Hepatology* 2004;39:188–96.

191. Kleiner DE, Brunt EM, Van Natta ML, et al. Nonalcoholic Steatohepatitis Clinical Research Network. Design and validation of a histologic scoring system for NAFLD. *Hepatology* 2005;41:1313–21.

192. Gastaldelli A, Kozakova M, Højlund K, et al. RISC Investigators. Fatty liver is associated with insulin resistance, risk of coronary

heart disease, and early atherosclerosis in a large European population. *Hepatology* 2009;49:1537–44.

193. Dunn W, Xu R, Wingard DL, et al. Suspected nonalcoholic fatty liver disease and mortality risk in a population-based cohort study. *Am J Gastroenterol* 2008;103:2263–71.

194. Ionnou GN, Weiss NS, Kowdley KV, Dominitz JA. Is obesity a risk factor for cirrhosis-related death or hospitalization? A population-based cohort study. *Gastroenterology* 2003;125:1053–9.

195. de Marco R, Locatelli F, Zoppini G, Verlato G, Bonora E, Muggeo M. Cause-specific mortality in type 2 diabetes. The Verona Diabetes Study. *Diabetes Care* 1999;22:756–61.

196. Sasaki A, Horiuchi N, Hasegawa K, Uehara M. Mortality and causes of death in type 2 diabetic patients. *Diabetes Res Clin Pract* 1989;7:33–40.

197. Caldwell S, Argo C. The natural history of non-alcoholic fatty liver disease. *Dig Dis* 2010;28:162–8.

198. Matteoni CA, Younossi ZM, Gramlich T, Boparai N, Liu YC, McCullough AJ. Nonalcoholic fatty liver disease: a spectrum of clinical and pathological severity. *Gastroenterology* 1999;116:1413–19.

199. Hilden M, Juhl E, Thomsen AC, Christoffersen P. Fatty liver persisting for up to 33 years. *Acta Med Scand* 1973;194:485–9.

200. Dixon JB, Bhathal PS, O'Brien PE. Nonalcoholic fatty liver disease: predictors of nonalcoholic steatohepatitis and liver fibrosis in the severely obese. *Gastroenterology* 2001;121:91–100.

201. Ong JP, Elariny H, Collantes R, et al. Predictors of nonalcoholic steatohepatitis and advanced fibrosis in morbidly obese patients. *Obes Surg* 2005;15:310–15.

202. Garcia-Monzon C, Martin-Perez E, Iacono OL, et al. Characterization of pathogenic and prognostic factors of nonalcoholic steatohepatitis associated with obesity. *J Hepatol* 2000;33:716–24.

203. Ekstedt M, Franzen LE, Mathiesen UL, et al. Long-term follow-up of patients with NAFLD and elevated liver enzymes. *Hepatology* 2006;44:865–73.

204. Lee RG. Nonalcoholic steatohepatitis: a study of 49 patients. *Hum Pathol* 1989;20:594–8.

205. Harrison SA, Torgerson S, Hayashi PH. The natural history of non-alcoholic fatty liver disease: a clinical histopathological study. *Am J Gastroenterol* 2003;98:2042–7.

206. Fassio E, Alvarez E, Dominguez N, Landeria G, Longo C. Natural history of nonalcoholic steatohepatitis: a longitudinal study of repeat liver biopsies. *Hepatology* 2004;40:820–6.

207. Adams LA, Sanderson S, Lindor KD, Angulo P. The histological course of nonalcoholic fatty liver disease: a longitudinal study of 103 patients with sequential liver biopsies. *J Hepatol* 2005;42:132–8.

208. Argo CK, Northup PG, Al-Osaimi AM, Caldwell SH. Systematic review of risk factors for fibrosis progression in non-alcoholic steatohepatitis. *J Hepatol* 2009;51:371–9.

209. Adams LA, Lymp JF, St Sauver J, et al. The natural history of non-alcoholic fatty liver disease: a population-based cohort study. *Gastroenterology* 2005;129:113–21.

210. Ekstedt M, Franzen LE, Mathiesen UL, et al. Long-term follow-up of patients with NAFLD and elevated liver enzymes. *Hepatology* 2006;44:865–73.

211. Ong JP, Pitts A, Younossi ZM. Increased overall mortality and liver-related mortality in non-alcoholic fatty liver disease. *J Hepatol* 2008;49:608–12.

212. Rafiq N, Bai C, Fang Y, et al. Long-term follow-up of patients with nonalcoholic fatty liver. *Clin Gastroenterol Hepatol* 2009;7:234–8.

213. Hui JM, Kench JG, Chitturi S, et al. Long-term outcomes of cirrhosis in nonalcoholic steatohepatitis compared with hepatitis C. *Hepatology* 2003;38:420–7.

214. Sanyal AJ, Banas C, Sargeant C, et al. Similarities and differences in outcomes of cirrhosis due to nonalcoholic steatohepatitis and hepatitis C. *Hepatology* 2006;43:682–9.

215. Malik SM, Devera ME, Fontes P, Shaikh O, Sasatomi E, Ahmad J. Recurrent disease following liver transplantation for nonalcoholic steatohepatitis cirrhosis. *Liver Transpl* 2009;15:1843–51.

216. Nair S, Mason A, Eason J, Loss G, Perrillo RP. Is obesity an independent risk factor for hepatocellular carcinoma in cirrhosis? *Hepatology* 2002;36:150–5.

217. El-Serag HB, Richardson PA, Everhart JE. The role of diabetes in hepatocellular carcinoma: a case–control study among United States veterans. *Am J Gastroenterol* 2001;96:2462–7.

218. Cotrim HP, Parana R, Braga E, Lyra L. Nonalcoholic steatohepatitis and hepatocellular cancer: natural history? *Am J Gastroenterol* 2000;95:3018–19.

219. Shimada M, Hashimoto E, Taniai M, et al. Hepatocellular carcinoma in patients with nonalcoholic steatohepatitis. *J Hepatol* 2002;37:154–60.

220. Yatsuji S, Hashimoto E, Tobari M, Taniai M, Tokushige K, Shiratori K. Clinical features and outcomes of cirrhosis due to non-alcoholic steatohepatitis compared with cirrhosis caused by chronic hepatitis C. *J Gastroenterol Hepatol* 2009;24:248–54.

221. Giannini EG, Marabotto E, Savarino V, et al. Hepatocellular carcinoma in patients with cryptogenic cirrhosis. *Clin Gastroenterol Hepatol* 2009;7:580–5.

222. Ratzui V, Bonyhay L, Di Martino V, et al. Survival, liver failure, and hepatocellular carcinoma in obesity-related cryptogenic cirrhosis. *Hepatology* 2002;35:1485–93.

223. Kawada N, Imanaka K, Kawaguchi T, et al. Hepatocellular cancer arising from non-cirrhotic alcoholic steatohepatitis. *J Gastroenterol* 2009;44:1190–4.

224. Paradis V, Zalinski S, Chelbi E, et al. hepatocellular carcinomas in patients with metabolic syndrome often develop without significant fibrosis: a pathological analysis. *Hepatology* 2009;49:851–9.

225. Roskams T, Yang SQ, Koteish A, et al. Oxidative stress and oval cell accumulation in mice and humans with alcoholic and nonalcoholic fatty liver disease. *Am J Pathol* 2003;163:1301–11.

226. Farrell GC. Animal models of steatohepatitis. In: Farrell GC, George J, Hall P, McCullough AJ, eds. *Fatty Liver Disease; NASH and Related Disorders.* Malden, MA: Blackwell Publishing: 2005:91.

227. Rinella ME, Green RM. The methionine-choline deficient dietary model of steatohepatitis does not exhibit insulin resistance. *J Hepatol* 2004;40:47–51.

228. de Lima VM, Oliveira CP, Alves VA, et al. A rodent model of NASH with cirrhosis, oval cell proliferation and hepatocellular carcinoma. *J Hepatol* 2008;49:1055–61.

229. Tetri LH, Basaranoglu M, Brunt EM, Yerian LM, Neuschwander-Tetri BA. Severe NAFLD with hepatic necroinflammatory changes in mice fed trans fats and a high-fructose corn syrup equivalent. *Am J Physiol Gastrointest Liver Physiol* 2008;295:G987–95.

230. Hölttä-Vuori M, Salo VT, Nyberg L, et al. Zebrafish: gaining popularity in lipid research. *Biochem J* 2010;429:235–42.

231. Nakagawa H, Oikawa S, Oohashi T, Katoh N. Decreased serum lecithin:cholesterol acyltransferase in spontaneous cases of fatty liver in cows. *Vet Res Commun* 1997;21:1–8.

232. Lee L, Alloosh M, Saxena R, et al. Nutritional model of steatohepatitis and metabolic syndrome in the Ossabaw miniature swine. *Hepatology* 2009;50:56–67.

233. Center SA, Guida L, Zanelli MJ, Dougherty E, Cummings J, King J. Ultrastructural hepatocellular features associated with severe hepatic lipidosis in cats. *Am J Vet Res* 1993;54:724–31.

234. Zomborszky Z, Husveth F. Liver total lipids and fatty acid composition of shot red and fallow deer males in various reproduction periods. *Comp Biochem Phys A* 2000;126:107–14.

235. Pelsers MM, Butler PJ, Bishop CM, Glatz JFC. Fatty acid binding protein in heart and skeletal muscles of the migratory barnacle goose throughout development. *Am J Physiol* 1999;276:R637–43.

236. Schlosberg A, Elkin N, Malkinson M, et al. Severe hepatopathy in geese and broilers associated with ochratoxin in their feed. *Mycopathologia* 1997;138:71–6.

237. Hermier D, Saadoun A, Salichon M-R, Sellier N, Rousselot-Paillet D, Chapman MJ. Plasma lipoproteins and liver lipids in two breeds of geese with different susceptibility to hepatic steatosis: changes induced by development and forced-feeding. *Lipids* 1991;26 331–9.

238. Mourot J, Guy G, Lagarrigue S, Peiniau P, Hermier D. Role of hepatic lipogenesis in the susceptibility to fatty liver in the goose (Anser anser). *Comp Biochem Phys B* 2000;126:81–7.

239. Caldwell SH, Ikura Y, Iezzoni JC, Liu Z. Has natural selection in human populations produced two types of metabolic syndrome (with and without fatty liver)? *J Gastroenterol Hepatol* 2007; 22(Suppl 1):S11–19.

240. Unger RH. Lipotoxic diseases. *Ann Rev Med* 2002;53:319–36.

241. Day CP, James OFW. Steatohepatitis: a tale of two hits. *Gastroenterology* 1998;114:842–5.

242. Wanless IR, Shiota K. The pathogenesis of nonalcoholic steatohepatitis and other fatty liver diseases: a four-step model including the role of lipid release and hepatic venular obstruction in the progression to cirrhosis. *Semin Liv Dis* 2004;24:99–106.

243. Leevy CM. Fatty liver: a study of 270 patients with biopsy proven fatty liver and a review of the literature. *Medicine* 1962;41: 249–76.

244. Diraison F, Moulin P, Beylot M. Contribution of hepatic de novo lipogenesis and reesterification of plasma non esterified fatty acids to plasma triglyceride synthesis during non-alcoholic fatty liver disease. *Diabetes Metab* 2003;29:478–85.

245. Mavrelis PG, Ammon HV, Gleysteen JJ, Komorowski RA, Charaf UK. Hepatic free fatty acids in alcoholic liver disease and morbid obesity. *Hepatology* 1983;2:226–31.

246. Bass NM, Merriman RB. Fatty acid metabolism and lipotoxicity in the pathogenesis of NAFLD/NASH. In: Farrell GC, George J, Hall P, McCullough AJ, eds. *Fatty Liver Disease; NASH and Related Disorders.* Malden, MA: Blackwell Publishing, 2005:109–22.

247. Li Z, Oben JA, Yang S, et al. Norepinephrine regulates hepatic innate immune system in leptin-deficient mice with nonalcoholic steatohepatitis. *Hepatology* 2004;40:434–41.

248. Romijn JA, Fliers E. Sympathetic and parasympathetic innervation of adipose tissue: metabolic implications. *Curr Opin Clin Nutr* 2005;8:440–4.

249. Browning JD, Horton JD. Molecular mediators of hepatic steatosis. *J Clin Invest* 2004;114:147–52.

250. Tamura S, Shimomura I. Contribution of adipose tissue and de novo lipogenesis to nonalcoholic fatty liver diseases. *J Clin Invest* 2005;115:1139–42.

251. Brown MS, Goldstein JL. The SREBP pathway: regulation of cholesterol metabolism by proteolysis of a membrane-bound transcription factor. *Cell* 1997;89:331–40.

252. Harvey RA, Champe PC. Lippincott's Illustrated Review: *Biochemistry*, 3rd edn. Philadelphia, PA: Lippincott Williams and Wilkins, 2005.

253. Donnelly KL, Smith CI, Schwarzenberg SJ, Jessurun J, Boldt MD, Parks EJ. Sources of fatty acids in liver and secreted via lipoproteins in patients with nonalcoholic fatty liver disease. *J Clin Invest* 2005;115:1343–51.

254. Debois D, Bralet M-P, Le Naour F, Brunelle A, Laprevote O. In situ lipidomic analysis of nonalcoholic fatty liver by cluster TOF-SIMS imaging. *Anal Chem* 2009;81:2823–31.

255. Cheng J, Fujita A, Ohsaki Y, Suzuki M, Shinohara Y, Fujimoto T. Quantitative electron microscopy shows uniform incorporation of triglycerides into existing lipid droplets. *Histochem Cell Biol* 2009;132:281–91.

256. Villanueva CJ, Monetti M, Shih M, et al. Specific role for acyl coA:diacylglycerol acyltransferase 1 (Dgat1) in hepatic steatosis due to exogenous fatty acids. *Hepatology* 2009;50:434–42.

257. Puri P, Baillie RA, Wiest MM, et al. A lipidomic analysis of nonalcoholic fatty liver disease. *Hepatology* 2007;46:1081–90.

258. Kolak M, Westerbacka J, Velagapudi VR, et al. Adipose tissue inflammation and increased ceramide content characterize subjects with high liver fat content independent of obesity. *Diabetes* 2007;56: 1960–8.

259. Bradbury MW, Berk PD. Lipid metabolism in hepatic steatosis. *Clin Liver Dis* 2004;8:639–71.

260. Charlton M, Sreekumar R, Rasmussen D, Lindor K, Nair KS. Apolipoprotein synthesis in nonalcoholic steatohepatitis. *Hepatology* 2002;35:898–904.

261. Fabbrini E, Mohammed BS, Magkos F, Korenblat KM, Patterson BW, Klein S. Alterations in adipose tissue and hepatic lipid kinetics in obese men and women with nonalcoholic fatty liver disease. *Gastroenterology* 2008;134:424–31.

262. Koruk M, Sava MC, Yilmer O, et al. Serum lipids, lipoproteins and apolipoprotein levels in patients with nonalcoholic steatohepatitis. *J Clin Gastroenterol* 2003;37:177–82.

263. Musso G, Gambino R, De Michieli F, Biroli G, Fagà E, Pagano G, Cassader M. Association of liver disease with postprandial large intestinal triglyceride-rich lipoprotein accumulation and pro/antioxidant imbalance in normolipidemic non-alcoholic steatohepatitis. *Ann Med* 2008;40:383–94.

264. Seki S, Kitada T, Sakaguchi H, Nakatani K, Wakasa K. In situ detection of lipid peroxidation and oxidative DNA damage in nonalcoholic fatty liver disease. *J Hepatol* 2002;37:56–62.

265. Ikura Y, Ohsawa M, Suekane T, et al. Localization of oxidized phosphatidyl-choline in nonalcoholic fatty liver disease: impact on disease progression. *Hepatology* 2006;43:506–14.

266. Garcia-Monzon C, Martin-Perez E, Lo Iacono O, et al. Characterization of pathogenic and prognostic factors of nonalcoholic steatohepatitis associated with obesity. *J Hepatol* 2000;33:716–24.

267. Malaguarnera L, Madeddu R, Palio E, Arena N, Malaguarnera M. Heme oxygenase-1 levels and oxidative stress-related parameters in non-alcoholic fatty liver disease patients. *J Hepatol* 2005;2: 585–91.

268. Puri P, Wiest MM. Cheung O, et al. The plasma lipidomic signature of nonalcoholic steatohepatitis. *Hepatology* 2009;50:1827–38.

269. Recknagle RO, Glende EA, Britton RS. Free radical damage and lipid peroxidation. In: Meeks RG, Harrison SD, Bull RJ, eds. *Hepatotoxicology.* Boca Raton, FL: CRC Press, 1991:401–36.

270. Tribble DL, Aw TY, Jones DP. The pathophysiological significance of lipid peroxidation in oxidative cell injury. Hepatology 1987;7:377–87.

271. Recknagle RO, Glende EA, Britton RS. Free radical damage and lipid peroxidation. In: Meeks RG, Harrison SD, Bull RJ, eds. *Hepatotoxicology.* Boca Raton, FL: CRC Press, 1991:401–36.

272. Hruszkewycz AM. Evidence for mitochondrial DNA damage by lipid peroxidation. *Biochem Bioph Res Co* 1988;153:191–7.

273. Bell M, Wang H, Chen H, et al. Consequences of lipid droplet coat protein down regulation in liver cells: abnormal lipid droplet metabolism and induction of insulin resistance. *Diabetes* 2008;57: 2037–45.

274. Puri V, Ranjit S, Konda S, et al. Cidea is associated with lipid droplets and insulin sensitivity in humans. *Proc Natl Acad Sci USA* 2008;105:7833–8.

275. Caldwell S, Ikura Y, Dias D, et al. Hepatocellular ballooning in NASH. *J Hepatol* 2010;53:719–23.

276. Tauchi-Sato K, Ozeki S, Houjou T, Taguchi R, Fujimoto T. The surface of lipid droplets is a phospholipid monolayer with a unique fatty acid composition. *J Biol Chem* 2002;277:44507–12.

277. Ohsaki Y, Chen J, Suzuki M, et al. Biogenesis of cytoplasmic lipid droplets: from the lipid ester globule in the membrane to visible structure. *Biochem Biophys Acta* 2009;1791:399–407.

278. Straub BK, Stoeffel P, Heid H, Zimbelmann R, Schirmacher P. Differential pattern of lipid droplet-associated proteins and de novo perilipin expression in hepatocyte steatogenesis. *Hepatology* 2008;47:1936–46.

279. Imai Y, Varela GM, Jackson MB, Graham MJ, Crooke RM, Ahima RS. Reduction of hepatosteatosis and lipid levels by an adipose differentiation-related protein antisense oligonucleotide. *Gastroenterology* 2007;132:1947–54.

280. Bickel PE, Tansey JT, Welte MA. PAT proteins, an ancient family of lipid droplet proteins that regulate cellular lipid stores. *Biochem Biophys Acta* 2009;1791:419–40.

281. Puri V, Ranjit S, Konda S, et al. Cidea is associated with lipid droplets and insulin sensitivity in humans. *Proc Natl Acad Sci USA* 2008: 105; 7833–8.

282. Welte MA, Cermelli S, Griner J, et al. Regulation of lipid-droplet transport by the perilipin homolog LSD2. *Curr Biol* 2005;15:1266–75.

283. Robenek H, Robenek MJ, Troyer D. PAT family proteins pervade lipid droplet cores. *J Lipid Res* 2005;46:1331–8.

284. Fujii H, Ikura Y, Arimoto J, et al. Expression of perilipin and adipophilin in nonalcoholic fatty liver disease: relevance to oxidative injury and hepatocyte ballooning. *J Athero Thromb* 2009;16:893–901.

285. Cairns SR, Peters TJ. Micromethods for quantitative lipid analysis of human liver needle biopsy specimens. *Clin Chim Acta* 1983;127:373–82.

286. Cairns SR, Peters TJ. Isolation of micro- and macro-droplet fractions from needle biopsy specimens of human liver and determination of the subcellular distribution of the accumulating liver lipids in alcoholic fatty liver. *Clin Sci* 1984;67:337–45.

287. Singh R, Kaushik S, Wang Y, et al. Autophagy regulates lipid metabolism. *Nature* 2009;458:1131–5.

288. Ohsaki Y, Cheng J, Suzuki M, Fujita A, Fujimoto T. Lipid droplets are arrested in the ER membrane by tight binding of lipidated apolipoprotein B-100. *J Cell Sci* 2008;121:2415–22.

289. Joshi-Barve S, Barve SS, Amancherla K, et al. Palmitic acid induces production of proinflammatory cytokine interleukin-8 from hepatocytes. *Hepatology* 2007;46:823–30.

290. Puri P, Mirshahi F, Cheung O, et al. Activation and dysregulation of the unfolded protein response in nonalcoholic fatty liver disease. *Gastroenterology* 2008;134:568–76.

291. Fujita K, Nozaki Y, Wada K, et al. Dysfunctional very-low-density lipoprotein synthesis and release is a key factor in nonalcoholic steatohepatitis pathogenesis. *Hepatology* 2009;50:772–80.

292. Su Q, Tsai J, Xu E, et al. Apolipoprotein B100 acts as a molecular link between lipid-induced endoplasmic reticulum stress and hepatic insulin resistance. *Hepatology* 2009;50:77–84.

293. Singh R, Wang R, Schattenberg JM, Xiang Y, Czaja MJ. Chronic oxidative stress sensitizes hepatocytes to death from hydroxynonenal by JNK/c-Jun overactivation. *Am J Physiol Gastrointest Liver Physiol* 2009;297:G907–17.

294. Dianzani MU. Uncoupling of oxidative phosphorylation in mitochondria from fatty livers. *Biochem Biophys Acta* 1954;14:514–32.

295. Cortez-Pinto H, Chatham J, Chacko VP, Arnold C, Rashid A, Diehl AM. Alterations in liver ATP homeostasis in human nonalcoholic steatohepatitis: a pilot study. *JAMA* 1999;282:1659–64.

296. Caldwell SH, Chang CY, Nakamoto RK, Krugner-Higby L. Mitochondria in nonalcoholic fatty liver disease. *Clin Liver Dis* 2004;8:595–618.

297. Vendemiale G, Grattagliano I, Caraceni P, et al. Mitochondrial oxidative injury and energy metabolism alteration in rat fatty liver: effect of the nutritional status. *Hepatology* 2001;33:808–15.

298. Caldwell SH, de Freitas LA, Park SH, et al. Intramitochondrial crystalline inclusions in nonalcoholic steatohepatitis. *Hepatology* 2009;49:1888–95.

299. Perez-Carrera M, Del Hoyo P, Martin MA, et al. Defective hepatic mitochondrial respiratory chain in patients with nonalcoholic steatohepatitis. *Hepatology* 2003;38:999–1007.

300. Diehl AM, Hoek JB. Mitochondrial uncoupling: role of uncoupling protein anion carriers and relationship to thermogenesis and weight control "the benefits of losing control". *J Bioenerg Biomembr* 1999;31:493–506.

301. Selzner M, Rudiger HA, Sindram D, Madden J, Clavien P-A. Mechanisms of ischemic injury are different in the steatotic and normal rat liver. *Hepatology* 2000;32:1280–8.

302. Marsman WA, Weisner RH, Rodriguez L, et al. Use of fatty donor liver is associated with diminished early patients and graft survival. *Transplantation* 1996;62:1246–51.

303. Schneider ARJ, Kraut C, Lindenthal B, Braden B, Caspary WF, Stein, J. Total body metabolism of 13C-octanoic acid is preserved in patients with non-alcoholic steatohepatitis, but differs between women and men. *Euro J Gastroenterol Hepatol* 2005;17:1181–4.

304. Iozzo P, Bucci M, Roivainen A, et al. Fatty acid metabolism in the liver, measured by positron emission tomography, is increased in obese individuals. *Gastroenterology* 2010;139:846–56.

305. Caballero F, Fernández A, De Lacy AM, Fernández-Checa JC, Caballería J, García-Ruiz C. Enhanced free cholesterol, SREBP-2 and StAR expression in human NASH. *J Hepatol* 2009;50:789–96.

306. Lemasters JJ. Dying a thousand deaths: redundant pathways from different organelles to apoptosis and necrosis. *Gastroenterology* 2005;129:351–60.

307. Charlton M, Viker K, Krishnan A, et al. Differential expression of lumican and fatty acid binding protein-1: new insights into the histologic spectrum of nonalcoholic fatty liver disease. *Hepatology* 2009;49:1375–84.

308. Feldstein AE, Canby A, Angulo P, et al. Hepatocyte apoptosis and FAS expression are prominent features of human nonalcoholic steatohepatitis. *Gastroenterology* 2003;125:437–43.

309. Ramalho RM, Cortez-Pinto H, Castro RE, et al. Apoptosis and Bcl-2 expression in the livers of patients with steatohepatitis. *Eur J Gastroenterol Hepatol* 2006;18:21–9.

310. Li Z, Berk M, McIntyre TM, Gores GJ, Feldstein AE. The lysosomal-mitochondrial axis in free fatty acid-induced hepatic lipotoxicity. *Hepatology* 2008;47:1495–503.

311. Amidi F, French BA, Chung D, Halsted CH, Medici V, French SW. M-30 and 4HNE are sequestered in different aggresomes in the same hepatocytes. *Exp Mol Pathol* 2007;83:296–300.

312. Feldstein AE, Wieckowska A, Lopez AR, Liu YC, Zein NN, McCullough AJ. Cytokeratin-18 fragment levels as noninvasive biomarkers for nonalcoholic steatohepatitis: a multicenter validation study. *Hepatology* 2009;50:1072–8.

313. Friedman SL. Hepatic stellate cells: protean, multifunctional, and enigmatic cells of the liver. *Physiol Rev* 2008;88:125–72.

314. Watanabe A, Hashmi A, Gomes DA, et al. Apoptotic hepatocyte DNA inhibits hepatic stellate cell chemotaxis via toll-like receptor 9. *Hepatology* 2007;46:1509–18.

315. Richardson MM, Jonsson JR, Powell EE, et al. Progressive fibrosis in nonalcoholic steatohepatitis: association with altered regeneration and a ductular reaction. *Gastroenterology* 2007;133:80–90.

316. Weltman MD, Farrell GC, Hall P, Ingelman-Sundberg M, Liddle C. Hepatic cytochrome P450 2E1 is increased in patients with nonalcoholic steatohepatitis. *Hepatology* 1998;27:128–33.

317. Niemela O, Parkkila S, Juvonen RO, Viitala K, Gelboin HV, Pasanen M. Cyotchromes P450 2 A6, 2 E1, and 3A and production of protein–aldehyde adducts in the liver patients with alcoholic and non-alcoholic liver disease. *J Hepatol* 2000;33:893–901.

318. Schattenberg JM, Wang Y, Rigoli RM, Koop DR, Czaja MJ. CYP2E1 over expression alters hepatocyte death from mendione and fatty acids by activation of ERK1/2 signaling. *Hepatology* 2004;39:444–55.

319. Rao MS, Reddy JK. Peroxisomal beta oxidation and steatohepatitis. *Semin Liver Dis* 2001;21:43–55.

320. De Craemer D, Pauwels M, Van den Branden C. Alterations of peroxisomes in steatosis of the human liver: a quantitative study *Hepatology* 1995;22:744–52.

321. Yeh MM, Brunt EM. Pathology of nonalcoholic fatty liver disease. *Am J Clin Pathol* 2007;128:837–47.

322. Contos MJ, Choudhury J, Mills AS, Sanyal AJ. The histological spectrum of nonalcoholic fatty liver disease. *Clin Liver Dis* 2004; 8:481–500.

323. Younossi ZM, Gramlich T, Liu YC, et al. Nonalcoholic fatty liver disease: assessment of variability in pathological interpretations. *Mod Pathol* 1998;11:560–5.

324. Arias IM. The hepatocyte organization. In: Arias IM, Jacoby WB, Popper H, Schachter D, Shafritz DA, eds. *The Liver: Biology and Pathobiology*, 2nd edn. New York: Raven Press, 1988:9.

325. Brunt EM, Neuschwander-Tetri BA, Oliver D, Wehmeier KR, Eacon BR. Nonalcoholic steatohepatitis: histologic features and clinical correlations with 30 blinded biopsy specimens. *Hum Pathol* 2004;35:1070–82.

326. Zatloukal K, French SW, Stumptner C, et al. From Mallory to Mallory–Denk bodies: what, how and why? *Exp Cell Res* 2007;313: 2033–49.

327. Lackner C, Gogg-Kamerer M, Zatloukal K, Stumptner C, Brunt EM, Denk H. Ballooned hepatocytes in steatohepatitis: the value of keratin immunohistochemistry for diagnosis. *J Hepatol* 2008;48: 821–8.

328. Amidi F, French BA, Chung D, Halsted CH, Medici V, French SW. M-30 and 4HNE are sequestered in different aggresomes in the same hepatocytes. *Exp Mol Pathol* 2007;83:296–300.

329. Tao GZ, Looi KS, Toivola DM, et al. Keratins modulate the shape and function of hepatocyte mitochondria: a mechanism for protection from apoptosis. *J Cell Sci* 2009;122:3851–5.

330. Taylor R. Causation of type 2 diabetes: The Gordian knot unravels. *N Engl J Med* 2004;350:639–41.

331. Roden M, Price TB, Perseghin G, et al. Mechanism of free fatty acid-induced insulin resistance in humans. *J Clin Invest* 1996;97:2859–65.

332. Korenblat KM, Fabbrini E, Mohammed BS, Klein S. Liver, muscle, and adipose tissue insulin action is directly related to intrahepatic triglyceride content in obese subjects. *Gastroenterology* 2008;134:1369–75.

333. Hotamisligil GS. Inflammation and endoplasmic reticulum stress in obesity and diabetes. *Int J Obes* 2008;32:S52–4.

334. Kintscher U, Hartge M, Hess K, et al. T-lymphocyte infiltration in visceral adipose tissue: a primary event in adipose tissue inflammation and the development of obesity-mediated insulin resistance. *Arterioscler Thromb Vasc Biol* 2008;28:1304–10.

335. Farrell GC. Signaling links in the liver: knitting SOCS with fat and inflammation. *J Hepatol* 2005;43:193–6.

336. Goldfine AB, Kahn CR. Adiponectin: Linking the fat cell to insulin sensitivity. *Lancet* 2003;362:1431–2.

337. Maeda K, Okubo K, Shimomura I, Funahashi T, Matsuzawa Y, Matsubara K. cDNA cloning and expression of a novel adipose specific collagen-like factor, apM1 (AdiPose Most abundant gene transcript 1). *Biochem Bioph Res Co* 1996;221:286–96.

338. Yamauchi T, Kamon J, Minokoshi Y, et al. Adiponectin stimulates glucose utilization and fatty-acid oxidation by activating AMP-activated protein kinase. *Nat Med* 2002;8:1288–95.

339. Cao H, Gerhold K, Mayers JR, Wiest MM, Watkins SM, Hotamisligil GS. Identification of a lipokine, a lipid hormone linking adipose tissue to systemic metabolism. *Cell* 2008;134:933–44.

340. Wigg AJ, Roberts-Thomson IC, Dymock RB, McCarthy PJ, Grose RH, Cummins AG. The role of small intestinal bacterial overgrowth, intestinal permeability, endotoxaemia, and tumour necrosis factor alpha in the pathogenesis of non-alcoholic steatohepatitis. *Gut* 2001;48:206–11.

341. Miele L, Valenza V, La Torre G, et al. Increased intestinal permeability and tight junction alterations in nonalcoholic fatty liver disease. *Hepatology* 2009;49:1877–87.

342. Bardella MT, Valenti L, Pagliari C, et al. Searching for coeliac disease in patients with non-alcoholic fatty liver disease. *Dig Liv Dis* 2004; 36:333–6.

343. Sharpe RM, Drake AJ. Bisphenol a and metabolic syndrome. *Endocrinology* 2010;151:2404–7.

344. van Marken Lichtenbelt WD, Vanhommerig JW, Smulders NM, et al. Cold-activated brown adipose tissue in healthy men. *N Engl J Med* 2009;360:1500–8.

345. Li Z, Oben JA, Yang S, et al. Norepinephrine regulates hepatic innate immune system in leptin-deficient mice with nonalcoholic steatohepatitis. *Hepatology* 2004;40:434–41.

346. Peters RL, Gay T, Reynolds TB. Post-jejunoileal bypass hepatic injury. Its similarity to alcoholic liver disease. *Am J Clin Pathol* 1975; 63:318–31.

347. Babany G, Uzzan F, Larrey D, et al. Alcohol-like liver lesions induced by nifedipine. *J Hepatol* 1989;9:252–5.

348. Chitturi S, Farrell GC. Etiopathogenesis of nonalcoholic steatohepatitis. *Semin Liver Dis* 2001;21:27–41.

349. Oien KA, Moffat D, Curry GW, et al. Cirrhosis with steatohepatitis after adjuvant tamoxifen. *Lancet* 1999;353:36–7.

350. Cotrim HP, Salles BR, Almeida CE, et al. Anabolic-androgenic steroids: a possible new risk factor of toxicant-associated fatty liver disease. *Liver Int* 2011;31:348–53.

351. Lewis JH, Mullick F, Ishak KG, et al. Histopathological analysis of suspected amiodarone hepatotoxicity. *Hum Pathol* 1990;21:59–67.

352. Gan SK, Samaras K, Thompson CH, et al. Altered myocellular and abdominal fat partitioning predict disturbance in insulin action in HIV protease inhibitor-related lipodystrophy. *Diabetes* 2002; 51:3163–9.

353. Zorzi D, Laurent A, Pawlik TM, Lauwers GY, Vauthey JN, Abdalla EK. Chemotherapy-associated hepatotoxicity and surgery for colorectal liver metastases. *Br J Surg* 2007;94:274–86.

354. Baker AL, Rosenberg IH. Hepatic complications of total parenteral nutrition. *Am J Med* 1987;82:489–97.

355. Cavicchi M, Beau P, Crenn P, Degott C, Messing B. Prevalence of liver disease and contributing factors in patients receiving home parenteral nutrition for permanent intestinal failure. *Ann Intern Med* 2000;132:525–32.

356. Kaminski DL, Adams A, Jellinek M. The effect of hyperalimentation on hepatic lipid content and lipogenic enzyme activity in rats and man. *Surgery* 1980;88:93–100.

357. Quigley EM, Zetterman RK. Hepatobiliary compliactions of malabsorption and malnutrition. *Semin Liver Dis* 1988;8:218–28.

358. Bardella MT, Valenti L, Pagliari C, et al. Searching for coeliac disease in patients with non-alcoholic fatty liver disease. *Dig Liv Dis* 2004;36:333–6.

359. Cullen JM, Ruebner BH. Histopathologic classification of chemical-induced injury of the liver. In: Meeks RG, Harrison SD, Bull RJ, eds. *Hepatotoxicology.* Boca Raton, FL: CRC Press, 1991:67–92.

360. Cotrim HP, Carvalho F, Siqueira AC, Lordelo M, Rocha R, De Freitas LA. Nonalcoholic fatty liver and insulin resistance among petrochemical workers. *JAMA* 2005;294:1618–20.

361. Cave M, Falkner KC, Ray M, et al. Toxicant-associated steatohepatitis in vinyl chloride workers. *Hepatology* 2010;51:474–81.

362. Scheinberg IH, Sternlieb I. Wilson disease and idiopathic copper toxicosis. *Am J Clin Nutr* 1996;63:S842–5.

363. Thomas GR, Forbes JR, Roberts EA, Walshe JM, Cox DW. The Wilson disease gene: spectrum of mutations and their consequences. *Nat Genet* 1995;9:210–17.

364. Tarugi P, Lonardo A, Ballarini G, et al. Fatty liver in heterozygous hypobetalipoproteinemia caused by a novel truncated form of apolipoprotein B. *Gastroenterology* 1996;111:1125–33.

365. Lonardo A, Tarugi P, Ballarini G, Bagni A. Familial heterozygous hypobetalipoproteinemia, extrahepatic primary malignancy and hepatocellular carcinoma. A case report. *Dig Dis Sci* 1998;43:2489–92.

366. Burt AD, Mutton A, Day CP. Diagnosis and interpretation of steatosis and steatohepatitis. *Semin Diagn Pathol* 1998;15:246–58.

367. Ioannou GN, Weiss NS, Kowdley KV, Dominitz JA. Is obesity a risk factor for cirrhosis-related death or hospitalization? A population based cohort study. *Gastroenterology* 2003;125:1053–9.

368. Suzuki A, Lindor K, St Saver J, et al. Effect of changes on body weight and lifestyle in nonalcoholic fatty liver disease. *J Hepatol* 2005;43:1060–6.

369. Clark JM, Brancati FL. Negative trials in nonalcoholic steatohepatitis: why they happen and what they teach us. *Hepatology* 2004;39:602–3.

370. Musso G, Gambino R, Cassader M, Pagano G. A meta-analysis of randomized trials for the treatment of nonalcoholic fatty liver disease. *Hepatology* 2010;52:79–104.

371. Feldstein AE, Papouchado BG, Angulo P, Sanderson S, Adams L, Gores GJ. Hepatic stellate cells and fibrosis progression in patients with nonalcoholic fatty liver disease. *Clin Gastroenterol Hepatol* 2005;3:384–9.

372. Tuomilehto J, Lindstrom J, Eriksson JG, et al. Prevention of type 2 diabetes mellitus by changes in lifestyle among subject with impaired glucose tolerance. *N Engl J Med* 2001;344:1343–50.

373. McTigue KM, Harris R, Hemphill B, et al. Screening and interventions for obesity in adults: summary of evidence for the US preventive services task force. *Ann Intern Med* 2003;139:933–49.

374. American Diabetes Association. Evidence-based nutrition principles and recommendations for the treatment and prevention of diabetes and related complications. *Diabetes Care* 2002;25:S50–60.

375. Kantartzis K, Thamer C, Peter A, et al. High cardiorespiratory fitness is an independent predictor of the reduction in liver fat during a lifestyle intervention in non-alcoholic fatty liver disease. *Gut* 2009;58:1281–8.

376. Rector RS, Thyfault JP, Laye MJ, et al. Cessation of daily exercise dramatically alters precursors of hepatic steatosis in Otsuka Long-Evans Tokushima Fatty (OLETF) rats. *J Physiol* 2008;586:4241–9.

377. Caldwell S, Lazo M. Is exercise an effective treatment for NASH? Knowns and unknowns. *Ann Hepatol* 2009;8(Suppl 1):S60–6.

378. Rector RS, Thyfault JP, Uptergrove GM, et al. Mitochondrial dysfunction precedes insulin resistance and hepatic steatosis and contributes to the natural history of non-alcoholic fatty liver disease in an obese rodent model. *J Hepatol* 2010;52:727–36.

379. Schrauwen P. High-fat diet, muscular lipotoxicity and insulin resistance. *Proc Nutr Soc* 2007;66:33–41.

380. Van Baak MA. Exercise training and substrate utilization in obesity. *Int J Obesity* 1999;23:S11–17.

381. Seip RL, Snead D, Pierce EF, Stein P, Weltman A. Perceptual responses and blood lactate concentration: effect of training state. *Med Sci Sport Exer* 1991;23:80–7.

382. Church TS, Earnest CP, Skinner JS, Blair SN. Effects of different doses of physical activity on cardiorespiratory fitness among sedentary, overweight or obese postmenopausal women with elevated blood pressure: a randomized controlled trial. *JAMA* 2007;297:2081–91.

383. Johnson NA, Sachinwalla T, Walton DW, et al. Aerobic exercise training reduces hepatic and visceral lipids in obese individuals without weight loss. *Hepatology* 2009;50:1105–12.

384. Clark JM. Weight loss as a treatment for nonalcoholic fatty liver disease. *J Clin Gastroenterol* 2005;39:S295–9.

385. Palmer M, Schaffner F. Effect of weight reduction on hepatic abnormalities in overweight patients. *Gastroenterology* 1990;99:1408–12.

386. Huang MA, Greenson JK, Chao C, et al. One-year intense nutritional counseling results in histological improvement in patients with nonalcoholic steatohepatitis: a pilot study. *Am J Gastroenterol* 2005;100:1072–81.

387. Hickman IJ, Jonsson JR, Prins JB, et al. Modest weight loss and physical activity in overweight patients with chronic liver disease results in sustained improvements in alanine aminotransferase, fasting insulin, and quality of life. *Gut* 2004;53:413–19.

388. Ueno T, Sugawara H, Sujaku K, et al. Therapeutic effects of restricted diet andexercise in obese patients with fatty liver. *J Hepatol* 1997;27:103–7.

389. Nobili V, Manco M, Devito R, et al. Lifestyle intervention and antioxidant therapy in children with nonalcoholic fatty liver disease: a randomized, controlled trial. *Hepatology* 2008;48:119–28.

390. Promrat K, Kleiner DE, Niemeier HM, et al. Randomized controlled trial testing the effects of weight loss on nonalcoholic steatohepatitis. *Hepatology* 2010;51:121–9.

391. Browning JD, Davis J, Saboorian MH, Burgess SC. A low-carbohydrate diet rapidly and dramatically reduces intrahepatic triglyceride content. *Hepatology* 2006;44:487–8.

392. Kechagias S, Ernersson A, Dahlqvist O, Lundberg P, Lindström T, Nystrom FH; Fast Food Study Group Gut. Fast-food-based hyperalimentation can induce rapid and profound elevation of serum alanine aminotransferase in healthy subjects. *Gut* 2008;57:649–54.

393. Borkman M, Storlien LH, Pan DA, Jenkins AB, Chisolm DJ, Campbell LV. The relationship between insulin sensitivity and the fatty acid composition of skeletal muscle. *N Engl J Med* 1993;328:238–44.

394. Zheng X, Rivabene R, Cavallari C, et al. The effects of chylomicron remnants enriched in n-3 or n-6 polyunsaturated fatty acids on the transcription of genes regulating their uptake and metabolism by the liver: influence of cellular oxidative state. *Free Radical Bio Med* 2002;32:1123–31.

395. Levy JR, Clore JN, Stevens W. Dietary n-3 polyunsaturated fatty acids decrease hepatic triglycerides in Fischer 344 rats. *Hepatology* 2004;39:608–16.

396. Nanji AA, Sadrzadeh SMH, Yang EK, Fogt F, Meydani M, Dannenberg AJ. Dietary saturated fatty acids: a novel treatment for alcoholic liver disease. *Gastroenterology* 1995;109; 547–54.

397. Masterton GS, Plevris JN, Hayes PC. Review article: omega-3 fatty acids – a promising novel therapy for non-alcoholic fatty liver disease. *Aliment Pharmacol Ther* 2010;31:679–92.

398. Abid A, Taha O, Nseir W, Farah R, Grosovski M, Assy N. Soft drink consumption is associated with fatty liver disease independent of metabolic syndrome. *J Hepatol* 2009;51:918–24.

399. Abdelmalek MF, Suzuki A, Guy C, et al. Nonalcoholic Steatohepatitis Clinical Research Network. Increased fructose consumption is associated with fibrosis severity in patients with nonalcoholic fatty liver disease. *Hepatology* 2010;51:1961–71.

400. Parks EJ, Skokan LE, Timlin MT, Dingfelder CS. Dietary sugars stimulate fatty acid synthesis in adults. *J Nutr* 2008;138:1039–46.

401. Harrison SA, Fecht W, Brunt EM, Neuschwander-Tetri BA. Orlistat for overweight subjects with nonalcoholic steatohepatitis: a randomized, prospective trial. *Hepatology* 2009;49:80–6.

402. Pillai AA, Rinella ME. Non-alcoholic fatty liver disease: is bariatric surgery the answer? *Clin Liver Dis* 2009;13:689–710.

403. Dixon JB, Bhathal PS, Hughes NR, O'Brien PE. Non-alcoholic fatty liver disease: improvement in liver histological analysis with weight loss. *Hepatology* 2004;39:1647–54.

404. Kral JG, Thung SN, Biron S, et al. Effects of surgical treatment of the metabolic syndrome on liver fibrosis and cirrhosis. *Surgery* 2004;135:48–58.

405. Brolin RE, Bradley LJ, Taliwal RV. Unsuspected cirrhosis discovered during elective obesity operations. *Arch Surg* 1998;133:84–8.

406. Mathurin P, Hollebecque A, Arnalsteen L, et al. Prospective study of the long-term effects of bariatric surgery on liver injury in patients without advanced disease. *Gastroenterology* 2009;137:532–40.

407. Trauner M, Graziadei W. Review article: mechanisms of action and therapeutic applications of ursodeoxycholic acid in chronic liver diseases. *Aliment Pharmacol Ther* 1999;13:979–95.

408. Laurin J, Lindor KD, Crippen JS, et al. Ursodeoxycholic acid or clofibrate in the treatment of non-alcohol-induced steatohepatitis: a pilot study. *Hepatology* 1996;23:1464–7.

409. Bauditz J, Schmidt J, Dippe P, Lochs H, Pirlich M. Non-alcohol induced steatohepatitis in non-obese patients: treatment with ursodeoxycholic acid. *Am J Gastroenterol* 2004;99:959–60.

410. Lindor KD, Kowdley KV, Heathcote EJ, et al. Ursodeoxycholic acid for treatment of nonalcoholic steatohepatitis: results of a randomized trial. *Hepatology* 2004;39:770–8.

411. Leuschner UF, Lindenthal B, Herrmann G, et al. NASH Study Group. High-dose ursodeoxycholic acid therapy for nonalcoholic steatohepatitis: a double-blind, randomized, placebo-controlled trial. *Hepatology* 2010;52:472–9.

412. Dufour JF, Oneta CM, Gonvers JJ, et al. Swiss Association for the Study of the Liver. Randomized placebo-controlled trial of ursodeoxycholic acid with vitamin e in nonalcoholic steatohepatitis. *Clin Gastroenterol Hepatol* 2006;4:1537–43.

413. Malaguarnera M, Gargante MP, Russo C, et al. L-carnitine supplementation to diet: a new tool in treatment of nonalcoholic steatohepatitis – a randomized and controlled clinical trial. *Am J Gastroenterol* 2010;105:1338–45.

414. Brigelius-Flohe R, Traber MG. Vitamin E: function and metabolism. *FASEB J* 1999;13:1145–55.

415. Hasegawa T, Yoneda M, Nakamura K, Makino I, Terano A. Plasma transforming growth factor β-1 level and efficacy of α-tocopherol in patients with non-alcoholic steatohepatitis: A pilot study. *Aliment Pharmacol Ther* 2001;15:1667–72.

416. Kugelmas M, Hill DB, Vivian B, Marsano L, McClain C. Cytokines and NASH: a pilot study of the effects of lifestyle modification and vitamin E. *Hepatology* 2003;38:413–19.

417. Chang CY, Argo CK, Al-Osaimi AMS, Caldwell SH. Therapy of NAFLD: antioxidants and cytoprotective agents. *J Clin Gastroenterol* 2005;39(Suppl 4):S307–16.

418. Harrison SA, Torgerson S, Hayashi P, Ward J, Schenker S. Vitamin E and vitamin C treatment improves fibrosis in patients with nonalcoholic steatohepatitis. *Am J Gastroenterol* 2003;98:2485–90.

419. Sanyal AJ, Chalasani N, Kowdley KV, et al. NASH CRN. Pioglitazone, vitamin E, or placebo for nonalcoholic steatohepatitis. *N Engl J Med* 2010;362:1675–85.

420. Dufour JF. Vitamin E for nonalcoholic steatohepatitis: ready for prime time? *Hepatology* 2010;52:789–92.

421. Miller ER 3rd, Pastor-Barriuso R, Dalal D, Riemersma RA, Appel LJ, Guallar E. Meta-analysis: high-dosage vitamin E supplementation may increase all-cause mortality. *Ann Intern Med* 2005;142:37–46.

422. Brown BG, Crowley J. Is there any hope for vitamin E? *JAMA* 2005;293:1387–90.

423. Neuschwander-Tetri BA. Betaine: an old therapy for a new scourge. *Am J Gastroenterol* 2001;96:2534–6.

424. Abdelmalek MF, Sanderson SO, Angulo P, et al. Betaine for nonalcoholic fatty liver disease: results of a randomized placebo-controlled trial. *Hepatology* 2009;50:1818–26.

425. Caldwell SH, Argo CK, Al-Osaimi AMS. Therapy of NAFLD: insulin sensitizing agents. *J Clin Gastroenterol* 2005;39(Suppl 4):S317–22.

426. Rigazio S, Lehto HR, Tuunanen H, et al. The lowering of hepatic fatty acid uptake improves liver function and insulin sensitiv-

ity without affecting hepatic fat content in humans. *Am J Physiol Endocrinol Metab* 2008;295:E413–19.

427. Shulman AI, Mangelsdorf DJ. Retinoid X receptor heterodimers in the metabolic syndrome. *N Engl J Med* 2005;353:604–15.

428. Vamecq J, Latruffe N. Medical significance of peroxisome proliferator-activated receptors. *Lancet* 1999;354:141–8.

429. Kelly IE, Han TS, Walsh K, Lean ME. Effects of a thiazolidinedione compound on body fat and fat distribution of patients with type 2 diabetes *Diabetes Care* 1999;22:288–93.

430. Parulkar AA, Pendergrass ML, Granda-Ayala R, Lee TR, Fonseca VA. Nonhypoglycemic effects of thiazolidinediones. *Ann Intern Med* 2001;134:61–71.

431. Belfort R, Harrison SA, Brown K, et al. A placebo-controlled trial of pioglitazone in subjects with nonalcoholic steatohepatitis. *N Engl J Med* 2006;355:2297–307.

432. Aithal GP, Thomas JA, Kaye PV, et al. Randomized, placebo-controlled trial of pioglitazone in nondiabetic subjects with nonalcoholic steatohepatitis. *Gastroenterology* 2008;135:1176–84.

433. Ratziu V, Giral P, Jacqueminet S, et al. LIDO Study Group. Rosiglitazone for nonalcoholic steatohepatitis: one-year results of the randomized placebo-controlled Fatty Liver Improvement with Rosiglitazone Therapy (FLIRT) Trial. *Gastroenterology* 2008;135:100–10.

434. Ratziu V, Charlotte F, Bernhardt C, et al. LIDO Study Group. Long-term efficacy of rosiglitazone in nonalcoholic steatohepatitis: results of the Fatty Liver Improvement by Rosiglitazone Therapy (FLIRT 2) extension trial. *Hepatology* 2010;51:445–53.

435. Ratziu V, Caldwell S, Neuschwander-Tetri B. Therapeutic trials in NASH: insulin sensitizers and related methodological issues. *Hepatology* 2010;52:2206–15.

436. Lutchman G, Modi A, Kleiner DE, et al. The effects of discontinuing pioglitazone in patients with nonalcoholic steatohepatitis. *Hepatology* 2007;46:424–9.

437. Argo CK, Iezzoni JC, Al-Osaimi AM, Caldwell SH. Thiazolidinediones for the treatment in NASH: sustained benefit after drug discontinuation? *J Clin Gastroenterol* 2009;43:565–8.

438. Caldwell SH, Argo CK. Divergent effects of peroxisome proliferator-activated receptor-gamma ligands in human and mouse nonalcoholic steatohepatitis. *Hepatology* 2007;46:285–7.

439. Gitlin N. Julie NL, Spurr CL, Lim KN, Juarbe HM. Two cases of severe clinical and histologic hepatotoxicity associated with troglitazone. *Ann Intern Med* 1998;129:36–8.

440. Forman LM, Simmons DA, Diamond RH. Hepatic failure in a patient taking rosiglitazone. *Ann Intern Med* 2000;132:118–21.

441. May LD, Lefkowitch JH, Kram MT, Mittal M. Mixed hepatocellular-cholestatic liver injury after pioglitazone therapy. *Ann Intern Med* 2002;136:449–52.

442. Nesto RW, Bell D, Bonow RO, et al. Thiazolidinedione use, fluid retention, and congestive heart failure: consensus statement from the American Heart Association and the American Diabetes Association. *Circulation* 2003;108:2941–8.

443. Nissen SE, Wolski K. Effect of rosiglitazone on the risk of myocardial infarction and death from cardiovascular causes. *N Engl J Med* 2007;356:2457–71.

444. Lincoff AM, Wolski K, Nicholls SJ, Nissen SE. Pioglitazone and risk of cardiovascular events in patients with type 2 diabetes mellitus: a meta-analysis of randomized trials. *JAMA* 2007;298:1180–8.

445. Misbin RI, Green L, Stadel BV, Guerguiguian JL, Gubbi A, Fleming GA. Lactic acidosis in patients with diabetes treated with metformin. *N Engl J Med* 1998;338:265–6.

446. Kirpichnikov D, McFarlane SI, Sowers JI. Metformin: an update. *Ann Intern Med* 2002;137:25–33.

447. Zhou G, Myers R, Li Y, et al. Role of AMP-activated protein kinase in mechanism of metformin action. *J Clin Invest* 2001;108:1167–74.

448. Bailey CJ. Biguanides and NIDDM. *Diabetes Care* 1992;15:755–72.

449. Tiikkainen M, Hakkinen A-M, Korsheninnikova E, Nyman T, Makimattila S, Yki-Jarvinen H. Effects of rosiglitazone and metformin on liver fat content, hepatic insulin resistance, insulin clearance, and gene expression in adipose tissue in patients with type 2 diabetes. *Diabetes* 2004;53:2169–76.

450. Bugianesi E, Gentilcore E, Manini R, et al. A randomized controlled trial of metformin versus vitamin E or prescriptive diet in nonalcoholic fatty liver disease. *Am J Gastroenterol* 2005;100:1082–90.

451. Uygun A, Kadayifci A, Isik AT, et al. Metformin in the treatment of patients with non-alcoholic steatohepatitis. *Aliment Pharmacol Ther* 2004;19:537–44.

452. Nair S, Diehl AM, Wiseman M, Farr GH, Perrillo RP. Metformin in the treatment of non-alcoholic steatohepatitis. *Aliment Pharmacol Ther* 2004;20:23–38.

453. Basaranoglu M, Acbay O, Sonsuz A. A controlled trial of gemfibrozil in the treatment of patients with nonalcoholic steatohepatitis. *J Hepatol* 1999;31:384.

454. Conjeevaram HS, McKenna BJ, Kang H, et al. A randomized placebo controlled study of PPAR-alpha agonist fenofibrate in patients with NASH (submitted).

455. Vuppalanchi R, Chalasani N. Statins for hyperlipidemia in patients with chronic liver disease: are they safe? *Clin Gastroenterol Hepatol* 2006;4:838–9.

456. Argo CK, Loria P, Caldwell SH, Lonardo A. Statins in liver disease: a molehill, an iceberg, or neither? *Hepatology* 2008;48:662–9.

457. Ekstedt M, Franzén LE, Mathiesen UL, Holmqvist M, Bodemar G, Kechagias S. Statins in non-alcoholic fatty liver disease and chronically elevated liver enzymes: A histopathological follow-up study. *J Hepatol* 2007;47:135–41.

458. Rallidis LS, Drakoulis CK. Pravastatin in patients with nonalcoholic steatohepatitis: Results of a pilot study. *Atherosclerosis* 2004;174: 193–6.

459. Nelson A, Torres DM, Morgan AE, Fincke C, Harrison SA. A pilot study using simvastatin in the treatment of nonalcoholic steatohepatitis: a randomized placebo-controlled trial. *J Clin Gastroenterol* 2009;43:990–4.

460. Anstee QM, Concas D, Kudo H, et al. Impact of pan-caspase inhibition in animal models of established steatosis and non-alcoholic steatohepatitis. *J Hepatol* 2010;53:542–50.

461. Witek RP, Stone WC, Karaca FG, et al. Pan-caspase inhibitor VX-166 reduces fibrosis in an animal model of nonalcoholic steatohepatitis. *Hepatology* 2009;50:1421–30.

462. Li Z, Oben JA, Yang S, et al. Norepinephrine regulates hepatic innate immune system in leptin-deficient mice with nonalcoholic steatohepatitis. *Hepatology* 2004;40:434–41.

463. Loomba R, Rao F, Zhang L, et al. Genetic covariance between gamma-glutamyl transpeptidase and fatty liver risk factors: role of beta2-adrenergic receptor genetic variation in twins. *Gastroenterology* 2010;139:836–45.

464. Yokohama S, Yoneda M, Haneda M, et al. Therapeutic efficacy of an angiotensin II receptor antagonist in patients with nonalcoholic steatohepatitis. *Hepatology* 2004;40:1222–5.

465. Dixon JB, Bhathal PS, Jonsson JR, Dixon AF, Powell EE, O'Brien PE. Pro-fibrotic polymorphisms predictive of advanced liver fibrosis in the severely obese. *J Hepatol* 2003;39:967–71.

466. Nair S, Verma S, Thuluvath PJ. Obesity and the effect on survival in patients undergoing orthotopic liver transplantation in the United States. *Hepatology* 2002;35:105–9.

467. Burke A, Lucey MR. Non-alcoholic fatty liver disease, non-alcoholic steatohepatitis and orthotopic liver transplantation. *Am J Transplant* 2004;4:686–93.

468. Seo S, Maganti K, Khehra M, et al. De novo nonalcoholic fatty liver disease after liver transplantation. *Liver Transpl* 2007;13: 844–7.

469. Bhagat V, Mindikoglu AL, Nudo CG, Schiff ER, Tzakis A, Regev A. Outcomes of liver transplantation in patients with cirrhosis due to nonalcoholic steatohepatitis versus patients with cirrhosis due to alcoholic liver disease. *Liver Transpl* 2009;15: 1814–20.

470. Malik SM, Devera ME, Fontes P, Shaikh O, Ahmad J. Outcome after liver transplantation for NASH cirrhosis. *Am J Transplant* 2009;9:782–93.

471. Yalamanchili K, Saadeh S, Klintmalm GB, Jennings LW, Davis GL. Nonalcoholic fatty liver disease after liver transplantation for cryptogenic cirrhosis or nonalcoholic fatty liver disease. *Liver Transpl* 2010;16:431–9.

472. Rinella ME, Alonsa E, Rao S, et al. Body mass index as a predictor of hepatic steatosis in living liver donors. *Liver Transpl* 2001;7: 409–14.

473. Caldwell SH. Cryptogenic cirrhosis: what are we missing? *Curr Gastroenterol Rep* 2009;12:40–8.

474. Sanyal AJ, Mofrad PS, Contos MJ, et al. A pilot study of vitamin E versus vitamin E and pioglitazone for the treatment of nonalcoholic steatohepatitis. *Clin Gastroenterol Hepatol* 2004;2:1107–15.

Multiple choice questions

32.1 NASH (nonalcoholic steatohepatitis) is the more severe form of NAFLD (nonalcoholic fatty liver disease). It is present in about one third of patients with NAFLD. Which of the following is true about NASH?

    a Steatosis exceeds 5–10% liver triglyceride by weight (estimated by light microscopic appearance)

    b NASH progresses to cirrhosis in 15–20% of patients.

    c NASH is characterized histologically by inflammation, cellular ballooning, and fibrosis, usually beginning as perisinusoidal fibrosis.

    d NASH currently requires biopsy to confirm and stage.

    e All of the above.

    f None of the above.

32.2 The treatment of NAFLD is evolving. Exercise and dietary changes are cornerstones. Pharmacologic therapy has been primarily aimed at NASH because of its greater risk of progression. Which of the following is correct?

    a Thiazolidinediones (pioglitazone) are the only agents approved for treating NASH.

    b Vitamin E and other antioxidants have been uniformly ineffective in treating NASH.

    c Exercise (with or without weight loss) can reduce liver fat.

    d Statin agents have been shown to ameliorate NASH in randomized controlled trials.

    e All of the above.

    f None of the above.

Answers to the multiple choice questions can be found in the Appendix at the end of the book.

These multiple choice questions are also available for you to complete online.
Visit http://www.schiffsdiseasesoftheliver.com/

PART VIII

Vascular Diseases of the Liver

CHAPTER 33
Vascular Diseases of the Liver

Ranjeeta Bahirwani, Mark A. Rosen, & Thomas W. Faust

Division of Gastroenterology, Department of Internal Medicine, The University of Pennsylvania School of Medicine, Philadelphia, PA, USA

Key concepts

- Budd–Chiari syndrome occurs as a consequence of thrombotic occlusion of hepatic venous outflow.
- Hypercoagulable states account for most cases of Budd–Chiari syndrome. Anticoagulation is the mainstay of medical management.
- Webs and membranes in the inferior vena cava develop from prior thrombosis and represent the most common subtype of Budd–Chiari syndrome in the Far East.
- Acute or subacute Budd–Chiari syndrome may present with abdominal pain, hepatomegaly, and ascites, whereas symptoms and signs of portal hypertension are prominent with chronic disease.
- Doppler ultrasonography is a useful noninvasive screening test for Budd–Chiari syndrome. Contrast-enhanced computed tomography and magnetic resonance imaging can also demonstrate hepatic vein occlusion and associated parenchymal abnormalities secondary to venous outflow obstruction. Venography and liver biopsy remain the gold standards for diagnosis.

- Angioplasty and thrombolysis may be of benefit in highly selected cases. Decompressive surgery and transjugular intrahepatic portosystemic shunting (TIPS) are often reserved for progressive liver disease despite medical management. Liver transplantation may be performed for patients with decompensated cirrhosis or acute liver failure.
- Hereditary hemorrhagic telangiectasia, also known as Rendu–Osler–Weber syndrome, is a multisystemic vascular disorder that may involve the liver.
- Peliosis hepatis is characterized by blood-filled cystic lesions in the hepatic parenchyma, which may occur in the setting of immunosuppression or human immunodeficiency virus (HIV) infection. *Bartonella henselae* is the cause of bacillary peliosis hepatis in patients with HIV infection.

Budd–Chiari syndrome and related disorders

Etiology

The most frequent causes of venous obstruction are prothrombotic disorders, particularly myeloproliferative diseases (Box 33.1) [1]. In one of the largest series, 45% of patients with Budd–Chiari syndrome had polycythemia rubra vera and 9% were diagnosed with essential thrombocythemia [2]. Occult myeloproliferative states, demonstrated by spontaneous endogenous erythroid colony formation in the absence of erythropoietin stimulation, are also common [3]. An increasing number of thrombotic disorders have been associated with Budd–Chiari syndrome [4–6]. In over 25% of cases, more than one thrombophilic state may be present [6]. Careful, systematic evaluation for prothrombotic disorders has lowered the proportion of cases labeled as idiopathic to less than 10% [3,6]. Factor V Leiden mutation is the most frequent cause of hereditary thrombophilia and is thought

to be the second most common cause of thrombotic occlusion of the hepatic veins and vena cava [4–9]. Other hypercoagulable states associated with Budd–Chiari syndrome include antiphospholipid antibody syndrome, paroxysmal nocturnal hemoglobinuria, prothrombin G mutation, methylene-tetrahydrofolate reductase mutation, antithrombin III deficiency, and deficiencies of protein C and protein S [6,7,10–15]. Patients who are pregnant or are taking oral contraceptives and develop Budd–Chiari syndrome usually also have an underlying thrombophilic state [4–9].

Local compression by adjacent tumor, abscess, or inflammation may lead to a secondary Budd–Chiari syndrome. Neoplasms associated with outflow obstruction include primary hepatocellular, renal, adrenal, pulmonary, pancreatic, and gastric carcinomas [16–19]. Benign and malignant vascular neoplasms arising within the hepatic veins or vena cava (e.g., cavernous hemangiomas, leiomyomas, and leiomyosarcomas) have also been associated with Budd–Chiari syndrome [20–22].

Schiff's Diseases of the Liver, Eleventh Edition. Edited by Eugene R. Schiff, Willis C. Maddrey and Michael F. Sorrell.
© 2012 John Wiley & Sons, Ltd. Published 2012 by John Wiley & Sons, Ltd.

Box 33.1 Etiology of Budd–Chiari syndrome.[a]

Myeloproliferative disorders
- Polycythemia rubra vera
- Essential thrombocytosis
- Occult myeloproliferative disorders

Local compression
- Neoplasms
- Infection

Systemic diseases
- Behçet's disease
- Inflammatory bowel disease
- Sarcoidosis
- Idiopathic

Other hypercoagulable states
- Factor V Leiden mutation
- Prothrombin G20210A gene mutation
- Antiphospholipid antibody syndrome
- Methylene-tetrahydrofolate reductase mutation
- Paroxysmal nocturnal hemoglobinuria
- Protein C and S deficiency
- Antithrombin III deficiency
- Oral contraceptives
- Pregnancy

[a] Frequently more than one condition may be present.

Box 33.2 Budd–Chiari syndrome subtypes and sinusoidal obstruction syndrome.

Classic Budd–Chiari syndrome
- Thrombosis principally of hepatic veins
- More common in western countries
- Thrombophilic state most common etiology

Obliterative hepatocavopathy
- Webs and membranes (representing prior thrombosis) in inferior vena cava
- More common in China, Nepal, India, Japan, and South Africa
- Thrombophilic state, idiopathic and hepatocellular cancer common

Sinusoidal obstruction syndrome
- Nonthrombotic fibrosis of hepatic sinusoids and small intrahepatic veins
- Almost exclusively seen in the setting of bone marrow transplantation
- Mainly caused by conditioning chemotherapy

Other rare causes of hepatic venous outflow obstruction have been identified. Bacterial, viral, and parasitic infections, collagen vascular diseases, and inflammatory bowel disease may all also result in venous occlusion [23–28].

Inferior vena cava thrombosis

Budd–Chiari syndrome includes thrombosis anywhere along the hepatic venous outflow tract. It has been proposed that obstruction principally affecting the inferior vena cava should be termed *obliterative hepatocavopathy* [29]. Primary inferior vena cava thrombosis appears to be more common in India, China, Japan, Nepal, and South Africa for unclear reasons. Compared to classic Budd–Chiari syndrome, obliterative hepatocavopathy is more often considered idiopathic [29–31]. It has also been found in association with hepatocellular carcinoma [29–31]. However, systematic investigation frequently reveals an underlying thrombophilic state [30,32]. The obstruction results from caval webs or membranes, which may also involve the ostia of the hepatic veins. Although the lesions were formerly thought to be congenital, it is now recognized that they represent the transformation of inferior vena cava thrombosis [29,33]. Widespread acceptance of obliterative hepatocavopathy as a distinct entity has not occurred because its etiology, prognosis, and management are similar to those of classic Budd–Chiari syndrome (Box 33.2) [34].

Occlusion of the terminal hepatic venules (sinusoidal obstruction syndrome)

Sinusoidal obstruction syndrome (previously called venoocclusive disease) refers to obstruction of the hepatic sinusoids or small intrahepatic veins. In contradistinction to Budd–Chiari syndrome, occlusion is not thrombotic but results from fibroobliterative endophlebitis (Box 33.2). Occasionally, Budd–Chiari syndrome may involve only small intrahepatic veins. Sparing of the large hepatic veins can be seen with allergic phlebitis, granulomatous disease, paroxysmal nocturnal hemoglobinuria, and other thrombophilic states [6,34]. Distinction from sinusoidal obstruction syndrome can generally be accomplished by recognition of etiology and in some cases by demonstration of clots. Outside the setting of bone marrow transplantation, the two conditions may be indistinguishable.

Initial reports of sinusoidal obstruction syndrome were attributed to ingestion of herbal teas containing large quantities of pyrrolizidine alkaloids [35,36]. Today, sinusoidal obstruction syndrome is seen almost exclusively in the setting of bone marrow transplantation. Hepatotoxic agents, particularly certain chemotherapeutic conditioning regimens, account for most cases (Box 33.2). Recipients of liver and renal allografts and patients exposed to azathioprine are also at risk for developing sinusoidal obstruction syndrome. Other rare conditions associated with sinusoidal obstruction syndrome include vitamin A toxicity, arsenic poisoning, exposure to insecticides, administration of 6-thioguanine, intra-arterial 5-fluoro-2′-deoxyuridine, and a combination of norethisterone with conditioning chemotherapeutic agents [35,37–40].

Pathology

Hepatic venous outflow obstruction is caused by thrombotic occlusion of the terminal hepatic venules, hepatic veins, or inferior vena cava. Generally, the disease is silent if only one hepatic vein is occluded. Obstruction may manifest as fibrous cord remnants of hepatic veins, short-length stenoses, membranes, webs, or occlusions of the hepatic venous ostia [10,29,33,41]. In acute Budd–Chiari syndrome, the liver appears enlarged, smooth, and red-purple because of congestion. In chronic disease, direct outflow from the caudate lobe to the inferior vena cava may compensate for venous outflow obstruction of the major hepatic veins, resulting in caudate lobe hypertrophy with atrophy and cirrhosis of the remaining segments [42]. In some cases caudate lobe hypertrophy may obstruct the intrahepatic portion of the inferior vena cava.

Histologic changes may be uneven and result in liver biopsy sampling errors. Centrilobular congestion and sinusoidal dilatation are seen with acute obstruction, whereas atrophy, necrosis, and centrizonal hepatocyte dropout with extension to periportal regions are associated with severe injury. Venous stasis and congestion lead to hypoxic damage and oxidative injury to hepatocytes [43,44]. In chronic disease, there is complete obliteration of the central veins associated with centrilobular fibrosis that may culminate in cirrhosis [45,46]. Periportal fibrosis may be more prominent if branches of the portal vein are concomitantly thrombosed because of stasis [47]. Large, regenerative nodules are also commonly reported in areas exposed to a compensatory increase in arterial blood flow [43,47].

Clinical presentation

About two thirds of patients with Budd–Chiari syndrome are women, with the onset of symptoms usually in the late thirties [2]. Clinical presentation is variable and depends on the extent and rate of outflow obstruction, as well as the development of collaterals (Box 33.3) [10]. Presentation may range from an asymptomatic state to fulminant hepatic failure, or to cirrhosis with complications of portal hypertension [7,48,49]. More than 85% of patients have hepatomegaly and ascites, whereas esophagogastric varices and splenomegaly may be seen in 40–60% of individuals [48]. The presence of dilated subcutaneous veins over the body and trunk are more often associated with inferior vena cava obstruction [29]. Acute obstruction is commonly accompanied by right upper quadrant abdominal pain, nausea, vomiting, hepatomegaly, and ascites [48]. Jaundice and splenomegaly may be present with acute occlusion but are usually mild. Rarely, massive hepatocellular necrosis with acute hepatic failure may follow rapid and complete occlusion of all major hepatic veins [48]. A subacute presentation of less than

> ### Box 33.3 Clinical manifestations of Budd–Chiari syndrome.
>
> - Right upper quadrant pain
> - Hepatomegaly
> - Ascites
> - Splenomegaly (rare)
> - Jaundice
> - Acute liver failure (rare)
> - Weight gain
> - Nausea and vomiting
> - Pleural effusions
> - Lower-extremity edema
> - Complications of portal hypertension

6 months is characterized by vague right upper quadrant discomfort, hepatomegaly, mild to moderate ascites, and splenomegaly [48,49]. Jaundice is either absent or mild. Chronic Budd–Chiari syndrome of greater than 6 months' duration generally presents with progressive ascites. It may also be accompanied by other complications of portal hypertension, such as bleeding varices, encephalopathy, coagulopathy, renal insufficiency, fatigue, and muscle wasting [10,48,49]. Generally, cirrhosis is found only in patients with chronic disease. However, the demonstration of cirrhosis in biopsy specimens taken from patients with acute outflow tract obstruction provides an argument that the current classification system leaves room for improvement [50].

Diagnostic evaluation

Laboratory investigation

Standard laboratory investigation is rarely helpful in patients with Budd–Chiari syndrome. Nonspecific mild transaminase level elevation can be seen in 25–50% of patients but does not aid in establishing the diagnosis [16]. Transaminase values over 1,000 IU/L are possible in acute outflow obstruction or hepatic failure, especially if there is accompanying portal vein thrombosis [16]. Serum bilirubin and alkaline phosphatase levels and prothrombin time are usually normal or mildly elevated and are also not specific [16,51]. Ascitic fluid analysis is consistent with portal hypertension. Myeloproliferative and thrombotic disorders are common. Therefore, systematic, comprehensive evaluation for hypercoagulable disorders should be undertaken. The following tests should be performed: plasma clotting factors and inhibitors, factor V Leiden factor mutation, prothrombin G gene analysis, antiphospholipid antibodies and lupus anticoagulant, flow cytometry for paroxysmal nocturnal hemoglobinuria, blood smear analysis, and in select cases determination of total red cell mass, bone marrow biopsy, and measurement of serum erythropoietin levels [34]. Caution must be exercised in the interpretation of protein C, protein S, and antithrombin III abnormalities because compromised hepatic synthetic function may provide alternative explanations.

Medical imaging

Doppler ultrasonography allows for noninvasive evaluation of the hepatic veins, inferior vena cava, and portal vein. In experienced hands the sensitivity of ultrasonography for detecting venous obstruction approaches 85–95% [7,10,52]. Real-time evaluation of acute venous occlusion reveals enlarged, stenotic, or tortuous hepatic veins, whereas the major hepatic veins of patients with chronic disease may not be seen [52,53]. Intrahepatic venous-to-venous spiderweb collaterals and/or the presence of intrahepatic or subcapsular hepatic venous collaterals are highly suggestive of Budd–Chiari syndrome [34,52]. Ultrasonography may also show caval compression by a hypertrophied caudate lobe or obstruction of the vena cava by thrombus, tumor, or membranes [52,53]. Visualization of a caudate vein is over 90% specific for Budd–Chiari syndrome, although only 50% sensitive [54]. The addition of Doppler to conventional ultrasonography increases sensitivity. Doppler is effective for evaluating not only the perihepatic vascular anatomy but also the direction of blood flow and site of obstruction. Loss of the normal triphasic wave variation in the vena cava or hepatic veins has a sensitivity of 88% for occlusion [55].

Computed tomography (CT) scan and magnetic resonance imaging (MRI) are complementary investigations to Doppler ultrasonography [56–58]. Abnormalities seen may include nonvisualization of vessels or obstruction by thrombus [52,53,59,60]. Acute thrombus may be demonstrated as an expanded nonenhancing vein (Fig. 33.1), whereas more chronic changes are suggested when vessels are narrowed or not visualized.

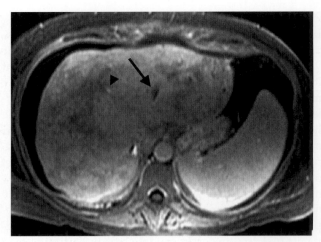

Figure 33.1 Gadolinium-enhanced magnetic resonance imaging of a 67-year-old woman with Budd–Chiari syndrome and acute hepatic decompensation. Delayed postgadolinium images demonstrate expanded nonenhancing left hepatic vein (arrow), representing acute thrombus. A narrowed but enhancing middle hepatic vein is also shown (arrowhead). Vessel narrowing suggests prior thrombosis with recanlization. Portal vein thrombus and ascites were also present. The patient decompensated and underwent transplantation. Explant pathology confirmed acute left hepatic vein thrombus. The middle and right hepatic veins with chronic thrombotic changes and recanalization were also demonstrated.

A "mosaic" pattern of abnormal parenchymal enhancement (Fig. 33.2), representing the effects of relative venous outflow obstruction, is commonly seen in contrast-enhanced CT and MRI. This pattern is not specific for Budd–Chiari syndrome and can also be seen in severe right-sided heart failure. In cases of chronic venous outflow obstruction, parenchymal changes of nodular regeneration (including macroregenerative nodules) and cirrhosis may ensue (Fig. 33.3) [53,55,60,61]. When portal hypertension develops, characteristic imaging findings (e.g., splenomegaly, ascites, collateral vessels) are often depicted as well.

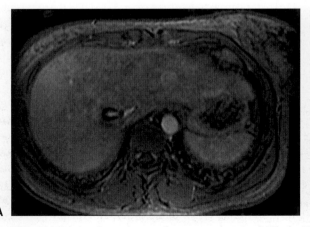

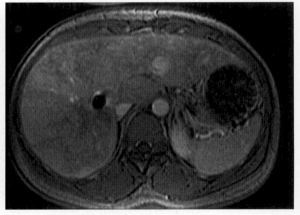

A   **B**

Figure 33.2 Gadolinium-enhanced magnetic resonance imaging (MRI) of a 57-year-old woman with chronic Budd–Chiari syndrome and a prior transjugular intrahepatic portosystemic shunt. The MRI demonstrates heterogeneous (mosaic) enhancement in the left lobe (A) and portions of the right lobe (B).

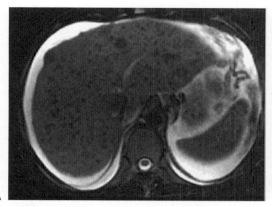
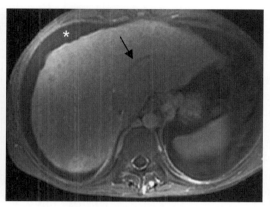

A   B

Figure 33.3 Magnetic resonance imaging of the liver of a 31-year-old man with longstanding Budd–Chiari syndrome. (A) In the T2-weighted image, liver parenchyma is abnormally edematous, with signal intensity elevation (comparable to that of the spleen). Multiple regenerative nodules characteristic of longstanding Budd–Chiari syndrome are hypointense to the edematous liver parenchyma. (B) In the postgadolinium image, nodular enhancement heterogeneity is shown. A portion of the thrombosed left hepatic vein is demonstrated (arrow); ascites is also seen (asterisk).

Venography remains the standard of reference for diagnosis and is key to planning optimal therapy. Typical venographic findings include narrowed, irregular hepatic veins with or without occlusive thrombi. Thrombi may be found either at the junction of the hepatic veins with the cava or just distal to the venous orifices [16,51]. The replacement of hepatic veins with the classic "spiderweb" appearance, intrahepatic collaterals, and recanalized veins can also be appreciated [16,51,55,62]. Angiographic assessment of the vena cava provides important information about the location and extent of obstruction, as well as its amenability to angioplasty and stenting [16,51,62]. Both catheter-based and magnetic resonance venography can be used to depict stenoses or webs of the inferior vena cava (Fig. 33.4). Local installation of thrombolytics may be performed at the time of venography in patients with fresh clots (less than 3–4 weeks) [63]. Liver biopsy may also be obtained at the time of catheter venography. Furthermore, pressure measurements obtained at the time of venography can provide useful information before surgical decompression [16,51,62].

Liver biopsy

Although not mandatory, liver biopsy is complementary to medical imaging and clinical patient assessment. Generally, the diagnosis can be established by medical imaging. In select patients, biopsy may be required to distinguish Budd–Chiari syndrome from sinusoidal obstruction syndrome or cirrhosis from other causes. Biopsy specimens may establish the presence of fibrosis and cirrhosis and may also grade the severity of hepatocellular necrosis. However, caution should be used when interpreting results because sampling error is common. Bilobar biopsy may provide a higher diagnostic yield [62]. However, it is not clear whether results from liver biopsy determine the prognosis [64,65]. In a multivariate

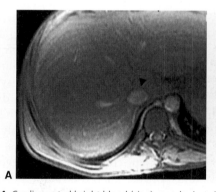
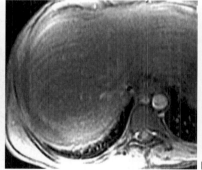
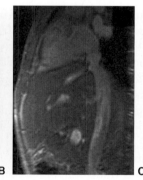

A   B   C

Figure 33.4 Cardiac-gated bright blood (cine) vascular imaging 2 cm below (A) and at (B) the level of the hepatic vein confluence of a 20-year-old man with lower extremity swelling and liver dysfunction showing (A) a patent inferior vena cava (IVC) with flow (arrowhead), and (B) a narrowed IVC. Dark areas within the IVC lumen represent turbulent (nonlaminar) flow. A cavogram (not shown) demonstrated IVC stenosis with thrombus, severely narrowing the lumen with a large pressure gradient. Angioplasty relieved both the lower extremity symptoms and the hepatic abnormalities. (C) Repeat cine magnetic resonance imaging in the sagittal plane after angioplasty demonstrating a patent IVC with mild structuring at the site of prior stenosis.

analysis, age, Child–Pugh score, responsiveness to diuretics, and creatinine were predictive of survival, whereas data from carefully documented biopsies were not [65].

Management

In the absence of prospective natural history studies of untreated and unselected patients and randomized, controlled trials of treatment options, firm management recommendations cannot be made; however, some general principles have emerged. Anticoagulation is recommended for most patients. Thrombolytics may be of benefit in acute thrombosis. Angioplasty with or without stenting may be considered for focal obstruction. If symptoms are progressive despite medical therapy, decompressive therapy with transjugular intrahepatic portosystemic shunting (TIPS) or surgical shunting is advised. Some investigators recommend decompressive procedures early in the course or if extensive necrosis is seen on liver biopsy. Generally, liver transplantation is reserved for acute liver failure or decompensated cirrhosis.

Medical therapy

Early series demonstrated poor survival in untreated Budd–Chiari syndrome; most patients died within 3 years of diagnosis [16,51]. More recent studies show an improvement in survival. In one study, 5-year survival was 50% before 1985 and 75% afterwards [65]. Widespread adoption of anticoagulation with warfarin is thought to be the cause of this improved trend. It seems prudent to recommend anticoagulation even in the absence of an identifiable prothrombotic state. It is possible that in some patients with myeloproliferative disorders, hydroxyurea and aspirin may be more appropriate [66]. Patients with ascites should be placed on a low-sodium diet and diuretics. Responsiveness to such measures is an independent predictor of survival [65]. For ascites uncontrolled after anticoagulation and medical therapy, decompressive therapy is recommended.

In carefully selected patients with clots no older than 3 or 4 weeks, the prompt administration of thrombolytics (e.g., streptokinase, urokinase, or recombinant tissue plasminogen activator) has been effectively used to dissolve thrombi and relieve hepatic congestion [63,67]. Thrombolysis may be more effective when thrombolytics are administered locally into the hepatic vein and combined with angioplasty with or without stenting [63].

Interventional radiology

Percutaneous transluminal balloon angioplasty has been used to treat focal stenoses of the inferior vena cava and/or hepatic vein [68]. Although excellent short-term results are achievable, sustained patency rates of only 50% are seen at 2 years [69]. Wire-, laser-, or needle-assisted angioplasty is appropriate for stenoses refractory

to standard techniques [70]. For salvage of failed angioplasty or as primary therapy for focal stenoses, percutaneous intraluminal stenting is an option [10,69,70]. More than 80% of stents remain patent 3 years after placement, with good control of symptoms [10,71]. Stenting has also been used to treat intrahepatic inferior vena cava obstruction caused by compression from caudate lobe hypertrophy, which would otherwise preclude portacaval shunting. After stenting, portacaval shunting has been successfully performed [72].

TIPS is being increasingly used as an alternative to decompressive surgical procedures because it is less invasive and does not carry the high perioperative mortality associated with surgical shunting. TIPS may have a role as a bridge to transplantation for patients with end-stage liver disease and ascites refractory to diuretics and sodium restriction [73–75] or in patients who present with fulminant hepatic failure [73–76]. The use of TIPS has been reported after progressive, symptomatic liver disease and ascites despite anticoagulation and medical therapy with successful control of symptoms, improvement of Child–Pugh class, and good 5-year survival without liver transplantation (74%) [50]. Survival after TIPS compares favorably with historical controls from surgical series. Shunt dysfunction often develops over time because of thrombotic occlusion. Therefore, surveillance with ultrasonography or angiography and chronic anticoagulation are recommended [50,76]. The introduction of polytetrafluoroethylene-coated stents may dramatically reduce TIPS thrombosis. In one study, only 33% of patients with covered stents experienced dysfunction after TIPS within 1 year of the procedure, compared to 87% of patients with bare stents [77].

Surgical decompression

There is currently a divergence of opinion about whether surgical decompressive procedures should be offered early in the course of Budd–Chiari syndrome or should be reserved for patients who have progressive symptomatic disease despite medical therapy. One approach emphasizes the role of liver biopsy in determining which patients should undergo early surgical shunting. Anticoagulation alone is recommended if biopsy reveals only centrilobular congestion and sinusoidal dilatation, whereas surgery is reserved for those with hepatocyte necrosis [78]. A second strategy advocates early surgical decompression, regardless of biopsy findings. Presumably, early relief of hepatic congestion may prevent ongoing necrosis and fibrosis. Such a strategy is supported by recent studies that found carefully collected data from liver biopsy to be not predictive of prognosis [64, 65]. Furthermore, in one retrospective study after adjustment for case severity, surgical shunting was associated with improved outcomes [64]. If biopsy does not predict outcome, but performance of a surgical shunt does, then perhaps early surgery is preferable. However, caution must be exercised because no rigorous prospective study has been performed to test this strategy.

A third treatment approach has been increasingly used. Patients are first treated medically with anticoagulation and diuretics if ascites is present. If symptoms and serum tests of hepatic synthetic function do not improve within days for subacute Budd–Chiari syndrome and within weeks for slower presentations, then decompressive shunting is advised [2]. Similar treatment strategies using TIPS in place of surgical decompression have achieved excellent results [50]. Success with TIPS has led to recommendations that decompressive surgery be relegated to third-line therapy. Moreover, surgical decompression is associated with high perioperative mortality (5–30%) and cannot be safely performed for patients with Child–Pugh class B or C cirrhosis [10,34,50]. A therapeutic algorithm is depicted in Fig. 33.5.

A variety of portosystemic shunts are available to relieve sinusoidal hypertension of Budd–Chiari syndrome. Side-to-side portacaval shunts have been successfully used to convert the portal vein into an outflow tract [7,16,58,79]. A pressure gradient of more than 10 mmHg between the portal vein and the inferior vena cava is required for adequate shunt flow. For patients with compression of the intrahepatic portion of the inferior vena cava by a hypertrophic caudate lobe, inferior vena cava shunting may not be possible. Mesocaval shunts between the superior mesenteric vein and vena cava provide effective portal decompression for these patients [16,78]. As with the side-to-side approach, caval pressure must be considerably lower than portal pressure. Shunt thrombosis remains a problem for 20–55% of patients who receive mesocaval shunts [7]. Other shunts have been described, including splenocaval, cavoatrial, hepaticoatrial, and mesojugular shunts [80]. Interposition synthetic grafts are also occasionally used. Finally, transatrial membranotomy with finger fracture or excision may be effective for patients with fenestrated membranes [81,82].

Liver transplantation

Liver transplantation is the preferred treatment for patients with Budd–Chiari syndrome and either acute liver failure or decompensated cirrhosis [7,62,79,83]. Patients with significant liver disease who decompensate after receiving decompressive shunts or those with shunt failure may be rescued with transplantation [81]. Excellent 5-year patient and graft survival have been achieved, with rates similar to those for patients undergoing

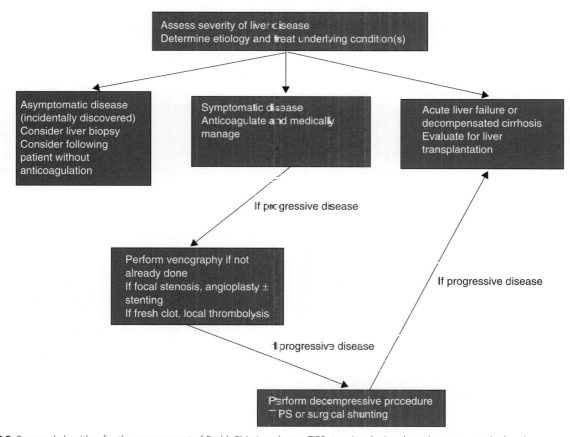

Figure 33.5 Proposed algorithm for the management of Budd–Chiari syndrome. TIPS, transjugular intrahepatic portosystemic shunting.

transplantation for other diseases [84]. Transplantation is curative for protein C, protein S, and antithrombin III deficiency. All patients should receive indefinite anticoagulation for hypercoagulable states not curable by liver replacement [83]. Aspirin and hydroxyurea effectively reduce platelet aggregation and number, respectively, and may be appropriate for preventing recurrent thrombosis after transplantation in patients with underlying myeloproliferative disorders [66,85]. Patient selection is critical because individuals with short life expectancies due to underlying medical conditions are not appropriate for transplantation. However, most underlying myeloproliferative and other disorders associated with Budd–Chiari syndrome have near normal 10-year life expectancies, which should not preclude transplantation [84].

Liver involvement in hereditary hemorrhagic telangiectasia

Hereditary hemorrhagic telangiectasia (HHT), also known as Rendu–Osler–Weber syndrome, is a multisystemic vascular disorder that variably affects the liver. The Curacao criteria require the presence of three of the four following criteria for definitive diagnosis: recurrent and spontaneous epistaxis, multiple mucocutaneous telangiectasias, visceral arteriovenous malformations, and diagnosis of HHT in a first-degree relative [86]. The disease is autosomal dominant and exhibits age-dependent penetrance. Identification of endoglin (*ENG*) and activin receptor-like kinase 1 (*ALK-1*) gene mutations have allowed subclassification of HHT into types 1 and 2 [87]. Both *ENG* and *ALK-1* encode membrane glycoproteins expressed on vascular endothelial cells involved in vascular remodeling [87]. Patients affected with HHT1 tend to have *ENG* mutations and are more likely to have pulmonary arteriovenous malformations. HHT2 is

associated with *ALK-1* mutations and is often clinically milder and more commonly associated with hepatic involvement. Additionally, mutations in the *MADH4* gene (encoding SMAD 4 protein) have been identified in individuals with combined juvenile poylposis and HHT syndrome [88].

Retrospective studies suggested radiologic evidence for hepatic involvement in only 8–30% of patients with HHT [89]. However, a more recent prospective study using multiphasic helical CT scans demonstrated hepatic vascular abnormalities, including arterioportal shunts, arteriosystemic shunts, telangiectasias, vascular masses, and parenchymal perfusion disorders, in up to 74% of 70 serial patients with HHT [90]. Hepatic vascular abnormalities may be visualized with Doppler ultrasonography, CT angiography (Fig. 33.6), direct catheter angiography, or magnetic resonance angiography [91]. Using contrast-enhanced CT or catheter angiography as the gold standard, sensitive and specific sonographic criteria for HHT have been defined. These include a dilated common hepatic artery (>7 mm) and the presence of intrahepatic hypervascularization on Doppler evaluation [92]. Therefore, absence of these findings on a sonographic study may obviate the need for additional imaging. Furthermore, screening for hepatic involvement in HHT is not generally required because most hepatic lesions remain asymptomatic and do not require treatment [90].

There are several possible symptomatic presentations of HHT with hepatic involvement (Table 33.1). High-output cardiac failure presenting with dyspnea and edema may be related to extensive hepatic artery to hepatic vein shunting [93]. Portal hypertension resulting from shunting between the hepatic artery and portal vein may present with ascites or variceal hemorrhage [93]. Hepatic encephalopathy may develop in the presence of portal vein to hepatic vein shunting [93]. Finally, cholestasis and biliary abnormalities may result from

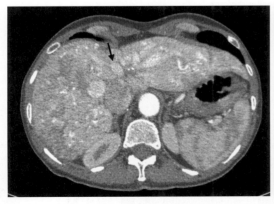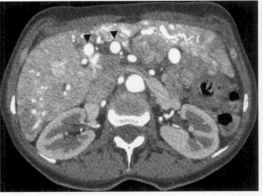

Figure 33.6 Contrast-enhanced computed tomography scan in a female patient with hereditary hemorrhagic telaniectasia and hepatic involvement. (A) Heterogeneous hypervascularity of the liver parenchyma in the upper liver. Hepatic veins are markedly dilated (arrow). (B) At the level of the porta hepatis, the dilated tortuous proper hepatic artery is shown (arrowheads).

Table 33.1 Hepatic involvement of hereditary hemorrhagic telangiectasia: clinical presentations.

Clinical presentation	Type of shunting
High-output cardiac failure	Hepatic artery to hepatic vein
Dyspnea	Hepatic artery to hepatic vein
Edema	Hepatic artery to hepatic vein
Portal hypertension	Hepatic artery to portal vein
Ascites	Hepatic artery to portal vein
Variceal bleeding	Hepatic artery to portal vein
Hepatic encephalopathy	Portal vein to hepatic vein
Biliary abnormalities	Hepatic artery to hepatic vein
Cholestasis	Hepatic artery to hepatic vein
Cholangitis	Hepatic artery to hepatic vein

ischemic injury related to hepatic artery to hepatic vein shunting [93]. Symptomatic disease can often be managed conservatively. Hepatic arterial embolization of vascular lesions was initially used with some success, but more recent reports have highlighted the high mortality rates associated with postembolization hepatic and biliary necrosis [94]. Hepatic arterial embolization can no longer be recommended for the treatment of hepatic HHT. Liver transplantation has been successfully performed despite technical difficulties with vascular reorganization [95].

Peliosis hepatis

Peliosis hepatis is characterized by blood-filled cystic cavities in the hepatic parenchyma lined by hepatocytes or endothelial cells [96]. Similar lesions may also develop in the spleen. Peliosis has been well described in immunosuppressed patients, including those with human immunodeficiency virus (HIV) infection, tuberculosis, and cancer, and after solid organ transplantation [97,98]. Medications associated with peliosis hepatis include anabolic and androgenic steroids, azathioprine, and cyclosporine [98].

Bartonella henselae, associated with catscratch disease, is the causative agent of bacillary peliosis hepatis in patients with HIV infection [97]. Exposure to cat bites, scratches, and fleas are risk factors for the acquisition of *B. henselae* [97]. This fastidious Gram-negative bacillus has a granular and purple appearance on a Warthin–Starry stain of affected hepatic specimens [96]. Infection with the bacteria may also be demonstrated by blood culture, serologies, and polymerase chain reaction-based tests, although no single test is reliable. Some patients with bacillary peliosis hepatis also develop bacillary angiomatosis, characterized by vascular lesions affecting the skin (most com-

monly red or purple papules), lymph nodes, bones, and central nervous system.

Imaging reports of peliosis hepatis are largely limited to isolated case reports [99]. On sonography, vague areas of slightly decreased heterogeneous echotexture have been described. On unenhanced CT scan, irregular areas of low attenuation are shown. On MRI, lesions are usually of low-signal intensity on T1-weighted imaging and high-signal intensity on T2-weighted imaging. However, appearance on MRI may vary if lesions are complicated by hemorrhage, with variable T1 brightening. On both CT scans and MRI, dynamic contrast enhancement demonstrates an early central enhancement, with gradual centripetal fill-in. This pattern is distinct from that of other vascular liver lesions, including hemangioma, adenoma, and focal nodular hyperplasia, and may be the key to diagnosis.

Peliosis hepatis is often an incidental finding. Among patients with HIV infection, fever, lymphadenopathy, anemia, elevated alkaline phosphatase level, and lower CD4 counts are more common in affected patients than in controls [100]. Treatment of bacillary peliosis hepatis consists of several months of administration of erythromycin (500 mg four times daily) or an alternative macrolide. Nonbacillary peliosis is best treated by stopping the offending medication or addressing the underlying etiology.

Conclusions

Budd–Chiari syndrome is an uncommon disease associated with thrombotic obstruction of the terminal hepatic venules, hepatic veins, vena cava, and/or right atrium. Sinusoidal congestion and centrilobular necrosis occur as a consequence of venous outflow obstruction and can lead to fibrosis and cirrhosis. Most patients present with chronic signs and symptoms of portal hypertension, although some may present subacutely or even acutely. Doppler sonography is an excellent screening test for evaluating the patency of the major hepatic veins and vena cava. CT scans and MRI are complementary studies. Venography remains the standard of reference for the diagnosis of venous occlusion and may either show the classic spider web appearance of hepatic vein obstruction or demonstrate intrahepatic or subcapsular collaterals. Liver biopsy and pressure measurements made during venography may also guide treatment selection.

Rigorous studies are not available to derive definitive treatment algorithms. Generally, anticoagulation is offered to all patients. Diuretics and a low-sodium diet are prescribed for those with ascites. If symptoms and hepatic synthetic dysfunction do not resolve after medical therapy, then decompressive procedures are offered.

Some investigators recommend the performance of surgical shunting or TIPS early in the course of disease. Thrombolytic therapy may be useful for acute thrombosis. Angioplasty with or without stenting may treat focal stenoses. TIPS can effectively decompress hepatic sinusoids with symptomatic improvement. Surgical shunting has been used successfully for those with adequate hepatic reserve, although perioperative mortality can be high. Liver transplantation is preferred for patients with acute liver failure or decompensated cirrhosis. Survival after transplantation is similar to that of patients undergoing transplantation for cirrhosis due to other causes.

HHT is characterized by epistaxis, mucocutaneous telangiectasias, and visceral arteriovenous malformations. Patients with hepatic lesions are generally asymptomatic; possible symptoms include high-output cardiac failure, complications of portal hypertension, hepatic encephalopathy, and symptoms related to cholestasis. Management is most often conservative, and hepatic arterial embolization has been associated with unacceptably high mortality.

Peliosis hepatis is often an incidental finding. Characteristic blood-filled cystic cavities may occur in the setting of immunosuppression or HIV infection. *Bartonella henselae* is the cause of bacillary peliosis hepatis in patients with HIV infection. Generally, treatment consists of addressing the underlying cause of immunosuppression or treating *Bartonella* infection.

Annotated references

Deleve LD, Valla DC, Garcia-Tsao G. Vascular disorders of the liver. AASLD Practice Guidelines. *Hepatology* 2009;5:1729–64.
An excellent overview of vascular disorders of the liver with guidelines by the American Association for the Study of Liver Diseases.

Denniger MH, **Chait Y**, **Casadevall N, et al.** Cause of portal or hepatic venous thrombosis in adults: the role of multiple concurrent factors. *Hepatology* 2000;31:587–91.
The authors suggest that the occurrence of multiple prothrombotic disorders is more common than expected. Evaluation for hypercoagualable states in patients with hepatic or portal venous occlusion is recommended.

Garcia-Tsao G, **Korzenik JR**, **Young L, et al.** Liver disease in patients with hereditary hemorrhagic telangiectasia. *N Engl J Med* 2000;343:931–6.
The authors describe and categorize symptomatic presentations in 19 patients with hereditary hemorrhagic telangiectasia involving the liver.

Janssen HL, **Garcia-Pagan JC**, **Elias E, et al.** European Group for the Study of Vascular Disorders of the Liver. Budd–Chiari syndrome: a review by an expert panel. *J Hepatol* 2003;38:364–71.
The authors discuss difficulties with nomenclature. They emphasize that in the absence of rigorous studies, aggressive early treatment can not currently be advised.

Klein AS, **Molmenti EP.** Surgical treatment of Budd–Chiari syndrome. *Liver Transpl* 2003;9:891–6.
A comprehensive review of surgical decompressive techniques. Patient selection and success with various procedures are discussed.

Koehler JE, **Sanchez MA**, **Garrido CS, et al.** Molecular epidemiology of *Bartonella* infections in patients with bacillary angiomatosis-peliosis. *N Engl J Med* 1997;337:1876–83.

This case–control study used molecular techniques to show that bacillary peliosis hepatis is associated exclusively with Bartonella henselae. Epidemiologic links to cat and flea exposures were identified.

Murad SD, **Valla DC**, **de Groen PC, et al.** Determinants of survival and the effect of portosystemic shunting in patients with Budd–Chiari syndrome. *Hepatology* 2004;39:500–8.
The authors present a large retrospective series of patients with Budd–Chiari syndrome (n = 237). On multivariate analysis encephalopathy, ascites, prothrombin time, and bilirubin were the only independent predictors of survival. Portosystemic shunting showed a trend towards improved survival in a select group of patients.

Okuda K. Inferior vena cava thrombosis at its hepatic portion (obliterative hepatocavopathy). *Semin Liver Dis* 2002;22:15–16.
Okuda proposes that inferior vena cava obstruction, characterized by webs and membranes, and typically seen in Nepal, South Africa, China, India, and Japan, should be considered a distinct disease from classic Budd–Chiari syndrome. He proposes a new term, obliterative hepatocavopathy.

References

1. Ganguli SC, Ramzan NN, McKusick MA, et al. Budd–Chiari syndrome in patients with hematological disease: a therapeutic challenge. *Hepatology* 1998;27:1157–61.
2. Murad SD, Valla DC, de Groen PC, et al. Determinants of survival and the effect of portosystemic shunting in patients with Budd–Chiari syndrome. *Hepatology* 2004;39:500–8.
3. De Stefano V, Teofili L, Leone G, et al. Spontaneous erythroid colony formation as the clue to an underlying myeloproliferative disorder in patients with Budd–Chiari syndrome or portal vein thrombosis. *Semin Thromb Hemost* 1997;23:411–18.
4. Gambaro G, Patrassi G, Pittarello F, et al. Budd–Chiari syndrome, during nephrotic relapse in a patient with resistance to activated protein C clotting inhibitor. *Am J Kidney Dis* 1998;92:657–60.
5. Mahmoud AEA, Elias E, Beauchamp N, et al. Prevalence of the factor V Leiden mutation in hepatic and portal vein thrombosis. *Gut* 1997;40:798–800.
6. Denniger MH, Chait Y, Casadevall N, et al. Cause of portal or hepatic venous thrombosis in adults: the role of multiple concurrent factors. *Hepatology* 2000;31:587–91.
7. Tilanus HW. Budd–Chiari syndrome. *Br J Surg* 1995;82:1023–30.
8. Gordon SC, Polson DJ, Shirkoda A. Budd–Chiari syndrome complicating preeclampsia: diagnosis by magnetic resonance imaging. *J Clin Gastroenterol* 1991;13:460–2.
9. Valla D, Le MG, Poynard T, et al. Risk of hepatic vein thrombosis in relation to recent use of oral contraceptives. A case–control study. *Gastroenterology* 1986;90:807–11.
10. Valla DC. Hepatic vein thrombosis (Budd–Chiari syndrome). *Semin Liver Dis* 2002;22:5–14.
11. Espinosa G, Font J, Garcia-Pagan JC, et al. Budd–Chiari syndrome secondary to antiphospholipid syndrome: clinical and immunologic characteristics of 43 patients. *Medicine* 2001;80:345–54.
12. Valla D, Dhumeaux D, Babany G, et al. Hepatic vein thrombosis in paroxysmal nocturnal hemoglobinuria. A spectrum from asymptomatic occlusion of hepatic venules to fatal Budd–Chiari syndrome. *Gastroenterology* 1987;93:569–75.
13. Langnas AN, Sorrell MF. The Budd–Chiari syndrome: a therapeutic gordian knot? *Semin Liver Dis* 1993;13:352–9.
14. Das M, Carroll SF. Antithrombin III deficiency: an etiology of Budd–Chiari syndrome. *Surgery* 1985;97:242–6.
15. Bourliere M, Le Treut YP, Arnoux D, et al. Acute Budd–Chiari syndrome with hepatic failure and obstruction of the inferior vena cava as presenting manifestations of hereditary protein C deficiency. *Gut* 1990;31:949–52.

16. Mitchell MC, Boitnott JK, Kaufman S, et al. Budd–Chiari syndrome:etiology, diagnosis and management. *Medicine* 1982;61: 199–218.

17. Ehrich DA, Widmann JJ, Berger RL, et al. Intracavitary cardiac extension of hepatoma. *Ann Thorac Surg* 1975;19:206–11.

18. Nakajima Y, Baba S, Nagahama T, et al. Renal cell carcinoma presenting as Budd–Chiari syndrome. *Urol Int* 1989;44:173–6.

19. Michael J, Desmond AD, Jackson BT, et al. Occlusion of the hepatic veins by an adrenal carcinoma. *Am J Gastroenterol* 1978;69:599–600.

20. Kim DY, Pantelic MV, Yoshida A, et al. Cavernous hemangioma presenting as Budd–Chiari syndrome. *J Am Coll Surg* 2005;200:470–1.

21. Lee PK, Teixeira OH, Simons JA, et al. Atypical hepatic vein leiomyoma extending into the right atrium: an unusual cause of Budd–Chiari syndrome. *Can J Cardiol* 1990;6:107–10.

22. Cacoub P, Piette JC, Wechsler B, et al. Leiomyosarcoma of the inferior vena cava. Experience with 7 patients and literature review. *Medicine* 1991;70:293–306.

23. Mehrotra G, Singh RP, Krishna A, et al. Pyogenic liver abscess causing acute Budd–Chiari syndrome. *Ann Trop Paediatr* 1992;12:451–3.

24. Khuroo MS, Datta DV, Khoshy A, et al. Alveolar hydatid disease of the liver with Budd–Chiari syndrome. *Postgrad Med* 1980;56:197–201.

25. Nakamura H, Uehara H, Okada T, et al. Occlusion of small hepatic veins associated with systemic lupus erythematosus with the lupus anticoagulant and anticardiolipin antibody. *Hepatogastroenterology* 1989;36:393–7.

26. Cosnes J, Robert A, Levy VG, et al. Budd–Chiari syndrome in a patient with mixed connective-tissue disease. *Dig Dis Sci* 1980;25:467–9.

27. Chesner IM, Muller S, Newman J. Ulcerative colitis complicated by Budd–Chiari syndrome. *Gut* 1986;27:1096–100.

28. Maccini DM, Berg JC, Bell GA. Budd–Chiari syndrome and Crohn's disease. An unreported association. *Dig Dis Sci* 1989;34:1933–6.

29. Okuda K. Inferior vena cava thrombosis at its hepatic portion (obliterative hepatocavopathy). *Semin Liver Dis* 2002;22:15–26.

30. Valla DC. The diagnosis and management of Budd–Chiari syndrome: consensus and controversies. *Hepatology* 2003;38:793–803.

31. Simson IW. Membranous obstruction of the inferior vena cava and hepatocellular carcinoma in South Africa. *Gastroenterology* 1982;82:171–8.

32. Mohanty D, Shetty S, Ghosh K, et al. Hereditary thrombophilia as a cause of Budd–Chiari syndrome: a study from Western India. *Hepatology* 2001;34:666–70.

33. Kage M, Arakawa M, Kojiro M, et al. Histopathology of membranous obstruction of the inferior vena cava in the Budd–Chiari syndrome. *Gastroenterology* 1992;102:2081–90.

34. Janssen HL, Garcia-Pagan JC, Elias E, et al. European Group for the Study of Vascular Disorders of the Liver. Budd–Chiari syndrome: a review by an expert panel. *J Hepatol* 2003;38:364–71.

35. DeLeve LD, Shulman HM, McDonald GB. Toxic injury to hepatic sinusoids: sinusoidal obstruction syndrome (veno-occlusive disease). *Semin Liver Dis* 2002;22:27–41.

36. Bras G, Jellife DB, Stuart KL. Veno-occlusive disease of the liver with nonportal type of cirrhosis, occurring in Jamaica. *Arch Pathol* 1954;57:285–300.

37. Hagglund H, Remberger M, Klaesson S, et al. Norethisterone treatment, a major risk-factor for veno-occlusive disease in the liver after allogeneic bone marrow transplant. *Blood* 1998;92:4568–72.

38. Russell RM, Boyer JL, Bagheri SA, et al. Hepatic injury from chronic hypervitaminosis a resulting in portal hypertension and ascites. *N Engl J Med* 1974;291:435–40.

39. Labadie H, Stoessel P, Callard P, et al. Hepatic venoocclusive disease and perisinusoidal fibrosis secondary to arsenic poisoning. *Gastroenterology* 1990;99:1140–3.

40. Nakhleh RE, Wesen C, Snover DC, et al. Venoocclusive lesions of the central veins and portal vein radicles secondary to intraarterial 5-fluoro-2'-deoxyuridine infusion. *Hum Pathol* 1989;20:1218–20.

41. Valla D, Hadengue A, el Younsi M, et al. Hepatic venous outflow block caused by short-length hepatic vein stenoses. *Hepatology* 1997;25 814–19.

42. Olzinski AT, Sanyal AJ. Treating Budd–Chiari syndrome: making rational choices from a myriad of options. *J Clin Gastroenterol* 2000; 30(2):155–61.

43. Cazals-Hatem D, Vilgrain V, Genin P, et al. Arterial and portal circulation and parenchymal changes in Budd–Chiari syndrome: a study in 17 explanted livers. *Hepatology* 2003;37:510–19.

44. McCuskey RS. Morphological mechanisms for regulating blood flow through hepatic sinusoids. *Liver* 2000;20:3–7.

45. Scheuer PJ, Lefkowitch JH. Vascular disorders. In: Scheuer PJ, Lefkowitch JH. *Liver Biopsy Interpretation*, Vol. 31. London: WB Saunders, 1994:182–93.

46. Ludwig J. Abnormal blood vessels and hemorrhages. In: Rogers P, ed. *Practical Liver Biopsy Interpretation: diagnostic algorithms*, Vol. 1, Chicago: ASCP Press, 1992:233–58.

47. Tanaka M, Wanless IR. Pathology of the liver in Budd–Chiari syndrome: portal vein thrombosis and the histogenesis of veno-centric cirrhosis, veno-portal cirrhosis, and large regenerative nodules. *Hepatology* 1998;27:488–96.

48. Bismuth H, Sherlock DJ. Portosystemic shunting versus liver transplantation for the Budd–Chiari syndrome. *Ann Surg* 1991;214: 581–9.

49. Mahmoud AE, Mendoza A, Meshikhes AN, et al. Clinical spectrum, investigations and treatment of Budd–Chiari syndrome. *Q J Med* 1996;89:37–43.

50. Fossle M, Olschewski M, Siegerstetter V, et al. The Budd–Chiari syndrome: outcome after treatment with the transjugular intrahepatic portosystemic shunt. *Surgery* 2004;135:394–403.

51. Tavill AS, Wood EJ, Kreel L, et al. The Budd–Chiari syndrome: correlation between hepatic scintigraphy and the clinical, radiological, and pathological findings in nineteen cases of hepatic venous outflow obstruction. *Gastroenterology* 1975;68:509–18.

52. Gupta S, Barter S, Phillips GW, et al. Comparison of ultrasonography, computed tomography, and 99mTc liver scan in diagnosis of Budd–Chiari syndrome. *Gut* 1987;28:242–7.

53. Lim JH, Park JH, Auh YH. Membranous obstruction of the inferior vena cava: comparison of findings at sonography, CT, and venography. *Am J Roentgenol* 1992;159:515–20.

54. Bargallo X, Gilabert R, Nicolau C, et al. Sonography of the caudate vein: value in diagnosing Budd–Chiari syndrome. *AJR Am J Roentgenol* 2003;181:1641–5.

55. Al-Damegh S. Budd–Chiari syndrome: a short radiological review. *J Gastroenterol Hepatol* 1999;14:1057–61.

56. Mulholland JP, Fong SM, Kafaghi FA, et al. Budd–Chiari syndrome: diagnosis with ultrasound and nuclear medicine calcium colloid liver scan following non-diagnostic contrasted CT scan. *Australas Radiol* 1997;41:53–6.

57. Mergo PJ, Ros PR. Imaging of diffuse liver disease. *Radiol Clin North Am* 1998 36:365–75.

58. Ueda K, Matsui O, Kadoya M, et al. CTAP in Budd–Chiari syndrome: evaluation of intrahepatic portal flow. *Abdom Imaging* 1998;23:304–8.

59. Mori H, Maeda H, Fukuda T, et al. Acute thrombosis of the inferior vena cava and hepatic veins in patients with Budd–Chiari syndrome: CT demonstration. *AJR Am J Roentgenol* 1989;153:987–91.

60. Stark DD, Hahn FF, Trey C, et al. MRI of the Budd–Chiari syndrome. *AJR Am J Roentgenol* 1986;146:1141–8.

61. Brancatelli G, Federle MP, Grazioli L, et al. Large regenerative nodules in Budd–Chiari syndrome and other vascular disorders of the

liver: CT and MR imaging findings with clinicopathologic correlation. *AJR Am J Roentgenol* 2002;178:877–83.

62. Henderson JM, Warren D, Millikan WJ, et al. Surgical options, hematologic evaluation, and pathologic changes in Budd–Chiari syndrome. *Am J Surg* 1990;159:41–88.

63. Sharma S, Texeira A, Texeira P, et al. Pharmacological thrombolysis in Budd Chiari syndrome: a single centre experience and review of the literature. *J Hepatol* 2004;40:172–80.

64. Tang TJ, Batts KP, de Groen PC, et al. The prognostic value of histology in the assessment of patients with Budd–Chiari syndrome. *J Hepatol* 2001;35:338–43.

65. Zeitoun G, Escolano S, Hadengue A, et al. Outcome of Budd–Chiari syndrome: a multivariate analysis of factors related to survival including surgical portosystemic shunting. *Hepatology* 1999;30:84–9.

66. Melear JM, Goldstein RM, Levy MF, et al. Hematologic aspects of liver transplantation for Budd–Chiari syndrome with special reference to myeloproliferative disorders. *Transplantation* 2002;74:1090–5.

67. Raju GS, Felver M, Olin JW, et al. Thrombolysis for acute Budd–Chiari syndrome: case report and literature review. *Am J Gastroenterol* 1996;91:1262–3.

68. Sparano J, Chang J, Trasi S, et al. Treatment of the Budd–Chiari syndrome with percutaneous transluminal angioplasty. Case report and review of the literature. *Am J Med* 1987;82:821–8.

69. Xu K, He FX, Zhang HG, et al. Budd–Chiari syndrome caused by obstruction of the hepatic inferior vena cava: immediate and 2-year treatment results of transluminal angioplasty and metallic stent placement. *Cardiovasc Intervent Radiol* 1996;19:32–6.

70. Witte AMC, Kool LJS, Veenendaal R, et al. Hepatic vein stenting for Budd–Chiari syndrome. *Am J Gastroenterol* 1997;92:498–501.

71. Zhang CQ, Fu LN, Xu L, et al. Long term effect of stent placement in 115 patients with Budd–Chiari syndrome. *World J Gastroenterol* 2003;9:2587–91.

72. Oldhafer KJ, Frerker M, Prokop M, et al. Two-step procedure in Budd–Chiari syndrome with severe intrahepatic vena cava stenosis: vena cava stenting and portocaval shunt. *Am J Gastroenterol* 1998;93:1165–6.

73. Ganger DR, Klapman JB, McDonald V, et al. Transjugular intrahepatic portosystemic shunt (TIPS) for Budd–Chiari syndrome and portal vein thrombosis. *Am J Gastroenterol* 1999;94:603–8.

74. Shresta R, Durham JD, Wachs M, et al. Use of transjugular intrahepatic portosystemic shunt as a bridge to transplantation in fulminant hepatic failure due to Budd–Chiari syndrome. *Am J Gastroenterol* 1997;92:2304–6.

75. Attwell A, Ludkowski M, Nash R, et al. Treatment of Budd–Chiari syndrome in a liver transplant unit, the role of transjugular intrahepatic porto-systemic shunt and liver transplantation. *Aliment Pharmacol Ther* 2004;20:867–73.

76. Blum U, Rossle M, Haag K, et al. Budd–Chiari syndrome: technical, hemodynamic, and clinical results of treatment with transjugular intrahepatic portosystemic shunt. *Radiology* 1995;197:805–11.

77. Hernandez-Guerra M, Turnes J, Rubinstein P, et al. PTFE-covered stents improve TIPS patency in Budd–Chiari syndrome. *Hepatology* 2004;40:1197–202.

78. Klein AS, Molmenti EP. Surgical treatment of Budd–Chiari syndrome. *Liver Transpl* 2003;9:891–6.

79. Orloff MJ, Daily PO, Orloff SL, et al. A 27-year experience with surgical treatment of Budd–Chiari syndrome. *Ann Surg* 2000;232:340–52.

80. Dang XW, Xu PQ, Ma XX. Splenocaval versus mesocaval shunt with artificial vascular graft for the treatment of Budd–Chiari syndrome. *Hepatobiliary Pancreat Dis Int* 2005;4:68–70.

81. Ringe B, Lange H, Oldhafer K, et al. Which is the best surgery for Budd–Chiari syndrome: venous decompression or liver trans-

plantation? A single-center experience with 50 patients. *Hepatology* 1995;21:1337–44.

82. Chang CH, Lee M-C, Shieh M-J, et al. Transatrial membranotomy for Budd–Chiari syndrome. *Ann Thorac Surg* 1989;48:409–12.

83. Campbell DA, Rolles K, Jamieson N, et al. Hepatic transplantation with perioperative and long term anticoagulation as treatment for Budd–Chiari syndrome. *Surg Gynecol Obstet* 1988;166:511–18.

84. Srinivasan P, Rela M, Prachalias A, et al. Liver transplantation for Budd–Chiari syndrome. *Transplantation* 2002;73:973–7.

85. Goldstein R, Clark P, Klintmalm G, et al. Prevention of recurrent thrombosis following liver transplantation for Budd–Chiari syndrome associated with myeloproliferative disorders: treatment with hydroxyurea and aspirin. *Transplant Proc* 1991;23:1559–60.

86. Shovlin CL, Guttmacher AE, Buscarinin E, et al. Diagnostic criteria for hereditary hemorrhagic telangiectasia (Rendu–Osler–Weber syndrome). *Am J Med Genet* 2000;91:66–7.

87. Kuehl HK, Caselitz M, Hasenkamp S, et al. Hepatic manifestation is associated with ALK1 in hereditary hemorrhagic telangiectasia: identification of five novel ALK1 and one novel ENG mutations. *Hum Mutat* 2005;25:320–7.

88. Gallione CJ, Repetto GM, Legius E, et al. A combined syndrome of juvenile polyposis and hereditary hemorrhagic telangiectasia associated with mutations in MADH4 (SMAD4). *Lancet* 2004;363:852–9.

89. Plauchu H, de Chadarevian JP, Bideau A, et al. Age-related clinical profile of hereditary hemorrhagic telangiectasia in an epidemiologically recruited population. *Am J Med Genet* 1989;32:291–7.

90. Stabile Ianora AA, Memeo M, Sabba C, et al. Hereditary hemorrhagic telangiectasia: multi-detector row helical CT assessment of hepatic involvement. *Radiology* 2004;230:250–9.

91. Saluja S, White RI. Hereditary hemorrhagic telangiectasia of the liver: hyperperfusion with relative ischemia – poverty amidst plenty. *Radiology* 2004;230:25–7.

92. Caselitz M, Bahr MJ, Bleck JS, et al. Sonographic criteria for the diagnosis of hepatic involvement in hereditary hemorrhagic telangiectasia (HHT). *Hepatology* 2003;37:1139–46.

93. Garcia-Tsao G, Korzenik JR, Young L, et al. Liver disease in patients with hereditary hemorrhagic telangiectasia. *N Engl J Med* 2000;343:931–6.

94. Whiting JH, Korzenik JR, Miller FJ Jr, et al. Fatal outcome after embolotherapy for hepatic arteriovenous malformations of the liver in two patients with hereditary hemorrhagic telangiectasia. *J Vasc Interv Radiol* 2000;11:855–8.

95. Thevenot T, Vanlemmens C, Di Martino V, et al. Liver transplantation for cardiac failure in patients with hereditary hemorrhagic telangiectasia. *Liver Transpl* 2005;11:834–8.

96. Perkocha LA, Geaghan SM, Yen TS, et al. Clinical and pathological features of bacillary peliosis hepatis in association with human immunodeficiency virus infection. *N Engl J Med* 1990;323:1581–6.

97. Koehler JE, Sanchez MA, Garrido CS, et al. Molecular epidemiology of *Bartonella* infections in patients with bacillary angiomatosis-peliosis. *N Engl J Med* 1997;337:1876–83.

98. Izumi S, Nishiuchi M, Kameda Y, et al. Laparoscopic study of peliosis hepatis and nodular transformation of the liver before and after renal transplantation: natural history and etiology in follow-up cases. *J Hepatol* 1994;20:129–37.

99. Gouya H, Vignaux O, Legmann P, et al. Peliosis hepatis: triphasic helical CT and dynamic MRI findings. *Abdom Imaging* 2001;26:507–9.

100. Mohle-Boetani JC, Koehler JE, Berger TG, et al. Bacillary angiomatosis and bacillary peliosis in patients infected with human immunodeficiency virus: clinical characteristics in a case–control study. *Clin Infect Dis* 1996;22:794–800.

Multiple choice questions

33.1 Which of the following is the most common prothrombotic disorder leading to Budd–Chiari syndrome?

   a   Polycythemia vera.
   b   Factor V Leiden.
   c   Antiphospholipid antibody syndrome.
   d   Paroxysmal nocturnal hemoglobinuria.
   e   Protein C deficiency.

33.2 Imaging findings in Budd–Chiari syndrome include all of the following except which one?

   a   Hepatomegaly.
   b   Caudate lobe hypertrophy.
   c   Ascites.
   d   Inferior vena cava obstruction by the caudate lobe.
   e   Cystic lesions in the liver.

Answers to the multiple choice questions can be found in the Appendix at the end of the book.

These multiple choice questions are also available for you to complete online.
Visit http://www.schiffsdiseasesoftheliver.com/

CHAPTER 34

The Liver in Circulatory Failure

Santiago J. Munoz[1,2], *Jonathan M. Fenkel*[3], *& Kiley Kolb*[1]

[1]Department of Medicine and [2]Division of Abdominal Organ Transplantation, Temple University Hospital and School of Medicine, Philadelphia, PA, USA
[3]Division of Gastroenterology and Hepatology, Thomas Jefferson University, Philadelphia, PA, USA

Key concepts

- The hepatic artery and portal vein provide a dual blood supply that makes the liver comparatively resistant to ischemic injury.
- Nonetheless, during acute and severe arterial hypotension, shock, or hemodynamic instability, hepatic perfusion may become compromised resulting in ischemic hepatic injury.
- Zone 3 of the hepatic lobule is the most susceptible to ischemic damage, but in severe cases the histology may reveal extension of the hepatocellular necrosis into zone 2 and even periportal areas.
- There is a spectrum of severity of ischemic hepatic injury. However, it is an uncommon cause of acute (fulminant) liver failure. In typical cases, serum aminotransferases rapidly increase within a few days, followed by an equally prompt decline after the inciting hypotensive episode is resolved.
- Passive congestion of the liver caused by heart failure results in abnormal serum aminotransferases and may include elevated serum bilirubin and coagulopathy. Ascites may be a presenting feature of passive hepatic congestion, even in the absence of cirrhosis. Chronic, severe, passive hepatic congestion may lead to hepatic fibrosis and a characteristic form of cirrhosis ("cardiac cirrhosis") with complications that include hepatocellular carcinoma.
- Cirrhotic preexisting to the ischemic injury may be particularly susceptible to ischemia, and acute-on-chronic liver failure may follow after severe hypotension or shock.
- The unique circulatory abnormalities of the Budd–Chiari syndrome include hepatocellular necrosis due to venous outflow obstruction. In severe Budd–Chiari syndrome with associated portal vein thrombosis, extensive hepatocellular necrosis with liver failure may result from the inability of the portal vein to serve as a secondary compensatory outflow tract from the liver.
- Hepatic arterial occlusion may result in ischemic cholangiopathy due to the exclusive arterial blood supply of the biliary ductal system. This may lead to biliary strictures developing long after the occlusive episode.
- Hepatic infarction may also result from occlusion of the main hepatic artery, particularly in the early postoperative period following liver transplantation.

The liver is abundantly perfused with blood from both the portal vein and hepatic artery. This dual blood supply mixes within the hepatic sinusoids and subsequently exits the liver through the three major hepatic veins. The dual blood supply dampens the effect of arterial hypotension or decreased cardiac output on the total hepatic blood flow. Nonetheless, marked and/or prolonged decreases in cardiac output or shock may lead to ischemic hepatic injury. Heart failure associated with arterial hypotension primarily affects arterial blood flow and oxygen delivery to the liver. If severe, this can lead to hepatocellular necrosis and prominent, at times towering, elevation in serum levels of liver-derived aminotransferases. Acute hepatic ischemic injury frequently occurs without affecting hepatic function or causing permanent liver damage. Less severe but chronic hepatic ischemia may exhibit mild to moderate elevations of aminotransferase levels but may lead to progressive hepatic fibrosis. Acute or chronic congestive heart causes elevated pressures in the vena cava and hepatic veins leading to passive hepatic congestion, ascites formation, and eventually the development of cirrhosis. Hepatic injury caused by circulatory failure may exhibit a broad array of biochemical, histologic, and pathophysiologic features.

This chapter discusses liver injury related to acute ischemia, passive hepatic congestion, ischemic cholangiopathy, hepatic infarction, obstruction to the venous outflow of the liver, and heatstroke. Liver cells may also be injured, as reflected by abnormal liver chemistries, by many other disorders affecting hepatic blood flow such as immunologic diseases and vasculitides, which are discussed in other chapters.

Anatomy and physiology of hepatic blood flow

The hepatic vascular anatomy and physiology of hepatic blood flow is reviewed in detail elsewhere. Certain aspects relevant to circulatory failure are summarized below.

About two thirds of the dual blood supply of the liver enters the organ through the main portal vein. The portal blood is a low-pressure system that contains nutrients absorbed from the intestine, including glucose, amino acids, water-soluble vitamins, and triglycerides; it has a relatively low oxygen content [1]. The remaining one third of the blood flow is derived from the hepatic artery. In contrast, hepatic arterial blood supplies about one third of the hepatic blood flow and is an oxygen-rich high-pressure system. More than half of the oxygen delivered to the liver is supplied by the hepatic artery blood flow, which is also the only blood supply for the entire biliary ductal system. The liver, including the biliary ductal system, is susceptible to ischemic injury due to a reduction in hepatic arterial blood flow. A comparable decrease in portal blood flow is less likely to cause ischemic injury to the liver. Inadvertent ligation of hepatic arterial branches during surgery or the embolization of hepatic arterial branches for treatment of hepatocellular carcinoma (HCC) may lead to hepatic infarction of the segment(s) supplied by the occluded vessel. Arterial hypotension may also result in partial or widespread hepatic infarction. Patients with portal vein thrombosis, in which the only hepatic blood supply is through the hepatic artery, are particularly susceptible to ischemic hepatic injury following a disruption in hepatic arterial blood

flow. This may occur after chemoembolization of HCC or simply with hypotension.

The functional unit of the liver is the hepatic acinus or lobule, a roughly pentagonal-shaped structure with a single central hepatic vein flanked by several portal tracts (Fig. 34.1). Each portal triad contains a small branch of the hepatic artery, portal vein, and one or two bile ducts. Sheets of hepatocytes, one to two cells thick and lined by hepatic sinusoids, extend between the portal triads and central vein. Both the portal and hepatic arterial blood enters the hepatic acinus through the portal tracts (zone 1 of the hepatic acinus in the Rappaport classification) and mixes within the hepatic sinusoids [2]. This admixed portal and arterial blood then flows to the center of the acinus (Rappaport zone 3), and ultimately exits the liver through the major hepatic veins. Therefore, zone 1 of the hepatic acinus contains oxygen- and nutrient-rich blood, and as blood flows through the sinusoids distally, it is progressively depleted of these components. Conversely, the zone 3 pericentral area receives less oxygen, and is more susceptible to ischemic injury.

The portal blood flowing into the liver is a low-pressure and relatively slow system, minimally affected by changes in systemic arterial blood pressure. In contrast, the hepatic arterial blood flow is a high-pressure system closely regulated to maintain a constant total hepatic blood flow (the sum of arterial and portal blood flows) [3]. Adenosine, a potent vasodilator of arterial smooth muscle cells, regulates hepatic arterial blood flow via local synthesis of nitric oxide. As portal blood flow increases, portal triad adenosine levels become diluted, leading to constriction of the hepatic arterioles and a decline in arterial blood flow [4,5]. The response of hepatic

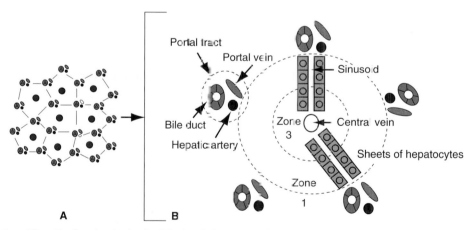

Figure 34.1 (A) A section of liver. The functional subunit of the liver is the hepatic lobule or acinus, a roughly pentagonal-shaped structure with a central vein in the center and portal triads at each corner. Each portal triad is shared by several hepatic lobules. (B) A hepatic lobule or acinus. Each portal triad contains a branch of the hepatic artery, portal vein, and bile duct. Sheets of hepatocytes extend between the central vein and portal triads at the edges of the lobule. Hepatic arterial and portal venous blood enters the acinus through the portal triad and then flows through hepatic sinusoids to the central vein. Zone 1 of the lobule lies at the periphery of the hepatic acinus (outer dashed circle). Zone 3 of the lobule lies in the center of the acinus (inner dashed circle).

arterial smooth muscle to adenosine is not impaired in patients with cirrhosis.

Ischemic hepatic injury

Ischemic hepatic injury, previously termed ischemic hepatitis, is caused by reduced oxygen delivery leading to hepatocellular dysfunction and necrosis [6–10]. This form of hepatic injury is most often seen in the setting of severe arterial hypotension leading to global hepatic hypoperfusion. The most common causes of ischemic hepatic injury are shown on Box 34.1. Events that cause abrupt and severe acute reductions in cardiac output (for instance, massive myocardial infarction, pulmonary embolus, or congestive heart failure) are common causes of ischemic hepatic injury. Hypovolemia from exsanguinating hemorrhage, dehydration, heatstroke, sepsis, or hypoxia associated with respiratory failure may also result in ischemic injury of the liver. The term *shock liver* is sometimes utilized when hepatic ischemic injury develops in the setting of severe hemodynamic instability.

Pathophysiology

The histologic hallmark of ischemic hepatic injury is zone 3 hepatocellular necrosis with little or no inflammatory response. In more severe cases, extensive lobular collapse may be observed (Figs 34.2 and 34.3). Fibrosis is absent unless there is chronic congestion or hypoxia, or an underlying unrelated chronic liver disease. Features of both acute passive congestion and ischemic hepatic injury may be simultaneously present in patients with congestive heart failure experiencing episodic reductions in car-

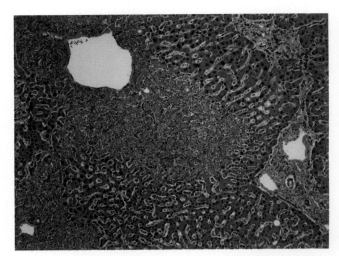

Figure 34.2 The liver in congestive hepatopathy. Zones 3 and 2 show sinusoidal congestion with necrosis of the hepatocytes; in contrast, periportal sinusoids and hepatocytes are spared. Hematoxylin and eosin (H&E), original ×100.

diac output and hypotension. Ischemic hepatic injury often resolves spontaneously following correction of the initial ischemic insult, with hepatocyte regeneration, and a return to normal histology and liver function. However, in patients with chronic passive congestion and fibrosis, these abnormalities remain after resolution of the ischemic hepatic injury.

Clinical features

Most patients with ischemic hepatic injury do not develop signs or symptoms of liver disease such as jaundice, ascites, or encephalopathy, but exhibit changes confined to the liver biochemistries (see below). Patients with ischemic hepatic injury often have changes in mental status but this is rarely due to fulminant liver failure as a

Box 34.1 Causes of ischemic hepatic injury.

Arterial hypotension
- Cardiac failure:
  - Myocardial infarction
  - Pulmonary embolus
  - Exacerbation of congestive heart failure
  - Cor pulmonale
  - Pericardial tamponade
- Hypovolemia:
  - Hemorrhage
  - Dehydration
  - Extensive burns
- Miscellaneous:
  - Septic shock
  - Heatstroke
  - Sickle cell crisis

Hypoxia
- Acute respiratory failure
- Acute exacerbation of chronic respiratory disease
- Obstructive sleep apnea

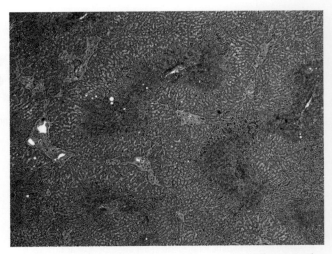

Figure 34.3 Zonal distribution of sinusoidal congestion and necrosis of hepatocytes in congestive heart failure. H&E, original ×40.

result of the ischemia. In a large prospective series, acute liver failure due to ischemic hepatic injury represented a very small proportion of cases (6%) [11]. Thus, true hepatic encephalopathy and associated hyperammonemia is uncommon in ischemic hepatic injury. In most cases, it is likely that the mental changes are related to the acute hypotensive event and hemodynamic derangements leading to cerebral hypoperfusion.

An abrupt elevation in serum levels of alanine aminotransferase (ALT), aspartate aminotransferase (AST), and lactate dehydrogenase (LDH) is the biochemical hallmark of ischemic hepatic injury. These enzymes, released from ischemic hepatocellular necrosis, generally peak 1–3 days following the ischemic insult (for instance, an episode of severe hypotension (Figs 34.2 and 34.3)). Patients with ischemic hepatic ischemic injury are often hospitalized and/or acutely ill. Given the greater abundance of ALT in hepatocytes, this aminotransferase generally exhibits higher serum levels than AST. When AST is the dominant aminotransferase elevation following ischemia, additional sources (extrahepatic) of AST and organ damage should be suspected, such as muscle, cardiac, brain, or hemolysis. In fact, ischemic hepatic injury is frequently associated with hypoxic or hypotensive injury to other organs, particularly the kidneys, as reflected by a rise in serum creatinine and other signs of acute kidney injury. Serum aminotransferase levels typically peak in the range of 500 to 5,000 IU/L and the values often rapidly improve and return to normal within a few days provided the initial hypotensive event has resolved. Serum bilirubin level may remain normal or begin to rise 2–5 days after the elevation of aminotransferases, peaking 5–10 days after the maximum rise in aminotransferase levels (Fig. 34.4). The extent of serum bilirubin elevation is quite variable as it depends not only on the severity of the inciting event but also on the use of blood transfusions for resuscitation, associated hemolysis, and the presence of any underlying chronic liver disease. Serum alkaline phosphates may remain normal or increase to a moderate extent. The prothrombin time, expressed as the international normalized ratio (INR), generally remains normal, but in severe ischemic hepatic injury mild to moderate prolongation in INR may be observed. Serum ammonia is often elevated in these gravely ill patients with multiorgan failure but it is generally associated with a hypercatabolic state rather than acute hepatic failure.

The rapid rise in serum aminotranferase levels brings up the differential diagnosis of acute viral or nonviral hepatitis. However, the abrupt rise and fall in AST and ALT levels typical of ischemic hepatic injury is highly uncommon in acute viral hepatitis. Furthermore, in the later aminotransferase levels gradually return to normal over several weeks rather than days. The systemic viremic syndrome (nausea, vomiting, anorexia, malaise, low-grade fever, and/or right upper quadrant discomfort), is absent in patients with hepatic ischemic injury. Nonetheless, acute hepatitis A, B, and C virus should be routinely excluded in patients with rapidly raising aminotransferases by the corresponding serologies. Inadvertent acetaminophen overdose is also an important differential diagnosis to keep in mind; the medical history and careful review of administered medications are key elements to identify this etiology. In the appropriate setting, causes of nonviral acute hepatitis such as Wilson disease and autoimmune hepatitis should be screened for as well.

The hypotensive event leading to hepatic ischemic injury is often readily apparent, but occasionally a transient or inapparent hypotensive event may lead to hepatic ischemia presenting as acute liver injury of unclear etiology. This scenario may be seen in patients with cirrhosis in whom hepatic blood flow is more dependent on hepatic arterial flow than under normal circumstances. Ischemic hepatic injury superimposed on cirrhosis may lead to lesser aminotransferase elevations and to an acute-on-chronic episode of liver failure associated with a mortality greater than 60% (see below). Likewise, in patients with chronic right or left heart failure, the liver is also more sensitive to changes in hepatic arterial blood flow caused by systemic arterial hypotension. Ischemic hepatic injury may occur in patients with hypoxic conditions including acute respiratory failure, decompensated chronic obstructive pulmonary disease (COPD), or sleep apnea in the absence of arterial hypotension [6–10].

The severity and prognosis of ischemic hepatic injury is related to the precipitating hypotensive or hypoxic event. If the episode of hypotension and/or hypoxia is brief and promptly reversed, the hepatic ischemic damage fully and rapidly resolves in most cases. In contrast, if hypotension is extremely severe or persistent, the ischemic hepatic injury eventually becomes part of irreversible multiorgan failure. Patients with chronic congestive heart

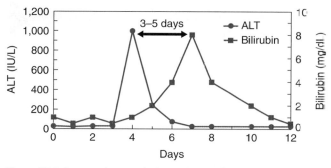

Figure 34.4 Pattern of serum alanine aminotransferase (ALT) and bilirubin level variation in patients with ischemic hepatitis. There is an abrupt and marked rise in serum aspartate aminotransferase (AST) (not shown) and ALT levels to values of 200–1,000 IU/L. This is followed by a delayed rise in serum bilirubin level, which usually reaches a maximum 3–5 days after the peak in serum AST and ALT levels.

failure associated with passive hepatic congestion or cirrhosis are at risk of developing liver failure due to episodic hypotension or hypoxia.

The management of ischemic hepatic injury consists of restoring hepatic blood perfusion by promptly and effectively correcting the arterial hypotension and hypoxia. No specific drugs or agents promoting hepatic recovery from ischemia are available.

Hepatic ischemia in the patient with cirrhosis

The circulatory system is compromised in patients with cirrhosis in parallel with the severity of the liver dysfunction. A hyperdynamic circulatory state with relative arterial hypotension, peripheral arterial vasodilatation, and pooling of blood in the mesenteric splanchnic territory are characteristic of advanced cirrhosis. To compensate for the increased intrahepatic resistance to portal vein inflow, there is often enlargement of the hepatic artery with a resulting greater proportion of arterial blood flow to the liver. This may lead to increased susceptibility of the cirrhotic liver to changes in systemic arterial blood pressure [12,13]. Thus, sepsis, general anesthesia, dehydration, hemorrhage, and other hypovolemic states may be followed by decompensation of the cirrhosis in a previously well-compensated patient. This is one of the mechanisms involved in the development of acute-on-chronic liver failure (AOCLF). Maintenance of adequate hepatic perfusion is, therefore, of paramount importance in preventing ischemic injury to the cirrhotic liver. The prevention of hepatic ischemic injury is important in patients with cirrhosis undergoing surgery under general anesthesia, in whom efforts should be made to avoid intraoperative arterial hypotension. Certain therapeutic agents such as β-blockers are commonly used in cirrhosis in the prophylaxis of esophagogastric variceal hemorrhage [14]. However, these agents may induce a decrease in cardiac output and additional hypotension, which may be deleterious in the setting of cirrhosis. For instance, β-blockers may not be safe in patients with the hepatorenal syndrome [15]. Moreover, a recent study found an increased mortality of patients with refractory ascites who were concomitantly treated with β-blockers [16]. Further work is necessary to ascertain the safety of hemodynamic active therapeutic agents in patients with cirrhosis.

Hepatic infarction

Hepatic infarction refers to a focal area of ischemic injury caused by a disruption in blood flow to a specific branch of the hepatic artery. Less often, a hepatic infarct can originate from hepatic or portal vein compromise. Unlike the lesions observed in ischemic hepatic injury, hepatic infarction is not usually reversible. Fortunately, the liver's dual blood supply makes this condition uncommon as the hepatocytes can augment their portal venous oxygen extraction during periods of hepatic arterial ischemia. However, the diagnosis of hepatic infarction may be on the rise as the result of more frequent use of computed tomography (CT) scans after interventional abdominal procedures.

Hepatic infarction generally occurs in three settings: iatrogenic injury, particularly after surgical or vascular interventions; secondary to a predisposing underlying disease; or related to an acute vascular event. The most common etiologies are detailed in Box 34.2.

Hepatic artery thrombosis complicates 2–6% of all liver transplants, and may result in hepatic infarction within the liver allograft [17]. Local ablative therapies for HCC and other liver lesions are risk factors for hepatic infarction, with an estimated incidence of 1.8% in patients undergoing radiofrequency ablation and 0.15% in patients after chemoembolization for HCC [18,19]. It occurs postoperatively in approximately 1% of all pancreaticobiliary surgeries, typically as a result of hepatic artery injury during lymph node dissection, inadvertent right hepatic artery ligation, or prolonged clamp time on the hepatic artery. Hepatic artery injury, particularly right hepatic artery, can also occur during cholecystectomy. Hepatic infarction has also been reported in

---

Box 34.2 Common etiologies for hepatic infarction.

Iatrogenic
- Liver transplantation
- Pancreaticobiliary surgery
- Cholecystectomy
- Embolization in acute GI bleeding
- Local ablative therapies for liver masses
- TIPS placement

Underlying disease
- Systemic lupus erythematosus
- Hypercoagulable states
- Polycythemia vera
- Vasculitis
- Sickle cell disease
- Hepatocellular carcinoma

Acute vascular injury
- Aortic dissection
- Septic emboli
- Cocaine
- Preeclampsia/HELLP syndrome in pregnancy
- Necrotizing pancreatitis

GI, gastrointestinal; HELLP, hemolysis, elevated liver enzymes, and low platelets; TIPS, transjugular intrahepatic portosystemic shunt.

association with embolization for acute gastrointestinal hemorrhage, aortic dissection, septic emboli, systemic lupus erythematosus, sickle cell disease, preeclampsia, and the HELLP syndrome (hemolysis, elevated liver enzymes, and low platelets) with or without coexisting antiphospholipid antibody syndrome, thrombotic angiitis, polyarteritis nodosa, necrotizing pancreatitis, and cocaine-induced hepatic artery vasospasm.

While most hepatic infarctions are the result of hepatic arterial impairment, they can also rarely occur in the setting of hepatic venous disease such as HCC itself invading the hepatic veins causing severe congestion and subsequent ischemia, or in combination with portal vein thrombosis in polycythemia vera and other procoagulative conditions. Hepatic infarction has also been reported in the Budd–Chiari syndrome and after transjugular intrahepatic portosystemic shunt (TIPS) placement [20–23].

The diagnosis of a large hepatic infarction should be suspected in patients with increasing serum aminotransferases, right upper quadrant abdominal pain, fever, nausea, vomiting, right shoulder pain following abdominal interventional procedures, or the presence of risk factors detailed above. Some patients may be asymptomatic and diagnosed incidentally during a postoperative CT scan or imaging for another condition. Serum aminotransferases may rise to the 500–1000 IU/L range and leukocytosis is also common. Acute liver failure may develop if the infarct is large, or if a major arterial branch is involved. A CT scan typically identifies hepatic infarction as a low attenuation, segmental lesion, which is often peripheral and wedge-shaped, but may also be rounded or oval. The shape can evolve over time to be more rounded or to contain liquefaction. Contrast images may discover the culprit vessel, as well, or detect infarcts in other organs suggestive of embolic disease. More than 30% of patients have more than one site of infarction on CT scan at presentation. Ultrasound is excellent to examine for hepatic artery thrombosis, but not very sensitive in distinguishing infarctions. Magnetic resonance imaging (MRI) can also be used to detect infarction, on which it will have low T1 signal intensity and may show increased T2 signal intensity. An involved vessel may also be seen on MRI or magnetic resonance angiography. The diagnosis can be made clinically with confirmatory imaging. A liver biopsy is not necessary unless the diagnosis is not evident or the patient has an ambiguous clinical presentation. If a liver biopsy is performed, areas of coagulative necrosis involving all three zones of the hepatic lobule surrounded by inflammation may be observed. This lesion is then itself surrounded by a zone of partial necrosis. The involvement of all three zones is characteristically different from the histologic pattern of ischemic hepatic injury, which is typically limited to zone 3.

The management of hepatic infarction is usually supportive. Infarcted areas heal over time with scar formation and parenchymal atrophy. Prostaglandin E1, hemodialysis, corticosteroids, and plasma exchange have all been tried in the acute setting with some presumed success, albeit this evidence is limited to a few case reports. Since abscess formation is common in large infarcted areas, broad spectrum systemic antibiotics may be used empirically. The presence of gas inside the infarct on CT is highly suspicious for abscess formation. Needle aspiration and drainage should be performed in situations where abscess is suspected and antibiotics initiated without delay until cultures return. For patients in whom the etiology of hepatic infarction is obvious, i.e., postsurgery or postembolization, no further workup is necessary after the patient has recovered. In patients with systemic disorders such as antiphospholipid antibody syndrome or polycythemia vera, treatment specific to those disorders should be implemented as well. In post-liver transplant recipients, retransplantation may be necessary if the infarction is extensive and occurs soon after transplantation. Retransplantation improves short-term survival, and 5-year survival is similar to patients who underwent a single liver transplant. In patients whose etiology for hepatic infarction remains obscure, a hypercoagulable state evaluation and infectious workup to exclude septic emboli are recommended.

Congestive hepatopathy

Hepatic congestion develops in patients with significant and persistent elevations in hepatic veins and right atrial pressure caused by heart failure [24–27]. The main etiologies of heart disease leading to heart failure and hepatic congestion are shown in Box 34.3. The elevated intracardiac pressures lead to increased central venous pressure, which is transmitted to the hepatic veins, into the central veins of the hepatic acinus, and ultimately into the hepatic sinusoids. Congestive hepatopathy causes characteristic histologic changes (Figs 34.3 and 34.5).

Box 34.3 Causes of congestive hepatopathy.

- Cardiomyopathies
- Tricuspid insufficiency
- Myocardial infarction
- Pulmonary hypertension
- Cor pulmonale
- Mitral stenosis
- Constrictive pericarditis
- Pericardial tamponade
- Pulmonary embolus
- Congenital heart disease

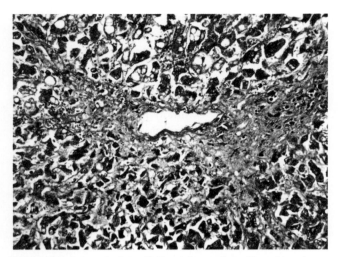

Figure 34.5 Perivenular (zone 3) fibrosis in a patient with prolonged hepatic congestion due to chronic congestive heart failure. Masson trichrome stain, original ×200. (Courtesy of Dr Rebecca Thomas, Director of Pathology and Clinical Laboratories, Temple University Hospital and School of Medicine.)

Chronic hepatic congestion ultimately leads to hepatic fibrosis, including bridging fibrosis and eventually "cardiac" cirrhosis [24–26]. In contrast to cirrhosis resulting from chronic active hepatitis, the bridges of fibrosis in cardiac cirrhosis connect the central veins to other central veins. In some cases, exuberant regeneration of the periportal hepatocytes may lead to the formation of noncirrhotic nodules known as nodular regenerative hyperplasia.

Prolonged passive congestion may lead to sinusoidal fibrosis, which may impair oxygen delivery to zone 3 hepatocytes, increasing their susceptibility to hypoxic injury. Furthermore, the elevated venous pressure causes enlargement of the sinusoidal fenestrae. In the setting of hepatic congestion, the passage of protein-rich fluid into the subendothelial space of Disse may cause the formation of ascites, yielding a low serum–ascites albumin gradient (SAAG) in the absence of portal hypertension. Once fibrosis and cardiac cirrhosis develop, the ascites protein content diminishes and the SAAG may increase above 1.0.

Patients with congestive hepatopathy may be asymptomatic and have only mild abnormalities in serum liver biochemical tests, including total and indirect bilirubin, and a modestly prolonged INR. In severe cases, right upper quadrant pain or discomfort and new-onset ascites may occur. Occasionally, the evidence of heart failure may not be obvious and the patient may be initially thought to have ascites due to cryptogenic cirrhosis.

The classic physical findings of right heart failure and congestive hepatopathy include jugular venous distension, pulsatile hepatomegaly, and hepatojugular reflex. Hepatic ultrasonography may reveal echogenic hepatomegaly. Enlarged hepatic veins and a reversal of flow may be detected by Doppler ultrasonography. CT scans and MRI may show a heterogeneous appearance of the liver consistent with the characteristic "nutmeg" macroscopic aspect of the congested liver.

If a liver biopsy is obtained because of diagnostic doubts, the transjugular route is preferred since the hepatic venous pressure gradient (HVPG) can be simultaneously determined to ascertain the role of the passive congestion, the existence of cirrhosis, and/or an independent liver disorder.

The management of congestive hepatopathy consists of therapy of the underlying congestive heart failure, which in turns depends on its specific etiology. Successful control of the heart failure improves the liver biochemical abnormalities and helps with ascites resolution. Prudent use of diuretics and occasional paracentesis may be necessary for symptomatic therapy of severe ascites. In contrast to noncardiac cirrhosis, the use of TIPS is contraindicated in the management of ascites caused by congestive hepatopathy. The increased preload on the heart brought about by TIPS installation may be excessive for these patients with heart failure. Patients with congestive hepatopathy may be unusually sensitive to warfarin (Coumadin®) and the INR may increase substantially on very low doses of warfarin. Additionally, the slower hepatic drug metabolism in congestive hepatopathy may lead to higher therapeutic drug levels and a lower threshold for toxicity.

The prognosis of patients with congestive hepatopathy is related to the severity of the underlying cardiac disease [24].

Hepatic outflow obstruction

Hepatic venous outflow obstruction may result in significant histologic changes and liver injury as a result of impaired drainage of blood from the liver [22,23,28,29]. Venoocclusive disease (sinusoidal obstruction syndrome, SOS) and the Budd–Chiari syndrome are examples of conditions limiting the hepatic venous outflow. SOS was initially described in a patient who ingested a drink that contained pyrrolizidine alkaloids. However, SOS may also develop in patients soon after hematopoietic stem cell transplantation, or after chemotherapy, abdominal radiotherapy, and liver or kidney transplantation. Common presenting symptoms include tender hepatomegaly, ascites, weight gain, and jaundice. The mechanism of injury is direct toxicity to the sinusoidal endothelial cells and loss of fenestration of the endothelial cell membrane. This damage allows red blood cells to penetrate into the space of Disse allowing the sinusoidal lining cells to slough and embolize downstream, obstructing sinusoidal blood flow. Early histologic changes include damage to the sinusoidal endothelial cell predominantly in the perivenular area (zone 3 of the liver acinus).

Subendothelial edema leads to sinusoidal congestion and hepatocellular necrosis. The endothelial injury to both the sinusoids and small hepatic venules may cause activation of the coagulation cascade and the formation of thrombi. These abnormalities cause an intrahepatic form of postsinusoidal portal hypertension and the clinical manifestations of hepatomegaly, weight gain, and ascites. Progression of venular collagen deposition ensues, ultimately leading to widespread hepatic fibrosis [22,23,28,29].

In the Budd–Chiari syndrome there is thrombotic or nonthrombotic hepatic outflow obstruction at the level of the hepatic venules, large hepatic veins, or the inferior vena cava at the junction of the right atrium [22]. Decompression via a "spider web" of collateral veins around the area of obstruction facilitates the diagnosis by a typical appearance on the hepatic venogram. The caudate lobe outflow is often not involved by the occlusive process, given its veins directly drain into the inferior retrohepatic vena cava. Sinusoidal congestion, portal vein hypertension, and reduced portal vein flow are the hemodynamic consequences of hepatic vein outflow obstruction. Indeed, a patent portal vein in Budd–Chiari syndrome may show a reversal of flow (away from the liver: hepatofugal) and may become the outflow tract from the liver. In cases of severe prothrombotic diathesis, the portal vein may also become occluded. The absence of any outflow tract leads to a particularly severe form of Budd–Chiari syndrome, with marked elevation of the serum aminotransferases and often acute liver failure.

Ischemic cholangiopathy

In contrast to the dual blood supply of the liver parenchyma, the biliary ductal system receives its entire blood supply through the hepatic artery alone [30]. The bile ducts are, in fact, the intended target of approximately 50% of the blood flowing through the hepatic artery. As such, the bile ducts are susceptible to ischemic injury (termed ischemic cholangiopathy (IC)) if the hepatic arterial flow is compromised [31,32]. This can occur in the setting of ischemic hepatic injury but, more commonly, it occurs as an isolated phenomenon and spares the parenchymal liver cells.

Understanding the anatomy of the biliary arterial supply helps to predict where IC is most likely to occur. The intrahepatic branches of the hepatic artery course nearby the ducts, terminating in the peribiliary plexus (PBP). This plexus is composed of an inner capillary layer and an outer vascular layer, which is intimately connected to the intrahepatic portal venules. The PBP is responsible for the blood supply to the proximal and mid common bile duct (CBD), the biliary hilum, as well as smaller bile duct branches. Thus, an ischemic condition of the PBP may preferentially cause IC of the mid to

proximal CBD, biliary hilum, and intrahepatic bile duct branches. The distal CBD, however, may be spared, as it receives substantial blood supply from small branches off the gastroduodenal artery.

The transplanted liver is more susceptible to IC than the native liver as transcapsular peripheral arteries are severed during the transplantation procedure, reducing the ability to utilize collateral blood flow.

Isolated IC is often iatrogenic. It commonly occurs after liver transplantation, particularly in recipients of organs procured after cardiac death where the incidence may be greater than 30%. Common conditions associated with isolated IC are outlined in Box 34.4. Other conditions implicated in IC include polyarteritis nodosa, hypercoagulable states such as paroxysmal nocturnal hemoglobinuria, atherosclerosis, cholesterol crystal embolization after cardiac catheterization, sickle cell disease, and hereditary hemorrhagic telangiectasia.

In post-liver transplant recipients, IC is the most common cause of nonanastomotic biliary strictures [33–35]. Early hepatic artery thrombosis can cause severe stricturing and some patients may eventually require retransplantation. Prolonged cold ischemia time, reperfusion injury, cytomegalovirus infection, and rejection all predispose patients to IC by increasing the likelihood of PBP damage. Approximately one third of liver recipients who develop IC may require retransplantation. The use of a transcystic tube and histidine tryptophan ketoglutarate preservation solution may decrease the risk of nonanastomotic biliary strictures in transplanted patients.

Patients with IC may present with symptoms of biliary obstruction including jaundice, dark urine, abdominal pain, and pruritus. Some patients are asymptomatic but have abnormal liver biochemical tests with a subsequent discovery of a new biliary stricture – the hallmark lesion of IC. A cholestatic biochemical pattern is typical. The most common location for an IC-related biliary stricture is in the mid CBD, followed by the hilum, and then the intrahepatic bile ducts. Less frequently, hepatic abscess or cholangitis may lead to the diagnosis of IC. Secondary sclerosing cholangitis can develop in intensive care patients with secondary bacteremia and biliary cast formation, leading to high morbidity.

Liver biopsy is generally not helpful in IC. The injury occurs in the medium to large ducts, while biopsy typically examines more peripheral, smaller branches of the bile ducts. When histology is available, the pathology is often consistent with biliary obstruction, including bile ductular proliferation, portal tract edema, and mixed inflammatory infiltrates. In more severe cases, hepatocellular ballooning and necrosis may be present, along with Kupffer cell hyperplasia and hypertrophy.

Patients suspected of having IC should have imaging to help confirm the diagnosis and treat the stricture. One must consider the etiology of the IC and the management of IC separately from an imaging standpoint. To determine the etiology, the first test should be a duplex ultrasound of the liver, which can effectively detect hepatic artery thrombosis. In suspected cases of hepatic artery thrombosis not confirmed by ultrasound, CT angiography or conventional angiography can be diagnostic. If the patient is nontransplant, has no hepatic artery thrombosis, and there is no obvious cause from the patient history for the IC, a hypercoagulable workup, human immunodeficiency virus (HIV) testing, and vasculitis workup are reasonable next steps.

Treatment depends on the inciting etiology. If hepatic artery thrombosis occurs in the first month after transplant, urgent retransplantation is often necessary. For hepatic artery thrombosis occurring later after transplantation, revascularization procedures including thrombolysis, thrombectomy, stent placement, or surgical repair may be required. The available data are mixed as to whether revascularization improves graft or patient survival [33–35].

The management of IC is generally based on the stricture(s) location. Cholangiography, either by magnetic resonance cholangiopancreatography (MRCP) or percutaneous cholangiogram, should be used to precisely determine the site of stricture and define the anatomy. The strictures can be long and often multiple, resembling primary sclerosing cholangitis or cholangiocarcinoma. Endoscopic retrograde cholangiopancreatography (ERCP) can provide long-term successful stricture management in 50–75% of post-transplant cases via the extraction of debris/casts, dilatation, and stent placement. Insufficient data exist regarding the success of endoscopic management of IC-related strictures in nontransplant patients. Surgical revision creating a Roux limb is an option for refractory strictures.

Heat stroke and the liver

Heat stroke is the most severe form of heat-related illness, with a mortality of 20–60%. The diagnosis is suspected when neurologic changes develop in the setting of an ele-vated core body temperature (>40°C) and is associated with multisystem organ dysfunction including disseminated intravascular coagulation. The two main variants of heat stroke include exertional heat stroke (EHS) and classic heat stroke (CHS), the latter typically occurring as a result of environmental exposure. The liver is frequently involved in heat stroke, ranging from moderately abnormal liver biochemical tests to the fully developed syndrome of acute (fulminant) liver failure, which occurs in 5–12% of cases [36–39].

The pathophysiology of liver injury in heat stroke is multifactorial. The three major pathways include: (i) a hyperthermia-induced increase in metabolic demands, causing a relatively hypoxic state with circulatory dysfunction; (ii) direct cytotoxic injury from excessive heat; and (iii) activation of systemic inflammatory mediators leading to endothelial cell activation and cytokine release. Arterial hypotension that occurs as part of the multiorgan dysfunction may also cause ischemic hepatic injury.

Macroscopically, the liver in heat stroke has a yellow-brown appearance, with conflicting descriptions of density. Histologically, the presence of extensive centrilobular (zone 3) necrosis without compensatory bile duct proliferation should suggest heat-related liver injury. Microvesicular steatosis is characteristically present in the remaining viable hepatocytes. The distribution of these changes is predominantly centrilobular (zone 3), suggestive of acute hypoxia. Acute nondestructive cholangitis may also be present in up to 20% cases. Histologic changes reverse completely within 4–5 weeks in those who recover.

Serum aminotransferases can be markedly elevated, reaching peak levels 24–48 hours after the development of heat stroke. They are often higher in EHS than CHS, and may reach levels greater than 25 times the upper limit of normal. Whereas aminotransferase recovery is rapid in ischemic hepatic injury, in heat stroke the serum aminotransferases may remain elevated for an average of 2 weeks. Alkaline phosphatase and serum bilirubin are usually not significantly altered, except in severe and fatal cases, where cholestasis can be present. In addition to hyperbilirubinemia, severe hypophosphatemia (<0.5 mmol/L) may be associated with acute liver failure. Lactate and lactate dehydrogenase are frequently significantly elevated in EHS, as well as, but less often, in CHS.

Patients with chronic liver disease may be more susceptible to heat stroke. Alcohol abuse, poor physical conditioning, psychiatric conditions, and diuretic use have all been associated with lowering the threshold for developing heat stroke.

Treatment is mainly supportive. Over half of patients who develop acute liver failure from heat stroke will spontaneously recover. Others may progress to death without urgent liver transplantation. Transplantation, however, is not an option for every patient with acute liver failure; irreversible neurologic injury and sepsis associated with heat stroke may preclude transplantation. There are four reports of patients with heat stroke-induced acute liver failure undergoing liver transplantation, including one allograft from a living donor. However, only one recipient survived 1 year after liver transplantation, underscoring the severity of heat-related liver injury. At present, conservative intensive medical management remains the standard of care. Considerable scrutiny should be used when determining liver transplant candidacy for a patient with acute liver failure due to heat stroke [39].

References

1. Lautt W, Greenway C. Conceptual review of the hepatic vascular bed. *Hepatology* 1987;7:952–63.
2. Rappaport AM. The microcirculatory hepatic unit. *Microvasc Res* 1973;6:212–28.
3. Lautt WW. Mechanism and role of intrinsic regulation of hepatic arterial blood flow: hepatic arterial buffer response. *Am J Physiol* 1985;249:G549–56.
4. Browse DJ, Mathie RT, Benjamin IS, et al. The action of ATP on the hepatic arterial and portal venous vascular networks of the rabbit liver: the role of adenosine. *Eur J Pharmacol* 1997;320:139–44.
5. Smits P, Williams SB, Lipson DE, et al. Endothelial release of nitric oxide contributes to the vasodilator effect of adenosine in humans. *Circulation* 1995;92:2135–41.
6. Seeto R, Fenn B, Rockey DC. Ischemic hepatitis: clinical presentation and pathogenesis. *Am J Med* 2000;109:109–13.
7. Bynum TE, Boitnott JK, Maddrey WC. Ischemic hepatitis. *Dig Dis Sci* 1979;24:129–35.
8. Ebert E. Hypoxic liver injury. *Mayo Clin Proc* 2006;81:1232–6.
9. Birrer R, Takuda Y, Takara T. Hypoxic hepatopathy: pathophysiology and prognosis. *Intern Med* 2007;46:1063–70.
10. Henrion J, Schapira M, Luwaert R, et al. Hypoxic hepatitis: clinical and hemodynamic study in 142 consecutive cases. *Medicine (Baltimore)* 2003;82:392–406.
11. Ostapowicz G, Fontana R, Schiodt F, et al. Results of a prospective study of acute liver failure at 17 tertiary care centers in the United States. *Ann Intern Med* 2002;137;947–54.
12. Zipprich A, Steudel N, Behrmann C, et al. Functional significance of hepatic arterial flow reserve in patients with cirrhosis. *Hepatology* 2003;37:385–92.
13. Henrion J, Colin L, Schmitz A, et al. Ischemic hepatitis in cirrhosis: rare but lethal. *J Clin Gastroenterol* 1993;16:35–9.
14. Garcia-Tsao G, Sanyal A, Grace N, et al. Prevention and management of gastroesophageal varices and variceal hemorrhage in cirrhosis. *Hepatology* 2007;46(3):922–38.
15. Munoz S. The hepatorenal syndrome. *Med Clin North Am* 2008;92:813–37.
16. Serste T, Melot C, Francoz C, et al: Deleterious effects of beta-blockers on survival in patients with cirrhosis and refractory ascites. *Hepatology* 2010;52:1017–22.
17. Tzakis AG, Gordon RD, Shaw BW, et al. Clinical presentation of hepatic artery thrombosis after liver transplantation. *Transplantation* 1985;40:667–71.
18. Cohen SE, Safadi R, Verstandig A, et al. Liver–spleen infarcts following transcatheter chemoembolization. *Dig Dis Sci* 1997;42:938–43.
19. Gates J, Hartnell GG, Stuart KE, et al. Chemoembolization of hepatic neoplasms: safety, complications, and when to worry. *Radiographics* 1999;19:399–414.
20. Mayan H, Kantor R, Rimon U, et al. Fatal liver infarction after transjugular intrahepatic portosystemic shunt procedure. *Liver* 2001;21:361–4.
21. Schmidt SC, Langrehr JM, Hintze RE, et al. Long-term results and risk factors influencing outcome of major bile duct injuries following cholecystectomy. *Br J Surg* 2005;92:76–82.
22. Menon KV, Shah V, Kamath PS. The Budd–Chiari syndrome. *N Engl J Med* 2004;350(6); 578–85.
23. Cazals-Hatem D, Vilgrain V, Genin P, et al. Arterial and portal circulation and parenchymal changes in Budd–Chiari syndrome: a study of 17 explanted livers. *Hepatology* 2003;37(3):510–18.
24. Gelow J, Desai A, Hoichberg C, et al. Clinical predictors of hepatic fibrosis in chronic advanced heart failure. *Circulation: Heart Failure* 2010;3:59–64.
25. Darkhom S, O'Reilly S, Gansukh L, Alfa A. Hepatocellular carcinoma in two patients with cardiac cirrhosis. *Eur J Gastroenterol Hepatol* 2010;22:889–91.
26. Kisloff B, Schaffer G. Fulminant hepatic failure secondary to congestive heart failure. *Am J Dig Dis* 1976;21:895–900.
27. Carez E, Ngoc E, Decoodt P. Fulminant hepatic necrosis resulting from heart failure. *Acta Cardiol* 2009;64:95–7.
28. Bayraktar Y, Bayraktar U, Seren S. Hepatic venous outflow obstruction: three similar syndromes. *World J Gastroenterol* 2007;13(13);1912–27.
29. Senzolo M, Germani G, Cholongitas E, Burra P, Burroughs AK. Veno occlusive disease: update on clinical management. *World J Gastroenterol* 2007;13(29); 3918–24.
30. Takasaki S, Hano H. Three-dimensional observations of the human hepatic artery (arterial system in the liver). *J Hepatol* 2001;34(3) 455–66.
31. Deltenre P, Valla DC. Ischemic cholangiopathy. *Semin Liver Dis* 2008;28(3) 235–46.
32. Chan EY, Olson LC, Kisthard JA, et al. Ischemic cholangiopathy following liver transplantation from donation after cardiac death donors. *Liver Transpl* 2008;14(5):604–10.
33. Welling TH, Heidt DG, Englesbe MJ, et al. Biliary complications following liver transplantation in the model for end-stage liver disease era: effect of donor, recipient, and technical factors. *Liver Transpl* 2008;14(1) 73–80.
34. Gelbmann CM, Rümmele P, Wimmer M, et al. Ischemic-like cholangiopathy with secondary sclerosing cholangitis in critically ill patients. *Am J Gastroenterol* 2007;102(6):1221–9.
35. Warnaar N, Polak W, de Jong K, et al. Long term results of urgent revascularization for hepatic artery thrombosis after pediatric liver transplantation. *Liver Transplant* 2010;16:847–55.
36. Kew M, Bersohn I, Seftel H, et al. Liver damage in heatstroke. *Am J Med* 1970;49:192–202.
37. Hassanein T, Razack A, Gavaler J, et al. Heatstroke: its clinical and pathological presentation with particular attention to the liver. *Am J Gastroenterol* 1992;87:1382–9.
38. Rubel LR, Ishak KG. The liver in fatal exertional heatstroke. *Liver* 1983;3:249–60.
39. Hadad E, Ben-Ari Z, Heled Y, et al. Liver transplantation in exertional heat stroke: a medical dilemma. *Int Care Med* 2004;30:1474–8.

Multiple choice questions

34.1 An abrupt raise in serum aminotransferases with a peak at 1–3 days and a subsequent rapid decline is characteristic of which of the following?

a Acute viral hepatitis.
b Passive hepatic congestion.
c Budd–Chiari syndrome.
d Acute hepatic ischemic injury.
e Portal vein thrombosis.

34.2 The following therapeutic modalities for hepatocellular carcinoma are considered risk factor for hepatic infarction, except for which of the following?

a Radioembolization with yttrium-90.
b Conventional transarterial chemoembolization (TACE).
c Segmental or lobar hepatic resection.
d Sorafenib chemotherapy.
e Radiofrequency ablation.

Answers to the multiple choice questions can be found in the Appendix at the end of the book.

These multiple choice questions are also available for you to complete online.
Visit http://www.schiffsdiseasesoftheliver.com/

PART IX

Benign and Malignant Tumors; Cystic Disorders

CHAPTER 35

Benign Tumors, Nodules, and Cystic Diseases of the Liver

Adrian M. Di Bisceglie & Alex S. Befeler

Division of Gastroenterology and Hepatology, Saint Louis University Liver Center, Saint Louis University School of Medicine, St Louis, MO, USA

Key concepts

- Hepatocellular adenoma is a rare benign neoplasm of the liver, often related to the use of oral contraceptives, that may be complicated by rupture, hemorrhage, and, rarely, development of malignancy.
- Hemangioma of the liver is the second most common benign focal hepatic lesion (simple cyst being the most common one) and the most common *solid* hepatic tumor (1–7.4% of the normal population). It is rarely of significant clinical consequence.
- Dysplastic nodules are defined as a nodular region of hepatocytes that are macroscopically different from surrounding cirrhotic nodules and have a significant risk of developing into hepatocellular carcinoma
- Focal nodular hyperplasia (FNH) is a benign tumor-like lesion of the liver considered to be hyperplastic rather than neoplastic in origin. This lesion is related to an abnormal blood supply and is rarely of clinical significance.
- There is rarely an indication for a surgical intervention in patients with a hemangioma, FNH, or most other benign solid lesions.
- Nodular regenerative hyperplasia is defined by hepatocellular nodules that are distributed throughout the liver in the absence of fibrous

- septae between the nodules. This condition is often associated with systemic diseases and is complicated by portal hypertension.
- Polycystic liver disease (PCLD) is an inherited disease in which multiple cysts develop within the parenchyma of the liver and produce disease from direct mechanical effects of the cysts.
- PCLD is often associated with other related diseases, such as autosomal dominant polycystic kidney disease, whereas the rarer congenital hepatic fibrosis and choledochal cysts may occur in association with autosomal recessive polycystic kidney disease.
- PCLD is usually asymptomatic but can be complicated by the development of abdominal pain, portal hypertension, hepatic venous outflow obstruction, obstructive jaundice, and cyst infection.
- Cystadenoma is a benign tumor of the liver that is hypothesized to arise from congenital defects of the bile ducts or gallbladder. This condition carries a high risk of development of malignancy.
- Echinococcal cysts are related to infection with the parasites *Echinococcus granulosus* and *E. multilocularis* and may affect many organs, including the liver.

Benign focal lesions of the liver are identified with increasing frequency because of the common use of imaging studies of the abdomen. They represent a relatively common reason for referral to the hepatologist or gastroenterologist. Most benign lesions are detected incidentally by imaging studies performed for unrelated reasons. Many of the lesions that present as a focal liver mass are true neoplasms, while others result from reactive proliferation of different cells.

Benign tumors

In general, benign tumors of the liver may arise from hepatocytes, bile duct epithelium, the supporting mesenchymal tissue, or a combination of two or more of these (Box 35.1). In addition to true neoplastic conditions of the

liver, a variety of nodular diseases may occur that resemble, and must therefore be differentiated from, tumors.

Although most patients with benign hepatic tumors are asymptomatic, a minority may present with symptoms that may be local or systemic. In these patients, the relationship between the symptoms and the hepatic lesions may be difficult to correlate, and additional evaluation is necessary to rule out other causes for the patients' complaints. In most cases patients with benign hepatic lesions have no preexisting liver disease, and the finding of a coexisting chronic liver disease such as cirrhosis, chronic hepatitis B or C, or hemochromatosis should raise a suspicion for a malignant tumor. A conclusive diagnosis of a focal hepatic lesion is essential because it may represent a primary or secondary malignancy, which may require immediate treatment. In addition, some benign lesions carry specific risks such as rupture, bleeding, malignant

Schiff's Diseases of the Liver, Eleventh Edition. Edited by Eugene R. Schiff, Willis C. Maddrey and Michael F. Sorrell.
© 2012 John Wiley & Sons, Ltd. Published 2012 by John Wiley & Sons, Ltd.

Box 35.1 Benign solid tumors of the liver.

Epithelial tumors
- Hepatocellular adenoma
- Bile duct adenoma
- Biliary cystadenoma
- Biliary papillomatosis
- Peribiliary gland hamartoma

Mesenchymal tumors
- Hemangioma
- Infantile hemangioendothelioma
- Fibroma
- Angiomyolipoma
- Lipoma
- Lymphangioma
- Mesenchymal hamartoma

Mixed tumors
- Teratoma

Tumor-like lesions
- Focal nodular hyperplasia
- Nodular regenerative hyperplasia
- Mesenchymal hamartoma
- Microhamartoma (von Meyenburg complex)
- Inflammatory pseudotumor
- Focal fatty change
- Pseudolipoma
- Macroregenerative nodule

transformation, consumptive coagulopathy, and disseminated intravascular coagulation. Often the clinical presentation provides important clues to a specific diagnosis and suggests whether the tumor is benign or malignant. Still, in many cases the clinical information and the first imaging study are nondiagnostic and the clinician must choose additional studies from an ever-increasing number of available options. Despite continuing advancement in sensitivity and accuracy, imaging studies fail to yield conclusive diagnosis in a sizable number of patients, and in these cases histopathologic assessment is necessary to characterize the lesion. A tissue sample may be obtained by an ultrasonography or computed tomography (CT)-guided percutaneous liver biopsy or by a laparoscopic liver biopsy. Histopathologic evaluation remains essential in the clinical management of a significant number of tumors or masses in the liver; possible exceptions include hemangioma, focal nodular hyperplasia (FNH), and focal fatty change, which may be unequivocally diagnosed by imaging studies. Unfortunately, in some benign lesions (e.g., hemangioma and hepatic adenoma) liver biopsy carries a high risk of bleeding and is therefore contraindicated. A fundamental knowledge of the various lesions and their characteristic features should help in the differential diagnosis.

Benign tumors of epithelial origin

Hepatocellular adenoma

Epidemiology and risk factors

Hepatocellular adenoma, also termed *liver cell adenoma, hepatic adenoma,* or *telangiectatic adenoma* is a benign tumor of epithelial origin occurring primarily in women of childbearing age. It is considerably less common than hemangioma or FNH, occurring in less than 0.004% of the population at risk. Adenomas may be solitary or multiple and may reach more than 20 cm in size. Hepatocellular adenoma has a very strong association with the oral contraceptive pill (OCP) and other estrogens, though it may rarely occur in the absence of exogenous estrogens and in men. The annual incidence in long-term users of OCPs is to 3–4 per 100,000 compared to 1–1.3 per million in nonusers [1]. The use of OCPs with high hormonal potency, use for more than 5 years, and age over 30 years may further increase the risk [1,2]. However, in 10% of patients diagnosed with hepatocellular adenoma, the exposure to OCPs may be as short as 6–12 months [3]. Other risk factors for hepatocellular adenomas include anabolic-androgen steroids and familial polyposis coli [4,5].

Hepatocellular adenomas (typically multiple lesions) are commonly encountered in association with type I and III glycogen storage diseases [6]; the incidence is 22–75% in type I and 25% in type III [6]. In sharp contrast to hepatocellular adenomas in general, which show a strong female preponderance, those associated with glycogen storage disease show a male predominance [6]. Furthermore, adenomas associated with glycogen storage diseases develop before the age of 20 years.

A condition in which more than ten lesions are present has been termed *liver adenomatosis* [7]. This condition has been reported in men and women in the absence of OCP use or glycogen storage disease [7–9]. It may not be an independent entity and maybe related to germline mutations in hepatocyte nuclear factor 1α (HNF-1α) [8,9]. It is also seen in adenomas with somatic mutations of HNF-1α (see below).

Pathogenesis and genotype/phenotype classification

The pathogenesis of hepatocellular adenoma is still unclear. Hepatocellular adenomas are a heterogeneous group of monoclonal tumors. The strong association with the OCP and pregnancy suggests a possible trophic effect of estrogen on this tumor [10]. Furthermore, regression of adenomas after discontinuation of OCPs is well documented [10,11]. More recently, a genotypic and phenotypic classification for hepatocellular adenoma has been

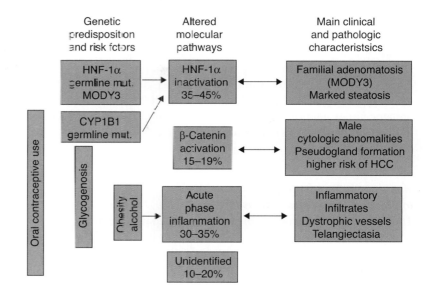

Figure 35.1 Pathogenesis and classification of hepatocellular adenoma. HCC, hepataocellular carcinoma; HNF-1α, hepatocyte nuclear factor 1α; MODY3, mature-onset diabetes of the young. (Adapted from Rebouissou et al. [280] with permission from Elsevier.)

proposed by the Bordeaux group that subdivides hepatocellular adenomas into four groups (Fig. 35.1) [12,13].

Hepatocyte nuclear factor 1α inactivated group

The HNF-1α inactivated group is characterized by biallelic inactivation of the tumor suppressor gene *HNF1A* and represents about 35% of cases [8,13]. HNF-1α is implicated in the regulation of gene expression in the liver associated with hepatocyte differentiation and liver development [8]. Most (approximately 85%) of the mutations in *HNF1A* are somatic, athough heterozygous germline mutations can occur [8]. The germline mutations are associated with mature-onset diabetes of the young (MODY3), which is an autosomal dominant form of non-ketotic diabetes mellitus that usually presents before the age of 25 years. Germline mutations are also associated with a family history of adenomatosis, a syndrome in which there are multiple adenomas, usually more than ten [9].

Grossly, the tumors have irregular lobulated borders with multiple small foci of hepatocellular adenomas surrounding the main tumor mass [12,13]. Pathologically, the adenomas have marked steatosis and a lack of cytologic abnormalities or inflammation [8,12,13]. HNF-1α inactivated hepatocellular adenomas can be recognized on immunohistochemistry by a lack of liver fatty acid-binding protein (LFABP) staining in the tumor compared with the surrounding liver [12]. LFABP is positively regulated by HNF-1α.

Beta-catenin mutations

Beta-catenin mutations are present in about 10% of hepatocellular adenomas and define a separate group for those hepatocellular adenomas that do not have features of the inflammatory group (see below) [13]. β-Catenin is a key molecule in the Wnt signaling pathway and can lead activation of genes that lead to cell proliferation and a variety of cancers including about a third of hepatocellular carcinomas [13].

The hepatocellular adenomas usually have pseudoglandular formation and cytologic abnormalities that may make it difficult to distinguish them histologically from well-differentiated hepatocellular carcinoma [13]. These tumors lack steatosis. β-Catenin staining can be demonstrated by immunohistochemistry, but it is usually patchy and unreliable so staining for glutamine synthetase, an enzyme upregulated by β-catenin, is preferred [13]. These adenomas are more likely to occur in male patients and are associated with male hormone ingestion, glycogen storage disease, and familial adenomatous polyposis [13, 14]. Most importantly, this group is responsible for most of the risk of developing hepatocellular carcinoma from hepatocellular adenoma.

Inflammatory hepatocellular adenoma

Inflammatory hepatocellular adenomas represent about 50% of all hepatic adenomas and include what was previously called telangiectatic focal nodular hyperplasia [12,13,15]. The patients have an inflammatory syndrome with elevated serum C-reative protein (CRP) and often are obese. Inflammatory hepatocellular adenomas appear to have activation of the interleukin 6 (IL6) inflammatory signaling pathway, including signal transducer and activator of transcription 3 (STAT3) [16]. In 60% this activation is due to a mutation in gp130, a co-receptor for IL6 [16].

The tumors have focal inflammatory infiltrates, sinusoidal dilatations, and thick-walled isolated arteries

[12,13]. There can be a variable amount of tumor steatosis, peliosis, and hemorrhage. Inflammatory hepatocellular adenomas can be classified by immunohistochemical staining for the inflammatory proteins, serum amyloid A (SAA), and CRP in the tumor hepatocytes, but not in the surrounding liver [12,13]. About 10% of inflammatory hepatocellular adenomas have a β-catenin mutation and thus are at increased risk for transformation into hepatocellular carcinoma.

Hepatocellular adenomas without genetic or phenotype markers (unclassified)

The tumors in this group represent 5% of hepatocellular adenomas and have no evidence of mutations in *HFNF1A* or β-catenin and have no inflammatory infiltrates [13].

Pathology

Hepatocellular adenoma is usually a large, well-circumscribed, yellow to light-brown tumor. It arises in an otherwise normal liver and a complete or partial capsule is frequently present, although it may occasionally be absent. It is typically solitary but may be multiple, and it ranges in size from 1 to 30 cm [17–19]. Adenomas tend to be larger in women taking OCPs. They occur more commonly in the right lobe and are usually subcapsular, projecting slightly from the surface. Occasionally, they may be pedunculated. Foci of central hemorrhage or necrosis are frequently observed.

Microscopically, this tumor is composed of cells closely resembling normal hepatocytes. They are arranged in plates separated by sinusoids, which may be focally dilated, particularly in the inflammatory group. The plates may be slightly thicker than those in normal liver tissues (more than two cells). β-Catenin mutated hepatocellular adenoma may have a relatively increased nuclear:cytoplasmic ratio, resembling well-differentiated hepatocellular carcinoma (HCC). They may also contain bile-containing acinar structures. A variety of cytoplasmic changes and inclusions can be seen, including Mallory hyaline, lipofuscin, and giant mitochondria. Typically, there are few or no portal tracts or central veins within the adenoma [17–19]. Vascular elements, particularly thick-walled arteries and arterioles, are seen at the periphery of the tumor [17–19]. Peliosis hepatis may also be seen, particularly in the inflammatory group [12].

An absence of Kupffer cells was initially reported in hepatocellular adenoma; however, studies using immunoperoxidase staining for lysozyme demonstrated the presence of Kupffer cells in variable numbers within the adenoma [18,19]. Nevertheless, hepatocellular adenomas usually do not demonstrate the uptake of ^{99m}Tc-sulfur colloid, which is typically taken up by Kupffer cells.

Adenomas are perfused predominantly by peripheral arterial feeders that are unaccompanied by bile ducts. The arterial perfusion and their hypervascular nature, with dilated sinusoids and poor connective tissue support, may explain their tendency to bleed. A percutaneous needle liver biopsy theoretically carries an increased risk of bleeding, but can be performed safely.

Clinical manifestations and complications

Hepatocellular adenoma may present in different ways, and there are conflicting numbers in the literature with regard to the frequency of each type of presentation. In most series, patients presented with abdominal symptoms, usually pain or discomfort in the epigastrium or right upper quadrant [12,14,20]. Typical, the patient is a woman between 20 and 50 years who has a history of more than 5 years of OCP use [21]. More recently, the tumor commonly may be detected as an incidental finding on abdominal imaging study or at surgery. These tend to be the smaller adenomas and are less likely to be associated with OCPs. Presentation can be with severe pain and associated with hypotension in the setting of an acute hemorrhage or rupture [12,14,20]. Liver chemistries are usually normal although serum alkaline phosphatase and γ-glutamyl transpeptidase may be elevated, particularly in patients with bleeding or rupture [14,22].

The general risk of bleeding and rupture appears to be more likely in the inflammatory group and in those patients taking OCPs [12,14,20]. Bleeding is generally limited to larger adenomas, usually >5 cm in diameter [12,14,20]. Mortality may be as high as 6%, but in more recent series is rare [12,14,20,23].

Malignant transformation of hepatocellular adenoma into carcinoma is uncommon but well documented. Unfortunately, there are no observational studies addressing the risk over time of an adenoma transforming into HCC. Most surgical resection series contain 5–8% of cases with associated HCC [12,14,20]. Size is a good predictor of malignancy risk with virtually all reported HCCs occurring in adenomas >5 cm. Multiple adenomas do not appear to confer additional risk of malignancy above the risk associated with size [14]. Transformation from adenoma to carcinoma may occur despite the discontinuation of OCPs [24]. β-Catenin mutations are associated with most HCCs [12,13]. The risk of malignant transformation appears to be significantly higher in men regardless of a β-catenin mutation [12,13]. An enlarging lesion, local or systemic symptoms, progressive abnormalities in liver chemistries, and rising blood levels of α-fetoprotein may all be signs of transformation to HCC.

Imaging studies

- *Ultrasonography* is nonspecific, often showing a well-demarcated mass with smooth borders and variable

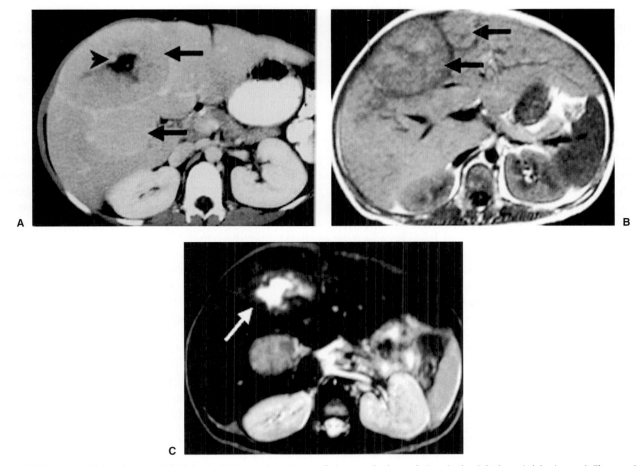

Figure 35.2 Hepatocellular adenoma. (A) Abdominal CT scan shows two well-circumscribed mass lesions in the right-hepatic lobe (arrows). The anterior lesion shows central necrosis (arrowhead). (B) Abdominal MRI (T1-weighted image) of the same patient shows two lesions with slightly decreased intensity and well-defined low-intensity capsule (arrows), which are suggestive of hepatocellular adenoma. (C) T2-weighted image shows a central high signal intensity (arrow), which is consistent with central hemorrhage.

echogenicity [25]. Color and power Doppler and particularly ultrasound with contrast may show vascular flow from the periphery to the center of the lesion (centripetal filling), though these findings are not diagnostic [26].

- *CT scanning* does not provide a diagnostic picture either, although findings on multiphasic contrast-enhanced CT scans can help in suggesting the diagnosis (Fig. 35.2A) [26]. On precontrast images, the adenoma appears as a hypo- or isodense mass, which may show high-density areas, consistent with intratumoral hemorrhage [26]. After contrast injection, in the arterial phase, the mass may show irregular enhancement with areas of normal, increased, and decreased density, which is characteristic for hepatocellular adenoma [27]. In the portal-venous phase, enhancement fades, becomes more uniform, and may be slightly hyperintense to isointense to the surrounding liver. There can be peripheral enhancement due to feeding vessels. On delayed imaging there can be "washout" similar to that

seen with hepatocellular carcinoma (Fig. 35.2A) [26]. In the setting of an acute hemorrhage, the center may be hyperdense in the arterial phase. In the presence of an old hemorrhage, the center usually remains hypodense after contrast injection, making the differential diagnosis from a central scar difficult.

- *Magnetic resonance imaging* (MRI) shows a well-demarcated lesion that on T1-weighted images may show a mildly hypointense to mildly hyperintense signal (Fig. 35.2B) [26]. T2-weighted images show an isointense to slightly hyperintense signal that may be heterogenous because of areas of bleeding. Central necrosis typically appears as low signal intensity on T2-weighted images, whereas a recent hemorrhage may show increased signal on T1 images (Fig. 35.2C). Gadolinium (Gd) enhancement is similar to the pattern described for CT with arterial phase blush followed by a rapid fading in the venous and delayed phases to hypointensity or isointensity, with persistence of an enhancing rim related to the capsule. MRI can identified HNF-1α mutated hepatocellular adenoma with reasonable reliability by demonstrating the combination of diffuse signal dropout on T1-weighted chemical shift due to steatosis, an isointense to slightly hyperintense signal on T2-weighted images, and moderate arterial enhancement without persistent enhancement in portal-venous and delayed phases [28]. Inflammatory hepatocellular adenoma show an absent to slight signal dropout on chemical shift, a marked hyperintense signal on T2, particularly on the edges from sinusoidal dilatations, and strong arterial enhancement with persisting enhancement in the portal-venous and delayed phases [28].

Hepatocyte-selective contrast agents such as Gd-BOPTA (gadobenate dimeglumine) have been shown to improve the differentiation between FNH and adenoma. This contrast agent is selectively taken up by functioning hepatocytes and excreted into the bile. It results in prolonged enhancement of the liver parenchyma. More than 1 hour after contrast injection, almost all FNH lesions appear hyper- or isointense, whereas almost all hepatocellular adenomas are hypointense [26].

- ^{99m}Tc-sulfur colloid scintigraphy may be helpful in the diagnosis of hepatocellular adenoma because it typically shows no uptake of the colloid due to decreased activity of Kupffer cells within the adenoma. This is in contrast to FNH, which shows normal to increased uptake [26].

Diagnosis

In the setting of a person without liver disease or a prior history of cancer, the main differential diagnosis of a mass in the liver is usually between hepatocellular adenoma and FNH. There are no completely reliable radiologic features for the diagnosis of hepatocellular adenoma though some enhancement patterns are suggestive. FNH can be reliably diagnosed, thereby removing hepatocellular adenoma from the differential. A tentative diagnosis of hepatocellular adenoma is usually made in the setting of women aged 20–50 years, with a his-

tory of OCP use, and a typical-appearing focal hepatic lesion or lesions. Although there is considerable overlap in the radiologic features of hepatocellular adenoma and HCC, the latter is usually associated with a background of chronic liver disease, usually with evidence of cirrhosis. In patients with chronic hepatitis B or cirrhosis, any suspicious focal lesion with radiologic features consistent with both HCC and adenoma should be regarded as HCC until proved otherwise. High or increasing serum levels of α-fetoprotein, significant increase in nodule size, abnormal hepatic biochemical test results, and involvement of the portal vein are highly suggestive of HCC. Despite the advances in imaging modalities, the diagnosis often remains uncertain and histologic examination may be necessary. In hepatocellular adenoma, a percutaneous needle liver biopsy may carry an increased but acceptable risk of bleeding, which can be potentially mitigated by a laparoscopic biopsy with direct hemostasis. Historically, needle biopsies have often been nondiagnostic and pathologic review of resected nodules may be needed for definitive diagnosis, though new immunohistochemical staining has improved diagnostic ability. Liver biopsy can reliably categorize hepatic nodules into definite HCC or high-risk hepatocellular adenomas and metastatic lesions. Hepatocellular adenoma is sometimes difficult to differentiate from FNH. The two conditions are compared in Table 35.1.

Management

Classically, surgical treatment is recommended, if possible based on anatomic location of the lesions and co-morbidities to avoid the risks of rupture, hemorrhage, and malignant transformation [29]. More modern series advocate that asymptomatic hepatocellular adenoma that are smaller than 4 or 5 cm in size are unlikely to rupture and bleed and, therefore, should not be resected, but should be followed by periodic imaging studies [12,14,20]. The interval and duration of imaging has not been clearly defined although one group recommends follow-up through menopause [12]. Blood α-fetoprotein levels are often followed, although there is scarce

Feature	Adenoma	Focal nodular hyperplasia
Sex	Female	Female
Oral contraceptive use	Strong association	Questionable
Symptoms	Occasional	Rare
Multiple	12–30%	Approximately 30%
Central arterial scar	No	Yes
Treatment	Resection	Resection only if symptomatic

Adapted from Rodes and Sherlock [279] with permission.

Table 35.1 Comparison of hepatocellular adenoma and focal nodular hyperplasia.

evidence to support the efficacy of this approach [6]. The development of symptoms, increasing size of the nodule, unexplained liver chemistry abnormalities, or rising α-fetoprotein levels should raise the suspicion of malignant transformation and should prompt a surgical intervention to remove the lesion. The data for this approach are stronger for hepatocellular adenoma with imaging and/or biopsy features of the HNF-1α mutated group than for the inflammatory and unclassified group. There are no prospective studies to confirm these recommendations, but there is long-term follow-up in a number of patients with residual hepatocellular adenoma after resection with only rare growth of the tumors requiring treatment [12,14]. Hepatocellular adenoma in men and with β-catenin mutations regardless of size should be resected because of the risk of HCC [12,14,20]. Some have recommended a period of observation after OCPs have been discontinued to assess whether the tumor size decreases or disappears [12]. However, there are rare reports of cancer occurring even in adenomas that have decreased in size or disappeared after the discontinuation of OCPs [24]. The risk : benefit ratio should be assessed for every case and the final decision should be made on an individual basis.

Surgical approaches for hepatocellular adenoma have included enucleation, resection, and liver transplantation. Enucleation is associated with less blood loss and preservation of normal liver tissue [30]. Both resection and enucleation are performed laparoscopically in many centers with excellent results, when technically feasible [12,14,20]. Almost all solitary lesions can be completely resected, but there is often residual hepatocellular adenoma if there were multiple lesions [12,14,20]. The mortality of an elective surgery is about 1%, but it increases to 5–8% for emergency resection [12,14,20,30,31]. Arterial embolization has been used to control bleeding, converting a high-risk emergency resection surgery into a low-risk elective case [14,20]. Embolization can also reduce the tumor size preoperatively, or relieve symptoms in patients with inoperable tumors [20,32–34]. Radiofrequency ablation (RFA) can also be used for small tumors [35]. There is only limited long-term follow-up of patients with hepatocellular adenoma having RFA and embolization as primary treatment for their hepatocellular adenomas.

In rare patients with multiple adenomas, orthotopic liver transplantation (OLT) may be the only way to remove all the lesions, though transplantation is generally reserved for patients with glycogen storage disease [6,36,37]. In type I glycogen storage disease, OLT also corrects the metabolic defect [36,37].

Generally, pregnancy should be avoided to prevent the risk of rapid tumor growth, rupture, and bleeding [38]. One series did have several successful pregnancies with occasional tumor growth but no cases of hemorrhage or rupture in women with a prior incomplete resection [14]. Women who have had hepatocellular adenoma, whether resected or not, should avoid the use of OCPs permanently. In patients with glycogen storage disease, pregnancy is probably safe. In the few reports of patients with glycogen storage disease and hepatocellular adenomas who became pregnant, there was no change in the size or number of the adenomas [39]. This observation supports the notion that the pathogenesis of hepatocellular adenoma in patients with glycogen storage disease may be different from that of adenomas occurring in healthy individuals.

Hepatocellular carcinoma

Hepatocellular carcinoma is a malignant neoplasm of hepatocytes and is described in Chapter 36. HCC has been described as occurring in association with several of the nodular lesions described earlier, including nodular regenerative hyperplasia (NRH), dysplastic nodules, hepatocellular adenoma, and FNH. The link between HCC and NRH or FNH probably involves compromise of blood supply to the liver because of the presence of the malignant tumor, which causes direct pressure or microvascular invasion, whereas dysplastic nodules and adenoma may give rise to HCC.

Intrahepatic bile duct adenoma

Intrahepatic bile duct adenoma is a rare non-neoplastic focal lesion that is usually discovered incidentally. Most cases are reported in men older than 40 years. Typically, it is a solitary subcapsular lesion measuring 0.5–2 cm in size [40]. Microscopically, it consists of numerous, uniform, normal appearing bile duct-like structures that are surrounded by a small amount of fibrous stroma. This lesion is occasionally confused with cholangiocarcinoma or metastatic adenocarcinoma on frozen sections. The distinction should be made by the absence of nuclear hyperchromasia, mitotic activity, and vascular invasion. Bile duct adenoma has also been referred to as peribiliary gland hamartoma [41].

Benign tumors of mesenchymal origin

Hemangioma

Epidemiology

Hemangioma is the most common benign *solid* lesion of the liver. The reported prevalence at autopsy ranges from 0.4% to 7.4% [42]. Among the benign focal hepatic lesions, it is second in prevalence only to simple cysts. Hemangiomas are most often found incidentally and have no major clinical implications. They are more prevalent in women and in the right hepatic lobe; the sex ratio is between 4 : 1 and 6 : 1. Hemangiomas may present at any age but are most common between the third and fifth decades and rare in young children. There is some controversy about the term *cavernous hemangioma*. Whereas some authors use it as a general name for hemangiomas, others use it to describe a stage of development of the lesion [43].

Pathogenesis

Hepatic hemangiomas are congenital vascular malformations. They enlarge by ectasia rather than hyperplasia or hypertrophy and are considered to be hamartomas [44]. They compress, rather than infiltrate, the surrounding liver parenchyma, which results in a dissectible plane between the hemangioma and liver tissue. There is an ongoing controversy about the role of estrogen in their growth. Although most researchers found no association [45], some have reported growth or initial symptoms during pregnancy or in women receiving OCPs [46–48]. These reports suggest that although hemangiomas are unrelated to estrogens in most women, they may play a role in individual cases.

Pathology

On gross examination the hemangioma appears as a dark purple, compressible, spongy lesion (Fig. 35.3A, B) that may replace considerable portions of liver parenchyma

(Fig. 35.3C, D). On microscopic examination, a hemangioma is typically composed of multiple vascular spaces of varying sizes, which are lined by a single layer of endothelial cells and are separated by fibrous septa (Fig. 35.3D). Intraluminal thrombi may be present and may lead to local calcifications. Nevertheless, biopsy is usually unnecessary and may be associated with significant morbidity because of bleeding.

Clinical manifestations

In most cases, hemangiomas are small and asymptomatic. Infrequently, they may grow to a large size, causing pressure or the displacement of adjacent structures. Hemangiomas larger than 4 cm in size have been referred to as *giant hemangiomas* [49]. Large hemangiomas are uncommon; however, they are more likely to cause symptoms. The most common complaints are of abdominal pain or discomfort; while early satiety, nausea, and vomiting may also occur [50,51]. Pain may be intermittent and is likely due to distension of the liver capsule or pressure on adjacent structures. Severe sudden pain may be caused by infarction, necrosis, or bleeding into the hemangioma. Other rare manifestations related to giant hemangiomas include gastric obstruction, obstructive jaundice [52], and symptoms resembling polymyalgia rheumatica [53]. The

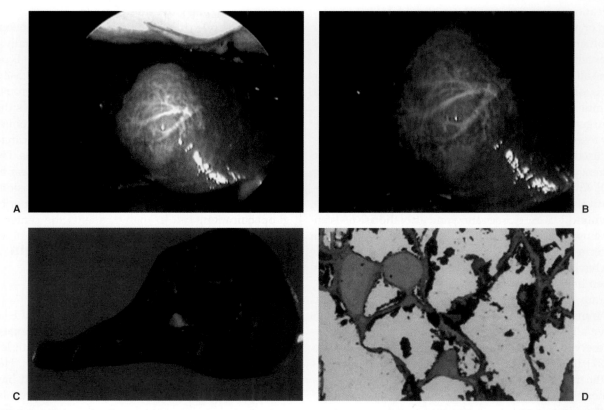

Figure 35.3 Hemangioma. (A, B) Laparoscopic appearance of a giant hemangioma showing a well-circumscribed soft lesion with dark colored areas. (C) A cut surface of a giant hemangioma occupying a large part of the right and left lobes. (D) Histologic examination exhibits numerous dilated vascular channels with thickened, acellular fibrous septa. (Courtesy of Dr P. A. Bejarano, Department of Pathology, University of Miami School of Medicine.)

relationship between symptoms and the hemangioma may be difficult to ascertain, and in many cases other causes are discovered, such as peptic ulcer, gastroesophageal reflux disease (GERD), hernias of the abdominal wall, or tumors of the gastrointestinal tact. In one series of 87 patients with hepatic hemangiomas, 54% of patients were ultimately found to have other causes for their symptoms [54]. In these cases, symptoms may resolve after treatment of the concomitant illness and therapy for the hemangioma is not required.

Physical examination is usually unremarkable. Occasionally, there is abdominal tenderness over the right upper quadrant and a palpable mass may be encountered. Rarely, a bruit may be heard over a large hemangioma.

Hepatic biochemical tests are usually normal and are therefore of little help in the diagnosis of hepatic hemangioma. On rare occasions, serum aminotransferases or alkaline phosphatase level may be mildly elevated. Serum levels of α-fetoprotein and carcinoembryogenic antigen (CEA) are invariably normal.

Complications and natural history

Spontaneous bleeding into a hemangioma, although extremely rare, has been reported [51]. This complication typically presents with abdominal pain in the right upper quadrant and declining hematocrit, in the absence of trauma. The diagnosis is usually made on an abdominal CT scan and in some cases treatment is the removal of the hemangioma by lobectomy or enucleation. Thrombosis within a hemangioma may also present with right abdominal pain and occasionally with fever and an increase of the erythrocyte sedimentation rate [52]. Spontaneous rupture of hepatic hemangiomas is exceedingly rare [54]; however, there are several reports of the rupture of giant hemangiomas of the right lobe after abdominal trauma [55]. A few patients have presented with obstructive jaundice due to pressure on the bile ducts [52,56] or portal hypertension due to pressure on the portal vein [57]. Hemangiomas have rarely been reported to grow rapidly during pregnancy, and after the use of estrogens; however, the effect of pregnancy and estrogens on growth is inconsistent. Rarely, patients with giant hemangiomas may develop consumption coagulopathy within the hemangioma and may present with evidence of disseminated intravascular coagulation (DIC), the so-called Kasabach–Merritt syndrome [46,51,58], which typically occurs in infants. The pathogenesis is likely platelet trapping in the hemangioma that leads to activation of the clotting cascade and consumption of both platelet and clotting factors.

Despite rare reports of complications, the long-term clinical course of most hepatic hemangiomas is benign [59], and most patients will never experience symptoms. When followed up for periods of 15–20 years, most patients remained asymptomatic and showed no significant changes in quality of life [44,60]. In one of the largest series, 158 hemangiomas in 123 subjects were followed up for 12–60 months. No complications were observed during the follow-up period. Only one patient developed new symptoms, and only one hemangioma showed a significant change in size [61].

Imaging studies

- The typical *ultrasonographic* appearance of a hemangioma is of an echogenic, well-demarcated homogenous lesion with well-defined borders, although approximately 20–30% of patients may present with an atypical sonographic appearance. Posterior acoustic enhancement is a common feature. Doppler does not usually detect flow within the hemangioma because of the slow blood flow [62]. Larger hemangiomas are more heterogenous and occasionally contain central fibrosis due to a previous hemorrhage. These usually require further imaging studies. A characteristic radiographic feature of hemangiomas with contrast-enhanced imaging is slow centripetal filling of the lesion by the contrast agent. This may be demonstrated by dynamic CT imaging, contrast-enhanced harmonic ultrasonography or multiphasic MRI [63,64].

- *Dynamic CT scans* offer a few advantages over ultrasonography in the diagnosis of hepatic hemangioma and are often performed to verify the diagnosis suggested by the ultrasonography. On CT prior to the administration of intravenous contrast, the typical appearance is that of a well-defined hypodense lesion (Fig. 35.4). Serial images in the arterial phase of contrast administration show early peripheral enhancement with subsequent progressive globular centripetal filling [65]. Globular enhancement in the arterial phase represents venous lakes within the hemangioma and may be seen in 94% of large lesions. It usually takes about 3 minutes for complete opacification of the lesion to occur; however, it may take 10–15 minutes to complete opacification, and in many patients the center of the lesion may remain hypodense because of a central hemorrhage or fibrosis [66]. Smaller lesions generally fill more rapidly and larger lesions are more likely to show slower central filling. Large hemangiomas (>4 cm) typically develop central areas that fail to fill in on the delayed enhanced images. The center of the hemangioma is more likely to remain hypodense as the size increases. The contrast agent classically remains within the hemangioma for a long time (as long as 60 minutes) after the injection. Occasionally, calcifications may be seen within a large hemangioma. The diagnostic sensitivity and specificity of dynamic CT scan are more than 90% in lesions larger than 2 cm in size, but are significantly lower in smaller lesions [66,67].

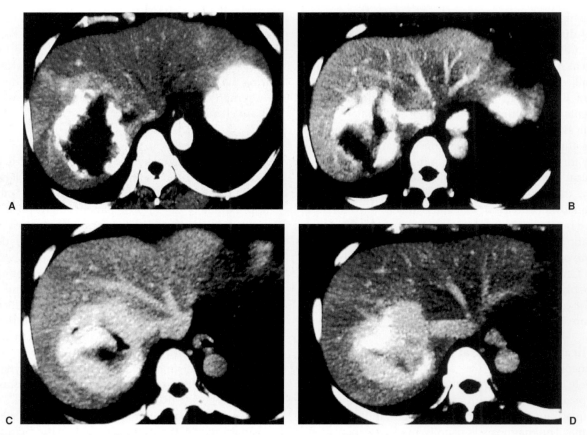

Figure 35.4 Hepatic hemangioma. Dynamic, contrast-enhanced computed tomography (CT) scan demonstrates globular peripheral enhancement with gradual diffusion of the contrast from the periphery to the center of the lesion: (A) 40 seconds, (B) 60 seconds, (C) 90 seconds, and (D) 120 seconds after intravenous contrast injection.

- *MRI* shows a high degree of sensitivity and specificity (both >90%) in the diagnosis of hemangioma and is generally considered to be superior to CT scan for this purpose [68,69]. It has a special value for the diagnosis of hemangiomas smaller than 2 cm in size and in patients with contraindications to the use of iodine-based intravenous contrast. A hemangioma usually appears as a well-circumscribed lesion that shows a moderately elevated signal on T2-weighted images and a low signal on T1-weighted images. The increased signal on T2-weighted images is typically less intense than that demonstrated by a simple cyst. Similar to the findings on CT scan, contrast enhancement with gadolinium shows a centripetal nodular filling on the arterial phase, which is considered by many to be a pathognomonic finding. Venous and delayed phases show progressive enlargement and coalescence of the peripheral nodules with variable degree of central filling.
- *^{99m}Tc-pertechnetate-labeled red blood cell (^{99m}Tc-RBC) pool scintigraphy* may occasionally be helpful in controversial cases, but the use of this technique is decreasing in most medical centers. It typically shows initial hypoperfusion during the arterial flow phase followed by a gradual increase in the isotope in the lesion, which

peaks at 30–50 minutes after the injection. Delayed images usually show retention of the tracer, which is typical of hemangioma. ^{99m}Tc-RBC scan has low sensitivity for lesions smaller than 2 cm in size. Single photon emission computed tomography (SPECT) using ^{99m}Tc-RBC has been shown to increase the resolution of planar scintigraphy [70] and has a clear advantage over ultrasonography in differentiating large hepatic hemangiomas from other solid masses [71]. The sensitivity and specificity of ^{99m}Tc-RBC SPECT may be as high as 90–97% in lesions larger than 2 cm in size, which is close to the accuracy of MRI, but the specificity may decrease to 50% in lesions with mixed echoic pattern. ^{99m}Tc-RBC SPECT is best used to clarify a doubtful lesion on CT or to confirm a suspected hemangioma seen as a hyperechoic lesion on ultrasonography.
- *Plain X rays* of the abdomen may show calcification within a hemangioma but are otherwise of little value.
- *Catheter angiography* is rarely used for the diagnosis of hepatic hemangioma. The contrast injected into the common hepatic artery rapidly fills the vascular spaces, creating a "starry night" appearance in the early phase and vascular lakes in later phases, which remain opacified beyond the venous phase (>40 seconds) [72]. The

borders may be irregular but are well defined, and the feeding vessels are typically displaced and curled at the margins of the lesion. Arteriovenous shunting is typically absent and its presence should raise suspicions of HCC. Still, hepatic hemangiomas may show atypical features mimicking HCC such as early fading after arterial enhancement [73], arteriovenous shunting [74], and centrifugal rather than centripetal enhancement pattern [75].

Discrepancy in different imaging studies should therefore warrant further follow-up and evaluation. A combination of ultrasonography, contrast-enhanced CT scan, and ^{99m}Tc-RBC scintigraphy was shown in one study to have a sensitivity of 86%, specificity of 100%, and accuracy of 91% in differentiating hepatic hemangioma from FNH and adenoma in 437 patients [76].

Management

Because most hemangiomas are asymptomatic, rarely enlarge in size or rupture, and have no malignant potential, surgical intervention is rarely indicated. When the diagnosis of hemangioma is conclusive, observation is sufficient and the rare risk of rupture should not be considered as an indication for surgery. Surgical therapy is indicated only in patients with severe symptoms, complications, or inconclusive diagnoses that cannot be resolved with imaging studies. Biopsy should be avoided because of a high risk of bleeding [77]. Overall, surgical resection is indicated in about 2% of diagnosed hemangiomas. This percentage may increase considerably in referral centers because of selection bias. The most common cause for surgical intervention in patients with hemangiomas is the presence of symptoms. The causative relationship between the hemangioma and symptoms should be confirmed and additional tests should be considered to rule out other potential causes such as gastroesophageal reflux disease, peptic ulcer, or gallstones. When symptoms are clearly related to the hemangioma, resolution may be observed in as many as 96% of the patients after surgical treatment. Another major reason for surgery is to exclude the presence of malignancy. In one case series from the Memorial Sloan–Kettering Cancer Center, suspicion or inability to exclude malignancy was the indication in 36% of the patients subjected to surgery [51]. The surgical mortality in experienced centers is zero or nearly zero [51,54,78,79]. Nevertheless, even in specialized centers the frequency of postoperative complications may be as high as 25% [51]. Enucleation is the preferred approach by many groups because it allows the resection of large hemangiomas with less blood loss and preservation of more hepatic parenchyma compared with resection. Enucleation is performed using the interface between the hemangioma and the surrounding normal liver tissue [51,76,80]. Laparoscopy is currently used as the procedure of choice in many centers when the diagnosis is well established.

Although surgical resection remains the main definitive treatment for symptomatic hemangioma, other less effective options are occasionally used. Transarterial embolization has been used for symptomatic lesions [48,49], acute bleeding [81], and consumption coagulopathy [82]. However, there are few data on its long-term efficacy, and the procedure may have to be repeated or may lead to liver abscesses [83]. Transarterial embolization was used preoperatively to decrease blood supply to the hemangioma and improve the safety of the surgery [82]. Hepatic artery ligation [51], radiation therapy [46,84], radiofrequency ablation [85], and liver transplantation [86,87] have been used on rare occasions for unresectable giant hemangiomas. Recurrence has been described after surgical, intra-arterial, and radiation therapy [47,83].

Infantile hemangioendothelioma

Infantile hemangioendothelioma is a tumor derived from vascular endothelial cells, which is the most common benign hepatic tumor in children. It accounts for approximately 12% of all childhood hepatic tumors and for more than 50% of benign tumors of the liver diagnosed in infancy and childhood [88]. It can be solitary (55% of patients) or multiple (45% of patients) and may vary in size from a few millimeters to more than 20 cm. More than 90% are diagnosed before the age of 6 years. The typical presentation is of hepatomegaly, hemangiomas of the skin, and heart failure resulting from massive arteriovenous shunting [89]. In addition to heart failure, this tumor may cause consumption coagulopathy (Kasabach–Merritt syndrome) and obstructive jaundice [90].

Although well circumscribed, this tumor is not encapsulated and often has scattered calcifications. Microscopically, this tumor consists of multiple small vessels lined by plump endothelial cells and surrounded by fibrous stroma. Two types of infantile hemangioendotheliomas exist. The more common, type I, has a prominent endothelium closely related to the portal tract and tends to displace, rather than infiltrate, the liver parenchyma. It consists of small vascular channels lined by flattened or rounded endothelial cells with rare mitotic figures. Extramedullary hematopoiesis may occasionally be seen. Type II lesions are composed of tortuous vascular channels, with endothelial cells proliferating into the adjacent hepatic tissue. They exhibit larger, irregular channels lined by pleomorphic endothelial cells. Differentiation of type II hemangioendothelioma and rare malignant angiosarcoma may be difficult. In many cases, infantile hemangioendothelioma is associated with extrahepatic hemangiomas that may be found in the skin, lung, lymph nodes, pancreas, retroperitoneum, and bone. The most frequently involved site is the skin, where single or multiple lesions may be present. Other associated abnormalities include atrial septal defect, patent ductus arteriosus, myelomeningocele, renal agenesis, and absent common bile duct [90]. Rarely, infantile hemangioendothelioma may undergo transformation to angiosarcoma [91].

The diagnosis is suggested when an infant presents with an enlarged liver, congestive heart failure, and cutaneous hemangiomas.

Ultrasonography usually shows hepatomegaly and solitary or multiple hepatic lesions, which may vary from anechoic to hyperechoic. The unenhanced CT scan demonstrates the lesion as a well-defined hypoattenuating mass, occasionally with calcifications. After contrast injection, the lesion may show enhancement resembling hemangioma and may become isodense on delayed images. Angiography shows dilated, irregular vascular lakes that commonly persist beyond the venous phase. ^{99m}Tc-sulfur colloid scintigraphy shows the lesion as a cold spot because of a lack of Kupffer cells within the tumor.

The prognosis of this lesion is dependent on its size and its effect on the heart function. Spontaneous regression is frequent but death may occur within the first 6 months of life because of cardiac failure or replacement of the normal hepatic parenchyma [92]. The prognosis is usually good if heart failure is managed successfully.

Treatment is dictated by tumor-related symptoms produced by tumor size. Management of congestive heart failure may be sufficient in some cases. If symptoms are not relieved, treatment should be aimed at decreasing the tumor size. Several studies have confirmed the success of steroid therapy [93]. However, failure of some tumors to respond to steroids has led to the use of other drugs such as cyclophosphamide [94] and interferon α2a [95]. Other treatments include hepatic artery ligation, transcatheter endovascular embolization, and radiation therapy [96–98]. Liver transplant is increasingly recognized as a viable treatment modality for infantile hemangioendothelioma when other treatments fail [99].

Epithelioid hemangioendothelioma

This tumor of low-grade malignant potential also has a vascular origin and occurs more frequently in adults. It may spread extensively within the liver and may metastasize beyond the liver.

Mesenchymal hamartoma

Mesenchymal hamartoma is a rare, slow-growing tumor of childhood that comprises approximately 5% of pediatric liver tumors. It has a male predominance and is diagnosed in most cases before the age of 3 years [100, 101], although it has been reported in adults [102]. The tumor is usually a solitary, large (average size of 16 cm), well-demarcated mass with a predilection for the right hepatic lobe. The cut surface shows multiple cysts separated by solid, pink-tan areas. The solid portions have a mixture of hepatic cells and mesenchymal cells with vascular proliferation and bile duct-like structures. The cystic spaces are filled with fluid or solid gelatinous material. The islands of hepatocytes within the mesenchymal stroma may show reactive and regenerative changes. Most patients present with abdominal enlargement or an abdominal mass. Few have pain or respiratory distress. Ultrasonography and CT demonstrate a large tumor, with central cystic changes showing internal septations [100]. Angiography reveals a hypovascular or avascular lesion. It is important to differentiate this tumor from embryonal sarcoma because both may demonstrate loose edematous myxoid stroma. In most cases of embryonal sarcoma, the cellularity of the tumor is readily evident, and the neoplastic cells show distinctive cytologic features of highly malignant cells. Resection is recommended when the tumor is large and compresses adjacent abdominal organs. It is curative in most cases. Simultaneous involvement of the liver by mesenchymal hamartoma and infantile hemangioendothelioma requiring liver transplantation has been reported [103].

Benign lipomatous tumors and tumor-like lesions

Focal fatty change

Focal fatty change is a localized area of steatosis that can sometimes be misinterpreted on imaging studies as a neoplastic growth. It is usually an ill-defined area that may be single or multiple. Multiple areas of fatty change may mimic metastatic disease on imaging studies. Focal fatty change is associated with alcoholism, obesity, malnutrition, total parenteral nutrition, corticosteroid treatment, cytotoxic chemotherapy, acquired immunodeficiency syndrome (AIDS), hypertriglyceridemia, and diabetes mellitus. Hepatic biochemical tests may be normal or mildly abnormal.

Ultrasonography shows a hyperechoic area with ill-defined borders. On CT scan, focal fatty change appears as a hypodense area, which is usually sharply demarcated without mass effect on the hepatic or portal veins [104]. The demonstration of normal-caliber vessels coursing through the hypodense lesion on CT scan is characteristic [105] and can help in distinguishing this lesion from primary or metastatic malignancy. MRI shows increased intensity on T1-weighted images. This finding is characteristic for focal fatty change, appearing in 100% of cases compared with less than 4% of other benign tumors. The differential diagnosis of a hyperintense focal hepatic lesion on T1-weighted images includes hemorrhage, malignant melanoma, and iron or copper overload [106]. Fat-suppressed T1-weighted images may be helpful in identifying fatty infiltration because the hyperdense area typically becomes hypodense in a fat-containing lesion [106]. ^{99m}Tc-sulfur colloid scintigraphy shows no focal lesion; however, areas of steatosis show retention of ^{133}Xe [107]. Biopsy is diagnostic but not always required. Microscopically, the lesion shows macrovesicular fatty change within the lesion, which is indistinguishable from other forms of steatosis.

The treatment of focal fatty change is directed against the underlying disease. Resolution has been described after weight loss and abstinence from alcohol [108]. Occasionally, the focal absence of fat in a liver that is otherwise fatty may also give the appearance of a tumorous lesion.

Angiomyolipoma

Angiomyolipoma is a rare, benign, lipomatous tumor resembling the more common renal angiomyolipoma. It is usually solitary, ranging in size from 0.3 to more than 20 cm. It is typically asymptomatic and is detected as an incidental finding between the second and eighth decades, predominantly in women [109,110]. It is composed of variable proportions of adipose tissue and smooth muscle with thick-walled blood vessels. Tumors with extensive extramedullary hematopoiesis have been termed myelolipoma or angiomyelolipoma [111].

Angiomyelolipoma is a homogenous well-circumscribed tumor that is highly echogenic on ultrasonography. On enhanced CT scan, the density measurements are characteristic of fat (−2 to −115 Hounsfield units) [112]; MRI is also diagnostic. The prognosis is usually excellent. Budd–Chiari syndrome related to compression of the hepatic veins by angiomyelolipoma has been described [113]. Malignant transformation has not been reported. For symptomatic lesions or lesions in which the diagnosis cannot be confirmed, resection is the treatment of choice [109].

Pseudolipoma

Pseudolipoma is a small encapsulated lesion located on the capsular surface of the liver or immediately under the capsule. It consists of mature lipocytes and is presumed to originate from adherent epiploic appendices that became detached. Fat necrosis and calcifications may occur. The importance of this rare and asymptomatic lesion lies in its differential diagnosis from primary or metastatic tumors. There are no clear predisposing factors [114].

Inflammatory pseudotumor

Inflammatory pseudotumor of the liver is a rare benign condition presenting as a localized parenchymal mass. It is considered by some to be secondary to an infectious process [115], although the exact pathogenesis remains

unclear, and few microscopic studies of hepatic tissue have disclosed pathogenic microorganisms. An association with extrahepatic infectious conditions and with Crohn disease [116,117] has been reported in a few patients. The lesion may be solitary or multiple and its size ranges from 1 to 25 cm. It is usually well circumscribed and may be encapsulated. It affects patients at any age and has a predilection for men with a male:female ratio of 3:1 to 8:1.

Patients usually present with fever, abdominal pain, and malaise. Jaundice and weight loss may occur. Elevated sedimentation rate, leukocytosis, and mildly abnormal hepatic biochemical tests are common. Ultrasonography reveals a heterogeneous lesion that may show a mosaic pattern. CT scan shows an irregular, clearly demarcated heterogeneous mass that is typically hypodense compared with surrounding liver parenchyma.

The differential diagnosis includes pyogenic hepatic abscess, as well as malignant and metastatic tumors. Needle liver biopsy is usually needed to establish the diagnosis. Histologically, the mass is composed of fibrous tissue and myofibroblasts and infiltrated by dense mixed inflammatory infiltrate with numerous plasma cells. Vascular invasion can sometimes be seen, and phlebitis may be present.

The prognosis of hepatic inflammatory pseudotumor is usually favorable. The lesion may regress and disappear spontaneously within a few weeks to months [118–120]. In a few cases antibiotic treatment was used and was followed by complete resolution. Response to steroids has also been reported. In some cases the lesion was treated successfully by local resection [120], but surgical removal is unnecessary in most patients. When the diagnosis is unequivocal, observation is the treatment of choice [118–120].

Other tumors of the liver

A variety of other very rare tumors of mesenchymal or mixed origin may occur in the liver, including fibroma, lymphangioma, benign mesenchymoma, and tertatoma.

Nodular diseases of the liver

In addition to the benign tumorous lesions of the liver described above, a series of nodular conditions may also affect the liver and need to be distinguished from neoplasms, benign or malignant. The classification and terminology of nodular diseases of the liver is somewhat confusing because different terms have been applied to the same type of lesion. In an attempt to standardize the terminology, the International Working Party proposed a new nomenclature, which has been widely adopted by pathologists [121]. However, this terminology does not always lend itself to everyday clinical use, and the following discussion represents an attempt to combine this new standard terminology with the clinical features of hepatic nodules. A key factor to considering in discussing nodular conditions of the liver is whether or not they are associated with cirrhosis.

Hepatocellular nodular lesions with cirrhosis

The definition of cirrhosis has three components based on gross or microscopic pathologic findings: (i) nodules of regenerating hepatocytes; (ii) bands of fibrosis that surround these nodules; and (iiic) the process by which this occurs, which is diffuse throughout the liver. Many of the other forms of nodules described later are differentiated from cirrhosis by not meeting one of these three criteria. Cirrhosis is usually classified on the basis of morphologic findings as being *micronodular*, *macronodular*, or *mixed*. These terms refer to the size of the nodules of regenerating hepatocytes that are present. Therefore, in micronodular cirrhosis, the nodules are usually 2–3 mm in diameter. This pattern is characteristic of the cirrhosis caused by alcohol and hemochromatosis, whereas most other causes of cirrhosis result in macronodular or mixed macronodular and micronodular cirrhosis, in which the nodules typically range between 3 and 10 mm in diameter.

Dysplastic nodules

Among cirrhotic nodules, some stand out as being unusual on gross or microscopic examination. Therefore, dysplastic nodules are defined as a nodular region of hepatocytes at least 1 mm in diameter with dysplasia but without definite criteria of malignancy. For nodules larger than 10 mm, the term *macroregenerative nodule* (MRN) has been applied. Although the International Working Party abandoned it, this term may still have some value because clinicians and radiologists often encounter large regenerative nodules that seem to have a propensity to become malignant. Synonyms for this lesion include large regenerative nodule and adenomatous hyperplasia.

In two series of cases, investigators examined the incidence of MRNs in liver explants. Ferrell et al. [122] examined 110 sequentially explanted cirrhotic livers and found that 19 of them (17.3%) had nodules between 0.8 and 3.5 cm in diameter (Fig. 35.5). Ten livers had more than one nodule, and a total of 40 nodules were detected. Twelve of the nodules were HCC and 28 were MRNs. Theise et al. [123] examined 44 explanted livers and identified 48 MRNs larger than 1 cm in diameter in 11 livers. Both these studies showed a close association between MRNs and HCC in the same liver (Fig. 35.5).

There is debate about the origin of dysplastic nodules. It was thought that they are simply "overgrown" cirrhotic

nodules. The observation that nearly all dysplastic nodules contain intact portal triads implies that these lesions are not derived from regenerating nodules but rather that they may represent the growth of nodules of transformed hepatocytes [124].

Dysplastic nodules rarely result in any clinical symptoms. Patients may have clinical features associated with cirrhosis, or the nodules may be detected radiographically if they are large enough, usually as an incidental finding. Nodules larger than 1 cm in diameter can be detected with either ultrasonographic examination or sensitive CT or MRI techniques. Unfortunately, large dysplastic nodules cannot be differentiated reliably from HCC by radiographic means; therefore, they present a challenge to the clinician caring for the patient. Biopsy of such nodules can be performed with CT or ultrasonographic guidance to rule out HCC, but if cancer is not present in the specimen, the possibility that the correct portion of the lesion has not been sampled cannot be excluded. Table 35.2 shows the high rate of development of malignant growth within large dysplastic nodules, ranging between 24% and 45% over a period of several years [125–128].

It may be difficult to distinguish dysplastic nodules from well-differentiated HCC. Their radiographic features are similar and even their histologic features may overlap and be difficult to distinguish, particularly on small needle biopsy specimens (Table 35.3) [17].

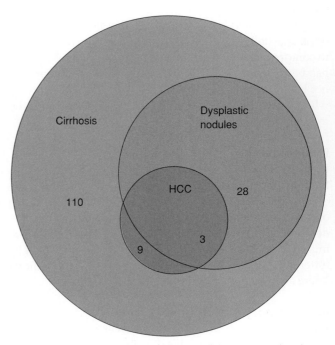

Figure 35.5 Dysplastic nodules and hepatocellular carcinoma (HCC) found in cirrhotic livers at the time of transplantation. (Data from Ferrell et al. [122].)

Table 35.2 Outcome of radiographically identified dysplastic nodules.

| Number of nodules | Outcome of nodules | | | Reference |
	Disappeared, n (%)	Hepatocellular carcinoma, n (%)	Unchanged, n (%)	
20	2 (10%)	9 (45%)	9 (45%)	Takayama et al. [125]
17	4 (24%)	4 (24%)	9 (52%)	Kondo et al. [126]
32	7 (22%)	3 (25%)	17 (53%)	Borzio et al. [127]
154	43 (28%	29 (19%)	82 (53%)	Kobayashi et al [128]

Macroregenerative nodules

There is ongoing discussion about the characterization and classification of hepatocellular nodules found in the cirrhotic liver. An improvement of imaging techniques has led to the frequent detection of focal lesions in cirrhotic livers, many of which are benign nodules with various degrees of atypia. They may occur in cirrhotic livers of any cause. Several groups have suggested nomenclatures and diagnostic criteria to describe these lesions; however, none of these is used consistently [129]. Terms such as regenerative nodules, MRNs, adenomatous hyperplastic nodules, dysplastic nodules, atypical adenomatous hyperplastic nodules, and borderline nodules [129–132] have been suggested by different authors to describe what is believed to be different stages of the same lesion.

An MRN is typically larger than 1.0 cm. MRNs may be seen in less than 2% of cases of acute massive necrosis and in 14–21% of patients with cirrhosis [133]. The expanding nodule typically compresses the surrounding liver tissue. It may be solitary but many livers contain multiple MRNs. It is separated from the rest of the liver parenchyma by fibrous connective tissue. Needle biopsy specimens from these lesions are commonly classified as benign, but in some cases they may demonstrate varying degrees of atypia and occasionally foci of overt HCC. The characteristic histologic findings of MRN include normal thin plates of hepatocytes (two cells thick) and a lack of cytologic atypia (normal nuclear : cytoplasmic ratio). The nodule may include multiple portal areas. Larger hepatocytes may be seen and are considered an acceptable finding as long as the normal nuclear : cytoplasmic ratio is maintained.

MRNs have been classified according to the degree of atypia into type I and type II [134]. Type I MRN shows no cell atypia and is probably an ordinary adenomatous hyperplasia, whereas type II MRN represents atypical adenomatous hyperplasia, which is probably a true precursor of HCC [134]. The clonality of MRNs suggests that at least some of them are neoplastic and probably premalignant [132]. The incidence of progression to malignancy is still unclear; however, some authors recommend

Table 35.3 Differential diagnosis of well-differentiated hepatocellular carcinoma (HCC) from benign hepatocellular nodules.

	HCC	Adenoma	Dyspastic nodule
Cirrhosis in surrounding liver	80%	0%	100%
Portal areas	Absent	Absent	Present
Growth patterns	Trabecular	Sheet-like	Two-cell thick plates
	Pseduoglandular	Nodule-in-nodule	Compact
N : C ratio	High	Low	Low
Nuclear pleomorhism	Present/absent	Absent	Absent
Nucleoli	Frequent	Absent	Absent
Mitoses	Occasional	Absent	Absent
Vascular invasion	Frequent	Absent	Absent
Stains:			
Reticulin	Decreased	Present	Present
CD34	Diffuse	Variable	Periseptal

From Goodman 2007 [17] with permission.

treating atypical (type II) MRN in a patient with cirrhosis as a malignant lesion [135]. In a study of 307 patients with cirrhosis, multivariate analysis showed dysplasia to be the most important independent risk factor for the development of HCC [136].

Imaging studies may be suggestive of MRN, although they may not be sufficient to establish the diagnosis or distinguish MRN from HCC. On T1-weighted MRI, MRNs are typically isointense to slightly hyperintense compared with the surrounding hepatic parenchyma. On T2-weighted images the lesions are hypointense. In contrast, HCC has variable diminished signal intensity on T1, becomes hyperintense on T2, and enhances during the arterial phase of gadolinium injection. HCC also has a characteristic capsule of low signal intensity [68], which is typically absent in MRNs. Magnetic resonance angiography usually shows sparse arterial supply in MRN. Uniform arterial opacification is seen without neovascularity. The transition of MRN to dysplastic nodule and subsequently to HCC is associated with vascular proliferation within the nodule and preferential blood supply from branches of the hepatic artery [68,137].

Hepatocellular nodular lesions without cirrhosis

Nodular regenerative hyperplasia

Nodular regenerative hyperplasia is defined by hepatocellular nodules distributed throughout the liver in the absence of fibrous septae between the nodules. Most reports have been of single cases or small series of cases. A recent autopsy study showed that NRH was present in 2.6% of 2,500 consecutive autopsies. NRH has been reported to occur in children and even in fetal liver. Familial occurrence has been documented. NRH has been described in association with a variety of hepatic and systemic diseases (Box 35.2) but appears to be a nonspecific tissue adaptation to heterogeneous distribution of blood flow rather than a distinct disease entity. What many of these conditions appear to have in common is the disturbance of blood flow to the liver, which can involve the portal vein (through thrombosis), the hepatic artery (with arteritis), and the hepatic outflow tract (as in the Budd–Chiari syndrome and congestive heart failure). Even some of the drugs associated with NRH probably act through their effect on blood vessels. For example, azathioprine may cause signs and symptoms that resemble those of venoocclusive disease, and the use of this agent is causally linked with NRH. It seems that insufficient blood supply to portions of the liver, caused by conditions such as portal-venous thrombosis, leads to atrophy of the parenchyma, with compensatory hyperplasia occurring in areas with adequate blood supply.

Box 35.2 Conditions associated with nodular regenerative hyperplasia.

- Vascular diseases:
    Budd–Chiari syndrome
    Portal-venous thrombosis
- Drugs and toxins:
    Azathioprine
    Thorotrast
    Toxic oil syndrome
    Thioguanine
- Collagen vascular disease:
    Systemic lupus erythematosus
    Scleroderma
    Mixed connective tissue disease
    Rheumatoid arthritis
    Felty syndrome
- Polymyalgia rheumatica
- Antiphospholipid antibody syndrome
- Other liver diseases:
    Primary biliary cirrhosis
    After liver transplantation
    Metastases from pancreatic cancer
    Hepatocellular carcinoma
- Neoplastic conditions:
    Myeloproliferative disorders
    After bone marrow transplantation
    Non-Hodgkin lymphoma
    Castleman disease
- Immunodeficiency syndromes:
    HIV infection
    Common variable immunodeficiency
- Miscellaneous:
    Primary pulmonary hypertension
    Glomerulonephritis
    Behçet disease
    Schnitzler syndrome
    Diabetes mellitus
    Congestive heart failure
- Idiopathic:
    Sporadic
    Familial

HIV, human immunodeficiency virus.

At gross examination of the liver, there is diffuse fine nodularity of the liver approximately 1–2 mm in diameter. Microscopic examination shows that the normal architecture has been replaced with monoacinar regenerative nodules, which often contain portal tracts [138]. The nodules are surrounded by compressed liver cell plates rather than fibrosis, and dilated sinusoids may be seen adjacent to nodules (Fig. 35.6). Although the nodularity may be visible with hematoxylin and eosin stain, it is best seen with a reticulin stain, which shows thick cell plates

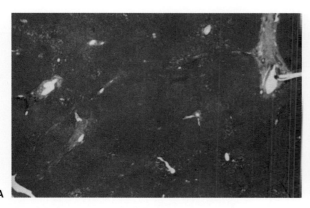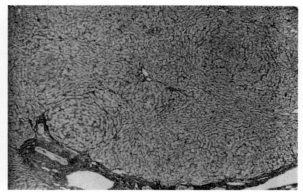

A   B

Figure 35.6 (A) Photomicrograph of the liver shows nodules of nodular regenerative hyperplasia without surrounding fibrosis. Hematoxylin and eosin (H&E). (B) Nodular regenerative hyperplasia. Reticulin stain. (Courtesy of D. Elizabeth M. Brunt.)

within the nodule and compressed plates surrounding the nodule.

The clinical features of NRH are variable, and many patients have no symptoms. Patients range widely in age, although NRH is rare among children. Patients often have a history of another medical illness, which was presumably a predisposing factor for NRH. The main clinical consequence of NRH is portal hypertension, which manifests as splenomegaly and gastroesophageal varices. Ascites is uncommon because in most patients the hepatic synthetic function is preserved and, therefore, serum albumin levels are normal. Serum aminotransferase levels are characteristically normal, as are bilirubin values, although alkaline phosphatase levels are usually moderately elevated [139]. Therapy is directed at removing the causative agent if possible and controlling portal hypertension. Patients with NRH who experience bleeding from varices usually tolerate this well because hepatic synthetic function is preserved. Surgical shunting or transjugular intrahepatic portosystemic shunt (TIPS) is rarely indicated, and the varices can often be controlled with injection, sclerotherapy, or endoscopic banding. Patients with NRH have mistakenly undergone liver transplantation because they were thought to have cirrhosis, and they have done well.

Unusual forms of nodular regenerative hyperplasia

Felty syndrome is a rare complication of rheumatoid arthritis consisting of leukopenia and splenomegaly [140]. Leukopenia may be associated with an increased risk of bacterial infection. The splenomegaly is thought to be caused by portal hypertension. Most biopsy specimens of the liver from patients with Felty syndrome show NRH, although a small proportion show only portal fibrosis or sinusoidal lymphocytosis. Felty syndrome carries an increased risk of non-Hodgkin lymphoma [141].

Partial nodular transformation

Partial nodular transformation (PNT) of the liver is a rare entity characterized by the formation of large hepatocellular nodules without marked fibrosis, particularly at the hepatic hilum or around large portal areas. It does not meet the criteria of cirrhosis because the condition is not diffuse and the nodules are not surrounded by fibrosis. It is similar to NRH, except that the nodules of NRH are diffuse throughout the liver and are usually much smaller (Table 35.4). PNT usually occurs as an isolated condition but has been reported in association with vascular abnormalities such as persistent ductus venosus, portal-venous thrombosis, and portal-venous emboli of HCC [142–144]. The pathogenesis is uncertain, but it has been suggested that PNT may represent a variant of NRH in which localized obstruction of blood flow causes the formation of localized hepatic nodules [141]. Because these nodules occur predominantly in or near the hepatic hilum, PNT often leads to presinusoidal portal hypertension.

PNT has been found in both adults and children. Patients usually have features of portal hypertension, such as bleeding from gastroesophageal varices and ascites. If the nodules are large enough, hepatomegaly resulting from portal hypertension may be present with splenomegaly. Serum aminotransferase activity is typically within the normal range. The diagnosis of PNT is often made only at autopsy or surgery, but it can be made with needle biopsy of the liver. No characteristic radiographic features of PNT have been described. Because PNT is such a rare condition, there are no specific treatment guidelines other than a recommendation for symptomatic management.

Focal nodular hyperplasia

Focal nodular hyperplasia is a benign, tumor-like lesion of the liver considered to be hyperplastic in origin rather than neoplastic. The exact frequency is not known, but

Table 35.4 Nodular diseases of the liver.

Lesion		Size	Single/multiple	Common underlying causes	Comment
Nodular regenerative hyperplasia		Usually <1 cm	Multiple	Immunologic disorders (e.g., rheumatoid arthritis) Myeloproliferative disorders	Pathogenesis related to portal venopathy and decreased blood flow; usually presents with portal hypertension
Focal nodular hyperplasia		Usually <5 cm	Single	None recognized	Often an incidental finding
Hepatocellular adenoma		May be very large	Usually single; occasionally multiple	Estrogen use	Requires resection because of risk of rupture or hemorrhage
Hepatocellular carcinoma		May be very large	Often multiple	Cirrhosis Chronic viral hepatitis	Probably arises from within dysplastic nodules
Partial nodular transformation		1–5 cm	Multiple but localized to perihilar area	None recognized	Rare entity; presents with portal hypertension

Reproduced from Di Bisceglie and Buetow [281] with permission from Current Science.

large series of cases have been reported. FNH occurs predominantly in women but has also been found in men and children. It rarely causes clinical complications, but its importance lies mainly in being differentiated from hepatocellular adenoma and HCC. FNH classically occurs in noncirrhotic liver, but a recent report suggests that similar lesions may be seen in cirrhosis as well [145]. In most cases, it is an incidental finding on abdominal imaging or surgery performed for unrelated reasons.

Pathogenesis

Focal nodular hyperplasia is considered to be hyperplastic rather than neoplastic in origin, although its exact pathogenesis remains a matter of controversy. It typically occurs in the background of a healthy liver. It is believed by many to be a hyperplastic response to a preexisting vascular anomaly in the location of the lesion. According to this theory, the initial injury may be arterial malformation, which leads to increased arterial blood flow to a specific region compared to the adjacent parenchyma, which in turn leads to high sinusoidal pressure, resulting in hepatocellular hyperperfusion. This may be followed by local angiogenesis, leading to hyperplasia and causing the typical arterial branching in the center of the FNH [146].

FNH typically occurs in isolation but may be associated with other liver diseases such as Budd–Chiari syndrome, pulmonary hypertension, primary sclerosing cholangitis, hemochromatosis, echinococcal cyst, and agenesis of the portal vein. Because of the female preponderance of this condition (female : male ratio approximately 8 : 1), a link with oral contraceptive use has been postulated. However, Mathieu et al. [147], in a study in which the subjects were 216 women with FNH, examined tumors in patients taking oral contraceptives and those not taking these agents. The investigators found that neither the size nor the number of FNH lesions was influenced by oral contraceptive use. A more recent study identified an odds ratio of 2.8 for using oral contraceptives at any point of time among patients with FNH compared with controls [148]. FNH may be associated with other vascular conditions affecting the liver, such as hemangioma and hereditary hemorrhagic telangiectasia [149,150].

A recent report of FNH diagnosed in the same hepatic segment in identical twins supports the theory of a congenital anomaly being an initial event in the pathogenesis of this lesion, at least in some patients [151]. Most FNHs are supplied by a single artery, which is typically enlarged. In contrast to the usual situation, this artery is not accompanied by a portal vein or a bile duct. Although some reports suggested that FNH may be a clonal lesion on the basis of a uniform pattern of X-chromosome inactivation, others have shown it to be of a clear polyclonal nature [152,153].

Pathology

The typical macroscopic appearance is of a firm, nodular mass with a dense central stellate scar and radiating fibrous septa that divide the lesion into lobules of various size (Fig. 35.7A–C) [154,155]. The lesion is sharply demarcated from the surrounding liver tissue but has no true capsule. The central scar is clearly seen macroscopically in approximately 50% of the cases [154]; however, in some of the cases it is absent and the fibrous septa may be poorly developed. The lesion is light brown or yellowish gray and usually occupies a superficial position. The average size is 5 cm and the lesion uncommonly exceeds 10 cm in diameter. Occasionally, it is exophytic or pedunculated. Larger lesions may have foci of hemorrhage or necrosis. FNH is solitary in most cases and is located in the right lobe more often than in the left [154]. Two or more lesions are encountered in approximately 20% of patients and a distinct minority may have more than five lesions [154–157]. The size may range from 1 mm to

more than 20 cm but most (64%) are smaller than 5 cm in diameter [154].

In a study of 168 patients with FNH, investigators examined the gross and microscopic pathologic features of this condition [155]. In 76% of patients, the mass was solitary and more often located in the right lobe than in the left. In 21% of patients, between two and five nodules were found, whereas in the other 3% of cases between 15 and 30 nodules were detected. The lesions ranged in size from 1 mm to 19 cm in diameter. In total, 64% of masses were smaller than 5 cm in diameter. A central scar was visible on gross examination of 138 of 305 lesions (45%), and a large vascular pedicle was found in the periphery of 22 lesions (7%) (Fig. 35.7). Microscopic examination showed that all the lesions consisted of nodular hyperplastic parenchyma, partially or completely surrounded by fibrous septae. Additional changes such as periodic acid–Schiff-positive globules and Mallory hyaline were sometimes found in hepatocytes within the lesion. A central scar was found on light microscopic examination of 153 lesions, and the lesions always contained malformed blood vessels of varying caliber. Histologic cholestasis was found in 36 cases, and some patients had hepatocellular steatosis. Portal tracts and terminal hepatic venules were not present.

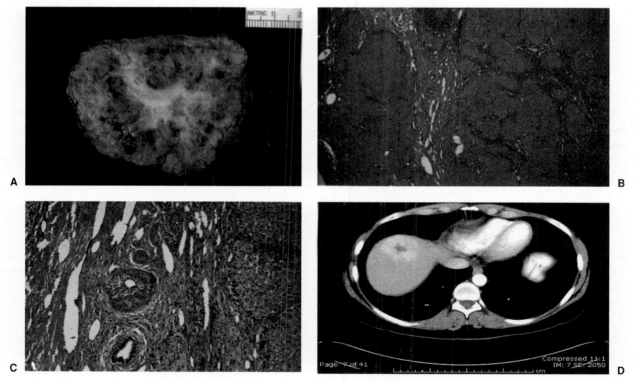

Figure 35.7 (A) Macroscopic appearance of resected focal nodular hyperplasia. The typical central scar is evident. (B) Photomicrograph of focal nodular hyperplasia shows regenerating nodules of hepatocytes surrounding a central core that contains abnormal blood vessels and a bile duct. (C) Focal nodular hyperplasia with an abnormal, thick-walled artery adjacent to the center of the lesion. (D) Dynamic computed tomography scan of the liver showing focal nodular hyperplasia. Note hypervascular area in right lobe of the liver with a darker central stellate scar. (A–C, Courtesy of Dr Elizabeth M. Brunt.)

Clinical manifestations and natural history

In most cases FNH is asymptomatic and detected incidentally on imaging studies performed for unrelated reasons or during surgery. Hepatic biochemical tests are typically normal and the serum level of α-fetoprotein is not elevated. Abdominal discomfort may be the presenting symptom in a minority of patients [158]. Abdominal pain is rare and should prompt an evaluation for other causes. Some patients may present with hepatomegaly, abdominal mass, or abdominal tenderness but most (approximately 85%) will have normal findings in the physical examination [159]. Sudden abdominal pain may be related to rupture or bleeding that is distinctly rare [160]. Fibrolamellar HCC may be mistaken for FNH [161] or may occur in the same liver [162]. However, malignant transformation has not been unequivocally described in FNH, and there is no evidence that FNH it is a precursor of HCC or fibrolamellar carcinoma.

The prognosis of patients with FNH is almost invariably excellent. Most patients remain asymptomatic and exhibit no significant changes in lesion size over time [163]. Occasionally, FNH may regress [90,164] and only a small minority (<10%) may show some increase in size [76]. Any significant increase in size should therefore prompt an evaluation for another diagnosis such as HCC or fibrolamellar carcinoma.

Diagnosis

Because these lesions are usually clinically silent, radiographic imaging is a key tool in the evaluation of hepatic lesions and the diagnosis of FNH is often made by certain characteristic radiographic features. In most imaging studies, the typical appearance of FNH is related to the characteristic central scar, the hypervascularity, and the distinctive arterial blood supply, which begins in the center of the lesion with peripheral ramification in a spoke wheel pattern [165]. Other lesions in the differential diagnosis that may have similar radiographic features include hepatocellular adenoma and fibrolamellar carcinoma, although FNH is by far the most frequent of these conditons.

- *Standard ultrasonography* is highly sensitive but nonspecific for the diagnosis of FNH. It usually demonstrates the lesion as a well-demarcated nodular mass but is frequently nondiagnostic [163,166]. Ultrasonography detects the central scar in approximately 20% of cases [165,167,168], although the addition of Doppler imaging may reveal arterial signals within the lesion in other cases [169].
- *Contrast-enhanced harmonic sonography* has recently been demonstrated to show the typical spoke wheel pattern of the central arteries during the vascular phase in more than 90% of individuals with FNH [170]. In addition, it produces a typical pronounced enhancement during the hepatic arterial phase and the early portal-venous phase that may help differentiate it from hepatic adenoma [171]. This technique, which is based on the injection of a microbubble contrast agent, has been used for various focal liver lesions and may be a promising modality for the diagnosis of FNH.
- *CT scan* should always be used in the multiphase contrast-enhanced mode for the evaluation of a possible FNH. The enhancement pattern may be helpful in suggesting the diagnosis or ruling it out [172]. On precontrast images, FNH can be hypodense or isodense to the surrounding normal liver parenchyma. It is typically hyperdense on arterial phase images (20–30 seconds after contrast injection), becoming less prominent on portal-venous phase images (70–90 seconds), and may become completely isodense [168,173]. A central scar is seen in 43–60% of cases on imaging [174]. It is typically hypodense on the precontrast and arterial phase, becoming hyperdense on the portal-venous phase [173, 175]. Occasionally, FNH may show imaging characteristics suggestive of a primary or metastatic malignancy. These may include the absence of a central scar, rapid washout, calcifications, or the presence of a capsule. The use of three-dimensional volume-rendered CT angiography (CTA) may demonstrate the characteristic anomalous feeding artery and may be helpful in distinguishing FNH from other lesions [176]. Calcifications have been reported in 1.4% of 295 patients with FNH [161]. This finding raises the suspicion of fibrolamellar carcinoma and usually mandates a surgical exploration to rule out this diagnosis.
- *MRI* usually shows FNH as a homogenous lesion that is isointense to mildly hypointense on T1-weighted images and isointense to slightly hyperintense on T2-weighted images. The margins are usually not well defined and the central scar may be identified by T2-weighted images in approximately 50% of cases [159, 173,177,178]. On gadolinium-enhanced imaging, the lesion shows an early homogenous enhancement in the arterial phase and becomes isointense or slightly hyperintense compared to the surrounding liver in the venous and delayed phases. The central scar shows slowly progressive enhancement, which becomes maximal on delayed images. This characteristic appearance may differentiate FNH from malignant vascular tumors [179] and has a sensitivity of 70–80% and specificity of 98% in lesions that are larger than 2 cm in size. Another distinguishing feature on gadolinium-enhanced images is the lack of capsule enhancement that is commonly seen in adenomas and HCCs. Small FNH (<1 to 2 cm) may appear more uniform in enhancement and the central scar may not be perceived.

- *Three-dimensional gadolinium-enhanced MR angiography* may increase the accuracy of the test for the diagnosis of FNH by demonstrating the characteristic vessels radiating from the center to the periphery of the lesion (the so-called star sign) [180]. The use of liver-specific MRI contrast agents (i.e., reticuloendothelial and hepatobiliary agents) offers greater lesion-to-liver contrast than the conventional extracellular contrast agent, gadolinium chelate, which has a nonspecific distribution [68, 181]. These agents may be helpful in a small fraction of cases that remain ambiguous. The administration of superparamagnetic iron oxide (SPIO) particles, which undergo phagocytosis by Kupffer cells, may help distinguish benign from malignant lesions [182]. Recently, the use of the hepatocyte-selective contrast agent gadobenate-dimeglumine (Gd-BOPTA) has been shown to improve the differentiation between FNH and adenoma with a sensitivity of 80% and specificity of more than 96% [174,183,184].
- *^{99m}Tc-sulfur colloid scintigraphy* is currently used less commonly by most centers for the diagnosis of FNH. FNH takes up ^{99m}Tc-sulfur colloid at the same or greater rate compared with the surrounding liver parenchyma in 50–70% of patients. Hyperconcentration of the colloid by the lesion is uncommon (approximately 7%) but is considered typical of FNH because of the highly active Kupffer cells within the lesion [164,185]. Nevertheless, the reliability of this modality is poor in lesions smaller than 3–4 cm in size, and this technology has largely been replaced by spiral CT and MRI. Positron emission tomography (PET) scans using ^{18}F-fluorodeoxyglucose (^{18}F-FDG) has been shown to be helpful for the differentiation of FNH from liver metastases in patients with cancer [186].

Although the diagnosis of FNH can be made by the examination of a needle biopsy specimen of the liver, this approach is less than ideal because of sampling error. Needle biopsy samples only a small portion of the lesion. The specimen may contain only a group of hepatocytes that cannot be reliably differentiated from hepatocellular adenoma. Furthermore, the presence of fibrous septae within the lesion may give the appearance of cirrhosis (referred to as pseudocirrhosis). Therefore, if the results of radiographic studies are convincing and the patient has no symptoms, no further testing is needed. However, if there is uncertainty about the diagnosis, surgical resection or large surgical biopsy may be needed for accurate diagnosis of FNH. A recent study suggests that the application of a rigorous scoring system to liver biopsy specimens can aid in the accurate diagnosis of FNH [187].

Management

Focal nodular hyperplasia rarely results in clinically important consequences or complications. Specifically,

the risk of bleeding or rupture is very low, as is the risk of the development of malignant changes. Few longitudinal studies have been done, but in one small series of 18 cases of FNH, the volume remained stable in six, decreased in ten, and increased in two [188]. Usually, no specific treatment is needed, but surgical resection is curative if the patient has symptoms. Resection is often performed in cases of diagnostic uncertainty.

When surgery is indicated, wedge resection and enucleation are generally the recommended approaches [76,139]. In many cases, they can be performed laparoscopically with excellent results because the lesions tend to be smaller and peripheral. In patients with a large FNH, a segmental resection or a formal lobectomy may be required. Angiographic embolization and hepatic artery ligation are alternative approaches for unresectable lesions [190].

Unusual forms of focal nodular hyperplasia

The International Working Party has designated multiple FNH syndrome as a distinct syndrome consisting of two or more FNH lesions in association with hemangioma of the liver, vascular malformations of the central nervous system, or tumors of meningeal or astrocytic origin [121]. Of course, FNH is multiple in approximately 30% of cases, but most of these do not have the other features associated with this syndrome.

Nguyen et al. [154] found that approximately 20% of cases of FNH are *nonclassic*. This term refers to lesions lacking some of the typical histologic features, such as malformed vessels, a central scar, or abnormal nodular architecture. Notwithstanding these histologic differences, these cases were clinically identical to those with classic features.

Another variant of FNH is the telangiectatic form, which differs from typical lesions by the absence of a central scar and lack of architectural nodular distortion. Instead, there is sinusoidal prominence with associated hepatic plate atrophy. Telangietactic FNH is more likely to be monoclonal in origin than is classic FNH and is more likely to be multiple and perhaps even more likely to result in hemorrhage than typical FNH, making it more like adenoma [191]. Recently, it has been suggested that telangiectatic FNH may be closer to hepatic adenoma and should be referred to as *telangiectatic hepatocellular adenoma* [17].

Clinical approach to a focal solid lesion of the liver

Focal solid hepatic lesions often represent a diagnostic challenge and frequently mandate an extensive evaluation and a multidisciplinary approach. Although there is a wide spectrum of conditions that needs to be considered when a focal lesion is detected in the liver, most lesions fall into a relatively small group of entities. The clinician must decide at an early stage whether the lesion is malignant or benign, whether a biopsy is indicated, and whether surgical intervention is required. In dealing with a patient with an unknown solid hepatic lesion, it is critical to determine whether the patient has underlying liver disease, and in particular whether cirrhosis is present. This involves serologic testing for various causes of liver disease and may even need liver biopsy away from the area of concern. If cirrhosis is present, HCC or dysplastic nodules are very likely to be found, whereas if there is no significant liver disease, FNH or adenoma should be considered. Imaging techniques have improved dramatically over the last decade and often allow excellent characterization of nodular lesions.

A detailed history should be obtained and should include questions about the history of cancer and previous use of OCPs, androgens, and anabolic steroids. The specific approach may vary according to the type of presentation, demographics of the patient, and medical history. The diagnostic approach in a young, asymptomatic, previously healthy woman should focus on the differential diagnosis of hemangioma, FNH, and adenoma. A history of prolonged treatment with OCPs will point toward a diagnosis of hepatocellular adenoma. In contrast, when the patient has a history of cancer, a focal hepatic lesion will often be a metastasis. In the presence of cirrhosis or chronic hepatitis B virus (HBV) infection, a focal solid lesion should be regarded as HCC until proved otherwise. A history of primary sclerosing cholangitis should point toward intrahepatic cholangiocarcinoma.

Presenting symptoms such as abdominal pain, weight loss, and malaise should raise the suspicion of malignancy. It should be remembered that most patients with benign hepatic lesions are asymptomatic, and the relationship between the symptoms and the focal lesion should be corroborated. Physical findings such as ascites, firm nodular liver, or splenomegaly should suggest the presence of a chronic liver disease and should point toward HCC. Hepatic biochemical tests are typically normal in patients with benign hepatic lesions, and a significant abnormality should raise the suspicion of a neoplastic lesion, a complication such as hemorrhage (usually in an adenoma), or an underlying liver disease. Tumor marker levels are also normal and are unhelpful in making the distinction between benign tumors. Nevertheless, any abnormality in tumor marker should prompt an evaluation for malignancy.

Imaging studies are commonly helpful in distinguishing between focal hepatic lesions (Fig. 35.8), but the differential diagnosis may be challenging because many of the lesions have overlapping radiographic features [68,192].

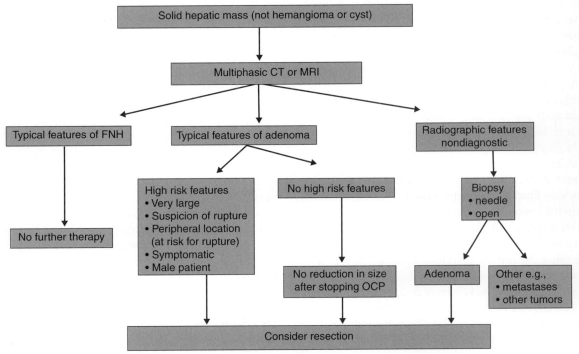

Figure 35.8 Algorithm for evaluation and management an incidental hepatic mass in patient without cirrhosis. Such masses may have been identified incidentally because of an imaging study being done for some other reason. Occassionally the mass itself may cause symptoms leading its discovery. Ultrasound examination may be used initially to assess for features of either hemangioma or cysts. CT, computed tomography; FNH, focal nodular hyperplasia; MRI, magnetic resonance imaging; OCP oral contraceptive pill.

Although ultrasonography is an excellent modality for the initial detection of lesions and for determining a solid versus cystic lesion, the sonographic appearance of a solid liver mass is often nonspecific and many patients will require additional hepatic imaging. CT is a reliable and easily reproducible method for the evaluation of focal hepatic lesions. It allows the characterization of lesions as small as 1.5 cm in size and may also help in the evaluation of the entire abdomen for signs of cirrhosis, portal hypertension, or malignancy [174]. Multiphasic CT scans using up-to-date equipment are capable of showing the vascularity of hepatic tumors and nodules in great detail. In a patient with cirrhosis or chronic HBV infection and a solid lesion, arterial enhancement on dynamic CT scan strongly supports the diagnosis of HCC [193]. When a hemangioma is suspected, triphasic dynamic CT with late images should be performed. A dynamic CT scan may conclusively establish the diagnosis of a hemangioma and, occasionally, FNH without any further workup [194].

However, the greatest advances appear to have occurred with MRI. Recent studies have demonstrated accurate differentiation of FNH from hepatic adenoma using contrast-enhanced MRI, or the distinction between adenoma or HCC and "nonsurgical" lesions such as FNH or regenerative nodules, although Krinsky and Israel found that dysplastic and nondysplastic nodules still cannot be separated [195–197].

Tagged RBC scan (^{99m}Tc-RBC pool scintigraphy) may be helpful in questionable hemangiomas, although gadolinium-enhanced MRI is superior to tagged RBC scan in most cases. ^{99m}Tc-RBC scan with SPECT is highly sensitive in hemangiomas larger than 2 cm in size and may be used to confirm the diagnosis. ^{99m}Tc-sulfur colloid scintigraphy is usually not helpful for the differential diagnosis of focal hepatic lesions, but it may assist in distinguishing between FNH and adenoma. If no focal defect is seen or if the uptake is increased, FNH should be suspected. In contrast, decreased uptake is more consistent with an adenoma.

In cases of uncertainty or when malignancy is suspected, a liver biopsy may be considered. A percutaneous liver biopsy is generally safe. The accuracy and safety of ultrasonography-guided biopsy of these lesions has been documented [198]. However percutaneous biopsy may be hazardous in hemangiomas and should be avoided when these tumors are suspected, or when imaging studies indicate hypervascularity. In these cases, laparoscopic liver biopsy may be considered as it has the advantage of hemostasis under direct vision.

In a minority of patients, an accurate diagnosis cannot be established despite histopathologic examination because of sampling error or inadequate sample size. In these cases, resection may be indicated. Similarly, persistent symptoms, increasing levels of tumor markers,

or evidence of tumor growth are indications for a surgical resection, regardless of the diagnosis. Benign hepatic lesions accounted for 5% of hepatic resections in a recent database review in the United States [199]. Resection of benign lesions is performed laparoscopically in many centers with excellent results.

Cystic diseases of the liver

Cystic diseases of the liver represent three groups of hepatic disorders that share the clinical feature of abnormal fluid-filled spaces in the liver and biliary tree (Fig. 35.9). The first and largest group is fibrocystic diseases of the liver and biliary tree. They are related hepatic disorders characterized by overgrowth of biliary epithelium leading to the production of fluid-filled dilated spaces, the formation of portal fibrosis, and the development of embryonic ductal plate malformations. The lesions result from malformations in different portions of the developing biliary tree and include polycystic liver disease (PCLD), simple hepatic cysts, congenital hepatic fibrosis (CHF), von Meyenburg complexes, and choledochal cysts (Table 35.5). The second group of disorders results from congenital defects of the embryonic foregut and includes ciliated foregut cyst, cystadenoma, and cystadenocarcinoma. The last group of disorders mimic the other cystic liver diseases and result from infection with the parasites *Echinococcus granulosus* or *E. multilocularis*.

Fibrocystic liver disease

Polycystic liver disease

Polycystic liver disease is a rare disease in which multiple cysts develop within the parenchyma of the liver. It is generally defined as the presence of four or more thin-walled cysts within the hepatic parenchyma because simple hepatic cysts are commonly characterized by one, two, or three cysts [200]. PCLD occurs both in association with autosomal dominant polycystic kidney disease (ADPKD) and in isolation (Fig. 35.10).

Epidemiology and course of disease

The true prevalence of PCLD is not known. Results in autopsy series suggest that the prevalence ranges from 0.05% to 0.13% [201,202]. The prevalence of multiple liver cysts in patients with ADPKD is 45–68% [202]. Cyst prevalence in ADPKD increases from approximately 24% in the third decade of life to 80% in the sixth decade of life [203]. The association of PCLD with ADPKD occurs in 16–93% of patients [204,205]. This range is wide because the prevalence of PCLD in ADPKD depends on age and the amount of renal dysfunction [206].

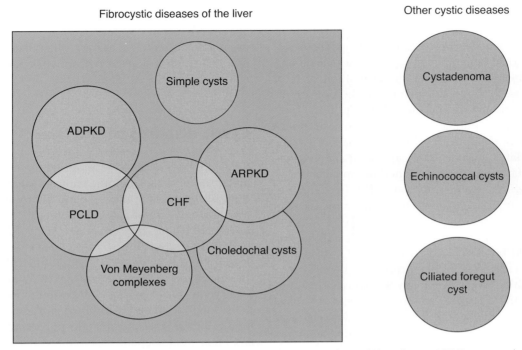

Figure 35.9 Interrelation between cystic diseases of the liver. ADPKD, autosomal dominant polycystic kidney disease; ARPKD, autosomal recessive polycystic kidney disease; CHF, congenital hepatic fibrosis; PCLD, polycystic liver disease.

When occurring with ADPKD, cysts generally begin to form in the liver after the onset of puberty. Although the proportion of men and women with liver cysts and ADPKD is the same, women tend to have both more and larger cysts [207]. Cyst formation is thought to be associated with estrogen exposure because the number and size of cysts correlate with the number of pregnancies, use of oral contraceptives, and use of female hormone replacement therapy [207]. Clinically relevant polycystic disease also correlates with advancing age, severity of renal cystic disease, and presence of renal dysfunction [206].

There are few published data on the frequency of symptomatic PCLD associated with ADPKD. Descriptions of symptomatic complications of PCLD are most often published in the form of case reports or reports of small series of patients over the course of many years. Most authors indicate that PCLD is predominantly a silent disease. The

frequency of symptoms may be increasing because of the success of hemodialysis and renal transplantation – larger numbers of older patients with renal insufficiency are likely to have more and larger cysts within the liver. One report indicated that as much as 10% of the mortality among patients with ADPKD who undergo hemodialysis may be related to PCLD [208].

There is even less understanding of the epidemiology and course of isolated PCLD. Reports of old autopsy and surgical series suggest that multiple hepatic cysts may be present in the absence of renal cysts in as many as 50% of all patients with multiple hepatic cysts [209]. This is probably an overestimation. Results of a more recent autopsy series suggested that only 7% of patients with PCLD did not have associated renal cysts [202]. Several kindreds of patients have been found to have multiple cysts in their livers and no evidence of ADPKD [201, 210–212]. Similar to ADPKD-associated PCLD, isolated PCLD is more severe in women and more severe disease is associated with pregnancy [213]. Many patients are likely asymptomatic with clinically silent disease [213]. Because these series represent small numbers of patients, there is no clear understanding of the clinical course of isolated PCLD.

Genetics and molecular pathogenesis

Autosomal dominant polycystic kidney disease is one of the most common genetic defects, with a disease

Table 35.5 Bile duct segment associated with fibrocystic disease of the liver and biliary tract.

Fibrocystic disease	Associated bile duct
Choledochal cysts	Common hepatic
Caroli disease	Segmental area
Congenital hepatic fibrosis	Interlobular
Polycystic liver disease	Intralobular
Simple cysts	Intralobular

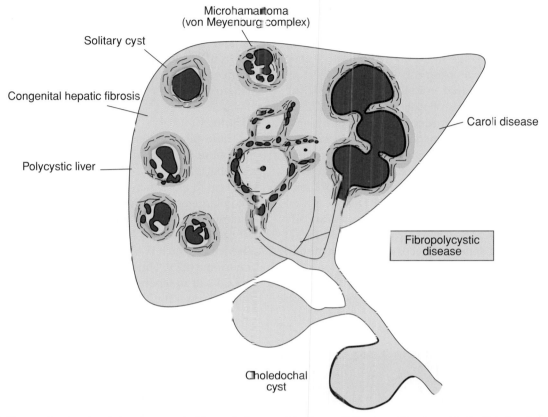

Figure 35.10 Diagram showing the relations between the fibrocystic diseases of the liver and biliary tract. (Courtesy of Dr Jay H. Lefkowitch.)

frequency of 1:1,000 in the white population [214]. There are two genes associated with ADPKD – *PKD-1* and *PKD-2* [215]. *PKD-1* is located on the short arm of chromosome 16 and is responsible for approximately 85% of cases of ADPKD [215]. *PKD-2* is located on the long arm of chromosome 4 and is responsible for about 15% of ADPKD [216]. There are numerous mutations known for the *PKD-1* and *PKD-2* genes. The gene products, polycystin-1 and polycystin-2, are transmembranous glycoproteins that are thought to be involved in cell–cell and cell–matrix interactions, cell cycle control, calcium ion regulation, and Wnt signaling [217]. Polycystin-1 appears to interact with a G protein signaling pathway that modulates calcium channels [216]. Polycystin-2 is an integral membrane protein with the characteristics of a cation channel [216]. Polycystin-1 and polycystin-2 complex in the cell membrane and localize in the primary cilium [216]. The primary cilium is a microtubule-based cellular structure found on the luminal surface of epithelium, including biliary and renal tubular epithelium, which acts as a flow sensor and regulates Ca^{2+} influx. Loss of flow sensing has been hypothesized to lead to dedifferentiation, cell proliferation, and loss of restriction in tubule size, resulting in cyst formation [218]. There is also evi-

dence that the cysts contain high numbers of receptors for estrogen and insulin growth factor 1 [219]. Cultured human cyst cells proliferate in response to estrogen and insulin growth factor 1, which may explain the higher prevalence of symptomatic disease in women [219]. One potential mechanism for cyst lining cell proliferation is a reduction in microRNA 15a, a modulator of Cdc25A, a cell cycle regulator [198]. Proliferation of cyst epithelium has also been linked to the cyclic adenosine monophosphate (cAMP)-mediated activation of the mitogen-activated protein kinase/extracellular regulated kinase pathway and mammalian target of rapamycin (mTOR) pathway [213]. Cyst fluid secretion appears to be controlled by a cAMP-dependent pathway [213]. Changes in cell adhesion mediated by matrix metalloproteins also seem to be important for cell growth [213]. Neovascularization mediated by a number of factors is likely important for cyst growth [213]. Although the genetic inheritance pattern is autosomal dominant, a cellular recessive two-hit model has been proposed. A germline mutation in *PKD-1* or *PKD-2* is not sufficient to produce disease, but a second somatic mutation in the functional *PKD* gene triggers monoclonally derived cyst formation [220,221].

Recent progress has been made in understanding the genetic basis of isolated PCLD. Reynolds et al. studied two large kindreds with autosomal dominant isolated PCLD and showed linkage to a putative causative gene on the long arm of chromosome 19 [212]. Drenth et al. and Li et al. identified that mutations in *PRKCSH* are responsible for some cases of isolated PCLD [222,223]. PRKCSH has been previously identified as protein kinase C substrate 80K-H, but the function of the protein product, hepatocystin, is unclear. Hepatocystin can function as the noncatalytic β-subunit of glucosidase II, which plays a major role in the regulation of proper folding and maturation of glycoproteins. PKD-1 and PKD-2 are glycoproteins, so it has been proposed that mechanistically there could be a link between ADPKD-associated PCLD and isolated PCLD if defective glycosylation from mutant glucosidase II results in improper functioning of polycystins [223,224]. There is a preliminary report that mutations in translocation protein SEC63 are associated with

isolated PCLD in persons who have normal PRKCSH [224]. SEC63 is also involved in the processing of integral and secreted proteins as a part of the multicomponent translocation involved in protein translocation [224]. A similar two-hit model of ADPKD-associated PCLD has been proposed for isolated PCLD.

Pathology

The fluid-filled cysts of PCLD are usually scattered throughout the liver, although they can be present in only one lobe (Fig. 35.11). The cysts vary in size from less than 1 cm to more than 10 cm in diameter and cause massive enlargement of the liver. Microscopically, the cysts are close to or actually within the portal tracts [225]. The cyst cavities are lined by flat or cuboidal epithelium, the presence of which is often associated with biliary microhamartoma [226]. Fluid within the cysts is consistent with the bile salt-independent fraction of bile and increases with secretin stimulation. Therefore, the cysts are lined

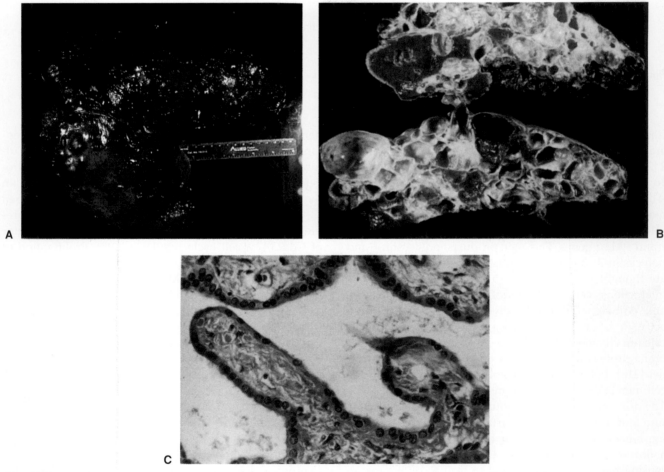

Figure 35.11 (A) Polycystic liver with massive enlargement of the liver. (B) Cut surface of a portion of a polycystic liver containing numerous cyst pockets. (C) Photomicrograph of polycystic liver stained with H&E showing cuboidal cyst lining. (B, C, courtesy of Dr Elizabeth M. Brunt.)

with biliary-type epithelium [227] and are hypothesized to form from the dilatation of biliary microhamartomata [203,226]. During their development the cysts become disconnected from the biliary tract [226]. It is not clear whether the biliary microhamartomata are congenital or develop as the patient ages [226].

Clinical features

The symptoms of isolated and ADPKD-associated PCLD are most often caused by the mechanical effects of the enlarged cystic liver. Most cases are asymptomatic [213] Some cases of PCLD may manifest as vague abdominal fullness or a palpable abdominal mass. Patients who underwent surgical intervention have been reported to have the following symptoms: abdominal pain, abdominal distension, early satiety, fatigue, orthopnea, jaundice, ascites, and variceal bleeding [228]. The right upper quadrant pain and shortness of breath experienced by patients with both PCLD and ADPKD correlate with larger liver volumes and not with kidney volume [229] Patients generally have preserved hepatic function on the basis of galactose elimination capacity and antipyrine clearance [229]. Total hepatocyte volume remains normal, according to calculations of hepatic mass from CT images (Fig. 35.12) [227]. Results of liver function tests are either normal or show a cholestatic pattern with usually mild elevations in alkaline phosphatase and total bilirubin

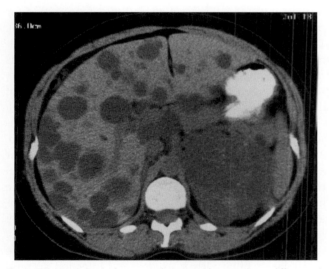

Figure 35.12 Abdominal computed tomography scan shows diffuse cystic involvement by polycystic liver disease involves obliteration of varices by means of repeated band ligation. Pharmacologic intervention with β-blockers or somatostatin analogs can also be attempted. TIPS is generally technically unfeasible because of the large cysts. Surgical debulking of the cysts can lead to relief of venous outflow tract obstruction and, therefore, of portal hypertension in some patients [62]. Surgical portocaval shunts can be helpful. Liver transplantation can be considered in cases of refractory disease.

levels. Serum albumin levels can be mildly depressed and prothrombin time elevated because of poor nutrition [213,228].

Complications

The development of portal hypertension in PCLD is rare. There are 19 case reports of variceal bleeding related to PCLD in the literature [230]. The pathophysiology of the development of varices is not clear. Some patients seem to have hepatic venous and/or inferior vena caval obstruction from direct compression of the cysts. Others may have associated CHF. Treatment involves obliteration of varices by means of repeated band ligation. Pharmacologic intervention with β-blockers or somatostatin analogs can also be attempted. TIPS is generally technically unfeasible because of the cysts. Surgical debulking of the cysts can lead to relief of venous outflow tract obstruction and, therefore, of portal hypertension in some patients [228]. Surgical portocaval shunts can be helpful. Liver transplantation can be considered for refractory cases.

Hepatic venous outflow tract obstruction has been reported in small case series [231]. These patients have a history of PCLD and new development of ascites. Hepatic function is usually preserved, and the ascitic fluid has a high protein content. Findings on CT or MRI may suggest hepatic venous outflow tract obstruction, which can be confirmed with hepatic venography. Abdominal surgery may precipitate hepatic venous outflow tract obstruction. If there is no evidence of thrombus in the hepatic veins or vena cava, percutaneous or surgical treatment can be directed at the obstructing cyst. If thrombosis of vessels or the presence of multiple small cysts is the cause, surgical portosystemic shunting or liver transplantation should be considered. Transplantation should probably be reserved for patients with evidence of hepatic decompensation. Patients should be screened for hypercoagulable states with the appropriate laboratory studies.

Obstructive jaundice is a rare complication of PCLD, being described only in case reports. It results from direct obstruction of the biliary tree by a cyst. Endoscopic retrograde cholangiopancreatography (ERCP) is helpful to rule out other causes of biliary obstruction and to help identify the culprit cyst, usually with the aid of an abdominal CT scan [232]. Therapy can be with percutaneous drainage and sclerosis or with surgery.

Infection of hepatic cysts is a rare complication of PCLD. It occurs in 1–3% of patients with PCLD and ADPKD and appears to be more common in patients with renal failure [208]. Most patients have fever and right upper quadrant abdominal or right flank pain [208]. Leukocytosis or left shift is usually present, but results of liver function tests have a cholestatic pattern in

Table 35.6 Selected series of patients who underwent open or laparoscopic surgery for polycystic liver disease: morbidity, mortality, and recurrence of symptoms.

No. of patients	Operation	Mean follow-up period (years)	Morbidity (%)	Mortality (%)	Rate of recurrent symptoms (%)	Reference
9	OF	1.4	56	11	0	Newman et al. 1990 [236]
10	OF	ns	20	10	30	Soravia et al. 1995 [237]
16	LF	2.2	63	0	73	Kabbej et al. 1996 [238]
9	OF	4.2	56	0	11	Gigot et al. 1997 [239]
1	LF	4.7	0	0	0	
6	OF	8	40	0	20	Martin et al. 1998 [240]
9	R	0.75	67	0	0	
7	LF	3.1	29	0	71	
8	LF	ns	38	0	13	Katkhounda et al. 1999 [241]
124	OR	8	63	3	11	Schnelldorfer et al. 2009 [228]
10	OLF	8	0	0	ns	
13	OF	4.9	8	8	0	Mazza et al. 2009 [242]
20	LF		25	0	5	
3	R		66	0	0	

F, fenestration; L, laparoscopic; ns, not significant; O, open; R, resection.

fewer than one half of patients [208]. Imaging with CT, ultrasonography, or MRI usually shows either a thickened cyst wall or different density of the cyst fluid [208]. If there is doubt, an indium leukocyte scan appears to be more sensitive than a gallium scan in the diagnosis of cyst infection [208]. Results of the culture of cyst fluid are almost always positive for single bacterial organisms, suggesting a hematogenous route of infection [208]. Treatment is with percutaneous or surgical drainage and intravenous broad-spectrum antibiotics.

Both ADPKD-associated PCLD and isolated PCLD are associated with the development of intracranial aneurysms [233,234]. Autopsy series show that 20% of patients with ADPKD have associated intracranial aneurysms [234]. Screening for aneurysms is probably prudent before considering anticoagulation or surgical therapy.

Management

The method of management of liver cysts depends on the size, number, and location of the cysts and on the clinical manifestations. Surgical therapy is generally reserved for patients with significant clinical symptoms that alter performance status given the relatively high morbidity and potential of mortality [228]. Surgical options include both open and laparoscopic fenestration (deroofing) of the cyst, hepatic resection and cyst fenestration, and OLT. Percutaneous drainage has no role in treatment because of the almost universal recurrence rate, but drainage followed by the addition of a sclerosing agent may be an alternative. Patients with one or a few cysts can be treated with laparoscopic fenestration or percutaneous drainage with sclerosis. The open surgical approach with cyst fenestration is more appropriate for deeper and larger numbers of cysts. Some surgeons have advocated open surgery with hepatic resection and cyst fenestration for patients with massive, highly symptomatic PCLD [228]. This procedure is most appropriate for patients with multiple cysts and areas of parenchymal sparing. OLT is reserved for patients with massive diffuse bilobar disease, who are homebound and unable to perform activities of daily living, or who have evidence of hepatic failure [235].

Table 35.6 lists selected series of both open and laparoscopic surgical results in the management of PCLD [228, 236–242]. In general, laparoscopic techniques have lower morbidity but higher rates of recurrence. Hepatic resection with cyst fenestration is the most effective technique in preventing recurrence, but it carries a high morbidity. Recurrence of symptoms is usually not caused by new cysts but by enlargement of the remaining cysts. Common postoperative complications include massive hemorrhage, biliary leaks, ascites, and infection. Careful patient selection is critical, especially with regard to the certainty that the symptoms are related to the liver cysts [243]. If there is doubt, consideration should be given to percutaneous cyst aspiration to assess clinical response.

Several small series with limited follow-up evaluation have shown successful sclerosis of hepatic cysts with alcohol and minocycline hydrochloride. This technique is generally more successful for the management of simple hepatic cysts than as therapy for PCLD. Complications include abdominal pain, fever, and ethanol intoxication. Care must be taken to avoid sclerosis of cysts that communicate with the biliary tree.

There are about 100 case reports of patients who have been have undergone liver transplantation for highly symptomatic PCLD [244]. Deceased-donor liver transplant with or without kidney transplantation is typical, but there are a few cases of living-donor transplantation. Symptom relief was nearly universal among the surviving patients. The outcome of OLT is similar to that of OLT performed for other typical indications at 1 year and probably superior with longer follow-up. Previous attempts at surgery may increase the risk of perioperative complications. Earlier series typically performed liver and kidney transplantation, but more recent series suggest that combined transplantation is only necessary if significant renal dysfunction is present.

While there is currently no clear role for medical therapy for PCLD, there is recent evidence that somatostatin analogs and mTOR inhibitors can decrease cyst size and potentially reduce symptoms.

Simple hepatic cysts

Simple hepatic cysts are thought to result from congenital defects of intrahepatic bile ducts. They are lined with biliary-type epithelium but do not generally connect with the biliary tree. These cysts are estimated to have an incidence of 2.5% among the general population, with increased frequency with advancing age [200]. They are most often asymptomatic incidental findings on abdominal imaging. When symptomatic, simple hepatic cysts can produce the same range of symptoms and complications as PCLD, although less frequently. Simple hepatic cysts can be differentiated from PCLD by lack of an autosomal dominant inheritance pattern, lack of associated renal

cysts, and smaller numbers of cysts, usually less than four [213]. Imaging with ultrasonography, CT, or MRI usually provides enough information for a diagnosis. On imaging the cysts appear as thin, smooth-walled, anechoic masses or water densities. Any septations or papillary projections should raise suspicion for cystadenoma or cystadenocarcinoma [245]. Management of symptomatic cysts is by percutaneous sclerosis, open surgical or laparoscopic fenestration, or resection. Percutaneous treatment with aspiration followed by alcohol or another sclerosing agent is successful in most cases, and the recurrence rate is low. Open and laparoscopic fenestration can be performed with similar success but higher morbidity.

Congenital hepatic fibrosis

Congenital hepatic fibrosis is a rare disorder that results in the fibrous destruction of interlobular bile ducts. The liver shows fibrous enlargement of the portal tracts; portal–portal bridging forms thick bands of scar that contain abnormal bile ducts. Normal-appearing cuboidal cells line the bile ducts in the scar (Fig. 35.13). CHF has been reported in association with other fibrocystic liver diseases, including adult PCLD, Caroli disease, choledochal cysts, and von Meyenburg complexes (see Fig. 35.9). CHF is most commonly associated with autosomal recessive polycystic kidney disease (ARPKD), which is caused by mutations in the PKHD1 gene [246]. It is not known whether the genetic defect in ARPKD is responsible for CHF, but the gene products localize to the primary cilium, the same location as the proteins associated with ADPKD [246]. At least one half and probably more of patients with CHF have associated renal disease. CHF also has been associated with a variety of rare pediatric syndromes, including renal dysplasia, nephronophthisis, Joubert syndrome, COACH syndrome (cerebellar vermis hypoplasia, oligophrenia, congenital

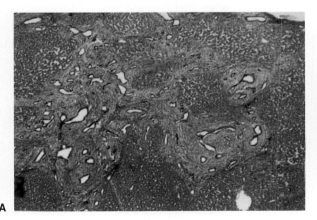
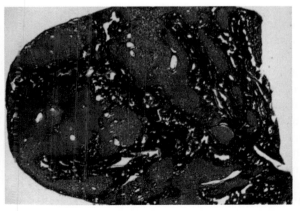

Figure 35.13 (A) Congenital hepatic fibrosis. Photomicrograph of the liver showing bands of scar with otherwise intact hepatic architecture and bile ducts in the scar lined by cuboidal epithelium. H&E. (B) Congenital hepatic fibrosis. Photomicrograph showing highlighting bands of scar with otherwise intact hepatic architecture. Masson trichrome stain. (Courtesy of Dr Elizabeth M. Brunt.)

*a*taxia, *c*oloboma, and *h*epatic fibrocirrhosis), Meckel syndrome type 1, Jeune syndrome, vaginal atresia, tuberous sclerosis, phosphomannose isomerase 1 deficiency, Ivemark syndrome type 2, short-rib syndrome, and osteochondrodysplasia [247].

The incidence of CHF is unknown. Because of the many clinical associations and the variable clinical presentation, some investigators believe that CHF is not a single entity but a spectrum of diseases. The cause of CHF is unknown. Desmet hypothesized that at birth, patients who will eventually have CHF have ductal plate malformations of the interlobular bile ducts. These immature bile ducts undergo destructive cholangitis that results in the loss of bile duct profiles and the formation of fibrous scar. The destructive cholangitis progresses at variable rates and may arrest, explaining the variety of clinical presentations of the disease [247]. The cause of the associated portal hypertension has been hypothesized to be hypoplasia or compression of the small branches of the portal vein [247].

The four patterns of clinical presentation of CHF are portal hypertensive, cholangitic, portal hypertensive–cholangitic, and latent. Serum aminotransferase levels are usually normal, although the alkaline phosphatase level is sometimes elevated. These patients usually do not have cirrhosis and maintain normal hepatic lobular architecture with normal hepatic function. The diagnosis is based on findings at liver biopsy. Surgical biopsy may be needed to obtain sufficient liver for diagnosis.

The portal hypertensive presentation is most common, representing approximately 70% of cases [248]. Portal hypertensive CHF usually manifests in childhood or young adulthood as complications of portal hypertension, especially variceal bleeding, with intact hepatic function. Hepatosplenomegaly may be present. Wedged hepatic venous pressure is normal, a finding consistent with presinusoidal portal hypertension. Symptomatic portal hypertension has traditionally been managed with surgical placement of a portosystemic shunt. Development of hepatic encephalopathy after shunting is extremely rare, probably because hepatic function is intact. Endoscopic variceal band ligation may be used to control acute bleeding. Endoscopic obliteration of esophageal varices is at least theoretically useful, although it would entail long-term endoscopic surveillance. Long-term follow-up evaluation of surgical shunts has shown that 39% of patients have jaundice, 17% have recurrent bleeding, and 17% have hepatic encephalopathy [249].

The cholangitic form of CHF manifests as fever, right upper quadrant pain, and a cholestatic pattern in the levels of the liver-associated enzymes. At least initially, patients with cholangitic CHF do not have evidence of portal hypertension. Treatment is with intravenous antibiotics. Either ERCP or percutaneous transhepatic cholangiography (PTC) can be used to image the biliary tree and relieve obstruction. These patients often have associated Caroli disease, which results in the cholangitic signs and symptoms. Repeated bouts of cholangitis can lead to secondary biliary cirrhosis and the need for liver transplantation. Patients should be treated for Caroli disease as described later.

The portal hypertensive–cholangitic or mixed presentation is a combination of symptoms of portal hypertension and cholangitis. Treatment is based on the presence of the symptoms described earlier. The latent form is typically discovered either at autopsy or during evaluation for other problems. It is generally asymptomatic and therefore requires no treatment.

Rare reported associations with CHF include disease isolated to one lobe of the liver, cholangiocarcinoma, ascites, and cavernous transformation of the portal vein.

Von Meyenburg complexes

Von Meyenburg complexes, also called *biliary microhamartomata*, are usually incidental and asymptomatic findings at liver biopsy. They are found in approximately 5% of adults and 1% of children in series of consecutive autopsies. The complexes consist of variable numbers of dilated bile ducts embedded in a fibrous stroma and occur in small groups adjacent to portal tracts (Fig. 35.14). The complexes may contain inspissated bile concretions and polypoid projections into the lumen. They are hypothesized to result from fibrosis and occasionally from the involution of remnant ductal plate malformations of peripheral interlobular bile ducts [225]. Von Meyenburg complexes are thought to be the origin of the cysts in PCLD. They are also found in association with Caroli disease, CHF, and in normal liver. There are rare

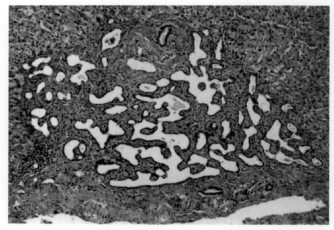

Figure 35.14 Photomicrograph of the liver showing a typical von Meyenburg complex with a group of dilated bile ducts in fibrous stroma. H&E. (Courtesy of Dr Elizabeth M. Brunt.)

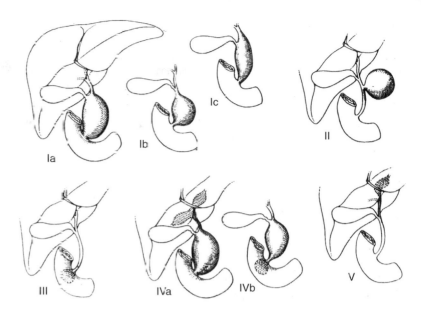

Figure 35.15 The Todani modification of the Alonso–Lej classification of choledochal cysts. (Adapted from Todani et al. [250] with permission from Elsevier.)

reports of cholangiocarcinoma developing within a von Meyenburg complex.

Choledochal cysts

Epidemiology, course of disease, and clinical features

Choledochal cysts are congenital dilatations of the intrahepatic and extrahepatic biliary tree. Vater and Elzer first described choledochal cysts in 1723. The Todani modification of the Alonso–Lej classification of choledochal cysts is the system most often used for planning the management of these cysts (Fig. 35.15) [250]. The estimated incidence varies from 1 in 13,000 in Japan to 1 in 2 million in England [251,252]. The frequency of diagnosis seems to be increasing, probably because of improvements in abdominal imaging [252]. Type I cysts represent approximately 85% of most series [253]. Type II cysts are rare, representing less than 2% of cases, and are sometimes called common bile duct diverticulum [254]. Type III cysts or choledochoceles also are rare, representing approximately 2% of cases, although they may be more common in tertiary referral endoscopy centers [255]. Type IV cysts represent the remaining approximately 10% of cases. Type V cysts are Caroli disease.

The cysts usually manifest themselves in childhood but may be diagnosed in the prenatal period through late adulthood. Only approximately 20% of cases manifest themselves in adults. There is a female predominance [256]. Neonates have jaundice and a palpable mass [257]. In the first decade of life, ascending cholangitis is a more likely manifestation. The diagnosis is made when ultrasonography, CT, hydroxy iminodiacetic acid (HIDA) imaging, endoscopic retrograde cholangiography, PTC, or magnetic resonance cholangiography shows characteris-

tic dilatation of the biliary tree. Liver function tests may show elevated alkaline phosphatase, total bilirubin, and γ-glutamyl transpeptidase levels consistent with biliary obstruction [257]. Manifestation in adulthood is often preceded by several years of vague right upper quadrant abdominal pain [258]. At diagnosis the patient usually has a complication such as jaundice, cholangitis, or pancreatitis [258]. CHF is often associated with choledochal cysts, especially Caroli disease.

Etiology

There are several theories about their etiology, although the true cause of choledochal cysts remains unclear. One theory suggests that failure of canalization of the fetal biliary tree results in obstruction and, later, dilatation of the common bile duct. Another theory suggests that obstruction occurs from anatomic kinking or external pressure on the developing bile ducts that results in cyst dilatation. Probably the most accepted theory was first proposed by Babbit, which stated that the high insertion of the common bile duct into the pancreatic duct leads to reflux of pancreatic juice into the biliary tree. This leakage causes weakening of the bile duct wall, inflammation, and fibrosis. The distal bile duct becomes obstructed and therefore results in proximal dilatation with cyst formation [259]. There appears to be a high rate of anomalous pancreaticobiliary duct junction in the range of 90% in most series [260].

Management

Management of choledochal cysts is based on the type of cyst according to the Todani classification (see Fig. 35.15). Some authors argue that the Todani classification scheme is misleading and overcomplicated [261]. They propose a simplified naming system matched to the treatment and risk of future malignant transformation, which is described at the end of this section. The first premise of treatment is to obtain adequate drainage and antibiotic coverage for any patient with signs and symptoms of cholangitis, as seen with PTC or ERCP.

The current standard of practice for type I and II choledochal cysts is complete cyst excision with anastomosis of the bifurcation of the hepatic ducts, common hepatic duct, or common bile duct with Roux-en-Y anastomosis to the jejunum or directly to the duodenum. The surgery can be performed either with an open or a laparoscopic approach. Biliary enteric anastomosis at the bifurcation of the hepatic ducts appears to offer the advantage of a lower rate of late strictures [262]. Cyst enterostomy is generally no longer performed because of the high rate of long-term complications, including anastomotic strictures that result in jaundice and cholangitis and the late development of cholangiocarcinoma [258,263]. Patients who have undergone previous cyst enterostomy and have late complications of surgery need complete cyst excision with Roux-en-Y hepaticojejunostomy. Patients with an asymptomatic cyst who are otherwise good surgical candidates should be considered for elective cyst excision and Roux-en-Y hepaticojejunostomy to prevent the development of cancer [258].

Type III choledochal cysts are also called *choledochoceles*. Patients have pancreatitis, obstructive jaundice, or biliary colic [264]. They may have a history of cholecystectomy for acalculous cholecystitis with continued symptoms after surgery [264]. The differential diagnosis includes papillary tumor, papillitis from an impacted stone, papillary fibrosis, pancreatitis, duodenal duplication, and submucosal contrast injection during ERCP [265]. This broad differential diagnosis warrants cholangiography and biopsy to rule out tumors [265]. Choledochoceles rarely develop into cancer, and therefore complete excision may not be mandatory [255,256]. Large cysts should be excised either partially or completely and the ducts reanastomosed to the duodenum [260]. Small choledochoceles can be managed with endoscopic sphincterotomy [256,261]. Endoscopic pancreatic sphincterotomy may be necessary if the pancreatic duct does not drain well [255].

Type IVa choledochal cysts with both intrahepatic and extrahepatic components make total cyst excision difficult. Total excision of the extrahepatic cysts can usually be accomplished, and anastomosis with the enteric tract should be performed at the hilum to prevent a high rate of anastomotic strictures. Formation of a Hutson loop, which provides easy percutaneous access to the reconstructed biliary tree, has been advocated, especially if intrahepatic cysts are not resected [266]. Partial hepatectomy, if technically feasible, has also been advocated for

the removal of intrahepatic cysts because of malignant potential. The risk of biliary cancer in the retained intrahepatic cysts is not known but is probably low, with only a few reported cases.

The presence of type V cysts, also known as *Caroli disease*, results in multiple intrahepatic biliary cysts and makes treatment more difficult. Complete resection of biliary cysts is usually impossible because of the location of the cysts. For this reason, conservative treatment of cholangitis with antibiotics is usually the initial choice. Rotating antibiotics to suppress episodes of cholangitis is advisable but is of unproven value. If the cysts are superficial and limited in number, hepatic resection can sometimes be curative. An alternative is to relieve obstruction with partial cyst excision and Roux-en-Y cyst jejunostomy. Liver transplantation is generally reserved for patients with hepatic failure. Prognosis is much worse for this type of choledochal cyst than for the others. Tsuchida et al. [267] found a 63% mortality in a survey of patients whose cases were reported in the literature.

Without therapy for choledochal cysts, biliary cancer, usually cholangiocarcinoma, develops in approximately 15–19% of patients older than 20 years and generally carries a dismal prognosis [258,263]. The most common site of the cancer is the cyst wall, but as many as 40% of cases occur at other sites in the liver or pancreas, especially the gallbladder [254]. For this reason and to prevent future gallbladder-related symptoms, cholecystectomy is usually performed during cyst surgery. There are rare case reports of late cholangiocarcinoma after initial resection, particularly if any cysts can not be resected or if there is persistent dilatation of a segment of the biliary tree.

Complications include jaundice, pancreatitis, spontaneous cyst rupture, biliary cirrhosis, and signs of portal hypertension, including variceal bleeding and ascites [268]. The postoperative rate of recurrence of symptoms can be as high as 32%, but the symptoms most often respond to conservative therapy with antibiotics [269].

The simplified system calls type I and IVa cysts "choledochal cysts" because they are variations of a single disease with dilatation of the extrahepatic biliary tree and varying levels of involvement of the intrahepatic tree. They represent the most common type of choledochal cysts, have the highest risk of malignant transformation, are associated with pancreaticobiliary maljunction, and require complete excision of the extrahepatic biliary tree with a high biliary enteric anastomosis. Type II cysts are rare diverticuli of the common bile duct that can be treated with simple excision of the cyst. Type III should be called choledochoceles because they are lined with duodenal mucosa, do not require complete excision, and rarely develop malignant transformation. Type V cysts should be called Caroli disease and differ from the other types by affecting only the intrahepatic ducts, being associated with ductal plate malformation, having low malignant potential, and being associated with CHF and portal hypertension.

Cystic neoplasms of the liver: cystadenoma

Cystadenoma, also called *biliary cystadenoma*, is a benign tumor of the liver in which an epithelial layer surrounds a large, fluid-filled cyst in the hepatic parenchyma or rarely in the extrahepatic biliary tree. It represents less than 5% of cystic lesions of the liver. Cystadenoma is hypothesized to arise from a congenital defect of the bile ducts or gallbladder. It may form out of rests of primitive foregut. It can be found in association with bile duct hamartoma.

Cystadenoma manifests itself any time from childhood onward, although 80–85% of cases occur among middle-aged women. The clinical manifestations are typically the result of compression of an expanding liver mass on adjacent structures. Approximately 70% of patients have epigastric or right upper quadrant pain, sometimes with radiation to the right shoulder. Approximately one half of patients have a palpable abdominal mass or increasing abdominal girth, and approximately one third of patients have compression of the biliary tree that leads to cholangitis or jaundice [270]. Some patients have symptoms of gastric compression, such as nausea, vomiting, bloating, and anorexia. In some patients, the cysts are incidental findings on imaging of the abdomen. Extrahepatic cystadenoma typically manifests as abdominal pain and jaundice [271].

Complications are rare and have been reported to include sepsis, hemorrhage, and rupture. Transformation into malignant cystadenocarcinoma can occur and result in local invasion and occasional distant metastasis. Nearly all the reported cases of malignant transformation occur in patients who have the stromal layer.

The diagnosis of cystadenoma is suggested by the ultrasonographic findings of a multilocular, anechoic, fluid-filled cyst with thickened walls and multiple septations or papillary projections [272]. The cyst is usually located in the hepatic parenchyma, although extrahepatic cysts have been reported. There is usually no connection with the biliary tree. Levels of liver-associated enzymes are usually normal unless there is biliary obstruction. The serum level of cancer antigen 19-9 (CA19-9) may be mildly elevated, but levels of carcinoembryonic antigen 125 (CA125) and α-fetoprotein are normal. Cyst fluid CA19-9 level is elevated, but aspiration carries a small risk of dissemination if carcinoma is present. The lesions should be differentiated from pyogenic abscess, amebic abscess, and echinococcal cysts on the basis of clinical manifestations and imaging findings.

Pathologic examination reveals cuboidal and columnar epithelial cells with vacuolizations lining the cysts. Usually adjacent to the epithelium is an area of spindle cell

stroma (also called mesenchymal stroma) surrounded by a layer of collagenous connective tissue. Mesenchymal stroma are exclusively found in female patients and may represent a different form of the disease than those without stroma [273]. The cyst fluid is usually mucinous, but it may contain bile or blood.

Treatment is complete surgical resection by means of either enucleation (excision of a mass with a thin layer of normal tissue) or anatomic resection. In the past, incomplete excision or drainage procedures led to a high recurrence rate and did not remove the risk of malignant transformation. There is a 50% rate of recurrence of extrahepatic cysts without sleeve resection with biliary enteric anastomosis [274].

Ciliated foregut cyst

Foregut cysts derive from the primitive foregut and may occur in the mediastinum, pancreas, tongue, and upper aerodigestive tract as well as in the liver and subhepatic space. They are filled with mucinous, sometimes bloody, fluid and their main clinical significance is that they can sometimes be confused with solid tumors [275,276].

Echinococcal cysts

Hydatid disease caused by *Echinococcus granulosus* cystic echinococcosis is endemic in parts of western and southern Europe, the Middle East, northern Africa, South and Central America, Russia, and China. The annual incidence ranges from less than one case to as many as 42 cases/100,000 persons in some regions [277]. Humans are accidental hosts who ingest eggs from contaminated dogs that were usually infected from sheep. The liver is involved in one half to three fourths of cases. The cysts range from 1 to >20 cm in size. Rarely, hydatid disease called *alveolar echinococcosis* can occur due to *E. multilocularis*. It is endemic in parts of North America, central Europe, and northern and central Eurasia. Incidence is generally less than 1/100,000 [277]. Humans are accidental hosts who ingest eggs from foxes or forest rodents.

Diagnosis is based on a high index of clinical suspicion and findings on imaging with ultrasonography, CT, or MRI. The initial symptoms are usually caused by complications of the cysts or physical compression of adjacent organs by the cysts. Symptoms such as epigastric or right upper quadrant pain, fatigue, fever, nausea, and dyspepsia may be present. Cyst rupture can produce jaundice, cholangitis, acute pancreatitis, and immune reactions such as anaphylaxis or asthma. Ultrasonography, CT, and MRI are sensitive and specific for hydatid disease, with cross-sectional imaging being superior in identifying the location of the cysts, including extrahepatic cysts, and the type of cyst. Serologic tests, including an indirect hemagglutination test and enzyme-linked immunosorbent assay for antibodies to *Echinococcus* antigens are approximately 90% sensitive but have variable specificity because of cross-reaction with other parasites and may not distinguish cystic from alveolar disease.

There is controversy about the most appropriate treatment for cystic echinococcosis. Some advocate treatment even in asymptomatic patients to prevent complications such as rupture, infection, or anaphylaxis. Others have shown that small, nonsuperficial, and asymptomatic cysts can remain stable for more than 10 years. The choice of treatment depends on the type of cyst (usually defined by ultrasonographic appearance), the location of the cyst, the general medical status of the patient, and local experience. Because of its potential for aggressive infiltration of the liver and other organs and high mortality, radical surgical resection and at least 2 years of chemotherapy is the first choice of treatment for alveolar echinocococcosis.

Open surgery with cyst removal or drainage and obliteration of the cyst cavity was until recently the primary mode of treatment for cystic echinococcosis. Although in the literature results of series of open surgical treatment are variable, they generally show a mortality ranging from 0% to 5%, morbidity from 8% to 25%, and long-term recurrence rates of 2–25%. Several series of laparoscopic cyst surgery have shown morbidity and mortality similar to those of open surgery but they generally involve less difficult cyst types and locations. Any surgical or percutaneous therapy carries a risk of dissemination of daughter cysts into the abdomen, but modern techniques and experienced surgeons significantly limit the risk.

Puncture, aspiration, introduction of protoscolicidal agent, and reaspiration (PAIR) is a percutaneous treatment developed by interventional radiologists in the mid-1980s. The connection of the cyst to the biliary tree is an absolute contraindication for this procedure, and only certain configurations of cysts are amenable to this treatment. Series of patients treated with PAIR and chemotherapy at experienced centers showed no mortality and less than 10% morbidity but the cysts were generally smaller, less complex, and amenable to a percutaneous approach. Long-term recurrence rates are not yet available but short-term results look promising.

Chemotherapy with benzimidazole compounds, mebendazole or albendazole, is generally reserved for patients not amenable to treatment by other means or as an adjunct to other treatment, especially PAIR [278]. Chemotherapy has approximately a 30% cure rate, but up to 70% of cysts will reduce in size. Relapse rates are about 25%.

Annotated references

Charny CK, Jarnagin WR, Schwartz LH, et al. Management of 155 patients with benign liver tumours. *Br J Surg* 2001;88:808–13.

A large retrospective study from the New York Presbyterian Hospital–Cornell Campus reviewing the indications and results of resection of benign hepatic lesions in 155 patients.

Desmet VJ. What is congenital hepatic fibrosis? *Histopathology* 1992;20:465–77.

A narrative description of CHF, a condition closely linked with several cystic liver diseases, by an expert hepatopathologist.

Dokmak S, Paradis V, Vilgrain V, et al. A single-center surgical experience of 122 patients with single and multiple hepatocellular adenomas. *Gastroenterology* 2009;137:1698–705.

A large case series that identifies features of high-risk adenomas.

Eckert, J, Deplazes P. Biological, epidemiological, and clinical aspects of echinococcosis, a zoonosis of increasing concern. *Clin Microbiol Rev* 2004;17(1):107–35.

A thorough review of echinococcosis.

Geller SA, Petrovic LM. Benign tumors and tumor-like conditions. In: Geller SA, Petrovic LM. *Biopsy Interpretation of the Liver*, 2nd edn. Philadelphia, PA: Lippincott Williams and Wilkins, 2003:281–304.

This chapter provides detailed illustrated descriptions of the macroscopic and microscopic appearance of hepatic tumors and tumor-like lesions.

International Working Party. Terminology of nodular hepatocellular lesions. *Hepatology* 1995;22:983–93.

An important paper that provides a pathology-based classification of nodular diseases of the liver.

Makhlouf HR, Abdul-Al HM, Goodman ZD. Diagnosis of focal nodular hyperplasia of the liver by needle biopsy. *Hum Pathol* 2005;36:1210–16.

Illustrated histologic review of 100 consecutive cases of FNH evaluated at the Armed Forces Institute of Pathology giving a broad summary of the typical pathologic features of FNH.

Martin DR, Danrad R, Hussain SM. MR imaging of the liver. *Radiol Clin North Am* 2005;43:861–98.

A recent extensive overview on MRI of diffuse and focal lesions of the liver. It discusses imaging techniques and characteristic features of focal hepatic lesions.

Nguyen BN, Flejou JF, Terris B, et al. Focal nodular hyperplasia of the liver: a comprehensive pathologic study of 305 lesions and recognition of new histologic forms. *Am J Surg Pathol* 1999;23:1441–54.

A large case series of patients with FNH. Clinical presentation and pathology are described.

Rebouissou S. Bioulac-Sage P. Zucman-Rossi J. Molecular pathogenesis of focal nodular hyperplasia and hepatocellular adenoma. *J Hepatol* 2008;48:163–70.

A review of the pathogenesis and classification of hepatocellular adenoma.

Todani T, Watanabe Y, Narusue M, et al. Congenital bile duct cysts: classification, operative procedures, and review of thirty-seven cases including cancer arising from choledochal cyst. *Am J Surg* 1977;134:263–9.

The classification of choledochal cysts described in the paper is still used today and plays an important role in planning therapy.

Torres VE. Polycystic liver disease. In: Watson M, Torres VE, eds. *Polycystic Kidney Disease*. Oxford: Oxford University Press, 1996:500–29.

A detailed review of the pathogenesis, pathology, clinical presentation, and management of PCLD.

Wanless IR. Micronodular transformation (nodular regenerative hyperplasia) of the liver: a report of 64 cases among 2,500 autopsies and a new classification of benign hepatocellular nodules. *Hepatology* 1990;11:787–97.

A very large autopsy series of patients with NRH and a proposed classification of this condition.

Yoon SS, Charny CK, Fong Y, et al. Diagnosis, management, and outcomes of 115 patients with hepatic hemangioma. *J Am Coll Surg* 2003;197:392–402.

A comprehensive review of 115 patients evaluated at the Memorial Sloan–Kettering Cancer Center for hepatic hemangiomas.

References

1. Rooks JB, Ory HW, Ishak KG, et al. Epidemiology of hepatocellular adenoma. The role of oral contraceptive use. *JAMA* 1979;242(7):644–8.

2. Edmondson HA, Henderson B, Benton B. Liver-cell adenomas associated with use of oral contraceptives. *N Engl J Med* 1976;294(9):470–2.

3. Cherqui D, Rahmouni A, Charlotte F, et al. Management of focal nodular hyperplasia and hepatocellular adenoma in young women: a series of 41 patients with clinical, radiological, and pathological correlations. *Hepatology* 1995;22(6):1674–81.

4. Sale GE, Lerner KG. Multiple tumors after androgen therapy. *Arch Pathol Lab Med* 1977;101(11):600–3.

5. Bala S, Wunsch PH, Ballhausen WG. Childhood hepatocellular adenoma in familial adenomatous polyposis: mutations in adenomatous polyposis coli gene and p53. *Gastroenterology* 1997;112(3):919–22.

6. Labrune P, Trioche P, Duvaltier I, et al. Hepatocellular adenomas in glycogen storage disease type I and III: a series of 43 patients and review of the literature. *J Pediatr Gastroenterol Nutr* 1997;24(3):276–9.

7. Grazioli L, Federle MP, Ichikawa T, et al. Liver adenomatosis: clinical, histopathologic, and imaging findings in 15 patients. *Radiology* 2000;216(2):395–402.

8. Bluteau O, Jeannot E, Bioulac-Sage P, et al. Bi-allelic inactivation of TCF1 in hepatic adenomas. *Nat Genet* 2002;32:312–15.

9. Bacq Y, Jacquemin E, Balabaud C, et al. Familial liver adenomatosis associated with hepatocyte nuclear factor 1α inactivation. *Gastroenterology* 2003;125:1470–5.

10. Wanless IR, Medline A. Role of estrogens as promoters of hepatic neoplasia. *Lab Invest* 1982;46(3):313–20.

11. Edmondson HA, Reynolds TB, Henderson B, et al. Regression of liver cell adenomas associated with oral contraceptives. *Ann Intern Med* 1977;86(2):180–2.

12. Bioulac-Sage P, Laumonier H, Couchy G, et al. Hepatocellular adenoma management and phenotypic classification: the Bordeaux experience. *Hepatology* 2009;50(2):481–9.

13. Bioulac-Sage P, Balabaud C, Zucman-Rossi J. Subtype classification of hepatocellular adenoma. *Dig Surg* 2010;27:39–45.

14. Dokmak S, Paradis V, Vilgrain V, et al. A single-center surgical experience of 122 patients with single and multiple hepatocellular adenomas. *Gastroenterology* 2009;137:1698–705.

15. Paradis V, Benzekri A, Dargere D, et al. Telangiectatic focal nodular hyperplasia: a variant of hepatocellular adenoma. *Gastroenterology* 2004;126:1323–9.

16. Rebouissou S, Amessou M, Couchy G, et al. Frequent in-frame somatic deletions activate gp130 in inflammatory hepatocellular tumors. *Nature* 2009;457:200–5.

17. Goodman ZD. Neoplasms of the liver. *Mod Pathol* 2007;20:S49–60.

18. Ishak KG. Benign tumors and pseudotumors of the liver. *Appl Patho* 1988;6(2):82–104.

19. Geller S, Petrovic L. Benign tumors and tumor-like conditions. In *Biopsy Interpretation of the Liver*, 3rd edn. Philadelphia, PA: Lippincott Williams and Wilkins, 2003:281–304.

20. Deneve JL, Pawlik TM, Cunningham S, et al. Liver cell adenoma: a multicenter analysis of risk factors for rupture and malignancy. *Ann Surg Oncol* 2009;16:640–8.

21. Reddy KR, Kligerman S, Levi J, et al. Benign and solid tumors of the liver: relationship to sex, age, size of tumors, and outcome. *Am Surg* 2001;67(2):173–8.

22. Kerlin P, Davis GL, McGill DB, et al. Hepatic adenoma and focal nodular hyperplasia: clinical, pathologic, and radiologic features. *Gastroenterology* 1983;84(5 Pt 1):994–1002.

23. Klatskin G. Hepatic tumors: possible relationship to use of oral contraceptives. *Gastroenterology* 1977;73(2):386–94.

24. Gordon SC, Reddy KR, Livingstone AS, et al. Resolution of a contraceptive-steroid-induced hepatic adenoma with subsequent evolution into hepatocellular carcinoma. *Ann Intern Med* 1986;105(4):547–9.

25. Niserbaum HL, Rowling SE. Ultrasound of focal hepatic lesions. *Semin Roentgenol* 1995;30(4):324–46.

26. van den Esschert JW, van Gulik TM, Phoa SSKS. Imaging modalities for focal nodular hyperplasia and hepatocellular adenoma. *Dig Surg* 2010;27:46–55.

27. Nino-Murcia M, Olcott EW, Jeffrey RB Jr, et al. Focal liver lesions: pattern-based classification scheme for enhancement at arterial phase CT. *Radiology* 2000;215(3):746–51.

28. Laumonier H, Bioulac-Sage P, Laurent C, et al. Hepatocellular adenomas: magnetic resonance imaging features as a function of molecular pathological classification. *Hepatology* 2008;48(3):808–18.

29. Gibbs JF, Litwin AM, Kahlenberg MS. Contemporary management of benign liver tumors. *Surg Clin North Am* 2004;84(2):463–80.

30. Eckhauser FE, Krol JA, Raper SE, et al. Enucleation combined with hepatic vascular exclusion is a safe and effective alternative to hepatic resection for liver cell adenoma. *Am Surg* 1994;60(7):466–71.

31. Descottes B, Glineur D, Lachachi F, et al. Laparoscopic liver resection of benign liver tumors. *Surg Endosc* 2003;17(1):23–30.

32. Erdogan D, van Delden OM, Busch OR, et al. Selective transcatheter arterial embolization for treatment of bleeding complications or reduction of tumor mass of hepatocellular carcinoma. *Cardiovasc Intervent Radiol* 2007;30(6):1252–8.

33. Stoot JHMB, van der Linden E, Terprstra OT, et al. Life-saving therapy for haemorrhaging liver adenomas using selective arterial embolization. *Br J Surg* 2007;94(10):1249–53.

34. Kim YI, Chung JW, Park JH. Feasibility of transcatheter arterial chemoembolization for hepatic adenoma. *J Vasc Intervent Radiol* 2007;18:862–7.

35. Rhim H, Lim HK, Kim Y-S, et al. Percutaneous radiofrequency ablation of hepatocellular adenoma: initial experience in 10 patients. *J Gastroenterol Hepatol* 2008;23:e422–7.

36. Selby R, Starzl TE, Yunis E, et al. Liver transplantation for type I and type IV glycogen storage disease. *Eur J Pediatr* 1993;152(Suppl 1):S71–6.

37. Reddy SK, Austin SL, Spencer-Manzon M, et al. Liver transplantation for glycogen storage disease type Ia. *J Hepatol* 2009;51:483–90.

38. Gyorffy EJ, Bredfeldt JE, Black WC. Transformation of hepatic cell adenoma to hepatocellular carcinoma due to oral contraceptive use. *Ann Intern Med* 1989;110(6):489–90.

39. Ryan IP, Havel RJ, Laros RK Jr. Three consecutive pregnancies in a patient with glycogen storage disease type IA (von Gierke's disease). *Am J Obstet Gynecol* 1994;170(6):1687–90.

40. Allaire GS, Rabin L, Ishak KG, et al. Bile duct adenoma. A study of 152 cases *Am J Surg Pathol* 1988;12(9):708–15.

41. Eathal PS, Hughes NR, Goodman ZD. The so-called bile duct adenoma is a peribiliary gland hamartoma. *Am J Surg Pathol* 1996;20:858–64.

42. Lubin RS, Mitchell DG. Evaluation of the solid hepatic mass. *Med Clin North Am* 1996;80(5):907–28.

43. Brunt EM. Benign tumors of the liver. *Clin Liver Dis* 2001;5(1):1–15.

44. Nichols FC III, van Heerden JA, Weiland LH. Benign liver tumors. *Surg Clin North Am* 1989;69(2):297–314.

45. Gemer O, Moscovici O, Ben-Horin CL, et al. Oral contraceptives and liver hemangioma: a case–control study. *Acta Obstet Gynecol Scand* 2004;83(12):1199–201.

46. Au WY, Liu CL. Growth of giant hepatic hemangioma after triplet pregnancy. *J Hepatol* 2005;42(5):781.

47. Conter RL, Longmire WP Jr. Recurrent hepatic hemangiomas. Possible association with estrogen therapy. *Ann Surg* 1988;207(2):115–19.

48. Graham E, Cohen AW, Soulen M, et al. Symptomatic liver hemangioma with intra-tumor hemorrhage treated by angiography and embolization during pregnancy. *Obstet Gynecol* 1993; 81(5(Pt 2):813–16.

49. Adam YG, Huvos AG, Fortner JG. Giant hemangiomas of the liver. *Ann Surg* 1970;172(2):239–45.

50. Deutsch GS, Yeh KA, Bates WB III, et al. Embolization for management of hepatic hemangiomas. *Am Surg* 2001;67(2):159–64.

51. Yoon SS, Charny CK, Fong Y, et al. Diagnosis, management, and outcomes of 115 patients with hepatic hemangioma. *J Am Coll Surg* 2003;197(3):392–402.

52. Pateron D, Babany G, Belghiti J, et al. Giant hemangioma of the liver with pain, fever, and abnormal liver tests. Report of two cases. *Dig Dis Sci* 1991;36(4):524–7.

53. Kadry Z, Mentha G, Cereda JM. Polymyalgia rheumatica as a manifestation of a large hepatic cavernous hemangioma. *J Hepatol* 2000;32(2):358–60.

54. Farges O, Daradkeh S, Bismuth H. Cavernous hemangiomas of the liver: are there any indications for resection? *World J Surg* 1995;19(1):19–24.

55. Hotokezaka M, Kojima M, Nakamura K, et al. Traumatic rupture of hepatic hemangioma. *J Clin Gastroenterol* 1996;23(1):69–71.

56. Roslyn JJ, Kuchenbecker S, Longmire WP, et al. Floating tumor debris. A cause of intermittent biliary obstruction. *Arch Surg* 1984;119(11):1312–15.

57. Takahashi T, Katoh H, Dohke M, et al. A giant hepatic hemangioma with secondary portal hypertension: a case report of successful surgical treatment. *Hepatogastroenterology* 1997;44(16):1212–14.

58. Hall GW. Kasabach–Merritt syndrome: pathogenesis and management. *Br J Haematol* 2001;112(4):851–62.

59. Yamagata M, Kanematsu T, Matsumata T, et al. Management of haemangioma of the liver: comparison of results between surgery and observation. *Br J Surg* 1991;78(10):1223–5.

60. Trastek VF, van Heerden JA, Sheedy PF, et al. Cavernous hemangiomas of the liver: resect or observe? *Am J Surg* 1983;145(1):49–53.

61. Gandolfi L, Leo P, Solmi L, et al. Natural history of hepatic haemangiomas: clinical and ultrasound study. *Gut* 1991;32(6):677–80.

62. Kim TK, Han JK, Kim AY, et al. Signal from hepatic hemangiomas on power Doppler US: real or artefactual? *Ultrasound Med Biol* 1999;25(7):1055–61.

63. Kim TK, Choi BI, Han JK, et al. Hepatic tumors: contrast agent-enhancement patterns with pulse-inversion harmonic US. *Radiology* 2000;216(2):411–17.

64. Bertolotto M, Dalla PL, Quaia E, et al. Characterization of unifocal liver lesions with pulse inversion harmonic imaging after Levovist injection: preliminary results. *Eur Radiol* 2000;10(9):1369–76.

65. Kim T, Federle MP, Baron RL, et al. Discrimination of small hepatic hemangiomas from hypervascular malignant tumors smaller than 3 cm with three-phase helical CT. *Radiology* 2001;219(3):699–706.

66. Freeny PC, Marks WM. Hepatic hemangioma: dynamic bolus CT. *AJR Am J Roentgenol* 1986;147(4):711–19.

67. van Leeuwen MS, Noordzij J, Feldberg MA, et al. Focal liver lesions: characterization with triphasic spiral CT. *Radiology* 1996;201(2):327–36.

68. Martin DR, Danrad R, Hussain SM. MR imaging of the liver. *Radiol Clin North Am* 2005;43(5):861–86, viii.

69. Semelka RC, Martin DR, Balci C, et al. Focal liver lesions: comparison of dual-phase CT and multisequence multiplanar MR imaging including dynamic gadolinium enhancement. *J Magn Reson Imaging* 2001;13(3):397–401.

70. Farlow DC, Chapman PR, Gruenewald SM, et al. Investigation of focal hepatic lesions: is tomographic red blood cell imaging useful? *World J Surg* 1990;14(4):463–7.

71. Tsai CC, Yen TC, Tzen KY. The value of Tc-99m red blood cell SPECT in differentiating giant cavernous hemangioma of the liver from other liver solid masses. *Clin Nucl Med* 2002;27(8):578–81.

72. Soulen MC. Angiographic evaluation of focal liver masses. *Semin Roentgenol* 1995;30(4):362–74.

73. Vilgrain V, Boulos L, Vullierme MP, et al. Imaging of atypical hemangiomas of the liver with pathologic correlation. *Radiographics* 2000;20(2):379–97.

74. Naganuma H, Ishida H, Konno K, et al. Hepatic hemangioma with arterioportal shunts. *Abdom Imaging* 1999;24(1):42–6.

75. Kim S, Chung JJ, Kim MJ, et al. Atypical inside-out pattern of hepatic hemangiomas. *AJR Am J Roentgenol* 2000;174(6):1571–4.

76. Weimann A, Ringe B, Klempnauer J, et al. Benign liver tumors: differential diagnosis and indications for surgery. *World J Surg* 1997;21(9):983–90.

77. Terriff BA, Gibney RG, Scudamore CH. Fatality from fine-needle aspiration biopsy of a hepatic hemangioma. *AJR Am J Roentgenol* 1990;154(1):203–4.

78. Belli L, de CL, Beati C, et al. Surgical treatment of symptomatic giant hemangiomas of the liver. *Surg Gynecol Obstet* 1992;174(6):474–8.

79. Iwatsuki S, Todo S, Starzl TE. Excisional therapy for benign hepatic lesions. *Surg Gynecol Obstet* 1990;171(3):240–6.

80. Gedaly R, Pomposelli JJ, Pomfret EA, et al. Cavernous hemangioma of the liver: anatomic resection vs. enucleation. *Arch Surg* 1999;134(4):407–11.

81. Yamamoto T, Kawarada Y, Yano T, et al. Spontaneous rupture of hemangioma of the liver: treatment with transcatheter hepatic arterial embolization. *Am J Gastroenterol* 1991;86(11):1645–9.

82. Suzuki H, Nimura Y, Kamiya J, et al. Preoperative transcatheter arterial embolization for giant cavernous hemangioma of the liver with consumption coagulopathy. *Am J Gastroenterol* 1997;92(4):688–91.

83. Reading NG, Forbes A, Nunnerley HB, et al. Hepatic haemangioma: a critical review of diagnosis and management. *Q J Med* 1988;67(253):431–45.

84. Gaspar L, Mascarenhas F, da Costa MS, et al. Radiation therapy in the unresectable cavernous hemangioma of the liver. *Radiother Oncol* 1993;29(1):45–50.

85. Zagoria RJ, Roth TJ, Levine EA, et al. Radiofrequency ablation of a symptomatic hepatic cavernous hemangioma. *AJR Am J Roentgenol* 2004;182(1):210–12.

86. Russo MW, Johnson MW, Fair JH, et al. Orthotopic liver transplantation for giant hepatic hemangioma. *Am J Gastroenterol* 1997;92(10):1940–1.

87. Ferraz AA, Sette MJ, Maia M, et al. Liver transplant for the treatment of giant hepatic hemangioma. *Liver Transpl* 2004;10(11):1436–7.

88. Ehren H, Mahour GH, Isaacs H Jr. Benign liver tumors in infancy and childhood. Report of 48 cases. *Am J Surg* 1983;145(3):325–9.

89. Zafrani ES. Update on vascular tumours of the liver. *J Hepatol* 1989;8(1):125–30.

90. Linderkamp O, Hopner F, Klose H, et al. Solitary hepatic hemangioma in a newborn infant complicated by cardiac failure, consumption coagulopathy, microangiopathic hemolytic anemia, and obstructive jaundice. Case report and review of the literature. *Eur J Pediatr* 1976;124(1):23–9.

91. Strate SM, Rutledge JC, Weinberg AG. Delayed development of angiosarcoma in multinodular infantile hepatic hemangioendothelioma. *Arch Pathol Lab Med* 1984;108(12):943–4.

92. Hobbs KE. Hepatic hemangiomas. *World J Surg* 1990;14(4):468–71.

93. Goldberg SJ, Fonkalsrud E. Successful treatment of hepatic hemangioma with corticosteroids. *JAMA* 1969;208(13):2473–4.

94. Hurvitz SA, Hurvitz CH, Sloninsky L, et al. Successful treatment with cyclophosphamide of life-threatening diffuse hemangiomatosis involving the liver. *J Pediatr Hematol Oncol* 2000;22(6):527–32.

95. Ezekowitz RA, Mulliken JB, Folkman J. Interferon alfa-2a therapy for life-threatening hemangiomas of infancy. *N Engl J Med* 1992;326(22):1456–63.

96. deLorimier AA, Simpson EB, Baum RS, et al. Hepatic-artery ligation for hepatic hemangiomatosis. *N Engl J Med* 1967;277(7):333–7.

97. Warmann S, Bertram H, Kardorff R, et al. Interventional treatment of infantile hepatic hemangioendothelioma. *J Pediatr Surg* 2003;38(8):1177–81.

98. Rotman M, John M, Stowe S, et al. Radiation treatment of pediatric hepatic hemangiomatosis and coexisting cardiac failure. *N Engl J Med* 1980;302(15):852.

99. Walsh R, Harrington J, Beneck D, et al. Congenital infantile hepatic hemangioendothelioma type II treated with orthotopic liver transplantation. *J Pediatr Hematol Oncol* 2004;26(2):121–3.

100. DeMaioribus CA, Lally KP, Sim K, et al. Mesenchymal hamartoma of the liver. A 35-year review. *Arch Surg* 1990;125(5):598–600.

101. Stocker JT, Ishak KG. Mesenchymal hamartoma of the liver: report of 30 cases and review of the literature. *Pediatr Pathol* 1983;1(3):245–67.

102. Dooley JS, Li AK, Scheuer PJ, et al. A giant cystic mesenchymal hamartoma of the liver: diagnosis, management, and study of cyst fluid. *Gastroenterology* 1983;85(4):958–61.

103. Bejarano PA, Serrano MF, Casillas J, et al. Concurrent infantile hemangioendothelioma and mesenchymal hamartoma in a developmentally arrested liver of an infant requiring hepatic transplantation. *Pediatr Dev Pathol* 2003;6(6):552–7.

104. Baker ME, Silverman PM. Nodular focal fatty infiltration of the liver: CT appearance. *AJR Am J Roentgenol* 1985;145(1):79–80.

105. Bluemke DA, Soyer P, Fishman EK. Helical (spiral) CT of the liver. *Radiol Clin North Am* 1995;33(5):863–86.

106. Mathieu D, Paret M, Mahfouz AE, et al. Hyperintense benign liver lesions on spin-echo T1-weighted MR images: pathologic correlations. *Abdom Imaging* 1997;22(4):410–17.

107. Lisbona R, Mishkin S, Derbekyan V, et al. Role of scintigraphy in focally abnormal sonograms of fatty livers. *J Nucl Med* 1988;29(6):1050–6.

108. Rich HG. Resolution of focal fatty infiltration of the liver. *South Med J* 1996;89(10):1024–7.

109. Hoffman AL, Emre S, Verham RP, et al. Hepatic angiomyolipoma: two case reports of caudate-based lesions and review of the literature. *Liver Transpl Surg* 1997;3(1):46–53.

110. Goodman ZD, Ishak KG. Angiomyolipomas of the liver. *Am J Surg Pathol* 1984;8(10):745–50.

111. Nishizaki T, Kanematsu T, Matsumata T, et al. Myelolipoma of the liver. A case report. *Cancer* 1989;63(5):930–4.

112. Jacobs JE, Birnbaum BA. Computed tomography imaging of focal hepatic lesions. *Semin Roentgenol* 1995;30(4):308–23.

113. Kelleher T, Staunton M, Malone D, et al. Budd Chiari syndrome associated with angiomyolipoma of the liver. *J Hepatol* 2004;40(6):1048–9.

114. Karhunen PJ. Hepatic pseudolipoma. *J Clin Pathol* 1985;38(8):877–9.

115. Horiuchi R, Uchida T, Kojima T, et al. Inflammatory pseudotumor of the liver. Clinicopathologic study and review of the literature. *Cancer* 1990;65(7):1583–90.

116. Amankonah TD, Strom CB, Vierling JM, et al. Inflammatory pseudotumor of the liver as the first manifestation of Crohn's disease. *Am J Gastroenterol* 2001;96(8):2520–2.

117. Papachristou GI, Wu T, Marsh W, et al. Inflammatory pseudotumor of the liver associated with Crohn's disease. *J Clin Gastroenterol* 2004;38(9):818–22.

118. Jackson RB, Gatling RR. Inflammatory pseudotumor of the liver. *Surgery* 1991;109(3 Pt 1):329–32.

119. Gollapudi P, Chejfec G, Zarling EJ. Spontaneous regression of hepatic pseudotumor. *Am J Gastroenterol* 1992;87(2):214–17.

120. Shek TW, Ng IO, Chan KW. Inflammatory pseudotumor of the liver. Report of four cases and review of the literature. *Am J Surg Pathol* 1993;17(3):231–8.

121. International Working Party. Terminology of nodular hepatocellular lesions. *Hepatology* 1995;22:983–93.

122. Ferrell L, Wright T, Lake J, et al. Incidence and diagnostic features of macroregenerative nodules vs. small hepatocellular carcinoma in cirrhotic livers. *Hepatology* 1992;16:1372–81.

123. Theise N, Schwartz M, Miller C, et al. Macroregenerative nodules and hepatocellular carcinoma in forty-four sequential adult liver explants with cirrhosis. *Hepatology* 1992;16:949–55.

124. Hytiroglou P, Theise N. Differential diagnosis of hepatocellular nodular lesions. *Semin Diagn Pathol* 1998;15:285–99.

125. Takayma T, Makuuchi M, Hirohashi S, et al. Malignant transformation of adenomatous hyperplasia to hepatocellular carcinoma. *Lancet* 1990;336:1150–3.

126. Kondo F, Ebara M, Wada H, et al. Histological features and clinical course of large regenerative nodules: evaluation of their precancerous potentiality. *Hepatology* 1990;12:592–8.

127. Borzio M, Borzio F, Croce A, et al. Ultrasonography-detected macroregenerative nodules in cirrhosis: a prospective study. *Gastroenterology* 1997;112:1617–23.

128. Kobayashi M, Ikeda K, Hosaka T et al. Dysplastic nodules frequently develop into hepatocellular carcinoma in patients with chronic viral hepatitis and cirrhosis. *Cancer* 2006;106;636–47.

129. Ferrell LD, Crawford JM, Dhillon AP, et al. Proposal for standardized criteria for the diagnosis of benign, borderline, and malignant hepatocellular lesions arising in chronic advanced liver disease. *Am J Surg Pathol* 1993;17(11):1113–23.

130. Arakawa M, Kage M, Sugihara S, et al. Emergence of malignant lesions within an adenomatous hyperplastic nodule in a cirrhotic liver. Observations in five cases. *Gastroenterology* 1986;91(1):198–208.

131. Rabinowitz JG, Kinkabwala M, Ulreich S. Macro-regenerating nodule in the cirrhotic liver. Radiologic features and differential diagnosis. *Am J Roentgenol Radium Ther Nucl Med* 1974;121(2):401–11.

132. Tsuda H, Hirohashi S, Shimosato Y, et al. Clonal origin of atypical adenomatous hyperplasia of the liver and clonal identity with hepatocellular carcinoma. *Gastroenterology* 1988;95(6):1664–6.

133. Theise ND. Macroregenerative (dysplastic) nodules and hepatocarcinogenesis: theoretical and clinical considerations. *Semin Liver Dis* 1995;15(4):360–71.

134. Hytiroglou P, Theise ND, Schwartz M, et al. Macroregenerative nodules in a series of adult cirrhotic liver explants: issues of classification and nomenclature. *Hepatology* 1995;21(3):703–8.

135. Nakanuma Y, Terada T, Ueda K, et al. Adenomatous hyperplasia of the liver as a precancerous lesion. *Liver* 1993;13(1):1–9.

136. Borzio M, Bruno S, Roncalli M, et al. Liver cell dysplasia is a major risk factor for hepatocellular carcinoma in cirrhosis: a prospective study. *Gastroenterology* 1995;108(3):812–17.

137. Kudo M. Imaging diagnosis of hepatocellular carcinoma and premalignant/borderline lesions. *Semin Liver Dis* 1999;19(3):297–309.

138. Wanless IR. Micronodular transformation (nodular regenerative hyperplasia) of the liver: a report of 64 cases among 2,500 autopsies and a new classification of benign hepatocellular nodules. *Hepatology* 1990;11(5):787–97.

139. Naber A, Van Haelst U, Yap S. Nodular regenerative hyperplasia of the liver: an important cause of portal hypertension in non-cirrhotic patients. *J Hepatol* 1991;12:94–9.

140. DeCoux R, Achord J. Portal hypertension in Felty's syndrome. *Am J Gastroenterol* 1980;73:315–18.

141. Gridley G, Klippel J, Hoover R, et al. Incidence of cancer among men with the Felty syndrome. *Ann Intern Med* 1994;120:35–9.

142. Wanless I, Lentz J, Roberts E. Partial nodular transformation of liver in an adult with persistent ductus venosus. *Arch Pathol Lab Med* 1985;109:427–32.

143. Hoso M, Terada T, Nakanuma Y. Partial nodular transformation of liver developing around portal venous emboli of hepatocellular carcinoma. *Histopathology* 1996;29:580–2.

144. Terayama N, Terada T, Hoso M, et al. Partial nodular transformation of the liver with portal vein thrombosis. *J Clin Gastroenterol* 1995;20:71–6.

145. Nakashima O, Kurogi M, Yamaguchi R, et al. Unique hypervascular nodules in alcoholic liver cirrhosis: identical to focal nodular hyperplasia-like nodules? *J Hepatol* 2004;41:992–8.

146. Wanless IR, Mawdsley C, Adams R. On the pathogenesis of focal nodular hyperplasia of the liver. *Hepatology* 1985;5(6):1194–200.

147. Mathieu D, Kobeiter H, Maison P, et al. Oral contraceptive use and focal nodular hyperplasia of the liver. *Gastroenterology* 2000;118:560–4.

148. Scalori A, Tavani A, Gallus S, et al. Oral contraceptives and the risk of focal nodular hyperplasia of the liver: a case–control study. *Am J Obstet Gynecol* 2002;186:195–7.

149. Vilgrain V, Uzan F, Brancatelli G, et al. Prevalence of hepatic hemangioma in patients with focal nodular hyperplasia: MR imaging analysis [see comment]. *Radiology* 2003;229:75–9.

150. Buscarini E, Danesino C, Plauchu H, et al. High prevalence of hepatic focal nodular hyperplasia in subjects with hereditary hemorrhagic telangiectasia. *Ultrasound Med Biol* 1089;30:1089–97.

151. Mindikoglu AL, Regev A, Levi JU, et al. Focal nodular hyperplasia in identical twins. *Am J Gastroenterol* 2005;100(7):1616–19.

152. Chen TC, Chou TB, Ng KF, et al. Hepatocellular carcinoma associated with focal nodular hyperplasia. Report of a case with clonal analysis. *Virchows Arch* 2001;438(4):408–11.

153. Gaffey MJ, Iezzoni JC, Weiss LM. Clonal analysis of focal nodular hyperplasia of the liver. *Am J Pathol* 1996;148(4):1089–96.

154. Nguyen BN, Flejou JF, Terris B, et al. Focal nodular hyperplasia of the liver: a comprehensive pathologic study of 305 lesions and recognition of new histologic forms. *Am J Surg Pathol* 1999;23(12):1441–54.

155. Finley AC, Hosey JR, Noone TC, et al. Multiple focal nodular hyperplasia syndrome: diagnosis with dynamic, gadolinium-enhanced MRI. *Magn Reson Imaging* 2005;23(3):511–13.

156. Nguyen B, Flejou J, Terris B, et al. Focal nodular hyperplasia of the liver: a comprehensive pathologic study of 305 lesions and recognition of new histologic form. *Am J Surg Pathol* 1999;23:1441–54.

157. Kim J, Nikiforov YE, Moulton JS, et al. Multiple focal nodular hyperplasia of the liver in a 21-year-old woman. *J Gastrointest Surg* 2004;8(5):591–5.

158. Fioole B, Kokke M, van Hillegersberg R, Rinkes IH. Adequate symptom relief justifies hepatic resection for benign disease. *BMC Surg* 2005;5:7.

159. Lee MJ, Saini S, Hamm B, et al. Focal nodular hyperplasia of the liver: MR findings in 35 proved cases. *AJR Am J Roentgenol* 1991;156(2):317–20.

160. Becker YT, Raiford DS, Webb L, et al. Rupture and hemorrhage of hepatic focal nodular hyperplasia. *Am Surg* 1995;61(3):210–14.

161. Caseiro-Alves F, Zins M, Mahfouz A-E, et al. Calcification in focal nodular hyperplasia: a new problem for differentiation from fibrolamellar hepatocellular carcinoma. *Radiology* 1996;198(3):889–92.

162. Imkie M, Myers SA, Li Y, et al. Fibrolamellar hepatocellular carcinoma arising in a background of focal nodular hyperplasia: a report of 2 cases. *J Reprod Med* 2005;50(8):633–7.

163. Di Stassi M, Caturelli E, De Sio I, et al. Natural history of focal nodular hyperplasia of the liver: an ultrasound study. *J Clin Ultrasound* 1996;24(7):345–50.

164. Welch TJ, Sheedy PF, Johnson CM, et al. Focal nodular hyperplasia and hepatic adenoma: comparison of angiography, CT, US, and scintigraphy. *Radiology* 1985;156(3):593–5.

165. Goodman ZD, Mikel UV, Lubbers PR, et al. Kupffer cells in hepatocellular adenomas. *Am J Surg Pathol* 1987;11(3):191–6.

166. Kehagias D, Moulopoulos L, Antoniou A, et al. Focal nodular hyperplasia: imaging findings. *Eur Radiol* 2001;11(2):202–12.

167. Shamsi K, De Schepper A, Degryse H, et al. Focal nodular hyperplasia of the liver: radiologic findings. *Abdom Imaging* 1993;18(1):32–8.

168. Hardwigsen J, Pons J, Veit V, et al. A life-threatening complication of focal nodular hyperplasia. *J Hepatol* 2001;35(2):310–12.

169. Wang LY, Wang JH, Lin ZY, et al. Hepatic focal nodular hyperplasia: findings on color Doppler ultrasound. *Abdom Imaging* 1997;22(2):178–81.

170. Kim MJ, Lim HK, Kim SH, et al. Evaluation of hepatic focal nodular hyperplasia with contrast-enhanced gray scale harmonic sonography: initial experience. *J Ultrasound Med* 2004;23(2):297–305.

171. Dietrich CF, Schuessler G, Trojan J, et al. Differentiation of focal nodular hyperplasia and hepatocellular adenoma by contrast-enhanced ultrasound. *Br J Radiol* 2005;78(932):704–7.

172. Brancatelli G, Federle MP, Grazioli L, et al. Focal nodular hyperplasia: CT findings with emphasis on multiphasic helical CT in 78 patients. *Radiology* 2001;219(1):61–8.

173. Buetow PC, Pantongrag-Brown L, Buck JL, et al. Focal nodular hyperplasia of the liver: radiologic-pathologic correlation. *Radiographics* 1996;16(2):369–88.

174. Kruskal JB, Kane RA. Imaging of primary and metastatic liver tumors. *Surg Oncol Clin North Am* 1996;5(2):231–60.

175. Brady MS, Coit DG. Focal nodular hyperplasia of the liver. *Surg Gynecol Obstet* 1990;171(5):377–81.

176. Brancatelli G, Federle MP, Katyal S, et al. Hemodynamic characterization of focal nodular hyperplasia using three-dimensional volume-rendered multidetector CT angiography. *AJR Am J Roentgenol* 2002;179(1):81–5.

177. Mortele KJ, Praet M, Van Vlierberghe H, et al. CT and MR imaging findings in focal nodular hyperplasia of the liver: radiologic-pathologic correlation. *AJR Am J Roentgenol* 2000;175(3):687–92.

178. Vilgrain V, Flejou JF, Arrive L, et al. Focal nodular hyperplasia of the liver: MR imaging and pathologic correlation in 37 patients. *Radiology* 1992;184(3):699–703.

179. Mahfouz AE, Hamm B, Taupitz M, et al. Hypervascular liver lesions: differentiation of focal nodular hyperplasia from malignant tumors with dynamic gadolinium-enhanced MR imaging. *Radiology* 1993;186(1):133–8.

180. Ko SF, Ng SH, Lee TY, et al. Hepatic focal nodular hyperplasia: the "star sign" on gadolinium-enhanced magnetic resonance angiography. *Hepatogastroenterology* 2002;49(47):1377–81.

181. Imam K, Bluemke DA. MR imaging in the evaluation of hepatic metastases. *Magn Reson Imaging Clin N Am* 2000;8(4):741–56.

182. Vogl TJ, Hammerstingl R, Schwarz W, et al. Superparamagnetic iron oxide-enhanced versus gadolinium-enhanced MR imaging for differential diagnosis of focal liver lesions. *Radiology* 1996;198(3):881–7.

183. Grazioli L, Morana G, Kirchin MA, et al. Accurate differentiation of focal nodular hyperplasia from hepatic adenoma at gadobenate dimeglumine-enhanced MR imaging: prospective study. *Radiology* 2005;236(1):166–77.

184. Balci NC, Semelka RC. Contrast agents for MR imaging of the liver. *Radiol Clin North Am* 2005;43(5):887–98, viii.

185. Kinnard MF, Alavi A, Rubin RA, et al. Nuclear imaging of solid hepatic masses. *Semin Roentgenol* 1995;30(4):375–95.

186. Kurtaran A, Becherer A, Pfeffel F, et al. 18F-fluorodeoxyglucose (FDG)-PET features of focal nodular hyperplasia (FNH) of the liver. *Liver* 2000;20(6):487–490.

187. Fabre A, Audet P, Vilgrain V, et al. Histologic scoring of liver biopsy in focal nodular hyperplasia with atypical presentation. *Hepatology* 2002;35:414–20.

188. Leconte I, Van Beers B, Lacrosse M, et al. Focal nodular hyperplasia: natural course observed with CT and MRI. *J Comput Assist Tomogr* 2000;24:61–6.

189. Aldinger K, Ben-Menachem Y, Whalen G. Focal nodular hyperplasia of the liver associated with high-dosage estrogens. *Arch Intern Med* 1977;137(3):357–9.

190. Gussick SD, Quebbeman EJ, Rilling WS. Bland embolization of telangiectatic subtype of hepatic focal nodular hyperplasia. *J Vasc Interv Radiol* 2005;16(11):1535–8.

191. Bioulac-Sage P, Rebouissou S, Sa Cunha A, et al. Clinical, morphologic, and molecular features defining so-called telangiectatic focal nodular hyperplasias of the liver. *Gastroenterology* 2005;128:1211–18.

192. Ito K, Honjo K, Fujita T, et al. Liver neoplasms: diagnostic pitfalls in cross-sectional imaging. *Radiographics* 1996;16(2):273–93.

193. Lee HM, Lu DS, Krasny RM, et al. Hepatic lesion characterization in cirrhosis: significance of arterial hypervascularity on dual-phase helical CT. *AJR Am J Roentgenol* 1997;169(1):125–30.

194. Oliver JH III, Baron RL. Helical biphasic contrast-enhanced CT of the liver: technique, indications, interpretation, and pitfalls. *Radiology* 1996;201(1):1–14.

195. Grazioli L, Morana G, Kirchin MA, et al. Accurate differentiation of focal nodular hyperplasia from hepatic adenoma at gadobenate dimeglumine-enhanced MR imaging: prospective study. *Radiology* 2005;236:166–77.

196. Scharitzer M, Schima W, Schober E, et al. Characterization of hepatocellular tumors: value of mangafodipir-enhanced magnetic resonance imaging. *J Comput Assist Tomogr* 2005;29:181–90.

197. Krinsky GA, Israel G. Nondysplastic nodules that are hyperintense on T1-weighted gradient-echo MR imaging: frequency in cirrhotic patients undergoing transplantation. *AJR Am J Roentgenol* 2003;180:1023–7.

198. Lee S-O, Masyuk T, Splinter P, et al. MicroRNA15a molecules expression of the cell-cycle regulator Cdc25A and affects hepatic cystogenesis in a rat model of polycystic kidney disease. *J Clin Invest* 2008;118(11):3714–24.

199. Dimick JB, Cowan JA Jr, Knol JA, et al. Hepatic resection in the United States: indications, outcomes, and hospital procedural volumes from a nationally representative database. *Arch Surg* 2003;138(2):185–91.

200. Gaines PA, Sampson MA. The prevalence and characterization of simple hepatic cysts by ultrasound examination. *Br J Radiol* 1989;62:335–7.

201. Karhunen PJ, Tenhu M. Adult polycystic liver and kidney diseases are separate entities. *Clin Genet* 1986;30:29–37.

202. Kwok MK, Lewin KJ. Massive hepatomegaly in adult polycystic liver disease. *Am J Surg Pathol* 1988;12:321–4.

203. Gabow PA, Johnson AM, Kaehny WD, et al. Risk factors for the development of hepatic cysts in autosomal dominant polycystic kidney disease. *Hepatology* 1990;11:1033–7.

204. Karhunen PJ, Tenhu M. Adult polycystic liver and kidney diseases are separate entities. *Clin Genet* 1986;30:29–37.

205. Kwok MK, Lewin KJ. Massive hepatomegaly in adult polycystic liver disease. *Am J Surg Pathol* 1988;12:321–4.

206. Milutinovic J, Fialkow PJ, Rudd TG, et al. Liver cysts in patients with autosomal dominant polycystic kidney disease. *Am J Med* 1980;68:741–4.

207. Gabow PA, Johnson AM, Kaehny WD, et al. Risk factors for the development of hepatic cysts in autosomal dominant polycystic kidney disease. *Hepatology* 1990;11:1033–7.

208. Grunfeld JP, Albouze G, Jungers P, et al. Liver changes and complications in adult polycystic kidney disease. *Adv Nephrol Necker Hosp* 1985;14:1–20.

209. Melnick F. Polycystic liver : analysis of seventy cases. *Arch Pathol* 1955;59:162–72.

210. Pirson Y, Lannoy N, Peters D, et al. Isolated polycystic liver disease as a distinct genetic disease, unlinked to polycystic kidney disease 1 and polycystic kidney disease 2. *Hepatology* 1996;23:249–52.

211. Iglesias DM, Palmitano JA, Arrizurieta E, et al. Isolated polycystic liver disease not linked to polycystic kidney disease 1 and 2. *Dig Dis Sci* 1999;44:385–8.

212. Reynolds DM, Falk CT, Li A, et al. Identification of a locus for autosomal dominant polycystic liver disease, on chromosome 19p13.2-13.1. *Am J Hum Genet* 2000;67:1598–604.

213. Qian Q. Isolated polycystic liver disease. *Adv Chronic Kid Dis* 2010;17:181–9.

214. Gabow PA. Autosomal dominant polycystic kidney disease. *N Engl J Med* 1993;329:332–42.

215. Koptides M, Deltas CC. Autosomal dominant polycystic kidney disease: molecular genetics and molecular pathogenesis. *Hum Genet* 2000;107:115–26.

216. Nauli SM, Alenghat FJ, Luo Y, et al. Polycystins 1 and 2 mediate mechanosensation in the primary cilium of kidney cells. *Nat Genet* 2003;33:129–37.

217. Ong ACM, Harris PC. Molecular pathogenesis of ADPKD: The polycystin complex gets complex. *Kidney Int* 2005;67:1234–47.

218. Nauli SM, Zhou J. Polycystins and mechanosensation in renal and nodal cilia. *Bioessays* 2004;26:844–56.

219. Alvaro D, Onori P, Alpini G, et al. Morphological and functional features of hepatic cyst epithelium in autosomal dominant polycystic kidney disease. *Am J Pathol* 172(2):321–32.

220. Qian F, Watnick TJ, Onuchic LF, et al. The molecular basis of focal cyst formation in human autosomal dominant polycystic kidney disease type I. *Cell* 1996;87:979–87.

221. Everson GT, Taylor MRG, Doctor RB. Polycystic disease of the liver. *Hepatology* 2004;40:774–82.

222. Drenth JPH, Martina JA, van de Kerkhof R, et al. Polycystic liver disease is a disorder of cotranslational protein processing. *Trends Mol Med* 2005;11:37–42.

223. Li A, Davila S, Furu L, et al. Mutations in PRKCSH cause isolated autosomal dominant polycystic liver disease. *Am J Hum Genet* 2003;72:691–703.

224. Davila S, Furu L, Gharavi AG, et al. Mutations in SEC63 cause autosomal dominant polycystic liver disease. *Nat Genet* 2004;36:575–7.

225. Desmet VJ. Ludwig symposium on biliary disorders – part I. Pathogenesis of ductal plate abnormalities. *Mayo Clin Proc* 1998;73:80–9.

226. Ramos A, Torres VE, Holley KE, et al. The liver in autosomal dominant polycystic kidney disease. Implications for pathogenesis. *Arch Pathol Lab Med* 1990;114:180–4.

227. Everson GT, Scherzinger A, Berger-Leff N, et al. Polycystic liver disease: quantitation of parenchymal and cyst volumes from computed tomography images and clinical correlates of hepatic cysts. *Hepatology* 1988;8:1627–34.

228. Schnelldorfer T, Torres VE, Zakaria S, et al. Polycystic liver disease. *Ann Surg* 2009;250(1):112–18.

229. Sherstha R, McKinley C, Russ P, et al. Postmenopausal estrogen therapy selectively stimulates hepatic enlargement in women with autosomal dominant polycystic kidney disease. *Hepatology* 1997;26:1282–6.

230. Srinivasan R. Polycystic liver disease: an unusual cause of bleeding varices. *Dig Dis Sci* 1999;44:389–92.

231. Uddin W, Ramage JK, Portmann B, et al. Hepatic venous outflow obstruction in patients with polycystic liver disease: pathogenesis and treatment. *Gut* 1995;36:142–5.

232. Lerner ME, Roshkow JE, Smithline A, et al. Polycystic liver disease with obstructive jaundice: treatment with ultrasound-guided cyst aspiration. *Gastrointest Radiol* 1992;17:46–8.

233. Pirson Y, Chauveau D, Torres V. Management of cerebral aneurysms in autosomal dominant polycystic kidney disease. *J Am Soc Nephrol* 2002;13:269–76.

234. Geevarghese SK, Powers T, Marsh JW, et al. Screening for cerebral aneurysm in patients with polycystic liver disease. *South Med J* 1999;92:1167–70.

235. Washburn WK, Johnson LB, Lewis WD, et al. Liver transplantation for adult polycystic liver disease. *Liver Transpl Surg* 1996;2: 17–22.

236. Newman KD, Tores VE, Rakela J, et al. Treatment of highly symptomatic polycystic liver disease. Preliminary experience with hepatic resection-fenestration procedure. *Ann Surg* 1990;212:30–7.

237. Soravia C, Mentha G, Giostra E, et al. Surgery for adult polycystic liver disease. *Surgery* 1995;117:272–5.

238. Kabbej M, Sauvanet A, Chauveau D, et al. Laparoscopic fenestration in polycystic liver disease. *Br J Surg* 1996;83:1697–701.

239. Gigot JF, Jadoul P, Que F, et al. Adult polycystic liver disease: is fenestration the most adequate operation for long-term management? *Ann Surg* 1997;225:286–94.

240. Martin IJ, McKinnley AJ, Currie EJ, et al. Tailoring the management of nonparasitic liver cysts. *Ann Surg* 1998;228:167–72.

241. Katkhounda N, Hurwitz M, Gugenheim J, et al. Laparoscopic management of benign solid and cystic lesions of the liver. *Ann Surg* 1999;229:460–6.

242. Mazza OM, Fernandez DL, Pekolj J, et al. Management of nonparasitic hepatic cysts. *J Am Coll Surg* 2009;209(6):733–9.

243. Gigot JF, Legrand M, Hubens G, et al. Laparoscopic treatment of nonparasitic liver cysts: adequate selection of patients and surgical technique. *World J Surg* 1996;20:556–61.

244. Krohn PS, Hillingso JG, Kirkegaard P. Liver transplantation in polycystic liver disease: a relevant treatment modality for adults? *Scand J Gastroenterol* 2008;43:89–94.

245. Mergo PJ, Rose PR. Hepatic imaging. *Radiol Clin North Am* 1998;36:319–31.

246. Al-Bhalal L, Akhtar M. Molecular basis of autosomal recessive polycystic kidney disease (ARPKD). *Adv Anat Pathol* 2008;15(1):54–8.

247. Desmet VJ. What is congenital hepatic fibrosis? *Histopathology* 1992;20:465–77.

248. Sommerschild HC, Langmark F, Maurseth K. Congenital hepatic fibrosis: report of two new cases and review of the literature. *Surgery* 1973;73:53–8.

249. Kerr DN, Okonkwo S, Choa RG. Congenital hepatic fibrosis: the long-term prognosis. *Gut* 1978;19:514–20.

250. Todani T, Watanabe Y, Narusue M, et al. Congenital bile duct cysts: classification, operative procedures, and review of thirty-seven cases including cancer arising from choledochal cyst. *Am J Surg* 1977;134:263–9.

251. Kasai M, Asakura Y, Taira Y. Surgical treatment of choledochal cyst. *Ann Surg* 1970;172:844–51.

252. Olbourne NA. Choledochal cysts. A review of the cystic anomalies of the biliary tree. *Ann R Coll Surg Engl* 1975;56:26–32.

253. O'Neill JA Jr. Choledochal cyst. *Curr Prob Surg* 1992;29:361–410.

254. Katyal D, Lees GM. Choledochal cysts: a retrospective review of 28 patients and a review of the literature. *Can J Surg* 1992;35:584–8.

255. Martin RF, Biber BP, Bosco JJ, et al. Symptomatic choledochoceles in adults. Endoscopic retrograde cholangiopancreatography recognition and management. *Arch Surg* 1992;127:536–8; discussion 538–9.

256. Lopez RR, Pinson CW, Campbell JR, et al. Variation in management based on type of choledochal cyst. *Am J Surg* 1991;161:612–15.

257. Rha SY, Stovroff MC, Glick PL. et al. Choledochal cysts: a ten year experience. *Am Surg* 1996;62:30–4.

258. Stain SC, Guthrie CR, Yellin AE, et al. Choledochal cyst in the adult. *Ann Surg* 1995;222:128–33.

259. Babbit D. Congenital choledochal cysts: new etiological concept based upon anomalous relationships of the common bile duct and pancreatic bulb. *Ann Radiol* 1969;12:231–40.

260. Komi N, Tamura T, Miyoshi Y, et al. Nationwide survey of cases of choledochal cyst. Analysis of coexistent anomalies, complications and surgical treatment in 645 cases. *Surg Gastroenterol* 1984;3:69–73.

261. Visser BC, Suh I, Way LW, et al. Congenital choledochal cysts in adults. *Arch Surg* 2004; 855–60; discussion 860–2.

262. Todani T, Watanabe Y, Urushihara N, et al. Biliary complications after excisional procedure for choledochal cyst. *J Pediatr Surg* 1995;30:478–81.

263. Todani T, Watanabe Y, Toki A, et al. Carcinoma related to choledochal cysts with internal drainage operations. *Surg Gynecol Obstet* 1987;164:61–4.

264. Sarris GE, Tsang D. Choledochocele: case report, literature review, and a proposed classification. *Surgery* 1989;105:408–14.

265. Venu RP, Geenen JE, Hogan WJ, et al. Role of endoscopic retrograde cholangiopancreatography in the diagnosis and treatment of choledochocele. *Gastroenterology* 1984;87:1144–9.

266. Scudamore CH, Hemming AW, Teare JP, et al. Surgical management of choledochal cysts. *Am J Surg* 1994;167:497–500.

267. Tsuchida Y, Sato T, Sanjo K, et al. Evaluation of long-term results of Caroli's disease: 21 years' observation of a family with autosomal "dominant" inheritance, and review of the literature. *Hepato-gastroenterology* 1995;42:175–81.

268. Stringer MD, Dhawan A, Davenport M, et al. Choledochal cysts: lessons from a 20 year experience. *Arch Dis Child* 1995;73:528–31.

269. Chen HM, Jan YY, Chen MF, et al. Surgical treatment of choledochal cyst in adults: results and long-term follow-up. *Hepatogastroenterology* 1996;43:1492–9.

270. Akwari OE, Tucker A, Seigler HF, et al. Hepatobiliary cystadenoma with mesenchymal stroma. *Ann Surg* 1990;211:18–27.

271. Davies W, Chow M, Nagorney D. Extrahepatic biliary cystadenomas and cystadenocarcinoma. Report of seven cases and review of the literature. *Ann Surg* 1995;222:619–25.

272. Korobkin M, Stephens DH, Lee JK, et al. Biliary cystadenoma and cystadenocarcinoma: CT and sonographic findings. *AJR Am J Roentgenol* 1989;153:507–11.

273. Wheeler DA, Edmondson HA. Cystadenoma with mesenchymal stroma (CMS) in the liver and bile ducts. A clinicopathologic study of 17 cases, 4 with malignant change. *Cancer* 1985;56:1434–45.

274. Davies CW, McIntyre AS. Treatment of a symptomatic hepatic cyst by tetracycline hydrochloride instillation sclerosis. *Eur J Gastroenterol Hepatol* 1996;8:173–5.

275. Murakami T, Imai A, Nakamura H, et al. Ciliated foregut cyst in cirrhotic liver. *J Gastroenterol* 1996;31(3):446–9.

276. Idress MT, Reid-Nicholson M, Unger P, et al. Subhepatic ciliated foregut cyst. *Ann Diag Path* 2005;9(1):54–6.

277. Eckert J, Deplazes P. Biological, epidemiological, and clinical aspects of echinococcosis, a zoonosis of increasing concern. *Clin Microbiol Rev* 2004; 107–35.

278. McManus DP, Zhang W, Li J, et al. Echinococcosis. *Lancet* 2003; 1295–304.

279. Rodes J, Sherlock S. Focal nodular hyperplasia in a young female. *J Hepatol* 1998;29:1005–9.

280. Rebouissou et al. *J Hepatol* 2008;48:163–70.

281. Di Bisceglie AM, Buetow PC. Tumors of the liver. In: Maddrey WC, Feldman M, eds. *Atlas of the Liver*, 2nd edn. Philadelphia, PA: Current Medicine, 2000:13.1–13.14.

Multiple choice questions

35.1 All of the following are risk factors for hepatocellular adenoma transforming into hepatocellular carcinoma except which one?

    a Beta-catenin mutation.
    b Male gender.
    c Diameter greater than 5 cm.
    d Hepatocyte nuclear factor 1α (HNF-1α) inactivation.
    e Enlarging nodules.

35.2 Indications for operative or percutaneous interventions in polycystic liver disease include all of the following except which one?

    a Right upper quadrant pain causing altered performance status.
    b Cyst compression of the biliary tree leading to jaundice.
    c Fever with evidence of infected cyst on imaging.
    d Massively enlarged cysts throughout all segments of the liver.
    e Hepatic venous outflow tract obstruction with ascites formation.

Answers to the multiple choice questions can be found in the Appendix at the end of the book.

These multiple choice questions are also available for you to complete online.
Visit http://www.schiffsdiseasesoftheliver.com/

CHAPTER 36

Hepatocellular Carcinoma

Alejandro Forner, Carmen Ayuso, & Jordi Bruix

Barcelona-Clínic Liver Cancer Group, Hospital Clinic Barcelona, CIBERehd, Institut d'Investigacions Biomediques Agusto Pi i Sunyer (IDIBAPS), University of Barcelona, Barcelona, Spain

Key concepts

- Hepatocellular carcinoma (HCC) is a neoplasm that has well-defined risk factors, such as chronic viral infection and excessive alcohol intake. These induce chronic liver disease, that is, cirrhosis, and induce genetic damage, leading to cancer development.
- HCC is the leading cause of death in patients with cirrhosis.
- The sole option to reduce cancer-related death is to detect cancer at an early stage and apply effective therapy. Patients with cirrhosis who are candidates for therapy if HCC is diagnosed should be encouraged to enter screening protocols.
- Early detection of HCC should be based on hepatic ultrasonography every 6 months. Unfortunately, tumor marker determination lacks precision and efficacy.
- Diagnosis of HCC can be done without histologic confirmation in patients with cirrhosis by imaging techniques.

- Effective therapies for HCC with potential long-term cure include surgical resection, liver transplantation, and percutaneous ablation. Among palliative approaches, the only two therapies with a positive impact on survival are transarterial chemoembolization and sorafenib.
- Positive results with sorafenib are proof of the potential efficacy of molecular targeted therapies in the treatment of HCC.
- Prevention of HCC should come from the avoidance of risk factors through vaccination for the prevention of hepatitis B and the maintenance of proper health standards and adequate lifestyle (limitation of exposure to alcohol). Antiviral therapy may cure chronic hepatitis B and C and hence prevent progression to cirrhosis and cancer.

Until very recently, it was common to consider hepatocellular carcinoma (HCC) as a cancer with a low incidence in the western world. However, recent data show that its incidence has increased in several western countries [1]. In addition, cohort studies have revealed that HCC is currently the leading cause of death in cirrhotic patients. The feasibility of early detection along with the availability of several effective therapies has permitted encouraging long-term survival after diagnosis. As a result, the interest in all aspects of diagnosis and treatment has sharply increased [2]. In that sense, it has been recognized that hepatologists play a key role in the management of patients with HCC. Hepatologists decide if HCC surveillance should be pursued in patients at risk and are responsible for disease staging and treatment indication. The most critical decision is the selection of candidates for liver transplantation and, once selected, their management before and after surgery. In some countries, mostly in Asia, even surveillance and percutaneous treatment (alcohol injection and radiofrequency ablation) are performed by hepatologists after they have received specific training to acquire the needed expertise.

In the present chapter we summarize the most relevant issues about epidemiology, diagnosis, and treatment of this neoplasm.

Epidemiology

Primary liver cancer is now the sixth most common cancer in the world and the third cause of cancer-related mortality [3]. More than half a million cases are diagnosed every year and there are major geographic differences in incidence. The annual incidence rates in eastern Asia and sub-Saharan Africa exceed 15/100,000 inhabitants, while figures are intermediate (between 5 and 15/100,000) in the Mediterranean basin and southern Europe, and very low (below 5/100,000) in northern Europe and America [1]. Vaccination against hepatitis B virus (HBV) has induced a decrease in HCC incidence in countries where this virus was highly prevalent [4], while the contrary is true in areas where viral dissemination (mostly hepatitis C virus (HCV)) has occurred in the last decades. These data suggest that the geographic heterogeneity is related

Schiff's Diseases of the Liver, Eleventh Edition. Edited by Eugene R. Schiff, Willis C. Maddrey and Michael F. Sorrell.
© 2012 John Wiley & Sons, Ltd. Published 2012 by John Wiley & Sons, Ltd.

to differences in the exposure rate to risk factors and time of acquisition, rather than to genetic predisposition. Studies in migrant populations have demonstrated that first-generation immigrants carry with them the high incidence of HCC that is present in their native countries, but in the subsequent generations the incidence decreases [5].

The age at which HCC appears varies according to gender, geographic area, and risk factor associated with cancer development. In high-risk countries with major HBV dissemination, the mean age at diagnosis is usually below 60 years, while it is not infrequent to observe HCC in childhood, underlying the impact of viral exposures early in life [1]. In intermediate or low incidence areas most cases appear beyond 60 years of age. In all areas, males have a higher prevalence than females, the gender ratio usually ranging between 2:1 and 4:1, and in most areas female age at diagnosis is higher than in males [1].

Risk factors for HCC

Cirrhosis underlies HCC in more than 80% of affected individuals [6,7]. Thus, any agent leading to chronic liver damage and ultimately cirrhosis should be considered as a risk factor for HCC. Obviously, the major causes of cirrhosis, and hence HCC, are HBV, HCV, and alcohol, but less prevalent conditions such as hemochromatosis, primary biliary cirrhosis, nonalcoholic steatohepatitis, and Wilson disease have also been associated with HCC development. The risk within cirrhosis increases in parallel to the impairment of liver function and is higher in males, in patients older than 50 years, and in subjects with increased α-fetoprotein (AFP) concentration [6]. Pathologic characteristics such as increased proliferation, the presence of dysplastic cells, or irregular regeneration have also been proposed as useful risk markers but are not fully validated.

Hepatitis B virus

The evidence linking HBV with HCC is unquestioned [8]. Active viral replication implies a higher risk and longstanding active infection resulting in cirrhosis is the major event resulting in increased risk [9]. The incidence of HCC in inactive HBV carriers without liver cirrhosis is less than 0.3% [6]. The role of specific genotypes or mutations is not well established. HBV can be integrated into the host cellular genome and induce genetic damage. DNA integration in nontumoral cells in patients with HCC suggests that genomic integration and damage precede the development of tumor. Thus, infection with HBV may be correlated with the emergence of HCC even in the absence of liver cirrhosis. In addition, some of the HBV proteins disrupt cellular functions and may favor neoplastic transformation, induce proliferation, and impede apoptosis [8].

Interestingly, occult HBV infection may become apparent if properly investigated by molecular techniques even in the absence of serologic markers of HBV itself [10]. Identification of the HBV genome has been reported in liver tumors of patients who are HCV-positive and hepatitis B surface antigen (HBsAg)-negative in the serum. The rate of occult infection in those patients can be as high as 63% [10]. Finally, the implementation of vaccination against HBV has resulted in a significant decrease of HCC incidence [4] and this is the final proof of the importance of this virus in the genesis of this cancer.

Hepatitis C virus

The prevalence of HCV in HCC cohorts varies according to the penetration of the agent in the population of each geographic area. There is a single prospective population-based study of the risk of HCC in patients with hepatitis C [11]. This study included 12,000 men and described a 20-fold increased risk of HCC in infected individuals, this figure being very close to the estimated risk obtained in a meta-analysis of 21 case–control studies [12]. The risk is clearly related to the degree of liver damage induced by the virus. There are some case reports of healthy HCV carriers with HCC, but several cohort studies have indicated that the incidence in patients with chronic hepatitis is low (below 1%) and that the risk sharply increases once cirrhosis develops [6,13]. At that time, the annual incidence ranged between 2% and 8% [6]. In addition, once the cirrhosis is established, the risk of HCC does not disappear after a sustained response to interferon for the treatment of chronic hepatitis C [14]. Finally, despite preliminary encouraging results, long-term treatment with interferon has not been shown to be efficacious for the prevention of HCC development in chronically infected HCV patients [15,16].

Patients infected with the human immunodeficiency virus (HIV) are now effectively treated with combined regimens and, if coinfected with HCV, manifest a faster evolution to cirrhosis and thus are at risk for HCC development. In fact, liver disease and/or HCC are the major cause of death in these patients [17].

Alcohol, tobacco, and coffee

A large proportion of alcoholic cirrhotics are infected by HCV, thus the risk based on studies done before the recognition of this virus are certain to have overestimated the role of alcohol. The risk for HCC increases linearly beyond an estimated intake of 40–60 g of alcohol per day and also with the period of alcohol consumption and with the presence of coinfection with HBV or HCV [18]. Upon the development of decompensated cirrhosis, the yearly incidence increases beyond 2%. Smoking slightly increases the oncogenic risk [19], while coffee consumption reduces the risk [20].

Pathogenesis

Active inflammation with oxidative damage is thought to be the key event leading to liver cancer, but the detailed molecular mechanisms are not known. Cumulative genetic changes occur and allow the appearance of high-grade dysplastic hepatocytes without an overt malignant phenotype, that in one third of cases may evolve into overt HCC after a follow-up of 5 years [21,22]. Intense neoangiogenic activity accompanies this transition and results in a well-known enhanced blood supply derived from the hepatic artery that permits radiologic characterization. The most frequently affected chromosomes are 1, 4, 8, 16, and 17, but none of these is abnormal in more than 60% of cases [23]. Downregulation of p53 is observed in up to 40% of cases and a G to T mutation reflects genetic damage due to aflatoxin intake.

The expression of several genes has been related to initiation, growth, and dissemination, but none of them has been strongly enough validated to become part of the decision-making process in clinical practice. Over the last few years, several groups have proposed molecular classifications of HCC based on genomic expression [24]. A recent meta-analysis has revealed that common transcriptome-based subclasses exist across different studies, supporting the idea that there is a certain commonality in the global molecular status of HCC tumors irrespective of the clinical heterogeneity [25].

Pathology

The appearance of HCC changes from the early to advanced stages [21]. It is common to use the Edmonson and Steiner criteria to grade the differentiation degree according to nuclear irregularity, hyperchromatism, and nuclear:cytoplasmic ratio. The cytoplasm shows a fine granular eosinophilia and may accumulate bile and fat, Mallory bodies, and α_1-antitrypsin globules. Fat deposition is seen in 30–40% of tumors about 1.5 cm in size and translates into increased echogenicity at ultrasonography [21]. Immunostaining can recognize numerous proteins such as cytokeratins 7, 8, 18, and 19, carcinoembryonic antigen, α-fetoprotein (AFP), and several others, and preliminary studies have suggested that the detection of glypican 3, heat-shock protein 70, clathrin heavy chain, and glutamyne synthetase may be highly specific for HCC diagnosis [26]. Malignant hepatocytes accumulate as thin (microtrabecular) or thick (macrotrabecular) layers separated by sinusoids that may contain Kupffer

and stellate cells. Gross appearance may be described as expansive, infiltrative, or diffuse. The first type shows distinct margins and a surrounding reticulin pseudocapsule. No distinct margins are seen in the infiltrative type and the diffuse type corresponds to a multinodular tumor that mimics a cirrhotic liver. Usually, HCC appears as a distinct nodule of varying size that increases in size together with the development of additional tumor sites, first in the vicinity and then in separate segments. Portal vein branches are invaded and at late stages all the liver may be occupied by malignant foci and the tumor spreads outside the liver (initially in lymph nodes, and then to adrenal glands, lung, and bone). The prevalence of portal vein invasion increases together with tumor size. Less than 20% of HCC under 2 cm in diameter have microscopic vascular invasion and well-differentiated HCC without such an invasive profile and the absence of minute satellite nodules has recently been named as very early HCC or carcinoma in situ [21]. This initial lesion does not have increased vascularization and, currently, is only confidently diagnosed after resection.

Clinical manifestations

Since most HCC cases appear in the setting of cirrhosis, a major part of the findings will be undistinguishable from the clinical picture observed in patients with advanced cirrhosis. Patients may present with jaundice, ascites, encephalopathy, or bleeding due to ruptured esophageal varices. Cancer-related symptoms such as abdominal pain or constitutional syndrome (weight loss, anorexia, malaise) reflect advanced tumor stage. Acute hemoperitoneum due to ruptured HCC or bone metastases is the first symptom in a minority of cases.

Advanced HCC is associated with increased bilirubin, alkaline phosphatase, and γ-glutamyl transpeptidase; alanine aminotransferase (ALT) and aspartate aminotransferase (AST) concentration have no diagnostic value. Paraneoplastic manifestations include diarrhea or severe hypoglycemia, which in some cases are the most relevant concerns. Other manifestations include hypercalcemia, sexual changes, polymyositis, thrombophlebitis, and skin rashes.

Diagnosis and staging

Diagnosis at an advanced stage when cancer-related symptoms are present and a large mass can be recognized even by physical examination is not difficult. The development of ultrasonography has permitted the detection of HCC at an asymptomatic stage, and its incorporation into the clinical workup of patients with known or suspected liver disease has sharply changed the diagnostic algorithm. This has prompted the establishment of early detection plans for HCC in the population at risk, namely patients with cirrhosis. The efficacy of surveillance depends on the level of risk and on the availability of effective therapy. Hence surveillance should be initiated upon the development of cirrhosis and be restricted to patients who would be treated if diagnosed with HCC. Thus, screening should be limited to Child–Pugh class A and B patients, while Child–Pugh class C patients should be evaluated for liver transplantation as HCC in them could become a contraindication [7]. There is a single randomized controlled trial of surveillance versus no surveillance [27]. It included more than 18,000 Chinese patients and showed a survival benefit following a strategy based on surveillance with AFP and ultrasound every 6 months. Several cohort studies have also shown that surveillance advances the tumor stage at diagnosis and suggest an improvement in patient survival. AFP has very low sensitivity and slight increases may also be observed in cirrhotics in the absence of malignancy [28–31]. Thus, the clinical role of AFP is none for screening and a reduced one for diagnosis, this probably being limited to patients with very advanced tumor stage in whom no treatment will be applied [7]. In these terminal patients, no imaging technique is needed after ultrasonography to confirm and stage the disease. Other tumor markers such as lectin-bound AFP [30], des-γ-carboxy-prothrombin [30], or glypican [32] have been proposed to surpass the efficacy of AFP but their clinical efficacy is yet to be unequivocally proven. All these data indicate that surveillance programs should be based on regular ultrasonography examination (Fig. 36.1).

Based on the data about tumor volume doubling time, most experts recommend cirrhotic patients should be screened by ultrasonography every 6 months; a prospective study in France has shown that shorter intervals of evaluation do not improve the performance of surveillance programs [33]. It is important to note that increased risk does not mean faster tumor progression and thus cirrhotic patients at higher risk do not require screening at shorter time periods.

Once a nodule in detect by ultrasonography, an active diagnostic workup should be initiated. However, the unequivocal diagnosis of those nodules within a cirrhotic liver represents a major clinical challenge. Biopsy is not always possible because of the location of the tumor, ascites, and clotting disorders that may impede needle insertion, and it is flawed by false-negative results due to sampling error or to the difficulties of confidently distinguishing between dysplastic changes and well-differentiated HCC. This raises the need for well-defined noninvasive criteria that would allow an accurate diagnosis based on the imaging characterization. Sev-

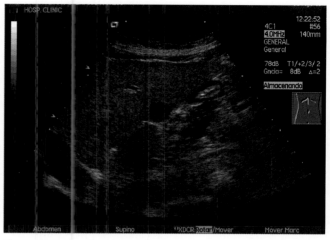

Figure 36.1 A small nodule measuring less than 20 mm detected during ultrasonography surveillance that corresponds to an early HCC site. Note its hypoechoic pattern as compared with the surrounding cirrhotic liver. This type of tumor is the target of early detection plans as it is at this stage that effective therapy (resection, transplantation, or percutaneous ablation) may provide long-term disease survival.

eral groups have demonstrated that the presence of arterial uptake followed by wash-out is highly specific for HCC [34–37]. Based on this specific feature, the American Association for the Study of Liver Diseases (AASLD) published a diagnostic algorithm following the detection of a nodule by screening ultrasonography, establishing diagnosis of HCC if a nodule within a cirrhotic liver exhibits intense arterial uptake followed by washout in the venous phase [7]. In the first proposal of the algorithm, in nodules between 1 and 2 cm in diameter, two coincidental imaging techniques showing a specific vascular pattern were requested. However, external validations have demonstrated that using a single contrast-enhanced modality has an outstanding positive predictive value [35,37]. Taking into account this information, the AASLD has updated the diagnostic algorithm and a confident HCC diagnosis can now be made in nodules larger than 1 cm when the specific vascular pattern is demonstrated by dynamic magnetic resonance imaging (MRI) (the preferred imaging technique) or computed tomography (CT) [38]. Contrast-enhanced ultrasound (CEUS) is unable to distinguish HCC from other primary neoplasia such as intrahepatic cholangiocarcinoma [39], so this imaging technique should not be used as the sole diagnostic tool for noninvasive diagnosis of HCC in cirrhosis. If the nodule displays an atypical vascular pattern on imaging techniques, a biopsy should be requested and a negative result should not discard the HCC diagnosis since sensitivity of percutaneous biopsy on these small nodules may be less than 70% [35]. Finally, in those nodules <1 cm, due to the low probability of malignancy and the difficulty of imaging and histologic characterization, a close follow-up before initiating an active workup is recommended [7].

Staging of HCC should be based on expert CT or MRI [34]. Both techniques confidently detect tumors larger than 2 cm while smaller tumors pose major difficulties in being accurately characterized as benign or malignant. Angiography has currently no role in diagnosis and staging, while lipiodol CT is not reliable [7]. The detection of additional tumor sites and of vascular invasion indicates an advanced tumor stage. Extrahepatic spread is infrequent at early stages but should be ruled out by chest CT. Bone metastases are usually symptomatic and should be ruled out if needed using bone scintigraphy.

Prognostic prediction

Since cirrhosis underlies HCC in most of the patients, prognosis depends not only on tumor burden, but also on the degree of liver function impairment and the treatment received. At the same time, liver function and tumor extent determines the feasibility of treatment and all parameters should be considered in making clinical predictions [2].

Therefore, systems that only consider one dimension such as the TNM (tumor, node, metastasis) classification, the Child–Pugh score, or the model for end-stage liver disease (MELD) score, will be inaccurate. Similarly, scores that just consider general health status and physical capacity, such as the performance status or the Karnofsky index, will have reduced value. In fact, the sole usefulness of all unidimensional systems is to identify patients with very advanced disease stage and poor short-term outcome. There are several scores that combine liver function and/or tumor stage and/or physical status, but the majority just stratify patients according to expected outcome. Only the Barcelona Clinic Liver Cancer (BCLC) system considers all evolving stages and links staging with treatment indication, while recent studies have validated its usefulness [40,41]. This system was constructed years ago, taking into account the outcome data of several cohort investigations and randomized clinical trials. Patients are divided into the relevant evolutionary stages according to tumor stage, liver function, and presence of symptoms, and within each strata patients are classified using specific prognostic tools, finally linking stage to therapy [2].

Treatment

The only options that can achieve long-term cure are surgical resection, liver transplantation, and percutaneous ablation. These are effective for patients diagnosed at early stages, which represents less than 40% of patients. In those cases with more advanced disease who cannot benefit from curative therapies, there are two available treatment options that have been shown to have a positive impact on survival in well-selected candidates: transarterial chemoembolization [42] and sorafenib [43].

Treatment indication requires a careful evaluation of tumor stage, degree of liver failure, and general health. Figure 36.2 shows the BCLC staging and treatment algorithm.

Surgical treatment

There are no trials comparing resection against liver transplantation, thus the decision as to which should be the first option is highly controversial and should take into account the available resources and the survival expected by applying either approach.

Resection

Resection is usually restricted to patients with solitary tumors and is the optimal approach for patients with normal liver. Unfortunately this represents less than 5% of HCC patients in the western world, and the presence of cirrhosis heavily limits surgical resection. The selection of candidates with cirrhosis for treatment should aim at identifying those with a likely perioperative mortality of less than 1%, a transfusion rate of <10%, and a 5-year survival rate of >50%, which requires careful evaluation [44]. Allocation into Child–Pugh class A is not sufficent to identify the best candidates for resection. Studies in Barcelona have shown that measurements of portal pressure and bilirubin concentration are the best parameters for this purpose. Patients with normal bilirubin and without clinically relevant portal hypertension – defined as either a hepatic vein pressure gradient of ≥ 10 mmHg, esophageal varices, or splenomegaly with a platelet count of $<100,000/mm^3$ – will achieve 5-year survival rates of 70%, whereas this decreases to 50% in patients with portal hypertension, and to 25% in those with portal hypertension and a raised bilirubin [45]. HCC recurrence may affect more than 50% of patients at 3 years and its appearance indicates a decreased long-term survival. Early recurrence is thought to correspond to tumor spread prior to resection, while recurrence beyond 2–3 years may be due to the emergence of metachronic HCC that originated in a separate cellular clone [44]. The most powerful predictors of postoperative recurrence due to dissemination are the presence of microvascular invasion, poor differentiation, and satellite lesions. Contrarily, late recurrence is closely associated with damaged liver parenchyma ("field effect") and can be predicted by gene expression profiling [46]. Unfortunately, despite promising reports using interferon, selective radiation, adaptive immunotherapy, retinoids, and heparanase inhibitors, to

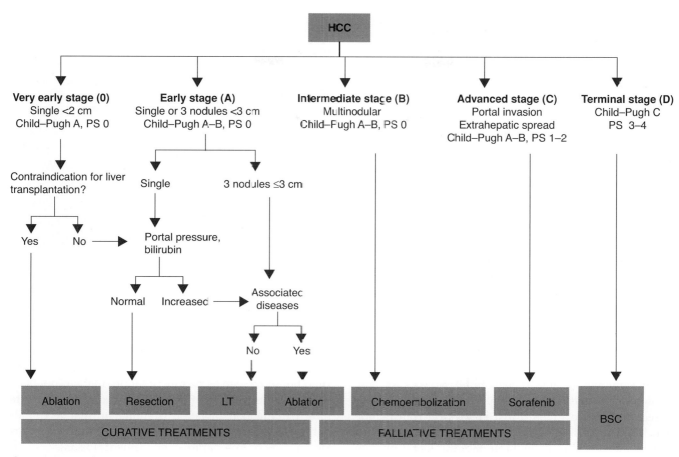

Figure 36.2 Barcelona Clinic Liver Cancer (BCLC) staging and treatment algorithm. BSC, best supportive care; HCC, hepatocellular carcinoma; LT, liver transplantation; PS, performance status. (Adapted from Forner et al. [2].)

date there is no effective method of diminishing recurrence rates after curative resection.

Transplantation

This option provides excellent outcomes if restricted to patients with early-stage disease, as defined by the Milano criteria: solitary HCC ≤5 cm or up to three nodules each measuring ≤3 cm (Fig. 36.3) [47]. The survival of patients selected according to this definition exceeds 70% at 5 years [47]. Disease recurrence is around 15% and affects mostly liver, lymph nodes, lung, and bones. Recurrence is more frequent if pathology discloses vascular invasion (macro- or microscopic) or additional tumor nests, characteristics that are highly prevalent in tumors exceeding 5 cm [48]. The main limitation for liver transplantation is the scarcity of livers. As a result, there is a waiting time between enlistment and transplantation. During this period of time the tumor may progress and impede successful therapy. Policies to prioritize patients with a high risk of exclusion because of tumor progression have been attempted but still have to be refined to insure equity between tumor and nontumor patients and

to avoid the transplantation of patients with more aggressive disease and poor outcomes. Locoregional treatment such as percutaneous ablation or chemoembolization are

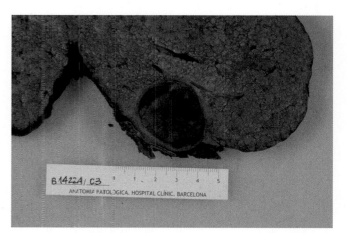

Figure 36.3 Explanted liver showing an HCC measuring 3 cm within a cirrhotic liver. The tumor has well-defined margins and exhibits a thin pseudocapsule. No satellite nodules are observed and the vessels appear free of invasion at macro- and microscopic examination. This pathology profile indicates a low recurrence risk during follow-up.

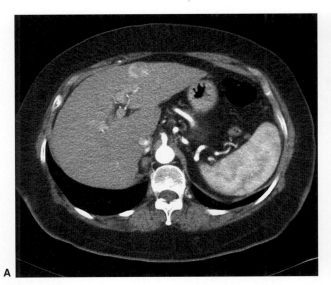
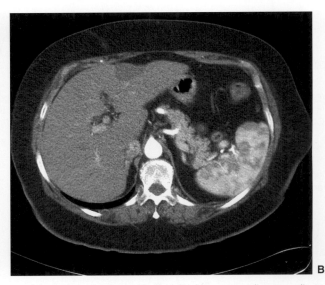

Figure 36.4 (A) Dynamic arterial CT scan showing a tumor with heterogeneous arterial vascularization located in the left lobe corresponding to a solitary HCC less than 20 mm in size. (B) Impaired liver function and associated conditions prevented resection or transplantation so the tumor was treated by percutaneous injection of ethanol. Dynamic CT evidence shows that no enhancement is present in the treated tumor, which now appears as a hypodense necrotic residual lesion.

considered when the waiting time exceeds 6 months as these techniques are able to delay tumor progression and, hence, decrease risk of exclusion [7]. The option that has raised most expectations is live donor liver transplantation. This requires a healthy donor to offer the right or left hepatic lobe to be implanted into the recipient. Donation implies a 0.5% mortality risk [49], and data from Korea suggest that outcome after live donation is very similar to that for cadaveric transplantation [50]. In recent years, several groups have reported excellent outcomes in transplantation in patients with HCC minimally exceeding the Milan criteria [48,51]. However, all these cohort studies are flawed by small sample size, short follow-up, and low applicability, and there is no reliable information regarding the impact of using the expanded criteria in the setting of scarce liver donations.

Percutaneous treatments

This is a therapeutic option that has rapidly grown during the last decade. Destruction or ablation of tumor cells can be achieved by the injection of chemical substances (ethanol, acetic acid, boiling saline) or by inserting a probe that modifies local tumor temperature (radiofrequency, microwave, laser, cryotherapy). The procedure can be done percutaneously with minimal invasiveness or during laparoscopy, and is currently considered the best option for patients with early HCC who are not candidates for surgery. Treatment is repeated on separate days and its efficacy is evaluated at 1 month by a dynamic imaging technique, where the absence of contrast uptake reflects tumor necrosis (Fig. 36.4). However, some of the tumors initially classified as having been completely

necrosed present intratumoral recurrence later on, and this should be seen as treatment failure that has not been detected immediately after therapy. The recurrence rate after percutaneous ablation is similar to that seen after surgical resection and presents as separate nodules occurring nearby or in separate liver segments [52,53].

For several years, percutaneous ethanol injection (PEI) under ultrasound guidance was the optimal approach. Complete tumor necrosis is achieved in 90–100% of HCCs smaller than 2 cm in diameter [53], while success is lower in larger tumors [54]. This is due to the presence of septa that prevent the diffusion of ethanol, a limitation that does not exist for radiofrequency ablation (RFA). RFA can be performed through single or multiple cooled-tip electrodes, percutaneously, laparoscopically, or intraoperatively. Its efficacy is similar to ethanol injection in HCC <2 cm and is superior in larger lesions [55]. In addition, the number of treatment sessions is reduced, and, overall, radiofrequency has become the preferred approach. However, there are specific locations (near to the main biliary tree, abdominal organs, or heart) where the application of RFA is contraindicated because of the risk or severe complications and this still leaves ethanol as a useful option. Several randomized controlled trials (RCTs) have confirmed this superiority for the local control of tumors. Although the impact in survival is less well established, recently published meta-analyses have suggested that RFA is superior to PEI in terms of survival, particularly in nodules >2 cm [55,56]. The 3-year survival of patients treated percutaneously exceeds 50% at 5 years and it has been shown that initial response to treatment is an independent predictor of better survival [52].

Transarterial chemoembolization

Since the blood supply to HCC comes mostly through the hepatic artery, any intervention that blocks this vessel will result in tumor ischemia and necrosis to a variable extent. Obviously, the absence of portal blood flow (portal vein obstruction, portosystemic anastomosis, or hepatofugal flow) is a contraindication for the procedure, which is also not indicated in patients with extrahepatic spread. Liver function should be preserved and this limits its application to patients in Child–Pugh class A.

Hepatic artery obstruction requires an angiographic procedure with the advancement of a catheter into the hepatic artery in order to interrupt blood flow to the tumor as selectively as possible, thus limiting the injury of surrounding nontumor liver. Mere obstruction of the hepatic artery is known as transarterial or bland embolization, while if combined with prior injection of chemotherapy (doxorubicin, mitomycin, or cisplatin) the procedure is known as transarterial chemoembolization (TACE) (Fig. 36.5). There are several agents that can be used for arterial obstruction. The most common is gelfoam prepared as 1 mm cubes, but active research is underway to develop more effective obstructing agents [57]. In this regard, a relevant advance has been the development of drug-eluting beads. These are particles that are loaded with chemotherapy as well as the embolization device to deliver the drug to the tumor without initial systemic washout release. This results in higher concentrations of drug over a longer time period, reaching the tumor, with minimal systemic passage and, therefore, significantly less drug-related side effects [58,59]. The intervention is

well tolerated but it is not free of side effects. The most frequent complication is the so-called "postembolization syndrome" that appears in nearly 50% of patients and consists of fever, abdominal pain, and a moderate degree of ileus. This is resolved in 48 hours and overlaps with the potential side effects of chemotherapy.

Objective responses as reflected by intratumoral necrosis and reduced tumor burden on dynamic CT scan or MRI are seen in nearly 75% of the patients [58,59]. Objective response is associated with delayed tumor progression and, as a whole, results in an improvement of survival as shown by two RCTs [60,61] and a cumulative meta-analysis [42].

In recent years, other potentially useful transarterial treatments have emerged. Radioembolization using yttrium-90 spheres stands out among them [62]. Preliminary phase II clinical trials on inoperable HCC subjects with portal vein thrombosis have shown a high tumor response rate and good clinical tolerance [63]. Despite the promising results, there are currently no conclusive data available regarding its benefits in terms of survival. It is an expensive and complex treatment, so at the moment its use is limited to experimental circumstances.

Systemic therapies: sorafenib

Conventional chemotherapy has no benefit (<10% objective responses) and is frequently associated with toxicity and hence is usually not recommended [7]. Estrogen blockade with tamoxifen has no benefit even if used at high doses when it can also become toxic [42]. Antiandrogenic therapy is also inactive and induces hepatic

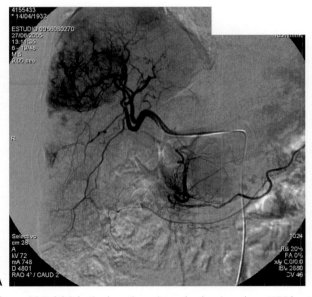 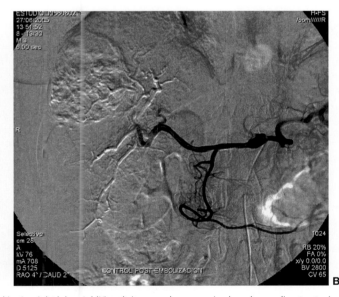

Figure 36.5 (A) Selective hepatic angiography showing a large HCC located in the right lobe. Additional sites are also recognized, and according to staging the appropriate treatment is chemoembolization. (B) After injection of chemotherapy suspended in lipiodol and arterial obstruction with gelfoam cubes, the tumor vascularization has been completely abolished. This combined therapy results in extensive tumor necrosis and improved patient survival.

toxicity that might even impair survival. Octreotide, vitamin D derivates, and interferon have also been tested with negative results [7].

Over the last few years, a great deal of progress has been made in understanding the molecular alterations that condition tumor initiation and progression [64]. This has allowed the development of several agents that act on the molecular pathways in specific ways. Several molecular treatments have been evaluated and in these studies the results are promising [65,66]. Until now, the only agent that has proven to be effective in terms of survival outcome in a phase III placebo-controlled study is sorafenib [43,67]. This is an oral, multikinase inhibitor that acts by blocking the different signaling pathways associated with hepatocarcinogenesis, especially the Raf/MEK/ERK pathway, by inhibiting Raf kinase and different tyrosine kinases (vascular endothelial growth factor receptor 2, platelet-derived growth factor receptor, and c-Kit receptors). Sorafenib basically acts by reducing angiogenesis and delaying cell proliferation. After obtaining positive results in preclinical studies [68] and in a phase II trial [69], two international, multicenter, randomized, controlled, double-blinded clinical studies were carried out. A dose of sorafenib 400 mg/12 h was compared with a placebo; both were administered to subjects with advanced HCC and compensated liver function. In both studies, sorafenib demonstrated a significant impact on survival (hazard ratio for survival compared with placebo of 0.69) and a delay of tumor progression measured by a significant increase of the time to progression (Table 36.1). The most common adverse events were diarrhea, weight loss, and hand/foot skin reaction. In most cases, the adverse events were mild and easy to manage so treatment was continued for 90% of subjects. Sorafenib has also been evaluated for treating subjects with compensated liver function (Child–Pugh grade A) but there are few data regarding its usefulness for treating Child–Pugh grade B subjects with regard to survival outcome. The pharmacokinetic profile is not significantly modified and there have been no reports of a significant increase in side effects. Therefore, the use of sorafenib in Child–Pugh grade B subjects should be evaluated on an individual basis. Contrarily, preliminary experience in Child–Pugh class C patients discourages the use of sorafenib in this population [70].

Table 36.1 Summary of the main results of the two randomized controlled trials assessing the benefit of sorafenib in advanced HCC.

	SHARP trial [50]	Asian-Pacific trial [67]
Number of patients	299 treated (303 placebo)	150 treated (76 placebo)
Median age	65 years	51 years
Liver function: Child–Pugh class A/B	95%/5%	97%/3%
BCLC stage B/C	18%/82%	4%/96%
Metastasis	51%	68%
Vascular invasion	36%	34%
PS 0–1/2	92%/8%	95%/5%
Failed previous treatment	67%	NA
Etiology of cirrhosis:		
HCV	29%	11%
HBV	19%	71%
Alcohol	26%	18%
Other	29%	NA
Response rate	DCR 43%	DCR 35%
CR/PR/SD/PD	0%/2%/71%/23%	0%/6%/54%/31%
TTP (control)	5.5 months (2.8 months)	2.8 months (1.4 months)
HR S/P (95% CI)	0.58 (0.45–0.74)	0.57 (0.42–0.79)
Median survival (control)	10.7 months (7.9 months)	6.5 months (4.2 months)
HR S/P (95% CI)	0.69 (0.55–0.87)	0.68 (0.50–0.93)

BCLC, Barcelona Clinic Liver Cancer; CI, confidence interval; CR, complete response; DCR, disease control rate; HBV, hepatitis B virus; HCV, hepatitis C virus; HR S/P, hazard ratio of sorafenib versus placebo; NA, not available; PD, progressive disease; PR, partial response; PS, performance status; SD, stable disease; TTP, time to progression.

Positive results with sorafenib provide a hope of molecular targeted therapy in HCC and open the possibility of multipathway blockade. Currently, there are several drugs, alone or in association, under evaluation as first- or second-line therapy in advanced disease or as adjuvants after surgical resection or locoregional therapies. Accordingly, in the near future we should witness a dramatic change in the therapeutic management of these patients [65].

References

1. Bosch FX, Ribes J, Diaz M, Cleries R. Primary liver cancer: worldwide incidence and trends. *Gastroenterology* 2004;127(5 Suppl 1):S5–16.
2. Forner A, Llovet JM, Bruix J. Hepatocellular carcinoma. *Lancet* 2011 (in press).
3. Ferlay J, Shin HR, Bray F, Forman D, Malthers C, Parkin DM. Estimates of worlwide burden of cancer in 2008: GLOBOCAN 2008. *Int J Cancer* 2010;127(12):2893–917.
4. Chang MH, Chen CJ, Lai MS, et al. Universal hepatitis B vaccination in Taiwan and the incidence of hepatocellular carcinoma in children. *Taiwan Childhood Hepatoma Study Group*. N Engl J Med 1997;336(26):1855–9.
5. McCredie M, Williams S, Coates M. Cancer mortality in East and Southeast Asian migrants to New South Wales, Australia, 1975–1995. *Br J Cancer* 1999;79(7–8):1277–82.
6. Fattovich G, Stroffolini T, Zagni I, Donato F. Hepatocellular carcinoma in cirrhosis: incidence and risk factors. *Gastroenterology* 2004; 127(5 Suppl 1):S35–50.
7. Bruix J, Sherman M. Management of hepatocellular carcinoma. *Hepatology* 2005;42(5):1208–36.
8. Brechot C. Pathogenesis of hepatitis B virus-related hepatocellular carcinoma: old and new paradigms. *Gastroenterology* 2004;127(5 Suppl 1):S56–61.
9. Yang HI, Lu SN, Liaw YF, et al. Hepatitis B e antigen and the risk of hepatocellular carcinoma. *N Engl J Med* 2002;347(3):168–74.
10. Pollicino T, Squadrito G, Cerenzia G, et al. Hepatitis B virus maintains its pro-oncogenic properties in the case of occult HBV infection. *Gastroenterology* 2004;126(1):102–10.
11. Sun CA, Wu DM, Lin CC, et al. Incidence and cofactors of hepatitis C virus-related hepatocellular carcinoma: a prospective study of 12,008 men in Taiwan. *Am J Epidemiol* 2003;157(8):674–82.
12. Goodgame B, Shaheen NJ, Galanko J, El-Serag HB. The risk of end stage liver disease and hepatocellular carcinoma among persons infected with hepatitis C virus: publication bias? *Am J Gastroenterol* 2003;98(11):2535–42.
13. Masuzaki R, Tateishi R, Yoshida H, et al. Risk assessment of hepatocellular carcinoma in chronic hepatitis C patients by transient elastography. *J Clin Gastroenterol* 2008;42(7):839–43.
14. Bruno S, Stroffolini T, Colombo M, et al. Sustained virological response to interferon-alpha is associated with improved outcome in HCV-related cirrhosis: a retrospective study. *Hepatology* 2007;45(3): 579–87.
15. Di Bisceglie AM, Shiffman ML, Everson GT, et al. Prolonged therapy of advanced chronic hepatitis C with low-dose peginterferon. *N Engl J Med* 2008;359(23):2429–41.
16. Bruix J, Poynard T, Colombo M, et al. Pegintron maintenance therapy in cirrhotic (METAVIR F4) HCV patients, who failed to respond to interferon/ribavirin (IR) therapy: Final results of the EPIC3 cirrhosis maintenance trial. *J Hepatol* 2009;50:49.
17. Salmon-Ceron D, Rosenthal E, Lewden C, et al. Emerging role of hepatocellular carcinoma among liver-related causes of deaths in HIV-infected patients: the French national Mortalite 2005 Study. *J Hepatol* 2009;50(4):736–45.
18. Bagnardi V, Blangiardo M, La Vecchia C, Corrao G. Alcohol consumption and the risk of cancer: a meta-analysis. *Alcohol Res Health* 2001;25(4):263–70.
19. Marrero JA, Fontana RJ, Fu S, Conjeevaram HS, Su GL, Lok AS. Alcohol, tobacco and obesity are synergistic risk factors for hepatocellular carcinoma. *J Hepatol* 2005;42(2):218–24.
20. Bravi F, Bosetti C, Tavani A, et al. Coffee drinking and hepatocellular carcinoma risk: a meta-analysis. *Hepatology* 2007;46(2):430–5.
21. Kojiro M, Roskams T. Early hepatocellular carcinoma and dysplastic nodules. *Semin Liver Dis* 2005;25(2):133–42.
22. Borzio M, Fargion S, Borzio F, et al. Impact of large regenerative, low grade and high grade dysplastic nodules in hepatocellular carcinoma development. *J Hepatol* 2003;39: 208–14.
23. Villanueva A, Newell P, Chiang DY, Friedman SL, Llovet JM. Genomics and signaling pathways in hepatocellular carcinoma. *Semin Liver Dis* 2007;27(1):55–76.
24. Hoshida Y, Toffanin S, Lachenmayer A, Villanueva A, Minguez B, Llovet JM. Molecular classification and novel targets in hepatocellular carcinoma: recent advancements. *Semin Liver Dis* 2010;30(1):35–51.
25. Hoshida Y, Nijman SM, Kobayashi M, et al. Integrative transcriptome analysis reveals common molecular subclasses of human hepatocellular carcinoma. *Cancer Res* 2009;69(18):7385–92.
26. Di Tommaso L, Destro A, Fabbris V, et al. Diagnostic accuracy of clathrin heavy chain staining in a marker panel for th diagnosis of small hepatocellular carcinoma. *Hepatology* 2011;53(5):1549–57.
27. Zhang BH, Yang BH, Tang ZY. Randomized controlled trial of screening for hepatocellular carcinoma. *J Cancer Res Clin Oncol* 2004;130(7):417–22.
28. Trevisani F, D'Intino PE, Morselli-Labate AM, et al. Serum alphafetoprotein for diagnosis of hepatocellular carcinoma in patients with chronic liver disease: influence of HBsAg and anti-HCV status. *J Hepatol* 2001;34(4):570–5.
29. Di Bisceglie AM, Sterling RK, Chung RT, et al. Serum alphafetoprotein levels in patients with advanced hepatitis C: results from the HALT-C Trial. *J Hepatol* 2005;43(3):434–41.
30. Marrero JA, Feng Z, Wang Y, et al. Alpha-fetoprotein, des-gamma carboxyprothrombin, and lectin-bound alpha-fetoprotein in early hepatocellular carcinoma. *Gastroenterology* 2009;137(1):110–18.
31. Singal A, Volk ML, Waljee A, et al. Meta-analysis: surveillance with ultrasound for early-stage hepatocellular carcinoma in patients with cirrhosis. *Aliment Pharmacol Ther* 2009;30(1):37–47.
32. Capurro M, Wanless IR, Sherman M, et al. Glypican-3: a novel serum and histochemical marker for hepatocellular carcinoma. *Gastroenterology* 2003;125(1):89–97.
33. Trinchet JC, Chaffaut C, Bourcier V, et al. Ultrasonographic surveillance of hepatocellular carcinoma in cirrhosis: A randomized trial comparing 3- and 6-month periodicities. *Hepatology* 2011. In press. DOI: 10.1002/hep.24545.
34. Burrel M, Llovet JM, Ayuso C, et al. MRI angiography is superior to helical CT for detection of HCC prior to liver transplantation: an explant correlation. *Hepatology* 2003;38(4):1034–42.
35. Forner A, Vilana R, Ayuso C, et al. Diagnosis of hepatic nodules 20 mm or smaller in cirrhosis: prospective validation of the non-invasive diagnostic criteria for hepatocellular carcinoma. *Hepatology* 2008;47(1):97–104.
36. Rimola J, Forner A, Reig M, et al. Cholangiocarcinoma in cirrhosis: absence of contrast washout in delayed phases by magnetic resonance imaging avoids misdiagnosis of hepatocellular carcinoma. *Hepatology* 2009;50(3):791–8.
37. Sangiovanni A, Manini MA, Iavarone M, et al. The diagnostic and economic impact of contrast imaging technique in the diagnosis of small hepatocellular carcinoma in cirrhosis *Gut* 2010;59(5):638–44.

38. Bruix J, Sherman M. Management of hepatocellular carcinoma: an update. *Hepatology* 2011;53(3):1020–2.

39. Vilana R, Forner A, Bianchi L, et al. Intrahepatic peripheral cholangiocarcinoma in cirrhosis patients may display a vascular pattern similar to hepatocellular carcinoma on contrast-enhanced ultrasound. *Hepatology* 2010;51(6):2020–9.

40. Grieco A, Pompili M, Caminiti G, et al. Prognostic factors for survival in patients with early-intermediate hepatocellular carcinoma undergoing non-surgical therapy: comparison of Okuda, CLIP, and BCLC staging systems in a single Italian centre. *Gut* 2005;54(3):411–18.

41. Marrero JA, Fontana RJ, Barrat A, et al. Prognosis of hepatocellular carcinoma: comparison of 7 staging systems in an American cohort. *Hepatology* 2005;41(4):707–16.

42. Llovet JM, Bruix J. Systematic review of randomized trials for unresectable hepatocellular carcinoma: chemoembolization improves survival. *Hepatology* 2003;37(2):429–42.

43. Llovet J, Ricci S, Mazzaferro V, et al. Sorafenib in advanced hepatocellular carcinoma. *N Engl J Med* 2008;359(4):378–90.

44. Llovet JM, Schwartz M, Mazzaferro V. Resection and liver transplantation for hepatocellular carcinoma. *Semin Liver Dis* 2005;25(2):181–200.

45. Llovet JM, Fuster J, Bruix J. Intention-to-treat analysis of surgical treatment for early hepatocellular carcinoma: resection versus transplantation. *Hepatology* 1999;30(6):1434–40.

46. Hoshida Y, Villanueva A, Kobayashi M, et al. Gene expression in fixed tissues and outcome in hepatocellular carcinoma. *N Engl J Med* 2008;359(19):1995–2004.

47. Mazzaferro V, Regalia E, Doci R, et al. Liver transplantation for the treatment of small hepatocellular carcinomas in patients with cirrhosis. *N Engl J Med* 1996;334(11):693–9.

48. Mazzaferro V, Llovet JM, Miceli R, et al. Predicting survival after liver transplantation in patients with hepatocellular carcinoma beyond the Milan criteria: a retrospective, exploratory analysis. *Lancet Oncol* 2009;10(1):35–43.

49. Ghobrial RM, Freise CE, Trotter JF, et al. Donor morbidity after living donation for liver transplantation. *Gastroenterology* 2008;135(2):468–76.

50. Hwang S, Lee SG, Joh JW, Suh KS, Kim DG. Liver transplantation for adult patients with hepatocellular carcinoma in Korea: comparison between cadaveric donor and living donor liver transplantations. *Liver Transpl* 2005;11(10):1265–72.

51. Herrero JI, Sangro B, Pardo F, et al. Liver transplantation in patients with hepatocellular carcinoma across Milan criteria. *Liver Transpl* 2008;14(3):272–8.

52. Sala M, Llovet JM, Vilana R, et al. Initial response to percutaneous ablation predicts survival in patients with hepatocellular carcinoma. *Hepatology* 2004;40(6):1352–60.

53. Livraghi T, Meloni F, Di Stasi M, et al. Sustained complete response and complications rate after radiofrequency ablation of very early hepatocellular carcinoma in cirrhosis. Is resection still the treatment of choice? *Hepatology* 2008;47(1):82–9.

54. Lencioni RA, Allgaier HP, Cioni D, et al. Small hepatocellular carcinoma in cirrhosis: randomized comparison of radio-frequency thermal ablation versus percutaneous ethanol injection. *Radiology* 2003;228(1):235–40.

55. Germani G, Pleguezuelo M, Gurusamy K, Meyer T, Isgro G, Burroughs AK. Clinical outcomes of radiofrequency ablation, percutaneous alcohol and acetic acid injection for hepatocellular carcinoma: a meta-analysis. *J Hepatol* 2010;52(3):380–8.

56. Cho YK, Kim JK, Kim MY, Rhim H, Han JK. Systematic review of randomized trials for hepatocellular carcinoma treated with percutaneous ablation therapies. *Hepatology* 2009;49(2):453–9.

57. Bruix J, Sala M, Llovet JM. Chemoembolization for hepatocellular carcinoma. *Gastroenterology* 2004;127(5 Suppl 1):S179–88.

58. Varela M, Real MI, Burrel M, et al. Chemoembolization of hepatocellular carcinoma with drug eluting beads: efficacy and doxorubicin pharmacokinetics. *J Hepatol* 2007;46(3):474–81.

59. Lammer J, Malagari K, Vogl T, et al. Prospective randomized study of doxorubicin-eluting-bead embolization in the treatment of hepatocellular carcinoma: results of the PRECISION V study. *Cardiovasc Intervent Radiol* 2010;33(1):41–52.

60. Llovet JM, Real MI, Montana X, et al. Arterial embolisation or chemoembolisation versus symptomatic treatment in patients with unresectable hepatocellular carcinoma: a randomised controlled trial. *Lancet* 2002;359(9319):1734–9.

61. Lo CM, Ngan H, Tso WK, et al. Randomized controlled trial of transarterial lipiodol chemoembolization for unresectable hepatocellular carcinoma. *Hepatology* 2002;35(5):1164–71.

62. Sangro B, Bilbao JI, Boan J, et al. Radioembolization using 90Y-resin microspheres for patients with advanced hepatocellular carcinoma. *Int J Radiat Oncol Biol Phys* 2006;66(3):792–800.

63. Kulik LM, Carr BI, Mulcahy MF, et al. Safety and efficacy of 90Y radiotherapy for hepatocellular carcinoma with and without portal vein thrombosis. *Hepatology* 2008;47(1):71–81.

64. Villanueva A, Minguez B, Forner A, Reig M, Llovet JM. Hepatocellular carcinoma: novel molecular approaches for diagnosis, prognosis and therapy. *Annu Rev Med* 2010;61: 317–28.

65. Llovet JM, Bruix J. Molecular targeted therapies in hepatocellular carcinoma. *Hepatology* 2008;48(4):1312–27.

66. Bruix J, Llovet JM. Major achievements in hepatocellular carcinoma. *Lancet* 2009;373(9664):614–16.

67. Cheng AL, Kang YK, Chen Z, et al. Efficacy and safety of sorafenib in patients in the Asia–Pacific region with advanced hepatocellular carcinoma: a phase III randomised, double-blind, placebo-controlled trial. *Lancet Oncol* 2009;10(1):25–34.

68. Wilhelm SM, Carter C, Tang L, et al. BAY 43-9006 exhibits broad spectrum oral antitumor activity and targets the RAF/MEK/ERK pathway and receptor tyrosine kinases involved in tumor progression and angiogenesis. *Cancer Res* 2004;64(19):7099–109.

69. Abou-Alfa GK, Schwartz L, Ricci S, et al. Phase II study of sorafenib in patients with advanced hepatocellular carcinoma. *J Clin Oncol* 2006;24(26):4293–300.

70. Worns MA, Weinmann A, Pfingst K, et al. Safety and efficacy of sorafenib in patients with advanced hepatocellular carcinoma in consideration of concomitant stage of liver cirrhosis. *J Clin Gastroenterol* 2009;43(5):489–95.

Multiple choice questions

36.1 **Which is the best treatment option for a 55-year-old patient with a history of chronic hepatitis C infection and a solitary, 4.5 cm hepatocellular carcinoma (HCC) located in segment 2 and diagnosed and staged by magnetic resonance imaging?**

   a Radiofrequency ablation.
   b Liver transplantation.
   c Surgical resection.
   d Transarterial chemoembolization.
   e Sorafenib.

36.2 **Which statement is not correct?**

   a Conclusive HCC diagnosis can be done without histologic confirmation.
   b AFP should not be used for the surveillance of HCC.
   c The main cause of HCC worldwide is chronic HBV infection.
   d Sorafenib increases survival in advanced HCC because it leads to tumor shrinkage demonstrated by dynamic imaging techniques.
   e Vascular invasion and the presence of symptoms are relevant prognostic factors that usually indicate advanced disease.

Answers to the multiple choice questions can be found in the Appendix at the end of the book.

These multiple choice questions are also available for you to complete online.
Visit http://www.schiffsdiseasesoftheliver.com/

CHAPTER 37

Surgical Options in Liver Cancers

B. Daniel Campos & Jean F. Botha

Division of Transplantation, Department of Surgery, University of Nebraska Medical Center, Omaha, NE, USA

Key concepts

- Hepatocellular carcinoma (HCC) is the third leading cause of cancer-related death worldwide. Surgical treatment (resection or transplantation) is the only form of curative treatment.
- The minority of patients with HCC are noncirrhotic; around 5% of patients are in western countries and around 40% in Asia. Nearly 75% of patients with HCC are not candidates for surgery because of advanced HCC stage or severity of underlying liver disease.
- In patients with underlying liver disease, imaging-based diagnosis of HCC can obviate the need of histologic diagnosis.
- Liver resection for HCC has good outcomes only when limited to noncirrhotic patients or patients with an early stage of cirrhosis (normal bilirubin, hepatic vein pressure gradient <10 mmHg, platelet count >100,000/mm^3).
- Liver transplantation provides the best chance of long-term survival, particularly when limited to patients who have a solitary HCC (less than 5 cm in diameter) or three or fewer tumors, none measuring more than 3 cm. The absence of vascular invasion is also associated with a better long-term prognosis.
- Preoperative ablative therapies (radiofrequency ablation, transarterial chemoembolization, percutaneous ethanol injection, etc.) are commonly performed in patients awaiting liver transplantation with the hope of improving long-term survival or preventing tumor growth while waiting. There is little evidence that these treatments are effective for either the prevention of dropout from the waiting list or improvement of long-term survival.
- Shortage of donor organs, which has traditionally limited the use of transplantation, has been partially addressed by the use of living

- donors. The definitive outcomes of living donor liver transplantation for HCC are still under scrutiny.
- Bile duct cancer is the second most common primary hepatic malignancy. Less than 20% of patients with hilar cholangiocarcinomas are candidates for a curative resection.
- Surgical resection is the standard of treatment. Intrahepatic tumors are treated by a partial hepatectomy, distal tumors are treated by a pancreatoduodenectomy, and hilar tumors are treated either by a hemihepatectomy or by a total hepatectomy with liver transplant if they are unresectable. Successful surgical treatment (resection or transplantation) remains the only hope for long-term survival. Surgical resection provides a 5-year survival ranging from 11% to 40% at best.
- Microscopic extension of bile duct cancer is always beyond the macroscopic margin. Superficial and submucosal infiltration often includes direct lymphatic and/or perineural invasion. A macroscopic surgical margin of at least 10 mm is recommended along with examination of frozen sections of the bile duct cut end.
- Portal vein embolization and biliary drainage are important and safe adjuncts to major hepatectomies in order to prevent liver failure.
- Liver transplantation in the setting of a rigorous protocol of neoadjuvant chemoradiation therapy has demonstrated a 5-year survival of 82% with a 5-year recurrence rate of 12%; which compares favorably with any other form of treatment for bile duct cancer.

The present chapter contains a detailed review of the variety of surgical options currently available to treat hepatocellular carcinoma (HCC) and cholangiocarcinoma (CC).

Hepatocellular carcinoma

Liver cancer, primarily HCC, is the third leading cause of death from cancer worldwide and the ninth leading cause of cancer deaths in the United States. Chronic hepati-

tis B virus (HBV) and hepatitis C virus (HCV) infections account for an estimated 80% of global HCC cases [1]. In the continued absence of effective nonsurgical means for either prevention or treatment of HCC, surgery remains the mainstay of cure. Although resection has long been advocated as the first choice for those patients whose general condition, degree of liver dysfunction, and total tumor burden allow it, patients with underlying chronic liver disease face a lifetime risk of developing additional malignancies in the diseased liver left behind. In this

Schiff's Diseases of the Liver, Eleventh Edition. Edited by Eugene R. Schiff, Willis C. Maddrey and Michael F. Sorrell.
© 2012 John Wiley & Sons, Ltd. Published 2012 by John Wiley & Sons, Ltd.

subset of patients, liver transplantation is currently viewed as the most effective form of treatment. Its application is tempered by an insufficient donor pool, the risks of lifetime immunosupression, and a high recurrence rate of hepatitis for those with chronic HCV.

Preoperative assessment

The outcome of patients with HCC undergoing surgical treatment is dependent on four major factors: (i) tumor grade and stage; (ii) severity of underlying liver disease; (iii) ability of the patient to withstand the treatment; and (iv) the proposed intervention. On the basis of an assessment of these factors, almost 80% of patients with HCC will be excluded from curative surgery (liver resection or transplantation) [2]. Patients deemed to have tumors not suitable for surgical treatment are offered one or more of the increasing number of available palliative therapies.

The need to establish a preoperative histologic diagnosis of HCC is controversial to some extent. It is generally agreed that in patients with evidence of cirrhosis, a definitive diagnosis of HCC can be made without tissue analysis in case of nodules >2 cm with a characteristic pattern on either computed tomography (CT) or magnetic resonance imaging (MRI) (hypervascularity in the arterial phase and washout in the early or delayed venous phase). Two concordant imaging techniques (triphasic CT and MRI) are needed to ascertain HCC in cases of nodules between 1 and 2 cm [3]. Biopsy is needed for making a diagnosis of HCC in patients with cirrhosis with nodules that do not fulfill the above criteria. Image-guided percutaneous needle biopsy is the most common approach to obtain tissue for histologic diagnosis despite evidence that aspiration cytology is both more accurate and more sensitive than standard histology [4]. The incidence of needle tract seeding is <2% in the largest series [5,6]. Multiple reports of late recurrences of HCC in subcutaneous tissue illustrate the risk associated with percutaneous needle biopsy [7,8].

Standard preoperative workup should include: complete blood count, comprehensive metabolic panel, coagulatory parameters, ultrasonography of the liver, and CT scan of the abdomen, pelvis, and thorax. Suspicious lesions found during metastatic evaluation should be biopsied using percutaneous techniques. Histologic documentation of extrahepatic disease obviates curative resection and is considered a contraindication to transplantation. Liver surgery inflicts significant physiologic stress on the patient. Patients should be carefully evaluated for possible cardiac disease with a screening electrocardiogram (ECG) and a careful evaluation of the patient's level of activity. Hepatic resection carries a high risk for cardiac events according to the classifications presented by Eagle and Boucher [9]. Further cardiac evaluations are usually required in patients with risk factors for coronary artery disease. Patients with unstable coronary syndromes, decompensated congestive heart failure, significant arrhythmias, or severe valvular disease often require extensive cardiac workup, medical management, and, potentially, cardiac surgery prior to hepatic resection. Patients with a known history of pulmonary disease should be evaluated with preoperative pulmonary function tests and an arterial blood gas.

Liver resection

Surgical resection for HCC is carried out with a curative intent. The minority of patients with HCC are noncirrhotic; around 5% of patients are in western countries and around 40% in Asia. In these patients, partial liver resection is without question the treatment of choice. The overwhelming majority of patients with HCC have different stages of cirrhosis, which makes the decision algorithm for resection far less straightforward. Despite the fact that any degree of portal hypertension along with hepatocellular dysfunction negatively impact on the outcome of resection, most experts would agree that patients with Child–Pugh class A cirrhosis, normal bilirubin, and minimal portal hypertension (e.g., platelet count >100,000/mm^3 and/or hepatic venous pressure gradient <10 mmHg) are excellent candidates for resection. This selected group of patients has almost no risk for postoperative liver failure and may achieve a 5-year survival of around 70%. The survival of those subjects with both adverse predictors (portal hypertension and elevated bilirubin) is less than 30% at 5 years, regardless of their Child–Pugh stage [10].

Improved patient selection in conjunction with advances in operative techniques and perioperative management have decreased the operative morbidity and mortality in patients undergoing liver resections. There is a large variation in survival, mortality, and recurrence rate following liver resections for HCC due to the lack of uniform definitions in the different series published. Table 37.1 presents the results of a number of published series of liver resection for HCC in the last two decades [11–24]. A recently published meta-analysis of the surgical outcomes of liver resections for the treatment of HCC reported a median perioperative (30 day in-hospital) mortality rate of 4.7%, median 1-, 3-, and 5-year overall survival rates of 80.1%, 55%, and 37.1%, respectively, and disease-free survivals of 64%, 38%, and 27% in the same time intervals [25]. Unfortunately, long-term survival is negatively affected by an overall tumor recurrence rate of well over 50%. Recurrence may occur in the liver or at extrahepatic sites. Recurrence occurs not only because of the biologic behavior of the tumor, but also because the remnant liver still has premalignant potential, with HCV-positive patients being at particular risk [26].

Table 37.1 Results of liver resection for hepatocellular carcinoma.

Number of patients	% cirrhotic	Overal survival (%)			Disease-free survival (%)			Recurrence (%)	Comments	Reference
		1 year	3 years	5 years	1 year	3 years	5 years			
76	23	71	47	33	–	–	–	50		Iwatsuki et al. 1991 [11]
131	30	67	42	35	–	–	–	32		Ringe et al. 1991 [12]
72	100	68	51	–	–	–	–	22		Franco et al. 1990 [130]
60	100	–	52	–	–	27	–	73		Bismuth et al. 1993 [14]
280	–	88	70	50	–	–	29	71		Takenaka et al. 1996 [15]
106	33	–	–	41	–	–	–	–		Vauthey et al. 1995 [16]
76	100	81	52	39	62	27	14	69	TACE in 35% of patients	Majno et al. 1997 [17]
37	100	–	35	24	69	26	9	78		Gouillat et al. 1999 [18]
35	100	83	57	51	70	44	31	–		Figueras et al. 2000 [19]
386	–	–	–	34	–	–	10	66	TACE in 36% of patients	Hanazaki et al. 2000 [20]
264	100	–	63	41	–	49	28	56		Grazi et al. 2001 [21]
303	55	84	67	51	–	–	27	–		Kanematsu et al. 2002 [22]
218	100	63	41	31	51	34	27	–		Yeh et al. 2002 [23]
98	50	81	58	26	–	–	–	–		Neeff et al. 2009 [24]

TACE, transarterial chemoembolization.

Tumor size appears not to be a mayor barrier to resection provided the tumor is circumscribed. Patients that have multiple tumors are not ideal candidates for resection due to the presence of intrahepatic metastasis. Macroscopic vascular invasion is a strong risk factor for recurrence; however, in selected cases with normal liver function, no portal hypertension, and with a unilateral intraportal tumor that does not completely occlude the bifurcation, resection and portal tumor extraction can be achieved with acceptable long-term survival [27].

The type of resection performed is dictated by the size and location of the tumor. Resections are usually segmental or lobar. Most commonly, a bilateral subcostal incision is used. Initial exploration of the abdomen should rule out extrahepatic disease. The arterial anatomy of the liver should be assessed to identify aberrant left or replaced right hepatic arteries. After the liver is mobilized, resectability of the tumor should be confirmed. The use of intraoperative ultrasound may give the surgeon information about the proximity of the tumor to hepatic veins and portal vessels. It also provides further assurance that no previously unidentified lesions are present in the liver. Traditionally, the hilar structures (hepatic artery, portal vein, and bile duct) leading to the lobe or segment(s) to be resected are identified and individually ligated prior to the parenchymal dissection. A Pringle maneuver may be used to occlude the inflow during the parenchymal division to minimize blood loss. Inflow can

be occluded for up to 60 minutes continuously or intermittently. An alternative approach is total vascular exclusion where the vena cava is isolated above and below the liver and a soft vascular clamp is placed across the hilum of the liver prior to parenchymal division. This technique is useful for segmental and lobar resections. Patients who do not tolerate the lack of venous return may be supported with veno-veno bypass. All patients undergoing a hepatic resection should have blood products available for the operating room. We do not routinely use autologous shed blood recovery techniques when resecting malignancies in the liver. Patients with liver disease and prolonged prothrombin times should receive fresh frozen plasma (FFP) to correct the coagulopathy early in the surgery. Midorikawa et al. advocate the use of FFP routinely, both in the operating room and postoperatively, in all hepatic resections [28].

Prognostic assessment

Prognostic risk factors for intra- and extrahepatic recurrence after resection for HCC have been extensively studied and reported; the conventional pathologic features of HCC tumors are the most widely cited in the literature. Tumor size, gross or microscopic tumor involvement at the resection margin, tumor grade, macro- and microscopic vascular invasion, multiple tumors or satellite lesions, and α-fetoprotein (AFP) levels have all being

Table 37.2 Child–Pugh score.

Criterion	1 point	2 points	3 points
Serum bilirubin (mg/dL)	<2	2–3	>3
Serum albumin (g/dL)	>3.5	3–3.5	<3
Ascites	None	Easily controlled	Poorly controlled
Encephalopathy	None	Minimal	Advanced
INR	<1.7	1.7–2.3	>2.3

5–6 points, Child–Pugh class A; 7–9 points, class B; 10–15 points, class C; INR, international normalized ratio.

shown to predict recurrence and therefore negatively impact the outcome after surgical treatment [29]

The risk of liver failure after surgical resection has been less easy to predict. Numerous tests and formulas to calculate liver function have been proposed but there is no uniformly accepted method to assess functional hepatic reserve. The bromsulfophthalein retention test, the ^{14}C-aminopyrine breath test, the indocyanine green (ICG) clearance test, and the monoethylglycinexylidide (MEGX) test are a few examples of these. The ICG clearance test is the most widely used test (particularly in Japan). ICG is actively and solely removed from plasma by the liver. Clearance of ICG is considered to be impaired when 15% or more of the dye remains within the plasma 15 minutes after intravenous injection. Patients with HCC most often have cirrhosis, and it therefore comes as no surprise that liver failure after resection is a major cause of morbidity and mortality. Bruix et al. showed that the presence of portal hypertension, defined as a wedged hepatic vein to portal vein pressure gradient of greater than 10 mmHg,

is associated with hepatic decompensation in up to 60% of patients with Child–Pugh class A cirrhosis after liver resection [30].

The Child–Pugh score is the first and most established predictive system. It is universally used to classify the degree of liver dysfunction (Table 37.2). This score was originally developed to predict the survival of patients with cirrhosis and variceal hemorrhage undergoing portocaval shunts. Numerous studies have failed to confirm its value in predicting morbidity and mortality after liver resection.

It is evident that current pathologic staging for HCC (pTNM) does not correlate with survival outcomes, mainly due to the fact that it does not take into account the severity of the underlying cirrhosis or the residual liver function. The TNM system was revised in 2002 and the new version has been demonstrated to be more accurate [31,32]. However, a recent Japanese cohort of over 900 patients failed to identify a correlation between their survival figures determined by Kaplan–Meyer analysis and those according to TNM staging and Child–Pugh classification [33]. Iwatsuki et al. reviewed a series of over 300 patients surgically treated for HCC [34]. They analyzed a number of clinical and pathologic variables to predict the risk of recurrence. Based on multivariate analysis they identified the following as risk factors of recurrence: bilobar distribution, tumor size either 2–5 cm or >5 cm, micro- and macrovascular invasion, and more than three tumors. A prognostic risk score (PRS) was calculated for each patient based the summation of each variable's relative risk of recurrence. This PRS system correlated extremely well with disease-free survival (Table 37.3) [34].

Table 37.3 Risk factors and prognostic risk score (PRS) for disease-free survival following liver transplantation for hepatocellular carcinoma. (a) Multivariate analysis of risk factors. (b) PRS and 5-year disease-free survival.

(a)				(b)					
Variable	RR	95% CI			Grade 1	Grade 2	Grade 3	Grade 4	Grade 5
Bilobar tumor	3.1	1.7, 5.4	PRS[a]		<7.5	7.5–11	11–15	15	LN, DM
Tumor size:			5-year disease-free survival (%)		100	61	40	5	0
2–5 cm	4.5	1.5, 13.0							
5 cm	6.7	2.2, 19.9							
Vascular invasion:									
Micro	4.4	2.1, 9.5							
Macro	15.0	6.7, 33.8							

CI, confidence interval; RR, relative risk.
[a]The PRS was calculated based on the addition of the relative risk of recurrence (based on multivariate analysis) identified for: bilobar distribution, tumor size 2–5 or >5 cm, and micro- and macrovascular invasion.
LN, lymph node; DM, distal metastasis.
From Iwatsuki et al. [34].

Many other prognostic staging systems have been developed in the last two decades: the Okuda staging system [35], Cancer of Liver Italian Program (CLIP) [36], Barcelona Clinic Liver Cancer (BCLC) [37], Groupe d'Etude du Treatment du Carcinome Hepatocellulaire (GRETCH) [38], Chinese University Prognostic System (CUPI), and Japan Integrated Staging Score (JIS) [39]. The Okuda staging system was developed in 1985. It is the first staging system to take into account variables related to liver function and tumor size on imaging or surgery. However, it failed to include important variables strongly associated with recurrence such as vascular invasion. It has been proven to be inaccurate for patients with early HCC. The BCLC system derived from the results of surgical treatment of early HCC and the natural history of untreated HCC. Several groups have validated it [41–43]. The CLIP uses four variables: the Child–Pugh score, tumor morphology, serum AFP level, and portal vein invasion. It appears likely that its broad inclusion criteria will reduce its value in cases of early HCC. The CUPI was based mainly on HBV-associated patients but only 10% of the patients received curative treatment. It appears to be complex and yet to be validated. The GRETCH system included mainly patients with alcoholic liver disease. Its validation in well debated [44]. The JIS system was proposed by Kudo et al. and combines the Child–Pugh score and the modified TNM classification according to the Liver Cancer Study Group of Japan (LCSGJ) [39]. This system is more suitable for patients with early HCC, and a recently modified JIS system proposed by Nanashima et al. was shown to be useful for predicting the prognosis of patients receiving resection [45].

The number of staging systems emphasizes the difficulty in adequately stratifying HCC based on different clinical, pathologic, and biochemical variables and produce a universally accepted system that reliably predicts survival outcomes of the current forms of treatment. It remains controversial as to which of these systems is best for staging HCC. It appears to this date that we do not have an adequate test to predict liver failure nor we have a staging system that reliably predicts outcomes after resection. No single test offers a better prediction of postoperative liver failure than the Child–Pugh score in conjunction with the judgment of an experienced liver surgeon.

In order to improve the outcomes of liver resection for HCC other adjuncts to resection have been theorized and studied. To date, preoperative chemoembolization of the tumor offers no benefit. The same is true for the general use of portal vein embolization of the hepatic lobe hosting the tumor to induce compensatory liver growth and to improve functional capacity in the nonaffected lobe prior to resection [46–48]. Additionally, there is no proven effective adjuvant postoperative therapy that can reduce recurrence rates.

Liver transplantation

The first patient to survive liver transplantation for more than a year was a child with HCC. Foreshadowing the failure of attempts to cure liver cancer reliably with total hepatectomy, the patient died with recurrent tumor 400 days following transplantation. The collected experience during the last two decades highlights a progression of improving outcomes. Today, total hepatectomy with transplantation is regarded as the best alternative for treating HCC in the cirrhotic patient. Liver transplantation removes the diseased liver, which is often associated with HCC, providing the widest surgical margins, which translates into the best survival outcomes and the lowest risk of recurrence.

In 1983, a National Institutes of Health consensus development conference endorsed the use of liver transplantation for the treatment of selected patients with HCC. As liver transplant centers proliferated throughout North America and Europe, wider experience underscored a serious concern. Although providing a chance for cure to patients with no other alternatives, when compared with the results for transplantation in the treatment of other liver diseases, the long-term survival probability for patients who underwent transplantation for HCC was disappointing in most and unacceptable in others. Five-year survival rates reported between 1985 and 1989 from three leading transplant centers were 25–40% [49–51]. In 1991, Penn, relying on data submitted by numerous transplant centers to the Transplant Tumor Registry, reported that the overall 5-year survival observed was 18%. These reports arrived at a time when the shortage of donor livers was beginning to drive waiting times for most patients beyond the 1-year mark, leading to an alarming increase in the risk of death for waiting candidates. With 5-year survival probabilities for other types of liver transplant recipients reportedly in excess of 80–85%, advocates for providing liver transplantation to patients with HCC were obliged to improve their results.

One approach involved better patient selection through examination of retrospective information about tumor staging and histologic grade. Others included a variety of pre- and post-transplant treatment regimens designed to lessen the risk of recurrence. Early reports suggested, and subsequent experience has confirmed, that the most favorable results are obtained in patients with so-called incidental HCC. In the experience reported by Iwatsuki et al. in 1991, no patients in this category experienced recurrence of tumor during the follow-up period [11]. The same report, as well as data from other authors, has confirmed that among patients with known HCC, those with small tumors fare better than those with larger ones. Remarkably, in 1996, Mazzaferro et al. from Milan reported a randomized controlled study demonstrating that restricting liver transplantation to patients diagnosed with a single tumor less than 5 cm in diameter or two to three tumors less than 3 cm in diameter by radiologic standards prior to transplantation resulted in a 4-year overall survival of 75%, a recurrence-free survival of 92%, and a overall recurrence rate of 8% [52]. Other groups around the world have reproduced these results [53–55]. In the United States, the United Network for Organ Sharing (UNOS) has adopted the so-called Milan criteria (Box 37.1) for the allocation of organs.

In 2002, the model of end-stage liver disease (MELD) system was implemented in the United States. Livers from cadaveric donors are now allocated according to a patient's score that is based on their international normalized ratio (INR), creatinine level, and bilirubin level. Patients with HCC usually do not have decompensation of their cirrhotic state so the transplant community decided to implement a separate point system that would provide HCC patients access to organs before their disease progressed beyond the point where they were eligible for transplantation. The Milan criteria have been used to define which patients are eligible for liver transplantation. Documentation of the presence of tumor is through imaging and a positive biopsy, an AFP of more than 200 ng/mL, or previous ablative therapy of the lesion. Points are assigned on the basis of prediction of survival for patients with stage I and II disease. With the introduction of the MELD system for liver allocation in adult patients who underwent transplant, the incidence of transplantation for HCC has risen dramatically. In 2001, 2.8% of liver transplants in the United States were for a diagnosis of HCC with or without cirrhosis, and this rose to 7% in 2004. Since the origination of the MELD system, the point allocation for patients with HCC has been adjusted and currently only patients with stage II disease are eligible for point upgrades. Patient survival rates after

liver transplantation for HCC are acceptable, with the 5-year survival being 61.1% in a review of patients transplanted between 1996 and 2001. This rate is lower than that for patients transplanted without HCC (5-year survival approximately 70%), but remains acceptable [54].

Expanding the transplantation criteria

The Barcelona group [56], The University of California at San Francisco (UCSF) group [57], and others have presented proposals for the expansion of the Milan criteria. None of these proposals are backed by rigorous prospective randomized data and their application has been a matter of debate [58,59]. The most common and studied proposal is the UCSF expanded criteria, which allows transplantation of patients with one tumor 6.5 cm or three or less tumors less than 4.5 cm, with the sum of the diameter of these tumors to be less than 8 cm, without compromising patient survival (Box 37.1) [59,60]. Multiple other studies have reproduced the UCSF results [60,61]. The largest retrospective review of HCC patients treated by liver transplantation published by the University of California at Los Angeles has validated the UCSF expanded criteria. In this report, patients meeting the Milan criteria had similar 5-year post-transplant survival compared to patients meeting the UCSF criteria by preoperative imaging and explant pathology [62].

The majority of patients within the UCSF criteria are also within the Milan criteria. The same group in Milan has recently published retrospective data regarding outcome in 1,112 patients exceeding the original Milan criteria. In this study, a 71.2% 5-year overall survival was achieved using expanded criteria (HCC with 7 as the sum of the size of the largest tumor (in centimeters) plus the number of tumors) [63]. This modest expansion of the Milan criteria does not appear to negatively impact post-transplant survival; however it only translates into a net increase of less than 10% to the potential recipient pool over conventional Milan transplant criteria. The true impact on the remainder of the waiting list is unknown and the broader application of expanded criteria is not yet accepted.

Salvage transplantation

Most agree that the best treatment strategy for small HCC, even in patients with preserved liver function (Child–Pugh class A), is liver transplantation. Some authors believe that small and resectable HCCs with preserved hepatic function should undergo liver resection as the first-line treatment, reserving transplantation in the event of HCC recurrence (salvage transplantation). This approach is a reasonable option in terms of saving valuable donated organs and sparing some patients from the burdens and risks associated with transplantation and immunosupression. However, this approach seems to result in higher recurrence and decreased survival when compared with primary liver transplantation [64,65]. On average, only one out of five patients who undergoes liver resection for HCC will receive a "salvage" liver transplant, as reported by the transplantability rates of the groups in Spain, Italy, and France 16.2%, 21.2%, and 25%, respectively [66].

Living donor liver transplantation

Treatment of HCC with liver transplantation is limited by the availability of deceased donor liver grafts, particularly in Asia, where the rate of deceased donors is negligible (five donors per 1 million population compared to 10–35 per 1 million in western countries). Living donor liver transplantation (LDLT) has been increasingly used to treat hepatic tumors worldwide in recent years, and is currently the most effective alternative to deceased donor liver transplantation to overcome the problem of organ shortage. The indications for LDLT are not clearly outlined. Most groups agree that if a HCC patient meets conventional Milan criteria and cannot undergo liver resection because of poor liver function, and a cadaveric graft is not available within 6 months, LDLT may be selected. The benefits of LDLT for HCC are clear in terms of eliminating the waiting list time and therefore preventing tumor progression and dropout from the waiting list. The results from LDLT appear to show good long-term survival rates with retrospective studies showing comparable rates to orthotopic liver transplantation (OLT). Using a statistical decision analysis technique that considered a cohort of hypothetical patients with compensated Child–Pugh A cirrhosis and an unresectable 3.5 cm HCC, Cheng et al. satisfied themselves that live donor adult-to-adult liver transplantation offered a 4.5-year increase in tumor-free survival as compared with waiting for cadaveric donor liver transplantation or no transplant. The advantage persisted in their model even in the face of varying severity of cirrhosis, age, tumor doubling time, tumor growth pattern, blood type, regional transplant volume, initial tumor size, and rate of progression of cirrhosis [67]. A similar experience was reported by the Mount Sinai Hospital during the period from 1998 to 2001, where the average waiting time for a deceased donor was 414 days as compared with 83 days for a living donor. They also proposed that HCC is an ideal indication for LDLT [68]. There are, however, a number of published retrospective studies that show a higher rate of tumor recurrence in LDLT than with conventional OLT [69–71]. The reasons for this are not entirely elucidated. A multi-center adult-to-adult LDLT study reported a statistically significant higher HCC recurrence rate after LDLT versus deceased donor liver transplantation [72–74]. More studies are needed to better define the role of LRLT for HCC. Another concern for the application of LDLT are the morbidity (14–21%) and mortality (0.25–1%) associated with donor hepatectomy. Recently, and despite its smaller size, the use of left lobe grafts with surgical portal inflow modulation has demonstrated enhanced donor safety with comparable outcomes [75,76].

Adjunctive therapy

The most common pattern of recurrence for HCC following liver transplantation is a multifocal spread in the newly transplanted liver. Kar and Carr showed that patients with HCC can have as many as 1 billion tumor cells in the systemic circulation each day [77]. It was speculated then that efforts directed at circulating tumor cells might effectively reduce the risk of recurrence. Therefore, the use of pretransplant adjunctive therapies has received widespread attention during the last decades; particularly because most transplant programs are reluctant to simply observe cirrhotic patients with HCC while they await transplantation because of the latent risk of disease progression and dropout from the waiting list.

Pretransplant neoadjuvant therapy in the form of radiofrequency ablation (RFA), transarterial chemoembolization (TACE), and percutaneous ethanol injection (PEI) is often recommended to patients with HCC and cirrhosis awaiting liver transplantation. Neoadjuvant therapy has three potential benefits: (i) to down-size existing tumors that are bigger than the Milan criteria, thus expanding the transplantability of some patients; (ii) halting disease progression and thus preventing dropout while on the transplant list; and (iii) potentially providing a survival benefit after transplant. Single-center studies have documented advantages for pretransplantation TACE [78,79] and RFA [80] in minimizing waiting list dropout rates. In 2006, an evidence-based review of all the available literature to that date concluded that TACE as a bridge to liver transplantation did not improve long-term survival nor decreased dropout rates on the waiting list [81]. More recently, however, Freeman et al. have shown a survival benefit after transplantation for patients receiving pretransplant locoregional therapy [82].

Downstaging hepatocellular carcinoma

Early in the experience with TACE, prior to liver transplantation and in nonrandomized applications, several authors believed they had obtained improved survival. In 1997, Majno et al. from Paris, found a benefit for disease-free survival in those patients who responded to TACE (50% reduction in size) prior to liver transplantation compared with those who did not [78]. More recent studies, though, have not shown a significant survival advantage to patients undergoing TACE and liver transplantation [83,84]. Effectively downstaging tumors that are beyond the Milan criteria is emerging as a viable alternative to simply expanding the transplantation criteria. A review of the UNOS database examined 1,377 histology reports from explanted livers and indicated that pretransplantation ablation treatment resulted in markedly more cases being downstaged than cases where no ablation was given, with TACE being more effective than RFA [85]. The UCSF group have recently reported excellent outcomes after liver transplantation in a strictly selected group of patients beyond the Milan criteria who were primarily downstaged by laparoscopic RFA and/or TACE. Tumor downstaging was successful in 70.5% of the patients. Survival rates at 1 and 4 years were 96.2% and 92.1%, respectively. No patient had HCC recurrence after a median follow-up of 25 months. Treatment failed in 29.5% mainly due to tumor progression. The authors inferred that successful downstaging dissects out those tumors with a more aggressive biologic behavior based on their progression despite treatment [86,87]. Pretransplantation neoadjuvant treatments remain an option for downstaging HCC tumors despite the absence of randomized data.

Most patients with HCC are not candidates for hepatic resection or transplantation. This is because of multifocal intrahepatic disease, extrahepatic disease, inadequate functional reserve, or involvement of the portal vein bifurcation. For these reasons, several techniques have been developed in order to provide therapeutic/palliative options for this subgroup of patients with HCC. Treatment modalities include systemic and regional chemotherapy, percutaneous ethanol or acetic acid injection, and cryotherapy and thermal ablative techniques such as laser, microwave, and RFA; most of these ablative therapies are applied percutaneously. It is not unusual to perform RFA or cryotherapy through laparotomy or laparoscopy. A detailed discussion of these techniques, indications, and outcomes escapes the scope of this chapter.

Cholangiocarcinoma

Bile duct cancer is the second most common primary hepatic malignancy. It is a slow growing and a highly aggressive malignancy difficult to diagnose in the early stage. Most patients with bile duct cancer have developed jaundice at presentation, and the tumor stage is already well advanced. Not surprisingly, less than 20% of patients with hilar cholangiocarcinomas are amenable to a potential curative resection. Successful surgical treatment remains the only hope for long-term survival. Those fortunate enough to undergo surgical resection have a 5-year survival ranging from 11% to 40%.

A detailed anatomic definition is necessary before discussing the role of surgical treatment in the management of bile duct cancer. Cholangiocarcinomas are divided into intrahepatic (5–10% of all cholangiocarcinomas) and

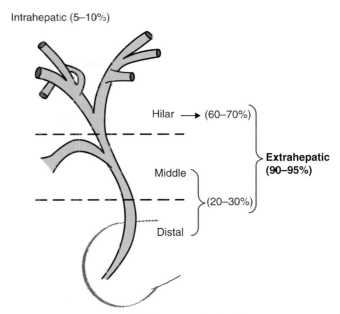

Figure 37.1 Distribution of bile duct cancer in the biliary tree.

extrahepatic (Fig. 37.1) Intrahepatic cholangiocarcinoma is treated as a hepatic tumor, because it requires liver resection alone. The surgical treatment of extrahepatic bile duct cancer is complex and depends on its location along the bile duct tree (hilar, middle, and distal bile duct cancer). Surgical resection by means of pancreatoduodenectomy is the choice of surgical treatment for middle and distal cholangiocarcinomas (20–30% of all bile duct cancers). Tumors arising high in the biliary tract above the cystic duct, in the territory of the confluence of the bile ducts (hilium), have been historically referred as hilar or perihilar cholangiocarcinomas or, if right at the confluence, Klatskin tumors. They represent approximately 60–70% of all cholangiocarcinomas. Determining resectability of these tumors is best guided by the Bismuth–Corlette classification (Fig. 37.2) [88,89]. Cholangiocarcinomas type I, II, and III are generally considered resectable by means of an extended hemihepatectomy. A type IV tumor, involving both sides of the bile duct confluence, is best resected by a total hepatectomy and could be considered an indication for liver transplantation.

Preoperative biliary drainage and portal vein embolization

Portal vein embolization has been used in the preoperative period in order to prevent liver failure after extended hemihepatectomy in patients with hilar cholangiocarcinoma [90]. Resecting a major portion of the liver results in a concomitant increase in the portal vein pressure. Excessive portal vein pressure can be detrimental to the function of a small remnant liver. Portal vein embolization can theoretically reduce the degree of portal

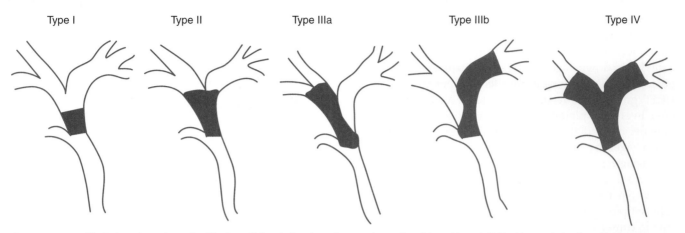

Figure 37.2 Modified Bismuth–Corlette classification of hilar cholangiocarcinomas. (Reproduced from Bismuth [82] with permission from Lippincott Williams and Wilkins.)

hypertensive damage and also improve the rate of liver volume loss due to the atrophy–hypertrophy theory. Kubota et al. delineated indication criteria for portal vein embolization according to the volume of liver to be resected [91]. Several recent reports have confirmed the safety of major hepatectomy following portal vein embolization [91–93]. The rate of liver volume to be preserved increased by 8–12% 2 weeks after portal vein embolization [94,95].

Preoperative biliary drainage aims to improve liver function and reduce morbidity and mortality after surgery. A major hepatectomy in a severely cholestatic liver (jaundiced patient) with a hilar cholangiocarcinoma is a set up for the development of postoperative liver failure. Multiple studies from Japan recommend that radical surgery be performed after complete recovery of liver function from cholestasis, which usually takes 4–6 weeks with a functioning biliary drain (bilirubin <2.0 mg/dL) [92–94]. Figure 37.3 shows a protocol for portal vein embolization and percutaneous biliary drainage in the management of hilar cholangiocarcinoma prior to surgical resection.

Many reports have emphasized the adverse effects of biliary drainage, i.e. infectious complications due to bile contamination and tract seeding [96–98]. A meta-analysis conducted by Sewnath et al. failed to show a definitive benefit of biliary drainage prior to surgery [99]. However, the rate of resection in the randomized controlled studies analyzed was only 15% on average, and pancreatico-duodenectomy composed nearly 90% of resected cases and hemihepatectomy only 2%. Strictly discussing biliary drainage in the treatment of hilar cholangiocarcinoma by a hemihepatectomy appears to our eyes to be a separate topic of discussion.

Particular attention has been given to bile contamination and suppurative cholangitis and its relation to postoperative infectious complications. We believe that

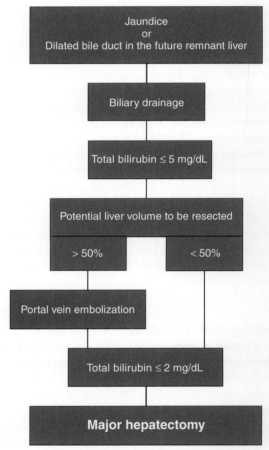

Figure 37.3 Protocol for percutaneous biliary drainage and portal vein embolization in the management of hilar cholangiocarcinoma prior to surgical resection.

infectious complications related to a biliary drain are, in the majority of cases, related to inadequate drain care, drainage tube failure, and particularly unnecessary cholangiography. Cholangitis is caused by pushing contaminated bile into the undrained area during cholangiography or by occlusion of the drainage tube. The most important means of preventing cholangitis is to not perform cholangiography in patients whose right and left bile ducts are not communicated due to tumor obstruction. In this subset of patients the future remnant liver should be preferentially drained percutaneously [100–103]. Cholangiography should be limited to the time of placement of the biliary drain (percutaneous transhepatic or endoscopic retrograde) or to the afternoon of the day before surgery. Biliary stents placed endoscopically should be exchanged every 2 weeks to prevent tube occlusion [104]. Bile cultures should be performed routinely, and isolates should be tested for antibiotic sensitivity.

Catheter tract seeding is a complication related to percutaneous transhepatic biliary drain placement. Its incidence has been reported to be 5–10%. Multiple drains and cholangiograms may increase the risk of seeding. Sakata et al. reported that resection of an isolated metastasis along the catheter tract may prolong survival [105].

Surgical management of middle and distal cholangiocarcinoma

A conventional pancreatoduodenectomy or a pylorus-preserving pancreatodudodenectomy are the treatment of choice for middle and lower bile duct cancer. Short- and long-term results of both procedures are comparable [106, 107]. It is important to understand the modes of infiltration and spread of bile duct cancer in order to insure adequate surgical treatment. Microscopic extension of bile duct cancer is always beyond the margin observed macroscopically. Longitudinal extension consists of superficial and submucosal infiltration and includes often direct, lymphatic, and/or perineural invasion. A macroscopic surgical margin of at least 10 mm is recommended. Intraoperative pathologic examination of frozen sections is necessary to confirm the margin of the cut end of the bile duct. When a middle bile duct cancer arises midway along the extrahepatic duct, the decision has to be made as to whether a pancreatoduodenectomy or extended hemihepatectomy is more appropriate according to the tumor location and extension.

The reported 5-year survival rates after pancreatoduodenectomy for middle and distal bile duct cancers have ranged from 24% to 39% [108–110]. Favorable prognostic factors following surgical resection are: R0 resection, absence of lymphatic metastatic disease, well-differentiated histology, and tumor location (middle and distal).

Surgical management of hilar cholangiocarcinomas

Because of the complex anatomic relations between structures at the hepatic hilium, an experienced surgeon with three-dimensional knowledge of this area is required to determine the extent of tumor invasion and the extent of resection needed. There are two critical points to a radical resection of a hilar cholangiocarcinoma. The first is removal of the liver parenchyma adjacent to the hepatic hilum together with the hilar plate; an extended right or left hepatectomy is preferable for this purpose. The second is caudate lobectomy and resection of the inferior area of segment IV to extirpate cancer infiltration to the thinner bile ducts near the hilum. The importance of a caudate lobectomy in the surgical treatment of hilar cholangiocarcinoma was established in a retrospective study that demonstrated a clear difference in patient survival (46% with caudate lobectomy versus 12% without caudate lobectomy) [111].

An extended hemihepatectomy is recognized as the standard surgical procedure for hilar cholangiocarcinoma [92,93,112,113]. Extended right hemihepatectomy consists of resection of the right liver, the inferior part of segment IV, and the caudate lobe. Extended left hemihepatectomy consists of resection of the left liver, the hilar part of the anterior segment, and most of the caudate lobe. Even in patients with Bismuth type I or type II, an extended hemihepatectomy is needed to achieve curative resection according to the mode of tumor extension discussed previously. If the tumor is predominantly on the right side or centrally located, extended right hepatectomy is selected. Extended left hemihepatectomy is indicated for left-side dominant tumor. If the tumor has spread diffusely into the intrapancreatic bile duct, a pancreatoduodenectomy should be performed simultaneously [113].

In selected cases when a cholangiocarcinoma widely invades the hepatic hilum (Bismuth type IV), a right or left trisegmentectomy could be used to completely resect the tumor. The extent of this intervention offers an advantage in obtaining a cancer-free margin in the hepatic ducts. It is clear that the operative risk of a hepatic trisegmentectomy is greater than that of extended hemihepatectomy. Proper patient selection and adequate preoperative treatment are required when radical high-risk operations, such as trisegmentectomy, are preformed for hilar cholangiocarcinoma.

As highlighted in this section, major hepatectomy is the standard surgical procedure for removing hilar cholangiocarcinomas with a curative intent. It is currently also viewed as the standard procedure. Table 37.4 shows the results of several reports of major hepatectomies for cholangiocarcinoma over the last 10 years [114–125].

Liver transplantation for hilar cholangiocarcinoma

The results of liver transplantation for cholangiocarcinoma have been historically discouraging and much inferior to the results of transplantation for other liver

Table 37.4 Results of major hepatectomy for cholangiocarcinoma.

Number of patients	Major hepatectomy	% R0	Biliary drainage	Portal vein embolization	Mortality (%)	5-year survival	Reference
138	109	78	Yes	Yes	9.7	25.8	Nagino et al. 1998 [114]
30	22	83	No	No	6.6	45	Burke et al. 1998 [115]
95	66	61	Yes	TAE	9.0	22	Neuhaus et al. 1999 [116]
93	66	70	No	Partial	12.0	36	Miyazaki et al. [117]
112	32	14	Yes	No	25.0	NA	Gerhards et al. 2000 [118]
80	62	78	Selective	No	11.0	39	Jarnagin et al. 2001 [119]
67	58	64	Yes	Yes	0.0	40	Seyama et al. 2003 [94]
79	69	68	Yes	Yes	1.3	40	Kawasaki et al. 2003 [93]
40	26	95	Yes	Yes	0.0	40	Kondo et al. 2004 [120]
53	52	80	Yes	Yes	9.0	35	Hemming et al. 2005 [121]
82	59	46	Yes	Selective	5.0	20	Baton et al. 2007 [122]
126	126	57	Yes	Yes	7.9	35	Sano et al. 2007 [123]
59	51	69	Yes	Selective	6.8	35	Konstadoulakis et al. 2008 [124]
149	43	77	Selective	Selective	6.9	36	Giuliante et al. 2010 [125]

NA, not available; TAE, transarterial embolization.

conditions. The early experience with liver transplantation for the treatment of cholangiocarcinoma reported a 5-year survival of 0–38%. In the present decade, the addition of neoadjuvant chemoradiation therapy in the treatment of cholangiocarcinoma has significantly improved the outcomes. In 2002, our group at the University of Nebraska reported a 5-year survival of 45% with the use of chemoradiation and liver transplantation [126]. In 2005, the group at the Mayo Clinic published an unprecedented report in the treatment of cholangiocarcinoma. A total of 38 patients underwent rigorous pretransplantation evaluation as well as neoadjuvant chemoradiation. This approach yielded a 5-year survival of 82%, which is not different to the results of liver transplantation for early HCC or other benign conditions. The 5-year recurrence rate reported was 12%. The intention to treat analysis of this group was 58% at 5-years which compares favorably to any other form of treatment for this disease [127].

These remarkable results are a reflection of meticulous pretransplantation evaluation and exclusion criteria. Nearly 50% of patients were excluded from transplantation during evaluation. Diagnosis was based on intraluminal brush cytology/biopsy or a carbohydrate antigen 19.9 (CA 19.9) >100 ng/mL in the setting of a radiographic malignant stricture or biliary aneuploidy demonstrated with digital image analysis (DIA) and fluorescent in situ hybridization (FISH). Staging studies included standard imaging plus endoscopic ultrasound with fine needle aspiration (FNA) of any suspicious lymph nodes. The neoadjuvant chemoradiation protocol was based on combination cycles of external beam radiation therapy (EBRT) and 5-fluorouracil (5-FU) followed by intraluminal iridium brachytherapy followed by infusional 5-FU. At the end of this protocol, an exploratory laparotomy with biopsies was performed on all patients. Of the total number of patients that completed neoadjuvant chemoradiation and reached operative staging, 23% were excluded because of intraoperative findings that precluded transplantation. A detailed algorithm of this protocol can be found in Fig. 37.4. The widespread application of their protocol awaits validation by other centers [127,128].

Resection and transplantation for hilar cholangiocarcinoma

Under the light of the most current results, a comparison between surgical resection and transplantation would be fundamentally inaccurate since the protocol of neoadjuvant therapy followed by transplantation is only applicable to patients with unresectable hilar cholangiocarcinoma. Historically, on average only 50% of patients that are explored with the intent of surgical resection are suitable for a potentially curative resection. The results of several published papers in the surgical treatment of cholangiocarcinoma by means of a major hepatectomy show a 5-year survival ranging from 20% to 45% (see Table 37.4) The Mayo Clinic group reported their results with liver resections as treatment for cholangiocarcinoma. Survival at 3 and 5 years was 53% and 18%, respectively, regardless of the presence of a node-negative R0 resection. The overall cumulative data of surgical resection as treatment of

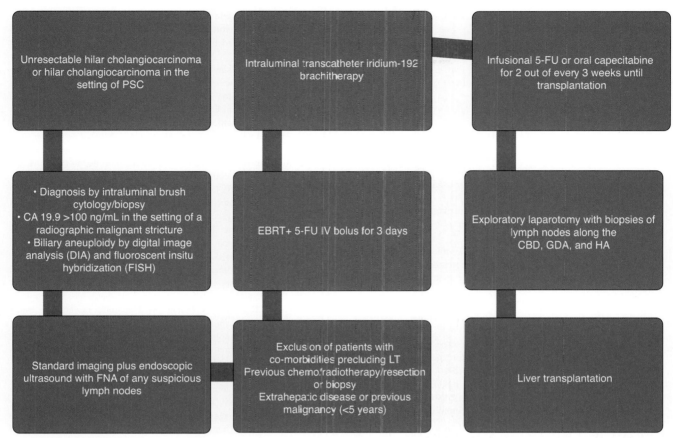

Figure 37.4 Mayo Clinic protocol for pretransplant evaluation and neoadjuvant chemoraciation therapy prior to liver transplantation. CA 19.9, carbohydrate antigen 19.9; CBD, common bile duct; EBRT, external beam radiation therapy; FNA, fine needle aspiration; 5-FU, 5-fluorouracil; GDA, gastroduodenal artery; HA, hepatic artery; LT, liver transplantation; PSC, primary sclerosing cholangitis.

cholangiocarcinoma denote persistent poor results. There are no reports of neoadjuvant therapy prior to resection as treatment for cholangiocarcinoma. Those patients with unresectable hilar cholangiocarcinoma enrolled in a protocol of neoadjuvant therapy followed by transplantation have, to this date, a better chance of survival. LDLT is an emerging viable option for the treatment of this disease. It overcomes the potential waiting list time as well as the limited supply of deceased donated organs. The introduction of neoadjuvant chemoradiation therapy has improved outcomes significantly. A rigorous pretransplant evaluation seems to be the key in order to reproduce comparable outcomes.

Annotated references

Bruix J, Sherman M. Practice Guidelines Committee, American Association for the Study of Liver Diseases. Management of hepatocellular carcinoma. *Hepatology* 2005;42(5):1208–36.
A summary of an important consensus regarding the treatment of HCC.

Durand F, Belghiti J, Paradis V. Liver transplantation for hepatocellular carcinoma: role of biopsy. *Liver Transpl* 2007;13(11 Suppl 2): S17–23.
A detailed review of the role of percutaneous biopsy in the diagnosis and treatment of HCC.

Gondolesi G, Munoz L, Matsumoto C, et al. Hepatocellular carcinoma: a prime indication for living donor liver transplantation. *J Gastrointest Surg* 2002;6(1):102–7.
Compelling data supporting the use of living donors for patients with HCC.

Iwatsuki S, Dvorchik I, Marsh JW, et al. Liver transplantation for hepatocellular carcinoma: a proposal of a prognostic scoring system. *J Am Coll Surg* 2000;191(4):389–94.
An accurate prognostic system of disease-free survival for HCC after transplantation.

Kawasaki S, Imamura H, Kobayashi A, Noike T, Miwa S, Miyagawa S. Results of surgical resection for patients with hilar bile duct cancer: application of extended hepatectomy after biliary drainage and hemihepatic portal vein embolization. *Ann Surg* 2003;238:84–92.
A report illustrating the safety, indications, and outcomes of biliary drainage and portal vein embolization prior to major hepatectomies in the treatment of cholangiocarcinoma.

Majno PE, Adam R, Bismuth H, et al. Influence of preoperative transarterial lipiodol chemoembolization on resection and transplantation for hepatocellular carcinoma in patients with cirrhosis. *Ann Surg* 1997;226:688–703.
Often-cited paper demonstrating the influence of preoperative TACE on resection and transplantation for HCC patients with cirrhosis.

Mazzaferro V, Regalia E, Doci R, et al. Liver transplantation for the treatment of small hepatocellular carcinomas in patients with cirrhosis. *N Engl J Med* 1996;334:693–9.
Landmark paper in the treatment of HCC by liver transplantation (using the Milan criteria).

Rea DJ, Heimbach JK, Rosen CB, et al. Liver transplantation with neoadjuvant chemoradiation is more effective than resection for hilar cholangiocarcinoma. *Ann Surg* 2005;242:451–61.

A rigorous evaluation and pretransplant chemoradiation protocol in the treatment of cholangiocarcinoma reporting the best long-term outcomes.

Seyama Y, Makuuchi M. Current surgical treatment for bile duct cancer. *World J Gastroenterol* 2007;13(10):1505–15.

A detailed review of the surgical management of bile duct cancer.

References

1. Centers for Disease Control and Prevention (CDC). Hepatocellular carcinoma – United States, 2001–2006. *MMWR* 2010;59(17):517–20.

2. Blum HE, Spangenberg HC. Hepatocellular carcinoma: an update. *Arch Iran Med* 2007;10(3):361–71.

3. Durand F, Belghiti J, Paradis V. Liver transplantation for hepatocellular carcinoma: role of biopsy. *Liver Transpl* 2007;13(11 Suppl 2):S17–23.

4. Caturelli E, Bisceglia M, Fusilli S, et al. Cytology versus micro-histological diagnosis of hepatocellular carcinoma. Comparative accuracies in the same fine-needle biopsy specimen. *Dig Dis Sci* 1996;41:2326–31.

5. Huang GT, Sheu JC, Yang PM, et al. Ultrasound-guided cutting biopsy for the diagnosis of hepatocellular carcinoma-a study based on 420 patients. *J Hepatol* 1996;25:334–8.

6. Durand F, Regimbeau JM, Belghiti J, et al. Assessment of the benefits and risks of percutaneous biopsy before surgical resection of hepatocellular carcinoma. *J Hepatol* 2001;35:254–8.

7. Chang S, Kim SH, Lim HK, et al. Needle tract implantation after percutaneous interventional procedures in hepatocellular carcinomas: lessons learned from a 10-year experience. *Korean J Radiol* 2008;9(3):268–74.

8. Silva MA, Hegab B, Hyde C, et al. Needle track seeding following biopsy of liver lesions in the diagnosis of hepatocellular cancer: a systematic review and meta-analysis. *Gut* 2008;57(11):1592–6.

9. Eagle KA, Boucher CA. Cardiac risk of noncardiac surgery. *N Engl J Med* 1989;321(19):1330–2.

10. Llovet JM, Fuster J, Bruix J. Intention-to-treat analysis of surgical treatment for early hepatocellular carcinoma: resection versus transplantation. *Hepatology* 1999;30:1434–40.

11. Iwatsuki S, Starzl TE, Sheahan DG, et al. Hepatic resection versus transplantation for hepatocellular carcinoma. *Ann Surg* 1991;214:221–9.

12. Ringe B, Pichlmayr R, Wittekind C, et al. Surgical treatment of hepatocellular carcinoma: experience with liver resection and transplantation in 198 patients. *World J Surg* 1991;15:270–85.

13. Franco D, Capussotti L, Smadja C, et al. Resection of hepatocellular carcinomas. Results in 72 European patients with cirrhosis. *Gastroenterology* 1990;98(3):733–8.

14. Bismuth H, Chiche L, Adam R, et al. Liver resection versus transplantation for hepatocellular carcinoma in cirrhotic patients. *Ann Surg* 1993;218(2):145–51.

15. Takenaka K, Kawahara N, Yamamoto K, et al. Results of 280 liver resections for hepatocellular carcinoma. *Arch Surg* 1996;131(1):71–6.

16. Vauthey JN, Klimstra D, Franceschi D, et al. Factors affecting long-term outcome after hepatic resection for hepatocellular carcinoma. *Am J Surg* 1995;169(1):28–34.

17. Majno PE, Adam R, Bismuth H, et al. Influence of preoperative transarterial lipiodol chemoembolization on resection and transplantation for hepatocellular carcinoma in patients with cirrhosis. *Ann Surg* 1997;226:688–703.

18. Gouillat C, Manganas D, Saguier G, et al. Resection of hepatocellular carcinoma in cirrhotic patients: long term results of a prospective study. *J Am Coll Surg* 1999;189(3):282–90.

19. Figueras J, Jaurrieta E, Valls C, et al. Resection or transplantation for hepatocellular carcinoma in cirrhotic patients: outcomes based on indicated treatment strategy. *J Am Coll Surg* 2000;190(5):580–7.

20. Hanazaki K, Kijikawa S, Shimozawa N, et al. Survival and recurrence after hepatic resection of 386 consecutive patients with hepatocellular carcinoma. *J Am Coll Surg* 2000;191(4):381–8.

21. Grazi GL, Ercolani G, Pierangeli F, et al. Improved results of liver resection for hepatocellular carcinoma on cirrhosis give the procedure added value. *Ann Surg* 2001;234(1):71–8.

22. Kanematsu T, Furui J, Yanaga K, et al. A 16-year experience in performing hepatic resection in 303 patients with hepatocellular carcinoma: 1985–2000. *Surgery* 2002;131(1):S153–8.

23. Yeh CN, Chen MF, Lee WC, Jeng LB. Prognostic factors of hepatic resection for hepatocellular carcinoma with cirrhosis: univariate and multivariate analysis. *J Surg Oncol* 2002;81(4):195–202.

24. Neeff H, Makowiec F, Harder J, et al. Hepatic resection for hepatocellular carcinoma – results and analysis of the current literature. *Zentralbl Chir* 2009;134(2):127–35.

25. Morris-Stiff G, Gomez D, de Liguori Carino N, Prasad KR. Surgical management of hepatocellular carcinoma: is the jury still out? *Surg Oncol* 2009;18(4):298–321.

26. Broelsch CE, Frilling A, Malago M. Hepatoma resection or transplantation. *Surg Clin North Am* 2004;84(2):495–511.

27. Ohkubo T, Yamamoto J, Sugawara Y, et al. Surgical results for hepatocellular carcinoma with macroscopic portal vein tumor thrombosis. *J Am Coll Surg* 2000;191(6):657–60.

28. Midorikawa Y, Kubota K, Takayama T, et al. A comparative study of postoperative complications after hepatectomy in patients with and without chronic liver disease. *Surgery* 1999;126(3):484–91.

29. Schwartz M, Roayaie S, Konstadoulakis M. Strategies for the management of hepatocellular carcinoma. *Nat Clin Pract Oncol* 2007;4(7):424–32.

30. Bruix J, Sherman M, Llovet JM, et al. EASL Panel of Experts on HCC. Clinical management of hepatocellular carcinoma. Conclusions of the Barcelona-2000 EASL conference. European Association for the Study of the Liver. *J Hepatol* 2001;35(3):421–30.

31. Ramacciato G, Mercantini P, Cautero N, et al. Prognostic evaluation of the new American Joint Committee on Cancer/International Union Against Cancer staging system for hepatocellular carcinoma: analysis of 112 cirrhotic patients resected for hepatocellular carcinoma. *Ann Surg Oncol* 2005;12:289–97.

32. Varotti G, Ramacciato G, Ercolani G, et al. Comparison between the fifth and sixth editions of the AJCC/UICC TNM staging systems for hepatocellular carcinoma: multicentric study on 393 cirrhotic resected patients. *Eur J Surg Oncol* 2005;31:760–7.

33. Saito H, Masuda T, Tada S, et al. Hepatocellular carcinoma in Keio affiliated hospitals – diagnosis, treatment, and prognosis of this disease. *Keio J Med* 2009;58(3):161–75.

34. Iwatsuki S, Dvorchik I, Marsh JW, et al. Liver transplantation for hepatocellular carcinoma: a proposal of a prognostic scoring system. *J Am Coll Surg* 2000;191(4):389–94.

35. Okuda K, Ohtsuki T, Obata H, et al. Natural history of hepatocellular carcinoma and prognosis in relation to treatment. Study of 850 patients. *Cancer* 1985;56:918–28.

36. Cancer of the Liver Italian Program (CLIP) Investigators. A new prognostic system for hepatocellular carcinoma: a retrospective study of 435 patients. *Hepatology* 1998;28:751–5.

37. Bruix J, Sherman M, Llovet JM, et al. Clinical management of hepatocellular carcinoma. Conclusions of the Barcelona-2000 EASL conference. European Association for the Study of the Liver. *J Hepatol* 2001;35:421–30.

38. Chevret S, Trinchet JC, Mathieu D, et al. A new prognostic classification for predicting survival in patients with hepatocellular

carcinoma. Groupe d'Etude et de Traitement du Carcinome Hepatocellulaire. *J Hepatol* 1999;31:133–41.

39. Liver Cancer Study Group of Japan. Predictive factors for long term prognosis after partial hepatectomy for patients with hepatocellular carcinoma in Japan. *Cancer* 1994;74(10):2772–80.

40. Kudo M, Chung H, Haji S, et al. Validation of a new prognostic staging system for hepatocellular carcinoma: the JIS score compared with the CLIP score. *Hepatology* 2004;40:1396–405.

41. Rapaccini GL, Gasbarrini G. Prognostic factors for survival in patients with early-intermediate hepatocellular carcinoma undergoing non-surgical therapy: comparison of Okuda, CLIP, and BCLC staging systems in a single Italian centre. *Gut* 2005;54:411–18.

42. Marrero JA, Fontana RJ, Barrat A, et al. Prognosis of hepatocellular carcinoma: comparison of 7 staging systems in an American cohort. *Hepatology* 2005;41:707–16.

43. Sala M, Forner A, Varela M, Bruix J. Prognostic prediction in patients with hepatocellular carcinoma. *Semin Liver Dis* 2005;25(2): 171–80.

44. Giannini E, Risso D, Botta F, et al. Prognosis of hepatocellular carcinoma in anti-HCV positive cirrhotic patients: a single-center comparison amongst four different staging systems. *J Intern Med* 2004;255:399–408.

45. Nanashima A, Sumida Y, Abo T, et al. Modified Japan Integrated Staging is currently the best available staging system for hepatocellular carcinoma patients who have undergone hepatectomy. *J Gastroenterol* 2006;41(3):250–6.

46. Yamasaki S, Hasegawa H, Kinoshita H, et al. A prospective randomized trial of the preventive effect of pre-operative transcatheter arterial embolization against recurrence of hepatocellular carcinoma. *Jpn J Cancer Res* 1996;87:206–11.

47. Tanaka H, Hirohashi K, Kubo S, et al. Preoperative portal vein embolization improves prognosis after right hepatectomy for hepatocellular carcinoma in patients with impaired hepatic function. *Br J Surg* 2000;87:879–82.

48. Farges O, Belghiti J, Kianmanesh R, et al. Portal vein embolization before right hepatectomy: prospective clinical trial. *Ann Surg* 2003;237:208–17.

49. Iwatsuki S, Gordon RD, Shaw BW Jr, et al. Role of liver transplantation in cancer therapy. *Ann Surg* 1985;202:401–7.

50. Ringe B, Wittekind C, Bechstein WO, et al. The role of liver transplantation in the treatment of liver cancer. *Cancer Chemother Pharmacol* 1989;23:S104–9.

51. Penn I. Hepatic transplantation for primary and metastatic cancers of the liver. *Surgery* 1991;110:726–35.

52. Mazzaferro V, Regalia E, Doci R, et al. Liver transplantation for the treatment of small hepatocellular carcinomas in patients with cirrhosis. *N Engl J Med* 1996;334:693–9.

53. Jonas S, Bechstein WO, Steinmuller T, et al. Vascular invasion and histopathologic grading determine outcome after liver transplantation for hepatocellular carcinoma in cirrhosis. *Hepatology* 2001;5:1080–6.

54. Befeler AS, Hyashi PH, Bisceglie AM. Liver transplantation for hepatocellular carinoma. *Gastroenterology* 2005;128:1752–64.

55. Bruix J, Fuster J, Llovet JM. Liver transplantation for hepatocellular carcinoma: Foucault pendulum versus evidence-based decision. *Liver Transpl* 2003;7:700–2.

56. Llovet JM, Bruix J, Fuster J, et al. Liver transplantation for small hepatocellular carcinoma: the tumor–node–metastasis classification does not have prognostic power. *Hepatology* 1998;27:1572–7.

57. Yao FY, Ferrell L, Bass NM, et al. Liver transplantation for hepatocellular carcinoma: expansion of the tumor size limits does not adversely impact survival. *Hepatology* 2001;33:1394–403.

58. Decaens T, Roudot-Thoraval F, Hadni-Bresson S, et al. Impact of UCSF criteria according to pre- and post-OLT tumor features: analysis of 479 patients listed for HCC with a short waiting time. *Liver Transpl* 2006;12:1761–9.

59. Leung JY, Zhu AX, Gordon FD, et al. Liver transplantation outcomes for early-stage hepatocellular carcinoma: results of a multi-center study. *Liver Transpl* 2004;11:1343–54.

60. Onaca N, Davis GL, Goldstein RM, et al. Expanded criteria for liver transplantation in patients with hepatocellular carcinoma: a report from the International Registry of Hepatic Tumors in Liver Transplantation. *Liver Transpl* 2007;13:391–9.

61. Sotiropoulos GC, Molmenti EP, Omar OS, et al. Liver transplantation for hepatocellular carcinoma in patients beyond the Milan but within the UCSF criteria. *Eur J Med Res* 2006;11:467–70.

62. Duffy JP, Vardanian A, Benjamin E, et al. Liver transplantation criteria for hepatocellular carcinoma should be expanded: a 22-year experience with 467 patients at UCLA. *Ann Surg* 2007;246(3):502–9.

63. Mazzaferro V, Llovet JM, Miceli R, et al. Predicting survival after liver transplantation in patients with hepatocellular carcinoma beyond the Milan criteria: a retrospective, exploratory analysis. *Lancet Oncol* 2009:10:35–43.

64. Adam R, Azoulay D, Castaing D, et al. Liver resection as a bridge to transplantation for hepatocellular carcinoma on cirrhosis: a reasonable strategy? *Ann Surg* 2004;238(4):508–18.

65. Del Gaudio M, Ercolani G, Ravaioli M, et al. Liver transplantation for recurrent hepatocellular carcinoma on cirrhosis after liver resection: University of Bologna experience. *Am J Transplant* 2008;8(6):1177–85

66. Botha JF, Campos BD. Salvage transplantation: does saving livers save lives? *Am J Transplant* 2008;8(6):1085–6.

67. Cheng SJ, Pratt DS, Freeman RB, et al. Living-donor versus cadaveric liver transplantation for unresectable small hepatocellular carcinoma and compensated cirrhosis: a decision analysis. *Transplantation* 2001;72(5):861–8.

68. Gondolesi G, Munoz L, Matsumoto C, et al. Hepatocellular carcinoma: a prime indication for living donor liver transplantation. *J Gastrointest Surg* 2002;6(1):102–7.

69. Lo CM, Fan ST, Liu CL, Chan SC, Wong J. The role and limitation of living donor liver transplantation for hepatocellular carcinoma. *Liver Transpl* 2004;10:440–7.

70. Hwang S, Lee SG, Joh JW, Suh KS, Kim DG. Liver transplantation for adult patients with hepatocellular carcinoma in Korea: comparison between cadaveric donor and living donor liver transplantations. *Liver Transpl* 2005;11:1265–72.

71. Thuluvath PJ, Yoo HY. Graft and patient survival after adult live donor liver transplantation compared to a matched cohort who received a deceased donor transplantation. *Liver Transpl* 2004;10:1263–8.

72. Fisher RA, Kulik LM, Freise CE, et al. Hepatocellular carcinoma recurrence and death following living and deceased donor liver transplantation. *Am J Transplant* 2007;7:1601–8.

73. Lo CM, Fan ST, Liu CL, et al. Living donor versus deceased donor liver transplantation for early irresectable hepatocellular carcinoma. *Br J Surg* 2007;94:78–86.

74. Umeshita K, Fujiwara K, Kiyosawa K et al. Operative morbidity of living liver donors in Japan. *Lancet* 2003;362:687–90.

75. Botha JF, Langnas AN, Campos BD, et al. Left lobe adult-to-adult living donor liver transplantation: small grafts and hemiportocaval shunts in the prevention of small-for-size syndrome. *Liver Transpl* 2010;16(5):649–57.

76. Ogura Y, Hori T, El Moghazy WM, et al. Portal pressure <15 mm Hg is a key for successful adult living donor liver transplantation utilizing smaller grafts than before. *Liver Transpl* 2010;16(6):718–28.

77. Kar S, Carr BI. Detection of liver cells in peripheral blood of patients with advanced stage hepatocellular carcinoma. *Hepatology* 1995;21:403–7.

78. Majno PE, Adam R, Bismuth H, et al. Influence of preoperative transarterial lipiodol chemoembolization on resection and transplantation for hepatocellular carcinoma in patients with cirrhosis. *Ann Surg* 1997;226:688–701.

79. Graziadei IW, Sandmueller H, Waldenberger P, et al. Chemoembolization followed by liver transplantation for hepatocellular carcinoma impedes tumor progression while on the waiting list and leads to excellent outcome. *Liver Transpl* 2003;9:557–63.

80. Mazzaferro V, Battiston C, Perrone S, et al. Radiofrequency ablation of small hepatocellular carcinoma in cirrhotic patients awaiting liver transplantation: a prospective study. *Ann Surg* 2004;240:900–9.

81. Lesurtel M, Müllhaupt B, Pestalozzi BC, Pfammatter T, Clavien PA. Transarterial chemoembolization as a bridge to liver transplantation for hepatocellular carcinoma: an evidence-based analysis. *Am J Transplant* 2006;6(11):2644–50.

82. Freeman RB Jr, Steffick DE, Guidinger MK, Farmer DJ, Berg CL, Merion RM. Liver and intestine transplantation in the United States, 1997–2006. *Am J Transplant* 2008;8(4 Pt 2):958–76.

83. Saborido BP, Meneu JC, Moreno E, et al. Is transarterial chemoembolization necessary before liver transplantation for hepatocellular carinoma? *Am J Surg* 2005;190:383–7.

84. Decaens T, Roudot-Thoraval F, Bresson-Hadni S, et al. Impact of pretransplantation transarterial chemoembolization on survival and recurrence after liver transplantation for hepatocellular carcinoma. *Liver Transpl* 2005;11(7):767–75.

85. Freeman RB Jr. Transplantation for hepatocellular carcinoma: the Milan criteria and beyond. *Liver Transpl* 2006;12(11 Suppl 2): S8–13.

86. Yao FY, Kerlan RK Jr, Hirose R, et al. Excellent outcome following down-staging of hepatocellular carcinoma prior to liver transplantation: an intention-to-treat analysis. *Hepatology* 2008;48(3):819–27.

87. Otto G, Herber S, Heise M, et al. Response to transarterial chemoembolization as a biological selection criterion for liver transplantation in hepatocellular carcinoma. *Liver Transpl* 2006;12:1260–7.

88. Bismuth H, Corlette MB. Intrahepatic cholangioenteric anastomosis in carcinoma of the hilus of the liver. *Surg Gynecol Obstet* 1975;140:170–8.

89. Bismuth H, Nakache R, Diamond T. Management strategies in resection for hilar cholangiocarcinoma. *Ann Surg* 1992;215:31–8.

90. Makuuchi M, Thai BL, Takayasu K, et al. Preoperative portal embolization to increase safety of major hepatectomy for hilar bile duct carcinoma: a preliminary report. *Surgery* 1990;107:521–7.

91. Kubota K, Makuuchi M, Kusaka K, et al. Measurement of liver volume and hepatic functional reserve as a guide to decision-making in resectional surgery for hepatic tumors. *Hepatology* 1997;26:1176–81.

92. Miyagawa S, Makuuchi M, Kawasaki S. Outcome of extended right hepatectomy after biliary drainage in hilar bile duct cancer. *Arch Surg* 1995;130:759–63.

93. Kawasaki S, Imamura H, Kobayashi A, et al. Results of surgical resection for patients with hilar bile duct cancer: application of extended hepatectomy after biliary drainage and hemihepatic portal vein embolization. *Ann Surg* 2003;238:84–92.

94. Seyama Y, Kubota K, Sano K, et al. Long-term outcome of extended hemihepatectomy for hilar bile duct cancer with no mortality and high survival rate. *Ann Surg* 2003;238:73–83.

95. Takayama T, Makuuchi M. Preoperative portal vein embolization: is it useful? *J Hepatobiliary Pancreat Surg* 2004;11:17–20.

96. Povoski SP, Karpeh MS Jr, Conlon KC, Blumgart LH, Brennan MF. Association of preoperative biliary drainage with postoperative outcome following pancreaticoduodenectomy. *Ann Surg* 1999;230:131–42.

97. Cherqui D, Benoist S, Malassagne B, Humeres R, Rodriguez V, Fagniez PL. Major liver resection for carcinoma in jaundiced patients without preoperative biliary drainage. *Arch Surg* 2000;135:302–8.

98. Mansfield SD, Barakat O, Charnley RM, et al. Management of hilar cholangiocarcinoma in the north of England: pathology, treatment, and outcome. *World J Gastroenterol* 2005;11:7625–30.

99. Sewnath ME, Karsten TM, Prins MH, Rauws EJ, Obertop H, Gouma DJ. A meta-analysis on the efficacy of preoperative biliary drainage for tumors causing obstructive jaundice. *Ann Surg* 2002;236:17–27.

100. Noie T, Sugawara Y, Imamura H, Takayama T, Makuuchi M. Selective versus total drainage for biliary obstruction in the hepatic hilus: an experimental study. *Surgery* 2001;130:74–81.

101. Neuhaus P, Jonas S, Bechstein WO, et al. Extended resections for hilar cholangiocarcinoma. *Ann Surg* 1999;230:808–18.

102. Liu CL, Lo CM, Lai EC, Fan ST. Endoscopic retrograde cholangiopancreatography and endoscopic endoprosthesis insertion in patients with Klatskin tumors. *Arch Surg* 1998;133:293–6.

103. Rerknimitr R, Kladcharoen N, Mahachai V, Kullavanijaya P. Result of endoscopic biliary drainage in hilar cholangiocarcinoma. *J Clin Gastroenterol* 2004;38:518–23.

104. Jagannath P, Dhir V, Shrikhande S, Shah RC, Mullerpatan P, Mohandas KM. Effect of preoperative biliary stenting on immediate outcome after pancreaticoduodenectomy. *Br J Surg* 2005;92: 356–61.

105. Sakata J, Shirai Y, Wakai T, Nomura T, Sakata E, Hatakeyama K. Catheter tract implantation metastases associated with percutaneous biliary drainage for extrahepatic cholangiocarcinoma. *World J Gastroenterol* 2005;11:7024–7.

106. Seiler CA, Wagner M, Sadowski C, Kulli C, Buchler MW. Randomized prospective trial of pylorus-preserving vs. classic duodenopancreatectomy (Whipple procedure): initial clinical results. *J Gastrointest Surg* 2000;4:443–52.

107. Tran KT, Smeenk HG, van Eijck CH, et al. Pylorus preserving pancreaticoduodenectomy versus standard Whipple procedure: a prospective, randomized, multicenter analysis of 170 patients with pancreatic and periampullary tumors. *Ann Surg* 2004;240:738–45.

108. Yeo CJ, Sohn TA, Cameron JL, Hruban RH, Lillemoe KD, Pitt HA. Periampullary adenocarcinoma: analysis of 5-year survivors. *Ann Surg* 1998;227:821–31.

109. Todoroki T, Kawamoto T, Koike N, Fukao K, Shoda J, Takahashi H. Treatment strategy for patients with middle and lower third bile duct cancer. *Br J Surg* 2001;88:364–70.

110. Yoshida T, Matsumoto T, Sasaki A, Morii Y, Aramaki M, Kitano S. Prognostic factors after pancreatoduodenectomy with extended lymphadenectomy for distal bile duct cancer. *Arch Surg* 2002;137:69–73.

111. Sugiura Y, Nakamura S, Iida S, et al. Extensive resection of the bile ducts combined with liver resection for cancer of the main hepatic duct junction: a cooperative study of the Keio Bile Duct Cancer Study Group. *Surgery* 1994;115:445–51.

112. Kosuge T, Yamamoto J, Shimada K, Yamasaki S, Makuuchi M. Improved surgical results for hilar cholangiocarcinoma with procedures including major hepatic resection. *Ann Surg* 1999;230:663–71.

113. Miyagawa S, Makuuchi M, Kawasaki S, et al. Outcome of major hepatectomy with pancreatoduodenectomy for advanced biliary malignancies. *World J Surg* 1996;20:77–80.

114. Nagino M, Nimura Y, Kamiya J, et al. Segmental liver resections for hilar cholangiocarcinoma. *Hepatogastroenterology* 1998;45:7–13.

115. Burke EC, Jarnagin WR, Hochwald SN, Pisters PW, Fong Y, Blumgart LH. Hilar cholangiocarcinoma: patterns of spread, the importance of hepatic resection for curative operation, and a presurgical clinical staging system. *Ann Surg* 1998;228:385–94.

116. Neuhaus P, Jonas S, Bechstein WO, et al. Extended resections for hilar cholangiocarcinoma. *Ann Surg* 1999;230:808–18.

117. Miyazaki M, Ito H, Nakagawa K, et al. Parenchyma-preserving hepatectomy in the surgical treatment of hilar cholangiocarcinoma. *J Am Coll Surg* 1999;189:575–83.

118. Gerhards MF, van Gulik TM, de Wit LT, Obertop H, Gouma DJ. Evaluation of morbidity and mortality after resection for hilar cholangiocarcinoma – a single center experience. *Surgery* 2000;127: 395–404.

119. Jarnagin WR, Fong Y, DeMatteo RP, et al. Staging, resectability, and outcome in 225 patients with hilar cholangiocarcinoma. *Ann Surg* 2001;234:507–17.

120. Kondo S, Hirano S, Ambo Y, et al. Forty consecutive resections of hilar cholangiocarcinoma with no postoperative mortality and no positive ductal margins: results of a prospective study. *Ann Surg* 2004;240:95–101.

121. Hemming AW, Reed AI, Fujita S, Foley DP, Howard RJ. Surgical management of hilar cholangiocarcinoma. *Ann Surg* 2005;241:693–9.

122. Baton O, Azoulay D, Adam DV, Castaing DJ. Major hepatectomy for hilar cholangiocarcinoma type 3 and 4: prognostic factors and longterm outcomes. *Am Coll Surg* 2007;204(2):250–60.

123. Sano T, Shimada K, Sakamoto Y, Esaki M, Kosuge T. Changing trends in surgical outcomes after major hepatobiliary resection for hilar cholangiocarcinoma: a single-center experience over 25 years. *J Hepatobiliary Pancreat Surg* 2007;14(5):455–62.

124. Konstadoulakis MM, Roayaie S, Gomatos IP, et al. Aggressive surgical resection for hilar cholangiocarcinoma: is it justified? Audit of a single center's experience. *Am J Surg* 2008;196(2):160–9.

125. Giuliante F, Ardito F, Vellone M, Nuzzo G. Liver resections for hilar cholangiocarcinoma. *Eur Rev Med Pharmacol Sci* 2010;14(4): 368–70.

126. Sudan D, DeRoover A, Chinnakotla S, et al. Radiochemotherapy and transplantation allow long-term survival for nonresectable hilar cholangiocarcinoma. *Am J Transplant* 2002;2:774–9.

127. Rea DJ, Heimbach JK, Rosen CB, et al. Liver transplantation with neoadjuvant chemoradiation is more effective than resection for hilar cholangiocarcinoma. *Ann Surg* 2005;242:451–61.

128. De Vreede I, Steers JL, Burch PA, et al. Prolonged disease-free survival after orthotopic liver transplantation plus adjuvant chemoirradiation for cholangiocarcinoma. *Liver Transpl* 2000;6: 309–16.

Infectious and Granulomatous Disease

CHAPTER 38

Amoebic and Pyogenic Liver Abscesses

Marco A. Olivera-Martínez[1] & David Kershenobich[2]

[1]Department of Internal Medicine, Section of Gastroenterology and Hepatology, University of Nebraska Medical Center, Omaha, NE, USA
[2]Experimental Research Unit, Universidad Nacional Autónoma de México, Hospital General de México, Mexico City, Mexico

Key concepts

- A liver abscess is a space-occupying suppurative lesion in the liver resulting from the invasion and proliferation of microorganisms, entering directly from an injury, through blood vessels, or by way of the bile ducts.
- The most common forms of liver abscesses are amoebic, pyogenic, or mixed in etiology.
- The invasive process of *Entamoeba histolytica* in the liver is driven by the motility of the parasite. The parasite relies on a dynamic actomyosin cytoskeleton and on surface adhesion molecules for dissemination in the tissue.

- Emerging new risk factors for amoebic liver abscess include the use of immunosuppressive drugs, sexual lifestyles, human immunodeficiency virus infection, traveling to endemic areas, and population migration.
- Risk factors for pyogenic liver abscess include aggressive treatment of liver and pancreas malignancies, intraluminal stent placement, sphincterotomy, tumor embolization, ethanol injection, or radiofrequency ablation.
- Distinguishing between amoebic or pyogenic liver abscess is crucial since the treatment and prognosis are different. Differential diagnosis relies on clinical history and laboratory and imaging findings.

A liver abscess is a space-occupying suppurative lesion in the liver resulting from the invasion of microorganisms entering directly from an injury, through the blood vessels, or through the bile ducts. The most common forms of liver abscesses are amoebic, pyogenic, or mixed in etiology. Approximately 60% are solitary and they are mainly located in the right lobe as a result of the streaming pattern of portal blood flow, secondary to the fact that the right lobe is supplied predominantly by the superior mesenteric vein and because most of the hepatic volume is in the right lobe. When multiple abscesses are present, pyogenic or mixed etiologies are the most likely. A detailed clinical history is useful in identifying risk factors that may suggest a possible etiology. Emerging new risk factors include the use of immunosuppressive drugs for neoplastic diseases or for organ transplantation, sexual lifestyles, human immunodeficiency virus (HIV) infection, history of traveling to endemic areas, and the population migration phenomena [1].

Amoebic liver abscess

Epidemiology

Entamoeba histolytica infection is the principal cause of liver abscess throughout the world, especially in tropical and subtropical regions. It is the most common form of extraintestinal invasive amoebiasis and its prevalence is higher in developing countries. It can be spread from person to person when polluted water is used to freshen vegetables and fruits sold by street vendors. The greatest risk is associated with cyst passers, especially if they are food handlers.

Landmark advances in the epidemiology of amoebiasis include the recognition that there are two distinct species: *E. histolytica*, which is the cause of dysentery, colitis, and liver abscess, and *E. dispar*, which is a nonpathogenic (commensal) form of amoeba [2]. Recent technologic advances exploring the genome of the different strains of *E. histolytica* may ultimately lead to the development of vaccines [3].

Specific probes derived from the analysis of repetitive DNA sequence in the *Entamoeba* genome have demonstrated possible candidates that distinguish between *E. histolytica* and *E. dispar*. For example, transposable elements that harbor non-long terminal repeat (non-LTR) retrotransposons (also called long interspersed repetitive elements or LINEs) [4] or short interspersed repetitive elements known as EhSINE1 [5].

More recently, a proteomic analysis of both species of amoebae showed that *E. dispar* has a lower activity of nicotinamide adenine dinucleotide phosphate

Schiff's Diseases of the Liver, Eleventh Edition. Edited by Eugene R. Schiff, Willis C. Maddrey and Michael F. Sorrell.
© 2012 John Wiley & Sons, Ltd. Published 2012 by John Wiley & Sons, Ltd.

(NADP)-dependent alcohol dehydrogenase (ADH), while *E. histolytica* expresses higher concentrations of ADH2 and ADH3. Other differences among species are amino acid substitutions, splice variants, post-translational modifications, truncations, insertions, and different protein expression as in the case of grainin 2, a calcium-binding protein. The latter (overexpression) is particularly characteristic of *E. dispar*, suggesting that protein expression, specifically granins, might be related to the microorganism's virulence. On the other hand, *E. histolytica* expresses a higher level of proteins containing cysteine- and histidine-rich, zinc-coordinating domains that mediate protein–DNA or protein–protein interactions (Lin11-lsl-1-Mec-3 or LIM domain), which has a role in regulating eukaryotic nucleic acid transcription [6]. Genotyping has revealed an extensive genetic diversity among *E. histolytica* isolates, preventing an association of a single genotype with hepatic disease [7]. The HM-1:IMSS strain of *E. histolytica*, isolated in Mexico 30 years ago, and those isolated in India and Bangladesh, cause disease in experimental animals and humans and have been used for nearly all immunologic, biochemical, and molecular biologic studies of amoebae [8].

Pathogenesis

The invasive process is driven importantly by the parasite's motility. The parasite relies on a dynamic acto-myosin cytoskeleton and on surface adhesion molecules for dissemination in the tissues. Myosin II is essential for *E. histolytica* intercellular motility through intestinal cell monolayers and for its motility in the liver, while surface galactose-binding lectins, mainly galactose acetyl-galactosamine (Gal/GalNAc), modulate the distribution of trophozoites in the liver and their capacity to migrate in the hepatic tissue [9]. Gal/GalNAc acts as a major cell surface antigen activating target epithelial cells and triggering subsequent disease pathology and parasite survival. This lectin favors the synthesis of tumor necrosis factor α (TNF-α), contributing to inflammatory cell recruitment and cytokine synthesis and release.

Gal/GalNAc also inhibits the assembly of C5b-9 in the complement cascade, preventing in this way the formation of membrane attack complexes by the host. These complexes lead to lysis of the trophozoite [10]. Lectin-stimulated cells show an immediate rise in Ca^+, which in turn activates cyclic nucleotides and other protein kinases, leading to activation of the mitogen-activated protein kinases (MAPK) cascade. Activation of MAPK pathway is implicated in events such as apoptosis, proliferation, cytoskeleton rearrangements, and permeability changes [11].

One of the initial steps in tissue invasion is the release of proteases by trophozoites, which are capable of degrading extracellular matrix components. *E. histolytica* is a cytotoxic effector cell with an extraordinary capacity to lyse surrounding cells. The inflammatory response (mainly neutrophils and macrophages) initiated by amoebic invasion may further contribute to tissue damage by added lysis of parenchymal cells [12]. When amoebae are inoculated in the liver, significant areas of apoptosis develop within the amoebic liver abscess [13]. A major role in this regard is played by the protozoan phosphoglycans contained in the parasite's glycocalix since they can build a physical barrier that protects the cells from membrane attack complexes after tissue invasion [10].

Virulence

There is evidence that the virulence of this parasite depends on the overexpression of several genes in some strains of *E. histolytica*. Among these are the genes that induce a thiol-specific antioxidant known as peroxiredoxin, which has both peroxidase and antioxidant activities. Peroxiredoxin seems to increase virulence by conferring the amoeba protection against reactive oxygen species (ROS) [14]. The tissue invasion capability of *E. histolytica* resides mainly in the amoebapores – intravesicular proteins with pore-forming activity essential for the bacterial phagocytic activity of the amoeba [15].

The sequencing of the genome of *E. histolytica* has allowed a reconstruction of its metabolic pathways. It appears that some amino acids may play roles in both adenosine triphosphate (ATP) synthesis and nicotinamide adenine dinucleotide (NAD) regeneration [16]. *E. histolytica* uses a complex mix of signal transduction systems in order to sense and interact with different environments and encounters. The analysis of its genome has reveled almost 270 putative protein kinases [17].

Clinical manifestations

Amoebic liver abscess is found more frequently in men aged between 20 and 40 years, but can occur at any age. Gender differences in abscess formation in adults have been related to alcohol consumption. Other risk factors have also been identified, including a history of prior travel or residency in endemic areas.

Patients almost always present with a constant, dull, and intense right upper quadrant abdominal pain that exacerbates with movement and frequently radiates to the scapular region and right shoulder. Patients usually have a fever between 38 and 40°C, chills, and sweating. Very frequently they will give a history of malaise and nausea in the previous 2 weeks and moderate weight loss. Some patients have cough and chest pain. Most of them do not have coexistent dysentery, although a past history of diarrhea or dysentery is present in approximately 50% of cases. On physical examination the patient appears pale and wasted, with painful hepatomegaly, and

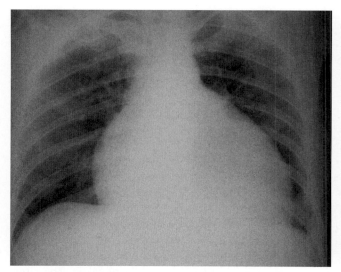

Figure 38.1 Amoebic liver abscess ruptured into the pericardium.

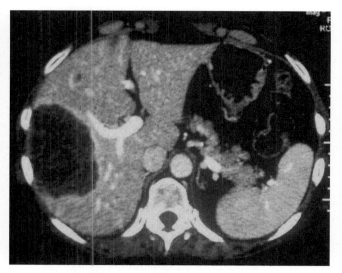

Figure 38.2 Liver metastases of colorectal cancer. No specific characteristics differentiate it from primary neoplasia, or pyogenic or amoebic liver abscess.

point tenderness over the liver, below the ribs, or in the intercostal spaces. When the abscess is located in the left lobe, the patient may have epigastric tenderness. Ventilation in the right lung is frequently restricted and respiratory sounds are reduced. Jaundice is infrequent. The pathophysiology of jaundice is not fully understood and multiple factors are involved; increased pressure within the biliary system posed by an expanding abscess [18] and, more recently, the presence of biliary vascular fistulas have been suggested as contributing factors [19].

Alarm signs include abdominal rebound tenderness, guarding, absence of bowel sounds, and pleural or pericardial rub. The abscess may extend to the peritoneum, abdominal organs, great vessels, pericardium (Fig. 38 1), pleura, bronchial tree, and lungs [20,21]. Common differential diagnoses include pyogenic liver abscess, primary hepatic carcinoma, liver metastases (Fig. 38.2), or hydatid cysts. The clinical presentation of amoebic liver abscess (ALA) among high-risk groups such as HIV patients or other immunosuppressed individuals is similar to that described for other patients [22].

Diagnosis

Leukocytosis ($>15 \times 10^9$ cells/L) with neutrophilia, an increased erythrocyte sedimentation rate, slight anemia, and elevated alkaline phosphatase are common (Table 38.1). Serum antibodies to *E. histolytica* are detected in >90% of patients. An indirect hemagglutination (IHA) test with a cutoff value of 1:512 is considered diagnostic. The enzyme immunoassay (EIA) test, with a sensitivity of 99% and specificity greater than 90%, is also commonly used. In those patients in whom an aspirate is obtained, either for diagnostic or therapeutic purposes, the material should also be sent for Gram staining and culture [23].

Imaging studies are very important in the workup of patients with suspected ALA and have reduced the delay in diagnosis. Ultrasound is the initial screening choice. The abscess appears as a hypoechoic, round or oval lesion with well-defined margins. More advanced imaging techniques such as computed tomography (CT) or magnetic resonance imaging (MRI) are indicated for differential diagnosis. Chest X-ray may reveal elevation of the right diaphragm, atelectasis, and pleural effusion [24].

Therapy

The drug of choice is metronidazole at an oral dose of 1 g twice daily for 10–15 days in adults and 30–50 mg/kg

Table 38.1 Diagnostic differences between amoebic and pyogenic liver abscesses.

Amoebic liver abscess	Pyogenic liver abscess
Leukocytosis $>15 \times 10^9$	Leukocytosis $>15 \times 10^9$
Serum antibodies to *Entamoeba histolytica* >1:512	Serum antibodies to *E. histolytica* negative
Aspirated pus shows no microorganisms	Aspirated pus shows bacteria
Jaundice uncommon (<8% of patients)	Jaundice common in presentation
Abnormal chest findings in physical examination uncommon	Abnormal chest findings in physical examination common
Younger patients (usually 20–40 years)	Older patients (usually 60–70 years)
Previously healthy	Presence of debilitating disease (cancer)

daily for 10 days divided into three doses for children. When given intravenously the dosage is 500 mg every 6 hours for adults and 7.5 mg/kg every 6 hours for children for 10 days. Other nitroimidazoles include tinidazole or ornidazole at a dose of 2 g PO per day for 10 days. Secondary drugs include chloroquine 1 g PO daily for 2 days, followed by 500 mg/day for 2–3 weeks. In children the dose is 15 mg/kg PO daily for 2–5 days followed by 5 mg/kg daily for 2 weeks. Percutaneous drainage is still controversial; a recent Cochrane collaborative review concluded that there is no advantage of adding percutaneous drainage to metronidazole therapy in uncomplicated ALA [25]. However, this approach may be necessary in nonresponders to anti-amoeba therapy to rule out a pyogenic abscess or when less than 1 cm of rim liver tissue remains around a liquefied abscess.

Vaccination

Studies are ongoing in experimental animals using *E. histolytica* galactose and *N*-acetylgalactosamine-inhibitable surface lectin either for systemic application or oral administration. Research has focused on how to fuse surface lectin to the β-subunit of cholera toxin, attenuated *Salmonella*, or *Yersinia enterocolitica* for antigen delivery [26].

Pyogenic liver abscess

Epidemiology

The incidence of pyogenic liver abscess (PLA) is 0.007–2.2% of hospital admissions, 11 per 1 million in the general population, and between 0.29% and 1.47% in autopsy series. A recent population-based study revealed an incidence of 3.6% in the United States between 1994 and 2005, suggesting an increasing incidence of the disease [27]. PLA varies among different geographic regions, influenced by the local prevalence of bacterial, parasitic, and helmintic infections, the age of the population, and the presence of chronic debilitating diseases. Benign or malignant biliary tract disease, diverticulitis, and Crohn disease are the most common predisposing factors. The frequency of PLA has increased as a complication of the more aggressive treatment of liver or pancreatic malignancies: stent placement, sphincterotomy, embolization, ethanol injection, or radiofrequency ablation. In the past PLA was primarily a complication of a ruptured appendix [28]. Accordingly, the age of presentation has moved from the second and third decades of life to the sixth and seventh [28,29]. Advances in imaging techniques and new antibiotics have decreased the morbidity and mortality of PLA [29,30].

Pathogenesis

Abscess formation, a host defense strategy to contain the spread of infection, is promoted by a combination of factors that impair phagocytosis and the clearance of microorganisms. Neutrophils and platelets attached to the endothelial surface, and endotoxins produced by Gram-negative bacteria, contribute to tissue injury by releasing proinflammatory cytokines and ROS. When bacteria reach the liver, endotoxins stimulate the proliferation of Kupffer cells that engorge and produce toxic mediators that modulate the microvascular response. After adhesion, the bacteria diapedese through cell junctions. The inflammation thus produced causes obstruction of the sinusoidal lumen and secondary obstruction of the blood flow. These phenomena inhibit sodium and potassium ATP activity, impair the generation of energy for bile excretion, and promote biliary stasis. The sinusoidal diameter is reduced and hence the velocity of the blood flow decreases; as the number of obstructed sinusoids increases and hydrostatic pressure rises, hepatic ischemia develops [31].

The source of infection determines to a certain degree the localization and number of abscesses. If infection reaches the liver via the portal system, several abscesses may develop, mostly confined to the right lobe. The left lobe is usually involved in septic thrombosis of the portal vein. When bacteria reach the liver via arterial circulation, several small abscesses develop, equally distributed in both lobes. Forty percent of patients with PLA have multiple liver abscesses [32].

Clinical manifestations

An early clinical diagnosis requires a high index of suspicion; fever, malaise, right upper quadrant abdominal pain, nausea, and vomiting for more than 2 weeks are the most common presentations [28]. Abdominal pain in patients with PLA is similar to that found in patients with ALA [32]. Other symptoms such as anorexia, jaundice, and painful hepatomegaly are less prevalent in PLA as compared with ALA [33–35]. Jaundice predicts a complicated clinical course but has no impact on mortality. Approximately 60% have an underlying debilitating condition or have had a recent interventional procedure (e.g., biliary stent placement, ethanol injection). PLA should be suspected in elderly patients, those taking steroids, or in patients with right-sided pulmonary abnormalities of unknown origin [35,36].

Diagnosis

When PLA is diagnosed, prognostic factors associated with increased mortality include low albumin, anemia, high BUN (blood urea nitrogen) and creatinine, prolonged prothrombin time, polymicrobial infection, pleural effusion, high APACHE II (acute physiology and chronic health evaluation II) score, disseminated intravascular coagulation, and septic shock. Multiple abscesses carry a high mortality independently of other risk factors [30]. Regarding PLA in cancer populations, morphology and topography are not different from that found in non-cancer patients [32,36].

Distinguishing characteristics

Distinguishing PLA from ALA is crucial since treatment and prognosis are different (see Table 38.1). The detection of PLA relies on laboratory and imaging findings. Abdominal ultrasound and CT scans have sensitivities >95% in detecting abscess formation [30], although PLA and ALA have similar imaging characteristics (Fig. 38.3) [33]. Patients with PLA are older than those with ALA, and are more likely to have debilitating diseases, which might explain the lower concentration of albumin found in patients with PLA. Abnormal chest findings are more prevalent in patients with PLA [33].

Laboratory and microbiology findings

These data include leukocytosis, anemia, elevated alkaline phosphatase, positive C-reactive protein, and negative *E. histolytica* antibodies. Other findings include increased total bilirubin, low albumin, and prolonged prothrombin time.

Microbiology studies are the gold standard in establishing the diagnosis of PLA. Specimens of pus and blood should be obtained for culture under strict anaerobic and microaerophilic techniques. Gram stain results should guide the selection of the antibiotic regimen pending the result of culture. One third of PLAs are caused by aer-

obic bacteria, one third by anaerobes, and one third by a mixture of both. Enteric Gram-negative rods are the most frequent isolates in either blood or pus aspirated from the abscess. In children *Staphylococcus aureus* is the most frequent organism. Only 50% of anaerobic PLAs are diagnosed by culture because of defective sampling or suboptimal laboratory techniques, but this should not delay the initiation of antibiotics. A combination of antibiotics against different microorganisms is the treatment of choice [28].

Bacteriology of PLA is evolving and in some areas of the world specific bacteria have been isolated. *Klebsiella pneumoniae* has been found in PLA in the Asian population in America suggesting either an epidemiologic transition or the continued prevalence of an endemic infection [29,32,33]. Resistant bacteria and fungi are opportunistic infections in patients with debilitating conditions [36]. The isolation of fungi is frequent in patients with manipulated biliary stents or with intermittent cholangitis treated with broad spectrum antibiotics. Immunocompromised individuals can develop PLA with other microorganisms such as *Salmonella* [35].

Imaging

Ultrasound is the screening test of choice. CT scans can detect collections as small as 0.5 cm in diameter and allow therapeutic interventions (e.g., needle aspiration/drainage). The presence of aggregates of multiple, small abscesses suggests coalescence into a larger abscess (cluster sign) and indicates PLA [28]. MRI using serial gadolinium-enhanced gradient-echo images can help differentiating PLA from other focal lesions [37]. Magnetic resonance cholangiograms can be useful in planning

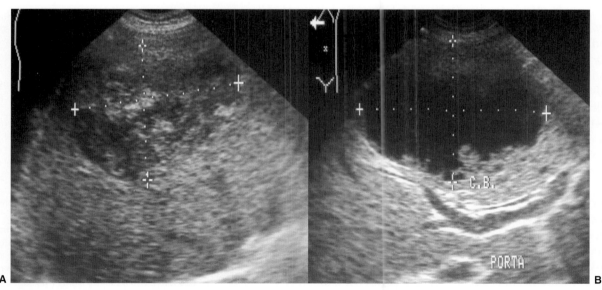

Figure 38.3 Pyogenic liver abscess. (A) Initial ultrasound showing debris inside the abscess cavity. (B) Liquefied pus inside the abscess.

possible resectional therapy. All of these modalities are able to demonstrate loculation and consistency of the contained pus in order to make therapeutic decisions.

Therapy

Antibiotic therapy choices involve combining broad spectrum antibiotics: third-generation cephalosporin plus clindamycin or metronidazole; broad spectrum penicillin plus aminoglycosides; and second-generation cephalosporin plus aminoglycosides. Treatment should be started immediately after specimens have been obtained for culture without waiting for definitive results. Imipenem, aztreonam, piperacillin, tazobactam, ticarcillin, clavulanate, and quinolones are active against almost all aerobic Gram-negative bacilli [28]. Antibiotics should be given before, during, and after drainage and surgical procedures. Parenteral therapy for 2–3 weeks followed by oral antibiotics for 4–6 weeks is recommended. For a solitary abscess <5 cm in diameter, confirmed by aspirate and with available antimicrobial sensitivity, resolution can be achieved with antibiotics alone [38,39]. For an abscess >5 cm with thick and viscous pus, or for large multiloculated abscesses, surgical drainage or continuous percutaneous drainage may be necessary [40].

Aspiration and drainage

Under imaging guidance, PLAs can be aspirated and drained. Drainage is most effective when well-liquefied pus is completely evacuated. If the abscess is not well liquefied or has a thick wall, it is impossible to remove the pus completely. In such cases, most of the drainable pus is removed by needle aspiration, after which antibiotic therapy is necessary to treat the residual abscess. Needle aspiration should be performed with an 18-gauge fine-walled needle. In multiloculated abscesses, the needle tip should be inserted into the various loculi to evacuate pus as completely as possible. Percutaneous needle aspiration is considered unsuccessful when patients fail to improve clinically or radiologically after the second aspiration. Factors affecting drainage include accessibility, the number and size of the abscesses, communication of the abscess with the biliary tree, and, finally, the patient's general condition [41,42]. Those abscesses most accessible to percutaneous drainage are posterior deep-seated lesions of the right lobe (Fig. 38.4), those adhered to the abdominal wall, and peripheral abscesses of the right lobe [43].

Surgery

Surgical therapy is necessary for multiple macroscopic or multiloculated abscesses, or those in the left lobe, after percutaneous drainage failure. Surgical drainage may be required in the presence of ascites or renal failure, when there is evidence of clinical deterioration, persistent jaundice, or concomitant steroid therapy, or when abscesses

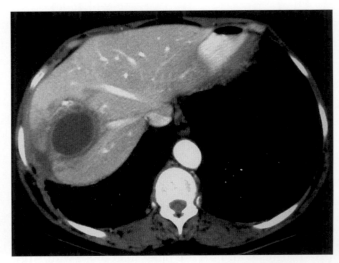

Figure 38.4 Pyogenic liver abscess in the right lobe showing a hypointense rim which is secondary to peripheral inflammation.

are not accessible to radiologic manipulation, and in the case of a ruptured abscess [39,40].

Endoscopic drainage

In patients with stones or strictures of the bile duct and abscess formation in continuity with the biliary system, endoscopic therapy provides biliary drainage, promoting abscess drainage [44].

Annotated references

Coudrier E, Amblard F, Zimmer C, et al. Myosin II and the Gal-GalNAc lectin play a crucial role in tissue invasion by *Entamoeba histolytica*. *Cell Microbiol* 2005;7:19–27.
The observations described in this article are in agreement with emerging studies that highlight marked differences in the way that cells migrate in vitro in two dimensions versus in vivo in three dimensions, that may be pivotal to the discovery of new therapeutic drugs based on Entamoeba histolytica motility and adhesion.

Lodhi S, Sarwari AR, Muzammil M, Salam A, Smego RA. Features distinguishing amoebic from pyogenic liver abscess: a review of 577 adult cases. *Trop Med Health* 2004;9:718–23.
An analysis of the largest population of patients with pyogenic liver abscess since 1938 and of the available current therapies.

Mezhir JJ, Fong Y, Jacks LM, et al. Current management of pyogenic liver abscess: surgery is now second-line treatment. *J Am Coll Surg* 2010;210:975–83.
This article analyzes the current therapeutic approaches to pyogenic liver abscesses and emphasizes those situations when surgery is advised in addition to antibiotics and drainage.

Olivera MA, Kershenobich D. Pyogenic liver abscess. *Curr Treat Options Gastroenterol* 1999;2(2):86–90.
This article includes a position statement regarding the therapeutic approach in pyogenic liver abscess. It is a review of the global experience regarding differences in etiologies and presentation in different age groups.

Santi-Rocca J, Rigothier MC, Guillén N. Host–microbe interactions and defense mechanisms in the development of amoebic liver abscess. *Clin Microbiol Rev* 2009;22(1):65–75.
An exhaustive review of the interactions between the amoeba and the liver. It also reviews the host's response to the injury posed by the parasite and the mechanism of action of virulence and adaptive immune response.

References

1. World Health Organization. *The World Health Report. Life in the 21st century: a vision for all.* Geneva: WHO, 1998.
2. Cox FEG. Taxonomy and classification of human parasites. In: Murray PR, Baron EJ, Jorgensen JH, Pfaller MA, Yolken RH, eds. *Manual of Clinical Microbiology*, 8th edn. Washington DC: ASM Press, 2003:1897–1902.
3. MacFarlane R, Bhattacharya D, Singh U. Genomic DNA microarrays for *Entamoeba histolytica*: applications for use in expression profiling and strain genotyping. *Exp Parasitol* 2005;110:196–202.
4. Srivastava S, Bhattacharya S, Paul J. Species- and strain-specific probes derived from repetitive DNA for distinguishing *Entamoeba histolytica* and *Entamoeba dispar*. *Exp Parasitol* 2005;110:303–8.
5. VanDellen K, Field J, Wang Z, Loftus B, Samuelson J. LINEs and SINE-like elements of the protest *Entamoeba histolytica*. *Gene* 2002;297:229–39.
6. Davis PH, Chen M, Zhang X, et al. Proteomic comparison of *Entamoeba histolytica* and *Entamoeba dispar* and the role of *E. histolytica* alcohol dehydrogenase 3 in virulence. *PLoS Negl Trop Dis* 2009;3(4):e415. doi:10.1371/journal.pntd.0000415.
7. Simonishvili S, Tsanava S, Sanadze K, et al. *Entamoeba histolytica*: the serine-rich gene polymorphism-based genetic variability of clinical isolates from Georgia. *Exp Parasitol* 2005;110:313–17.
8. Diamond LS, Clark CG. A re-description of *Entamoeba histolytica* Schaudinn, 1903 (emended Walker, 1911) separating it from *Entamoeba dispar* Brumpt, 1925. *J Eukaryot Microbiol* 1993;40:340–4.
9. Coudrier E, Amblard F, Zimmer C, et al. Myosin II and the Gal-GalNAc lectin play a crucial role in tissue invasion by *Entamoeba histolytica*. *Cell Microbiol* 2005;7:19–27.
10. Santi-Rocca J, Rigothier MC, Guillén N. Host–microbe interactions and defense mechanisms in the development of amoebic liver abscess. *Clin Microbiol Rev* 2009;22(1):65–75.
11. Tavares P, Rigothier MC, Khun H, et al. Roles of cell adhesion and cytoskeleton activity in *Entamoeba histolytica* pathogenesis: a delicate balance. *Infect Immun* 2005;73:1771–8.
12. Quintanar-Quintanar ME, Jarillo-Luna A, Rivera-Aguilar V, et al. Immunosuppressive treatment inhibits the development of amebic liver abscesses in hamsters. *Med Sci Monit* 2004;10:B317–24.
13. Seydl KB, Stanley SL Jr. *Entamoeba histolytica* induces host cell death in amebic liver abscess by non-Fas dependent, non-tumor necrosis factor alfa-dependent pathway of apoptosis. *Infect Immun* 1998;66:2980–3.
14. Choi MH, Sajed D, Poole L, et al. An unusual surface peroxiredoxin protects invasive *Entamoeba histolytica* from oxidant attack. *Mol Biochem Parasitol* 2005;143:80–9.
15. Zhang X, Zhang Z, Alexander D, et al. Expression of amoebapores is required for full expression of *Entamoeba histolytica* virulence in amebic liver abscess but is not necessary for the induction of inflammation or tissue damage in amebic colitis. *Infect Immun* 2004;72:678–33.
16. Anderson IJ, Loftus BJ. *Entamoeba histolytica*: observations on metabolism based on the genome sequence. *Exp Parasitol* 2005;110:173–7.
17. Loftus B, Anderson I, Davies R, et al. The genome of the protist parasite *Entamoeba histolytica*. *Nature* 2005;433:865–8.
18. Nigam P, Gupta AK, Kapoor KK, et al. Cholestasis in amoebic liver abscess. *Gut* 1985;26(2):140–5.
19. Singh V, Bhalla A, Sharma N, et al. Pathophysiology of jaundice in amoebic liver abscess. *Am J Trop Med Hyg* 2008;78:556–9.
20. Hughes MA, Petri WA Jr. Infections of the liver. Amebic liver abscess. *Infect Dis Clin North Am* 2000;14:565–82.
21. Mortele KJ, Segatto E, Ros PR. The infected liver: radiologic-pathologic correlation. *RadioGraphics* 2004;24:937–55.
22. Myoung-don O, Kwanghyuck L. Amebic liver abscess on HIV infected patients. *AIDS* 2000;14:1872–3.
23. Khanna D, Chaudhary D, Kumar A, Vij JC. Experience with aspiration in cases of amebic liver abscess in an endemic area. *Eur J Clin Microbiol Infect Dis* 2005;24:428–30.
24. Shamsuzzaman SM, Hashiguchi Y. Thoracic amebiasis. *Clin Chest Med* 2002;23:479–92.
25. Chavez-Tapia NC, Hernandez-Calleros J, Tellez-Avila FI, Torre A, Uribe M. Image-guided percutaneous procedure plus metronidazole versus metronidazole alone for uncomplicated amoebic liver abscess. *Cochrane Database Syst Rev* 2009;1:CD004886. doi:10.1002/14651858.
26. Lotter H, Russman H, Heesemann J, Tannich E. Oral vaccination with recombinant *Yersinia enterocolitica* expressing hybrid type III proteins protects gerbils from amebic liver abscess. *Infect Immun* 2004;72:7318–21.
27. Meddings L, Myers RP, Hubbard J, et al. A population-based study of pyogenic liver abscess in the United States: incidence, mortality and temporal trends. *Am J Gastroenterol* 2010;105:117–24.
28. Olvera MA, Kershenobich D. Pyogenic liver abscess. *Curr Treat Options Gastroenterol* 1999;2:86–90.
29. Rahimian J, Wilson T, Oram V, Holzman RS. Pyogenic liver abscess: recent trends in etiology and mortality. *Clin Infect Dis* 2004;39:1654–9.
30. Alvarez-Pérez JA, González JJ, Baldonedo RF, et al. Clinical course, treatment and multivariate analysis of risk factors for pyogenic liver abscess. *Am J Surg* 2001;181:177–86.
31. Kaita NI, Nichitalio ME, Kotenko OG, et al. Etiology, pathogenesis and clinic-diagnostic aspects of hepatic abscess. *Klin Khir* 2004;10:54–8.
32. Nan BK, Kim YS, Moon HS, et al. Recent changes of organism and treatment in pyogenic liver abscess. *Taehan Kan Hokohe Chi* 2003;9:275–83.
33. Lodhi S, Sarwari AR, Muzammil M, et al. Features distinguishing amoebic from pyogenic liver abscess: a review of 577 adult cases. *Trop Med Health* 2004;9:718–23.
34. Ahsan T, Jehangir MU, Mahmood T, et al. Amoebic versus pyogenic liver abscess. *J Pak Med Assoc* 2002;52:497–501.
35. Lee CC, Poon SK, Chen GH. Spontaneous gas-forming liver abscess caused by salmonella within hepatocellular carcinoma. A case report and review of the literature. *Dig Dis Sci* 2002;47:586–9.
36. Alvarez-Pérez JA, González-González JJ, Baldonedo-Cernuda RF, et al. Pyogenic liver abscess in cancer patients. *Rev Clin Esp* 2001;201:632–7.
37. Balci NC, Semelka RC, Noone TC, et al. Pyogenic hepatic abscesses. MRI findings on T-1 and T-2 weighted and serial gadolinium enhanced gradient echo images. *J MRI* 1999;9:285–90.
38. Calvo-Romero JM, Lima-Rodriguez EM. Favourable outcome of multiple pyogenic liver abscesses with conservative treatment. *Scand J Infect Dis* 2005;37:141–57.
39. Bergert H, Kersting S, Pyrc J, et al. Therapeutic options in the treatment of pyogenic liver abscess. *Ultraschall Med* 2004;25:356–62.
40. Tan YM, Chung AY, Chow PK, et al. An appraisal of surgical and percutaneous drainage for pyogenic liver abscess larger than 5 cm. *Ann Surg* 2005;241:435–90.
41. Mezhir JJ, Fong Y, Jacks LM, et al. Current management of pyogenic liver abscess: surgery is now second-line treatment. *J Am Coll Surg* 2010;210:975–83.
42. Chen SC, Huang CC, Tsai SJ, et al. Severity of disease as main predictor for mortality in patients with pyogenic liver abscess. *Am J Surg* 2009;198:164–72.
43. Yu SC, Ho SS, Lau WY, et al. Treatment of pyogenic liver abscess: prospective randomized comparison of catheter drainage and needle aspiration. *Hepatology* 2004;42:2783–5.
44. Dull JS, Topa L, Balgha V, Pap A. Non-surgical treatment of biliary liver abscesses: efficacy of endoscopic drainage and local antibiotic lavage with nasobiliary catheter. *Gastrointest Endosc* 2000;51(1):55–9.

Multiple choice questions

38.1 All of the following are features useful to identify *Entamoeba histolytica* from *E. dispar* except for which one?

a Differences in non-LTR retrotransposons.
b Differences in the activity of NADP-dependent alcohol dehydrogenase.
c Differences in protein expression, specifically grainin.
d Differences in the membrane's lipid arrangement on electron microscopy.
e All of the above.

38.2 In the pathogenesis of amoebic liver abscess which of the following is the most accurate statement?

a Myosin I and III are important in the parasites' motility in the intestine.
b Gal/GalNAc inhibits the synthesis of TNF-α, thus favoring parasite clearance.
c Gal/GalNAc inhibits the assembly of C5b-9 preventing the formation of the membrane attack complex.
d All of the above.
e None of the above.

38.3 The following are potential causes of pyogenic liver abscess except which one?

a Radiofrequency ablation of hepatocellular carcinoma.
b A perforated appendicitis.
c Bile duct manipulation and stenting of a cholangiocarcinoma.
d Active Crohn disease treated with biologic drugs.
e All of the above.

Answers to the multiple choice questions can be found in the Appendix at the end of the book.

**These multiple choice questions are also available for you to complete online.
Visit http://www.schiffsdiseasesoftheliver.com/**

CHAPTER 39
Parasitic Diseases

Michael A. Dunn

Division of Gastroenterology, Hepatology and Nutrition, University of Pittsburgh, Pittsburgh, PA, USA

Key concepts

- Liver parasites span a wide range of complexity, from intracellular protozoa to visible multicellular helminths with highly evolved life cycles. Different species mature and reproduce within hepatocytes, reticuloendothelial cells, the portal venous system, and the bile ducts.
- Well-adapted parasites cause minimal acute injury to the host organ as they generate enormous numbers of progeny that pass into the blood or bile with the potential to infect other hosts. Examples include the malaria parasites, the schistosome worms, and the bile duct flukes.
- When a parasite enters a species or an organ to which it is poorly adapted, acute or severe injury is likely: *Echinococcus* tapeworms,

well adapted to canine–herbivore or canine–rodent life cycles, cause severe cystic liver disease in accidental human hosts. The protozoan *Entamoeba histolytica* and the roundworm *Ascaris*, both well suited to the human intestinal lumen, cause acute injury when they invade the liver parenchyma or bile ducts, respectively.
- Successful parasites have evolved to evade or to accommodate the effects of the defenses and immunologic responses of healthy hosts. Hosts with abnormal or compromised responses are at risk for severe disease manifestations, such as the reactivation of subclinical *Leishmania* infection with the development of advanced visceral leishmaniasis in human immunodeficiency virus-infected persons.

Protozoal diseases

Malaria, one of the world's most serious and widespread infectious diseases, is intimately involved with the liver during its preerythrocytic and exoerythrocytic stages of development. Visceral leishmaniasis is a cause of severe debility and hepatosplenomegaly in the tropics and a growing concern for immunosuppressed persons in temperate climates. In addition to these obligatory intracellular parasites, *Entamoeba histolytica*, an extracellular protozoan cause of liver abscess, is considered in Chapter 33.

Malaria

Malaria, the world's most prevalent fatal parasitic disease, is caused in humans by intracellular protozoa of four species: *Plasmodium falciparum*, *P. vivax*, *P. ovale*, and *P. malariae*. All are transmitted by mosquito bite, and involve the entry of mosquito-borne sporozoites into hepatocytes, where a preerythrocytic stage of the parasite multiplies and is subsequently released to invade erythrocytes. Malaria continues to kill 2 million persons a year and to frustrate eradication efforts because of the parasite's capacity to develop drug resistance. There is, therefore, great interest in defining the events within the

liver that may account for complete protection of animals with vaccines directed against genetically attenuated sporozoites [1]. Protective immunity against preerythrocytic parasites binding to and entering hepatocytes involves a complex interaction of antibody-mediated and both innate and adaptive cellular responses [2].

The cyclic fevers, hemolysis, vascular stasis, shock, and multiple organ failure of severe malaria are the clinical end results of synchronized multiplication and release of the parasite's erythrocytic stage. Kupffer cells take up released hemoglobin degradation products known as malarial pigments, which appear as dark cytoplasmic granules in liver specimens from persons with a history of malaria. Humans with intact host defenses normally recover from acute episodes of malaria. The highest risk for severe illness and death is with *P. falciparum* infection. Falciparum malaria often produces clinical and laboratory evidence of multiple organ dysfunction. Patients often show modest elevations in serum bilirubin, aminotransferase, or alkaline phosphatase levels. Severe liver injury in malaria is infrequently seen in patients with heavy *P. falciparum* infections, and is commonly associated with acute renal failure and encephalopathy. In a report from India, seven such patients presented with the acute onset of jaundice, asterixis or impaired

Schiff's Diseases of the Liver, Eleventh Edition. Edited by Eugene R. Schiff, Willis C. Maddrey and Michael F. Sorrell.
© 2012 John Wiley & Sons, Ltd. Published 2012 by John Wiley & Sons Ltd.

sensorium, bleeding with prolonged prothrombin and partial thromboplastin times, and aminotransferase elevations at four-fold the normal [3]. *P. falciparum* infection was evident in their blood smears. The three survivors responded to intravenous quinine and supportive care that included lactulose and bowel cleansing. One of the four patients who died had submassive hepatic necrosis; focal steatonecrosis was present in postmortem liver specimens from the other three. As with earlier similar reports, it is unclear to what extent liver injury contributed to morbidity in these patients. The key message remains, however, that a clinical presentation suggesting acute hepatic failure in persons at risk for malaria infection should prompt consideration of this readily diagnosed and treatable illness.

Leishmaniasis

Visceral leishmaniasis, or kala-azar, is an infection of the reticuloendothelial cells of the liver, spleen, bone marrow, and other organs with an intracellular protozoan parasite, *Leishmania* [4]. Common throughout the tropics, visceral leishmaniasis has been increasingly recognized elsewhere as a potential problem for immunosuppressed persons with human immunodeficiency virus (HIV) disease or after organ transplantation. As an experimental disease model, leishmanial infection provides an opportunity to study liver inflammation and fibrosis with the same methods that have advanced our knowledge of these important processes in other diseases, such as hepatic schistosomiasis.

Infections with different species of *Leishmania* cause visceral, cutaneous, and mucocutaneous patterns of disease. Visceral leishmaniasis, involving the liver, normally results from infection of children and young adults with *L. donovani*. In the Indian subcontinent, the parasite is transmitted by sandflies that have bitten infected humans. Elsewhere – in South America, southern Europe, Africa, the Middle East, and China – *L. donovani* transmission to humans by sandflies is primarily enzootic, involving canine and rodent reservoir hosts. Visceral involvement with *L. tropica*, a species that normally causes cutaneous disease, occurred in veterans of the 1991 Persian Gulf War [5], and disease due to *L. donovani* has been seen in American soldiers exposed to infection in Iraq and Afghanistan [6]. Other than infection from the bite of sandflies in endemic areas, *Leishmania* can be transmitted by blood transfusion or needles shared for drug abuse, by sexual contact, and by transplantation of infected organs.

After bloodstream infection and uptake of the parasite by reticuloendothelial cells, its amastygote stage, shown in Fig. 39.1, multiplies within Kupffer cells and macrophages, infects new cells, and triggers cellular and humoral host responses. Immunocompetent persons

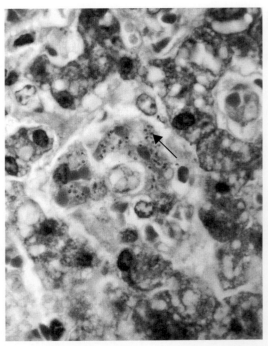

Figure 39.1 Visceral leishmaniasis showing dot-like organisms (arrow) present in several hypertrophied Kupffer cells. Hematoxylin and eosin (H&E), original ×1,000. (Armed Forces Institute of Pathology (AFIP) negative 87-5647.)

respond to infection with a successful combined T helper cell 1 (Th1) and Th17 cell-mediated host defense that prevents clinical disease and suppresses, but may not eliminate, the infection [7]. Such a cellular response, akin to that seen in tuberculoid leprosy or successfully contained initial *Mycobacterium tuberculosis* infection, involves the same T4 cells and cytokines – interferon-γ, interleukin 2 (IL2), IL12, IL17, IL22, and tumor necrosis factor (TNF) – as well as nitric oxide synthesis, that are critical for dealing with other intracellular organisms. Humoral antibody responses, also regularly present, do not appear to modify the course of leishmanial infection; nor do the Th2-type cellular responses seen in persons who develop clinically severe disease.

Pathologic examination of liver specimens shows findings that parallel the predominant host response [8]. In persons with minimal disease and few parasites visible in liver specimens, epithelioid granulomas (including fibrin-ring granulomas similar to those described in Q fever) may be present. Numerous parasites multiplying within activated Kupffer cells and macrophages, the appearance of myofibroblasts, deposition of intralobular collagen, and effacement of the space of Disse with connective tissue all accompany an ineffective response in persons with overt disease. A pattern of severe intralobular liver fibrosis as a predominant finding was described by Rogers [9] in 1908 as a "peculiar cirrhosis" in Indian patients with visceral leishmaniasis. So-called Rogers cirrhosis, however, shows normal liver architecture and no regenerative nodules. Visceral leishmaniasis has attracted investigative interest because of its association with severe intralobular liver fibrosis, which appears to be fully reversible after treatment of the infection. When experimental animal systems for the study of liver fibrosis in visceral leishmaniasis are defined, we may gain information of comparable significance to that which has already been gained for the immunopathology of this disease.

The major clinical manifestations of visceral leishmaniasis include fever, weight loss, hepatomegaly, splenomegaly, lymphadenopathy, pancytopenia, and hypergammaglobulinemia. All organs with reticuloendothelial cells may be involved, including the entire gastrointestinal tract. Laboratory abnormalities may include modest elevations in serum aminotransferases and alkaline phosphatase levels and depressed albumin levels, as well as skin test anergy to common delayed hypersensitivity antigens. Although hepatic and splenic enlargement from cellular infiltration may be truly massive and intralobular liver fibrosis may be pronounced, overt ascites is uncommon, and the very rare occurrence of either hepatocellular failure or of clinically evident portal hypertension suggests another etiology. Persons with advanced disease are at risk of death from intercurrent infections or severe malnutrition. Conversely, malnutrition, immunosuppressive therapy, or an immunosuppressive disease such as HIV infection can precipitate the development of overt visceral leishmaniasis in previously healthy persons with latent infections acquired as long as 20 years earlier.

Severe HIV-associated visceral leishmaniasis has been described in reports from Spain, a *Leishmania* endemic area, as well as from nonendemic countries such as France and Germany [10]. Visceral leishmaniasis should be sought as a treatable cause of fever, hepatosplenomegaly, and rapid deterioration in HIV-infected persons with even a remotely positive travel history or risk factors for non-sandfly-transmitted blood-borne infection. Intracellular parasites may be seen in liver or intestinal biopsy specimens obtained during the evaluation of HIV-infected persons for persistent fever or diarrhea. Most such patients have CD4 cell counts less than $400/mm^3$, consistent with the importance of an intact Th1 cellular response for dealing with leishmanial infection. This relationship supports the suggestion that visceral leishmaniasis in HIV-infected persons should be considered as an acquired immune deficiency syndrome (AIDS)-defining illness [11]. Most HIV-positive patients with visceral leishmaniasis respond well to initial therapy; however, relapse after cessation of treatment is common, so that long-term suppressive therapy with fluconazole, ketoconazole, pentamidine, or intermittent liposomal amphotericin B is often used.

Visceral leishmaniasis may also become manifest in immunosuppressed solid organ transplant recipients; in one report, the donor liver was considered the likely source of parasite infection [12]. The reduction of immunosuppressive regimens to the minimum needed to support graft function, combined with long-term suppressive antiparasitic therapy, is the recommended management. New biologic therapies for chronic inflammatory diseases, such as the anti-TNF agent adalimumab, may also reactivate latent infection, as shown in a patient from Italy with rheumatoid arthritis [13].

The diagnostic procedure for visceral leishmaniasis with the highest accuracy, close to 100%, is the examination and culture of a needle splenic aspirate. In nonendemic areas where experience levels to safely perform splenic aspiration are lacking, examination and culture of bone marrow and liver biopsy specimens are more often performed. Either method provides a 50–80% yield. Polymerase chain reaction (PCR)-based detection of leishmanial DNA in peripheral blood has diagnostic accuracy comparable with that of bone marrow aspiration.

Until recently, therapy for visceral leishmaniasis usually involved intramuscular or intravenous administration of pentavalent antimonial compounds for 3 weeks or longer. Second-line anti-leishmanials have included pentamidine, amphotericin B, allopurinol, paromomycin, ketoconazole, and related azole compounds. A newer drug, miltefosine, is administered orally for 28 days. Intravenous liposomal amphotericin B represents a new drug delivery strategy that targets the intracellular location of the parasite. It has now become the preferred treatment for initial or relapsed disease because of its high efficacy, approaching 100%, its short duration of therapy, ranging from a single infusion to five daily infusions at a total dose of 10–20 mg/kg, and its minimal toxicity [14]. It is US Food and Drug Administration (FDA) approved for treatment of visceral leishmaniasis. Response to therapy is assessed by resolution of fever, regression of splenomegaly, and weight gain; serologic testing is not helpful.

Although the clinical manifestations of visceral leishmaniasis resolve with antiparasitic therapy, it remains unclear, especially in persons with underlying immunologic deficits, whether the infection is ever truly eliminated or only suppressed below detectable limits. The successful use of highly active antiretroviral therapy (HAART) in HIV-infected patients, for example, is thought to be responsible for recent major decreases in the incidence of clinically overt visceral leishmaniasis in France and Spain, although HIV-infected persons with inapparent leishmanial infection remain at lifelong risk for the occurrence of clinical illness [15].

Helminthic liver diseases

- *Schistosomiasis.* Schistosomes are blood flukes that are well adapted to long survival as male and female adults in the venous circulations of human hosts. Human disease involves host responses to the deposition of schistosome eggs in tissues.
- *Fascioliasis* is caused by flukes that primarily infect sheep and other herbivores. When humans are infected, a biphasic liver disease results from maturation of the parasite as it migrates through the liver parenchyma followed by an extended life span in the bile ducts.
- *Clonorchiasis* and *opisthorchiasis* are biliary infections by trematode flukes that are well adapted to humans. Asymptomatic or minimally symptomatic for many years in most infected persons, these infections are of major concern because of their potential for the development of cholangiocarcinoma.
- *Echinococcosis* is a potentially life-threatening cystic liver disease caused by the infection of humans as accidental intermediate hosts of three species of canine cestode tapeworms.
- *Biliary ascariasis.* Intestinal infection with the nematode roundworm *Ascaris lumbricoides* affects one quarter of the world's population. Biliary ascariasis, which is relatively uncommon, manifests as biliary colic, cholangitis, or pancreatitis induced by the migration of one or more of these large (up to 20 cm) adult worms into the ductal system [16]. Biliary ascariasis usually occurs in children or in adults with an abnormal, open ampullary orifice produced by preexisting biliary tract disease or after surgical or endoscopic sphincterotomy. *Ascaris* worms in the ductal system are readily visualized on ultrasonography or computed tomography (CT). If the worms do not spontaneously clear from the duct after antihelminthic treatment with mebendazole or an alternative agent, they may be removed endoscopi-

cally. Chronic biliary ascariasis has been implicated in the development of Oriental cholangiohepatitis, as discussed later for clonorchiasis and opisthorchiasis. Abdominal imaging methods may show characteristic findings in helminthic liver diseases, as summarized in Table 39.1. The laboratory diagnosis of helminthic infections, as shown in Table 39.2, relies primarily on demonstrating eggs in the stool when the parasite's life cycle involves egg excretion by the human host. Serologic examinations, especially enzyme-linked immunosorbent assay (ELISA) methods, have become established for most infections as diagnostic adjuncts. Serologic diagnosis is especially helpful when positive in the acute stage of fascioliasis and in echinococcosis, situations in which fecal egg excretion does not take place. Eosinophilia is such a regular accompaniment of most helminthic infections that its occurrence should prompt their diagnostic consideration, and its persistence after presumed parasitologic cure may signal treatment failure.

Schistosomiasis

Schistosomes are trematode flukes that infect more than 200 million persons worldwide. Schistosomiasis has attracted more study and effort than all the other parasitic liver diseases combined. Few other diseases of any cause have posed the intensity and breadth of challenges in molecular biology, immunology, economic development, pharmacology, and surgical therapy that have been overcome and others that remain for this disease [17].

Disease mechanisms

Schistosomes begin their life cycles with the passage of eggs by adult females that live, paired with male worms, in the mesenteric or vesical venous beds. Viable eggs erode through the intestinal or bladder mucosa, are passed in feces or urine, hatch in water, and infect an intermediate snail host. Snails shed free-swimming

Table 39.1 Imaging characteristics in helminthic liver diseases.

Infection	Imaging methods	Findings	Reversibility
Schistosomiasis	Ultrasonography	Portal fibrosis	Years to permanent
Fascioliasis, acute	CT	Serpiginous linear subcapsular abscess tracts	Months
Fascioliasis, chronic	Ultrasonography, CT, cholangiography	Dilated ducts, visible adult worms	Months to years
Clonorchiasis and opisthorchiasis	Ultrasonography, CT, cholangiography	Dilated irregular ducts, stones, associated cholangiocarcinoma	Years to permanent
Cystic and alveolar echinococcosis	Ultrasonography, CT, magnetic resonance imaging	Cysts with variable wall calcification, complex internal structures, and daughter cysts	Years to permanent
Ascariasis	Ultrasonography, CT, cholangiography	Dilated ducts obstructed by worms	Months

CT, computed tomography.

Table 39.2 Diagnosis of helminthic liver diseases.

Infection	Stool examination for eggs	Serology
Schistosomiasis	Method of choice in active infection, may be supplemented with rectal mucosal biopsy	ELISA available
Fascioliasis, acute	Negative	ELISA highly sensitive and specific, serial testing useful to monitor response to therapy
Fascioliasis, chronic	Often positive but egg production may be intermittent	ELISA method useful in addition to stool examination
Clonorchiasis and opisthorchiasis	Method of choice in active infection, stool PCR may be useful in mass screening	ELISA available; limited utility
Echinococcosis	Negative	IHA or ELISA positive in 90% of cases, serial testing useful to monitor response to therapy
Ascariasis	Method of choice	Not applicable

ELISA, enzyme-linked immunosorbent assay; IHA, indirect hemagglutination assay; PCR, polymerase chain reaction.

ceracariae, the infectious stage for humans, which have the ability to penetrate human skin and transform into immature worms. The worms mature over a period of approximately 6 weeks as they traverse the venous, pulmonary, and systemic circulations and localize in their species-specific target vessels to form male–female copulating adult worm pairs and to initiate egg production that may continue for decades.

Five species of schistosomes, listed in Table 39.3, develop to maturity in humans. The great majority of schistosomal liver disease is caused by infections with *Schistosoma mansoni* in Africa and South America and *S. japonicum* in Asia. Although portal tract egg deposition, granuloma formation, and fibrosis have been reported in persons infected with *S. hematobium*, these findings are minor compared with urinary tract egg deposition and disease. *S. mekongi* and *S. intercalatum* have limited geographic distributions in Asia and Africa, respectively.

The preferential homing and predilection of maturing schistosomes of all species other than *S. hematobium* is to concentrate in the mesenteric venous system, and of the latter species to concentrate in the vesical plexus. This is central to the pattern of subsequent injury that their infections produce. Immature worms make several passes through the circulation before remaining at their preferred location. The mechanism that signals this remarkable preference for specific vascular beds is unknown. One potential localizing signal was suggested by the finding that human portal serum, but not peripheral blood, contains material of molecular weight greater than 1,000 that stimulates cell proliferation in immature *S. mansoni* worms [18].

Mature worm pairs in the mesenteric veins continuously produce large numbers of viable eggs that are carried to the intestine or the liver. Eggs deposited in the vessels of the intestinal mucosa may remain trapped within inflammatory granulomas, or erode into the lumen and be excreted. Liver disease in schistosomiasis results from the entrapment of eggs that lodge in portal venules. Eggs in the liver remain viable for approximately 3 weeks and secrete products that elicit a characteristic initial response, the schistosome egg granuloma, as shown in Fig. 39.2A. In some persons with heavy infections, the end result of hepatic schistosomiasis is severe portal fibrosis, as shown in Fig. 39.2B. Advanced schistosomal hepatic fibrosis gives a gross appearance of greatly enlarged fibrotic

Table 39.3 Human schistosomes.

Species	Geographic range	Preferred vascular bed	Main target organs
Schistosoma mansoni	Middle East, Africa, Central and South America	Mesenteric	Liver, colon
Schistosoma japonicum	Far East	Mesenteric	Liver, small intestine, colon
Schistosoma hematobium	Middle East, Africa	Vesical	Bladder, ureters
Schistosoma mekongi	Southeast Asia	Mesenteric	Liver, small intestine, colon
Schistosoma intercalatum	Central Africa	Mesenteric	Colon, less severe liver and small intestinal disease

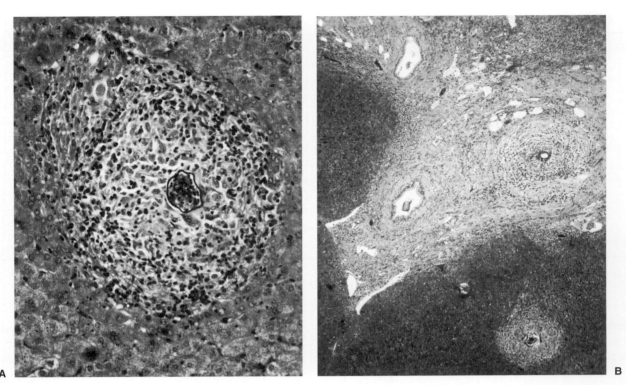

Figure 39.2 (A) A *Schistosoma mansoni* egg granuloma in the liver. The schistosome egg has lodged in a portal venule, with the formation of an epithelioid granuloma. H&E, original ×250. (AFIP negative 79-16805.) (B) Hepatic schistosomiasis. The large area of scarring corresponds grossly to pipestem portal fibrosis. A *Schistosoma mansoni* egg granuloma is at the lower right margin of the field. H&E, original ×60. (AFIP negative 79-16808.)

portal tracts, described by Symmers [19] in 1904 as resembling clay pipestems thrust through the liver, and now termed Symmers pipestem fibrosis.

Schistosomiasis has become a valuable model disease, in both clinical and experimental animal studies, for advancing our understanding of the key processes of hepatic inflammation and fibrosis [20]. Important control points and mechanisms of immune regulation and collagen gene expression are more clearly defined in schistosomiasis than in other chronic liver diseases. The antigenic products secreted by living schistosome eggs first elicit a predominant Th1-type cellular response, marked by an influx of mononuclear cells and formation of highly cellular egg granulomas, with the initiation of increased collagen formation. Over time, from several weeks to months depending on the specific experimental model or human infection, a modulation of the initial cellular reaction takes place as egg deposition continues. There is a diminution of the intensity of inflammation and a shift to a predominantly Th2-type cellular response with prominent eosinophilic infiltration of granulomas and continuing deposition of fibrous tissue. Of the mediators associated with the Th2 response, IL13 appears to have strong potential as a pivotal mediator of fibrogenesis, based on studies in *S. mansoni*-infected gene knock-out mice that fail to express either IL13 or its receptor complex [21].

As the shift from a predominant Th1 to Th2 response takes place, the Th17 pathway associated with the production of IL17 and IL23 also appears important in helping to drive inflammation and fibrosis [22]. In humans, there appears to be a genetic component of susceptibility of infected persons to severe fibrotic disease, as suggested by a reported association of a codominant gene with an allele frequency of 0.16 in a heavily infected community in Sudan with severe schistosomal hepatic fibrosis. The gene, located on chromosome 6, was closely linked to the interferon-γ receptor gene [23]. In general, however, the most important single determinant of the severity of disease in hepatic schistosomiasis appears to be the intensity of egg deposition in the liver over time.

Hepatic fibrosis

The synthesis, deposition, remodeling, and turnover of collagen types I and III and basement membrane-associated collagen components, as well as that of fibronectin and accompanying matrix substances such as glycosaminoglycans, are greatly increased in hepatic schistosomiasis, as are the plasma levels of multiple markers of collagen deposition. Experimental schistosomiasis has been an especially useful model for the study of the specific inflammatory cytokines proposed to have an influence on fibrogenesis.

In schistosomiasis, cells in granulomas and in adjacent fibrotic portal tracts show the appearance of stellate cells known to produce collagen and other connective tissue components in other chronic liver diseases [24]. The potential interactions among granuloma macrophages, cytokines, and stellate cells, and angiogenesis within granulomas, appear to parallel those described in other experimental model systems and human diseases [25]. As disease progresses from initial egg deposition to advanced fibrosis, the portal tracts become less prominently involved with inflammatory cells, and prominent cellular infiltrates diminish and disappear. The portal tracts in persons with Symmers fibrosis are markedly expanded with broad, dense-appearing bands of relatively acellular, mature fibrous tissue (Fig. 39.2B).

Because normal liver architecture is preserved in hepatic schistosomiasis, the reversal of portal tract inflammation and fibrosis should allow resolution of the disease and restoration of normal function. Reversal of fibrosis has been well described after the cure of early *S. mansoni* and *S. japonicum* infections in mice. Murine schistosomiasis is one of the best studied examples of the increased activity of two competing processes, collagen biosynthesis versus collagenolysis, in inflammatory fibrotic liver disease. In this model system, cure of infection with cessation of new egg deposition in the liver appears to allow collagenolysis to predominate over continued collagen synthesis, with a resolution of fibrosis. It is unclear, however, to what extent the advanced dense portal collagen deposition associated with chronic human hepatic fibrosis might be subject to the same outcome. Two lines of evidence suggest that even dense pipestem fibrosis may be reversible, at least in part. First, rabbits infected with *S. japonicum* provide an animal model of dense portal collagen deposition that resembles human pipestem fibrosis morphologically and biochemically and shows slow reversibility of fibrosis over a 40-week period after cure of the infection [26]. Second, serial ultrasonographic examination of persons with schistosome infection has become a standard method of assessing pipestem hepatic fibrosis in population-based treatment studies. The ultrasonographic appearance of pipestem fibrosis is shown in Fig. 39.3. Ultrasonography in persons with acute nonfibrotic liver diseases may show a modest degree of portal tract expansion that cannot be distinguished from early schistosomal fibrosis, and the imaging method is not reliable for assessing fibrosis in persons with schistosomiasis and coexisting conditions such as chronic viral hepatitis. Taking these precautions into account, multiple reports now clearly document the partial or complete resolution over several years of the ultrasonographic findings of pipestem fibrosis after parasitologic cure of human infection [27]. In children and in adults treated after relatively short durations of infection, ultrasonographic resolution

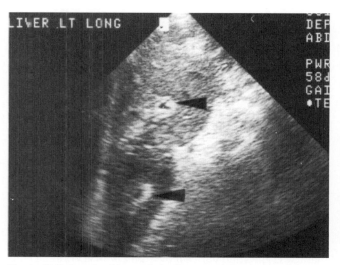

Figure 39.3 Hepatic schistosomiasis. Ultrasonography showing echogenic deposits of pipestem portal fibrosis (arrowheads). (Courtesy of Colonel Michael P. Brazaitis, Department of Radiology, Walter Reed Army Medical Center.)

is more likely to be complete and accompanied by a reversal of hepatomegaly and splenomegaly as assessed on physical examination.

Clinical manifestations

The cercariae of all schistosomes, including those that die on skin penetration in humans, such as the avian schistosome species, may cause a hypersensitivity dermatitis called swimmer's itch. A potentially fatal acute illness, Katayama fever, is a serum sickness-like syndrome triggered by the onset of tissue egg deposition in heavy infections [17]. The cardinal characteristic manifestations of advanced hepatic schistosomiasis are related to portal fibrosis and the development of presinusoidal portal hypertension, with passive congestion of the portal system, hepatomegaly, potentially marked splenomegaly, and the enlargement of collateral vessels such as esophageal and gastric varices. Patients classically present with a history of one or multiple variceal bleeding episodes, accompanied by prominent splenomegaly, no ascites, and normal or nearly normal indices of synthetic liver function and other biochemical laboratory values. It has become increasingly evident from careful longitudinal study of the populations of endemic areas, however, that the greatest health and economic impact of chronic schistosomiasis may not be its dramatic end state with variceal bleeding, but retardation of growth and development, malnutrition, and generalized debility in heavily infected children and adults [28]. Growth retardation in children with schistosomiasis is specifically associated with the infection rather than other potential causes and is only partially overcome after parasitologic cure.

The prominent splenomegaly of persons with hepatic schistosomiasis is caused both by infiltration with inflammatory cells and by passive congestion. The spleen is firm, normally nontender on palpation, and may be the site of sufficient sequestration to produce clinically important reductions in red blood cells, leukocytes, and platelets, as well as significant discomfort attributed to the bulk of the enlarged organ. Symptomatic splenomegaly may persist after the cure of infection, so that simple splenectomy is one of the most common surgical procedures in endemic areas. Segmental splenectomy, with removal of the bulk of an enlarged organ and preservation of a functional remnant of approximately normal size, is safe and effective in experienced hands when hypersplenism in schistosomiasis requires surgical therapy [29]. When variceal bleeding is an additional concern, portal variceal disconnection may be added [30], although as discussed in the subsequent text, optimal therapy to prevent recurrent variceal bleeding in schistosomiasis is far from clear. Massive splenomegaly may suggest the presence of follicular lymphoma of the spleen, the only malignant tumor clearly associated with hepatic schistosomiasis. Follicular lymphoma was reported to occur in 1% of *S. mansoni*-infected Brazilian patients who required splenectomy [31].

Bacterial infections associated with schistosomiasis include pyogenic liver abscesses, predominantly caused by *Staphylococcus aureus* and chronic *Salmonella* bacteremia [32]. Liver abscesses tend to occur in persons with early schistosome infections, perhaps coincident with the effects of initial egg deposition and the initial formation of highly cellular and vascular egg granulomas. Chronic *Salmonella* bacteremia appears related to the sequestration of living bacteria in the integument of adult worms and may be permanently cured only after elimination of the parasitic infection. HIV and schistosome infections now coexist in a growing number of persons as the HIV epidemic spreads through areas endemic for schistosomiasis. HIV-infected persons treated for an active schistosome infection had a less rapid increase in HIV viral load and improved CD4 cell counts compared with those in whom antiparasitic therapy was delayed [33].

Schistosomiasis and viral hepatitis

The accepted clinical findings of hepatic schistosomiasis – normal liver architecture and cellular function in the presence of portal fibrosis and portal hypertension – are present only in a minority of schistosome-infected persons who require hospitalization for liver disease. Because testing for the markers of hepatitis B and C infections has become widespread, it is now evident that regions with a high prevalence of *S. mansoni* and *S. japonicum* infections also tend to have high endemicity for chronic viral hepatitis. In most populations studied, there is no higher occurrence of coinfection with schistosomiasis and hepatitis B or C than would be expected by their independent prevalence [34]. An increased risk for acquiring both infections has been reported, however, in persons with schistosomiasis who required transfusions, and a major increase in the risk for hepatitis C infection has now become evident as the unintended consequence of mass treatment programs for schistosomiasis prior to 1980 that used injections with inadequately sterilized, nondisposable syringes and needles. For example, in communities in Egypt with an overall prevalence of antihepatitis C virus (anti-HCV) of 15–20%, up to 50% of persons in age groups with a history of such mass parenteral therapy are now anti-HCV-positive. The intensive viral transmission attributed to these mass parenteral treatment programs, with the formation of a large reservoir of chronic HCV infection, is thought to be responsible for the high current prevalence and transmission rates of hepatitis C in these areas [35].

In persons who develop both hepatic schistosomiasis and chronic viral hepatitis, severe illness is common. Most of the subset of persons living in schistosomiasis endemic areas who are hospitalized for variceal bleeding, management of ascites, or decompensated hepatocellular failure do, in fact, have both schistosomiasis and chronic viral hepatitis, frequently with cirrhosis. Whether co-morbidity involves specific interactions of the pathologic mechanisms of both diseases or is simply a summation of their effects is unclear. When acute hepatitis C infection occurred in health care providers with preexisting chronic *S. mansoni* infection, they showed a uniform inability to clear viremia and an accelerated histologic progression of chronic hepatitis C compared with the course of hepatitis C infection in their colleagues without schistosome infection [36]. Persons with coexisting *S. mansoni* infection and chronic hepatitis C appear less likely than others to respond to interferon therapy and *S. mansoni*-infected persons respond less consistently to hepatitis B vaccination, although vaccination should be a high priority in schistosome endemic areas to prevent as much comorbidity as possible. Antiviral therapy for chronic hepatitis B or C should be considered for persons who have been cured of active schistosome infection and who would otherwise meet treatment criteria, bearing in mind that the predominant HCV genotype transmitted in Egypt is type 4 [35].

Diagnosis

The detection of schistosome eggs in the stool is the most useful diagnostic method for documenting active infection. Quantitative studies have shown generally strong relationships between the extent of fecal egg output, the host's worm burden, and the extent of pathology in both *S. mansoni* and *S. japonicum* infections [17]. Stool examinations for eggs become negative after parasitologic cure of infection. Some persons with active untreated *S. japonicum* infections causing significant morbidity may also show few or no eggs on stool examination. Low-power examination of fresh rectal mucosal biopsies may show schistosome eggs that were not apparent in stool specimens. Serologic ELISA methods to detect the antibody to parasitic antigens show excellent sensitivity and are of value in population surveys, but may not be helpful in assessing the activity of infection in an individual patient. Of the standard abdominal imaging methods, ultrasonography, as discussed earlier, is by far the most practical for field application and appears to be of better diagnostic utility than CT or magnetic resonance imaging (MRI) for assessment of the extent of portal fibrosis.

Medical therapy

Praziquantel is an effective drug against all human schistosomes, producing parasitologic cures in approximately 90% of persons. It is orally administered, preferably in three doses of 20 mg/kg body weight given over 8 hours for a total of 60 mg/kg. Single-dose therapy of 40 and 50 mg/kg has been used in some community mass treatment programs for *S. mansoni* and *S. japonicum* infections, respectively. Praziquantel is approved by the US FDA for use in schistosomiasis. Gastrointestinal irritation is the major side effect of this generally well-tolerated drug. Another drug effective for *S. mansoni* infection is oxamniquine, used in mass treatment programs in Africa and South America.

Mass treatment programs have become a central element in the efforts of many countries to combat schistosomiasis. For *S. mansoni* infection, a community-based strategy of mass chemotherapy followed by periodic surveillance with stool examinations and prompt treatment of any reinfections has reduced morbidity and promoted resolution of ultrasonographic evidence of portal fibrosis [27]. Reducing new transmission by largely eliminating the contamination of water with shed parasite eggs underlies this approach. Although promising results have also been achieved in some *S. japonicum* endemic areas, adults in other treated communities show a persistence of hepatosplenomegaly and fibrosis even with decreased prevalence of infection [37]. The existence of numerous animal reservoirs of *S. japonicum* in other communities, coupled with the inability of stool examinations to detect all *S. japonicum* reinfections, suggests that in these locations, frequent mass retreatment would be more effective than surveillance by stool examination for reinfection. In addition, parasitologic cure followed by prompt reinfection might produce a rebound of the relatively severe inflammatory and fibrotic events that accompany acute infection rather than the persistence of a modulated, relatively less damaging long-term response. In such a situation, it may be especially important to maintain effective mass retreatment once a decision has been made to begin community-based therapy.

There are no clinical data to suggest that specific therapy directed at fibrosis promotes any greater degree of resolution of schistosomal liver fibrosis in humans beyond what would normally be expected after the cure of active infection, as discussed in the preceding text. However, administration of the immunomodulating Th1 cytokine interferon-γ to schistosome-infected mice, or promotion of its release by the inhibition of IL4, diminishes liver collagen deposition [38,39]. Schistosomes, along with all other multicellular parasites, continue to defy efforts to produce an effective antiparasitic vaccine. However, a combined antigen–cytokine vaccination concept may help limit parasite-induced host injury: sensitization of mice with *S. mansoni* eggs administered together with IL12 appears to prime the animals to respond with markedly diminished liver fibrosis when they are subsequently challenged with a schistosome infection [40].

Surgical therapy

Four major factors contribute to portal hypertension, increased collateral blood flow, and variceal enlargement in schistosomiasis [41]. They include: (i) portal fibrosis that produces presinusoidal obstruction of portal inflow; (ii) arterialization of abnormal vessels within the portal fibrous tissue that promotes increased hepatic arterial inflow; (iii) cellular infiltration of the spleen that adds to passive congestion to produce marked splenomegaly and increased splenic blood flow; and (iv) poorly understood functional disturbances that diminish splanchnic resistance and promote a hyperdynamic splanchnic circulation.

Nearly every form of medical and surgical therapy for bleeding varices has been advocated in schistosomiasis. Solid information to support evidence-based treatment decisions remains as elusive in schistosomiasis as it is for other causes of variceal bleeding. In the era before widespread variceal banding and transjugular intrahepatic portosystemic shunting (TIPS), the results of a randomized trial of schistosomal variceal bleeding treated with proximal splenorenal shunt, distal splenorenal shunt, and splenectomy with esophagogastric devascularization in schistosomiasis were reported [42] and critically reviewed [43]. Now that surgical shunts have been largely superseded by variceal banding [44] and TIPS, the remaining open surgical procedure that may be considered in experienced centers is splenectomy-devascularization for variceal bleeding refractory to endoscopic therapy. Devascularization may also be an appropriate option for persons at risk for variceal bleeding who require splenectomy for other indications. Propranolol decreases recurrent variceal bleeding in patients with schistosomiasis. In a report from Sudan, sustained-release propranalol at a single daily dose of 160 mg showed a 40% reduction in mortality after 2 years [45].

The general movement toward medical, endoscopic, and nonshunting surgical therapy for variceal bleeding in schistosomiasis shares common ground with the same trends and uncertainties that apply to other liver diseases. Key considerations in schistosomiasis include the frequent occurrence of marked splenomegaly, which has attracted interest in evaluating the potential benefits of complete or partial splenectomy, as well as concern about encephalopathy after shunting. Shunted patients require lifelong vigilant prevention of reinfection to avoid iatrogenic pulmonary egg deposition and the development of schistosomal-induced pulmonary hypertension and cor pulmonale. Pulmonary hypertension is a known problem even in nonshunted persons with hepatic schistosomiasis, potentially related to incomplete hepatic clearance of vasoactive compounds and mediators [46].

Fascioliasis

Fasciola hepatica is a trematode bile duct fluke with a worldwide distribution in sheep and cattle [47]. The leaf-shaped male and female adult worms reach a size of approximately 2 cm and may remain viable in the bile ducts for more than a decade. They produce eggs that pass in feces, hatch in water, and infect a snail as an intermediate host. Snails release a cercarial stage of the parasite that contaminates aquatic plants ingested by sheep, cattle, or humans. When ingested, transformed metacercariae penetrate the intestine, traverse the peritoneal cavity and liver capsule, and burrow through the liver parenchyma for 1–3 months while maturing, finally entering the bile ducts to become mature adults and complete the cycle. Heavy infection of sheep and cattle, called *liver rot*, is an important economic cause of livestock loss in areas where animals regularly consume aquatic vegetation. Humans with fascioliasis generally give a history of eating watercress or drinking potentially contaminated water. Human fascioliasis is prevalent in developing countries with humid climates and largely agrarian populations and is less frequently seen in Europe and North America. In the Nile delta of Egypt, there is a positive association between *Fasciola* and *S. mansoni* infections [48].

Acute fascioliasis is a febrile illness, typically of up to 3 months duration, presenting with right upper quadrant discomfort and hepatomegaly. As immature flukes continue their course through the liver parenchyma, they leave behind a track of coagulation necrosis infiltrated by an intense eosinophilic inflammatory response. In sheep with experimental fascioliasis, the ability of the parasite to keep moving ahead of the host inflammatory response appears to allow it to literally outrun what would otherwise be an effective host defense [49]. The resulting tracks show a characteristic appearance of yellow-white serpiginous subcapsular cords at laparoscopy [50]. On CT, the tracks appear as tortuous linear arrays of small, 1–3 cm abscess-like lesions [51].

In acute fascioliasis, fever, leukocytosis, and right upper quadrant pain are each present in approximately two thirds of patients, and eosinophilia in the 15–65% range is a regular finding. Atypical manifestations of acute fascioliasis may result when penetration of the ductal system causes hemobilia or discrete abscess formation [52], or as reported in a Chilean patient, when a multisystem vasculitis occurred that resolved with cure of the infection [53]. Immature flukes that fail to migrate into the liver can produce ectopic masses or abscesses in many locations, most commonly appearing as subcutaneous nodules with an eosinophilic infiltrate surrounding the degenerating parasite tissues. In addition, a syndrome of eosinophilic pleuritis and pericarditis without direct parasitic involvement of these structures may accompany acute fascioliasis.

After bile duct penetration by mature flukes, egg production initiates chronic fascioliasis. Host responses to adult worms are limited to local inflammation, ductal epithelial proliferation, and fibrous thickening of the duct wall. *Fasciola* produces proline, a key precursor of collagen, as a major nitrogen excretion product. Animal experiments suggest that high local concentrations of proline in fascioliasis may promote ductal hyperplasia and fibrosis [54]. Large numbers of adult flukes in the ductal system may precipitate episodes of acute biliary obstruction and cholangitis. In addition to visualization of the adult flukes, dilated ducts may be seen by ultrasonography, CT, or cholangiography. CT is the preferred imaging study during the acute intrahepatic phase and ultrasonography is most effective for visualization of the mature flukes in the bile ducts [55].

Fever and right upper quadrant abdominal pain in acute fascioliasis, or biliary symptoms in chronic infection, coupled with a consistent dietary history, suggest the possibility of fascioliasis. Eosinophilia and consistent imaging findings strongly support the diagnosis. An ELISA test has high diagnostic accuracy and is especially useful during the initial stage of infection before adult flukes appear in the bile ducts and begin egg production [56]. Stool examination for eggs is useful only in chronic disease and may be negative when egg output is intermittent.

Bithionol has been the most widely used antihelminthic compound for fascioliasis. It is given in courses of 10–30 days for acute and chronic infections. Gastrointestinal irritation is common; rash, leukopenia, and hepatotoxicity are less frequent; and retreatment may be attempted for nonresponders to an initial course of therapy.

Triclabendazole, a benzamidazole compound widely used in veterinary practice, appears to be more effective and less toxic than bithionol in humans with fascioliasis [57]. Limited quantities of bithionol are available in the United States from the Centers for Disease Control and Prevention parasitic drug service as an investigational drug. Triclabendazole, the preferred agent, may now be imported for investigational human use in the United States with FDA approval of an expedited individual use request.

Clonorchiasis and opisthorchiasis

Clonorchis sinensis, Opisthorchis viverrini, and *O. felineus* are bile duct flukes acquired by humans who eat raw fish containing the parasite's infective metacercaria stage. Human hosts excrete eggs that hatch in water and pass through snail and fish stages to infect new humans and animals. With a size of approximately 1 cm and a ventral sucker that permits attachment to the intrahepatic bile duct epithelium, male and female adult flukes have life spans of 10 years or more. *C. sinensis* infects persons in China, Korea, and elsewhere in East Asia. *O. viverrini* has a more limited range in Thailand, Laos, and Cambodia but shows very high prevalence in northeast Thailand, where one third of the population is infected [58]. *O. felineus* infects cats and humans in limited areas of Russia and eastern Europe.

Most infected persons have relatively light parasite burdens of 100 or fewer worms. For *O. viverrini* infection, there is a strong quantitative relationship between the number of eggs excreted per gram of stool and a host's burden of adult worms. A new PCR-based fecal test as an alternative for microscopic stool examination may facilitate the screening of large populations. Study of the intensity of infection in population-based samples has provided strong evidence to support the linkage of bile duct fluke infection with chronic biliary tract abnormalities and with the ultimate development of cholangiocarcinoma, a leading cause of cancer deaths in endemic areas. In surveys using ultrasonography, the intensity of infection is strongly correlated with the occurrence of gallbladder enlargement and wall irregularity, biliary sludge, and enhanced portal tract echogenicity [59]. For cholangiocarcinoma in northeastern Thailand, a locality-adjusted odds ratio of 14.1 was found for male residents with the highest intensity of *O. viverrini* infection; 4% of the surveyed male population with more than 6,000 eggs/g feces had the malignancy [60].

The bile ducts that harbor adult *Clonorchis* or *Opisthorchis* worms can show dilatation, irregular thickening, and adenomatous epithelial hyperplasia (Fig. 39.4). Some of these changes may be reversible, especially after treatment of light or early infection. Ten months after eliminating *O. viverrini* infection with praziquan-

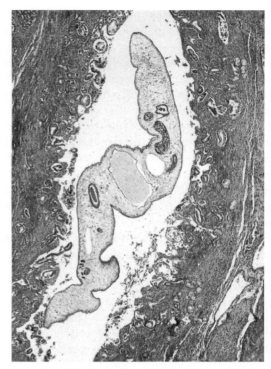

Figure 39.4 Clonorchiasis, showing a dilated intrahepatic bile duct containing an adult worm cut in cross-section. The ductal epithelium shows adenomatous hyperplasia. H&E, original ×40. (AFIP negative 72-11587.)

tel treatment, repeated ultrasonographic study of 72 persons showed resolution of gallbladder enlargement, improved gallbladder contractility, and decreases in visible sludge and portal tract echogenicity [61]. However, repeat endoscopic cholangiography at an average interval of 32 months in persons treated for *C. sinensis* infection showed some improvement in the appearance of the intrahepatic ducts and loss of the filling defects caused by the presence of adult worms but no changes in measured duct enlargement or the presence of duct wall irregularities [62]. Adenomatous hyperplasia of the papilla in chronic clonorchiasis can produce radiographic duct abnormalities indistinguishable from those of cholangiocarcinoma.

The development of cholangiocarcinoma appears to reflect the interaction of multiple processes. For example, *O. viverrini*-infected persons with ultrasonographic biliary abnormalities have increased activity of cytochrome P450 2A6, an enzyme that promotes activation of carcinogenic nitrosamines [63]. Administration of the carcinogen dimethylnitrosamine to *C. sinensis*-infected hamsters resulted in the development of cholangiocarcinomas that did not occur in uninfected animals or in infected animals not exposed to dimethylnitrosamine [64]. In a comparison of the histopathology of fluke-associated and sporadic cholangiocarcinomas, the fluke-associated tumors more frequently showed cells with an intestinal goblet cell phenotype by immunostaining and overexpression of p53 antigenic protein compared with sporadic cancers occurring in persons outside endemic areas [65]. Although the morbidity associated with biliary fluke infection before the development of cholangiocarcinoma appears to be slight in most persons, the outlook is very poor in those who present with the tumor with expected survival measured in months, similar to that for sporadically occurring cholangiocarcinoma. With the currently available information, prevention would appear to depend both on persuading residents of areas with high prevalence of infection and cholangiocarcinoma to modify their dietary habits, and eliminating existing infection with praziquantel, an easily administered and effective curative drug [58]. Screening and parasitologic cure of immigrants to western countries, who are at high risk for infection, is also warranted.

Oriental cholangiohepatitis is a chronic illness marked by episodes of cholangitis with the formation of multiple pigment stones, irregular bile duct dilatation with a predilection for disproportionate severity in the left hepatic ductal system, and the formation of multiple strictures [66,67]. Its geographic range corresponds roughly to that of bile duct flukes and *Ascaris* infection. Figure 39.5 shows a cholangiogram from a patient with this condition and associated clonorchiasis. In many patients with severe distortion of the ductal system, recurrent

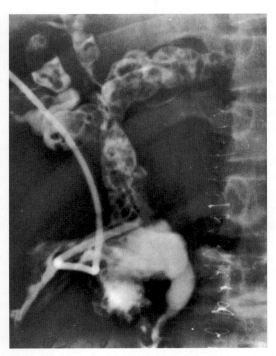

Figure 39.5 Oriental cholangiohepatitis associated with clonorchiasis. The cholangiogram shows a dilated, distorted intrahepatic ductal system with contrast material outlining numerous filling defects that represent adult *Clonorchis sinensis* flukes. (AFIP negative 96-22949.)

episodes of cholangitis appear to be self-perpetuating in the absence of active parasitic infection. Helminth infection should be sought and eliminated in persons with the disease. In addition, recurrences due to obstructing stones were reported to be more easily managed in patients who had placement of a Roux-en-Y jejunal conduit for biliary access [68]. When hepatolithiasis and strictures mainly involve the left hepatic lobe, laparoscopic left hepatectomy combined with choledoscopic removal of right lobe stones is reported to be effective [69].

Echinococcosis

Echinococcosis, or hydatid disease, develops in humans when they become accidental hosts for a cystic intermediate stage of one of three canine tapeworms, *Echinococcus granulosus*, *E. multilocularis*, or *E. vogeli*. Humans become infected by eating food contaminated with eggs excreted by domestic or wild dogs or other canines such as foxes, coyotes, and wolves [70]. The parasite normally multiplies as a larval scolex stage within cysts in the solid organs of herbivores or rodents that have consumed excreted eggs. Consumption of the cyst-containing viscera of these animals by new canines completes the cycle.

Hydatid disease most often affects humans in contact with sheep-herding dogs infected with *E. granulosus*. The resulting cystic hydatid disease has a worldwide distribution. *E. multilocularis* infection, concentrated mainly in the Arctic and sub-Arctic regions of the northern hemisphere, causes human alveolar hydatid disease. *E. vogeli*, the cause of human polycystic hydatid disease, has a very limited range in Central and South America.

Hydatid liver cysts caused by *E. granulosus*, as shown in Fig. 39.6, are most often asymptomatic. They are fluid-filled structures delimited by a parasite-derived membrane (Fig. 39.7A) that contain germinal epithelium that buds viable scoleces (Fig. 39.7B). Imaging by ultrasonography, CT (see Fig. 39.6), or MRI may demonstrate the formation of daughter cysts, cyst wall calcification, and compression and fibrous reaction of the surrounding liver parenchyma. Imaging may also show in complicated disease communication of the cyst with the biliary system or external leakage of cyst material. The cysts formed in *E. multilocularis* infection are less well delimited. They tend to invade the liver parenchyma and seed adjacent organs and structures with scoleces and daughter cysts [71]. The polycystic hydatid disease of *E. vogeli* infection shows well-delimited multiple cysts.

Cystic hydatid disease now most often presents as a hepatic mass with a typical appearance on abdominal imaging, coupled with confirmatory serologic testing by indirect hemagglutination or ELISA, which is positive in approximately 90% of hydatid cysts. As discussed above, no fecal eggs are present in human hosts. Eosinophilia is usually present. Biliary or peritoneal extension or

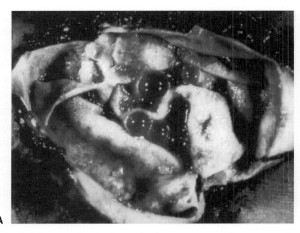
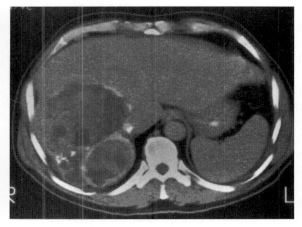

Figure 39.6 (A) Hepatic hydatid cyst of *Echinococcus granulosus*, opened to show folds of the pale, thickened germinal membrane associated with translucent budding daughter cysts. (AFIP negative 95-82642.) (B) Hepatic hydatid cyst of *Echinococcus granulosus*. A computed tomographic image showing a large cyst in the posterior right lobe of the liver with a complex internal structure similar to the cyst shown in (A) and areas of wall calcification. (AFIP negative 92-84646.)

pulmonary cystic disease is usually easily recognized; however, ectopic cysts in the kidney, spleen, brain, orbit, heart, and bone may produce unusual findings. Uncommon presentations of hydatid disease include segmental portal hypertension due to splenic vein compression by a cyst in the splenic hilum, with adjacent perihilar varix formation [72], and rupture of a hepatic cyst causing inferior vena cava thrombosis [73].

Until recently, most hydatid cysts came to clinical attention because of symptomatic enlargement, so that their management by surgical excision was a straightforward decision. Palliative resections for the spreading, poorly contained cysts of *E. multilocularis*-induced alveolar hydatid disease were often inadequate to deal with this frequently lethal disease. Now that many hydatid cysts are detected as incidental findings during abdominal imaging, and newer forms of medical and surgical therapy for hydatid disease are being reported, therapeutic options are at once more promising and more challenging.

After initial evaluation of the benzimidazole antihelminthic compound mebendazole, a related compound, albendazole, has become the current standard for medical therapy of hydatid disease [74]. Albendazole has strong scolicidal activity for *E. granulosus* and *E. multilocularis* and superior absorption, bioavailability, and distribution into hydatid cysts compared with mebendazole. Albendazole is an effective preoperative adjunct for disrupting the viability of *E. granulosus* and *E. multilocularis* cysts and in improving resectability in the latter disease. Albendazole as primary therapy, either alone or in combination with praziquantel, has been advocated for

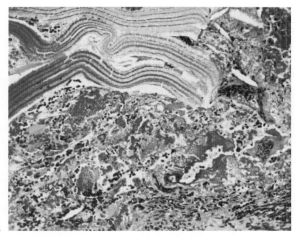
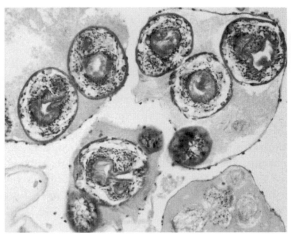

Figure 39.7 (A) Hepatic hydatid cyst of *Echinococcus granulosus* showing a laminated membrane at the top, and debris within the cyst. H&E, original ×160. (AFIP negative 82-12615.) (B) Hepatic hydatid cyst of *E. granulosus* showing viable scoleces cut in cross-section. H&E, original ×250. (AFIP negative 82-12530.)

noninvasive therapy of small uncomplicated *E. granulosus* cysts [75]. In an extensive series of 929 cysts in 448 persons treated with mebendazole or albendazole with up to 14 years follow-up, approximately one in four cysts recurred after initial resolution or regression [76]. Recurrence was greatest within 2 years of resolution. Albendazole, approved for use in the United States, is generally administered two to three times daily with food at doses ranging from 10 to 50 mg/kg per day, for 12–24 weeks or longer, with or without intervening rest periods. Toxicity includes variable alopecia and, in many patients, minor elevations in aminotransferase levels as well as transient pain perceived at the location of a cyst on the initiation of treatment. Elevation of aminotransferase levels more than four times normal or leukopenia requires discontinuing albendazole.

Traditional surgical therapy for hepatic *E. granulosus* cysts at laparotomy includes: isolation by packing; careful aspiration of cyst fluid to avoid spillage of viable scoleces or anaphylaxis; injection of the cyst with hypertonic saline, alcohol, or dilute silver nitrate to kill the scolices if the aspirated fluid is crystal clear; and resection of either the cyst alone or both the cyst and its pericystic rim of compressed liver tissue [77]. Aspiration of turbid cyst fluid suggests a biliary communication so that injection with potential sclerosants is avoided. The use of percutaneous drainage, described in the subsequent text, for an increasing proportion of patients with relatively simple cysts, has left the remaining patients who now come to open surgery as a population with relatively greater aggregate complexity and technical challenge than those of earlier surgical series.

Laparoscopic evacuation [78] and ultrasound-guided percutaneous drainage [79] are reported to be safe and effective for treating uncomplicated cystic hydatid disease. Percutaneous drainage has become the first-line management for cystic hydatid disease in many centers. The most extensive current experience is with an ultrasound-guided four-step PAIR process of: (i) *p*uncture; (ii) *a*spiration; (iii) *i*njection with hypertonic saline, silver nitrate, or other scolicidal solution; and (iv) *r*e-aspiration, with one or more days of subsequent percutaneous catheter drainage for large cysts. Patients normally receive a 10-day preprocedure course of oral albendazole, and are given antihistamine and steroid coverage for the procedure to minimize anaphylaxis in the event of cyst leakage at puncture, followed by continued albendazole for 2 months after the procedure. Advantages of the PAIR technique include minimal disability and early return to full activity, with a 1–2-day length of hospital stay compared to a typical 2-week stay after open cyst evacuation. In contrast to primary medical therapy without aspiration and drainage, the PAIR technique has the advantages of a much shorter duration of 2 months of adjunctive albendazole therapy postprocedure, compared with up to 6 months or more for albendazole as the primary treatment, as well as a minimal recurrence rate compared with a recurrence of 25% of cysts treated medically alone. PAIR and laparoscopic cyst evacuation in experienced centers have both shown low morbidity, with anaphylaxis being the most significant problem in the 1–2% range, which is generally easily managed in pretreated patients, and the potential for bleeding or duct injury common to all liver punctures. Communication of cysts with the biliary system due to rupture may be suspected when cholestasis or cholangitis are present. This problem, which tends to occur more often in larger cysts of 7.5 cm or greater diameter, may be identified by endoscopic cholangiopancreatography (ERCP) or magnetic resonance cholangiopancreatography (MRCP), and can often be managed with endoscopic drainage [80,81].

Patients with alveolar hydatid disease due to *E. multilocularis* have an infection whose biologic behavior resembles that of a malignant tumor as its complex cystic structures invade the liver parenchyma and spread by direct extension to adjacent sites. Albendazole therapy is administered in an effort to stabilize unresectable disease, or as an adjunct to liver resection, which may cure early localized disease. Alveolar hydatid disease may require multiple surgical procedures in an attempt to deal with severe complications such as hepatic vein compression and thrombosis, and secondary sclerosing cholangitis. Similar major problems occur much less frequently in cystic hydatid disease. Liver transplantation for patients with end-stage alveolar or cystic hydatid disease often presents a technical challenge related to extensive prior surgery, but transplantation may produce a good long-term outcome in patients whose disease has progressed beyond the point of cure or control by other methods [82,83].

Annotated references

Arjona R, Riancho JA, Aguado JM, et al. Fascioliasis in developed countries: a review of classic and aberrant forms of the disease. *Medicine* 1995;74:13–23.
An excellent clinical review including 20 patients from the authors' hospital showing the full spectrum of acute and chronic fascioliasis.

Khuroo MS, Wani NA, Javid G, et al. Percutaneous drainage compared with surgery for hepatic hydatid cysts. *N Engl J Med* 1997;337:881–7.
Well-conducted comparative study showing the advantage of percutaneous drainage combined with adjunctive albendazole therapy.

Murray HW, Berman JD, Davies CR, et al. Advances in leishmaniasis. *Lancet* 2005;366:1561–77.
Concise review of mechanisms, clinical manifestations, and management of visceral leishmaniasis.

Ross AGP, Bartley PB, Sleigh AC, et al. Current concepts: schistosomiasis. *N Engl J Med* 2002;346:1212–20.
A review of the epidemiology, transmission, clinical manifestations, therapy, and prospects for public health control of schistosomiasis.

Shah OJ, Ali Zargar S, Robbani I. Biliary ascariasis: a review. *World J Surg* 2006;30:1500–6.
Clinical review of the occurrence, presentation, and medical, endoscopic, and surgical therapy of an ubiquitous intestinal roundworm infection that occasionally involves an abnormal biliary system.

References

1. Mueller AK, Labaied M, Kappe SH, et al. Genetically modified *Plasmodium* parasites as a protective experimental malaria vaccine. *Nature* 2005;433:164–7.
2. Roland J, Soulard V, Sellier C, et al. NK cell responses to *Plasmodium* infection and control of intrahepatic parasite development. *J Immunol* 2006;177:1229–39.
3. Srivastava A, Khanduri A, Lakhtakia S, et al. Falciparum malaria with acute liver failure. *Trop Gastroenterol* 1996;17:172–4.
4. Murray HW, Berman JD, Davies CR, et al. Advances in leishmaniasis. *Lancet* 2005;366:1561–77.
5. Magill AJ, Grogl M, Gasser RA Jr, et al. Visceral infection caused by *Leishmania tropica* in veterans of operation desert storm. *N Engl J Med* 1993;328:1383–7.
6. Myles O, Wortmann G, Cummings JF, et al. Visceral leishmaniasis: clinical observations in 4 US Army soldiers deployed to Afghanistan or Iraq, 2002–2004. *Arch Intern Med* 2007;167:1899–901.
7. Pitta MGR, Romano A, Cabantous S, et al. IL-17 and IL-22 are associated with protection against human kala azar caused by *Leishmania donovani*. *J Clin Invest* 2009;119:2379–87.
8. El Hag IA, Hashim FA, El Toum IA, et al. Liver morphology and function in visceral leishmaniasis (kala-azar). *J Clin Pathol* 1994;47:547–51.
9. Rogers L. A peculiar intralobular cirrhosis of the liver produced by the protozoal parasite of kala-azar. *Ann Trop Med Parasitol* 1908;2:147–52.
10. Pintado V, Martin-Rabadan P, Rivera ML, et al. Visceral leishmaniasis in human immunodeficiency virus (HIV)-infected and non-HIV-infected patients. A comparative study. *Medicine* 2001;80:54–73.
11. Albrecht H, Sobottka I, Emminger C, et al. Visceral leishmaniasis emerging as an important opportunistic infection in HIV-infected persons living in areas nonendemic for *Leishmania donovani*. *Arch Pathol Lab Med* 1996;120:189–98.
12. Horber FF, Lerut JP, Reichen J, et al. Visceral leishmaniasis after orthotopic liver transplantation: impact of persistent splenomegaly. *Transplant Int* 1993;6:55–7.
13. Bassetti M, Pizzorni C, Gradoni L, et al. Visceral leishmaniasis infection in a rheumatoid arthritis patient treated with adalimumab. *Rheumatology* 2006;45:1446–8.
14. Sundar S, Chakravarty J, Agarwal D, et al. Single-dose liposomal amphotericin B for visceral leishmaniasis in India. *N Engl J Med* 2010;362:504–12.
15. del Guidice P, Mary-Krause M, Paradier C, et al. Impact of highly active antiretroviral therapy on the incidence of visceral leishmaniasis in a French cohort of patients infected with human immunodeficiency virus. *J Infect Dis* 2002;186:1366–70.
16. Shah OJ, Ali Zargar S, Robbani I. Biliary ascariasis: a review. *World J Surg* 2006;30:1500–6.
17. Ross AGP, Bartley PB, Sleigh AC, et al. Current concepts: schistosomiasis. *N Engl J Med* 2002;346:1212–20.
18. Shaker YM, Wu CH, El-Shobaki FA, et al. Human portal serum stimulates cell proliferation in immature *Schistosoma mansoni*. *Parasitology* 1998;117:293–9.
19. Symmers WSC. Note on a new form of liver cirrhosis due to the presence of ova of *Bilharzia haematobium*. *J Pathol Bacteriol* 1904;9:237–9.
20. Pearce EJ, MacDonald AS. The immunobiology of schistosomiasis. *Nat Rev Immunol* 2002;2:499–511.
21. Wynn TA, Thompson RW, Cheever AW, et al. Immunopathogenesis of schistosomiasis. *Immunol Rev* 2004;201:156–67.
22. Rutitzky LI, Bazzone L, Shainheit MG, et al. IL-23 is required for the development of severe egg-induced immunopathology in schistosomiasis and for lesional expression of IL-17. *J Immunol* 2008;180:2486–95.
23. Dessein AJ, Hillaire D, Elwali NE, et al. Severe hepatic fibrosis in *Schistosoma mansoni* infection is controlled by a major locus that is closely linked to the interferon-gamma receptor gene. *Am J Hum Genet* 1999;65:709–21.
24. Bartley PB, Ramm GA, Jones MK, et al. A contributory role for activated hepatic stellate cells in the dynamics of *Schistosoma japonicum* egg-induced fibrosis. *Int J Parasitol* 2006;36:993–1001.
25. Friedman SL. Mechanisms of hepatic fibrogenesis. *Gastroenterology* 2008;134:1655–69.
26. Dunn MA, Cheever AW, Paglia LM, et al. Reversal of advanced liver fibrosis in rabbits with schistosomiasis japonica. *Am J Trop Med Hyg* 1994;50:499–505.
27. Homeida MA, El Tom I, Nash T, et al. Association of the therapeutic activity of praziquantel with the reversal of Symmers' fibrosis induced by *Schistosoma mansoni*. *Am J Trop Med Hyg* 1991;45:360–5.
28. King CH, Dickman K, Tisch DJ. Reassessment of the cost of chronic helminthic infection: a meta-analysis of disability-related outcomes in endemic schistosomiasis. *Lancet* 2005;365:1561–9.
29. Kamel R, Dunn MA, Skelly RR, et al. Clinical and immunologic results of segmental splenectomy in schistosomiasis. *Br J Surg* 1986;73:544–7.
30. Petroianu A. Subtotal splenectomy and portal variceal disconnection in the treatment of portal hypertension. *Can J Surg* 1993;36:251–4.
31. Andrade ZA, Neves Abreu W. Follicular lymphoma of the spleen in patients with hepatosplenic schistosomiasis mansoni. *Am J Trop Med Hyg* 1971;20:237–43.
32. Lambertucci JR, Rayes AA, Serufo JC, et al. Schistosomiasis and associated infections. *Mem Inst Oswaldo Cruz* 1998;93(Suppl 1):135–9.
33. Kallestrup P, Zinyama R, Gomo E, et al. Schistosomiasis and HIV-1 infection in rural Zimbabwe: effect of treatment of schistosomiasis on CD4 cell count and plasma HIV-1RNA load. *J Infect Dis* 2005;152:1956–61.
34. Kamel MA, Miller FD, El Masry AG, et al. The epidemiology of *Schistosoma mansoni*, hepatitis B and hepatitis C infection in Egypt. *Ann Trop Med Parasitol* 1994;88:501–9.
35. Strickland GT. Liver disease in Egypt: hepatitis C superseded schistosomiasis as a result of iatrogenic and biological factors. *Hepatology* 2006;43:915–22.
36. Kamal SM, Rasenack JW, Bianchi L, et al. Acute hepatitis C without and with schistosomiasis: correlation with hepatitis C-specific CD4+ T-cell and cytokine response. *Gastroenterology* 2001;121:646–56.
37. West PM, Wu G, Zhong S, et al. Schistosomiasis on Jishan Island, Jiangxi Province, People's Republic of China: prevalence of hepatic fibrosis after reduction of the prevalence of infection with age. *Trans R Soc Trop Med Hyg* 1993;87:290–4.
38. Czaja MJ, Weiner FR, Takahashi S, et al. γ-Interferon treatment inhibits collagen deposition in murine schistosomiasis. *Hepatology* 1989;10:795–800.
39. Cheever AW, Finkelman FD, Cox TM. Anti-interleukin-4 treatment diminishes secretion of Th2 cytokines and inhibits hepatic fibrosis in murine schistosomiasis japonica. *Parasite Immunol* 1995;17:103–9.
40. Wynn TA, Cheever AW, Jankovic D, et al. An IL-12-based vaccination method for preventing fibrosis induced by schistosome infection. *Nature* 1995;376:594–6.
41. Denie C, Vachiery F, Elman A, et al. Systemic and splanchnic hemodynamic changes in patients with hepatosplenic schistosomiasis. *Liver* 1996;16:309–12.
42. Raia S, Da Silva LC, Gayotto LCC, et al. Portal hypertension in schistosomiasis: a long-term follow-up of a randomized trial comparing three types of surgery. *Hepatology* 1994;20:398–403.

43. Conn HO. A randomized comparison of three types of surgery in schistosomal portal hypertension: many fewer answers than questions. *Hepatology* 1994;20:526–8.

44. Siqueira ES, Rohr MR, Libera ED, et al. Band ligation or sclerotherapy as endoscopic treatment for oesophageal varices in schistosomotic patients: results of a randomized study. *HPB Surg* 1998;11:27–32.

45. El Tourabi H, El Amin AA, Shaheen M, et al. Propranolol reduces mortality in patients with portal hypertension secondary to schistosomiasis. *Ann Trop Med Parasitol* 1994;88:493–500.

46. Lapa M, Dias B, Jardim C, et al. Cardiopulmonary manifestations of hepatosplenic schistosomiasis. *Circulation* 2009;119:1518–23.

47. Arjona R, Riancho JA, Aguado JM, et al. Fascioliasis in developed countries: a review of classic and aberrant forms of the disease. *Medicine* 1995;74:13–23.

48. Esteban JG, Gonzalez C, Curtale F, et al. Hyperendemic fascioliasis associated with schistosomiasis in villages in the Nile Delta of Egypt. *Am J Trop Med Hyg* 2003;69:429–37.

49. Meeusen E, Rickard MD, Brandon MR. Cellular responses during liver fluke infection in sheep and its evasion by the parasite. *Parasite Immunol* 1995;17:37–45.

50. Moreto M, Barron J. The laparascopic diagnosis of the liver fascioliasis. *Gastrointest Endosc* 1980;26:147–9.

51. Van Beers B, Pringot J, Geubel A, et al. Hepatobiliary fascioliasis: noninvasive imaging findings. *Radiology* 1990;174:809–10.

52. Kim JB, Kim DJ, Huh S, et al. A human case of invasive fascioliasis associated with liver abscess. *Korean J Parasitol* 1995;33:395–8.

53. Llanos C, Sabugo F, Gallegos I, et al. Systemic vasculitis associated with *Fasciola hepatica* infection. *Scand J Rheumatol* 2006;35:143–6.

54. Isseroff H, Sawma JT, Reino D. Fascioliasis: role of proline in bile duct hyperplasia. *Science* 1977;198:1157–9.

55. Kabaalioglu A, Ceken K, Alimoglu E, et al. Hepatobiliary fascioliasis: sonographic and CT findings in 87 patients during the initial phase and long-term follow-up. *Am J Roentgenol* 2007;189:824–8.

56. O'Neill SM, Parkinson M, Strauss W, et al. Immunodiagnosis of *Fasciola hepatica* infection (fascioliasis) in a human population in the Bolivian Altiplano using purified cathepsin L cysteine proteinase. *Am J Trop Med Hyg* 1998;58:417–23.

57. Fairweather I. Triclabendazole progress report, 2005–2009: an advancement of learning? *J Helminthol* 2009;83:139–50.

58. Sithithaworn P, Haswell-Elkins M, Mairiang P, et al. Parasite-associated morbidity: liver fluke infection and bile duct cancer in northeast Thailand. *Int J Parasitol* 1994;24:833–43.

59. Elkins DB, Mairiang E, Sithithaworn P, et al. Cross-sectional patterns of hepatobiliary abnormalities and possible precursor conditions of cholangiocarcinoma associated with *Opisthorchis viverrini* infection in humans. *Am J Trop Med Hyg* 1996;55:295–301.

60. Haswell-Elkins MR, Mairiang E, Mairiang P, et al. Cross-sectional study of *Opisthorchis viverrini* infection and cholangiocarcinoma in communities within a high-risk area in northeast Thailand. *Int J Cancer* 1994;59:505–9.

61. Mairiang E, Haswell-Elkins MR, Mairiang P, et al. Reversal of biliary tract abnormalities associated with *Opisthorchis viverrini* infection following praziquantel treatment. *Trans R Soc Trop Med Hyg* 1993;87:194–7.

62. Leung JWC, Sung Y, Banez VP, et al. Endoscopic cholangiopancreatography in hepatic clonorchiasis – a follow-up study. *Gastrointest Endosc* 1990;36:360–3.

63. Satarug S, Lang MA, Yongvanit P, et al. Induction of cytochrome P450 2A6 expression in humans by the carcinogenic parasite infection, opisthorchiasis viverrini. *Cancer Epidemiol Biomarkers Prev* 1996;5:795–800.

64. Lee J-H, Rim H-J, Bak U-B. Effect of *Clonorchis sinensis* infection and dimethylnitrosamine administration on the induction of cholangiocarcinoma in Syrian golden hamsters. *Korean J Parasitol* 1993;31:21–30.

65. Hughes NR, Pairojkul C, Royce SG, et al. Liver fluke-associated and sporadic cholangiocarcinoma: an immunohistochemical study of bile duct, peribiliary gland and tumour phenotypes. *J Clin Pathol* 2006;59:1073–8.

66. Lim JH. Oriental cholangiohepatitis: pathologic, clinical and radiologic features. *Am J Roentgenol* 1991;157:1–8.

67. Sperling RM, Koch J, Sandlin JS, et al. Recurrent pyogenic cholangitis in Asian immigrants to the United States: natural history and role of therapeutic ERCP. *Dig Dis Sci* 1997;42:865–71.

68. Gott PE, Tieva MH, Barcia PJ, et al. Biliary access procedure in the management of oriental cholangiohepatitis. *Am Surg* 1996;62:930–4.

69. Tu JF, Jiang FZ, Zhu HL, et al. Laparoscopic vs open hepatectomy for hepatolithiasis. *World J Surg* 2010;16:2818–23.

70. Bastani B, Dehdashti F. Hepatic hydatid disease in Iran, with review of the literature. *Mt Sinai J Med* 1995;62:62–9.

71. Ammann RW. Swiss Echinococcosis Study Group. Improvement of liver resectional therapy by adjuvant chemotherapy in alveolar hydatid disease. *Parasitol Res* 1991;77:290–3.

72. El Fortia M, Bendaoud M, Taema S, et al. Segmental portal hypertension due to a splenic *Echinococcus* cyst. *Eur J Ultrasound* 2000;11:21–3.

73. Anuradha S, Agarwal SK, Khatri S, et al. Spontaneous rupture of hepatic hydatid cyst causing inferior vena cava thrombosis. *Indian J Gastroenterol* 1999;18:34.

74. Falagas ME, Bliziotis JA. Albendazole for the treatment of human echinococcosis: a review of comparative clinical trials. *Am J Med Sci* 2007;334:171–9.

75. Mohamed AE, Yasawy MI, Al Karawi MA. Combined albendazole and praziquantel versus albendazole alone in the treatment of hydatid disease. *Hepatogastroenterology* 1998;45:1690–4.

76. Franchi C, Di Vico B, Teggi A. Long-term evaluation of patients with hydatidosis treated with benzimidazole carbamates. *Clin Infect Dis* 1999;29:304–9.

77. Alonso Casado O, Moreno Gonzalez E, Loinaz Segurola C, et al. Results of 22 years of experience in radical surgical treatment of hepatic hydatid cysts. *Hepatogastroenterology* 2001;48:235–43.

78. Chen W, Xusheng BA. Laparoscopic techniques in patients with hydatid cysts. *Am J Surg* 2007;194:243–7.

79. Khuroo MS, Wani NA, Javid G, et al. Percutaneous drainage compared with surgery for hepatic hydatid cysts. *N Engl J Med* 1997;337:881–7.

80. Kilic M, Yoldas O, Koc M., et al. Can biliary-cyst communication be predicted before surgery for hepatic hydatid disease: does size matter? *Am J Surg* 2008;196:732–5.

81. Erden A, Ormeci N, Fitoz S, et al. Intrabiliary rupture of hydatid cysts: diagnostic accuracy of MR cholangiopancreatography. *Am J Roentgenol* 2007;189:W84–9.

82. Bresson-Hadni S, Franza A, Miguet JP, et al. Orthotopic liver transplantation for incurable alveolar echinococcosis of the liver: report of 17 cases. *Hepatology* 1991;13:1061–70.

83. Moreno-Gonzalez E, Loinaz Segurola C, Garcia Urena MA, et al. Liver transplantation for *Echinococcus granulosus* hydatid disease. *Transplantation* 1994;58:797–800.

Multiple choice questions

39.1 Factors that cause portal hypertension and predispose to variceal bleeding in hepatic schistosomiasis include which combination of the following?

1 Presinusoidal obstruction of portal inflow.
2 Cellular infiltration of the spleen with passive congestion and increased splenic blood flow.
3 Arterialization of abnormal vessels within portal fibrous tissue.
4 Functional decrease in splanchic resistance with a hyperdynamic splanchnic circulation.
   a 1 and 3 only.
   b 1, 2, and 3.
   c 2 and 4 only.
   d 1, 2, 3, and 4.

39.2 This parasitic liver disease can persist as a latent asymptomatic infection for many years in immunocompetent hosts. Within its geographic range it is recognized as an AIDS-defining illness in HIV-infected persons who develop immunosuppression. Choose the one correct answer.

a Fascioliasis.
b Alveolar echinococcosis.
c Visceral leishmaniasis.
d Clonorchiasis.

Answers to the multiple choice questions can be found in the Appendix at the end of the book.

These multiple choice questions are also available for you to complete online.
Visit http://www.schiffsdiseasesoftheliver.com/

CHAPTER 40

Granulomas of the Liver

James H. Lewis

Department of Hepatology, Georgetown University Medical Center, Washington, DC, USA

Key concepts

- Hepatic granulomas are found in 2–10% of liver biopsy series, and represent a localized inflammatory response to a variety of infectious, immunologic, drug-induced, neoplastic, and nonmicrobial chemical and foreign body irritants. Both genders and all ages can be affected.
- While dozens of causes have been reported, worldwide the most common are tuberculosis and sarcoidosis, reflecting geographic differences in disease prevalence. Primary biliary cirrhosis represents the predominant cause of granulomas in several western population studies. More than 60 drugs have been associated with a granulomatous reaction, many of which are associated with a hypersensitivity reaction (e.g., allopurinol, sulfonamides, phenylbutazone, phenothiazines, carbamazepine).
- Two main types of granulomas are found: lipogranulomas that form around fat droplets associated with the ingestion of mineral oil, waxes, and other lipid materials, and epithelioid granulomas that are often formed in response to a hypersensitivity reaction. A special form of lipogranuloma is the fibrin-ring granuloma seen with Q fever, allopurinol, and a few other causes. Necrotizing epithelioid granulomas are usually caused by mycobacteria or other infectious agents.
- Granulomas may be found as a coincidental lesion or may serve to confirm a variety of infectious or other disorders associated with their

development. They may be the only clue to the presence of certain infectious or neoplastic diseases, and occasionally are found as part of fever of unknown origin (FUO). Recent series still report that about 10% are considered "idiopathic" with no specific etiology able to be identified, even utilizing modern serologic and immunohistochemical methods.
- While biochemical tests are generally nonspecific, jaundice is unusual with most causes of granulomas, and should prompt a search for other etiologies. Certain histopathologic clues to the etiology of granulomas continue to be emphasized, such as sarcoidosis having multiple noncaseating granulomas of different ages; tuberculosis having caseating granulomas; many drugs and parasites being associated with surrounding eosinophils; and fibrin-ring granulomas suggesting Q fever or allopurinol exposure.
- Treatment of hepatic granulomas depends on their etiology and the degree of symptomatology. Chronic cholestatic liver disease leading to biliary cirrhosis may be seen in a small percentage of sarcoidosis patients. In general, however, granulomatous hepatic involvement due to most causes is nonprogressive. Drug-induced granulomas often resolve after the offending agent is withdrawn. Corticosteroid therapy has been helpful in certain cases of idiopathic granulomatous hepatitis causing FUO.

Granulomas are focal collections of epithelioid cells, including macrophages, mononuclear cells, and other inflammatory cells, that fuse together to form multinucleated giant cells in response to a variety of infectious, immunologic and neoplastic disorders, drugs, and nonmicrobial chemical irritants [1–3]. They are the end result of a complex interplay of inflammatory and immunologic factors [4], depending on the nature of the infectious or antigenic stimulus. The liver is a common location for granulomas due to its prominent blood supply that exposes most drugs, many infectious organisms, and other materials to its large numbers of reticuloendothelial (Kupffer) cells. When found, granulomas usually prompt a search for a specific etiology from a list that has grown

to include dozens of causes, as will be discussed. Hepatic granulomas are present in only approximately 3% of large modern-day liver biopsy series, with a range of 1–15%, varying by geographic location and disease prevalence (Table 40.1) [5–22]. This also appears to apply to pediatric populations from around the globe [23,24]. Granulomas may be an anticipated or incidental finding, reflecting either a primary hepatic disorder (approximately 5%), or seen as part of a systemic disease process with hepatic involvement (70–75%), including fever of unknown origin (FUO) [1,25–28].

A variety of disorders are associated with a granulomatous histologic response that can involve one or more organ systems [3,4]. Infections are the most common

Schiff's Diseases of the Liver, Eleventh Edition. Edited by Eugene R. Schiff, Willis C. Maddrey and Michael F. Sorrell.
© 2012 John Wiley & Sons, Ltd. Published 2012 by John Wiley & Sons, Ltd.

Table 40.1 Causes of hepatic granulomas by geographic location.

Study location	Years covered	Number of cases (% of liver bx)[a]	Etiology						Reference
			TB	Sarcoidosis	DILD	Miscellaneous[b]	PBC	Idiopathic[c]	
Cleveland	1966–1971	50 (2.4% of 2,086)	10%	22%	Up to 18%	14–32% (histoplasmosis 12%, cirrhosis 8%, lymphoma 6%)	–	36%	Mir-Madjlessi et al. 1973 [5]
London	1965–1975	138	2.5%	54%	–	17% (CLD 9%)	19%	10%	Neville et al. 1975 [6]
Spain	1971–1977	107	28%	18%	–	47% (Mediterrean fever 12%, infectious 15%)	–	7.4%	Vilaseca et al. 1979 [7]
South Carolina	1969–1978	95 (6% of 1,500)	8.5%	33%	29%	12% (visceral larva migrans 2%, fungal 1%, ceoplasm 3%)	–	12%	McMaster & Hennigar 1981 [8]
Glasgow	1970–1979	77	10%	10%	–	48% (CLD 15%, bile duct obstruction 9%, eoplasm 8%)	Excluded	11–31%	Cunningham et al. 1982 [9]
Australia	1968–1984	59	7%	12%	7%	45% (Q fever 5%, CLD 20%, neoplasm 8%, biliary tract disease 5%)	Excluded	29%	Anderson et al. 1988 [10]
Mayo Clinic	1976–1985	88	3%	22%	6%	25% (histoplasmosis 1%)	6%	50%	Sartin & Walker 1991 [11]
Northern Ireland	1980–1992	163	2%	18%	1.5%	14% (psoriasis 4%, Crohn disease 1.5%, CLD 1.5%)	55%	11%	McCluggage & Sloan 1994 [12]
India	1985–1995	51 (4% of 1,234)	55%	–	–	33%	–	12%	Sabharwal et al. 1995 [13]
Italy	1989–1994	15 (1%)	7%	15%	20%	58% (HBV or HCV 20%)	–	–	Guglielmi et al. 1994 [14]
France	1984	73	–	33%	20%	47% (Q fever 20%, Hodgkin disease)	–	–	Voigt et al. 1984 [15]
Scotland	1991–2001	63 (4% of 1,662)	5%	11%	9.5%	39% (HCV 9.5%, AIH 6.3%, Hodgkin disease 6.3%, resolving obstruction 3%)	24	11	Gaya et al. 2003 [16]

(Continued)

Table 40.1 Causes of hepatic granulomas by geographic location. (*Continued*)

Study location	Years covered	Number of cases (% of liver bx)[a]	TB	Sarcoidosis	DILD	Miscellaneous[b]	PBC	Idiopathic[c]	Reference
Saudi Arabia	1990	59	32%	–	3.5%	65% (schistosomiasis 54%, brucellosis 6%)	–	–	Satti et al. 1990 [17]
USC	1990	169	27%	29%	1.2%	28% (leprosy 5.3%, brucellosis 5.3%, Hodgkin disease 4%, Q fever 3.5%)	–	15%	Reynolds et al. 1990 [18]
France	2000–2008	21 (4.5% or 471)	4.7%	9.5%	–	52% (schistosomiasis 4.7%, Hodgkin disease 9.5%, Sjogren syndrome 4.7%, Behcet disease 4.7%, HCV 4.7%)	24%	14.3%	Martin-Blondel et al. 2009 [19]
Greece	1999–2004	66 (3.7% or 1,768)	1.5%	7.5%	3.0%	19.5% (AIH 6%, viral hepatitis 7.5%, *Leishmania* 1.5%, schistosomiasis 1.5%, vasculitis 1.5%, HCC 1.5%)	62%	6%	Dourakis et al. 2007 [20]
Saudi Arabia	Over 13 years	66 (1.2% or 5,531)	42.6%	5%	1.6%	26.3% (HCV 14.8%, HBV 3.3%, *Brucella* 1.6%, Crohn disease 3.3%, HCC 1.6%)	–	14.8%	Sanai et al. 2008 [21]
Germany	1996–2004	442 (3.63% or 12,161)	0.7%	8.4%	2.5%	2.7% (Q fever, miscellaneous infections)	48.6%	36%	Drebber et al. 2008 [22]

[a]% of liver bx is the frequency of finding granulomas in the series of liver biopsies being reported.

[b]Percent of total number of granulomas in the series listed under miscellaneous.

[c]Cause not established.

AIH, autoimmune hepatitis; CLD, chronic liver disease (not specified); DILD, drug-induced liver disease; HBV, hepatitis B virus; HCC, hepatocellular carcinoma; HCV, hepatitis C virus; PBC, primary biliary cirrhosis; TB, tuberculosis; –, not listed.

cause of disseminated granulomas, and previously unrecognized etiologic agents have been identified by improved diagnostic techniques [28]. Nevertheless, granulomas often still present a diagnostic challenge to the clinician. In the recent series by Drebber et al. from Germany, more than one third of the granulomas were considered idiopathic, despite the availability of polymerase chain reaction (PCR) testing for infections and the use of a diagnostic algorithm [22].

Men and women have been nearly equally represented in several large series of granulomas, although women not unexpectedly predominate when primary biliary cirrhosis (PBC) accounts for a significant percentage of cases [16,20,22]. The age of adult patients with hepatic granulomas generally has been in their forties to fifties, but children are affected as well [23,24].

Histopathology

Histologically, two main types (and three subtypes) of granulomas are described based on their appearance as lipogranulomas or epithelioid granulomas (Box 40.1). *Microgranulomas*, as described by Kleiner [3], are small collections of macrophages 3–7 cells across, admixed with lymphocytes (Fig. 40.1). They stain purple with periodic acid–Schiff (PAS) after diastase, and are nonspecific, forming in response to a wide spectrum of chronic inflammatory conditions. As a result, they are regarded as clinically insignificant in most instances.

Lipogranulomas are composed mainly of loose aggregates of lymphocytes and macrophages surrounding lipid droplets, and are secondary to the ingestion of mineral oil or other lipid material (Fig. 40.2) [29,30]. They stain positively with oil red O. In a series of 44 cases in nonfatty livers reported by Dinscoy et al. [31], lipogranulomas were attached to or were closely associated with the walls of hepatic venules, and were most likely a reaction to absorbed mineral oils or other other saturated hydrocarbon foodstuffs. Lipogranulomas comprise a relatively smaller percentage of all granulomas, ranging up to 26% [16], but have been described as having nearly tripled in incidence between the early 1950s and the late 1970s in one series. This is attributed to the increasing

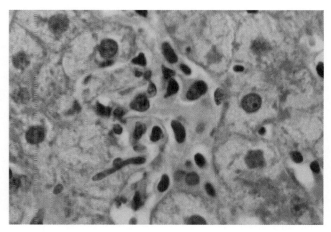

Figure 40.1 Microgranulomas are nonspecific small collections of macrophages, 3 to 7 cells across admixed with lymphocytes. (Reproduced from Kleiner [3] with permission from Elsevier.)

use of mineral oils and saturated hydrocarbons used in processed foods [3,31]. Among autopsy specimens, lipogranulomas have been found in 48%, often in association with lipogranulomas in the spleen [29]. In the series by Dourakis et al. [20], lipogranulomas were found with nearly equal frequency to epithelioid granulomas (2.9% versus 3.7%). They may be discovered incidentally and are generally of little, if any, clinical significance [30,32]. However, reports of venous outflow obstruction have been published [33] and a case of prolonged fever associated with lipogranulomas from paraffin oil has appeared [34].

A distinctive subtype of lipogranulomas is that characterized by an eosinophilic *fibrin ring* enclosing a vacuolar clear space of necrosis [3,35]. These "doughnut"-shaped granulomas have traditionally been associated with Q fever (Fig. 40.3A) [36] and with allopurinol toxicity (Fig. 40.3B) [37]. However, this pathologic appearance is

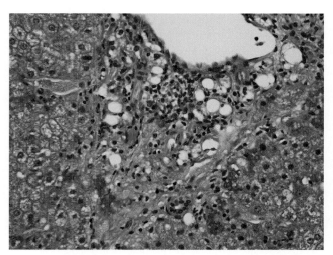

Figure 40.2 Lipogranuloma secondary to mineral oil. Hematoxylin and eosin (H&E), original ×250. (Courtesy of Dr K. G. Ishak, Armed Forces Institute of Pathology.)

Box 40.1 Types of hepatic granulomas.

- Lipogranulomas:
    Fibrin-ring subtype
- Epithelioid granulomas:
    Non-necrotizing
    Necrotizing
- Microgranulomas (nonspecific)

Adapted from Kleiner [3].

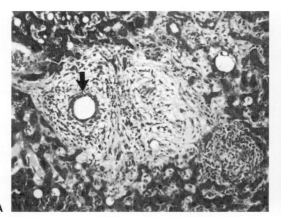 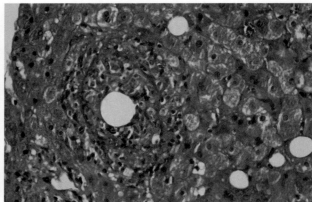

Figure 40.3 (A) Fibrin-ring granulomas secondary to Q fever. A fat globule is surrounded by a ring of fibrin (arrow). H&E, original ×160. (B) "Doughnut" type of fibrin-ring granuloma associated with allopurinol toxicity. H&E, original ×150. (Courtesy of Dr K. G. Ishak, Armed Forces Institute of Pathology.)

not limited to these causes, and several other infections and etiologies have been described (Box 40.2) [35,38–41]. The pathogenesis of fibrin-ring granulomas may be the result of endotheiliitis of sinusoidal cells [3].

Epithelioid granulomas are the predominant histologic form in most series. The name is derived from their polygonal shape and abundant cytoplasm (Fig. 40.4) [18]. They generally develop in response to delayed hypersensitivity reactions [4]. Cytokines mediating the T helper cell 1 (Th1) immune response attract CD4+ and CD8+ T lymphocytes and fibrocytes that form the periphery of many granulomas. Activation of the Th2 immune response occurs as a result of antigenic sensitization, leading to necrosis or caseation, depending on the nature of the antigenic stimulus [4,42].

The non-necrotizing (noncaseating) subtype is composed of either well-circumscribed, tight collections of cells, as in sarcoidosis, or by poorly formed granulomas consisting of macrophages admixed with lymphocytes and other inflammatory cells, such as seen in PBC. As noted by Kleiner [3] and other others [1,43], at times the edges of these granulomas are indistinct, giving rise to the term "granulomatous inflammation." Both subtypes are generally small (100–300 μm in diameter), but may coalesce to form larger macroscopic lesions.

Box 40.2 Causes of fibrin-ring granulomas.

- Q fever
- Allopurinol
- Hodgkin disease
- Giant cell arteritis
- Hepatitis A
- Visceral leishmaniasis
- Epstein–Barr virus
- Toxoplasmosis
- Boutonneuse fever (*Rickettsia conorii*)
- Systemic lupus erythematosus
- Staphylococcal infection

Necrotizing epithelioid granulomas are generally larger (several hundred micrometers) and may form cavitary granulomatous abscesses rimmed by giant cells and often surrounded by connective tissue [3]. The necrotic material in the center is eosinophilic and granular (hence the term "caseating") and may contain calcifications.

Pathophysiology

Both foreign body-type granulomas (nonimmunologic) and hypersensitivity-mediated granulomas can be seen in the liver [44]. Granulomas are most likely to be seen when macrophages drawn to the site of acute inflammation are unable to clear antigens and inflammatory by-products. As a result, monocytes are attracted from the blood and bone marrow and help transform macropahges into epithelioid histiocytes that fuse together to become multinucleated (Langhans type) giant cells [2,44–46]. Such cells lose their phagocytic function and develop secretory

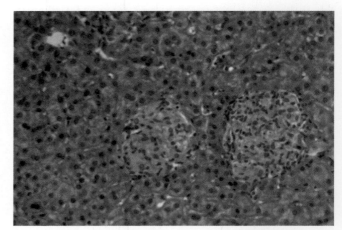

Figure 40.4 Noncaseating epithioid granuloma characterized by giant cell transformation. H&E, original ×300. (Courtesy of Dr K. G. Ishak, Armed Forces Institute of Pathology.)

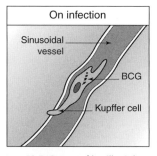
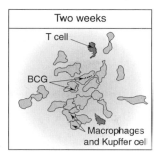
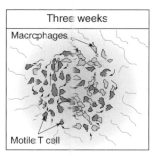
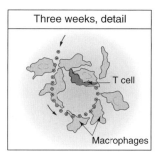

Figure 40.5 Stages of bacille Calmette–Guérin (BCG) granuloma formation: 2 weeks after BCG organisms are phagocytosed by resident Kupffer cells, infected Kupffer cells attract local macrophages and monocyte-derived macrophages and T lymphocytes arrive. By 3 weeks, T cells are plentiful and migrate in constant contact with macrophages, forming the "scaffold" of the granuloma. (Reproduced from Davis et al. [51] with permission from Elsevier.)

properties [47], such as sarcoid granulomas producing angiotensin-converting enzyme (ACE) [48]. The cytokine network and immunology associated with granuloma formation has been reviewed in detail by James [4].

Macrophages must be immunologically activated in order to encircle and destroy infectious organisms [2]. In the presence of T lymphocytes (CD4+ cells) with certain Th1 and Th2 cytokine profiles, they become bacteriocidal and aggregate to form granulomas [3]. Interferon γ plays an important role in the aggregation process [49]. Blocking tumor necrosis factor γ (TNF-γ) has been shown to cause regression of granulomas, but at the cost and risk of increasing a host's susceptibility to mycobacterial infections [3].

Elegant studies performed by Egen and colleagues [50] have demonstrated that granulomas are not merely participating in a passive defense reaction to "wall off" an infectious organism, foreign body, or other antigenic stimulus that cannot otherwise be destroyed. Utilizing blood-borne bacille Calmette–Guérin (BCG) as a model for tuberculosis (TB), these investigators have shown that granulomas form as part of a dynamic process, with T lymphocytes being in constant motion within and around each granuloma, in order to make direct contact with the macrophages that comprise all parts of the structure (Fig. 40.5) [51]. As a result, both innate and adaptive immune cells play an integral part in the development of granulomas, and the work of Egen et al. provides an important insight into the events involved in the containment and escape of mycobacteria [50].

Etiology

Depending on the geographic locale, the causes of granulomas vary according to the prevalence of diseases encountered (see Table 40.1). For example, in India and Saudi Arabia, most are due to TB [13,21]; in Europe, PBC tends to predominate [12,16,19,20,22]. In the midwest of the United States, histoplasmosis is seen more often than in other areas [5,52]; schistosomiasis is important in the

Middle East and the tropics [17], Mediterranean fever in Spain [7], and brucellosis and Q fever in sheep- and cattle-raising regions and in slaughterhouse workers [53,54]. In many series, infectious disorders are the leading causes of hepatic granulomas, consistent with the notion that granulomas form in response to intracellular pathogens that trigger active cell-mediated immunity, or to the persistence of nondegradable (foreign body) products [4]. Table 40.1 lists several representative series of hepatic granulomas from diverse geographic areas that attest to their spectrum of causes. The etiopathogenesis of hepatic granulomas often depends on the extent to which a specific diagnosis is sought, although no cause was identified in up to half of the cases in the older series. However, with the advanced diagnostic testing currently at our disposal, including serologic tests and the use of PCR analyses for a variety of infectious agents, the percentage of truly "idiopathic" (unexplained) granulomas has been reduced; in more recent series it is found to be about 10% [9,52]. A complete listing of the causes of hepatic granulomas is given in Box 40.3.

Clinical consequences

Granulomas come to attention based on the clinical setting in which they arise – either as part of an acute generalized hypersensitivity reaction or infection, during the evaluation of FUO, or as part of the workup for abnormal liver-associated enzymes (usually alkaline phosphatase, γ-glutamyltransferase (GGT), or hyperglobulinemia). In a Mayo Clinic series [11], 74% of patients had unexplained symptoms (including fever) present for a mean of 19 months, with the remainder of granulomas being discovered on liver biopsy for abnormal liver function tests (LFTs). While granulomas are often associated with a classic inflammatory response, significant hepatocellular dysfunction is unusual; hence the term "granulomatous hepatitis" [5] less commonly applies. The term favored by most authorities is "hepatic

Box 40.3 Causes of hepatic granulomas.[a]

Infections

- Bacteria:
    Brucellosis
    Catscratch disease (*Bartonella henselae*)
    Yersinia enterocolitica
    Melioidosis
    Nocardiosis
    Tularemia (*Pasturella tularensis*)
    Salmonellosis
    Staphylococcus
- Mycobacteria:
    Mycobacterium tuberculosis
    Mycobacterium avium complex
    Mycobacterium leprae (leprosy, Hansen disease)
    Atypical mycobacteria
    BCG vaccination
- Fungi:
    Histoplasmosis (*Histoplasma capsulatum*)
    Coccidioidomycosis (*Coccidioides immitis*)
    Candidiasis
    Blastomycosis
    Aspergillosis
    Mucormycosis
- Parasites:
    Schistosomiasis
    Visceral larval migrans (*Toxacara canis*)
    Toxocariasis (visceral larva migrans)
    Visceral leishmaniasis (*L. donovani*, kala-azar)
    Strongyloidosis
    Fascioliasis
    Giardiasis
- *Chlamydia*:
    Psittacosis (*Chlamydia psittaci*)
- Rickettsiae:
    Q fever (*Coxiella burnetti*)
    Boutonneuse fever (*Rickettsia conorii*)
    Scrub typhus (*Orientia tsutsugamushi*)
- Spirochetes:
    Syphilis (*Treponema pallidum*)
- Viruses:
    Hepatitis A
    Hepatitis B
    Hepatitis C
    Cytomegalovirus
    Epstein–Barr virus (mononucleosis)
    Varicella

Neoplasms

- Hodgkin disease
- Lymphoma
- Hairy cell leukemia
- Renal cell carcinoma

Drugs

See Box 40.7

Metals

- Beryllium
- Copper sulfate
- Gold
- Aluminum
- Thorotrast (thorium dioxide)

Foreign materials

- Silica
- Talc (IV drug use, glove powder)
- Silicone (spallation of dialysis tubing, ball-valve prostheses)
- Mineral oil
- Barium sulfate
- Suture material
- Cement, mica dust
- Polyvinyl pyrrolidone

Miscellaneous causes

- Sarcoidosis
- Jejunoileal bypass
- Primary biliary cirrhosis
- Primary sclerosing cholangitis
- Chronic biliary obstruction
- Hypogammaglobulinemia
- Wegener granulomatosis
- Chronic granulomatous disease
- Giant cell arteritis
- Rheumatoid arthritis
- Crohn disease
- Postliver transplant rejection, recurrent disease

Idiopathic (no cause established)

Factitious

- Quinine

[a] Based on references [18,44,55,56,57].

granulomas" as used by my predecessor of this chapter [55] and others [2,56]. Despite the relative absence of overt hepatic dysfunction with most granulomas, several clinicopathologically significant lesions are described in association with granulomatous involvement (Table 40.2).

Clinical evaluation

Clinical and historical clues

The extent to which a specific cause of granulomas in the liver is sought often corresponds to the frequency with which certain diagnoses are found in various geographic locales. A patient's travel history, drug history, occupation, presence of household pets, and proximity or exposure to domesticated farm or feral animals may provide useful clues as to the diagnosis (Table 40.3).

granulomatous hepatitis includes nodules 0.5–4.5 cm in diameter; with caseating granulomas being intermediate to high signal on T2-weighted images and low signal on T1. Noncaseating granulomas were found to have an increased enhancement on arterial phase images that persisted into late phases [64]. On ultrasound, multiple echogenic lesions 3–5 mm in size surrounded by a hypoechoic halo have been described [65]. Diagnostic laparoscopy is described as revealing a range of liver capsule findings, including exudative, pinpoint, granular, macular, and cord-like features. TB was most often granular, while brucellosis was exudative [66].

Histopathologic appearance

Granulomatous reactions may take one of several forms as described by Goodman [43] and Kleiner [3]: (i) simple (bland) granulomas without other associated injury; (ii) granulomatous hepatitis with hepatocellular injury, including apoptosis and parenchymal inflammation; and (iii) granulomatous cholangitis or vasculitis. The pathologic appearance and location of the granulomas may offer important clues to their cause, as listed in Box 40.5. Special stains for acid-fast bacilli (AFB) and fungi, the use of polarizing microscopy looking for talc, and immunohistochemical stains for hematogenous malignancies, etc., may be helpful. The culture of liver biopsy material has a relatively low yield in terms of *Mycobacterium tuberculosis* and other infections, but is often performed, especially in patients with FUO. Kleiner [3] has emphasized the need to avoid mistaking isolated, incidental granulomas for a generalized disease process, such as sarcoidosis or hepatitis C.

Specific causes

A number of the most common causes of hepatic granulomas listed in Box 40.3 are described in the following section.

Sarcoidosis

Sarcoidosis is a chronic multisystem granulomatous disease that is seen in all races and ages, and is the leading cause of hepatic granulomas in the United States. It preferentially affects young African-Americans, who have a ten-fold higher prevalence compared with Caucasians, and tends to have a more severe clinical course [67]. The liver is the third most common site of involvement after the lungs and lymphatics. The diagnosis requires the presence of noncaseating granulomas in at least two organs, with negative staining for AFB and being able to exclude other causes [68]. The presence of systemic symptoms (fever, weight loss, malaise) may occur without pulmonary disease. Hepatic involvement generally

---

Box 40.5 Histopathologic clues to the etiology of hepatic granulomas.

- Large number of granulomas: sarcoidosis, miliary TB
- Lipogranulomas: mineral oil, food stuffs containing waxes or other saturated hydrocarbons
- Associated bile duct injury: PBC, sarcoidosis
- Well-formed granulomas: sarcoidosis, TB, schistosomiasis, histoplasmosis, coccidioidomycosis, chronic brucellosis, phenylbutazone
- Poorly formed granulomas (granulomatous inflammation/necrosis): *Mycobacterium avium*, acute brucellosis, Q fever, many drugs, PBC
- Caseation (central necrosis): TB
- Non-necrotizing but AFB positive: BCG
- Uniform age of granulomas: drug injury
- Noncaseating granulomas of different ages: sarcoidosis
- Multinucleated giant cells: sarcoidosis, TB
- Inclusions (stellate-shaped (asteroid bodies) and lamellar (Schaumann bodies)): sarcoidosis
- Fibrin-ring granulomas (central vacuole surrounded by a ring of fibrin) often staining positive for PTAH: Q fever, allopurinol, Hodgkin disease, other causes listed in Box 40.2
- Eosinophils: drug injury, schistosomiasis, toxocariasis, visceral larva migrans, catscratch disease, Hodgkin disease, non-Hodgkin lymphoma (excludes TB and sarcoidosis)
- Positive AFB stain: TB, *Mycobacterium avium*
- Positive silver stain: fungi
- Foamy macrophages/histiocytes: *Mycobacterium avium*
- Foreign body reaction: talc, silica, schistosome eggs, etc
- Pigment/crystals:
  - Black granules: gold, titanium
  - Grey-tan birefringent material in RES: barium
  - Coarse, pink-brown granules: thorium dioxide
  - Colorless amorphous birefringent crystals: silicone
- Location/distribution of granulomas:
  - Lobular: drugs, sarcoidosis, brucellosis
  - Portal/periportal: sarcoid, TB, Q fever, drugs
  - Periductal: PBC
  - Perivenous: mineral oil
  - Periarterial: phenytoin

AFB, acid-fast bacilli; BCG, bacille Calmette–Guérin; PBC, primary biliary cirrhosis; PTAH, phosphotungistic acid hematoxylin; RES, reticuloendothelial system; TB, tuberculosis.

---

does not cause significant morbidity, but a small subset may develop progressive cholestatic disease that can lead to cirrhosis and portal hypertension [58,59]. Serum alkaline phosphatase levels can reach very high levels (>1,000 IU/L), but aminotransferases and bilirubin levels are generally normal.

Sarcoid granulomas are compact aggregates of large epithelial cells, often with multinucleated giant cells and a rim of lymphocytes and macrophages (Fig. 40.6). They occur diffusely throughout the liver, but are most prominent in the portal and periportal zones. Klatskin [1]

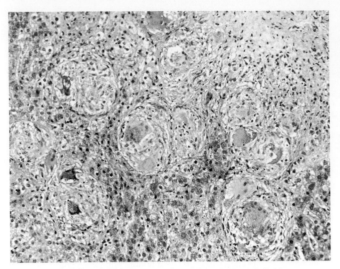

Figure 40.6 Sarcoidosis with multiple noncaseating epithelioid granulomas with multinucleated giant cells. H&E, original ×150. (Courtesy of Dr K. G. Ishak, Armed Forces Institute of Pathology.)

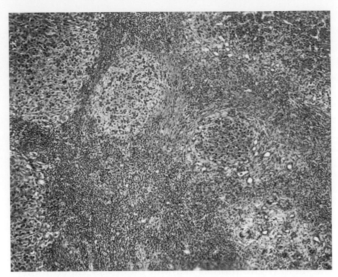

Figure 40.7 Chronic cholestasis of sarcoidosis with micronodular biliary cirrhosis. H&E, original ×60. (Courtesy of Dr K. G. Ishak, Armed Forces Institute of Pathology.)

estimated that there were as many as 75 million granulomas in the liver at various stages of maturation. Inclusions in giant cells (Schaumann and asteroid bodies) are characteristic, but not pathognomonic [69,70]. The pathogenesis of sarcoid granulomas involves their transformation from tissue macrophages that are derived from circulating blood monocytes. According to Okabe [71], they are under the control of colony-stimulating factors and possibly vitamin D3, which promote their proliferation. Their transformation to secretory cells, producing ACE, was described by Gronhagen-Riska and others [48].

Three stages of development were described by Klatskin [1]: early on the granulomas are small, later on they become well defined and ovoid in shape with associated Kupffer cell hyperplasia, and finally they form fibrinoid nodules. Sarcoid granulomas tend to segment as they enlarge, forming multilobulated granulomas [18] that may persist for long periods of time. Confluent granulomas may result in extensive, irregular scarring [72]. They are never caseating (in contrast to TB) and should not be confused with the fibrinoid necrosis that can occasionally be seen [70,72]. Tissue eosinophilia is also absent (in contrast to drug-induced granulomas). Bile duct damage may be seen, although less commonly and with less severity than in PBC. Large sarcoid nodules situated in the hilum may produce biliary obstruction. Chronic cholestasis resembling PBC is a well-described but less common clinical outcome (Fig. 40.7) [58,60,61]. Progression to frank biliary cirrhosis with portal hypertension (from occlusion of intrahepatic portal vein branches) requiring transplant is relatively uncommon, but the disease may recur in allografts [62]. Moreno-Merlo et al. [73] suggested that cirrhosis and focal fibrosis may be

caused by ischemia secondary to primary granulomatous phlebitis of portal and hepatic veins, with portal hypertension occurring secondary to portal vein thrombosis, as cirrhosis was absent at the onset of variceal bleeding in two patients they described.

Sarcoidosis may be present in association with untreated hepatitis C [74] and can reactivate during interferon therapy [75,76], possibly through the stimulation of the Th1 immune response [77].

In a series of 100 patients with hepatic sarcoidosis studied by the Armed Forces Institute of Pathology (AFIP) [70], the volume of granulomas was estimated from <1% to 90%; 99% of which were noncaseating. Three biochemical patterns were found: cholestatic in 58% (nearly half of whom had bile duct lesions similar to PBC or primary sclerosing cholangitis (PSC)); necroinflammatory in 41% (with spotty necrosis and/or chronic portal inflammation); and vascular in 20% (with sinusoidal dilatation and nodular regenerative hyperplasia). Ductopenia was found in 37 of 58 individuals with chronic cholestasis. Another 12 had acute cholangitis changes without clinical evidence of ductal obstruction. Fibrosis was seen in 21 patients (periportal in 13, bridging in two, and cirrhosis in six).

The therapeutic options for sarcoidosis have been reviewed by others [67]. Treatment of hepatic granulomas is usually administered only when the patient has systemic symptoms from granulomatous hepatitis or cholestatic liver disease, or other symptomatic organ involvement [68]. There is no evidence that corticosteroids prevent progression of hepatic disease in asymptomatic individuals [78], although alkaline phosphatase levels may decline. Granulomas may heal without a trace

[70]. In a series by Gottlieb et al. [79], patients with hepatic involvement had a three-fold higher risk of relapse after a course of steroids compared with those without liver disease. Ursodiol may be beneficial in patients with the cholestatic form of the disease [80,81].

Mycobacterium tuberculosis

Granulomas are the most common histologic feature of TB involving the liver, but a wide spectrum of nonspecific histopathologic lesions may be present [81–85]. Granulomas are seen in approximately 20% of patients with pulmonary TB (depending on how many sections are examined) and are seen nearly universally in those with miliary TB [85]. Isolated hepatic involvement is also well described [86]. As many as two thirds of patients with acquired immune deficiency syndrome (AIDS) coinfection have extrapulmonary involvement, that frequently involves the liver (as described below) [87].

The granulomas associated with *Mycobacterium tuberculosis* are composed of mononuclear (epithelioid) cells surrounded by lymphocytes, with or without Langhans-type multinucleated giant cells (Fig. 40.8). They are generally 1–2 mm in size, but large tuberculomas up to 12 cm are reported [87]. Caseation (central necrosis surrounded by peripheral macrophages) is considered a hallmark finding of TB granulomas, and is present in 33–100% of liver biopsy specimens from various series [85]. Caseation is thought to occur as a result of overwhelming acute dissemination of mycobacterial organisms, and therefore occurs more commonly in miliary TB. It is characteristically granular and "cheesy" in appearance, hence the term "caseous" (Fig. 40.9A). Giant cells are often present and AFB stains are positive in about 60% (Fig. 40.9B), in contrast to cultures often being negative [85]. PCR assays are diagnostic in most patients with TB granulomas in the liver [88,89].

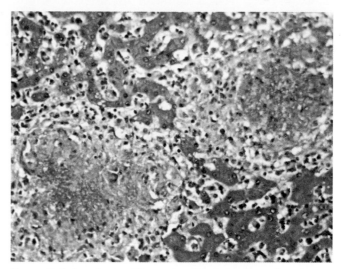

Figure 40.8 Granulomas with caseation necrosis in miliary tuberculosis. H&E, original ×100. (Courtesy of Dr K. G. Ishak, Armed Forces Institute of Pathology.)

Clinical and biochemical clues to the presence of hepatic TB are nonspecific [85]. Hyperglobulinemia is often seen and serum alkaline phosphatase levels are often raised, while aminotransferase values remain normal in pulmonary disease and mildly elevated in miliary TB [90,91]. Jaundice is unusual and should prompt a search for biliary obstruction or associated hepatotoxicity from anti-TB drug therapy. An uncommon form of acute miliary TB described by Essop et al [92], called "tuberculous hepatitis," was accompanied by fever, tender hepatomegaly, and splenomegaly, and had a very high incidence (96%) of hepatic granulomas, with caseation seen in 83%. However, tubercle bacilli were found in only 9% of cases. The demonstration of AFB has generally been low in pulmonary TB, and higher in military disease, but

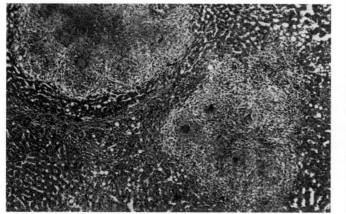 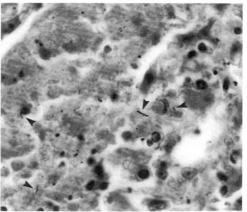

Figure 40.9 (A) Caseous necrosis with multinucleated Langhans giant cells in granulomas associated with *Mycobacterium tuberculosis*. H&E, original ×100. (B) Higher magnification demonstrated acid-fast organisms (arrows) in a caseating granuloma. Ziehl=Neelson stain, original ×1,000. (Courtesy of Dr K. G. Ishak, Armed Forces Institute of Pathology.)

positive cultures have been rare in the literature [85]. Following successful anti-TB treatment, complete resolution of hepatic granulomas is described as occurring within a few months [92,93].

TB rarely affects liver allografts in contrast to renal and other solid organ transplants [94]. In a series of 42 post orthotopic liver transplantation (OLT) patients with granulomas on liver biopsy, Ferrel et al. [95] found only one patient with documented TB (a prevalence of 2.4%). Granulomatous hepatitis has been attributed to isoniazid and pyrazinamide, although one wonders whether the underlying TB may have been responsible for the finding of granulomas in this setting. In general, hepatotoxicity from isoniazid and pyrazinamide takes the form of acute hepatocellular injury, including fulminant hepatic failure [85,96].

Rarely is a mycobacterium other than *M. tuberculosis* isolated from the liver. *M. kansasii*, *M. mucogenicum*, and other atypical mycobacterial organisms have been found [85].

Granulomatous hepatitis caused by BCG is reported in 12–28% of patients receiving BCG as immunotherapy for neoplastic disease [97,98], often several months after the last inoculation. A role for both BCG bacilli and a hypersensitivity reaction has been proposed as the mechanism. O'Brien and Hyslop [99] note that BCG organisms may remain viable for weeks to months. BCG preparations are antigenic, with granulomas forming as a result of a hypersensitivity response [98].

Leprosy (*Mycobacterium leprae*)

Granulomas are common in lepromatous leprosy, but symptoms and signs of hepatic involvement are generally absent, apart from hyperglobulinemia [100]. Histologically, a spectrum of epithelioid, tubercular, and foam cell granulomas is seen [101]; the first two suggesting the tuberculoid form of the disease and the latter lepromatous leprosy. Foam cells consist of Kupffer cells that are filled with *M. leprae* organisms. The *M. leprae* bacteria are much less common in epithelioid granulomas. Hepatic granulomas in leprosy correlated with cutaneous involvement in the series by Chen et al. [102].

Granulomas in HIV and AIDS

Hepatic granulomas were seen in 37% of 501 liver biopsies in one large series [103] and in 16–48% of smaller series [87,104,105]. A microbiologic diagnosis was apparent only after liver biopsy in over 50% of a series of patients presenting with fever and elevated alkaline phosphatase and GGT levels [106]. The most common cause of granulomas appears to be due to *M. avium* complex (MAC), which was present in 20–50% of all autopsy series in fatal AIDS cases and in 10–70% of those undergoing liver biopsy for suspected AIDS hepatopathy [87,107].

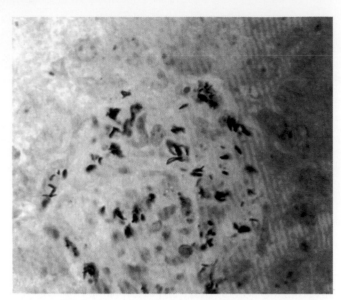

Figure 40.10 *Mycobacterium avium* in a poorly formed granuloma in a patient with AIDS. Numerous acid-fast bacteria are seen in distended histiocytes. H&E, original ×630. (Courtesy of Dr K. G. Ishak, Armed Forces Institute of Pathology.)

MAC has been reported to develop in up to 20% of patients after an AIDS-defining illness has occurred. The granulomas are generally poorly formed and composed of foamy histiocytes with a paucity of other cells, but they contain numerous AFB (Fig. 40.10). Granulomas may be absent in a severely immunosuppressed host. In a series of liver biopsies and autopsies from 71 AIDs patients from 1982 to 1986 in Paris, Astagneau et al. [108] found granulomatous hepatitis in 22 patients, half of which were associated with opportunistic infections and the remainder remained unexplained. Well-formed necrotizing and non-necrotizing granulomas are described in immunocompetent patients infected with MAC [109].

M. tuberculosis has been described in 60% of AIDS patients with pulmonary disease and in 7.5% with extra-pulmonary disease, often as a result of reactivated disease from a previous focus [87,110]. These granulomas tend to be better formed and occur earlier in the course of HIV infection compared with those in MAC. However, fewer AFB are present on immunohistochemical stains. In contrast to *M. tuberculosis*, MAC is usually the result of a primary infection, typically in the late stages of AIDS with CD4+ counts <200/mm^3 [87]. An improved response to multidrug regimens has correlated with improved survival. Alkaline phosphatase values, reflecting hepatic involvement, may normalize after successful therapy.

A number of parasites can cause granulomatous disease in the HIV population. *Pneumocystis carinii* pneumonia (PCP) with extrapulmonary spread is seen in over

30% of cases at autopsy. Toxoplasmosis, leishmaniasis, and schistosomiasis are described in this population. Fungal causes of granulomas may also be seen [55].

Schistosomiasis

Schistosomiasis (*Schistosoma mansoni, S. japonicum, S. mekongi*) is acquired by contact with fresh water infested by the parasitic larvae (cercariae) carried by their host snails. Several hundred million persons are affected worldwide, mostly in tropical regions of the Middle East, the Caribbean (Puerto Rico), Central America, Africa, and Southeast Asia. The life cycle of schistosomes is well described [63]. The adult worms can survive in the host for up to 35 years, depositing hundreds to thousands of eggs daily. Most eggs find their way to the portal circulation and become trapped in several organs, notably the liver. Constant deposition of eggs results in a CD4+ T-helper-cell-mediated granulomatous response to egg antigens (e.g., Sm-p40 and the presence of interleukin 23 (IL23)) [111–113]. This can cause a chronic hepatic reaction with large granulomas in portal areas (hepatosplenic involvement) that become surrounded by fibrosis leading to noncirrhotic portal hypertension (Fig. 40.11) [114]. Following the death of the ova, a dense portal fibrosis may be the only histologic remnant of the infection [18].

Clinically, a serum sickness-like illness from circulating immune complexes produces fever, myalgias, arthralgias, cough, diarrhea (sometimes bloody), and eosinophilia [115]. Eggs may be found in the stool, but an enzyme-linked immunosorbent assay (ELISA) test to detect schistosome antibodies is more reliable. Features of periportal fibrosis and portal hypertension on abdominal imaging tests may also be helpful in making the diagnosis [28]. Several groups of researchers have found that zinc admin-

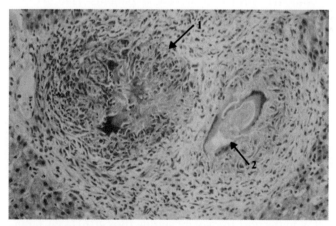

Figure 40.11 Schistosomiasis (*Schistosoma mansoni*) granuloma (arrow 1) next to an ovum blocking an intrahepatic portal vein branch (arrow 2) in a patient with portal hypertension. H&E, original ×400. (Courtesy of Dr K. G. Ishak, Armed Forces Institute of Pathology.)

istration leads to a reduction in the number and size of hepatic granulomas in animal studies [116,117].

Q fever

This worldwide zoonosis among ruminants and birds is caused by tick-borne *Coxiella burnetti*, an obligate intracellular Gram-negative bacterium forming spore-like forms that inhabits monocytes and macrophages [118]. Acute infection in humans occurs primarily by inhalation of contaminated aerosols and dusts from domestic animals, particularly after contact with partuent females and their birth products as the placenta harbors millions of the bacteria [119]. Q fever may present as a community-acquired pneumonia with high fever, cough, headache, and myalgias [119,120], or as a self-limited febrile illness without pulmonary symptoms [119]. Up to 50% of patients present with acute hepatitis-like symptoms, several of which have hyperbilirubinemia, including jaundice [121]. Hepatic involvement also presents as fever of unknown origin and as an incidental finding in patients with pneumonia. Industrial outbreaks (from aerosolized spores) have been described [122], but the infection occurs most frequently among workers on sheep [54] and cattle farms or in slaughterhouses [123] outside the United States. A chronic form of the disease can result in endocarditis, myocarditis, pericarditis, and chronic fatigue syndrome [124]. Hepatitis generally affects younger patients, while pneumonia is seen in older individuals [53].

The characteristic histologic appearance is a fibrin-ring granuloma [36], previously referred to as a "doughnut" granuloma (125) (see Fig. 40.3) [125]. They are usually in portal areas and accompanied by prominent lymphoid hyperplasia. Toll-like receptor 4 appears to play a role in the uptake of virulent organisms and the development of granulomas [118]. In mice, the intraperitoneal route of infection led to hepatic involvement, while the intranasal route was more often associated with pneumonitis [126]. Serology and PCR testing are available to confirm the diagnosis. Treatment has been successful with the use of doxycycline and steroids [53,127]. A preventative vaccine is also available [53].

Other infectious causes

- *Syphilis.* Secondary lues (*Treponema pallidum*) involves the liver in up to 50% of cases, often with tender hepatomegaly and sometimes overt jaundice. Elevated alkaline phosphatase with lesser elevations in aminotransferases is the most common biochemical finding. Spirochetes have been demonstrated by appropriate staining in up to half of affected liver specimens [128]. Following successful antibiotic treatment, resolution of granulomas and other hepatic abnormalities can be expected. In tertiary syphilis, single or multiple hepatic gummas are seen that may give rise to a lobulated appearance (hepar lobatum). Although much larger than granulomas, gummas may also resolve following treatment [28].

- *Yersinia enterocolitica.* Diffuse granulomas of the liver and spleen are seen in the septicemic form. Twelve percent of infections may involve the liver, in some cases causing chronic hepatitis [129].
- *Bartonella henselae* (catscratch fever) develops after a scratch or bite by a cat or kitten and usually results in regional lymphadenitis, although peripheral adenopathy is not always present [130,131]. Scattered granulomas with central necrosis may coalesce to form abscesses. It has been diagnosed in a liver transplant patient with FUO [132]. Warthin–Starry silver staining may identify the Gram-negative bacillus early in the course of infection. An antigen skin test is positive in 90%, but PCR tests are now available [133].
- *Visceral leishmaniasis* (*Leishmania donovani*, kala-azar) is transmitted by the bite of the sandfly, causing a papular or ulcerative skin lesion with systemic symptoms occurring after a latent period of 2–6 months or longer. Intermittent fever, weight loss, tender hepatosplenomegaly, and occasional jaundice are seen. Phagocytosis of the parasite by macrophages in the reticuloendothelial system allows the organism to multiply in the affected liver, spleen, bone marrow, and lymph nodes. The diagnosis is based on the finding of amastigotes in aspirates or promastigotes in culture from these tissues as well as serologic testing [39,134].
- *Visceral larva migrans*, caused by *Toxacara canis*, typically produces hepatic granulomas containing numerous eosinophils. In a series of 43 cases reviewed by Kaplan et al. from the AFIP [135], 30% were under the age of 20 years and 60% were asymptomatic with the disease discovered incidentally. Fever and/or abdominal pain were the most common symptoms reported in the remainder. Granulomas were multiple in 61% of cases and central necrosis was characteristically surrounded by eosinophils and neutrophils, often with Charcot–Leyden crystals. Remnants of the parasite were detected in 23%, and immunohistochemical staining and serology confirmed the diagnosis in many others.
- *Brucellosis.* Acquired from infected cattle (*Brucella abortus*), pigs (*B. suis*), sheep (*B. ovis*), and goats (*B. melitensis*), often from raw, unpasteurized milk and dairy products, brucellosis typically presents as an acute febrile illness with hepatic involvement [136–139]. Jaundice is fairly common [136,137], as is relapsing (undulant) fever. Epithelioid granulomas are most often seen in the chronic form of the disease, with a lobular location more common that the portal tracts. Central necrosis, a polymorphic infiltrate, relatively few giant cells, and peripheral fibrosis is typically seen. The

diagnosis is confirmed by serology, positive *Brucella* PCR [138,140], or culture of liver tissue [140]. Untreated, the clinical course is usually one of spontaneous resolution within 3–12 months, although antibiotics may shorten the illness [28,136].

- *Histoplasmosis* (*Histoplasma capsulatum*) is found most commonly in the midwest and central parts of the United States, especially in river valleys, and usually affects young children more than adults [52]. Four to 8.5% of patients have rare well-formed granulomas [52,141]. Rarely they are caseating, resembling tuberculosis. Clinically, adrenal insufficiency may be a diagnostic clue [141].
- *Coccidioidomycosis* (*Coccidioides immitis*) is most likely to be found in the deserts of the southwest United States. Granulomas are more likely to be found in the liver compared with histoplasmosis, and eosinophilia is often present [142].

Granulomas associated with chronic viral hepatitis and its therapy

Several reports have described granulomas in patients with hepatitis C infection [143–147], although some of these may be related to suspected or unsuspected sarcoidosis [77,148] or PBC [149]. As noted by Kleiner [3], granulomas are not usually considered part of the normal histopathologic spectrum of acute or chronic hepatitis C. Emile et al. [144] described multiple epithelioid granulomas in 10% of cirrhotic livers due to hepatitic C virus (HCV) without any other cause identified. These granulomas were located within cirrhotic nodules and not in portal areas suggesting that they were most likely unrelated to the viral infection. Nevertheless, a small percentage of granulomas in this setting do not have another readily identifiable etiology [150].

In contrast, interferon (IFN) has been associated with granuloma formation in HCV patients [143,144,151] although the exact pathogenesis is not always certain. IFN-induced cutaneous sarcoid has been described in hepatitis C patients [79], and induction [80] and reactivation [78] of systemic sarcoidosis has also occurred, possibly through the production of inflammatory cytokines mediated by IFN [152] or entanercept [153].

Granulomas have been seen in a small percentage of chronic hepatitis B patients; 1.5% among 663 patients in one series [154], although the cause is uncertain.

Granulomas after liver transplantation are reported to occur in 3–9% of allografts [95], and may reflect recurrence of the original disorder, such as PBC, sarcoidosis, etc., or possibly de novo formation from IFN therapy for HCV in the post-transplant setting (Box 40.6) [155]. Granulomatous cholangitis may be seen in acute cellular rejection or a delayed vanishing bile duct syndrome (VBDS) [156]. Infections with opportunistic agents, including TB

Box 40.6 Causes of granulomas in the postliver transplant setting.

- Recurrence of primary disease: primary biliary cirrhosis, sarcoidosis, HCV, HBV
- Interferon therapy-induced
- Acute cellular rejection: granulomatous cholangitis
- Chronic ductopenic rejection: VBDS
- Post-transplant opportunistic infections: cytomegalovirus, tuberculosis, fungi, toxoplasmosis

HBV, hepatitis B virus; HCV, hepatitis C virus; VBDS, vanishing bile duct syndrome.

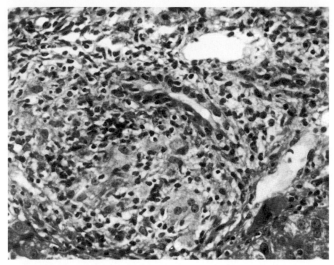

Figure 40.12 Granulomatous cholangitis in primary biliary cirrhosis. H&E, original ×400. (Courtesy of Dr K. G. Ishak, Armed Forces Institute of Pathology.)

[85] and *Toxoplasma gondii*, is described. Toxoplasmosis appears as within the first 3 months with fever, pneumonia, and possibly meningitis or encephalitis, usually from activation of a latent infection [157].

Granulomas in other chronic cholestatic liver diseases

Primary biliary cirrhosis

Epithelioid granulomas are found in at least 25% of PBC patients, usually in the early stages of the disease [158]. PBC typically affects middle-aged women who may present with subclinical alkaline phosphatase elevations or with symptoms reflecting chronic cholestasis, including pruritus. The disease is associated with positive antimitochondrial antibodies in >95% of cases and this may serve to differentiate PBC from sarcoidosis. In addition, PBC often occurs in association with other autoimmune disorders, such as the sicca syndrome, Sjogren syndrome, and CREST (calcinosis, Raynaud phenomenon, esophageal dysfunction, sclerodactyly, and telangiectasia) syndrome among others [158]. Granulomas in the portal areas are in close proximity to injured bile ducts, and may give the appearance of being germinal centers (Figs 40.12 and 40.13). It is thought that they form as part of the immune-mediated ductal injury, but the release of bile acids and phospholipids from injured ducts may also contribute to their development [159,160].

Granulomas located in the hepatic lobules are non-caseating and show less central matrix deposition than is usually seen in sarcoidosis [72]. The highest prevalence of granulomas is seen in the early stages of the disease [70,72] and generally confer a favorable prognosis [3,158]. As PBC progresses, granulomas become less frequent [161]. Treatment with ursodiol therapy may also be associated with a reduction in granulomas through its beneficial effects on the histologic features of cholestasis [162,163]. The presence of granulomatous bile duct lesions can help differentiate and confirm the diagnosis of recurrent PBC from chronic rejection after liver transplant [161].

Primary sclerosing cholangitis

Granulomas have also been reported in PSC [159,164]. Thirteen percent of 100 patients undergoing liver transplant for PSC had noncaseating, non-necrotizing epithelioid granulomas, some with giant cells [164]. They were found in the portal areas, in scars, and in the hepatic parenchyma, and were present in all stages of the disease, but do not represent granulomatous cholangitis (in contrast to PBC where the granulomas are a feature of duct destruction). Ludwig et al. [164] surmise that the granulomas in PSC form in response to bile acid leakage as perigranulomatous lymphocytic infiltrates were common.

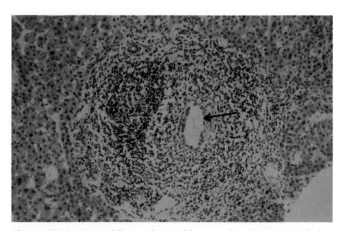

Figure 40.13 Primary biliary cirrhosis with a granuloma in an expanded portal area near a damaged bile duct (arrow). H&E, original ×160. (Courtesy of Dr K. G. Ishak, Armed Forces Institute of Pathology.)

Drug-induced granulomas

More than 60 drugs have been implicated (Box 40.7) although most are isolated case reports [165,166]. A few agents appear to be well documented as causing granulomatous hepatitis, usually as part of a hypersensitivity syndrome, e.g., phenylbutazone (Fig. 40.14) [167], sulfonamides, allopurinol (see Fig. 40.3B) [37], phenothiazines, and penicillins. Drug-induced granulomas have been reported with a frequency of up to 29% of all causes of hepatic granulomas [8], although the prevalence has usually been far lower. In the McMaster case series [8] the drugs that were listed as probably or possibly related were predominantly from antihypertensive, antirheumatic, anticonvulsant, and antimicrobial drug classes, and included methyldopa, hydralazine, phenytoin, isoniazid, cephalexin, penicillin, sulfonamides, procainamide, etc. Up to 9.5% of granulomas in other series were due to many of the same drug classes [10,11,16,20,22] and included chlorpropamide, allopurinol, phenylbutazone, synthetic penicillins, quinidine, carbamazepine, and phenothiazines, among others.

The most frequent clinical presentation is an acute febrile illness, with or without a rash and peripheral eosinophilia, followed by jaundice and biochemical evidence of hepatic dysfunction [8]. A latency period of 1–16 weeks is described by McMaster et al. [8], which is consistent with the time frame for other hypersensitivity reactions from drugs [96,166]. Histologic features suggesting a drug-induced cause include the relatively uniform age of the granulomas, and the present of eosinophils, apoptotic bodies, acute cholangitis, and/or vasculitis [3,43]. In contrast, tissue eosinophilia is not seen in sarcoidosis or TB. The prognosis is generally good with recovery after the offending agent is withdrawn. Healing without sequellae is the rule [8,43]. Histopathologic clues to drug-induced granulomas are given in Table 40.5.

Granulomas associated with metals and minerals

- *Beryllium poisoning* uncommonly involves the liver, as the chronic form of the disease is primarily a pulmonary granulomatosis with dyspnea and cough [168]. It should be suspected in occupational exposure where beryllium is employed, such as in the manufacture of ceramics and alloys, and in atomic energy workers. The granulomas seen in beryllium disease may contain Schaumann and asteroid inclusion bodies, which are the end-products of actively secreting epithelioid cells [4] and may be confused with those seen in sarcoidosis [169]. Tissue analysis for beryllium may be confirmatory.
- *Talc* microcrystals are commonly seen in intravenous drug users, many of whom "cut" their heroin with

---

Box 40.7 Drugs associated with granulomas and granulomatous reactions.

- Allopurinol
- Amiodarone
- Amoxicillin–clavulanic acid
- Aprindine
- Carbamazepine
- Chlorpromazine
- Chlorpropamide
- Dapsone
- Diazepam
- Dicloxacillin
- Diltiazem
- Disopyramide
- Glyburide
- Glibenclamide
- Gold salts
- Green juice
- Halothane
- Hydralazine
- Interferon α
- Isoniazid
- Mebendazole
- Mesalamine
- Methimazole
- Methotrexate
- Methyl dopa
- Mineral oil
- Nitrofurantoin
- Norfloxacin
- Oral contraceptives
- Oxacillin
- Oxyphenbutazone
- Papaverine
- Penicillin
- Phenbutazone
- Phenprocoumon
- Phenytoin
- Procainamide
- Procarbazine
- Pronestyl
- Pyrazinamide
- Pyrimethamine-chloroquine
- Quinidine
- Quinine
- Rantidine
- Rosiglitazone
- Saridon
- Seatone (green-lipped mussel extract)
- Sulfanilamide and other sulfa drugs
- Sulfasalazine
- Tetrabamate (atrium)
- Tetrahydroaminoacridine (tacrine)
- Tolbutamide

Based on references contained in references [43,55,96,165,166].

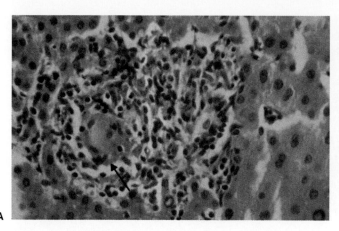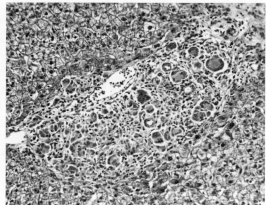

Figure 40.14 Granulomas associated with an acute hypersensitivity reaction to phenylbutazone. (A) Two epithelioid granulomas similar in size and age. H&E, original ×100. (B) Epithelioid granuloma containing several multinucleated giant cells. H&E, original ×150. (Courtesy of Dr K. G. Ishak, Armed Forces Institute of Pathology.)

talcum powder. They are found in hypertrophied portal macrophages, but generally do not develop into well-formed granulomas [170], in contrast to silica, which forms foreign body-type giant cells that contain the birefringent crystals [171]. The presence of talc in the liver, however, may be an important clue as to the etiology of chronic hepatitis C in IV drug users [172].

- Refractile *silicone* particles (confirmed by X-ray energy dispersive spectroscopy) were described in association with sarcoid-like granulomas, some with giant cells, in hemodialysis patients where embolization (spallation) of silicone was traced back to tubing traumatized in the roller pump [173]. Abnormalities in liver-associated enzymes persisted more than 4 years later in two patients [174].
- Multiple granulomas were described in long-term hemodialysis patients [175] with *aluminum* found in the cytoplasm of macrophages in the liver, spleen, and lymph nodes.

Table 40.5 Histopathologic clues to the cause of drug-induced granulomas.

Feature	Drug causing granuloma
Associated cholestatic hepatitis	PBZ, quinidine, allopurinol
Associated cholangitis	CPZ, methyldopa, allopurinol
Associated vasculitis	PCN, sulfonamides, DPH, allopurinol, glibenclamide
Fibrin-ring granulomas	Allopurinol

Adapted from Kleiner [3].
CPZ, chlorpromazine; DPH, diphenylhydantoin; PBZ, phenylbutazone; PCN, penicillin.

Granulomas associated with malignancy and immunodefieciency states

Hodgkin disease, lymphomas and certain hematogenous malignancies (e.g., *hairy cell leukemia*) are associated with granulomas. Granulomas are seen in approximately 10% of those with Hodgkin disease (Fig. 40.15) [176,177], and were present in 31% of those with hairy cell leukemia [178]. Granulomas in the liver may precede the diagnosis of Hodgkin disease or lymphoma [179], and may be a source of diagnostic confusion with sarcoidosis [4]. Rarely, the granulomas associated with Hodgkin disease are caseating [180]. The presence of granulomas does not appear to convey any clinical advantage as suggested by early reports [181]. Mimics of lymphomas that may be associated with hepatic granulomas include *Kikuchi lymphadenitis*, among others [182].

Common variable immunodeficiency is associated with noncaseating granulomas in the liver and spleen [183]. *Chronic granulomatous disease* [184] may appear in adults as well as children [185]. Hepatic involvement was found in nearly one third of 429 patients in a European series [186].

Miscellaneous causes

- *Jejunoileal bypass.* Granulomas were among several hepatic lesions, including steatohepatitis, that were seen following jejunoileal bypass surgery for morbid obesity; 24% of patients undergoing jejunoileal bypass in a series of 25 patients reported by Banner et al. developed granulomas [187]. They developed within 3 months to 4 years after the surgery and were much more common than the incidence (4%) of granulomas seen in obese patients prior to surgery. Their exact etiopathogenesis is unclear.
- *Rheumatoid arthritis* is a rare cause of granulomas [188], as are other rheumatic disorders.

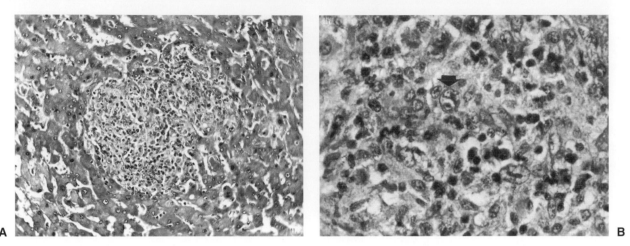

Figure 40.15 Hodgkin disease granulomas. (A) Focal granulomatous infiltrate. H&E. original ×180. (B) Higher magnification showing a pleomorphic infiltrate with a Reed–Sternberg cell (arrow). H&E, original ×750. (Courtesy of Dr K. G. Ishak, Armed Forces Institute of Pathology.)

Idiopathic granulomatous hepatitis and fever of unknown origin

Up to 74% of hepatic granulomas in early series were not identified with a specific diagnosis [27]. Many of these patients had FUO (Table 40.6) or other systemic symptoms or hypersensitivity features, and were designated as "granulomatous hepatitis" [25]. Sarcoidosis has been found in a number of such patients [189], and infectious agents in some of the others [190,193] although no cause was apparent in many [22,26]. Aderka et al. [191] found that certain clinical parameters could differentiate idiopathic granulomas from those that are secondary to lymphoma and other malignancies – namely smaller spleen size, small liver size (<4 cm below the respective costal margin), lower number of eosinophils (<4%), and fever lasting <4 weeks. The spectrum of hepatic candidiasis includes granulomas, especially among patients with

hematologic mailgignancies presenting with fever, and elevated alkaline phosphatase levels [192]. In a series by Cunningham and colleagues [9], 31% of granulomas that were considered initially to be "idiopathic" were subsequently diagnosed as having a specific cause based on more in-depth study. In contrast, the etiology of more than one third of the granulomas reported in the series by Drebber et al. from Germany remained obscure [22]. Schlegel [57] described what he termed "factitious" granulomatous hepatitis in a health care worker who had hepatic granulomas and leukopenia attributed to quinine ingestion that was likely being taken surreptiously.

Treatment of hepatic granulomas and granulomatous hepatitis

General principles

Granulomas that are found incidentally are often asymptomatic but should prompt a workup for the most common causes of granulomas (see Box 40.2, Tables 40.2 and 40.5). They may may not require treatment if involvement is isolated to the liver. Individuals presenting with granulomatous hepatitis, including those with FUO and other systemic symptoms, can be treated for a specific cause, if found. Those that are considered *idiopathic* may respond to an empirical course of corticosteroids [5,25–27]. In a series of 23 cases reported by Zoutman et al. [27] presenting with FUO, 74% were considered idiopathic. Forty-one percent of this group resolved spontaneously, while the remaining 59% received corticosteroids or indomethacin, 18% short term and 41% long term (mean 33 months). All were described as having remained afebrile and healthy after a 5-year follow-up. A similarly good prognosis after long-term corticosteroid therapy of up to 10 years was described by Telenti and Hermans [26] with no

Table 40.6 Hepatic granulomas as a cause of fever of unknown origin.

Number of cases	Diagnoses	Reference
60	Sarcoidosis 47%; tuberculosis 25%; idiopathic 17%	Terplan 1971 [193]
25	36% "positive" diagnosis	Bruguera et al. 1981 [190]
15	Sarcoidosis 100%	Israel et al. 1984 [189]
20	Idiopathic 100%	Telenti & Hermans 1989 [26]
23	Idiopathic 74% (41% spontaneous regression), 26% specific diagnosis (Q fever, tuberculosis, histoplasmosis)	Zoutman et al. 1991 [27]

progression or dissemination of an unrecognized infectious process.

In sarcoidosis, corticosteroids are usually given when there is evidence of extrahepatic sarcoidosis as most experts do not believe that isolated hepatic involvement requires therapy unless there is evidence of severe cholestasis [67]. Methotrexate has also been utilized in this disorder [194], as has ursodiol [67], especially for the cholestatic form. Liver transplantation has been required to treat some patients with end-stage chronic cholestatic sarcoidosis [62].

Specific antibiotic therapy for various infectious causes and other treatment options directed at specific causes of hepatic granulomas are reviewed elsewhere (see Table 40.4) [28]. Empirical treatment for TB has been offered in some instances [194]. Drug-induced causes generally resolve spontaneously once the medication has been discontinued.

In cases of symptomatic idiopathic granulomatous hepatitis (such as FUO), corticosteroids have been the mainstay of treatment [26]. Longstreth and Bender [195] described the use of cyclophosphamide as a steroid-sparing maintenance agent in preventing the recurrence of idiopathic hepatic granulomatosis. Methotrexate was described as being effective in seven patients presenting with fever and anorexia in a series by Knox et al. [194]. Nonsteroidal anti-inflammatory drugs were used successfully in a child with necrotizing granulomatous inflammation [196].

Conclusions

Hepatic granulomas are not infrequently encountered in the evaluation of a variety of infectious, chronic cholestatic, inflammatory, hypersensitivity-mediated, and neoplastic disorders. Granulomas can be expected to be present in 3–10% of routine liver biopsies, and in a substantially higher percentage of patients with suspected localized or systemic granulomatous diseases. Both genders and all ages can be affected. The list of possible etiologies, including dozens of drug-related causes, has been expanding, although certain causes still predominate, namely sarcoidosis, tuberculosis, PBC, and certain drugs (especially those acting through hypersensitivity mechanisms), often relating to the geographic location of the patient. Less common causes remain a diagnostic challenge, but are being found more frequently, commensurate with the wider availability of serologic and other PCR-based test systems. Hepatic granulomas may be the only histologic clue as to the presence of several infections, such as tuberculosis and Q fever, among others. Once found, a decision regarding the extent of a further diagnostic evaluation must be made and, ultimately, what treatment, if any, is required. The cause of up to 36% of granulomas remains undefined (idiopathic), some of which are associated with unexplained fever and other symptoms (including arthralgias and rash) that define "granulomatous hepatitis." These cases are arguably the most challenging, often having to rely on empirical treatment regimens. It is anticipated that further advances in clinical and histopathologic diagnostic methodologies will help identify even the most refractory causes of hepatic granulomas in the future.

Annotated references

Collins MH, Jiang B, Croffie JM, Chong SK, Lee CH. Hepatic granulomas in children. A clinicopathologic analysis of 23 cases including polymerase chain reaction for histoplasma. *Am J Surg Pathol* 1996;20:332–8.
One of the largest reviews of granulomas in a pediatric population. In comparison to adults where the most common causes are sarcoidosis, tuberculosis, drugs, neoplasms, and chronic cholestatic liver diseases, in this series, histoplasmosis accounted for 65% of granulomas with an identifiable etiology. The authors emphasize the usefulness of PCR-based testing to improve diagnostic accuracy.

Denk H, Scheuer PJ, Baptista A, et al. Guidelines for the diagnosis and interpretation of hepatic granulomas. *Histopathology* 1994;25:209–18.
A preeminent group of hepatopathologists define four diagnostic groups based on the pathologic, clinical, historical, and serologic findings in patients found to have granulomas in the liver.

Devaney K, Goodman ZD, Epstein MS, Zimmerman HJ, Ishak KG. Hepatic sarcoidosis. Clinicopathologic features of 100 patients. *Am J Surg Pathol* 1993;17:1272–80.
One of the largest series of hepatic granulomas due to sarcoidosis from the experts at the Armed Forces Institute of Pathology. They describe three main categories of hepatic sarcoidosis based on biochemical and histologic features: cholestatic in 58% (often with bile duct injury and ductopenia similar to PBC), necroinflammatory in 41%, and those with associated vascular changes of sinusoidal dilatation or nodular regenerative hyperplasia in 20%.

Drebber U, Kasper HU, Ratering J, et al. Hepatic granulomas: histological and molecular pathological approach to differential diagnosis – a study of 442 cases. *Liver Int* 2008;28:828–34.
In a large series of patients with granulomas, the cause was unknown in more than one third despite using all available serologic and histologic approaches to the diagnosis.

Egen JG, Rothfuchs AG, Feng CG, et al. Macrophage and T cell dynamics during the development and disintegration of mycobacterial granulomas. *Immunity* 2008;28:271–84.
Elegant studies in BCG-induced granulomas demonstrate the dynamic movement of T cells in and around macrophages.

Ishak KG, Zimmerman HJ. Drug-induced and toxic granulomatous hepatitis. *Baillieres Clin Gastroenterol* 1988;2:463–80.
The most comprehensive review of drugs and chemical toxins associated with hepatic granulomas from two of the leading experts in the fields of drug-induced hepatotoxicity and hepatopathology, emphasizing the role of liver biopsy in this setting. Histologic lesions that suggested a drug etiology included associated tissue eosinophilia, acute cholangitis, and the uniform age of the granulomas. Special stains and other histopathologic analyses may also play an important role in helping to confirm the diagnosis and assigning causality to a drug.

James DG. A clinicopathological classification of granulomatous disorders. *Postgrad Med J* 2000;76:457–65.
An excellent review of the pathophysiology and immunology of granuloma formation. The author describes the interplay of the invading organism, drug, chemical, or other irritants and the cytokines and other biologic mediators

involved in the transformation of macrophages to epithelioid cells that comprise a majority of granulomas. An overview of many infectious, chemical, and other causes of granulomas is provided.

Kleiner DE. Granulomas in the liver. *Semin Diagn Pathol* 2006;23:161–9.
A comprehensive review of the histopathology of granulomas, including pathologic clues to their various etiologies.

Taylor TH, Lewis JH. Tuberculosis of the liver, biliary tract and pancreas. In: Schlossberg D, ed. *Tuberculosis and Nontuberculous Mycobacterial Infections*, 6th edn. Washington, DC: ASM Press, 2011:372–408.
A comprehensive review of tuberculous infections of the liver and the spectrum of granulomatous disease they produce. Hepatic granulomas are found most often in miliary TB and less often in pulmonary and extrapulmonary disease. Caseating necrosis is seen most commonly in association with the acute disseminating infections of miliary TB. The yield of special stains and culture remains low, but PCR-based tests of TB have improved disgnostic yields.

Raoult D, Tissot-Dupont H, Foncault C, et al. Q fever 1985–1998. Clinical and epidemiologic features of 1,383 infections. *Medicine (Baltimore)* 2000;79:109–23.
A comprehensive review of Q fever from France. This organism (Coxiella burnetti) is responsible for a characteristic fibrin-ring type of granuloma. Acute hepatitis was the most common clinical presentation, seen in 40% of cases, often associated with Q fever pneumonitis. The authors describe a number of patient host factors that appear to dictate the clinical expressions of the disease.

Wanless IR, Geddie WR. Mineral oil lipogranulomata in liver and spleen. A study of 465 autopsies. *Arch Pathol Lab Med* 1985;109: 283–6.
Lipogranulomas are less common than epithelioid granulomas, but were found in 48% of livers examined in this large series. The authors describe the clinicohistologic features of lipogranulomas, which are generally clinically silent. They appear most often in older adults, particularly men, and are associated with the ingestion of mineral oil in most instances.

Zoutman DE, Ralph ED, Frei JV. Granulomatous hepatitis and fever of unknown origin. An 11-year experience of 23 cases with three years' follow-up. *J Clin Gastroenterol* 1993;17:89.
One of the largest series that helps to define the natural history of idiopathic granulomatous hepatitis associated with FUO. The authors were able to identify a specific diagnosis in only 26% of their patients. Among the cases without a precise etiology, 41% eventually resolved spontaneously, 18% resolved after short-term treatment with corticosteroids and anti-inflammatory drugs, while the remaining 41% required long-term corticosteroid therapy to maintain clinical remission and prevention of fever over nearly 6 years of follow-up.

References

1. Klatskin G. Hepatic granulomata: problems in interpretation. *Mt Sinai J Med* 1977;44:798–812.
2. Denk H, Scheuer PJ, Baptista A, et al. Guidelines for the diagnosis and interpretation of hepatic granulomas. *Histopathology* 1994; 25:209–18.
3. Kleiner DE. Granulomas in the liver. *Semin Diagn Pathol* 2006; 23:161–9.
4. James DG. A clinicopathological classification of granulomatous disorders. *Postgrad Med J* 2000;76:457–65.
5. Mir-Madjlessi SH, Farmer RG, Hawk WA. Granulomatous hepatitis. A review of 50 cases. *Am J Gastroenterol* 1973;60:122–34.
6. Neville E, Piyasena KHG, James GD. Granulomas of the liver. *Postgrad Med J* 1975;51:361–5.
7. Vilaseca J, Guardia J, Cuxart A, et al. Granulomatous hepatitis. Etiologic study of 107 cases. *Med Clin (Barc)* 1979;72:272–5.
8. McMaster KR 3rd, Hennigar GR. Drug–induced granulomatous hepatitis. *Lab Invest* 1981;44:61–73.
9. Cunningham D, Mills PR, Quigley EM, et al. Hepatic granulomas: experience over a 10-year period in the West of Scotland. *Q J Med* 1982;51:162–70.
10. Anderson CS, Nicholls J, Rowland R, LaBrooy JT. Hepatic granulomas: a 15-year experience in the Royal Adelaide Hospital. *Med J Aust* 1988;148:71–4.
11. Sartin JS, Walker RC. Granulomatous hepatitis: a retrospective review of 88 cases at the Mayo Clinic. *Mayo Clin Proc* 1991;6: 914–18.
12. McCluggage WG, Sloan JM. Hepatic granulomas hepatitis in Northern Ireland: a thirteen year review. *Histopathology* 1994;25:219–28.
13. Sabharwal BD, Malholtra N, Garg R, Malholtra V. Granulomatous hepatitis: a retrospective study. *Indian J Pathol Microbiol* 1995;38:413–16.
14. Guglielmi V, Manghisi OG, Pirrelli M, Caruso ML. Granulomatous hepatitis in a hospital population in southern Italy. *Pathologica* 1994;86:271–4.
15. Voigt JJ, Cassigul J, Delsol G, Vinel JP, Pau H, Fabre J. Granulomatous hepatitis. Apropos of 112 cases in adults. *Ann Pathol* 1984;4:78–80.
16. Gaya DR, Thorburn D, Oien KA, Morris AJ, Stanley AJ. Hepatic granulomas: a 10 year single centre experience. *J Clin Pathol* 2003;56:850–3.
17. Satti MB, al-Freihi H, Ibrahim EM, et al. Hepatic granuloma in Saudi Arabia: a clinicopathological study of 59 cases. *Am J Gastroenterol* 1990;85:669–74.
18. Reynolds TB, Campra JL, Peters RL. Hepatic granulomata. In: Zakim D, Boyer TD, eds. *Hepatology. A textbook of liver disease*, 2nd edn. Philadelphia, PA: WB Saunders, 1990: 998–1114.
19. Martin-Blondel G, Camara B, Selves J, et al. Etiology and outcome of liver granulomatosis: a retrospective study of 21 cases. *Rev Med Interne* 2010;31(2):97–106.
20. Dourakis SP, Saramadou R, Alexopoulou A, et al. Hepatic granulomas: a 6-year experience in a single center in Greece. *Eur J Gastroenterol Hepatol* 2007;19:101–4.
21. Sanai FM, Ashraf S, Abdo AA, et al. Hepatic granuloma: decreasing trend in a high-incidence area. *Liver Int* 2008;28:1402–7.
22. Drebber U, Kasper HU, Ratering J, et al. Hepatic granulomas: histological and molecular pathological approach to differential diagnosis – a study of 442 cases. *Liver Int* 2008;28:828–34.
23. Ahmad M, Afzal S, Roshan E, et al. Usefulness of needle biopsy in the diagnosis of paediatric liver disorders. *J Pak Med Assoc* 2005;55:24–8.
24. Zhang HF, Yang XJ, Zhu SS, et al. Pathological changes and clinical manifestations of 1020 children with liver diseases confirmed by biopsy. *Hepatobiliary Pancreat Dis Int* 2004;3:395–8.
25. Simon HB, Wolff SM. Granulomatous hepatitis and prolonged fever of unknown origin: a study of 13 patients. *Medicine (Baltimore)* 1973;52:1–21.
26. Telenti A, Hermans PE. Idiopathic granulomatosis as fever of unknown origin. *Mayo Clin Proc* 1989;64:44–50.
27. Zoutman DE, Ralph ED, Frei JV. Granulomatous hepatitis and fever of unknown origin. An 11-year experience of 23 cases with three years' follow-up. *J Clin Gastroenterol* 1993;17:89.
28. Mandell GL, Bennett JE, Dolin R, eds. *Mandell, Douglas, and Bennett's Principles and Practice of Infectious Diseases*, 6th edn. Philadelphia, PA: Elsevier Churchill Livingstone, 2005.
29. Wanless IR, Geddie WR. Mineral oil lipogranulomata in liver and spleen. A study of 465 autopsies. *Arch Pathol Lab Med* 1985; 109:283–6.
30. Fleming KA, Zimmermann H, Shubik P. Granulomas in the livers of humans and Fischer rats associated with the ingestion of mineral hydrocarbons: a comparison. *Regul Toxicol Pharmacol* 1998;27: 75–81.
31. Dinscoy HP, Weesner RE, MacGee J. Lipogranulomas in non-fatty human livers. A mineral oil induced environmental disease. *Am J Clin Pathol* 1982;78:35–41.

32. Carlton WW, Boitnott JK, Dungworth DL, et al. Assessment of the morphology and significance of the lymph nodal and hepatic lesions produced in rats by the feeding of certain mineral oils and waxes. Proceedings of a pathology workshop held at the Fraunhofer Institute of Toxicology and Aerosol Reasearch, Hannover Germany, May 7–9, 2001. *Exp Toxicol Pathol* 2001;53:247–55.

33. Keen ME, Engstrand DA, Hafez GR. Hepatic lipogranulomatosis simulating veno-occlusive disease of the liver. *Arch Pathol Lab Med* 1985;109:70–2.

34. Trivalle C, Profit P, Bonnet B, et al. Liver lipogranulomas with long-term fever caused by paraffin oil. *Gastroenterol Clin Biol* 1991;15:551–3.

35. Marazuela M, Moreno A, Yebra M, Cerezo E, Gomez-Gesto C, Vargas JA. Hepatic fibrin-ring granulomas: a clinicopathologic study of 23 patients. *Hum Pathol* 1991;22:607–13.

36. Pellegrin M, Delsol G, Auvergnat JC, et al. Granulomatous hepatitis in Q fever. *Hum Pathol* 1980;11:51–7.

37. Stricker BH, Blok AP, Babany G, Benamou JP. Fibrin ring granulomas and allopurinol. *Gastroenterology* 1989;96:1199–203.

38. Ponz E, Garcia-Pagan JC, Bruguera M, Bruix J, Rodes J. Hepatic fibrin-ring granulomas in a patient with hepatitis A. *Gastroenterology* 1991;100:268–70.

39. Moreno A, Marazuela M, Yebra M, et al. Hepatic finbrin-ring granulomas in visceral leishmaniasis. *Gastroenterology* 1988;95;1123–6.

40. Nenert M, Mavier P, Dubuc N, Deforges L, Zafrani ES. Epstein–Barr virus infection and hepatic fibrin-ring granulomas. *Hum Pathol* 1988;19:608–10.

41. de Bayser L, Roblot P, Ramassamy A, Silvain C, Levillain P, Becq-Giraudon B. Hepatic fibrin-ring granulomas in giant cell arteritis. *Gastroenterology* 1993;105:272–3.

42. Iizasa H, Yoneyama H, Mukaida N, et al. Exaccerbation of granuloma formation in IL-1 receptor antagonist-deficient mice with impaired dendritic cell maturation associated with Th2 cytokine production. *J Immunol* 2005;174:3273–80.

43. Goodman ZD. Drug hepatotoxicity. *Clin Liver Dis* 2002;6:381–97.

44. Ishak KG. Granulomas in the liver. *Adv Pathol Lab Med* 1995;8:247–361.

45. Papadimiotriou JM, can Bruggen I. Evidence that multinucleate giant cells are examples of mononuclear phagocytic differentiation. *J Pathol* 1986;148:149–57.

46. Seitzer U, Haas H, Gerdes J. A human in vitro granuloma model for the investigation of multinucleated giant cell and granuloma formation. *Histol Histopathol* 2001;16:645–53.

47. Turk JL, Narayanan RB. The origin, morphology, and function of epithelioid cells. *Immunobiology* 1982;161:274–82.

48. Gronhagen-Riska C, Fyhrquist F. von Willebrand E. Angiotensin I-converting enzyme. A marker of highly differentiated monocytic cells. *Ann NY Acad Sci* 1986;465:242–9.

49. Sneller MC. Granuloma formation, implications for the pathogenesis of vasculitis. *Cleve Clin J Med* 2002;69(Suppl 2);SII40–3.

50. Egen JG, Rothfuchs AG, Feng CG, et al. Macrophage and T cell dynamics during the development and disintegration of mycobacterial granulomas. *Immunity* 2008;28:271–84.

51. Davis JM, Ramakrishnan L. "The very pulse of the machine": the tuberculous granuloma in motion. *Immunity* 2008;28:146–8.

52. Collins MH, Jiang B, Croffie JM, Chong SK, Lee CH. Hepatic granulomas in children. A clinicopathologic analysis of 23 cases including polymerase chain reaction for histoplasma. *Am J Surg Pathol* 1996;20:332–8.

53. Raoult D, Tissot-Dupont H, Foncault C, et al. Q fever 1985–1998. Clinical and epidemiologic features of 1,383 infections. *Medicine (Baltimore)* 2000;79:109–23.

54. Lyytikainen O, Ziese T, Schwartlander B, et al. An outbreak of sheep-associated Q fever in a rural community in Germany. *Eur J Epidemiol* 1998;14:193–9.

55. Maddrey WC. Granulomas of the liver. In: Schiff ER, Sorrell MF, Maddrey WC, eds. *Schiff's Diseases of the Liver*, 8th edn. Philadelphia, PA: Lippincott Raven Publishers, 1999: 1571–85.

56. Burt AD, Portmann BC, MacSween RNM. Liver pathology associated with diseases of other organs or systems. In: MacSween RNM, Burt AD, Portmann BC, Ishak KG, Scheuer PJ, Anthony PP, eds. *Pathology of the Liver*, 4th edn. London: Churchill Livingstone, 2002: 829–38.

57. Schlegel A. Factitious granulomatous hepatitis? *Am J Med* 2004;116:500–1

58. Rudzki C, Ishak KG, Zimmerman HJ. Chronic intraheptic cholestasis of sarcoidosis. *Am J Med* 1975;59:373–87.

59. Valla D, Pessegueiro-Miranda H, Degott C, Lebrec D, Rueff B, Benhamou JP. Hepatic sarcoidosis with portal hypertension: a report of seven cases with a review of the literature. *Q J Med* 1987;242:531–44.

60. Pereira-Lima, J, Schaffner F. Chronic cholestasis in hepatic sarcoidosis with clinical features resembling primary biliary cirrhosis. Report of two cases. *Am J Med* 1987;83:144–8.

61. Bass NM, Burroughs AK, Scheuer PJ, James DG, Sherlock S. Chronic intrahepatic cholestasis due to sarcoidosis. *Gut* 1982;23:417–21.

62. Lipson EJ, Fiel MI, Florman SS, Korenblat KM. Patient and graft outcomes following liver transplantation for sarcoidosis. *Clin Transplant* 2005;19:487–91.

63. Lucey DR, Maguire JH. *Schistosomiasis*. Infect Dis Clin North Am 1993;7:635–53.

64. Balci NC, Tunaci A, Akinci A, Cevikbas U. Granulomatous hepatitis: MRI findings. *Magn Reson Imaging* 2001;19:1107–11.

65. Mills P, Saverymuttu S, Fallowfield M, Nussey S, Joseph AE. Ultrasound in the diagnosis of granulomatous liver disease. *Clin Radiol* 1990;41:113–15.

66. Moreto M, Testillano M, Zaballa M, Suarez M, Ibanez. Diagnostic yield and endoscopic patterns of laparoscopy in the diagnosis of granulomatous hepatitis. *Endoscopy* 1988;20:294–7.

67. Johns CJ, Michele TM. The clinical management of sarcoidosis: a 50-year experience at the Johns Hopkins Hospital. *Medicine (Baltimore)* 1999;78:65–111.

68. Ebert EC, Kierson M, Hagspiel KD. Gastrointestinal and hepatic manifestations of sarcoidosis. *Am J Gastroenterol* 2008;103:3184–92.

69. Gadde PS, Moscovic EZ. Asteroid bodies: products of unusual microtubule dynamics in monocyte-derived giant cells. An immunohistochemical study. *Histol Histopathol* 1994;9:633–42.

70. Devaney K, Goodman ZD, Epstein MS, Zimmerman HJ, Ishak KG. Hepatic sarcoidosis. Clinicopathologic features of 100 patients. *Am J Surg Pathol* 1993;17:1272–80.

71. Okabe T. Origin of epithelioid cells in sarcoid granuloma. *Nippon Rinsho* 2002;60:1714–19.

72. Ishak KG. Sarcoidosis of the liver and bile ducts. *Mayo Clin Proc* 1998;73:467–72.

73. Moreno-Merlo F, Wanless IR, Shimamatsu K, Sherman M, Greig P, Chiasson D. The role of granulomatous phlebitis and thrombosis in the pathogenesis of cirrhosis and portal hypertension in sarcoidosis. *Hepatology* 1997;26:554–60.

74. Bonnett F, Morlat P, Dubuc J, et al. Sarcoidosis-associated hepatitis C virus infection. *Dig Dis Sci* 2002;467:794–6.

75. Li SD, Yong S, Srinivas D, Van Thiel DH. Reactivation of sarcoidosis during interferon therapy. *J Gastroenterol* 2002;37:50–4.

76. Cogrel O, Doutre MS, Marliere V, Beylot-Barry M, Couzigou P, Beylot J. Cutaneous sarcoidosis during interferon alpha and ribavirin treatment of hepatitis C virus infection: two cases. *Br J Dermatol* 2002;146:320–4.

77. Butnor, KJ. Pulmonary sarcoidosis induced by interferon-alpha therapy. *Am J Surg Pathol* 2005;29:976–9.

78. Murphy JR, Sjogren MH, Kikendall JW, Peura DA, Goodman Z. Small bile duct abnormalities in sarcoidosis. *J Clin Gastroenterol* 1990;12:555–61.

79. Gottlieb JE, Isreal HL, Steiner RM, Triolo J, Patrick H. Outcome in sarcoidosis. The relationship of relapse to corticosteroid therapy. *Chest* 1997;111:623–31.

80. Becheur H, Dall'osto H, Chatellier G, et al. Effect of ursodeooxy-cholic acid on chronic intrahepatic cholestasis due to sarcoidosis. *Dig Dis Sci* 1997;42:789–91.

81. Amarapurkar DN, Patel ND, Amarapurkar AD. Hepatobil-iary tuberculosis in western India. *Indian J Pathol Microbiol* 2008;51:175–81.

82. Maharaj B, Leary WP, Pudifin DJ. A prospective study of hepatic tuberculosis in 41 black patients. *Q J Med* 1987;63:517–22.

83. Huang WT, Wang CC, Chen WJ, Cheng YF, Eng HL. The nodu-lar form of hepatic tuberculosis: a review with five additional new cases. *J Clin Pathol* 2003;56:835–9.

84. Alenezi B, Lamoureux E, Alpert L, Azilagyi A. Effect of ursodeooxy-cholic acid on granulomatous liver disease due to sarcoidosis. *Dig Dis Sci* 2005;50:196–200.

85. Taylor TH, Lewis JH. Tuberculosis of the liver, biliary tract and pan-creas. In: Schlossberg D, ed. *Tuberculosis and Nontuberculous Mycobac-terial Infections*, 6th edn. Washington, DC: American Society for Microbiology Press, 2011: 372–408.

86. Alvarez SZ. Hepatobiliary tuberculosis. *Gastroenterol Hepatol* 1998;13:833–9.

87. Amarapurkar AD, Sangle NA. Histological spectrum of liver in HIV – autopsy study. *Ann Hepatol* 2005;4:47–51.

88. Alcantara-Payawal DE, Matsumura M, Shiratori Y, et al. Direct detection of *Mycobacterium* tuberculosis using polymerase chain reaction assay among patients with hepatic granuloma. *J Hepatol* 1997;27:620–7.

89. Vilaichone RK, Vilaichone W, Tumwasorn S, Suwanagool P, Wilde H, Mahachai V. Clinical spectrum of hepatic tuberculosis: compar-ison between immunocompetent and immunocompromised hosts. *J Med Assoc Thai* 2003;86:S432–8.

90. Chien RN, Lin PY, Liw YF. Hepatic tuberculosis comparison of mil-itary and local form. *Infection* 1995;23:5–8.

91. Gupta S, Meena HS, Chopra R. Hepatic involvement in tuberculosis. *J Assoc Physicians India* 1993;41:20–2.

92. Essop AR, Posen J, Hodkinson JG, et al. Tuberculosis hepatitis: a clinical review of 96 cases. *Q J Med* 1984;53:465–77.

93. Okuda K, Kimura K, Takara K, et al. Resolution of diffuse granu-lomatous fibrosis of the liver with antituberculous chemotherapy. *Gastroenterology* 1986;91:456–60.

94. Lopez de Castilla D, Schluger NW. Tuberculosis following solid organ transplantation. *Transpl Infect Dis* 2010;12:106–12.

95. Ferrell LD, Lee R, Brixko C, et al. Hepatic granulomas follow-ing liver transplantation. Clinicopathologic features in 42 patients. *Transplantation* 1995;60:926–33.

96. Lewis JH. Drug-induced liver disease. *Med Clin North Am* 2000;84:1275–311.

97. Flippin T, Mukherji B, Dayal Y. Granulomatous hepatisits as a late complication of BCG immunotherapy. *Cancer* 1980;46:1959–62.

98. Gottke MU, Wong P, Muhn C, Jabbari M, Morin S. Hepatitis in dis-seminated bacillus Calmette–Guerin infection. *Can J Gastroenterol* 2000;14:333–6.

99. O'Brien TF, Hyslop NE Jr. Case records of the Massachusetts Gen-eral Hospital, case 34-1975. *N Engl J Med* 1975;293:443–8.

100. Ferrari TC, Araujo, MG, Riberio MM. Hepatic involvement in lep-romatous leprosy. *Lepr Rev* 2002;73:72–5.

101. Patnaik JK, Saha PK, Satpathy SK, Das BS, Bose TK. Hepatic mor-phology in reactional states of leprosy. *Int J Lepr Other Mycobact Dis* 1989;57:499–505.

102. Chen TS, Drutz DJ, Whelan GE. Hepatic granulomas in leprosy. Their relation to bacteremia. *Arch Pathol Lab Med* 1976;100:182–5.

103. Lefkowitch JH. The liver in AIDS. *Semin Liver Dis* 1997;17:335–44.

104. Kahn SA, Saltzman BR, Klein RS, Mahadevia PS, Friedland GH, Brandt LJ. Hepatic disorders in the acquired immune deficiency syndrome: a clinical and pathological study. *Am J Gastroenterol* 1986;81:1135–8.

105. Dworkin BM, Stahl RE. Giardina MA, et al. The liver in acquired immune deficiency syndrome: emphasis on patients with intra-venous drug abuse. *Am J Gastroenterol* 1987;82:231–6.

106. Cavicchi M, Pialoux G, Carnot F, et al. Value of liver biopsy for the rapid diagnosis of infection in human immunodeficiency virus-infected patients who have unexplained fever and elevated serum levels of alkaline phosphatase or gamma-glutamyl transferase. *Clin Infect Dis* 1995;20:606–10.

107. Garcia-Ordonez MA, Colmenero JD, Jimenez-Onate F, Martos F, Martinez J, Juarez C. Diagnostic usefulness pf percutaneous liver biopsy in HIV-infected patients with fever of unknown origin. *J Infect* 1999;38:94–8.

108. Astagneau P, Michon C, Marche C, et al. Heatic involvement in AIDS. A retrospective clinical study in patients. *Ann Med Interne (Paris)* 1990;141:459–63.

109. Farhi DC, Mason UG 3rd, Hordburgh CR Jr. Pathologic findings in disseminated *Mycobacterium avium-intracellulare* infection. A report of 11 cases. *Am J Clin Pathol* 1986;85:67–72.

110. Poles MA, Dieterich DT. Infections of the liver in HIV-infected patients. *Infect Dis Clin North Am* 2000;14:741–59.

111. Rutitzky LI, Bazzone L, Shainheit MG, et al. IL-23 is required for the development of severe egg-induced immunopathology in schistosomiasis and for lesional expression of of IL-17. *J Immunol* 2008;180:2486–95.

112. Ashahi H, Stadecker MJ. Analysis of egg antigens inducing hepatic lesions in schistosome infection. *Parasitol Int* 2003;52:361–7.

113. Burke ML, Jones MK, Gobert GN, et al. Immunopathogenesis of human schistosomiasis. *Parasite Immunol* 2009;31:163–76.

114. Andrade ZA. Schistosomiasis and liver fibrosis. *Parasite Immunol* 2009;31:656–63.

115. Caldas IR, Campi-Azevedo AC, Oliveira LF, et al. Human schis-tosomiasis mansoni: immune responses during acute and chronic phases of the infection. *Acta Trop* 2008;108:109–17.

116. Friis H, Andersen CB, Vennervald BJ, Christesen NO, Pakkenberg B. The use of a stereological method to estimate the volume of *Schistosoma mansoni* granulomas: the effect of zinc deficiency. *Ann Trop Med Parasitol* 1998;92:785–92.

117. Helmy MM, Mahmoud SS, Fahmy ZH. *Schistosoma mansoni*: effect of dietary zinc supplement on egg granuloma in Swiss mice treated with praziqantal. *Exp Parasitol* 2009;122:310–17.

118. Honstettre A, Ghigo E, Moynault A, et al. Lipopolysaccharide from *Coxiella burnetti* is involved in bacterial phagocyosis, filamentous actin reorganization, and inflammatory responses though Toll-like receptor 4. *J Immunol* 2004;172:3695–703.

119. Maurin M, Raoult D. Q fever. *Clin Microbiol Rev* 1999;12:518–53.

120. Takahashi H, Tokue Y, Kikuchi T, et al. Prevalence of community-acquired respiratory tract infections associated with Q fever in Japan. *Diagn Microbiol Infect Dis* 2004;48; 247–52.

121. Chang K, Yan JJ, Lee HC, Liu KH, Lee NY, Ko WC. Acute hepati-tis with or without jaundice: a predominant presentation of acute Q fever in southern Taiwan. *J Microbiol Immunol Infect* 2004;37:103–8.

122. van Woerden HC, Mason BW, Nehaul LK, et al. Q fever outbreak in industrial setting. *Emerg Infect Dis* 2004;10:1828–9.

123. Gilroy N, Formica N, Beers M, Egan A, Conaty S, Marmion B. Abattoir-associated Q fever: a Q fever outbreak during a Q fever vaccination program. *Aust NZ J Public Health* 2001;25:362–7.

124. Marmion BP, Storm PA, Ayres JG, et al. Long-term persistence of *Coxiella burnetti* after acute primary Q fever. *Q J Med* 2005;98:7–20.

125. Travis LB, Travis WD, Li CY, Pierre RV. Q fever. A clinicopathologic study of five cases. *Arch Pathol Lab Med* 1986;110:1017–20.

126. Marrie TJ, Stein A, Janigan D, Raoult, D. Route of infection determines the clinical manifestations of acute Q fever. *J Infect Dis* 1996;173:484–7.

127. Raoult D, Houpikian P, Tissot Dupont H, Riss JM, Arditi-Djiane J, Brouqui P. Treatment of Q fever endocarditis: comparison of 2 regimens containing doxycycline and ofloxacin or hydrooxychloroquine. *Arch Intern Med* 1999;159:167–73.

128. Murray FE, O'Loughlin S, Dervan P, Lennon JR, Crowe J. Granulomatous hepatitis in secondary syphilis. *Ir J Med Sci* 1990;159:53–4.

129. Saebo A, Lassen J. Acute and chronic liver disease associated with *Yersinia enterocolitica* infection: a Norwegian 10-year follow-up study of 458 hospitalized patients. *J Intern Med* 1992;231:531–5.

130. Lenoir AA, Storch GA, DeSchryver-Kecskemeti K, et al. Granulomatous hepatitis associated with cat scratch disease. *Lancet* 1988;1:1132–6.

131. Malatack JJ, Jaffe R. Granulomatous hepatitis in three children due to cat-scratch disease without peripheral adenopathy. An unrecognized cause of fever of unknown origin. *Am J Dis Child* 1993;147:499–53.

132. Humar S, Salit I. Disseminated *Bartonella* infection with granulomatous hepatitis a liver transplant recipient. *Liver Transpl Surg* 1999;5:249–51.

133. Margolis B, Kuzu I, Herrmann M, Raible MD, His E, Alkan S. Rapid polymerase chain reaction-based confirmation of cat scratch disease and *Bartonella henselae* infection. *Arch Pathol Lab Med* 2003;127:706–10.

134. Zijlstra EE, el-Hassan AM. Leishmaniasis in Sudan. Visceral leishmaniasis. *Trans R Soc Trop Med Hyg* 2001;95(Suppl 1):S27–58.

135. Kaplan KJ, Goodman ZD, Ishak KG. Eosinophilic granuloma of the liver: a characteristic lesion with relationship to visceral larva migrans. *Am J Surg Pathol* 2001;25:1316–21.

136. Lulu AR, Araj GF, Khateeb MI, Mustafa MY, Yusuf AR, Fenech FF. Human brucellosis in Kuwait: a prospective study of 400 cases. *Q J Med* 1988;66:39–54.

137. Talley NJ, Eckstein RP, Gattas MR, Stiel D. Acute hepatitis and *Brucella melitensis* infection: clinicopathological findings. *Med J Aust* 1988;148:587–8, 590.

138. Colmenero J de D, Queipo-Ortuno MI, Maria Reguera J, Angel Suarez-Munoz M, Martin-Carballino S, Morata P. Chronic hepatosplenic abscesses in brucellosis. Clinico-therapeutic features and molecular diagnostic approach. *Diagn Microbiol Infect Dis* 2002;42:159–67.

139. Akritidis N, Tzivras M, Delladetsima I, et al. The liver in brucellosis. *Clin Gastroenterol Hepatol* 2007;5(9):1109–12.

140. Al Dahouk S, Tomaso H, Nockler K, Neubauer H, Frangoulidis D. Laboratory-based diagnosis of brucellosis – a review of the literature. Part II: serological tests for brucellosis. *Clin Lab* 2003;49:577–89.

141. Lamps LW, Molina CP, West AB, Haggitt RC, Scott MA. The pathologic spectrum of gastrointestinal and hepatic histoplasmosis. *Am J Clin Pathol* 2000;113:64–72.

142. Craig JR, Hillberg RH, Balchum OJ. Disseminated coccidioidomycosis. Diagnosis by needle biopsy of liver. *West J Med* 1975;122:171–4.

143. Harada K, Minato H, Hiramatsu K, Nakanuma Y. Epithelioid cell granulomas in chronic hepatitis C: immunohistochemical character and histological marker of favourable response to interferon-alpha therapy. *Histopathology* 1998;33:216–21.

144. Emile JF, Sebagh M, Feray C, David F, Reynes M. The presence of epithelioid granulomas in hepatitis C virus-related cirrhosis. *Hum Pathol* 1993;24:1095–7.

145. Ryan BM, McDonald GS, Pilkington R, Kelleher D. The development of hepatic granulomas following interferon-alpha2b therapy for chronic hepatitis C infection. *Eur J Gastroenterol Hepatol* 1998;10:349–51.

146. Goldin RD, Levine TS, Foster GR, Thomas HC. Granulomas and hepatitis C. *Histopathology* 1996;28:265–7.

147. Ozaras R, Tahan V, Mert A, et al. The prevalence of hepatic granulomas in chronic hepatitis C. *J Clin Gastroenterol* 2004;38:449–52.

148. Tsimpoukas F, Goritsas C, Papdopoulos N, Trigidou R, Ferti A. Sarcoidosis in untreated chronic hepatitis C virus infection. *Scand J Gastroenterol* 2004;39:401–3.

149. Hoso M, Nakamuna Y, Kawano M, et al. Granulomatous cholangitis in chronic hepatitis C; a new diagnostic problem in liver pathology. *Pathol Int* 1996;46:301–5.

150. Snyder N, Martinez JG, Xiao SY. Chronic hepatitis C is a common association with hepatic granulomas. *World J Gastroenterol* 2008;14(41):6366–9.

151. Yamamoto S, Iguchi Y, Ohomoto K, Mitsui Y, Shimabara M, Mikami K. Epitheloid granuloma formation in type C chronic hepatitis: report of two cases. *Hepatogastroenterology* 1995;42:291–3.

152. Moller DR, Forman JD, Liu MC, et al. Enhanced expression of IL-12 associated with Th1 cytokine profiles in active pulmonary sarcoidosis. *J Immunol* 1996;156:4952–60.

153. Farah M, Rashidi A, Owen DA, et al. Granulomatous hepatitis associated with etanercept therapy. *J Rheumatol* 2008;35:349–51.

154. Tahan V, Ozaras R, Lacevic N, et al. Prevalence of hepatic granulomas in chronic hepatitis B. *Dig Dis Sci*. 2004;49:1575–7.

155. Fiel MI, Shukla D, Saraf N, et al. Development of hepatic granulomas in patients receiving pegylated interferon therapy for recurrent hepatitis C virus post liver transplantation. *Transpl Infect Dis* 2008;10:184–9.

156. Anania FA, Howell CD, Laurin JM, Drachenberg CI. Delayed granuloma formation in a patient with vanishing bile duct syndrome 7 years post-liver transplantation. *Liver Transpl* 2001;7:999–1001.

157. Botterel F, Ichai P, Feray C, et al. Disseminated toxoplasmosis, resulting from infection of allograft, after orthotopic liver transplantation: usefulness of quantitative PCR. *J Clin Microbiol* 2002;40:1648–50.

158. Scheuer PJ. Ludwig Symposium on biliary disorders – part II. Pathologic features and evolution of primary biliary cirrhosis and primary sclerosing cholangitis. *Mayo Clin Proc* 1998;73:179–83.

159. Burt AD. Primary biliary cirrhosis and other ductopenic diseases. *Clin Liver Dis* 2002;6:363–80.

160. Wiesner R, LaRusso N, Ludwig J, et al. Comparison of the clinicopathologic features of primary sclerosing cholangitis and primary biliary cirrhosis. *Gastroenterology* 1985;88:108–14.

161. Matheus T, Munoz S. Granulomatous liver disease and cholestasis. *Clin Liver Dis* 2004;8:229–46.

162. Degott C, Zafrani ES, Callard P, Balkau B, Poupon RE, Poupon R. Histopathological study of primary biliary cirrhosis and the effect of ursodeoxycholic acid treatment on histology progression. *Hepatology* 1999;29:1007–12.

163. Paumgartner G, Beuers U. Mechanisms of action and therapeutic efficacy of ursodeoxycholic acid in cholestatic liver disease. *Clin Liver Dis* 2004;8:67–81.

164. Ludwig J, Colina F, Poterucha JJ. Granulomas in primary sclerosing cholangitis. *Liver* 1995;15:307–12.

165. Ishak KG, Zimmerman HJ. Drug-induced and toxic granulomatous hepatitis. *Baillieres Clin Gastroenterol* 1988;2:463–80.

166. Zimmerman HJ. *Hepatotoxicity. The adverse effects of drugs and other chemicals on the liver*, 2nd edn. Philadelphia, PA: Lippincott Williams and Wilkins, 1999.

167. Benjamin SB, Ishak KG, Zimmerman HJ, Grushka A. Phenylbutazone liver injury: a clinical-pathologic survey of 23 cases and review of the literature. *Hepatology* 1981;1:255–63.

168. Rossman MD. Chronic beryllium disease: a hypersensitivity disorder. *Appl Occup Environ Hyg* 2001;16:615–18.

169. Fireman E, Haimsky E, Noiderfer M, Priel I, Lerman Y. Misdiagnosis of sarcoidosis in patients with chronic beryllium disease. *Sarcoidosis Vasc Diffuse Lung Dis* 2003;20:144–8.

170. Allaire GS, Goodman ZD, Ishak KG, Rabin L. Talc in liver tissue of intravenous drug abusers with chronic hepatitis. A comparative study. *Am J Clin Pathol* 1989;92:583–8.

171. Liu YC, Tomashefski J Jr, McMahon JT, Petrelli M. Mineral-associated hepatic injury: a report of seven cases with X-ray microanalysis. *Hum Pathol* 1991;22:1120–7.

172. Sherman KE, Lewey SM, Goodman ZD. Talc in the liver of patients with chronic hepatitis C infection. *Am J Gastroenterol* 1995;90:2164–6.

173. Leong AS, Disney AP, Gove DW. Spallation and migration of silicone from blood-pump tubing in patients on hemodialysis. *N Engl J Med* 1982;306:135–40.

174. Hunt J, Farthing MJ, Baker LR, Crocker PR, Levison DA. Silicone in the liver: possible late effects. *Gut* 1989;30:239–42.

175. Kurumaya H, Kono N, Nakanuma Y, Tomoda F, Takazakura E. Hepatic granulomatra in long-term hemodialysis patients with hyperaluminumemia. *Arch Pathol Lab Med* 1989;113:1132–4.

176. Sacks EL, Donaldson SS, Gordon J, Dorfman RF. Epithelioid granulomas associated with Hodgkin's disease: clinical correlations in 55 previously untreated patients. *Cancer* 1978;41:562–7.

177. Chopra R, Rana R, Zachariah A, Mahajan MK, Prabhakar BR. Epithelioid granulomas in Hodgkin's disease – prognostic significance. *Indian J Pathol Microbiol* 1995;38:427–33.

178. Bendix-Hansen K, Bayer Kristensen I. Granulomas of spleen and liver in hairy cell leukaemia. *Acta Pathol Microbiol Immunol Scand A* 1984;92:157–60.

179. Bergter W, Fetzer IC, Sattler B, Ramadori G. Granulomatous hepatitis preceding Hodgkin's disease (case-report and review on differential dDiagnosis). *Pathol Oncol Res* 1996;2:177–80.

180. Johnson LN, Iseri O, Knodell RG. Caseating hepatic granulomas in Hodgkin's lymphoma. *Gastroenterology* 1990;99:1837–40.

181. Abrams J, Pearl P, Moody M, Schimpff SC. Epithelioid granulomas revisited: long-term follow-up in Hodgkin's disease. *Am J Clin Oncol* 1988;11:456–60.

182. Brown JR, Skarin AT. Clinical mimics of lymphoma. *Oncologist* 2004;9:406–16.

183. Spickett GP, Zhang JG, Green T, Shrimankar J. Granulomatous disease in common variable immunodeficiency: effect on immunoglobulin replacement therapy and response to steroids and splenectomy. *J Clin Pathol* 1996;49:431–4.

184. Glaser J, Gahr M, Munnetha A, Mann O, von Eiff M, Pausch J. Chronic granulomatosis: a rare differential diagnosis in liver granulomas in adulthood. *Dtsch Med Wochenschr* 1995;120:646–8.

185. Nakhleh RE, Glock M, Snover DC. Hepatic pathology of chronic granulomatous disease of childhood. *Arch Pathol Lab Med* 1992;116:71–5.

186. van den Berg JM, van Koppen E, Ahlin A, et al. Chronic granulomatous disease: the European experience. *PLoS One* 2009;4(4):e5234.

187. Banner BF, Banner AS. Hepatic granulomas following ileal bypass for obesity. *Arch Pathol lab Med* 1978;102:655–7.

188. Ruderman EM, Crawford JM, Maier A, Liu JJ, Gravallese EM, Weinblatt ME. Histologic liver abnormalities in an autopsy series of patients with rheumatoid arthritis. *Br J Rheumatol* 1997;36:210–13.

189. Israel HL, Margolis ML, Rose LJ. Hepatic granulomatosis and sarcoidosis. Further observations. *Dig Dis Sci* 1984;29:353–6.

190. Bruguera M, Torres-Salinas M, Bordas JM, Bru C, Rodes J. The role of liver biopsy in the study of patients with fever of unknown origin. *Med Clin (Barc)* 1981;77:115–17.

191. Aderka D, Kraus M, Weinberger A, Pinkhas J. Parameters which can differentiate patients with "idiopathic" from patients with lymphoma-induced liver granulomas. *Am J Gastroenterol* 1985;80:1004–7.

192. Lewis JH, Patel HR, Zimmerman HJ. The spectrum of hepatic candidiasis. *Hepatology* 1982;2:479–87.

193. Terplan M. Hepatic granulomas of unknown cause presenting with fever. *Am J Gastroenterol* 1971;55:43–9.

194. Knox TA, Kaplan MM, Gelfand JA, Wolff SM. Methotrexare treatment on idiopathic granulomatous hepatitis. *Ann Intern Med* 1995;122:592–5.

195. Longstreth GF, Bender RA. Cyclophosphamide therapy of idiopathic hepatic granulomatosis. *Dig Dis Sci* 1989;34:1615–16.

196. Berlin CM Jr, Boal DK, Zaino RJ, Karl SR. Hepatic granulomata. Presenting with prolonged fever. Resolution with anti-inflammatory treatment. *Clin Pediatr (Phila)* 1990;29:339–42.

Multiple choice questions

40.1 Match the most likely etiology of hepatic granulomas with the appropriate histologic feature from the following lists.

Feature:
a Lipogranuloma.
b Fibrin ring granuloma.
c Non-necrotising granulomas.
d Acid-fast bacilli positive.
e Periductal granulomas.

Etiology:
1 Q fever.
2 Sarcoidosis.
3 Primary biliary cirrhosis
4 BCG.
5 Mineral oil.

40.2 Which one of the following statements regarding the granulomas of sarcoidosis is false?

a Sarcoidosis is associated with the greatest number of hepatic granulomas.
b Granulomas tend to be in different stages of development.
c Granulomas are most prominent in portal and periportal areas.
d Granulomas are non-necrotizing.
e Giant cell inclusions (asteroid bodies) are pathognomonic of sarcoidosis.

Answers to the multiple choice questions can be found in the Appendix at the end of the book.

These multiple choice questions are also available for you to complete online.
Visit http://www.schiffsdiseasesoftheliver.com/

CHAPTER 41

Hepatobiliary Manifestations of Human Immunodeficiency Virus

Marie-Louise Vachon, Ponni Perumalswami, & Douglas T. Dieterich

Division of Liver Diseases, Department of Medicine, Mount Sinai School of Medicine, New York, NY, USA

Key concepts

- Liver disease is the second most common cause of death among patients with human immunodeficiency virus (HIV) after acquired immune deficiency syndrome-related mortality because of the increased life expectancy as a result of antiretroviral therapy (ART).
- Coinfection with hepatitis B virus (HBV) and hepatitis C virus (HCV) is common. HIV accelerates the natural history of HBV and HCV infections. Chronic HBV and HCV infections are responsible for the increasing morbidity and mortality due to liver disease in this population.
- Treatment of chronic HCV with pegylated interferon and ribavirin results in a cure in about 40% of patients. The use of HCV direct-acting antivirals to increase cure rates is under study.

- The HIV population is aging. New complications of HIV and ART are recognized and include noncirrhotic portal hypertension. This adds to the burden of liver disease in this population.
- Hepatic steatosis is common in patients with HIV, and long-term ART use is associated with metabolic changes including lipodystrophy.
- ART has substantially decreased the incidence of opportunistic infections, although in immunosuppressed HIV patients the liver and biliary tract are frequent sites of infection.
- Hepatocellular carcinoma is a growing problem and presents at a younger age and most often with coinfection with HCV and/or HBV.
- Early referral, a lower model for end-stage liver disease score at the time of transplantation, and well-controlled HIV disease are predictors of successful outcomes after liver transplant in HIV-infected patients.

Since its recognition nearly three decades ago, the natural history of infection with human immunodeficiency virus (HIV) has undergone a vast change, from a disease associated with high mortality due to opportunistic infections, to a chronic illness that may last for decades associated with age- rather than HIV-related morbidities. The introduction of antiretroviral therapy (ART) in the mid-1990s was responsible for the dramatic prolongation of survival of patients diagnosed with HIV. Along with acquired immune deficiency syndrome (AIDS)-related complications, liver diseaseve has now become one of the most important factors affecting survival, quality of life, and health care costs among HIV-infected patients. HIV-infected patients experience an array of hepatobiliary manifestations. Most liver diseases in these patients are due to hepatitis C virus (HCV) or hepatitis B virus (HBV) coinfection, but other entities such as steatosis, steatohepatitis, and drug hepatotoxicity add to the burden of liver disease in this population. Aging of the HIV population facilitates the development of liver disease and allows for the recognition of long-term com-

plications of HIV and ART such as noncirrhotic portal hypertension (NCPH). Liver transplantation is a promising option for HIV-infected patients with end-stage liver disease (ESLD). HIV has become a disease of older adults and represents a completely different challenge.

Human immunodeficiency virus and viral coinfections

Hepatitis B virus coinfection

Prevalence and importance

Human immunodefiency virus and HBV share common risk factors for transmission. As a result, evidence of prior exposure to HBV can be found in as many as 90% of HIV-infected patients, and the prevalence of chronic HBV infection in HIV-infected patients is around 7–10%. Testing for the presence of HBV infection should thus be part of the initial evaluation of all HIV-infected patients, as should screening for the presence of chronic HCV infection and immunity to hepatitis A virus (HAV). The likelihood of spontaneous clearance after acute HBV infection is lower in HIV-infected patients compared with HIV-uninfected patients. HIV/HBV coinfection is associated with higher HBV DNA levels, lower aminotransferase levels, decreased spontaneous loss of hepatitis B e antigen (HBeAg), and decreased seroconversion rates of antibodies to hepatitis B e antigen (anti-HBe). HIV accelerates progression to cirrhosis, ESLD, development of hepatocellular carcinoma (HCC), and liver-related mortality [1]. The high coinfection prevalence coupled with the aggressive course of liver disease and the increased life expectancy with effective ART among HIV-infected patients have led to an increase in the burden of hepatitis B (and C) coinfections in all age groups.

Chronic liver disease, driven by the high prevalence of viral hepatitis coinfections, has emerged as one of the leading causes of morbidity and mortality in HIV-infected patients in the post-ART era [2,3]. In a European prospective cohort study of HIV-infected patients, liver disease was the second most common cause of death among patients with HIV/HBV coinfection (22% versus 38% AIDS-related deaths) [2]. In other studies, liver-related mortality has been found to be 3–14 times higher in HIV/HBV-coinfected patients compared with HBV-monoinfected patients [1,4,5]. An increase in the CD4+ T-cell count reduces the risk of liver-related mortality. HCC development is a frequent cause of liver-related death in these patients and can present in the absence of cirrhosis. In HIV/HBV-coinfected patients, HCC development has been shown to be significantly associated with a lower absolute CD4+ T-cell count and percentage [6], and a longer survival is observed in patients with undetected HIV RNA [7].

The effects of HBV on the natural history of HIV are less clear. Although previous studies indicated that HBV had no effect on the course of HIV and its response to ART [1], recent data suggest that coinfection may be associated with lower CD4+ T-cell counts at the time of ART initiation and that response to ART may be slower in patients with HBeAg-positive HBV compared to HBeAg-negative HBV infection [8].

Diagnosis and prevention in susceptible individuals

All HIV-infected patients should be tested for HBV markers at the time of initial evaluation with a minimum of hepatitis B surface antigen (HBsAg), antibodies to hepatitis B surface antigen (anti-HBs), and antibodies to hepatitis B core antigen (anti-HBc). In patients with a positive HBsAg, the HBV DNA level, HBeAg, and anti-HBe markers will characterize the status of infection [9–11]. As for HBV monoinfection, HIV/HBV-coinfected patients should have a close follow-up of HBV DNA and alanine aminotransferase (ALT), in addition to periodic HCC

screening. When to perform a liver biopsy is an area of controversy. Most experts agree it should be done only when treatment indications are not clear, to rule out necroinflammation and/or significant fibrosis that would argue toward the need for treatment. In no way is it a requirement for treatment. Alternative methods of fibrosis assessment such as transient elastography are not US Food and Drug Administration (FDA) approved although transient elastography is standard of care in Europe and Canada.

In the setting of HIV infection, HBV serologic testing often shows an isolated anti-HBc in the absence of other markers of HBV exposure. Isolated anti-HBc is more common among HIV-infected patients compared with HIV-uninfected patients. The prevalence is estimated to lie between 17% and 81% depending on the cohorts studied, compared with 2–5% in HIV-uninfected patients [12]. Isolated anti-HBc represents either the result of a false-positive test, past HBV infection with loss of or undetectable levels of anti-HBs, or occult HBV infection. The clinical significance of isolated anti-HBc is unclear and the need for HBV vaccination is controversial in these cases. Occult HBV infection is defined as the presence of HBV DNA in the absence of HBsAg; usually an isolated anti-HBc is found at serology testing [10]. Occult HBV infection occurs predominantly in HIV-infected patients. In one study, patients with HIV RNA levels >1,000 copies/mL and without HCV coinfection were more likely to have occult HBV infection [13]. The exact significance of occult HBV and its long-term consequences are not well characterized, although it has the potential to reactivate secondary to immunosuppression or the interruption of ART containing active anti-HBV agents [14].

When serologic testing does not show any evidence of prior HBV exposure, the complete HBV vaccination series should be given and repeated a second time if no immune response is elicited 1 month after the third dose. The response rate to HBV single-dose vaccine is between 18% and 56% compared with 90% of immunocompetent individuals. Efforts should be made to increase the CD4+ T-cell count to >200 cells/mm^3 to optimize the immunologic response to the vaccine. Some studies have found a higher response rate to the double-dose vaccine (40 μg) when the CD4+ T-cell count was above 350 cells/mm^3 [15]. However, HBV vaccination should not be deferred while waiting for the CD4+ T-cell count to reach that threshold. The use of granulocyte–macrophage colony-stimulating factor (GM-CSF) as a vaccine adjuvant did not increase response rates [16].

Treatment

The goals of HBV therapy in patients with HIV/HBV coinfection are the suppression of HBV DNA, the normalization of ALT, seroconversion from HBeAg to anti-HBe, and ideally the loss of HBsAg and seroconversion to anti-HBs to prevent liver disease progression and reduce the risk of potential complications such as the development of HCC. Because of the close interactions between HIV and HBV, any treatment decision for hepatitis B should take into account the possible impact on HIV and vice versa. Recent evidence of a benefit for earlier initiation of ART in HIV-infected patients has led to a change in the HIV treatment recommendations issued by the US Department of Health and Human Services (DHHS) [17]. The recommendations are now to initiate ART with anti-HBV active agents whether treatment is needed for HBV (independent of the CD4+ T-cell count), HIV, or both. At the time of ART initiation and change of ART, it is important to use agents active against HBV to reduce the risk of immune reconstitution inflammatory syndrome and hepatic flare, which can be life threatening. Drugs approved for the treatment of chronic HBV infection are interferon (IFN), pegylated interferon α-2a (pegIFN-α-2a), lamivudine, adefovir dipivoxil, entecavir, and tenofovir disoproxil fumarate (TDF). Emtricitabine, approved for HIV therapy, is active against HBV but not FDA approved for the treatment of chronic HBV infection yet. Most studies in HBV treatment have been done using lamivudine and results have shown histologic and clinical improvement, and a significant reduction of liver-related death per year of treatment. Emergence of resistance is frequent and the highest with lamivudine use. After 4 years of lamivudine use, 90% of HIV/HBV-coinfected patients develop resistance mutations. The combination of two drugs active against HBV is recommended to prevent the emergence of resistance in HIV/HBV-coinfected patients. The antivirals that have activity against both HIV and HBV viruses are TDF, emtricitabine, lamivudine, and entecavir. Entecavir is not used to treat HIV but has some activity against it and has the ability to select for the M184V resistance mutation in HIV [18]. The preferred regimens are the combination of TDF and emtricitabine or TDF and lamivudine. TDF is a potent agent active against lamivudine-resistant HBV strains [19]. The mutation rtA194T has been reported to be associated with TDF resistance in one report, but not confirmed in other studies [20]. In the rare cases where HIV treatment is not desirable and HBV treatment is indicated, pegIFN and adefovir 10 mg are recommended to avoid HIV resistance development. In these cases, the criteria used to evaluate the need to treat HBV do not differ from those used in HBV-monoinfected patients, although some experts recommend treating HBeAg-positive and HBeAg-negative HBV at any HBV DNA level in all HIV-infected patients due to their accelerated liver disease progression. ALT levels, HBeAg status, and HBV DNA levels with or without fibrosis assessment determine the indication of HBV treatment. Guidelines for HIV-uninfected individuals with HBeAg-positive HBV infection recommend that treatment be considered for patients with serum HBV DNA above 20,000 IU/mL. For HBeAg-negative patients, a threshold of 2,000 IU/mL is used [10,21].

HCV coinfection

Prevalence, transmission, and importance

Human immunodeficiency virus and chronic HCV infection are two major public health problems. An estimated 170 million people are infected with HCV worldwide and 4–5 million are coinfected with HIV. In addition to both being major health issues, HIV and HCV have many similarities. Both viruses possess a single-stranded RNA genome and result in subclinical chronic infection. Each virus is able to evade the host's immune system because of high genetic variability, and the replication rate of both viruses is extremely high. Approximately 25–30% of HIV-infected patients are coinfected with HCV. Coinfection rates vary depending on the country and the region under study, the population, and the risk factors for HIV acquisition. The most efficient mode of HCV transmission is by direct exposure to blood or blood products. The main risk factor for acquisition in the United States is intravenous drug use. In this high-risk group, the rate of coinfection can reach 95%. HCV is not transmitted efficiently during heterosexual relationships, however HIV-infected men who have sex with men are emerging as a group at risk for sexual transmission of HCV. Several recent outbreaks of acute hepatitis C in Europe, Australia, and the United States have been reported [22]. In one of these reports, the majority of patients with acute HCV had stage 2/4 liver fibrosis at liver biopsy [23]. The vast majority of these patients share the same risk factors –high-risk sexual behavior, concomitant ulcerative sexually transmitted infections, and the use of recreational, IV or non-IV drugs such as methamphetamine. Vertical transmission of HCV is infrequent and increases in the setting of coinfection.

The improvement in HIV control with ART is evidenced by the emergence of chronic illnesses such as liver disease in this population and its associated complications. Liver-related death is now the most frequent cause of non-AIDS-related death among patients with HIV [3]. In a European prospective cohort study of HIV-infected patients, liver disease was the first cause of death among HIV/HCV-coinfected patients (31% of deaths versus 29% AIDS-related) [2]. In a prospective cohort study of 3,730 HIV-infected patients followed between 1995 and 2003, hospitalization rates decreased significantly in HIV-monoinfected patients but increased significantly in HIV/HCV-coinfected patients [24]. In the coinfected group, hospitalization rates increased for liver-related complications and HCV coinfection was an independent predictor of hospitalization.

Impact of human immunodeficiency virus and antiretroviral therapy on hepatitis C virus

Human immunodeficiency virus significantly affects the natural history of HCV-related liver disease. HIV-infected patients have a lower likelihood of spontaneous clearance of HCV compared with HIV-uninfected ones. Recent data in HCV-monoinfected patients have shown that the C/C genotype at a single nucleotide polymorphism (SNP) near the *IL28B* gene is associated with spontaneous clearance of HCV [25]. The same study among HIV/HCV-coinfected patients has not yet been published [26]. Serum and liver HCV viral loads are higher in HIV/HCV-coinfected patients compared with HCV-monoinfected patients because of greater HCV replication reflecting the immunosuppressed state. Liver fibrosis progression is accelerated compared to HCV monoinfection. Coinfected patients have an increased rate of progression to cirrhosis, ESLD, HCC, and death compared with monoinfected individuals [27–29]. As in HCV-monoinfected patients, liver fibrosis at baseline predicts the development of significant liver disease and death in HIV/HCV-coinfected patients [30]. In a study of 637 HIV/HCV-coinfected patients followed over a median duration of 5 years, the incidence rates of ESLD, HCC, or death increased in a stepwise manner according to the baseline fibrosis stage (METAVIR scoring system). Figure 41.1 shows Kaplan–Meier curves of ESLD/HCC/liver death-free survival according to the baseline METAVIR score in this study. Fibrosis stages 2 and above were significant predictors of ESLD, HCC, or death from any cause.

The incidence of HCC in the United States is rising overall and among the HIV-infected population. HCC is more aggressive in HIV with a higher frequency of infiltrating tumors, extranodal metastases at presentation, and portal invasion. HIV/HCV-coinfected individuals seem to be younger at the time of HCC diagnosis and have a faster progression from initial HCV infection to HCC development (26 versus 34 years) [7]. Data are contradictory as to whether HIV infection is independently associated with shorter survival in these patients [7,31].

The impact of ART on the evolution of HCV-related liver disease is contradictory. ART has been shown to slow the rate of fibrosis progression. One study showed that coinfected patients on ART with undetectable HIV RNA (<400 copies/mL) had a slower rate of fibrosis progression compared to those with HIV viremia and similar to HCV-monoinfected individuals [32]. A meta-analysis looking at the natural history of chronic hepatitis C in the HIV-infected population found that HIV/HCV-coinfected patients had a 2.1-fold higher risk of cirrhosis compared with HCV-monoinfected patients [33]. The increase was 2.5-fold in those not receiving ART and 1.7-fold in those receiving ART. This study suggests a partially protective role of ART against development of cirrhosis in this population. ART was found to reduce liver-related mortality in a retrospective study [34], although the same beneficial effect was not found in prospective studies [3,35]. In other reports, ART was associated with fibrosis progression and was dependent on the regimen used [36,37]. Hepatotoxicity of ART has been shown to be more likely to occur in patients with underlying HCV [38]. Effective treatment of HCV in coinfected individuals reduces ART related hepatotoxicity [39]. These contradictions in study results are likely due to the opposing effects of immune restoration and hepatotoxicity of ART regimens.

The presence of steatosis has been observed in up to 40% of patients with HIV/HCV coinfection. Patients with steatosis are more likely to have a higher stage of liver fibrosis and more severe HCV-related liver disease.

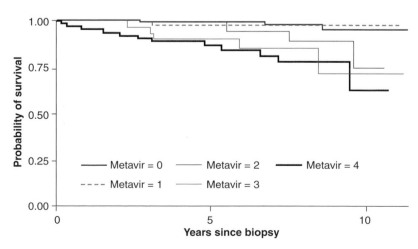

Figure 41.1 Probability of ESLD/HCC/liver death-free survival according to baseline METAVIR score. (Reproduced from Sulkowski et al. [30] with permission.)

Obesity, insulin resistance (IR), and the use of stavudine have been identified as modifiable risk factors for steatosis in this population.

Impact of hepatitis C virus on human immunodeficiency virus

Data regarding the influence of HCV on the natural history of HIV disease are conflicting. Overall, HCV does not seem to affect HIV disease progression, HIV RNA suppression following ART initiation, CD4+ T-cell count recovery, or the risk of AIDS. However, some studies have found a more rapid HIV disease progression and increased mortality in HIV/HCV-coinfected patients compared with HIV-monoinfected ones. HCV may negatively impact HIV disease by influencing ART tolerability and ART discontinuation.

Diagnosis

All patients with HIV should be screened for HCV. There is an estimated 3–4% false-negative rate with enzyme-linked immunosorbent assay (ELISA) testing in coinfected patients because of impaired HCV antibody production with immunosuppression, a rapid decline in HCV antibody titer, and a possible interaction between the two viruses. Therefore, screening with HCV RNA is useful in some high-risk coinfected patients such as those with low CD4+ T-cell counts, those on chronic hemodialysis, those who have hemophilia, or those who are former intravenous drug users. HCV screening is warranted at least at the time of initial evaluation and thereafter depending on risk factors for acquisition. The evaluation of elevations of ALT levels in HIV-infected patients should always include HCV testing, but HIV-infected patients are less likely to present with elevated ALT than HIV-uninfected patients [40]. Liver biopsy is the gold standard in staging liver fibrosis in the United States. Serologic biomarkers such as APRI and FIB-4 can be useful in discriminating advanced fibrosis from no fibrosis, but are less accurate than liver biopsy, especially in the intermediate stages of fibrosis. Transient elastography (FibroScan®), a noninvasive technique, seems more accurate but has not been approved by the FDA although it is standard of care in Europe and Canada.

In HIV-infected patients, staging of liver fibrosis with liver biopsy is not mandatory to guide treatment decisions in any HCV genotype and should not be a barrier to HCV treatment. There is every reason to treat HCV in HIV-infected patients. This includes patients with compensated (Child class A) cirrhosis. Patients who are willing to start therapy and who do not have contraindications to pegIFN and ribavirin (RBV) should be encouraged to undergo treatment based on the rapid progression of HCV-related liver disease, acceptable sustained virologic response (SVR) rates, and availability of early viral monitoring (weeks 4 and 12) to identify rapid responders and nonresponders.

The indication for HCV treatment is clear in those with stage 2 and above on the METAVIR fibrosis scale. When the liver biopsy indicates fibrosis stage 0 or 1 and the decision is made to postpone treatment, repeat fibrosis assessment is recommended at 3-year intervals [41].

Treatment

Given the impact of HIV on the natural history of HCV disease, HCV should be managed aggressively. HCV treatment is aimed at achieving viral eradication to slow the progression of liver disease and to prevent liver-related complications such as HCC. Successful treatment of HCV results in a reduced incidence of complications as demonstrated by several studies [43]. The simultaneous treatment of HCV and HIV is associated with the occurrence of drug interactions, overlapping toxicities, and increased incidence and severity of side effects. HIV/HCV-coinfected patients are in need of treatment, however state-of-the-art management requires different strategies in order to achieve cure with minimal adverse events. Viral eradication of HCV is termed SVR. SVR is defined as undetectable HCV RNA 24 weeks after completion of HCV treatment. When SVR is achieved, both in HCV-monoinfected patients and HIV/HCV-coinfected patients, this translates to a cure, and subsequent positive HCV RNA may reflect reinfection rather than HCV relapse [42]. Achievement of SVR reduces liver-related complications and mortality in HIV/HCV-coinfected patients [43].

SVR rates are lower in HIV/HCV-coinfected individuals compared with HIV-uninfected ones. Until recently, the best predictors of SVR were HCV genotype 2 and 3 and a low baseline HCV RNA. HCV RNA levels less than or equal to 400,000 IU/mL are predictive of treatment success [44]. Other factors have been found to be associated with SVR (Box 41.1) Recently, a strong association between a SNP near the *IL28B* gene and SVR in HCV-monoinfected and HIV/HCV-coinfected patients

---

Box 41.1 Favorable predictors of sustained virologic response (SVR).

- IL28B CC genotype
- Hepatitis C virus (HCV) genotype 2 or 3
- Low baseline HCV RNA (<400,000–800,000 IU/mL)
- Naïve to HCV treatment
- White race
- Younger age
- Low-stage fibrosis
- Absence of steatosis on liver biopsy
- Absence of insulin resistance
- Low body mass index

was found [45,46]. Individuals who carry the homozygous C/C genotype at this SNP have a significantly higher chance of achieving SVR with the standard of care. The study performed in HIV/HCV-coinfected patients has found that 65% of patients infected with HCV genotype 1 carrying the C/C genotype achieved SVR compared with 30% of those with the C/T or the T/T genotype [46]. The C/C allele is unevenly distributed among races and explains in part the lower response rate to HCV treatment among blacks. The C/C allele is most commonly found in Asia and Europe and is uncommon in Africa. A test for genotyping this SNP is now available in the United States to help predict treatment response. It is unclear to what extent the baseline CD4+ T-cell count influences SVR rates. In a recent study, patients infected with HCV genotype 1 had better SVR rates with higher baseline CD4+ T-cell counts [47]. No such association was found in HCV genotype 2 and 3 infected patients. When HCV treatment is considered, the best approach is to attempt to increase the CD4+ T-cell count before starting HCV treatment, but to avoid deferring treatment when the expected rise does not occur. There is no CD4+ T-cell threshold under which HCV treatment should not be attempted as long as HIV is optimally controlled.

The standard of care for HCV treatment in HIV/HCV-coinfected patients is pegIFN plus weight-based RBV for HCV genotypes 1 and 4 [41]. A 800 mg/day fixed-dose of RBV is recommended in HCV genotypes 2 and 3.

The present treatment recommendations are based on four main randomized controlled trials [48–51]. APRICOT enrolled 868 patients, of all genotypes and naïve to HCV treatment [48]. They were randomized to one of the three treatment arms to receive either: (i) pegIFN-α-2a 180 μg + RBV 800 mg; (ii) pegIFN-α-2a 180 μg + placebo; or (iii) standard IFN (3 million IU three times a week) + RBV 800 mg – all for 48 weeks. The pegIFN and RBV combination showed superiority with an overall SVR of 40% compared to 20% with pegIFN monotherapy and 12% with standard IFN. Higher baseline HCV RNA levels (>800,000 IU/mL) led to lower rates of SVR. The absence of early virologic response (EVR) (at least a 2 $\log_{10}$ decrease in HCV RNA at week 12) had a high negative predictive value to predict virologic failure as in HCV monoinfection. During HCV treatment, the absolute CD4+ T-cell count decreased but the mean CD4+ T-cell percentage increased. Safety issues were mostly hematologic and comparable to HCV-monoinfected patients.

The RIBAVIC trial compared standard IFN (3 million IU three times a week) + RBV to pegIFN-α-2b + RBV (1.5 μg/kg/week) [50]; 412 patients were enrolled. The overall SVR rate was 27% in the pegIFN group. Bridging fibrosis or cirrhosis were present in 40% of the patients. Many patients experienced adverse events not related to treatment and discontinued therapy. Serious adverse events, although similar in both groups, were higher than reported in the monoinfected population. Eleven cases of pancreatitis/hyperlactatemia were diagnosed in patients taking didanosine as part of their ART regimen.

The AIDS Clinical Trials Group (ACTG) A5071 study randomized 133 subjects to receive either pegIFN-α-2a (180 μg/week) + RBV or standard IFN-α-2a + RBV in a dose escalation schedule: 600 mg for 4 weeks, then 800 mg for 4 weeks, and then 1,000 mg for a total of 48 weeks [49]. PegIFN showed superiority over standard IFN with a reported SVR rate of 27% compared with 12%. A liver biopsy was performed at week 24 of treatment in patients with no virologic response; 35% of them had histologic improvement suggesting that benefits from the therapy extend beyond virologic control. In this study, the inadequate schedule of RBV may have explained the low SVR (high relapse) rates observed.

Laguno et al. [51] randomized patients to receive either standard IFN (3 million IU three times a week) or pegIFN-α-2b (100–150 μg/week) with weight-based RBV 800–1200 mg for 48 weeks. Patients with HCV genotype 2 and 3 infections who had HCV RNA <800,000 IU/ml were treated for 24 weeks only. Ninety-five patients, of whom 30% had bridging fibrosis or cirrhosis, were randomized. Overall, 44% achieved a SVR. This was the first randomized trial to use weight-based RBV and it yielded an increase in SVR. Patients with HCV genotype 2 and 3 infections experienced a high relapse rate after 24 weeks of treatment. Side effects were frequently reported, including depressive symptoms in 43% patients. There were nine cases of mitochondrial toxicity in patients receiving didanosine and/or stavudine.

The nonrandomized PRESCO trial sought to determine the role of weight-based RBV and extension of the duration of therapy in 389 coinfected patients [52]. These patients received pegIFN-α-2a (180 μg/week) + RBV (1,000 or 1,200 mg according to weight). Participants were treated for 48 versus 72 weeks. They achieved an overall SVR rate of 49.6%. SVR rates were significantly greater in the 72-week arm but with a withdrawal rate of 36/45 (80%) in patients with HCV genotype 1 infection. Higher dosage of RBV was well tolerated.

Overall, the expected SVR rates are 14–38% with HCV genotype 1 and 4 and 44–73% with HCV genotypes 2 and 3. State-of-the-art treatment of HCV involves individualizing treatment based on HCV viral kinetics. In the coinfected individuals, the kinetics of response is slower compared with HCV monoinfection. Response is first assessed at week 4 and undetectable viremia is termed rapid virologic response (RVR). In a substudy from RIBAVIC, authors reported no chance of SVR when HCV RNA could not be suppressed below 460,000 IU/mL at week 4 (negative predictive value of 100%) [53]. A similar analysis from APRICOT showed that RVR was the best predictor of SVR [54]. In a retrospective review of HCV genotype 2 and 3 coinfected patients from two prospective studies, Shea et al. reported a 100% (39 patients) SVR rate after a 24-week treatment with optimal doses of pegIFN and RBV when RVR was achieved [55]. Response is later assessed at week 12 and is termed EVR. EVR can either be partial (decrease of at least 2 logs from baseline viral load with detectable viremia) or complete (undetectable viremia). Coinfected patients who fail to achieve EVR have a 2% likelihood of SVR and thus treatment is discontinued when EVR is not achieved [48]. When partial EVR occurs and HCV RNA is still detectable at week 24, treatment should also be discontinued. Both RVR and EVR correlate with SVR in mono- and coinfected patients [52,53,56].

The two formulations of pegIFN (α-2a and α-2b) have been shown to have comparable safety in the treatment

of HCV in HIV-infected patients in the recently published GESIDA study [57]. Weight-based RBV was not found to be superior in the treatment of HCV genotype 1 in the randomized clinical trial PARADIGM; however, the study was powered to study safety of weight-based RBV and not efficacy [58].

In the nonrandomized PRESCO trial, 72% of patients with HCV genotypes 2 or 3 coinfected with HIV achieved SVR [52]. The use of a higher dose of RBV was not associated with an increased incidence of adverse events. Although not demonstrated to be superior in randomized controlled trials, most experts recommend weight-based RBV dosing for all HCV genotypes in HIV-infected patients. The treatment duration should be individualized to the treatment response (Fig. 41.2).

The use of pegIFN and RBV in coinfected patients is associated with many toxicities and drug interactions

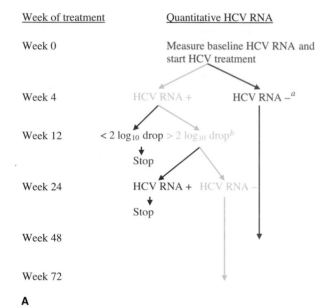

A

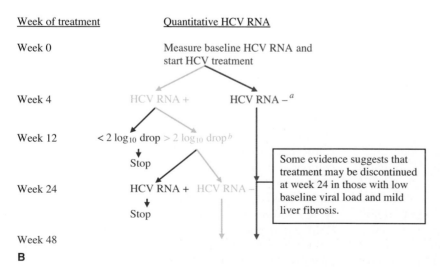

B

Figure 41.2 (A) Treatment algorithm for HIV/HCV genotype 1 and 4 infected patients. (B) Treatment algorithm for HIV/HCV genotype 2 and 3 infected patients. [a]HCV RNA under the limit of detection at week 4 is termed rapid virologic response (RVR) and its positive predictive value for achieving SVR is around 90%. [b]HCV RNA under the limit of detection at week 12 is termed complete early virologic response (cEVR). >2 log$_{10}$ drop of HCV RNA at week 12 with HCV RNA that remains above the limit of detection is termed partial early virologic response (pEVR). HCV, hepatitis C virus.

with ART. Mitochondrial toxicity and its clinical manifestations have been reported and are mainly due to the simultaneous use of RBV and the HIV nucleoside reverse transcriptase inhibitors (NRTIs), mostly didanosine and stavudine. This has led to the current recommendation to avoid the use of didanosine and stavudine with RBV. Zidovudine should also be avoided due to the occurrence of severe anemia when used with RBV. There is a possibility that some ART may impact SVR rates. A few studies have reported a better response to pegIFN and RBV in those with TDF-based regimens compared to abacavir [59,60]. Other studies did not support these findings.

HCV drug development is the subject of active research in HCV-monoinfected subjects. Over 30 compounds are under development. The first two direct-acting antivirals (DAAs), the HCV protease inhibitors boceprevir and telaprevir, have been recently approved by the FDA in May 2011. Both are presently being studied in HIV/HCV-coinfected patients. Other clinical trials of DAAs in HIV/HCV-coinfected are expected to start soon. Drug–drug interactions with ART will be a challenge in this population.

Acute hepatitis C virus in HIV-infected men who have sex with men

Acute HCV in HIV-infected individuals differs in many ways from acute HCV monoinfection in non-HIV-infected patients. This has been the focus of a recent review article [22]. Diligence in diagnosis is essential to identify these patients. When ALT levels increase in HIV-infected men who have sex with men, HCV RNA load and HCV antibody testing should be included in the initial blood tests. Toxicity secondary to ART is a diagnosis of exclusion. Data on treatment effectiveness in acute HCV in the setting of coinfection are limited. Treatment of acute HCV leads to higher SVR rates compared with the chronic stage; SVR rates are around 60–90%. The treatment recommendation is pegIFN (±RBV) for 24 weeks, for all genotypes when RVR is achieved according to recent European guidelines. If HCV RNA is still detectable at week 4 of treatment, a total of 48 weeks should be considered [136]. There should be 12 weeks of observation before starting HCV therapy allow for spontaneous clearance to occur. When HCV RNA levels are monitored every other week, treatment can be instituted at the time viremia establishes a plateau or starts to increase.

Adverse effects of hepatitis C virus treatment

Common side effects of IFN and RBV therapy include fatigue, influenza-like symptoms, hematologic abnormalities, gastrointestinal disturbances, and neuropsychiatric symptoms. Both standard IFN and pegIFN have similar side effect profiles and discontinuation rates. In the major trials in HIV/HCV-coinfected patients, discontinu-

ation rates with pegIFN and RBV were 12–17% [48–50]. In APRICOT, pegIFN dosage was reduced in 34% of patients secondary to neutropenia and thrombocytopenia [48]. The dose of RBV was reduced in 16% secondary to anemia. In the RIBAVIC trial, serious side effects were seen in 32% cases [50]. The toxicities observed in this population are due to their co-morbidities and drug interactions. A clinically significant interaction is seen between IFN and zidovudine, leading to anemia from bone marrow suppression. The more profound anemia seen during HCV therapy in coinfected patients is a combined effect of hemolytic anemia caused by RBV and the failure of the suppressed marrow to compensate for the loss of red blood cells. Anemia in this setting can be managed by reducing the dose of RBV and avoiding zidovudine. Erythropoietin is effective in treating anemia in coinfected patients undergoing anti-HCV therapy and has an efficacy similar to that in monoinfected patients. PegIFN-induced neutropenia does not lead to a higher rate of infection in the group of HIV/HCV-coinfected patients without cirrhosis or with well-compensated cirrhosis. RBV enhances the phosphorylation of didanosine, resulting in an increased risk of mitochondrial toxicity, pancreatitis, lactic acidosis, and fulminant hepatic failure. Therefore RBV is not used with didanosine and the FDA has issued a black box warning regarding their interaction. Toxicity may also be seen with other NRTIs, particularly those with a high affinity for the mitochondrial enzyme DNA polymerase-γ, such as stavudine and zalcitabine. Liver decompensation during HCV treatment is a possible complication. In HIV/HCV-coinfected patients with cirrhosis, hepatic decompensation occurs in 8–10% [48,50] and is associated with increased total bilirubin, anemia, and the use of didanosine. Therefore, it is recommended to monitor these patients closely and avoid the use of didanosine. Active psychiatric illness and active alcohol and drug use are possible barriers to anti-HCV treatment in coinfected patients. In general, current treatment with pegIFN and RBV is well tolerated with adverse events similar to those observed in HCV-monoinfected patients. Benefits of HCV treatment must be weighed against the risks of therapy, and individualization of treatment is the key to success. Judicious use of erythropoietin, granulocyte colony-stimulating factor (GCSF), and antidepressants can improve tolerance to treatment and outcome of therapy.

Retreatment of prior relapsers and nonresponders

Patients who are nonresponders to HCV therapy have a significantly higher frequency of overall death, liver-related death, and liver decompensation compared with those who achieve SVR [43]. Retreatment decisions should be individualized. Those who received a suboptimal treatment in the past (standard IFN, IFN, or pegINF monotherapy, suboptimal RBV dosage due to poor adherence or limiting toxicities) should be retreated adequately. Prior relapsers may have a higher chance of SVR than nonresponders, especially with extended treatment durations. Studies of retreatment in HIV/HCV-coinfected patients have reported overall SVR rates of 16–30% [61–65]. Predictors of SVR in retreatment have not been well studied. We found that in a population of HIV/HCV-coinfected patients carrying multiple negative predictive factors of response to HCV treatment, the strongest predictor of failure to achieve SVR at retreatment was insulin resistance, and the highest SVR rate of 35% was seen in patients with a homeostatic model of assessment of IR (HOMA-IR) of less than 2 [65]. When negative predictive factors of SVR can be modified, such as weight loss in IR and decreased steatosis/steatohepatitis at liver biopsy, retreatment may lead to SVR although it has not been demonstrated in HIV/HCV-coinfected patients. Maintenance therapy with pegIFN monotherapy has not been proven effective in prior nonresponders. New direct-acting antiviral agents are being developed and tested in HIV/HCV-coinfected patients and should significantly improve SVR rates compared with standard of care. For nonresponders, the current approach is to wait until these new antivirals are available.

Hepatitis B virus and hepatitis D virus coinfection

Hepatitis delta virus (HDV, delta agent) is a defective RNA virus that requires HBsAg in order to replicate. The prevalence of antibodies to HDV, ranging from 15% to 50% of HIV-infected patients, depends on the risk factors for acquisition and geography [66]. HDV and HBV can infect the liver simultaneously (coinfection) or HDV can occur in a HBV carrier (superinfection); the latter is more likely in HIV-infected patients [66]. HDV superinfection causes a more severe liver disease than HBV infection alone, with progression to cirrhosis in 70–80% of immunocompetent patients. Evolution towards cirrhosis tends to be faster, and the outcome worse in patients with coinfections compared with monoinfection. Results of studies in patients with HIV/HBV/HDV triple infection are limited by the small samples of patients studied. One group compared liver fibrosis in patients with HIV/HBV/HDV triple infection with those with HIV/HBV alone [67]. They found a significant association between advanced fibrosis (METAVIR stage 3–4) in those with HIV/HBV/HDV triple infection. In a case–control study of 26 HIV/HBV/HDV triple-infected patients and 78 HDV-uninfected patients with a median follow-up of 55 months, those with triple infection had higher rates of hepatitis flares, hyperbilirubinemia, liver cirrhosis, hepatic decompensation, and death [68]. No studies have

been published on treatment of HDV in HIV/HBV triple infection except for two case reports of the use of pegIFN, one in a case of quadruple infection (HIV/HBV/HDV and HCV) [69,70]. One group evaluated the impact of treatment of HBV infection with potent nucleos(t)ide analogs on HDV replication in HIV/HBV/HDV triple infection and reported a decrease in HDV RNA in 13 out of 16 patients and HDV RNA undetectability in three of them [71].

Hepatitis A virus, hepatitis E virus, and GB virus C

The prevalence, morbidity, and mortality of HAV infection are not altered by HIV infection. Despite this, vaccination of HIV-infected patients is recommended, particularly for men who have sex with men who are at a higher risk of transmission through person-to-person sexual contact. A few studies have compared the presentation of HAV infection in HIV-infected men with uninfected controls. In one study, 15 HIV-infected men with acute HAV were compared with 15 HIV-uninfected men with acute HAV and found no difference in the severity of symptoms [72]. The main differences were that HIV-infected men had a higher HAV viral load, longer period of viremia, and less elevation of ALT, suggesting these patients might be more infectious and for a longer period of time then HIV-uninfected patients. The impact of HIV on the clinical presentation of HAV infection is unclear but does not seem to be significant. However, it is important to bear in mind that HIV-infected patients are at a high risk of contracting HAV because of shared risk factors for acquisition. HIV is not a risk factor for fulminant HAV infection, but coinfection with chronic HCV is [73,74]. Patients with HIV have poorer immune responses to the HAV vaccine. The response rates range from 48% to 95% with an overall response rate of 64% [75,76]. A three-dose schedule at 0–4 and 24 weeks of inactivated vaccine might be superior to the standard two-dose schedule at 0 and 24 weeks (83% versus 69% response at 1 month after the last dose) [77].

Hepatitis E virus (HEV) is a water-borne or fecal–orally transmitted virus. Its prevalence has been reported to be higher in HIV-infected patients compared with uninfected individuals – between 5% and 11% compared to <2% of the general population [78]. Until recently, HEV was known to cause acute infection only. Chronic infection has been shown to occur in recipients of solid organ transplants, in an immunosuppressed patient with lymphoma, and in patients with HIV infection, along with progressive liver disease [79,80].

GB virus C (GBC) is a flavivirus that, although closely related to HCV, has not been reported to cause hepatitis or other disease in humans. Transmission is parenteral, sexual, and vertical. Infection with GBC is common and higher among intravenous drug users compared with those with sexual risk exposure [81]. GBC, like HIV, is lymphotropic and replicates in CD4+ T cells. Inhibition of HIV replication has been shown to occur when lymphocytes were previously infected with GBC. Clinically, GBC has been shown to slow HIV disease progression. GBC viremia has been associated with increased survival among HIV-infected men and loss of GBV viremia has been associated with an increased hazard ratio of death 5–6 years after HIV seroconversion [82]. GBC testing is not routinely done in clinic.

Steatosis and lipodystrophy in HIV-infected patients

Nonalcoholic fatty liver disease (NAFLD) is characterized by the accumulation of lipid in the liver. The spectrum of fatty liver disease ranges from mild steatosis to nonalcoholic steatohepatitis (NASH), which may in turn lead to progressive fibrosis, cirrhosis, and even HCC. The prevalence of NAFLD in the HIV population is not known exactly due to lack of histologic data, but the estimated prevalence of NAFLD in patients with HIV has been shown to be 31% by ultrasound [83]. The classic risk factors for hepatic steatosis such as obesity, diabetes, and alcohol are also valid in HIV-infected patients. A recent cohort analysis suggested that more than a quarter of Danish patients infected with HIV met criteria for the metabolic syndrome [84]. ART can cause a variety of liver injuries, including hepatic steatosis, which may be associated with lipodystrophy or result from direct hepatotoxicity. HIV-related lipodystrophy (HIVLD) is a disorder of adipose tissue characterized by selective peripheral fat wasting or lipoatrophy (in the face, limbs, and buttocks) and central fat accumulation or lipohypertrophy (enlarged dorsocervical fat pad, circumferential expansion of neck, breast enlargement, and abdominal visceral fat accumulation). HIVLD is strongly associated with IR, glucose intolerance, and dyslipidemia and is characterized by hypertriglyceridemia, elevated total low-density lipoprotein (LDL) cholesterol, reduced high-density lipoprotein (HDL) cholesterol, and increased levels of nonesterified fatty acids. The latter are identical to the risk factors for development of the metabolic syndrome that is associated with NAFLD. In essence, lipodystrophy is an accelerated aging process characterized by metabolic syndrome effects on the body, including the liver. HIVLD represents a moderate-to long-term complication of ART, reported in at least 40–50% of patients with HIV taking ART. The combination of NRTIs and a protease inhibitor (PI) acting synergistically are primarily responsible for HIVLD [85]. Large cohort studies found a correlation between the duration of therapy with PIs or NRTIs and the development

of HIVLD. In vitro studies have demonstrated that PIs induce the inhibition of adipocyte maturation as well as apoptosis and increase lipolysis. PIs have also been associated with hyperlipidemia, IR, and consequent hepatic steatosis. The proposed mechanism of action for PIs inducing lipoatrophy is via inhibition of SREBP1 (sterol regulatory enhancer-binding protein 1)-mediated activation of the nuclear hormone receptor, PPARγ (peroxisome proliferator-activated receptor γ). While there is no definite therapy for HIVLD, exercise and resistance training reduce visceral adiposity and improve lipid parameters. However, the effects on liver histology are still unknown. In several studies, the use of metformin decreased IR and visceral adipose tissue [86]. Among the currently available therapies, pioglitazone seems to be the best option as it increases insulin sensitivity and subcutaneous adipose tissue while decreasing visceral adipose tissue [87]. Switching from a PI regimen to another regimen offers very little clinical benefit [88].

Direct hepatotoxicity from ART can manifest in a variety of patterns including fat accumulation. NRTIs have been the cornerstone for ART but carry the risk of inducing severe microsteatosis along with lactic acidosis through the impairment of mitochondrial β-oxidation. Stavudine, didanosine, zalcitabine (now removed from the market), and zidovudine are/were the most common culprits. Whether NRTI-induced chronic mitochondrial toxicity and lactic acidosis play a role in the development of NASH in patients with HIV infection is unknown, but it represents a plausible hypothesis [89]. The mechanism of NRTI-related mitochondrial toxicity appears to involve inhibition or alteration of the human RNA-dependent DNA polymerase γ, which is a key regulatory enzyme of mitochondrial DNA replication. Inhibition of this polymerase leads to complex alterations in mitochondrial function including in adipose tissue [85]. Rarely, this type of mitochondrial hepatotoxicity can lead to an acute, severe lactic acidosis, hepatic steatosis, and multiorgan failure with high mortality [90]. A common milder form, often chronic, is characterized by mild hyperlactatemia with nonspecific symptoms, mild hepatomegaly, and mild aminotransaminase elevations.

Several recent studies point to steatohepatitis as a major cause of chronic liver enzyme elevations in HIV-infected patients. A French study prospectively enrolled 30 HIV-monoinfected patients with unexplained elevations in serum transaminases for more than 6 months and correlated them with liver biopsies [91]. It is noteworthy that these patients were older HIV-infected individuals with a mean age of 46 years, mean duration of HIV infection of 13 years, and all with extensive exposure to ART. Histologic abnormalities were present in 22/30 patients. Eighteen patients had steatosis (severe in 9/18) and 16 of them also showed features of steatohepatitis. Six of 30 had liver fibrosis stage ≥2 (METAVIR scale) and 3/30 had cirrhosis. A similar study performed in the United States prospectively enrolled 24 HIV-infected adults with chronic transaminase elevations while on ART [92]. In this study, patients had a mean age of 50 years, mean duration of HIV infection of 17 years, and mean duration on ART of 12 years. On liver biopsy, 9/24 (37.5%) had steatohepatitis with 6/9 presenting bridging fibrosis. Steatohepatitis correlated with a higher body mass index (BMI) and IR. These two studies clearly demonstrate the high prevalence of steatosis and steatohepatitis in this subgroup of older, treatment-experienced HIV-infected patients. Other cofactors, more common in the HIV population, are associated with the development of steatosis and steatohepatitis, including alcohol and drug exposure and chronic viral hepatitis.

There is increasing evidence that hepatic steatosis and associated steatohepatitis contribute to the advanced hepatic fibrosis in HIV/HCV-coinfected patients. Recent biopsy data on HIV/HCV-coinfected patients on ART show rates of steatosis of 40–61% [93–95]. Investigators from the APRICOT study have demonstrated an association between hepatic steatosis and genotype 3 HCV, higher triglyceride levels, increased hip circumference, and advanced fibrosis in patients who are coinfected with HIV and HCV [96]. Furthermore, steatohepatitis with the associated histologic features of cytologic ballooning and pericellular fibrosis was found in 30% of HIV/HCV-coinfected patients in a North American cohort [97]. IR and the incidence of lipoatrophy are significantly increased in HIV/HCV-coinfected patients compared with those with HIV alone. In addition, IR is also significantly associated with steatosis and fibrosis in this group of patients and has an important role in histologic progression of the disease [98,99]. A recent Spanish multicentre cross-sectional study examined the relationship between IR as measured by the HOMA-IR method and hepatic fibrosis as determined by transient elastography in a cohort of patients coinfected with HIV/HCV and demonstrated that 60% of those with evidence of IR had elastography scores in the significant fibrosis range [98]. These data also suggest that hepatic steatosis is associated with more severe HCV-related liver disease in HIV/HCV-coinfected patients than has been shown previously for HCV-monoinfected patients.

All HIV-infected patients with NAFLD should be encouraged to pursue dietary and lifestyle modification that encourage maintenance of normal body weight. The treatment of associated conditions such as diabetes mellitus, hypertension, and hyperlipidemia is advised although the effects on liver histology have not been studied. For patients with ART-induced lipodystrophy and IR, the benefits of changing ART regimens might be minimal and must be balanced against the risk of HIV disease progression. The effects of using insulin sensitizers, either metformin or pioglitazone, in this setting have yielded inconclusive results without any data on liver histology improvement, although both drugs have been used in fatty liver disease in HIV-uninfected patients.

Interactions between HIV, age, and the liver

Older individuals represent a higher proportion of patients infected with HIV. In 2005, 15% of new HIV infections were in persons aged 50 years and older compared with 6% in 2000 and 4% in 1995 in the United States. Persons aged 50 and older represented 24% of those living with HIV/AIDS compared with 17% in 2001. Liver diseases are now a leading cause of death in the HIV-infected population and are significantly associated with older age, among other factors [3]. Aging is associated with decreased cellular immunity or immunosenescence. Older age at infection with HIV is a predictor of accelerated HIV disease progression [100,101]. Besides the natural aging process on the CD4+ T-cell compartment, there is evidence that HIV itself accelerates aging of both naïve and memory CD4+ T cells and CD8+ T cells [102]. Aging and HIV seem to share common mechanisms by which they alter cellular immunity. Aging of the immune system and HIV disease both lead to reductions in naïve CD4+ and CD8+ T cells. Aging is also associated with a decrease in expression of CD28 on CD8+ T cells. In HIV, decreased CD28 expression on CD4+ and CD8+ T cells has been linked to accelerated progression to AIDS [103]. The effect of age on CD4+ T cells has not been clearly determined, while CD4+ T-cell depletion is the hallmark of HIV infection.

An important and recently recognized consequence of HIV targeting the immune system is the alteration of mucosal immunity [104]. Acute HIV infection leads to a drastic destruction of CD4+ T cells, mainly in gut-associated lymphoid tissue (GALT), which is an extralymphoid CD4+ T-cell reservoir [105,106]. The depletion of gut CD4+ T cells persists during the chronic phase of HIV, despite ART [107]. This breach in the integrity of the gut mucosa allows bacteria and bacterial products to cross over and reach the portal and systemic circulations. This process, called microbial translocation, contributes to the proinflammatory state characterizing chronic HIV infection [108]. Microbial translocation may also accelerate liver disease progression in HIV/HCV coinfection, as suggested by one retrospective study [109]. The impact of aging on gut immunity is not known.

Decreased immunity and age both have an impact on liver disease progression. Advanced immunosuppression (CD4+ T-cell count ≤ 200 cells/mm^3) is a risk factor for accelerated progression of liver fibrosis in HIV/HCV coinfection. Aging has also been associated with faster fibrosis progression. The degree of immunodeficiency is an independent predictor of liver-related death. In the Data Collection on Adverse Events of Anti-HIV Drugs (D:A:D) study, the risk of liver-related death was inversely proportional to the CD4+ T-cell count. Those with a count lower than 50 cells/mm^3 had a 16-fold increased risk of death compared to those with a CD4+ T-cell count over 500 cells/mm^3. Other predictors of liver-related deaths in this population were coinfection with HCV and/or HBV, intravenous drug use as a risk factor for HIV acquisition, and older age [3]. The latter was found to have a relative risk of 1.3 (95% CI 1.2–1.4) per 5 years, meaning that an individual 10 years older has a 60% increased risk of death compared with the younger patients.

There is some evidence to suggest that HIV directly infects hepatocytes. For example, the detection of HIV antigen and RNA in hepatic cell lines in vivo, the detection of HIV proviral DNA in vivo, HIV infection of different cell lines with the production of infectious HIV particles in vitro, and the detection of hepatotropic variants of HIV in liver tissues [110]. HIV has also been found to infect and replicate within hepatic stellate cells leading to cell activation and fibrogenesis, suggesting a role in liver fibrosis progression in HIV/HCV-coinfected patients [111]. The role of HIV infection of the liver as well as how it relates to liver disease progression in this population needs further study.

Long-term complications of HIV and antiretroviral therapy

The HIV-infected elderly have increased co-morbidities compared with younger patients and are more likely to be taking multiple drugs besides ART, resulting in an increase in the likelihood of drug interaction and toxicity. Many potential factors contribute to the risk of hepatotoxicity in the HIV-infected individuals undergoing ART. The type of ART, coinfection with HBV and HCV, CD4+ T-cell count, alcohol intake, baseline elevated levels of transaminases, female sex, older age, and other factors have all been shown to influence the occurrence of hepatotoxicity. Among the mechanisms of liver injury in HIV-infected patients undergoing ART, mitochondrial toxicity has attracted much attention leading to potentially severe complications such as hepatic steatosis, lactic acidosis, and hepatic failure. The liver demonstrates mitochondrial toxicity by the accumulation of microvesicular steatosis and depletion of mitochondria; it is the signature toxicity of NRTIs. The toxicity is delayed and occurs after cumulative exposure during treatment with one or more NRTIs. In decreasing order of frequency, the NRTIs that cause lactic acidosis are: zalcitabine, didanosine, stavudine, zidovudine, lamivudine, abacavir, and TDF (with the latter three having the same effect) [112,

113]. Persistent, unexplained liver enzyme elevations in HIV-monoinfected individuals on ART are being reported at an increasing frequency. In some studies, it mostly affects individuals with longer duration of HIV infection and longer exposure to ART. In the Swiss HIV Cohort Study, chronic ALT elevation had an incidence of 3.7/100 person-years in HIV-monoinfected patients [114]. Multivariate analysis found prolonged ART exposure (NRTI and protease inhibitor), increased BMI, and high alcohol intake to be predictive of ALT elevation. In another study, using transient hepatic elastometry in 258 consecutive HIV-monoinfected patients (ALT variable not mentioned), Spanish investigators reported abnormal liver stiffness (defined as measurement $\geq$7.2 kPa) in 11.2% of patients [115]. Independent factors associated with liver stiffness were time on didanosine and abacavir, alcohol consumption, and a CD4+ T-cell count <200 cells/mm^3.

Some studies have failed to show a link between cryptogenic liver disease (CLD) and exposure to ART. A recent retrospective study of 13 HIV-monoinfected persons who met the definition of CLD (persistent elevated hepatic transaminase levels for more than 6 months in the absence of common causes of chronic liver disease) and had a liver biopsy performed, showed no association between the development of CLD and prolonged use of ART [116]. The mean age of patients was 45 years (39–65 years), the median CD4+ T-cell count was 187 cells/mm^3, HIV was undetectable except in one patient, and all were ART experienced. However two of the 13 patients showed features of nodular regenerative hyperplasia (NRH; see below) and both had been on didanosine for 59 and 102 months, respectively.

A few studies have relied on liver biopsies to elucidate the cause of CLD in HIV-monoinfected individuals. Among the liver lesions identified in these patients, hepatic steatosis and steatohepatitis [91,92], fibrosis [91,116,117], cirrhosis [91,116], cholangiopathy [116], sclerosing cholangitis [116], NRH [116–119], and hepatoportal sclerosis [120] have all been reported.

Noncirrhotic portal hypertension in HIV-infected patients

Nodular regenerative hyperplasia and hepatoportal sclerosis have been recently described in the HIV-monoinfected population and may now represent the most striking manifestations of the long-term consequences of HIV and its treatment on the liver. They are likely to be different liver histologic lesions on the same spectrum of disease. Our knowledge about these conditions, their exact risk factors, and pathogenesis are, however, limited. Both manifest clinically as NCPH, and esophageal variceal bleeding is the most frequent complication. A case series of 12 patients with HIV on

ART with abnormal liver function tests and/or symptomatic portal hypertension of unknown cause has been recently published [121]. NRH was defined as the finding of diffuse, small, regenerative liver nodules in the absence of significant fibrosis and HPS was characterized by varying degrees of portal fibrosis, sclerosis of portal vein branches, and dilatation of sinusoidal spaces. Out of 11 biopsies, NRH was found in three of them and HPS was found in the remaining eight. The median age of these patients was 47 years (28–67 years) and the median duration of HIV infection was 11 years. Out of the 12 patients, six experienced variceal bleeding. Liver biopsy did not show cirrhosis despite the presence of portal hypertension and its complications. Didanosine was reported as the sole drug received by all subjects and was thought to be the cause of the NCPH. Prior to this report, a case series of four HIV-infected patients presenting with NCPH was reported. The histologic diagnosis was also consistent with HPS. Another case series of six HIV-infected patients with unexplained portal hypertension showed similar histologic findings in five of the six patients with exposure to didanosine [119]. A nested case–control study inside the Swiss HIV Cohort Study identified 15 HIV-monoinfected patients with NCPH who were matched with 75 HIV-monoinfected controls for duration of HIV infection and time of follow-up [122]. All 15 had esophageal varices, splenomegaly, and no cirrhosis on liver biopsy, seven had a history of variceal bleeding, eight had ascites, five had portal thrombosis, two had hepatic encephalopathy, and four died of hepatic complications. The only independent risk factor associated with NCPH in bivariate models was prolonged exposure to didanosine.

A proposed mechanism for NCPH is that an initial endothelial cell injury, likely caused by didanosine, might lead to occlusion of the terminal branches of the portal venules and result in portal hypertension. A direct effect of HIV has been suggested but is less likely since most of the patients have undetectable HIV RNA levels and a CD4+ T-cell count above 200 cells/mm^3 at the time of diagnosis.

Liver infections in HIV-infected patients with severe immunosuppression

In the era of ART, HIV infection for those with access to medication and who are adherent to treatment has turned into a well-controlled chronic disease with relatively preserved CD4+ T-cell counts. As a consequence of this, the incidence of opportunistic infections has declined substantially in patients with HIV. However, in immunosuppressed HIV-infected patients, the liver and biliary tract are frequent sites of infection. Opportunistic infections have been seen in 33–78% of cases in autopsy series in patients with AIDS, and in liver biopsy of almost 90% of HIV-infected patients with abnormal liver function tests. A thorough clinical and diagnostic workup is warranted, which may include liver biopsy with appropriate cultures and staining, provided that less invasive tests are not conclusive.

Viral infections

Hepatitis B virus and HCV infections in HIV are discussed elsewhere in this chapter and therefore will not be discussed in this section. Opportunistic viral infections of the liver are often members of the Herpesviridae family. Although clinically significant hepatitis secondary to cytomegalovirus (CMV) or herpes simplex virus (HSV) is rare, CMV is detected frequently in autopsies of severely immunosuppressed patients with CD4+ T-cell counts <100 cells/mm^3 and is often a component of systemic involvement. Serum transaminases may be markedly elevated. Liver histology typically shows large intranuclear and cytoplasmic owl's eye inclusions with significant inflammation of portal and periportal regions and sparse necrosis. CMV infects every type of cell within the liver. CMV infection is being detected earlier now owing to pp65 antigen flow cytometry and CMV polymerase chain reaction. In addition, the development of ganciclovir (both IV and oral) has reduced the morbidity and mortality of CMV infection [123]. The major toxicity of ganciclovir and valganciclovir is bone marrow suppression. Resistance can also be a problem with ganciclovir, which may require switching to foscarnet. The major side effect limiting the use of foscarnet is its nephrotoxicity. Patients with HSV hepatitis may develop submassive hepatic necrosis with severe transaminitis and liver failure. Pathologically, HSV hepatitis is characterized by multinucleated hepatocytes and Cowdry A intranuclear inclusion bodies, which may be differentiated from those of CMV by specific immunohistochemistry. HSV hepatitis may be treated with IV aciclovir, ganciclovir, or foscarnet. However, hepatitis secondary to either CMV or HSV responds poorly to current treatments. Varicella-zoster virus (VZV), Epstein–Barr virus (EBV), and adenovirus are other agents responsible for viral hepatitis in patients with HIV.

Mycobacterial infections

Mycobacterium avium complex (MAC) is the most common opportunistic pathogen affecting the liver. However, with the introduction of ART the incidence of disseminated MAC infection has declined, and the prognosis has significantly improved. Infection with MAC manifests with systemic symptoms and signs, such as fever,

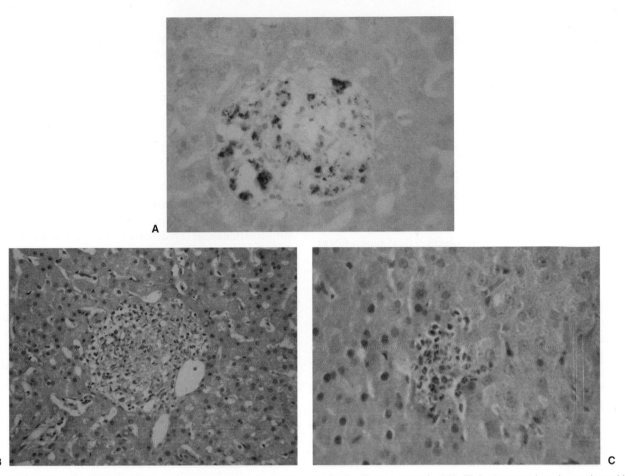

Figure 41.3 (A) An epithelioid granuloma containing *Mycobacterium avium*. Acid-fast bacilli stain, original ×200. (B) A microgranuloma in a patient with mycobacterial infection. Hematoxylin and eosin (H&E), original ×200. (C) A microabscess in the liver of a patient with acquired immunodeficiency syndrome (AIDS) and cytomegalovirus (CMV) infection. H&E, original ×200.

abdominal pain, wasting, and biliary obstruction secondary to enlarged lymph nodes at the porta hepatis. It is seen in late-stage AIDS patients when the CD4+ T-cell count is less than 50 cells/mm^3. MAC is detected in 20–55% of autopsies and in 10–30% of liver biopsies in patients with AIDS. Typical laboratory features include severe cholestasis with marked elevations in alkaline phosphatase (ALP) levels, although high transaminases may be the only abnormality. Icterus is rare. Blood cultures are the most sensitive test for diagnosis of MAC. However, liver biopsy showing diffuse, poorly formed, noncaseating granulomas is necessary for definitive diagnosis of liver involvement. Abundant acid-fast bacilli (AFB) may be seen on staining (Fig. 41.3), but liver tissue culture is needed to distinguish between different *Mycobacterium* species. Liver biopsy has been reported to be more sensitive than bone marrow biopsy in diagnosing disseminated mycobacterial infection in AIDS.

The long-term prognosis of disseminated mycobacterial infection is poor with a median survival of only 6 months. Combination therapy with a macrolide such as clarithromycin or azithromycin, rifampin, and ethambutol is the most common treatment. Ciprofloxacin or amikacin may be added in more severe cases. Previous data suggest that 12 months of therapy may suffice for patients who are on ART with a sustained CD4+ T-cell count >100 cells/mm^3 [124]. Primary prophylaxis with azithromycin or clarithromycin is indicated in patients with a CD4+ T-cell count of less than 50 cells/mm^3.

Extrapulmonary *Mycobacterium tuberculosis* infection involving the liver occurs in 5–10% of HIV-related tuberculosis cases and may present with tuberculous liver abscess in severely immunocompromised patients. However, ART and rifampicin-containing antitubercular therapy have decreased the incidence, recurrence, and mortality rate of tuberculosis [125]. Hepatic involvement of tuberculosis is usually because of the reactivation of a latent infection. Liver tuberculosis is associated with fever, abdominal pain, hepatosplenomegaly, and wasting similar to that found in MAC infection. However, as the virulence of *M. tuberculosis* is greater than in the other species of *Mycobacterium*, it may infect patients who have higher CD4+ T-cell counts, of more than 200 cells/mm^3. Cholestasis is seen with significantly elevated ALP and mild increases in bilirubin and transaminases. The specific diagnosis is made by culture and polymerase chain reaction of blood, urine, or tissue specimens including liver. AFB may be seen in the liver histology, which is typically characterized by the presence of caseating granulomas. As this infection often occurs in the setting of lesser immunosuppression, hepatic granulomas are better formed than those of MAC. The combination of isoniazid, rifampin, ethambutol, and pyrazinamide for 9–12 months is the treatment of choice for tuberculosis of the liver. Liver chemistry tests should be closely monitored during treatment, especially in elderly patients. Rarely, liver infections with other mycobacterial species such as *M. kansasii*, *M. xenopi*, and *M. genavense* have also been reported.

Fungal infections

Major fungal pathogens infecting the liver are *Cryptococcus neoformans*, *Histoplasma capsulatum*, *Coccidioides immitis*, and *Candida* species. They are uncommon, and are ordinarily seen in the setting of disseminated disease and in patients with less than 100 CD4+ T cells/mm^3. Fungal pathogens typically cause cholestasis, and imaging studies often demonstrate focal or diffuse liver lesions. Liver histology often reveals poorly formed granulomas with minimal inflammatory reaction. Meningitis is the most common manifestation of cryptococcal disease in HIV-infected patients. Liver involvement occurs as a result of hematogenous spread. The common presenting features are fever and hepatosplenomegaly. Histoplasmosis is particularly common in the midwestern United States, Central and South America, and the Caribbean, including Puerto Rico. Disseminated histoplasmosis is often the first sign of immunodeficiency in patients with AIDS in endemic areas. Constitutional symptoms along with hepatosplenomegaly and lymphadenopathy are the common features. *Coccidioides immitis* infection usually occurs in patients infected with HIV who are living in endemic areas such as the southwestern United States. The disease typically presents as a subacute illness with pulmonary involvement; hepatic infection is again secondary to disseminated disease. Despite the frequent esophageal involvement of candidiasis in AIDS, systemic infection and liver involvement are quite rare in the absence of neutropenia. The symptoms are nonspecific and include nausea, vomiting, abdominal pain, and hepatomegaly. The most common laboratory findings of hepatic candidiasis include neutropenia and elevated ALP. Imaging may demonstrate a single lesion, classically described as having a bull's eye appearance. *Cryptococcus neoformans* and *H. capsulatum* may be rapidly detected by polysaccharide capsular antigenemia; other causes of fungal hep-

atitis need special staining and culture of liver tissue for definitive diagnosis. There are also rare reports of *Aspergillus fumigatus* causing liver abscess and disseminated *Sporothrix schenckii* involving the liver. Treatment consists mainly of amphotericin B for fungal hepatitis; however, as the relapse rate is high for most of the fungal infections in immunocompromised patients, fluconazole or itraconazole have been suggested as suppression therapy indefinitely in most cases.

Protozoal infections

Protozoa are rare pathogens causing infections in patients with AIDS. Routine prophylaxis with trimethoprim/sulfamethoxazole (TMP-SMX) has reduced the incidence of *Pneumocystis jirovecii*, *Toxoplasma gondii*, and *Listeria monocytogenes*. In the past, *P. jirovecii* (formerly *Pneumocystis carinii*) hepatitis was associated with the prophylactic use of aerosolized pentamidine for *Pneumocystis* pneumonia. Inhalation failed to provide adequate drug levels to extrapulmonary sites and up to 39% of such patients developed extrapulmonary spread. A mixed pattern of elevated liver enzymes is usually seen. Abdominal computed tomography (CT) scans may demonstrate diffuse and punctuate calcifications in the liver. Liver biopsy shows foamy nodules that are periportal or diffuse containing numerous *Pneumocystis* cysts that stain with Gomori methenamine silver. Treatment is with IV TMP-SMX or pentamidine. *T. gondii* also involves the liver rarely through hematogenous dissemination and may present with granulomatous disease or hepatitis. Diagnosis is made by culture or microscopic examination of Giemsa-stained specimens. TMP-SMX is the drug of choice for toxoplasmosis. Microsporidial infection of the liver is rare and is associated with a rise in bilirubin, transaminases, and high ALP levels. Light microscopy reveals focal granulomatous and suppurative necrosis, mainly in the portal area, accompanied by characteristic spores. Although there is no established therapy for microsporidial hepatitis, treatment with albendazole may be efficacious for *Encephalitozoon intestinalis*. *Strongyloides stercoralis*, a helminth of the nematode family, may result in a hyperinfection syndrome in the immunocompromised patient. The liver is involved through the hematogenous spread of the larvae from the gastrointestinal tract. *Entamoeba histolytica* may invade the bowel wall and spread to the liver, forming an abscess. Reactivated leishmaniasis is another rare infection of the liver.

Infections of the biliary tract

The biliary tree, including the gallbladder, is a common site of infection in HIV-infected patients with immunosuppression. It may be involved in the form of cholangiopathy or acalculous cholecystitis.

Cholangiopathy

Cholangiopathy in AIDS is a form of secondary sclerosing cholangitis that occurs because of opportunistic infections in advanced stages of HIV infection, particularly in patients with a CD4+ T-cell count of less than 135 cells/mm^3. Affected patients develop right upper quadrant pain, fever, and cholestasis. ALP is often elevated up to 10–20 times above normal. Icterus is seldom seen as biliary obstruction is usually partial. There are multiple opportunistic organisms that have been identified in the biliary tree of patients with AIDS cholangiopathy including CMV, *Cryptosporidium* sp., and *Microsporidium* sp., and less often MAC, *Isospora belli*, and *Enterocytozoon bieneusi*. However, no pathogen is isolated in up to 50% of cases. Although liver ultrasonography may show biliary dilatation, and magnetic resonance cholangiopancreatography (MRCP) may demonstrate characteristic findings of cholangiopathy, endoscopic retrograde cholangiopancreatography (ERCP) is more sensitive and has the advantage of allowing both tissue biopsy and sphincterotomy to be performed when necessary. Four patterns of abnormalities shown by ERCP have been described: (i) stenosis of the papilla of Vater with dilated extrahepatic bile ducts; (ii) sclerosing cholangitis; (iii) combined sclerosing cholangitis and papillary stenosis; and (iv) long extrahepatic strictures with or without sclerosing cholangitis. Duodenal and papillary biopsies and biopsies from inside the biliary ducts may be sent for both culture and pathologic examinations. Endoscopic sphincterotomy may provide benefit for symptomatic patients with papillary stenosis. Prognosis depends on the degree of underlying HIV-related immunosuppression rather than the hepatobiliary disease [126]. A review of 94 HIV-infected patients over a period of almost two decades in the era of ART demonstrated a median survival of patients with AIDS cholangiopathy to be 9 months. Poor prognostic factors were opportunistic infections (especially cryptosporidiosis) and markedly elevated serum ALP. ART has significantly improved the survival of patients with AIDS cholangiopathy [126].

Acalculous cholecystitis

Acalculous cholecystitis usually occurs in later stages of HIV infection with a CD4+ T-cell count of less than 50 cells/mm^3. Concurrent cholangitis is commonly seen. Patients usually present with abdominal pain, fever, nausea, and vomiting. Icterus is rare, but ALP and γ-glutamyltransferase (GGT) are markedly elevated in most cases. In acalculous cholecystitis, the gallbladder wall appears thickened and edematous on imaging without any gallstones. Pericholecystic fluid may be present. Gallbladder histology often reveals an opportunistic organism as a cause. The spectrum of responsible pathogens is similar to that identified in AIDS cholangiopathy.

Complications of acalculous cholecystitis include perforation and peritonitis. Cholecystectomy can be performed in most patients; in the remaining cases, CT or ultrasonography-guided percutaneous cholecystostomy may be an option to decompress the gallbladder.

Hepatic mass lesions in HIV-infected patients

The most common hepatic neoplastic mass lesion is Kaposi sarcoma (KS) caused by human herpesvirus type 8 (HHV-8). The incidence of KS in HIV-infected patients may be 10–20%, more than 100,000 times that in the general population. Fortunately, its incidence in AIDS continues to decrease and the lesions often respond to ART. Among HIV-infected individuals, KS occurs predominantly in men who have sex with men. Despite the presence of hepatic KS in approximately one third of patients with cutaneous involvement, it is seldom diagnosed on antemortem biopsy. Patients may present with abdominal pain and hepatosplenomegaly with an elevated ALP level, but most commonly it is asymptomatic. There is no specific finding on CT scan; however, the lesions are hypoattenuated and enhance after a bolus of IV contrast. The tumor appears to be a vascular proliferation characterized by the presence of spindle cells, vascular channels, and a mixed cellular infiltrate on histology.

B-cell lymphoma is the second most common neoplasm in patients with HIV infection after KS. It is controversial whether the incidence of non-Hodgkin lymphoma has changed since the introduction of ART. Non-Hodgkin lymphomas in patients with AIDS are often of B-cell phenotype with high grade and advanced stage, and predominantly extranodal, involving most frequently the central nervous system and the gastrointestinal system. They appear to be a late manifestation of HIV disease with rates rising directly with the duration of infection. The liver is involved in approximately 10% of cases. The CD4+ T-cell count is usually less than 200 cells/mm^3. Primary hepatic lymphoma usually presents with multiple masses and involvement of other abdominal organs or lymph nodes. Persistent fever, tender hepatomegaly, and mildly abnormal liver chemistry tests combined with an elevated lactate dehydrogenase (LDH) level may give a clue to the diagnosis. The lesions appear hypodense on both noncontrast and contrast-enhanced CT imaging. Diagnosis can be established by laparoscopic or CT-guided biopsy. However, as bone marrow involvement is frequent, a bone marrow aspirate or biopsy should be considered before a more invasive liver or retroperitoneal lymph node biopsy. AIDS-associated lymphomas have generally an aggressive course and respond poorly to treatment.

Bacillary peliosis hepatis is a vascular lesion caused by *Bartonella henselae*, a fastidious Gram-negative bacillus. It usually occurs in patients with CD4+ T-cell counts of less than 200 cells/mm³. Peliosis hepatis may be found incidentally on liver biopsy or occasionally can present with abdominal pain, hepatosplenomegaly, liver failure, and portal hypertension in extensive cases. Systemic symptoms such as fever, anemia, and cutaneous lesions of bacillary angiomatosis may be observed. Laboratory analysis may reveal an elevated ALP level and prothrombin time. Abdominal CT scans display multiple, small, low-attenuation lesions scattered in the liver parenchyma. Biopsy shows cystic blood-filled spaces within the liver that are usually a few millimeters in size. They are associated with fibromyxoid stroma containing clumps of bacilli that can be detected by Warthin–Starry stain. Erythromycin is the drug of first choice for the treatment of peliosis. Other options include clarithromycin, tetracycline, or doxycycline. Liver abscess secondary to mycobacterial infections and HCC that may be seen in the setting of HCV or HBV coinfection are other mass lesions observed in HIV-infected patients. The incidence of mycobacterial liver abscess is decreasing since the introduction of ART and effective antimycobacterial therapy. On the other hand, the incidence of HCC in HIV-infected patients is increasing because of improved survival with ART and the rising incidence of end-stage liver disease because of HCV and/or HBV coinfection and alcohol abuse [127].

Hepatocellular carcinoma in HIV-infected patients

Increased survival of HIV-infected patients in the era of ART has lead to an increase in liver-related mortality in this group of patients. A French survey on the causes of death in HIV-infected patients confirmed the increasing role of HCC as a non-AIDS-related cause of death: the prevalence rate increased from 4.7% in 1995 to 11% in 1997 and 25% in 2001 [128]. Additionally, an estimated 25–30% of patients with HIV are coinfected with HCV and the accelerated progression of HCV-related liver disease places this group of patients at extremely high risk of liver disease and its complications including HCC [129]. A retrospective European study of 41 patients with HCC in HIV-infected persons found most patients to be coinfected with HCV, to have a younger age at onset, a shorter estimated duration of disease, and a more aggressive clinical course when compared with HIV-uninfected patients with HCC [31]. A multicenter, US/Canadian study of 63 HIV-infected patients with HCC found similar results of younger age and more frequent infection with HCV or HBV than in HIV-uninfected patients. They also found

tumor staging and survival to be similar between the HIV-infected and HIV-uninfected cohorts [7]. Additionally, other causes of liver disease including hepatic steatosis and steatohepatitis that are increasing in frequency may pose additional risks for HCC development and will need to be studied in the future. Despite the increasing number of patients with HCC and the prolonged survival of HIV-infected patients, there are no updated guidelines on screening for HCC in this population [130]. Current screening guidelines for patients with cirrhosis should apply to HIV-infected patients with cirrhosis, and should at a minimum include imaging of the liver every 6 months.

Liver transplantation in HIV-infected patients

The introduction of ART has dramatically reduced disease progression and death among patients with HIV infection. As the life expectancy for HIV-infected individuals has increased, liver disease has become a leading cause of non-AIDS-related death in those infected with HIV [3,5,130]. A French study found 28% of non-AIDS-related deaths were attributed to ESLD [130]. Prior to ART, HIV with or without AIDS was considered a contraindication to liver transplantation (LT) by most centers due to poor outcomes with a high incidence of opportunistic infections post-transplant resulting in higher mortality and 3-year survival rates of 45%. Even in the era of ART, until recently, the presence of AIDS was an absolute contraindication to LT, and asymptomatic HIV infection remained a relative contraindication. However, in recent years, with widespread use of ART and increased numbers of HIV-infected patients living with chronic liver disease, LT has been reconsidered as a possible therapeutic option for these patients.

In 2003, Ragni and colleagues prospectively studied the survival rates of 24 HIV-infected LT recipients. With 1-, 2- and 3-year survival rates of 87.1%, 72.8%, and 72.8%, respectively, in these HIV-infected patients, the results were not statistically different to the rates of 86.6%, 81.6%, and 77.9% found among 5,225 age- and race-matched HIV-uninfected patients from the United Network of Organ Sharing (UNOS) database [131]. In HIV-infected patients the etiology of liver disease was chronic HCV infection in 63%, chronic HBV infection in 29%, and acute liver failure in 13% of subjects. However, in the HIV/HCV-coinfected group, survival was worse compared with the HCV-monoinfected group. In this study, worse outcome was associated with post-transplant ART intolerance, a CD4+ T-cell count of less than 200 cells/mm³, an HIV viral load of greater than 400 copies/mL, and HCV coinfection. In another early series from King's College Hospital in London, 14 HIV-infected liver allograft recipients were evaluated [132]. HCV was the etiology of liver disease in seven patients, HBV in four patients, alcohol in two patients, and acute liver failure in one patient. In the non-HCV group ($n = 7$), all patients were still alive with a survival range of 668 to 2,661 days after transplantation, none experienced HBV recurrence, and graft function was normal in all patients. However, five of the seven HCV-infected patients died after transplantation at 95–784 days (median 161 days). Most deaths were because of complications of recurrent HCV and sepsis. This study demonstrated a poor outcome in the HIV/HCV-coinfected patients, but more recent studies have shown better results.

A recent Spanish study by Murillas revealed that the model for end-stage liver disease (MELD) score and the inability to reach an undetectable plasma HIV-1 RNA viral load at any time during follow-up were the only variables independently associated with the risk of death ($P < 0.001$) [133]. While 104 patients were included in the study, only 14% met inclusion criteria for listing for LT and five patients were transplanted. The waiting list mortality rate in patients with a MELD score <20 and in patients with a MELD score >20 was 58% and 100%, respectively (median follow-up of 5 months). A recent US cohort of HIV in Solid Organ Transplantation Multi-Site Study (HIVTR) enrolled patients with HIV infection and ESLD who were candidates for LT at 20 transplant centers in the United States between February 2003 and September 2007. Patients were required to meet standard site criteria for placement on the LT waiting list as well as HIV-specific study inclusion criteria. The latter included a CD4+ T-cell count of >100 cells/mm^3, or >200 cells/mm^3 if there was a history of prior opportunistic infection or HIV-1 RNA <50 copies/mL or >50 copies/mL in those with hepatotoxicity or ART intolerance in whom HIV suppression was predicted post-transplantation. HIV-infected subjects ($n = 167$) were matched with HIV-uninfected LT candidate controls ($n = 792$) without HCC from the UNOS database. It should be noted that 75% of cases and controls were HCV-infected patients. Pretransplantation mortality characteristics were similar between HIV-infected and HIV-uninfected candidates. The authors concluded that although lower CD4+ T-cell counts and detectable levels of HIV RNA might be associated with a higher rate of pretransplantation mortality, the baseline MELD score (cutoff value of 25) was the only significant independent predictor of pretransplantation mortality in HIV-infected LT candidates. These recent findings suggest that survival of HIV-infected LT recipients does not differ from that of HIV-uninfected recipients and that HIV should not be a contraindication to LT, provided patients meet the current inclusion and exclusion criteria for listing.

While there has been a significant decline in LT in patients with chronic HBV due to improvement in antiviral therapy, HBV coinfection remains an important cause of liver failure in HIV-infected patients [5]. In patients transplanted for HIV/HBV coinfection, post-transplant survival was not limited by HBV reinfection of the allograft because of effective prophylaxis using hepatitis B immune globulin and antivirals such as lamivudine, adefovir, or TDF [5,132,134].

All HIV-infected patients with ESLD should be considered as candidates for LT provided they do not have advanced HIV disease. Those with severe immunosuppression (<100 CD4+ T cells/mm^3) should be treated with ART to control viral replication before they are evaluated for transplantation. Patients with a good response to ART, but with prior AIDS-related opportunistic infections and neoplasm, have a higher risk of relapse while on immunosuppressive medication after transplantation. These findings highlight the importance of early referral and multidisciplinary care to expand the number of HIV-infected patients with ESLD who could be candidates for successful LT and to minimize the number of deaths occurring whilst on the waiting lists. The essential condition for LT in patients with HIV is that the patient must be able to undergo effective and long-lasting ART during the post-transplant period. The ideal situation is one in which the patient tolerates ART before transplant and is ready for the transplant with undetectable plasma HIV viral load by ultrasensitive techniques (<50 copies/mL).

There are some important pharmacokinetic drug interactions between protease inhibitors and non-NRTIs and immunosuppressive agents like tacrolimus and ciclosporin. Protease inhibitors can increase the levels of tacrolimus and ciclosporine through the inhibition of cytochrome P450, whereas non-NRTIs can reduce their levels. Therefore, some ways to improve survival after LT in HIV-infected patients is to optimize the dose of immunosuppressive medication to prevent toxicity secondary to drug interactions with ART agents, the use of ART to suppress HIV RNA, and to maintain CD4+ T-cell counts >200 cells/mm^3 to decrease the risk of opportunistic infections [135]. Therefore, while LT in HIV-infected patients is complex and requires a multidisciplinary approach, it is a promising treatment option.

Conclusions

The HIV/AIDS epidemic is changing. The HIV population is aging and with older age comes the increased risk of chronic disease development. In the field of liver diseases, we are faced with the increasing incidence of metabolic complications leading to hepatic steatosis and steatohepatitis. As the HIV population ages, we see complications of long-term ART of which NCPH is the newest. Opportunistic infections are becoming rarer. The aging population coinfected with HBV and/or HCV has a considerable impact on the burden of liver-related morbidity and mortality. LT is an option to consider in HIV/HCV-coinfected patients. The importance of primary prevention of transmission of chronic viral illnesses cannot be overemphasized. Effective treatment of HBV with TDF-containing regimens has altered the landscape of liver diseases in patients infected with HBV and HIV. HCV treatment has clearly demonstrated survival benefits when SVR is achieved and should be considered for all HIV/HCV-coinfected patients. The year 2011 is the dawn of a new era in HCV treatment in both mono and coinfected patients. In May 2011, the first direct-acting antiviral agents, the two protease inhibitors boceprevir and telaprevir were approved by the FDA for use in HCV-monoinfected patients. The results are awaited in HIV/HCV-coinfected patients. Combination treatment with direct antiviral agents of different classes with nonoverlapping resistance mutations is clearly the way of the future. Whether pegIFN and RBV will be part of the new direct antiviral agent regimens has yet to be determined. We all eagerly anticipate the new decade where we will see great leaps forward in antiviral treatment of HCV.

References

1. Konopnicki D, Mocroft A, de Wit S, et al. Hepatitis B and HIV: prevalence, AIDS progression, response to highly active antiretroviral therapy and increased mortality in the EuroSIDA cohort. *AIDS* 2005;19:593–601.
2. Salmon-Ceron D, Lewden C, Morlat P, et al. Liver disease as a major cause of death among HIV infected patients: role of hepatitis C and B viruses and alcohol. *J Hepatol* 2005;42:799–805.
3. Weber R, Sabin CA, Friis-Moller N, et al. Liver-related deaths in persons infected with the human immunodeficiency virus: the D:A:D study. *Arch Intern Med* 2006;166:1632–41.
4. Thio CL. Hepatitis B in the human immunodeficiency virus-infected patient: epidemiology, natural history, and treatment. *Semin Liver Dis* 2003;23:125–36.
5. Thio CL, Seaberg EC, Skolasky R Jr, et al. HIV-1, hepatitis B virus, and risk of liver-related mortality in the Multicenter Cohort Study (MACS). *Lancet* 2002;360:1921–6.
6. Clifford GM, Rickenbach M, Polesel J, et al. Influence of HIV-related immunodeficiency on the risk of hepatocellular carcinoma. *AIDS* 2008;22:2135–41.
7. Brau N, Fox RK, Xiao P, et al. Presentation and outcome of hepatocellular carcinoma in HIV-infected patients: a US–Canadian multicenter study. *J Hepatol* 2007;47:527–37.
8. Idoko J, Meloni S, Muazu M, et al. Impact of hepatitis B virus infection on human immunodeficiency virus response to antiretroviral therapy in Nigeria. *Clin Infect Dis* 2009;49:1268–73.
9. Lok AS, McMahon BJ. Chronic hepatitis B. *Hepatology* 2007;45:507–39.
10. Keeffe EB, Dieterich DT, Han SH, et al. A treatment algorithm for the management of chronic hepatitis B virus infection in the United States: 2008 update. *Clin Gastroenterol Hepatol* 2008;6:1315–41.
11. Rockstroh JK, Bhagani S, Benhamou Y, et al. European AIDS Clinical Society (EACS) guidelines for the clinical management and treatment of chronic hepatitis B and C coinfection in HIV-infected adults. *HIV Med* 2008;9:82–8.
12. Liang SH, Chen TJ, Lee SS, et al. Risk factors of isolated antibody against core antigen of hepatitis B virus: association with HIV infection and age but not hepatitis C virus infection. *J Acquir Immune Defic Syndr* 2010;54:122–8.
13. Lo Re V 3rd, Frank I, Gross R, et al. Prevalence, risk factors, and outcomes for occult hepatitis B virus infection among HIV-infected patients. *J Acquir Immune Defic Syndr* 2007;44:315–20.
14. Bagaglio S, Porrino L, Lazzarin A, et al. Molecular characterization of occult and overt hepatitis B (HBV) infection in an HIV-infected person with reactivation of HBV after antiretroviral treatment interruption. *Infection* 2010;38(5):417–21.
15. Fonseca MO, Pang LW, De Paula Cavalheiro N, et al. Randomized trial of recombinant hepatitis B vaccine in HIV-infected adult patients comparing a standard dose to a double dose. *Vaccine* 2005;23:2902–8.
16. Overton ET, Kang M, Peters MG, et al. Immune response to hepatitis B vaccine in HIV-infected subjects using granulocyte–macrophage colony-stimulating factor (GM-CSF) as a vaccine adjuvant: ACTG study 5220. *Vaccine* 2010;28:5597–604.
17. Panel on Antiretroviral Guidelines for Adults and Adolescents. *Guidelines for the use of Antiretroviral Agents in HIV-1-infected Adults and adolescents.* Department of Health and Human Services, 2009: 1–161. Available at http://www.aidsinfo.nih.gov/ContentFiles/AdultandAdolescentGL.pdf.
18. McMahon MA, Jilek BL, Brennan TP, et al. The HBV drug entecavir – effects on HIV-1 replication and resistance. *N Engl J Med* 2007;356:2614–21.
19. Benhamou Y, Fleury H, Trimoulet P, et al. Anti-hepatitis B virus efficacy of tenofovir disoproxil fumarate in HIV-infected patients. *Hepatology* 2006;43:548–55.
20. Sheldon J, Camino N, Rodes B, et al. Selection of hepatitis B virus polymerase mutations in HIV-coinfected patients treated with tenofovir. *Antivir Ther* 2005;10:727–34.
21. Ghany MG, Strader DB, Thomas DL, et al. American Association for the Study of Liver Diseases. Diagnosis, management, and treatment of hepatitis C: an update. *Hepatology* 2009;49:1335–74.
22. Van de Laar TJ, Matthews GV, Prins M, et al. Acute hepatitis C in HIV-infected men who have sex with men: an emerging sexually transmitted infection. *AIDS* 2010;24:1799–812.
23. Fierer DS, Uriel AJ, Carriero DC, et al. Liver fibrosis during an outbreak of acute hepatitis C virus infection in HIV-infected men: a prospective cohort study. *J Infect Dis* 2008;198:683–6.
24. Bica I, McGovern B, Dhar R, et al. Increasing mortality due to end-stage liver disease in patients with human immunodeficiency virus infection. *Clin Infect Dis* 2001;32:492–7.
25. Thomas DL, Thio CL, Martin MP, et al. Genetic variation in IL28B and spontaneous clearance of hepatitis C virus. *Nature* 2009;461:798–801.
26. Di Iulio J, Bochud PY, Rotger M, et al. Association of IL28B haplotypes with chronic hepatitis C virus infection in HIV/HCV coinfected individuals. In: *17th Conference on Retroviruses and Opportunistic Infections, February 16–19, 2010, San Francisco, California.* Abstract no. 163.
27. Giordano TP, Kramer JR, Souchek J, et al. Cirrhosis and hepatocellular carcinoma in HIV-infected veterans with and without the hepatitis C virus: a cohort study, 1992–2001. *Arch Intern Med* 2004;164:2349–54.
28. Martinez-Sierra C, Arizcorreta A, Diaz F, et al. Progression of chronic hepatitis C to liver fibrosis and cirrhosis in patients

coinfected with hepatitis C virus and human immunodeficiency virus. *Clin Infect Dis* 2003;36:491–8.

29. Merchante N, Giron-Gonzalez JA, Gonzalez-Serrano M, et al. Survival and prognostic factors of HIV-infected patients with HCV-related end-stage liver disease. *AIDS* 2006;20:49–57.

30. Sulkowski M, Mehta S, Sutcliffe CEA. Baseline liver disease is independently associated with risk of death in 631 HIV/HCV co-infected adults with histologic staging. In: *17th Conference on Retroviruses and Opportunistic Infections, February 16–19, 2010, San Francisco, California.* Abstract no. 166.

31. Puoti M, Bruno R, Soriano V, et al. Hepatocellular carcinoma in HIV-infected patients: epidemiological features, clinical presentation and outcome. *AIDS* 2004;18:2285–93.

32. Brau N, Salvatore M, Rios-Bedoya CF, et al. Slower fibrosis progression in HIV/HCV-coinfected patients with successful HIV suppression using antiretroviral therapy. *J Hepatol* 2006;44:47–55.

33. Thein HH, Yi Q, Dore GJ, e al. Natural history of hepatitis C virus infection in HIV-infected individuals and the impact of HIV in the era of highly active antiretroviral therapy: a meta-analysis. *AIDS* 2008;22:1979–91.

34. Qurishi N, Kreuzberg C, Luchters G, et al. Effect of antiretroviral therapy on liver-related mortality in patients with HIV and hepatitis C virus coinfection. *Lancet* 2003;362:1708–13.

35. Mocroft A, Soriano V, Rockstroh J, et al. Is there evidence for an increase in the death rate from liver-related disease in patients with HIV? *AIDS* 2005;19:2117–25.

36. Bani-Sadr F, Lapidus N, Bedossa P, et al. Progression of fibrosis in HIV and hepatitis C virus-coinfected patients treated with interferon plus ribavirin-based therapy: analysis of risk factors. *Clin Infect Dis* 2008;46:768–74.

37. Macias J, Castellano V, Merchante N, et al. Effect of antiretroviral drugs on liver fibrosis in HIV-infected patients with chronic hepatitis C: harmful impact of nevirapine. *AIDS* 2004;18:767–74.

38. Nunez M, Soriano V. Hepatotoxicity of antiretrovirals: incidence, mechanisms and management. *Drug Saf* 2005;28:53–66.

39. Labarga P, Soriano V, Vispo ME, et al. Hepatotoxicity of antiretroviral drugs is reduced after successful treatment of chronic hepatitis C in HIV-infected patients. *J Infect Dis* 2007;196:670–6.

40. Vogel M, Deterding K, Wiegand J, et al. Initial presentation of acute hepatitis C virus (HCV) infection among HIV-negative and HIV-positive individuals – experience from 2 large German networks on the study of acute HCV infection. *Clin Infect Dis* 2009;49:317–19.

41. Soriano V, Puoti M, Sulkowski M, et al. Care of patients coinfected with HIV and hepatitis C virus: 2007 updated recommendations from the HCV-HIV International Panel. *AIDS* 2007;21:1073–89.

42. Swain MG, Lai MY, Shiffman ML, et al. A sustained virologic response is durable in patients with chronic hepatitis C treated with peginterferon alfa-2a and ribavirin. *Gastroenterology* 2010;139(5):1593–601.

43. Berenguer J, Alvarez-Pellicer J, Martin PM, et al. Sustained virological response to interferon plus ribavirin reduces liver-related complications and mortality in patients coinfected with human immunodeficiency virus and hepatitis C virus. *Hepatology* 2009;50:407–13.

44. Dore GJ, Torriani FJ, Rodriguez-Torres M, et al. Baseline factors prognostic of sustained virological response in patients with HIV–hepatitis C virus co-infection. *AIDS* 2007;21:1555–9.

45. Ge D, Fellay J, Thompson AJ, et al. Genetic variation in IL28B predicts hepatitis C treatment-induced viral clearance. *Nature* 2009;461:399–401.

46. Rallon NI, Naggie S, Benito JM, et al. Association of a single nucleotide polymorphism near the interleukin-28B gene with response to hepatitis C therapy in HIV/hepatitis C virus-coinfected patients. *AIDS* 2010;24:F23–9.

47. Opravil M, Sasadeusz J, Cooper DA, et al. Effect of baseline CD4 cell count on the efficacy and safety of peginterferon alfa-2a (40KD) plus ribavirin in patients with HIV/hepatitis C virus coinfection. *J Acquir Immune Defic Syndr* 2008;47:36–49.

48. Torriani FJ, Rodriguez-Torres M, Rockstroh JK, et al. Peginterferon alfa-2a plus ribavirin for chronic hepatitis C virus infection in HIV-infected patients. *N Engl J Med* 2004;351:438–50.

49. Chung RT, Andersen J, Volberding P, et al. Peginterferon alfa-2a plus ribavirin versus interferon alfa-2a plus ribavirin for chronic hepatitis C in HIV-coinfected persons. *N Engl J Med* 2004;351:451–9.

50. Carrat F, Bani-Sadr F, Pol S, et al. Pegylated interferon alfa-2b vs standard interferon alfa-2b, plus ribavirin, for chronic hepatitis C in HIV-infected patients: a randomized controlled trial. *JAMA* 2004;292:2839–48.

51. Laguno M, Murillas J, Blanco JL, et al. Peginterferon alfa-2b plus ribavirin compared with interferon alfa-2b plus ribavirin for treatment of HIV/HCV co-infected patients. *AIDS* 2004;18:F27–36.

52. Nunez M, Miralles C, Berdun MA, et al. Role of weight-based ribavirin dosing and extended duration of therapy in chronic hepatitis C in HIV-infected patients: the PRESCO trial. *AIDS Res Hum Retroviruses* 2007;23:972–82.

53. Payan C, Pivert A, Morand P, et al. Rapid and early virological response to chronic hepatitis C treatment with IFN alpha2b or PEG-IFN alpha2b plus ribavirin in HIV/HCV co-infected patients. *Gut* 2007;56:1111–16.

54. Rodriguez-Torres M. On-treatment responses at week 4 and 12 can be used to predict sustained virologic response rates in HIV-HCV co-infected patients with peginterferon alfa-2a (40KD) (PEGASYS) and ribavirin (COPEGUS). In: *15th CROI, Boston, 2008.* Abstract no. 1073.

55. Shea DO, Tuite H, Farrell G, et al. Role of rapid virological response in prediction of sustained virological response to peg-IFN plus ribavirin in HCV/HIV co-infected individuals. *J Viral Hepat* 2008;15:482 9.

56. Carrat F, Bani-Sadr F, Pol S, et al. Pegylated interferon alfa-2b vs standard interferon alfa-2b, plus ribavirin, for chronic hepatitis C in HIV-infected patients: a randomized controlled trial. *JAMA* 2004;292:2839–48.

57. Berenguer J, Gonzalez-Garcia J, Lopez-Aldeguer J, et al. Pegylated interferon {alpha}2a plus ribavirin versus pegylated interferon {alpha}2b plus ribavirin for the treatment of chronic hepatitis C in HIV-infected patients. *J Antimicrob Chemother* 2009;63:1256–63.

58. Rodriguez-Torres M, Slim J, Bhatti Lea. Standard versus high dose ribavirin in combination with peginterferon alfa-2a (40KD) in genotype 1 (G1) HCV patients coinfected with HIV: final results of the PARADIGM study. In: *60th AASLD, 2009.* Abstract no. 1561.

59. Mira JA, Lopez-Cortes LF, Barreiro P, et al. Efficacy of pegylated interferon plus ribavirin treatment in HIV/hepatitis C virus co-infected patients receiving abacavir plus lamivudine or tenofovir plus either lamivudine or emtricitabine as nucleoside analogue backbone. *J Antimicrob Chemother* 2008;62:1365–73.

60. Vispo E, Barreiro P, Pineda JA, et al. Low response to pegylated interferon plus ribavirin in HIV-infected patients with chronic hepatitis C treated with abacavir. *Antivir Ther* 2008;13:429–37.

61. Myers RP, Benhamou Y, Bochet M, et al. Pegylated interferon alpha 2b and ribavirin in HIV/hepatitis C virus-co-infected non-responders and relapsers to IFN-based therapy. *AIDS* 2004;18:75–9.

62. Rodriguez-Torres M, Rodriguez-Orengo JF, Rios-Bedoya CF, et al. Efficacy and safety of peg-IFN alfa-2a with ribavirin for the treatment of HCV/HIV coinfected patients who failed previous IFN based therapy. *J Clin Virol* 2007;38:32–8.

63. Crespo M, Mira JA, Pineda JA, et al. Efficacy of pegylated interferon and ribavirin for retreatment of chronic HCV infection in HIV

co-infected patients failing a previous standard interferon-based regimen. *J Antimicrob Chemother* 2008;62:1365–73.

64. Labarga P, Vispo E, Barreiro P, et al. Rate and predictors of success in the retreatment of chronic hepatitis C virus in HIV/hepatitis C virus coinfected patients with prior nonresponse or relapse. *J Acquir Immune Defic Syndr* 2010;53:364–8.

65. Vachon M, Factor S, Branch A, et al. Insulin resistance predicts retreatment failure in an efficacy study of peginterferon-α-2a and ribavirin in HIV/HCV co-infected patients. *J Hepatol* 2011;54(1):41–7.

66. Soriano V, Vispo E, Labarga P, et al. Viral hepatitis and HIV co-infection. *Antiviral Res* 2010;85:303–15.

67. Lacombe K, Boyd A, Desvarieux M, et al. Impact of chronic hepatitis C and/or D on liver fibrosis severity in patients co-infected with HIV and hepatitis B virus. *AIDS* 2007;21:2546–9.

68. Sheng WH, Hung CC, Kao JH, et al. Impact of hepatitis D virus infection on the long-term outcomes of patients with hepatitis B virus and HIV coinfection in the era of highly active antiretroviral therapy: a matched cohort study. *Clin Infect Dis* 2007;44: 988–95.

69. Rosa I, Costes L, Garrait V, et al. Efficacy of pegylated interferon alpha-2b for the treatment of chronic delta hepatitis in a patient co-infected with HIV. *AIDS* 2005;19:2177–8.

70. Gozlan J, Lacombe K, Gault E, et al. Complete cure of HBV-HDV co-infection after 24 weeks of combination therapy with pegylated interferon and ribavirin in a patient co-infected with HBV/HCV/HDV/HIV. *J Hepatol* 2009;50:432–4.

71. Sheldon J, Ramos B, Toro C, et al. Does treatment of hepatitis B virus (HBV) infection reduce hepatitis delta virus (HDV) replication in HIV-HBV-HDV-coinfected patients? *Antivir Ther* 2008;13: 97–102.

72. Ida S, Tachikawa N, Nakajima A, et al. Influence of human immunodeficiency virus type 1 infection on acute hepatitis A virus infection. *Clin Infect Dis* 2002;34:379–85.

73. Vento S, Garofano T, Renzini C, et al. Fulminant hepatitis associated with hepatitis A virus superinfection in patients with chronic hepatitis C. *N Engl J Med* 1998;338:286–90.

74. Keeffe EB. Acute hepatitis A and B in patients with chronic liver disease: prevention through vaccination. *Am J Med* 2005;118(Suppl 10A):S21S–7.

75. Weissman S, Feucht C, Moore BA. Response to hepatitis A vaccine in HIV-positive patients. *J Viral Hepat* 2006;13:81–6.

76. Shire NJ, Welge JA, Sherman KE. Efficacy of inactivated hepatitis A vaccine in HIV-infected patients: a hierarchical bayesian meta-analysis. *Vaccine* 2006;24:272–9.

77. Overton ET, Nurutdinova D, Sungkanuparph S, et al. Predictors of immunity after hepatitis A vaccination in HIV-infected persons. *J Viral Hepat* 2007;14:189–93.

78. Pischke S, Ho H, Urbanek F, et al. Hepatitis E in HIV-positive patients in a low-endemic country. *J Viral Hepat* 2010;17:598–9.

79. Dalton HR, Bendall RP, Keane FE, et al. Persistent carriage of hepatitis E virus in patients with HIV infection. *N Engl J Med* 2009;361:1025–7.

80. Renou C, Lafeuillade A, Cadranel JF, et al. Hepatitis E virus in HIV-infected patients. *AIDS* 2010;24:1493–9.

81. Ramezani A, Mohraz M, Vahabpour R, et al. Frequency of hepatitis G virus infection among HIV positive subjects with parenteral and sexual exposure. *J Gastrointestin Liver Dis* 2008;17:269–72.

82. Williams CF, Klinzman D, Yamashita TE, et al. Persistent GB virus C infection and survival in HIV-infected men. *N Engl J Med* 2004;350:981–90.

83. Crum-Cianflone N, Dilay A, Collins G, et al. Nonalcoholic fatty liver disease among HIV-infected persons. *J Acquir Immune Defic Syndr* 2009;50:464–73.

84. Hansen BR, Petersen J, Haugaard SB, et al. The prevalence of metabolic syndrome in Danish patients with HIV infection: the effect of antiretroviral therapy. *HIV Med* 2009;10:378–87.

85. Villarroya F, Domingo P, Giralt M. Drug-induced lipotoxicity: lipodystrophy associated with HIV-1 infection and antiretroviral treatment. *Biochim Biophys Acta* 2010;1801:392–9.

86. Hadigan C, Corcoran C, Basgoz N, et al. Grinspoon S. Metformin in the treatment of HIV lipodystrophy syndrome: a randomized controlled trial. *JAMA* 2000;284:472–7.

87. Gelato MC, Mynarcik DC, Quick JL, et al. Improved insulin sensitivity and body fat distribution in HIV-infected patients treated with rosiglitazone: a pilot study. *J Acquir Immune Defic Syndr* 2002;31:163–70.

88. Carr A, Workman C, Smith DE, et al. Abacavir substitution for nucleoside analogs in patients with HIV lipoatrophy: a randomized trial. *JAMA* 2002;288:207–15.

89. Ristig M, Drechsler H, Powderly WG. Hepatic steatosis and HIV infection. *AIDS Patient Care STDS* 2005;19:356–65.

90. Ogedegbe AE, Thomas DL, Diehl AM. Hyperlactataemia syndromes associated with HIV therapy. *Lancet Infect Dis* 2003;3: 329–37.

91. Ingiliz P, Valantin MA, Duvivier C, et al. Liver damage underlying unexplained transaminase elevation in human immunodeficiency virus-1 mono-infected patients on antiretroviral therapy. *Hepatology* 2009;49:436–42.

92. Morse C, Jones A, McLaughlin M, et al. High prevalence of hepatic fibrosis and steatosis in HIV/AIDS patients without chronic viral hepatitis but with chronically elevated transaminases on ART [Poster]. CROI Meeting, Montreal, 2009. Poster no. 748.

93. Sulkowski MS, Mehta SH, Torbenson M, et al. Hepatic steatosis and antiretroviral drug use among adults coinfected with HIV and hepatitis C virus. *AIDS* 2005;19:585–92.

94. Bani-Sadr F, Carrat F, Bedossa P, et al. Hepatic steatosis in HIV-HCV coinfected patients: analysis of risk factors. *AIDS* 2006;20: 525–31.

95. Marks KM, Petrovic LM, Talal AH, et al. Histological findings and clinical characteristics associated with hepatic steatosis in patients coinfected with HIV and hepatitis C virus. *J Infect Dis* 2005;192:1943–9.

96. Rodriguez-Torres M, Govindarajan S, Sola R, et al. Hepatic steatosis in HIV/HCV co-infected patients: correlates, efficacy and outcomes of anti-HCV therapy: a paired liver biopsy study. *J Hepatol* 2008;48:756–64.

97. Sterling RK, Contos MJ, Smith PG, et al. Steatohepatitis: risk factors and impact on disease severity in human immunodeficiency virus/hepatitis C virus coinfection. *Hepatology* 2008;47:1118–27.

98. Merchante N, Rivero A, De Los Santos-Gil I, et al. Insulin resistance is associated with liver stiffness in HIV/HCV-coinfected patients. *Gut* 2009;62:1365–73.

99. Agarwal K, Fiel M, Uriel AJ. Correlation of insulin resistance with steatosis and fibrosis in hepatitis C and HIV co-infection: cross-sectional analysis of 101 patients. *Hepatology* 2004;40:587A.

100. Darby SC, Ewart DW, Giangrande PL, et al. Importance of age at infection with HIV-1 for survival and development of AIDS in UK haemophilia population. UK Haemophilia Centre Directors' Organisation. *Lancet* 1996;347:1573–9.

101. Egger M, May M, Chene G, et al. Prognosis of HIV-1-infected patients starting highly active antiretroviral therapy: a collaborative analysis of prospective studies. *Lancet* 2002;360:119–29.

102. Cao W, Jamieson BD, Hultin LE, et al. Premature aging of T cells is associated with faster HIV-1 disease progression. *J Acquir Immune Defic Syndr* 2009;50:137–47.

103. Effros RB. Replicative senescence: the final stage of memory T cell differentiation? *Curr HIV Res* 2003;1:153–65.

104. Effros RB, Fletcher CV, Gebo K, et al. Aging and infectious diseases: workshop on HIV infection and aging: what is known and future research directions. *Clin Infect Dis* 2008;47:542–53.

105. Mehandru S, Poles MA, Tenner-Racz K, et al. Primary HIV-1 infection is associated with preferential depletion of CD4+ T lymphocytes from effector sites in the gastrointestinal tract. *J Exp Med* 2004;200:761–70.

106. Poles MA, Boscardin WJ, Elliott J, et al. Lack of decay of HIV-1 in gut-associated lymphoid tissue reservoirs in maximally suppressed individuals. *J Acquir Immune Defic Syndr* 2006;43:65–8.

107. Mehandru S, Poles MA, Tenner-Racz K, et al. Lack of mucosal immune reconstitution during prolonged treatment of acute and early HIV-1 infection. *PLoS Med* 2006;3:e484.

108. Brenchley JM, Price DA, Schacker TW, et al. Microbial translocation is a cause of systemic immune activation in chronic HIV infection. *Nat Med* 2006;12:1365–71.

109. Balagopal A, Philp FH, Astemborski J, et al. Human immunodeficiency virus-related microbial translocation and progression of hepatitis C. *Gastroenterology* 2008;135:226–33.

110. Blackard JT, Sherman KE. HCV/ HIV co-infection: time to re-evaluate the role of HIV in the liver? *J Viral Hepat* 2008;15:323–30.

111. Tuyama AC, Hong F, Saiman Y, et al. Human immunodeficiency virus (HIV)-1 infects human hepatic stellate cells and promotes collagen I and monocyte chemoattractant protein-1 expression: implications for the pathogenesis of HIV/hepatitis C virus-induced liver fibrosis. *Hepatology* 2010;52:612–22.

112. Birkus G, Hitchcock MJ, Cihlar T. Assessment of mitochondrial toxicity in human cells treated with tenofovir: comparison with other nucleoside reverse transcriptase inhibitors. *Antimicrob Agents Chemother* 2002;46:716–23.

113. Maida I, Nunez M, Rios MJ, et al. Severe liver disease associated with prolonged exposure to antiretroviral drugs. *J Acquir Immune Defic Syndr* 2006;42:177–82.

114. Kovari H, Ledergerber B, Battegay M, et al. Incidence and risk factors for chronic elevation of alanine aminotransferase levels in HIV-infected persons without hepatitis B or C virus co-infection. *Clin Infect Dis* 2010;50(4):502–11.

115. Merchante N, Perez-Camacho I, Mira JA, et al. Prevalence and risk factors for abnormal liver stiffness in HIV-infected patients without viral hepatitis coinfection: role of didanosine. *Antivir Ther* 2010;15(5):753–63.

116. Stebbing J, Wong N, Tan L, et al. The relationship between prolonged antiretroviral therapy and cryptogenic liver disease. *J Acquir Immune Defic Syndr* 2009;50:554–6.

117. Maida I, Garcia-Gasco P, Sotgiu G, et al. Antiretroviral-associated portal hypertension: a new clinical condition? Prevalence, predictors and outcome. *Antivir Ther* 2008;13:103–7.

118. Mallet V, Blanchard P, Verkarre V, et al. Nodular regenerative hyperplasia is a new cause of chronic liver disease in HIV-infected patients. *AIDS* 2007;21:187–92.

119. Garvey LJ, Thomson EC, Lloyd J, et al. Response to Mallet et al., 'Nodular regenerative hyperplasia is a new cause of chronic liver disease in HIV-infected patients'. *AIDS* 2007;21:1494–5.

120. Schiano TD, Kotler DP, Ferran E, et al. Hepatoportal sclerosis as a cause of noncirrhotic portal hypertension in patients with HIV. *Am J Gastroenterol* 2007;102:2536–40.

121. Vispo E, Moreno A, Maida I, et al. Noncirrhotic portal hypertension in HIV-infected patients: unique clinical and pathological findings. *AIDS* 2010;24:1171–6.

122. Kovari H, Ledergerber B, Peter U, et al. Association of non-cirrhotic portal hypertension in HIV-infected persons and ART with didanosine. *CROI, Montreal, 2009.* Abstract no. 751.

123. Razonable RR, Paya CV. Valganciclovir for the prevention and treatment of cytomegalovirus disease in immunocompromised hosts. *Expert Rev Anti Infect Ther* 2004;2:27–41.

124. Aberg JA, Williams PL, Liu T, et al. A study of discontinuing maintenance therapy in human immunodeficiency virus-infected subjects with disseminated *Mycobacterium avium* complex: AIDS Clinical Trial Group 393 Study Team. *J Infect Dis* 2003;187:1046–52.

125. Santoro-Lopes G, de Pinho AM, Harrison LH, et al. Reduced risk of tuberculosis among Brazilian patients with advanced human immunodeficiency virus infection treated with highly active antiretroviral therapy. *Clin Infect Dis* 2002;34:543–6.

126. Ko WF, Cello JP, Rogers SJ, et al. Prognostic factors for the survival of patients with AIDS cholangiopathy. *Am J Gastroenterol* 2003;98:2176–81.

127. Murillas J, Del Rio M, Riera M, et al. Increased incidence of hepatocellular carcinoma (HCC) in HIV-1 infected patients. *Eur J Intern Med* 2005;16:113–15.

128. Rosenthal E, Poiree M, Pradier C, et al. Mortality due to hepatitis C-related liver disease in HIV-infected patients in France (Mortavic 2001 study). *AIDS* 2003;17:1803–9.

129. Monforte A, Abrams D, Pradier C, et al. HIV-induced immunodeficiency and mortality from AIDS-defining and non-AIDS-defining malignancies. *AIDS* 2008;22:2143–53.

130. Rosenthal E, Pialoux G, Bernard N, et al. Liver-related mortality in human-immunodeficiency-virus-infected patients between 1995 and 2003 in the French GERMIVIC Joint Study Group Network (MORTAVIC 2003 Study). *J Viral Hepat* 2007;14:183–8.

131. Ragni MV, Belle SH, Im K, et al. Survival of human immunodeficiency virus-infected liver transplant recipients. *J Infect Dis* 2003;188:1412–20.

132. Norris S, Taylor C, Muiesan P, et al. Outcomes of liver transplantation in HIV-infected individuals: the impact of HCV and HBV infection. *Liver Transpl* 2004;10:1271–8.

133. Murillas J, Rimola A, Laguno M, et al. The model for end-stage liver disease score is the best prognostic factor in human immunodeficiency virus 1-infected patients with end-stage liver disease: a prospective cohort study. *Liver Transpl* 2009;15:1133–41.

134. Tateo M, Roque-Afonso AM, Antonini TM, et al. Long-term follow-up of liver transplanted HIV/hepatitis B virus coinfected patients: perfect control of hepatitis B virus replication and absence of mitochondrial toxicity. *AIDS* 2009;23:1069–76.

135. Eisenbach C, Merle U, Stremmel W, et al. Liver transplantation in HIV-positive patients. *Clin Transplant* 2009;23(Suppl 21):68–74.

136. European AIDS Treatment Network (NEAT) Acute Hepatitis C Infection Consensus Panel. Acute hepatitis C in HIV-infected individuals: recommendations from the European AIDS Treatment Network (NEAT) consensus conference. *AIDS* 2011;25(4):399–409.

Multiple choice questions

41.1 Noncirrhotic portal hypertension (NCPH) has been most consistently associated with the use of which antiretroviral?

    a Lamivudine.
    b Zidovudine.
    c Zalcitabine.
    d Nevirapine.
    e Didanosine.

41.2 Predictors of successful outcomes after liver transplant in HIV-infected patients include all the following except which one?

    a Well-controlled HIV disease.
    b Lower model for end-stage liver disease (MELD) score.
    c Early referral to transplant team.
    d HCV coinfection.

Answers to the multiple choice questions can be found in the Appendix at the end of the book.

These multiple choice questions are also available for you to complete online.
Visit http://www.schiffsdiseasesoftheliver.com/

PART XI

Elements of Liver Transplantation

Overview

Michael F. Sorrell

The success of liver transplantation has transformed the discipline of hepatology. The potential role of liver replacement has changed how physicians approach the care of end-stage liver disease. Because of the centrality of transplantation, the practice of liver disease is now intertwined in a multidisciplinary manner with multiple other specialties. Much of the success of liver transplantation in the past 30 plus years can be attributed to advances in these sister disciplines. This is particularly true with regard to radiologic imaging and intervention. Now that liver transplantation is firmly established as a proven treatment option, attention has shifted to the long-term consequences of transplantation and the central role of post-hospital care with an emphasis on the resultant quality of life. Not withstanding the success of liver transplantation, new challenges and controversies surface as would be expected in such a dynamic and changing field.

Perhaps the most prominent of the challenges and controversies remains that of donor liver distribution and to some degree allocation. The challenge of allocation was met by the development of the model for end-stage liver disease (MELD) score, with subsequent modifications termed MELD exception scores. The move to MELD with its objective criteria substantially eliminated many of the disparities surrounding organ allocation and reduced deaths on the waiting list. However, marked disparities in organ distribution remain because of variation in the number of available organs between individual organ procurement organizations. The US Institute of Medicine recommendation that access to organs be more equitably distributed by the development of regional sharing has been stoutly resisted by transplant physicians who would be adversely affected by the adoption of these recommendations. Further changes in organ allocation will require a political solution.

In response to the shortage of donor organs, transplant surgeons have responded by expanding the donor organ pool in several ways. The use of living donor grafts was at one time thought to be a partial answer both to donor organ shortage and optimal timing of liver grafting. The absence of a living donor death registry does not allow for an accurate assessment of the risk of live donor donation. Within the United States, the wide dissemination within the popular press of live donor deaths has contributed to a halving of live donor grafting. It is estimated that at least 23 donor deaths directly attributed to the surgical procedure have occurred in the United States and Europe. The use of deceased cardiac donors has been another approach to increasing the organ donor pool. Although short-term graft survival in some centers is similar using deceased donors, the surgical complications, particularly diffuse biliary strictures, have lessened the appeal of using such donors.

The value of liver transplantation as a life-saving modality is firmly established. The technical aspects of the transplant procedure itself have been largely worked out and only minor emendations appear in the literature; however, long-term management challenges remain. The major indication for liver transplantation is chronic hepatitis C followed closely by nonalcoholic steatohepatitis (NASH). Recurrence following transplantation is the rule. The lack of a predictably effective treatment for recurrent hepatitis C has resulted in a decreased 5-year survival rate when compared to primary biliary cirrhosis, primary sclerosing cholangitis, and alcoholic liver disease. NASH recurrence is common, and in a similar vein, effective drug therapy for recurrent disease is lacking.

The increased incidence of vascular disease, cancer, metabolic complications, and renal failure influence not only morbidity and mortality but also quality of life. Many of the long-term complications are caused by immunization protocols required to maintain graft survival. The development of new immunosuppressive drugs and solving the puzzle of tolerance remain the best hope for the future of improved survival and enhanced quality of life.

PART XI

Elements of Liver Transplantation

Overview

CHAPTER 42
Selection and Timing of Liver Transplantation

Richard B. Freeman Jr.

Department of Surgery, Dartmouth-Hitchcock Medical Center, Lebanon, NH, USA

Key concepts

- The selection of candidates for liver transplantation is not necessarily linked to the timing of liver transplantation due to the severely constrained organ donor resource. This means that individual candidates cannot always receive a transplant at the optimal time for his or her benefit.
- For most patients with chronic liver disease, selection for transplantation depends on their risk of dying from the liver disease weighed against their risk of dying from the transplant procedure and attendant medications. Mortality risk scores have been helpful in determining when the risk of death without a transplant is greater than the risk of the procedure. Survival benefit, or the life gained with a transplant compared with lifetime gained staying on the list without a transplant, is an increasingly accepted concept for selecting liver transplant recipients.
- For some liver conditions, the benefit of liver transplantation cannot be weighed against the mortality risk from intrinsic liver disease. Thus

- other methods, such as estimates of disease progression, must be used for proper selection of waiting candidates. Disease progression estimates are limited by lack of good natural history data.
- Pediatric patients with liver disease face unique problems and mortality risk models utilizing variables specific for children have been developed to address these differences.
- Efficient selection of liver transplant candidates with acute liver failure is especially challenging because of the need to rapidly assess the probable natural course of the disease so that patients not likely to recover will receive transplant priority but those more likely to recover do not receive needless organs.
- Living donor liver transplantation improves the ability of the clinician to "time" the transplant at the most advantageous point in the disease process for the waiting candidate. However, donor risks and informed consent must not be subjugated in an effort to maximize the timing benefit.

Inhabitants in the developed world are fortunate that, in large measure, effective treatments for most medical conditions are generally available, with access to these treatments limited mostly by socioeconomic, or distributive, problems rather than scarcity of the therapeutic substrate itself. This is not the case for transplantation. Unlike any other field in medicine, the clinician's ability to apply transplantation therapy is not completely defined by the risk–benefit ratio of that therapy for the patient in question. For patients who could potentially benefit from liver transplantation, the constrained donor liver resource problem is acutely severe since alternative liver support technologies are not perfected. Thus, the application of liver transplant therapy depends not only on the diagnosis of a problem for which liver transplantation is likely to provide more benefit than harm, but also on the availability of the therapeutic substrate – the liver itself. Consequently, and in contrast to most other medical conditions, determining if a patient diagnosed with progressive liver disease will receive benefit from liver trans-

plantation is not sufficient for initiation of delivery of the treatment. This makes the optimal timing for liver transplantation a two-sided proposition: (i) determining when a patient's disease has advanced far enough that he or she will receive more benefit than harm from the transplant procedure and subsequent maintenance treatments; and (ii) determining who, among all those who are deemed to likely receive benefit, should come first when donor constraints allow only one patient at a time to be treated. The former patient-based issue can be categorized as the selection of appropriate candidates for transplantation. The second topic, timing of liver transplantation, is not entirely under the control of the treating physician or patient but is much more influenced by allocation and distribution rules. Only in the case of living liver donor transplantation can treating clinicians completely control the timing of liver transplantation for candidates they have deemed appropriate. This chapter addresses the selection of patients for liver transplantation, the optimal timing of liver transplantation absent

Schiff's Diseases of the Liver, Eleventh Edition. Edited by Eugene R. Schiff, Willis C. Maddrey and Michael F. Sorrell.
© 2012 John Wiley & Sons, Ltd. Published 2012 by John Wiley & Sons, Ltd.

organ donor constraints, the timing of liver transplantation in the context of living donor liver transplantation, and finally organ allocation priorities and their influence on the timing of liver transplantation.

Selection of candidates for liver transplantation

Mortality risk
Liver transplantation, like all therapies, should be offered when the risks are outweighed by the benefits. Quantifying risk and benefit, however, is no easy proposition and is fraught with subjective interpretations of need for transplantation. For any candidate, co-morbid conditions such as cardiopulmonary disease [1], renal function, chronic or active acute infections, neurologic and psychiatric impairments, as well as the social support system available to the patient must be assessed and considered in the overall determination of surgical risk. Caregivers and patients must weigh mortality risks, disease progression, and the impact of deterioration in quality of life for those with liver disease who may be candidates for liver transplantation. In the past, most patients were deemed reasonable candidates for transplantation based on the development of signs or symptoms of decompensation usually related to portal hypertension. These original assessments of liver transplant candidacy were subsequently incorporated into minimal listing criteria based on an anticipated 1-year survival of 90% or less if no transplant was performed [2]. This 1-year waiting list survival criterion was equated to a Child–Turcotte–Pugh (CTP) [3] score of greater than or equal to 7. However, the use of subjective variables, and differences in cholestatic versus noncholestatic liver diseases, as well as a "ceiling effect" inherent in the CTP score for more advanced chronic liver disease, led investigators to look to other models to predict mortality. To this end, Malinchoc et al. defined a mathematical model to predict mortality risk in any patient with portal hypertensive complications undergoing a transjugular intrahepatic portosystemic shunt (TIPS) procedure regardless of the underlying chronic liver disease [4] and without using the subjective variables employed by the CTP score (Box 42.1). The model for end-stage liver disease (MELD) score has subsequently been shown to be highly predictive of 3-month mortality for a variety of cohorts of patients with chronic liver disease [5,6] and for a cohort of US patients waiting for liver transplantation [7]. The MELD model has been widely accepted as a measure of chronic liver disease severity where severity of disease is defined as 3-month mortality risk and has been incorporated in liver allocation systems in the United States and many other areas around the world. Thus, if one defines need for liver

> **Box 42.1 Model for end-stage liver disease (MELD) and pediatric end-stage liver disease (PELD) scores.[a]**
>
> **MELD score**
> - $R = 0.957 \times \log_e(\text{creatinine mg/dL}) + 0.378 \times \log_e(\text{bilirubin mg/dL}) + 1.120 \times \log_e(\text{INR}) + 0.643 \times (\text{disease etiology}^b)$
>
> **MELD score, UNOS/OPTN policy**
> - $R = [0.957 \times \log_e(\text{creatinine mg/dL}) + 0.378 \times \log_e(\text{total bilirubin mg/dL}) + 1.120 \times \log_e(\text{INR}) + 0.643] \times 10$
>
> **PELD score**
> - $R = [0.463 \times (\text{age}^c) - 0.687 \times \log_e(\text{albumin g/dL}) + 0.480 \times \log_e(\text{total bilirubin mg/dL}) + 1.857 \times \log_e(\text{INR}) + 0.667 (\text{growth failure}^d)] \times 10$
>
> [a]MELD score as originally reported by Malinchoc et al. [4] and as modified for US organ allocation. PELD score as reported by McDairmid et al. [67] and as is currently used for US pediatric liver allocation policy.
> [b]1 for noncholestatic disease; 0 for cholestatic disease.
> [c]1 for <1 year of age; 0 for ≥1 year of age.
> [d]1 for 2 standard deviations below the mean for age; 0 for ≤2 standard deviations below the median for age.
>
> OPTN, Organ Procurement and Transplantation Network; UNOS, United Network for Organ Sharing.

transplant in terms of risk of dying of liver disease, the MELD score provides an objective, readily available, easily applied measure for the selection of liver transplant candidates with chronic liver disease.

Health-related quality of life
Mortality risk, however, may not be the only measure of need for liver transplantation. Numerous studies have documented that health-related quality of life (HRQOL) is poor for patients with progressive chronic liver disease [8–10] and that measures of mortality risk may not necessarily correlate with measures of HRQOL for these patients [11]. Nonetheless, when weighing quality of life considerations, physicians must account for mortality risk because, for patients who die, there can be no *quality* of life. Thus, mortality risk usually takes precedence in determining appropriate timing of liver transplantation for individual patients when the risks of death from transplantation surgery and immunosuppression are relatively low in relation to the mortality risk without transplantation even though the patient's quality of life may be poor. For example, offering liver transplantation to patients with limitations in their HRQOL who face a higher risk of dying due to the surgery and post-transplant treatments than they face if they wait until their disease becomes more severe, may not be in the best interest of that patient. Interestingly, however, in one

Table 42.1 Health-related quality of life indices in 20-year liver transplant survivors.

Category	20-year survivors (n = 68)	US population (n = 2,474)	P	Chronic liver disease (n = 210)	P
Physical functioning	79 ± 26	84 ± 23	0.038	51 ± 29	<0.001
Role–physical	67 ± 42	81 ± 34	<0.001	38 ± 31	<0.001
Bodily pain	72 ± 28	75 ± 24	0.315	50 ± 32	<0.001
General health	62 ± 23	72 ± 20	<0.001	54 ± 27	0.033
Vitality	63 ± 22	61 ± 21	0.329	52 ± 28	0.002
Social functioning	77 ± 26	83 ± 23	0.026	33 ± 21	<0.001
Role–emotional	75 ± 39	81 ± 33	0.098	58 ± 20	<0.001
Mental health	80 ± 20	74 ± 18	0.029	34 ± 22	<0.001
Physical component summary	46 ± 12	50 ± 10	<0.001	—	—
Mental component summary	52 ± 11	50 ± 10	0.124	—	—

study of end-stage liver disease patients, subjects were frequently willing to accept a reduction in life expectancy in return for improved health and onehalf of the subjects would accept a 50% mortality risk in exchange for perfect health [12]. Almost all studies have shown significant improvements in HRQOL after transplant [13], and the HRQOL outcome is not associated with the severity of illness before transplant [14]. Moreover, even 20 years after transplant, recipients have acceptable quality of life and achieve many of the important life events that the general population enjoys (Table 42.1) [15]. Thus, regardless of how ill patients are before the transplant, if they survive, most can expect a reasonable HRQOL or functional status afterwards. Therefore, there does not seem to be justification for selecting one group of patients

for liver transplantation because they are likely to achieve a better HRQOL afterwards, than another. The available literature suggests that all recipients report relatively similar and significantly improved HRQOL afterwards.

Transplant benefit

The concept of selecting patients based on estimates of transplant benefit, as measured in number of life years gained, has garnered increasing attention. Merion et al. compared the mortality risk for liver transplant candidates remaining on the list with mortality risk for recipients of deceased donor liver transplants and stratified their results by MELD score at listing (Fig. 42.1). These investigators found that recipients with MELD scores <15 experienced a higher hazard for death than the

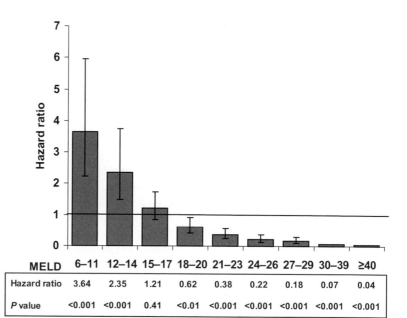

Figure 42.1 Comparison of mortality risk expressed as hazard ratio by MELD score for recipients of liver transplants compared to candidates on the liver transplant waiting list. (Reproduced from Merion et al. [16] with permission from Wiley-Blackwell.)

MELD	6–11	12–14	15–17	18–20	21–23	24–26	27–29	30–39	≥40
Hazard ratio	3.64	2.35	1.21	0.62	0.38	0.22	0.18	0.07	0.04
P value	<0.001	<0.001	0.41	<0.01	<0.001	<0.001	<0.001	<0.001	<0.001

candidates who remained on the list without transplantation at 1 year of follow-up. The authors concluded that, "liver transplants are being performed for some candidates who have a higher risk of dying from the transplant procedure than they have from dying from their underlying liver disease" [16]. It is interesting to note that, in this study, there was no MELD score beyond which a benefit in survival was obtainable. Therefore, even for candidates with very high pretransplant mortality risks as defined by their MELD score, a significant benefit was achieved by liver transplantation because the success rate was still acceptable and their survival probability without transplant was essentially zero. However, the posttransplant survival results were based only on candidates for whom liver transplantation was performed and many more patients with high MELD scores were removed from the waiting list for reasons of death or being too sick than patients with lower MELD scores [17]. These results indicate that there is a selection process by which centers are choosing candidates with high MELD scores for whom they expect a good chance of success. The transplant benefit concept has been further analyzed by stratifying recipient benefit across donor quality indices. Transplanting livers with higher risks of failure confers even more risk on recipients who have low risks of dying without the transplant. These high-risk livers, or so-called extended criteria donor livers, still confer a survival benefit to patients with the highest risks of dying without the transplant because the increased risk of the organ and surgery is still considerably less compared with the near 100% mortality risk for patients with the highest MELD scores [18]. From these data the optimal timing of liver transplantation for patients with chronic liver disease can be estimated based on their mortality risk as defined by their MELD score. Most patients with chronic cirrhosis who have MELD scores >15 will receive a benefit from liver transplantation even when using grafts from higher risk donors, whereas those with lower MELD scores have a better chance of surviving without a transplant. Giving these low-risk candidates higher risk grafts reduces the survival benefit for these candidates because the risks of surgery and graft failure are higher than remaining on the list and continuing to wait for a lower risk graft.

Clearly, however, there are diagnostic groups of patients with chronic liver disease for whom the MELD score may not accurately reflect mortality risk. Patients with human immunodeficiency virus (HIV) and hepatitis C virus (HCV) coinfection [19], patients with intestinal failure [20], and perhaps patients with severe ascites [21] may have higher mortality risks than their MELD score defines. Attempts to better calibrate the MELD score for patients with ascites and hyponatremia have produced mathematical models that incorporate serum sodium along with other laboratory values, and these may be more accurate in predicting death for such patients [22]. Overall, for individual patients with severe symptoms or poor HRQOL but low mortality risks, transplantation must be carefully weighed to determine if there is sufficient justification to accept greater hazards of death for potential improvement in HRQOL.

Other disease progression end-points

For some patients with liver diseases treatable by transplantation, mortality or HRQOL risk may not be the correct metrics to judge need. Examples of such conditions are hepatocellular carcinoma (HCC), metabolic liver diseases, and hepatopulmonary and portopulmonary hypertension syndromes. Patients with these disorders usually do not have significant mortality risks due to their underlying liver disease but face risks of disease progression beyond a point at which liver transplantation can be offered with a reasonable chance of success. Unfortunately, risk models for disease progression for these conditions have not been derived, making evidence-based selection problematic.

Hepatocellular cancer

Since HCC is increasingly recognized as a worldwide health problem, much more attention has been focused on its natural history and treatment. Excellent short and longer term results have been achieved with liver transplantation for patients with small HCC lesions arising in cirrhotic livers. Specifically, cirrhotic patients with a single HCC lesion less than 5 cm in diameter or three or fewer lesions, the largest of which is less than 3 cm in diameter – the so-called Milan criteria [23] – have 4-year survival rates in excess of 80%. These rates are comparable to liver transplant recipients with nonmalignant primary liver diseases [24] and are better than surgical resection [25]. These excellent results depend on timing the transplantation for patients before the tumor extends to a larger size and/or disseminates. Thus, more accurate selection of appropriate candidates with HCC for liver transplantation requires the development of prognostic models of tumor progression. Increasingly, clinicians have recognized that HCC can progress at variable rates and that some tumors beyond the Milan criteria have favorable recurrence patterns after transplantation. Investigators at the University of California at San Francisco (UCSF) demonstrated that selecting HCC candidates for liver transplantation with single tumors <6.5 cm in size, or three or fewer tumors with the largest being <4.5 cm and the total tumor diameter of <8 cm, can achieve 5-year survival results comparable to patients selected using the Milan criteria [26]. Extending this concept, European investigators assessed post liver transplantation outcome for HCC patients with various tumor numbers and sizes and developed the Metro ticket

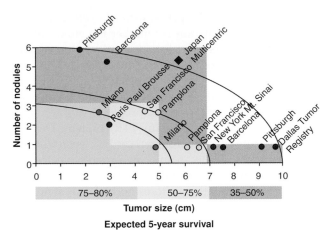

Figure 42.2 Metro ticket concept for hepatocellular cancer.

concept (Fig. 42.2) [27]. More recent single center studies have suggested that the probability of progression for HCC tumors that are less than 3 cm in size is approximately 10% within 1 year after listing, while larger tumors have an approximately 60% chance of progressing beyond Milan criteria within a year of listing [28]. The concept of downstaging tumors presenting beyond Milan criteria has gained acceptance as a criterion of selection for liver transplantation. Patients responding to local treatment whose tumors do not progress for 3–6 months after treatment appear to be associated with favorable long-term results after transplantation [29].

Diagnostic accuracy for HCC, however, confounds optimal timing of liver transplantation for these candidates. Screening high-risk populations for HCC and subsequent confirmatory computed tomography (CT) or magnetic resonance imaging (MRI) scans can achieve sensitivity and specificity of 70–80% [30–32]. The accuracy of imaging tests is further reduced for lesions less than 2 cm in size (Table 42.2). Liver biopsy has been advocated to overcome some of these problems [33], but risks of bleeding, needle tract seeding by tumor, and sampling errors have limited its widespread use [34]. Liver transplantation for patients with false-positive diagnoses of HCC who otherwise do not have severe

underlying liver disease, exposes these patients to increased surgical and immunosuppressive risks relative to medical management and diverts scarce organs away from those who could benefit more (see discussion below regarding timing of liver transplantation in the context of liver allocation).

The available evidence suggests that patients with documented HCC within the Milan criteria who otherwise are acceptable liver transplant candidates should be selected for transplantation. Diagnostic inaccuracy compels caregivers to confirm the diagnosis with complementary modalities [35]. In the future, improved genomic or proteomic testing may be widely available and may provide much more accurate diagnostic [36] as well as prognostic information to optimize the selection of patients for surgical resection or transplantation [37].

Pulmonary syndromes

Some patients with chronic liver disease develop pulmonary symptoms that impair their HRQOL and increase their risk for surgical intervention [38]. These patients may or may not have severe intrinsic liver disease [39] and may not have advanced CTP or MELD scores [40]. Hepatopulmonary syndrome (HPS) defines a constellation of symptoms including dyspnea, hypoxia, reduced diffusion capacity, and increased pulmonary arteriovenous shunting in the presence of chronic liver disease. Recent reports have better characterized patients at risk for death on the waiting list who would also have significant benefit if they receive liver transplantation in a timely fashion [41]. These data along with others have led to changes in the Organ Procurement and Transplantation Network (OPTN) policy that assigns increased priority to patients with HPS and have helped to define mortality risk and more precisely define the disease. Results for HPS patients selected for transplantation have been acceptable, with a majority of patients experiencing improvement or resolution of their pulmonary condition [42]. For these reasons, patients with signs and symptoms of HPS who do not have severe pulmonary hypertension should be considered for transplantation before their

Table 42.2 Comparison of radiologic sensitivity for diagnosing HCC in candidates for liver transplantation.

Modality	N	Nodule <10 mm	Nodule 10–20 mm	Nodule >20 mm	Reference
CT scan	76	10	65	100	Burrel et al. 2003 [30]
CT scan	83	50	96	100	Kim et al. 2009 [31]
MRI	83	70	92	100	Kim et al. 2003 [31]

CT, computed tomography; MRI, magnetic resonance imaging.

pulmonary function deteriorates to a point where anesthetic and surgical risks become prohibitive.

Individuals with cirrhosis also can present with pulmonary hypertension or so-called portopulmonary hypertension (PPH). In some cases these patients are asymptomatic, and their increased pulmonary resistance is discovered only at the time of invasive monitoring for the transplant procedure. Patients with PPH have an increased mortality risk above that expected from their underlying liver disease, and increased perioperative cardiovascular mortality has been reported for patients with elevated pulmonary artery pressures who undergo liver transplantation [43]. Nonetheless, many of these cases can be managed effectively with medical therapy [44] and outcomes for selected candidates, though sparsely reported, have been reasonable [45]. These patients have to be carefully selected with multidisciplinary evaluation by transplant hepatology, pulmonology, anesthesiology, and surgical specialists. Patients with elevated pulmonary artery pressures who respond to pulmonary vasodilator treatment have better results after liver transplantation than those who do not, making a trial of medical management a reasonable diagnostic and therapeutic choice prior to selection for transplantation [46,47]. At this time, the available literature suggests that patients with moderate PPH or those who respond to vasodilator treatment should be selected for liver transplantation since their outcomes are acceptable and transplantation may improve their PPH afterward [48].

Metabolic liver diseases

Individuals with metabolic liver disease may also have legitimate indications for liver transplantation but may not have significant synthetic liver failure. Diseases such as Wilson disease, porphyria-associated liver disease, hemachromatosis, cystic fibrosis, and α_1-antitrypsin disease generally cause cirrhosis, portal hypertension, and hepatic synthetic failure. Consequently, mortality risk and existing measures of HRQOL should function well for these patients because they can be selected for transplantation using a mortality risk-based need for transplantation defined by their intrinsic liver disease. However, patients with conditions such as familial amyloid polyneuropathy (FAP), hereditary oxalosis, and inborn errors of hepatic metabolism – such as urea cycle defects, Crigler–Najjar syndrome, tyrosinemia, and other rare enzymatic diseases – may not develop hepatic fibrosis, portal hypertensive symptoms, or deterioration in hepatic synthetic function as is normally captured in measurements of bilirubin, coagulation factors, albumin synthesis, or assessment of portal hypertensive signs and symptoms. Nonetheless, particularly for metabolic defects that are intrinsic to the liver, liver transplantation has offered excellent short- and long-term results for properly

selected individuals. The prime factor in selecting these patients for transplantation is whether the effects of the disease will be reversed by liver transplantation regardless of the anatomic location of the metabolic defect.

In adults, the best example of such a condition is FAP, where the enzymatic defect occurs in an otherwise normal liver but causes severe systemic problems due to deposition of a mutant transthyretin (TTR) protein. Deposition of these fibrils in neurologic, cardiac, gastrointestinal, and urinary tissues results in progressive loss of function, and an untreated median survival of 9–13 years [49]. Liver transplantation restores normal TTR synthesis with the disappearance of the mutant protein from the blood of affected recipients and a slowing or partial resolution of symptoms in successful cases [50,51]. Thus, the extent of secondary manifestations of FAP at the time of presentation, especially myocardial dysfunction and progressive neuropathy, limits successful recovery after liver transplantation. Optimal selection of liver transplantation candidates with FAP requires early identification and assessment of the severity of end-organ involvement so that the candidate has sufficient cardiopulmonary reserve to survive the surgery and before these complications become irreversible. In some cases, the end-organ disease does not improve after restoring normal TTR synthesis with transplantation.

Children with primary hyperoxaluria type 1 (PH-1) develop severe renal calculi and resultant renal failure but the metabolic defect resides in the alanine glycoxalate aminotransferase gene that is exclusively expressed in hepatic peroxisomes. Thus liver transplantation cures the enzyme defect because the deficient genes are replaced with the newly transplanted liver's enzymes, although established renal damage does not resolve after liver transplantation. Thus, most PH-1 patients are selected for liver transplantation after conservative measures have failed and renal disease has progressed. Consequently, many PH-1 patients are treated with combined liver–kidney transplants [52]. Preemptive liver transplant, performed before renal complications have progressed, has been advocated for some PH-1 cases [53] but the morbidity and mortality risks incurred by liver transplantation and immunosuppression must be considered carefully for these minimally symptomatic patients with relatively preserved renal function who may enjoy a good HRQOL and survival with nonoperative management for many years [54].

Other examples of diseases intrinsic to the liver are the urea cycle disorders [55], other hyperammoniemic syndromes [56,57], maple syrup urine disease [58], and hereditary tyrosinemia type 1 [59] where defects cause extremely elevated ammonia levels, neurologic disease and coma, all of which can be reversed with liver transplantation if recognized early. In some cases, the neurologic consequences of these diseases progress to a point where they cannot be reversed by liver transplantation, making early recognition the most critical aspect in selection of patients with these conditions for liver transplantation.

Pediatric considerations

As alluded to above, selecting children for liver transplantation is complicated by the fact that growth retardation, delayed development, and neurologic impairment are all deleterious sequelae of many of the liver diseases and metabolic disorders presenting in childhood. There is evidence that liver transplantation can help reverse some of the growth retardation [60,61] and developmental delay [62] but may not completely do so [63–65]. Most children do not return to the same level of functioning as the general, unaffected, population [66]. For these reasons, pediatricians have emphasized the need to select children at a stage early enough in their disease so that liver transplantation will provide a reasonable chance for some catch-up growth and development [66]. However, it clear that striving to achieve these desirable outcomes must be weighed against the mortality risks of the surgery and immunosuppression, as children who do not survive the transplant procedure cannot possibly achieve catch-up growth, accelerate their mental and physical development, or improve their HRQOL.

Mortality risk factors for children with liver disease differ from mortality risk variables in adults. The pediatric end-stage liver disease (PELD) score (see Box 42.1) utilizes bilirubin, international normalized ratio (INR), albumin, age, and growth failure factors to predict 3-month mortality in patients less than 19 years of age, with reasonable accuracy [67]. Other prognostic scores such as the Wilson disease index employ white blood cell count and serum aspartate aminotransferase (AST) levels in addition to albumin, bilirubin, and INR levels [68]. Since children often present with metabolic diseases for which liver transplantation can be beneficial but without intrinsic liver synthetic failure, selection of these candidates requires early diagnosis and identification of extrahepatic manifestations before they become irreversible.

Acute liver failure

Acute liver failure, also known as fulminant hepatic failure, remains a vexing and lethal clinical problem for pediatric and adult liver specialists, although there is evidence that the incidence is decreasing. The diverse etiologies and difficulty in predicting which patients will recover spontaneously from those who will die without timely liver transplantation contribute to the complexity of selecting these patients for transplantation. Liver transplantation remains the best option for long-term recovery, but predicting who will recover without liver trans-

> **Box 42.2 King's College and Clichy criteria for probability of death from acute liver failure.**
>
> **King's College criteria**
> - INR >6.5
>
> *Or any three of the following:*
> - Age <10 or >40 years
> - Etiology of drug toxicity or viral hepatitis
> - Duration of jaundice before onset of encephalopathy >7 days
> - INR >3.5
> - Bilirubin >17.5 mg/dL
>
> **Clichy criteria**
> - Portosystemic encephalopathy
> - Factor V <20% for age <30 years or <30% for age >30 years

plantation and who will not remains the critical issue for clinicians caring for these patients. Several prognostic scores have been developed to assist decision-making in this regard. The King's College group [69] and a French group [70] each published models for the prediction of death from acute liver failure (Box 42.2). Both of these models have excellent positive predictive value for determining which patients will die from acute liver failure but, in subsequent studies, both models have been shown to have relatively low negative predictive values [71–73]. While it may be desirable to err on the side of transplantation when the consequences of failure to transplant a patient destined to die of liver failure are so extreme, use of these models can result in inappropriate utilization of donor organs for patients who would otherwise recover without engraftment. More recently, in a study where patients with acetaminophen toxicity were excluded, the MELD score was shown to have superior positive and negative predictive value and a higher concordance for predicting which patients would die and which would recover with acute liver failure [74]. These results have been further supported by a recent study of the US liver transplant database in which the MELD score for patients with nonacetaminophen-induced acute liver failure was highly predictive of mortality risk [75]. Prognostic indicators for early mortality in patients with acetaminophen toxicity such as acetaminophen plasma half-life levels [76], coagulation factor levels [77], Gc protein levels [78], APACHE II score [79], phosphate levels [80], or addition of serum lactate [81] to the King's College models have been reported. However, a recent meta-analysis found that these prognostic models have limited sensitivity and specificity, making them of questionable usefulness for the selection of patients with acetaminophen-induced liver failure for transplantation [82]. Other prognostic scores for specific causes of acute liver failure have been developed that may have better predictive value for those disease etiologies [83] and several new biomarkers have been identified as potentially useful in preliminary studies [84].

Accurate prognostic information is essential for the selection of patients with acute liver failure for transplantation. The King's College criteria, Clichy criteria, MELD score, and disease-specific scores may be helpful tools for patients with nonacetaminophen-induced fulminant failure but their low negative predictive value should be kept in mind. The selection of patients with acetaminophen-induced liver failure remains more problematic, and careful clinical observation for encephalopathy and trends in hepatic synthetic function remain indispensable in the selection of these and all patients with acute liver failure.

Timing of liver transplantation

Living donor liver transplantation

The advent of living donor liver transplantation (LDLT) in the late 1980s for children [85] and early 1990s for adults [86] introduced the possibility of electively timing liver transplantation. With this innovation, it became possible for those patients with liver disease treatable with liver transplantation who are fortunate enough to have a suitable and willing donor, to receive their transplant at a point where the risks of the surgery are outweighed by the risks of not doing the transplant. This was the main justification for the application of LDLT to children [87] since pediatric deceased donor organs are even more scarce than adult organs and, as discussed previously, the timing of transplantation for children may not always be best estimated by mortality risk derived from the intrinsic liver disease. Patients selected for LDLT have included children with most indications for liver transplantation including acute liver failure, and adults with HCC [88,89] and other conditions that do not consistently receive enough priority on the waiting list. In general, LDLT has been reserved for patients with less severe liver disease and estimates of mortality risk can be helpful in selecting candidates who will derive benefit from the transplant [90]. A report from Japan used the MELD score to identify candidates who could receive the smaller left lobe graft and still achieve an acceptable outcome [91]. A concern for more rapid recurrence of HCV in regenerating liver segments transplanted from living donors limited the early use of living donors for patients with HCV. More recent data suggest that HCV recurrence is no more frequent or aggressive in recipients of living donor grafts when compared with recipients of deceased donor livers [92,93].

Although there are limited reports of LDLT being performed for acute liver failure in adults [94], most clini-cians reserve the living donor procedure for patients with moderately severe chronic liver disease. There is then sufficient time for a complete donor evaluation and informed consent without the added coercion of an acute, potentially immediately fatal liver disease in the recipient candidate. Conversely, LDLT for pediatric candidates, where an adult donor donates a smaller portion of his or her liver and thus faces a lower operative risk, seems applicable for nearly all indications for liver transplantation in children.

Paramount to the selection of recipient candidates for LDLT is a thorough assessment of the donor's risks for donation, estimation of the potential of success for the recipient, and fully informed consent for both donor and recipient. There are several recent reviews compiling these risks, which should be used to inform potential living liver donors [95].

Timing of liver transplantation in the context of organ allocation

In an ideal world all patients would receive the most effective treatment at the time when they are most likely to gain the most benefit and suffer the least harm from that intervention. However, since liver transplantation is severely limited by the availability of the therapeutic substrate, there must be some method for selection from all those who could potentially benefit, the few individuals who will receive the treatment. Thus, the timing of liver transplantation for individual patients will be determined in large part by this allocation selection process regardless of the presence of the beneficial potential a transplant may pose for any of the waiting patients. Living donor transplantation introduces some flexibility for the timing of these cases, but since only about 3% of liver transplant procedures were from living donors in 2009 [96], the timing of the vast majority of liver transplants procedures depends on the allocation system. Timing for these patients, then, is not so much determined by what is most appropriate for that individual to maximize success and minimize complications and/or failures, but is much more determined by what is the most equitable for all users of the organ donor pool. Equitability is difficult to define, but prioritization of measures of equitable outcomes is possible. Since deceased individuals cannot have a quality of life or growth or development or other improvement in their burden of disease, it is difficult to accept any form of liver allocation where nonmortality end-points supersede the risk of death. Consequently, prioritizing an individual with a very poor quality of life or delayed growth and development before someone with a higher mortality risk is difficult to justify. However, risk of disease progression as is conceptualized in liver allocation for HCC patients in the United States can also serve as an equitable prioritization tool.

Thus, timing of deceased donor liver transplantation will depend mostly on which individual from among all the waiting candidates has the highest mortality risk (or risk of disease progression) if he or she continues to wait even though there may be many other individuals on the list for whom transplantation at that point time would also be beneficial.

Annotated references

Freeman RB. MELD and quality of life. *Liver Transplant* 2005;11:134–6.
A discussion on the balance between health-related quality of life and mortality risk in selecting candidates for liver transplantation.

Krowka MJ, Mandel MS, Ramsay MA, et al. Heptopulmonary syndrome and portopulmonary hypertension: a report from a multicenter liver transplant database. *Liver Transplant* 2004;10:174–82.
This is the largest report of patients with hepatopulmonary and portopulmonary syndromes.

Lucey MR, Brown KA, Everson GT, et al. Minimal criteria for placement of adults on the liver transplant waiting list: a report of a national conference organized by the American Society of Transplant Physicians and the American Association for the Study of Liver Diseases. *Liver Transplant Surg* 1997;3:628–37.
This is the first consensus document regarding minimal listing criteria for liver transplant candidates. These minimal listing criteria can be defined as minimal "selection" criteria since listing and selection are more or less synonymous.

Mazzaferro V, Regalio E, Doci R, et al. Liver transplantation for the treatment of small hepatocellular carcinomas in patients with cirrhosis. *N Engl J Med* 1996;334:693–9.
This study documented the excellent survival rates attainable for patients with early stage hepatocellular cancer with liver transplantation. In this paper, tumor stage criteria were proposed for which these excellent survival rates could be obtained that have served as the basis for most liver transplant centers acceptance criteria for patients with hepatocellular cancer.

McDairmid SV, Anand R, Linblad A. Development of a pediatric end-stage liver disease score to predict poor outcome awaiting liver transplantation. *Transplantation* 2002;74:173–81.
Excellent description of the development of a mortality risk model for children with chronic liver disease.

Merion RM, Schaubel DE, Dykstra DM, Freeman RB, Port FK, Wolfe RA. The survival benefit of liver transplantation. *Am J Transplant* 2005;2:307–13.
A carefully executed study comparing the risk of remaining on the waiting list with the risk of liver transplantation for patients with various MELD scores. This study clearly shows that there is no survival benefit in offering liver transplantation to patients with low MELD scores as measured by 1-year survival rates.

Pauwels A, Mostefa-Kara N, Florent C, et al. Emergency liver transplantation for acute liver failure; evaluation of London and Clichy criteria. *J Hepatol* 1993;17:124–7.
This study compares the King's College and Clichy criteria for their ability to predict outcome for patients with acute liver failure.

Wiesner RH, Edwards EB, Freeman RB, et al. Model for end stage liver disease (MELD) and allocation of donor livers. *Gastroenterology* 2003;124:91–6.
A description of how the MELD score, a model to predict mortality risk for patients with chronic liver disease, can be used to "select" which patients should receive the first organ offer for transplant.

References

1. Epstein SK, Freeman RB, Khayat A, Unterborn J, Pratt DS, Kaplan MM. Aerobic capacity is associated with 100-day outcome after hepatic transplantation. *Liver Transplant* 2004;10:418–24.

2. Lucey MR, Brown KA, Everson GT, et al. Minimal criteria for placement of adults on the liver transplant waiting list: a report of a national conference organized by the American Society of Transplant Physicians and the American Association for the Study of Liver Diseases. *Liver Transpl Surg* 1997;3:628–37.

3. Child CG II, Turcotte JG. Surgery and portal hypertension. In: Child CG III, ed. *The Liver and Portal Hypertension.* Philadelphia, PA: WB Saunders, 1964:50–8.

4. Malinchoc M, Kamath PS, Gordon FD, Peine CJ, Rank J, terBorg PL. A model to predict poor survival in patients undergoing transjugular intrahepatic portosystemic shunts. *Hepatology* 2000;31:864–71.

5. Kamath PS, Wiesner RH, Malinchoc M, et al. A model to predict survival in patients with end-stage liver disease. *Hepatology* 2001;33:464–70.

6. Wiesner RH, McDiarmid SV, Kamath PS, et al. MELD and PELD: application of survival models to liver allocation. *Liver Transplant* 2001;7:567–80.

7. Wiesner RH, Edwards EB, Freeman RB, et al. Model for end stage liver disease (MELD) and allocation of donor livers. *Gastroenterology* 2003;124:91–6.

8. Younissi ZM, Guyatt G, Kiwi M, Moparai N, King D, Development of a disease specific questionnaire to measure health-related quality of life in patients with chronic liver disease. *Gut* 1999;45:295–300.

9. Gralnek IM, Hays RD, Kilbourne A, et al. Development and evaluation of the liver disease quality of life instrument in persons with advanced, chronic liver disease – the LDQOL 1.0. *Am J Gastroenterol* 2000;95:3552–65.

10. Marchesini G, Bianchi G, Amodio P, et al. and the Italian Study Group for Quality of Life in Cirrhosis. Factors associated with poor health-related quality of life of patients with cirrhosis. *Gastroenterology* 2001;120:170–8.

11. Saab S, Ibrahim AB, Shpaner A, et al. MELD fails to measure quality of life in liver transplant candidates. *Liver Transplant* 2005;11:218–23.

12. Bryce CL, Angus DC, Switala J, Roberts MS, Tsevat J. Health status versus utilities of patients with end-stage liver disease. *Qual Life Res* 2004;13:773–82.

13. Bravata DM, Olkin I, Barnato AE, Keeffe EB, Owens DK. Health related quality of life after liver transplantation; a meta-analysis. *Liver Transpl Surg* 1999;5:318–31.

14. O'Carroll RE, Couston M, Cossar J, Masterton G, Hayes PC. Psychological outcome and quality of life following liver transplantation: a prospective, national, single-center study. *Liver Transplant* 2003;9:712–20.

15. Duffy JP, Kao K, Ko CY, et al. Long-term patient outcome and quality of life after liver transplantation: analysis of 20-year survivors. *Ann Surg* 2010;252:652–61.

16. Merion RM, Schaubel DE, Dykstra DM, Freeman RB, Port FK, Wolfe RA. The survival benefit of liver transplantation. *Am J Transplant* 2005;2307–13.

17. Merion RM. When is a patient too well and when is a patient too sick for a liver transplant? *Liver Transplant* 2004;10:S69–73.

18. Schaubel DE, Sima CS, Goodrich NP, Feng S, Merion RM. The survival benefit of decreased donor liver transplantation as a function of candidate disease severity and donor quality. *Am Transplant* 2008;8:419–25.

19. El-Serag HB, Giordano TP, Kramer J, Richardson P, Souchek J. Survival in hepatitis C and HIV co-infection: a cohort study of hospitalized veterans. *Clin Gastroenterol Hepatol* 2005;3:175–83.

20. Fryer J, Pellar S, Ormond D, Koffron A, Abecassis M. Mortality in candidates waiting for combined liver–intestine transplants exceeds that for other candidates waiting for liver transplants. *Liver Transplant* 2003;9:748–53.

21. Heuman DM, Abou-Assi SG, Habib A, et al. Persistent ascites and low serum sodium identify patients with cirrhosis and low MELD scores who are at high risk for early death. *Hepatology* 2004;40:802–10.

22. Biggins SW, Kim WR, Terrault NA, et al. Evidence-based incorporation of serum sodium concentration into MELD. *Gastroenterology* 2006;130:1652–60.

23. Mazzaferro V, Regalio E, Doci R, et al. Liver transplantation for the treatment of small hepatocellular carcinomas in patients with cirrhosis. *N Engl J Med* 1996;334:693–9.

24. Hemming AW, Cattral MS, Reed AI, et al. Liver transplantation for hepatocellular carcinoma. *Ann Surg* 2001;233:652–9.

25. Figueras J, Jaurrieta E, Valls C, et al. Resection or transplantation for hepatocellular carcinoma in cirrhotic patients: outcomes based on indicated treatment strategy. *J Am Coll Surg* 2000;190:580–7.

26. Yao FY, Ferrell L, Bass NM, et al. Liver transplantation for hepatocellular carcinoma: expansion of the tumor size limits does not adversely impact survival. *Hepatology* 2001;33:1394–403.

27. Mazzaferro V, Llovet JM, Miceli R, et al, and the Metroticket Investigator Study Group. Predicting survival after liver transplantation in patients with hepatocellular carcinoma beyond the Milan criteria: a retrospective, exploratory analysis. *Lancet Oncol* 2009;10:35–4.

28. Yao FY, Bass NM, Nikolai B, et al. Liver transplantation for hepatocellular carcinoma: analysis of survival according to the intention-to-treat principle and dropout from the waiting list. *Liver Transplant* 2002;8:873–83.

29. Yao, FY, Kaplan RK, Hirose R, et al. Excellent outcome following down-staging of hepatocellular carcinoma prior to liver transplantation: an intention to treat analysis. *Hepatology* 2008;48:819–27.

30. Burrel M, Llovet JM, Ayuso C, et al. MRI angiographically is superior to helical CT for detection of HCC prior to liver transplantation: an explant correlation. *Hepatology* 2003;38:1034–42.

31. Kim SH, Kim SH, Lee J, et al. Gadoxetic acid-enhanced MRI versus triple phase MDCT for the pre-operative detection for of hepatocellular cancer. *Am J Roentgenol* 2009;192:1675–81.

32. Fung KT, Li FT, Raimondo MvL, et al. Systematic review of radiological imaging for hepatocellular carcinoma in cirrhotic patients. *Br J Radiol* 2004;77:633–40.

33. Durand F, Regimbeau JM, Belghiti J, et al. Assessment of the benefits and risks of percutaneous biopsy before surgical resection of hepatocellular carcinoma. *J Hepatol* 2001;35:254–8.

34. Torzilli G, Minagawa M, Takayama T, et al. Accurate preoperative evaluation of liver mass lesions without fine-needle biopsy. *Hepatology* 1999;30:889–93.

35. Bruix J, Llovet JM. Prognostic prediction and treatment strategy in hepatocellular carcinoma. *Hepatology* 2002;315:519–24.

36. Iizuka N, Oka M, Yamada-Okabe H, et al. Oligonucleotide microarray for prediction of early intrahepatic recurrence of hepatocellular carcinoma after curative resection. *Lancet* 2003;361(9361):923–9.

37. Villanueva A, Hoshida Y, Toffanin S, et al. New strategies in hepatocellular carcinoma: genomic prognostic markers. *Clin Cancer Res* 2010;16:4688–94.

38. Schenk P, Schoninger-Hekele M, Fuhrmann V, Maadl C, Silberhumer G, Muller C. Prognostic significance of the hepatopulmonary syndrome in patients with cirrhosis. *Gastroenterology* 2003;125:1042–52.

39. Krowka MJ, Wiseman GA, Burnett OL, et al. Heptapulmonary syndrome: a prospective study of relationships between severity of liver disease, PaO$_2$, response to 100% oxygen, and brain uptake after (99m)Tc MAA lung scanning. *Chest* 2000;118:615–24.

40. Krowka MJ, Mandel MS, Ramsay MA, et al. Heptopulmonary syndrome and portopulmonary hypertension: a report from a multicenter liver transplant database. *Liver Transplant* 2004;10:174–82.

41. Fallon MB, Krowka MJ, Brown RS, et al. and Pulmonary Vascular Complications of Liver Disease Study Group. Impact of hepatopul-

monary syndrome on quality of life and survival in liver transplant candidates. *Gastroenterology* 2008;135:1168–75.

42. Rodriguez-Roisin R, Krowka MJ, Herve P, et al. on behalf of the ERS Task Force Pulmonary-Hepatic Vascular Disorders Scientific Committee ERS Task Force PHD Scientific Committee. Pulmonaryhepatic vascular disorders (PHD). *Eur Respir J* 2004;24:861–80.

43. Krowka MJ, Plevak DJ, Findlay JY, Rosen CB, Wiesner RH, Krom RA. Pulmonary hemodynamics and peri-operative cardiopulmonary-related mortality in patients undergoing liver transplantation. *Liver Transplant* 2000;6:443–50.

44. Gough MS, White RJ. Sildenafil therapy is associated with improved hemodynamics in liver transplantation candidates with pulmonary arterial hypertension. *Liver Transplant* 2009;15:30–6.

45. Starkel P, Vera A, Gunson B, Mutimer D. Outcome of liver transplantation for patients with portopulmonary hypertension. *Liver Transplant* 2002:8:382–8.

46. Kuo P, Johnson L, Plotkin J, Howell C, Bartlett S, Rubin L. Continuous intravenous infusion of epoprostenol for the treatment of portopulmonary hypertension. *Transplantation* 1997;63:604–6.

47. Plotkin J, Kuo P, Rubin L, et al. Successful use of chronic epoprostenol as a bridge to liver transplantation in severe portopulmonary hypertension. *Transplantation* 1998;65:457–9.

48. Swanson KL, Wiesner RH, Nyberg SL, Rosen CB, Krowka MJ. Survival in portopulmonary hypertension: Mayo Clinic experience categorized by treatment subgroups. *Am J Transplant* 2008;8: 2445–53.

49. Anderson R. Familial amyloidosis with polyneuropathy: a clinical study based on patients living in northern Sweden. *Acta Med Scand* 1976;198(Suppl 590):S1–76.

50. Pomfret EA, Lewis WD, Jenkins RL, et al. Effect of orthotopic liver transplantation on progression of familial amyloidotic polyneuropathy. *Transplantation* 1998;65:918–25.

51. Suhr OB, Herlenius G, Friman S, Ericzon BG. Liver transplantation for hereditary transthyretin amyloidosis. *Liver Transplant* 2000;6: 263–76.

52. Jamieson NV, Watts RW, Evans DB, Williams R, Calne RY. Liver and kidney transplantation in the treatment of primary hyperoxaluria. *Transplant Proc* 1991:23;1557–8.

53. Nolkemper D, Kemper MJ, Burdelski M, et al. Long-term results of pre-emptive liver transplantation in primary hyperoxaluria type 1. *Pediatr Transplant* 2000;4:177–81.

54. Leumann E, Hoppe B. Pre-emptive liver transplantation in primary hyperoxaluria type 1: a controversial issue. *Pediatr Transplant* 2004;4:161–4.

55. Leonard JV, McKiernan PJ. The role of liver transplantation in urea cycle disorders. *Mol Genet Metab* 2004;81(Suppl 1):S74–8,

56. Ensenauer R, Tuchman M, El-Youssef M, et al. Management and outcome of neonatal-onset ornithine transcarbamylase deficiency following liver transplantation at 60 days of life. *Mol Genet Metab* 2005;84(4):363–6.

57. Nyhan WL, Khanna A, Barshop BA, et al. Pyruvate carboxylase deficiency – insights from liver transplantation. *Mol Genet Metab* 2002; 77(1–2):143–9.

58. Bodner-Leidecker A, Wendel U, Saudubray JM, et al. Branched-chain L amino acid metabolism in classcal maple syrup urine disease after orthotopic liver transplantation. *J Inherited Metab Dis* 2000;23: 805.

59. Mohan N, Mekiernan P, Preece MA, et al. Indications and outcome of liver transplantation in tyrosinemia type 1. *Eur J Pediatr* 1999;158:159.

60. Maes M, Sokal E, Otte JB. Growth factors in children with end-stage liver disease before and after liver transplantation: a review. *Pediatr Transplant* 1997;1(2):171.

61. Superina RA, Zangari A, Acal L, et al. Growth in children following liver transplantation. *Pediatr Transplant* 1998;2(1):70.

62. Tornqvist J, Van Broeck N, Finkenauer C, et al. Long-term psychosocial adjustment following pediatric liver transplantation. *Pediatr Transplant* 1999;3(2):115.

63. Kennard BD, Stewart SM, Phelan-McAuliffe D, et al. Academic outcome in long-term survivors of pediatric liver transplantation. *J Dev Behav Pediatr* 1999;20(1):17.

64. Krull K, Fuchs C, Yurk H, et al. Neurocognitive outcome in pediatric liver transplant recipients. *Pediatr Transplant* 2003;7(2):111.

65. Schulz KH, Wein C, Boeck A, Rogiers X, Burdelski M. Cognitive performance of children who have undergone liver transplantation. *Transplantation* 2003;75:1236–40.

66. Weissberg-Benchell J, Zielinski TE, Rodgers S, et al. Pediatric health-related quality of life: feasibility, reliability and validity of the PedsQL transplant module. *Am J Transplant* 2010;10(7):1677–85.

67. McDairmid SV, Anand R, Linblad A. Development of a pediatric end-stage liver disease score to predict poor outcome awaiting liver transplantation. *Transplantation* 2002;74:173–81.

68. Dhawan A, Taylor RM, Cheeseman P, De Silva P, Katsiyiannakis L, Mieli-Vergani G. Wilson's disease in children: 37-year experience and revised King's score for liver transplantation. *Liver Transplant* 2005;11:441–8.

69. O'Grady JG, Alexander GJ, Hayllar KM, Williams R. Early indicators of prognosis in fulminant hepatic failure. *Gastroenterology* 1989;97:439–45.

70. Bernuau J, Samuel D, Durand F. Criteria for emergency liver transplantation in patients with acute viral hepatitis and factor V below 50% of normal. *Hepatology* 1991;14:49A.

71. Bernal W, Donaldson N, Wyncoll D, et al. Blood lactate as an early predictor of outcome in paracetamol induced acute liver failure: a cohort study. *Lancet* 2002;359:558–63.

72. Pauwels A, Mostefa-Kara N, Florent C, et al. Emergency liver transplantation for acute liver failure; evaluation of London and Clichy criteria. *J Hepatol* 1993;17:124–7.

73. Anand AC, Nightingale P, Neuberger J. Early indicators of prognosis in fulminant hepatic failure: an assessment of the King's criteria. *J Hepatol* 1997;26:62–8.

74. Yaterno SET, Trentadue JJ, Ruf AE, et al. The model for end stage liver disease (MELD): a useful tool to assess prognosis in fulminant liver failure. *Liver Transplant* 2004;10;C36.

75. Kremers WK, van Ijperen M, Kim RW, et al. MELD score as a predictor of pre and post transplant survival in OPTN/UNOS status 1 patients. *Hepatology* 2004;39:764–9.

76. Schiodt FV, Ott P, Christensen E, Bondesen S. The value of plasma acetaminophen half-life in antidote-treated acetaminophen overdosage. *Clin Pharmacol Ther* 2002;71(4):221–5.

77. Pereira L, Langley P, Hayllar K, et al: Coagulation factor V and VIII/V ratio as predictors outcome in paracetamol induced fulminant hepatic failure: relation to other prognostic indicators. *Gut* 1992;33:98–102.

78. Lee W, Galbraith R, Watt G, et al. Predicting survival in fulminant hepatic failure using serum Gc protein concentrations. *Hepatology* 1995;21:101–5.

79. Bernal W, Wendon J, Rela M, et al. Use and outcome of liver transplantation in acetaminophen-induced acute liver failure. *Hepatology* 1998;27:1050–5.

80. Schmidt LE, Dalhoff K. Serum phosphate is an early predictor of outcome in severe acetaminophen-induced hepatotoxicity. *Hepatology* 2002;36:659–65.

81. Bernal W, Donaldson N, Wyncoll D, et al. Blood lactate as an early predictor of outcome in paracetamol induced acute liver failure: a cohort study. *Lancet* 2002;359:558–63.

82. Bailey B, Amre DK, Gaudreault P. Fulminant hepatic failure secondary to acetaminophen poisoning: a systematic review and meta-analysis of prognostic criteria determining the need for liver transplantation. *Crit Care Med* 2003;31:299–305.

83. Taylor RM, Davern T, Munoz S, et al. Fulminant hepatitis A virus infection in the United States: incidence, prognosis, and outcomes. *Hepatology* 2006;44:1589–97.

84. Polson AJ. Assessment of prognosis in acute liver failure. *Semin Liver Dis* 2008;28(2):218–25.

85. Broelsch CE, Emond JC, Whitington PF, Thistlethwaite JR, Baker AL, Lichtor JL. Application of reduced-size liver transplants as split grafts, auxiliary orthotopic grafts, and living related segmental transplants. *Ann Surg* 1990;212(3):368–75.

86. Tanaka K, Uemoto S, Tokunaga Y, et al. Surgical techniques and innovations in living related liver transplantation. *Ann Surg* 1993;217:82–91.

87. Singer PA, Siegler M, Whitington PF, et al. Ethics of liver transplantation with living donors. *N Engl J Med* 1989;321(9):620–2.

88. Roberts JP. Role of adult living liver donation in patients with hepatocelluar cancer. *Liver Transplant* 2003;9:S60–3.

89. Cheng S, Pratt D, Freeman RB, Kaplan MM, Wong J. Living-related versus orthotopic liver transplant for small hepatocellular carcinoma: a decision analysis. *Transplantation* 2001;72:861–8.

90. Freeman RB. The impact of the model for end stage liver disease on recipient selection for adult living liver donation. *Liver Transplant* 2003;9(Suppl 2):54–9.

91. Sugarawa Y, Makuuchi M, Kaneko J, Kokudo N. MELD score for selection of patients to receive left liver graft. *Transplantation* 2003;75:573–4.

92. Shiffman ML, Stravitz RT, Contos MJ, et al. Histologic recurrence of chronic hepatitis C virus in patients after living donor and deceased donor liver transplantation. *Liver Transplant* 2004;10:1248–55.

93. Bozorgzadeh A, Jain A, Ryan C, et al. Impact of hepatitis C viral infection in primary cadaveric liver allograft versus primary living-donor allograft in 100 consecutive liver transplant recipients receiving tacrolimus. *Transplantation* 2004;77:1066–70.

94. Nishizaki T, Hiroshige S, Ikegami T, et al. Living-donor liver transplantation for fulminant hepatic failure in adult patients with a left-lobe graft. *Surgery* 2002;131(1 Suppl):S182–9.

95. Adcock L, Macleod C, Dubay D, et al. Adult living liver donors have excellent long-term medical outcomes: the University of Toronto Liver Transplant Experience. *Am J Transplant* 2010;10:364–71.

96. From the OPTN website http://www.optn.org/latestData/rptData.asp, accessed November 30, 2010.

CHAPTER 43

Immunosuppression: The Global Picture

Russell H. Wiesner

Transplant Center, Mayo Clinic, Rochester, MN, USA

Key concepts

- Advances in immunosuppression in recent years have led to impressive patient and graft survival rates and reduced rejection rates in liver transplantation.
- The administration of immunosuppression remains an art in that there are few markers of overall immunosuppression, tolerance, or measurements of alloreactivity.
- There is a poor correlation between rejection and degree of abnormalities of liver function tests and immunosuppressive levels.
- Graft loss related to rejection occurs in less than 7% of patients undergoing liver transplantation.
- The major challenge with immunosuppression has been long-term complications, particularly renal dysfunction, hypertension, hyperlipidemia, diabetes mellitus, and de novo cancers.

- Data suggest that liver transplant patients are overimmunosuppressed and that reducing the side effects of immunosuppression today is a major goal.
- The goals of immunosuppression are to control alloreactivity rather than eliminating it and thus minimize toxicity using larger number of agents with smaller doses.
- Individualization of immunosuppressive therapy, when possible, should be utilized for patients undergoing transplant for alcoholic liver disease, hepatitis C, autoimmune liver disease, and hepatocellular cancer.
- The ultimate goal is the development of therapeutic strategies to promote tolerance or a state in which the allograft is specifically accepted without the need for chronic immunosuppression.

New developments in immunosuppression, along with advances in surgical and anesthetic techniques, have led to continued improvements in patient and graft survival following liver transplantation. Recent data indicate that patient survival at 1 and 5 years following liver transplantation approaches 90% and 75%, respectively [1]. Today, over 40,000 patients in the United States are living with a hepatic allograft, and survival of greater than 30 years following the procedure has been reported [2]. Thus liver transplant has become overwhelmingly the best therapeutic option for patients suffering from end-stage liver disease.

Historical perspective

After multiple unsuccessful attempts, the first successful liver transplantation was performed by Dr Thomas Starzl in 1967 on an 18-month-old child with hepatoblastoma [2]. Immunosuppression was achieved using corticosteroids, azathioprine, and antilymphocyte globulin, which enabled the child to survive over 1 year without the development of major hepatic allograft dysfunction related to rejection. However, it was not until 1979 with the discovery of cyclosporine and its potent immunosuppressive properties that markedly diminished the incidence and severity of hepatic allograft rejection. Liver transplantation now truly became a realistic therapeutic option. Using cyclosporine-based immunosuppression Dr Starzl was able to obtain a 1-year patient survival of over 60%, which was a major achievement at the time [3]. Indeed, cyclosporine-based immunosuppression rapidly became the standard of care for all solid organ transplants, and paved the way for the recommendation by the National Institutes of Health (NIH) in 1983 to make liver transplantation an acceptable and financially reimbursable therapeutic option for patients with end-stage liver disease [4].

The next advancement in immunosuppressive therapy came nearly a decade later in the discovery and development of a drug named FK506. This drug also had potent immunosuppressive properties and was demonstrated in a controlled clinical trial to be associated with a lower incidence of acute rejection and a decreased incidence of

Schiff's Diseases of the Liver, Eleventh Edition. Edited by Eugene R. Schiff, Willis C. Maddrey and Michael F. Sorrell.
© 2012 John Wiley & Sons, Ltd. Published 2012 by John Wiley & Sons, Ltd.

steroid resistant rejection [5,6]. Over the ensuing years, FK506 (also known as tacrolimus) became the calcineurin inhibitor of choice and is presently being used in over 85% of patients undergoing liver transplantation in the United States [7].

Immunosuppression was further refined by the development and introduction of other immunosuppressive agents that could be used in combination with corticosteroids and calcineurin inhibitors. Some of these agents included mycophenolate acid mofetil, rapamycin, and a number of cytokine antibodies antagonistic to specific targets in the antigen recognition pathway such as OKT3 and antithymocyte globulin [8]. As immunosuppressive therapy further evolved, it became clear that combination therapy with lower doses of each agent, which were able to control rejection, and reduce and prevent the development of immunosuppression related side effects, became the standard of care. Even today, the minimization of immunosuppressive therapy to control alloreactivity and to lower the severity of related side effects remains a persistent challenge.

Immunologic mechanisms of rejection response (three-signal pathway of lymphocyte activation)

Hepatic allograft rejection relates to the recipient immunologic response precipitated by donor recipient mismatches of a major histocompatibility complex (MHC), which leads to what is referred to as an alloimmune response. In the hepatic allograft and its surrounding tissue, dendritic cells or antigen-presenting cells of donor and recipient origin become activated by their interaction with foreign antigens and subsequently migrate to the T-cell areas of secondary lymphoid organs [9].

There, the antigen-bearing cells engage alloantigen, reactive naïve T cells and memory cells and trigger lymphocyte activation transduced through the T-cell receptor (CD3 complex) which is often referred to as *signal 1* [10,11]. Dendritic cells provide co-stimulation or *signal 2* when CD80 and CD86 markers on the surface of dendritic cells engage CD28 receptors on T lymphocytes [12, 13]. Signals 1 and 2 activate signal transduction pathways including: (i) the calcium–calcineurine pathway; and (ii) the Ras–mitogen-activated protein kinase (MAPK) pathway and the nuclear factor κB (NF-κB) pathway. These pathways activate transcription factors that trigger the expression of many new molecules including interleukin 2 (IL2) and other cytokines that are able to activate the target of rapamycin pathway providing *signal 3* or the trigger for cell proliferation [12]. Lymphocyte proliferation also requires nucleotide synthesis. This proliferation

of T cells leads to the differentiation and production of large numbers of effecter T and B cells. Effecter cells that emerge from lymphoid organs infiltrate the hepatic allograft and orchestrate an inflammatory response [13]. In T-lymphocyte-mediated rejection, the graft is infiltrated by effector T cells, activated macrophages, secretory B cells, and plasma cells, which leads ultimately to organ damage (Fig. 43.1). T-cell-mediated damage results from the secretion of numerous factors such as tumor necrosis factor α (TNF-α) and TNF-β, fas ligand expression, as well as the secretion of cytotoxins such as perforin and granzyme F. The diagnostic pathology of lymphocyte-mediated rejection is mononuclear cells invading the liver that target small arteries, veins, and bile duct epithelium [13–15].

In addition, antibodies against donor antigens are also produced through these mechanisms. However, antibody-mediated rejection in liver transplantation appears to be a rare phenomenon and rarely thought to be of clinical significance.

Classification of immunosuppressive drugs

Immunosuppressive drugs can be broadly classified into two categories: (i) pharmacologic or small molecule drugs (Table 43.1); and (ii) biologic agents consisting of polyclonal and monoclonal antilymphocyte antibodies (Table 43.2). The latter can be further classified as lymphocyte depleting and nonlymphocyte depleting.

Most small molecule immunosuppressive agents are derived from microbial products and target proteins that are important in the alloimmune response (Fig. 43.2) These agents include corticosteroids, cyclosporine, tacrolimus, mycophenolate acid, azathioprine, and rapamycin (Table 43.1).

Biologic immunosuppressive drugs include lymphocyte-depleting immunosuppressive agents, which are antibodies that destroy T cells, B cells, or both (Fig. 43.2). T-cell depletion is often accompanied by the release of cytokines, which produce severe systemic symptoms, especially after the first dose (Table 43.2). The use of depleting antibodies reduces the risk of early rejection but increases the risk of infection with cytomegalovirus (CMV), fungi, and the development of post-transplantation lymphoproliferative disease. Recovery from immune-depleting lymphocyte antibodies takes months to years and may never be complete in older individuals. The depletion of antibody-producing cells is better tolerated than T-cell depletion, because it is not usually accompanied by cytokine release, and immunoglobulin levels are usually maintained. However, depletion of antibody-producing cells is incomplete

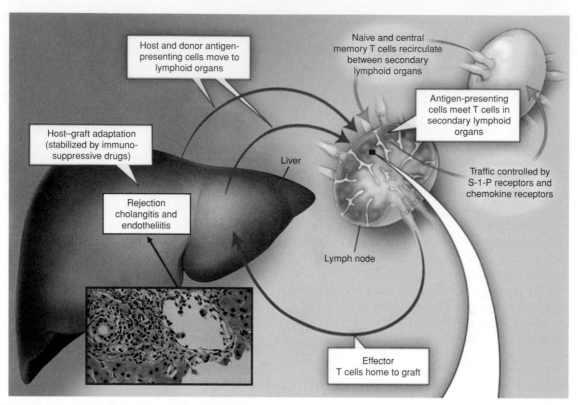

Figure 43.1 Antigen-presenting cells and the activation of T cells leading to hepatic allograft rejection.

because many plasma cells are resistant to available antibodies that target B cells such as anti-CD20 antibody (rituximab).

Nonlymphocyte-depleting immunosuppressive agents are monoclonal antibodies or fusion proteins that reduce responsiveness without compromising lymphocyte populations (Table 43.2). These drugs have low nonimmune toxicity because they target proteins that are expressed only on immune cells and trigger little release of cytokines. They typically target mechanisms such as IL2 receptors, which explains their limited efficacy and the absence of immune deficiency complications. They are generally used in combination with corticosteroids, calcineurin inhibitors, and antimetabolites.

Table 43.1 Classification of pharmacologic (small molecule) immunosuppressive agents.

Agent	Effects
Corticosteroids	Inhibits cytokine transcription by antigen-presenting cell
Calcineurin inhibitors:	Inhibits signal 2 transduction
Cyclosporine	
Tacrolimus	
Azathioprine	Inhibits purine and DNA synthesis
	Prevents T-cell proliferation
Mycophenolic acid:	Inhibits purine and DNA synthesis
Cellcept	Prevents T-cell proliferation
Myfortic	
Rapamycin (mTOR inhibitors):	Inhibits signal 3 transduction
Sirolimus	Prevents T-cell proliferation
Everolimus	

mTOR, mammalian target of rapamycin.

Table 43.2 Classification of biologic immunosuppressive agents.

Agent	Effects
T-cell depleting agents	
Anti-CD3 (monoclonal): OKT3	Interferes with signal 1
Antithymocyte globulin: Horse and rabbit ATG, ALG	Interferes with signals 1, 2, and 3
Anti-CD52 monoclonal: Campath 1-H (alemtuzumab)	Depletion of thymocytes, T cells, B cells, and monocytes
Non-T-cell depleting	
Anti-IL2 receptor: Basiliximab Daclilumumab	Inhibits T-cell proliferation Inhibits signal 3
Belatacept Daclizumab	Inhibits signal 2 Competes with CD28 for CD80/86 binding

Small molecule immunosuppressive agents

Corticosteroids

Corticosteroids were one of the earliest agents used for immunosuppression, first developed in the late 1940s and introduced into immunosuppressive regimens in the late 1950s [16]. They have been applied in a variety of ways in liver transplantation. These include: (i) as induction immunosuppression by way of bolus corticosteroid therapy at the time of organ implantation; (ii) as maintenance therapy to prevent rejection; and (iii) in the treatment of established acute cellular rejection. Although their chronic, long-term use is somewhat disputed in recent years, they continue to be widely used both in induction and during short-term maintenance therapy in liver transplant recipients.

The most common agents used in liver transplantation include prednisone, prednisolone, and methylprednisolone. These corticosteroid agents possess a

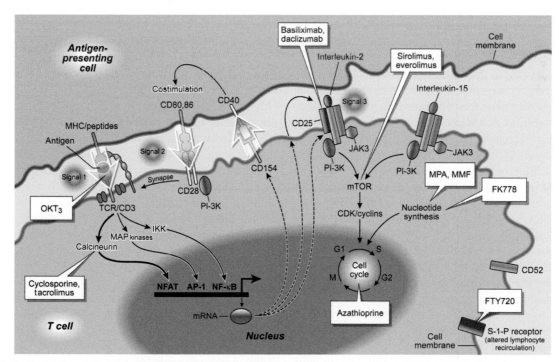

Figure 43.2 T-cell activation via three signals and site of activation of immunosuppressive drugs. AP-1, activator protein 1; JAK3, janus kinase 3; MAP, mitogen-activated protein; MHC, major histocompatibility complex; MMF, mycophenolate mofetil; MPA, mycophenolic acid; NF-κB, nuclear factor κB; TCR, T-cell receptor.

predominantly anti-inflammatory immunosuppressive potency with relatively low mineralocorticoid activity. Prednisone is rapidly absorbed from the gastrointestinal tract; however, it needs to be metabolized by the liver to prednisolone for biologic activity. Following absorption, corticosteroids are primarily metabolized into inactive compounds by the liver and excreted in the urine.

Corticosteroids exert their effects through their actions on a wide variety of white cells including lymphocytes, granulocytes, macrophages, and monocytes. Glucocorticoids circulate either in a free form or in association with cortisol-binding globulin in the blood. The free form of the steroid readily diffuses through the plasma membrane of lymphocytes and binds with high affinity to intracellular glucocorticoid receptors. This ligand–receptor complex, following activation, modulates transcription both positively and negatively, in the nucleus of specific genes and coding factors critical in the generation and maintenance of the immune and inflammatory responses. In addition to modulating transcription, glucocorticoids can also influence later cellular events including RNA translation and protein synthesis and secretion [17]. Leukocytes, through their mechanism of localization and activation, generate numerous products that play a key role in cellular rejection, and glucocorticoids therefore modulate this function. On lymphocytes, the major mechanism of action of corticosteroids seems to be a negative regulation of cytokine gene expression. Regulation of cytokine gene production occurs through the inhibitory action of glucocorticoid on gene transcription through the inhibition of activator protein 1 (AP-1) and NF-κB. Glucocorticoids also affect other cells such as macrophages, neutrophils, eosinophils, basophils, mast cells, and endothelial cells. Glucocorticoids antagonize macrophage differentiation and inhibit many of their functions that promote inflammation. Glucocorticoids inhibit neutrophil adhesions to endothelial cells, thereby decreasing their extravasation to the site of inflammation. This process may partly explain the neutrophilia that is seen with glucocorticoid therapy. Additionally, glucocorticoids downregulate endothelial cell function including expression of class II MHC antigen, expression of adhesion molecule 1 (ELAM-1), and the intracellular cell adhesion molecule 1 (ICAM-1) formation of IL1 and arachidonic acid metabolites, thereby inhibiting the expression of cyclooxygenase type 2.

Corticosteroids are administered at various stages of liver transplantation. In general, high-dose methylprednisolone is usually administered intravenously around the time the liver is implanted and is continued for several days postoperatively. Induction doses range from 300 to 1,000 mg intravenously per day. Initially thought to be essential, trials have now demonstrated that corticosteroid-free regimens do not necessarily lead to increased rejection. These trials have used other induction agents such as antithymocyte globulin or IL2 receptor antibodies [18–20].

For maintenance therapy, steroids are rapidly tapered from the time of surgery to a daily maintenance dose of 5–10 mg per day. Many centers now taper and stop prednisone after 3–6 months. Indeed 50% of liver recipients are off corticosteroids 1 year after transplantation [7]. Prednisone cessation does not seem to adversely affect the hepatic graft in most instances and may be beneficial in ameliorating some of the side effects of long-term prednisone use such as osteoporosis, diabetes, weight gain, hypertension, cataracts, hyperuricemia, and cosmetic problems.

In patients who have undergone transplantation for autoimmune liver diseases such as primary biliary cirrhosis, primary sclerosing cholangitis, or autoimmune hepatitis, the continuation of low-dose prednisone indefinitely may be prudent [21]. In addition, patients who have ulcerative colitis have been reported to have a major flare following discontinuation of prednisone.

Corticosteroids have been used in the context of treating acute cellular rejection [22]. In this context, intravenous methylprednisolone is given in a dose of 1,000 mg on alternate days for a total of three doses. Some centers use what is called a recycle, which involves giving high oral doses of prednisone (i.e., 60 mg) and tapering down to 10 mg over a 7-day period. Excellent responses to these regimens in patients with acute rejection have been reported in that 75–80% of patients have histologic resolution following high-dose IV bolus corticosteroid therapy [23].

Corticosteroid therapy is not without side effects. Short-term corticosteroid use such as IV boluses to treat acute cellular rejection may cause transient hyperglycemia, and infections can be unmasked or exacerbated. In patients with hepatitis C, the use of bolus high-dose IV corticosteroids to treat acute rejection has been associated with high hepatitis C RNA levels and early and more severe recurrence of hepatitis C [24,25]. Long-term corticosteroid therapy is associated with a number of side effects, some of which may be reversed by steroid withdrawal (Box 43.1). Cosmetic side effects such as acne and hirsutism may adversely affect compliance, especially in the younger population undergoing transplantation.

Azathioprine

Azathioprine, which is derived from 6-mercaptopurine (6-MP), was the first immunosuppressive agent to achieve widespread use in organ transplantation. The developers of azathioprine, Gertrude Elion and George Hitchings, were acknowledged by a share of the 1988 Nobel Prize. Azathioprine is thought to act by releasing 6-MP, which interferes with DNA synthesis. Azathioprine is

Box 43.1 Side effects of corticosteroids.
- Impaired wound healing
- Hypertension
- Weight gain
- Hyperglycemia
- Hyperlipidemia
- Osteoporosis
- Fluid retention
- Hirsutism
- Acne
- Myopathy
- Cataracts
- Infection

absorbed readily from the gastrointestinal tract, and peak plasma concentrations are achieved 1–3 hours after oral administration. Azathioprine is rapidly cleared from the circulation, but approximately 30% is bound to serum proteins. The half-life of azathioprine is approximately 3 hours with normal kidney function and up to 50 hours in patients with anuria. The active metabolite acts as a purine analog, which is incorporated into cellular DNA and inhibits purine nucleotide synthesis and metabolism. The resultant alteration in RNA synthesis and function prevents mitosis and proliferation. 6-MP undergoes two major inactivation routes. The main metabolite route is thiomethylation, which is catalyzed by the enzyme thiopurine S-methyltransferase (TPMT) to form the inactive metabolite methyl-6-MP. TPMT activity is controlled by a genetic polymorphism. For Caucasians and African-Americans, approximately 10% of the populations inherit one nonfunctional TPMT allele (heterozygous) conferring intermediate TPMT activity. In addition, 0.3% of the population inherit two TPMT nonfunctional alleles (homozygous) for low or absent TPMT activity. Patients with intermediate TPMT activity may be at increased risk of myelotoxicity if receiving conventional doses of azathioprine. Patients with low or absent TPMT activity are at increased risk of developing severe, life-threatening myelotoxicity if receiving conventional doses of azathioprine. TPMT genotyping or phenotyping can help identify patients who are at increased risk for developing azathioprine toxicity and is recommended particularly in the transplant population. One note of caution: accurate phenotyping may give unreliable results in patients who have received recent blood transfusions.

Azathioprine was first used in combination with corticosteroids for renal transplantation and was found to be highly efficacious. It is currently used in combination with a calcineurin inhibitor and corticosteroids. Daily doses vary between 1 and 2 mg/kg and are generally used in combination therapy. More recently, azathioprine has been replaced by mycophenolic acid in a large num-

ber of liver transplant recipients, as reported by the United Network for Organ Sharing (UNOS) registry from their analysis of the UNOS database [7]. Use of azathioprine at the time of discharge from the hospital is noted in only 1% of patients compared with mycophenolic acid, which is used in 65% of patients undergoing liver transplant [7].

Azathioprine is associated with well-established side effects, which include myelosuppression, reversible hepatotoxicity, alopecia, and gastrointestinal side effects such as nausea, dyspepsia, and acute pancreatitis. Other short-term side effects include the development of fever, skin rash, arthralgias, myalgias, and acute hypersensitivity reactions. During long-term therapy, an increased incidence of malignancy of the skin such as squamous cell carcinoma and non-Hodgkin's lymphoma has been reported. Xanthine oxidase, a major enzyme in the metabolism of azathioprine metabolites, is blocked by allopurinol and, hence, when used concurrently with allopurinol, the dose of azathioprine must be decreased by 25–30%. Other drugs that interact with azathioprine and worsen its bone marrow suppression include methotrexate and angiotensin-converting enzyme inhibitors.

Cyclosporine

Cyclosporine is a highly aliphatic, cyclic, undecapeptide molecule. It was originally isolated from the soil fungus of *Cylindrocarpon lucidum*. Since its discovery, cyclosporine has remained the cornerstone of immunosuppression, not only for liver transplantation but also for kidney, heart, and other solid organ transplantations. Cyclosporine came into widespread clinical use in the early 1980s, and in liver transplantation Starzl et al. reported the first use of cyclosporine and prednisone in 1981, achieving an 83% patient survival after 8–14.5 months of follow-up [3].

Cyclosporine enters cells and lymphocytes through diffusion and at high concentrations by active transport through the low-density lipoprotein cholesterol receptor. In the cell, cyclosporine binds to a number of carrier proteins, including cyclophilin, which are important for protein folding. The cyclosporine–cyclophilin complex binds to calcium-activated calcineurin, a serine/threonine phosphatase important in the lymphocyte activation cascade, preventing the dephosphorylation of the transcription factor NFAT (nuclear factor of activated T cells) [26,27]. This prevents NFAT from engaging to specific DNA-binding sites in the promoter region of several T-cell growth factors and the synthesis cytokines such as IL2, interferon-γ, TNF-α, and co-stimulation molecules such as CD40. This lack of engagement downregulates the expression of these various cytokines essential for the alloimmune response. Therefore, cyclosporine enables the activated T cells to potentially return to their quiescent state inhibiting early antigen recognition, reducing clonal expansion, and inhibiting the synthesis of multiple cytokines necessary for the alloimmune response. Cyclosporine is not cytotoxic and does not inhibit myeloid or erythroid cell lines.

An earlier formulation of cyclosporine (Sandimmune®) was notable for very low absorption and bioavailability. However, with the recent introduction of a microemulsion nonaqueous form (Neoral®), absorption and bioavailability had become more predictable [28]. Cyclosporine in generic forms has become widely available, and in switching to generic forms of the drug, blood levels should be checked.

Cyclosporine is absorbed primarily in the proximal jejunum and achieves peak blood levels in 2–4 hours. It is widely distributed with the highest concentrations found in adipose, kidney, adrenal, pancreatic, and liver tissues. Cyclosporine is metabolized primarily through the liver, occurring through the cytochrome P450 system, and is excreted predominantly through the bile. Therefore, with liver failure, or in the case of split liver transplantation, the propensity to develop toxic cyclosporine concentrations should be recognized. Cyclosporine has an average half-life of approximately 27 hours (range, 10–40 hours) [28]. Various drugs that stimulate or inhibit the hepatic cytochrome P450 enzyme system may increase or decrease blood levels and can result in under-immunosuppression or toxicity (Box 43.2). These agents include calcium channel blockers, antifungal agents, macrolide antibiotics, prokinetic agents such as cisapride and metoclopramide, and a variety of miscellaneous agents such as amiodarone, cimetidine, omeprazole, and protease inhibitors. Of note, the new protease antihepatitis C drugs including telaprevir and boceprevir are potent cytochrome P450 inhibitors, and close monitoring of calcineurin inhibitors will be needed when these drugs become available and utilized in liver transplant patients.

Dosing of cyclosporine is generally regulated by examining a 12-hour trough level, as this is convenient for patients. However, it has been shown that trough concentrations do not actually reflect the area under the curve for cyclosporine exposures in all individuals. More recently, peak cyclosporine levels at 2 hours after oral administration is thought to be a better measure of the area under the curve and may be more useful in controlling toxicity and enhancing efficacy. However, this causes a tremendous inconvenience to the patient.

Target trough and peak levels vary with respect to time after liver transplantation. Within the immediate posttransplant period, 12-hour trough levels between 250 and 300 ng/mL are desirable. With time, however, 12-hour trough levels between 100 and 125 ng/mL are sufficient to prevent rejection and minimize toxicities.

Cyclosporine is commonly used in conjunction with prednisone and mycophenolic acid. With time, prednisone and other agents may be withdrawn leaving cyclosporine as the sole immunosuppressive agent.

The main side effects of cyclosporine include nephrotoxicity and hypertension (Box 43.3). With long-term follow-up of liver transplant recipients, it is becoming apparent that up to 20% of patients on calcineurin inhibitors will end up with chronic renal insufficiency requiring dialysis and/or a renal transplantation after 10 years of follow-up [29,30]. The nephrotoxicity of cyclosporine was thought to result from vasoconstrictor effects on renal blood vessels. Although early toxicity resulting in renal dysfunction may be reversible, late stages of cyclosporine nephrotoxicity resulting in

---

Box 43.2 Drug interactions with cyclosporine, tacrolimus, and sirolimus.

Increased levels (of cyclosporine, tacrolimus)

- Azithromycin
- Boceprevir
- Diltiazem
- Doxycycline
- Erythromycin
- Fluconazole
- Grapefruit juice
- HAART regimen
- Itraconazole
- Metoclopramide
- Protease inhibitors
- Telaprevir

Decreased levels (of cyclosporine, tacrolimus)

- Barbiturates
- Carbamazepine
- Phenytoin
- Rifampin

HAART, highly active antiretroviral therapy.

Box 43.3 Side effects of calcineurin inhibitors.

- Nephrotoxicity
- Hypertension
- Neurologic (tremors)
- Seizures, headaches
- Hyperkalemia
- Hyperlipidemia
- Diabetes
- Hirsutism, hypertrichosis[a]
- *Gingival hyperplasia[a]

[a]Specific to cyclosporine.

advanced tubular interstitial fibrosis and scarring may be irreversible.

Other significant side effects from cyclosporine include neurologic sequelae that occur in 10–20% of patients, usually in the earlier post-transplant course. These include paresthesias, tremors, hallucinations, confusions, migraine headaches, and rarely seizures. Cyclosporine may also cause hirsutism and gingival hyperplasia, which can lead to significant cosmetic problems in younger patients undergoing liver transplantation. Cyclosporine can also induce hyperlipidemia, post-transplantation diabetes mellitus, and rarely the hemolytic uremic syndrome.

Tacrolimus

Tacrolimus (FK506) is a metabolite of a fungus, *Streptomyces tsukubaensis*, and was isolated in 1986. Tacrolimus engages another immunophilin, FK506-binding protein 12, to create a complex that inhibits calcineurin with greater molar potency than does cyclosporine. Tacrolimus has been shown to be 10–100 times more powerful than cyclosporine. The first successful use was reported by Dr Starzl in 1989 as a rescue therapy for liver grafts failing conventional therapy with cyclosporine [31]. Subsequently, tacrolimus was evaluated for routine use in liver transplantation. Multicenter trials that compared the efficacy and safety of tacrolimus with cyclosporine showed that tacrolimus was associated with significantly less rejection, in particular corticosteroid-resistant rejection [32–36]. Similar results were also demonstrated in a European multicenter trial with an additional finding that there was a lower incidence of chronic rejection and infection. However, like cyclosporine, tacrolimus was associated with significant nephrotoxicity and neurotoxicity. Furthermore, tacrolimus compared with cyclosporine was associated with less hyperlipidemia, hypertension, and cosmetic problems such as hirsutism and gingival hyperplasia. On the other hand, it has a slightly higher incidence of post-transplant-induced diabetes mellitus [37].

Tacrolimus is absorbed in the duodenum and jejunum, and, unlike cyclosporine, does not require the presence of bile for absorption. The recommended initial dose is 0.1 mg/kg per 24 hours administrated in divided dose every 12 hours. Initial blood levels after liver transplantation are maintained between 10 and 15 ng/mL whole blood trough levels. With time, 12-hour trough levels may be lowered to between 5 and 10 ng/mL to reduce side effects, particularly nephrotoxicity. Although initially used in combination with other immunosuppressant agents, most commonly corticosteroids and mycophenolic acid, tacrolimus monotherapy in the later stages of liver transplant is more widely practiced. Today, tacrolimus is the primary immuno-

suppressive agent used in the United States, with over 85% of patients dismissed after liver transplant being on a tacrolimus-based immunosuppressive regimen [7]. Like cyclosporine, tacrolimus is metabolized by the cytochrome P450 enzyme system and is subject to blood variation when administered simultaneously with drugs known to stimulate or inhibit the cytochrome P450 enzyme system (Box 43.2). In patients with hepatitis C, the reduced incidence and severity of acute rejection episodes associated with tacrolimus appears to be associated with less severe recurrence of hepatitis C compared to cyclosporine-based immunosuppressive regimens [37].

Mycophenolic acid

Both mycophenolate mofetil (MMF) and mycophenolate sodium (MPS) undergo immediate first-past metabolism in the liver into the active compound mycophenolic acid. Mycophenolic acid was first discovered in 1893; however, the immunosuppressive properties were not recognized until the 1990s. Mycophenolic acid is a noncompetitive inhibitor of inosine 5'-monophosphate dehydrogenase (IMPDH), which is the rate-limiting enzyme in the de novo synthesis of guanine nucleotides. Inhibition of the IMPDH pathway results in selective blockade of lymphocyte proliferation. Mycophenolic acid is metabolized to mycophenolic acid glucuronide, which is excreted in bile and has an enterohepatic circulation [38,39]. It is excreted in the urine in humans and to a lesser extent in the bile. There may be larger variations of pharmacokinetics in liver transplant recipients related to fluctuations in serum albumin, unlike that seen in renal transplant recipients.

The major advantage of using mycophenolic acid is the lack of renal toxicity. In patients with preexisting renal disease [40] mycophenolic acid has been used in conjunction with low-dose calcineurin inhibitors as part of a renal-sparing protocol with promising results. The use of MMF in conjunction with corticosteroids and tacrolimus has been shown to be superior in preventing rejection and improving renal function as compared with tacrolimus and corticosteroid therapy alone [41]. Patients discharged home on immunosuppressive therapy that included MMF appear to have better long-term patient and graft survival. It is possible that the use of MMF may enable a lower dose of calcineurin inhibitor to be used in an attempt to preserve renal function. Therefore, MMF may be particularly useful in patients who may be at higher risk of rejection, such as younger patients undergoing liver transplant for fulminant liver failure and patients undergoing transplant for autoimmune liver diseases. MMF monotherapy after calcineurin inhibitor withdrawal has been associated with a high incidence of acute cellular rejection and steroid-resistant rejection

[42,43]. Therefore, the use of MMF alone may not be sufficient to prevent rejection in liver transplantation.

The usual dose is 1,000 mg administered orally twice daily. Dose reductions are made depending on toxicity. An enteric-coated preparation (Myfortic®) is available that allows delayed release of the active drug in the small intestine rather than the stomach. This may help alleviate some of the gastrointestinal side effects presently seen with MMF therapy.

Significant side effects of MMF are related to gastrointestinal disorders and bone marrow suppression. Indeed, reduction of dosage or discontinuation of MMF therapy is common in liver recipients. Diarrhea is the most common dose-limiting adverse effect, although abdominal pain, nausea, and vomiting can frequently occur. Studies have also shown an increased incidence of CMV, herpes simplex virus, *Candida* infections, and rarely progressive multifocal leukoencephalopathy with the use of mycophenolic acid. In pregnant patients, there is an increased risk of spontaneous abortions during the first trimester and serious congenital malformations have also been reported. Therefore, mycophenolic acid must be discontinued in liver transplant recipients who wish to bear children.

While we are able to measure mycophenolic acid levels, these assays are generally not employed in clinical practice in liver transplant recipients. In many instances, these side effects appear to be dose dependent. Side effects may require dose reduction or withdrawal in up to 50% of patients. Gastrointestinal side effects may be reduced by acid reduction using proton pump inhibitors. Bone marrow suppression usually responds to dose reduction, but in some instances it may require drug discontinuation or the use of granulocyte-stimulating factor.

Sirolimus

Sirolimus (rapamycin, Rapamune®) is a macrolide antibiotic isolated from the fungus *Streptomyces hygroscopicus*, first discovered in soil samples from Easter Island. It is structurally similar to the calcineurin inhibitor tacrolimus and has proved to have potent immunosuppressive properties.

Like calcineurin inhibitors cyclosporine and tacrolimus, rapamycin acts by binding to the immunophilin FKB12. However, this does not affect calcineurin activity, but instead the complex binds and inhibits the protein called mammalian target of rapamycin (mTOR). Inhibition of mTOR results in selective inhibition of synthesis of new ribosomal proteins that are essential for progression of the cells from the G1 to the S phase. In addition, rapamycin has also been associated with diminished fibroblastic activity [44,45]. While in vitro studies have suggested that sirolimus and tacrolimus might compete for FKBP12 protein and act as antagonists, studies have subsequently confirmed that sirolimus augments the immunosuppressive activity of tacrolimus.

Sirolimus is absorbed rapidly from the small intestine with mean peak blood concentrations occurring 1–2 hours after administration. Bioavailability is approximately 15% [46]. Time to maximum concentration can be reduced by the ingestion of a fatty meal or with the use of a liquid formulation. The drug is excreted in the feces (50%) with very little urinary excretion. The mean half-life is approximately 60 hours in patients with normal renal function. The long half-life has allowed once-daily administration. A loading dose of approximately three times the maintenance dose has been recommended at the initiation of therapy. Drug monitoring of trough levels is recommended. Clinical studies suggest that efficacy and toxicity are related to sirolimus concentrations, and there is high interpatient variability. Whole blood concentrations of the drug must be measured since 95% of the drug is sequestered in red blood cells. Drugs that induce or inhibit cytochrome P4503A enzymes have been shown to interact significantly with sirolimus.

Sirolimus was first reported for use in liver transplantation from the United Kingdom by Watson et al. [47]. McAllister et al. used sirolimus with low-dose tacrolimus and reported a very low incidence of acute rejection at 14% [48]. However, two international randomized controlled clinical trials combining rapamycin and cyclosporine with rapamycin with tacrolimus revealed some disturbing results [49]. In the rapamycin–cyclosporine combination group versus cyclosporine and prednisone group, rates of biopsy-confirmed rejection were lower in the sirolimus group (45.5% versus 59.6%) but there was no significant difference in patient survival. There was a significantly higher incidence of wound infections in the sirolimus group (16.2% versus 0%) and there was a higher incidence of hepatic artery/portal-venous thrombosis in the sirolimus group (12.8% versus 3.8%). In the rapamycin–tacrolimus combination group there was no difference in the incidence of rejection compared to the tacrolimus/prednisone group but there was a significantly higher incidence of graft loss (22.7% versus 8.9%; $P < 0.006$) and death (14.5% versus 5.4%; $P < 0.025$). Here again a higher incidence of hepatic artery thrombosis was found in the sirolimus group (5.4% versus 0.9%; $P < 0.06$) [50]. Both of these studies were terminated prematurely and led to a black box warning from the US Food and Drug Administration (FDA) stating that sirolimus in combination with tacrolimus and cyclosporine is associated with excess mortality and graft loss.

Other single center studies have not supported these findings [51,52]. Today, rapamycin is primarily used as an immunosuppressive agent for its renal-sparing effect in patients experiencing calcineurin nephrotoxicity.

However, recent studies have questioned the renal toxic-sparing effect of sirolimus in randomized controlled trials [53]. In addition, uncontrolled trials have suggested that rapamycin may have antineoplastic effects and may be effective in hepatocellular cancer [54–56]. While a number of studies have suggested an antineoplastic effect of rapamycin in hepatocellular carcinoma (HCC) patients, this finding has not been confirmed as yet in controlled trials [57].

Finally, rapamycin has been shown in some studies to have a positive effect on the recurrence of hepatitis C [58,59]. However, a recent analysis of the Scientific Registry of Transplant Recipients (SRTR) database shows that sirolimus use in hepatitis C patients is associated with a significantly increased risk of patient death following liver transplantation [60]. Other studies have shown that pretreatment with sirolimus attenuated the anti-hepatitis C virus (HCV) replication effect of interferon-α in the HCV replication model. It has also shown that ribavirin activates mTOR which in turn enhances the interferon signaling pathway. Rapamycin, on the other hand, is an inhibitor of mTOR. Thus, the true effect of rapamycin on hepatitis C recurrence needs further assessment.

Rapamycin has a number of side effects that currently restrict its usage in liver transplantation. Adverse effects of rapamycin include thrombocytopenia, leukopenia, anemia requiring blood transfusions, arthralgias, and pneumonitis. Rapamycin is also associated with a high incidence of hyperlipidemia with up to one third of patients requiring treatment for hyperlipidemia. Delayed wound healing and oral ulcers which are quite painful are also frequently seen and often limit continued use of this agent. In addition to the side effects noted above, there have been reports of an increased risk of nephrotoxicity when combining rapamycin with high doses of calcineurin inhibitors. Thus, the future role of sirolimus in the liver transplant recipient remains undefined, and further data with regard to its antineoplastic effect will be forthcoming [57].

Biologic immunosuppressive agents

Immunosuppression with antibody therapy in liver transplantation may consist of either polyclonal antibodies or monoclonal antibodies. Polyclonal antibodies include antithymocyte globulin and antilymphocyte globulin. Polyclonal preparations may be obtained by immunizing either a horse or rabbit with different immunogens, whereas monoclonal antibodies are produced in response to a single antigen. The advent of hybridoma technology to fuse two cell lines, one capable of specific antibody production and the other capable of permanent cell growth, was a key breakthrough in monoclonal antibody production.

Depleting antibodies

Polyclonal antithymocyte globulin is prepared by immunizing animals such as horses or rabbits with immunogens from different sources, followed by harvesting the immunoglobulin G (IgG) and absorbing out the toxic antibodies, i.e., those against platelets and erythrocytes. Antithymocyte globulin is produced by using human thymocytes as immunogens, whereas antilymphocyte globulin is produced using human lymphocytes. Polyclonal agents have been in use since the early 1960s. The initial agents, termed antilymphocyte serum, consist of unfractioned serum obtained from animals after immunization with human lymphocytes. Subsequently this preparation is purified, and the immunoglobin is concentrated since the immunosuppressive properties of the serum are contained in the immunoglobulin fraction. Various preparations of polyclonal antibodies are available throughout the world. In the United States, the commonly used polyclonal preparations are antithymocyte globulins derived either from the horse (Atgam®) or the rabbit (Thymoglublin®). The polyclonal antibodies exert their action through various mechanisms that include complement-mediated cell lysis, increased uptake of T cells by the reticuloendothelial system, and also by modulation of surface receptors of lymphocytes thus blocking their function. As an induction agent, polyclonal antithymocyte globulin is usually used for 3–10 days to produce "profound and durable" lymphopenia that can last often beyond 1 year. In addition to immunodeficiency complications, toxic effects of polyclonal antithymocyte globulin include thrombocytopenia, the cytokine release syndrome, and occasionally serum sickness or allergic reactions [61,62]. Concerns remain about an increase in infectious complications and an increase in the incidence of post-transplant lymphoproliferative disorders when these antibodies are utilized.

Monoclonal antibodies

Muromonab-CD3 (OKT3) is a mouse monoclonal antibody against the T-cell receptor (CD3), and has been used for 20 years for immunosuppressive induction and to treat rejection [62,63]. OKT3 binds to the T-cell receptor-associated CD3 complex and triggers a massive cytokine release syndrome before both depleting and functionally altering T cells. Administration of OKT3 results in rapid depletion and extravasation of most T cells from the blood stream and peripheral lymphoid organs such as lymph nodes and spleen. This depletion is secondary to both cell death and margination of the T lymphocytes into the vascular endothelial walls and redistribution to nonlymphoid organs such as the lung. More recently, OKT3 has been used in liver transplant to treat steroid-resistant cellular rejection episodes [64].

OKT3 has been associated with a high incidence of adverse effects related to the cytokine release phenomena, and premedication with steroids, antihistamines, and analgesics is generally advised. This syndrome usually occurs within an hour of drug administration during the first two to three doses [61]. Additionally, during OKT3 administration to treat rejection, prophylaxis against infections such as with CMV, pneumocystis, and fungi is advised. The use of OKT3 has also been associated with early and severe recurrence of hepatitis C and has been associated with an increased incidence of lymphoproliferative disease in liver transplant recipients [65, 66]. The total lymphocyte counts and CD3 counts are usually monitored during therapy, and dose adjustment may be needed to ensure adequate suppression of the CD3 count. Humans can make neutralizing antibodies against OKT3 that terminate its effects and limit its use, thus the importance of following CD3 counts.

A second depleting monoclonal antibody, alemtuzumab or Campath®, is a humanized recombinant anti-CD52 monoclonal antibody. Campath produces profound depletion of circulating lymphoctyes that can last for months to up to a year. It has been approved for treating refractory B-cell chronic lymphocytic leukemia but has not been approved for immunosuppression in solid organ transplantation [67,68]. Side effects of alemtuzumab include first-dose reactions, profound neutropenia, anemia, and rarely pancytopenia and autoimmunity (i.e., hemolytic anemia, thrombocytopenia, and hyperthyroidism). The risk of immunodeficiency complications, i.e., infectious complications, is high, and severe recurrence of hepatitis C has been reported [69,70]. Currently, the use of alemtuzumab remains experimental in liver transplantation, and while initially it was thought to invoke tolerance, this theory has been not substantiated.

Nondepleting antibodies and fusion proteins

Interleukin 2 receptor antibodies (anti-CD25) daclizumab and basiliximab have been used in liver transplantation. The exact mechanism of action is still incompletely understood but likely results from their binding to the IL2 receptor on the surface of activated, but not resting, T cells. Because the expression of CD25 (IL2 receptor α-chain) requires T-cell activation, anti-CD25 antibody causes little depletion of T cells and is only moderately effective in preventing rejection. Anti-CD25 antibody has been used for induction immunosuppression, especially in patients with renal failure, to provide a window of opportunity for the kidneys to recover before commencing calcineurin inhibitors [70–72]. It has also been used for induction immunosuppression in corticosteroid-free

protocols [73]. One of the two IL2 receptor antibodies, daclizumab, has been discontinued in the United States by the manufacturer. Its noted side effects are uncommon, but a high incidence of hepatic allograft rejection has been reported when these antibodies are utilized without the use of a calcineurin inhibitor. Two recent studies have questioned whether or not anti-CD25 antibody use has a renal-sparing effect [74,75].

Co-stimulation blockade

T-cell activation requires interaction of the T-cell receptor with an MHC molecule on an antigen-presenting cell and a second costimulatory signal (signal 2). One costimulatory signal is between the CD28 receptor on T cells and CD80 and CD86 on the antigen-presenting cell. Importantly, cytotoxic T-lymphocyte-associated antigen 4 (CTLA-4) is a natural homolog to CD28 that is transiently expressed on T cells and acts as a negative regulator by competing with CD28 for CD80/86 binding. As such, the immune response can be inhibited by stimulating CTLA-4 activity through therapeutic induction of soluble CTLA-4. In organ transplantation, the most well-developed soluble CTLA agent is belatacept, which is a soluble recombinant immunoglobulin fusion protein comprised of the extracellular CTLA-4 domain and the FC portion of IgG1. It is administered once a month by injection. Reports from early trials thus far have been reported in renal transplantation, and belatacept in combination with MMF, corticosteroids, and basiliximab has shown significant improvement in renal function when compared with calcineurin inhibitor use [76]. In liver transplantation, the initial assessment has been less promising with a significantly increased incidence of rejection being reported in the calcineurin-free belatacept arms as compared with the calcineurin inhibitor arms. Further studies in liver transplant will be forthcoming.

Goals of immunosuppression

Today, the administration of immunosuppression remains as much an art as a science. While we have made great strides in developing new immunosuppressive agents, the use of combination therapy remains to be refined. There are few markers of overall immunosuppression, tolerance, rejection, or degree of alloreactivity. In addition, there remains a poor correlation between rejection and degree of abnormality of liver function tests and immunosuppressive levels. Thus, today, liver biopsy remains the gold standard guide to diagnosing and treating rejection. However, in the future there remains hope of monitoring alloreactivity using transcriptional profiling and developing diagnostic tests to assess overall immunosuppression and operational tolerance in liver transplant recipients [77].

Today we achieve excellent patient and graft survival, with an incidence of rejection of 35–40%. However, graft loss related to rejection occurs in less than 5% of patients. The main challenge is that patients continue to suffer from complications related to immunosuppression including metabolic complications such as diabetes mellitus, cardiovascular risk and coronary disease, an increase in de novo malignancies, a renal failure rate of 20% at 15 years, and severe recurrence of hepatitis C, frequently leading to graft failure and need for retransplantation. These findings all suggest liver transplant recipients are over-immunosuppressed.

The strategy for future immunosuppressive therapy appears to be changing. Today, the goal is to control alloreactivity using low-dose combination therapy that will prevent rejection yet minimize side effects. Tailoring immunosuppressive therapy in the individual transplant recipient is a concept that has evolved in recent times. Today, we are attempting to administer immunosuppression that best meets the needs of individual patients, i.e., delaying the introduction of calcineurin inhibitors to allow renal function to improve, corticosteroid avoidance for patients with osteoporosis or hepatitis C, and increased immunosuppression and continuance of corticosteroid therapies in young patients undergoing a liver transplant for acute liver failure or autoimmune liver disease where rejection rates are the highest. In addition, we know that alloreactivity is highest within the first few weeks following liver transplantation but subsides thereafter and, thus, the need for immunosuppression decreases with time (Fig. 43.3). Indeed, over 20% of patients can be completely withdrawn from immunosuppression without experiencing a detrimental effect [78,79]. Thus, the development of therapeutic strategies to promote tolerance or a state in which the allograft is specifically accepted without the need for chronic immunosuppression remains our ultimate goal [80,81].

With the advent of unlocking human DNA, new avenues have opened to true individualization based on drug metabolism. Pharmacogenetic typing offers the possibility of significant improvement in the individualization of immunosuppressive drug prescribing with reduced rates of rejection and, more importantly, in minimizing toxicity.

References

1. Thuluvath PJ, Guidinger MK, Fung JJ, et al. Liver transplantation in the United States 1999–2008. *Am J Transplant* 2010;10:1003–19.
2. Groth CG. Forty years of liver transplantation: personal recollections. *Transplant Proc* 2008;40:1127–9.
3. Starzl TE, Klintmalm GBG, Porter KA, Iwatsuki S, Schroter GP. Liver transplantation with use of cyclosporin A and prednisone. *N Engl J Med* 1981;305(5):266–9.
4. Liver transplantation. National Institutes of Health Consensus Development. *Natl Inst Health Consens Dev Conf Summ* 1983;4:15.
5. US Multicenter FK506 Liver Study Group. A comparison of tacrolimus (FK506) and cyclosporine for immunosuppression in liver transplantation. *N Engl J Med* 1994;331:1110.
6. Wiesner RH. A long-term comparison of tacrolimus (FK506) versus cyclosporine in liver transplantation: a report of the United States FK506 Study Group. *Transplantation* 1998;66:493–9.
7. Meier-Kreischo HU, Li S, Griessner RWG, et al. Immunosuppression evolution in practice and trends 1994–2004. *Am J Transplant* 2006;6(2):1111–31.
8. Pillai A, Levitsky J. Overview of immunosuppression in liver transplantation. *World J Gastroenterol* 2009;15(34):4225–4233.
9. Von Andrian UH, Mackay CR. T-cell function and migration: two sides of the same coin. *N Engl J Med* 2000;343:1020–34.
10. Choudhuri K, Wiseman D, Brown MH, Gould K, van der Merwe PA. T-cell receptor triggering is critically dependent on the dimensions of its peptide-MHC ligand. *Nature* 2005;436:578–82.
11. Zheng H, Hin B, Henrickson SE, Perelson AS, von Andrian UH, Chakraborty AK. How antigen quantity and quality determine T cell decisions in lymphoid tissue. *Mol Cell Biol* 2008;28:4040–51.
12. Wang D, Matsumoto R, You Y, et al. CD3/CD28 costimulation-induced NF-kappaB activation is mediated by recruitment of protein kinase C-theta, Bcl10, and IkappaB kinase beta to the immunological synapse through CARMA1. *Mol Cell Biol* 2004;24:164–71.
13. Martinez OM, Rosen HR. Basic concepts in transplant immunology. *Liver Transpl* 2005;11:370–81.
14. Wiesner RH, Ludwig J, van Hoek B, Krom RAF. Current concepts in cell-mediated hepatic allograft rejection leading to ductopenia and liver failure. *Hepatology* 1991;14:721–9.
15. Demetris AJ, Batts KP, Dhillon AP, et al. Banff schema for grading liver allograft rejection: an International Consensus Document. *Hepatology* 1997;25:658–63.
16. Morgan JA. The influence of cortisone on the survival of homografts of skin in the rabbit. *Surgery* 1951;30:506–15.
17. Boumpas DT, Chrousos GP, Wilder RL, et al. Glucocorticoid therapy for immune mediated diseases: basic and chemical correlates. *Ann Intern Med* 1993;119:1198–208.
18. Eason JD, Nair S, Cohen AJ, et al. Steroid-free liver transplantation using rabbit antithymocyte globulin and early tacrolimus monotherapy. *Transplantation* 2003;75:1396–9.
19. Eason JD, Loss GE, Blazek J, et al. Steroid free liver transplantation using rabbit antithymocyte globulin induction: results of a prospective randomized trial. *Liver Transpl* 2001;7:693–7.

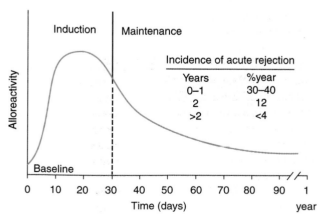

Figure 43.3 Alloreactivity with time following liver transplantation.

20. Tector AJ, Fridell JA, Mangus S, et al. Promising early results using delayed introduction of tacrolimus and rabbit antithymocyte globulin in adult liver transplant recipients. *Liver Transpl* 2004;10: 404–7.

21. Gautam M, Cheruvattath R, Balan V. Recurrence of autoimmune liver disease after liver transplantation: a systematic review. *Liver Transpl* 2006;12:1813–24.

22. Wiesner RH, Ludwig J, Krom RA, et al. Treatment of early cellular rejection following liver transplantation with intravenous methylprednisolone, the effect on dose response. *Transplantation* 1994;58:1053–6.

23. Wiesner RH, Demetris J, Belle SH, et al. Acute hepatic allograft rejection: incidence, risk factors, and impact on outcome. *Hepatology* 1998;28:638–45.

24. Berenguer M, Prieto M, Cordoba J, et al. Early development of chronic active hepatitis in recurrent hepatitis C virus infection after liver transplantation: association with treatment of rejection. *J Hepatol* 1998;28:756–63.

25. Vivarelli M, Burra P, La Barba G, et al. Influence of steroids on HCV recurrence after liver transplantation: a prospective study. *J Hepatol* 2007;47:793–8.

26. Clipstone NA, Crabtree GR. Identification of calcineurin as a key signaling enzyme in T-lymphocyte activation. *Nature* 1992;357: 695–7.

27. Borel JF, Feurer C, Gubler HJ, Stahelin H. Biological effects of cyclosporin A: a new antilymphocytic agent. *Agents Actions* 1976;6: 468–75.

28. Noble S, Markhan A. Cyclosporine: a review of the pharmacokinetic properties, chemical efficacy, and tolerability of a microemulsion based formulation (Neoral). *Drugs* 1995;50:924–41.

29. Gonwa TA, Mai ML, Melton LB, et al. End-stage renal disease (ESRD) after orthotopic liver transplantation (OLTX) using calcineurin-based immunotherapy: risk of development and treatment. *Transplantation* 2001;72:1934–9.

30. Ojo AO, Held PJ, Port FK, et al. Chronic renal failure after transplantation of a nonrenal organ. *N Engl J Med* 2003;349:931–40.

31. Starzl TE, Todo S, Fung J, et al. FK506 for liver, kidney, and pancreas transplantation. *Lancet* 1989;2:1000.

32. US Multicenter FK506 Liver Study Group. A comparison of tacrolimus (FK506) and cyclosporine for immunosuppression in liver transplantation. *N Engl J Med* 1994;331:1110–15.

33. European FK506 Multicenter Liver Study Group. Randomized trial comparing tacrolimus (FK506) and cyclosporin in prevention of liver allograft rejection. *Lancet* 1994;344:423–8.

34. O'Grady JG, Hardy P, Burroughs AK, Elbourne D, UK and Ireland Liver Transplant Study Group. Randomized controlled trial of tacrolimus versus microemulsified cyclosporine (TMC) in liver transplantation: poststudy surveillance to 3 years. *Am J Transplant* 2007;7:137–41.

35. McAlister VC, Haddad E, Renouf E, Malthaner RA, Kjaer MS, Gluud LL. Cyclosporin versus tacrolimus as a primary immunosuppressant after liver transplantation: a meta-analysis. *Am J Transplant* 2006;6:1578–85.

36. Haddad EM, McAlister VC, Renouf E, Malthaner R, Kjaer MS, Gluud LL. Cyclosporin versus tacrolimus for liver transplanted patients. *Cochrane Database Syst Rev* 2006;4:CD005161.

37. Wiesner RH, FK506 Study Group. A long-term comparison of tacrolimus (FK506) versus cyclosporine in liver transplantation: a report of the United States FK506 Study Group. *Transplantation* 1998;66:493–9.

38. Fultin B, Markham A. Mycophenolate mofetil: a review of its pharmacodynamic and pharmacokinetic properties and clinical efficacy in renal transplantation. *Drugs* 1996;51:278–98.

39. Jain A, Venkataramanan R, Hamad IS, et al. Pharmacokinetics of mycophenolic acid after mycophenolate mofetil administration in liver transplant patients treated with tacrolimus. *J Clin Pharmacol* 2001;41:268–76.

40. Barkmann A, Nashan B, Schmidt HH, et al. Improvement of acute and chronic renal dysfunction in liver transplant patients after substitution of calcineurin inhibitors by mycophenolate mofetil. *Transplantation* 2000;69:1886–90.

41. Wiesner RH, Shorr JS, Steffen BJ, et al. Mycophenolate mofetil combination therapy improves long-term outcomes after liver transplantation in patients with and without hepatitis C. *Liver Transpl* 2005;11:750–9.

42. Schlitt HJ, Barkmann A, Boker KH, et al. Replacement of calcineurin inhibitors with mycophenolate mofetil in liver transplant patients with renal dysfunction: a randomized controlled study. *Lancet* 2001;357:587–91.

43. Stewart SF, Hudson M, Talbot D, et al. Mycophenolate mofetil monotherapy in liver transplantation. *Lancet* 2001;357:609–10.

44. Sehgal SN. Sirolimus: its discovery, biological properties, and mechanism of action. *Transplant Proc* 2003;35(Suppl 3):75–145.

45. Augustine JJ, Bodziak KA, Hricik DE. Use of sirolimus in solid organ transplantation. *Drugs* 2007;67(3):369–91.

46. Neuhaus P, Klupp J, Langrehr JM. mTOR inhibitors: an overview. *Liver Transpl* 2001;7(6):473–84.

47. Watson CJ, Friend PJ, Jamieson NV, et al. Sirolimus: a potent new immunosuppressant for liver transplantation. *Transplantation* 1999;67(4):505–9.

48. McAlister VC, Peltekian KM, Malatjalian DA, et al. Orthotopic liver transplantation using low-dose tacrolimus and sirolimus. *Liver Transpl* 2001;7(8):701–8.

49. Wiesner RH, Klintmalm G, McDiarmid SV, Rapamune Liver Transplant Study Group. Sirolimus immunotherapy results in reduced rates of acute rejection in de novo orthotopic liver transplant recipients. *Am J Transplant* 2002;2(Suppl 3):464.

50. Camici GG, Steffel J, Amanovic I, et al. Rapamycin promotes arterial thrombosis in vivo: implications for everolimus and zotarolimus eluting stents. *Eur Heart J* 2010;31:236–42.

51. Molinari M, Berman K, Meeberg G, et al. Multicentric outcome analysis of sirolimus-based immunosuppression in 252 liver transplant recipients. *Transpl Int* 2010;23(2):155–68.

52. Levy G, Schmidli H, Panch J, et al. Safety, tolerability, and efficacy of everolimus in de novo liver transplant recipients: 12- and 36-month results. *Liver Transpl* 2006;12(11):1640–8.

53. Asrani SK, Leise MD, West CP, et al. Use of sirolimus in liver transplant recipient with renal insufficiency: a systematic review and meta-analysis. *Hepatology* 2010;52:1360–70.

54. Zimmerman MA, Trotter JF, Wachs M, et al. Sirolimus-based immunosuppression following liver transplantation for hepatocellular carcinoma. *Liver Transpl* 2008;14(5):633–8.

55. Chinnakotla S, Davis GL, Vasani S, et al. Impact of sirolimus on the recurrence of hepatocellular carcinoma after liver transplantation. *Liver Transpl* 2009;15(12):1834–42.

56. Toso C, Merani S, Bigam DL, et al. Sirolimus-based immunosuppression is associated with increased survival after liver transplantation for hepatocellular carcinoma. *Hepatology* 2010;51(4):1237–43.

57. Schnitzbauer AA, Zuelke C, Graeb C, et al. A prospective randomized, open-labeled trial comparing sirolimus-containing versus mTOR-inhibitor-free immunosuppression in patients undergoing liver transplantation for hepatocellular carcinoma. *BMC Cancer* 2010;10:190.

58. Samonakis DN, Vargas CL, Manzarbeitia C, et al. Sustained, spontaneous disappearance of serum HCV-RNA under immunosuppression after liver transplantation for HCV cirrhosis. *J Hepatol* 2005;43(6):1091–3.

59. Wagner D, Kniepeiss D, Schaffenllner S, et al. Sirolimus has a potential to influence viral recurrence in HCV positive liver transplant candidates. *Int Immunopharmacol* 2010;10(8):990–3.

60. Watt KD, Bruak K, Deschenes M, et al. Impact of sirolimus on post-liver transplant patient and graft survival – an analysis of the SRTR database. Presented at the International Liver Transplant Society Congress 2010, Hong Kong.

61. Jeyarajah DR, Thistlethwaite JR Jr. General aspects of cytokine release syndrome: timing and incidence of symptoms. *Transplant Proc* 1993;25(2 Suppl 1):16–20.

62. Cosimi AB. The clinical value of antilymphocyte antibodies. *Transplant Proc* 1981;13:462.

63. Fung JJ, Demetris AJ, Porter KA, et al. Use of OKT3 with cyclosporin and steroids for reversal of acute kidney and liver allograft rejection. *Nephron* 1987;46(Suppl 1):19–33.

64. Cosimi AB, Cho SI, Delmonico FL, et al. A randomized clinical trial comparing OKT3 and steroids for treatment of hepatic allograft rejection. *Transplantation* 1987;43:91–5.

65. Rosen HR, Shackleton CR, Higa L, et al. Use of OKT3 is associated with early and severe recurrence of hepatitis C after liver transplantation. *Am J Gastroenterol* 1997;92:1453–7.

66. Swinnen LJ, Costanzo-Nordin MR, Fisher SG, et al. Increased incidence of lymphoproliferative disorder after immunosuppression with the monoclonal antibody OKT3 in cardiac-transplant recipients. *N Engl J Med* 1990;323:1723–8.

67. Marcos A, Eghtesad B, Fung JJ, et al. Use of alemtuzumab and tacrolimus monotherapy for cadaveric liver transplantation: with particular reference to hepatitis C virus. *Transplantation* 2004;78: 966–71.

68. Tryphonopoulos P, Weppler D, Nishida S, et al. Six year experience with campath-1H (C1H) induction in adult liver transplantation. *Am J Transplant* 2008;8(Suppl 2):307.

69. Levitsky J, Thudi K, Ison MG, Wang E, Abecassis M. Alemtuzumab induction in non-hepatitis C positive liver transplant recipients. *Liver Transpl* 2011;17:32–7.

70. Dhesi S, Boland B, Colquhoun S. Alemtuzumab and liver transplantation: a review. *Curr Opin Organ Transplant* 2009;14:245–9.

71. Eckhoff DE, McGuire B, Sellers M, et al. The safety and efficacy of a two-dose daclizumab (Zenapax) induction therapy in liver transplant recipients. *Transplantation* 2000;69:1867–172.

72. Emre S, Gondolesi G, Polat K, et al. Use of daclizumab as initial immunosuppression in liver transplant recipients with impaired renal function. *Liver Transpl* 2001;7:220–5.

73. Liu CL, Fan ST, Lo CM, et al. Interleukin-2 receptor antibody (basiliximab) for immunosuppressive induction therapy after liver transplantation: a protocol with early elimination of steroids and reduction of tacrolimus dosage. *Liver Transpl* 2004;10: 728–33.

74. Hirose R, Roberts JP, Quan D, et al. Experience with daclizumab in liver transplantation: renal transplant dosing without calcineurin inhibitors is insufficient to prevent acute rejection in liver transplantation. *Transplantation* 2000;69:307–11.

75. Asrani SK, Kim WR, Pedersen RA. Daclizumab induction therapy in liver transplant recipients with renal insufficiency. *Alimentary Pharmacol Ther* 2010;32(6):776-86.

76. Vincenti F, Larsen C, Durrbach A, et al. Costimulation blockade with belatacept in renal transplantation. *N Engl J Med* 2005;353: 770–81.

77. Martinez M, Lozano J, Puig-Pey I, et al. Using transcriptional profiling to develop a diagnostic test of operational tolerance in liver transplant recipients. *J Clin Invest* 2008;118:2845–57.

78. Sanchez-Fueyo A. Identification of operationally tolerant liver transplant recipients. *Liver Transpl* 2010;16:S82–6.

79. Martinez-Llordella M, Puig-Pey I, Orlando G, et al. Multiparameter immune profiling of operational tolerance in liver transplantation. *Am J Transplant* 2007;7:309–19.

80. Halloran PF. Immunosuppressive drugs for kidney transplantation. *N Engl J Med* 2004;351(26):2715–29.

81. Sanchez-Fueyo A, Strom TB. Immunologic basis of graft rejection and tolerance following transplantation of liver or other solid organs. *Gastroenterology* 2011;140(1):51–64.

CHAPTER 44

The First Six Months Following Liver Transplantation

Rajender Reddy[1] & Manuel Mendizabal[2]

[1]Department of Hepatology, Hospital of the University of Pennsylvania, Philadelphia, PA, USA
[2]Unidad de Hígado y Trasplante Hepático, Hospital Universitario Austral, Pilar, Argentina

Key concepts

- Initial postoperative assessment of liver transplant recipients should focus on careful evaluation and management of hemodynamic stability. Assessment of renal and pulmonary function is mandatory and continuous neurologic examination is essential. Within the first few days following liver transplantation, profound graft dysfunction suggests primary nonfunction or hepatic artery thrombosis and early diagnosis is critical as this entails consideration of retransplantation.

- Throughout the first few weeks, allograft function should be monitored closely in order to recognize acute cellular rejection (ACR) so that it can be treated promptly. Full knowledge and understanding of the side effects of immunosuppressants is essential so as to avoid adverse events.

- Initial immunosuppression consists of corticosteroids associated with a calcineurin inhibitor (CNI) (tacrolimus or cyclosporine). Careful attention should be paid to potential drug–drug interactions leading to variability in the blood levels of CNIs. Not uncommonly some centers use OKT3, thymoglobulin, or interleukin 2 antibody receptors (e.g., basiliximab, dacluzimab) for induction, whereas others restrict their use to patients with renal failure.

- Common side effects related to immunosuppression agents include hypertension, renal insufficiency, diabetes, and hyperlipidemia and these have a high impact on post-transplant morbidity and mortality if left untreated.

- Biliary tract abnormalities have been described in as high as 30% of liver transplant recipients and these include biliary leak and stenosis. Diagnosis and potential treatment is best pursued with endoscopic retrograde cholangiopancreatography.

- ACR mostly occurs within the first 3 months following transplantation, but can be encountered at any time. Distinguishing it from recurrent disease, particularly hepatitis C, is crucial since management is different. In recipients transplanted for hepatitis C, prolonged or high-dose corticosteroid administration may accelerate allograft hepatitis and result in poorer long-term outcomes.

Over the past several years the postoperative care of liver transplantation (LT) has improved dramatically. Most life-threatening complications following LT occur within the perioperative period and include primary nonfunction of the allograft (PNF), acute cellular rejection (ACR), technical complications related to the surgery such as biliary leaks and hepatic artery thrombosis (HAT), and a variety of medical complications (Fig. 44.1). Better understanding of the pathophysiology of some of these complications and improved diagnostic tools has allowed us to differentiate and appropriately manage these often critically ill patients.

Intensive care unit management

Following LT, patients are transferred from the operating room to the intensive care unit (ICU), where care is provided by a multidisciplinary team including an intensivist, a transplant surgeon, a hepatologist, and an experienced nursing team. Patients with an uncomplicated transplant operation, those who have a rapid reversal of anesthetic effects, and those who have a functioning allograft and are hemodynamically stable are usually good candidates for early extubation in the recovery room. As with any patient undergoing major abdominal surgery, careful and frequent assessment of the patient's level of consciousness and hemodynamic status, including cardiopulmonary function and urinary output, is done. Periodic assessment of intra-abdominal drainage through drains is essential. The quantity and character of the drainage is determined and particular note is made of whether it is clear or bloody. In some centers, a T tube is placed at the donor–recipient anastomosis, allowing easy appraisal of bile quantity and quality with pale and low

Schiff's Diseases of the Liver, Eleventh Edition. Edited by Eugene R. Schiff, Willis C. Maddrey and Michael F. Sorrell.
© 2012 John Wiley & Sons, Ltd. Published 2012 by John Wiley & Sons, Ltd.

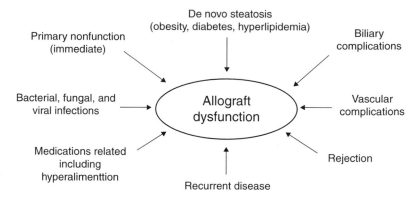

Figure 44.1 Causes for allograft dysfunction following liver transplantation.

output being associated with poor graft function. It is well described that when larger volumes of blood products are used intraoperatively, complications after transplantation increase [1]. Physicians must be aware of potential issues including pulmonary problems, infectious complications, renal failure, and cardiac complications. Neurologic abnormalities are not infrequent in the immediate postoperative period. Brachial plexus palsy as a result of compression injury secondary to the use of retractors and extremity position during the surgery can be seen. Mental status changes ranging from anxiety to delusional states and encephalopathy can be expected, but most resolve with no intervention [2,3].

General management

Assessment of the allograft function is initiated in the operating room at the time of graft reperfusion, mainly by observation of the bile production and its characteristics. The degree of elevation of serum aminotransferases levels indicates the extent of liver parenchymal injury due to a variety of factors, including reperfusion injury and graft ischemia time, defined mainly by two variables – cold ischemia time (CIT) and warm ischemia time (WIT). CIT is defined as the time interval that begins when an organ is cooled with a cold perfusion solution after organ procurement surgery and ends when the organ is implanted. On the other hand, WIT begins when the organ reaches physiologic temperature before the completion of surgical anastomosis and ends with reestablishment of the blood circulation in the graft. The duration of ischemia correlates with the degree of hepatocyte injury characterized by apoptosis, necrosis, and inflammation. Serum aminotransferase elevation peaks at 1–2 days after the transplant but should rapidly decline along with the prothrombin time if graft function is satisfactory. This may be followed by a cholestatic picture with increases in alkaline phosphatase (AP), γ-glutamyltransferase (GGT), and bilirubin; these slowly improve if the preservation injury is not severe.

Graft function

During the immediate postoperative period, three major complications can cause profound graft dysfunction, which in most cases requires prompt liver retransplantation (Table 44.1). PNF, HAT, and hyperacute rejection remain a great challenge for the transplant team and have a major impact on postoperative morbidity and mortality. PNF is an extreme form of preservation injury occurring in 3–6% of allografts. PNF manifests as acute liver failure (encephalopathy, elevated serum aminotransferases, coagulopathy, jaundice) and may be associated with multiorgan failure (renal dysfunction, pulmonary complications) [4,5]. Risk factors include donor age older than 50 years, donor liver steatosis greater than 30%, donation after cardiac death (DCD) graft, reduced size graft, severe donor hypernatremia ([Na+] greater than 170 mEq/L), severely ill recipient, and protracted CIT [4,6]. Urgent retransplantation is usually required.

HAT can occur early after transplantation or in the late postoperative period and can be a devastating

Table 44.1 Expected complications following liver transplantation.

Time	Medical complications	Surgical complications
First week	Hyperacute rejection Neurologic complications Primary nonfunction	Intra-abdominal bleeding HAT Biliary leak
Second to fourth week	ACR Neurologic complications Renal failure	HAT Portal vein thrombosis Biliary leak
First to sixth month	ACR Recurrent HCV Hypertension CMV infection Renal failure	Delayed HAT Biliary strictures/casts Portal vein thrombosis

ACR, acute cellular rejection; CMV, cytomegalovirus; HAT, hepatic artery thrombosis; HCV, hepatitis C virus.

complication. It is reported to occur in 4–15% of LT recipients and is generally more frequent after pediatric LT [7,8]. When present within the first few days to 2 weeks after transplantation, HAT manifests with profound graft dysfunction, along with biliary strictures, sepsis, and liver abscesses. Color Doppler ultrasonography is the preferred method to evaluate hepatic artery patency with a reported sensitivity of approximately 90% for acute HAT [9]. Multidetector computed tomography (CT) angiography or magnetic resonance angiography are alternative options for the diagnosis of HAT in patients with difficult or indeterminate sonographic examinations [10, 11]. Angiography provides the opportunity to administer thrombolytics and perform thrombectomy or stenting of the hepatic artery. Early diagnosis and treatment of HAT can avoid liver retransplantation [12]. On the other hand, late unrecognized HAT can lead to biliary tract problems, manifested by either leaks or obstruction, and intrahepatic bilomas. In these cases the treatment of HAT depends on the extension of the graft damage, and has included urgent revascularization or prompt liver retransplantation [12].

At the present time, hyperacute rejection is extremely rare post-LT. This type of rejection becomes apparent within hours post-transplantation and is caused by preformed humoral antibodies against the allograft endothelial cells [13]. Clinical signs and symptoms usually resemble PNF and liver biopsy is necessary for accurate diagnosis in that it reveals congestion and hemorrhagic necrosis within the graft sinusoids. Thus far, no effective treatment has been described other than retransplantation.

Infectious complications

Infectious complications are a continuous threat to every immunosuppressed patient [14]. During the early postoperative period, infections are related to a difficult and prolonged surgical procedure or technical complications of surgery, poor nutritional status, large amounts of blood products intraoperatively, prolonged ICU stay, and poor graft function [15]. Prophylactic strategies include preoperative cultures and antibiotics covering a broad spectrum of organisms, especially enteric Gram-negative and Gram-positive bacteria. Intravenous antibiotics are generally administered before transplantation in the operating room and for 24–48 hours after surgery. Bacterial infections due to an indwelling catheter source (30%), pneumonia (25%), and surgical wounds (10%) dominate the first week. Gram-negative bacteremia should prompt investigation of a biliary tract source and are more common in those with diabetes or with a poor nutritional status [16]. Viral and opportunistic infections are not a major concern during the first few weeks in uncomplicated liver transplant recipients.

Immediate surgical complications

Postoperative bleeding is the most common surgical complication following LT. Approximately 5–15% of posttransplant recipients require reoperation to control early postoperative hemorrhage [17]. However, in approximately half of the patients no specific site of bleeding is found, and after careful examination of the vascular bed is completed such bleeding is usually attributed to coagulopathy. Importantly, it has been reported that two thirds of the patients with poor graft function undergoing reoperation for hemorrhage will die within 6 months of transplantation [17]. Renal failure secondary to postoperative hemorrhage and hemodynamic instability may evolve but usually resolves after controlling the bleeding and with careful hemodynamic monitoring. Biliary complications can occur at any time after transplantation. The vast majority, however, occur within the first 3 months of transplantation, requiring reoperation in 10–20% of patients [18]. Biliary leaks and stenosis are the most common complications. In general, early bile leak is related to technical complications at the biliary anastomotic site. On the other hand, late bile leaks are caused by either ischemic injury from HAT or by removal of T tubes and poor anastomotic healing. Patients with early bile leak can present with bile in the abdominal drains, hyperbilirubinemia, and abdominal pain. Management of small, contained leaks is primarily via endoscopic retrograde cholangiopancreatography (ERCP) and internal stent placement or internal/external biliary drains by percutaneous transhepatic cholangiography (PTC). Over the long term, reoperation and surgical revision may be required for a focal stricture or one not responsive to endoscopic therapy.

Immunsuppression management

A key component of postoperative management of a liver transplant recipient is the regulation of immunosuppressant drugs and it varies widely among centers. The primary goal of immunosuppression is to avoid rejection and graft loss and a secondary objective is to diminish adverse side effects of the antirejection therapy. Significant advances have been achieved in pharmacologic immunosuppression, allowing a wide array of immunosuppressive agents to be used [19]. Induction therapy with high-dose steroids is initiated intraoperatively, and then slowly tapered off. A calcineurin inhibitor (CNI), either tacrolimus or cyclosporine, is usually introduced during the first postoperative day. However, in patients with preexisting renal insufficiency, some centers may delay CNI use and initiate OKT3 or interleukin 2 (IL2) antibody receptors (i.e., basiliximab) during the initial phase. Over the past decade, azathioprine has been substituted by mycophenolate mofetil in some centers as a CNI-sparing strategy, not only in those patients with renal failure but in those who develop CNI-related nervous system toxicity as well. However, in LT, the clinical benefit of mycophenolate mofetil over azathioprine is questionable [20]. During the ICU stay, rejection is generally not a concern.

Hepatitis B prophylaxis

Prior to the introduction of hyperimmune hepatitis B immunoglobulin (HBIg), patients transplanted with a diagnosis of chronic or fulminant hepatitis B virus (HBV) infection had an approximate 75% rate of recurrent HBV [21]. Recurrence of HBV infection is associated with reduced graft and patient survival [22]. Although there is extreme variation in immunoprophylaxis protocols among transplant centers, current prophylactic post-transplant strategies include HBIg and nucleos(t)ide analogs. Most protocols use HBIg intravenously initially during the anhepatic phase and for a variable period post-transplant. Thereafter, some transplant centers administer HBIg monthly and some others, as needed, maintain high and variable anti-hepatitis B surface (HBs) serum titers. With current strategies that also include effective antiviral nucleos(t)ide analogs, the HBV recurrence rate is less than 10% [23]. Newer strategies with much lower doses of HBIg have shown similar results at far less cost in patients with low viral load or HBV DNA-negative status prior to transplantation [24].

Floor care

Monitoring for rejection and treatment

Uncomplicated patients are usually ready to be transferred from the ICU to the floor 24–48 hours after transplant, where close monitoring of the hepatic function should be continued, concurrently with immunosuppression titration into the therapeutic range. Careful and thorough patient and care giver education by transplant coordinators and physicians should be clearly addressed.

Daily performance of liver function tests is used for surveillance of proper engraftment. Prothrombin time (PT) is a particular sensitive index to monitor hepatocellular function. Serum albumin is a good index of graft synthetic function but not in the immediate post-transplant period because of its prolonged half-life and unstable fluid shifts. A few variables associated with early allograft dysfunction have been described as indicators of poor long-term graft and patient survival. These include donors older than 50 years, a CIT greater than 15 hours, donor preprocurement acidosis, and recipient PT or bilirubin that stays steadily elevated [1,25]. Abnormalities of the liver function tests in this phase of the post-transplant period are frequently a manifestation of preservation injury or ACR. Preservation injury usually

presents with an elevation of AP and GGT and without a significant increase in total bilirubin. In contrast, an elevation of transaminases (alanine transaminase (ALT) and aspartate transaminase (AST)) together with rising bilirubin level and/or GGT should raise concern for ACR. However, changes in hepatic biochemical tests are non-specific and reflect injury from any cause, making liver biopsy essential for accurate diagnosis. Biopsy-proven acute rejection occurs in 50% of liver allografts within the first 6 weeks after transplantation [26]. Reported rates of rejection vary because of differences in the reason for a liver biopsy, such as a biopsy triggered by abnormal liver function tests or done routinely as per transplant center protocol. Histologic findings consistent with ACR without significant biochemical abnormalities can be seen in a third of protocol biopsies. The clinical significance of these findings remains unclear; however, most of the transplant centers performing protocol biopsies may treat rejection based solely on histology [27,28]. Rejection reveals portal inflammation with a mixed cellular infiltrate characterized by lymphocytes, neutrophils, and eosinophils (Fig. 44.2). Venous endothelium and biliary ducts are the targets of the inflammatory reaction (Tables 44.2 and 44.3) [29,30]. An adequate level of immunosuppression decreases the risk of ACR. Young and relatively healthy recipients without renal insufficiency and prolonged CIT have been described to have higher incidences of graft rejection [26].

Treatment consists of augmented immunosuppression. Milder rejection episodes may resolve by increasing the dosage of the maintenance immunosuppressant, such as

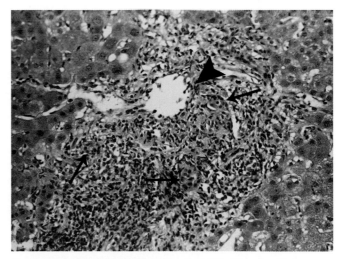

Figure 44.2 Histopathologic findings associated with acute cellular rejection. This core needle biopsy specimen shows portal inflammatory infiltrate containing lymphocytes (predominantly), eosinophils, and neutrophils. Endothelitis characterized by subendothelial localization of the inflammatory cells in a portal vein branch (arrow head) and bile duct inflammation/damage (arrows) can also be seen.

Table 44.2 Grading of acute allograft rejection. A global assessment of the rejection grade is made on a review of the biopsy and after the diagnosis of rejection has been established.

Global assessment[a]	Criteria
Indeterminate	Portal inflammatory infiltrate that fails to meet the criteria for the diagnosis of acute rejection
Mild	Rejection infiltrate in a minority of the triads that is generally mild, and confined within the portal space
Moderate	Rejection infiltrate, expanding most or all of the triads
Severe	As above for moderate to severe perivenular inflammation that extends into the hepatic parenchyma and is associated with perivenular hepatocyte necrosis

[a]Verbal description of mild, moderate, or severe acute rejection could also be labeled as grade I, II, and III, respectively.
Reproduced from Demetris et al. [29] with permission from Plenum.

a CNI, especially if trough levels are suboptimal. More severe episodes require corticosteroid pulse therapy and recycle, and in steroid-refractory cases antilymphocyte preparations or monoclonal antibodies (i.e., OKT3) may be used. In contrast to other solid organ transplants, the liver allograft might be relatively protected after an ACR episode [31]. In allograft recipients with hepatitis C virus (HCV) infection, cellular rejection can be sometimes difficult to distinguish from recurrent HCV. Liver biopsy in recurrent hepatitis C may demonstrate a few similar histologic findings to ACR such as portal inflammatory reaction and lymphocyte predominance [32]. Distinction between these two entities is essential, because the use of antirejection therapy, especially steroids, might accelerate allograft hepatitis and result in poorer long-term outcomes.

Medical complications

In those who have pretransplant ascites, the ascites present before transplantation may continue after LT but usually resolves over days to weeks with sodium restriction and conservative use of diuretics. If large ascites persists, other causes, such as venous outflow anastomosis obstruction, should be considered. Nowadays, with the piggyback technique, caval obstruction is rare and outflow obstruction usually results from suprahepatic anastomoses, manifested as acute outflow obstruction with coagulopathy, jaundice, and ascites. Late

Table 44.3 Rejection activity index using criteria that can be used to score liver allograft biopsies with acute rejection, as defined by the World Gastroenterology Consensus document.

Category	Criteria	Score
Portal inflammation	Mostly lymphocytic inflammation involving, but not noticeably expanding, a minority of the triads	1
	Expansion of most or all of the triads by a mixed infiltrate containing lymphocytes with occasional blasts, neutrophils, and eosinophils	2
	Marked expansion of most or all of the triads by a mixed infiltrate containing numerous blasts and eosinophils with inflammatory spillover into the periportal parenchyma	3
Bile duct inflammation damage	A minority of the ducts are cuffed and infiltrated by inflammatory cells and show only mild reactive changes such as an increased nuclear cytoplasmic ratio of the epithelial cells	1
	Most or all of the ducts are infiltrated by inflammatory cells. More than occasional ducts show degenerative changes such as nuclear pleomorphism, disordered polarity, and cytoplasmic vacuolization of the epithelium	2
	As above for score 2, with most or all of the ducts showing degenerative changes or focal luminal disruption	3
Venous Endothelial Inflammation	Subendothelial lymphocytic infiltration involving some, but not a majority, of the portal and/or hepatic venules	1
	Subendothelial infiltration involving most or all of the portal and/or hepatic venules	2
	As above for score 2, with moderate or severe perivenular inflammation that extends into the perivenular parenchyma and is associated with perivenular hepatocyte necrosis	3

Reproduced from Demetris et al. [29] with permission from Plenum.

presentation of hepatic outflow obstruction manifests as hepatomegaly and persistent ascites resistant to medical therapy. Diagnosis can be made with Doppler ultrasonography in some cases, but hepatic venography and assessment of a gradient between the pre- and postanastomotic site remains the gold standard. Findings on liver biopsy include central lobular congestion and necrosis with cholestasis and the absence of other features of rejection. Management of outflow obstruction is dictated by the severity of allograft dysfunction and the timing of presentation. Emergent revision of the outflow anastomosis and even retransplantation may be required within the first days after LT. Chronic outflow obstruction with preservation of the graft function can be handled conservatively with diuretics. However, radiologic revision of outflow anastomoses followed by venous stenting or angioplasty of the obstruction might be required.

During this phase of hospitalization, many patients develop variable degrees of psychiatric or neurologic abnormalities. Anxiety and psychosis with delusions and hallucinations are frequent, but most resolve gradually without any specific therapy. Seizures, encephalopathy, and tremors are not uncommon at this stage; they are usually multifactorial in origin. Precipitating factors associated with neurotoxicity include metabolic causes (i.e., electrolyte abnormalities, uremia), sleep deprivation, adverse effects of immunosuppressants, and infections. CNIs and steroids have known neurologic side effects; adding mycophenolate mofetil or azathioprine allows for a reduction in the dose of the CNI. LT recipients are not exempt from suffering cerebrovascular events. In the setting of thrombocytopenia and coagulopathy, intracerebral hemorrhage or subdural hematoma may occur spontaneously. Ischemic cerebrovascular events are less common in this setting. Central pontine myelinolysis (CPM) is a devastating neurologic complication associated with variable symptoms including coma, ataxia, dysarthria, and dysphagia. CPM has been classically associated with rapid serum sodium shifts in the perioperative period, potentiated by high CNI levels [33]. Treatment is supportive, with protracted neurologic rehabilitation. Patients transplanted for acute liver failure present a higher risk of neurologic complications. These patients usually present with cerebral edema, and in those cases where an intracranial pressure monitor is in place careful intraoperative monitoring is warranted to reduce the risk of pre and post-transplant neurologic complications.

Several other medical complications can occur during the course of hospitalization. These can be exacerbations of preexisting conditions, but more often are side effects of the immunosuppressive drugs (Table 44.4). Arterial hypertension is the most common cardiovascular complication and is seen in 50–60% of LT recipients [34]. Hypertension is due to a number of factors, including volume overload, preoperative stress, impaired glomerular filtration rate, glucocorticoids, and CNI administration [35]. The first line of therapy is to ensure an appropriate CNI trough level. In the absence of toxic immunosuppressant drug levels, antihypertensive pharmacotherapy is necessary. The mechanism underlying CNI-induced hypertension is vasoconstriction of renal and systemic vessels and, therefore, calcium channel blockers that do not interfere with CNI metabolism, such as amlodipine and nifedipine, are preferred over diltiazem or verapamil. Thiazide diuretics may be effective to treat volume overload. When a second agent is required, β-blockers such as atenolol can be added, but generally are less effective than amlodipine. In the early postoperative period angiotensin-converting enzyme (ACE) inhibitors and angiotensin II receptor blockers are not preferred due to their potential to aggravate hyperkalemia and renal dysfunction. Nevertheless, ACE inhibitors can be very effective in the long term, especially in patients with diabetes and/or proteinuria [36].

New-onset diabetes mellitus (DM) can be seen in approximately 15% of LT recipients [34]. HCV seropositivity and, in particular, the use of corticosteroids and CNIs (mainly tacrolimus) may predispose recipients to insulin resistance and glucose intolerance [37, 38]. Preexisting or new-onset DM is associated with an increased incidence of cardiovascular morbidity and mortality, infections, renal impairment, rejection episodes, and decreased graft survival. Corticosteroid withdrawal and switching from tacrolimus to the less diabetogenic drug cyclosporine can be effective [39]. Treatment does not differ from that for the nontransplant population. Lifestyle and diet modifications, including oral hypoglycemic agents and/or insulin administration, might be necessary. Sulfonylureas, such as glimepiride or glyburide, are preferred as the initial agent. In patients with renal dysfunction metformin is to be avoided because of the potential risk of developing lactic acidosis [36].

Cytomegalovirus and *Pneumocystis jirovecii* prophylaxis

An antiviral prophylactic regimen against cytomegalovirus (CMV) is essential in high-risk patients (CMV-positive donor for a CMV-negative recipient (D+/R–)) since CMV infection following LT is associated with poorer graft survival [40]. Other risk factors for CMV infection include the use of antilymphocyte antibodies and retransplantation. Several agents have been suggested for CMV prophylaxis although the recommended regimen in D+/R– patients is oral ganciclovir 5 mg/kg/day or valganciclovir 900 mg/day immediately after transplantation and continued for 3–6 months. These protocols reduce the risk of CMV disease in the recipient by 90–95% [41–43]. When prophylaxis is used in CMV-positive recipients (with either D+ or D–), 3 months of antiviral agents is recommended [43]. CMV infection

Table 44.4 Adverse effects of common immunosuppressive drugs.

Drug	Adverse effect									
	Hypertension	Diabetes	Nephrotoxicity	Neurotoxicity	Headaches	Hyperlipidemia	Hirsutism	Gingival hyperplasia	GI symptoms	Impaired wound healing
Tacrolimus	++	++	++	++	++	+	-	-	+	-
Cyclosporine	+++	+	+++	++	++	+	+	+	+	-
Corticosteroids	+++	+++	-	+	++	++	++	-	+	+
Mycophenolate	-	-	-	-	+	-	-	-	+++	+
Sirolimus	+	-	+	-	-	+++	-	-	+	+++

GI, gastrointestinal.

can be asymptomatic or manifest between 2 and 12 months after LT with one or more features of: mild increase in aminotransferases, leukopenia, thrombocytopenia, retinitis, pneumonitis, and diarrhea [40]. Diagnosis is made from tissue samples and/or blood (CMV DNA and/or CMV antigenemia). Liver biopsy findings include microabscesses, lobular hepatitis, and giant cells with viral inclusions. It is important to differentiate CMV hepatitis from ACR because treatment of CMV hepatitis involves the reduction of immunosuppression. CMV infection can also result from the reactivation of a prior infection in the recipient; in such cases, treatment again includes intravenous ganciclovir 5 mg/kg every 12 hours for 2–4 weeks with conversion to oral valganciclovir for completion of therapy [43].

Prior to the introduction of prophylactic regimens, the risk of *Pneumocystis* pneumonia (PCP) in LT recipients ranged from 5% to 15% [44]. Prophylaxis with trimethoprim-sulfamethoxazole (TMP-SMX) is effective in preventing PCP [45]. In patients with sulfa allergy or TMP-SMX intolerance, pentamidine or atovaquone are also effective. The length of time of prophylaxis is for 6–12 months after transplantation, coincident with the highest immunosuppression requirements and greatest risk of infection.

Another important objective while the patient is still in the transplant unit is education of the recipient and care giver with respect to the administration of medications over the long term, and proper health care practices. A member of the transplantation team should spend time instructing the patient and family about medication side effects, signs and symptoms of infection, rejection, diet, and general rules of medical care. Patients should also be instructed in the care of the surgical wound, T tube (if one is placed), and any drains that remain. This time can also be used to emphasize the importance of communication with the liver transplant center regarding unexpected clinical situations that may occur at home. A good knowledge of medications and health care issues is vital for a successful outcome over the long run.

Clinic visits

General management

Following discharge from the hospital after LT, patients must continue medical care in the transplant clinic. The frequency of visits varies among centers but it is mostly dictated by the patient's overall condition. Usually during the first 1–2 months, visits are weekly, twice a month thereafter, and monthly up to 1 year. During clinic visits, attention is paid to nutrition, diet, medical compliance, and overall health. Patients should continue to be monitored closely for signs of graft dysfunction and a continued low threshold for suspicion of rejection needs to be maintained. Any reportable abnormal result from hepatic biochemical tests, especially serum aminotransferases, should prompt a liver biopsy to rule out ACR or other causes of ALT or AST elevation such as HCV recurrence or CMV infection. Acute rejection episodes not diagnosed in time or refractory to treatment can lead to chronic rejection, which is characterized by the disappearance of small intrahepatic bile ducts and obliterative angiopathy (Table 44.5) [46]. Chronic rejection is an uncommon complication occurring mostly after 6 months of transplantation. Left untreated, chronic rejection can

Table 44.5 Grading of chronic allograft rejection.

Structure	Early chronic rejection	Late chronic rejection
Small bile ducts (<60 μm)	Degenerative changes involving a majority of ducts; eosinophilic transformation of the cytoplasm; increased N:C ratio; nuclear hyperchromasia; uneven nuclear spacing; ducts only partially lined by biliary epithelial cells	Degenerative changes in the remaining bile ducts
	Bile duct loss in <50% of portal tracts	Loss in ≥50% of portal tracts
Terminal hepatic venules and zone 3 hepatocytes	Intimal/luminal inflammation	Focal obliteration
	Lytic zone 3 necrosis and inflammation	Variable inflammation
	Mild perivenular fibrosis	Severe (bridging) fibrosis
Portal tract hepatic arterioles Other	Occasional loss involving <25% of portal tracts	Loss involving >25% of portal tracts
	So-called "transition" hepatitis with spotty necrosis of hepatocytes	Sinusoidal foam cell accumulation; marked cholestasis
Large perihilar hepatic artery branches	Intimal inflammation; focal foam cell deposition without luminal compromise	Luminal narrowing by subintimal foam cells; fibrointimal proliferation
Large perihilar bile ducts	Inflammation damage and focal foam cell deposition	Mural fibrosis

Reproduced from Demetris et al. [46] with permission from Plenum.

result in graft failure and the need for retransplantation. However, after retransplantation, the risk of recurrent chronic rejection can be as high 90% [47]. Monitoring of immunosuppression levels is necessary at every clinic visit. CNIs and mammalian target of rapamycin (mTOR) inhibitors (i.e., sirolimus) are metabolized by cytochrome P450 3A4 (CYP3A4). A large number of drugs are metabolized by CYP3A4 as well; thus, the possibility of drug–drug interactions exists, especially in the early post-transplant period when patients usually take a large number of medications (Box 44.1). A pharmacist particularly dedicated to the transplant program can help in sorting out the drug–drug interactions for the patients,

---

Box 44.1 Medications with significant interactions with calcineurin Inhibitors.[a]

Decreased CNI levels

Antibiotics
- Isoniazid
- Rifabutin
- Rifampicin

Anticonvulsants
- Carbamazepine
- Phenobarbital
- Phenytoin

Others
- St John's wort (herbal preparation)

Increased CNI levels

Antibiotics
- Azithromycin
- Clarithromycin
- Erythromycin

Antifungals
- Caspofungin
- Fluconazole
- Itraconazole
- Ketocanzole
- Voriconazole

Calcium channel blockers
- Diltiazem
- Nicardipine
- Verapamil

Others
- Atorvastatin
- Cisapride
- Grapefruit juice
- HIV protease inhibitors

[a]This is not a complete list. The pharmacy should be consulted for other drug–drug interactions.
CNI, calcineurin inhibitor; HIV, human immunodeficiency virus.

---

families, and heath care providers, and can help facilitate proper care.

Late surgical complications

Biliary tract complications are more frequent within the first 6 months following transplantation. Hyperbilirubinemia and GGT and/or AP elevation are usually early signs of biliary complications, and when clinically suspected a cholangiographic evaluation is indicated. If a T tube is still in place, cholangiography through the tube allows rapid diagnosis. ERCP or PTC not only permit diagnosis but potentially offer a therapeutic avenue as well. In cases where a Roux-en-Y anastomosis is performed, magnetic resonance retrograde cholangiopancreatography (MRCP) is being increasingly used. At this stage, biliary tract abnormalities include intra- or extrahepatic strictures and casts/sludge formation. First-line therapy of extrahepatic biliary strictures includes either ERCP or PTC balloon dilatation and stenting (Fig. 44.3). Surgical management with Roux-en-Y biliary reconstruction is reserved for patients who fail endoscopic or percutaneous therapy. Nonanastomotic strictures frequently develop secondary to vascular insufficiency; however in a small group the pathogenesis remains unclear. Known risk factors for nonanastomotic strictures include prolonged graft ischemia time, older donor age, recurrence of primary sclerosing cholangitis (PSC), and DCD organs [48,49]. Surgical therapy ranging from Roux-en-Y reconstruction to retransplantation may be required. Biliary stones and casts may develop late after LT, commonly presenting with cholangitis. Endoscopic treatment is usually effective in extracting stones but fails to treat biliary casts. Surgical treatment or even retransplantation may be required in such cases.

Complications of the hepatic vasculature can emerge late after LT. While early HAT has a fulminant presentation, late HAT often manifests in an indolent manner. Delayed HAT is a serious complication and patients can present with liver abscesses, bile leak or stricture, and recurrent cholangitis [50]. These patients might be eligible for vascular or biliary endoscopic treatment; however, as with early HAT, most of these patients will ultimately require retransplantation. Hepatic artery aneurysms are an infrequent complication commonly associated with fungal infections and can rupture with resultant intra-abdominal bleeding requiring surgical hepatic artery reconstruction. Portal vein thrombosis (PVT) is also an infrequent vascular complication of LT, occurring in 1–3% of the recipients [7]. As with HAT, PVT occurs primarily in the early postoperative period, but it can also manifest several months to years following transplantation. Common clinical manifestations include hepatic decompensation and complications of portal hypertension such as ascites and variceal hemorrhage. In contrast to HAT, PVT

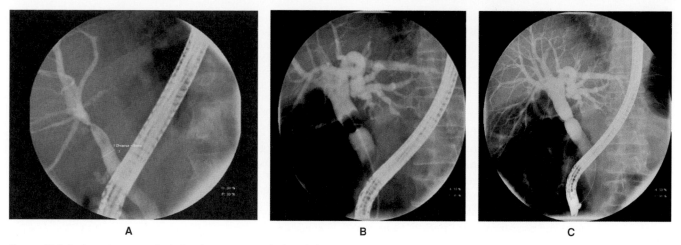

Figure 44.3 Endoscopic retrograde cholangiopancreatography (ERCP) showing an anastomotic biliary stricture at the choledochocholedochostomy (A), followed by dilatation (B) and stenting (C).

technically challenges retransplantation. Extensive PVT might involve the superior mesenteric vein as well, making retransplantation technically more difficult [7]. Treatment for PVT is recommended for symptomatic patients. If PVT occurs in the immediate postoperative period, reoperation and thrombectomy or vascular reconstruction yields excellent results. Direct repair of the portal vein in patients with chronic PVT is particularly difficult. Decompressive shunt surgery has been used with success; however, retransplantation may be required if the various nontransplant modalities fail to alleviate complications of portal hypertension [51].

Immunosuppresion-related complications

Special attention should be paid to the potential medical complications that can emerge following LT, most of which are related to long-term use of immunosuppression. Dyslipidemia develops in up to 47% of LT recipients [52,53]. Corticosteroids, cyclosporine, and especially mTOR inhibitors have a significant effect on serum lipid levels [36]. Lowering cholesterol is an important intervention to prevent long-term cardiovascular disease. As with nontransplant patients, implementing lifestyle modifications is the first-line treatment. If serum lipids remain elevated, pharmacologic therapy with "statins" can be safely initiated. Myopathy, hepatotoxicity, and rhabdomyolysis are uncommon side effects. In patients on CNIs, hydrophilic statins (i.e., fluvastatin, pravastatin) are preferred because they are not metabolized through CYP3A4 [53]. Switching from cyclosporine or mTOR inhibitor to tacrolimus can be considered if cholesterol level remains elevated. Bile acid sequestrants, fibrates, and nicotinic acid should be avoided because of their potential interference with other drugs. Preventing the development of atherosclerotic disease is essential in the transplant recip-

ients since cardiovascular disease is a significant cause of morbidity and mortality [54].

Early recurrent disease

Recurrence of the original liver disease is another important cause of graft dysfunction. Virtually all conditions for which a LT was done can recur; however, this is almost invariably seen with hepatitis C. HCV recurrence usually evolves during the first 6 months following LT and typically manifests with serum aminotransferase elevation. Histologic findings at times are similar to those of ACR and therefore distinction between these two entities may be challenging. A constellation of clinical and histologic features may help differentiate them, otherwise steroid boluses given for "diagnosed" ACR can promote fibrosis progression in the event the patient has recurrent HCV [55]. Importantly, there is a cholestatic variant of recurrent HCV characterized by extremely high HCV RNA levels and a cholestatic clinical picture. It occurs early in the post-transplant period in approximately 5% of transplanted patients with hepatitis C and generally results in graft failure [56]. Treatment remains uncertain; reducing immunosuppression and interferon therapy are usually ineffective. Most centers consider cholestatic HCV recurrence a contraindication for retransplantation. Reported recurrence rates for autoimmune hepatitis (AIH) after LT are approximately 20–40% [57,58]. Steroids, azathioprine, and/or mycophenolate mofetil have been successfully used to treat recurrent AIH [59]. Overall post-transplant recurrence rates of primary biliary cirrhosis can reach 50% and range from 10% to 27% for those transplanted for PSC [60,61]. Therapy with ursodeoxycholic acid in the post-transplant setting has not been defined although it is routinely used. Patients transplanted for hepatocellular carcinoma (HCC) that exceeded the Milan criteria and/or with vascular invasion present a higher risk of recurrence [62]. Periodic and often semiannual chest CT and liver magnetic resonance imaging is recommended for surveillance for recurrence. More commonly, HCC recurrence is diagnosed beyond 6 months post-transplant.

Cancer

All transplant recipients are at higher risk than the general population of developing de novo malignancies (i.e., hematologic, skin, lung, colon, genitourinary tract, and oropharynx) [63] or having a recurrence of previous cancers. Prolonged exposure to immunosuppressive therapy has been described as the main risk factor for developing malignancies in the post-transplant period. Skin cancers, especially squamous cell carcinoma, basal cell carcinomas, and melanoma, account for 39% of malignancies that develop after LT [64]. Although, the peak incidence of cutaneous malignancies is 3–5 years after organ transplantation, patients should always be instructed to use effective sunscreen, and an annual follow-up by a dermatologist is highly recommended. Post-transplant lymphoproliferative disorder (PTLD) occurs in about 2% of LT recipients and most cases develop during the first year after transplantation [65]. Early PTLD is usually associated with Epstein–Barr virus (EBV) reactivation or primary infection. Risk factors for PTLD in LT recipients are young age, pretransplant EBV naivety, and a high degree of immunosuppression [66,67]. Symptoms include fever, weight loss, malaise, and night sweats. First-line treatment consists of immunosuppression reduction while monitoring for allograft dysfunction. Patients who do not respond or are intolerant to this first step should be treated with rituximab or chemotherapy.

Long-term follow-up

Liver transplant recipients should always be motivated to continue medical follow-up. Preventive measures must be emphatically implemented by the transplant center and primary care physician. Transplanted patients should be encouraged to maintain routine dental care, and discontinue tobacco or cannabis smoking. Vaccines are recommended in the post-transplant setting, especially inactivated vaccines such as pneumococcus, influenza, and tetanus. Immunosuppressed patients overall have lower seroconversion rates. Most centers recommend against live-attenuated vaccines. Obesity is a major problem after transplantation and approximately a fifth of patients become obese within 2 years after LT [68]. Pretransplant obese patients tend to gain more weight after LT. Patients should be counseled about lifestyle modifications, including diet and exercise programs.

References

1. Bennett-Guerrero E, Feierman DE, Barclay GR, et al. Preoperative and intraoperative predictors of postoperative morbidity, poor graft function, and early rejection in 190 patients undergoing liver transplantation. *Arch Surg* 2001;136:1177–83.
2. Bronster DJ, Emre S, Boccagni P, et al. Central nervous system complications in liver transplant recipients – incidence, timing, and long-term follow-up. *Clin Transplant* 2000;14:1–7.
3. Lewis MB, Howdle PD. Neurologic complications of liver transplantation in adults. *Neurology* 2003;61:1174–8.
4. Johnson SR, Alexopoulos S, Curry M, et al. Primary nonfunction (PNF) in the MELD era: an SRTR database analysis. *Am J Transplant* 2007;7:1003–9.
5. Kemmer N, Secic M, Zacharias V, et al. Long-term analysis of primary nonfunction in liver transplant recipients. *Transplant Proc* 2007;39:1477–80.
6. Ploeg RJ, D'Alessandro AM, Knechtle SJ, et al. Risk factors for primary dysfunction after liver transplantation – a multivariate analysis. *Transplantation* 1993;55:807–13.
7. Duffy JP, Hong JC, Farmer DG, et al. Vascular complications of orthotopic liver transplantation: experience in more than 4,200 patients. *J Am Coll Surg* 2009;208:896–903; discussion 5.
8. Silva MA, Jambulingam PS, Gunson BK, et al. Hepatic artery thrombosis following orthotopic liver transplantation: a 10-year experience from a single centre in the United Kingdom. *Liver Transpl* 2006;12:146–51.
9. Flint EW, Sumkin JH, Zajko AB, et al. Duplex sonography of hepatic artery thrombosis after liver transplantation. *AJR Am J Roentgenol* 1988;151:481–3.
10. Glockner JF, Forauer AR, Solomon H, et al. Three-dimensional gadolinium-enhanced MR angiography of vascular complications after liver transplantation. *AJR Am J Roentgenol* 2000;174:1447–53.
11. Kayahan Ulu EM, Coskun M, Ozbek O, et al. Accuracy of multidetector computed tomographic angiography for detecting hepatic artery complications after liver transplantation. *Transplant Proc* 2007;39:3239–44.
12. Maruzzelli L, Miraglia R, Caruso S, et al. Percutaneous endovascular treatment of hepatic artery stenosis in adult and pediatric patients after liver transplantation. *Cardiovasc Intervent Radiol* 2010;33:1111–19.
13. Knechtle SJ, Kwun J. Unique aspects of rejection and tolerance in liver transplantation. *Semin Liver Dis* 2009;29:91–101.
14. Fishman JA. Infection in solid-organ transplant recipients. *N Engl J Med* 2007;357:2601–14.
15. Garcia S, Roque J, Ruza F, et al. Infection and associated risk factors in the immediate postoperative period of pediatric liver transplantation: a study of 176 transplants. *Clin Transplant* 1998;12:190–7.
16. Singh N, Paterson DL, Gayowski T, et al. Predicting bacteremia and bacteremic mortality in liver transplant recipients. *Liver Transpl* 2000;6:54–61.
17. Lebeau G, Yanaga K, Marsh JW, et al. Analysis of surgical complications after 397 hepatic transplantations. *Surg Gynecol Obstet* 1990;170:317–22.
18. Verdonk RC, Buis CI, Porte RJ, et al. Biliary complications after liver transplantation: a review. *Scand J Gastroenterol Suppl* 2006:89–101.
19. Geissler EK, Schlitt HJ. Immunosuppression for liver transplantation. *Gut* 2009;58:452–63.
20. Germani G, Pleguezuelo M, Villamil F, et al. Azathioprine in liver transplantation: a reevaluation of its use and a comparison with mycophenolate mofetil. *Am J Transplant* 2009;9:1725–31.
21. Davies SE, Portmann BC, O'Grady JG, et al. Hepatic histological findings after transplantation for chronic hepatitis B virus infection,

including a unique pattern of fibrosing cholestatic hepatitis. *Hepatology* 1991;13:150–7.

22. Todo S, Demetris AJ, Van Thiel D, et al. Orthotopic liver transplantation for patients with hepatitis B virus-related liver disease. *Hepatology* 1991;13:619–26.

23. Marzano A, Salizzoni M, Debernardi-Venon W, et al. Prevention of hepatitis B virus recurrence after liver transplantation in cirrhotic patients treated with lamivudine and passive immunoprophylaxis. *J Hepatol* 2001;34:903–10.

24. Angus PW, Patterson SJ. Liver transplantation for hepatitis B: what is the best hepatitis B immune globulin/antiviral regimen? *Liver Transpl* 2008;14(Suppl 2): S15–22.

25. Deschenes M, Belle SH, Krom RA, et al. Early allograft dysfunction after liver transplantation: a definition and predictors of outcome. National Institute of Diabetes and Digestive and Kidney Diseases Liver Transplantation Database. *Transplantation* 1998;66: 302–10.

26. Wiesner RH, Demetris AJ, Belle SH, et al. Acute hepatic allograft rejection: incidence, risk factors, and impact on outcome. *Hepatology* 1998;28:638–45.

27. Bartlett AS, Ramadas R, Furness S, et al. The natural history of acute histologic rejection without biochemical graft dysfunction in orthotopic liver transplantation: a systematic review. *Liver Transpl* 2002;8:1147–53.

28. Mells G, Neuberger J. Protocol liver allograft biopsies. *Transplantation* 2008;85:1686–92.

29. Demetris AJ, Batts KP, Dhillon AP, et al. Banff schema for grading liver allograft rejection: an international consensus document. *Hepatology* 1997;25:658–63.

30. Ormonde DG, de Boer WB, Kierath A, et al. Banff schema for grading liver allograft rejection: utility in clinical practice. *Liver Transpl Surg* 1999;5:261–8.

31. Neuberger J, Adams DH. What is the significance of acute liver allograft rejection? *J Hepatol* 1998;29:143–50.

32. Burton JR Jr, Rosen HR. Acute rejection in HCV-infected liver transplant recipients: the great conundrum. *Liver Transpl* 2006;12:S38–47

33. Fryer JP, Fortier MV, Metrakos P, et al. Central pontine myelinolysis and cyclosporine neurotoxicity following liver transplantation. *Transplantation* 1996;61:658–61.

34. Sheiner PA, Magliocca JF, Bodian CA, et al. Long-term medical complications in patients surviving > or − 5 years after liver transplant. *Transplantation* 2000;69:781–9.

35. Guckelberger O. Long-term medical comorbidities and their management: hypertension/cardiovascular disease. *Liver Transpl* 2009;15(Suppl 2): S75–8.

36. Desai S, Hong JC, Saab S. Cardiovascular risk factors following orthotopic liver transplantation: predisposing factors, incidence and management. *Liver Int* 2010;30:948–57.

37. Heisel O, Heisel R, Balshaw R, et al. New onset diabetes mellitus in patients receiving calcineurin inhibitors: a systematic review and meta-analysis. *Am J Transplant* 2004;4:583–95.

38. Saliba F, Lakehal M, Pageaux GP, et al. Risk factors for new-onset diabetes mellitus following liver transplantation and impact of hepatitis C infection : an observational multicenter study. *Liver Transpl* 2007;13:136–44.

39. Dumortier J, Bernard S, Bouffard Y, et al. Conversion from tacrolimus to cyclosporine in liver transplanted patients with diabetes mellitus. *Liver Transpl* 2006;12:659–64.

40. Limaye AP, Bakthavatsalam R, Kim HW, et al. Impact of cytomegalovirus in organ transplant recipients in the era of antiviral prophylaxis. *Transplantation* 2006;81:1645–52.

41. Hodson EM, Barclay PG, Craig JC, et al. Antiviral medications for preventing cytomegalovirus disease in solid organ transplant recipients. *Cochrane Database Syst Rev* 2005;1:CD003774.

42. Sampathkumar P, Paya CV. Management of cytomegalovirus infection after liver transplantation. *Liver Transpl* 2000;6:144–56.

43. Kotton CN, Kumar D, Caliendo AM, et al. International consensus guidelines on the management of cytomegalovirus in solid organ transplantation. *Transplantation* 2010;89:779–95.

44. Sepkowitz KA. Opportunistic infections in patients with and patients without acquired immunodeficiency syndrome. *Clin Infect Dis* 2002;34:1098–107.

45. Green H, Paul M, Vidal L, et al. Prophylaxis for Pneumocystis pneumonia (PCP) in non-HIV immunocompromised patients. *Cochrane Database Syst Rev* 2007;1:CD005590.

46. Demetris A, Adams D, Bellamy C, et al. Update of the International Banff Schema for Liver Allograft Rejection: working recommendations for the histopathologic staging and reporting of chronic rejection. An international panel. *Hepatology* 2000;31:792–9.

47. Neuberger J. Incidence, timing, and risk factors for acute and chronic rejection. *Liver Transpl Surg* 1999;5:S30–6.

48. Buis CI, Verdonk RC, Van der Jagt EJ, et al. Nonanastomotic biliary strictures after liver transplantation. Part 1: Radiological features and risk factors for early vs. late presentation. *Liver Transpl* 2007;13:708–18.

49. Maheshwari A, Maley W, Li Z, et al. Biliary complications and outcomes of liver transplantation from donors after cardiac death. *Liver Transpl* 2007;13:1645–53.

50. Gunsar F, Rolando N, Pastacaldi S, et al. Late hepatic artery thrombosis after orthotopic liver transplantation. *Liver Transpl* 2003;9: 605–11.

51. Krebs-Schmitt D, Briem-Richter A, Grabhorn E, et al. Effectiveness of Rex shunt in children with portal hypertension following liver transplantation or with primary portal hypertension. *Pediatr Transplant* 2009;13:540–4.

52. Gisbert C, Prieto M, Berenguer M, et al. Hyperlipidemia in liver transplant recipients: prevalence and risk factors. *Liver Transpl Surg* 1997;3:416–22.

53. Imagawa DK, Dawson S 3rd, Holt CD, et al. Hyperlipidemia after liver transplantation: natural history and treatment with the hydroxy-methylglutaryl-coenzyme A reductase inhibitor pravastatin. *Transplantation* 1996;62:934–42.

54. Pruthi J, Medkiff KA, Esrason KT, et al. Analysis of causes of death in liver transplant recipients who survived more than 3 years. *Liver Transpl* 2001;7:811–15.

55. Berenguer M, Prieto M, Cordoba J, et al. Early development of chronic active hepatitis in recurrent hepatitis C virus infection after liver transplantation: association with treatment of rejection. *J Hepatol* 1998;28:756–63.

56. Dixon LR, Crawford JM. Early histologic changes in fibrosing cholestatic hepatitis C. *Liver Transpl* 2007;13:219–26.

57. Duclos-Vallee JC, Sebagh M, Rifai K, et al. A 10 year follow up study of patients transplanted for autoimmune hepatitis: histological recurrence precedes clinical and biochemical recurrence. *Gut* 2003;52:893–7.

58. Molmenti EP, Netto GJ, Murray NG, et al. Incidence and recurrence of autoimmune/alloimmune hepatitis in liver transplant recipients. *Liver Transpl* 2002;8:519–26.

59. Salcedo M, Vaquero J, Banares R, et al. Response to steroids in de novo autoimmune hepatitis after liver transplantation. *Hepatology* 2002;35:349–56.

60. Duclos-Vallee JC, Sebagh M. Recurrence of autoimmune disease, primary sclerosing cholangitis, primary biliary cirrhosis, and autoimmune hepatitis after liver transplantation. *Liver Transpl* 2009;15(Suppl 2): S25–34.

61. Gautam M, Cheruvattath R, Balan V. Recurrence of autoimmune liver disease after liver transplantation: a systematic review. *Liver Transpl* 2006;12:1813–24.

62. Parfitt JR, Marotta P, Alghamdi M, et al. Recurrent hepatocellular carcinoma after transplantation: use of a pathological score on explanted livers to predict recurrence. *Liver Transpl* 2007;13: 543–51.

63. Watt KD, Pedersen RA, Kremers WK, et al. Long-term probability of and mortality from de novo malignancy after liver transplantation. *Gastroenterology* 2009;137:2010–17.

64. Herrero JI, Lorenzo M, Quiroga J, et al. De Novo neoplasia after liver transplantation: an analysis of risk factors and influence on survival. *Liver Transpl* 2005;11:89–97.

65. Opelz G, Dohler B. Lymphomas after solid organ transplantation: a collaborative transplant study report. *Am J Transplant* 2004;4:222–30.

66. Kremers WK, Devarbhavi HC, Wiesner RH, et al. Post-transplant lymphoproliferative disorders following liver transplantation: incidence, risk factors and survival. *Am J Transplant* 2006;6:1017–24.

67. Jacobson CA, LaCasce AS. Lymphoma: risk and response after solid organ transplant. *Oncology (Williston Park)* 2010;24:936–44.

68. Everhart JE, Lombardero M, Lake JR, et al. Weight change and obesity after liver transplantation: incidence and risk factors. *Liver Transpl Surg* 1998;4:285–96.

Multiple choice questions

44.1 Histopathologic diagnosis of acute cellular rejection includes all except which one of the following?

   a Subendothelial localization of inflammatory cells in portal vein branches.
   b Small bile ducts inflammation and damage.
   c Presence of lobular microabscesses.
   d Portal inflammatory infiltrate including lymphocytes, eosinophils, and neutrophils.

44.2 Common complications associated with graft loss in the first few weeks after liver transplantation include all of the following except which one?

   a Hepatic artery thrombosis (HAT).
   b Primary nonfunction of graft (PNF).
   c Acute cellular rejection (ACR).
   d Cytomegalovirus (CMV) infection.

44.3 Common complications associated with immunosuppressants include all of the following except which one?

   a Diabetes mellitus.
   b Hypertension.
   c Infections.
   d Parkinson disease.
   e Renal insufficiency.

Answers to the multiple choice questions can be found in the Appendix at the end of the book.

These multiple choice questions are also available for you to complete online.
Visit http://www.schiffsdiseasesoftheliver.com/

CHAPTER 45

Long-term Management of the Liver Transplant Patient

Timothy M. McCashland

Department of Hepatology, University of Nebraska Medical Center, Nebraska Medical Center, Omaha, NE, USA

Key concepts

- Preventive care is paramount in the liver transplant recipient and includes vaccination, dental care, and counseling to abstain from smoking.
- Common medical problems in the long-term liver transplant recipient include metabolic syndrome (obesity, hyperlipidemia, diabetes mellitus), osteoporosis, cardiovascular disease, and renal disease – all of which may result in increased morbidity and mortality.
- Technical-related problems of biliary complications may be corrected by endoscopic therapy. However, living related biliary complications are common both in the donor and recipient and require a multidiscipline team approach.

- Common causes of deaths in survivors of more than 1 year include development of de novo malignancy, cardiovascular causes, renal failure, and recurrent disease. Diligent surveillance for these diseases may lead to early detection and lower morbidity.
- Renal impairment is common in long-term survivors. The development of end-stage renal disease is reported up to 18%, with markedly decreased survival in these patients.
- Quality of life post liver transplantation is improved but many times does not reach the level of the general population

The traditional model of care in most transplant centers is for the transplant surgeon to manage the immediate postoperative care, with gradual incorporation of transplant hepatologists and primary care physicians [1,2]. With increasing success in liver transplantation, a major shift in the prevention and management of a patient's medical-related complications secondary to liver transplantation has become the principle management focus. Distinct differences exist among transplant centers as to who becomes the primary physician in charge of long-term management [3–5]. The majority of transplant centers rely on transplant hepatologists for the management of long-term care [3–5]. However, a recent study noted that transplant hepatologists support a shift toward incorporating primary care physicians as integral members of the transplant team to manage metabolic complications [5]. In actuality, this rarely happens and the transplant hepatologists are managing the patients. Transplant centers nevertheless do not favor primary care physicians managing immunosuppression, acute allograft rejection, recurrent disease, and biliary complications.

Several comprehensive reviews of medical complications and the management of liver transplant recipients have been published previously [6–10]. The American Society of Transplantation also has published guidelines for the long-term management of the liver transplant patient [11]. This chapter will address management of long-term care of the liver transplant patient divided into topics of quality of life, preventive care (vaccinations, dental care), metabolic complications (obesity, diabetes mellitus, cardiovascular disease, bone disease, gout), inflammatory bowel disease, renal dysfunction, transplant-related diseases (biliary complications, de novo neoplasia), and causes of death in long-term survivors,

Quality of life

The immediate goal of liver transplantation is to improve survival of the recipient. However, the secondary goal is to improve the quality of life (QOL) and return the patient to a productive life. Bownik and Saab provide a comprehensive review of this topic [12]. Health-related quality of life (HRQOL) is the measurement of a patient's self-assessment of their physical, functional, social and

Schiff's Diseases of the Liver, Eleventh Edition. Edited by Eugene R. Schiff, Willis C. Maddrey and Michael F. Sorrell.
© 2012 John Wiley & Sons, Ltd. Published 2012 by John Wiley & Sons, Ltd.

psychological health. A recent review of instruments used to assess QOL in the adult liver transplant population noted that generic assessment questionnaires are most common and include: the Medical Outcomes Study short form 36 (SF-36), the Hospital Anxiety and Depression Scale (HADS), and the Beck Depression Inventory (BDI) [13]. The SF-36 remains the most popular instrument and has advantage of being able to compare scores with the general population and those with chronic diseases. Interestingly, Saab et al. found that the model for end-stage liver disease (MELD) score was not predictive of HRQOL scores post transplant [14]. In contrast, Castaldo et al. noted improved physical HRQOL post transplant with increasing MELD scores [15]. Early studies with follow-up of less than 2 years noted liver recipients achieve very satisfactory levels of HRQOL in the mental and physical components [16–18]. However, the HRQOL levels were below that of the general population. A prospective multicenter study assessing pretransplant and post-transplant HRQOL using the SF-36 and EuroQol (EQ-5D) instruments with follow-up of 2 years showed a significant improvement in all dimensions of the SF-36 including the role emotion dimension and the EQ-5D scores [18]. Longer survival after transplantation, younger age, and patients from larger transplant centers were independent predictive variables of higher QOL scores. A cross-sectional study from Finland with exceptional follow-up discovered that liver transplant patients had slightly worse HRQOL than the general population, especially in those with increasing age and transplantation for acute liver failure [19]. Unfortunately, with longer follow-up sustained growth in HRQOL does not happen and in fact may decrease, especially in the mental health and role emotion/anxiety domains [20]. Painter et al. however showed that patients up to 5 years after transplant who participated in physical activity and had fewer comorbid conditions improved their HRQOL [21]. Desai et al. in a single center study evaluated QOL in patients 10–30 years post transplant. Patients had an overall good QOL, but reduced physical function was associated with age >60 years, female gender, post-transplant complications, and recurrent disease [22]. A meta-analysis by Bravata et al. on HRQOL concluded improvements in general health, physical health, daily activity function, and sexual function [23]. A more recent study incorporating 44 longitudinal studies and 19 studies using the SF-36 showed the general public had higher rating in physical functioning, role physical, role emotional, social functioning, energy, and general health than liver transplant patients [20]. Therefore, improvement in QOL may be overstated by previous studies. As for specific etiology of liver disease and decreased QOL, conflicting results have been reported. Cowling et al. noted no difference in QOL between Laennec versus non-Laennec patients with

follow-up to 5 years [24]. However, other studies found impaired lower global QOL and physical functioning in hepatitis C patients with recurrent disease [25].

Psychologic improvement after liver transplantation has also been shown to begin immediately after surgery. More recent long-term studies tend to show that depression coping skills, anxiety, and social environments are more relevant in liver transplant recipients' QOL than other somatic factors [26]. Not surprisingly, elevated levels of anxiety and neuroticism prior to transplant were associated with worse psychologic health after transplantation [27]. A concerning and interesting investigation by Lewis et al. using multiple tests in cognitive function in 36 patients 10 years after transplantation showed patients scored significantly lower than healthy controls across a wide range of cognitive functions [28]. Unfortunately the reason for this lower function is unknown and needs further study. Blanch et al., using the psychosocial-adjustment-to-illness scale, found that women had poorer adjustment to orthotopic liver transplantation (OLT) than men; the proportion of women with poor adjustment was higher (31.5% versus 16.7%) [26]. Women showed a greater dysfunction in health care orientation, sexual relations, extended family relationships, and psychologic distress. Therefore women may need more psychologic intervention after transplant than men. Thus, psychologic factors are important contributors to QOL issues in the long-term management of liver transplant recipients.

Return to employment after liver transplantation is achieved by 25–60% of patients within the first 6 months' post transplant [10]. Factors associated with return to work include younger age, better general health, pretransplant employment, private insurance, and higher physical conditioning [29].

Preventive care

As the concerns of allograft rejection and infections lessen in the patient with long-term survival after liver transplantation, the physician care giver still must be diligent in adherence to preventive care. This should include a yearly review of vaccinations, dental care, smoking history, and weight, and surveillance for bone disease and malignancy.

Vaccines

Influenza is a seasonal infection that disproportionately affects those who are immunocompromised. Harris et al. brought to light that solid organ transplant recipients unfortunately remain underimmunized against influenza [30]. Using a vaccine safety dataset from three large health maintence organization systems, 49% of pretransplant or post-transplant liver recipients were found to be vaccinated for influenza. Variables associated with higher rates of vaccinations included older age (odds ratio (OR), 1.8) and prior vaccination (OR, 4.5). Previously published studies reported influenza vaccination response in adult liver transplant recipients to be from 50% to 95% seroconversion [31,32]. Duchini et al. studied 20 post-transplant patients at baseline and 6 weeks after vaccination [33]. Side effects were well tolerated, but all had significantly lower titers than normal individuals.

Invasive pneumococcal disease has a 13-fold greater incidence in solid organ transplant recipients compared with the general population. We have previously reported on pneumococcccal vaccination before transplantation with post-transplantation follow-up. Antibody levels were equal to or less than baseline at 3 months' post transplantation [34]. The American Society of Transplantation has published guidelines recommending a single dose of pneumococcal polysaccharide vaccine, with an additional dose given 3–5 years later [35]. A very interesting recent study tried to enhance immunogenicity by priming the liver transplant recipient with a 7-valent pneumoccoccal conjugate vaccine followed by boosting with the standard 23-valent vaccine [36]. At 16 weeks' post vaccination, 86% and 91% of patients in primed and unprimed groups responded to the pneumococcal vaccines. Therefore, priming with conjugated vaccine did not improve the response rate. Thus, recipients should continue with a standard single dose of 23-valent vaccine with revaccination 3–5 years later.

Inactivated vaccines are safe to administer to liver transplant patients. These include hepatitis A and B, diphtheria, *Haemophilus influenza*, human papillomavirus, pertussis, pneumococcus, meningococcus, and tetanus. Investigators have shown that the licensed live attenuated varicella-zoster virus was well tolerated, with 87% developing humoral and cellular immunity in liver transplant pediatric patients [37].

In 1996, the Advisory Committee on Immunization Practices recommended all patients with chronic liver disease be vaccinated for hepatitis A virus (HAV). Unfortunately, some patients are not vaccinated pre transplant and may require the vaccine after transplant. A Mayo Clinic study of 39 patients evaluated HAV seroconversion rates at 1 and 7 months after the first dose, utilizing two standard doses given at 6 months apart [38]. Seroconversion rates were dramatically lower in the OLT patients compared to patients with chronic liver disease and healthy controls at 1 month (8% OLT versus 83% chronic liver disease versus 93% controls) and 6 months (21% versus 97% versus 98%).

Prevention of hepatitis B after liver transplantation is evolving. Strategies include short-term use of hepatitis B immunoglobulin (HBIg) and long-term use of nucleos(t)ide analog medications. Several investigators have tried hepatitis B vaccination as another alternative tactic [39,40]. Sanchez-Fueyo et al. in a pilot trial of recombinant HBV vaccine in liver transplant patients reported anti-hepatitis B surface (HBs) titers greater than 10 IU/L in 14 of 17 patients. The Berlin group evaluated antibody response to hepatitis B surface antigen (HBsAg) in 10 patients 2 years after transplantation [39]. In contrast to other studies, patients were continued on HBIg during the study. They additionally received 20 µg of recombinant HBV antigen with a novel adjuvant (monophosphoryl lipid A) at weeks 0, 2, 4, 16, and 18. Five of ten patients developed antibody titers greater than 500 IU/L. Others have reported markedly poorer results, even with the use of double doses (40 µg in up to 12 doses) [41]. Gunther et al. reported the results of using a double dose revaccination booster 2 years after the initial vaccination. After the booster vaccination anti-HBs titers increased significantly in all patients [42]. Regrettably, at this time use of vaccination as a sole means of protection has not proven to be the strategy of choice.

Recommendations

- Vaccinate patients prior to liver transplantation if possible for HAV, hepatitis B virus (HBV), and pneumococcus.
- Give a yearly influenza vaccination to liver transplant recipients.
- All personnel associated with care of liver transplant patients should receive an annual influenza vaccination.
- If a patient is unvaccinated for HAV prior to transplantation, consider vaccination post transplant.
- The discontinuation of passive immunoprophylaxis of HBIg with HBV vaccination has not become common practice.

Dental care

A common question asked in transplant programs is if antibiotic prophylaxis is needed with any dental care in liver transplant recipients. The American Heart Association does not recommend antibiotics, unless the patient has a high-risk condition of prior endocarditis, prosthetic valves, or congenital heart disease [43].

Metabolic complications

The metabolic syndrome is the constellation of diseases related to insulin resistance and increased risk of diabetes mellitus and cardiovascular diseases (Box 45.1) [44]. The prevalence of the metabolic syndrome in post liver transplant patients has jumped to the forefront in long-term management. Two comprehensive recent reviews eloquently describe the details and management of this

Box 45.1 Metabolic syndrome.

Defined by the presence of any three of the follow five characteristics:
- Abdominal obesity, which is defined as a waist circumference in men >102 cm (40 inches) and in women >80 cm (>35 inches)
- Serum triglycerides >150 mg/dL (1.7 mmol/L) or drug treatment for elevated triglycerides
- Serum high-density lipoprotein cholesterol <40 mg/dL (1 mmol/L) in men and <50 mg/dL (1.3 mmol/L) in women or drug treatment for low high-density lipoprotein cholesterol
- Blood pressure >130/85 mmHg or drug treatment for elevated blood pressure
- Fasting plasma glucose >100 mg/dL (5.6 mmol/L) or drug treatment for elevated blood glucose

common syndrome [45,46]. The prevalence of the metabolic syndrome in several studies has reported to be 45–58% [47,48]. Each component of the syndrome will be reviewed in detail.

Obesity

Weight gain is also common after liver transplantation. Studies have detailed that by 1 and 3 years' post transplantation, 24–60% of patients had a body mass index (BMI) of >30 kg/m^2 [49,50]. Predictive factors included age >50 years and a BMI >30 kg/m^2 before transplantation. Appetite stimulation from corticosteroids, change to a less restrictive diet, lack of exercise, and higher cumulative doses of prednisone lead to increased weight. Nair et al., using the Scientific Registry of Transplant Recipients database, assessed the morbidity and mortality in obese patients after liver transplantation [51]. Primary graft nonfunction and immediate, 1-year, and 2-year mortality were significantly higher in the morbidly obese group. Five-year mortality was higher in the severely obese (28%) and morbidly obese patients (27%) mainly due to infections and cardiovascular events. These results were confirmed by a more recent study using the United Network for Organ Sharing (UNOS) database [52]. In contrast, analysis of the National Institute of Diabetes and Digestive and Kidney Diseases Liver Transplantation database, when the BMI was corrected for ascites, showed similar patient and graft survival in obese patients when compared with those of normal weight [53]. These studies have led many centers to institute weight-restriction guidelines prior to liver transplantation. Bariatric surgery for morbid obesity remains minimally documented as only a small case report of two successful patients with steatohepatitis noted improvement [54].

Recommendations

- Patients should have yearly evaluation for weight gain and evaluation of immunosuppression.

- If obesity develops, the target weight loss should be approximately 0.5–1 kg/week (1–2 lb/week). This requires multiple clinical visits and the supervision of a nutritionist.

Hyperlipidemia

Hyperlipidemia is common after liver transplantation, with an incidence in up to 50–75% of patients post transplant [55]. Mixed hyperlipidemia (types 2a, 2b, and 4) with high cholesterol and triglyceride levels is the common pattern after transplantation. The etiology of hyperlipidemia is multifactoral [55]. Immunosuppressant medications, steroids, calcineurin inhibitors, and mammalian target of rapamycin (mTOR) inhibitors all can lead to elevations of total cholesterol, low-density lipoprotein cholesterol, and triglycerides. Steriods increase the secretion of very low-density lipoproteins (VLDLs) and the conversion of low-density lipoproteins (LDLs). Cyclosporine inhibits 26-hydroxylase, reducing the transport of cholesterol into bile, and binding to LDL receptors, increasing the levels of LDL cholesterol. Sirolimus use can result in severe dyslipidemia, especially hypertriglyceridemia, in liver transplantation [56]. The proposed mechanism of sirolimus-induced hyperlipidemia is thought to be related to elevated apoCIII levels, which inhibit lipoprotein lipase activity [57]. Use of the National Cholesterol Education Program (NCEP) III lipid guideline goals should be employed for liver transplant patients: total cholesterol <200 mg/dL, LDLs <100 mg/dL, high-density lipoproteins >60 mg/dL, and triglycerides <150 mg/dL [58]. Surprisingly, few data exist on the use of statins for hyperlipidemia in liver transplant patients. In a small study of 16 patients, cerivastatin and pravastatin decreased cholesterol by 21% and 15%, and LDLs by 27% and 17%, respectively [59]. Atorvastatin and ezetimibe have been shown to be safe in renal transplant patients [60,61]. One underlining concern has been the risk of myopathy with the use of statins and calcineurin inhibitors. This potential drug–drug interaction may theoretically be reduced with the use of pravastatin, which is not extensively metabolized by cytochrome P450 3A4 (CYP3A4). The usual starting doses of statins are simvastatin 40 mg/day, atorvastatin 40 mg/day, and pravastian 20 mg/day. The addition of fenofibrates and niacin for severe hypertriglycerides may be needed to reach target triglyceride goals.

Recommendations

- Patients should have an annual evaluation of total cholesterol, low-density lipoprotein, high-density lipoprotein, and triglyceride levels.
- Use NCEP III lipid guidelines for treatment.

Hypertension

Earlier hypertension studies within the first year noted hypertension ranging from 17% to 82% [62,63]. More recent studies using a standard definition of hypertension readings of greater than 140/85, reported that the incidence at 3 months was 82% in cyclosporine patients and 32% of tacrolimus patients; at 6 months 50% of patients were hypertensive [64]. In studies with longer follow-up, from 3 to 5 years after transplant, overall incidence was around 50%. Detailed analysis in the Rabkin et al. study noted 58% required a single antihypertensive agent, 29% required two agents, and 10% needed three agents [65]. Galioto et al. found that nifedipine was effective in only 22% of patients, whereas 33% of carvedilol-treated patients after liver transplant responded favorably [66]. In a large study, Neal et al. reported 46% of patients responded to amlodipine with a decrease in systolic blood pressure from 154 to 130 mmHg [67]. Those patients unresponsive or intolerant to amlodipine were randomized to bioprolol or lisinopril. Lisinopril was successful in 84% of patients, reducing the systolic blood pressure from 154 to 130 mmHg. Galioto and colleagues compared nifedipine (30–60 mg/day) and carvedilol (12.5–25 mg/day) in 50 patients post liver transplant for up to 1 year [68]. Monotherapy therapy was successful in 21% in nifedipine patients and 29% in carvedilol patients. Carvediol was better tolerated, and the addition of an angiotensin-converting enzyme (ACE) inhibitor increased response in 20% of the cases.

Recommendations

- The early treatment of hypertension incorporates the use of diuretics, clonidine, and calcium channel blockers followed by β-blockers and ACE inhibitors.
- The target blood pressure is <140/90 mmHg.
- ACE inhibitors, especially in patients with diabetes, are a good choice for the treatment of hypertension.

Diabetes

The incidence of new-onset diabetes mellitus (NODM) remains difficult to estimate due to discrepancies in diagnostic criteria and definitions in the post-transplant setting. However, a reasonable estimate would be around 25% within 3–6 months post transplant. Consensus guidelines on the definition of NODM after transplantation have been developed based on definitions from the American Diabetes Association, World Health Organization, and American College of Endocrinology [69]. Two recent comprehensive reviews detail this topic in detail [70,71].

Immunosuppressive medications are diabetogenic. Corticosteroids induce insulin resistance. Calcineurin inhibitors decrease insulin synthesis and secretion and induce insulin resistance [72]. Cyclosporine and tacrolimus appear to increase diabetic risk, although a systematic review of multiple studies noted a higher risk with tacrolimus [73]. Other immunosuppression medications including azathioprine, myophenolate mofetil, and sirolimus do not induce diabetes. In a large study comparing tacrolimus plus steroids to those receiving tacrolimus plus daclizumab (steroid free), the incidence of NODM was 15.3% versus 5.7% [74].

Several risk factors for the development of NODM after transplantation have been characterized: family history of diabetes, African-American or Hispanic race, age over 40 years, obesity, steroid-resistant rejection, hepatitis C, alcoholic cirrhosis, and male gender [71]. Hepatitis C is the leading indication for liver transplantation and, with its higher association of diabetes mellitus (both pre and post transplantation), a planned and concerted effort of management with immunosuppression and risk of accelerated fibrosis should be discussed.

An early study by John and Thuluvath from Johns Hopkins University found that 46/435 (10.5%) of post-transplant patients developed NODM, of which 18 patients were insulin dependent and 28 patients were treated by oral hypoglycemic medications [75]. Using the UNOS database, Yoo et al. found 7.6% were insulin-dependent diabetics and another 7.6% were noninsulin-dependent diabetics at 1 year after transplant [76]. A more recent study using the UNOS database from 2004 to 2008 reported an incidence of 26.4% NODM [77]. Independent predictors were age >50 years, African-American race, BMI >25 kg/m^2, donor age >60 years, diabetic donor, tacrolimus use, and steroid use at discharge. Conversely, Ahn and colleagues have shown that patients with younger age, longer time before development of NODM, non-hepatitis C virus (HCV) patients, and use of mycophenolate were factors that predicted reversal of NODM [78].

The overall impact of NODM on morbidity and mortality in liver transplantation recipients has had mixed results, but with longer follow-up a trend is developing toward worse outcomes. Khalili et al. reported that overall infectious episodes in the presence of diabetes were five-fold higher [79]. Higher morbidity in diabetic versus nondiabetic patients from cardiac (48% versus 24%), major infective (41% versus 25%), minor infections (28% versus 5%), neurologic (22% versus 9%), and neuropsychiatric (22% versus 6%) episodes were seen a Baltimore study [75]. A UNOS database study reported that 5-year patient survival was lower in patients with type 1 (insulin-dependent) diabetes compared with those without diabetes (63% versus 75%) [76]. Patients with diet-controlled diabetes had a minimally decreased 5-year survival compared with nondiabetics. Furthermore, patients with type 1 diabetes or coronary artery disease were 40% more likely to die within 5 years compared with those without these risk factors. In agreement, investigators from Miami in a large single center study confirmed that patients with sustained NODM had lower survival rates at 10 years (69% versus 78%) and higher rates of death due to infection (9.5% versus 4.3%) [80]. Veldt et al. added further concerns by illustrating that patients with hepatitis C and insulin resistance post transplant had a significantly higher probability of developing advanced fibrosis [81].

Scant information is available on the proper treatment of NODM in liver transplant patients. One study reported dismal management with less than 40% being referred to endocrinology and only 15% of patients having glycosylated hemoglobin level monitoring. Of those receiving treatment for NODM, 39% were on insulin and 39% were on oral antiglycemia medications, and 21% on both [82]. There are no studies in the transplant setting that show that tight glycemic control reduces morbidity and mortality. NODM usually resembles type 2 diabetes mellitus, thus a management approach of lifestyle modifications (weight control, exercise, proper diabetic diet) are the first line of treatment. The second step is the use of oral antidiabetic drugs with normal renal and graft function. For those still in poor control, the final management step is long-term insulin use in consultation with a diabetologist, consideration of altering the calcineurin inhibitor, and a minimal or steroid-free regimen.

Recommendations
- Standard immunosuppression is associated with a higher risk of NODM.
- The management of patients who develop NODM is similar to recommendations for patients with type 2 diabetes.
- Those with a hemoglobin A1C level >6.5% should start treatment.
- The initial treatment is lifestyle modifications (exercise, weight loss) and education (dietary and natural history).
- If glycemic control is unsuccessful with dietary modification, the use of oral diabetic agents may be considered.
- Insulin should be used if blood glucose levels do not fall below 120 mg/dL before meals or <160 mg/dL after meals.
- A liberal use of endocrinology consultation is recommended for patients difficult to control with consideration of altered immunosuppression.

Bone disease
Osteoporosis is characterized by reduced bone mass and altered architecture, increasing the risk of fracture, typically in the spine, hip, rib, or wrist areas. Risk factors pre transplantation include cholestatic liver disease, alcoholic liver disease, lower body weight, and older age [83].

Within 6 months' post transplantation, bone loss reaches the nadir of bone mass index with gradual recovery over years. Guichelaar et al. reported a gradual improvement of osteoporosis with follow-up 8 years post transplant [84]. Fractures are common in the high-risk group, most commonly in the hip, pelvis, spine, ribs, and wrist with frequently reported risks ranging from 5% to 35% [85]. Hardinger et al. from St Louis followed 153 patients over 10 years [86]. The prevalence of symptomatic fractures was 15% at a mean of 2.2 years' post transplantation. The only factor associated with risk of fracture was being female. Age, time from transplant, race, menopause, renal insufficiency, family history of osteoporosis, bone mineral density (BMD), and T score did not predict either osteoporosis or fractures after liver transplantation.

Immunosuppressive medications are also thought to contribute to osteoporosis. Glucocorticoids increase bone resorption by the inhibition of osteoblast activity even at low doses of less than 7.5 mg per day. A histomorphometric analysis of 33 patients after liver transplantation by the Mayo Clinic suggested that patients with tacrolimus therapy have an earlier recovery of bone formation and trabecular structure by 4 months compared with cyclosporine-treated patients [87]. Secondary causes of osteoporosis are common in patients with end-stage liver disease. They include hyperparathyroidism, hypogonadism, smoking, loop diuretics, low dietary calcium, and vitamin D deficiency (<30 ng/mL).

Treatment of osteoporosis after liver transplant has usually been reported in small uncontrolled series. A randomized, multicenter, Austalian, double blind trial compared infusions of zoledronic acid 4 mg versus placebo given within 7 days of transplantation and at 1, 3, 6, and 9 months. At 12 months, the BMD percentage of change in the treatment groups was +2–4% from baseline [88]. In contrast in a study from Austria, the use of prophylactic treatment with alendoronate, calcium, and vitamin D prevented further bone loss in the first 4 months after liver transplant. Continued use lead to increased BMD during up to 48 months of study [89].

Two comprehensive reviews by Crippin and Compston provide excellent guidelines on the management of bone disease in liver transplant patients [90,91].

Recommendatons
- Pretransplant evaluation should be done with a dual-energy X-ray absorptiometry (DEXA) bone scan and serum tests of calcium, phosphorous, parathyroid hormone, testosterone (men), estradiol (women), and 25-hydroxyvitamin D levels.
- All patients should be treated with 1500 mg of calcium per day and any deficiencies corrected.
- Vitamin D deficiency should be corrected to a serum 25-hydroxyvitamin D level of >30 ng/mL.

- If severe osteoporosis is noted by a T score >2 SD below normal, then consider starting oral bisphosphanates.
- Those under treatment for osteoporosis should have yearly DEXA scans, measurement of calcium, phosphorous, 25-hydroxyvitamin D levels, and a check of thyroid function.

Inflammatory bowel disease

Conflicting results have been published on the prevalence and severity of inflammatory bowel disease (IBD) after liver transplantation [92]. Differences may be attributed to variations in immunosuppression and/or maintenance IBD medications, duration of IBD, and length of follow-up. IBD can be either the exacerbation of preexisting disease or de novo disease. Haagsma et al., in a single center study, reported 36% of patients with pre-OLT IBD experienced excerbations at a median of 1 year after transplant [93]. Additionally, 11% of patients developed de novo IBD, with risks of 4% (3 years), 11% (5 years), and 14% (10 years) after transplantation. Interestingly, none of the patients were continued on IBD medications such as aminosalicylates. A study from Nebraska reviewed 40 patients with IBD [94]. Recurrence of IBD was seen in 65% of these patients post transplant with 16% having flares that responded poorly to medical management and required colectomy. De novo IBD developed in eight patients. Overall cumulative risk for IBD was 15%, 39%, and 54% at 1, 5, and 10 years post transplant. De novo IBD has been associated with CMV infection, CMV mismatch, and transplantation of autoimmune hepatitis. Risk factors for the exacerbation of preexisting IBD post transplantation include the use of tacrolimus, active disease at transplantation, a long duration of disease, and early discontinuation of steroids. Most transplant centers now continue specific IBD medications along with immunosupressants. From a different perspective, Dvorchik from Pittsburgh analyzed 303 patients to look at the risk of colectomy after transplantation in patients with inflammatory bowel disease [95]. Twenty-two patients (7%) had a colectomy due to refractory disease in follow-up to 12 years post transplant. Surprisingly, only OLT was the significant risk factor for colectomy (hazard ratio (HR), 3.1).

Patients with primary sclerosing cholangitis (PSC) and IBD may have an increased risk of developing colorectal cancer after liver transplantation. Vera et al. from Birmingham, UK studied 82 patients with PSC and IBD to identify risk factors for colorectal cancer [96]. Colorectal cancer developed in 9.6% of these patients with a mean interval between liver transplantation and cancer of 46 months (21–68 months). The cumulative risk of developing colorectal cancer was 14% and 17%, 5 and 10 years after transplantation. Multivariate analysis identified three variables significantly related to colorectal cancer: dysplasia post transplant, duration of colitis for more than 10 years, and pancolitis. When all three variables were present the risk of colorectal cancer was 100% within 5 years post transplant. Proctocolectomy and ileal pouch–anal anastomosis for severe ulcerative colitis after liver transplantation has been reported in several small case series with excellent outcomes, and a slightly higher rate of prouchitis [97].

Recommendations
- Maintenance use of IBD medications after transplantation (i.e., aminosalicylates) is recommended.
- Patients transplanted for PSC should have yearly colonoscopy with surveillance biopsies.
- If dysplasia is found, colectomy is warranted.

Renal dysfunction

The development of renal dysfunction is becoming more of a major problem after liver transplantation coupled with greater long-term patient survival. Renal dysfunction in relationship to liver transplantation was recently reviewed by a multidisciplined group [98]. Calcineurin inhibitor (CNI) medications (cyclosporine and tacrolimus) remain the cornerstone of immunosuppression in liver transplantation; however, they remain the principle cause of renal dysfunction. A decrease in glomeruloar filtration rate of 30–50% within 6 months after transplantation is commonly seen [99]. Renal biopsies in those with chronic renal failure (CRF) associated the CNIs demonstrate interstitial fibrosis, tubular atrophy, arteriolar hyalinosis and sclerosis, and collapse of the glomeruli.

The incidence of CRF and end-stage renal disease (ESRD) after liver transplantation has been variably described, likely due to differences in definition, method of measurement, and duration of follow-up. The most frequently cited early study, by Gonwa et al. from Dallas, studied 834 patients with a follow-up of up to 13 years after liver transplant using a definition of CRF of serum creatinine >2.5 mg/dL [100]. The incidence of ESRD gradually rose from 1.6% at year 1 to 3% at year 5 and 9.5% at year 13; the total incidence of severe renal dysfunction (CRF + ESRD) at year 13 was 18.1%. A significant difference in the development of CRF and ESRD was seen in patients with pretransplant hepatorenal syndrome (HRS) compared to those without (HRS group: CRF, 8%, ESRD, 11%; versus non-HRS group: CRF, 4%, ESRD, 4%). Postoperative 1-year, 3-month, and 4-week serum creatinine levels were predictive of CRF and ESRD. Additionally, a profound difference in survival

(27% versus 71%) was noted by year 6 after transplant in patients who developed ESRD on chronic hemodialysis compared with those who received a kidney transplant. The sentinel study by Ojo et al. using registry data of transplant recipients in the United States found a 5-year risk of chronic kidney disease (glomerular filtration rate (GFR), 15–29 mL/min/1.73 m^2) at 18% in liver transplant patients [101]. Risk factors associated with CRF included advanced age, female sex, pretransplantation hepatitis C infection, hypertension, diabetes mellitus, and postoperative acute renal failure. Those that developed CRF had a five-fold greater risk of death compared with those without CRF. This study concluded that an enormous financial burden of treatment of ESRD in this population is likely in the future, if not currently. Patients who proceed to liver transplantation with HRS present a complex decision regarding the potential of renal function recovery. Patient who have been on renal replacement for more than 8 weeks due to HRS prior to transplantation will likely benefit with a combined liver–kidney transplant for long-term survival [102]. This conclusion was validated in a study of renal replacement treatment (RRT) pre transplantation and long-term results [103]. Only 11% of patients with RRT for >90 days before the transplant recovered renal function, and for those who did not recover renal function their survival was only 38% at 1 year post transplant.

What can be done to reduce this risk of CRF in liver transplant recipients? Marotta described three strategies: reduction or withdrawal of CNIs by addition of an adjuvant agent, conversion of CNI to non-CNI therapy (sirolimus/everolimus + mycophenolate mofetil (MMF)), and lastly antibody induction with delayed CNI therapy [104]. A reduction of CNIs by up to 75% and the addition of MMF led to an improvement in GFR at 1 year from 59 to 64 mL/min in a recent study [105]. In a study comparing two immunosuppression groups – those started and continued on a CNI versus those started on a CNI in combination with MMF [106] – the decrease in GFR was less in the MMF group when compared with the CNI alone group (at 3 years: –15% versus –33%, respectively). Conversion from a CNI to everolimus (mTOR inhibitor) resulted in renal function improvement; however, side effects of hyperlipidemia and proteinuria were of concern [107]. Lastly, induction therapy with daclizumab and MMF followed by delayed administration up until the fifth day post transplantation with lower dose tacrolimus was studied in a mulicenter, prospective, randomized trial compared with groups given immunosuppression of tacrolimus and corticosteroids and MMF and reduced dose tacrolimus and corticosteroids. The estimated GFR decrease at 1 year post liver transplantation was –13.6 mL/min in the induction/delayed dose tacrolimus group versus –23.6 mL/min in the tacrolimus/corticosteroid group versus –21.2 mL/min in the MMF/reduced dose tacrolimus/corticosteroid group [108]. The optimum strategy to prevent or reduce renal dysfunction remains a difficult task in liver transplantation. New immunosuppression agents will have to be discovered as CNIs continue to be the leading cause of CRF. In the United States, the number of combined liver–kidney transplantations over the last 10 years has increased by 279% (from 100 to 379) [109]. The most likely reasons for the increase in kidney transplantation are acute renal failure and HRS associated with end-stage liver disease. Those with a combined liver–kidney transplantation had a survival of 85% at 1 year.

Recommendations

- Those with a known high risk of development of CRF should be considered for nontraditional immunosuppression and careful monitoring.
- Consider a CNI-free immunosuppression regimen for patients who develop renal insufficiency.
- If progressive renal dysfunction is seen, evaluation by ultrasound and consultation by nephrology is warranted.
- Kidney transplantation offers a significant survival difference compared to chronic dialysis. Therefore patients should be counseled regarding these differences.

Transplant-related diseases

Biliary complications

Biliary tract complications remain a common postoperative complication after liver transplantation and three excellent recent review articles discuss this topic in detail [110–112]. Liver transplantation is associated with postoperative biliary complications such as biliary strictures, leaks, sludge, stone casts, mucoceles, biloma, hemobilia, and sphincter of Oddi dysfunction [112]. Endoscopic or interventional radiologic treatment is now the standard of care, replacing initial management of bile duct complications with surgical revision. The two most common categories of biliary complications are strictures (anastomotic and nonanastomotic) and leaks (T tube, anastomotic, cut edge). In addition, stricture or leaks can be classified as early (<30 days) or late and they may be associated with hepatic artery thrombosis. Risk factors for the development of biliary complications after transplantation are shown in Box 45.2. Leaks may be associated with T-tube migration or T-tube removal. Poor healing of the choledochocholedochostomy anastomosis can also result in stricturing. The use of T tubes is rapidly declining. Living-related transplantation has been reported to double biliary complications due to the challenging technical

Box 45.2 Risk factors for biliary complications.

- Roux-en-Y anastomosis
- Ischemia/reperfusion
- T tube
- Duct mismatch size
- Cytomegalovirus infection
- Hepatic artery thrombosis
- ABO mismatch
- Non-heart-beating donor
- Primary sclerosing cholangitis
- Chronic ductopenic rejection
- Older age donor
- Prolonged cold ischemic time donor
- Prolonged warm ischemic time

reconstruction of either a Roux-en-Y hepaticojejunostomy or duct-to-duct anastomosis [110]. The challenge can be an inability to traverse the stricture, complex anastomosis, or sharp angulation or "crane neck" deformed bile ducts.

Patients typically present with elevations of serum aminotransferase, bilirubin, and alkaline phosphatase. Fevers, pruritus, and right upper abdominal pain are frequent symptoms. Diagnosis of biliary complication may be made by endoscopic retrograde cholangiopancreatography (ERCP), percutaneous transhepatic cholangiogram (PTC), or more recently magnetic resonance cholangiopancreatography (MRCP). The Barcelona group verified in a group of 63 patients that MRCP made the correct diagnosis of biliary complication in 91% of patients with a sensitivity of 95% and positive predictive value of 97% [113]. However, with a high incidence of abnormal findings many physicians proceed directly to ERCP with PTC reserved for unsuccessful endoscopic cases.

Overall, biliary stricture rates of 4–15% are reported for deceased donor liver transplantation and in living related transplantation of up to 30% [112]. Anastomosis strictures most often require three to five endoscopic interventions with progressively larger dilatations/stents with long-term success rates of 70–100% in OLT, but with a 25% lower success rate in living related transplantation [112]. Nonanastomotic strictures are more difficult to treat than anastomositic strictures. Only 50–70% of patients have long-term success with dilatation and stent placement and require the use of PTC more often and have a higher risk of graft loss.

Leaks are equally common (4–11%), with anastomic or T-tube leaks occurring early after transplantation. Endoscopic cholangiography with biliary sphincterotomy and stent placement are universally used, with successful outcomes of over 90% [111].

Recommendations

- Diagnosis of biliary complication may be obtained by ERCP, PTC, or MRCP.
- Biliary strictures are treated with dilatation and the placement of progressively larger stents for longer periods (>6 months).
- Biliary leaks are treated with biliary stents (usually <6 weeks' duration).
- Living related donor transplantation biliary complications requires a multidiscipline team approach.

De novo malignancy

Transplant recipients are at risk for development of de novo malignancies due to multiple factors including etiology of liver disease, viral infection, inflammatory bowel disease, behavior, age, and immunosuppression exposure. The overall risk of malignancy is two to four times higher than an age- and sex-matched population [114]. Unfortunately, more than 30% of late deaths in liver transplant recipients are due to de novo malignancy [115]. The most frequently diagnosed cancers are non-melanoma skin cancer, post-transplant lymphoproliferative disease (Epstein–Barr virus (EBV) driven), colorectal cancer, lung cancer, oropharyngeal cancer, Kaposi sarcoma, and urologic tumors. Breast, cervical, and prostate cancers seem to have similar rates as found in the general population [115]. The relative risk of neoplasia in this patient population is illustrated in Table 45.1. Earlier studies showed that liver transplant recipients have a high rate of lymphoma occurrence. These are commonly EBV-driven lymphomas, predominately of B-cell origin. Higher risks of oropharyngeal and lung cancers are noted in patients transplanted for alcoholic cirrhosis and who smoke. Watt et al. have provided the most recent comprehensive study of long-term probability and mortality of de novo malignancy after

Table 45.1 Relative risks of de novo malignancy after liver transplantation.

Malignancy	Relative risk
Skin (basal/squamous)	20–70
Lymphoma	10–30
Kaposi sarcoma	100
Head and neck	4–7
Lung	1.5–2.5
Colorectal overall	3–12
Colorectal in ulcerative colitis	25–30
Kidney	5–30
Hepatocellular	3.5
Breast	1
Prostate	1
Cervical	1

transplantation using a multicenter dataset with greater than 10-year follow-up [116]. One hundred and seventy-one patients were studied, who developed 271 malignancies (147 skin, 92 solid organ, and 29 hematologic). Patients transplanted for primary sclerosing cholangitis (22% at 10 years) and alcoholic liver disease (18% at 10 years) had the highest risks. Risk factors for de novo malignancy were age by decade (HR, 1.33), history of smoking (HR, 1.6), PSC (HR, 2.5), and alcoholic liver disease (HR, 2.1). The long-term prognosis was extremely poor for solitary organ cancers, with death rates at 1 year of 40% and 55% at 5 years after diagnosis.

The role of immunosuppression influence on de novo malignancy remains uncertain. Antilymphocyte antiglobulin therapy increases lymphoproliferative disorders and azathiprine may increase cutaneous cancers. The risk of de novo cancers with newer immunosuppressant medications such as mycophenolate or rapamycin remains unknown, but may lower the risk due to its antiproliferative effects. However, Toso et al., using the Scientific Registry of Transplant Recipients, evaluated maintenance immunosuppression for at least 6 months comparing sirolimus versus CNI in patients transplanted for hepatocellular carcinoma [117]. Anti-CD25 antibody induction and sirolimus-based maintenance therapy was associated with higher survival due to lower hepatocellular carcinoma recurrence in this study.

Screening recommendation strategies have not been studied in this population and recommendations are inferred by screening of the general public. However, an alarming study reported only 40% of patients had dermatologic and oral examinations or mammograms within 2 years of transplant [118]. Eleven percent had a gynecologic examination in the follow-up period and only 50% had either sigmoidoscopy or colonoscopy.

Recommendations
- Patients should cease smoking and using alcohol.
- Similar screening protocols to those used in the general population should be utilized.
- There should be an annual examination for skin cancer and the use of sunscreen lotion of SP 50 or greater when exposed to sunlight.
- Mammograms and gynecological evaluation should be biannual for women.
- A yearly measurement of prostate-specific antigen in males more than 50 years of age is recommended
- Patients transplanted for alcoholic cirrhosis may benefit from an annual examination of the mouth and throat combined with a chest X-ray.
- Patients with inflammatory bowel disease must have annual colonoscopy with surveillance biopsies for dysplasia. Colonoscopy every 5–10 years for liver trans-

plant recipients without inflammatory bowel disease is recommended.

Causes of mortality

The most comprehensive recent study evaluating the long-term causes of death was analyzed by Watt et al. noting a shift at more than 1 year post transplant: 28% hepatic, 22% malignancy, 11% cardiovascular, 9% infectious, and 6% renal related [119]. Risk factors for a higher risk of death beyond 1 year were age in decades (HR, 1.23), diabetes prior to liver transplant (HR, 1.48), renal dysfunction (HR, 3.59), cholangiocarcinoma (HR, 3.22), hepatocellular carcinoma (HR, 1.79), and retransplantation (HR, 4.79). This study illustrated the shift in hepatic- and renal-related deaths as main causes of late mortality. The authors proposed that diligent medical management of diabetes, hypertension, and renal insufficiency, treatment of viral hepatitis, and improved immunosuppression may impact long-term mortality.

In summary, with a longer survival of patients after transplant there are more frequent complications related to medical, immunosuppression, and surgical treatment of these patients. However, the quality of life appears to improve in the long-term survivor. Common complications secondary to the transplantation procedure include the development of de novo malignancy and metabolic syndrome (cardiovascular disease or diabetes) and these require annual evaluations and surveillance to prevent or lower the risk of morbidity or mortality. Renal dysfunction appears to be increasing with often dire consequences.

References
1. Weisner RH, Martin P, Stribling R. Post-transplant care/medical complications. In: Norman D, Suki W, eds. *Primer on Transplantation.* Thorofare, NJ: American Society of Transplantation, 1998:343–62.
2. O'Grady JG, Williams R. Postoperative care: long-term. In: Maddrey WC, Sorrell MF, eds. *Transplantation of the Liver*, 2nd edn. East Norwolk, CT: Appleton and Lange, 1998:207–24.
3. McCashland T. Posttransplantation care: role of the primary care physician versus transplant center. *Liver Transpl* 2001;7(Suppl 1): S2–12.
4. Shiffman ML, Rockey DC. Role and support for hepatologist at liver transplant programs in the United States. *Liver Transpl* 2008;14: 1092–9.
5. Heller JC, Prochazka AV, Everson GT, Forman LM. Long-term management after liver transplantation: primary care physicians versus hepatologist. *Liver Transpl* 2009;15:1330–5.
6. Zetterman RK, McCashland TM. Long-term follow-up of the orthotopic liver transplantation patient. *Semin Liver Dis* 1995;15:173–80.
7. Munoz SJ. Long-term management of the liver transplant recipient. *Med Clin North Am* 1996;80:1103–20.
8. Reich D, Rothstein K, Manzarbeitia C, et al. Common medical disease after liver transplantation. *Semin Gastrointest Dis* 1998;9: 110–25.

9. Liu LU, Schiano TD. Long-term care of the liver transplant recipient. *Clin Liver Dis* 2007;11:397–416.

10. Mells G, Neuberger J. Long-term care of the liver allograft recipient. *Semin Liver Dis* 2009;29:102–20.

11. McGuire BM., Rosenthal P, Brown CC, et al. Long-term management of the liver transplant patient: recommendations for the primary care doctor. *Am J Transplant* 2009;9:1988–2003.

12. Bownik H, Saab S. Health-related quality of life after liver transplantation for adult recipients. *Liver Transpl* 2009;15:S42–9.

13. Jay CL, Butt Z, Ladner DP, et al. A review of quality of life instruments used in liver transplantation. *J Hepatol* 2009;51:949–59.

14. Saab S, Ibrahim AB, Shpaner A, et al. MELD fails to measure quality of life in liver transplant candidates. *Liver Transpl* 2005;11:218–23.

15. Castaldo ET, Feurer ID, Russell RT, Pinson W. Correlation of health-related quality of life after liver transplantation with the model for end-stage liver disease score. *Arch Surg* 2009;144:167–72.

16. Caccamo L, Azara M, Doglia M, et al. Longitudinal prospective measurement of the quality of life before and after liver transplantation among adults. *Transplant Proc* 2001;33:1880–1.

17. Telles-Correia D, Barbosa A, Mega I, et al. When does quality of life improve after liver transplantation? A longitudinal prospective study. *Transplant Proc* 2009;41:904–5.

18. Ratcliffe J, Longworth L, Young T, et al. Asessing health related quality of life pre and post liver transplantation: a prospective multicenter study. *Liver Transpl* 2002;8:262–70.

19. Aberg F, Rissanen AM, Sintonen H, et al. Health-related quality of life and employment status of liver transplant patients. *Liver Transpl* 2009;15:64–72.

20. Tome S, Wells JT, Said A, Lucey MR. Quality of life after liver transplantation. A systematic review. *J Hepatol* 2008;48:567–77.

21. Painter P, Krasnoff J, Paul SM, et al. Physical activity and health-related quality of life in liver transplantation. *Liver Transpl* 2001;7:213–19.

22. Desai R, Jamieson NV, Gimson AE, et al. Quality of life up to 30 years following liver transplantation. *Liver Transpl* 2008;14:1473–9.

23. Bravata DM, Olkin I, Barnato AE, et al. Health-related quality of life after liver transplantation: a meta-analysis. *Liver Transpl Surg* 1999;5:318–31.

24. Cowling T, Jennings LW, Jung GS, et al. Comparing quality of life following liver transplantation for laennec's versus non-laennec's patients. *Clin Transpl* 2000;14:115–20.

25. De Bona M, Panton P, Emani M, The impact of liver disease and medical complications on quality of life and psychological distress before and after liver transplantation. *J Hepatol* 2000;33:609–15.

26. Blanch J, Sureda B, Flavia M, et al. Psychosocial adjustment to orthotopic liver transplantation in 266 recipients. *Liver Transpl* 2004;10:228–34.

27. Nickel R, Wunsch A, Enle UT, et al. The relevance of anxiety, depression, and coping in patients after liver transplantation. *Liver Transpl* 2002;8:63–71.

28. Lewis MB, Howdle PD. Cognitive dysfunction and health-related quality of life in long-term liver transplant survivors. *Liver Transpl* 2003;9:1145–8.

29. Rongey C, Bambha K, Vanness D, et al. Employment and health insurance in long-term liver transplant recipients. *Am J Transplant* 2005;5:1901–8.

30. Harris K, Baggs J, Davis RL, et al. Influenza vaccination coverage among adult solid organ transplant recipients at three health maintence organizations 1995–2005. *Vaccine* 2009;27:2335–41.

31. Burbach G, Bienzle U, Stark K, et al. Influenza vaccination in liver transplant recipients. *Transplantation* 1999;67:753–5.

32. Soesman NMR, Rimmelzwaan GF, Nieuwkoop NJ, et al. Efficacy of influenza vaccination in adult liver transplant recipients. *J Med Virol* 2000;61:85–93.

33. Duchini A, Hendry M, Nyberg LM, et al. Immune response to influenza vaccine in adult liver transplant recipients. *Liver Transpl* 2001;7:311–13.

34. McCashland T, Preheim L, Gentry-Nielsen MJ. Pneumococcal vaccine response in cirrhosis and liver transplantation. *J Infect Dis* 2000;181:757–60.

35. Guidelines for vaccination of solid organ transplant candidates and recipients. *Am J Transplant* 2004;4(Suppl 10):160–3.

36. Kumar D, Chen MH, Wong G, et al. A randomized, double-blind, placebo-controlled trial to evaluate the prime-boost strategy for pneumococcal vaccination in adult liver transplant recipients. *Clin Infect Dis* 2008;47:885–92.

37. Weinberg A, Horslen SP, Kaufman SS, et al. Safety and immunogenicity of varicella-zoster virus vaccine in pediatric liver and intestine transplant recipients. *Am J Transplant* 2006;6:565–568.

38. Arslan M, Wiesner R, Poterucha J, et al. Safety and efficacy of hepatitis A vaccination in liver transplantation recipients. *Transplantation* 2001;72:272–6.

39. Sanchez-Fueyo A, Rimola A, Grande L, et al. Hepatitis B immunoglobulin discontinuation followed by hepatitis B virus vaccination; a new strategy in the prophylaxis of hepatitis B virus recurrence after liver transplantation. *Hepatology* 2000;31:496–501.

40. Bienzle U, Gunther M, Neuhaus R, et al. Successful hepatitis B vaccination in patients who underwent transplantation for hepatitis B virus-related cirrhosis: preliminary results. *Liver Transpl* 2002;8:562–4.

41. Rosenau J, Hooman N, Hadem J, et al. Failure of hepatitis B vaccination with conventional HBsAg vaccine in patients with continuous HBIG prophylaxis after liver transplantation. *Liver Transpl* 2007;13:367–73.

42. Gunther M, Neuhaus R, Bauer T, et al. Immunization with an adjuvant hepatitis B vaccine in liver transplant recipients: antibody decline and booster vaccination with conventional vaccine. *Liver Transpl* 2006;12:316–19.

43. Wilson W, Taubert Ka, Gewitz M, et al. Prevention of infective endocarditis: guidelines from the American Heart Association: a guideline from the American Heart Association Rheumatic Fever, Endocarditis and Kawasaki Disease Committee, Council on Cardiovascular Disease in the Young, and the Council on Clinical Cardiology, Council on Cardiovascular Surgery and Anesthesia and Quality of Care and Outcomes Research Interdisciplinary Working Group. *J Am Dent Assoc* 2007;138:739–45.

44. Ford ES, Giles Wh, Dietz Wh. Prevalence of the metablic syndrome among US adults: findings from the third National Health and Nutrition Examination Survey. *JAMA* 2002;287:356–9.

45. Charlton M. Obesity, hyperlipidemian and metabolic syndrome. *Liver Transpl* 2009;15:S83–9.

46. Pagadala M, Dasarathy S, Eghtesad B, McCullough A. Posttransplant metabolic syndrome: an epidemic waiting to happen. *Liver Transpl* 2009;15:1662–70.

47. Laryea M, Watt KD, Molinari M, et al. Metabolic syndrome in liver transplant recipients; prevalence and association with major vascular events. *Liver Transpl* 2007;13:1109–14.

48. Bianchi G, Marchesini G, Marzocchi R, et al. Metabolic syndrome in liver transplantation; relation to etiology and immunosuppression. *Liver Transpl* 2008;14:1648–54.

49. Richards J, Gunson B, Johnson J, et al. Weight gain and obesity after liver transplantation. *Transplant Int* 2005;18:461–6.

50. Munoz SL, Deems RO, Moritz MJ, et al. Hyperlipidemia and obesity after orthotopic liver transplantation. *Transplant Proc* 1991;21:1480–3.

51. Nair S, Verma S, Thuluvath P. Obesity and its effect on survival in patients undergoing orthotopic liver transplantation in the United States. *Hepatology* 2002;35:105–9.

52. Dick AAS, Spitzer AL, Seifert CF, et al. Liver transplantation at the extremes of the body mass index. *Liver Transpl* 2009;15:968–77.

53. Leonard J, Heimbach JK, Malinchoc M, et al. The impact of obesity on long-term outcomes in liver transplant recipients-results of the NIDDK liver transplant database. *Am J Transplant* 2008;8:667–72.

54. Duchini A, Brunson ME. Rou-en-Y gastric bypass for recurrent non-alcoholic steatohepatitis in liver transplant recipients with morbid obesity. *Transplantation* 2001;72:156–9.

55. Munoz SJ. Hyperlipidemia and other coronary risk factors after orthotopic liver transplantation: pathogenesis, diagnosis and management. *Liver Transpl Surg* 1995;1(Suppl 1):S29–38.

56. Trotter J, Wachs M, Trouillot T, et al. Dyslipidemia during sirolimus therapy in liver transplant recipients occurs with concomitant cyclosporine but not tacrolimus. *Liver Transpl* 2001;7:401–8.

57. Hoogeveen R, Ballantyne C, Pownall H, et al. Effect of sirolimus on the metabolism of ApoB100-containing lipoproteins in renal transplant patients. *Clin Transplant* 2001;72:1244–50.

58. Lipsy RJ. The National Cholesterol Education Program Adult Treatment Panel III. *Circulation* 2002;106:3143–421.

59. Zachoval R, Gerbes A, Schwandt P, et al. Short-term effects of statin therapy in patients with hyperlipoproteinemia after liver transplantation: results of a randomized cross-over trial. *J Hepatol* 2001;35:86–91.

60. Taylor PJ, Kubler PA, Lynch SV, et al. Effect of atorvastatin on cyclosporine pharmacokinetics in liver transplant recipients. *Ann Pharmacother* 2004;38:205–8.

61. Kohnle M, Pietruck F, Kribben A, et al. Ezetimibe for the treatment of uncontrolled hypercholesterolemia in patients with high-dose statin therapy after renal transplantation. *J Transplant* 2006;6:205–8.

62. Guckelberger O, Bechstein WO, Neuhaus R, et al. Cardiovascular risk factors in long-term follow-up after orthotopic liver transplantation. *Clin Transplant* 1997;11:60–5.

63. Johnson SD, Morris JK, Cramb R, et al. Cardiovascular morbidity and mortality after orthotopic liver transplantation. *Transplantation* 2002;73:901–6.

64. Neal D, Brown M, Wilkinson I, et al. Mechanisms of hypertension after liver transplantation. *Transplantation* 2005;79:935–40.

65. Rabkin J, Corless C, Rosen H, et al. Immunosuppression impact on long-term cardiovascular complications after liver transplantation. *Am J Surg* 2002;183:595–9.

66. Galioto A, Angeli P, Guarda S, et al. Comparison between nifedipine and carvedilol in the treatment of de novo arterial hypertension after liver transplantation; preliminary results of a controlled clinical trial. *Transplant Proc* 2005;37:1245–7.

67. Neal D, Brown M, Wilkinson I, et al. Hemodynamic effects of amlodipine, bisoprolol and lisinopril in hypertensive patients after liver transplantation. *Transplantation* 2004;77:748–66.

68. Galioto A, Semplicini A, Zanus G, et al. Nifedipine versus carvedilol in the treatment of de novo arterial hypertension after liver transplantation: results of a controlled clinical trial. *Liver Transpl* 2008;14:1020–8.

69. Davidson J, Wilkinson A, Dantal J, et al. New-onset diabetes after transplantation; 2003 international consensus guidelines. *Transplantation* 2003;75(Suppl 1):S3–24.

70. Marchetti P. New-onset diabetes after liver transplantation from pathogenesis to management. *Liver Transpl* 2005;11:612–20.

71. Pageeaux GP, Faure S, Bouyabrine H, et al. Long-term outcomes of liver transplantation; diabetes mellitus. *Liver Transpl* 2009;15(Suppl 2):S79–82.

72. Alejandro R, Feldman E, Bloom A, et al. Effects of cyclosporine on insulin and C-peptide secretion in healthy beagles. *Diabetes* 1989;38:698–703.

73. Heisel O, Heisel R, Balshaw R, et al. New onset diabetes mellitus in patients receiving calcineurin inhibitors: a systematic review and meta-analysis. *Am J Transplant* 2004;4:583–95.

74. Boillot O, Mayer DA, Boudjema K, et al. Corticosteroid-free immunosuppression with tacrolimus following induction with daclizumab: a large randomized clinical study. *Liver Transpl* 2005;11:61–7.

75. John P, Thuluvath P. Outcome of patients with new-onset diabetes mellitus after liver transplantation compared with those without diabetes mellitus. *Liver Transpl* 2002;8:708–13.

76. Yoo H, Thuluvath P. The effect of insulin-dependent diabetes mellitus on outcome of liver transplantation. *Transplantation* 2002;74:1007–12.

77. Oufroukhi L, Kamar N, Muscari F, et al. Predictive factors for post-transplant diabetes mellitus within one year of liver transplantation. *Transplantation* 2008;85:1436–42.

78. Ahn HY, Cho YM, Yi NJ, et al. Reversibility of posttransplantation diabetes mellitus following liver transplantation. *J Korean Med Sci* 2009;24:567–70.

79. Khalili M, Lim J, Bass N, et al. New onset diabetes mellitus after liver transplantation; the critical role of hepatitis C infection. *Liver Transpl* 2004;10:349–55.

80. Moon JI, Barbeito R, Faradji RN, et al. Negative impact of new-onset diabetes mellitus on patient and graft survival after liver transplantation: long-term follow up. *Transplantation* 2006;82:1625–8.

81. Veldt BJ, Poterucha JJ, Watt KD, et al. Insulin resistance, serum adipokines and risk of fibrosis progression in patients transplanted for hepatitis C. *Am J Transplant* 2009;9:1406–13.

82. Saliba F, Lakehal M, Pageaux GP, et al. Risk factors for new-onset diabetes mellitus following liver transplantation and impact of hepatitis C infection: an observational mulicenter study. *Liver Transplant* 2007;13:136–44.

83. Stein E, Ebeling P, Shane E. Post-transplantation osteoporosis. *Endocrinol Metab Clin North Am* 2007;36:937–63.

84. Guichelaar M, Kendall R, Malinchoc M, Hay JE. Bone mineral density before and after OLT: long-term follow-up and predictive factors. *Liver Transpl* 2006;12:1390–402.

85. Ebling PR. Approach to the patient with transplantation-related bone loss. *J Clin Endocrinol Metab* 2009;94:1483–90.

86. Hardinger K, Ho B, Schnitzler M, et al. Serial measurements of bone density at the lumbar spine do not predict fracture risk after liver transplantation. *Liver Transpl* 2003;9:857–62.

87. Guichelaar M, Malinchoc M, Sibonga J, et al. Immunosuppressive and postoperative effects of orthotopic liver transplantation on bone metabolism. *Liver Transpl* 2004;10:638–47.

88. Crawford BA, Kam C, Pavlovic J, et al. Zoledronic acid prevents bone loss after liver transplantation. *Ann Intern Med* 2006;144:239–48.

89. Millonig G, Graziadei IW, Eichler D, et al. Alendronate in combination with calcium and vitamin D prevents bone loss after orthotopic liver transplantation: a prospective single-center study. *Liver Transpl* 2005;11:960–6.

90. Crippin JS. Bone disease after liver transplantation. *Liver Transpl* 2001;7(Suppl 1):S27–35.

91. Compston JE. Osteoporosis after liver transplantation. *Liver Transpl* 2003;9:321–30.

92. Hampton D, Poleski M, Onken J. Inflammatory bowel disease following solid organ transplantation. *Clin Immunol* 2008;128:287–93.

93. Haagsma E, Van den Berg A, Kleibeuker J, et al. Inflammatory bowel disease after liver transplantation; the effect of different

immunosuppressive regimens. *Aliment Pharmacol Ther* 2003;18: 33–44.

94. Verdonk RC, Dijkstra G, Haagsma EB. Inflammatory bowel disease after liver transplantation: risk factors for recurrence and de novo disease. *Am J Transplant* 2006;6:1422–9.

95. Dvorchik I, Subotin M, Demetris A, et al. Effect of liver transplantation on inflammatory bowel disease in patients with primary sclerosing cholangitis. *Hepatology* 2002;35:380–4.

96. Vera A, Gunson B, Ussafoff V, et al. Colorectal cancer in patients with inflammatory bowel disease after liver transplantation for primary sclerosing cholangitis. *Transplantation* 2003;75:1983–8.

97. Rowley S, Candinas D, May AD, et al. Restorative proctocolectomy and pouch anal anastomosis for ulcerative colitis following orthotopic liver transplantation. *Gut* 1995;37:845–7.

98. Charlton MR, Wall WJ, Ojo AO, et al. Report of the First International Liver Transplantation Society expert panel consensus conference on renal insufficiency in liver transplantation. *Liver Transpl* 2009;15:S1–34.

99. Gonwa T, Klintmalm G, Levy M, et al. Impact of pretransplant renal function on survival after liver transplanatation. *Transplantation* 1995;59:361–5.

100. Gonwa T, Mai M, Melton L, et al. End-stage renal disease (ESRD) after orthotopic liver transplantation (OLTX) using calcineurin-based immunotherapy. *Transplantation* 2001;72:1934–9.

101. Ojo A, Held P, Port F, et al. Chronic renal failure after transplantation of a nonrenal organ. *N Engl J Med* 2003;349:931–40.

102. Eason JD, Gonwa TA, Davis CL, et al. Proceedings of consensus conference on simultaneous liver kidney transplantation. *Am J Transplant* 2008;8:2243–51.

103. Northup PG, Argo CK, Bakhru MR, et al. Pretransplant predictors of recovery of renal function after liver transplantation. *Liver Transpl* 2010;16:440–6.

104. Marotta PJ. Renal-sparing protocols in liver transplantation. *Liver Transpl* 2009;15:S14–16.

105. Dale C, Marotta P. Continuous improvement in measured GFR with tapering CNI and the introduction of MMF in liver transplant recipients. *Can J Gastroenterol* 2008;22:44–5.

106. Kari-Guigues S, Janus N, Saliba F, et al. Long-term renal function in liver transplant recipients and impact of immunosuppressive regimens (calcineurin inhibitors alone or in combination with mycophenolate mofetil): the TRY study. *Liver Transpl* 2009;15:1083–91.

107. De Simone P, Carrai P, Precisi A, et al. Conversion to everolimus monotherapy in maintenance liver transplantation: feasibility, safety, and impact on renal function. *Transpl Int* 2009;22:279–86.

108. Neuberger JM, Mamelok RD, Neuhaus P, et al. Delayed introduction of reduced-dose tacrolimus, and renal function in liver transplantation: the ReSpECT study. *Am J Transpl* 2009;9:327–36.

109. Thuluvath PJ, Guidinger MK, Fung JJ, et al. Liver transplantation in the United States, 1999–2008. *Am J Transpl* 2010;10(Part 2):1003–19.

110. Sharma S, Gurakar A, Jabbour N. Biliary strictures following liver transplantation: past, present and preventive strategies. *Liver Transpl* 2008;14:759–69.

111. Londono M, Balderramo D, Cardenas A. Management of biliary complications after orthotopic liver transplantation: the role of endoscopy. *World J Gastroenterol* 2008;14:493–7.

112. Williams ED, Draganov PV. Endoscopic management of biliary strictures after liver transplantation. *World J Gastroenterol* 2009;15: 3725–33.

113. Valls C, Alba E, Cruz M, et al. Biliary complications after liver transplantation: diagnosis with MR cholangiopancreatography. *AJR Am J Roentgenol* 2005;184:812–20.

114. Herrero JI. De novo malignancies following liver transplantation: impact and recommendations. *Liver Transpl* 2009;15:S90–4.

115. Penn I. Post-transplantation de novo tumors in liver allograft recipients. *Liver Transpl Surg* 1996;2:52–9.

116. Watt KDS, Pedersen RA, Kremers WK, et al. Long-term probability of and mortality from de novo malignancy after liver transplantation. *Gastroenterology* 2009;137:2010–17.

117. Toso C, Merani S, Bigam DL, et al. Sirolimus-based immunosuppression is associated with increased survival after liver transplantation for hepatocellular carcinoma. *Hepatology* 2010;51:1237–43.

118. Zeldin G, Maygers J, Klein A, et al. Vaccination, screening for malignancy, and health maintenance of the liver transplant recipient. *J Clin Gastroenterol* 2001;32:148–50.

119. Watt KDS, Pedersen RA, Kremers WK, et al. Evolution of causes and risk factors for mortality post-liver transplant: results of the NIDDK long-term follow-up study. *Am J Transpl* 2010;10:1420–7.

CHAPTER 46

The Liver Transplant Procedure

Bijan Eghtesad & John J. Fung

Department of General Surgery, The Cleveland Clinic, Cleveland, OH, USA

Key concepts

- The transplant operation has been standardized in the past 25 years. However, technical refinements continue to be introduced.
- The biliary anastomosis remains the Achilles heel of the recipient operation.
- Donor graft shortage remains a critical issue. Extended criteria donors have been increasingly utilized.

- Major complications after liver transplantation include: primary nonfunction, portal vein thrombosis, bleeding, hepatic artery thrombosis, and hepatic outflow obstruction.
- Biliary complications continue to be a major problem with an incidence of about 15–20%.

Orthotopic liver transplantation (LTX) has become an accepted means for the treatment of end-stage liver disease (ESLD). Although the technique of LTX has been refined to a relatively standardized approach, the operation still remains a formidable surgical challenge. As such, LTX is associated with numerous potential surgical complications, in which the recipient's pretransplant condition, anatomy, and diagnosis, as well as donor and immunologic factors, may all contribute. These risks can be minimized by fully appreciating anomalous anatomic variations, performing appropriate ABO matching, size matching of the donor liver to the recipient habitus, adequate maintenance of donor liver function, attention to organ procurement, and minimization of cold ischemic time. The purpose of this chapter is to review the operative procedure and to highlight some of the more important intraoperative and early and late postoperative complications.

Historical background

Although attempts at orthotopic liver transplantation were performed in large animals as early as 1956 [1], the technical aspects of the operation, including the critical need for portal-venous blood flow, were elucidated by Thomas Starzl in 1960 [2] prior to the first attempt at clinical LTX in 1963 [3]. The 3-year-old boy with biliary atresia ultimately died of hemorrhage and coagulopathy.

This was followed by six more unsuccessful LTXs in Denver, Boston, and Paris [3–5]. The poor outcomes of the first human LTX attempts resulted in a moratorium that extended into the summer of 1967 when a child finally underwent successful LTX in Denver [6]. This was followed in 1968 by the opening of a LTX unit in Cambridge, United Kingdom by Roy Calne [7]. The first 33 LTX, of which 25 were performed in Denver and four in Cambridge, were later described in 1969 in a book entitled *Experience in Hepatic Transplantation* [8].

Terminology

Orthotopic LTX replaces the removed liver with the transplanted allograft liver in the anatomically correct position. Heterotopic LTX places the liver allograft in an extrahepatic site, usually at the root of the mesentery, but is of historical significance only due to poor outcomes. Auxiliary LTX is the placement of the donor liver in the presence of the native liver. Such transplants can be either orthotopic, after removal of part of the native liver, or heterotopic, with placement of a portion of the donor liver in a heterotopic position.

Segmental LTX places only a portion of the donor liver into the recipient – this utilizes a reduced size liver allograft, sometimes referred to as a "technical variant" liver allograft. The source of segmental grafts can be cadaveric, living donor, or both (in the case of dual donor segmental

Schiff's Diseases of the Liver, Eleventh Edition. Edited by Eugene R. Schiff, Willis C. Maddrey and Michael F. Sorrell.
© 2012 John Wiley & Sons, Ltd. Published 2012 by John Wiley & Sons, Ltd.

transplants). In the case of cadaveric segments, the graft can be a split liver graft, where the cadaveric whole liver is reduced to one or two smaller grafts. In each case, the segmental allograft maintains its own venous drainage, portal-venous inflow, hepatic artery inflow, and biliary drainage. In practice, these structures must be partitioned in a way so as to maximize the likelihood of survival, but this entails added risk compared with a whole cadaveric graft. Living donor segmental LTX is similar to split livers in terms of technical issues and complications.

Donor considerations

As noted above, the source for donor organs can be from living donors or deceased donors. The nuances of options in both are complex; for example, living donor allografts can be segmental (as noted above) or whole grafts (in the case of a domino liver transplant). The options for sources of liver allografts will differ according to the age and size of the recipient, diagnosis, geographic location, waiting list size, and technical expertise. The use of a living donor segmental graft (living adult-to-child left lateral segment) for a pediatric recipient was first successfully reported by the transplant team from Brisbane, Australia in 1989 [9]. The adoption of this innovative approach, along with other technical variant livers, to addressing the organ shortage in the pediatric ESLD population has significantly reduced waiting list deaths in this historically high mortality while-waiting group with outcomes that match those of using whole pediatric grafts [10]. However, with the increasing mortality in adult candidates, the development of living adult-to-adult lobar donation has generated greater interest due to a potentially larger beneficiary pool. The principal concern is the demand for a larger volume of functional transplanted liver and the added technical skill and experience needed to minimize the substantially greater risk to the donor and recipient. Since the first report of an adult-to-adult living donor lobar liver transplant in Japan [11], an increasingly clearer assessment of the risk to the donor, using a standardized approach to the collection and categorization of complications, has been achieved.

In spite of dependence on the use of living donors in many parts of Asia, the overwhelming contribution of liver allografts in Europe and North and South America are from deceased donors. The majority of livers are from brain-dead donors (referred to as donation after brain death or DBD), although the use of classic, nonheart-beating donors (currently referred to as donation after cardiac death or DCD) is increasing. For DBD, following the declaration of death and consent for donation, careful management of donor physiologic parameters optimizes allograft function and thus recipient outcomes fol-

lowing LTX. The goal is to maintain adequate circulation, oxygenation, and metabolism prior to organ procurement [12]. This can be difficult in the face of cardiac instability, neurogenic shock, volatile intravascular fluid status, loss of the normal hormonal milieu, and depletion of high-energy stores for liver function.

As the number of waiting list patients exceeds the number of livers available for transplantation, the utilization of donors that in the past were not considered has been reassessed. An "expanded criteria donor" (ECD) is one in whom certain characteristics impart either real or perceived short- and/or long-term risks to the recipient. In particular, efforts have focused on identifying and defining ECDs [13]. Although there is no universally accepted definition of an ECD liver, the following is a brief list of some possible characteristics of an expanded criteria liver donor:

- A medical history of systemic malignancy in the donor, particularly lung, central nervous system, and melanoma.
- A predonation course of hemodynamic instability, reflected by high donor serum sodium and high levels of vasopressor use.
- Serologic and molecular evidence of active viral infection, e.g. rabies, West Nile virus.
- Evidence of less than optimal liver function prior to surgical recovery, including liver biopsy findings of steatosis.
- Adverse intraoperative recovery events, including iatrogenic surgical injury during procurement.
- Advanced donor age.
- Cause of death other than traumatic.

Donor operation

The key to successful LTX starts with the procurement of an optimally functioning donor liver allograft. In general, maximizing the number of organs procured and transplanted for each donor, while maintaining optimal function of those organs, is the goal to donor management and selection. Since wide exposure to the abdominal and thoracic organs is required, as well as access to the aorta and the provision of sufficient venous venting, a long midline incision, including median sternotomy, is generally preferred and allows for inspection of all organs that are to be procured (Fig. 46.1). The decision regarding the division of the vasculature should be decided prior to procurement and must be coordinated with the multiorgan donor team to prevent conflicts during the actual procedure.

As the basic principle of current organ preservation is as rapid as possible exsanguination and core cooling at the time of circulation cessation, early access to the

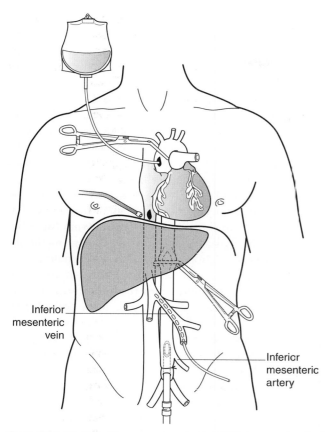

Inferior mesenteric vein

Inferior mesenteric artery

Figure 46.1 Classic multiorgan procurement in a DBD donor as described by Starzl et al. [14]. (Reproduced from Starzl et al. [14] with pemission from Elsevier.)

aorta (infrarenal aorta for abdominal organs and arch of the aorta for thoracic organs) is critical, particularly in an unstable patient or when immediate procurement is necessary. Simultaneously, preparing a site for venting of the venous blood and preservation solution can be achieved by preparing the vena cava for transection. The type of preservation solution has evolved, initially from lactated Ringer solution, to Collins solution, to University of Wisconsin solution (Viaspan®), to histidine-ketogluterate-tryptophan (Custodial®) and others, which has extended preservation times while maintaining optimal structural and metabolic functions of the liver. In addition, the practice of meticulous in vivo dissection has given way to more rapid techniques, designed to shorten the time in the operating room, reducing the risk of hemodynamic instability and bleeding and increasing the likelihood of multiorgan utilization. This is particularly important in situations where rapid exsanguination and core cooling is necessary in an uncontrolled fashion, e.g., DCD donors.

Once the liver is visualized and the decision is made to move forward with procurement, the liver is separated from its ligamentous attachments by division of the falci-

form, round, and triangular ligaments. At this point, the insertion of the diaphragmatic crux should be divided, exposing the celiac trunk and aorta. The aorta should be encircled at this point to allow for clamping to optimize flushing of abdominal organs. Care should be given before division of the hepatogastric ligament – inspection of the arterial supply of the liver can be performed at this time, paying close attention to anatomic variants, such as an accessory or aberrant right hepatic artery from the superior mesenteric artery (10% incidence) or an accessory left hepatic artery from the left gastric artery (13% incidence). In addition, after identification of the gastroduodenal artery, a trial clamp should be performed before division, in the event that there is significant celiac stenosis due to atherosclerotic disease or from median arcuate ligament syndrome, in which case the gastroduodenal artery should not be transected until aortic perfusion is completed. The gallbladder is incised and irrigated and the distal common bile duct is transected close to the pancreatic head. The aorta is encircled above the iliac artery bifurcation and cannulated. Some centers will choose to cannulate the inferior mesenteric vein at this point for simultaneous portal-venous perfusion. At this point, the liver is ready for exsanguination. Shortly before infusion of preservation solution, a dose of 300–500 U/kg of heparin should be given intravenously. Immediately before the infusion of preservation solution, the aorta at the diaphragmatic crux should be clamped and cold preservation solution infused under some pressure. The vena cava should be transected, either through an incision in the abdominal vena cava or immediately above the diaphragm (depending on whether thoracic organs are to be procured or not). If the heart is to be procured, cardioplegia infusion is started simultaneously. Ice-cold saline slush, prepared earlier, is then used topically to cool the organs in situ. After the allotted amount of preservation solution is used, the organs are then removed in order of heart, lungs, liver/pancreas/intestine, and finally kidneys. The organs are then placed into separate basins and further divided, characterized, and bagged for transport. It is usual practice to send a segment of donor iliac or carotid artery and donor iliac vein, in case of the need for alternative revascularization (see below).

Recipient operation

The technique of LTX has been progressively refined since its introduction in humans in 1963, with several variations that are applied selectively according to the patient's specific situation and/or the transplant center's routine practice. The initially described conventional LTX involves resection of the recipient native liver (hepatectomy) along with the retrohepatic inferior vena cava (IVC) and a short anhepatic phase, followed by the implantation of a whole deceased donor liver graft with the interposed donor IVC. Restoration of venous continuity during the implantation is achieved by an upper subdiaphragmatic and a lower suprarenal end-to-end donor-to-recipient IVC anastomosis. The donor-to-recipient portal vein and hepatic artery anastomoses are also performed in an end-to-end fashion. The biliary continuity is reestablished using either a primary duct-to-duct technique or the performance of a hepaticojejunostomy.

Hepatectomy

The "standard incision" for LTX has historically been a bilateral subcostal incision with an upper midline extension to the xiphoid (sometimes called an inverted Y or Mercedes incision) (Fig. 46.2). Other incisions have been used, however the principle in determining the type of incision is to gain adequate exposure to the liver and to other intra-abdominal structures, such as the infrarenal aorta, should the need arise. The type of incision is of paramount importance and choosing the wrong incision can make the operation difficult. The presence of previous incisions may require modifications to the planned incision in order to avoid flap necrosis from devascular-

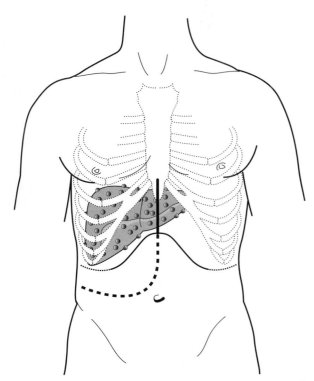

Figure 46.2 Types of incisions utilized in liver transplantation, classically utilizing a bilateral subcostal incision with an upper midline incision. Alternatively, a bilateral subcostal incision without an upper midline incision, or right subcostal with an upper midline extension, can be utilized.

ization. In the case of preceding surgery in the LTX recipient, particular attention must be paid upon entering the abdominal cavity, as the presence of vascular adhesions can lead to both significant blood loss and/or violation of the gastrointestinal tract.

Usually, the hepatectomy is the most difficult part the LTX procedure. Consequently, technical misadventures during this phase of the operation may result in significant complications. This is particularly true during the hepatectomy in patients with previous upper abdominal surgery. Excessive bleeding is the most common complication. This can be the result of carelessness, massive portal hypertension, and the presence of unusual collaterals (especially in the presence of portal vein thrombosis) and/or vascularized adhesions. Deliberate, methodic, and bloodless dissection translates to a much smoother operation and, ironically, a considerably shorter total case time. It is particularly difficult to perform surgical hemostasis once the allograft is in place, especially if there is any degree of post-reperfusion coagulopathy and if the graft is relatively large compared with the recipient abdominal compartment. In addition, early portal decompression with the veno-venous by-pass (see below) may aid in reducing the risk of massive bleeding.

Careful dissection of the hilum of the liver is critical during the hepatectomy. This is true especially in case of hepatectomy for segmental LTX, in cases of previous surgical procedures in the hilum of the liver, and in cases where there are anatomic variants. The goal in hepatectomy is preservation of the hilar structures, especially the hepatic artery and portal vein needed to revascularize the new liver allograft, as well as preservation of a sufficient length of the common bile and hepatic ducts for biliary reconstruction. Approaches to the hilum can commence either from the right side with dissection of the cystic duct and common bile duct or from the left with dissection of the hepatic artery. After identification of the common bile duct, it is good practice to preserve the surrounding soft tissue so as not to cause damage to the bile duct blood supply (Fig. 46.3). This is important to prevent postoperative bile duct ischemia and necrosis or stricture formation. An important technical issue in dissection of the hepatic artery is to start dissection of the artery at the level of the right and left branches and to proceed to the confluence and then to the gastroduodenal artery, and finally to the common hepatic artery. The surgeon should avoid too much traction of the artery to prevent intimal dissection in the artery, which can predispose the artery to postoperative thrombosis. Dissection of the branches of the common hepatic artery will allow the surgeon to select which part of the artery will provide a better size match with the donor hepatic artery. In addition, recognition of variations in the recipient anatomy of the hepatic artery is

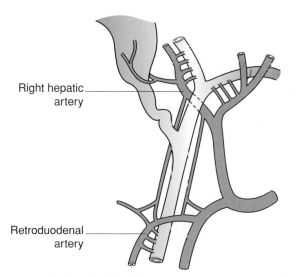

Figure 46.3 Blood supply of the biliary system. The unique nature of the blood supply for the bile duct depends solely on a hepatic artery blood supply via a vascular plexus to assure bile duct viability.

helpful to prevent the possibility of damage to the artery at the time of dissection.

Portal vein dissection is usually done after division of the hepatic artery and bile duct. All the soft tissue around the portal vein should be dissected and removed from the hilar plate to the level of the head of the pancreas. The avulsion of small pancreatic branches entering the portal vein or injury to the left gastric vein can cause massive bleeding in light of portal hypertension.

A potentially serious complication during hepatectomy is injury to the right adrenal gland, which results in severe bleeding, that is difficult to control and may require adrenalectomy. Another feared complication is injury to the right renal vein during mobilization of the infrahepatic vena cava. Dissection of the vena cava at too low a level must be avoided. Injury of the suprahepatic vena cava is an uncommon but potentially disastrous complication. Rarely, injury of the suprahepatic vena cava, with a resulting cuff that is too short, in patients with Budd–Chiari syndrome or in patients undergoing liver retransplantation in the face of a previous suprahepatic vena caval stenosis, may require control of the vena cava at the level of the diaphragm or within the pericardium. This allows placement of the vascular clamp close to or at the level of the right heart atrium. If necessary, the suprahepatic vena cava may need to be sutured closed, and venous outflow of the hepatic allograft may require a caval–atrial anastomosis.

Another potential complication is injury to the right phrenic nerve. This occurs when an excessive amount of diaphragm is included in the suprahepatic vascular clamp, particularly in the pediatric patient. This injury is usually reversible, but on occasion it can lead to permanent paralysis of the right hemidiaphragm. In addition, excessive diathermy to the right diaphragm may lead to necrosis and subsequently a diaphragmatic hernia.

Anhepatic phase

During classic LTX simultaneous complete occlusion of the recipient IVC and portal vein can lead to hemodynamic instability (Fig. 46.4). As a result, veno-venous by-pass was developed to allow diversion of blood from the recipient IVC and portal vein directly to the patient's superior vena cava during the anhepatic phase, using heparin-bonded cannulae and a motor-driven by-pass system (Fig. 46.5) [14]. Veno-venous by-pass can be used either routinely or selectively in patients showing hemodynamic instability after a trial of clamping the IVC and portal vein, prior to the total removal of the recipient liver [15,16]. Advantages of veno-venous by-pass include the following:

- The avoidance of cardiovascular instability resulting from reduced venous return to the heart during venous cross-clamping, particularly in patients with acute liver failure or in patients with noncirrhotic indications for LTX who have not developed portosystemic venous collaterals.
- The reduction of blood loss due to decompression of the portal circulation, minimizing transfusion and volume requirements.

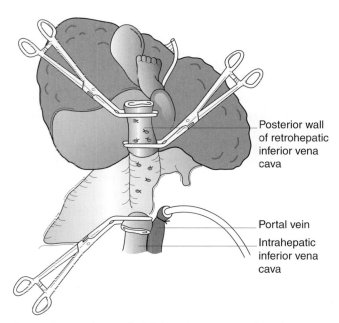

Posterior wall of retrohepatic inferior vena cava

Portal vein

Intrahepatic inferior vena cava

Figure 46.4 Requirement for infrahepatic vena cava and portal vein clamping during classic standard liver transplantation. In this case a veno-venous by-pass is being utilized, as evidenced by the portal-venous cannulae in place to decompress the mesenteric venous system.

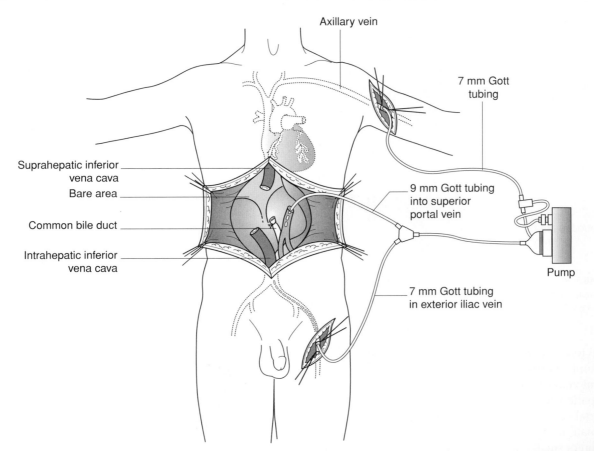

Figure 46.5 Veno-venous by-pass in liver transplantation, shown in the anhepatic phase with removal of the recipient vena cava, using the right axillary vein as the inflow. Alternatively, the by-pass may utilize percutaneously placed cannulae through the femoral vein and jugular vein.

- The avoidance of mesenteric stasis and bowel edema, and the subsequent development and release of anaerobic metabolic products and bacterial translocation into the circulation after reperfusion.
- The protection of renal function by avoiding renal-venous hypertension with a reduction of renal perfusion.
- Decompression of the portal system pressures and the avoidance of hemodynamic instability, thus allowing a safe prolongation of the anhepatic phase. This allows meticulous hemostasis and any necessary dissection as well as facilitating the correction of any complications arising during this phase of the operation.

Another advantage of the veno-venous by-pass is to allow a methodic approach to teaching trainees the complex procedure of LTX. However, the veno-venous by-pass can cause complications, some of them fatal. Complications associated with veno-venous by-pass have been described as occurring in 10–30% of cases [17–19]. These include seroma at the site of cannulae insertion, hematoma, wound infection, deep venous thrombosis, and nerve injury. The most frequent complications are wound lymphocoeles, both in the inguinal and axillary incisions. They can be avoided by careful dissection and ligation of all lymphatics. Lymphocoeles are usually self-limiting and self-healing, but occasionally chronic lymphorrhea can be quite disabling and requires surgical correction. Newer approaches to percutaneous cannulation of the femoral vein and internal jugular vein may obviate wound complications associated with cutdowns [20], however the risk of hematoma formation or venous perforation exists with these techniques. Mortality has also been described with an air embolus at the time of decannulation as well as intracircuit clots and a subsequent pulmonary embolus, the latter having occurred mainly when nonheparin-bonded tubing was used [21].

Over the past two decades there has been a trend towards avoiding the use of veno-venous by-pass, with an increasing number of transplant surgeons questioning its need [22,23]. This is due in part to the improved intraoperative hemodynamic management of the patient by the anesthesiology team and in part to the improved technical skills of the surgeons. The preservation of the entire retrohepatic vena cava and anastomosis of the new liver to a cuff formed from one or more of the main suprahepatic veins, has been advocated as a method of

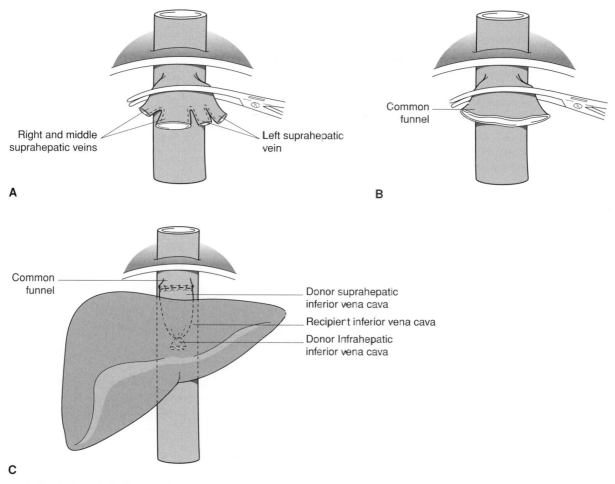

Figure 46.6 Piggyback method of recipient hepatectomy preserving the intrahepatic vena cava for liver allograft implantation utilizing end-to-side cavo-hepatic venous anastomosis. A. Following removal of liver with origins of individual hepatic veins; B. creating a common orifice by dividing the septa between individual hepatic veins; C. end-to-side cavo-cavostomy using suprahepatic vena cava of donor to common funnel orifice of recipient hepatic veins.

avoiding veno-venous by-pass. The advantages of preserving the vena cava can be significant, but this technique (also known as the "piggyback technique") requires additional skills and complete knowledge of and confidence with standard LTX with veno-venous by-pass [24]. Essentially, the technique consists of the dissection of the caudate process and right lobe of the liver from the retrohepatic vena cava, until only the right, middle, and left hepatic veins remain. Subsequently, the major hepatic veins are clamped and interconnected, thus forming a cuff that can then be anastomosed to the suprahepatic vena cava of the donor liver, in an end-to-side fashion (Fig. 46.6). After flushing the liver to clear the preserving solution, the infrahepatic cava of the allograft can be simply ligated. The new liver will then lie on top of the recipient's vena cava, but can also result in compression of the recipient's vena cava with the development of thrombosis [25,26].

There are several potential advantages of the piggyback technique, including less bleeding, less chance of adrenal gland and renal vein injury, shortening the anhepatic phase by eliminating the lower caval anastomosis, protection of the renal-venous outflow and function, and potentially less hemodynamic instability. In this situation, if portal cross-clamping in the patient with existing portal hypertension is well tolerated, it may be appropriate not to utilize a veno-venous by-pass. There have been many modifications to the caval-preserving methods used in different conditions and indications at the time of transplantation. The essential part of all these methods is to preserve the inferior vena cava with or without the use of veno-venous by-pass. In cases without preexisting portal hypertension (e.g., fulminant hepatitis), a temporary portacaval shunt can be fashioned during the initiation of the anhepatic phase to achieve mesenteric vein decompression without veno-venous by-pass (Fig. 46.7) [27]. In addition, modifications to implantation, using a side-to-side cavo-cavostomy, either handsewn [28,29] or by stapler [30], have been described.

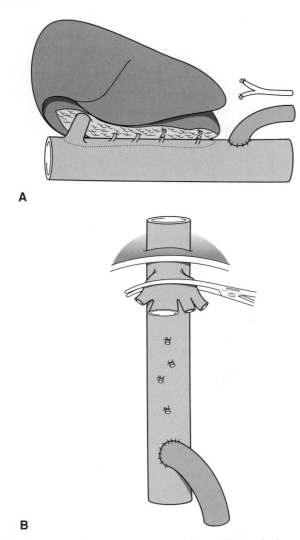

Figure 46.7 Use of a temporary portacaval shunt with piggyback vena cava preservation. A. Lateral view of portocaval shunt prior to mobilization of liver from short hepatic veins; B. frontal illustration of recipient inferior vena cava with portocaval shunt after removal of liver.

It is important to take advantage of the anhepatic phase and perform a thorough hemostasis of the operative area. At times, after the implantation of the new liver, there is not enough exposure to get a good hemostasis in the retrohepatic space. This is especially true in cases when the allograft is large and difficult to mobilize.

Implantation

Implantation of the new liver consists of several vascular anastomoses, reperfusion of the liver with the recipient blood, and biliary reconstruction. The conventional method of implanting the new liver consists of end-to-end anastomoses of the supra- and infrahepatic vena cava of the donor liver to the corresponding vena caval cuffs in the recipient, followed by end-to-end anastomosis of the portal vein of the donor liver to the recipient por-

tal vein. Usually, after completion of these anastomoses, the liver is reperfused with the recipient's blood and the clamps are removed and the recipient's venous circulation is reestablished through the new liver. Reperfusion of the liver can be one of the more unstable parts of the procedure. This is mainly due to the potential risk of cardiac arrhythmias, hypotension, and pulmonary edema secondary to the release of effluent from the liver allograft, which contains relatively high concentrations of potassium, necrotic debris, and cytokines, into the circulation. The use of preservative solutions with a high potassium content, such as the University of Wisconsin solution, and the use of livers from expanded criteria donors or livers with a prolonged cold ischemia time can exaggerate the magnitude of these complications. To potentially lessen or prevent these problems many surgeons flush the liver with lactated Ringer solution, 5% albumin, or recipient portal blood before full reperfusion.

In describing the surgical techniques involved in LTX, variations in the approach to recipients with preexisting underlying portal vein thrombosis should be mentioned. The incidence of portal vein thrombosis in patients with cirrhosis has been reported to vary between 0.6% and 64.1% depending upon the diagnostic study used and on patient selection [31,32]. The presence of portal vein thrombosis was previously considered a relative contraindication for LTX, a viewpoint that has since changed. Therapeutic options in the approach during LTX to preexisting portal vein thrombosis include eversion thromboendartectomy of the recipient portal vein (Fig. 46.8), the use of either interposition or jump venous grafts between the donor portal vein and the recipient portal or superior mesenteric vein (Fig. 46.9), cavoportal hemitransposition [33], anastomosis of the donor portal vein to an alternative recipient vein or venous collateral, and rarely arterialization of the portal vein [34]. Cavoportal hemitransposition is an option utilized when extensive thrombosis of the recipient portomesenteric venous system is present and its use is rarely indicated [35].

Arterial anastomosis between the donor and recipient arteries is usually end-to-end and the site usually varies depending on the arterial anatomy of the donor and recipient and the surgeon's preference. One must recognize that patients with an anomalous hepatic arterial anatomy may not have a large enough common hepatic artery to use as inflow. Patients with celiac axis stenosis may also have inadequate inflow. The median arcuate ligament syndrome has been described as affecting arterial inflow in LTX [36]. In these circumstances, the use of a donor iliac arterial conduit from the infrarenal (Fig. 46.10) (or occasionally supraceliac) (Fig. 46.11) aorta to the allograft may be necessary. Artificial conduits, e.g., polytetrafluoroethylene (PTFE) (Gortex®) grafts, should be avoided due to the risk of thrombosis and infection.

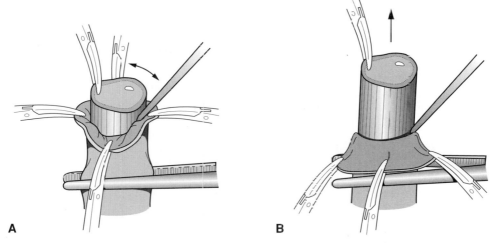

Figure 46.8 Eversion portal-venous thromboendarterectomy to reestablish the blood flow in portal vein thrombosis.

The biliary anastomosis has been referred to as the "Achilles heel" of the LTX operation [37]. There are currently two commonly practised biliary reconstructions after LTX. The most common is the choledochocholedochostomy (duct-to-duct anastomosis) and the other is the choledochojejunostomy (to a Roux-en-Y defunctionalized intestinal loop) (Fig. 46.12). The duct-to-duct anastomosis is usually done over a T tube, which remains as a stent in the duct for a few months (Fig. 46.12, insert). The advantages of leaving a T tube are the ability to quantify and characterize bile production as an early sign of hepatic allograft function; and to provide ready cholangiographic access to the biliary system in cases of abnormal liver function tests to rule out biliary problems. The disadvantage of the T tube is the risk of bile leak after removal of the tube, requiring emergent endoscopic retrograde cholangiopancreatography (ERCP) and decompression of the duct. Recently some transplant surgeons have questioned the need for a T tube in duct-to-duct anastomosis [38–40]. The use of stents in Roux-en-Y choledochojejunostomy is also a matter of controversy and some surgeons have stopped using them because of complications such as retention of the stent and obstruction of the biliary system. Other "historic" types

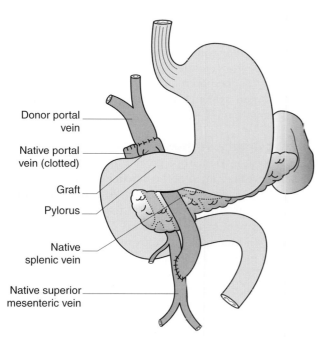

Figure 46.9 Use of an interposition vein graft from the recipient's superior mesenteric vein to the allograft portal vein in the setting of portal vein thrombosis.

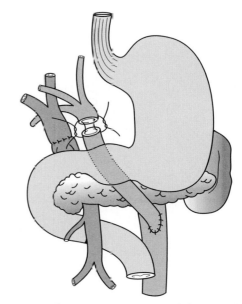

Figure 46.10 Use of an interposition arterial graft from the infrarenal aorta to the allograft hepatic artery in the setting of inadequate recipient hepatic artery inflow.

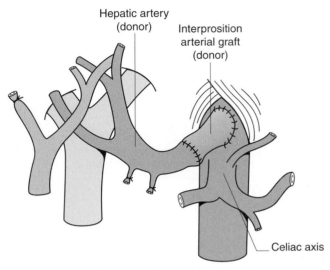

Figure 46.11 Use of an interposition arterial graft from the supraceliac aorta to the allograft hepatic artery in the setting of inadequate recipient hepatic artery inflow.

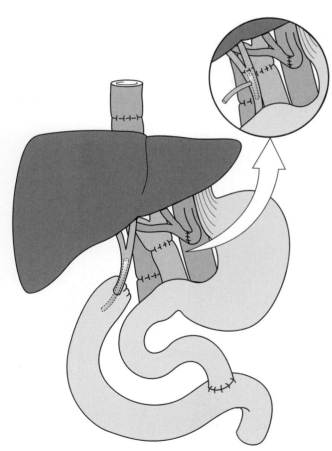

Figure 46.12 Options for establishing biliary continuity using a hepaticojejunostomy over a temporary indwelling biliary stent or alternatively a primary duct-to-duct technique over a T tube (insert).

of biliary reconstructions include choledochoduodenostomy and the now defunct cholecystoduodenostomy (the "Wadell–Calne" biliary reconstruction) [37].

Complications

Complications after LTX have a significant impact on outcome and cost of the procedure. The postoperative course in patients can range from straightforward to extremely complicated, and the outcome depends on the status of the recipient, the donor organ, and technical issues in the operation. Timely diagnosis of alterations in the normal postoperative course is the critical factor to minimize morbidity and mortality and to have a better outcome.

Primary nonfunction

Primary nonfunction (PNF) is characterized by encephalopathy, coagulopathy, minimal bile output, and progressive renal and multisystem failure with increasing serum lactate levels and rapidly rising liver enzymes and histologic evidence of hepatocyte necrosis in the absence of any vascular complications. With better donor management and selection, improved operative techniques, and newer preservation solutions, the risk of PNF has decreased but still occurs in somewhere between 4% and 6% of LTX procedures. Various donor risk factors can be implicated in primary graft dysfunction; these include prolonged cold ischemia time, an unstable donor, high level of steatosis in the liver allograft, older donor, high serum sodium level in the donor, preformed lymphocytotoxic antibodies, ABO incompatibility, and recovered organs from DCD donors. Patients with initial dysfunction may recover with support but those who progress to show evidence of extrahepatic complications such as hemodynamic instability, renal failure, or other organ system dysfunction may require urgent retransplantation [41–43].

Hepatic artery stenosis/thrombosis

Angiographic evidence of a greater than 50% reduction in the caliber of the lumen of the hepatic artery is defined as hepatic artery stenosis. This occurs in about 5% of cases after LTX. Clinically, these patients may show an increase in liver numbers or no sign at all. Sonographically, the presence of a low resistive index of less than 0.5 with an increase in focal peak velocity is suggestive of the pathology [44–46]. The detection of hepatic artery stenosis early after LTX can usually be managed by surgical intervention, when the risk for anastomotic disruption by angioplasty is highest [47]. Percutaneous angioplasty is generally reserved for stenosis occurring several weeks after the transplant procedure with an over 90% success rate [48,49].

Intimal dissection of the artery can result from too vigorous manipulation during surgery, either in the donor or the recipient, or from direct trauma to the artery from too forceful clamping. If not recognized early, intimal flaps will lead to arterial thrombosis. Complete thrombosis of the hepatic artery (HAT) is usually more symptomatic and dramatic when it occurs early in the post-transplant period and it occurs more often in adults than in children. It can lead to acute, massive necrosis, the formation of a central biloma secondary to intrahepatic duct necrosis, multiple biliary structures, or intermittent bacteremia [50–52]. Occasionally, rarely in adults but more often in children, HAT can be asymptomatic. The factors that determine whether a liver fails or survives in the face of complete HAT are not known, however the presence of collateral circulation (e.g., from the phrenic artery via vascularized adhesions to the liver) is usually associated with a more benign course after HAT. Segmental or lobar HAT has also been described. Left HAT (usually associated with an injury to an unrecognized anomalous left hepatic artery arising from the left gastric artery) is generally benign. However, right HAT (usually associated with an injury to an unrecognized anomalous right hepatic artery arising from the superior mesenteric artery, or from technically imperfect reconstruction of the anomalous right hepatic artery at the back table) is associated with the development of biliary strictures, due to the dependence of biliary viability on hepatic artery blood flow. Angiography is the gold standard for diagnosis, and in the case of early documentation of HAT urgent revascularization may result in restoration of arterial patency [47,53,54]. However, a significant number of patients treated in this manner may still require retransplantation due to biliary complications and persistent biliary sepsis [55,56].

Portal vein stenosis/thrombosis

Portal vein strictures can present shortly after LTX characterized by an increased production of ascites and liver allograft dysfunction. Ultrasonography and computed tomography (CT) angiography are usually diagnostic, while superior mesenteric artery angiography with late films is the confirmatory test [57]. Treatment is by surgical intervention in early post transplantation and by percutaneous transhepatic dilatation or stenting of the stricture later after LTX. If left untreated, it can progress to complete thrombosis of the vein or severe graft dysfunction and hemodynamic instability secondary to a massive production of ascites.

Portal vein thrombosis is an uncommon but significant complication after adult LTX, but is more common following pediatric LTX. It can manifest by rapid graft dysfunction with production of massive ascites. The differential diagnosis of portal-venous insufficiency includes technical errors such as kinking or redundancy of the

vein, poor mesenteric flow secondary to the open collateral venous system (steal syndrome), and anastomotic stricture or twist. Treatment is immediate surgical revascularization of the graft by thrombectomy and correction of the technical problem, ligation of large collaterals in the portal-venous system, by-pass grafting via the superior mesenteric vein, or percutaneous portal vein stenting. Otherwise, retransplantation may be the only therapeutic option.

Hepatic outflow obstruction

Complications associated with vena cava stenosis include a 2.5–6% incidence of venous outflow obstruction (iatrogenic Budd–Chiari syndrome), caused by either rotation of the liver graft or anastomotic stricture [58]. Stenosis of the suprahepatic cava anastomosis can present with hepatic outflow obstruction in the form of liver allograft dysfunction, ascites formation, and impairment of renal function. The problem carries a high risk for morbidity and mortality. Although hepatic outflow obstruction occurs following both standard and piggyback techniques, it is more common with the piggyback procedure. One study showed a reduction in the incidence of venous outflow obstruction from 6% to 1% when the caval anastomosis was performed using the termination of the three native hepatic veins rather than only two hepatic veins [26]. Others have adapted a side-to-side cavo-cavoplasty in order to reduce the risk of stenosis [25,26].

Diagnosis can be made by cavagram and measurements of the venous pressure gradients proximal and distal to the anastomosis. Treatment options are by angioplasty, stent placement, or surgical correction of the strictured area [59–61]. Anastomosis between the infrahepatic donor cava and the recipient cava with the piggyback technique can decompress the liver in patients with outflow obstruction secondary to anastomotic narrowing between the suprahepatic donor cava and the confluence of the hepatic vein in the recipient [62]. When all these measures fail, retransplantation may be the only option.

Biliary complications

Biliary complications continue to be a major problem after LTX with an overall incidence of about 15–20% [63–65]. These complications range from early anastomotic leak to late stricture and obstruction, both in the extrahepatic or intrahepatic biliary system. The associated mortality rate with biliary complications is about 10% and this is mainly due to delays in diagnosis or misdiagnosis of the problem and secondary infectious complications and graft dysfunction [66]. The biochemical abnormalities with elevation of bilirubin and canalicular enzymes (alkaline phosphatase and γ-glutamyltransferase) are not specific. These indicators of biliary obstruction are also seen in ischemic graft injury, rejection, recurrent hepatitis C virus (HCV), and sepsis. In order to make an accurate diagnosis, it is helpful to use imaging modalities like cholangiography, both transhepatic and endoscopic, to evaluate strictures, obstruction, or leak; ultrasonography for the detection of biliary dilatation; and radioisotope studies to evaluate anastomotic or cut surface leaks [67–69].

The most common biliary complication is biliary stenosis. This is the result of either an imperfect anastomotic technique or ischemia of the bile duct, which as it heals leads to a stenotic area in the common bile duct, either at or slightly proximal to the biliary anastomosis, with proximal biliary dilatation. Recurrent bouts of cholangitis or persistent abnormal liver function tests may indicate an obstruction to bile outflow. In these cases, endoscopic or percutaneous balloon dilatation of the bile duct stricture and stenting have been successful. In cases with no response, revision of the choledochojejunostomy or conversion of the duct-to-duct anastomosis to a choledochojejunostomy with a Roux-en-Y loop is the treatment of choice [70–72].

It has been hypothesized that the papilla of Vater is innervated by fibers coursing through the hepatic branch of the vagus, and that the hepatectomy can result in a syndrome known as "ampullary dysfunction" [66]. The radiologic examination of the biliary tree reveals dilatation of both the donor and recipient bile ducts, distal to the choledochocholedochostomy. The treatment consists of conversion to a choledochojejunostomy, although the alternative treatment, endoscopic papillotomy, has been attempted with some success.

Multiple intrahepatic strictures of the biliary tree have been described by various groups [73]. The causes and pathophysiology of these intrahepatic strictures have not been clearly elucidated. In many cases, the strictures seem to be associated with a hepatic artery thrombosis or stenosis, and ischemia of the biliary tree is probably the etiology, especially in nonheart-beating donors [74]. Preservation damage of the allograft may result in multiple intrahepatic biliary strictures, with or without biliary sludge and casts [73]. An immunologic association to a positive lymphocytotoxic-positive crossmatch has also been hypothesized. In some patients who were originally transplanted for primary sclerosing cholangitis, recurrence of the disease seems a possibility [75–79]. While some patients with multiple intrahepatic strictures eventually need to be retransplanted, others can live for years with minimal difficulties, especially if they receive chronic antibiotic prophylaxis. Recently, a grading system for intrahepatic biliary strictures and their projections for outcomes based on a large number of DCD liver transplant recipients was described [80].

The most feared complication of the biliary anastomosis is an anastomotic biliary leak. This complication is particularly lethal in choledochojejunostomies since the bile collection is rapidly infected with enteric organisms, which results in an inflamed and friable operative site during attempted repair. The presence of continued enteric leak may result in mycotic rupture of the hepatic artery anastomosis. In choledochocholedochostomies the leaks usually occur at the exit site of the T tube. In order to avoid this, a purse-string suture should be placed around the exit site. Leakage at the T-tube exit site is usually self-containing and no treatment is necessary so long as the distal bile duct empties well. Some surgeons have advocated not using any stenting following choledochocholedochostomy in an attempt to avoid the risk of T-tube site leakage [81–83].

When a Roux-en-Y loop is used, bleeding can occur at the jejunojejunostomy. In about half of the cases this is a self-limiting problem. In the other half, endoscopic intervention with a pediatric colonoscope with a heater probe or epinephrine injection or the need for surgical exploration for hemostasis may be necessary. This can be avoided by using a hemostatic running suture to approximate the mucosa and submucosa. A potentially lethal complication of Roux-en-Y biliary drainage is an unrecognized internal hernia through the mesentery at the jejunojejunostomy, unexplained abdominal distention, and vomiting due to small bowel volvulus that can progress to vascular compromise and loss of intestinal viability. Prompt recognition is critical and CT scans may reveal findings of a closed loop obstruction. Careful closure of the defect in the mesentery can reduce this complication [84].

Bleeding

Poor graft function, coagulopathy, imperfect hemostasis, or slippage of a tie may result in postoperative bleeding requiring reexploration. Postoperative bleeding is reported in between 7% and 15% of patients and requires reexploration in approximately half of them [85]. Even if easily controlled, postoperative bleeding leads to increased cost, morbidity, and mortality. Thus meticulous attention to intraoperative hemostasis and correction of coagulopathy will reduce the likelihood of postoperative hemorrhage. Early reexploration is indicated when the volume of blood transfusions exceeds 4 units within 24 hours.

Survey of liver transplantation practices

Recently, an international survey of the practice of performing deceased donor LTX was conducted by Alexis Laurent, Riccardo Memeo, and Daniel Cherqui

Table 46.1 Summary of the SALT survey on the practice of liver transplantation.

Technique used	World	United States	Europe
IVC preservation (piggyback):			
Always		4%	29%
Never		0%	4%
Selectively		4%	18%
Temporary portacaval shunt used:			
Yes		0%	58%
Type of caval anastomosis:			
Piggyback – three hepatic veins		22%	36%
Piggyback – two hepatic veins		33%	13%
Side-to-side		22%	38%
Other		23%	13%
Placement of aortic conduit:			
Supraceliac		17%	30%
Infrarenal		33%	49%
Either		50%	41%
Biliary anastomosis			
Use of stents			
Duct-to-duct without T tube	75%	86%	72%
Duct-to-duct with T tube	24%	14%	26%
Suture technique:			
Posterior running & anterior interrupted	16%	10%	14%
Interrupted	47%	50%	46%
Running	37%	40%	40%
Use of drains:			
None	10%		
One drain	20%		
Two drains	43%		
Three drains	18%		
Other	9%		
Closure:			
Full thickness		25%	10%
By layer		75%	90%

(http://hopital-mondor.imadiff.net/fmi/iwp/res/iwp_auth.html). This survey, Survey on Adult Liver Transplantation (SALT), encompassed 50 centers in Europe, eight centers in North America, two in South America, one in South Africa, and three in the Middle East. As shown in Table 46.1, there is considerable intercontinental variation in some specific aspects of the LTX procedure outlined in this chapter.

Of note was that preservation of the IVC (for piggyback implantation) was the most frequently used technique, used routinely by 57% of the teams and selectively by 38%. The use of venous by-pass was in 15% of cases of IVC preservation and in 58% when the IVC was resected. Several types of venous outflow reconstruction were used – the most common being piggyback on the stump of two or three hepatic veins followed by a side-to-side caval anastomosis. Lastly, the duct-to-duct biliary anastomosis was most often used as the standard biliary reconstructive technique, with a T tube being used in 25% of the programs on a routine basis.

Given the excellent outcomes obtained around the world, it suggests that these modifications are rather insignificant in the hands of experienced surgeons in the current era of LTX.

Conclusions

While the results of LTX have improved dramatically over the past 50 years, many of the same technical considerations have plagued the procedure since its inception. With the increasing complexity of candidates undergoing LTX, an improved understanding of the pathophysiology of donor organ preservation, reperfusion injury, improved immunosuppression, more effective diagnostic tools, and new anti-infective agents, have all contributed to a smoother post-transplant course. Nevertheless, all of these advances cannot negate a poorly performed technical procedure.

References

1 Cannon JA. Brief report. *Transplant Bull* 1956;3:7.
2 Starzl TE, Kaupp HA, Brock DR, Lazarus RE, Johnson RV. Reconstructive problems in canine homotransplantations with special reference to the postoperative role of hepatic venous flow. *Surg Gynecol Obstet* 1960;111:733–43.
3 Starzl TE, Marchioro TL, von Kaulla KN, Hermann G, Brittain RS, Waddell WR. Homotransplantaion of the liver in humans. *Surg Gynecol Obstet* 1963;117:659–76.
4 Moore FD, Dagher F, Veith F, et al. Immunosuppression and vascular insufficiency in liver transplantation. *Ann NY Acad Sci* 1964;102:729–38.
5 Kuss R, Bourget P. *An Illustrated History of Organ Transplantation.* Rueil–Malmaison, France: Sandoz, 1992.
6 Starzl TE, Groth CG, Brettschneider L, et al. Orthotopic homotransplantation of the human liver. *Ann Surg* 1968;168:392–415.
7 Calne RY, Williams R. Liver transplantation in man. I. Observations of technique and organization in five cases. *Br Med J* 1968;4:535–40.
8 Starzl TE, Putnam CW. *Experience in Hepatic Transplantation.* Philadelphia, PA: WE Saunders, 1969: 131–5.
9 Strong RW, Lynch SV, Ong TH, Matsunami H, Koido Y, Balderson GA. Successful liver transplantation from a living donor to her son. *N Engl J Med* 1990;322:1505–7.
10 Diamond IR, Fecteau A, Millis JM, et al.; SPLIT Research Group. Impact of graft type on outcome in pediatric liver transplantation. A report from Studies of Pediatric Liver Transplantation (SPLIT). *Ann Surg* 2007;245:301–10.
11 Hashikura Y, Makuuchi M, Kawasaki S, et al. Successful living-related partial liver transplantation to an adult patient. *Lancet* 1994;343:1233–4.
12 Marino IR, Doyle HR, Fung JJ. Liver. In: Higgins RSD, Sanchez JS, Lorber MI, Baldwin JC, eds. *The Multi-organ Donor. Selection and Management.* Oxford: Blackwell Science, 1997:241–64.
13 Feng S, Goodrich NP, Bragg-Gresham JL, et al. Characteristics associated with liver graft failure. The concept of a donor risk index. *Am J Transplant* 2006;6:783–90.

14. Starzl TE, Miller C, Broznick B, Makowka L. An improved technique for multiple organ harvesting. *Surg Gynecol Obstet* 1987;165:343–8.

15. Shaw BW, Marquez JM, Kang YG, et al. Venous bypass in clinical liver transplantation. *Ann Surg* 1984;200:524–34.

16. Chari RS, Gan TJ, Robertson KM, et al. Venovenous bypass in adult orthotopic liver transplantation. routine or selective use? *J Am Coll Surg* 1998;186:683–90.

17. Khoury GF, Mann ME, Porot MJ, Abdul-Rasool IH, Busuttil RW. Air embolism associated with venovenous bypass during orthotopic liver transplantation. *Anaesthesiology* 1987;67:848–51.

18. Navalgund AA, Kang Y, Sarner JB, Jahr JS, Gieraerts R. Massive pulmonary thromboembolism during liver transplantation. *Anesth Analg* 1988;67:400–2.

19. Katirji MB. Brachial plexus injury following liver transplantation. *Neurology* 1989;39:736–8.

20. Ozaki CF, Langnas AN, Bynon JS, et al. A percutaneous method for venovenous bypass in liver transplantation. *Transplantation* 1994;57:472–3.

21. Budd JM, Isaac JL, Bennet J, Freeman JW. Morbidity and mortality associated with large-bore percutaneous venovenous bypass cannulation for 312 orthotopic liver transplantations. *Liver Transpl* 2001;7:359–62.

22. Wall WJ, Grant DR, Duff JH, Kutt JL, Ghent CN, Bloch MS. Liver transplantation without venous bypass. *Transplantation* 1987;43: 56–61.

23. Stock PG, Payne WD, Ascher NL, et al. Rapid infusion technique as a safe alternative to veno-venous bypass in orthotopic liver transplant. *Transplant Proc* 1989;21:2322–5.

24. Tzakis A, Todo S, Starzl TE. Orthotopic liver transplantation with preservation of the inferior vena cava. *Ann Surg* 1989;210:649–52.

25. Parrilla P, Sánchez-Bueno F, Figueras J, et al. Analysis of the complications of the piggyback technique in 1,112 liver transplants. *Transplantation* 1999;67:1214–17.

26. Robles R, Parrilla P, Acosta F, et al. Complications related to hepatic venous outflow in piggyback liver transplantation. Two versus three suprahepatic vein anastomosis. *Transplant Proc* 1999;31:2390–1.

27. Belghiti J, Noun R, Sauvanet A. Temporary portocaval anastomosis with preservation of caval flow during orthotopic. *Am J Surg* 1995;169:277–9.

28. Bismuth H, Castaing D, Sherlock DJ. Liver transplantation by face-a-face vena cavaplasty. *Surgery* 1992;111:151–5.

29. Belghiti J, Panis Y, Sauvanet A, Gayet B, Fékété F. A new technique of side to side caval anastomosis during orthotopic hepatic transplantation without inferior vena caval occlusion. *Surg Gynecol Obstet* 1992;175:270–2.

30. Quintini C, Miller CM, Hashimoto K, et al. Side-to-side cavocavostomy with an endovascular stapler. Rescue technique for severe hepatic vein and/or inferior vena cava outflow obstruction after liver transplantation using the piggyback technique. *Liver Transpl* 2009;15:49–53.

31. Yerdel MA, Gunson B, Mirza D, et al. Portal vein thrombosis in adults undergoing liver transplantation. Risk factors, screening, management, and outcome. *Transplantation* 2000;69:1873–81.

32. Stieber AC, Zetti G, Todo S, et al. The spectrum of portal vein thrombosis in liver transplantation. *Ann Surg* 1991;213 (3): 199–206.

33. Tzakis AG, Kirkegaard P, Pinna AD, et al. Liver transplantation with cavoportal hemitransposition in the presence of diffuse portal vein thrombosis. *Transplantation* 1998;65(5):619–24.

34. Erhard J, Lange R, Giebler R, Rauen U, de Groot H, Eigler FW. Arterialization of the portal vein in orthotopic and auxiliary liver transplantation. A report of three cases. *Transplantation* 1995;60: 877–9.

35. Gerunda GE, Merenda R, Neri D, et al. Cavoportal hemitransposition. A successful way to overcome the problem of total por-

36. tosplenomesenteric thrombosis in liver transplantation. *Liver Transpl* 2002;8:2–5.

36. Jurim O, Shaked A, Kiai K, Millis JM, Colquhoun SD, Busuttil RW. Celiac compression syndrome and liver transplantation. *Ann Surg* 1993;218:10–12.

37. Calne RY. A new technique for biliary drainage in orthotopic liver transplantation utilizing the gall bladder as a pedicle graft conduit between the donor and recipient common bile ducts. *Ann Surg* 1976;184:605–9.

38. Koivusalo A, Isoniemi H, Salmela K, Edgren J, von Numers H, Höckerstedt K. Biliary complications in one hundred adult liver transplantations. *Scand J Gastroenterol* 1996;31:506–11.

39. Shimoda M, Saab S, Morrisey M, et al. A cost effectiveness analysis of biliary anastomosis with or without T-tube after orthotopic liver transplantation. *Am J Transplant* 2001;1:157–61.

40. Scatton O, Meunier B, Cherqui D, et al. Randomized trial of choledochocholedocostomy with or without T-tube in orthotopic liver transplantation. *Ann Surg* 2001;233:432–7.

41. Busuttil RW, Tanaka K. The utility of marginal donors in liver transplantation. *Liver Transpl* 2003;9:651–63.

42. González FX, Rimola A, Grande L, et al. Predictive factors of early postoperative graft function in human liver transplantation. *Hepatology* 1994;20:565–73.

43. Bezeizi KI, Jalan R, Plevris JN, Hayes PC. Primary graft dysfunction after liver transplantation. From pathogenesis to prevention. *Liver Transpl* 1997;3:137–48.

44. Stange BJ, Glanemann M, Nuessler NC, Settmacher U, Steinmuller T, Neuhaus P. Hepatic artery thrombosis after adult liver transplantation. *Liver Transpl* 2003;9:612–20.

45. Dodd GD 3rd, Memel DS, Zajko AB, Baron RL, Santaguida LA. Hepatic artery stenosis and thrombosis in transplant recipients. Doppler diagnosis with resistive index and systolic acceleration time. *Radiology* 1994;192:657–61.

46. Nolten A, Sproat IA. Hepatic artery thrombosis after liver transplantation. Temporal accuracy of diagnosis with duplex-US and the syndrome of impending thrombosis. *Radiology* 1996;198:553–9.

47. Sheiner PA, Varma CV, Guarrera JV, et al. Selective revascularization of hepatic artery thrombosis after liver transplantation improves patient and graft survival. *Transplantation* 1997;64:1295–9.

48. Mondragon RS, Karani JB, Heaton ND, et al. The use of percutaneous transluminal angioplasty in hepatic artery stenosis after liver transplantation. *Transplantation* 1994;57:228–31.

49. Orons PD, Zajko AB, Bron KM, Trecha GT, Selby RR, Fung JJ. Hepatic artery angioplasty after liver transplantation. experience in 21 allografts. *J Vasc Interv Radiol* 1995;6:523–9.

50. Tzakis AG, Gordon RD, Shaw BW Jr, Iwatsuki S, Starzl TE. Clinical presentation of hepatic artery thrombosis after liver transplantation in the cyclosporine era. *Transplantation* 1985;40:667–71.

51. Bhattacharjya S, Gunson BK, Mirza DF, et al. Delayed hepatic artery thrombosis in adult orthotopic liver transplantation. a 12-year experience. *Transplantation* 2001;71:1592–6.

52. Tzakis AG. The dearterialized liver graft. *Semin Liver Dis* 1985;5: 375–6.

53. Pinna AD, Smith CV, Furukawa H, Starzl TE, Fung JJ. Urgent revascularization of liver allografts after early hepatic artery thrombosis. *Transplantation* 1996;62:1584–7.

54. Yanaga K, Lebeau G, Marsh JW. Hepatic artery reconstruction for hepatic artery thrombosis after liver transplantation. *Arch Surg* 1990;125:628–31.

55. Rabin JM, Roof SL, Cordless CL, et al. Hepatic allograft abscess with hepatic arterial thrombosis. *Am J Surg* 1998;175:354–9.

56. Tarzan K, Shacked A, Although KM. Etiology and management of symptomatic adult hepatic artery thrombosis after orthotopic liver transplantation. *Am Surg* 1996;62:237–40.

57. Crossing JD, Mirada D, Wilson SR. Ultrasound of liver transplants. normal and abnormal. *Radiographic* 2003;23:1093–114.

58. Settmacher U, Nussler NC, Glanemann M, et al. Venous complications after orthotopic liver transplantation. *Clin Transplant* 2000;14:235–41.

59. Tsiotos GG, Nagorney DM, de Groen PC. Selective management of hepatic venous outflow obstruction. *J Gastrointestinal Surg* 1997;1:377–85.

60. Althaus SJ, Perkins JD, Soltes G, Glickerman D. Use of a Wallstent in successful treatment of IVC obstruction following liver transplantation. *Transplantation* 1996;61:669–72.

61. Simó G, Echenagusia A, Camúñez F, et al. Stenosis of the inferior vena cava after liver transplantation. Treatment with Gianturco expandable metallic stent. *Cardiovasc Interv Radiol* 1993;18: 212–16.

62. Stieber AS, Gordon RD, Bassi N. A simple solution to a technical complication in "piggy back" liver transplantation. *Transplantation* 1997;64:654–5.

63. O'Connor TP, Lewis WD, Jenkins RL. Biliary tract complications after liver transplantation. *Arch Surg* 1995;130:312–17.

64. Qian YB, Liu CL, Lo CM, Fan ST. Risk factors for biliary complications after liver transplantation. *Arch Surg* 2004;139:1101–5.

65. Nemec P, Ondrásek J, Studeník P, Hökl J, Cern J. Biliary complications in liver transplantation. *Ann Transplant* 2001;6:24–8.

66. Greif F, Bronsther OL, Van Thiel DH, et al. The incidence, timing, and management of biliary tract complications after orthotopic liver transplantation. *Ann Surg* 1994;219:40–5.

67. Kurzawinski TR, Selves L, Farouk M. Prospective study of hepatobiliary scintigraphy and endoscopic cholangiography for the detection of early biliary complications after orthotopic liver transplantation. *Br J Surg* 1997;84:620–3.

68. Sung RS, Campbell DA Jr, Rudich SM, et al. Long-term follow-up of percutaneous transhepatic balloon cholangioplasty in the management of biliary strictures after liver transplantation. *Transplantation* 2004;77:110–15.

69. Thuluvath PJ, Atassi T, Lee J. An endoscopic approach to biliary complications following orthotopic liver transplantation. *Liver Int* 2003;23:156–62.

70. Shah S, Dooley J, Agarwal R, et al. Routine endoscopic retrograde cholangiography in the detection of early biliary complications after liver transplantation. *Liver Transpl* 2002;8:491–4.

71. Mata A, Bordas JM, Llach J, et al. ERCP in orthotopic liver transplanted patients. *Hepatogastroenterology* 2004;51:1801–4.

72. Rizk RS, McVicar JP, Emond MJ, et al. Endoscopic management of biliary strictures in liver transplant recipient: effect on patient and graft survival. *Gastrointest Endosc* 1998;47:128–35.

73. Nakamura N, Nishida S, Neff GR, et al. Intrahepatic biliary strictures without hepatic artery thrombosis after liver transplantation. An analysis of 1113 liver transplants at a single center. *Transplantation* 2005;79:427–32.

74. Abt P, Crawford M, Desai N, Markmann J, Olthoff K, Shaked A. Liver transplantation from controlled non-heart-beating donors. an increased incidence of biliary complications. *Transplantation* 2003;75:1659–63.

75. Khettry U, Keaveny A, Goldar-Najafi A, et al. Liver transplantation for primary sclerosing cholangitis. A long-term clinicopathologic study. *Hum Pathol* 2003;34:1127–36.

76. Gopal DV, Corless CL, Rabkins JM, Olyaei AJ, Rosen HR. Graft failure from severe recurrent primary sclerosing cholangitis following orthotopic liver transplantation. *J Clin Gastroenterol* 2003;37: 344–7.

77. Balan V, Abu-Elmagd K, Demetris AJ. Autoimmune liver disease. Recurrence after liver transplantation. *Surg Clin North Am* 1999;79:147–52.

78. Neuberger J. Recurrence of primary biliary cirrhosis, primary sclerosing cholangitis and autoimmune hepatitis. *Liver Transpl* 1995;1:109–15.

79. Vera A, Mcledina S, Gunson B, et al. Risk factors for recurrence of primary sclerosing cholangitis of liver allograft. *Lancet* 2002;360:1943–4.

80. Lee HW, Suh KS, Shin WY, et al. Classification and prognosis of intrahepatic biliary stricture after liver transplantation. *Liver Transpl* 2007;13:1736–42.

81. Koivusalo A, Isoniemi H, Salmela K, Edgren J, von Numers H, Höckerstedt K. Biliary complications in one hundred adult liver transplantations. *Scand J Gastroenterol* 1996;31:506–11.

82. Shimoda M, Saab S, Morrisey M, et al. A cost-effectiveness analysis of biliary anastomosis with or without T-tube after orthotopic liver transplantation. *Am J Transplant* 2001;1:157–61.

83. Scatton O, Meunier B, Chercui D, et al. Randomized trial of choledochocholedocostomy with or without T-tube in orthotopic liver transplantation. *Ann Surg* 2001;233:432–7.

84. Khanna A, Newman B, Reyes J, Fung JJ, Todo T, Starzl TE. Internal hernia and volvulus of the small bowel following liver transplantation. *Transplant Int* 1997;10:133–6.

85. Ozaki CF, Katz SM, Monsour HP. Surgical complications of liver transplantation. *Surg Clin North Am* 1994;74:1155–67.

CHAPTER 47

Recurrent Disease Following Liver Transplantation

Kymberly D. S. Watt[1] & Marie A. Laryea[2]

[1] Division of Gastroenterology and Hepatology, Mayo Clinic Rochester, MN, USA
[2] Hepatology/Multi-Organ Transplant Program, Dalhousie University, Halifax Nova Scotia, Canada

Key concepts

- Recurrent liver disease can occur for virtually all indications of liver transplantation.
- Hepatitis C virus (HCV) recurrence is almost universal, with up to 30% developing allograft cirrhosis by the fifth year post transplant.
- HCV-related allograft cirrhosis is associated with a high risk of decompensation and death.
- Hepatitis B virus recurrence is less common and the outcome of recurrence is substantially improved by the use of human immunoglobulin and nucleos(t)ide analogs.
- Recurrent primary biliary cirrhosis and autoimmune hepatitis do not have a substantial impact on patient and graft survival rates;
- however, recurrent primary sclerosing cholangitis is associated with reduced graft survival.
- Although recurrent alcohol use after transplantation for alcoholic liver disease is common, direct or indirect negative effects of recurrent alcohol use on the allograft is uncommon.
- Recurrent nonalcoholic fatty liver disease is common, but only 2.5–5% of patients experience graft loss due to recurrence.
- Recurrent Budd–Chiari syndrome can occur days to years after transplantation, despite adequate anticoagulation.

Recurrence of liver disease can occur for many of the primary indications for liver transplantation (LTX) (Table 47.1). The timing and natural history of recurrent disease can vary depending on the underlying disease and its course may differ from the original disease. A subset of patients with recurrent disease will develop allograft failure and may require retransplantation. Survival after LTX continues to improve. With this, it is anticipated that the proportion of patients requiring retransplantation will grow and concern exists that the need may outgrow the current donor supply. This chapter will review recurrent diseases after transplantation with a focus on recurrent viral hepatitis as it is the most clinically relevant recurrent disease in the transplant population. Retransplantation and recurrent malignancies will be covered in their respective chapters.

Recurrent hepatitis C

Hepatitis C virus (HCV) associated liver failure is the most common indication for liver transplantation and the infection recurs nearly universally following transplantation. Although the impact of HCV infection on the allograft varies substantially between recipients, allograft failure secondary to recurrence of HCV infection is a common cause of death and retransplantation among recipients with HCV infection [1–3]. In a large multicentered cohort study with over 10 years of follow-up, HCV infection was a specific risk factor for long-term liver-related mortality [4]. Recurrent HCV is a common indication for late retransplant (>3 months after primary transplant) and is a factor in up to 40% of retransplants [5]. Survival after retransplant may be lower for HCV patients but many variables interplay to make these survival rates lower [3].

Natural history

Hepatitis C virus infection of the allograft occurs at the time of transplantation [6]. HCV RNA is cleared rapidly from serum during the anhepatic phase and following reperfusion the rate of decrease in HCV RNA accelerates, believed to be related to intrahepatic uptake of

Schiff's Diseases of the Liver, Eleventh Edition. Edited by Eugene R. Schiff, Willis C. Maddrey and Michael F. Sorrell.
© 2012 John Wiley & Sons, Ltd. Published 2012 by John Wiley & Sons, Ltd.

Table 47.1 Recurrent disease rates following liver transplantation

Disease	Recurrence rate (5 years)
Hepatitis C	100%
Hepatitis B	9–10%
Autoimmune hepatitis	20–25%
Primary biliary cirrhosis	30–35%
Primary sclerosing cholangitis	9–30%
Alcoholic liver disease	Up to 24%
Nonalcoholic steatohepatitis	30–50%
Budd–Chiari syndrome	1–7%
Metabolic disease	None/unknown

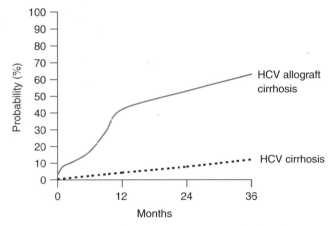

Figure 47.1 Probability of developing decompensated cirrhosis (ascites, encephalopathy, or variceal hemorrhage) from the time of diagnosis of hepatitis C virus (HCV) cirrhosis (pre transplant) and HCV allograft cirrhosis (post transplant). (Adapted from Berenguer et al. [13] and Fattovich et al. [130].)

the virus particles. Unfortunately, hepatocellular production of virions increases thereafter and HCV RNA levels increase rapidly from week 2 post transplantation, peaking by the fourth postoperative month. At the end of the first postoperative year HCV RNA levels are, on average, 10–20-fold greater than pretransplant levels [7]. Acute lobular hepatitis develops in approximately 75% of HCV recipients in the first 6–12 months following liver transplantation and generally (but not always) manifests as increased serum aminotransferase levels. By the fifth postoperative year, 80–100% of HCV-infected liver transplant recipients will have histologic evidence of chronic allograft injury secondary to hepatitis C [7].

Recurrent viral hepatitis is of limited significance unless associated with the development of fibrosis within the allograft. Neither the viral load nor liver enzyme abnormalities are predictive of intrahepatic injury or fibrosis progression. Liver biopsy is required to determine accurate grading of inflammation and staging of fibrosis. A median fibrosis progression rate of 0.8 units of fibrosis stage per year has been suggested [8], but is not applicable to individual patients. Predictors of more rapid progression (>0.8 units fibrosis per year) include warm ischemic time >60 minutes and donor age >55 years. Other studies suggest fibrosis progression is not linear over time, but shows a rapid and exponential increase during the first 3 years after LTX. After this period, progression slows and is nearly linear [9,10]. A 12-month protocol biopsy allows for stratification of fibrosis progression. Twenty-one percent of patients with Ishak fibrosis scores of 2–3, and 36% of patients with a hepatitis activity index score >4, at the 12-month biopsy progressed to cirrhosis within 3–5 years in one study [8]. A fibrosis stage greater than 2 confers a 15-fold increased risk of HCV-related graft loss, with a graft survival of only 55% at 5 years in another study [9]. Fibrosis progression has been shown to decrease, and established fibrosis improve, in transplant patients treated with antiviral medications with a sustained virologic response to treatment [10–12].

The natural history of recurrent HCV is greatly accelerated in some patients when compared with that of immunocompetent patients, whereby a disease course of decades is frequently telescoped to a few years. Up to 30% of patients can develop cirrhosis within 5 years, compared with 30% developing cirrhosis over 20–30 years in the immunocompetent population [7]. Once cirrhosis has developed in the allograft, 30–40% decompensate within 1 year and up to 60–70% by 3 years, compared with the nontransplant cirrhotic population where only 10% decompensate within 3 years (Fig. 47.1) [13,14]. Once a patient decompensates with HCV allograft cirrhosis, 54% die within 1 year and less than 10% survive 3 years (Fig. 47.2) [13,14]. Thus intervention early in the course of recurrent advanced fibrosis is needed to change this bleak natural history. Interventions may include antiviral medication or retransplantation.

A small proportion of HCV transplant patients (4–7%), develop an even more accelerated course of liver injury (fibrosing cholestatic hepatitis C) with subsequent rapid allograft failure, generally within 3–6 months. These patients are notable for very high HCV RNA levels with a predominantly cholestatic liver profile (bilirubin typically >6 mg/dL and alkaline phosphatase > 5 times normal). Bilirubin levels tend to be disproportionately elevated relative to serum alkaline phosphatase. Histologic confirmation is required and is depicted by ballooning hepatocytes (with preponderance to the perivenular region), sinusoidal fibrosis, paucity of inflammation with bile ductular proliferation, and cholestasis [15]. Once the diagnosis is established, prompt establishment of antivirals *may* be associated with improved clinical status but no data exist to confirm this.

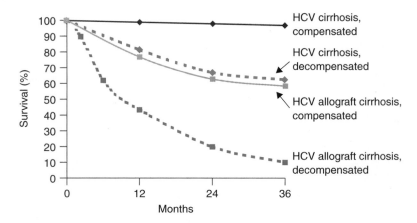

Figure 47.2 Survival rates for compensated and decompensated hepatitis C virus (HCV) cirrhosis and HCV allograft cirrhosis. (Adapted from Berenguer et al. [13] and Fattovich et al. [130].)

Risk factors

Many risk factors associated with severe recurrence and accelerated fibrosis progression have been identified (Fig. 47.3). Viral factors that impact disease progression include higher viral load both pre and post transplant. The impact of genotype is less clear. Recent data by Charlton et al. [16] demonstrated the TT haplotype of the interleukin 28b (IL28b) gene polymorphism, rs12979860, to be associated with worse outcomes post transplant. The likelihood of viral response to interferon-based treatment is also impaired in those patients with a TT genotype conferring a higher likelihood of failed treatment response both pre and post transplant. It is likely that the transplant population will predominantly have a TT genotype in the future, as they are less likely to respond to antiviral medication in the pretransplant phase and thus more likely to progress to end-stage liver disease and transplant need. Post-transplant tracking of HCV quasi-species emergence has suggested a strong correlation between genetic diversification in the viral envelope region and asymptomatic or mild disease patterns [17].

Recipient variables have been associated with more severe recurrence of HCV, and include increased age, non-

Caucasian race, and female gender but the data have not been compelling enough to alter clinical practice. Data on human leucocyte antigen (HLA) compatibility between donor and recipient has been conflicting and more study is needed to determine its true impact. Insulin resistance and diabetes have been shown to be associated with more rapid fibrosis progression and worse patient and graft outcomes [18]. Combining other known risk factors with diabetes will increase the risk of allograft cirrhosis exponentially. In one study, the combination of receiving a donor liver older than 55 years and having diabetes post transplant was associated with an 8.38-fold risk of progression to severe fibrosis ($P = 0.000124$) when compared with patients not diabetic post transplant who received livers from donors aged <55 years [19]. Cytomegalovirus (CMV) infection in the HCV patient is a known risk for worse outcomes and most centers now administer antiviral prophylaxis to prevent CMV infection.

Human immunodeficiency virus (HIV) coinfection has been associated with poor survival among liver transplant recipients with HCV infection. One year patient mortality in coinfected recipients ranges between 27% and 54% [20]. Reduced response rates to treatment

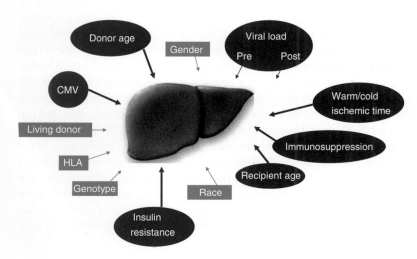

Figure 47.3 Risk factors for progressive fibrosis and worse outcomes in HCV patients after liver transplantation. *Note:* circles indicate factors with significant supporting evidence; squares indicate factors with conflicting or limited substantiating evidence. CMV, cytomegalovirus; HLA, human leucocyte antigen.

of HCV with interferon and ribavirin attenuate post-transplant outcomes in HIV–HCV coinfected liver transplant recipients. Strategies for improving outcomes in this fragile population are evolving.

Donor factors and operative factors also impact the severity of recurrence of HCV. Donor age is irrefutably linked to HCV recurrence. The exact donor age whereby the risk increases is unclear. Donor age >55–65 years are most frequently cited, but donor age >40 years is the lower range that has been implicated in worse outcomes in numerous studies [21]. Donor race in general has not been a factor in liver transplant outcomes, but when specifically analyzed in HCV recipients, if a donor:recipient race mismatch exists it may impact HCV recurrence and outcomes [22]. More study into this recent finding is needed to definitively alter practice specifically for HCV recipients. Donor liver steatosis has been inconsistently associated with HCV recurrence and the degree above which the risk increases is unclear. Warm and cold ischemic time, as reflected by preservation injury in the allograft, has important implications in the severity of HCV recurrence and has been associated with worse outcomes [23]. Living donor liver transplantation reduces the impact of ischemic time, donor age, and donor steatosis. The outcomes for living donor recipients in the recent era demonstrate at least equivalent outcomes as cadaveric donor recipients, and in some centers living donor recipients may experience less fibrosis progression than deceased donor recipients [24].

Immunosuppression impacts viral recurrence and progression of disease. The use of bolus steroid treatment for acute cellular rejection is associated with transient 1–2 log increases in HCV RNA levels [7]. In addition to being proviral, treatment of acute cellular rejection with corticosteroids is associated with increased mortality and graft loss in LTX recipients with HCV infection (relative risk, 2.9; $P = 0.04$) [25]. It has been suggested, though not proven, that a slow steroid taper is better than a rapid taper [26]. Although steroid-sparing regimens appear to be safe, a large randomized controlled study has found no difference in the rate of recurrence of HCV nor in patient or graft survival between steroid-free and steroid-utilizing arms, thus there is no compelling basis for avoiding corticosteroids in the early postoperative period [27].

Antilymphocyte agents, in particular muromonab (OKT3, a monoclonal anti-CD3 antibody) and alemtuzumab (a monoclonal anti-CD52 antibody), are strong T-cell-depleting agents associated with severe recurrence of HCV and worse short-term survival in HCV patients and are not recommended in this patient population [28, 29]. Polyclonal antilymphocyte agents and IL2 receptor blockers appear to have minimal impact on the severity of HCV recurrence in the allograft, but these studies are limited to retrospective analysis of induction regimens, which may reduce acute cellular rejection, thus interpretation on the direct effects on HCV disease cannot be made.

Conflicting data exist for the risk of worse outcomes based on calcineurin inhibitor use. Overall, there has been no major difference in outcomes of HCV patients using tacrolimus as first-line immunosuppression compared with cyclosporine use. A clinically relevant effect associated with mycophenolate mofetil in the HCV patient has not been found either. Sirolimus has conflicting data relating specifically to HCV patients and more study into the risks and benefits of the mammalian target of rapamycin (mTOR) inhibitors as a class is needed before any definitive recommendations can be made.

Treatment

Treatment regimens for recurrent HCV continue to be centered on pegylated interferons and ribavirin. Protease inhibitors have yet to be studied in the transplant population but can be expected to have drug interactions with the immunosuppressive drugs. Sustained virologic response (SVR) rates are less frequent in the transplant population than the general hepatology population, with an average response rate of approximately 30% in most studies [30]. SVR has been associated with histologic improvement and improved long-term outcomes [12,31]. Renal insufficiency and cytopenias limit doses in many instances and growth factors are frequently employed during antiviral treatment. Although uncommon, antiviral treatment has been associated with precipitating immune dysfunction, which can manifest as acute cellular rejection, chronic rejection, or autoimmune hepatitis [32–34]. These events appear to occur more commonly after seroconversion to a HCV RNA-negative state. The true frequency of this is presently being investigated in a multicentered study.

Optimal timing for antiviral medications is unclear but a fibrosis score of 2 or greater is a frequent starting point. Patients with high grades of inflammation early post transplant with stage 1 fibrosis may benefit from earlier initiation of treatment, but no definitive guideline exists. Achieving SVR prior to transplant is the ideal circumstance but is difficult to achieve in cirrhotic patients, and unsafe to attempt in decompensated patients. Attempts at treating HCV using a low accelerated dosing schedule prior to transplant have resulted in an SVR rate of 24%, but only 13% in genotype 1 patients (50% in genotypes 2 and 3) [35]. Significant adverse events and even death were documented, particularly in patients with decompensated liver disease. In patients able to achieve SVR in this study, 12/15 remained virus-negative by 6 months post transplant. The risk:benefit ratio must be weighed for each individual cirrhotic patient, before proceeding with antiviral treatment. Consensus guidelines recommend attempting treatment only in patients with a model for end-stage liver disease (MELD) score of less than 19, or in select cases when the MELD score ranges from 19 to 25 [36].

Unlike in hepatitis B management, the development of an effective immunoglobulin has been unsuccessful to date, but studies are ongoing. Preemptive treatment with interferon and ribavirin (within the first 3–4 weeks of transplant), is fraught with difficulty and adverse side effects without any real advantage, as only 8% SVR has been documented [37]. These investigators did demonstrate reduced histologic scores at 72 weeks but, due to the small numbers of biopsies obtained, no statistical significance was found. Prophylactic therapy (treatment initiated within 6–12 weeks of transplant) has been attempted as well, but once again proved difficult with poor treatment tolerance and no histologic improvement or significant benefit in SVR [37,38]. Cases of fibrosing cholestatic hepatitis or rapidly progressive HCV may warrant attempted preemptive or prophylactic treatment, but data to support this recommendation do not exist.

Treating patients later after transplant, once histologic evidence of advancing disease is apparent, is the standard approach to treating recurrent HCV. General recommendations are for treatment once stage 2 (periportal) fibrosis has been reached. A meta-analysis of four randomized (two only in abstract form) and two nonrandomized controlled trials of antiviral treatment in liver transplant recipients found an SVR of approximately 40% [39]. These trials are quite heterogeneous and difficult to compare. The two published randomized controlled trials of pegylated interferon and ribavirin performed in liver transplant recipients demonstrated an SVR rate between 33% and 48% [40,41]. These trials had suboptimal dosing of ribavirin, but so few transplant patients achieve optimal dosing it is likely closer to "real world" treatment. Studies have demonstrated an improvement in long-term survival in patients achieving SVR compared with those patients who do not [26,42]. In addition, interferon/ribavirin therapy, whether a remission was achieved or not, may also confer potential improvement in patient survival [31].

Baseline immunosuppression may impact the likelihood of SVR on antiviral treatment, with cyclosporine possibly associated with an increased SVR compared with tacrolimus. Small case series studies suggest higher rates of SVR in patients treated with antiviral medications and cyclosporine compared with those on tacrolimus. However, a small, pilot, randomized controlled trial showed only a trend toward improved SVR rates in cyclosporine-treated patients undergoing antiviral therapy (but was not powered for statistical significance) [43]. There is a large multicentered study now underway to answer this important question.

Recurrent hepatitis B

In the United States, 2,000–4,000 deaths each year are directly related to hepatitis B virus (HBV) infection. One million US residents are chronically infected and therefore at risk for cirrhosis, end-stage liver disease, and hepatocellular carcinoma. These manifestations of HBV infection, along with fulminant hepatic failure, can be cured by liver transplantation and account for approximately 4% of liver transplants in the United States. Historically, HBV infection carried a worse prognosis post-LTX than other indications, with a 5-year survival of 53% in US patients transplanted between 1987 and 1991 [44]. Preventing the recurrence of HBV infection in the graft has lead to dramatically improved outcomes, with 5-year survival greater than 80% globally [45–47].

Before the advent of prophylaxis and highly effective antiviral agents against hepatitis B, recurrence was nearly universal, frequently leading to rapid graft failure [48,49]. The publication of the seminal work by the European Concerted Action on Viral Hepatitis (EuroHep) in 1993 marked a turning point in transplantation for HBV-related disease by demonstrating that long-term (defined as greater than 6 months) immunoprophylaxis with hepatitis B immunoglobulin (HBIg) was associated with lower rates of recurrence when compared with patients who received short-term HBIg and those who received none (~36% and 75%, respectively) [50]. More importantly, this study showed that, with proper prophylaxis, HBV recurrence was not inevitable and good outcomes were possible for these patients.

When post-transplantation prophylaxis is used rates of recurrence are consistently below 10% [45,47,51,52] even though regimens vary widely amongst centers. In 2010 the National Institutes of Health (NIH) Hepatitis B Virus Orthotopic Liver Transplantation (NIH HBV-OLT) Study Group reported the overall probability of post-transplant HBV recurrence in 15 US transplant centers to be 3%, 7%, and 9% at 1, 3, and 5 years respectively [45]. The study centers represented the spectrum of prophylaxis regimens currently in use, giving a real-life evaluation of HBV recurrence in the United States. A lower rate of recurrence had been found previously in an Australasian study of low-dose intramuscular HBIg and lamivudine (LAM), where 4% of patients were affected by recurrent HBV at 5 years [47]. The difference is unlikely to be due to superiority of the prophylaxis regimen but to differences in study populations, notably length of treatment with LAM prior to LTX and the number of patients with detectable HBV DNA at the time of LTX

(64% in the NIH study versus 0% in the Australasian study).

Definitions and diagnosis

It is crucial when reviewing literature on recurrent HBV post-LTX to understand how it is defined by the authors. Differences in assays and their limit of detection also need to be taken into account. The term *recurrence* is most often used to describe infection of an HBV-naïve graft once implanted in a hepatitis B surface antigen (HBsAg) positive patient. Given the current standard of care in HBV-positive recipients, recurrence is defined as failure of prophylaxis.

Recurrence of HBV is different from *reactivation*, where viral replication resumes after a graft containing HBV DNA (anti-hepatitis B core (HBc) positive donor) is transplanted into a recipient without immune mechanisms capable of keeping the virus in check. It is also different from *de novo infection* in a transplant recipient. Reactivation and de novo HBV infection are beyond the scope of this chapter.

A diagnosis of recurrent HBV is made when circulating HBsAg is detected in the serum after transplantation, even in the absence of hepatic inflammation or abnormal liver enzymes. *Viral breakthrough* occurs when HBV DNA is detected in the serum, even in the absence of a positive HBsAg. Patients with detectable HBV DNA and negative HBsAg do not have true recurrence as low level viral replication can occur even with prophylaxis. Viral breakthrough can herald significant viral replication but is often transient, with viral loads promptly returning to undetectable levels without intervention.

Prophylaxis is the term used to describe measures put in place post-LTX to avoid graft infection and recurrent HBV liver disease. It can involve passive immunization with HBIg, antiviral treatment with nucleos(t)ide analogs or, most commonly, a combination of measures.

Pathophysiology

One postulated mechanism for HBV recurrence is infection of the allograft by circulating viral particles present at the time of transplantation. HBV virions have a half-life between 24 seconds and 224 minutes [53]. There is therefore a period, however brief, where preformed circulating virions can infect the new graft. However, recurrence that emerges later, post transplant, is thought to be caused by virions stored in extrahepatic sites, particularly peripheral blood mononuclear cells that are released and lead to graft infection. These extrahepatic reservoirs may also cause recurrence in patients with active viral replication at the time of transplantation [54,55]. They are known to persist up to 10 years post-

LTX and explain why prophylaxis must be continued long term [56].

After transplantation, additional mechanisms enhance the ability of HBV to infect the graft. Immunosuppression makes virus clearance more difficult by blunting or eliminating the immune response. Use of corticosteroids in particular appears to enhance replication, presumably by binding to a steroid-responsive nuclear element [57].

In the era of universal prophylaxis post-LTX, recurrent HBV is almost always a failure of prophylaxis, although imperfect patient adherence to prescribed therapeutic measures can render otherwise adequate prophylaxis ineffective. In compliant patients, failure is due to the emergence of viral escape mutants or inadequate dose and/or duration of prophylaxis.

When HBIg was used as monotherapy for prophylaxis, escape preS/S HBsAg mutants emerged in some patients and eventually led to viral breakthrough and HBV recurrence. With LAM monotherapy, LAM-resistant mutants at the tyrosine, methionine, aspartate, aspartate (YMDD) nucleotide-binding locus of the HBV DNA polymerase can emerge and lead to recurrence [58]. Combination therapy minimizes the selection pressure exerted on the HBV and thereby minimizes recurrence. However, mutants carrying both the preS/S and YMDD mutations have been isolated in patients with recurrent HBV receiving HBIg and LAM [45,58]. Mutants resistant to adefovir have also been seen post transplant and this resistance can be associated with recurrence as well [59]. In fact, mutants resistant to all three agents (HBIg, LAM, and adefovir) have been detected [60].

Risk factors

In the era of HBIg and highly effective nucleos(t)ide analogs, the literature defines two groups of patients: those at high risk of HBV recurrence and those at low risk (Table 47.2). This separation allows for the tailoring of post-transplantation prophylaxis relative to viral and patient factors [61].

Table 47.2 Patient characteristics associated with a high or low rate of recurrent hepatitis B virus (HBV) infection after liver transplantation.

High risk for recurrence	Low risk for recurrence
Viral load ≥100,000 copies/mL at time of LTX [45,63]	Undetectable HBV DNA at time of LTX [45,50,62]
HBeAg-positive at LTX [45,52]	HBeAg-negative at LTX [45]
	Hepatitis D coinfection [45,50,63]
	Acute hepatitis B [45,50,63]

HBeAg, hepatitis B e antigen; LTX, liver transplantation.
Data from references [45,50,52,62,63].

High-risk patients

One of the earliest studies looking at passive immunization post-LTX for HBV found that patients HBV DNA-positive at the time of LTX had higher rates of recurrence than HBV DNA-negative patients (96% versus 29% at 2 years) [62]. Although subsequent studies found various factors associated with post-LTX HBV recurrence, these are largely surrogate markers for active viral replication at the time of transplantation (Table 46.2) [63]. The NIH HBV-OLT Study Group has published studies where the presence of hepatitis B e antigen (HBeAg) at listing [44] and serum HBV DNA $>10^5$ copies/mL at the time of transplant [45,52] were the only factors associated with post-transplant HBV recurrence.

When LAM was the only antiviral medication available for treatment of HBV, pretransplant resistance to LAM was a risk factor for HBV recurrence [64,65]. These patients tended to have higher viral loads at the time of transplant, which was thought to explain the higher rate of recurrence. However, a recent study of 160 patients found the detection of the YMDD mutation after LTX to be the only significant risk factor for recurrence, irrespective of the degree of viral replication at the time of LTX [66]. Even so, other studies have shown that when adefovir is given to patients with LAM resistance prior to transplant as rescue therapy [45,67], or as prophylaxis at time of transplant [68], the risk of recurrence is low.

Low-risk patients

In the 1993 EuroHep study, independent predictors of a lower risk of HBV recurrence after liver transplantation by multivariate analysis were hepatitis D virus superinfection, acute HBV, and long-term prophylaxis [50]. These are the most likely surrogate markers for low HBV viral loads at the time of LTX, as patients with an undetectable viral load at the time of transplant are known to have less recurrence as well. Hepatitis D infection is usually accompanied by a suppression of HBV replication due to unknown interference mechanisms. Fulminant HBV is caused by immune-mediated hepatolysis and most patients do not have obvious viral replication at the time of presentation. Many studies have since confirmed these to be predictive of low rates of recurrence along with other patient factors (Table 46.2).

Prevention

Analysis of early experiences in liver transplantation for HBV-related disease was crucial in proving the effectiveness of passive immunization with HBIg in preventing post-transplantation recurrence, allowing experts to advocate transplantation for HBV in the face of great reticence in the liver transplant community [69]. The prevention of HBV recurrence involves pretransplantation, intraoperative, and post-transplantation measures that help minimize risk to the graft.

Treatment of hepatitis B virus before liver transplantation

As previously mentioned, early studies proved that HBV-infected patients with undetectable levels of HBV DNA at the time of liver transplantation had better outcomes. This is the rational for treating patients with antiviral therapy prior to transplantation [70]. This is usually done by administering long-term oral nucleos(t)ide analogs, as these are very effective and well tolerated by decompensated patients. Pre-LTX interferon therapy has been attempted but is poorly tolerated by cirrhotic patients [71] and is contraindicated in decompensated patients [72,73]. In patients with hepatic dysfunction as the principal indication for transplantation, treatment with a nucleos(t)ide analog can also lead to regression of disease and significant improvement in liver function to the point where LTX may no longer be necessary [72].

The choice of nucleos(t)ide analog pretransplantation can be a difficult one but treatment guidelines for chronic hepatitis B should be followed when possible. Given that life-long prophylaxis post-LTX is recommended, and that patients may be treated for extended periods pre transplantation, entecavir and tenofovir are highly potent agents with a high genetic barrier to resistance and are recommended as first-line treatment [72–74]. The high rates of resistance associated with LAM (50% at 5 years in chronic hepatitis B and 50% at 2 years in LTX patients) make it a lesser choice in this context. However, LAM is less expensive and is best studied in advanced liver disease. It still has a role pre transplantation when and where resources are limited. Renal fragility in cirrhotic patients awaiting transplantation make adefovir, with its known nephrotoxicity, a less appealing choice than LAM, entecavir, or tenofovir.

Studies show that if virologic breakthrough occurs on therapy prior to LTX, rescue therapy should be started at least perioperatively to minimize recurrence [45,59,67,68].

Post-transplantation prophylaxis

Prophylaxis against recurrent HBV was initially based on HBIg alone [75]. It has evolved in parallel with treatment for chronic HBV, first with the advent of LAM approved in 1998, then with adefovir in 2002. Entecavir, a cyclopentyl guanosine analog, and the nucleotide reverse transcriptase inhibitor tenofovir, both highly potent antivirals, promise to further change standard practice in LTX.

Monotherapy with HBIg is associated with high rates of recurrence long term, especially in patients with ongoing viral replication at the time of transplant [62]. This is in large part due to the emergence over time of preS/S

Review: lamivudine and adefovir for prevention of recurrence of HBV after liver transplantation (7.09)
Comparision: 04 lamivudine or adefovir and HBIg versus HBIg alone
Outcome: 04 Reappearance of HBsAg

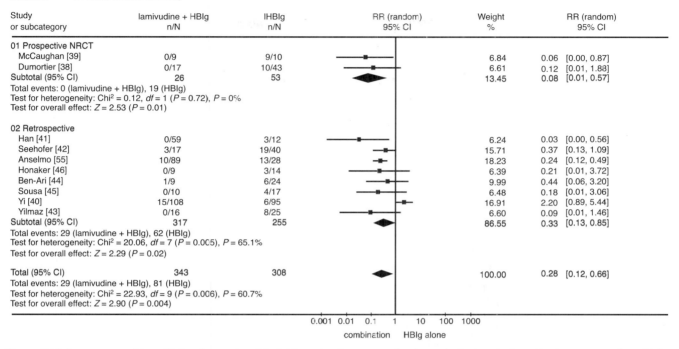

Study or subcategory	lamivudine + HBIg n/N	IHBIg n/N	RR (random) 95% CI	Weight %	RR (random) 95% CI
01 Prospective NRCT					
McCaughan [39]	0/9	9/10		6.84	0.06 [0.00, 0.87]
Dumortier [38]	0/17	10/43		6.61	0.12 [0.01, 1.88]
Subtotal (95% CI)	26	53		13.45	0.08 [0.01, 0.57]

Total events: 0 (lamivudine + HBIg), 19 (HBIg)
Test for heterogeneity: Chi² = 0.12, df = 1 (P = 0.72), I² = 0%
Test for overall effect: Z = 2.53 (P = 0.01)

02 Retrospective					
Han [41]	0/59	3/12		6.24	0.03 [0.00, 0.56]
Seehofer [42]	3/17	19/40		15.71	0.37 [0.13, 1.09]
Anselmo [55]	10/89	13/28		18.23	0.24 [0.12, 0.49]
Honaker [46]	0/9	3/14		6.39	0.21 [0.01, 3.72]
Ben-Ari [44]	1/9	6/24		9.99	0.44 [0.06, 3.20]
Sousa [45]	0/10	4/17		6.48	0.18 [0.01, 3.06]
Yi [40]	15/108	6/95		16.91	2.20 [0.89, 5.44]
Yilmaz [43]	0/16	8/25		6.60	0.09 [0.01, 1.46]
Subtotal (95% CI)	317	255		86.55	0.33 [0.13, 0.85]

Total events: 29 (lamivudine + HBIg), 62 (HBIg)
Test for heterogeneity: Chi² = 20.06, df = 7 (P = 0.005), I² = 65.1%
Test for overall effect: Z = 2.29 (P = 0.02)

Total (95% CI)	343	308		100.00	0.28 [0.12, 0.66]

Total events: 29 (lamivudine + HBIg), 81 (HBIg)
Test for heterogeneity: Chi² = 22.93, df = 9 (P = 0.006), I² = 60.7%
Test for overall effect: Z = 2.90 (P = 0.004)

0.001 0.01 0.1 1 10 100 1000
combination   HBIg alone

Figure 47.4 Reappearance of hepatitis B surface antigen (HbsAg) in studies that compared patients who had received combination treatment (hepatitis B immunoglobulin (HBIg) plus nucleos(t)ide analog) versus HBIg alone. CI, confidence interval; HBV, hepatitis B virus; NRCT, nonrandomized clinical trial; RR, relative risk. Original references can be obtained from Katz et al. [48]. (Reproduced from Katz et al. [48] with permission from Wiley.)

mutants [76]. For this reason, monotherapy with HBIg is no longer recommended in liver transplantation [74,77].

Standard practice for the first year post-LTX involves the use of nucleos(t)ide analogs, most commonly in combination therapy with HBIg, or, less commonly, as monotherapy or in combination with a second nucleos(t)ide analog. Combined HBIg and nucleos(t)ide analog prophylaxis is most often used long term, but some centers withdraw HBIg and transition patients to monotherapy with a nucleos(t)ide analog at a set interval that varies according to center [45]. A meta-analysis published in 2010 showed that few randomized controlled trials exist to show superiority of one regimen over the other, and highlighted the fact that practice in this area cannot truly be evidence-based [48]. However, nonrandomized trials favor combination therapy with HBIg and nucleos(t)ide analogs over nucleos(t)ide analog monotherapy (Figs 47.4 and 47.5).

Hepatitis B immunoglobulin

Passive immunization with HBIg has long been used in postexposure prophylaxis, most notably peripartum in the offspring of HBV-infected mothers. HBIg has also been the cornerstone of prevention of HBV recurrence in LTX for decades.

It is well documented that hepatitis B polyclonal immunoglobulins protect the graft from HBV infection. However, the exact mechanism is poorly understood. One hypothesis is that HBIg protects naïve hepatocytes from extrahepatic reservoirs of HBV by blocking a putative HBV receptor. Hepatitis B surface antibodies (anti-HBs) help clear circulating viral particles and induce lysis of infected hepatocytes via cell-mediated immunity [78]. HBIg does not, however, eradicate HBV infection and HBV DNA is detectable in the tissues, including liver biopsies, of patients long after transplantation [56] but may neutralize circulating virions through the formation of immune complexes and immune precipitation [79].

The use of HBIg varies widely between and within LTX centers. The original approach was to use a loading dose in the anhepatic phase with 10,000 units of HBIg IV followed by 10,000 units IV daily for the first 7 days post-LTX [45]. This phase helped clear circulating virions and rendered all patients HBsAg-negative after 7 days [75]. However, centers now opt for daily low-dose IV or low-dose IM HBIg from the time of transplant onward, especially in patients on nucleos(t)ide analogs at the time of transplant and at a low risk of recurrence [45,80].

HBIg is usually well tolerated with few side effects. Reports of osmotic nephrosis associated with some HBIg

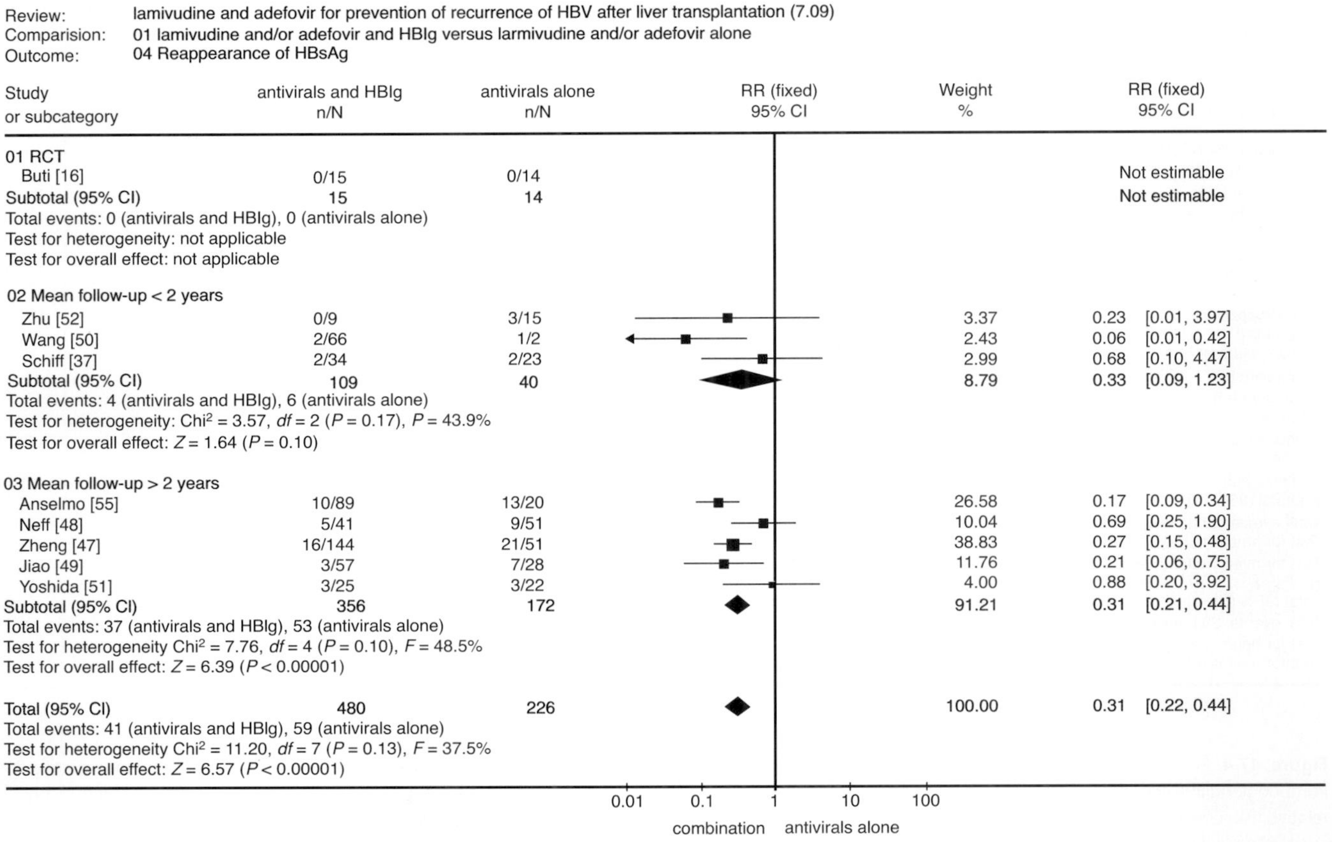

Review: lamivudine and adefovir for prevention of recurrence of HBV after liver transplantation (7.09)
Comparison: 01 lamivudine and/or adefovir and HBIg versus larmivudine and/or adefovir alone
Outcome: 04 Reappearance of HBsAg

Study or subcategory	antivirals and HBIg n/N	antivirals alone n/N	RR (fixed) 95% CI	Weight %	RR (fixed) 95% CI
01 RCT					
Buti [16]	0/15	0/14			Not estimable
Subtotal (95% CI)	15	14			Not estimable
Total events: 0 (antivirals and HBIg), 0 (antivirals alone)					
Test for heterogeneity: not applicable					
Test for overall effect: not applicable					
02 Mean follow-up < 2 years					
Zhu [52]	0/9	3/15		3.37	0.23 [0.01, 3.97]
Wang [50]	2/66	1/2		2.43	0.06 [0.01, 0.42]
Schiff [37]	2/34	2/23		2.99	0.68 [0.10, 4.47]
Subtotal (95% CI)	109	40		8.79	0.33 [0.09, 1.23]
Total events: 4 (antivirals and HBIg), 6 (antivirals alone)					
Test for heterogeneity: Chi² = 3.57, df = 2 (P = 0.17), I² = 43.9%					
Test for overall effect: Z = 1.64 (P = 0.10)					
03 Mean follow-up > 2 years					
Anselmo [55]	10/89	13/20		26.58	0.17 [0.09, 0.34]
Neff [48]	5/41	9/51		10.04	0.69 [0.25, 1.90]
Zheng [47]	16/144	21/51		38.83	0.27 [0.15, 0.48]
Jiao [49]	3/57	7/28		11.76	0.21 [0.06, 0.75]
Yoshida [51]	3/25	3/22		4.00	0.88 [0.20, 3.92]
Subtotal (95% CI)	356	172		91.21	0.31 [0.21, 0.44]
Total events: 37 (antivirals and HBIg), 53 (antivirals alone)					
Test for heterogeneity Chi² = 7.76, df = 4 (P = 0.10), I² = 48.5%					
Test for overall effect: Z = 6.39 (P < 0.00001)					
Total (95% CI)	480	226		100.00	0.31 [0.22, 0.44]
Total events: 41 (antivirals and HBIg), 59 (antivirals alone)					
Test for heterogeneity Chi² = 11.20, df = 7 (P = 0.13), I² = 37.5%					
Test for overall effect: Z = 6.57 (P < 0.00001)					

0.01   0.1   1   10   100
combination   antivirals alone

Figure 47.5 Reappearance of hepatitis B surface antigen (HbsAg) in studies that compared patients who had received combination treatment (hepatitis B immunoglobulin (HBIg) plus nucleos(t)ide analog) versus nucleos(t)ide analog alone. CI, confidence interval; HBV, hepatitis B virus; RCT, randomized clinical trial; RR, relative risk. Original references can be obtained from Katz et al. [47]. (Reproduced from Katz et al. [48] with permission from Wiley.)

preparations are unconfirmed but have raised some concern in the transplant population already at risk for renal injury [81]. To maintain anti-HBs levels, HBIg can be administered intravenously, intramuscularly and, as recently shown, subcutaneously (SC) [82]. SC administration of HBIg requires higher doses to achieve the desired titers, as absorption is decreased by 20% when compared with IM administration [83]. However, SC injections may be better tolerated by patients. HBIg can be administered at fixed intervals regardless of anti-HBs titers, or on demand according to antibody levels. Different protocols aim for different titers where higher titers (>500 IU/L) may protect more patients from recurrence but at greater cost. Most protocols aim for titers greater than 100 IU/L long term [45,83]. Lower titers of anti-HBs may be sufficient and trials in this area are necessary.

Since all combination prophylaxis regimens are associated with similar rates of HBV recurrence [45,51], choice of therapy is often driven by cost. The current trend is to minimize HBIg to reduce cost, first by lowering the dose, then the target anti-HBs titers, and now by HBIg-withdrawal strategies. By decreasing the amount of HBIg given and negating the charge associated with IV admin-

istration, low-dose IM HBIg offers significant cost savings [47]. Another cost-cutting measure is finite duration HBIg, where the transition to nucleos(t)ide analog-only prophylaxis usually takes place well after the first year post transplantation [45,46,84,85]. Some centers withdraw HBIg as early as 7 days post-LTX in low-risk patients (as defined in Table 47.2) [84,85]. More data on this approach are needed.

Nucleos(t)ide analogs

While HBIg is thought to prevent infection of hepatocytes and help in immune clearance of circulating virions, it has no impact on viral replication, specifically on extrahepatic reservoirs of HBV. Alternatively, nucleos(t)ide analogs (NAs) inhibit extrahepatic viral replication, thereby reducing and sometimes eradicating circulating virions capable of infecting hepatocytes and triggering an inflammatory response in the graft [77].

Most of the literature on NAs in liver transplantation focuses on LAM, the first agent found to be effective against HBV. The advantages of LAM are its safety profile in liver patients and the relatively low cost. Its greatest pitfall is the high rate of recurrence at (25% at 1 year in chronic hepatitis B), making it an imperfect choice in patients likely to require prolonged treatment. Although some centers use LAM monoprophylaxis in patients who are HBV DNA-negative at the time of transplant with good results [84], resistance must be cause for concern in the long-term management of these patients. Close follow-up and prompt administration of rescue therapy when mutants emerge are essential.

Adefovir has also been studied, mostly as a rescue agent when LAM resistance emerges [67,68,74]. It has a lower rate of resistance than LAM (2% at 1 year) and is effective in treating viral breakthrough secondary to LAM-resistant mutants [59,74]. Its pitfalls are potential resistance and nephrotoxicity. Combination therapy adefovir/LAM without HBIg was found to be equivalent to LAM/HBIg therapy in patients at least 12 months post-LTX without HBV recurrence. This randomized open-label trial also showed the combination of adefovir/LAM to be the more cost-effective measure.

Entecavir and tenofovir (along with the tenofovir/emtricitabine combination Truvada®) are highly effective antiviral agents that have very favorable resistance profiles and are recommended as first-line monotherapy in chronic hepatitis B [72,73]. Their role in post-LTX prophylaxis has been demonstrated in small studies that confirm their safety and efficacy [86]. Current practice guidelines recommend these agents be considered for prophylaxis given their profound viral suppression and low rates of resistance (B1 recommendation) [73]. However, few data currently exist to truly argue for superiority of these agents in LTX. These agents may become the backbone of HBIg-free prophylaxis, with HBIg-withdrawal strategies, NA monoprophylaxis regimens, and dual NA therapy all currently under investigation.

Vaccines

Many studies have looked at triggering active immunization in transplant recipients with purified recombinant HBsAg vaccines, with mixed results. In the general population, anti-HBs titers of >10 IU/L are sufficient to confer immunity. However, in transplantation, current goals are to maintain titers >100 IU/L long term to minimize recurrence. The failure of early vaccination strategies was two-fold: most patients failed to respond due to a blunted immune reaction from immunosuppression, and those that did were unable to maintain appropriate titers long term [87]. Adjuvants and concomitant HBIg were felt to be necessary to ensure response to vaccination. A novel strategy of combining recombinant vaccine and immune-modulating agents has shown promise in a trial published in 2010 whereby patients received HBIg, LAM, and monthly vaccination for 6 months, followed by LAM and monthly vaccination for 6 months, and then LAM alone

for 12 months of follow-up [88]. Twelve months after vaccination, 44% of patients continued to have titers >100 IU/L and no recurrence of HBV had been detected.

Treatment

The goal of treatment is to maintain graft function and arrest the progression of chronic HBV hepatitis. Once recurrence occurs and HBsAg is once again detected in the patient's serum post-LTX, HBIg can be discontinued, as its role is to prevent but not treat recurrence.

In chronic HBV, some advocate interferon-α therapy. However, in LTX, it is poorly tolerated and associated with an increased risk of rejection [70]. Recurrence is most commonly triggered by emerging resistance in adherent patients and treatment should be guided by known principles of HBV treatment (see Chapter 24). Rapid suppression of viral replication is desirable, and therefore tenofovir and entecavir are better rescue agents in recurrence, although adefovir has been shown effective when used to treat YMDD-mediated recurrence post-LTX [59,67,74]. With effective rescue therapy, HBV recurrence has a much more benign course than historically. Most patients respond promptly to therapy with no long-term graft-related issues.

Recurrent HBV should not be an absolute contraindication to retransplantation [70]. Should graft dysfunction arise and retransplantation be deemed necessary, the cause of HBV recurrence must be identified to determine whether retransplantation is an option. In cases where nonadherence is the main issue, candidates would need in-depth evaluation to ensure improved adherence with the next transplantation. In cases where prophylaxis failed, transplant physicians must carefully analyze the cause and determine if it is remediable. More powerful agents, longer use of HBIg with higher titers, or other novel strategies may be necessary to protect the new allograft from recurrent HBV disease.

Recurrent primary biliary cirrhosis

Primary biliary cirrhosis (PBC) is a disease characterized by progressive cholestasis secondary to immune-mediated destruction of cholangiocytes in the interlobular bile ducts. It accounts for 5% of all transplants in the United States.

In 1982, three UK patients who had undergone liver transplantation for PBC developed recurrent pruritus and jaundice post-LTX and were found to have histologic changes consistent with PBC [89]. Since then, recurrent PBC (rPBC) has become a well-recognized entity with a reported recurrence rate of 18% post-LTX [90,91]. Transplant centers that do not perform protocol post-LTX biopsies underestimate the prevalence of rPBC, leading to a variation in reported recurrence rates. The expansion of histologic criteria to include more subtle changes has also lead to more diagnosis of recurrence. Given the cumulative incidence of rPBC, studies with longer follow-up periods tend to report more recurrence, with rates as high as 30–35% [92,93]. In spite of significant recurrence, patients transplanted for PBC have the best outcomes after LTX [94].

Diagnosis

Whereas the diagnosis of native-liver PBC is supported by a clinical picture of classic symptoms, cholestasis, pathognomonic serology, and well-defined histologic findings, rPBC can be a much more subtle disease entity. The usual symptoms of pruritus, fatigue, and sicca are often absent, affecting only 12% of patients [94]. Recurrent disease can also be seen in patients with normal liver enzymes, further complicating diagnosis [95], although approximately one half will have an elevated alkaline phosphatase [91,93,96]. Antimitochondrial antibodies (AMAs), the serologic marker of PBC, are unhelpful in detecting rPBC as their presence or measured titers fail to predict recurrence [96]. Titers often fall after LTX only to reappear later in the post-LTX course, even in patients without histologic evidence of disease recurrence.

Recurrent PBC is therefore a histologic diagnosis best described in studies conducted in centers with protocol biopsies post-LTX. The presence of a *florid duct lesion* (granulomatous cholangitis) is the major diagnostic criteria for rPBC and is present in two thirds of patients at diagnosis [93]. Some degree of fibrosis is often present on the index biopsy, though it tends to be early stage [93,95]. Often more subtle inflammatory changes are seen in patients that either had, or went on to develop, the florid duct lesion [96]. Almost one third of rPBC patients have a dense lymphoplasmacytic infiltrate, defined as "a mononuclear infiltrate that filled at least one of the portal tracts, with or without expansion of the portal tract, containing ≥4 plasma cells," while none of the controls had this infiltrate. With this histologic finding included in the diagnostic criterion, rPBC prevalence may be as high as 30–35% [96,97]. By using set diagnostic criteria for rPBC, a diagnosis of definite or probable rPBC can be made relatively easily (Table 47.3). It should be noted, however, that similar to native-liver PBC, rPBC is patchy, leading to sampling errors and false-negative biopsies.

Natural history

Recurrent PBC is a progressive disease that can lead in some patients to advanced fibrosis, cirrhosis, eventual graft failure, and death [92,93,97] though most patients with rPBC do not develop graft dysfunction. Although early data failed to show the clinical impact of rPBC

[98], one study with longer follow-up revealed a negative effect on graft and patient survival with up to 22% of patients with rPBC decompensating or dying of their disease during 6 years of follow-up post diagnosis [92]. However, not all patients experience recurrence, and only 1.3% of all PBC patients lost their graft to disease recurrence in a study with 22 years of follow-up [99]. In general, time to rPBC-related graft loss is around 7 years. When compared with other recurrent diseases post-LTX, it progresses more slowly and carries the lowest risk of graft failure [92,99]. Retransplantation for rPBC is still a rare occurrence [92,93,98]. Recurrent PBC in the second graft has been described but does not necessarily follow the same course as rPBC in the first graft [90].

Risk factors

As post-LTX survival lengthens, and recurrent disease becomes a greater threat to graft survival, identifying modifiable donor and recipient risk factors for rPBC may lead to even better outcomes in this patient population.

Conflicting data on the influence of recipient age and HLA status exist in the literature and more work is needed to determine whether or not these are true risk factors for recurrence [100]. Some studies have shown longer cold ischemia time and donor age >65 years to be associated with higher rates of rPBC [94] but other studies failed to confirm these findings. Overall, no recipient or donor factors have consistently been shown to be associated with rPBC, largely due to a lack of available data rather than true epidemiologic evidence.

Recurrent PBC occurs regardless of immunosuppression regimen used, although rates of recurrence and time to rPBC appear affected by the agents chosen. The first hint that immunosuppression affected recurrence rates in PBC came in 1996 when a prospective trial comparing tacrolimus with cyclosporine head-to-head found higher rates of recurrence with shorter times to recurrence in patients on tacrolimus [101]. Later trials confirmed this finding while others failed to show an association between tacrolimus and increased rates of recurrence. A systematic review of four trials that had data on immunosuppression found no difference between the two agents, although a nonsignificant trend towards less rPBC in the cyclosporine group was found. A more recent retrospective study published in 2010 looking at 103 consecutive transplants for PBC found no difference in recurrence when tacrolimus or cyclosporine was used alone. By multivariate analysis, less recurrence occurred in patients receiving combination immunosuppression with azathioprine, with the lowest rates of rPBC in patients receiving cyclosporine and azathioprine [92]. No clear mechanism for this difference has been identified and prospective studies are needed to further determine the effect of immunosuppression on rPBC.

Table 47.3 Diagnostic criteria for recurrent autoimmune diseases after liver transplantation.

Disease	Diagnostic criteria
Recurrent autoimmune hepatitis (AIH)	Patient transplanted for AIH Autoantibodies in titers >1:80 Chronic elevation of transaminases Elevated serum IgG immunoglobulins Corticosteroid dependency Rule out rejection, viral or drug-induced hepatitis Diagnostic or compatible histology: 　Plasma cell-rich inflammation in portal tracts and the parenchyma 　Interface hepatitis 　Confluent/bridging necrosis (in more severe cases)
Recurrent primary biliary cirrhosis (PBC)	Patient transplanted for PBC AMA seropositivity after LTX Diagnostic or compatible histology:* 　Mononuclear inflammatory infiltrate 　Lymphoid aggregates 　Epithelioid granuloma formation 　Florid duct lesion
Recurrent primary sclerosing cholangitis (PSC)	Patient transplanted for PSC Multiple nonanastomotic biliary stricturing on cholangiography Diagnostic or compatible liver histology: 　Fibrous cholangitis with bile duct obliteration 　Ductopenia 　Secondary features of chronic cholestasis

*Three of four portal tract lesions: definite recurrent PBC. Two of four portal tract lesions: probable recurrent PBC.
AMA, antimitochondrial antibody; IgG, immunoglobulin G; LTX, liver transplantation.
Adapted from Schreuder et al. 2009 [90].

Treatment

The cornerstone of treatment in native-liver PBC is ursodeoxycholic acid (UDCA) and its use has been credited for the decreased number of PBC patients requiring transplantation [102]. UDCA has the greatest impact when used in patients with early disease. Given that most rPBC is diagnosed at an early stage in centers with post-LTX biopsy protocols, one can reasonably assume UDCA has a role to play in this population. However, UDCA in rPBC has not been studied in large randomized controlled trials. Some centers empirically treat patients with UDCA and retrospective analysis of their experience offers some data on efficacy. One of these retrospective studies demonstrated improved liver enzymes with no impact on liver function in 52% of UDCA-treated patients, where only 22% of untreated patients had improved enzymes [93]. No improvement in histologic progression, death, or need for retransplantation was seen in the treated groups, but follow-up in this study was relatively short (36 months) given the slow progression of rPBC. Furthermore, the patchy nature of rPBC makes assessing histologic regression challenging and prone to sampling errors. The efficacy of UDCA needs to be studied in long randomized prospective studies with hard clinical end-points (jaundice, death, decompensation, and retransplantation).

Given the apparent effect of immunosuppression on the natural history of rPBC, patients' drug regimens are sometimes modified upon diagnosis of rPBC. These strategies have not been systematically studied and are not yet supported by randomized clinical trial data.

Recurrent primary sclerosing cholangitis

Primary sclerosing cholangitis (PSC) is thought to be an immunologically mediated chronic disease marked by progressive scarring of the intra- and extrahepatic bile ducts, leading to end-stage liver disease requiring liver transplantation. PSC accounts for approximately 6% of all transplants in the United States. Unfortunately, the disease recurs in 9–30% of patients transplanted for PSC by 3–5 years [91,103–105], with six times the risk of graft loss due to recurrent disease compared with the risk of graft loss for rPBC [99]. Recurrence of PSC has been described before 3 months post transplant but usually ranges between 6 and 120 months after transplant. The difficulty with assessing recurrent disease timing and frequency is the lack of protocol biopsies in most studies. In many circumstances histologic disease may occur earlier than clinical disease is picked up. Patients having received a transplant for PSC generally have a hepatico-jejunostomy (Roux-en-Y anastomosis) for near complete removal of the native bile duct, and thus are prone to biliary reflux and intermittent fluctuating liver enzyme abnormalities. In patients with a sustained alkaline phosphatase level greater than 250 U/L after 1 year, recurrent PSC should be considered and a cholangiogram and/or liver biopsy obtained [104].

Diagnosis

Imaging studies and/or histology are required for the diagnosis of recurrent disease. Cholangiographic features of intrahepatic and/or extrahepatic strictures and beading along with histologic findings including biliary fibrosis, fibro-obliterative lesions, cholangitis, and ductopenia are required for an accurate diagnosis of recurrent PSC (Table 47.3) [105,106]. The diagnosis of recurrent PSC requires the exclusion of other causes of biliary stricturing including ABO incompatibility, early and late hepatic artery thrombosis, prolonged cold ischemic time, and infectious causes. Differentiating recurrent disease from other biliary complications is dependent on the clinical picture and the timing and location of the biliary strictures (Box 47.1). Recurrent intrahepatic PSC is difficult to discern from chronic rejection and it is not clear that the two entities are mutually exclusive [107,108]. The diagnosis requires experienced pathologists and supporting clinical and radiographic evidence.

Risk factors

Risk factors for recurrent disease have not been well established, but are thought to include age, male gender, gender mismatch, inflammatory bowel disease (IBD), presence of an intact colon, presence of cholangiocarci-

---

Box 47.1 Differential diagnosis for recurrent primary sclerosing cholangitis.

- ABO incompatibility
- Preservation/reperfusion injury
- Hepatic artery thrombosis
- Anastomotic stricture
- Malignant stricture
- Chronic rejection
- Cytomegalovirus infection
- Cryptosporidium infection

---

noma prior to transplant, steroid exposure, and acute cellular rejection [103,109]. It has been suggested that patients who receive maintenance corticosteroids or orthoclone (OKT3) post transplant appear to be at higher risk of recurrent PSC, but recurrence does not appear related to other immunosuppressant medications [110]. The risk associated with steroid use, however, may reflect active IBD, which has been thought to be associated with recurrent disease. A meta-analysis of 18 published studies, however, could not confirm IBD as a risk factor for the recurrence of PSC after liver transplantation [91], but these studies were quite heterogenous. Since that meta-analysis, however, further data have suggested that the absence of ulcerative colitis post transplant (whether there was pretransplant colectomy or not) was protective for recurrent PSC, and the presence of severe or de novo ulcerative colitis was associated with recurrent PSC [109]. Pre- or post-transplant colectomy appears to be associated with fewer cases of recurrent PSC [109,111]. PSC is a risk factor for cholangiocarcinoma but the risk in recurrent PSC, although reported, is unknown [112]. Although the recipient bile duct is resected at transplant, a tiny residual native bile duct is frequently retained within the pancreas. The risk of malignancy in this retained duct has not been studied.

Treatment

As in the nontransplant population, no effective treatments exist for PSC recurrence in the allograft. A randomized controlled trial of high-dose UDCA in nontransplant patients demonstrated worse outcomes [113]. Trials of moderate-dose ursodiol did not show significant benefit to patients, thus consensus guidelines do not advocate ursodiol use in nontransplant patients (and this has been extrapolated to include transplant patients).

Recurrent autoimmune hepatitis

Autoimmune hepatitis (AIH) is an inflammatory condition that may lead to cirrhosis and liver failure. Autoimmune cirrhosis, and less commonly fulminant AIH, account for around 5% of liver transplants worldwide. Like PBC, it is associated with excellent outcomes post-LTX. However, recurrence of disease post-LTX can lead to graft loss, retransplantation, or death in those affected. Patients transplanted for other indications can develop de novo AIH post-LTX but this is beyond the scope of this chapter.

The recurrence rate of AIH post-LTX is approximately 22% [91]. As in rPBC, centers that perform protocol biopsies have higher rates of recurrent AIH, detecting biochemically silent cases. Whether or not these cases are clinically relevant is still unclear. Median time to recurrence is approximately 2 years [114]. Graft loss due to recurrent disease has been demonstrated in 6% of patients in one study [99]. In general, however, recurrent AIH does not impact on overall patient survival, with survival rates similar to those of patients without recurrence at 5 and 10 years [115].

Diagnosis

The diagnosis of recurrent AIH depends heavily on histology, but serologic and biochemical markers must be taken into account as well (Table 47.3). In a patient transplanted for AIH, increased serum transaminases, autoantibodies, and γ-globulins, as well as histologic evidence of lobular and/or periportal hepatitis (in the absence of rejection, viral infection, or drug-induced hepatitis), are features consistent with a diagnosis of recurrent AIH [91]. Some have also suggested steroid dependence as a marker for recurrent disease [116] but this is unhelpful in distinguishing it from steroid-responsive entities that mimic recurrent AIH such as late cellular rejection and alloimmune hepatitis.

Risk factors

Most studies have failed to find any clear donor factors that influence the rate of recurrence. There are conflicting data on whether HLA status (particularly HLA-DR3 positivity in recipients) is associated with recurrent AIH [91] and further studies are needed to evaluate this risk factor definitively. A recent study in a center without protocolized post-LTX biopsies found by multivariate analysis that the presence of moderate to severe inflammation in the explanted liver and high immunoglobulin G (IgG) levels before LTX were both independently associated with recurrent AIH [115]. Whether the immunosuppression regimen used is tacrolimus or cyclosporine based does not appear to have an impact on the rate of recurrence post-LTX [115].

Treatment

The goal of treatment in recurrent AIH is to intensify immunosuppression. Increasing or reinstating steroids, adding mycophenolate, or increasing calcineurin-inhibitor levels are all rational approaches that have been successful [90]. With increased immunosuppression, biochemical abnormalities and histologic features of recurrence quickly resolve in most patients with minimal impact on graft survival. Severe, refractory, or untreated cases can lead to graft failure and retransplantation may be necessary [116].

Recurrent nonalcoholic steatohepatitis

Nonalcoholic steatohepatitis (NASH) is increasingly common in patients undergoing liver transplantation. It may even overtake hepatitis C as the leading indication for transplantation in the coming decades. NASH is associated strongly with the metabolic syndrome (hypertension, diabetes, hyperlipidemia, and truncal obesity), which is highly prevalent in the post liver transplant population. These metabolic parameters infrequently resolve after transplant and in fact the prevalence increases dramatically after transplant. Diabetes is present in 30–40% of patients after transplantation, with hypertension affecting 60–70% and hyperlipidemia found in 50–70% of patients after transplant [4]. Metabolic syndrome has been described in 44–58% of patients after transplantation [117] whether transplanted for NASH or not. It is thus not surprising that NASH recurs after transplantation.

Approximately 60% of transplant patients with NASH developed steatosis grade 2 or higher within 1–2 years post transplant [118,119]. The probability of steatosis at 5 years post-LTX was 100% in comparison to 25% probability observed in patients of similar age and weight with PBC or alcoholic liver disease [119]. Of the NASH recipients with recurrent steatosis, >50% developed overt recurrent NASH within 2 years post transplant [118]. Between 5% and 10% of patients undergoing liver transplantation for NASH had recurrence that progressed to cirrhosis in long-term follow-up, with graft failure reported in about half of patients with cirrhotic stage recurrence (i.e., long-term absolute NASH recurrence-associated graft loss rate of 2.5–5%) [118]. A more recent retrospective analysis had similar overall findings but observed no NASH recurrence-associated graft loss [120].

Metabolic syndrome may not be the only risk factor for recurrent steatosis. Certainly steroid treatment can have direct and indirect effects. Steroids are known to promote fatty changes within the hepatocytes, as well as increase insulin resistance and worsen diabetes. Steroid-free protocols reduce the frequency of diabetes after transplant, but the effect on steatosis post transplant has not been adequately studied.

As in the pretransplant patient population there is no treatment other than weight loss and medical management of hypertension, diabetes, and hyperlipidemia.

Recurrent alcohol-related liver disease

Alcohol is not only the cause of end-stage liver disease in genetically susceptible individuals but can act as a cofactor accelerating the disease progression of other liver disease. Although liver transplantation can successfully cure alcohol-related liver disease (ALD), alcoholism, when present, remains after transplantation. However, the allograft may no longer have the same susceptibility to alcohol-induced liver injury, thereby making recurrent ALD a separate, rarer entity than post-LTX recidivism of alcohol use and abuse. Patient selection for LTX and treatment of alcoholism is beyond the scope of this chapter.

It is difficult to determine the true rate of recurrent alcohol use/abuse post-LTX given the absence of a reliable marker of alcohol consumption with a long half-life. Recurrent alcohol use is estimated to be 20%, but definitions generally include "any use" even if infrequent or of small quantity [121]. Recurrent ALD, defined as patients actively consuming alcohol and the presence of steatosis or graft injury (as a direct alcohol effect or secondary to chronic rejection due to documented noncompliance), resulted in a rate of recurrent ALD of 24% over 22 years of follow-up [99]. Three percent of patients transplanted for ALD lost their graft to recurrent disease with a median time to graft loss of nearly 7 years in this study.

Recurrent alcohol use/abuse impacts long-term patient survival, with 5- and 10-year survival rtes of 92% and 45%, respectively, in recidivistic patients compared with 92% and 86% in abstinent patients [122]. The increased mortality at 10 years in these patients may be due to higher rates of cardiovascular events and cancers in patients that consume significant amounts of alcohol. Patients transplanted for ALD are also more likely to smoke pre and post-LTX [123] and suffer from higher rates of tobacco-associated malignancies after transplant [124].

It is clear that severe recurrent ALD can occur in recidivistic patients, leading to alcoholic hepatitis, cirrhosis, and liver failure, sometimes very soon after the transplant. These patients are usually not considered candidates for retransplantation and die of their disease. Abstinence really is the only hope for most of these patients. Treatment of alcoholic hepatitis in the allograft is similar to that in nontransplant patients, but no studies exist specifically addressing the transplant patient.

Recurrent vascular diseases

Hepatic venous outflow obstruction can be due to thrombosis (Budd–Chiari syndrome), right heart failure, and sinusoidal obstruction syndrome (SOS, or previously known as venoocclusive disease). As patients with right heart failure and SOS rarely receive a liver transplant, the discussion on recurrent vascular disease will focus on recurrent Budd–Chiari syndrome.

Budd–Chiari syndrome

Budd–Chiari syndrome can include thrombosis along any portion of the venous outflow tract and is usually attributed to a prothrombotic disorder requiring lifelong anticoagulation (although transplant is curative for protein C, protein S, and antithrombin III deficiency). Despite anticoagulation, Budd–Chiari syndrome has been reported to recur in up to 2–27% percent of patients [125–128]. One study [125], suggested a high rate of thrombus post transplant in patients transplanted for Budd–Chiari despite early post-transplant anticoagulation. Three of 11 patients (27%) developed early recurrent thrombus of the hepatic veins and an additional three patients developed other major vessel thrombi, whereas most other larger studies demonstrated much lower recurrence rates (1–7%) [127,128]. An alternative to anticoagulation in patients with Budd–Chiari syndrome secondary to myeloproliferative disease is the use of antiplatelet agents and hydroxyurea, since patients experienced equally low recurrence rates (1/10 patients, 10%) on this regimen [126].

Recurrent metabolic disease

Metabolic diseases comprise approximately 3–5% of all transplants performed in the United States (http://www.ustransplant.org/annual_reports/). The majority of metabolic diseases (tyrosinemia, urea cycle disorders, α_1-antitrypsin deficiency, etc.) are cured by transplantation. Hereditary hemochromatosis is a metabolic disorder of iron accumulation. A genetic predisposition underlies this iron accumulation, as described elsewhere in this textbook (see Chapters 29–31). It is unknown if the inadequate hepcidin response to iron levels is purely liver related, in which case transplantation can offer a cure. If the abnormal hepcidin response is a secondary reaction to a genetically predetermined trigger elsewhere in the iron metabolism event series, then transplantation would simply reset the clock, without altering the disease course. A recent study suggests the latter is more likely [129], but more data are needed. Recurrent disease, as defined by the iron accumulation within the liver, would then take decades to accumulate. Continued iron accumulation within other organs would be unaffected by transplantation, and thus more likely to impact longevity. Further ferritin and iron studies are recommended in these patients.

Conclusions

In summary, many of the most common indications for liver transplantation can recur following transplantation. The natural history of the disease in the allograft is not always the same as in the immunocompetent patient. Risk factors may help identify those patients at highest risk of recurrence, but we cannot reliably predict who will have a worse outcome relating to this recurrence. Recurrent disease, particularly hepatitis C, PSC, and possibly NASH, may increase the burden on liver retransplantation. With the limit on organ availability, more study into the prevention and management of recurrent disease is needed.

Annoted references

Berenguer M. Systematic review of the treatment of established recurrent hepatitis C with pegylated interferon in combination with ribavirin. *J Hepatol* 2008;49:274–87.

This paper summarizes the high-quality papers focused on pegylated interferon and ribavirin treatment protocols in the transplant patient.

Charlton M, Kasparova P, Weston S, et al. Frequency of nonalcoholic steatohepatitis as a cause of advanced liver disease. *Liver Transpl* 2001;7:608–14.

These authors determined the frequency of steatosis and steatohepatitis in the transplant allograft and established that patients transplanted for NASH have significantly higher rates of NASH than other patients who develop steatosis.

Cholongitas E, Shusang V, Papatheodoridis GV, et al. Risk factors for recurrence of primary sclerosing cholangitis after liver transplantation. *Liver Transpl* 2008;14:138–43.

This paper establishes risk factors, including active ulcerative colitis (and steroid use for management), as well as the influence of colectomy on recurrent PSC after liver transplantation.

Degertekin B, Han SH, Keeffe EB, et al. Impact of virologic breakthrough and HBIG regimen on hepatitis B recurrence after liver transplantation. *Am J Transplant* 2010;10(8):1823–33.

Study by the NIH HBV-OLT Study Group that reports the rate of HBV recurrence in 15 US transplant centers. This study also looked at HBIg regimens and found no statistically significant difference between them in terms of rates of recurrence, even in patients with virologic breakthrough as long as nucleos(t)ide analogs were used as rescue therapy pre- and post-LTX.

Duclos-Vallee JC, Sebagh M. Recurrence of autoimmune disease, primary sclerosing cholangitis, primary biliary cirrhosis, and autoimmune hepatitis after liver transplantation. *Liver Transpl* 2009;15(Suppl 2):S25–34.

Review of recurrent autoimmune diseases post transplantation including pictures of pathological findings and covering treatment.

Gane EJ. The natural history of recurrent hepatitis C and what influences this. *Liver Transpl* 2008;14(Suppl 2):S36–44.

A summary of all of the literature determining the natural history of recurrent HCV after liver transplantation.

Katz LH, Tur-Kaspa R, Guy DG, Paul M. Lamivudine or adefovir dipivoxil alone or combined with immunoglobulin for preventing hepatitis B recurrence after liver transplantation. *Cochrane Database Syst Rev* 2010;7:CD006005.

Systematic review of clinical trials of prophylaxis regimens for HBV recurrence that revealed the paucity of randomized clinical trial data in this area. It did show that nonrandomized trials favored combination prophylaxis with HBIg and a nucleos(t)ide analog versus monotherapy.

Wiesner RH, Sorrell M, Villamil F. Report of the first International Liver Transplantation Society expert panel consensus conference on liver transplantation and hepatitis C. *Liver Transpl* 2003;9:S1–9.

A summary of a consensus conference focusing on recurrent HCV. They define the natural history, risk factors predictive of worse outcomes, and management strategies to optimize these outcomes.

References

1. Gane EJ, Portmann BC, Naoumov NV, et al. Long-term outcome of hepatitis C infection after liver transplantation. *N Engl J Med* 1996;334(13):815–20.
2. Neumann UP, Berg T, Bahra M, et al. Long-term outcome of liver transplants for chronic hepatitis C: a 10-year follow-up. *Transplantation* 2004;77(2):226–31.
3. Forman LM, Lewis JD, Berlin JA, Feldman HI, Lucey MR. The association between hepatitis C infection and survival after orthotopic liver transplantation. *Gastroenterology* 2002;122(4):889–96.
4. Watt K, Pedersen R, Kremers W, Heimbach J, Charlton M. Evolution of causes and risk factors for mortality post liver transplant: Results of the NIDDK long term follow-up study. *Am J Transplant* 2010;10:1–8.
5. Watt KD, Lyden ER, McCashland TM. Poor survival after liver retransplantation: is hepatitis C to blame? *Liver Transpl* 2003;9(10):1019–24.
6. Garcia-Retortillo M, Forns X, Feliu A, et al. Hepatitis C virus kinetics during and immediately after liver transplantation. *Hepatology* 2002;35(3):680–7.
7. Gane EJ, Naoumov NV, Qian KP, et al. A longitudinal analysis of hepatitis C virus replication following liver transplantation. *Gastroenterology* 1996;110(1):167–77.
8. Firpi RJ, Abdelmalek MF, Soldevila-Pico C, et al. One-year protocol liver biopsy can stratify fibrosis progression in liver transplant recipients with recurrent hepatitis C infection. *Liver Transpl* 2004;10(10):1240–7.
9. Neumann U, Berg T, Bahra M, et al. Fibrosis progression after liver transplantation in patients with recurrent hepatitis C. *J Hepatol* 2004;41(5):830–6.
10. Walter T, Dumortier J, Guillaud O, Hervieu V, Scoazec JY, Boillot O. Factors influencing the progression of fibrosis in patients with recurrent hepatitis C after liver transplantation under antiviral therapy: a retrospective analysis of 939 liver biopsies in a single center. *Liver Transpl* 2007;13(2):294–301.
11. Bahra M, Neumann U, Jacob D, et al. Fibrosis progression in hepatitis C positive liver recipients after sustained virologic response to antiviral combination therapy (interferon-ribavirin therapy). *Transplantation* 2007;83(3):351–3.
12. Berenguer M, Palau A, Aguilera V, Rayón J, Juan F, Prieto M. Clinical benefits of antiviral therapy in patients with recurrent hepatitis C following liver transplantation. *Am J Transplant* 2008;8(3):679–87.
13. Berenguer M, Prieto M, Rayon JM, et al. Natural history of clinically compensated hepatitis C virus-related graft cirrhosis after liver transplantation. *Hepatology* 2000;32(4 Pt 1):852–8.
14. Firpi RJ, Clark V, Soldevila-Pico C, et al. The natural history of hepatitis C cirrhosis after liver transplantation. *Liver Transpl* 2009;15(9):1063–71.
15. Dixon L, Crawford J. Early histologic changes in fibrosing cholestatic hepatitis C. *Liver Transpl* 2007;13(2):219–26.
16. Charlton MR, Thompson A, Veldt BJ, et al. Interleukin-28B polymorphisms are associated with histological recurrence and treatment response following liver transplantation in patients with hepatitis C virus infection. *Hepatology* 2011;53(1):317–24.
17. Schvoerer E, Soulier E, Royer C, et al. Early evolution of hepatitis C virus (HCV) quasispecies after liver transplant for HCV-related disease. *J Infect Dis* 2007;196(4):528–36.
18. Veldt BJ, Poterucha JJ, Watt KD, et al. Insulin resistance, serum adipokines and risk of fibrosis progression in patients transplanted for hepatitis C. *Am J Transplant* 2009;9(6):1406–13.
19. Foxton M, Quaglia A, Muiesan P, et al. The impact of diabetes mellitus on fibrosis progression in patients transplanted for hepatitis C. *Am J Transplant* 2006;6(8):1922–9.
20. de Vera ME, Dvorchik I, Tom K, et al. Survival of liver transplant patients coinfected with HIV and HCV is adversely impacted by recurrent hepatitis C. *Am J Transplant* 2006;6(12):2983–93.
21. Mutimer DJ, Gunson B, Chen J, et al. Impact of donor age and year of transplantation on graft and patient survival following liver transplantation for hepatitis C virus. *Transplantation* 2006;81(1):7–14.
22. Pang PS, Kamal A, Glenn JS. The effect of donor race on the survival of black Americans undergoing liver transplantation for chronic hepatitis C. *Liver Transpl* 2009;15(9):1126–32.
23. Watt KD, Lyden ER, Gulizia JM, McCashland TM. Recurrent hepatitis C posttransplant: early preservation injury may predict poor outcome. *Liver Transpl* 2006;12(1):134–9.

24. Selzner N, Girgrah N, Lilly L, et al. The difference in the fibrosis progression of recurrent hepatitis C after live donor liver transplantation versus deceased donor liver transplantation is attributable to the difference in donor age. *Liver Transpl* 2008;14(12):1778–86.

25. Charlton M, Seaberg E. Impact of immunosuppression and acute rejection on recurrence of hepatitis C: results of the National Institute of Diabetes and Digestive and Kidney Diseases Liver Transplantation Database. *Liver Transpl Surg* 1999;5(4 Suppl 1):S107–14.

26. Berenguer M, Aguilera V, Prieto M, et al. Significant improvement in the outcome of HCV-infected transplant recipients by avoiding rapid steroid tapering and potent induction immunosuppression. *J Hepatol* 2006;44(4):717–22.

27. Klintmalm GB, Washburn WK, Rudich SM, et al. Corticosteroid-free immunosuppression with daclizumab in HCV(+) liver transplant recipients: 1-year interim results of the HCV-3 study. *Liver Transpl* 2007;13(11):1521–31.

28. Marcos A, Eghtesad B, Fung JJ, et al. Use of alemtuzumab and tacrolimus monotherapy for cadaveric liver transplantation: with particular reference to hepatitis C virus. *Transplantation* 2004; 78(7):966–71.

29. Rosen HR, Shackleton CR, Higa L, et al. Use of OKT3 is associated with early and severe recurrence of hepatitis C after liver transplantation. *Am J Gastroenterol* 1997;92(9):1453–7.

30. Berenguer M. Systematic review of the treatment of established recurrent hepatitis C with pegylated interferon in combination with ribavirin. *J Hepatol* 2008;49(2):274–87.

31. Veldt BJ, Poterucha JJ, Watt KD, et al. Impact of pegylated interferon and ribavirin treatment on graft survival in liver transplant patients with recurrent hepatitis C infection. *Am J Transplant* 2008; 8(11):2426–33.

32. Berardi S, Lodato F, Gramenzi A, et al. High incidence of allograft dysfunction in liver transplanted patients treated with pegylated-interferon alpha-2b and ribavirin for hepatitis C recurrence: possible de novo autoimmune hepatitis? *Gut* 2007;56(2):237–42.

33. Fernandez I, Ulloa E, Colina F, et al. Incidence, risk factors, and outcome of chronic rejection during antiviral therapy for posttransplant recurrent hepatitis C. *Liver Transpl* 2009;15(8):948–55.

34. Stravitz RT, Shiffman ML, Sanyal AJ, et al. Effects of interferon treatment on liver histology and allograft rejection in patients with recurrent hepatitis C following liver transplantation. *Liver Transpl* 2004; 10(7):850–8.

35. Everson GT, Trotter J, Forman L, et al. Treatment of advanced hepatitis C with a low accelerating dosage regimen of antiviral therapy. *Hepatology* 2005;42(2):255–62.

36. Wiesner RH, Sorrell M, Villamil F. Report of the first International Liver Transplantation Society expert panel consensus conference on liver transplantation and hepatitis C. *Liver Transpl* 2003;9(11):S1–9.

37. Chalasani N, Manzarbeitia C, Ferenci P, et al. Peginterferon alfa-2a for hepatitis C after liver transplantation: two randomized, controlled trials. *Hepatology* 2005;41(2):289–98.

38. Bzowej N, Nelson DR, Terrault N, et al. PHOENIX: a randomized controlled trial of peginterferon alfa-2a/ribavirin prophylactic treatment after liver transplant for hepatitis C. *Liver Transpl* 2010; 16(6 Suppl 1):S118.

39. Xirouchakis E, Triantos C, Manousou P, et al. Pegylated-interferon and ribavirin in liver transplant candidates and recipients with HCV cirrhosis: systematic review and meta-analysis of prospective controlled studies. *J Viral Hepatitis* 2008;15(10):699–709.

40. Angelico M, Petrolati A, Lionetti R, et al. A randomized study on peg-interferon alfa-2a with or without ribavirin in liver transplant recipients with recurrent hepatitis C. *J Hepatol* 2007;46(6):1009–17.

41. Carrion JA, Navasa M, Garcia-Retortillo M, et al. Efficacy of antiviral therapy on hepatitis C recurrence after liver transplantation: a randomized controlled study. *Gastroenterology* 2007;132(5):1746–56.

42. Kornberg A, Kupper B, Tannapfel A, et al. Sustained clearance of serum hepatitis C virus-RNA independently predicts long-term survival in liver transplant patients with recurrent hepatitis C. *Transplantation* 2008;86(3):469–73.

43. Firpi RJ, Soldevila-Pico C, Morelli GG, et al. The use of cyclosporine for recurrent hepatitis C after liver transplant: a randomized pilot study. *Dig Dis Sci* 2010;55(1):196–203.

44. Kim WR, Poterucha JJ, Kremers WK, Ishitani MB, Dickson ER. Outcome of liver transplantation for hepatitis B in the United States. *Liver Transpl* 2004;10(8):968–74.

45. Degertekin B, Han SH, Keeffe EB, et al. Impact of virologic breakthrough and HBIG regimen on hepatitis B recurrence after liver transplantation. *Am J Transplant* 2010;10(8):1823–33.

46. Yuefeng M, Weili F, Wenxiang T, et al. Long-term outcome of patients with lamivudine after early cessation of hepatitis B immunoglobulin for prevention of recurrent hepatitis B following liver transplantation. *Clin Transplant* 2010 (Epub ahead of print).

47. Gane EJ, Angus PW, Strasser S, et al. Lamivudine plus low-dose hepatitis B immunoglobulin to prevent recurrent hepatitis B following liver transplantation. *Gastroenterology* 2007;132(3):931–7.

48. Katz LH, Tur-Kaspa R, Guy DG, Paul M. Lamivudine or adefovir dipivoxil alone or combined with immunoglobulin for preventing hepatitis B recurrence after liver transplantation. *Cochrane Database Syst Rev* 2010;7: CD006005.

49. Konig V, Hopf U, Neuhaus P, et al. Long-term follow-up of hepatitis B virus-infected recipients after orthotopic liver transplantation. *Transplantation* 1994;58(5):553–9.

50. Samuel D, Muller R, Alexander G, et al. Liver transplantation in European patients with the hepatitis B surface antigen. *N Engl J Med* 1993;329(25):1842–7.

51. Chen J, Yi L, Jia JD, Ma H, You H. Hepatitis B immunoglobulins and/or lamivudine for preventing hepatitis B recurrence after liver transplantation: a systematic review. *J Gastroenterol Hepatol* 2010; 25(5):872–9.

52. Bzowej N, Han S, Degertekin B, et al. Liver transplantation outcomes among Caucasians, Asian Americans, and African Americans with hepatitis B. *Liver Transpl* 2009;15(9):1010–20.

53. Dandri M, Murray JM, Lutgehetmann M, Volz T, Lohse AW, Petersen J. Virion half-life in chronic hepatitis B infection is strongly correlated with levels of viremia. *Hepatology* 2008;48(4):1079–86.

54. Feray C, Zignego AL, Samuel D, et al. Persistent hepatitis B virus infection of mononuclear blood cells without concomitant liver infection. The liver transplantation model. *Transplantation* 1990; 49(6):1155–8.

55. Pontisso P, Vidalino L, Quarta S, Gatta A. Biological and clinical implications of HBV infection in peripheral blood mononuclear cells. *Autoimmun Rev* 2008;8(1):13–7.

56. Roche B, Feray C, Gigou M, et al. HBV DNA persistence 10 years after liver transplantation despite successful anti-HBS passive immunoprophylaxis. *Hepatology* 2003;38(1):86–95.

57. Chou CK, Wang LH, Lin HM, Chi CW. Glucocorticoid stimulates hepatitis B viral gene expression in cultured human hepatoma cells. *Hepatology* 1992;16(1):13–18.

58. Zheng S, Chen Y, Liang T, et al. Prevention of hepatitis B recurrence after liver transplantation using lamivudine or lamivudine combined with hepatitis B immunoglobulin prophylaxis. *Liver Transpl* 2006;12(2):253–8.

59. Schiff E, Lai CL, Hadziyannis S, et al. Adefovir dipivoxil for wait-listed and post-liver transplantation patients with lamivudine-resistant hepatitis B: final long-term results. *Liver Transpl* 2007; 13(3):349–60.

60. Villet S, Pichoud C, Villeneuve JP, Trepo C, Zoulim F. Selection of a multiple drug-resistant hepatitis B virus strain in a liver-transplanted patient. *Gastroenterology* 2006;131(4):1253–61.

61. Nath DS, Kalis A, Nelson S, Payne WD, Lake JR, Humar A. Hepatitis B prophylaxis post-liver transplant without maintenance hepatitis B immunoglobulin therapy. *Clin Transplant* 2006;20(2):206–10.

62. Samuel D, Bismuth A, Mathieu D, et al. Passive immunoprophylaxis after liver transplantation in HBsAg-positive patients. *Lancet* 1991;337(8745):813–15.

63. Marzano A, Gaia S, Ghisetti V, et al. Viral load at the time of liver transplantation and risk of hepatitis B virus recurrence. *Liver Transpl* 2005;11(4):402–9.

64. Seehofer D, Rayes N, Naumann U, et al. Preoperative antiviral treatment and postoperative prophylaxis in HBV-DNA positive patients undergoing liver transplantation. *Transplantation* 2001;72(8):1381–5.

65. Rosenau J, Bahr MJ, Tillmann HL, et al. Lamivudine and low-dose hepatitis B immune globulin for prophylaxis of hepatitis B reinfection after liver transplantation possible role of mutations in the YMDD motif prior to transplantation as a risk factor for reinfection. *J Hepatol* 2001;34(6):895–902.

66. Xie SB, Zhu JY, Ying Z, Zeng LJ, Chao M, Lu MQ. Prevention and risk factors of the HBV recurrence after orthotopic liver transplantation: 160 cases follow-up study. *Transplantation* 2010;90(7):786–90.

67. Marzano A, Lampertico P, Mazzaferro V, et al. Prophylaxis of hepatitis B virus recurrence after liver transplantation in carriers of lamivudine-resistant mutants. *Liver Transpl* 2005;11(5):532–8.

68. Lo CM, Liu CL, Lau GK, Chan SC, Ng IO, Fan ST. Liver transplantation for chronic hepatitis B with lamivudine-resistant YMDD mutant using add-on adefovir dipivoxil plus lamivudine. *Liver Transpl* 2005;11(7):807–13.

69. Samuel D, Alexander G. Liver transplantation for hepatitis B virus infection. *Liver Transpl Surg* 1995;1(4):270–4.

70. Jiang L, Yan LN. Current therapeutic strategies for recurrent hepatitis B virus infection after liver transplantation. *World J Gastroenterol* 2010;16(20):2468–75.

71. Marcellin P, Samuel D, Areias J, et al. Pretransplantation interferon treatment and recurrence of hepatitis B virus infection after liver transplantation for hepatitis B-related end-stage liver disease. *Hepatology* 1994;19(1):6–12.

72. Lok AS, McMahon BJ. Chronic hepatitis B: update 2009. *Hepatology* 2009;50(3):661–2.

73. Pawlotsky JM. EASL clinical practice guidelines. *J Hepatol* 2009; 50(2):243.

74. Patterson SJ, Angus PW. Post-liver transplant hepatitis B prophylaxis: the role of oral nucleos(t)ide analogues. *Curr Opin Organ Transplant* 2009;14(3):225–30.

75. Muller R, Samuel D, Fassati LR, Benhamou JP, Bismuth H, Alexander GJ. 'EUROHEP' consensus report on the management of liver transplantation for hepatitis B virus infection. European concerted action on viral hepatitis. *J Hepatol* 1994;21(6):1140–3.

76. Shields PL, Owsianka A, Carman WF, et al. Selection of hepatitis B surface "escape" mutants during passive immune prophylaxis following liver transplantation: potential impact of genetic changes on polymerase protein function. *Gut* 1999;45(2):306–9.

77. Terrault N, Roche B, Samuel D. Management of the hepatitis B virus in the liver transplantation setting: a European and an American perspective. *Liver Transpl* 2005;11(7):716–32.

78. Yi NJ, Suh KS, Cho JY, et al. Recurrence of hepatitis B is associated with cumulative corticosteroid dose and chemotherapy against hepatocellular carcinoma recurrence after liver transplantation. *Liver Transpl* 2007;13(3):451–8.

79. Shouval D, Samuel D. Hepatitis B immune globulin to prevent hepatitis B virus graft reinfection following liver transplantation: a concise review. *Hepatology* 2000;32(6):1189–95.

80. Jiang L, Yan L, Li B, et al. Prophylaxis against hepatitis B recurrence posttransplantation using lamivudine and individualized low-dose hepatitis B immunoglobulin. *Am J Transplant* 2010;10(8):1861–9.

31. Angeli P, Scaglione F. Nephrotoxicity of intravenous immunoglobulin in the setting of liver transplantation or HBV-related cirrhosis: an undervalued topic. *Minerva Gastroenterol Dietol* 2008;54(3):259–75.

82. Powell JJ, Apiratpracha W, Partovi N, et al. Subcutaneous administration of hepatitis B immune globulin in combination with lamivudine following orthotopic liver transplantation: effective prophylaxis against recurrence. *Clin Transplant* 2006;20(4):524–5.

83. Singham J, Greanya ED, Lau K, Erb SR, Partovi N, Yoshida EM. Efficacy of maintenance subcutaneous hepatitis B immune globulin (HBIG) post-transplant for prophylaxis against hepatitis B recurrence. *Ann Hepatol* 2010;9(2):166–71.

84. Yoshida H, Kato T. Levi DM, et al. Lamivudine monoprophylaxis for liver transplant recipients with non-replicating hepatitis B virus infection. *Clin Transplant* 2007;21(2):166–71.

85. Wong SN, Chu CJ, Wai CT, et al. Low risk of hepatitis B virus recurrence after withdrawal of long-term hepatitis B immunoglobulin in patients receiving maintenance nucleos(t)ide analogue therapy. *Liver Transpl* 2007;13(3):374–81.

86. Xi ZF, Xia Q, Zhang JJ, et al. The role of entecavir in preventing hepatitis B recurrence after liver transplantation. *J Dig Dis* 2009;10(4):321–7.

87. Rosenau J, Hooman N, Hadem J, et al. Failure of hepatitis B vaccination with conventional HBsAg vaccine in patients with continuous HBIG prophylaxis after liver transplantation. *Liver Transpl* 2007;13(3):367–73.

88. Di Paolo D, Lenci I, Cerocchi C, et al. One-year vaccination against hepatitis B virus with a MPL-vaccine in liver transplant patients for HBV-related cirrhosis. *Transpl Int* 2010;23(11):1105–12.

89. Neuberger J, Portmann B, Macdougall BR, Calne RY, Williams R. Recurrence of primary biliary cirrhosis after liver transplantation. *N Engl J Med* 1982;306(1):1–4.

90. Schreuder TC, Hubscher SG. Neuberger J. Autoimmune liver diseases and recurrence after orthotopic liver transplantation: what have we learned so far? *Transpl Int* 2009;22(2):144–52.

91. Gautam M, Cheruvattath R. Balan V. Recurrence of autoimmune liver disease after liver transplantation: a systematic review. *Liver Transpl* 2006;12(12):1813–24.

92. Manousou P, Arvaniti V, Tsochatzis E, et al. Primary biliary cirrhosis after liver transplantation: influence of immunosuppression and human leukocyte antigen locus disparity. *Liver Transpl* 2010;16(1):64–73.

93. Charatcharoenwitthaya P, Pimentel S, Talwalkar JA, et al. Long-term survival and impact of ursodeoxycholic acid treatment for recurrent primary biliary cirrhosis after liver transplantation. *Liver Transpl* 2007;13(9):1236–45.

94. Silveira MG, Talwalkar JA, Lindor KD, Wiesner RH. Recurrent primary biliary cirrhosis after liver transplantation. *Am J Transplant* 2010;10(4):720–6.

95. Abraham SC, Poterucha JJ, Rosen CB, Demetris AJ, Krasinskas AM. Histologic abnormalities are common in protocol liver allograft biopsies from patients with normal liver function tests. *Am J Surg Pathol* 2008;32(7):965–73.

96. Sylvestre P. Recurrence of primary biliary cirrhosis after liver transplantation: histologic estimate of incidence and natural history. *Liver Transpl* 2003;9(10):1086–93

97. Khettry U, Anand N, Faul PN, et al. Liver transplantation for primary biliary cirrhosis: a long-term pathologic study. *Liver Transpl* 2003;9(1):87–96.

98. Liermann Garcia RF, Evangelista Garcia C, McMaster P, Neuberger J. Transplantation for primary biliary cirrhosis: retrospective analysis of 400 patients in a single center. *Hepatology* 2001;33(1):22–7.

99. Rowe IA, Webb K, Gunson BK, Mehta N, Haque S, Neuberger J. The impact of disease recurrence on graft survival following liver transplantation: a single centre experience. *Transpl Int* 2008;21(5):459–65.

100. Silveira MG, Talwalkar JA, Lindor KD, Wiesner RH. Recurrent primary biliary cirrhosis after liver transplantation. *Am J Transplant* 2010;10(4):720–6.

101. Dmitrewski J, Hubscher SG, Mayer AD, Neuberger JM. Recurrence of primary biliary cirrhosis in the liver allograft: the effect of immunosuppression. *J Hepatol* 1996;24(3):253–7.

102. Poupon R. Primary biliary cirrhosis: a 2010 update. *J Hepatol* 2010; 52(5):745–58.

103. Campsen J, Zimmerman MA, Trotter JF, et al. Clinically recurrent primary sclerosing cholangitis following liver transplantation: a time course. *Liver Transpl* 2008;14(2):181–5.

104. Graziadei IW. Recurrence of primary sclerosing cholangitis after liver transplantation. *Liver Transpl* 2002;8(7):575–81.

105. Harrison RF, Davies MH, Neuberger JM, Hubscher SG. Fibrous and obliterative cholangitis in liver allografts: evidence of recurrent primary sclerosing cholangitis? *Hepatology* 1994;20(2):356–61.

106. Kubota T, Thomson A, Clouston AD, et al. Clinicopathologic findings of recurrent primary sclerosing cholangitis after orthotopic liver transplantation. *J Hepatobiliary Pancreat Surg* 1999;6(4):377–81.

107. Brandsaeter B, Schrumpf E, Bentdal O, et al. Recurrent primary sclerosing cholangitis after liver transplantation: a magnetic resonance cholangiography study with analyses of predictive factors. *Liver Transpl* 2005;11(11):1361–9.

108. McPartland KJ, Lewis WD, Gordon FD, et al. Post-liver transplant cholestatic disorder with biliary strictures: de novo versus recurrent primary sclerosing cholangitis. *Pathol Int* 2009;59(5):312–16.

109. Cholongitas E, Shusang V, Papatheodoridis GV, et al. Risk factors for recurrence of primary sclerosing cholangitis after liver transplantation. *Liver Transpl* 2008;14(2):138–43.

110. Kugelmas M, Spiegelman P, Osgood MJ, et al. Different immunosuppressive regimens and recurrence of primary sclerosing cholangitis after liver transplantation. *Liver Transpl* 2003;9(7):727–32.

111. Vera A, Moledina S, Gunson B, et al. Risk factors for recurrence of primary sclerosing cholangitis of liver allograft. *Lancet* 2002; 360(9349):1943–4.

112. Heneghan MA, Tuttle-Newhall JE, Suhocki PV, et al. De-novo cholangiocarcinoma in the setting of recurrent primary sclerosing cholangitis following liver transplant. *Am J Transplant* 2003;3(5): 634–8.

113. Lindor KD, Kowdley KV, Luketic VA, et al. High-dose ursodeoxycholic acid for the treatment of primary sclerosing cholangitis. *Hepatology* 2009;50(3):808–14.

114. Czaja AJ. Recurrent autoimmune hepatitis after liver transplantation: a disease continuum or a fresh start? *Liver Transpl* 2009; 15(10):1169–71.

115. Montano-Loza AJ, Mason AL, Ma M, Bastiampillai RJ, Bain VG, Tandon P. Risk factors for recurrence of autoimmune hepatitis after liver transplantation. *Liver Transpl* 2009;15(10):1254–61.

116. Duclos-Vallee JC, Sebagh M. Recurrence of autoimmune disease, primary sclerosing cholangitis, primary biliary cirrhosis, and autoimmune hepatitis after liver transplantation. *Liver Transpl* 2009; 15(Suppl 2):S25–34.

117. Laryea M, Watt KD, Molinari M, et al. Metabolic Syndrome in Liver Transplant Recipients:Prevalence and Association with Cardiovascular Events. *Liver Transpl* 2007;13(8):1109–14.

118. Charlton M, Kasparova P, Weston S, et al. Frequency of nonalcoholic steatohepatitis as a cause of advanced liver disease. *Liver Transpl* 2001;7(7):608–14.

119. Contos MJ, Cales W, Sterling RK, et al. Development of nonalcoholic fatty liver disease after orthotopic liver transplantation for cryptogenic cirrhosis. *Liver Transpl* 2001;7(4):363–73.

120. Malik SM, Gupte PA, de Vera ME, Ahmad J. Liver transplantation in patients with nonalcoholic steatohepatitis-related hepatocellular carcinoma. *Clin Gastroenterol Hepatol* 2009;7(7):800–6.

121. Lim JK, Keeffe EB. Liver transplantation for alcoholic liver disease: current concepts and length of sobriety. *Liver Transpl* 2004;10(10 Suppl 2):S31–8.

122. Cuadrado A, Fabrega E, Casafont F, Pons-Romero F. Alcohol recidivism impairs long-term patient survival after orthotopic liver transplantation for alcoholic liver disease. *Liver Transpl* 2005;11(4): 420–6.

123. DiMartini A, Javed L, Russell S, et al. Tobacco use following liver transplantation for alcoholic liver disease: an underestimated problem. *Liver Transpl* 2005;11(6):679–83.

124. Jain A, DiMartini A, Kashyap R, Youk A, Rohal S, Fung J. Long-term follow-up after liver transplantation for alcoholic liver disease under tacrolimus. *Transplantation* 2000;70(9):1335–42.

125. Cruz E, Ascher NL, Roberts JP, Bass NM, Yao FY. High incidence of recurrence and hematologic events following liver transplantation for Budd–Chiari syndrome. *Clin Transplant* 2005;19(4):501–6.

126. Melear JM, Goldstein RM, Levy MF, et al. Hematologic aspects of liver transplantation for Budd–Chiari syndrome with special reference to myeloproliferative disorders. *Transplantation* 2002; 74(8):1090–5.

127. Mentha G, Giostra E, Majno PE, et al. Liver transplantation for Budd–Chiari syndrome: a European study on 248 patients from 51 centres. *J Hepatol* 2006;44(3):520–8.

128. Ulrich F, Pratschke J, Neumann U, et al. Eighteen years of liver transplantation experience in patients with advanced Budd–Chiari syndrome. *Liver Transpl* 2008;14(2):144–50.

129. Garuti C, Tian Y, Montosi G, et al. Hepcidin expression does not rescue the iron-poor phenotype of Kupffer cells in Hfe-null mice after liver transplantation. *Gastroenterology* 2010;139(1):315–22, e1.

130. Fattovich G, Giustina G, Degos F, et al. Morbidity and mortality in compensated cirrhosis type C: a retrospective follow-up study of 384 patients. *Gastroenterology* 1997;112: 463–472.

Multiple choice questions

47.1 An individual patient undergoing liver transplantation for hepatitis C virus (HCV)-related end-stage liver disease has a risk of cirrhosis by 5 years after transplant of how much?

    a 1–2%.
    b 3–5%.
    c 10–15%.
    d 20–30%.
    e 40–50%.

47.2 A patient with hepatitis B end-stage liver disease has a liver transplant. The hepatitis B virus (HBV) DNA level is detectable at 10,000 copies/mL at the time of transplant. Management prophylaxis is initiated to prevent recurrence of HBV after transplant. You would recommend which of the following prophylactic regimens?

    a Hepatitis B immunoglobulin (HBIg) monotherapy.
    b Lamivudine monotherapy.
    c HBIg × 1 month with indefinite lamivudine.
    d HBIg and tenofovir combination therapy.
    e Tenofovir monotherapy.

Answers to the multiple choice questions can be found in the Appendix at the end of the book.

These multiple choice questions are also available for you to complete online.
Visit http://www.schiffsdiseasesoftheliver.com/

CHAPTER 48
The Role of Retransplantation

Peter L. Abt & Kim M. Olthoff

Department of Surgery, Division of Transplant Surgery, The Hospital of the University of Pennsylvania, Philadelphia, PA, USA

Key concepts

- Retransplantation after primary orthotopic liver transplantation (OLT) accounts for approximately 7–10% of all liver transplants in the United States.
- Overall graft and patient survival is lower following retransplantation compared with results after one transplant. The best outcome is achieved if retransplantation is undertaken immediately in the first week or at a much later stage after transplantation.
- Care should be taken in the decision to retransplant for recurrent disease. Severely decompensated patients who have poor functional status, high model for end-stage liver disease scores, advanced age, ventilator dependence, or require dialysis have relatively poor outcomes with retransplantation.

- Retransplantation for recurrent hepatitis C remains controversial; however the presence of hepatitis C virus in and of itself should not be a contraindication to retransplantation.
- Models to predict the outcome after retransplantation that take into account patient status, disease severity, and donor graft characteristics should be further developed and validated.
- Although retransplantation offers outcomes that are inferior to primary transplantation, it should still be offered as potential life-saving therapy in cases of acute graft dysfunction, and in well-selected cases of recurrent disease and chronic graft failure.

The great success of liver transplantation since the 1980s led to a rapid increase in the number of patients on the waiting list during the 1990s, with an unmatched increase in the number of deceased donor or living donors available. With the introduction of the model for end-stage liver disease (MELD) scoring system for organ allocation, the importance of waiting time for recipient priority was removed. Subsequently the waiting list size has stabilized, with slightly more than 26,000 patients alive on the waiting list at any time during the year for each of the last 8 years. The number of liver transplants performed each year in the United States peaked in 2006 at 6,363 and for the last published year (2008) was 6,069. Unfortunately wait list mortality, defined as dropout rate due to death or illness, has remained stable at 160 per 1,000 patient-years at risk since the inception of MELD [1]. Because of this disparity, the process of prioritizing individual patients for organ allocation is a constant source of debate, and is critical in the discussion of appropriate allocation of livers to patients with a failed first graft.

Despite increasing improvements in medical decision making, surgical technique, intensive care, and immunosuppression, a certain percentage of patients still experience acute or chronic graft failure and therefore require retransplantation – accounting for approximately 8–10% of all transplants performed in the United States per year. For the 12 months between July 2008 and June 2009, 7.5% of 11,089 new wait list registrants had a previous liver transplant and 8.4% of liver transplants were performed in patients with a prior transplant. The outcome after retransplantation in general is not as successful as with primary transplantation, with long-term survival decreasing with each successive transplant (Table 48.1 and Fig. 48.1) [2]. When considering retransplantation, it should be recognized that 7.7% of the newly listed patients from July 2008 to June 2009 died awaiting a transplant [3].

Liver retransplantation not only poses a clinical and technical challenge, but also brings to bear serious financial and ethical issues because of increased costs and a finite number of available donors. Hospital charges are significantly higher and the length of stay is longer for patients receiving a second transplant and there is an obligatory net loss from the donor organ pool for patients who may have a greater chance of survival [4,5]. In this chapter we will address the reasons for retransplantation,

Table 48.1 Unadjusted graft survival of deceased donor liver transplants, primary versus retransplants.

	3-month transplants (2005–2006)			1-year transplants (2005–2006)			5-year transplants (2001–2006)			10-year transplants (1996–2006)		
	N	%	SE	*N*	%	SE	*N*	%	SE	*N*	%	SE
Total	11,503	90.1%	0.3%	11,503	82.4%	0.4%	31,137	67.6%	0.3%	51,910	53.4%	0.3%
Previous liver transplant												
No	10,533	91.0%	0.3%	10,533	83.7%	0.4%	28,428	68.9%	0.3%	47,082	55.0%	0.4%
Yes	970	80.2%	1.3%	970	68.7%	1.5%	2,709	54.2%	1.1%	4,828	38.2%	1.0%

Data from the OPTN/SRTR 2008 Annual Report, Table 9.10a. Data as of May 1, 2008. The data and analyses reported in the *2008 Annual Report of the US Procurement and Transplantation Network and the Scientific Registry of Transplant Recipients* have been supplied by UNOS and URREA under contract with HHS. The authors alone are responsible for reporting and interpreting these data. Available at http://www.ustransplant.org/annual_reports/current/910a_prevorg_li.htm.

Rate of retransplantation and indications

The overall reported rate of retransplantation in individual centers seems to vary between 7% and 17% [2,5–14]. These rates have not remained constant over the years. The University of Pittsburgh studied the rates and causes of retransplantation in three eras – the early eighties, late eighties, and nineties. The overall rate of retransplantation declined significantly over time: from 33% in the early 1980s to 13% in the 1990s [11], likely the result of improved clinical judgment, immunosuppression, advanced technical skills, and better antiviral medications. The overall rate of retransplantation in the United States is decreasing, from 9.6% to 7.6% from 1999 to 2008 [1].

Just as the overall rate of retransplantation has changed over time, so have the indications for it. There has been a marked decrease in the rate of retransplantation for acute and chronic rejection. According to a series of 114 retransplants performed in Germany, the major causes of retransplantation during the early 1980s were acute and chronic rejection, with an incidence of 27% in each [15]. However, in a more recent series, the University of California at Los Angeles (UCLA) identified primary nonfunction (PNF) as the main cause, accounting for over 25% of all retransplantation cases [16]. According to data from a retrospective study of retransplantation at Pittsburgh over a 19-year period, the rate of retransplantation for rejection declined from 13.2% to 1%, and the rate of retransplantation for hepatic artery thrombosis (HAT) declined from 8.1% to 3.8%, with the rate for PNF increasing from 4.6% to 6.0% [11].

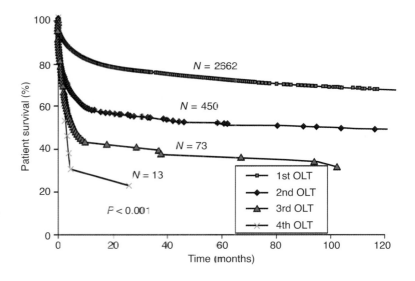

Figure 48.1 Survival estimates of recipients undergoing multiple liver transplantations. Recipient survival after primary orthotopic liver transplantation (OLT) was compared with survival after transplantation with second, third, or fourth OLTs in a single center series from the University of California at Los Angeles (UCLA) spanning two decades [2]. (Reproduced from Busuttil et al. [2] with permission from Lippincott Williams & Wilkins.)

Table 48.2 Indications for retransplant by time from first transplant to retransplant (*n* = 3969) for recipients with a first transplant between 1999 and 2008.

Cause of graft failure[a]	Quartile 1, 0–14 days		Quartile 2, 15–222 days		Quartile 3, 223–1,307 days		Quartile 4, >1,308 days	
	N	%	N	%	N	%	N	%
Primary graft failure	653	64.1	204	21.1	100	10.1	88	8.9
Vascular thrombosis	283	27.8	318	32.9	114	11.5	53	5.3
Biliary tract complication	14	1.4	142	14.7	146	14.7	53	5.3
Hepatitis: de novo	0	0.0	1	0.1	10	1.0	10	1.0
Hepatitis: recurrent	5	0.5	51	5.3	243	24.5	200	20.2
Recurrent disease	1	0.1	12	1.2	103	10.4	175	17.6
Acute rejection	42	4.1	67	6.9	50	5.0	22	2.2
Chronic rejection	1	0.1	34	3.5	183	18.5	204	20.6
Infection	15	1.5	83	8.6	51	5.1	25	2.5
Patient noncompliance	0	0.0	0	0.0	8	0.8	6	0.6
Missing	126	12.4	265	27.4	277	27.9	367	37.0

[a]Cause of graft failure of the primary transplant. Some patients may have multiple causes of graft failure.
Reproduced from Thuluvath et al. [1] with permission from Wiley-Blackwell.

There are several recipient characteristics that have been identified that predict a greater likelihood for retransplantation. Over the past 10 years the highest rate of retransplantation was observed in African-American recipients, who have a ratio of primary liver transplants to liver retransplants of 7.8:1. Asian recipients have the greatest utility of liver use, with one retransplant for every 15.1 allografts used. Woman have a slightly higher rate of retransplant of 1:10.5 compared with 1:11.6 livers utilized in males. The ratio of primary liver transplants to liver retransplants was lowest for acute hepatic necrosis where one of every 6.2 grafts were used for a retransplant and was greatest for malignant neoplasms where one of 40.1 grafts was used for retransplant. Interestingly, over the last 10 years there has been almost a three-fold difference in the rate of retransplantation among United Network for Organ Sharing (UNOS) regions. The region with the greatest risk of retransplantation was region 7, with one of 7.3 grafts being used for retransplant. Region 6 had the lowest rate of retransplant at a ratio of 1:20.4. The reasons for the disparity between geographic regions are unknown, but may reflect regional imbalances between the number of individuals awaiting transplant and the number of donors [1].

Retransplantation is also a significant event after pediatric liver transplantation, usually for different indications than adults, and often for technical reasons. The incidence of retransplantation in children is higher than in adults, with a range of 14–29% [17–20]. The use of split and reduced size grafts, the small size of donors and recipients, and noncompliance in the teen years are predisposing factors for an increased retransplantation rate in this population. The willingness of transplant surgeons and hepatologists to give more than one graft to children, or even more than two grafts, is greater, and, fortunately, outcome is significantly better in the pediatric population as well.

The indications for retransplantation for adults and children can essentially be divided into two groups – those patients needing emergent retransplantation in the early days and weeks following transplant due to graft failure secondary to graft dysfunction or technical complications, and those requiring late retransplantation due to chronic rejection, recurrence of disease, or late technical complications from vascular or biliary issues (Table 48.2).

Indications for early retransplantation

Primary graft dysfunction
Early graft dysfunction is a term that is used to describe a spectrum of clinical conditions in which the transplanted allograft fails to provide adequate metabolic and/or synthetic function. These patients present with various degrees of hemodynamic and metabolic instability, and the potential for the development of multiorgan system failure. The severity of global hepatic dysfunction may be assessed by biochemical and metabolic markers including elevated transaminases, persistence of metabolic acidosis, an elevated international normalized ratio (INR),

and rising bilirubin. A diagnosis of PNF is a diagnosis of exclusion made if a graft shows complete lack of initial function and its dysfunction cannot be attributed to technical or other recipient causes, and is the most common cause of retransplantation in the initial days after orthotopic liver transplantation (OLT). A more stringent definition is used for the allocation of a second organ, where PNF is defined as graft dysfunction within the first week post transplant leading to the death of the patient or retransplantation. Requirements include an aspartate aminotransferase (AST) of 3,000 U/L or more, and either an INR of 2.5 or more, a pH of less than 7.3, or a lactate value of 4.0 mmol/L or more. This allows for the rapid relisting of patients as status 1, which places the patient at the top of the allocation list. Other grafts may present with a less dramatic picture, demonstrating prolonged cholestasis, evidence of ischemic/harvest injury on biopsy, and slow or inadequate restoration of function. Termed *early allograft dysfunction* (EAD) or delayed nonfunction (DNF) these grafts may require retransplantation if they fail to recover, although they often do not meet status 1 criteria. These patients often have prolonged intensive care unit stays with an increased risk of serious infectious complications [21,22]. While many of these grafts recover, approximately one quarter of grafts exhibiting EAD criteria (high transaminases, prolonged cholestasis or coagulapathy) are lost in the first 6 months [23].

The use of "marginal" or extended criteria donor (ECD) grafts – that is, grafts from higher risk donors based on demographic, clinical, laboratory, or histologic data – may increase the risk for early graft dysfunction. Although the definition of ECD is not clearly defined, grafts that may have an increased risk of graft dysfunction usually include livers from older donors, donation after cardiac death (DCD) donors, steatotic livers, split liver grafts, and those with prolonged cold ischemic times. Each of these factors has been associated with decreased graft survival, thereby leading to an increased potential need for retransplantation. The donor risk index (DRI) is a more recent measure of donor quality assessed in terms of the risk of graft loss, which incorporates these and other donor variables [24]. There is an increasing risk of retransplantation as DRI increases [1].

Over the last decade there has been a 36% increase in the use of donors with a higher DRI value (>1.8) (Fig. 48.2). For example, there were 663 donor liver grafts from persons over 65 years (9.6% of all liver grafts) in 2007, compared with only 164 older grafts (4% of all grafts) in 1994. An increased rate of PNF has been associated with an increase in the utilization of donor organs from donors above 50 years of age [11]. There has also been an increase in the number of DCD livers over the last decade. In 1998, 24 (0.54%) deceased donor liver transplants were DCD, in 2009 this had increased to 290 (4.75%) (data from UNOS). Recipients of a DCD organ have a 13.0% risk of retransplant compared with 7.1% for donation after brain death (DBD) organ recipients. From an ethical perspective, it is precisely the availability of retransplantation organs of a high status that allows the use of these ECD donors by providing a safety net if the ECD liver does not function properly. Previously, these grafts were used in patients in desperate situations and

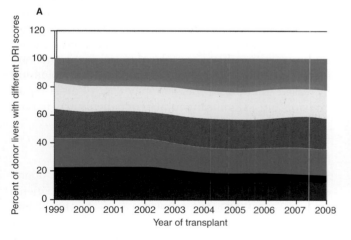
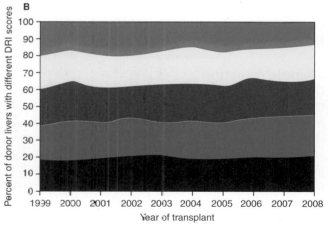

Figure 48.2 The donor risk index (DRI) for livers used for primary transplant (A) and retransplantation (B) for transplants performed between 1999 and 2008. (A) There has been a decrease in the percentage of donors with a DRI of <1.3 (17% decrease) and an increase in donors with a DRI of >1.8 (36% increase). (B) The DRI of livers used for retransplantation decreased with an 18% increase in donors with a DRI of <1.3 and a decrease in donors with a DRI of >1.8 (36%). (Reproduced from Thuluvath [1] with permission from Wiley-Blackwell. Data as of May 2009 from the Scientific Registry of Transplant Recipient (SRTR) database.)

were associated with dismal graft and patient survival. There is some debate as to which patients are acceptable candidates for these grafts, but in general less critically ill recipients are appropriate, as more stable patients may be able to better tolerate a period of relative graft dysfunction or the need for a retransplant procedure [25]. Although this matching of donor to recipient is ideal, it is often not possible with our current allocation system, which does not factor in graft quality.

Hepatic artery thrombosis

Acute HAT, despite a decreasing incidence (approximately 5%), is still a devastating problem that often requires retransplantation and is associated with markedly increased morbidity and mortality. In a review of 15 European liver transplant centers, the incidence of HAT was less than 5% but the mortality rate was as high as 55% and the retransplantation rate was approximately 80% [26]. The use of fibrinolysis, surgical thrombectomy, and immediate revascularization may avoid the necessity of retransplantation in some instances, but most patients still need a second graft. Previously, patients with HAT were designated as status 1 if diagnosed in the first week. However, recent data have shown that patients with HAT have a significantly lower risk of death while awaiting retransplantation than those requiring transplantation for other status 1 designations (fulminant failure or PNF) [27]. Therefore, HAT can only be given status 1A in adults if associated with a fulminant type of hepatic failure in the first 7 days (up to 14 days in children). In those not expressing signs of fulminant failure and those diagnosed beyond 7 days, increased MELD exception points up to 40 may be requested.

Indications for late retransplantation

Chronic rejection

Current modalities in immunosuppression have essentially eliminated the need for retransplantation for acute rejection, and the incidence of retransplantation for chronic rejection has declined significantly. However, it still remains a significant cause in the late retransplant group. In a large series from Gainesville, Florida, 27% of late retransplants in both children and adults were for chronic rejection [4], and the Kyoto group reported a 35% rate of chronic rejection in a series of living donor liver transplants as a cause for primary graft loss requiring retransplantation [28].

Primary biliary cirrhosis

Although there was initially some controversy, the recurrence of primary biliary cirrhosis (PBC) has been reported and is estimated at about 10–20%, occurring on average 3–6 years after transplantation. Pathology is considered the gold standard to diagnose recurrent PBC with the hallmark feature of granulomatous bile duct destruction. There is no correlation between antimitochondrial antibody (AMA) titer and clinical or histologic recurrence of PBC [29]. Progression of recurrent PBC is often slow and may not necessitate retransplantation [30]. In a series from the University of California, San Francisco (UCSF), recurrence of PBC was seen in eight patients with three graft failures that resulted in one death, one relisting for transplant, and one successful retransplant [31]. Ursodeoxycholic acid therapy for recurrent PBC is associated with biochemical improvement, but its role in delaying histologic progression remains unknown. [32].

Primary sclerosing cholangitis

Evidence of the recurrence of primary sclerosing cholangitis (PSC) has been documented with rates ranging from 14% to 41% post-OLT [33]. Cholangiographic and biochemical evidence along with histologic findings support the diagnosis of recurrence. Injury to the bile ducts due to anastomotic, ischemic, and infection-related strictures may present similarly to PSC, therefore these causes of bile duct damage must first be ruled out. In a study of the UNOS database of 2,154 patients with PSC, 315 (14.6%) required retransplantation [34]. It was postulated that the reasons behind this were not just disease recurrence, but also a high rate of biliary complications and chronic rejection.

Autoimmune hepatitis

Liver transplantation for autoimmune hepatitis (AIH) is highly successful; however, there is a high risk of rejection and severe recurrent AIH. Recurrence rates range from 16% to 46%. Recurrence is characterized by clinical deterioration, histology, elevated transaminases, and increased immunoglobulins. Treatment with steroids and increased immunosuppression may control disease progression, but a significant number of patients may require retransplantation [35].

Nonalcoholic steatohepatitis

Small case series have demonstrated recurrent nonalcoholic steatohepatitis (NASH) in 10–47% of patients post-OLT [36,37]. Diabetes mellitus, hyperlipidemia, and obesity, often associated with NASH, are common after transplantation and progression from fatty liver to cirrhosis post-OLT has been documented in serial biopsies, with cumulative steroid use being a potential risk factor [37]. There are very few, if any, data on retransplantation for recurrent NASH, but as the percentage of patients that are transplanted for this disease increases in the United States it may become a very significant concern.

Alcoholic liver disease

Alcoholic liver disease is the second most common cause of liver failure leading to OLT. Multiple studies have looked at recidivism rates that may be as high as 30–40%, but the recurrence of alcohol-induced cirrhosis and liver failure is rare [38]. Earlier arguments that suggested that alcohol recidivism would lead to poor adherence to immunosuppressive regimens and premature graft loss have also been proven false [39]. Obviously, resumption of alcohol use would be a contraindication for re-OLT and careful assessment of the psychosocial situation is necessary before approval in this patient group.

Hepatitis B virus

Historically, recurrent hepatitis B virus (HBV) after OLT resulted in rapidly progressive hepatic deterioration and extremely high mortality rates [40]. Prophylaxis with hepatitis B immunoglobulin (HBIg) and oral nucleoside therapy has greatly decreased the recurrence rate and made survival following OLT for patients with hepatitis B comparable to those with other causes of liver disease [41]. However, occasional recurrence evolves (approximately 5%), mainly due to acquired HBV mutations [42], although retransplantation for recurrent disease is now rare.

Hepatitis C virus

Cirrhosis from hepatitis C virus (HCV) is now the most common indication for liver transplantation in the United States [43]. After liver transplantation, HCV can be detected in the serum of nearly all patients who had HCV before transplant, although the degree of histologic recurrence is highly variable [44]. Hepatitis C viral RNA levels may increase to up to ten times those of pre-OLT levels at 4 weeks after transplantation and hepatic fibrosis may have an accelerated course [45–48]. Unlike HBV, no therapy has been conclusively shown to alter HCV recurrence or disease progression, although some progress has been made in antiviral therapy [49,50]. The natural history of post-transplant HCV infection is generally indolent but approximately 10–30% may have continuing graft damage progressing to cirrhosis in 5–10 years, and this percentage may be increasing [51,52]. However, once cirrhosis develops complications are common. Within 1 year of the finding of recurrent cirrhosis, 40% of patients develop evidence of hepatic decompensation and less than 50% survive a year from the time of decompensation [53].

Results of retransplantation

Comparison with primary transplantation

Early studies in liver transplantation showed significantly worse patient and graft survival after retransplantation when compared with primary transplants. Improvements in the results of primary grafting as well as the outcome of retransplantation have been noted. Between 1999 and 2008, the 1-year primary liver transplant survival rate improved by 4.1%, but the survival for first retransplants increased by 13% [1] (Fig. 48.3). However, when all patients are included, the results with retransplantation still fall short of primary grafting [54,55].

Timing of retransplantation

Several analyses have shown that timing plays an important role in the outcome of retransplantation [6,54,56,57]. The series from UCLA demonstrated that the survival of patients who underwent transplantation within 1 week is nearly equivalent to that seen in patients who underwent retransplantation at a much later date. It was the patients who underwent retransplantation in the period between 8 and 30 days who had a significantly worse outcome, emphasizing the need for early recognition of patients who require early retransplantation.

There is a clear differential outcome between those requiring early urgent retransplantation and those who require an "elective" second graft. In some cases, patients who underwent retransplantation many months after the primary transplant exhibited survival curves similar to those receiving a single transplant. For urgent retransplantation, which likely coincides with the first 30 days after surgery and is likely due to primary graft dysfunction, hospital charges are higher, the length of stay longer, and survival worse [5]. Although easier from a technical point of view, the mortality is likely high because of the poor clinical condition of the recipient [10].

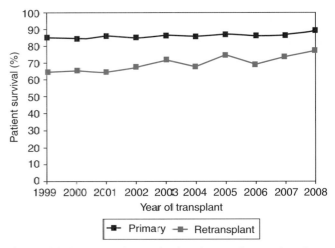

Figure 48.3 One-year patient survival for primary and retransplantation by year of transplant. (Reproduced from Thuluvath et al. [1] with permission from Wiley-Blackwell.)

Outcomes of retransplantation in hepatitis C virus patients

This remains a controversial subject with a great difference of opinion between centers. Early reports suggested that retransplant in HCV patients had a significantly worse outcome compared with other diseases, with the presence of HCV being an independent risk factor for increased mortality [47,58–61]. The presence of early fibrosing cholestatic hepatitis was considered a contraindication for retransplantation by many centers. Looking carefully at some of the earlier reports, it is found that many of the postoperative deaths were in the first 90 days, perhaps reflecting not just death from severe recurrent HCV, but also the poor perioperative condition of patients with recurrent HCV undergoing retransplantation. Some centers have supported retransplantation for recurrent HCV if retransplantation was performed early in the course of the recurrent disease [58]. Others have reported that it is the physical condition of the HCV-infected patient at the time of retransplantation that is most predictive of outcome [62]. An analysis with data from the Scientific Registry of Transplant Recipients (SRTR) assessed the relative effect of HCV diagnosis on mortality after retransplantation, demonstrating that retransplant recipients with HCV had a 30% higher covariate-adjusted mortality risk than those without HCV (Fig. 48.4) [63]. Of concern was the fact that the increased risk associated with mortality was concentrated in younger patients (age 18–39 years) and in patients transplanted in more recent years (2000 to 2002), perhaps reflecting a willingness of transplant centers to perform retransplantation in younger patients who may be more severely ill. This study, however, did not compare outcomes between recipients with HCV and other specific disorders, and inherent differences between cohorts may have less importance than the degree of illness at the time of re-OLT [64].

Positive HCV status is the most common diagnosis in retransplant patients, with an increase from 36% to 40.6% of all retransplant patients between 1994 and 2005 [1]. Survival among HCV patients who undergo retransplant is increasing, with a 1-year survival of 70.7% [65]. In some reports there appears to be little difference in the survival rate for HCV patients undergoing re-OLT when compared with other causes of re-OLT, if all other variables are kept equal [66,67], and therefore retransplantation should be considered a potential option for the treatment of recurrent disease [68]. A more recent analysis with national data demonstrated the importance of timing of retransplant in HCV. Patients with HCV who undergo retransplant within 90 days have similar survival rates as those with other diagnoses undergoing retransplant. However beyond 90 days, patients with HCV continue to have inferior outcomes (Fig. 48.5). The equivalent sur-

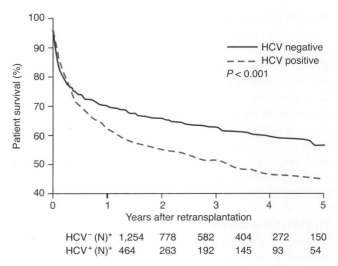

HCV⁻ (N)*	1,254	778	582	404	272	150
HCV⁺ (N)*	464	263	192	145	93	54

Figure 48.4 Kaplan–Meier curves comparing unadjusted mortality between hepatitis C virus (HCV) positive and HCV-negative liver retransplant recipients in a cohort of patients who underwent retransplantation between 1997 and 2002 using the Scientific Registry of Transplant Recipient (SRTR) database. (Reproduced from Pelletier et al. [63] with permission from American Association for the Study of Liver Diseases.)

vival for those who undergo retransplantation within a short interval from the primary transplant likely reflects non-HCV causes of graft dysfunction as compared with those who undergo retransplant beyond 90 days [65]. HCV patients require a more careful decision-making process when compared with non-HCV patients, and re-OLT is best performed before severe decompensation

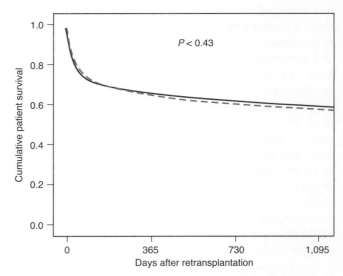

Figure 48.5 Kaplan–Meier curves comparing patient mortality between hepatitis C virus (HCV) positive and HCV-negative liver retransplant recipients from 1994 and 2005 using OPTN (Organ Procurement and Transplantation Network) data. There is no difference in survival for HCV-positive (dashed line) and HCV-negative (solid line) patients if the retransplant is performed within 90 days of the prior transplant. (Reproduced from Ghabril et al. [65] with permission from Wiley-Blackwell.)

[55,69]. This can be a difficult task in the current system of liver allocation that provides grafts to the "sickest first."

Cause of death following retransplantation

The development of sepsis and multiorgan failure accounts for most of the deaths in patients undergoing retransplantation, and the largest proportion of deaths occur in the first few weeks after transplant [70]. The incidence of death secondary to sepsis is twice as high in patients undergoing retransplantation compared with those receiving just one graft, with a 50% incidence of fungal infection [59,71]. In a series from UCSF, 28% of patients who underwent retransplantation experienced serious infections in the first month, and 17.5% died within the first 6 months from multiorgan dysfunction associated with sepsis or poor graft function [72]. Roayaie et al. reported that approximately two thirds of deaths after retransplant for HCV recurrence were associated with infection [61]. The high incidence of graft loss due to sepsis in these patients may reflect the immunosuppressed status of the patients prior to retransplantation, as well as their deteriorated functional status. In light of these findings, it may be prudent to reduce immunosuppression perioperatively and initiate more effective antimicrobial prophylaxis for patients undergoing retransplantation. Less frequent causes of death following retransplantation include technical problems such as intraoperative mortality, arterial and portal vein thrombosis, and postoperative complications such as cardiac events, neurologic complications, recurrent disease, and persistent liver failure.

Predictors of mortality after retransplantation

In an attempt to maximize the use of valuable organs, there have been many efforts to determine which factors are associated with the outcome in order to develop a model that might accurately predict survival in patients undergoing liver retransplantation. It has become increasingly apparent that it is not just the quality of the donor but also the status of the recipient that contributes most to the outcome after retransplantation. A multivariate analysis performed at UCLA determined that donor cold ischemia time over 12 hours, preoperative mechanical ventilator requirement, preoperative serum creatinine greater than 1.6 mg/dL, and serum total bilirubin over 13 mg/dL were all independent risk factors predictive of a patient's poor outcome [57,71]. Rosen and Martin identified bilirubin and creatinine as predictive of poor outcome in HCV patients [60]. The University of Pittsburgh identified older donor age, gender, and choice of immunosuppression as predictive of poor outcome [56]. In a series from Mount Sinai Medical Center, recipient age over 50 years, a preoperative creatinine greater

than 2 mg/dL, and the use of intraoperative blood products significantly impacted the survival of those patients requiring retransplantation within 6 months of the primary transplant [59].

Models to predict survival after retransplantation

The critical shortage of donor organs and the resultant prolonged patient waiting periods before transplantation have prompted many to define a mathematic model that adequately predicts survival after retransplantation. Rosen et al. assigned a mortality risk score based on preoperative variables in patients undergoing retransplantation, which included recipient age, creatinine, bilirubin, non-PNF diagnosis, and UNOS status [73]. Individual patients were then stratified into low-, medium-, and high-risk groups, in an attempt to predict survival; recipient age, creatinine and bilirubin levels, and timing of transplant between 15 and 60 days were found to be predictive of outcome. These findings were validated in a multicenter international study [74]. Another model put forward by Markmann et al. from the UCLA database similarly employed a scoring system utilizing five noninvasive and readily available clinical parameters: recipient age, creatinine, bilirubin, cold ischemia time, and ventilatory status [71]. Patients having four out of a possible five points had a 1-year survival of only 27%. This classification system adequately discriminated high-risk and low-survival patients in three databases to which it was applied. A universal model for predicting survival was proposed by Ghobrial et al. for both primary transplants and retransplants, hoping to provide guidance for tailoring specific organ needs to specific recipients on the basis of the severity of disease and expected outcomes. The model incorporated MELD score, recipient age, and timing of transplantation [69].

Interestingly, none of these models found the diagnosis of HCV as a poor prognostic indicator in multivariate analysis. More recent work has focused on the importance of donor factors to recipient survival after retransplant. The addition of the cause of graft failure to the DRI to create the retransplant donor risk index was highly predictive of death after retransplant [75]. Applications of models such as these can theoretically result in better decision making, improved survival, and an increased efficacy in organ utilization.

MELD score and retransplantation

In primary transplantation, MELD score has not correlated with post-transplant outcome except at the very highest MELD scores [76]. However, in the population who undergo retransplantation, MELD score may have a more significant impact, although there is some disagreement here as well (Table 48.3) [67,77]. MELD scores

Table 48.3 Survival after liver retransplantation based upon MELD score.

MELD score	1 year	5 year
<10	83%	55%
11–20	65%	55%
21–25	62%	47%
26–30	57%	37%
>30	42%	21%

Adapted from Zimmerman and Ghobrial [81] and Watt et al. [67].

correlated with survival outcome in patients who underwent retransplantation at the University of Nebraska [78]. In the multicenter study by Rosen, the MELD score was predictive of survival in patients undergoing retransplantation after 15 days [74]. Yao et al. noted a trend for a correlation between the Child–Turcotte–Pugh (CTP) and MELD scores with 1-year post-OLT mortality, with CTP values of 10+ and MELD scores of 25+ having worse outcomes at 1 and 5 years [72]. These studies demonstrate that using MELD scores for liver allocation in this patient population may have distinct disadvantages, because patients undergoing retransplantation would need to be quite ill before reaching the top of the allocation list, thereby losing their "window of opportunity" to have a good outcome after retransplantation. Other models have been proposed to determine which MELD score is associated with the greatest utility for retransplantation in patients with HCV and those without HCV. The optimal outcome for retransplantation appears to be achieved at MELD scores of less than 28, with the maximal utility achieved at a MELD score of 21 for patients with HCV, and a MELD score of 24 for patients without HCV [79]. Unfortunately, this is not an option in many parts of the United States where the mean MELD score at transplant is significantly higher.

Living donor liver transplantation and retransplantation

With the use of right lobe grafts for adult liver transplants, transplant surgeons and hepatologists are faced with technical decisions regarding the use of living donors for retransplants, and ethical issues whether retransplantation should be performed in living donor recipients transplanted outside UNOS criteria, such as for large hepatocellular carcinoma. In a series of living donor liver transplants (LDLTs) from the A2ALL consortium, 37 of 385 (9.6%) recipients of adult to adult LDLTs required retransplantation, mostly for technical reasons [80]. These technical issues markedly decreased as experience improved, and it may be that there will be less

retransplantation in this group as technical complications decrease.

The vast majority of retransplants are done with whole deceased donor grafts due to the technical demands of retransplantation and anatomic limitations of LDLTs. Data provided from UNOS demonstrated that from January 1999 until December of 2009 4,656 retransplants were performed in adults, and only 45 (0.97%) were with living donor liver allografts. During the same period of time, 758 retransplants were performed in children, 57 (7.5%) of whom received a living donor allograft.

Conclusions

The outcome of retransplantation is improving; however, survival after retransplantation is currently less than after primary OLT. Certain clinical criteria have been found to affect the outcome of retransplantation. The most important factors appear to be the preoperative status of the recipient as indicated by ventilator dependence, renal failure, physical condition, age, and MELD score. The time interval to retransplantation, donor cold ischemia time, and donor quality also contribute to the overall outcome. The overall impact of retransplantation on the survival of all patients awaiting liver transplantation and the cost-effectiveness of this procedure are issues of current debate. What also remains controversial and unanswered is retransplantation for recurrent HCV. National data demonstrate poorer outcomes when retransplantation is done beyond 90 days of the primary transplant, but other studies have demonstrated similar outcomes compared with other diagnoses [68]. Patient medical status is predictive in this population, and it may be that improved judgment ensures better outcomes in this patient population [64].

Despite continued improvements, the generally inferior outcome has prompted many to question the appropriateness of hepatic retransplantation on both economic and ethical grounds. On the other hand, an outright prohibition of hepatic retransplantation raises its own ethical questions of patient abandonment. In addition, limiting retransplantation would impede current efforts to expand the organ pool by the utilization of marginal donors. The safety net of retransplantation is needed if an aggressive donor organ acceptance strategy is to be adopted by all transplant centers. Retransplantation is an essential treatment for patients undergoing liver transplant who experience liver failure after their primary transplant. However, it must be applied with some discretion and careful decision making so that futility is avoided and maximal utility is achieved. Relying on the MELD score alone to allocate organs seems insufficient in this patient population and needs to be studied. Futile transplants and retransplantation in subgroups of patients with little chance of successful outcome should be avoided.

Annotated references

Burton JR Jr, Sonnenberg A, Rosen HR. Retransplantation for recurrent hepatitis C in the MELD era: maximizing utility. *Liver Transpl* 2004;10(Suppl 2):S59–64.
An excellent review of studies evaluating prognostic criteria with retransplantation and proposals for achieving maximal utility in the face of donor shortages in HCV patients.

Busuttil RW, Farmer DG, Yersiz H, et al. Analysis of long-term outcomes of 3200 liver transplantations over two decades: a single-center experience. *Ann Surg* 2005;241(6):905–16; discussion 916–18.
A single center review from a large US transplant center, including indications and outcomes with retransplantation.

Markmann JF, Gornbein J, Markowitz JS, et al. A simple model to estimate survival after retransplantation of the liver. *Transplantation* 1999;67(3):422–30.
A model that incorporates pretransplant factors to predict survival after retransplantation.

Pelletier SJ, Schaubel DE, Punch JD, et al. Hepatitis C is a risk factor for death after liver retransplantation. *Liver Transpl* 2005;11(4):434–40.
This paper presents outcomes in patients who underwent retransplantation with HCV from the SRTR database.

Thuluvath PJ, Guidinger MK, Fung JJ, et al. Liver transplantation in United States, 1999–2008. *Am J Transplant* 2010;10(Part 2):1003–19
This paper summarizes the SRTR database with an excellent section about retransplantation.

References

1. Thuluvath PJ, Guidinger MK, Fung JJ, et al. Liver transplantation in United States, 1999–2008. *Am J Transplant* 2010;10(Part 2):1003–19.
2. Busuttil RW, Farmer DG, Yersiz H, et al. Analysis of long-term outcomes of 3200 liver transplantations over two decades: a single-center experience. *Ann Surg* 2005;241(6):905–16; discussion 916–18.
3. http://www.ustransplant.org/.
4. Reed A, Howard RJ, Fujita S, et al. Liver retransplantation: a single-center outcome and financial analysis. *Transplant Proc* 2005;37(2):1161–3.
5. Azoulay D, Linhares MM, Huguet E, et al. Decision for retransplantation of the liver: an experience- and cost-based analysis. *Ann Surg* 2002;236(6):713–21; discussion 721.
6. Powelson JA, Cosimi AB, Lewis WD, et al. Hepatic retransplantation in New England – a regional experience and survival model. *Transplantation* 1993;55(4):802–6.
7. Wong T, Devlin J, Rolando N, et al. Clinical characteristics affecting the outcome of liver retransplantation. *Transplantation* 1997;64(6):878–82.
8. Kumar N, Wall WJ, Grant DR, et al. Liver retransplantation. *Transplant Proc* 1999;31(1–2):541–2.
9. Lerut J, Laterre PF, Roggen F, et al. Adult hepatic retransplantation. UCL experience. *Acta Gastroenterol Belg* 1999;62(3):261–6.
10. De Carlis L, Slim AO, Giacomoni A, et al. Liver retransplantation: indications and results over a 15-year experience. *Transplant Proc* 2001;33(1-2):1411–13.
11. Kashyap R, Jain A, Reyes J, et al. Causes of retransplantation after primary liver transplantation in 4000 consecutive patients: 2 to 19 years follow-up. *Transplant Proc* 2001;33(1–2):1486–7.
12. Dudek K, Nyckowski P, Zieniewicz K, et al. Liver retransplantation: indications and results. *Transplant Proc* 2002;34(2):638–9.
13. Jimenez M, Turrion VS, Alvira LG, et al. Indications and results of retransplantation after a series of 406 consecutive liver transplantations. *Transplant Proc* 2002;34(1):262–3.
14. Meneu Diaz JC, Vicente E, Moreno Gonzalez E, et al. Indications for liver retransplantation: 1087 orthotopic liver transplantations between 1986 and 1997. *Transplant Proc* 2002;34(1):306.
15. Fangmann J, Ringe B, Hauss J, et al. Hepatic retransplantation: the Hanover experience of two decades. *Transplant Proc* 1993;25:1077.
16. Markmann J, Markowitz J, Yersiz H, et al. Long-term survival after retransplantation of the liver. *Ann Surg* 1997;226(4):408–20.
17. Newell KA. Mills JM, Bruce DS, et al. An analysis of hepatic retransplantation in children. *Transplantation* 1998;65(9):1172–8.
18. Achilleos OA, Mirza DF, Talbot D, et al. Outcome of liver retransplantation in children. *Liver Transpl Surg* 1999;5(5):401–6.
19. Deshpande RR, Rela M, Girlanda R, et al. Long-term outcome of liver retransplantation in children. *Transplantation* 2002;74(8):1124–30.
20. Bourdeaux C, Brunati A, Janssen M, et al. Liver retransplantation in children. A 21 year single-center experience. *Trans Int* 2009;22:416–22.
21. Deschenes M, Belle SH, Krom EA, et al. Early allograft dysfunction after liver transplantation: a definition and predictors of outcome. National Institute of Diabetes and Digestive and Kidney Diseases Liver Transplantation Database. *Transplantation* 1998;66(3):302–10.
22. Yersiz H, Shaked A, Olthoff K, et al. Correlation between donor age and the pattern of liver graft recovery after transplantation. *Transplantation* 1995;60(8):790–4.
23. Olthoff KM, Kulik L, Samstein B, et al. Validation of a current definition of early graft dysfunction in liver transplant recipients and an analysis of risk factors. *Liver Transpl* 2010;16:943–9.
24. Feng S, Goodrich NP, Bragg-Gresham JL, et al. Characteristics associated with liver graft failure: the concept of a donor risk index. *Am J Transplant* 2006;6(4):783–90.
25. Cameron A, Busuttil RW. AASLD/ILTS transplant course: is there an extended donor suitable for everyone? *Liver Transpl* 2005;11(11 Suppl 2):S2–5.
26. Stange B, Glanemann M, Nuessler N, et al. Hepatic artery thrombosis after adult liver transplantation. *Liver Transpl* 2003;9(6):612–20.
27. Wiesner RH. MELD/PELD and the allocation of deceased donor livers for status 1 recipients with acute fulminant hepatic failure, primary nonfunction, hepatic artery thrombosis, and acute Wilson disease. *Liver Transpl* 2004;10(10 Suppl 2):S17–22.
28. Ogura Y, Kaihara S, Haga H, et al. Outcomes for pediatric liver retransplantation from living donors. *Transplantation* 2003;76(6):943–8.
29. Sanchez EQ, Levy MF, Goldstein RM, et al. The changing clinical presentation of recurrent primary biliary cirrhosis after liver transplantation. *Transplantation* 2003;76(11):1583–8.
30. Neuberger J. Liver transplantation for primary biliary cirrhosis: indications and risk of recurrence. *J Hepatol* 2003;39(2):142–8.
31. Renz JF, Ascher NL. Liver transplantation for nonviral, nonmalignant diseases: problem of recurrence. *World J Surg* 2002;26(2):247–56.
32. Charatcharoenwitthaya P, Pimentel S, Talwalkar JA, et al. Long-term survival and impact of ursodeoxycholic acid treatment for recurrent primary biliary cirrhosis after liver transplantation. *Liver Transpl* 2007;13:1236–45.
33. Graziadei IW. Recurrence of primary sclerosing cholangitis after liver transplantation. *Liver Transpl* 2002;8(7):575–81.
34. Maheshwari A, Yoo HY, Thuluvath PJ. Long-term outcome of liver transplantation in patients with PSC: a comparative analysis with PBC. *Am J Gastroenterol* 2004;99(3):538–42.
35. Neuberger J. Transplantation for autoimmune hepatitis. *Semin Liver Dis* 2002;22(4):379–86.
36. Kim WR, Poterucha JJ, Porayko MK, et al. Recurrence of nonalcoholic steatohepatitis following liver transplantation. *Transplantation* 1996;62(12):1802–5.
37. Contos MJ, Cales W, Sterling RK, et al. Development of nonalcoholic fatty liver disease after orthotopic liver transplantation for cryptogenic cirrhosis. *Liver Transpl* 2001;7(4):363–73.

38. Bravata DM, Olkin I, Barnato AE, et al. Employment and alcohol use after liver transplantation for alcoholic and nonalcoholic liver disease: a systematic review. *Liver Transpl* 2001;7(3):191–203.

39. Pageaux G, Michel J, Coste V, et al. Alcoholic cirrhosis is a good indication for liver transplantation, even for cases of recidivism. *Gut* 1999;45:421–6.

40. Ishitani M, McGory R, Dickson R, et al. Retransplantation of patients with severe posttransplant hepatitis B in the first allograft. *Transplantation* 1997;64(3):410–14.

41. Anselmo DM, Ghobrial RM, Jung LC, et al. New era of liver transplantation for hepatitis B: a 17-year single-center experience. *Ann Surg* 2002;235(5):611–19; discussion 619–20.

42. Schiff ER, Lai CL, Hadziyannis S, et al. Adefovir dipivoxil therapy for lamivudine-resistant hepatitis B in pre- and post-liver transplantation patients. *Hepatology* 2003;38(6):1419–27.

43. Brown RS. Hepatitis C and liver transplantation. *Nature* 2005; 436(7053):973–8.

44. Van Vlierberghe H, Troisi R, Colle I, et al. Hepatitis C infection-related liver disease: patterns of recurrence and outcome in cadaveric and living-donor liver transplantation in adults. *Transplantation* 2004;77(2):210–14.

45. Machicao VI, Bonatti H, Krishna M, et al. Donor age affects fibrosis progression and graft survival after liver transplantation for hepatitis C. *Transplantation* 2004;77(1):84–92.

46. Forman LM, Lewis JD, Berlin JA, et al. The association between hepatitis C infection and survival after orthotopic liver transplantation. *Gastroenterology* 2002;122(4):889–96.

47. Berenguer M, Prieto M, Palau A, et al. Severe recurrent hepatitis C after liver retransplantation for hepatitis C virus-related graft cirrhosis. *Liver Transpl* 2003;9(3):228–35.

48. Berenguer M. Host and donor risk factors before and after liver transplantation that impact HCV recurrence. *Liver Transpl* 2003; 9(11):S44–7.

49. Berenguer M. Treatment of hepatitis C after liver transplantation. *Clin Liver Dis* 2005;9(4):579–600.

50. Everson GT, Trotter J, Forman L, et al. Treatment of advanced hepatitis C with a low accelerating dosage regimen of antiviral therapy. *Hepatology* 2005;42(2):255–62.

51. Berenguer M, Ferrell L, Watson J, et al. HCV-related fibrosis progression following liver transplantation: increase in recent years. *J Hepatol* 2000;32(4):673–84.

52. Rosen HR, Gretch DR, Oehlke M, et al. Timing and severity of initial hepatitis C recurrence as predictors of long-term liver allograft injury. *Transplantation* 1998;65(9):1178–82.

53. Berenguer M, Prieto M, Rayon JM, et al. Natural history of clinically compensated hepatitis C virus-related graft cirrhosis after liver transplantation. *Hepatology* 2000;32(4 Pt 1):852–8.

54. Yoo HY, Maheshwari A, Thuluvath PJ. Retransplantation of liver: primary graft nonfunction and hepatitis C virus are associated with worse outcome. *Liver Transpl* 2003;9(9):897–904.

55. Biggins SW, Beldecos A, Rabkin JM, et al. Retransplantation for hepatic allograft failure: prognostic modeling and ethical considerations. *Liver Transpl* 2002;8(4):313–22.

56. Doyle HR, Morelli F, McMichael J, et al. Hepatic retransplantation – an analysis of risk factors associated with outcome. *Transplantation* 1996;61(10):1499–505.

57. Markmann JF, Markowitz JS, Yersiz H, et al. Long-term survival after retransplantation of the liver. *Ann Surg* 1997;226(4):408–18; discussion 418–20.

58. Ghobrial RM. Retransplantation for recurrent hepatitis C. *Liver Transpl* 2002;8(10 Suppl 1):S38–43.

59. Facciuto M, Heidt D, Guarrera J, et al. Retransplantation for late liver graft failure: predictors of mortality. *Liver Transpl* 2000;6(2):174–9.

60. Rosen HR, Martin P. Hepatitis C infection in patients undergoing liver retransplantation. *Transplantation* 1998;66(12):1612–16.

61. Roayaie S, Schiano TD, Thung SN, et al. Results of retransplantation for recurrent hepatitis C. *Hepatology* 2003;38(6):1428–36.

62. Neff GW, O'Brien CB, Nery J, et al. Factors that identify survival after liver retransplantation for allograft failure caused by recurrent hepatitis C infection. *Liver Transpl* 2004;10(12):1497–503.

63. Pelletier SJ, Schaubel DE, Punch JD, et al. Hepatitis C is a risk factor for death after liver retransplantation. *Liver Transpl* 2005;11(4):434–40.

64. Charlton M. Retransplantation for HCV – the view through a broken crystal ball. *Liver Transpl* 2005;11(4):382–3.

65. Ghabril M, Dickson R, Wiesner R. Improving outcomes of liver retransplantation: an analysis of trends and the impact of hepatitis C infection. *Am J Transpl* 2008;8:404–11.

66. McCashland TM. Retransplantation for recurrent hepatitis C: positive aspects. *Liver Transpl* 2003;9(11):S67–72.

67. Watt KD, Lyden ER, McCashland TM. Poor survival after liver retransplantation: is hepatitis C to blame? *Liver Transpl* 2003;9(10): 1019–24.

68. McCashland T, Watt K, Lyden E, et al. Retransplantation for hepatitis C: results of a U.S. multicenter retransplant study. *Liver Transpl* 2007;13:1246–53.

69. Ghobrial RM, Gornbein J, Steadman R, et al. Pretransplant model to predict posttransplant survival in liver transplant patients. *Ann Surg* 2002;236(3):315–22; discussion 322–3.

70. Pfitzmann R, Benscheidt B, Langrehr JM, et al. Trends and experiences in liver retransplantation over 15 years. *Liver Transpl* 2007; 13:248–57.

71. Markmann JF, Gornbein J, Markowitz JS, et al. A simple model to estimate survival after retransplantation of the liver. *Transplantation* 1999;67(3):422–30.

72. Yao FY, Saab S, Bass NM, et al. Prediction of survival after liver retransplantation for late graft failure based on preoperative prognostic scores. *Hepatology* 2004;39(1):230–8.

73. Rosen HR, Madden JP, Martin P. A model to predict survival following liver retransplantation. *Hepatology* 1999;29(2):365–70.

74. Rosen HR, Prieto M, Casanovas-Taltavull T, et al. Validation and refinement of survival models for liver retransplantation. *Hepatology* 2003;38(2):460–9.

75. Northup PG, Pruett TL, Kashner DM, et al. Donor factors predicting recipient survival after liver retransplantation: the retransplant donor risk index. *Am J Transpl* 2007;7:1984–8.

76. Desai NM, Mange KC, Crawford MD, et al. Predicting outcome after liver transplantation: utility of the model for end-stage liver disease and a newly derived discrimination function. *Transplantation* 2004;77(1):99–106.

77. Edwards E, Harper A. Does MELD work for relisted candidates? *Liver Transpl* 2004;10(10 Suppl 2):S10–16.

78. Watt KDS, Menke T, Lyden E, et al. Mortality while awaiting liver retransplantation: predictability of MELD scores. *Transplant Proc* 2005;37(5):2172–3.

79. Burton JR Jr, Sonnenberg A, Rosen HR. Retransplantation for recurrent hepatitis C in the MELD era: maximizing utility. *Liver Transpl* 2004;10(Suppl 2):S59–64.

80. Olthoff KM, Merion RM, Ghobrial RM, et al. Outcomes of 385 adult-to-adult living donor liver transplant recipients: a report from the A2ALL consortium. *Ann Surg* 2005;242(3):314–23; discussion 323–5.

81. Zimmerman MA, Ghobrial RM. When shouldn't we retransplant? *Liver Transpl* 2005;11(11 Suppl 1):S14–20.

CHAPTER 49

Controversies in Liver Transplantation

James F. Trotter

Division of Transplant Hepatology, Baylor University Medical Center, Dallas, TX, USA

Key concepts

- The institution of liver allocation based on the model for end-stage liver disease (MELD) score was created to alleviate problems that developed under previous liver allocation schemes.
- Liver allocation based on the MELD score has improved the triage of liver candidates by reducing the waiting list mortality rate.
- Despite these improvements, problems remain with regard to liver allocation and distribution.
- While the MELD score is an objective scoring system, relevant variation in the MELD score exists related largely to interlaboratory

- variation in measuring the serum creatinine and international normalized ratio.
- The institution of donation after cardiac death organs has increased the number of deceased donor organs available for transplantation.
- The application of living donor liver transplantation has decreased by more than half in the past several years.
- The definition of the expanded criteria donor has helped to identify specific donor and transplant characteristics associated with poor outcome.

Controversy is synonymous with liver transplantation where the stakes are high and the resources, in terms of donors, are limited. Through the years, medical advances in the field of transplantation have vastly improved the outcomes for recipients and the availability of donors. In such a dynamic field, disputes over the most effective application of this procedure are commonplace. Therefore, this chapter will focus on some of the most important current controversies in liver transplantation including liver allocation and distribution, variations in model for end-stage liver disease (MELD) score, donation after cardiac death (DCD), living donor liver transplantation (LDLT), expanded criteria donor (ECD), and MELD exception scores.

Liver allocation and distribution

The equitable allocation and distribution of donor livers has been a controversial issue since liver transplantation became widely available more than a quarter of a century ago. The terms "allocation" and "distribution" reflect different processes and for the purposes of this discussion will be defined as follows. *Allocation* is the process by which liver candidates are prioritized for transplantation.

The allocation scheme is dictated and overseen nationally by the United Network for Organ Sharing (UNOS) and is currently based almost entirely on the MELD score [1,2]. In addition, some patients may also receive a MELD score based on exception diagnoses as described below. Prioritizing patients for transplant has been one of the most controversial areas in the field and is continuously evolving to meet the changing requirements of liver transplant candidates. *Distribution* is essentially the delivery process; that is, the system by which donor livers are procured, matched, and delivered (transplanted) into prioritized patients within a geographic region. Perhaps more complex than liver allocation, distribution involves the supply (number of donor organs) and demand (number of transplant candidates) within a geographic area, as well as acceptance of specific organs for transplant based on their quality (or lack thereof) and policies regarding organ retention or sharing within the area.

Much of the ongoing controversy related to prioritizing patients and distributing donor organs for transplantation is the result of the increasing demand for the procedure. Since the inception of liver transplantation, the demand for organs has outpaced the supply. Consequently, as the liver transplant list grew over time, the disparity widened between the number of transplant

Schiff's Diseases of the Liver, Eleventh Edition. Edited by Eugene R. Schiff, Willis C. Maddrey and Michael F. Sorrell.
© 2012 John Wiley & Sons, Ltd. Published 2012 by John Wiley & Sons, Ltd.

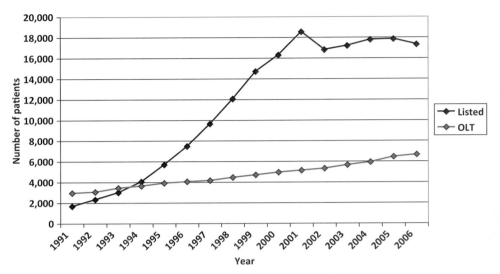

Figure 49.1 Number of listed and transplanted patients versus year. OLT, orthotopic liver transplant.

candidates and the limited donor pool. As a result, the competition for organs became increasingly intense and the prioritization of liver candidates and distribution of donor organs, in turn, more complicated. Through the years, three fundamental principles have formed the basis for liver allocation and distribution: (i) triage – the sickest liver candidates receive a higher priority for transplant compared with less sick patients; (ii) "first come, first served" – patients listed earlier receive a higher priority than patients listed later; and (iii) local organ utilization – donor organs are transplanted preferentially in the area of procurement. Most of the disputes about liver allocation and the distribution system over time are reflected in the relative importance given to each of these three principles. To understand the current controversies one must understand how the current system evolved [3].

Liver allocation is in a constant state of evolution. In the early 1990s when fewer patients were listed and competition for donor organ was less intense, liver allocation was less complicated. Candidates were prioritized based on only two criteria: waiting time and severity of illness as determined by the Child–Turcotte–Pugh (CTP) score; the higher the score, the higher the priority for transplant. There were only four gradations of illness (or statuses): status 3 for stable chronic patients (CTP score <10), status 2B for decompensated patients (CTP score ≥10), status 2A for critically ill patients (expected to die in less than 7 days), and status 1 for acute liver failure. Within each status, patients with the longest waiting time had the highest priority. Consequently, waiting time was an important determinant in prioritization for transplant. This system functioned relatively well during the time when the waiting list was small. In fact, in the early 1990s, the number of liver transplants exceeded the number of listed patients. However, during that decade, the size of

the transplant list increased nearly ten-fold from 1,676 in 1991 to 16,292 in 2000 (Fig. 49.1). With the growing number of patients listed for transplant, three specific allocation problems became manifest. First, there were too few grades (statuses) of illness to adequately differentiate and prioritize thousands of patients. Therefore, physicians recognized the need for a more precise and complex prioritization scheme, especially for patients with decompensated disease whose need for transplant was greatest. Second, the inclusion of subjective variables in the CTP score (i.e., degree of ascites and encephalopathy) led to widespread "gaming" of the system. That is, physicians could describe the severity of ascites and encephalopathy in the worst possible terms, thereby increasing a patient's priority for transplantation. Third, waiting time was given too much emphasis. This was especially true for the lower priority statuses, status 2B and 3 (which accounted for two thirds of liver transplant recipients), where patients with longer waiting times were frequently transplanted ahead of sicker patients. In addition, because of the importance of waiting time, patients sought early listing to increase their priority for transplant. Consequently, the transplant list swelled with candidates whose need for transplant was quite low.

These problems in allocation were further compounded by flaws that developed in liver distribution. Until 15 years ago, liver transplantation was primarily performed in a relatively few, selected, large centers. Consequently, liver recipients traveled great distances and, in turn, since many regions did not have a transplant center, all locally procured donor organs were distributed out of the local area to these larger transplant centers. However, as more and more physicians became trained in transplantation during the 1980s and 1990s, they set up new transplant centers across the United States. While increasing access to transplantation, these centers created novel challenges in liver distribution. Start-up centers began to compete with the larger, more established centers for the limited donor pool. The allocation and distribution of these donor livers is directed nationally by UNOS, although the functional unit is the local organ procurement organization (OPO) of which there are 50 across the United States. With few exceptions, preference is given to distributing donor livers to recipients listed within the local OPO. In fact, 70% of donor livers are transplanted into local recipients.

With the proliferation of liver transplant centers, a fundamental debate emerged regarding two competing interests in liver distribution: (i) retaining organs within the OPO of procurement based on considerations of efficiency and local organ ownership, versus (ii) sharing organs over a wider geographic region to expand the potential recipient pool, allowing sicker patients greater access to donor livers. In the debate over liver distribution, the new, smaller centers argued that they could provide excellent local transplant care obviating the need for patients relocating to larger centers. Local distribution of donor livers also has the advantage of faster and more efficient transplantation, which may improve recipient outcomes. In addition, it may permit greater use of ECD livers. Since these organs are particularly sensitive to prolonged cold ischemic time (the time between organ procurement and transplantation), they are less well adapted to regional sharing, which requires time to transport organs over great distances. On the other hand, the larger centers contended that distributing livers to their sicker patients would make better use of a precious resource, especially if the transplant was performed by their experienced team. Local ownership of donor organs was another factor that became a critical component in the debate. The establishment of a new transplant center within a state became an issue of local pride and retention of donor organs a requirement to maintain the center's viability. As a result, some states attempted to pass laws restricting the transport of organs outside their boundaries. Finally, the debate was further fueled by differences that emerged in the types of patients listed at small and large centers. Compared to the large centers, smaller programs had shorter lists with fewer sick patients. The established larger centers had built long lists with critically ill patients through years of national and international referrals. These differences in patient populations along with the local retention of donor organs led to wide disparities in transplant access across the United States. Less sick patients at small centers were transplanted much faster than sicker patients waiting in larger hospitals.

These systemic problems became increasingly acute as the national waiting list grew and more patients required access to donor organs. The inherent flaws in the liver allocation and distribution scheme led to a national perception amongst professionals and even the lay public that the system did not work properly. By the late 1990s, the discourse grew so intense that the federal government stepped in to perform an independent review of the entire process through the Institute of Medicine [4]. Their conclusions were expressed in regulatory terms through the "final rule" that stipulated three major revisions in allocation (points 1 and 2) and distribution (point 3):

1 Since it was determined to be irrelevant to a patient's need for transplant, waiting time should be eliminated as a determinant for prioritization.
2 The prioritization of liver candidates for transplantation should be based on an objective and more precise scoring system.
3 In order to provide equitable access to liver transplantation across the country, uniform and larger organ distribution areas, each serving a population base of at least 9 million people, should be established. Organs should be allocated and distributed based on patients' medical needs with less emphasis placed on keeping organs in the local area where they are procured.

Two of these three recommendations were fully implemented. Most notable, the MELD score was established as the means for prioritizing candidates for transplantation. The MELD score is based on a mathematical model predictive of 90-day mortality and defined by the following equation, which includes only three objective variables (serum creatinine, bilirubin, and international normalized ratio (INR)):

$$0.957 \times \ln(\text{creatinine mg/dL}) + 0.378$$
$$\times \ln(\text{bilirubin mg/dL}) + 1.120 \times \ln(\text{INR}) + 0.6431.$$

The higher each determinant value, the higher the MELD score and 90-day mortality, and the higher the priority for transplant. Each patient is awarded a MELD score, expressed in whole numbers; the minimum score is 6 and the maximum value is capped at 40. Thus, there are 35 possible MELD scores, compared to four under the prior system. While remaining as a determinant, waiting time serves as a "tie breaker" for candidates with the same MELD score. Since the number of gradations of status increased from four to 35, waiting time was greatly devalued under the MELD system compared with the earlier allocation scheme. In addition, the MELD score offered the possibility of achieving national parity in prioritizing patients for transplantation. Since it was determined solely by objective variables, the MELD score should be the same across the country with little of the subjective variability that plagued earlier allocation schemes.

Following implementation of MELD-based liver allocation in 2002 in the United States, several important changes occurred. First, the triage of transplant candidates improved and sicker patients were more effectively prioritized and transplanted than under the prior allocation system [5,6]. As a result, sicker patients were transplanted faster and correspondingly the number of patients dying on the waiting list dropped by 16% between 2001 and 2006. As expected, patients were sicker at the time of transplant, and the average MELD score of liver transplant recipients increased from 14 before MELD-based allocation to 22 afterwards. Second, the emphasis on waiting time was greatly reduced. As a result, fewer patients sought early listing and some of those with compensated liver disease were removed from the list. Therefore, the number of listed patients dropped by 13%, from 11,126 in 2001 to 9,646 the following year [7]. Third, unrelated to the implementation of MELD-based allocation, the donor supply improved. The total number of donors increased 30% from 2001 to 2006 due to activity on several fronts (as discussed below) including a nationwide initiative aimed at increasing donor awareness and more aggressive utilization of previously untapped sources of donors. Finally, the allocation system was further amended in 2005 to reduce the transplant priority for less sick patients. The basis for this amendment was the observation that many low MELD score patients (MELD score <15) were still able to receive a liver transplant, particularly in regions of the country with an ample donor supply.

In fact, between September 2001 and June 2003, 24% of all US liver recipients had a MELD score <15. Since many of these recipients had compensated liver disease, two concerns were raised. For a patient with compensated liver disease, the benefit of receiving a transplant is not as evident compared to sicker patients. The risk of transplantation in these low MELD recipients could be higher compared with the relatively low mortality risk of remaining on the transplant list. In an analysis from the Scientific Registry of Transplant Recipients (SRTR), the benefit of transplant was analyzed by comparing the 1-year waiting list and post-transplant mortality rates for liver transplant candidates and recipients based on MELD score [8]. This study showed that for low MELD patients (MELD score <15), the 1-year recipient mortality risk was much higher for recipients (who received transplantation) compared with candidates (who remained on the list) (hazard ratio (HR) = 3.64 at MELD 6–11, HR = 2.35 at MELD 12–14; both P <0.001). In response to these data, UNOS amended the allocation scheme to reduce the priority of patients with a MELD score <15. While status 1 patients remain at highest priority, organs are subsequently offered locally within the procuring OPO and then within the UNOS region to patients with MELD scores ≥15. Listed patients with MELD scores <15 are only eligible for deceased donor (DD) livers after these

status 1 and MELD ≥15 candidates have been exhausted. After this change, the proportion of low MELD liver recipients dropped by about one fifth [9]. In summary, these improvements in the prioritization of liver candidates along with the increase in donor supply helped to alleviate disparities in access to transplantation and, to a certain extent, quelled the national debate about liver transplantation.

However, despite the advancements, some problems have persisted. Of the three recommendations by the US Institute of Medicine, only the two regarding liver allocation (the creation of an objective scoring system and the de-emphasis of waiting time) were implemented. There has been no change in liver distribution relative to increasing the organ allocation area, simply because the liver transplant community could not reach a consensus on this topic. Consequently, some disparities in access to transplantation have persisted. A recent analysis demonstrated a wide geographic variation in the severity of illness of liver recipients [10]. This analysis found that OPOs serving a small population transplant significantly less sick patients. Twelve of the nation's 50 OPOs have fewer than 100 patients listed, representing the bottom quartile in OPO size. In fact, the mean number of patients listed in these small OPOs (43) is less than one tenth that of the remaining larger OPOs (462). However, the distribution of MELD scores within all of these OPOs is the same, with only 2% of listed patients with a MELD score >24. Therefore, in small OPOs in which a mean of 43 patients are listed for transplantation, none or only one patient is likely to have a MELD score >24 at any given time. However, in large OPOs, where more than 400 patients on average are listed, the number of patients with a MELD score >24 is likely to be eight or more. The national distribution policy dictates that, in general, livers should be allocated to the patient with the highest MELD score within the OPO where the organs are procured. Therefore, when an organ becomes available, large OPOs are more likely to have a patient with a higher MELD score (>24) compared with a small OPO. Consequently, the proportion of patients who received a transplant with a MELD score >24 is more than 2.5 times higher in large OPOs than in small OPOs (49% versus 19%; P <0.001). In addition, patients are transplanted faster within the small OPOs. The rate of transplantation (per years listed) was 2.5-fold higher for patients listed in small OPOs versus large OPOs (1.03 versus 0.41; P <0.001). Despite transplanting less sick patients faster, the 1-year patient and graft survival rates for small OPOs and large OPOs are not statistically different and waiting list mortality rates are similar in both. The consequences of this disparity have important implications for individual patients as well as for the liver distribution system as a whole. For the individual patient, selection of a transplant center within a small OPO will result in a faster transplant at a lower MELD score, but no better outcome in terms of pretransplant waiting list mortality rate or post-transplant survival. For the liver distribution and allocation system, transplantation of less sick patients within these selected OPOs represents a failure to fulfill the Institute of Medicine mandate, which states that organs should be distributed based on patients' medical needs with less emphasis placed on keeping organs in the local area where they were procured.

In response to this problem, UNOS is in active discussion with the liver community about widening the area of organ distribution; that is, regional sharing. While most transplant professionals support the concept of regional sharing, there is no consensus on its implementation.

Another problem in implementing regional sharing is that in general, smaller programs in remote regions are less supportive of increasing the organ distribution area because their local organs would preferentially be shared over a larger base of patients. On the other hand, big transplant programs in large metropolitan cities are more favorably inclined towards regional sharing since they could access more organs from a larger catchment area. Lack of consensus is the result of each center supporting the regional sharing system that would provide its center with the greatest number of transplants. Another problem in implementing regional sharing is the disparity in the distribution of patients and transplant centers across the United States. The large metropolitan population centers (mainly on the east and west coasts) have more transplant candidates and transplant centers compared to smaller cities, mostly located within the middle of the country. In addition, the largest cities have more transplant candidates per population because of better access to medical care and the relocation of sick patients to large, inner-city transplant centers. Were the Insitute of Medicine mandate followed, creating uniform organ distribution areas of 9 million people would encompass an area as small as metropolitan New York City (with five liver programs and 1,500 listed patients) and a region as large as 1 million square miles in the Rocky Mountain West (with one program and 120 listed patients). Establishing uniform allocation areas with such stark differences in geographic characteristics and population density is obviously difficult and probably impossible. In addition, there are significant logistic problems in sharing organs across wide expanses of sparsely populated regions. The time, and attendant cost, required to transport organs over vast areas are of particular concern since cold ischemic time is an important determinant of graft function. Therefore, at the time of this writing, the likelihood of adopting a national system for regional sharing of all donor livers in the near future seems remote. However, in the near future, there will likely be implementation of an incre-

mental shift towards a limited regional sharing plan, e.g., for the relatively few liver candidates with extremely high priority for transplant (i.e., MELD score >34). Ultimately, most transplant professionals believe that some form of regional sharing will likely be implemented throughout the country. Because of the inability of the liver community to reach a consensus on this important issue, development of a regional sharing plan may require a governmental mandate following an independent review, similar to what was required prior to the implementation of the MELD system.

Another potential improvement under consideration by UNOS is liver allocation based on the survival benefit of transplant [11]. Transition to such a system would represent a fundamental change in organ allocation, but has many attractive features. There are essentially three means by which liver candidates may be prioritized for transplantation, each with distinct advantages and disadvantages. The current allocation system is devised to prioritize patients based on their need or urgency for transplant independent of transplant outcome. The advantage of this system is that the patients with the greatest risk of death receive the highest priority for transplant. However, the disadvantage is that some patients with a high pretransplant priority have a high post-transplant mortality risk. Allocating livers to such patients would not represent the most utilitarian use of organs. A second means of prioritization is based on a utilitarian approach. That is, patients with the greatest chance of post-transplant survival would receive the highest transplant priority. The benefit of this allocation scheme is that only the best transplant candidates would receive organs thereby maximizing the lifespan of each patient and organ. However, many of the ideal candidates for transplant have a low urgency for transplant. Therefore, adoption of this system would likely increase the pretransplant waiting list mortality.

The third organ allocation scheme, and the one under current consideration, would be a combination of the two systems and is termed "transplant benefit" or "survival benefit." Under this proposed system, for each donor liver that becomes available, the transplant survival benefit score would be computed for each candidate on the waiting list based on their specific characteristics as well as those of the particular donor. This benefit is calculated based on the difference in 5-year mean survival with the transplant compared to the survival rate of remaining on the list. Proponents of this system contend that survival-based allocation makes the best use of each donor organ. In addition, they point to modeling projections that 2,000 life-years would be saved were such a scheme implemented. However, there are problems with this system, the greatest of which is that the current means of predicting post-transplant survival is inaccurate. The r^2

statistic for survival benefit liver allocation is only 0.6 (where 1 is the perfect prediction of the modeling for post-transplant survival). Many experts believe that this is too low to permit its implementation for liver allocation. (By comparison, the r^2 statistic for the predictive capacity of MELD is approximately 0.82.) In addition, opponents contend that the projected number of lives saved by survival benefit liver allocation each year (102) is minimal compared to the nearly 17,000 patients listed for transplant. Finally, changing the entire allocation scheme would likely create new unforeseen problems that could be worse. While survival-based organ allocation has been implemented for lung transplantation, its application in liver transplantation remains under intense review and consideration. As the financial resources in all fields of medicine are becoming increasingly restricted, expensive medical procedures such as liver transplantation will be required to demonstrate sufficient benefit to warrant continued funding from payors. Allocating and distributing livers under a "survival benefit" system could potentially provide for a more effective application of liver transplantation in such a financially constrained environment.

Variation in MELD score

Since it was developed more than 10 years ago, the MELD score has received intense scrutiny on virtually every aspect of its effect on liver allocation. One area of interest is the variation in two of its determinants (INR and serum creatinine) and the potential impact on liver allocation. The INR was devised primarily to standardize the anticoagulation effects of warfarin and not to provide a reproducibly precise assessment of severity of illness in patients with end-stage liver disease. Standardization of therapeutic anticoagulation became necessary when clinicians noted that the various thromboplastin reagents used to determine prothrombin time differed markedly in their responsiveness to the anticoagulant effects of warfarin. To rectify this problem, the World Health Organization (WHO) proposed the INR, which is a correction formula that adjusts for the variable sensitivities of different thromboplastin reagents. The INR can be defined by the following equation:

INR = (patient's prothrombin time/

mean normal prothrombin time)^x,

where x is the international sensitivity index. The INR allows for the standardization of the prothrombin time ratio (determined by any thromboplastin reagent) to a reference WHO thromboplastin standard. With this standardization, the INR allows safe and effective dosing of warfarin, independent of the sensitivity of the thromboplastin reagent.

In liver patients, however, there has never been a formal demonstration of reproducibly precise INR values. In fact, wide INR variations in liver patients have been recognized for years based on the selection of the thromboplastin reagent [12]. (Whether this interlaboratory INR variation was recognized when MELD was developed is unclear.) The reason(s) for the wide variation in INR in liver patients compared with patients receiving oral anticoagulants is not known. One explanation may be the different mechanisms of prothrombin time elevation caused by warfarin and liver disease. Warfarin causes prolonged prothrombin time through inhibition of the vitamin K-dependent γ-carboxylation of coagulation factors II, VII, IX, and X. In liver disease, the elevated prothrombin time is due in large part to a decreased production of coagulation factors. A recent study evaluated the effect of INR variation on MELD score in liver transplant candidates. These investigators found that based on the selection of clinical laboratory, the same blood sample can yield up to a 2.1-fold difference in INR, which corresponds to a change in MELD score of up to 9 points (Fig. 49.2) [13]. The importance of these findings is underscored by the observation that the greatest variations in INR (and corresponding MELD score) occurred in the patients with the highest INR and highest MELD score. That is, the patients with the highest priority for transplant have the greatest variation in MELD score. Similar findings have been replicated in other studies [14–16]. The fundamental problem with this interlaboratory variation in INR and MELD score is its impact of parity, especially since the greatest differences are noted in patients with the highest MELD scores. Patients with an urgent need for transplant could be advantaged or penalized by changes in their MELD score based on the selection of the clinical laboratory where the INR is measured. Similarly, if one center were using an INR assay yielding lower INR values than another center, all of its patients would be correspondingly disadvantaged. Several possible responses regarding this issue have been proposed [17]:

1 The problem could be ignored, with the recognition that clinically relevant variations in the MELD score are acceptable. This seems to be the most likely response.
2 Uniform reagents and measuring devices could be utilized by all laboratories across the country measuring the INR for the MELD score. Given the virtually infinite variety in the combination of regents and devices, such a response seems impractical.
3 A central laboratory for measuring INR could be developed within the local allocation area to minimize the INR variation. While possible, this solution would be logistically difficult especially when MELD scores are urgently required for ill patients.
4 A correction factor could be devised to normalize the MELD score between different clinical laboratories.

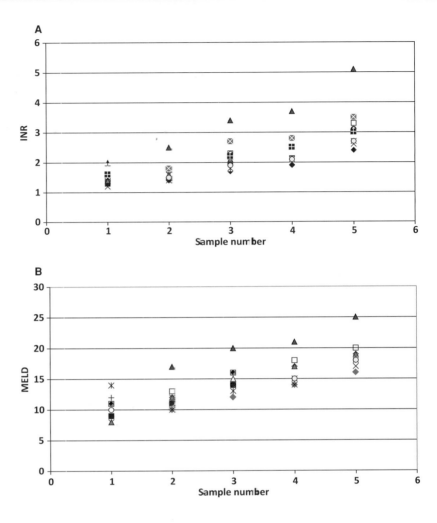

Figure 49.2 (A) International normalized ratio (INR) versus standardized blood sample number. (B) Model for end-stage liver disease (MELD) score versus standardized blood sample number.

Again, similar to point 2 above, this is likely impractical.

5 The INR could be removed from the MELD score. An analysis has demonstrated that removal of the INR from the MELD score would only minimally impact its predictive capacity; the *c*-statistic of the MELD-XI (without the INR) was comparable (0.829) to the MELD (0.842) [18].

6 The maximum INR value in the calculation of the MELD score could be capped, similar to the serum creatinine (Cr), which is capped at 4.0. Capping the INR would minimize the contribution of high values to the MELD score and would help to reduce interlaboratory variation [19]. This solution is currently under consideration and would likely be an important and easily implemented remediation of the INR problem.

The serum Cr is also subject to variation relative to the methodology selected for its measurement as well as patient gender. In particular, investigators have shown that elevated bilirubin levels may interfere with colorimetric assays for Cr [20]. They evaluated four different Cr assays in liver patients to assess changes in MELD score.

Agreement was found to be poor among all Cr assays and the variation in MELD score was greatest for the patients with the highest bilirubin. For those whose bilirubin was <5.8 mg/dL, only 3% had a difference of ≥2 MELD points. However, in patients with higher values (bilirubin ≥23.4 mg/dL), 78% had a difference of ≥3 MELD points. This variability among different assays, especially in patients with high bilirubin levels (and therefore high MELD scores and transplant priority) could have a relevant impact on prioritization for liver transplantation. The same investigators also reported the importance of the differences in Cr relative to the glomerular filtration rate (GFR) between the genders [21]. Compared to men, women have long been recognized to have lower serum Cr for the same GFR. Therefore, for the same degree of renal impairment, females would have a lower Cr, a lower corresponding MELD score, and lower priority for transplantation. These investigators used a correction formula to compensate for this difference and reported that correcting the Cr increases MELD score by 2 or 3 points in 65% of female liver candidates. Whether this variation in Cr relative to MELD score is sufficiently important to address through changes in the allocation system is unclear. However, the variation in MELD score relative to serum Cr and INR point out potential flaws in this carefully constructed allocation system.

Donation after cardiac death

Despite an overall shortage of donor organs, the number of donor livers has increased dramatically over the past decade due to changes in medical as well as administrative practice. Between 2000 and 2006 the number of donor livers increased by 33% from 4,997 to 6,651 in the United States [7]. Perhaps the most important reason for this increase was a change in administrative practices promulgated by the Organ Donation Breakthrough Collaborative in 2003, which facilitated the creation of systems within acute care hospitals and OPOs to ensure accurate and timely referral, screening, consent, organ recovery, and successful placement of organs [22].

In addition to these administrative changes, there have been three important medical innovations that have tapped into previously unavailable or underutilized sources of donors: DCD, ECD, and LDLT. The conventional deceased donor, donation after brain death (DBD), is a patient on a ventilator with a devastating brain injury whose death is declared based on the fulfillment of the strict criteria for brain death. On the other hand, DCD donors, while on a mechanical ventilator with irrecoverable brain injury (usually from trauma or hemorrhage), do not meet the strict criteria for brain death [23]. Prior to the development of DCD, such patients had not been eligible for donation. The protocol for DCD was therefore developed as a very controlled and regulated process through which these patients could be legally utilized for donation. Such patients are extubated and subsequently die (usually within 30 minutes) with the declaration of death occurring after the cessation of cardiac activity.

While utilization of such donors increases the overall donor pool, the means of acquiring DCD donors fundamentally compromises the quality and function of the donor organ. Between the time of extubation and cessation of heart function (donor warm ischemic time), there is a period of hypotension and hypoperfusion of the donor organ that negatively impacts its viability and function. While quite variable, the donor warm ischemic time is the single most important determinant of donor organ quality. In some cases, the warm time is so prolonged that the quality of the donor organs is compromised to the extent that the donor organ is discarded. In general, the outcomes with DCD liver recipients are inferior to those in DBD liver recipients. Specifically, two analyses from the SRTR (one between 1993 and 2001 and another from 1996 to 2003) reported virtually identical results with a mean 50% higher 1-year graft loss rate with DCD compared with DBD (29.4% versus 19.8 %; P <0.01) [24,25]. Perhaps the greatest progress towards improving outcomes is the identification of risk factors associated with graft loss with DCD. These include donor age >35 years (HR = 1.17), donor warm ischemia time >30 minutes (HR = 2.34), and donor cold ischemia time >10 hours (HR = 1.18); as well as recipient factors of age >60 years (HR = 1.17), life support (HR = 1.54), prior transplant (HR = 1.84), hemodialysis (HR = 1.26), and Cr >2.0 mg/dL (HR = 1.23) (P < 0.001). As these risk factors became recognized, the protocols for DCD procurement improved along with better selection of recipients for these marginal organs.

With these changes, some investigators found that patient outcomes with DCD are similar to DBD. For example, in a study where low-risk recipients were paired with low-risk DCD donors (warm ischemic time <30 minutes and cold ischemic time <10 hours), 1-year graft survival rates (81%) were not significantly different from those in DBD recipients (80%). However, despite these favorable results, the overall performance of DCD grafts is clearly inferior to DBD. The most important clinical complication associated with DCD is biliary strictures. Because the cause of biliary disease in DCD recipients is different to that in DBD recipients, so is the characteristic distribution of strictures within the liver. The biliary tree receives its critical perfusion through the arterial system and is therefore quite sensitive to hypoperfusion that may occur during DCD organ procurement. Consequently, DCD recipients are more likely to develop diffuse biliary stricturing throughout the liver, whereas most strictures in DBD recipients are at the biliary anastomosis. In fact, biliary disease is twice as common in DCD compared to DBD recipients and may frequently lead to significant graft dysfunction or failure [26,27]. The diffuse nature of the strictures in many DCD recipients makes them less amenable to interventional drainage and patients may be rendered as "biliary cripples," with serious chronic intractable biliary disease .

Implementation of DCD has expanded the total number of donor livers available for transplantation. The number of DCD donors in the United States increased more than ten-fold from just 23 in 1999 (<1% of liver transplants) to 307 in 2007 (4.9% of liver transplants) (Fig. 49.3). However, there was a slight decrease in the number of cases in 2008 to 276 cases (4.5% of all liver transplants) [28]. The reason(s) for the slight decline is not known, but is likely due to increased awareness of the associated risks and perhaps more careful selection of donors and recipients. Due to the higher risk of graft failure associated with DCD as well as the inherent complexities in organ procurement, some centers have not fully embraced the concept of DCD as a source of additional

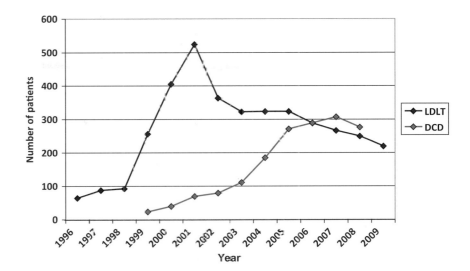

Figure 49.3 Numbers of living donor liver transplantation (LDLT) and donation after cardiac death (DCD) transplants versus year.

donor livers. Consequently, the application of DCD is quite variable amongst transplant centers across the country. In some regions of the United States, DCD accounts for nearly 10% of all adult deceased donor liver transplantation (DDLT) and in other areas fewer than 1%. DCD will likely remain as an important, but limited, means of expanding the donor pool, especially in areas where the donor supply is most limited. The effective application of DCD for liver transplantation requires cooperation between the OPO and the local transplant center(s) to ensure maximal utilization of these higher risk organs as well as careful application of the donor procurement protocols.

Living donor liver transplantation

The use of living donors has been another important development to partially alleviate the shortage of donor organs [29]. The first successful case was reported in 1989 and over the subsequent decade the procedure was largely limited to Asia where cultural mores prohibit the widespread application of deceased donation. At that time, the procedure utilized the left hepatic lobe or one of its segments. In the United States, relatively few cases were performed until 1999, largely in pediatric recipients where the parental donors readily accepted the procedural risk of donation and the small size of the left hepatic lobe provided a sufficient hepatic reserve. After 1999, LDLT was more widely applied and its rapid growth was due primarily to two factors. First, the growing shortage of deceased donors intensified in the late 1990s, forcing transplant centers to seek innovative strategies to increase the donor pool. Second, selected centers reported successful LDLT with the right hepatic lobe, which is larger than the left lobe and provided adequate hepatic volume to

support full-size adults. The subsequent growth in LDLT was rapid; in 1998, fewer than 100 cases were performed while the number increased to 524 in 2001, remarkably accounting for 11% of adult liver transplants in the United States (Fig. 49.3) [7]. There were initial projections that LDLT would constitute up to 50% of all liver transplants, although this has never been realized.

The choice to pursue LDLT for a specific patient is a complex consideration of the advantages and disadvantages of the procedure. The primary advantage associated with LDLT is speed and timing. Patients with an urgent need for transplant and no immediate prospects for DDLT are the best candidates for LDLT – such as patients with low MELD scores with hepatocellular carcinoma or primary sclerosing cholangitis with recurrent sepsis. While awaiting a deceased donor, such patients are at risk for dying or suffering decompensation, thereby jeopardizing the success of the DDLT. The primary risk for the LDLT recipient is associated with the immediate perioperative risk of complications, which are higher compared with DDLT, including death. In short, the patient who chooses to pursue LDLT incurs a potentially higher short-term risk related to an expedited transplant with the potential benefit of improved long-term survival by avoiding the risk of death while on the waiting list or decompensation which could ultimately jeopardize the success of DDLT. In fact, a recent study by the Adult-to-Adult Living Donor Liver Transplant Study Group (A2ALL) compared outcomes of LDLT versus DDLT [30]. The starting point for this study (from the time of donor evaluation) was carefully selected to encompass the clinical scenario (described above) related to the risks and benefit associated with the procedure. Of the 807 potential living donor recipients, 389 underwent LDLT, 249 underwent DDLT, 99 died without transplantation, and 70 were awaiting transplantation at last follow-up. Compared to waiting for DDLT, the receipt of an LDLT organ was associated with a significant survival benefit with an adjusted mortality HR of 0.56 (P <0.001). The benefits were even greater at centers performing more than 20 LDLTs, with a mortality HR of 0.35 (P <0.001). Therefore, this study demonstrated for the first time that the choice to pursue LDLT is associated with at least a 44% reduction in mortality risk compared to waiting for DDLT.

Despite these data supporting its use, LDLT has been negatively impacted by several recent developments. Consequently, the initial enthusiasm surrounding the procedure has waned, the number of cases in the United States has dropped significantly, and its role in the field of liver transplantation is being reconsidered. After the implementation of MELD-based liver allocation in 2002, there was less need for LDLT. As discussed above, better access to DDLT, due to improvements in liver allocation along with better donor supply, obviated the need for a living donor. In fact, a recent study found that 11% of LDLT donor candidates could not even finish their evaluation, because the recipient underwent DDLT prior to its completion [31]. Another reason for the decline in LDLT is the emergence of data showing inferior outcomes compared to DDLT. The rate of allograft failure in a risk-adjusted analysis was shown to be increased with LDLT (HR = 1.66; P <0.05) compared with DDLT [32]. In addition, the complication rate was significantly higher with LDLT. Data from the A2ALL study found that the following complications occurred at a higher rate after LDLT versus DDLT: biliary leak (31.8% versus 10.2%), reexploration (26.2% versus 17.1%), hepatic artery thrombosis (6.5% versus 2.3%), and portal vein thrombosis (2.9% versus 0.0%) (P <0.05) [33]. The reduction in LDLT cases over time was also due in part to a front-loaded effect. That is, at the inception of LDLT at each center, the most ideal donor–recipient pairs were identified and transplanted. However, after these cases were expended, it became apparent that many potential LDLT recipients were unable to identify a suitable donor and therefore were ultimately rejected for the procedure. This is reflected in the A2ALL study where the overall rate of donor acceptance was significantly higher during the early experience (47% in 1998–2000) compared with a later era (35% in 2001–2003; P <0.0002) [31]. Finally, the full extent of donor risk did not become apparent until several years after the widespread application of the procedure. Initial reports of donor complications were relatively low (less than 20%) [34]. However, a more comprehensive report of donor complications reported a complication rate of 38% that was nearly twice as high. While 27% of complications were minor, the remaining 11% were more serious, including 2% that were considered life threatening and 0.8% that led to death [35]. Reports began to surface of donor deaths and aborted donations (patients who underwent anesthesia in the operating room, but had the donor operation aborted prior to successful donation). Twelve (3%) aborted donors were reported from the A2ALL series and an additional 12 (4.7%) from Toronto [35,36]. While the risk of donor death is not known due to the absence of a comprehensive database, there are at least 13 worldwide donor deaths "definitely" related to the donor operation, making an estimated risk of 0.15% [37]. Because of all of these concerns, the number of LDLTs performed in the United States decreased by one half from its peak year of 2001 when 524 cases were performed, to only 219 adult recipients in 2009, representing just 3.5% of all liver transplants.

What does the future hold for LDLT? It will likely remain a viable procedure where the supply of DD organs is limited. In Asia, where LDLT remains the predominant means of providing liver transplantation, its application remains robust. In fact, the Asan Medical Center in Seoul, Korea – a country with less than one quarter the population of the United States – performs over 300 cases annually, which is more than the entire volume of LDLTs in the United States. In the latter, LDLT may remain a viable means to provide access to liver transplantation in selected patients, particularly in regions where the donor shortage is especially acute such as Boston, New York, Chicago, and California. However, in most other parts of the United States, the application of LDLT will likely remain quite limited. In addition, unless a program performs approximately ten or more cases each year, it seems unlikely that they would be able to maintain adequate performance standards for this technically complex procedure. In 2009, only seven hospitals in the United States had performed such a volume.

Expanded criteria donors

The use of ECDs, defined as donors who are not ideal or standard, is another strategy to increase the donor pool. While marginal liver grafts have been transplanted for decades, the concept of ECD is to objectively define the characteristics and associated risk of using these organs. By doing so, clinicians may learn how to mitigate these factors and select the best recipients for these marginal grafts, thereby maximizing organ utility. Perhaps the most detailed description of the ECD procedure was by Feng et al., who identified seven donor and graft factors associated with graft failure: donor age >40 years, DCD, split/partial grafts, African-American race, less height, cerebrovascular accident, and "other" causes of brain death [38]. Using these specific features, they devised the donor risk index (DRI), which is the relative risk of graft loss for an organ with a specific set of donor

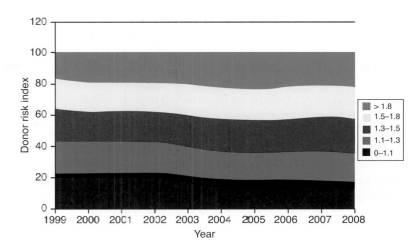

Figure 49.4 Donor risk index in primary liver recipients. (Reproduced from Thuluvath et al. [28] with permission from Wiley-Blackwell. Data as of May 2009.)

and transplant characteristics compared with a reference case, where DRI = 1.0. The higher the DRI, the higher is the 1-year graft loss rate. For example, the 1-year graft loss rate for a high DRI liver (DRI >2.0) is 28.6%, which is more than twice that of an ideal donor (DRI <1.0) at 12.4%.

Over the past decade, transplant centers have utilized an increasingly high proportion of marginal or high DRI livers. Between 1999 and 2008, there was a 36% increase in donors with a DRI of >1.8, with a corresponding 17% decrease in donors with a DRI of <1.3 (Fig. 49.4) [28]. When selecting recipients to receive a high DRI liver, transplant centers have developed a utilitarian approach towards graft disposition. Surgeons have learned through experience that transplanting high DRI livers into high MELD score patients is associated with higher rates of graft loss. Specifically, when using a liver with DRI ≥1.7, the 1-year graft loss rate is 37% higher in recipients with a MELD score ≥27 compared with a better liver (DRI <1.7) [39]. Therefore, high DRI organs are frequently rejected for use in high MELD recipients and are utilized in low MELD recipients where graft loss rates are lower. One-year graft loss rates in these low-risk patients (MELD score <15) are 21% lower than in high-risk recipients (MELD score ≥27) (20.9% and 26.6%, respectively). A recent SRTR analysis confirmed the widespread use of this strategy where investigators demonstrated an inverse relationship between DRI and recipient MELD score [40]. The liver DRI decreased as MELD score increased and the highest median DRI (1.50) was in patients transplanted in the lowest MELD categories (score <12). Conversely, the lowest median DRI (1.22) occurred in patients transplanted with a MELD score of 40. While this strategy may provide the most utilitarian use of a wide spectrum of donor livers, the benefit to specific recipients is less clear. Low MELD recipients (MELD score <12) receiving a high DRI liver suffer a significantly higher mortality

with transplant, compared to remaining on the waiting list. In fact, the highest relative risk of mortality occurred in recipients with the lowest MELD scores (score 6–8) who received high DRI organs (HR = 3.70; P <0.0005). So, which patients benefit the most from receiving high DRI livers? All recipients with a MELD score ≥20 had a significant survival benefit from transplantation, regardless of DRI. However, the patients who had the greatest relative benefit from high DRI organs were those with the highest MELD scores, due to their significant risk of death without transplantation. Even with the highest quartile risk DRI, recipients with the highest MELD score (score = 40) had a significantly lower mortality rate with transplant compared to remaining on the list. However, the impact of implementing such a practice would probably not have its intended result. In Schaubel et al.'s analysis, only 1% of all recipients had a MELD score of 40 and received a high DRI graft [40]. Therefore, these donor–recipient matches were likely selected for favorable outcome. Without selection mechanisms in place, the outcomes of high MELD/high DRI transplants might be very poor.

Currently, the liver transplant list is filled with a wide range of liver candidates, from those with minimal or no decompensation, to patients whose 90-day mortality is virtually 100%. The spectrum of quality in donor organs is equally wide. One of the greatest unmet challenges is devising a system that effectively matches specific organs and recipients to maximize the utilization of marginal grafts without impacting recipient outcomes.

MELD exception scores

Another area of considerable controversy is that of MELD exception scores. MELD exception scores are awarded to patients whose mortality risk is not adequately reflected by their laboratory MELD score. Assignment of MELD exception scores occurs through the regional review board for one of two broad indications: hepatocellular carcinoma (HCC) and non-HCC diagnoses. For HCC, candidates within the Milan criteria (or, in some regions, other similar specified criteria) receive a standard MELD exception score (22 points) to limit the risk of removal from the waiting list due to cancer progression. The number of transplant recipients with HCC increased from 999 in 2002 to 1,656 in 2008 or 27% of all liver transplants. Patients beyond the Milan criteria are also awarded MELD exception scores if approved by their regional review board. Some of these candidates meet prespecified tumor specifications – International Registry of Hepatic Tumors in UNOS region 4 [41] or University of California, San Francisco (UCSF) criteria [42] – both of which are slightly over the Milan criteria. Other patients with nonstandardized criteria for HCC are evaluated on a case-by-case basis by the regional review boards. The proportion of HCC patients on the waiting list (at the year's end) with a nonstandard HCC MELD exception score increased from 1.0% in 2002 to 20.6% in 2008 [28]. Many such patients may have been successfully downstaged with loco-regional therapies.

MELD exception scores are also awarded by the regional review board for indications other than HCC. Such patients have a risk of death, as subjectively judged by their transplant team, that is not reflected by their laboratory MELD score. These may be recognized diagnoses that include specific disorders (e.g., familial amyloidosis, hepatopulmonary syndrome, portpulmonary hypertension) or complications of liver disease (e.g., ascites, encephalopathy, biliary complications). The number and percentage of liver candidates with non-HCC MELD exception scores has increased every year since the institution of MELD-based allocation, from 382 in 2002 to 890 in 2008 [28]. However, the number of candidates with MELD exceptions on the waiting list (at the year's end, 2008) varies widely between UNOS regions, with only 16 in region 10 compared to 48 in region 5. Special concern relates to patients receiving non-HCC MELD exception points, particularly in regions where organs are in the highest demand, namely region 5 (California) and region 9 (New York), because these patients receive a very high priority for transplantation. For example, in New York, which runs a single list for the entire state (and region), there are 33 such patients, whose mean score is 27.2 points. In region 5, 48 patients have a mean score of 24.3. The high MELD scores awarded to these patients enhance the likelihood of them receiving a transplant. In fact, the rate of transplant is nearly three-fold higher than for patients with standard laboratory MELD scores [43]. There is concern that these non-HCC MELD exclusion scores may reflect another version of subjective upgrading that plagued previous allocation scheme (as described above).

To address this concern, UNOS organized a conference (MELD Exception Study Group and Conference (MESSAGE)) where standard criteria were developed and published for 17 exceptional medical conditions frequently encountered by the US regional review boards. The recommendations were researched, discussed utilizing an evidenced-based format, and ultimately published in 2006 to provide guidelines for regional review boards [44]. While these recommendations are not binding, they have been implemented in varying degrees within each region. The national impact of the MESSAGE guidelines on non-HCC MELD exception points is difficult to assess, but an analysis shows some improvement after their publication in 2006. There was a slight increase in the percentage of patients receiving a DDLT with a MELD exception other than HCC, from 7.6% in 2003 to 8.6% in 2007 [45]. The fraction of each region's total DDLTs with non-HCC exceptions has become more uniform. In 2003, the percentage of regional DDLTs with non-HCC exceptions ranged from 2% to 21%. By 2007, this range had narrowed to between 5% and 10% for all regions. There have been discussions about creating a national review board to ensure national uniformity in the diagnosis and scoring of these patients as well as normalizing the points awarded to each patient, but none has been formed as yet. One of the problems related to implementing a national review board is the wide disparity in MELD scores for liver recipients between regions. In regions that transplant at lower MELD scores, the number of MELD points requested for non-HCC MELD exception points would be lower than in regions where MELD scores are higher. This is reflected in the wide range of MELD scores given for non-HCC MELD exceptions, which range from a mean of 19.1 in UNOS region 3 to 28.5 in region 2.

Annotated references

Berg CL, Gillespie BW, Merion RM, et al. Improvement in survival associated with adult-to-adult living donor liver transplantation. *Gastroenterology* 2007;133:1806–13.

This is the first study that demonstrated the potential benefit for LDLT recipients compared with the option of remaining on the transplant list for a DD transplantation.

Feng S, Goodrich NP, Bragg-Gresham JL, et al. Characteristics associated with liver graft failure: the concept of a donor risk index. *Am J Transplant* 2006;6:783–90.

The authors describe specific risk factors associated with graft loss in liver transplant recipients and in doing so define the donor risk index (DRI, which serves as a yardstick to objectively assess the quality of a donor graft in liver transplantation.

Mateo R, Cho Y, Singh G, et al. Risk factors for graft survival after liver transplantation from donation after cardiac death donors: an analysis of OPTN/UNOS data. *Am J Transplant* 2006;6:791–6.

This paper describes the significant risk factors for graft loss associated with liver transplant recipients of DCD organs. The authors describe a means to match the recipients and DCD donors to maximize patient outcomes.

Merion RM, Schaubel DE, Dykstra DM, Freeman RB, Port FK, Wolfe RA. The survival benefit of liver transplantation. *Am J Transpl* 2005;5:307–13.

This study demonstrates the lower limit for the survival benefit for liver transplantation at a MELD score of 15. The findings in this study changed the liver allocation policy known as the "share 15" rule.

Schaubel DE, Guidinger MK, Biggins SW, et al. Survival benefit-based deceased-donor liver allocation. *Am J Transplant* 2009;9:970–81.
The development of a liver allocation system based on the survival benefit is described. While such a system has been adopted for lung transplantation, the liver allocation scheme remains under review.

References

1. Kamath PS, Wiesner RH, Malinchoc M, et al. A model to predict survival in patients with end-stage liver disease. *Hepatology* 2001;33:464–70.
2. Wiesner RH, McDiarmid SV, Kamath PS, et al. MELD and PELD: application of survival models to liver allocation. *Liver Transpl* 2001;7:567–80.
3. Coombes JM, Trotter JF. Development of the allocation system for deceased donor liver transplantation. *Clin Med Res* 2005;3:87–92.
4. Institute of Medicine Committee on Organ Procurement and Transplantation Policy. *Organ Procurement and Transplantation: assessing current policies and the potential impact of the DHHS final rule*. Washington, DC: National Academy Press, 1999:1–29.
5. Freeman RB Jr, Wiesner RH, Roberts JP, McDiarmid S, Dykstra DM, Merion RM. Improving liver allocation: MELD and PELD. *Am J Transplant* 2004;S9:114–31.
6. Freeman RB, Wiesner RH, Edwards E, Harper A, Merion R, Wolfe R; United Network for Organ Sharing Organ Procurement and Transplantation Network Liver and Transplantation Committee. Results of the first year of the new liver allocation plan. *Liver Transpl* 2004;10:7–15.
7. *UNOS Annual Report*. http://www.ustransplant.org/annual reports/current/401 opo.htm. Accessed July 1, 2010.
8. Merion RM, Schaubel DE, Dykstra DM, Freeman RB, Port FK, Wolfe RA. The survival benefit of liver transplantation. *Am J Transplant* 2005;5:307–13.
9. Freeman RB. The share 15 rule. In: Everson GT, Trotter JF. eds. *Liver Transplantation Challenging Controversies and Topics*. Totowa, NJ: Humana Press, 2009:91–101.
10. Trotter JF, Osgood MJ. MELD scores of liver transplant recipients according to size of waiting list: impact of organ allocation and patient outcomes. *JAMA* 2004;291:1871–4.
11. Schaubel DE, Guidinger MK, Biggins SW, et al. Survival benefit-based deceased-donor liver allocation. *Am J Transplant* 2009;9:970–81.
12. Robert A, Chazouillères O. Prothrombin time in liver failure: time, ratio, activity percentage, or international normalized ratio? *Hepatology* 1996;24:1392–4.
13. Trotter JF, Olson J, Lefkowitz J, Smith AD, Arjal R, Kenison J. Changes in international normalized ratio (INR) and model for endstage liver disease (MELD) based on selection of clinical laboratory. *Am J Transplant* 2007;7:1624–8.
14. Trotter JF, Brimhall B, Arjal R, Phillips C. Specific laboratory methodologies achieve higher model for endstage liver disease (MELD) scores for patients listed for liver transplantation. *Liver Transpl* 2004;10:995–1000.
15. Xiol X, Gines P, Castells L, et al. Clinically relevant differences in the model for end-stage liver disease and model for end-stage liver disease-sodium scores determined at three university-based laboratories of the same area. *Liver Transpl* 2009;15:300–5.
16. Lisman T, van Leeuwen Y, Adelmeijer J, et al. Interlaboratory variability in assessment of the model of end-stage liver disease score. *Liver Int* 2008;28:1344–51.
17. Porte RJ, Lisman T, Tripodi A, Caldwell SH, Trotter JF; Coagulation in Liver Disease Study Group. The international normalized ratio

18. Heuman DM, Mihas AA, Habib A, et al. MELD-XI: a rational approach to "sickest first" liver transplantation in cirrhotic patients requiring anticoagulant therapy. *Liver Transpl* 2007;13:30–7.
19. Leise MD, Kim WR, Kremers WK, Larson JJ, Benson JT, Therneau TM. A revised model for end-stage liver disease optimizes prediction of mortality among patients awaiting liver transplantation. *Gastroenterology* 2011;140:1952–60.
20. Cholongitas E, Marelli L, Kerry A, et al. Different methods of creatinine measurement significantly affect MELD scores. *Liver Transpl* 2007;13:523–9.
21. Cholongitas E, Marelli L, Kerry A, et al. Female liver transplant recipients with the same GFR as male recipients have lower MELD scores – a systematic bias. *Am J Transplant* 2007;7:685–92.
22. Howard DH, Siminoff LA, McBride V, Lin M. Does quality improvement work? Evaluation of the Organ Donation Breakthrough Collaborative. *Health Serv Res* 2007;42:2160–73.
23. Steinbrook R. Organ donation after cardiac death. *N Engl J Med* 2007;357:209–13.
24. Merion RM, Pelletier SJ, Goodrich N, Englesbe MJ, Delmonico FL. Donation after cardiac death as a strategy to increase deceased donor liver availability. *Ann Surg* 2006;244:555–62.
25. Mateo R, Cho Y, Singh G, et al. Risk factors for graft survival after liver transplantation from donation after cardiac death donors: an analysis of OPTN/UNOS data. *Am J Transplant* 2006;6:791–6.
26. Skaro AI, Jay CL, Baker TB, et al. The impact of ischemic cholangiopathy in liver transplantation using donors after cardiac death: the untold story. *Surgery* 2009;146:543–52.
27. de Vera ME, Lopez-Solis R, Dvorchik I, et al. Liver transplantation using donation after cardiac death donors: long-term follow-up from a single center. *Am J Transplant* 2009;9:773–81.
28. Thuluvath PJ, Guidinger MK, Fung JJ, Johnson LB, Rayhill SC, Pelletier SJ. Liver transplantation in the United States, 1999–2008. *Am J Transplant* 2010;10:1003–19.
29. Trotter JF, Wachs M, Everson GT, Kam I. Adult-to-adult transplantation of the right hepatic lobe from a living donor. *N Engl J Med* 2002;346:1074–82.
30. Berg CL, Gillespie BW, Merion RM, et al. Improvement in survival associated with adult-to-adult living donor liver transplantation. *Gastroenterology* 2007;133:1806–13.
31. Trotter JF, Wisniewski KA, Terrault NA, et al. Outcomes of donor evaluation in adult-to-adult living donor liver transplantation. *Hepatology* 2007;46:1476–84.
32. Abt PL, Mange KC, Olthoff KM, Markmann JF, Reddy KR, Shaked A. Allograft survival following adult-to-adult living donor liver transplantation. *Am J Transplant* 2004;4:1302–7.
33. Freise CE, Gillespie BW, Koffron AJ, et al. Recipient morbidity after living and deceased donor liver transplantation: findings from the A2ALL Retrospective Cohort Study. *Am J Transplant* 2008;8:2569–79.
34. Brown RS Jr, Russo MW, Lai M, et al. A survey of liver transplantation from living adult donors in the United States. *N Engl J Med* 2003;348:818–25.
35. Ghobrial RM, Freise CE, Trotter JF, et al. Donor morbidity after living donation for liver transplantation. *Gastroenterology* 2008;135:468–76.
36. Guba M, Adcock L, MacLeod C, et al. Intraoperative 'no go' donor hepatectomies in living donor liver transplantation. *Am J Transplant* 2010;10:612–18.
37. Trotter JF, Adam R, Lo CM, Kenison J. Documented deaths of hepatic lobe donors for living donor liver transplantation. *Liver Transpl* 2006;12:1485–8.
38. Feng S, Goodrich NP, Bragg-Gresham JL, et al. Characteristics associated with liver graft failure: the concept of a donor risk index. *Am J Transplant* 2006;6:783–90.

39. Maluf DG, Edwards EB, Kauffman HM. Utilization of extended donor criteria liver allograft: is the elevated risk of failure independent of the model for end-stage liver disease score of the recipient? *Transplantation* 2006;82:1653–7.

40. Schaubel DE, Sima CS, Goodrich NP, Feng S, Merion RM. The survival benefit of deceased donor liver transplantation as a function of candidate disease severity and donor quality. *Am J Transplant* 2008;8:419–25.

41. Onaca N, Davis GL, Goldstein RM, Jennings LW, Klintmalm GB. Expanded criteria for liver transplantation in patients with hepatocellular carcinoma: a report from the International Registry of Hepatic Tumors in Liver Transplantation. *Liver Transpl* 2007;13:391–9.

42. Yao FY, Ferrell L, Bass NM, Bacchetti P, Ascher NL, Roberts JP. Liver transplantation for hepatocellular carcinoma: comparison of the proposed UCSF criteria with the Milan criteria and the Pittsburgh modified TNM criteria. *Liver Transpl* 2002;8:765–74.

43. Rodriguez-Luna H, Vargas HE, Moss A, et al. Regional variations in peer reviewed liver allocation under the MELD system. *Am J Transplant* 2005;5:2244–7.

44. Freeman RB Jr, Gish RG, Harper A, et al. Model for end-stage liver disease (MELD) exception guidelines: results and recommendations from the MELD Exception Study Group and Conference (MESSAGE) for the approval of patients who need liver transplantation with diseases not considered by the standard MELD formula. *Liver Transpl* 2006;12:S128–36.

45. Berg CL, Steffick DE, Edwards EB, et al. Liver and intestine transplantation in the United States 1998–2007. *Am J Transplant* 2009;9:907–31.

Multiple choice questions

49.1 Which of the three following determinants in the model for end-stage liver disease (MELD) score has the highest multiplicative factor?

   a   Bilirubin.
   b   International normalized ratio (INR).
   c   Serum creatinine.
   d   Both b and c

49.2 Which of the following have helped to increase the number of deceased donor organs for liver transplantation?

   a   Expanded criteria donors (ECDs).
   b   Donation after cardiac death (DCD).
   c   Living donors.
   d   a, b, and c.
   e   a and b.

49.3 Which of the following factors is associated with the decline in the number of living donor liver transplantations (LDLTs) performed in the United States?

   a   The availability of deceased donor livers.
   b   Donor complication rates.
   c   Recipient complication rates.
   d   All of the above.

49.4 As a means to increase access to transplantation for sick patients, the United Network for Organ Sharing has implemented a widely accepted regional sharing plan for deceased donor livers across the United States.

   a   True.
   b   False.

49.5 The donor risk index (DRI) is which of the following?

   a   The ratio of observed versus expected graft loss.
   b   The relative risk of graft loss for an organ with a specific set of donor characteristics compared with reference case.
   c   Is only applicable to kidney transplantation.
   d   The relative risk of graft loss for an organ with a specific set of donor and graft characteristics compared with a reference case.

49.6 What is the basis for the liver allocation currently under active consideration?

   a   Pretransplant survival.
   b   Utilitarian.
   c   Survival benefit of the transplant.
   d   The donor risk index.

Answers to the multiple choice questions can be found in the Appendix at the end of the book.

These multiple choice questions are also available for you to complete online.
Visit http://www.schiffsdiseasesoftheliver.com/

APPENDIX
Multiple Choice Answers

Chapter 1 History Taking and Physical Examination for the Patient with Liver Disease

1.1 The correct answer is **e**, 200 mg.

1.2 The correct answer is **b**, Wilson disease.

Chapter 6 Bilirubin Metabolism and Jaundice

6.1 The correct answer is **c**, Urine dipstick for bilirubin: negative.

Comment: The negative urine dipstick despite obvious jaundice indicates that the patient has a purely unconjugated hyperbilirubinemia.

6.2 The correct answer is **c**, A decrease in total bilirubin from 4.0 to 0.4 mg/dL.

Comment: Unconjugated hyperbilirubinemia, reticulocytosis, and anemia often occur together in the presence of hemolysis. The unconjugated hyperbilirubinemia is a direct consequence of the breakdown of hemoglobin in hemolyzed red blood cells, and will diminish very quickly with a decrease in the rate of red blood cell destruction. The reticulocytosis is the bone marrow's response to the anemia induced by hemolysis, and will persist until the anemia has been repaired. This may require several weeks after cessation of the hemolytic process.

Reference

- Berk PD, Martin JF, Blaschke TF, Scharschmidt BF, Plotz PH. Unconjugated hyperbilirubinemia. Physiologic evaluation and experimental approaches to therapy. *Ann Intern Med* 1975;82:552–70.

6.3 The correct answer is **d**, Dubin–Johnson syndrome.

Comment: The progressive familial and benign recurrent intrahepatic cholestasis syndromes are both characterized by defects in bile secretion, with cholestasis and accumulation of bile acids in the serum. Conjugated hyperbilirubinemia is a secondary consequence of disordered bile secretion and consequent structural damage to the biliary tract. In contrast, conjugated hyperbilirubinemia in Dubin–Johnson syndrome is the consequence of a specific defect in secretion of bilirubin glucuronides into the bile. Bile secretion, including that of bile acids is normal, and there is no cholestasis.

Reference

- Thompson R, Jansen PLM. Genetic defects in hepatocanalicular transport. *Semin Liver Dis* 2000;20(3):365–72. DOI: 10.1055/s-2000-9384.

Chapter 8 Mechanisms of Liver Injury

8.1 The correct answer is **c**, FasL and Fas.

Comment: FasL was given intravenously in this experiment and resulted in massive hepatocyte apoptosis and fulminant hepatic failure. FasL binds and activates its cognate cell surface receptor Fas with subsequent activation of caspase 8, cleavage of Bid, activation of Bak and Bax, mitochondrial permeabilization, and apoptosis.

8.2 The correct answer is **c**, The innate immune system is a critical component of pathways that perpetuate liver injury and inflammation.

Comment: The innate immune system is a critical component of pathways that perpetuate liver injury and inflammation. Kupffer cells, natural killer cells, and natural killer T cells are vital components of the innate immune system in the liver. They secrete inflammatory cytokines such as TNF-α and interleukin-6, as well as death ligands such as Fas and TRAIL. Hepatocyte cell death can occur via apoptosis or necrosis, however the role of necroptosis, if any, is unknown. Caspase inhibition was associated with a decrease in aminotransferase levels in patients with chronic hepatitis C. Hepatocyte apoptosis is dependent on mitochondria, but can be initiated from the cell surface via death receptors, or from intracellular perturbations.

Chapter 9 Hepatic Manifestations of Systemic Disorders

9.1 The correct answer is **e**, All of the above.

Comment: The initial manifestations of hepatobiliary tuberculosis include a remarkable variety of presentations. Although traditionally considered in the presence of fever and raised serum alkaline phosphatase levels, clinicians should consider the possibility of tuberculosis in other settings, including all of the options noted above.

Reference

- Alvarez SZ. Hepatobiliary tuberculosis. *J Gastroenterol Hepatol* 1998;13:833–9.

9.2 The correct answer is **b**, Current guidelines advise antibiotic prophylaxis for exposed individuals in endemic regions.

Comment: Leptospirosis may present with acute abdominal pain, and doxycycline is the treatment of choice, but is not recommended as a prophylactic measure.

Reference

- Brett-Major DM, Lipnick RJ. Antibiotic prophylaxis for leptospirosis. *Cochrane Database Syst Rev* 2009:1; CD007342.

9.3 The correct answer is **c**, Increased levels of protoporphyrin in erythroid cells and feces helps establish the diagnosis.

Comment: Hepatic involvement is relatively uncommon in cases of erythropoietic protophoryria, and because the primary enzyme defect is in the erythroid cell line, liver transplantation is not curative. Phlebotomy is the treatment for porphyria cutanea tarda; alcoholic beverages may exacerbate acute intermittent porphyria.

Reference

- Kauppinen R. Porphyrias. *Lancet* 2005;365:241–52.

9.4 The correct answer is **c**, A gluten-free diet may improve the disease course of primary biliary cirrhosis when underlying celiac disease is present.

Comment: Although celiac disease is frequently associated with a wide variety of liver disorders, the elimination of gluten from the diet has no effect on the natural course of these other conditions.

Reference

- Rubio-Tapia A, Murray JA. The liver in celiac disease. *Hepatology* 2007;46:1650–8.

Chapter 10 Hepatobiliary Complications of Hematopoietic Cell Transplantation

10.1 The correct answer is **d**, Matched donor/recipient HCT.

Comment: HLA mismatched donor/recipient pairs are a higher risk clinical scenario for the development of GVHD compared to autologous or greater HLA matching. The presence of HBV and HCV in the donor or recipient or the presence of recipient iron overload increases the risk of acute and chronic liver disease following HCT.

Reference

- Strasser SI, Sullivan KM, Myerson D, et al. Cirrhosis of the liver in long-term marrow transplant survivors. *Blood* 1999;93:3259–66.

10.2 The correct answer is **b**, Terminal hepatic venule occlusion on biopsy.

Comment: Sinusoidal obstruction syndrome occurs early after transplant and presents classically with hepatomegaly, ascites, weight gain, and hyperbilirubinemia. Because of the sinusoidal portal hypertension, the hepatic venous pressure gradient is characteristically elevated and often >10 mmHg. Terminal hepatic venule occlusion is a late feature of SOS and is not necessary for the diagnosis. Thus the term venoocclusive disease (VOD) has been replaced with SOS.

References

- Shulman HM, Fisher LB, Schoch HG, Henne KW, McDonald GB. Veno-occlusive disease of the liver after marrow transplantation: histological correlates of clinical signs and symptoms. *Hepatology* 1994;19:1171–81.
- Shulman HM, McDonald GB, Matthews D, et al. An analysis of hepatic venocclusive disease and centrilobular hepatic degeneration following bone marrow transplantation. *Gastroenterology* 1980;79:1178–91.

Chapter 11 The Liver in Pregnancy

11.1 The correct answer is **d**.

Comment: Answer d is not associated with ICP and is therefore the correct answer. ICP occurs during the second or third trimester and is characterized by pruritus and an elevation of serum aminotransferases and bile acid concentrations. The main complications are prematurity and sudden intrauterine fetal death (1–2 % of cases currently). ICP is never associated with liver failure or encephalopathy. Ursodesoxycholic acid improves liver tests and pruritus. ICP recurs in 60–70% of cases during subsequent pregnancies.

Reference

- Pusl T, Beuers U. Intrahepatic cholestasis of pregnancy. *Orphanet J Rare Dis* 2007;2:26.

11.2 The correct answer is **a**.

Comment: Answer a is not associated with AFLP is therefore the correct answer. AFLP is a rare disease unique to pregnancy that occurs typically during the third trimester. If the diagnosis is delayed, AFLP may lead to acute liver failure with hepatic encephalopathy. The primary therapy of AFLP is early delivery, which has dramatically improved both maternal and fetal prognosis. An association has been found between AFLP and a defect of long-chain 3-hydroxyacyl coenzyme A dehydrogenase (LCHAD) in the fetus. Women in whom AFLP develops and their offspring should undergo DNA testing for the main associated genetic mutation (G1528C) in the gene coding for LCHAD. AFLP may recur during subsequent pregnancies, although recurrence is not the rule.

Reference

- Ibdah JA. Acute fatty liver of pregnancy: an update on pathogenesis and clinical implications. *World J Gastroenterol* 2006;12:7397–404.

Chapter 13 Preoperative Evaluation of the Patient with Liver Disease

13.1 The correct answer is **e**, Cancel the surgery.

Comment: The liver biochemical abnormalities in this patient are most consistent with alcoholic liver disease. The patient may have alcoholic hepatitis, which is associated with a high surgical mortality rate. Until the diagnosis is clear and, if necessary, the patient is abstinent from alcohol for 12 weeks, elective surgery should be deferred.

References

- Greenwood SM, Leffler CT, Minkowitz S. The increased mortality rate of open liver biopsy in alcoholic hepatitis. *Surg Gynecol Obstet* 1972;134:600–4.
- O'Leary JG, Yachimski PS, Friedman LS. Surgery in the patient with liver disease. *Clin Liver Dis* 2009;13:211–31.

13.2 The correct answer is **c**, A serum bilirubin level >50 μmol/L plus a prothrombin time index <50%.

Comment: Post-resectional liver failure is defined as a prothrombin time index (control prothrombin time divided by the patient's prothrombin time) of less than 50% (corresponding to an INR of >1.7) and a serum bilirubin level >50 μmol/L (2.9 mg/dL). When these criteria are met, the postoperative mortality rate has been reported to be 59%, compared with 1.2% when they are not met.

Reference

- van den Broek MA, Olde Damink SW, Dejong CH, et al. Liver failure after partial hepatic resection: definition, pathophysiology, risk factors and treatment. *Liver Int* 2008;28:767–80.

Chapter 14 Portal Hypertension: Nonsurgical and Surgical Management

14.1 The correct answer is **c**, Nonselective β-blocker.

Comment: Bleeding esophageal varices should be treated by pharmacologic and endoscopic treatments. The former should be intravenous administration of terlipressin or somatostatin, and the latter should be endoscopic sclerotherapy or band ligation. Oral administration of nonselective β-blockers is applied for primary or secondary prophylaxis of variceal bleeding.

Reference

- Sanyal AJ, Bosch J, Blei A, Arroyo V. Portal hypertension and its complications. *Gastroenterology* 2008;134:1715–28.

14.2 The correct answer is **a**, Small esophageal varices in Child–Pugh class A patients.

Comment: Varices with a high risk factor of bleeding are those found in Child–Pugh class C patients, and varices with a large size and/or red signs.

Reference

- Krawitt EL. *Medical Management of Liver Disease*. New York: Marcel Dekker, 1999.

Chapter 15 Renal Complications of Liver Disease and the Hepatorenal Syndrome

15.1 The correct answer is **a**, Renal failure where there is no structural damage in the kidneys.

Comment: Functional renal failure is a type of renal failure where there is no structural damage in the kidneys. It can be acute or chronic. Hepatorenal syndrome is only one type of functional renal failure. The cutoff value for the diagnosis of functional renal failure is 1.5 mg/dL.

Reference

- Montoliu S, Ballesté B, Planas R, et al. Incidence and prognosis of different types of functional renal failure in cirrhotic patients with ascites. *Clin Gastroenterol Hepatol* 2010;8:616–22.

15.2 The correct answer is **b**, It can include conditions such as glomerulonephritis in cirrhosis.

Comment: Acute kidney failure differs from functional renal failure in that the term denotes acute renal failure from whatever cause, whether there is structural damage in the kidneys or not, whereas the term functional renal failure requires that there is no structural damage in the kidneys. Therefore the causes of acute kidney injury are not specific to cirrhosis. It is a term that is well versed within the nephrology communities, but it has only just started to be used amongst hepatologists. The first stage of acute kidney injury requires a rise of 0.3 mg/dL for diagnosis even when the serum creatinine is still within the normal range.

Reference

- Mehta RL, Kellum JA, Shah SV, et al. Acute Kidney Injury Network: report of an initiative to improve outcomes in acute kidney injury. *Crit Care* 2007;11:R31.

15.3 The correct answer is **b**, The patient usually has signs to suggest a hyperdynamic circulation.

Comment: Type 1 hepatorenal syndrome is a form of functional renal failure. It occurs acutely, but is a condition that evolves over 2 weeks rather than 2 days. Hepatorenal syndrome is a consequence of the hemodynamic changes that occur in advanced cirrhosis, so the patient usually manifests signs of hemodynamic changes such as those associated with a hyperdynamic circulation. Although patients with acute hepatorenal syndrome usually have severe renal sodium retention, it is not a sine qua non diagnostic criterion, as patients with hepatorenal syndrome have been known to have high renal sodium excretion.

References

- Dudley FJ, Kanel GC, Wood LJ, et al. Hepatorenal syndrome without avid sodium retention. *Hepatology* 1986;6:248–51.
- Salerno F, Gerbes A, Gines P, et al. Diagnosis, prevention and treatment of hepatorenal syndrome in cirrhosis. *Gut* 2007;56:1310–8.

15.4 The correct answer is **a**, It should start as soon as all other cause of acute renal failure have been excluded.

Comment: The treatment for acute or type 1 hepatorenal syndrome should start as soon as all other causes of acute renal failure have been excluded. The usual first-line treatment is vasoconstrictor therapy. There have not been any randomized controlled trials to support the recommendation of the insertion of a transjugular intrahepatic portosystemic stent shunt as a first-line treatment. Vasoconstrictor therapy should continue for as long as the patient shows a response in terms of a reduction in serum creatinine levels. For terlipressin and norepinephrine, this should be less than 15 days; for a combination of midodrine and octreotide, this can be several weeks long. Although empirical antibiotic use is recommended in patients who present with acute renal failure, once bacterial infection is excluded, antibiotics should be stopped.

Reference

- Garcia-Tsao G, Parikh CR, Viola A. Acute kidney injury in cirrhosis. *Hepatology* 2008;48:2064–77.

15.5 The correct answer is **d**, Correcting the renal failure pre transplant can significantly improve patient survival post transplant.

Comment: Since the graft and patient survival are lower for patients with hepatorenal syndrome who receive a combined liver–kidney transplant when compared with those who receive a liver transplant alone, it is recommended that a liver transplant alone should be done first, unless the patient has been on renal replacement therapy for over 3 months, when the reverse is true. The presence of hepatorenal syndrome pre transplant increases post-transplant morbidity and reduces post-transplant graft and patient survival, hence it is recommended that the renal failure is corrected before the patient receives a liver transplant.

References

- Locke JE, Warren DS, Singer AL, et al. Declining outcomes in simultaneous liver–kidney transplantation in the MELD era: ineffective usage of renal allografts. *Transplantation* 2008;85:935–42.
- Restuccia T, Ortega R, Guevara M, et al. Effects of treatment of hepatorenal syndrome before transplantation on post-transplantation outcome. A case–control study. *J Hepatol* 2004;40:140–6.

Chapter 16 Pulmonary Manifestations of Liver Disease

16.1 The correct answer is **b**, Contrast Doppler echocardiography.

Comment: This patient has worsening dyspnea on exertion without evidence of significant intrinsic lung disease or fluid overload in addition to a low diffusing capacity for carbon monoxide. This clinical picture is suggestive of hepatopulmonary syndrome. The most appropriate next test is contrast echocardiography to assess intrapulmonary shunting.

16.2 The correct answer is **c**, Right heart catheterization.

Comment: This patient has decompensated cirrhosis with a high MELD score. He has marked lower extremity edema out of proportion to ascites, and echocardiographic findings suggestive of portopulmonary hypertension. Right heart catheterization is needed to define whether portopulmonary hypertension is present and to assess its severity. This would guide further management including medical therapy and candidacy for transplantation.

Chapter 17 Ascites and Spontaneous Bacterial Peritonitis

17.1 The correct answer is **d**, Oral spironolactone and furosemide.

Comment: In general oral spironolactone and furosemide constitute first-line treatment of patients with cirrhosis and ascites. Normokalemia is maintained and natriuresis is optimized. Intravenous furosemide causes azotemia and hypokalemia. Oral furosemide without spironolactone causes hypokalemia. Large-volume paracentesis is reserved for tense ascites and diuretic-resistant ascites.

Reference
- Runyon BA. Management of adult patients with ascites due to cirrhosis: an update. *Hepatology* 2009;49:2087–107.

17.2 The correct answer is **c**, Cefotaxime 2 g intravenously every 8 hours for 5 days.

Comment: Patients with cirrhosis do not tolerate the nephrotoxicity of gentamicin. Ceftriaxone 1 g intravenously daily prevents bacterial infections in patients with cirrhosis and gut hemorrhage, but does not treat SBP well at this dose due to its high protein binding and the low protein nature of ascitic fluid that develops SBP. At least 2 g of ceftriaxone must be used to treat SBP. Anaerobes seldom cause SBP; therefore anaerobic coverage is not needed.

Reference
- Runyon BA. Management of adult patients with ascites due to cirrhosis: an update. *Hepatology* 2009;49:2087–107.

Chapter 18 Hepatic Encephalopathy

18.1 The correct answer is **a**, True: a significant proportion of portal vein ammonia is generated by intestinal ammonia.

18.2 The correct answer is **b**, False: HE does not primarily arise because of large portosystemic shunts.

18.3 The correct answer is **a**, True: the correction of precipitating factors for HE is effective therapy.

18.4 The correct answer is **b**, False: prophylaxis with lactulose after TIPS has not been shown to reduce episodes of HE.

18.5 The correct answer is **a**, True: decreased brain myoinositol levels on NMR spectroscopy support the presence of cerebral edema in HE.

18.6 The correct answer is **a**, True: the presence of minimal HE predicts the development of overt HE.

18.7 The correct answer is **b**, False: blood ammonia levels are not useful for the diagnosis of HE.

18.8 The correct answer is **a**, True: neomycin inhibits intestinal glutaminase activity.

18.9 The correct answer is **a**, True: the treatment of minimal HE is associated with improved driving ability.

18.10 The correct answer is **b**, False: asterixis is not highly specific for the diagnosis of HE.

Chapter 19 Acute Liver Failure

19.1 The correct answer is **b**, True: the use of *N*-acetylcysteine in the setting of ALF not due to acetaminophen has been shown to improve transplant-free survival if given prior to the development of stage 1–2 hepatic encephalopathy.

Comment: A recent prospective, randomized, double-blind, placebo-controlled trial in the setting of ALF not due to acetaminophen showed a significant improvement in transplant-free survival in patients with early-stage encephalopathy (stages 1 and 2) who received NAC. There was no difference in overall survival in the entire group (all stages of encephalopathy). Thus NAC use early in the course of ALF may prevent progression to deeper encephalopathy with its associated complications.

Reference
- Lee WM, Hynan LS, Rossaro L, et al. Intravenous N-acetylcysteine improves transplant-free survival in early stage non-acetaminophen acute liver failure. *Gastroenterology* 2009;137:856–64.

19.2 The correct answer is **b**, The most common cause of death in the setting of acute liver failure is cerebral edema and brainstem herniation.

Comment: Cerebral edema and brainstem herniation remain the major cause of death in the setting of acute liver failure (nearly 50%). This is closely followed by infection/sepsis and multiorgan system failure.

Reference
- Ritt DJ, Whelan G, Werner DJ, Eigenbrodt EH, Schenker S, Combes B. Acute hepatic necrosis with stupor or coma. An analysis of thirty-one patients. *Medicine (Baltimore)* 1969;48:151–72.

19.3 The correct answer is **b**, Viral hepatitis is the most common cause of ALF worldwide.

Comment: Worldwide, the hepatitis viruses, particularly hepatitis B virus, make up the majority of cases of ALF. In western countries, drug-induced liver injury is more often seen. Acetaminophen is the most common drug implicated and is associated with overdosage.

References
- Acharya SK, Panda SK, Saxena A, Gupta SD. Acute hepatic failure in India: a perspective from the East. *J Gastroenterol Hepatol* 2000;15:473–9.
- Ayonrinde OT, Phelps GJ, Hurley JC, Ayonrinde OA. Paracetamol overdose and hepatotoxicity at a regional Australian hospital: a 4-year experience. *Intern Med J* 2005;35:655–60.
- Makin AJ, Wendon J, Williams R. A 7-year experience of severe acetaminophen-induced hepatotoxicity (1987–1993). *Gastroenterology* 1995;109:1907–16.
- Ostapowicz G, Fontana RJ, Schiodt FV, et al. Results of a prospective study of acute liver failure at 17 tertiary care centers in the United States. *Ann Intern Med* 2002;137:947–54.

Chapter 20 Primary Sclerosing Cholangitis
20.1 The correct answer is **d**, Generally, IBD is diagnosed prior to liver disease.
20.2 The correct answer is **c**, Liver transplantation has been consistently shown to improve outcomes in patients with PSC.

Chapter 21 Primary Biliary Cirrhosis
21.1 The correct answer is **c**, Serum antimitochondrial antibody.
21.2 The correct answer is **c**, Ursodeoxycholic acid.

Chapter 23 Hepatitis A and E
23.1 The correct answer is **c**, Detectable IgM anti-HAV.
23.2 The correct answer is **c**, Be told that immunologic memory exists despite absence of anti-HAV.

Chapter 26 Alcoholic Liver Disease
26.1 The correct answer is **b**, Corticosteroids.
26.2 The correct answer is **a**, The graft and patient survival are similar to that in nonalcoholic cirrhosis.

Chapter 27 Drug-induced Liver Disease
27.1 The correct answer is **b**, Concomitant use of statins does not increase the risk of acetaminophen hepatotoxicity

Comment: Co-prescription of medications can influence the risk of acetaminophen hepatotoxicity. In both sexes, the risk of liver injury is decreased with statin use and increased with ethanol. NAC remains the cornerstone of treatment in all patients with significant acetaminophen hepatotoxicity. More recently, when used in patients with grades I and II hepatic encephalopathy, it was shown to confer a survival benefit even in cases of acute liver failure resulting from drugs other than acetaminophen.

References
- Lee WM, Hynan LS, Rossaro L, et al. Intravenous N-acetylcysteine improves transplant-free survival in early stage non-acetaminophen acute liver failure. *Gastroenterology* 2009;137:856–64.
- Suzuki A, Yuen N, Walsh J, et al. Co-medications that modulate liver injury and repair influence clinical outcome of acetaminophen-associated liver injury. *Clin Gastroenterol Hepatol* 2009;7:882–8.

27.2 The correct answer is **d**, Atorvastatin.

Comment: Genetic factors have been linked to drug hepatotoxicity. While the risk of hepatic injury with nevirapine, abacavir, and flucloxacillin have been linked to specific HLA alleles, polymorphisms of the mitochondrial DNA polymerase-γ 1 (POLG1) gene confer a predisposition to sodium valproate hepatotoxicity in children.

References
- Daly AK. Drug-induced liver injury: past, present and future. *Pharmacogenomics* 2010;11:607–11.
- McFarland R, Hudson G, Taylor RW, et al. Reversible valproate hepatotoxicity due to mutations in mitochondrial DNA polymerase gamma (POLG1). *Arch Dis Child* 2008;93:151–3.

Chapter 29 Wilson Disease
29.1 The correct answer is **f**, All of the above.
29.2 The correct answer is **f**, Living donor transplant using a parent as a donor is never possible for these patients.
29.3 The correct answer is **d**, Desferrioxamine is not useful as a treatment for Wilson disease.

Chapter 30 Hemochromatosis and Iron Storage Disorders
30.1 The correct answer is **b**, Hepcidin.

Comment: The iron transporter, ferroportin, is located on the basolateral surface of duodenal enterocytes, and is responsible for egress of iron from enterocytes into the blood. Hepcidin is the major iron regulatory hormone and it acts to downregulate iron absorption by binding to ferroportin, resulting in its internalization and degradation.

Reference
- Nemeth E, Ganz T. The role of hepcidin in iron metabolism. *Acta Haematol* 2009;122:78–86.

30.2 The correct answer is **d**.

Comment: In cases of *HFE*-related hereditary hemochromatosis, liver biopsy is usually not indicated if the patient has normal liver enzyme levels and a serum ferritin level below 1,000 ng/mL (e.g., patients a and b). Such patients would be treated by phlebotomy to deplete their excess iron stores. Patient d is homozygous for the C282Y mutation and has a serum ferritin level above 1,000 ng/mL and elevated ALT activity – liver biopsy is indicated based on either of these findings.

Reference

• Olynyk JK, Trinder D, Ramm GA, Britton RS, Bacon BR. Hereditary hemochromatosis in the post-HFE era. *Hepatology* 2008;48:991–1001.

Chapter 31 Alpha-1 Antitrypsin Deficiency
31.1 The correct answer is **c**, PAS-positive, diastase-resistant globules in hepatocytes.
31.2 The correct answer is **a**, Liver transplantation.

Chapter 32 Nonalcoholic Fatty Liver Disease
32.1 The correct answer is **e**, All of the above.
32.2 The correct answer is **c**, Exercise (with or without weight loss) can reduce liver fat.

Chapter 33 Vascular Diseases of the Liver
33.1 The correct answer is **a**, Polycythemia vera.

Comment: Polycythemia vera is the most common prothrombotic disorder leading to Budd–Chiari syndrome, seen in up to 45% of patients. It must be considered in the diagnostic evaluation for hypercoagulable disorders in patients presenting with Budd–Chiari syndrome.

33.2 The correct answer is **e**, Cystic lesions in the liver.

Comment: Budd–Chiari syndrome may present on imaging with hepatomegaly and ascites; caudate lobe hypertrophy is seen with chronic disease and may obstruct the intrahepatic portion of the inferior vena cava. Regenerative nodules may also be seen due to compensatory increase in arterial blood flow; however, cystic lesions are not observed in Budd–Chiari syndrome.

Chapter 34 The Liver in Circulatory Failure
34.1 The correct answer is **d**, Acute hepatic ischemic injury.

Comment: The typical time course of serum aminotransferases in acute hepatic ischemic injury consists of a rapid raise and early peak followed by prompt decline after resolution of the hypotensive event. The time course of acute viral hepatitis is slower, and the remainder entities generally do not exhibit marked elevation of the serum aminotransferases.

34.2 The correct answer is **d**, Sorafenib chemotherapy.

Comment: With the exception of the oral agent sorafenib, all other modalities either directly embolize branches of the hepatic artery or carry a risk of hepatic artery injury and the potential for hepatic infarction.

Chapter 35 Benign Tumors, Nodules, and Cystic Diseases of the Liver
35.1 The correct answer is **d**. Hepatocyte nuclear factor 1 α (HNF-1α) inactivation.

Comment: Transformation from hepatocellular adenoma to hepatocellular carcinoma is strongly associated with β-catenin, male gender, size of nodules particularly if greater than 5 cm, and enlarging nodules. Hepatocellular adenomas with HNF-1α inhibition do not appear to develop hepatocellular carcinoma.

35.2 The correction answer is **d**, Massively enlarged cysts throughout all segments of the liver.

Comment: Treatment of polycystic liver disease is only offered to patients with significant symptoms or complications from cyst compression including severe pain, direct compression of the bile ducts or hepatic veins causing jaundice or ascites, or cyst infection because of the potential for significant morbidity and mortality with intervention.

Chapter 36 Hepatocellular Carcinoma
36.1 The correct answer is **c**, Surgical resection.

Comment: Surgical resection is the best option for those patients with normal liver or with compensated cirrhosis with normal bilirubin and an absence of clinically relevant portal hypertension.

Reference

• Bruix J, Sherman M. Management of hepatocellular carcinoma. *Hepatology* 2005;42:1208–36.

36.2 The correct answer is **d**, Sorafenib increases survival in advanced HCC because it leads to tumor shrinkage as demonstrated by dynamic imaging techniques.

Comment: Sorafenib is currently the only approved treatment for advanced HCC. It has shown survival benefit in two randomized controlled trials and it acts in delaying the tumor progression. However, in a few cases (less than 5%), sorafenib induces tumor response. AFP has a very low diagnostic accuracy and its use is not recommended for HCC surveillance. Once a liver nodule is detected by ultrasonography in a cirrhotic liver, conclusive HCC diagnosis can be done without histologic confirmation if the nodule displays a specific vascular pattern (contrast uptake during the arterial phase followed by washout in the venous phases). The main cause of HCC worldwide is, by far, chronic HBV infection. Finally, vascular invasion, extrahepatic spread, and the presence of symptoms are parameters associated with poor prognosis and define advanced disease.

References

- Bruix J, Sherman M. Management of hepatocellular carcinoma. *Hepatology* 2005;42:1208–36.
- Llovet J, Ricci S, Mazzaferro V, et al. Sorafenib in advanced hepatocellular carcinoma. *N Engl J Med* 2008; 359:378–90.
- Cheng AL, Kang YK, Chen Z, et al. Efficacy and safety of sorafenib in patients in the Asia-Pacific region with advanced hepatocellular carcinoma: a phase III randomised, double-blind, placebo-controlled trial. *Lancet Oncol* 2009;10:25–34.

Chapter 38 Amoebic and Pyogenic Liver Abscesses

38.1 The correct answer is **d**, Differences in the membrane's lipid arrangement on electron microscopy.

38.2 The correct answer is **c**, Gal/GalNAc inhibits assembly of C5b-9 preventing the formation of the membrane attack complex.

38.3 The correct answer is **e**, All of the above are potential causes of pyogenic liver abscess.

Chapter 39 Parasitic Diseases

39.1 The correct answer is **d**, 1, 2, 3 and 4.

39.2 The correct answer is **c**, Visceral leishmaniasis.

Chapter 40 Granulomas of the Liver

40.1 The correct answers are: a – 5; b – 1; c – 2; d – 4; e – 3.

40.2 The correct answer is **e**, Giant cell inclusions (asteroid bodies) are pathognomonic of sarcoidosis.

Comment: Giant cell inclusions such as asteroid or Schaumann bodies are often present but are not specific to sarcoidosis.

Reference

- Devaney K, Goodman ZD, Epstein MS, et al. Hepatic sarcoidosis: clinicopathologic features of 100 patients. *Am J Surg Pathol* 1993;17:1272–80.

Chapter 41 Hepatobiliary Manifestations of Human Immunodeficiency Virus

41.1 The correct answer is **e**, Didanosine.

Comment: NCPH has been recently described in the HIV-monoinfected population and may represent the most striking manifestation of long-term consequences of HIV and its treatment on the liver. Didanosine use has been consistently reported to be associated with it. The characteristic liver histologic lesions are either nodular regenerative hyperplasia or hepatoportal sclerosis. Both manifest clinically as NCPH, and esophageal variceal bleeding is the most frequent complication.

Reference

- Vispo E, Moreno A, Maida I, et al. Noncirrhotic portal hypertension in HIV-infected patients: unique clinical and pathological findings. *AIDS* 2010;24:1171–6.

41.2 The correct answer is **d**, HCV coinfection.

Comment: Early referral to transplant, MELD score at the time of transplantation, and inability to control HIV (reach CD4+ T-cell count above 100 and undetectable plasma HIV-1 RNA viral load) are the most important variables associated with death in HIV-infected patients undergoing a liver transplant. HCV coinfection has been reported to be associated with worse outcome in some studies of HIV-infected patients undergoing liver transplantation.

References

- Murillas J, Rimola A, Laguno M, et al. The model for end-stage liver disease score is the best prognostic factor in human immunodeficiency virus 1-infected patients with end-stage liver disease: a prospective cohort study. *Liver Transpl* 2009;15:1133–41.
- Norris S, Taylor C, Muiesan P, et al. Outcomes of liver transplantation in HIV-infected individuals: the impact of HCV and HBV infection. *Liver Transpl* 2004; 10:1271–8.
- Ragni MV, Belle SH, Im K, et al. Survival of human immunodeficiency virus-infected liver transplant recipients. *J Infect Dis* 2003;188:1412–20.

Chapter 44 The First Six Months Following Liver Transplantation

44.1 The correct answer is **c**, The histopathologic diagnosis of acute cellular rejection does not includes the presence of lobular microabscesses.

Comment: Acute cellular rejection of the hepatic allograft frequently manifests during the first 3 months following liver transplantation. Laboratory findings include nonselective elevation of total bilirubin, transaminases, and alkaline phosphatase. Diagnosis is confirmed by examination of a core needle biopsy.

Reference

- Demetris AJ, Batts KP, Dhillon AP, et al. Banff schema for grading liver allograft rejection: an international consensus document. *Hepatology* 1997;25:658–63.

44.2 The correct answer is **d**, Cytomegalovirus (CMV) infection.

Comment: Common causes of graft loss following the first few weeks after liver transplantation are HAT, PNF, and ACR. CMV infection can be associated with poor graft and patient outcomes, however, in the era of antiviral prophylaxis, it is typically encountered after the first month.

Reference

- Limaye AP, Bakthavatsalam R, Kim HW, et al. Impact of cytomegalovirus in organ transplant recipients in the era of antiviral prophylaxis. *Transplantation* 2006;81:1645–52.

44.3 The correct answer is **d**, Parkinson disease.

Comment: Immunosuppressive medications prescribed to prevent graft rejection result in short- and long-term morbidity and mortality. Therefore, special attention should be paid to the prevention and treatment of these complications.

Reference

- McGuire BM, Rosenthal P, Brown CC, et al. Long-term management of the liver transplant patient: recommendations for the primary care doctor. *Am J Transplant* 2009;9:1988–2003.

Chapter 47 Recurrent Disease Following Liver Transplantation

47.1 The correct answer is **d**, An individual patient undergoing liver transplantation for HCV-related end-stage liver disease has a risk of 20–30% of developing cirrhosis by 5 years after transplant.

Comment: Histologic HCV recurrence is nearly universal after liver transplantation. Fibrosis is progressive in many and approximately 20–30% of patients will develop cirrhosis within 5 years of transplant. Once cirrhosis develops, 30% will decompensate within 1 year and half of those will die within a year of decompensation.

47.2 The correct answer is **d**, HBIg and tenofovir combination therapy.

Comment: Prophylaxis for HBV recurrence after liver transplant is recommended for all patients with HBV, whether HBV DNA positive or not at the time of transplant. A patient with a detectable viral load is at higher risk for recurrence than those with undetectable levels at the time of transplant. Patients with high viral levels at the time of transplant are at the highest risk. Optimal prophylaxis consists of HBIg in combination with a nucleos(t)ide analog. Lamivudine therapy has a higher risk of viral resistance and thus is not the recommended first-line agent. Short-term HBIg therapy would not be recommended for patients with HBV DNA-positive status at the time of transplant. More data are required to know if short-term HBIg therapy is acceptable for HBV DNA-negative patients.

Chapter 49 Controversies in Liver Transplantation

49.1 The correct answer is **b**, The international normalized ratio (INR).

Comment: The MELD score is described by the following equation: [0.957 × ln(creatinine mg/dL) + 0.378 × ln(bilirubin mg/dL) + 1.120 × ln(INR) + 0.6431] × 10. The INR has the highest associated multiplicative factor (1.12) and as such has the greatest weight of the three determinants.

References

- Kamath PS, Wiesner RH, Malinchoc M, et al. A model to predict survival in patients with end-stage liver disease. *Hepatology* 2001;33:464–70.
- Wiesner RH, McDiarmid SV, Kamath PS, et al. MELD and PELD: application of survival models to liver allocation. *Liver Transpl* 2001;7:567–80.

49.2 The correct answer is **e**, Expanded criteria donors (ECDs) and donation after cardiac death (DCD).

Comment: Only ECD and DCD organs are from deceased donors. However, the combined utilization of ECDs, DCD, and living donor liver transplantation has increased the total donor pool for liver transplantation.

References

- Mateo R, Cho Y, Singh G, et al. Risk factors for graft survival after liver transplantation from donation after cardiac death donors: an analysis of OPTN/UNOS data. *Am J Transplant* 2006;6:791–6.
- Trotter JF, Wachs M, Everson GT, Kam I. Adult-to-adult transplantation of the right hepatic lobe from a living donor. *N Engl J Med* 2002;346:1074–82.

49.3 The correct answer is **d**, The availability of deceased donor livers, the donor complication rate, and the recipient complication rate are all relevant.

Comment: Each of the above factors has been associated with the decline in the number of LDLTs performed in the United States. Although the number of cases has dropped, LDLT will likely remain a viable means to provide transplantation especially in areas where the supply of deceased donor livers is critically limited.

Reference

- Trotter JF. Living donor liver transplantation: is the hype over? *J Hepatol* 2005;42:20–5.

49.4 The correct answer is **b**, The statement is false.

Comment: Regional sharing of deceased donor livers is one of the most controversial issues in liver transplantation. While many transplant professionals favor its development, regional sharing has not been widely accepted by the liver transplant community. Consequently, there is currently no regional sharing plan except in a very limited fashion.

49.5 The correct answer is **d**, The donor risk index (DRI) is the relative risk of graft loss for an organ with a specific set of donor and graft characteristics compared with a reference case.

Comment: The DRI was developed to identify objective donor and transplant characteristics associated with graft loss. Identification of these specific factors may help to understand the risk of using transplant organs. By doing so, clinicians may learn how to mitigate these factors and select the best recipients for marginal grafts, thereby maximizing organ utility.

Reference

- Feng S, Goodrich NP, Bragg-Gresham JL, et al. Characteristics associated with liver graft failure: the concept of a donor risk index. *Am J Transplant* 2006;6:783–90.

49.6 The correct answer is **c**, The basis for liver allocation currently under active consideration is the survival benefit of the transplant.

Comment: Liver allocation based on the survival benefit of the transplant is under active consideration by the liver transplant community. Under this proposed system, for each donor liver that becomes available, the transplant survival benefit score would be computed for each candidate on the waiting list based on their specific characteristics as well as those of the particular donor. Such a national allocation system has already been adopted for lung transplantation.

Reference

- Schaubel DE, Guidinger MK, Biggins SW, et al. Survival benefit-based deceased-donor liver allocation. *Am J Transplant* 2009;9:970–81.

Index

Page numbers in *italics* denote figures, thos in **bold** denote tables.